# Length of Stay by Operation

## United States, 2000

# LOS

# *Length of Stay*

RA981
A2
L4552
2000

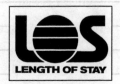

ISBN: 1-57372-236-7

ISSN: 1099-3320

Statistics reported in the 2000 edition are drawn from individual patient discharge records for the time period October 1, 1998, through September 30, 1999. This volume is one of the books in the *Length of Stay by Diagnosis and Operation* series:

Length of Stay by Diagnosis and Operation, United States
ISSN 0895-9824

Length of Stay by Diagnosis and Operation, Northeastern Region
ISSN 0895-9838

Length of Stay by Diagnosis and Operation, North Central Region
ISSN 0895-9846

Length of Stay by Diagnosis and Operation, Southern Region
ISSN 0895-9854

Length of Stay by Diagnosis and Operation, Western Region
ISSN 0895-9862

Pediatric Length of Stay by Diagnosis and Operation, United States
ISSN 0891-1223

**HCIA-Sachs, L.L.C.**
300 East Lombard Street
Baltimore, Maryland 21202
(800) 568-3282

Length of Stay by Diagnosis and Operation, United States, 2000

**Limitations of HCIA-Sachs (The Publisher) Liability**

**Publications Return Policy**

Printed books may be returned, in good condition, for a full refund within 10 **business** days of receipt. Electronic files (i.e., CDs, tapes, diskettes) are not refundable but are guaranteed against physical defects. If your publication arrives damaged, or you need to return it for another reason, please call HCIA-Sachs Customer Service immediately at (800) 568-3282.

Hard Copy Price: $295

ISSN 0895-9824
ISBN 1-57372-250-2

# CONTENTS

# INTRODUCTION

## HCIA-Sachs' *Length of Stay* Series: Real Patient Data for Powerful Decision Making

Today's health care professionals are challenged to reduce unnecessary stays and services without sacrificing quality of care. As a result, medical management continues to move toward a more aggressive style of managing inpatient care. This approach makes it essential to establish *Length of Stay* targets that are not only realistic, but based on real benchmark data that reflect the complexity of your patient population.

HCIA-Sachs' *Length of Stay* (LOS) series is unique. It is the only resource based solely on objective, quantitative data that are consistent and complete across the United States. This methodology ensures that the focus is on statistical rather than anecdotal evidence. HCIA-Sachs provides empirical data based on millions of discharges, enabling you to identify true utilization and achieve benchmark performance.

HCIA-Sachs' *Length of Stay* series was created to help you provide quality care while reducing health care costs—by efficiently managing inpatient cases. With LOS percentiles and demographic breakdowns, HCIA-Sachs' product is the industry's most powerful tool to determine stays by any sizable patient population—from the lowest realistic level to median stays, and stays at the highest outlier levels. While HCIA-Sachs' percentiles are based on real data from actual inpatient records, other products' panel-determined goals are based on subjective analysis.

Each patient is unique, and HCIA-Sachs' *Length of Stay* series allows you to factor in those differences. HCIA-Sachs LOS standards address the illness complexity and age of your patients by providing norms for both simple and more complex patients. Unlike some panel-determined goals, which address only the simple uncomplicated patient, HCIA-Sachs LOS provides figures for multiple diagnosis patients who have had a significant procedure performed and those who have not.

## Designed for Easy Use

HCIA-Sachs designed the *Length of Stay by Diagnosis and Operation* series to be user-friendly. The front section of each book includes information on practical applications of the data, a step-by-step guide to using the tables, and a description of the data source. The LOS tables themselves include data organized by ICD-9-CM code and represent every diagnosis and procedure group. The tables examine average, median, and percentile length of stay for patients in five age groups, with single and multiple diagnoses or procedures, and according to whether the patient's stay included a significant procedure.

The appendices include counts of U.S. hospitals by bed size, region, census division, setting (rural or urban), and teaching intensity; a list of the states included in each LOS comparative region; and a table showing operative status of every procedure code included in the book. The glossary defines all of the terms used in the tables. An alphabetical index of diagnoses and procedures grouped according to classification categories can assist users who do not know the ICD-9-CM code for a particular diagnosis.

## Length of Stay Data for a Variety of Needs

There are 11 different editions of *Length of Stay*, making it easy to find the information you need. Each book in the series is updated annually.

*Length of Stay by Diagnosis and Operation* provides data representing every ICD-9-CM diagnosis and procedure group.

- National and regional (Northeastern, North Central, Southern, and Western) editions
- National Pediatric edition, with data for patients 19 years old and younger

*Psychiatric Length of Stay by Diagnosis* catalogs diagnoses unique to psychiatric and substance abuse treatment.

- National and regional (Northeastern, North Central, Southern, and Western available in electronic format only) editions

Each title is available electronically for efficient analysis. The files load easily onto virtually any system, and give you the convenience to review, set LOS targets, and plan your utilization management quickly. With these files, you can generate custom reports and incorporate the data into your own decision support systems. Call HCIA-Sachs at 800-568-3282 for details.

## About HCIA-Sachs

HCIA-Sachs leads the health care industry in providing payors, providers, employers, and pharmaceutical companies with strategic consumer and patient intelligence. Armed with the largest health care information databases, HCIA-Sachs supplies clients with effective and innovative products and services for planning, marketing, quality improvement, and cost control. HCIA-Sachs' solutions include relationship marketing, data warehousing, benchmarking, and Internet-based information systems that streamline business decision-making.

For more information about HCIA-Sachs, send e-mail to info@hciasachs.com or call (800) 568-3282.

# DESCRIPTION OF THE DATABASE

HCIA-Sachs LOS standards are based on all-payor data gathered from more than 11 million actual inpatient records, representing one of every three discharges from U.S. hospitals annually. This detail-rich database is HCIA-Sachs' Projected Inpatient Database (PIDB), the largest all-payor inpatient database available in the marketplace. The PIDB supports publications, products, and custom studies, the results of which are applicable to all short-term, general, nonfederal (STGNF) hospitals in the United States. This exclusive database combines data from both public and proprietary state data as well as individual and group hospital contracts. Updated quarterly, HCIA-Sachs uses its PIDB to create the *Length of Stay* series, the *National Inpatient Profile*, the *National Link Study*, and other products.

## Data Projection Methodology

The PIDB was created as an external, stable, consolidated database to enable users to make accurate projections about the entire universe of U.S. short-term, general, nonfederal (STGNF) hospitals. To make this possible, HCIA-Sachs projects the data in the PIDB so that it accurately represents this universe. First, we standardize data from all sources to create an aggregated patient record database. We then assign each discharge record a weight (or projection factor) to indicate the number of discharges it represents. In this way, HCIA-Sachs projects the data to represent the universe of all inpatient episodes.

To create the projection factors, HCIA-Sachs uses two accurate external sources that describe the target universe of hospitals: the National Hospital Discharge Survey (NHDS) and the Medicare Provider Analysis and Review File (MedPAR). NHDS is a survey produced and published by the National Center for Health Statistics (NCHS) that has itself been projected to represent the entire universe of nonfederal, general (medical or surgical) or children's general, short stay hospitals in the United States. MedPAR is produced by the Health Care Financing Administration (HCFA) and contains 100 percent of all Medicare inpatient discharges. When the projection factors are summed over all discharges, they match the STGNF universe and are known as a weighted sum. Similarly, a count of the number of discharges in a particular patient subgroup would equal the estimated number of such patients in the STGNF universe, not just those in the database. Also, when the weights are properly applied, a mean length of stay (LOS), for example, represents the mean LOS for all such patients in the STGNF universe, rather than just those in the database. This measure is a weighted mean. The projection process takes into account the age and sex of the patient; the HCIA-Sachs-assigned bed service of the inpatient episode; and the census region, bed size, and teaching status of the hospital.

The universe of inpatients discharged from all short-term, general, nonfederal U.S. hospitals is defined using HCFA's MedPAR and the NHDS. These hospital characteristics are defined according to the American Hospital Association criteria:

**Short-Term:** The average length of stay for all patients at the facility is less than 30 days, or more than 50 percent of all patients are admitted to units in which the average length of stay is less than 30 days.

**General:** The primary function of the institution is to provide patient services, diagnostic and therapeutic, for a variety of medical conditions.

**Nonfederal:** The facility is controlled by a state, county, city, city-county, hospital district authority, or church.

U.S. hospitals include those in the 50 states and the District of Columbia. Data from long-term specialty institutions, e.g., long-term psychiatric or rehabilitation facilities, are excluded. To eliminate discharge records that do not represent a typical short-term inpatient stay, we exclude admissions from other short-term hospitals, discharges to other short-term hospitals, discharges against medical advice, and death.

## Data Quality and Validation

The PIDB is the cleanest consolidated source of data available. To ensure quality, HCIA-Sachs runs all data through a set of standard edit screens. Examples of discrepancies detected by the audit include records with invalid diagnosis or procedure codes, invalid or unrecorded principal diagnosis, sex- or age-specific diagnosis or procedure inconsistencies, and incalculable age or length of stay. All records from hospitals with more than 5 percent of discharges failing any screen are deleted from the database.

The projection methodology ensures that the PIDB is representative of the inpatient universe defined by NHDS and MedPAR. By comparing PIDB data with NHDS and MedPAR, the validity of the PIDB has been demonstrated on the ICD-9-CM diagnosis and procedure level, as well as on the DRG level.

To perform a comparison between PIDB data and NHDS and MedPAR data, the weighted discharges in the PIDB were grouped within ICD-9-CM diagnosis and procedure chapters, as were the discharges in NHDS and MedPAR. PIDB patients under the age of 65 were compared with NHDS patients for the same age range, and PIDB patients aged 65 and older were compared with MedPAR patients for the same age range. The findings show that the chapter distributions of the PIDB were highly representative of NHDS and MedPAR. In fact, HCIA-Sachs studies have proven the correlation between the PIDB and MedPAR to be 99.9 percent. And because the PIDB projection methodology incorporates payor data, the validity of the PIDB applies not only to the Medicare population, but across all payors.

# BENEFITS AND APPLICATIONS

HCIA-Sachs' *Length of Stay* series is an invaluable standard reference for health care professionals who want to measure inpatient utilization. Using the hospital stay data found in this series, you can compare regional and national norms to an individual institution or a special population. Specifically, the *Length of Stay* series allows you to:

- establish baselines (benchmarking);
- pre-authorize procedures;
- identify candidates for utilization review;
- project extended stay reviews;
- develop forecasts;
- and report lengths of stay versus benchmarks.

Patient severity, managed care market presence, and varying practice patterns all have significant impact on actual LOS statistics. As technological advances and financial pressures reduce inpatient days and increase outpatient volumes, only the most severely ill patients are left in the hospitals. Consequently, health care professionals must have detailed measurement criteria to make truly accurate, patient-focused assessments of appropriate lengths of stay.

Because HCIA-Sachs' *Length of Stay* series is based on real patient data, you can tailor your LOS analyses to a particular patient age group, or compare the norms for patients with single or multiple diagnoses. You may also study regional variations, as well as specialized groups including pediatric and psychiatric patient populations. And the 10th, 25th, 50th, 75th, 95th, and 99th percentile groups enhance the average length of stay data by allowing you to pick a realistic goal for an individual patient. HCIA-Sachs' LOS data can help pinpoint whether patients are being cared for efficiently, targeting areas that may need further clinical analysis.

The recent proliferation of new laws regulating utilization management procedures—in part, by requiring the disclosure of criteria used—is fueling the demand for high quality data. To comply with these new legal stipulations and to track fluctuating LOS trends, utilization managers must have reliable, industry-accepted criteria sets. Because HCIA-Sachs updates the *Length of Stay* series annually with millions of new patient records, it provides extremely useful trend information—including significant developments from one year to the next and over even longer periods of time. Compiled from HCIA-Sachs' exclusive Projected Inpatient Database (PIDB), the largest all-payor inpatient database available in the marketplace, this series is the most comprehensive, current source for length of stay data available.

# HOW TO USE THE TABLES

The data in each HCIA-Sachs *Length of Stay* volume are organized numerically by the International Classification of Diseases, 9th Revision, Clinical Modification (ICD-9-CM) coding system. Each Diagnosis volume contains every three-digit diagnosis code (including both summary and valid detail codes) and the nearly 1,200 four- and five-digit codes highest in projected volume. Each Operation volume contains every three-digit procedure code (including both summary codes and valid detail codes) and the nearly 850 four-digit codes highest in projected volume.

Data are categorized by number of observed patients, average length of stay, variance, and distribution percentiles. In addition, two subtotals and a grand total are included. All data elements except the number of observed patients are calculated using the projection methodology described on page vii.

Determining length of stay would be easy if all patients were identical, but they are not. Illness, complexity, age, and region of the country will cause some variation in the LOS of patients admitted with the same diagnosis or procedure. HCIA-Sachs recognizes those differences and our data tables let you to do the same. HCIA-Sachs' *Length of Stay* series gives you detailed length of stay breakdowns—by individual ICD-9-CM code—listed by age groups, single versus multiple diagnosis patient, and operated versus non-operated status. You can find specific length of stay norms by taking the following steps:

**Step 1:** Find the desired ICD-9-CM code in the tables in one of the *Length of Stay* volumes. If you do not know a patient's ICD-9-CM code, refer to the index, which provides an alphabetical listing of the descriptive titles for all codes included in the book.

The **Observed Patients** column gives you the number of patients in the stratified group as reported in HCIA-Sachs' projected inpatient database. "Observed" means that this data element, unlike the other elements in the LOS tables, is not projected. Patients with stays longer than 99 days (indicated as ">99") are not included.

**Step 2:** For each diagnosis code, patients are stratified by single or multiple diagnoses, operated or not operated status, and age. For each procedure code, patients are stratified by single or multiple diagnoses and age. Find the appropriate portion of the table for review by using the following patient information:

- Number of diagnoses
- Operated status
- Age

## Single or Multiple Diagnoses

More than 80 percent of all admissions are complicated (have more than one diagnosis). The data tables include rows for patients with single and multiple diagnoses. This enables you to identify stays that are realistic and on-target with the patient's unique characteristics.

Patients are classified in the multiple diagnoses category if they had at least one valid secondary diagnosis in addition to the principal one. The following codes are not considered valid secondary diagnoses for purposes of this classification:

1.  Manifestation codes (conditions that evolved from underlying diseases [etiology] and are in italics in ICD-9-CM, Volume 1)

2.  Codes V27.0-V27.9 (outcome of delivery)

3.  E Codes (external causes of injury and poisoning)

### Operated or Not Operated

In the diagnosis tables, operated patients are those who had at least one procedure that is classified by the Health Care Financing Administration (HCFA) as an operating room procedure. HCFA physician panels classify every ICD-9-CM procedure code according to whether the procedure would in most hospitals be performed in the operating room. This classification system differs slightly from that used in *Length of Stay* publications published before 1995, in which patients were categorized as "operated" if any of their procedures were labeled as Uniform Hospital Discharge Data Set (UHDDS) Class 1. Appendix C contains a list of procedure codes included in this series and their HCFA-defined operative status.

### Patient's Age

The data tables illustrate the impact of age by providing five age group breakouts. These ages are from the day of the patient's admission.

For diagnosis codes V30-V39, which pertain exclusively to newborns, age is replaced by birth weight in grams. Newborns with unrecorded birth weights with secondary diagnosis codes in the 764.01-764.99 and 765.01-765.19 ranges have been assigned to the appropriate birth weight category on the basis of the fifth digit of these codes. (Data for patients whose birth weights cannot be determined by using this method are included only in the Subtotal and Total rows of the table.)

**Step 3:** Choose from the average stay or the 10th, 25th, 50th, 75th, 95th, and 99th percentile columns to find the appropriate length of stay for your patient. HCIA-Sachs LOS standards document the statistical range of stays for each patient group. These ranges are represented as percentiles, so that you can determine a more aggressive (benchmark) or less aggressive (norm) LOS for your patient, depending on individual variables, and are all backed by actual patient data.

### Average Length of Stay

The average length of stay is calculated from the admission and discharge dates by counting the day of admission as the first day; the day of discharge is not included. The average is figured by adding the lengths of stay for each patient and then dividing by the total number of patients. Patients discharged on the day of admission are counted as staying one day. Patients with stays over 99 days (>99) are excluded from this calculation.

## Median and Percentiles

A statistical range of stays are presented for each patient group. These ranges are represented as percentiles, so that you can determine a more aggressive or less aggressive LOS for your patient, depending on individual variables such as illness complications, age, etc. A length of stay percentile for a stratified group of patients is determined by arranging the individual patient stays from low to high. Counting up from the lowest stay to the point where one-half of the patients have been counted yields the value of the 50th percentile. Counting one-tenth of the total patients gives the 10th percentile, and so on.

The 10th, 25th, 50th, 75th, 90th, 95th, and 99th percentiles of stay are displayed in days. If, for example, the 10th percentile for a group of patients is four, then 10 percent of the patients stayed four days or fewer. The 50th percentile is the median. Any percentile with a value of 100 days or more is listed as >99. Patients who were hospitalized more than 99 days (>99) are not included in the total patients, average stay, and variance categories. The percentiles, however, do include these patients.

**Step 4:** Consult the total patient sample (**Observed Patients** column) and variance to consider the homogeneity of the data (i.e., to what extent length of stay averages are clustered or spread out within a particular patient group).

The **Total** row represents a subtotal for each of the patient groups. The **Grand Total** row represents the total number of patients in the specified diagnosis or procedure category.

The **variance** is a measure of the spread of the data (from the lowest to the highest value) around the average. As such, it shows how much individual patient stays ranged around the average. The smallest variance is zero, indicating that all lengths of stay are equal. In tables in which there is a large variance and the patient group size is relatively small, the average stay may appear high. This sometimes occurs when one or two patients with long hospitalizations fall into the group.

# FEATURES OF A DIAGNOSIS TABLE

*ICD-9-CM* diagnosis code and title ⎯⎯⎯

Diagnosis group(s) previously used in HCIA-Sachs' former "List A and B" coding system

**008.8: VIRAL ENTERITIS NOS. Formerly included in diagnosis group(s) 001.**

| Type of Patients | Observed Patients | Avg. Stay | Vari-ance | Percentiles | | | | | | |
|---|---|---|---|---|---|---|---|---|---|---|
| | | | | 10th | 25th | 50th | 75th | 90th | 95th | 99th |
| **1. SINGLE DX** | | | | | | | | | | |
| *A. Not Operated* | | | | | | | | | | |
| 0–19 Years | 1346 | 1.9 | 2 | 1 | 1 | 2 | 2 | 3 | 4 | 5 |
| 20–34 | 416 | 1.7 | <1 | 1 | 1 | 2 | 2 | 3 | 3 | 5 |
| 35–49 | 213 | 2.3 | 3 | 1 | 1 | 2 | 3 | 3 | 5 | 10 |
| 50–64 | 89 | 2.0 | 3 | 1 | 1 | 1 | 3 | 3 | 4 | 12 |
| 65+ | 55 | 2.8 | 3 | 1 | 2 | 2 | 3 | 6 | 6 | 9 |
| *B. Operated* | | | | | | | | | | |
| 0–19 Years | 24 | 2.5 | 1 | 1 | 2 | 2 | 3 | 4 | 5 | 6 |
| 20–34 | 21 | 2.6 | <1 | 1 | 2 | 3 | 3 | 3 | 3 | 4 |
| 35–49 | 6 | 4.2 | 2 | 2 | 4 | 5 | 5 | 5 | 5 | 6 |
| 50–64 | 1 | 2.0 | 0 | 2 | 2 | 2 | 2 | 2 | 2 | 2 |
| 65+ | 0 | | | | | | | | | |
| **2. MULTIPLE DX** | | | | | | | | | | |
| *A. Not Operated* | | | | | | | | | | |
| 0–19 Years | 5020 | 2.3 | 5 | 1 | 1 | 2 | 3 | 4 | 5 | 8 |
| 20–34 | 1625 | 2.2 | 3 | 1 | 1 | 2 | 3 | 4 | 5 | 7 |
| 35–49 | 1453 | 2.7 | 3 | 1 | 1 | 2 | 3 | 5 | 6 | 9 |
| 50–64 | 1301 | 2.9 | 3 | 1 | 2 | 2 | 4 | 5 | 6 | 9 |
| 65+ | 2964 | 3.6 | 7 | 1 | 2 | 3 | 4 | 7 | 9 | 13 |
| *B. Operated* | | | | | | | | | | |
| 0–19 Years | 35 | 4.3 | 9 | 2 | 2 | 4 | 4 | 8 | 9 | 13 |
| 20–34 | 32 | 3.8 | 9 | 1 | 2 | 3 | 4 | 8 | 12 | 12 |
| 35–49 | 23 | 5.7 | 20 | 1 | 3 | 4 | 8 | 11 | 20 | 20 |
| 50–64 | 10 | 8.0 | 50 | 3 | 4 | 6 | 7 | 25 | 25 | 28 |
| 65+ | 27 | 14.0 | 92 | 4 | 7 | 10 | 18 | 30 | 31 | 43 |
| **SUBTOTALS:** | | | | | | | | | | |
| **1. SINGLE DX** | | | | | | | | | | |
| *A. Not Operated* | 2119 | 1.9 | 2 | 1 | 1 | 2 | 2 | 3 | 4 | 7 |
| *B. Operated* | 52 | 2.9 | 1 | 1 | 2 | 3 | 3 | 5 | 5 | 6 |
| **2. MULTIPLE DX** | | | | | | | | | | |
| *A. Not Operated* | 12363 | 2.7 | 5 | 1 | 1 | 2 | 3 | 5 | 6 | 10 |
| *B. Operated* | 127 | 6.7 | 46 | 2 | 3 | 4 | 8 | 15 | 20 | 31 |
| **1. SINGLE DX** | **2171** | **2.0** | **2** | **1** | **1** | **2** | **2** | **3** | **4** | **7** |
| **2. MULTIPLE DX** | **12490** | **2.7** | **6** | **1** | **1** | **2** | **3** | **5** | **7** | **10** |
| **A. NOT OPERATED** | **14482** | **2.6** | **5** | **1** | **1** | **2** | **3** | **5** | **6** | **9** |
| **B. OPERATED** | **179** | **5.2** | **31** | **2** | **2** | **3** | **5** | **10** | **15** | **30** |
| **TOTAL** | | | | | | | | | | |
| 0–19 Years | 6425 | 2.3 | 4 | 1 | 1 | 2 | 3 | 4 | 5 | 8 |
| 20–34 | 2094 | 2.1 | 3 | 1 | 1 | 2 | 3 | 4 | 4 | 7 |
| 35–49 | 1695 | 2.7 | 4 | 1 | 1 | 2 | 3 | 5 | 6 | 10 |
| 50–64 | 1401 | 2.8 | 4 | 1 | 2 | 2 | 3 | 5 | 6 | 9 |
| 65+ | 3046 | 3.7 | 8 | 1 | 2 | 3 | 5 | 7 | 9 | 15 |
| **GRAND TOTAL** | **14661** | **2.6** | **5** | **1** | **1** | **2** | **3** | **5** | **6** | **10** |

Because each patient is unique, we stratify patients by single or multiple diagnoses, operated or not operated, status, and age.

Length of stay (in days) by percentile document the statistical range of stays for each patient group, so you can determine the right length of stay for your patient.

Total number of patients

Observed Patients is the actual number of patient discharges. HCIA-Sachs derives length of stay figures from real patient data projected to represent the inpatient universe. See "Description of the Database" for further explanation.

The variance shows how much the individual patient lengths of stay ranged around the average.

Average length of stay, in days, calculated from the admission and discharge dates

# FEATURES OF AN OPERATION TABLE

ICD-9-CM procedure code and title ⌐

Operation group(s) used in HCIA-Sachs' former "List A and B" coding system ⌐

**01.1: SKULL/BRAIN DX PROCEDURE. Formerly included in operation group(s) 501, 512.**

| Type of Patients | Observed Patients | Avg. Stay | Vari-ance | Percentiles | | | | | | |
|---|---|---|---|---|---|---|---|---|---|---|
| | | | | 10th | 25th | 50th | 75th | 90th | 95th | 99th |
| **1. SINGLE DX** | | | | | | | | | | |
| 0–19 Years | 78 | 4.4 | 20 | 1 | 1 | 3 | 6 | 11 | 11 | 28 |
| 20–34 | 62 | 2.6 | 8 | 1 | 1 | 1 | 3 | 5 | 7 | 14 |
| 35–49 | 82 | 4.1 | 21 | 1 | 1 | 4 | 4 | 7 | 10 | 18 |
| 50–64 | 92 | 3.5 | 17 | 1 | 1 | 2 | 4 | 7 | 9 | 26 |
| 65+ | 68 | 5.6 | 32 | 1 | 1 | 2 | 10 | 15 | 15 | 17 |
| **2. MULTIPLE DX** | | | | | | | | | | |
| 0–19 Years | 425 | 15.6 | 236 | 2 | 4 | 11 | 21 | 38 | 56 | 71 |
| 20–34 | 429 | 14.1 | 238 | 1 | 3 | 7 | 19 | 42 | 49 | 71 |
| 35–49 | 471 | 11.0 | 137 | 1 | 3 | 6 | 15 | 29 | 35 | >99 |
| 50–64 | 471 | 8.5 | 77 | 1 | 3 | 5 | 9 | 21 | 31 | 37 |
| 65+ | 665 | 10.8 | 120 | 1 | 3 | 7 | 14 | 25 | 33 | 48 |
| **TOTAL SINGLE DX** | **382** | **4.1** | **21** | **1** | **1** | **2** | **5** | **10** | **15** | **18** |
| **TOTAL MULTIPLE DX** | **2,337** | **11.7** | **159** | **1** | **3** | **7** | **16** | **29** | **40** | **62** |
| **TOTAL** | | | | | | | | | | |
| 0–19 Years | 503 | 14.1 | 222 | 1 | 3 | 9 | 21 | 34 | 56 | 71 |
| 20–34 | 409 | 12.6 | 223 | 1 | 2 | 7 | 17 | 39 | 49 | 67 |
| 35–49 | 511 | 9.6 | 121 | 1 | 2 | 6 | 14 | 27 | 31 | 77 |
| 50–64 | 563 | 7.7 | 71 | 1 | 2 | 5 | 9 | 18 | 28 | 37 |
| 65+ | 733 | 10.4 | 115 | 1 | 3 | 7 | 14 | 25 | 30 | 48 |
| **GRAND TOTAL** | **2,719** | **10.7** | **147** | **1** | **2** | **7** | **14** | **28** | **37** | **59** |

Because each patient is unique, we stratify patients by single or multiple diagnoses and age.

Length of stay (in days) by percentile document the statistical range of stays for each patient group, so you can determine the right length of stay for your patient.

Total number of patients

Observed Patients is the actual number of patient discharges. HCIA-Sachs derives length of stay figures from real patient data projected to represent the inpatient universe. See "Description of the Database" for further explanation.

The variance shows how much individual patient lengths of stay ranged around the average.

Average length of stay, in days, calculated from the admission and discharge dates

## HCIASachs
### eHealthIntelligence

# Find the Health Care Resources You Need

---

**The Comparative Performance of U.S. Hospitals: The Sourcebook**
Search comprehensive information on the performance of the U.S. hospital industry for the latest five-year period. Included in the book are 59 key measures of hospital performance, with median and quartile values presented for 157 hospital comparison groups. Published with Deloitte & Touche. $399*

**The DRG Handbook: Comparative Clinical and Financial Benchmarks**
Focus on key clinical and financial measures for the 100 highest volume Diagnosis-Related Groups (DRGs). For each DRG, *The Handbook* provides data on clinical characteristics, resource consumption, costs, reimbursement, and charge levels. Includes all-payor data. Published with Ernst & Young. $399*

**Profiles of U.S. Hospitals**
Evaluate the performance for nearly every U.S. hospital using more than 50 key measures of financial, clinical, and operating data. Decile rankings for financial indicators such as profitability, leverage, and liquidity are also included. In addition, *Profiles of U.S. Hospitals* lists the number of cases, average charge, and average length of stay for each of the hospital's top five DRGs. $299*

\* Also available electronically.
Please call for prices.

*(continued on other side)*

# www.hciasachs.com

---

# 4 WAYS TO ORDER

❶ Call **(800) 568-3282**
❷ Fax your order to **(410) 752-6309**
❸ Return the attached order card(s)
❹ E-mail to **pubs@hciasachs.com**

---

## Order data on today's health care industry
### HCIASachs

| Item | Qty. | Price | Total |
|------|------|-------|-------|
| ❏ The Comparative Performance of U.S. Hospitals: The Sourcebook | | $ 399 | |
| ❏ The DRG Handbook: Comparative Clinical and Financial Benchmarks | | 399 | |
| ❏ Profiles of U.S. Hospitals | | 299 | |
| ❏ The Guide to the Managed Care Industry | | 245 | |
| ❏ The Guide to the Nursing Home Industry | | 249 | |

*Call for PDF and database prices*

(AL, CA, CO, CT, FL, GA, IL, KY, LA, MA, MD, MI, NC, NV, NY, OH, RI, SC, TN, TX, UT, VA, WA)

Subtotal _____
Sales Tax _____
Shipping and Handling (up to 6 items) ___$15.00___
Total _____

Name_____
Title_____
Company_____
Address_____
*(cannot be delivered to a P.O. box)*
City_____ State_____ Zip_____
Telephone_____
E-mail_____
Fax_____

❏ Enclosed is a check
 made payable to HCIA-Sachs for $_____

❏ Please bill my: ❏ VISA ❏ MasterCard ❏ AmEx
Account #_____
Expiration Date_____
Purchase Order #_____
Signature_____

---

## Target selected markets with HCIA-Sachs directories
### HCIASachs

| Item | Qty. | Price | Total |
|------|------|-------|-------|
| ❏ The Directory of Nursing Homes | | $ 249 | |
| ❏ The Directory of Retirement Facilities | | 249 | |
| ❏ The Directory of Health Care Professionals | | 299 | |

*Call for PDF and database prices*

(AL, CA, CO, CT, FL, GA, IL, KY, LA, MA, MD, MI, NC, NV, NY, OH, RI, SC, TN, TX, UT, VA, WA)

Subtotal _____
Sales Tax _____
Shipping and Handling (up to 6 items) ___$15.00___
Total _____

Name_____
Title_____
Company_____
Address_____
*(cannot be delivered to a P.O. box)*
City_____ State_____ Zip_____
Telephone_____
E-mail_____
Fax_____

❏ Enclosed is a check
 made payable to HCIA-Sachs for $_____

❏ Please bill my:
 ❏ VISA ❏ MasterCard ❏ AmEx
Account #_____
Expiration Date_____
Purchase Order #_____
Signature_____
*(required)*

---

## Receive specialized decision support products and service information
### HCIASachs

*All HCIA-Sachs products and services are supported by the industry's most sophisticated and reliable databases.*

**Yes!** Please send me information about the solutions HCIA-Sachs provides for: *(check all that apply)*

❏ **Providers,** such as hospitals, physician groups, and integrated delivery systems.

❏ **Buyers,** such as managed care organizations, indemnity insurers, and employers.

❏ **Suppliers,** such as pharmaceutical, biotechnology, and medical supply and device companies.

❏ **Free** publications catalog.

Name_____
Title_____
Company_____
Address_____
City_____ State____ Zip_____
Telephone_____
E-mail_____
Fax_____

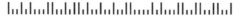
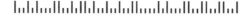
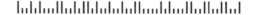
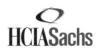
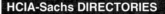
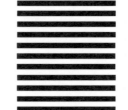

# LENGTH OF STAY TABLES
# OPERATION CODES

**United States, October 1998–September 1999 Data, by Operation**

## SUMMARY OF ALL PATIENTS IN OPERATION CODES

| Type of Patients | Observed Patients | Avg. Stay | Variance | Percentiles | | | | | | |
|---|---|---|---|---|---|---|---|---|---|---|
| | | | | 10th | 25th | 50th | 75th | 90th | 95th | 99th |
| **1. SINGLE DX** | | | | | | | | | | |
| 0–19 Years | 371,032 | 2.1 | 3 | 1 | 1 | 2 | 2 | 3 | 4 | 8 |
| 20–34 | 387,923 | 2.0 | 2 | 1 | 1 | 2 | 2 | 3 | 4 | 7 |
| 35–49 | 138,621 | 2.4 | 5 | 1 | 1 | 2 | 3 | 4 | 6 | 11 |
| 50–64 | 66,957 | 2.7 | 6 | 1 | 1 | 2 | 3 | 5 | 6 | 11 |
| 65+ | 49,704 | 3.1 | 8 | 1 | 1 | 2 | 4 | 6 | 7 | 14 |
| **2. MULTIPLE DX** | | | | | | | | | | |
| 0–19 Years | 723,186 | 4.7 | 64 | 1 | 2 | 2 | 4 | 9 | 16 | 49 |
| 20–34 | 875,178 | 3.4 | 18 | 1 | 2 | 2 | 3 | 6 | 9 | 21 |
| 35–49 | 813,850 | 4.6 | 32 | 1 | 2 | 3 | 5 | 9 | 14 | 29 |
| 50–64 | 840,381 | 5.6 | 41 | 1 | 2 | 4 | 7 | 11 | 16 | 33 |
| 65+ | 1,637,035 | 6.7 | 44 | 2 | 3 | 5 | 8 | 13 | 18 | 34 |
| **TOTAL SINGLE DX** | 1,014,237 | 2.2 | 3 | 1 | 1 | 2 | 2 | 4 | 5 | 9 |
| **TOTAL MULTIPLE DX** | 4,889,630 | 5.2 | 41 | 1 | 2 | 3 | 6 | 11 | 16 | 33 |
| **TOTAL** | | | | | | | | | | |
| 0–19 Years | 1,094,218 | 3.8 | 44 | 1 | 2 | 2 | 3 | 7 | 11 | 37 |
| 20–34 | 1,263,101 | 3.0 | 13 | 1 | 2 | 2 | 3 | 5 | 7 | 18 |
| 35–49 | 952,471 | 4.3 | 28 | 1 | 2 | 3 | 5 | 8 | 13 | 27 |
| 50–64 | 907,338 | 5.4 | 38 | 1 | 2 | 4 | 6 | 11 | 16 | 32 |
| 65+ | 1,686,739 | 6.5 | 43 | 1 | 3 | 5 | 8 | 13 | 18 | 33 |
| **GRAND TOTAL** | 5,903,867 | 4.7 | 35 | 1 | 2 | 3 | 5 | 10 | 14 | 30 |

# United States, October 1998–September 1999 Data, by Operation

## 01.0: CRANIAL PUNCTURE. Formerly included in operation group(s) 501.

| Type of Patients | Observed Patients | Avg. Stay | Variance | 10th | 25th | 50th | 75th | 90th | 95th | 99th |
|---|---|---|---|---|---|---|---|---|---|---|
| **1. SINGLE DX** | | | | | | | | | | |
| 0–19 Years | 23 | 2.5 | 6 | 1 | 1 | 3 | 3 | 3 | 4 | 22 |
| 20–34 | 7 | 2.8 | 11 | 1 | 1 | 1 | 4 | 11 | 11 | 11 |
| 35–49 | 5 | 2.9 | 9 | 1 | 1 | 1 | 6 | 11 | 8 | 8 |
| 50–64 | 7 | 2.1 | 4 | 1 | 1 | 1 | 3 | 4 | 4 | 10 |
| 65+ | 7 | 2.6 | 2 | 2 | 2 | 2 | 2 | 4 | 7 | 7 |
| **2. MULTIPLE DX** | | | | | | | | | | |
| 0–19 Years | 488 | 6.0 | 151 | 1 | 1 | 3 | 5 | 12 | 18 | 88 |
| 20–34 | 68 | 6.9 | 238 | 1 | 1 | 3 | 5 | 12 | 21 | 92 |
| 35–49 | 83 | 8.6 | 138 | 2 | 3 | 4 | 9 | 15 | 49 | 53 |
| 50–64 | 70 | 6.4 | 31 | 1 | 3 | 5 | 6 | 13 | 21 | 36 |
| 65+ | 111 | 7.8 | 41 | 2 | 4 | 7 | 9 | 15 | 19 | 34 |
| **TOTAL SINGLE DX** | 49 | 2.5 | 6 | 1 | 1 | 2 | 3 | 4 | 6 | 11 |
| **TOTAL MULTIPLE DX** | 820 | 6.6 | 133 | 1 | 2 | 4 | 7 | 13 | 20 | 86 |
| **TOTAL** | | | | | | | | | | |
| 0–19 Years | 511 | 5.8 | 143 | 1 | 2 | 3 | 5 | 12 | 18 | 86 |
| 20–34 | 75 | 6.6 | 225 | 1 | 1 | 2 | 5 | 12 | 21 | 92 |
| 35–49 | 88 | 8.4 | 134 | 2 | 3 | 4 | 9 | 15 | 49 | 53 |
| 50–64 | 77 | 5.9 | 30 | 1 | 2 | 5 | 6 | 13 | 20 | 36 |
| 65+ | 118 | 7.4 | 40 | 2 | 4 | 6 | 8 | 15 | 19 | 34 |
| **GRAND TOTAL** | 869 | 6.4 | 126 | 1 | 2 | 3 | 6 | 13 | 20 | 86 |

## 01.1: DXTIC PX ON SKULL/BRAIN. Formerly included in operation group(s) 501, 512.

| Type of Patients | Observed Patients | Avg. Stay | Variance | 10th | 25th | 50th | 75th | 90th | 95th | 99th |
|---|---|---|---|---|---|---|---|---|---|---|
| **1. SINGLE DX** | | | | | | | | | | |
| 0–19 Years | 70 | 4.1 | 11 | 1 | 2 | 3 | 5 | 8 | 11 | 17 |
| 20–34 | 51 | 4.7 | 19 | 1 | 3 | 3 | 7 | 12 | 12 | 25 |
| 35–49 | 86 | 2.2 | 3 | 1 | 1 | 1 | 3 | 4 | 8 | 10 |
| 50–64 | 82 | 3.4 | 6 | 1 | 1 | 4 | 4 | 6 | 7 | 12 |
| 65+ | 60 | 2.3 | 5 | 1 | 1 | 1 | 2 | 6 | 8 | 11 |
| **2. MULTIPLE DX** | | | | | | | | | | |
| 0–19 Years | 531 | 11.8 | 180 | 2 | 4 | 6 | 16 | 31 | 38 | 76 |
| 20–34 | 338 | 8.3 | 85 | 1 | 3 | 6 | 12 | 18 | 26 | 50 |
| 35–49 | 568 | 9.0 | 87 | 1 | 2 | 6 | 13 | 21 | 28 | 41 |
| 50–64 | 541 | 8.9 | 76 | 1 | 2 | 6 | 13 | 21 | 22 | 42 |
| 65+ | 797 | 8.7 | 70 | 2 | 3 | 7 | 11 | 18 | 28 | 46 |
| **TOTAL SINGLE DX** | 349 | 3.4 | 9 | 1 | 1 | 2 | 4 | 7 | 10 | 17 |
| **TOTAL MULTIPLE DX** | 2,775 | 9.3 | 100 | 1 | 3 | 6 | 12 | 21 | 29 | 49 |
| **TOTAL** | | | | | | | | | | |
| 0–19 Years | 601 | 10.3 | 157 | 1 | 3 | 5 | 14 | 26 | 38 | 67 |
| 20–34 | 389 | 8.0 | 80 | 1 | 3 | 5 | 11 | 16 | 25 | 49 |
| 35–49 | 654 | 8.2 | 83 | 1 | 2 | 4 | 12 | 20 | 26 | 39 |
| 50–64 | 623 | 8.2 | 70 | 1 | 2 | 6 | 12 | 18 | 21 | 42 |
| 65+ | 857 | 8.3 | 68 | 2 | 3 | 7 | 10 | 17 | 28 | 43 |
| **GRAND TOTAL** | 3,124 | 8.6 | 93 | 1 | 2 | 6 | 12 | 20 | 28 | 47 |

## 01.02: VENTRICULOPUNCT VIA CATH. Formerly included in operation group(s) 501.

| Type of Patients | Observed Patients | Avg. Stay | Variance | 10th | 25th | 50th | 75th | 90th | 95th | 99th |
|---|---|---|---|---|---|---|---|---|---|---|
| **1. SINGLE DX** | | | | | | | | | | |
| 0–19 Years | 8 | 1.4 | <1 | 1 | 1 | 1 | 1 | 3 | 4 | 4 |
| 20–34 | 1 | 11.0 | 0 | 11 | 11 | 11 | 11 | 11 | 11 | 11 |
| 35–49 | 0 | | | | | | | | | |
| 50–64 | 0 | | | | | | | | | |
| 65+ | 1 | 2.0 | 0 | 2 | 2 | 2 | 2 | 2 | 2 | 2 |
| **2. MULTIPLE DX** | | | | | | | | | | |
| 0–19 Years | 408 | 4.0 | 28 | 1 | 2 | 3 | 5 | 8 | 13 | 20 |
| 20–34 | 53 | 4.0 | 23 | 1 | 2 | 4 | 5 | 9 | 16 | 21 |
| 35–49 | 43 | 10.9 | 224 | 3 | 4 | 4 | 8 | 49 | 49 | >99 |
| 50–64 | 34 | 6.0 | 24 | 2 | 4 | 6 | 6 | 8 | 13 | 36 |
| 65+ | 44 | 7.3 | 28 | 2 | 4 | 6 | 9 | 12 | 22 | 27 |
| **TOTAL SINGLE DX** | 10 | 1.8 | 3 | 1 | 1 | 1 | 2 | 3 | 4 | 11 |
| **TOTAL MULTIPLE DX** | 582 | 4.9 | 46 | 1 | 2 | 3 | 6 | 9 | 16 | 49 |
| **TOTAL** | | | | | | | | | | |
| 0–19 Years | 416 | 4.0 | 27 | 1 | 2 | 3 | 5 | 8 | 13 | 20 |
| 20–34 | 54 | 4.0 | 23 | 1 | 1 | 2 | 5 | 11 | 16 | 21 |
| 35–49 | 43 | 10.9 | 224 | 3 | 4 | 4 | 8 | 49 | 49 | >99 |
| 50–64 | 34 | 6.0 | 24 | 2 | 2 | 6 | 6 | 8 | 13 | 36 |
| 65+ | 45 | 6.6 | 28 | 2 | 2 | 5 | 8 | 12 | 22 | 27 |
| **GRAND TOTAL** | 592 | 4.8 | 45 | 1 | 2 | 3 | 5 | 9 | 15 | 49 |

## 01.13: CLSD (PERC) BRAIN BX. Formerly included in operation group(s) 501.

| Type of Patients | Observed Patients | Avg. Stay | Variance | 10th | 25th | 50th | 75th | 90th | 95th | 99th |
|---|---|---|---|---|---|---|---|---|---|---|
| **1. SINGLE DX** | | | | | | | | | | |
| 0–19 Years | 26 | 3.1 | 8 | 1 | 1 | 2 | 4 | 8 | 11 | 11 |
| 20–34 | 33 | 2.3 | 3 | 1 | 1 | 2 | 3 | 5 | 8 | 8 |
| 35–49 | 62 | 2.0 | 3 | 1 | 1 | 1 | 2 | 3 | 5 | 10 |
| 50–64 | 57 | 1.9 | 3 | 1 | 1 | 1 | 2 | 3 | 5 | 8 |
| 65+ | 48 | 2.1 | 5 | 1 | 1 | 2 | 2 | 6 | 7 | 11 |
| **2. MULTIPLE DX** | | | | | | | | | | |
| 0–19 Years | 62 | 5.2 | 47 | 1 | 2 | 2 | 6 | 6 | 24 | 30 |
| 20–34 | 115 | 7.2 | 42 | 1 | 2 | 7 | 16 | 16 | 16 | 26 |
| 35–49 | 283 | 5.3 | 74 | 1 | 2 | 6 | 6 | 16 | 24 | 79 |
| 50–64 | 308 | 6.2 | 58 | 1 | 4 | 8 | 8 | 14 | 21 | 42 |
| 65+ | 524 | 6.1 | 44 | 1 | 5 | 8 | 8 | 12 | 16 | 32 |
| **TOTAL SINGLE DX** | 226 | 2.3 | 5 | 1 | 1 | 1 | 3 | 4 | 7 | 11 |
| **TOTAL MULTIPLE DX** | 1,292 | 6.1 | 54 | 1 | 4 | 4 | 8 | 15 | 19 | 42 |
| **TOTAL** | | | | | | | | | | |
| 0–19 Years | 88 | 4.4 | 33 | 1 | 2 | 3 | 4 | 11 | 17 | 28 |
| 20–34 | 148 | 6.4 | 39 | 1 | 3 | 3 | 9 | 16 | 16 | 23 |
| 35–49 | 345 | 4.8 | 64 | 1 | 2 | 2 | 5 | 12 | 20 | 78 |
| 50–64 | 365 | 5.7 | 54 | 1 | 3 | 3 | 7 | 12 | 19 | 42 |
| 65+ | 572 | 5.7 | 42 | 1 | 4 | 4 | 8 | 12 | 16 | 30 |
| **GRAND TOTAL** | 1,518 | 5.5 | 49 | 1 | 3 | 3 | 7 | 13 | 17 | 36 |

Length of Stay by Diagnosis and Operation, United States, 2000

# United States, October 1998–September 1999 Data, by Operation

## 01.14: OPEN BIOPSY OF BRAIN. Formerly included in operation group(s) 501.

| Type of Patients | Observed Patients | Avg. Stay | Vari-ance | Percentiles | | | | | | |
|---|---|---|---|---|---|---|---|---|---|---|
| | | | | 10th | 25th | 50th | 75th | 90th | 95th | 99th |
| **1. SINGLE DX** | | | | | | | | | | |
| 0–19 Years | 16 | 5.1 | 12 | 2 | 2 | 3 | 8 | 9 | 12 | 13 |
| 20–34 | 8 | 9.1 | 47 | 7 | 7 | 8 | 8 | 25 | 25 | 25 |
| 35–49 | 16 | 2.5 | 5 | 1 | 1 | 2 | 2 | 5 | 8 | 10 |
| 50–64 | 17 | 5.4 | 7 | 3 | 4 | 6 | 6 | 7 | 12 | 14 |
| 65+ | 7 | 3.4 | 4 | 2 | 2 | 3 | 5 | 5 | 10 | 10 |
| **2. MULTIPLE DX** | | | | | | | | | | |
| 0–19 Years | 64 | 17.2 | 437 | 3 | 4 | 8 | 24 | 39 | 90 | >99 |
| 20–34 | 50 | 6.8 | 176 | 1 | 1 | 2 | 6 | 15 | 24 | 94 |
| 35–49 | 147 | 8.4 | 88 | 2 | 3 | 4 | 12 | 19 | 30 | 47 |
| 50–64 | 138 | 9.2 | 92 | 2 | 3 | 7 | 11 | 18 | 27 | 42 |
| 65+ | 170 | 9.9 | 60 | 3 | 4 | 9 | 13 | 19 | 25 | 37 |
| **TOTAL SINGLE DX** | 64 | 4.7 | 13 | 1 | 2 | 4 | 6 | 9 | 12 | 14 |
| **TOTAL MULTIPLE DX** | 569 | 9.7 | 134 | 2 | 3 | 6 | 13 | 21 | 30 | 82 |
| **TOTAL** | | | | | | | | | | |
| 0–19 Years | 80 | 14.7 | 373 | 2 | 3 | 8 | 16 | 36 | 90 | >99 |
| 20–34 | 58 | 7.0 | 166 | 1 | 1 | 2 | 7 | 16 | 24 | 94 |
| 35–49 | 163 | 7.9 | 83 | 2 | 3 | 4 | 10 | 16 | 27 | 41 |
| 50–64 | 155 | 8.6 | 80 | 3 | 4 | 6 | 10 | 17 | 23 | 42 |
| 65+ | 177 | 9.6 | 59 | 2 | 3 | 8 | 12 | 19 | 25 | 37 |
| **GRAND TOTAL** | 633 | 9.1 | 123 | 2 | 3 | 6 | 12 | 19 | 28 | 64 |

## 01.2: CRANIOTOMY & CRANIECTOMY. Formerly included in operation group(s) 502.

| Type of Patients | Observed Patients | Avg. Stay | Vari-ance | Percentiles | | | | | | |
|---|---|---|---|---|---|---|---|---|---|---|
| | | | | 10th | 25th | 50th | 75th | 90th | 95th | 99th |
| **1. SINGLE DX** | | | | | | | | | | |
| 0–19 Years | 368 | 3.5 | 4 | 2 | 3 | 3 | 4 | 5 | 7 | 10 |
| 20–34 | 119 | 4.8 | 12 | 1 | 3 | 3 | 6 | 9 | 12 | 15 |
| 35–49 | 122 | 4.2 | 6 | 2 | 3 | 4 | 5 | 7 | 7 | 16 |
| 50–64 | 85 | 6.1 | 28 | 1 | 2 | 4 | 8 | 16 | 16 | 16 |
| 65+ | 60 | 4.1 | 7 | 2 | 3 | 3 | 4 | 8 | 11 | 11 |
| **2. MULTIPLE DX** | | | | | | | | | | |
| 0–19 Years | 738 | 7.6 | 107 | 3 | 3 | 4 | 8 | 15 | 23 | 76 |
| 20–34 | 388 | 9.2 | 105 | 3 | 3 | 6 | 10 | 18 | 36 | 45 |
| 35–49 | 566 | 12.0 | 113 | 3 | 4 | 8 | 18 | 28 | 36 | 40 |
| 50–64 | 545 | 9.2 | 74 | 2 | 4 | 7 | 12 | 20 | 25 | 46 |
| 65+ | 919 | 9.2 | 70 | 3 | 4 | 7 | 12 | 18 | 23 | 45 |
| **TOTAL SINGLE DX** | 754 | 4.1 | 9 | 2 | 3 | 3 | 4 | 7 | 10 | 16 |
| **TOTAL MULTIPLE DX** | 3,156 | 9.4 | 94 | 3 | 4 | 6 | 11 | 20 | 28 | 47 |
| **TOTAL** | | | | | | | | | | |
| 0–19 Years | 1,106 | 6.1 | 73 | 2 | 3 | 4 | 6 | 11 | 17 | 56 |
| 20–34 | 507 | 8.1 | 86 | 2 | 3 | 5 | 9 | 15 | 26 | 44 |
| 35–49 | 688 | 10.8 | 104 | 2 | 3 | 6 | 15 | 25 | 31 | 40 |
| 50–64 | 630 | 8.8 | 68 | 2 | 3 | 6 | 12 | 18 | 24 | 46 |
| 65+ | 979 | 8.9 | 68 | 3 | 4 | 6 | 11 | 17 | 23 | 45 |
| **GRAND TOTAL** | 3,910 | 8.3 | 81 | 2 | 3 | 5 | 10 | 18 | 25 | 45 |

## 01.18: DXTIC PX BRAIN/CEREB NEC. Formerly included in operation group(s) 512.

| Type of Patients | Observed Patients | Avg. Stay | Vari-ance | Percentiles | | | | | | |
|---|---|---|---|---|---|---|---|---|---|---|
| | | | | 10th | 25th | 50th | 75th | 90th | 95th | 99th |
| **1. SINGLE DX** | | | | | | | | | | |
| 0–19 Years | 21 | 4.6 | 12 | 2 | 3 | 4 | 5 | 5 | 17 | 17 |
| 20–34 | 9 | 8.4 | 11 | 4 | 7 | 7 | 12 | 12 | 12 | 14 |
| 35–49 | 3 | 2.8 | <1 | 1 | 3 | 3 | 3 | 3 | 3 | 3 |
| 50–64 | 5 | 4.3 | 2 | 4 | 4 | 4 | 4 | 5 | 9 | 9 |
| 65+ | 3 | 4.0 | 10 | 1 | 1 | 5 | 8 | 8 | 8 | 8 |
| **2. MULTIPLE DX** | | | | | | | | | | |
| 0–19 Years | 394 | 12.2 | 156 | 2 | 4 | 7 | 17 | 32 | 38 | 56 |
| 20–34 | 169 | 9.0 | 86 | 3 | 3 | 6 | 12 | 19 | 31 | 51 |
| 35–49 | 123 | 13.4 | 69 | 4 | 7 | 12 | 19 | 26 | 29 | 36 |
| 50–64 | 67 | 14.7 | 57 | 6 | 8 | 14 | 19 | 21 | 21 | 55 |
| 65+ | 68 | 13.7 | 91 | 4 | 8 | 10 | 16 | 28 | 36 | 39 |
| **TOTAL SINGLE DX** | 41 | 4.8 | 11 | 2 | 3 | 4 | 5 | 9 | 12 | 17 |
| **TOTAL MULTIPLE DX** | 821 | 12.1 | 109 | 3 | 4 | 9 | 17 | 26 | 35 | 52 |
| **TOTAL** | | | | | | | | | | |
| 0–19 Years | 415 | 11.1 | 142 | 2 | 4 | 5 | 14 | 29 | 38 | 55 |
| 20–34 | 178 | 9.0 | 84 | 3 | 3 | 7 | 12 | 19 | 31 | 50 |
| 35–49 | 126 | 13.1 | 70 | 4 | 7 | 12 | 18 | 26 | 29 | 36 |
| 50–64 | 72 | 13.3 | 62 | 4 | 8 | 14 | 18 | 21 | 21 | 45 |
| 65+ | 71 | 13.6 | 91 | 4 | 8 | 10 | 16 | 28 | 36 | 39 |
| **GRAND TOTAL** | 862 | 11.5 | 105 | 3 | 4 | 8 | 16 | 26 | 33 | 50 |

## 01.24: OTHER CRANIOTOMY. Formerly included in operation group(s) 502.

| Type of Patients | Observed Patients | Avg. Stay | Vari-ance | Percentiles | | | | | | |
|---|---|---|---|---|---|---|---|---|---|---|
| | | | | 10th | 25th | 50th | 75th | 90th | 95th | 99th |
| **1. SINGLE DX** | | | | | | | | | | |
| 0–19 Years | 280 | 3.6 | 5 | 2 | 3 | 3 | 4 | 6 | 7 | 11 |
| 20–34 | 74 | 4.4 | 9 | 2 | 3 | 3 | 5 | 9 | 10 | 15 |
| 35–49 | 87 | 4.5 | 7 | 2 | 3 | 4 | 5 | 7 | 7 | 16 |
| 50–64 | 66 | 3.7 | 6 | 1 | 2 | 3 | 5 | 7 | 8 | 12 |
| 65+ | 44 | 4.5 | 8 | 2 | 3 | 4 | 5 | 11 | 11 | 14 |
| **2. MULTIPLE DX** | | | | | | | | | | |
| 0–19 Years | 570 | 7.0 | 61 | 3 | 3 | 4 | 8 | 14 | 21 | 42 |
| 20–34 | 270 | 8.8 | 62 | 3 | 4 | 7 | 10 | 16 | 23 | 44 |
| 35–49 | 397 | 12.9 | 124 | 3 | 4 | 8 | 20 | 28 | 36 | 40 |
| 50–64 | 393 | 10.1 | 83 | 3 | 4 | 7 | 14 | 22 | 28 | 47 |
| 65+ | 770 | 9.2 | 68 | 3 | 4 | 7 | 11 | 18 | 23 | 45 |
| **TOTAL SINGLE DX** | 551 | 3.9 | 6 | 2 | 3 | 3 | 4 | 7 | 9 | 14 |
| **TOTAL MULTIPLE DX** | 2,400 | 9.4 | 81 | 3 | 4 | 6 | 12 | 21 | 27 | 44 |
| **TOTAL** | | | | | | | | | | |
| 0–19 Years | 850 | 5.8 | 44 | 2 | 3 | 4 | 6 | 12 | 15 | 33 |
| 20–34 | 344 | 7.9 | 54 | 3 | 3 | 6 | 9 | 15 | 21 | 44 |
| 35–49 | 484 | 11.6 | 116 | 2 | 4 | 7 | 18 | 28 | 36 | 40 |
| 50–64 | 459 | 9.1 | 77 | 3 | 3 | 6 | 12 | 20 | 25 | 46 |
| 65+ | 814 | 9.0 | 66 | 3 | 4 | 7 | 11 | 17 | 23 | 43 |
| **GRAND TOTAL** | 2,951 | 8.3 | 71 | 2 | 3 | 5 | 10 | 18 | 25 | 40 |

Length of Stay by Diagnosis and Operation, United States, 2000

# United States, October 1998–September 1999 Data, by Operation

## 01.25: OTHER CRANIECTOMY. Formerly included in operation group(s) 502.

| Type of Patients | Observed Patients | Avg. Stay | Variance | Percentiles | | | | | | |
|---|---|---|---|---|---|---|---|---|---|---|
| | | | | 10th | 25th | 50th | 75th | 90th | 95th | 99th |
| **1. SINGLE DX** | | | | | | | | | | |
| 0–19 Years | 83 | 3.2 | 2 | 2 | 3 | 3 | 3 | 4 | 6 | 7 |
| 20–34 | 36 | 2.9 | 3 | 1 | 1 | 3 | 4 | 6 | 6 | 7 |
| 35–49 | 26 | 3.3 | 1 | 2 | 3 | 3 | 3 | 5 | 5 | 8 |
| 50–64 | 12 | 5.1 | 13 | 1 | 3 | 5 | 6 | 7 | 15 | 15 |
| 65+ | 12 | 2.7 | 2 | 1 | 2 | 2 | 3 | 4 | 5 | 8 |
| **2. MULTIPLE DX** | | | | | | | | | | |
| 0–19 Years | 141 | 9.5 | 254 | 3 | 3 | 5 | 7 | 19 | 73 | 76 |
| 20–34 | 88 | 9.7 | 199 | 1 | 3 | 4 | 6 | 44 | 44 | 44 |
| 35–49 | 118 | 9.2 | 66 | 3 | 3 | 6 | 10 | 18 | 28 | 31 |
| 50–64 | 92 | 6.4 | 37 | 2 | 3 | 4 | 7 | 13 | 18 | 40 |
| 65+ | 99 | 9.2 | 89 | 2 | 4 | 6 | 12 | 18 | 22 | 58 |
| **TOTAL SINGLE DX** | 169 | 3.2 | 2 | 1 | 2 | 3 | 4 | 5 | 6 | 8 |
| **TOTAL MULTIPLE DX** | 538 | 9.0 | 138 | 2 | 3 | 5 | 9 | 19 | 31 | 76 |
| **TOTAL** | | | | | | | | | | |
| 0–19 | 224 | 6.8 | 155 | 2 | 3 | 4 | 5 | 8 | 29 | 76 |
| 20–34 | 124 | 8.1 | 161 | 1 | 3 | 5 | 5 | 44 | 44 | 44 |
| 35–49 | 144 | 8.1 | 60 | 3 | 3 | 5 | 10 | 18 | 28 | 31 |
| 50–64 | 104 | 6.3 | 35 | 2 | 3 | 4 | 7 | 13 | 18 | 35 |
| 65+ | 111 | 8.7 | 85 | 2 | 3 | 6 | 12 | 18 | 21 | 58 |
| **GRAND TOTAL** | 707 | 7.6 | 111 | 2 | 3 | 4 | 7 | 18 | 28 | 63 |

## 01.3: INC BRAIN/CEREB MENINGES. Formerly included in operation group(s) 501.

| Type of Patients | Observed Patients | Avg. Stay | Variance | Percentiles | | | | | | |
|---|---|---|---|---|---|---|---|---|---|---|
| | | | | 10th | 25th | 50th | 75th | 90th | 95th | 99th |
| **1. SINGLE DX** | | | | | | | | | | |
| 0–19 Years | 88 | 3.7 | 5 | 2 | 3 | 3 | 5 | 5 | 8 | 13 |
| 20–34 | 57 | 5.1 | 8 | 3 | 4 | 4 | 6 | 6 | 9 | 21 |
| 35–49 | 91 | 5.6 | 17 | 2 | 3 | 4 | 6 | 14 | 14 | 16 |
| 50–64 | 107 | 4.4 | 4 | 2 | 3 | 4 | 5 | 7 | 8 | 11 |
| 65+ | 157 | 4.5 | 9 | 1 | 2 | 4 | 6 | 9 | 9 | 17 |
| **2. MULTIPLE DX** | | | | | | | | | | |
| 0–19 Years | 429 | 12.9 | 143 | 2 | 5 | 9 | 16 | 28 | 35 | 57 |
| 20–34 | 293 | 13.9 | 121 | 3 | 6 | 13 | 18 | 29 | 34 | 66 |
| 35–49 | 587 | 13.2 | 130 | 3 | 5 | 9 | 18 | 31 | 37 | 56 |
| 50–64 | 935 | 11.5 | 121 | 3 | 5 | 8 | 14 | 24 | 35 | 64 |
| 65+ | 3,383 | 10.6 | 70 | 4 | 5 | 8 | 13 | 21 | 26 | 43 |
| **TOTAL SINGLE DX** | 500 | 4.6 | 9 | 2 | 3 | 4 | 6 | 9 | 10 | 16 |
| **TOTAL MULTIPLE DX** | 5,627 | 11.4 | 95 | 3 | 5 | 8 | 15 | 23 | 31 | 49 |
| **TOTAL** | | | | | | | | | | |
| 0–19 | 517 | 11.3 | 132 | 2 | 4 | 8 | 14 | 25 | 35 | 49 |
| 20–34 | 350 | 12.6 | 114 | 3 | 5 | 10 | 16 | 26 | 34 | 63 |
| 35–49 | 678 | 12.1 | 120 | 3 | 4 | 9 | 17 | 28 | 37 | 49 |
| 50–64 | 1,042 | 10.9 | 114 | 3 | 4 | 7 | 13 | 24 | 32 | 58 |
| 65+ | 3,540 | 10.3 | 69 | 3 | 5 | 8 | 13 | 21 | 26 | 43 |
| **GRAND TOTAL** | 6,127 | 10.8 | 91 | 3 | 4 | 7 | 14 | 23 | 30 | 49 |

## 01.31: INC CEREBRAL MENINGES. Formerly included in operation group(s) 501.

| Type of Patients | Observed Patients | Avg. Stay | Variance | Percentiles | | | | | | |
|---|---|---|---|---|---|---|---|---|---|---|
| | | | | 10th | 25th | 50th | 75th | 90th | 95th | 99th |
| **1. SINGLE DX** | | | | | | | | | | |
| 0–19 Years | 46 | 3.0 | 4 | 2 | 2 | 2 | 4 | 5 | 5 | 17 |
| 20–34 | 39 | 4.9 | 9 | 2 | 3 | 4 | 6 | 8 | 10 | 21 |
| 35–49 | 64 | 4.3 | 6 | 2 | 3 | 4 | 5 | 6 | 8 | 16 |
| 50–64 | 81 | 4.1 | 5 | 2 | 3 | 5 | 6 | 6 | 8 | 11 |
| 65+ | 133 | 4.8 | 7 | 2 | 3 | 5 | 6 | 9 | 9 | 11 |
| **2. MULTIPLE DX** | | | | | | | | | | |
| 0–19 Years | 248 | 13.4 | 151 | 3 | 5 | 12 | 15 | 32 | 35 | 65 |
| 20–34 | 157 | 14.4 | 113 | 3 | 8 | 14 | 20 | 26 | 34 | 88 |
| 35–49 | 366 | 13.0 | 125 | 3 | 5 | 9 | 18 | 31 | 37 | 49 |
| 50–64 | 634 | 10.4 | 111 | 3 | 4 | 7 | 11 | 23 | 28 | 58 |
| 65+ | 2,751 | 10.1 | 66 | 4 | 5 | 7 | 12 | 21 | 26 | 42 |
| **TOTAL SINGLE DX** | 363 | 4.4 | 6 | 2 | 3 | 4 | 5 | 8 | 9 | 15 |
| **TOTAL MULTIPLE DX** | 4,156 | 10.8 | 88 | 3 | 5 | 8 | 13 | 22 | 29 | 46 |
| **TOTAL** | | | | | | | | | | |
| 0–19 | 294 | 11.8 | 143 | 2 | 4 | 9 | 15 | 28 | 35 | 57 |
| 20–34 | 196 | 13.1 | 110 | 3 | 5 | 13 | 17 | 23 | 34 | 74 |
| 35–49 | 430 | 11.4 | 115 | 3 | 4 | 7 | 15 | 29 | 37 | 43 |
| 50–64 | 715 | 9.9 | 104 | 3 | 4 | 7 | 11 | 21 | 27 | 49 |
| 65+ | 2,884 | 9.8 | 64 | 3 | 5 | 7 | 12 | 20 | 26 | 42 |
| **GRAND TOTAL** | 4,519 | 10.3 | 84 | 3 | 5 | 7 | 13 | 22 | 28 | 44 |

## 01.39: OTHER BRAIN INCISION. Formerly included in operation group(s) 501.

| Type of Patients | Observed Patients | Avg. Stay | Variance | Percentiles | | | | | | |
|---|---|---|---|---|---|---|---|---|---|---|
| | | | | 10th | 25th | 50th | 75th | 90th | 95th | 99th |
| **1. SINGLE DX** | | | | | | | | | | |
| 0–19 Years | 38 | 4.3 | 6 | 2 | 3 | 4 | 5 | 5 | 11 | 13 |
| 20–34 | 17 | 5.4 | 7 | 3 | 3 | 6 | 9 | 9 | 9 | 9 |
| 35–49 | 26 | 4.8 | 13 | 2 | 3 | 4 | 6 | 10 | 11 | 19 |
| 50–64 | 26 | 5.0 | 3 | 3 | 4 | 5 | 6 | 7 | 9 | 9 |
| 65+ | 24 | 3.6 | 17 | 1 | 1 | 2 | 4 | 8 | 17 | 17 |
| **2. MULTIPLE DX** | | | | | | | | | | |
| 0–19 Years | 165 | 12.2 | 135 | 2 | 4 | 8 | 18 | 28 | 34 | 49 |
| 20–34 | 131 | 13.1 | 133 | 3 | 5 | 9 | 18 | 30 | 36 | 61 |
| 35–49 | 219 | 13.5 | 136 | 3 | 5 | 10 | 18 | 30 | 33 | 77 |
| 50–64 | 298 | 14.2 | 133 | 4 | 6 | 11 | 19 | 35 | 42 | >99 |
| 65+ | 629 | 12.7 | 82 | 4 | 6 | 11 | 17 | 24 | 29 | 50 |
| **TOTAL SINGLE DX** | 131 | 4.5 | 9 | 1 | 3 | 4 | 5 | 5 | 9 | 17 |
| **TOTAL MULTIPLE DX** | 1,442 | 13.1 | 113 | 3 | 6 | 10 | 18 | 26 | 35 | 56 |
| **TOTAL** | | | | | | | | | | |
| 0–19 | 203 | 10.7 | 120 | 2 | 3 | 7 | 12 | 24 | 33 | 49 |
| 20–34 | 148 | 11.9 | 122 | 3 | 5 | 8 | 16 | 30 | 34 | 61 |
| 35–49 | 245 | 13.0 | 133 | 3 | 4 | 10 | 18 | 28 | 33 | 67 |
| 50–64 | 324 | 13.3 | 128 | 3 | 6 | 10 | 17 | 31 | 41 | >99 |
| 65+ | 653 | 12.2 | 83 | 3 | 6 | 10 | 16 | 23 | 28 | 49 |
| **GRAND TOTAL** | 1,573 | 12.3 | 109 | 3 | 5 | 9 | 17 | 25 | 33 | 50 |

Length of Stay by Diagnosis and Operation, United States, 2000

# United States, October 1998–September 1999 Data, by Operation

## 01.4: THALAMUS/GLOBUS PALL OPS. Formerly included in operation group(s) 501.

| Type of Patients | Observed Patients | Avg. Stay | Variance | 10th | 25th | 50th | 75th | 90th | 95th | 99th |
|---|---|---|---|---|---|---|---|---|---|---|
| **1. SINGLE DX** | | | | | | | | | | |
| 0–19 Years | 6 | 2.8 | <1 | 2 | 3 | 3 | 3 | 3 | 3 | 3 |
| 20–34 | 1 | 1.0 | 0 | 1 | 1 | 1 | 1 | 1 | 1 | 1 |
| 35–49 | 10 | 1.9 | 1 | 1 | 1 | 2 | 2 | 3 | 6 | 6 |
| 50–64 | 26 | 2.1 | <1 | 1 | 1 | 2 | 3 | 3 | 4 | 4 |
| 65+ | 27 | 2.1 | 2 | 1 | 1 | 2 | 3 | 3 | 6 | 6 |
| **2. MULTIPLE DX** | | | | | | | | | | |
| 0–19 Years | 1 | 41.0 | 0 | 41 | 41 | 41 | 41 | 41 | 41 | 41 |
| 20–34 | 4 | 4.1 | 3 | 3 | 3 | 5 | 5 | 7 | 7 | 7 |
| 35–49 | 16 | 2.5 | 1 | 2 | 2 | 2 | 3 | 3 | 4 | 8 |
| 50–64 | 43 | 3.5 | 7 | 1 | 2 | 2 | 5 | 8 | 9 | 10 |
| 65+ | 79 | 3.3 | 7 | 1 | 1 | 2 | 4 | 7 | 8 | 16 |
| **TOTAL SINGLE DX** | 70 | 2.1 | 1 | 1 | 1 | 2 | 3 | 3 | 4 | 6 |
| **TOTAL MULTIPLE DX** | 143 | 3.8 | 27 | 1 | 2 | 2 | 4 | 7 | 9 | 41 |
| **TOTAL** | | | | | | | | | | |
| 0–19 Years | 7 | 15.2 | 343 | 2 | 3 | 3 | 41 | 41 | 41 | 41 |
| 20–34 | 5 | 3.9 | 3 | 2 | 3 | 3 | 5 | 7 | 7 | 7 |
| 35–49 | 26 | 2.3 | 2 | 1 | 2 | 2 | 3 | 3 | 4 | 8 |
| 50–64 | 69 | 3.0 | 5 | 1 | 1 | 2 | 4 | 7 | 8 | 10 |
| 65+ | 106 | 3.0 | 6 | 1 | 1 | 2 | 3 | 7 | 8 | 10 |
| **GRAND TOTAL** | 213 | 3.3 | 20 | 1 | 1 | 2 | 3 | 7 | 8 | 41 |

## 01.5: EXC/DESTR BRAIN/MENINGES. Formerly included in operation group(s) 501.

| Type of Patients | Observed Patients | Avg. Stay | Variance | 10th | 25th | 50th | 75th | 90th | 95th | 99th |
|---|---|---|---|---|---|---|---|---|---|---|
| **1. SINGLE DX** | | | | | | | | | | |
| 0–19 Years | 461 | 5.1 | 9 | 3 | 3 | 4 | 7 | 9 | 11 | 13 |
| 20–34 | 339 | 4.6 | 7 | 2 | 3 | 4 | 5 | 8 | 9 | 14 |
| 35–49 | 476 | 4.6 | 5 | 2 | 3 | 4 | 5 | 7 | 8 | 13 |
| 50–64 | 402 | 4.7 | 6 | 2 | 3 | 4 | 6 | 8 | 8 | 14 |
| 65+ | 192 | 5.5 | 14 | 2 | 3 | 4 | 7 | 13 | 13 | 15 |
| **2. MULTIPLE DX** | | | | | | | | | | |
| 0–19 Years | 1,346 | 9.7 | 94 | 3 | 4 | 7 | 12 | 20 | 28 | 57 |
| 20–34 | 857 | 6.6 | 36 | 2 | 3 | 5 | 8 | 13 | 18 | 34 |
| 35–49 | 2,009 | 7.5 | 48 | 3 | 4 | 5 | 9 | 14 | 20 | 38 |
| 50–64 | 2,642 | 7.6 | 46 | 3 | 4 | 6 | 9 | 15 | 19 | 42 |
| 65+ | 2,731 | 9.2 | 61 | 3 | 4 | 7 | 11 | 17 | 22 | 44 |
| **TOTAL SINGLE DX** | 1,870 | 4.8 | 7 | 2 | 3 | 4 | 6 | 8 | 10 | 13 |
| **TOTAL MULTIPLE DX** | 9,585 | 8.2 | 57 | 3 | 4 | 6 | 10 | 16 | 21 | 43 |
| **TOTAL** | | | | | | | | | | |
| 0–19 Years | 1,807 | 8.4 | 74 | 3 | 4 | 6 | 10 | 17 | 23 | 50 |
| 20–34 | 1,196 | 6.0 | 28 | 2 | 3 | 5 | 7 | 11 | 15 | 30 |
| 35–49 | 2,485 | 6.8 | 40 | 3 | 3 | 5 | 8 | 13 | 18 | 36 |
| 50–64 | 3,044 | 7.3 | 42 | 3 | 4 | 5 | 9 | 14 | 19 | 39 |
| 65+ | 2,923 | 8.9 | 59 | 3 | 4 | 7 | 11 | 16 | 22 | 43 |
| **GRAND TOTAL** | 11,455 | 7.6 | 50 | 3 | 4 | 6 | 9 | 15 | 20 | 40 |

## 01.51: EXC CEREB MENINGEAL LES. Formerly included in operation group(s) 501.

| Type of Patients | Observed Patients | Avg. Stay | Variance | 10th | 25th | 50th | 75th | 90th | 95th | 99th |
|---|---|---|---|---|---|---|---|---|---|---|
| **1. SINGLE DX** | | | | | | | | | | |
| 0–19 Years | 22 | 4.6 | 10 | 1 | 2 | 4 | 6 | 9 | 9 | 15 |
| 20–34 | 36 | 4.3 | 14 | 2 | 3 | 4 | 4 | 8 | 9 | 17 |
| 35–49 | 122 | 4.7 | 4 | 2 | 3 | 4 | 6 | 7 | 9 | 9 |
| 50–64 | 118 | 4.4 | 4 | 2 | 3 | 4 | 6 | 7 | 7 | 11 |
| 65+ | 57 | 4.2 | 5 | 2 | 3 | 3 | 5 | 7 | 7 | 16 |
| **2. MULTIPLE DX** | | | | | | | | | | |
| 0–19 Years | 54 | 9.1 | 104 | 2 | 3 | 6 | 12 | 19 | 23 | 64 |
| 20–34 | 72 | 4.7 | 14 | 3 | 3 | 5 | 5 | 7 | 10 | 20 |
| 35–49 | 373 | 6.2 | 41 | 2 | 3 | 4 | 7 | 11 | 14 | 38 |
| 50–64 | 532 | 7.8 | 61 | 3 | 4 | 5 | 9 | 13 | 20 | 46 |
| 65+ | 683 | 9.2 | 63 | 3 | 4 | 7 | 12 | 18 | 24 | 40 |
| **TOTAL SINGLE DX** | 355 | 4.5 | 5 | 2 | 3 | 4 | 6 | 7 | 8 | 11 |
| **TOTAL MULTIPLE DX** | 1,714 | 8.0 | 59 | 3 | 4 | 6 | 9 | 16 | 21 | 46 |
| **TOTAL** | | | | | | | | | | |
| 0–19 Years | 76 | 7.5 | 74 | 1 | 3 | 5 | 8 | 17 | 19 | 38 |
| 20–34 | 108 | 4.6 | 12 | 3 | 3 | 4 | 4 | 8 | 9 | 20 |
| 35–49 | 495 | 5.7 | 28 | 3 | 3 | 4 | 7 | 9 | 12 | 38 |
| 50–64 | 650 | 7.3 | 54 | 3 | 4 | 5 | 9 | 13 | 16 | 46 |
| 65+ | 740 | 9.0 | 62 | 3 | 4 | 7 | 11 | 18 | 24 | 36 |
| **GRAND TOTAL** | 2,069 | 7.4 | 51 | 3 | 4 | 5 | 9 | 14 | 19 | 42 |

## 01.53: BRAIN LOBECTOMY. Formerly included in operation group(s) 501.

| Type of Patients | Observed Patients | Avg. Stay | Variance | 10th | 25th | 50th | 75th | 90th | 95th | 99th |
|---|---|---|---|---|---|---|---|---|---|---|
| **1. SINGLE DX** | | | | | | | | | | |
| 0–19 Years | 26 | 5.0 | 8 | 3 | 4 | 4 | 5 | 7 | 12 | 19 |
| 20–34 | 28 | 6.0 | 12 | 2 | 3 | 5 | 9 | 11 | 12 | 14 |
| 35–49 | 29 | 5.2 | 7 | 3 | 3 | 4 | 6 | 10 | 10 | 13 |
| 50–64 | 11 | 4.8 | 5 | 2 | 3 | 4 | 8 | 8 | 8 | 8 |
| 65+ | 5 | 6.3 | 14 | 4 | 4 | 4 | 7 | 15 | 15 | 15 |
| **2. MULTIPLE DX** | | | | | | | | | | |
| 0–19 Years | 58 | 9.8 | 204 | 3 | 4 | 6 | 8 | 15 | 29 | 72 |
| 20–34 | 63 | 7.4 | 55 | 3 | 4 | 5 | 6 | 15 | 25 | 32 |
| 35–49 | 100 | 6.4 | 41 | 3 | 3 | 4 | 7 | 12 | 16 | 40 |
| 50–64 | 62 | 8.0 | 57 | 2 | 3 | 5 | 10 | 20 | 20 | 38 |
| 65+ | 47 | 7.1 | 21 | 2 | 3 | 7 | 10 | 14 | 14 | 19 |
| **TOTAL SINGLE DX** | 99 | 5.3 | 9 | 3 | 4 | 4 | 6 | 10 | 11 | 15 |
| **TOTAL MULTIPLE DX** | 330 | 7.6 | 77 | 3 | 3 | 5 | 8 | 14 | 20 | 54 |
| **TOTAL** | | | | | | | | | | |
| 0–19 Years | 84 | 8.3 | 147 | 3 | 4 | 5 | 6 | 12 | 18 | 72 |
| 20–34 | 91 | 7.1 | 46 | 3 | 4 | 5 | 7 | 13 | 18 | 32 |
| 35–49 | 129 | 6.2 | 35 | 3 | 3 | 4 | 7 | 10 | 15 | 40 |
| 50–64 | 73 | 7.6 | 52 | 2 | 3 | 5 | 8 | 19 | 20 | 38 |
| 65+ | 52 | 7.0 | 21 | 2 | 3 | 7 | 9 | 14 | 14 | 19 |
| **GRAND TOTAL** | 429 | 7.2 | 64 | 3 | 3 | 5 | 8 | 14 | 19 | 45 |

Length of Stay by Diagnosis and Operation, United States, 2000

# United States, October 1998–September 1999 Data, by Operation

## 01.59: EXC/DESTR BRAIN LES NEC. Formerly included in operation group(s) 501.

| Type of Patients | Observed Patients | Avg. Stay | Variance | 10th | 25th | 50th | 75th | 90th | 95th | 99th |
|---|---|---|---|---|---|---|---|---|---|---|
| **1. SINGLE DX** | | | | | | | | | | |
| 0–19 Years | 410 | 5.1 | 8 | 3 | 3 | 4 | 7 | 9 | 11 | 13 |
| 20–34 | 274 | 4.6 | 6 | 2 | 3 | 4 | 5 | 7 | 9 | 13 |
| 35–49 | 325 | 4.5 | 5 | 2 | 3 | 4 | 5 | 7 | 8 | 13 |
| 50–64 | 273 | 4.7 | 7 | 2 | 3 | 4 | 6 | 8 | 10 | 13 |
| 65+ | 130 | 5.8 | 16 | 2 | 3 | 4 | 7 | 13 | 13 | 14 |
| **2. MULTIPLE DX** | | | | | | | | | | |
| 0–19 Years | 1,188 | 9.6 | 86 | 3 | 4 | 7 | 12 | 20 | 27 | 54 |
| 20–34 | 720 | 6.8 | 36 | 2 | 3 | 5 | 8 | 13 | 19 | 35 |
| 35–49 | 1,531 | 7.8 | 50 | 3 | 4 | 6 | 9 | 15 | 20 | 38 |
| 50–64 | 2,047 | 7.6 | 42 | 3 | 3 | 6 | 9 | 15 | 19 | 32 |
| 65+ | 1,999 | 9.2 | 61 | 3 | 4 | 7 | 11 | 16 | 22 | 46 |
| **TOTAL SINGLE DX** | 1,412 | 4.9 | 8 | 2 | 3 | 4 | 6 | 8 | 10 | 14 |
| **TOTAL MULTIPLE DX** | 7,485 | 8.3 | 56 | 3 | 4 | 6 | 10 | 16 | 21 | 42 |
| **TOTAL** | | | | | | | | | | |
| 0–19 Years | 1,598 | 8.3 | 67 | 3 | 4 | 6 | 10 | 16 | 22 | 46 |
| 20–34 | 994 | 6.1 | 28 | 2 | 3 | 5 | 7 | 11 | 15 | 31 |
| 35–49 | 1,856 | 7.2 | 43 | 2 | 4 | 5 | 9 | 13 | 19 | 32 |
| 50–64 | 2,320 | 7.3 | 39 | 3 | 3 | 6 | 9 | 14 | 19 | 30 |
| 65+ | 2,129 | 9.0 | 58 | 3 | 4 | 7 | 11 | 16 | 22 | 46 |
| **GRAND TOTAL** | 8,897 | 7.7 | 49 | 3 | 4 | 6 | 9 | 15 | 20 | 39 |

## 02.0: CRANIOPLASTY. Formerly included in operation group(s) 503.

| Type of Patients | Observed Patients | Avg. Stay | Variance | 10th | 25th | 50th | 75th | 90th | 95th | 99th |
|---|---|---|---|---|---|---|---|---|---|---|
| **1. SINGLE DX** | | | | | | | | | | |
| 0–19 Years | 721 | 3.0 | 2 | 1 | 2 | 3 | 4 | 4 | 5 | 8 |
| 20–34 | 100 | 2.8 | 2 | 1 | 2 | 3 | 4 | 4 | 6 | 7 |
| 35–49 | 85 | 2.6 | 4 | 1 | 1 | 2 | 2 | 5 | 6 | 11 |
| 50–64 | 36 | 2.8 | 4 | 1 | 2 | 3 | 4 | 5 | 8 | 9 |
| 65+ | 3 | 2.2 | 1 | 1 | 3 | 3 | 3 | 3 | 3 | 3 |
| **2. MULTIPLE DX** | | | | | | | | | | |
| 0–19 Years | 1,128 | 6.2 | 47 | 2 | 3 | 4 | 7 | 12 | 17 | 44 |
| 20–34 | 413 | 7.3 | 63 | 1 | 2 | 4 | 10 | 19 | 19 | 36 |
| 35–49 | 392 | 7.2 | 57 | 1 | 2 | 5 | 10 | 15 | 18 | 35 |
| 50–64 | 206 | 5.5 | 42 | 1 | 2 | 3 | 7 | 10 | 19 | 40 |
| 65+ | 93 | 5.7 | 50 | 2 | 3 | 3 | 6 | 12 | 15 | 38 |
| **TOTAL SINGLE DX** | 945 | 2.9 | 3 | 1 | 2 | 3 | 4 | 4 | 5 | 8 |
| **TOTAL MULTIPLE DX** | 2,232 | 6.5 | 52 | 1 | 2 | 4 | 8 | 15 | 19 | 36 |
| **TOTAL** | | | | | | | | | | |
| 0–19 Years | 1,849 | 4.9 | 31 | 2 | 2 | 3 | 5 | 9 | 13 | 26 |
| 20–34 | 513 | 6.2 | 52 | 1 | 3 | 3 | 8 | 16 | 19 | 36 |
| 35–49 | 477 | 5.7 | 44 | 1 | 2 | 3 | 7 | 15 | 18 | 31 |
| 50–64 | 242 | 5.1 | 38 | 1 | 2 | 3 | 6 | 10 | 17 | 40 |
| 65+ | 96 | 5.6 | 49 | 2 | 3 | 3 | 6 | 12 | 15 | 38 |
| **GRAND TOTAL** | 3,177 | 5.3 | 39 | 1 | 2 | 3 | 6 | 12 | 17 | 34 |

## 01.6: EXCISION OF SKULL LESION. Formerly included in operation group(s) 501.

| Type of Patients | Observed Patients | Avg. Stay | Variance | 10th | 25th | 50th | 75th | 90th | 95th | 99th |
|---|---|---|---|---|---|---|---|---|---|---|
| **1. SINGLE DX** | | | | | | | | | | |
| 0–19 Years | 95 | 1.9 | 2 | 1 | 1 | 1 | 3 | 4 | 5 | 7 |
| 20–34 | 20 | 2.3 | 3 | 1 | 1 | 1 | 3 | 6 | 6 | 6 |
| 35–49 | 26 | 2.0 | 3 | 1 | 1 | 1 | 2 | 4 | 5 | 8 |
| 50–64 | 11 | 2.4 | 4 | 1 | 1 | 2 | 2 | 5 | 9 | 9 |
| 65+ | 7 | 1.2 | <1 | 1 | 1 | 1 | 1 | 1 | 4 | 5 |
| **2. MULTIPLE DX** | | | | | | | | | | |
| 0–19 Years | 51 | 6.3 | 47 | 1 | 2 | 4 | 10 | 10 | 13 | 40 |
| 20–34 | 34 | 4.8 | 30 | 1 | 1 | 2 | 9 | 13 | 17 | 22 |
| 35–49 | 62 | 5.2 | 19 | 1 | 3 | 4 | 7 | 15 | 19 | 32 |
| 50–64 | 66 | 13.2 | 210 | 1 | 1 | 4 | 35 | 35 | 35 | 35 |
| 65+ | 60 | 6.9 | 37 | 1 | 2 | 6 | 9 | 14 | 17 | 33 |
| **TOTAL SINGLE DX** | 159 | 1.9 | 2 | 1 | 1 | 1 | 3 | 4 | 6 | 7 |
| **TOTAL MULTIPLE DX** | 273 | 7.7 | 87 | 1 | 2 | 4 | 9 | 17 | 35 | 35 |
| **TOTAL** | | | | | | | | | | |
| 0–19 Years | 146 | 3.6 | 24 | 1 | 1 | 2 | 4 | 10 | 10 | 38 |
| 20–34 | 54 | 3.9 | 22 | 1 | 1 | 2 | 4 | 9 | 17 | 22 |
| 35–49 | 88 | 4.2 | 16 | 1 | 1 | 3 | 7 | 8 | 9 | 23 |
| 50–64 | 77 | 12.4 | 202 | 1 | 1 | 3 | 35 | 35 | 35 | 35 |
| 65+ | 67 | 5.4 | 34 | 1 | 1 | 3 | 9 | 11 | 16 | 33 |
| **GRAND TOTAL** | 432 | 5.5 | 63 | 1 | 1 | 3 | 7 | 11 | 33 | 35 |

## 02.01: OPENING CRANIAL SUTURE. Formerly included in operation group(s) 503.

| Type of Patients | Observed Patients | Avg. Stay | Variance | 10th | 25th | 50th | 75th | 90th | 95th | 99th |
|---|---|---|---|---|---|---|---|---|---|---|
| **1. SINGLE DX** | | | | | | | | | | |
| 0–19 Years | 206 | 2.7 | <1 | 2 | 2 | 3 | 3 | 4 | 4 | 5 |
| 20–34 | 0 | | | | | | | | | |
| 35–49 | 1 | 6.0 | 0 | 6 | 6 | 6 | 6 | 6 | 6 | 6 |
| 50–64 | 0 | | | | | | | | | |
| 65+ | 0 | | | | | | | | | |
| **2. MULTIPLE DX** | | | | | | | | | | |
| 0–19 Years | 177 | 4.0 | 11 | 2 | 3 | 4 | 4 | 5 | 6 | 22 |
| 20–34 | 1 | 19.0 | 0 | 19 | 19 | 19 | 19 | 19 | 19 | 19 |
| 35–49 | 1 | 9.0 | 0 | 9 | 9 | 9 | 9 | 9 | 9 | 9 |
| 50–64 | 0 | | | | | | | | | |
| 65+ | 0 | | | | | | | | | |
| **TOTAL SINGLE DX** | 207 | 2.7 | <1 | 2 | 2 | 3 | 3 | 3 | 4 | 6 |
| **TOTAL MULTIPLE DX** | 179 | 5.6 | 31 | 2 | 3 | 4 | 5 | 19 | 19 | 22 |
| **TOTAL** | | | | | | | | | | |
| 0–19 Years | 383 | 3.3 | 5 | 2 | 2 | 3 | 4 | 5 | 5 | 8 |
| 20–34 | 1 | 19.0 | 0 | 19 | 19 | 19 | 19 | 19 | 19 | 19 |
| 35–49 | 2 | 7.5 | 3 | 6 | 6 | 9 | 9 | 9 | 9 | 9 |
| 50–64 | 0 | | | | | | | | | |
| 65+ | 0 | | | | | | | | | |
| **GRAND TOTAL** | 386 | 4.0 | 17 | 2 | 2 | 3 | 4 | 5 | 19 | 19 |

Length of Stay by Diagnosis and Operation, United States, 2000

# United States, October 1998–September 1999 Data, by Operation

## 02.02: ELEVATION SKULL FX FRAG. Formerly included in operation group(s) 503.

| Type of Patients | Observed Patients | Avg. Stay | Variance | 10th | 25th | 50th | 75th | 90th | 95th | 99th |
|---|---|---|---|---|---|---|---|---|---|---|
| **1. SINGLE DX** | | | | | | | | | | |
| 0–19 Years | 171 | 2.6 | 4 | 1 | 2 | 2 | 3 | 4 | 5 | 14 |
| 20–34 | 42 | 3.6 | 5 | 1 | 2 | 3 | 5 | 6 | 7 | 14 |
| 35–49 | 28 | 4.2 | 10 | 2 | 3 | 4 | 4 | 6 | 11 | 20 |
| 50–64 | 5 | 5.1 | 3 | 4 | 4 | 5 | 5 | 9 | 9 | 9 |
| 65+ | 0 | | | | | | | | | |
| **2. MULTIPLE DX** | | | | | | | | | | |
| 0–19 Years | 333 | 9.4 | 77 | 3 | 4 | 6 | 11 | 19 | 26 | 48 |
| 20–34 | 253 | 9.8 | 76 | 2 | 3 | 7 | 15 | 19 | 25 | 36 |
| 35–49 | 177 | 9.1 | 87 | 2 | 4 | 7 | 11 | 18 | 23 | 73 |
| 50–64 | 55 | 9.8 | 101 | 2 | 3 | 6 | 13 | 21 | 25 | 50 |
| 65+ | 26 | 9.7 | 69 | 3 | 5 | 7 | 12 | 16 | 38 | 38 |
| **TOTAL SINGLE DX** | 246 | 2.9 | 5 | 1 | 2 | 2 | 4 | 5 | 6 | 14 |
| **TOTAL MULTIPLE DX** | 844 | 9.5 | 79 | 2 | 4 | 7 | 12 | 19 | 26 | 48 |
| **TOTAL** | | | | | | | | | | |
| 0–19 Years | 504 | 7.1 | 63 | 2 | 2 | 4 | 10 | 14 | 24 | 48 |
| 20–34 | 295 | 9.1 | 72 | 2 | 3 | 6 | 14 | 19 | 25 | 36 |
| 35–49 | 205 | 8.4 | 78 | 2 | 4 | 6 | 9 | 18 | 21 | 54 |
| 50–64 | 60 | 9.6 | 97 | 2 | 4 | 6 | 13 | 21 | 25 | 49 |
| 65+ | 26 | 9.7 | 69 | 3 | 5 | 7 | 12 | 16 | 38 | 38 |
| **GRAND TOTAL** | 1,090 | 8.0 | 70 | 2 | 3 | 5 | 11 | 18 | 23 | 47 |

## 02.1: CEREBRAL MENINGES REPAIR. Formerly included in operation group(s) 505.

| Type of Patients | Observed Patients | Avg. Stay | Variance | 10th | 25th | 50th | 75th | 90th | 95th | 99th |
|---|---|---|---|---|---|---|---|---|---|---|
| **1. SINGLE DX** | | | | | | | | | | |
| 0–19 Years | 44 | 3.1 | 3 | 1 | 2 | 3 | 4 | 5 | 5 | 13 |
| 20–34 | 23 | 3.1 | 3 | 1 | 3 | 3 | 3 | 6 | 7 | 11 |
| 35–49 | 36 | 4.2 | 6 | 2 | 2 | 3 | 6 | 7 | 10 | 10 |
| 50–64 | 18 | 3.3 | 1 | 2 | 3 | 3 | 3 | 5 | 6 | 7 |
| 65+ | 5 | 5.9 | <1 | 6 | 6 | 6 | 6 | 6 | 6 | 6 |
| **2. MULTIPLE DX** | | | | | | | | | | |
| 0–19 Years | 175 | 6.7 | 57 | 2 | 3 | 4 | 8 | 12 | 17 | 47 |
| 20–34 | 89 | 7.9 | 94 | 3 | 4 | 6 | 8 | 14 | 17 | 48 |
| 35–49 | 179 | 6.4 | 22 | 2 | 4 | 5 | 8 | 14 | 14 | 21 |
| 50–64 | 153 | 6.5 | 30 | 2 | 4 | 5 | 8 | 13 | 16 | 31 |
| 65+ | 51 | 7.0 | 20 | 1 | 4 | 8 | 8 | 11 | 17 | 27 |
| **TOTAL SINGLE DX** | 126 | 3.9 | 4 | 2 | 3 | 3 | 6 | 6 | 7 | 10 |
| **TOTAL MULTIPLE DX** | 647 | 6.8 | 45 | 2 | 3 | 5 | 8 | 13 | 16 | 31 |
| **TOTAL** | | | | | | | | | | |
| 0–19 Years | 219 | 6.1 | 49 | 2 | 3 | 4 | 7 | 12 | 14 | 47 |
| 20–34 | 112 | 6.7 | 76 | 2 | 3 | 5 | 8 | 10 | 16 | 48 |
| 35–49 | 215 | 6.0 | 20 | 2 | 3 | 5 | 7 | 13 | 14 | 21 |
| 50–64 | 171 | 6.2 | 28 | 2 | 3 | 5 | 7 | 12 | 15 | 26 |
| 65+ | 56 | 6.6 | 14 | 3 | 5 | 6 | 8 | 10 | 14 | 18 |
| **GRAND TOTAL** | 773 | 6.3 | 38 | 2 | 3 | 5 | 8 | 12 | 15 | 27 |

## 02.06: CRANIAL OSTEOPLASTY NEC. Formerly included in operation group(s) 503.

| Type of Patients | Observed Patients | Avg. Stay | Variance | 10th | 25th | 50th | 75th | 90th | 95th | 99th |
|---|---|---|---|---|---|---|---|---|---|---|
| **1. SINGLE DX** | | | | | | | | | | |
| 0–19 Years | 254 | 3.3 | 2 | 1 | 3 | 3 | 4 | 5 | 5 | 8 |
| 20–34 | 43 | 2.4 | <1 | 1 | 2 | 2 | 3 | 4 | 4 | 4 |
| 35–49 | 41 | 2.4 | 3 | 1 | 1 | 2 | 2 | 6 | 6 | 6 |
| 50–64 | 24 | 3.0 | 5 | 1 | 1 | 3 | 4 | 7 | 9 | 9 |
| 65+ | 2 | 3.0 | 0 | 3 | 3 | 3 | 3 | 3 | 3 | 3 |
| **2. MULTIPLE DX** | | | | | | | | | | |
| 0–19 Years | 429 | 4.7 | 26 | 2 | 3 | 4 | 5 | 8 | 14 | 21 |
| 20–34 | 101 | 3.1 | 13 | 1 | 1 | 2 | 3 | 8 | 11 | 18 |
| 35–49 | 141 | 3.8 | 18 | 1 | 2 | 2 | 4 | 8 | 13 | 22 |
| 50–64 | 109 | 3.6 | 11 | 1 | 1 | 3 | 5 | 7 | 10 | 21 |
| 65+ | 38 | 4.5 | 18 | 2 | 3 | 3 | 4 | 11 | 12 | 17 |
| **TOTAL SINGLE DX** | 364 | 2.9 | 2 | 1 | 2 | 3 | 4 | 5 | 6 | 8 |
| **TOTAL MULTIPLE DX** | 818 | 4.1 | 21 | 1 | 2 | 3 | 5 | 8 | 12 | 22 |
| **TOTAL** | | | | | | | | | | |
| 0–19 Years | 683 | 4.1 | 16 | 2 | 3 | 4 | 4 | 6 | 9 | 17 |
| 20–34 | 144 | 2.8 | 7 | 1 | 1 | 2 | 3 | 4 | 8 | 16 |
| 35–49 | 182 | 3.1 | 12 | 1 | 1 | 2 | 4 | 6 | 8 | 18 |
| 50–64 | 133 | 3.5 | 10 | 1 | 1 | 3 | 5 | 7 | 10 | 21 |
| 65+ | 40 | 4.5 | 17 | 2 | 3 | 3 | 3 | 11 | 12 | 17 |
| **GRAND TOTAL** | 1,182 | 3.6 | 13 | 1 | 2 | 3 | 4 | 6 | 9 | 17 |

## 02.12: REP CEREBRAL MENING NEC. Formerly included in operation group(s) 505.

| Type of Patients | Observed Patients | Avg. Stay | Variance | 10th | 25th | 50th | 75th | 90th | 95th | 99th |
|---|---|---|---|---|---|---|---|---|---|---|
| **1. SINGLE DX** | | | | | | | | | | |
| 0–19 Years | 44 | 3.1 | 3 | 1 | 2 | 3 | 4 | 5 | 5 | 13 |
| 20–34 | 22 | 3.0 | 3 | 1 | 3 | 3 | 3 | 6 | 7 | 11 |
| 35–49 | 34 | 4.0 | 6 | 2 | 2 | 3 | 5 | 9 | 10 | 10 |
| 50–64 | 18 | 3.3 | 1 | 2 | 3 | 3 | 3 | 5 | 6 | 7 |
| 65+ | 5 | 5.9 | <1 | 6 | 6 | 6 | 6 | 6 | 6 | 6 |
| **2. MULTIPLE DX** | | | | | | | | | | |
| 0–19 Years | 157 | 6.8 | 59 | 2 | 3 | 4 | 8 | 12 | 17 | 47 |
| 20–34 | 78 | 7.2 | 39 | 2 | 4 | 6 | 8 | 10 | 17 | 36 |
| 35–49 | 168 | 6.3 | 22 | 2 | 4 | 5 | 8 | 14 | 14 | 21 |
| 50–64 | 144 | 6.8 | 31 | 2 | 4 | 6 | 8 | 13 | 16 | 31 |
| 65+ | 45 | 7.0 | 17 | 2 | 4 | 8 | 8 | 10 | 14 | 27 |
| **TOTAL SINGLE DX** | 123 | 3.9 | 4 | 2 | 3 | 3 | 6 | 6 | 6 | 10 |
| **TOTAL MULTIPLE DX** | 592 | 6.7 | 36 | 2 | 3 | 5 | 8 | 13 | 16 | 28 |
| **TOTAL** | | | | | | | | | | |
| 0–19 Years | 201 | 6.1 | 51 | 2 | 3 | 4 | 6 | 12 | 14 | 47 |
| 20–34 | 100 | 6.1 | 33 | 2 | 3 | 5 | 8 | 9 | 16 | 36 |
| 35–49 | 202 | 6.0 | 20 | 2 | 3 | 4 | 7 | 14 | 14 | 21 |
| 50–64 | 162 | 6.4 | 29 | 2 | 3 | 5 | 7 | 13 | 16 | 26 |
| 65+ | 50 | 6.6 | 12 | 3 | 6 | 6 | 8 | 10 | 11 | 27 |
| **GRAND TOTAL** | 715 | 6.2 | 31 | 2 | 3 | 5 | 8 | 11 | 14 | 27 |

Length of Stay by Diagnosis and Operation, United States, 2000

# United States, October 1998–September 1999 Data, by Operation

## 02.2: VENTRICULOSTOMY. Formerly included in operation group(s) 504.

| Type of Patients | Observed Patients | Avg. Stay | Variance | Percentiles | | | | | | |
|---|---|---|---|---|---|---|---|---|---|---|
| | | | | 10th | 25th | 50th | 75th | 90th | 95th | 99th |
| **1. SINGLE DX** | | | | | | | | | | |
| 0–19 Years | 70 | 2.3 | 5 | 1 | 1 | 2 | 2 | 5 | 7 | 9 |
| 20–34 | 25 | 19.0 | 400 | 1 | 2 | 4 | 44 | 44 | 44 | 44 |
| 35–49 | 29 | 3.4 | 20 | 1 | 2 | 2 | 3 | 4 | 15 | 22 |
| 50–64 | 17 | 2.6 | 3 | 1 | 2 | 2 | 3 | 6 | 9 | 9 |
| 65+ | 21 | 3.6 | 11 | 1 | 1 | 2 | 7 | 8 | 9 | 14 |
| **2. MULTIPLE DX** | | | | | | | | | | |
| 0–19 Years | 487 | 14.6 | 233 | 2 | 5 | 11 | 18 | 31 | 51 | >99 |
| 20–34 | 208 | 14.9 | 172 | 2 | 5 | 13 | 25 | 30 | 43 | >99 |
| 35–49 | 305 | 15.8 | 163 | 2 | 7 | 13 | 20 | 30 | 45 | 71 |
| 50–64 | 398 | 14.4 | 160 | 1 | 4 | 12 | 21 | 29 | 38 | 56 |
| 65+ | 366 | 17.3 | 202 | 3 | 7 | 15 | 23 | 36 | 44 | 64 |
| **TOTAL SINGLE DX** | 162 | 5.4 | 106 | 1 | 1 | 2 | 4 | 9 | 44 | 44 |
| **TOTAL MULTIPLE DX** | 1,764 | 15.3 | 191 | 2 | 5 | 13 | 21 | 32 | 44 | 83 |
| **TOTAL** | | | | | | | | | | |
| 0–19 Years | 557 | 13.1 | 222 | 1 | 3 | 9 | 17 | 31 | 47 | >99 |
| 20–34 | 233 | 15.3 | 195 | 2 | 4 | 13 | 25 | 35 | 44 | >99 |
| 35–49 | 334 | 14.7 | 163 | 2 | 5 | 13 | 20 | 29 | 44 | 71 |
| 50–64 | 415 | 14.1 | 160 | 1 | 3 | 12 | 21 | 28 | 38 | 56 |
| 65+ | 387 | 16.6 | 201 | 2 | 7 | 14 | 22 | 36 | 44 | 64 |
| **GRAND TOTAL** | 1,926 | 14.5 | 192 | 1 | 4 | 11 | 20 | 31 | 44 | 83 |

## 02.3: EXTRACRANIAL VENT SHUNT. Formerly included in operation group(s) 504.

| Type of Patients | Observed Patients | Avg. Stay | Variance | Percentiles | | | | | | |
|---|---|---|---|---|---|---|---|---|---|---|
| | | | | 10th | 25th | 50th | 75th | 90th | 95th | 99th |
| **1. SINGLE DX** | | | | | | | | | | |
| 0–19 Years | 343 | 3.0 | 9 | 1 | 1 | 2 | 4 | 6 | 8 | 18 |
| 20–34 | 49 | 3.7 | 4 | 1 | 2 | 3 | 6 | 6 | 6 | 9 |
| 35–49 | 56 | 2.9 | 7 | 1 | 2 | 3 | 6 | 6 | 5 | 18 |
| 50–64 | 39 | 4.5 | 10 | 1 | 2 | 4 | 6 | 9 | 10 | 13 |
| 65+ | 87 | 2.9 | 4 | 1 | 2 | 2 | 4 | 5 | 6 | 14 |
| **2. MULTIPLE DX** | | | | | | | | | | |
| 0–19 Years | 1,241 | 11.8 | 242 | 1 | 2 | 5 | 14 | 33 | 53 | >99 |
| 20–34 | 253 | 10.1 | 319 | 2 | 3 | 5 | 8 | 19 | 33 | 95 |
| 35–49 | 363 | 9.8 | 162 | 2 | 2 | 5 | 11 | 26 | 39 | 55 |
| 50–64 | 415 | 11.0 | 141 | 2 | 3 | 6 | 15 | 29 | 35 | 65 |
| 65+ | 1,186 | 8.4 | 74 | 2 | 3 | 5 | 11 | 23 | 26 | 39 |
| **TOTAL SINGLE DX** | 574 | 3.2 | 8 | 1 | 1 | 2 | 4 | 6 | 7 | 18 |
| **TOTAL MULTIPLE DX** | 3,458 | 10.1 | 167 | 2 | 3 | 5 | 12 | 26 | 36 | 85 |
| **TOTAL** | | | | | | | | | | |
| 0–19 Years | 1,584 | 9.7 | 201 | 1 | 2 | 4 | 11 | 31 | 41 | >99 |
| 20–34 | 302 | 9.1 | 275 | 2 | 4 | 4 | 8 | 17 | 29 | 95 |
| 35–49 | 419 | 8.5 | 140 | 2 | 3 | 3 | 9 | 23 | 39 | 53 |
| 50–64 | 454 | 10.4 | 132 | 2 | 6 | 6 | 14 | 29 | 34 | 62 |
| 65+ | 1,273 | 8.2 | 72 | 2 | 3 | 5 | 11 | 23 | 26 | 38 |
| **GRAND TOTAL** | 4,032 | 9.1 | 150 | 1 | 2 | 4 | 11 | 23 | 34 | 76 |

## 02.34: VENT SHUNT TO ABD CAVITY. Formerly included in operation group(s) 504.

| Type of Patients | Observed Patients | Avg. Stay | Variance | Percentiles | | | | | | |
|---|---|---|---|---|---|---|---|---|---|---|
| | | | | 10th | 25th | 50th | 75th | 90th | 95th | 99th |
| **1. SINGLE DX** | | | | | | | | | | |
| 0–19 Years | 322 | 2.5 | 3 | 1 | 1 | 2 | 3 | 4 | 6 | 9 |
| 20–34 | 46 | 3.7 | 4 | 1 | 2 | 3 | 6 | 6 | 6 | 9 |
| 35–49 | 51 | 2.7 | 2 | 1 | 2 | 2 | 4 | 4 | 4 | 8 |
| 50–64 | 37 | 4.4 | 7 | 1 | 2 | 4 | 6 | 7 | 10 | 10 |
| 65+ | 83 | 2.9 | 4 | 1 | 2 | 2 | 3 | 5 | 5 | 14 |
| **2. MULTIPLE DX** | | | | | | | | | | |
| 0–19 Years | 1,052 | 10.2 | 228 | 1 | 2 | 4 | 11 | 31 | 53 | >99 |
| 20–34 | 216 | 9.7 | 349 | 2 | 2 | 4 | 7 | 17 | 36 | 95 |
| 35–49 | 324 | 7.5 | 108 | 2 | 2 | 4 | 8 | 17 | 28 | 53 |
| 50–64 | 358 | 9.6 | 128 | 2 | 3 | 6 | 12 | 27 | 29 | 74 |
| 65+ | 1,098 | 7.2 | 57 | 2 | 3 | 4 | 8 | 16 | 23 | 35 |
| **TOTAL SINGLE DX** | 539 | 2.8 | 4 | 1 | 1 | 2 | 4 | 6 | 6 | 9 |
| **TOTAL MULTIPLE DX** | 3,048 | 8.6 | 149 | 2 | 2 | 4 | 10 | 21 | 31 | 88 |
| **TOTAL** | | | | | | | | | | |
| 0–19 Years | 1,374 | 8.2 | 181 | 1 | 3 | 3 | 9 | 23 | 38 | >99 |
| 20–34 | 262 | 8.7 | 296 | 2 | 3 | 4 | 7 | 13 | 32 | 95 |
| 35–49 | 375 | 6.6 | 92 | 2 | 3 | 3 | 7 | 16 | 24 | 53 |
| 50–64 | 395 | 9.1 | 118 | 2 | 3 | 6 | 10 | 23 | 29 | 74 |
| 65+ | 1,181 | 6.9 | 55 | 2 | 3 | 4 | 8 | 16 | 23 | 35 |
| **GRAND TOTAL** | 3,587 | 7.7 | 131 | 1 | 2 | 4 | 8 | 18 | 30 | 80 |

## 02.4: VENT SHUNT REV/RMVL. Formerly included in operation group(s) 505.

| Type of Patients | Observed Patients | Avg. Stay | Variance | Percentiles | | | | | | |
|---|---|---|---|---|---|---|---|---|---|---|
| | | | | 10th | 25th | 50th | 75th | 90th | 95th | 99th |
| **1. SINGLE DX** | | | | | | | | | | |
| 0–19 Years | 537 | 2.5 | 7 | 1 | 1 | 2 | 3 | 5 | 7 | 13 |
| 20–34 | 69 | 2.8 | 8 | 1 | 1 | 2 | 3 | 8 | 8 | 16 |
| 35–49 | 24 | 2.2 | 2 | 1 | 2 | 2 | 3 | 5 | 6 | 8 |
| 50–64 | 23 | 2.7 | 5 | 1 | 2 | 2 | 3 | 7 | 8 | 9 |
| 65+ | 11 | 1.7 | 1 | 1 | 1 | 1 | 2 | 4 | 4 | 4 |
| **2. MULTIPLE DX** | | | | | | | | | | |
| 0–19 Years | 4,270 | 5.6 | 73 | 1 | 1 | 3 | 5 | 15 | 23 | 43 |
| 20–34 | 686 | 5.6 | 64 | 1 | 1 | 3 | 6 | 14 | 20 | 49 |
| 35–49 | 347 | 7.7 | 81 | 1 | 2 | 5 | 9 | 19 | 24 | 47 |
| 50–64 | 241 | 8.6 | 122 | 2 | 2 | 5 | 10 | 17 | 27 | 67 |
| 65+ | 287 | 7.9 | 82 | 1 | 2 | 4 | 10 | 21 | 28 | 42 |
| **TOTAL SINGLE DX** | 664 | 2.6 | 7 | 1 | 1 | 2 | 3 | 5 | 7 | 13 |
| **TOTAL MULTIPLE DX** | 5,831 | 6.0 | 76 | 1 | 1 | 3 | 6 | 16 | 23 | 43 |
| **TOTAL** | | | | | | | | | | |
| 0–19 Years | 4,807 | 5.3 | 66 | 1 | 1 | 3 | 5 | 14 | 22 | 42 |
| 20–34 | 755 | 5.4 | 60 | 1 | 1 | 3 | 6 | 13 | 19 | 48 |
| 35–49 | 371 | 7.5 | 79 | 1 | 2 | 5 | 9 | 19 | 24 | 44 |
| 50–64 | 264 | 8.3 | 117 | 2 | 2 | 5 | 9 | 17 | 27 | 67 |
| 65+ | 298 | 7.7 | 81 | 1 | 2 | 4 | 9 | 21 | 28 | 42 |
| **GRAND TOTAL** | 6,495 | 5.7 | 70 | 1 | 1 | 2 | 6 | 15 | 22 | 43 |

Length of Stay by Diagnosis and Operation, United States, 2000

# United States, October 1998–September 1999 Data, by Operation

## 02.42: REPL VENTRICLULAR SHUNT. Formerly included in operation group(s) 505.

| Type of Patients | Observed Patients | Avg. Stay | Vari-ance | 10th | 25th | 50th | 75th | 90th | 95th | 99th |
|---|---|---|---|---|---|---|---|---|---|---|
| **1. SINGLE DX** | | | | | | | | | | |
| 0–19 Years | 512 | 2.5 | 6 | 1 | 1 | 2 | 3 | 5 | 6 | 10 |
| 20–34 | 64 | 2.5 | 4 | 1 | 1 | 2 | 3 | 5 | 8 | 10 |
| 35–49 | 23 | 2.1 | 2 | 1 | 1 | 2 | 2 | 3 | 6 | 6 |
| 50–64 | 21 | 2.6 | 4 | 1 | 2 | 2 | 2 | 7 | 7 | 8 |
| 65+ | 10 | 1.7 | 1 | 1 | 1 | 1 | 2 | 4 | 4 | 4 |
| **2. MULTIPLE DX** | | | | | | | | | | |
| 0–19 Years | 3,845 | 4.5 | 49 | 1 | 1 | 2 | 4 | 10 | 18 | 36 |
| 20–34 | 593 | 4.7 | 50 | 1 | 1 | 2 | 5 | 11 | 18 | 49 |
| 35–49 | 280 | 6.8 | 75 | 1 | 2 | 3 | 8 | 19 | 24 | 44 |
| 50–64 | 187 | 8.0 | 131 | 1 | 2 | 4 | 9 | 14 | 26 | 67 |
| 65+ | 238 | 6.4 | 56 | 1 | 2 | 4 | 7 | 15 | 23 | 42 |
| **TOTAL SINGLE DX** | 630 | 2.5 | 6 | 1 | 1 | 2 | 3 | 5 | 6 | 10 |
| **TOTAL MULTIPLE DX** | 5,143 | 4.9 | 55 | 1 | 1 | 2 | 5 | 12 | 19 | 40 |
| **TOTAL** | | | | | | | | | | |
| 0–19 Years | 4,357 | 4.3 | 44 | 1 | 1 | 2 | 4 | 9 | 17 | 34 |
| 20–34 | 657 | 4.5 | 46 | 1 | 1 | 2 | 4 | 10 | 16 | 48 |
| 35–49 | 303 | 6.5 | 72 | 1 | 2 | 3 | 8 | 18 | 24 | 44 |
| 50–64 | 208 | 7.7 | 125 | 1 | 2 | 3 | 9 | 14 | 24 | 67 |
| 65+ | 248 | 6.2 | 55 | 1 | 2 | 4 | 6 | 15 | 23 | 42 |
| **GRAND TOTAL** | 5,773 | 4.7 | 50 | 1 | 1 | 2 | 4 | 10 | 18 | 37 |

## 02.43: RMVL VENTRICLULAR SHUNT. Formerly included in operation group(s) 505.

| Type of Patients | Observed Patients | Avg. Stay | Vari-ance | 10th | 25th | 50th | 75th | 90th | 95th | 99th |
|---|---|---|---|---|---|---|---|---|---|---|
| **1. SINGLE DX** | | | | | | | | | | |
| 0–19 Years | 25 | 3.5 | 19 | 1 | 1 | 1 | 3 | 13 | 13 | 17 |
| 20–34 | 4 | 5.9 | 33 | 2 | 2 | 2 | 10 | 16 | 16 | 16 |
| 35–49 | 1 | 8.0 | 0 | 8 | 8 | 8 | 8 | 8 | 8 | 8 |
| 50–64 | 2 | 5.8 | 19 | 2 | 2 | 9 | 9 | 9 | 9 | 9 |
| 65+ | 1 | 1.0 | 0 | 1 | 1 | 1 | 1 | 1 | 1 | 1 |
| **2. MULTIPLE DX** | | | | | | | | | | |
| 0–19 Years | 416 | 16.8 | 187 | 2 | 7 | 14 | 22 | 38 | 43 | 81 |
| 20–34 | 91 | 12.8 | 121 | 3 | 4 | 10 | 18 | 25 | 34 | 67 |
| 35–49 | 66 | 11.8 | 90 | 3 | 5 | 9 | 15 | 25 | 31 | 51 |
| 50–64 | 53 | 11.1 | 76 | 2 | 4 | 9 | 16 | 20 | 27 | 40 |
| 65+ | 48 | 16.4 | 141 | 2 | 7 | 15 | 28 | 31 | 32 | 61 |
| **TOTAL SINGLE DX** | 33 | 4.2 | 23 | 1 | 1 | 2 | 5 | 13 | 16 | 17 |
| **TOTAL MULTIPLE DX** | 674 | 15.1 | 158 | 2 | 6 | 13 | 19 | 31 | 41 | 81 |
| **TOTAL** | | | | | | | | | | |
| 0–19 Years | 441 | 16.0 | 187 | 2 | 6 | 14 | 20 | 38 | 43 | 81 |
| 20–34 | 95 | 12.3 | 117 | 2 | 4 | 10 | 17 | 24 | 31 | 43 |
| 35–49 | 67 | 11.7 | 89 | 2 | 5 | 9 | 15 | 25 | 31 | 51 |
| 50–64 | 55 | 11.0 | 75 | 2 | 4 | 9 | 16 | 20 | 27 | 40 |
| 65+ | 49 | 16.3 | 141 | 2 | 7 | 15 | 28 | 31 | 31 | 61 |
| **GRAND TOTAL** | 707 | 14.6 | 157 | 2 | 5 | 12 | 19 | 31 | 41 | 72 |

## 02.9: SKULL & BRAIN OPS NEC. Formerly included in operation group(s) 505.

| Type of Patients | Observed Patients | Avg. Stay | Vari-ance | 10th | 25th | 50th | 75th | 90th | 95th | 99th |
|---|---|---|---|---|---|---|---|---|---|---|
| **1. SINGLE DX** | | | | | | | | | | |
| 0–19 Years | 137 | 4.8 | 19 | 1 | 2 | 3 | 7 | 9 | 14 | 25 |
| 20–34 | 145 | 6.3 | 7 | 3 | 4 | 5 | 7 | 9 | 12 | 14 |
| 35–49 | 119 | 6.1 | 7 | 2 | 4 | 7 | 7 | 9 | 9 | 12 |
| 50–64 | 58 | 4.8 | 7 | 1 | 2 | 4 | 7 | 7 | 8 | 12 |
| 65+ | 53 | 2.1 | 10 | 1 | 1 | 2 | 2 | 3 | 4 | 14 |
| **2. MULTIPLE DX** | | | | | | | | | | |
| 0–19 Years | 268 | 10.4 | 93 | 2 | 4 | 7 | 13 | 28 | 28 | 43 |
| 20–34 | 333 | 6.9 | 37 | 2 | 3 | 6 | 8 | 12 | 16 | 35 |
| 35–49 | 400 | 7.1 | 33 | 2 | 4 | 6 | 9 | 12 | 15 | 30 |
| 50–64 | 259 | 6.8 | 50 | 1 | 2 | 5 | 8 | 14 | 23 | 36 |
| 65+ | 399 | 6.6 | 48 | 1 | 2 | 5 | 8 | 12 | 19 | 40 |
| **TOTAL SINGLE DX** | 512 | 5.4 | 11 | 1 | 3 | 6 | 7 | 9 | 11 | 15 |
| **TOTAL MULTIPLE DX** | 1,659 | 7.4 | 50 | 2 | 3 | 6 | 9 | 13 | 21 | 39 |
| **TOTAL** | | | | | | | | | | |
| 0–19 Years | 405 | 8.1 | 71 | 1 | 3 | 6 | 10 | 17 | 28 | 39 |
| 20–34 | 478 | 6.6 | 24 | 3 | 4 | 6 | 7 | 11 | 14 | 25 |
| 35–49 | 519 | 6.8 | 25 | 2 | 4 | 7 | 8 | 11 | 13 | 27 |
| 50–64 | 317 | 6.3 | 40 | 2 | 2 | 5 | 7 | 12 | 22 | 36 |
| 65+ | 452 | 5.8 | 44 | 1 | 2 | 5 | 7 | 12 | 17 | 36 |
| **GRAND TOTAL** | 2,171 | 6.8 | 38 | 2 | 3 | 6 | 8 | 12 | 16 | 34 |

## 02.93: IMPL IC NEUROSTIMULATOR. Formerly included in operation group(s) 505.

| Type of Patients | Observed Patients | Avg. Stay | Vari-ance | 10th | 25th | 50th | 75th | 90th | 95th | 99th |
|---|---|---|---|---|---|---|---|---|---|---|
| **1. SINGLE DX** | | | | | | | | | | |
| 0–19 Years | 48 | 5.3 | 40 | 1 | 1 | 2 | 9 | 15 | 18 | 25 |
| 20–34 | 41 | 9.5 | 19 | 1 | 7 | 11 | 14 | 14 | 14 | 14 |
| 35–49 | 40 | 3.8 | 20 | 1 | 2 | 2 | 5 | 10 | 12 | 25 |
| 50–64 | 29 | 3.0 | 9 | 1 | 1 | 2 | 3 | 8 | 12 | 13 |
| 65+ | 37 | 1.7 | <1 | 1 | 1 | 1 | 2 | 2 | 3 | 3 |
| **2. MULTIPLE DX** | | | | | | | | | | |
| 0–19 Years | 73 | 15.0 | 117 | 4 | 8 | 12 | 28 | 28 | 35 | 41 |
| 20–34 | 54 | 8.8 | 31 | 1 | 3 | 10 | 13 | 14 | 18 | 23 |
| 35–49 | 68 | 6.3 | 40 | 1 | 2 | 4 | 9 | 14 | 16 | 28 |
| 50–64 | 72 | 3.9 | 12 | 1 | 1 | 3 | 6 | 6 | 12 | 16 |
| 65+ | 117 | 2.6 | 6 | 1 | 1 | 2 | 3 | 6 | 7 | 8 |
| **TOTAL SINGLE DX** | 195 | 4.8 | 27 | 1 | 1 | 2 | 9 | 13 | 14 | 25 |
| **TOTAL MULTIPLE DX** | 384 | 7.7 | 74 | 1 | 2 | 4 | 10 | 17 | 28 | 39 |
| **TOTAL** | | | | | | | | | | |
| 0–19 Years | 121 | 11.0 | 108 | 1 | 1 | 9 | 15 | 28 | 28 | 39 |
| 20–34 | 95 | 9.2 | 24 | 1 | 5 | 10 | 13 | 14 | 14 | 21 |
| 35–49 | 108 | 5.4 | 34 | 1 | 2 | 3 | 8 | 9 | 16 | 28 |
| 50–64 | 101 | 3.6 | 11 | 1 | 1 | 3 | 5 | 9 | 12 | 16 |
| 65+ | 154 | 2.3 | 4 | 1 | 1 | 2 | 2 | 4 | 7 | 7 |
| **GRAND TOTAL** | 579 | 6.5 | 57 | 1 | 1 | 3 | 10 | 14 | 25 | 35 |

Length of Stay by Diagnosis and Operation, United States, 2000

## United States, October 1998–September 1999 Data, by Operation

### 02.94: INSERT/REPL SKULL TONGS. Formerly included in operation group(s) 505.

| Type of Patients | Observed Patients | Avg. Stay | Variance | 10th | 25th | 50th | 75th | 90th | 95th | 99th |
|---|---|---|---|---|---|---|---|---|---|---|
| **1. SINGLE DX** | | | | | | | | | | |
| 0–19 Years | 43 | 3.7 | 3 | 2 | 3 | 3 | 4 | 7 | 7 | 9 |
| 20–34 | 48 | 4.1 | 4 | 2 | 3 | 3 | 7 | 7 | 7 | 9 |
| 35–49 | 35 | 3.3 | 1 | 2 | 3 | 3 | 4 | 4 | 6 | 6 |
| 50–64 | 17 | 3.9 | 9 | 1 | 2 | 2 | 6 | 9 | 9 | 9 |
| 65+ | 13 | 7.5 | 77 | 2 | 2 | 4 | 7 | 31 | 31 | 31 |
| **2. MULTIPLE DX** | | | | | | | | | | |
| 0–19 Years | 143 | 8.4 | 69 | 2 | 3 | 6 | 11 | 19 | 28 | 48 |
| 20–34 | 211 | 7.1 | 70 | 2 | 3 | 5 | 8 | 15 | 21 | 54 |
| 35–49 | 243 | 7.5 | 53 | 2 | 3 | 5 | 10 | 13 | 18 | 38 |
| 50–64 | 158 | 8.1 | 69 | 1 | 3 | 5 | 9 | 22 | 26 | 38 |
| 65+ | 257 | 7.9 | 62 | 2 | 4 | 6 | 9 | 14 | 22 | 44 |
| **TOTAL SINGLE DX** | 156 | 4.0 | 7 | 2 | 3 | 3 | 4 | 7 | 7 | 10 |
| **TOTAL MULTIPLE DX** | 1,012 | 7.7 | 63 | 2 | 3 | 5 | 9 | 15 | 24 | 45 |
| **TOTAL** | | | | | | | | | | |
| 0–19 Years | 186 | 6.6 | 50 | 2 | 3 | 4 | 7 | 13 | 27 | 43 |
| 20–34 | 259 | 6.3 | 52 | 2 | 3 | 4 | 7 | 11 | 17 | 50 |
| 35–49 | 278 | 7.1 | 50 | 2 | 3 | 5 | 9 | 13 | 18 | 34 |
| 50–64 | 175 | 7.8 | 66 | 1 | 3 | 5 | 9 | 22 | 25 | 38 |
| 65+ | 270 | 7.9 | 62 | 2 | 4 | 6 | 9 | 14 | 22 | 44 |
| **GRAND TOTAL** | 1,168 | 7.1 | 55 | 2 | 3 | 5 | 8 | 13 | 22 | 43 |

### 03.0: SPINAL CANAL EXPLORATION. Formerly included in operation group(s) 506.

| Type of Patients | Observed Patients | Avg. Stay | Variance | 10th | 25th | 50th | 75th | 90th | 95th | 99th |
|---|---|---|---|---|---|---|---|---|---|---|
| **1. SINGLE DX** | | | | | | | | | | |
| 0–19 Years | 100 | 3.5 | 4 | 1 | 2 | 3 | 4 | 5 | 8 | 12 |
| 20–34 | 352 | 2.1 | 3 | 1 | 1 | 2 | 3 | 3 | 5 | 9 |
| 35–49 | 1,563 | 2.1 | 2 | 1 | 1 | 2 | 3 | 4 | 5 | 7 |
| 50–64 | 1,835 | 2.2 | 4 | 1 | 1 | 2 | 3 | 4 | 5 | 11 |
| 65+ | 1,555 | 2.6 | 3 | 1 | 2 | 2 | 3 | 4 | 5 | 7 |
| **2. MULTIPLE DX** | | | | | | | | | | |
| 0–19 Years | 362 | 6.5 | 61 | 2 | 3 | 4 | 8 | 14 | 18 | 35 |
| 20–34 | 653 | 5.5 | 45 | 1 | 2 | 3 | 6 | 12 | 22 | 24 |
| 35–49 | 3,581 | 3.5 | 17 | 1 | 1 | 2 | 4 | 6 | 9 | 21 |
| 50–64 | 6,981 | 3.2 | 12 | 1 | 1 | 2 | 4 | 6 | 8 | 18 |
| 65+ | 12,519 | 4.2 | 16 | 1 | 2 | 3 | 5 | 8 | 11 | 20 |
| **TOTAL SINGLE DX** | 5,405 | 2.3 | 3 | 1 | 1 | 2 | 3 | 4 | 5 | 8 |
| **TOTAL MULTIPLE DX** | 24,096 | 3.9 | 17 | 1 | 2 | 3 | 4 | 7 | 10 | 22 |
| **TOTAL** | | | | | | | | | | |
| 0–19 Years | 462 | 5.9 | 51 | 2 | 3 | 4 | 6 | 13 | 17 | 35 |
| 20–34 | 1,005 | 4.3 | 33 | 1 | 1 | 2 | 5 | 10 | 16 | 22 |
| 35–49 | 5,144 | 3.0 | 13 | 1 | 1 | 2 | 3 | 6 | 8 | 17 |
| 50–64 | 8,816 | 3.0 | 11 | 1 | 1 | 2 | 3 | 6 | 8 | 16 |
| 65+ | 14,074 | 4.1 | 15 | 1 | 2 | 3 | 5 | 7 | 10 | 20 |
| **GRAND TOTAL** | 29,501 | 3.6 | 15 | 1 | 2 | 3 | 4 | 7 | 9 | 20 |

### 03.02: REOPEN LAMINECTOMY SITE. Formerly included in operation group(s) 506.

| Type of Patients | Observed Patients | Avg. Stay | Variance | 10th | 25th | 50th | 75th | 90th | 95th | 99th |
|---|---|---|---|---|---|---|---|---|---|---|
| **1. SINGLE DX** | | | | | | | | | | |
| 0–19 Years | 0 | | | | | | | | | |
| 20–34 | 19 | 2.9 | 4 | 1 | 2 | 2 | 4 | 5 | 6 | 10 |
| 35–49 | 70 | 2.3 | 3 | 1 | 1 | 2 | 3 | 4 | 5 | 11 |
| 50–64 | 36 | 3.9 | 7 | 1 | 2 | 3 | 6 | 6 | 7 | 14 |
| 65+ | 13 | 2.0 | 6 | 1 | 1 | 1 | 2 | 4 | 4 | 13 |
| **2. MULTIPLE DX** | | | | | | | | | | |
| 0–19 Years | 3 | 6.6 | 74 | 2 | 4 | 4 | 4 | 26 | 26 | 26 |
| 20–34 | 68 | 4.8 | 14 | 2 | 3 | 4 | 6 | 7 | 11 | 22 |
| 35–49 | 249 | 4.6 | 28 | 1 | 1 | 3 | 6 | 9 | 12 | 23 |
| 50–64 | 241 | 4.7 | 26 | 1 | 1 | 3 | 6 | 9 | 14 | 27 |
| 65+ | 195 | 6.7 | 42 | 1 | 3 | 4 | 10 | 14 | 17 | 29 |
| **TOTAL SINGLE DX** | 138 | 2.7 | 5 | 1 | 1 | 2 | 3 | 6 | 6 | 11 |
| **TOTAL MULTIPLE DX** | 756 | 5.2 | 30 | 1 | 2 | 4 | 7 | 11 | 14 | 27 |
| **TOTAL** | | | | | | | | | | |
| 0–19 Years | 3 | 6.6 | 74 | 2 | 4 | 4 | 4 | 26 | 26 | 26 |
| 20–34 | 87 | 4.3 | 12 | 1 | 2 | 4 | 6 | 7 | 10 | 22 |
| 35–49 | 319 | 4.0 | 22 | 1 | 1 | 3 | 5 | 9 | 11 | 23 |
| 50–64 | 277 | 4.6 | 24 | 1 | 1 | 3 | 6 | 9 | 14 | 27 |
| 65+ | 208 | 6.2 | 40 | 1 | 2 | 4 | 9 | 14 | 16 | 27 |
| **GRAND TOTAL** | 894 | 4.7 | 26 | 1 | 1 | 3 | 6 | 10 | 14 | 24 |

### 03.09: SPINAL CANAL EXPLOR NEC. Formerly included in operation group(s) 506.

| Type of Patients | Observed Patients | Avg. Stay | Variance | 10th | 25th | 50th | 75th | 90th | 95th | 99th |
|---|---|---|---|---|---|---|---|---|---|---|
| **1. SINGLE DX** | | | | | | | | | | |
| 0–19 Years | 100 | 3.5 | 4 | 1 | 2 | 3 | 4 | 5 | 8 | 12 |
| 20–34 | 330 | 2.1 | 3 | 1 | 1 | 1 | 3 | 3 | 5 | 8 |
| 35–49 | 1,491 | 2.1 | 2 | 1 | 1 | 2 | 2 | 4 | 5 | 7 |
| 50–64 | 1,798 | 2.2 | 3 | 1 | 1 | 2 | 2 | 4 | 5 | 10 |
| 65+ | 1,542 | 2.6 | 2 | 1 | 2 | 2 | 3 | 4 | 5 | 7 |
| **2. MULTIPLE DX** | | | | | | | | | | |
| 0–19 Years | 350 | 6.5 | 61 | 2 | 3 | 4 | 7 | 14 | 17 | 35 |
| 20–34 | 570 | 5.3 | 49 | 1 | 2 | 3 | 6 | 12 | 22 | 24 |
| 35–49 | 3,317 | 3.4 | 17 | 1 | 1 | 2 | 4 | 6 | 9 | 21 |
| 50–64 | 6,726 | 3.2 | 12 | 1 | 1 | 2 | 4 | 6 | 8 | 17 |
| 65+ | 12,320 | 4.2 | 16 | 1 | 2 | 3 | 5 | 8 | 11 | 20 |
| **TOTAL SINGLE DX** | 5,261 | 2.3 | 3 | 1 | 1 | 2 | 3 | 4 | 5 | 8 |
| **TOTAL MULTIPLE DX** | 23,283 | 3.9 | 17 | 1 | 2 | 3 | 4 | 7 | 10 | 22 |
| **TOTAL** | | | | | | | | | | |
| 0–19 Years | 450 | 5.9 | 51 | 2 | 3 | 4 | 6 | 13 | 17 | 35 |
| 20–34 | 900 | 4.1 | 34 | 1 | 1 | 2 | 4 | 11 | 18 | 22 |
| 35–49 | 4,808 | 3.0 | 13 | 1 | 1 | 2 | 3 | 5 | 8 | 17 |
| 50–64 | 8,524 | 3.0 | 10 | 1 | 1 | 2 | 3 | 5 | 8 | 15 |
| 65+ | 13,862 | 4.0 | 15 | 1 | 2 | 3 | 5 | 7 | 10 | 19 |
| **GRAND TOTAL** | 28,544 | 3.6 | 15 | 1 | 2 | 3 | 4 | 7 | 9 | 20 |

Length of Stay by Diagnosis and Operation, United States, 2000

# United States, October 1998–September 1999 Data, by Operation

## 03.1: INTRASPIN NERVE ROOT DIV. Formerly included in operation group(s) 507.

| Type of Patients | Observed Patients | Avg. Stay | Vari-ance | 10th | 25th | 50th | 75th | 90th | 95th | 99th |
|---|---|---|---|---|---|---|---|---|---|---|
| **1. SINGLE DX** | | | | | | | | | | |
| 0–19 Years | 83 | 6.2 | 6 | 4 | 5 | 6 | 6 | 11 | 11 | 14 |
| 20–34 | 2 | 2.0 | 0 | 2 | 2 | 2 | 2 | 2 | 2 | 2 |
| 35–49 | 4 | 4.0 | 2 | 2 | 3 | 5 | 5 | 5 | 5 | 5 |
| 50–64 | 2 | 1.0 | 0 | 1 | 1 | 1 | 1 | 1 | 1 | 1 |
| 65+ | 1 | 4.0 | 0 | 4 | 4 | 4 | 4 | 4 | 4 | 4 |
| **2. MULTIPLE DX** | | | | | | | | | | |
| 0–19 Years | 126 | 6.4 | 16 | 4 | 5 | 6 | 6 | 9 | 14 | 29 |
| 20–34 | 10 | 1.5 | 2 | 1 | 1 | 1 | 1 | >99 | >99 | >99 |
| 35–49 | 22 | 3.2 | 7 | 1 | 1 | 2 | 4 | 7 | 11 | 11 |
| 50–64 | 12 | 3.3 | 15 | 1 | 2 | 3 | 2 | 7 | 17 | 17 |
| 65+ | 13 | 3.7 | 12 | 1 | 1 | 3 | 5 | 9 | 14 | 14 |
| **TOTAL SINGLE DX** | 92 | 5.7 | 7 | 2 | 4 | 6 | 6 | 11 | 11 | 14 |
| **TOTAL MULTIPLE DX** | 183 | 5.1 | 17 | 1 | 3 | 5 | 6 | 9 | 14 | >99 |
| **TOTAL** | | | | | | | | | | |
| 0–19 Years | 209 | 6.3 | 12 | 4 | 5 | 6 | 6 | 10 | 12 | 18 |
| 20–34 | 12 | 1.5 | 2 | 1 | 1 | 1 | 2 | 7 | >99 | >99 |
| 35–49 | 26 | 3.3 | 7 | 1 | 2 | 2 | 4 | 5 | 11 | 11 |
| 50–64 | 14 | 2.4 | 10 | 1 | 1 | 1 | 2 | 6 | 7 | 7 |
| 65+ | 14 | 3.7 | 12 | 1 | 1 | 3 | 5 | 9 | 14 | 14 |
| **GRAND TOTAL** | 275 | 5.3 | 14 | 1 | 4 | 5 | 6 | 9 | 14 | >99 |

## 03.2: CHORDOTOMY. Formerly included in operation group(s) 507.

| Type of Patients | Observed Patients | Avg. Stay | Vari-ance | 10th | 25th | 50th | 75th | 90th | 95th | 99th |
|---|---|---|---|---|---|---|---|---|---|---|
| **1. SINGLE DX** | | | | | | | | | | |
| 0–19 Years | 6 | 3.0 | <1 | 3 | 3 | 3 | 3 | 3 | 3 | 4 |
| 20–34 | 1 | 1.0 | 0 | 1 | 1 | 1 | 1 | 1 | 1 | 1 |
| 35–49 | 3 | 3.2 | 1 | 2 | 2 | 4 | 4 | 4 | 4 | 4 |
| 50–64 | 0 | | | | | | | | | |
| 65+ | 3 | 2.0 | 0 | 2 | 2 | 2 | 2 | 2 | 2 | 2 |
| **2. MULTIPLE DX** | | | | | | | | | | |
| 0–19 Years | 25 | 4.6 | 9 | 3 | 3 | 4 | 5 | 6 | 8 | 28 |
| 20–34 | 10 | 6.3 | 14 | 1 | 3 | 8 | 9 | 9 | 14 | 14 |
| 35–49 | 19 | 6.7 | 51 | 1 | 1 | 4 | 7 | 19 | 19 | 27 |
| 50–64 | 20 | 7.8 | 44 | 2 | 3 | 7 | 10 | 17 | 27 | 27 |
| 65+ | 10 | 10.9 | 89 | 2 | 4 | 9 | 14 | 33 | 33 | 33 |
| **TOTAL SINGLE DX** | 13 | 2.9 | <1 | 2 | 3 | 3 | 3 | 3 | 4 | 4 |
| **TOTAL MULTIPLE DX** | 84 | 5.7 | 25 | 3 | 3 | 4 | 7 | 9 | 16 | 28 |
| **TOTAL** | | | | | | | | | | |
| 0–19 Years | 31 | 4.2 | 7 | 3 | 3 | 4 | 4 | 6 | 8 | 8 |
| 20–34 | 11 | 6.0 | 15 | 1 | 3 | 8 | 9 | 9 | 14 | 14 |
| 35–49 | 22 | 6.2 | 45 | 1 | 3 | 7 | 7 | 16 | 19 | 27 |
| 50–64 | 20 | 7.8 | 44 | 2 | 3 | 8 | 10 | 17 | 27 | 27 |
| 65+ | 13 | 9.1 | 83 | 2 | 4 | 8 | 9 | 20 | 33 | 33 |
| **GRAND TOTAL** | 97 | 5.2 | 21 | 2 | 3 | 4 | 6 | 8 | 14 | 28 |

## 03.3: DXTIC PX ON SPINAL CANAL. Formerly included in operation group(s) 507, 512.

| Type of Patients | Observed Patients | Avg. Stay | Vari-ance | 10th | 25th | 50th | 75th | 90th | 95th | 99th |
|---|---|---|---|---|---|---|---|---|---|---|
| **1. SINGLE DX** | | | | | | | | | | |
| 0–19 Years | 9,847 | 2.8 | 3 | 1 | 2 | 2 | 3 | 4 | 6 | 10 |
| 20–34 | 1,665 | 3.1 | 6 | 1 | 2 | 2 | 4 | 6 | 8 | 14 |
| 35–49 | 1,074 | 3.0 | 4 | 1 | 3 | 2 | 4 | 5 | 7 | 10 |
| 50–64 | 273 | 3.7 | 6 | 1 | 3 | 3 | 4 | 8 | 9 | 12 |
| 65+ | 115 | 4.8 | 16 | 1 | 4 | 4 | 7 | 9 | 13 | 17 |
| **2. MULTIPLE DX** | | | | | | | | | | |
| 0–19 Years | 28,968 | 4.8 | 31 | 2 | 3 | 3 | 5 | 10 | 13 | 28 |
| 20–34 | 6,318 | 4.9 | 29 | 1 | 2 | 3 | 6 | 10 | 14 | 28 |
| 35–49 | 8,412 | 5.4 | 33 | 1 | 3 | 4 | 6 | 11 | 14 | 28 |
| 50–64 | 5,751 | 6.6 | 41 | 2 | 3 | 5 | 8 | 13 | 18 | 32 |
| 65+ | 8,721 | 7.6 | 38 | 2 | 4 | 6 | 10 | 15 | 20 | 29 |
| **TOTAL SINGLE DX** | 12,974 | 2.8 | 4 | 1 | 2 | 2 | 3 | 5 | 6 | 10 |
| **TOTAL MULTIPLE DX** | 58,170 | 5.5 | 34 | 2 | 2 | 4 | 7 | 11 | 15 | 29 |
| **TOTAL** | | | | | | | | | | |
| 0–19 Years | 38,815 | 4.2 | 24 | 1 | 2 | 3 | 5 | 8 | 11 | 25 |
| 20–34 | 7,983 | 4.5 | 25 | 1 | 2 | 3 | 5 | 9 | 12 | 26 |
| 35–49 | 9,486 | 5.1 | 30 | 2 | 3 | 4 | 6 | 10 | 14 | 26 |
| 50–64 | 6,024 | 6.5 | 39 | 2 | 3 | 5 | 8 | 13 | 17 | 31 |
| 65+ | 8,836 | 7.6 | 37 | 2 | 4 | 6 | 10 | 15 | 20 | 29 |
| **GRAND TOTAL** | 71,144 | 4.9 | 29 | 1 | 2 | 3 | 6 | 10 | 14 | 27 |

## 03.31: SPINAL TAP. Formerly included in operation group(s) 512.

| Type of Patients | Observed Patients | Avg. Stay | Vari-ance | 10th | 25th | 50th | 75th | 90th | 95th | 99th |
|---|---|---|---|---|---|---|---|---|---|---|
| **1. SINGLE DX** | | | | | | | | | | |
| 0–19 Years | 9,837 | 2.8 | 3 | 1 | 2 | 2 | 3 | 4 | 6 | 10 |
| 20–34 | 1,658 | 3.0 | 6 | 1 | 2 | 2 | 4 | 5 | 7 | 14 |
| 35–49 | 1,061 | 3.0 | 4 | 1 | 3 | 3 | 4 | 5 | 7 | 10 |
| 50–64 | 269 | 3.7 | 6 | 1 | 3 | 3 | 4 | 8 | 9 | 12 |
| 65+ | 113 | 4.8 | 16 | 1 | 4 | 4 | 6 | 10 | 13 | 17 |
| **2. MULTIPLE DX** | | | | | | | | | | |
| 0–19 Years | 28,950 | 4.8 | 31 | 2 | 3 | 3 | 5 | 10 | 13 | 28 |
| 20–34 | 6,295 | 4.9 | 29 | 1 | 2 | 3 | 6 | 10 | 14 | 28 |
| 35–49 | 8,361 | 5.4 | 32 | 1 | 3 | 4 | 6 | 11 | 14 | 27 |
| 50–64 | 5,691 | 6.6 | 40 | 2 | 3 | 5 | 8 | 13 | 18 | 31 |
| 65+ | 8,622 | 7.6 | 37 | 2 | 4 | 6 | 10 | 15 | 20 | 29 |
| **TOTAL SINGLE DX** | 12,938 | 2.8 | 4 | 1 | 2 | 2 | 3 | 5 | 6 | 10 |
| **TOTAL MULTIPLE DX** | 57,919 | 5.4 | 33 | 2 | 2 | 4 | 7 | 11 | 15 | 28 |
| **TOTAL** | | | | | | | | | | |
| 0–19 Years | 38,787 | 4.2 | 24 | 1 | 2 | 3 | 5 | 8 | 11 | 25 |
| 20–34 | 7,953 | 4.5 | 24 | 1 | 2 | 3 | 5 | 9 | 12 | 25 |
| 35–49 | 9,422 | 5.1 | 29 | 2 | 3 | 4 | 6 | 10 | 14 | 26 |
| 50–64 | 5,960 | 6.4 | 38 | 2 | 3 | 5 | 8 | 13 | 17 | 30 |
| 65+ | 8,735 | 7.6 | 37 | 2 | 4 | 6 | 10 | 15 | 20 | 29 |
| **GRAND TOTAL** | 70,857 | 4.9 | 29 | 1 | 2 | 3 | 6 | 10 | 14 | 26 |

Length of Stay by Diagnosis and Operation, United States, 2000

# United States, October 1998–September 1999 Data, by Operation

## 03.4: EXC SPINAL CORD LESION. Formerly included in operation group(s) 507.

| Type of Patients | Observed Patients | Avg. Stay | Variance | 10th | 25th | 50th | 75th | 90th | 95th | 99th |
|---|---|---|---|---|---|---|---|---|---|---|
| **1. SINGLE DX** | | | | | | | | | | |
| 0–19 Years | 91 | 4.7 | 10 | 2 | 3 | 4 | 5 | 8 | 15 | 15 |
| 20–34 | 95 | 3.7 | 6 | 1 | 2 | 3 | 4 | 6 | 8 | 17 |
| 35–49 | 156 | 4.8 | 12 | 2 | 2 | 4 | 6 | 11 | 11 | 13 |
| 50–64 | 128 | 3.7 | 6 | 1 | 2 | 3 | 5 | 8 | 8 | 9 |
| 65+ | 54 | 3.8 | 8 | 1 | 2 | 3 | 5 | 6 | 7 | 19 |
| **2. MULTIPLE DX** | | | | | | | | | | |
| 0–19 Years | 297 | 6.9 | 55 | 3 | 3 | 4 | 7 | 15 | 15 | 44 |
| 20–34 | 146 | 6.7 | 23 | 2 | 4 | 6 | 8 | 11 | 17 | 27 |
| 35–49 | 389 | 6.8 | 45 | 2 | 3 | 5 | 8 | 14 | 18 | 51 |
| 50–64 | 504 | 6.3 | 34 | 2 | 3 | 5 | 8 | 13 | 16 | 30 |
| 65+ | 561 | 7.4 | 35 | 2 | 3 | 6 | 9 | 15 | 20 | 29 |
| **TOTAL SINGLE DX** | 524 | 4.2 | 9 | 1 | 2 | 3 | 5 | 8 | 11 | 15 |
| **TOTAL MULTIPLE DX** | 1,897 | 6.8 | 39 | 2 | 3 | 5 | 8 | 14 | 18 | 30 |
| **TOTAL** | | | | | | | | | | |
| 0–19 Years | 388 | 6.2 | 43 | 3 | 3 | 4 | 7 | 15 | 15 | 36 |
| 20–34 | 241 | 5.5 | 19 | 2 | 3 | 5 | 6 | 10 | 14 | 25 |
| 35–49 | 545 | 6.2 | 36 | 2 | 3 | 5 | 8 | 11 | 17 | 29 |
| 50–64 | 632 | 5.5 | 27 | 1 | 3 | 5 | 7 | 10 | 15 | 27 |
| 65+ | 615 | 7.1 | 34 | 2 | 3 | 6 | 8 | 14 | 19 | 29 |
| **GRAND TOTAL** | 2,421 | 6.2 | 33 | 2 | 3 | 5 | 7 | 12 | 16 | 29 |

## 03.5: SPINAL CORD PLASTIC OPS. Formerly included in operation group(s) 507.

| Type of Patients | Observed Patients | Avg. Stay | Variance | 10th | 25th | 50th | 75th | 90th | 95th | 99th |
|---|---|---|---|---|---|---|---|---|---|---|
| **1. SINGLE DX** | | | | | | | | | | |
| 0–19 Years | 144 | 4.7 | 14 | 2 | 3 | 3 | 5 | 9 | 10 | 16 |
| 20–34 | 50 | 5.3 | 9 | 2 | 3 | 5 | 7 | 9 | 10 | 19 |
| 35–49 | 91 | 4.1 | 4 | 2 | 3 | 3 | 6 | 7 | 8 | 9 |
| 50–64 | 62 | 3.9 | 6 | 1 | 3 | 3 | 4 | 6 | 9 | 16 |
| 65+ | 18 | 4.1 | 7 | 2 | 3 | 3 | 5 | 8 | 10 | 12 |
| **2. MULTIPLE DX** | | | | | | | | | | |
| 0–19 Years | 757 | 7.9 | 75 | 3 | 4 | 5 | 9 | 17 | 23 | 56 |
| 20–34 | 216 | 8.4 | 99 | 2 | 4 | 6 | 9 | 15 | 25 | 76 |
| 35–49 | 344 | 8.0 | 53 | 2 | 4 | 7 | 9 | 15 | 22 | 42 |
| 50–64 | 254 | 7.3 | 30 | 2 | 4 | 5 | 9 | 14 | 18 | 23 |
| 65+ | 272 | 7.4 | 36 | 2 | 4 | 6 | 9 | 12 | 17 | 33 |
| **TOTAL SINGLE DX** | 365 | 4.5 | 9 | 2 | 3 | 3 | 6 | 9 | 10 | 12 |
| **TOTAL MULTIPLE DX** | 1,843 | 7.8 | 62 | 2 | 3 | 6 | 9 | 16 | 22 | 44 |
| **TOTAL** | | | | | | | | | | |
| 0–19 Years | 901 | 7.3 | 65 | 2 | 3 | 5 | 8 | 16 | 22 | 44 |
| 20–34 | 266 | 7.7 | 82 | 2 | 4 | 6 | 9 | 14 | 20 | 76 |
| 35–49 | 435 | 6.9 | 43 | 2 | 3 | 6 | 8 | 13 | 19 | 40 |
| 50–64 | 316 | 6.7 | 27 | 2 | 3 | 5 | 8 | 14 | 18 | 22 |
| 65+ | 290 | 7.2 | 34 | 2 | 3 | 6 | 9 | 12 | 17 | 33 |
| **GRAND TOTAL** | 2,208 | 7.2 | 53 | 2 | 3 | 5 | 9 | 14 | 20 | 42 |

## 03.53: VERTEBRAL FX REPAIR. Formerly included in operation group(s) 507.

| Type of Patients | Observed Patients | Avg. Stay | Variance | 10th | 25th | 50th | 75th | 90th | 95th | 99th |
|---|---|---|---|---|---|---|---|---|---|---|
| **1. SINGLE DX** | | | | | | | | | | |
| 0–19 Years | 9 | 7.6 | 8 | 2 | 7 | 9 | 9 | 9 | 11 | 11 |
| 20–34 | 22 | 6.8 | 10 | 4 | 5 | 6 | 7 | 7 | 10 | 19 |
| 35–49 | 14 | 4.0 | 5 | 1 | 3 | 3 | 6 | 7 | 8 | 8 |
| 50–64 | 7 | 4.2 | 11 | 1 | 1 | 3 | 7 | 9 | 9 | 9 |
| 65+ | 1 | 10.0 | 0 | 10 | 10 | 10 | 10 | 10 | 10 | 10 |
| **2. MULTIPLE DX** | | | | | | | | | | |
| 0–19 Years | 71 | 9.3 | 42 | 5 | 5 | 8 | 8 | 18 | 22 | >99 |
| 20–34 | 103 | 10.1 | 62 | 4 | 6 | 8 | 12 | 20 | 35 | >99 |
| 35–49 | 109 | 11.7 | 92 | 4 | 6 | 8 | 14 | 25 | 32 | 51 |
| 50–64 | 64 | 8.8 | 41 | 3 | 4 | 8 | 12 | 20 | 20 | 26 |
| 65+ | 121 | 8.5 | 50 | 3 | 5 | 7 | 9 | 14 | 19 | 47 |
| **TOTAL SINGLE DX** | 53 | 6.2 | 10 | 2 | 3 | 6 | 9 | 9 | 10 | 19 |
| **TOTAL MULTIPLE DX** | 468 | 9.7 | 60 | 3 | 5 | 8 | 11 | 20 | 25 | 51 |
| **TOTAL** | | | | | | | | | | |
| 0–19 Years | 80 | 8.9 | 36 | 4 | 5 | 8 | 9 | 18 | 22 | >99 |
| 20–34 | 125 | 9.4 | 53 | 4 | 5 | 7 | 11 | 19 | 29 | >99 |
| 35–49 | 123 | 10.7 | 88 | 3 | 5 | 9 | 13 | 22 | 32 | 51 |
| 50–64 | 71 | 8.6 | 41 | 3 | 4 | 7 | 11 | 20 | 20 | 26 |
| 65+ | 122 | 8.5 | 49 | 3 | 5 | 7 | 10 | 13 | 19 | 47 |
| **GRAND TOTAL** | 521 | 9.3 | 55 | 3 | 5 | 8 | 11 | 18 | 22 | 51 |

## 03.59: SPINAL STRUCT REPAIR NEC. Formerly included in operation group(s) 507.

| Type of Patients | Observed Patients | Avg. Stay | Variance | 10th | 25th | 50th | 75th | 90th | 95th | 99th |
|---|---|---|---|---|---|---|---|---|---|---|
| **1. SINGLE DX** | | | | | | | | | | |
| 0–19 Years | 115 | 4.0 | 6 | 2 | 3 | 3 | 5 | 6 | 10 | 12 |
| 20–34 | 26 | 3.8 | 4 | 2 | 3 | 3 | 5 | 6 | 7 | 10 |
| 35–49 | 64 | 3.6 | 3 | 2 | 3 | 3 | 4 | 6 | 8 | 9 |
| 50–64 | 44 | 3.9 | 7 | 1 | 3 | 3 | 4 | 6 | 9 | 16 |
| 65+ | 13 | 3.6 | 4 | 2 | 3 | 3 | 4 | 6 | 6 | 12 |
| **2. MULTIPLE DX** | | | | | | | | | | |
| 0–19 Years | 514 | 5.2 | 19 | 2 | 3 | 4 | 6 | 9 | 14 | 21 |
| 20–34 | 86 | 7.5 | 150 | 2 | 4 | 4 | 7 | 10 | 18 | 76 |
| 35–49 | 190 | 5.8 | 19 | 2 | 3 | 5 | 7 | 10 | 12 | 24 |
| 50–64 | 144 | 6.6 | 23 | 2 | 3 | 5 | 9 | 14 | 15 | 23 |
| 65+ | 118 | 7.2 | 23 | 2 | 4 | 7 | 9 | 11 | 14 | 26 |
| **TOTAL SINGLE DX** | 262 | 3.9 | 5 | 2 | 3 | 3 | 4 | 6 | 9 | 12 |
| **TOTAL MULTIPLE DX** | 1,052 | 5.9 | 33 | 2 | 3 | 4 | 7 | 11 | 14 | 24 |
| **TOTAL** | | | | | | | | | | |
| 0–19 Years | 629 | 4.9 | 17 | 2 | 3 | 4 | 5 | 8 | 13 | 21 |
| 20–34 | 112 | 6.6 | 119 | 2 | 3 | 4 | 7 | 9 | 14 | 76 |
| 35–49 | 254 | 5.1 | 15 | 2 | 3 | 4 | 7 | 9 | 10 | 23 |
| 50–64 | 188 | 6.0 | 20 | 2 | 3 | 6 | 8 | 14 | 14 | 18 |
| 65+ | 131 | 6.8 | 22 | 2 | 3 | 6 | 9 | 11 | 14 | 26 |
| **GRAND TOTAL** | 1,314 | 5.4 | 27 | 2 | 3 | 4 | 6 | 10 | 14 | 23 |

Length of Stay by Diagnosis and Operation, United States, 2000

# United States, October 1998–September 1999 Data, by Operation

## 03.6: SPINAL CORD ADHESIOLYSIS. Formerly included in operation group(s) 507.

| Type of Patients | Observed Patients | Avg. Stay | Vari-ance | Percentiles | | | | | | |
|---|---|---|---|---|---|---|---|---|---|---|
| | | | | 10th | 25th | 50th | 75th | 90th | 95th | 99th |
| **1. SINGLE DX** | | | | | | | | | | |
| 0–19 Years | 13 | 2.3 | <1 | 2 | 2 | 2 | 3 | 3 | 3 | 3 |
| 20–34 | 9 | 2.7 | 2 | 1 | 2 | 3 | 3 | 5 | 5 | 5 |
| 35–49 | 19 | 2.3 | <1 | 1 | 2 | 2 | 3 | 3 | 4 | 6 |
| 50–64 | 12 | 1.6 | <1 | 1 | 1 | 1 | 2 | 3 | 3 | 3 |
| 65+ | 5 | 1.8 | <1 | 1 | 2 | 2 | 2 | 2 | 2 | 2 |
| **2. MULTIPLE DX** | | | | | | | | | | |
| 0–19 Years | 26 | 3.2 | 4 | 2 | 2 | 2 | 4 | 8 | 8 | 8 |
| 20–34 | 22 | 3.9 | 10 | 1 | 2 | 3 | 5 | 11 | 11 | 13 |
| 35–49 | 100 | 3.8 | 11 | 1 | 2 | 3 | 4 | 11 | 11 | 11 |
| 50–64 | 79 | 4.1 | 21 | 1 | 2 | 2 | 4 | 10 | 14 | 28 |
| 65+ | 85 | 3.2 | 8 | 1 | 2 | 2 | 4 | 7 | 9 | 16 |
| **TOTAL SINGLE DX** | 58 | 2.3 | 1 | 1 | 2 | 2 | 3 | 3 | 5 | 5 |
| **TOTAL MULTIPLE DX** | 312 | 3.7 | 13 | 1 | 2 | 2 | 4 | 9 | 11 | 16 |
| **TOTAL** | | | | | | | | | | |
| 0–19 Years | 39 | 2.9 | 3 | 2 | 2 | 2 | 3 | 5 | 8 | 8 |
| 20–34 | 31 | 3.4 | 7 | 1 | 2 | 3 | 4 | 6 | 11 | 13 |
| 35–49 | 119 | 3.6 | 10 | 1 | 2 | 2 | 4 | 11 | 11 | 11 |
| 50–64 | 91 | 3.9 | 20 | 1 | 2 | 2 | 4 | 10 | 14 | 28 |
| 65+ | 90 | 3.1 | 8 | 1 | 2 | 2 | 4 | 7 | 9 | 16 |
| **GRAND TOTAL** | 370 | 3.5 | 11 | 1 | 2 | 2 | 4 | 8 | 11 | 16 |

## 03.7: SPINAL THECAL SHUNT. Formerly included in operation group(s) 507.

| Type of Patients | Observed Patients | Avg. Stay | Vari-ance | Percentiles | | | | | | |
|---|---|---|---|---|---|---|---|---|---|---|
| | | | | 10th | 25th | 50th | 75th | 90th | 95th | 99th |
| **1. SINGLE DX** | | | | | | | | | | |
| 0–19 Years | 25 | 3.5 | 6 | 1 | 2 | 3 | 4 | 6 | 7 | 13 |
| 20–34 | 29 | 2.5 | 3 | 1 | 1 | 2 | 3 | 6 | 6 | 7 |
| 35–49 | 31 | 4.4 | 3 | 2 | 3 | 5 | 6 | 6 | 6 | 8 |
| 50–64 | 7 | 4.4 | 5 | 2 | 3 | 3 | 7 | 7 | 7 | 7 |
| 65+ | 11 | 3.6 | 6 | 1 | 2 | 3 | 4 | 8 | 8 | 8 |
| **2. MULTIPLE DX** | | | | | | | | | | |
| 0–19 Years | 77 | 6.1 | 53 | 1 | 3 | 4 | 6 | 11 | 26 | 32 |
| 20–34 | 76 | 4.9 | 35 | 1 | 2 | 3 | 5 | 10 | 13 | 39 |
| 35–49 | 99 | 5.0 | 22 | 1 | 2 | 3 | 7 | 11 | 14 | 25 |
| 50–64 | 49 | 7.2 | 73 | 2 | 3 | 5 | 7 | 12 | 14 | 45 |
| 65+ | 69 | 6.0 | 31 | 1 | 2 | 5 | 7 | 13 | 18 | 26 |
| **TOTAL SINGLE DX** | 103 | 3.6 | 5 | 1 | 2 | 3 | 6 | 6 | 7 | 8 |
| **TOTAL MULTIPLE DX** | 370 | 5.8 | 43 | 1 | 2 | 4 | 7 | 11 | 19 | 32 |
| **TOTAL** | | | | | | | | | | |
| 0–19 Years | 102 | 5.7 | 46 | 1 | 2 | 4 | 6 | 9 | 26 | 32 |
| 20–34 | 105 | 4.3 | 28 | 1 | 2 | 3 | 4 | 8 | 12 | 39 |
| 35–49 | 130 | 4.8 | 16 | 2 | 3 | 5 | 6 | 9 | 14 | 25 |
| 50–64 | 56 | 6.8 | 66 | 2 | 3 | 5 | 7 | 12 | 13 | 45 |
| 65+ | 80 | 5.7 | 28 | 1 | 2 | 4 | 7 | 12 | 18 | 26 |
| **GRAND TOTAL** | 473 | 5.3 | 36 | 1 | 2 | 4 | 6 | 9 | 15 | 32 |

## 03.8: DESTR INJECT-SPINE CANAL. Formerly included in operation group(s) 507.

| Type of Patients | Observed Patients | Avg. Stay | Vari-ance | Percentiles | | | | | | |
|---|---|---|---|---|---|---|---|---|---|---|
| | | | | 10th | 25th | 50th | 75th | 90th | 95th | 99th |
| **1. SINGLE DX** | | | | | | | | | | |
| 0–19 Years | 27 | 7.3 | 52 | 1 | 2 | 6 | 7 | 24 | 24 | 24 |
| 20–34 | 2 | 1.8 | <1 | 1 | 2 | 4 | 2 | 2 | 2 | 2 |
| 35–49 | 2 | 5.3 | 6 | 4 | 4 | 4 | 9 | 9 | 9 | 9 |
| 50–64 | 4 | 1.4 | <1 | 1 | 1 | 1 | 1 | 3 | 3 | 3 |
| 65+ | 1 | 1.0 | 0 | 1 | 1 | 1 | 1 | 1 | 1 | 1 |
| **2. MULTIPLE DX** | | | | | | | | | | |
| 0–19 Years | 807 | 4.2 | 22 | 1 | 2 | 3 | 5 | 7 | 11 | 27 |
| 20–34 | 44 | 4.6 | 16 | 2 | 2 | 3 | 5 | 9 | 10 | 17 |
| 35–49 | 44 | 13.8 | 182 | 2 | 4 | 7 | 36 | 36 | 36 | 36 |
| 50–64 | 55 | 6.7 | 35 | 3 | 3 | 5 | 6 | 12 | 22 | 36 |
| 65+ | 31 | 12.2 | 71 | 3 | 5 | 12 | 17 | 24 | 30 | 34 |
| **TOTAL SINGLE DX** | 36 | 6.1 | 45 | 1 | 1 | 4 | 7 | 24 | 24 | 24 |
| **TOTAL MULTIPLE DX** | 981 | 5.0 | 37 | 1 | 2 | 3 | 5 | 10 | 15 | 36 |
| **TOTAL** | | | | | | | | | | |
| 0–19 Years | 834 | 4.3 | 23 | 1 | 2 | 3 | 5 | 7 | 11 | 24 |
| 20–34 | 46 | 4.6 | 16 | 2 | 2 | 4 | 5 | 9 | 10 | 17 |
| 35–49 | 46 | 13.5 | 178 | 2 | 4 | 7 | 15 | 36 | 36 | 36 |
| 50–64 | 59 | 6.1 | 34 | 2 | 3 | 4 | 6 | 12 | 18 | 36 |
| 65+ | 32 | 11.8 | 73 | 3 | 4 | 12 | 17 | 24 | 30 | 34 |
| **GRAND TOTAL** | 1,017 | 5.0 | 37 | 1 | 2 | 3 | 5 | 10 | 15 | 36 |

## 03.9: SPINAL CORD OPS NEC. Formerly included in operation group(s) 507, 512.

| Type of Patients | Observed Patients | Avg. Stay | Vari-ance | Percentiles | | | | | | |
|---|---|---|---|---|---|---|---|---|---|---|
| | | | | 10th | 25th | 50th | 75th | 90th | 95th | 99th |
| **1. SINGLE DX** | | | | | | | | | | |
| 0–19 Years | 153 | 2.9 | 4 | 1 | 1 | 2 | 4 | 6 | 7 | 9 |
| 20–34 | 649 | 2.7 | 2 | 1 | 2 | 2 | 4 | 5 | 5 | 7 |
| 35–49 | 858 | 3.2 | 10 | 1 | 2 | 2 | 4 | 6 | 10 | 14 |
| 50–64 | 387 | 3.9 | 7 | 1 | 3 | 3 | 5 | 7 | 10 | 10 |
| 65+ | 258 | 3.7 | 7 | 1 | 2 | 3 | 5 | 7 | 9 | 12 |
| **2. MULTIPLE DX** | | | | | | | | | | |
| 0–19 Years | 503 | 5.0 | 37 | 1 | 2 | 3 | 6 | 10 | 15 | 24 |
| 20–34 | 1,418 | 3.5 | 12 | 1 | 2 | 3 | 4 | 7 | 8 | 17 |
| 35–49 | 2,855 | 4.4 | 22 | 1 | 2 | 3 | 5 | 8 | 12 | 22 |
| 50–64 | 2,671 | 4.8 | 18 | 1 | 3 | 4 | 6 | 9 | 11 | 21 |
| 65+ | 5,482 | 6.3 | 23 | 2 | 3 | 5 | 8 | 12 | 15 | 23 |
| **TOTAL SINGLE DX** | 2,305 | 3.3 | 7 | 1 | 2 | 3 | 4 | 6 | 8 | 14 |
| **TOTAL MULTIPLE DX** | 12,929 | 5.2 | 22 | 1 | 2 | 4 | 7 | 10 | 14 | 22 |
| **TOTAL** | | | | | | | | | | |
| 0–19 Years | 656 | 4.6 | 31 | 1 | 2 | 3 | 6 | 9 | 14 | 24 |
| 20–34 | 2,067 | 3.3 | 9 | 1 | 2 | 3 | 4 | 6 | 7 | 14 |
| 35–49 | 3,713 | 4.1 | 19 | 1 | 2 | 4 | 5 | 8 | 12 | 19 |
| 50–64 | 3,058 | 4.6 | 16 | 1 | 2 | 4 | 6 | 9 | 11 | 19 |
| 65+ | 5,740 | 6.2 | 23 | 2 | 3 | 5 | 8 | 12 | 15 | 22 |
| **GRAND TOTAL** | 15,234 | 4.9 | 20 | 1 | 2 | 4 | 6 | 10 | 13 | 21 |

Length of Stay by Diagnosis and Operation, United States, 2000

# United States, October 1998–September 1999 Data, by Operation

## 03.90: INSERT SPINAL CANAL CATH. Formerly included in operation group(s) 512.

| Type of Patients | Observed Patients | Avg. Stay | Variance | 10th | 25th | 50th | 75th | 90th | 95th | 99th |
|---|---|---|---|---|---|---|---|---|---|---|
| **1. SINGLE DX** | | | | | | | | | | |
| 0–19 Years | 61 | 3.8 | 5 | 2 | 2 | 3 | 6 | 6 | 8 | 13 |
| 20–34 | 206 | 2.3 | 1 | 1 | 2 | 2 | 3 | 4 | 6 | 6 |
| 35–49 | 157 | 2.6 | 3 | 1 | 2 | 3 | 3 | 4 | 5 | 9 |
| 50–64 | 81 | 2.6 | 3 | 1 | 2 | 2 | 3 | 6 | 6 | 7 |
| 65+ | 49 | 2.6 | 2 | 2 | 2 | 2 | 3 | 4 | 5 | 8 |
| **2. MULTIPLE DX** | | | | | | | | | | |
| 0–19 Years | 178 | 5.1 | 24 | 2 | 2 | 4 | 6 | 8 | 13 | 24 |
| 20–34 | 379 | 3.8 | 13 | 2 | 2 | 3 | 4 | 7 | 10 | 20 |
| 35–49 | 676 | 5.1 | 28 | 2 | 2 | 3 | 6 | 10 | 13 | 27 |
| 50–64 | 646 | 5.2 | 27 | 1 | 2 | 3 | 7 | 10 | 13 | 27 |
| 65+ | 863 | 7.2 | 46 | 2 | 3 | 5 | 9 | 14 | 18 | 35 |
| **TOTAL SINGLE DX** | 554 | 2.6 | 3 | 1 | 2 | 2 | 3 | 4 | 6 | 8 |
| **TOTAL MULTIPLE DX** | 2,742 | 5.6 | 32 | 2 | 2 | 4 | 7 | 12 | 15 | 27 |
| **TOTAL** | | | | | | | | | | |
| 0–19 Years | 239 | 4.9 | 21 | 2 | 2 | 4 | 6 | 8 | 11 | 24 |
| 20–34 | 585 | 3.4 | 10 | 1 | 2 | 2 | 3 | 6 | 8 | 19 |
| 35–49 | 833 | 4.7 | 25 | 1 | 2 | 2 | 6 | 9 | 14 | 27 |
| 50–64 | 727 | 4.9 | 25 | 1 | 2 | 3 | 7 | 9 | 13 | 27 |
| 65+ | 912 | 7.0 | 45 | 2 | 3 | 5 | 9 | 14 | 18 | 32 |
| **GRAND TOTAL** | 3,296 | 5.1 | 29 | 1 | 2 | 3 | 6 | 11 | 14 | 27 |

## 03.91: INJECT ANES-SPINAL CANAL. Formerly included in operation group(s) 512.

| Type of Patients | Observed Patients | Avg. Stay | Variance | 10th | 25th | 50th | 75th | 90th | 95th | 99th |
|---|---|---|---|---|---|---|---|---|---|---|
| **1. SINGLE DX** | | | | | | | | | | |
| 0–19 Years | 39 | 2.7 | 3 | 1 | 2 | 2 | 3 | 7 | 7 | 8 |
| 20–34 | 179 | 2.6 | 2 | 1 | 2 | 2 | 3 | 4 | 5 | 7 |
| 35–49 | 146 | 2.6 | 5 | 1 | 2 | 2 | 3 | 4 | 7 | 12 |
| 50–64 | 60 | 4.9 | 7 | 2 | 3 | 4 | 5 | 10 | 10 | 10 |
| 65+ | 43 | 3.8 | 5 | 1 | 2 | 3 | 5 | 5 | 8 | 13 |
| **2. MULTIPLE DX** | | | | | | | | | | |
| 0–19 Years | 55 | 3.1 | 6 | 1 | 2 | 2 | 3 | 7 | 8 | 14 |
| 20–34 | 263 | 3.4 | 8 | 1 | 2 | 2 | 4 | 7 | 7 | 14 |
| 35–49 | 420 | 4.9 | 14 | 2 | 3 | 4 | 6 | 9 | 11 | 18 |
| 50–64 | 469 | 5.0 | 13 | 2 | 3 | 4 | 6 | 10 | 11 | 17 |
| 65+ | 1,141 | 6.2 | 18 | 3 | 3 | 5 | 8 | 11 | 15 | 21 |
| **TOTAL SINGLE DX** | 467 | 3.4 | 6 | 1 | 2 | 3 | 4 | 6 | 10 | 10 |
| **TOTAL MULTIPLE DX** | 2,348 | 5.3 | 16 | 2 | 3 | 4 | 7 | 10 | 13 | 19 |
| **TOTAL** | | | | | | | | | | |
| 0–19 Years | 94 | 3.0 | 5 | 1 | 2 | 2 | 3 | 7 | 7 | 11 |
| 20–34 | 442 | 3.1 | 6 | 1 | 2 | 2 | 4 | 7 | 7 | 10 |
| 35–49 | 566 | 4.2 | 12 | 1 | 2 | 4 | 5 | 8 | 10 | 16 |
| 50–64 | 529 | 5.0 | 12 | 2 | 3 | 4 | 6 | 10 | 11 | 17 |
| 65+ | 1,184 | 6.1 | 18 | 2 | 3 | 5 | 7 | 11 | 14 | 21 |
| **GRAND TOTAL** | 2,815 | 4.9 | 14 | 2 | 2 | 4 | 6 | 10 | 12 | 18 |

## 03.92: INJECT SPINAL CANAL NEC. Formerly included in operation group(s) 512.

| Type of Patients | Observed Patients | Avg. Stay | Variance | 10th | 25th | 50th | 75th | 90th | 95th | 99th |
|---|---|---|---|---|---|---|---|---|---|---|
| **1. SINGLE DX** | | | | | | | | | | |
| 0–19 Years | 28 | 1.4 | 1 | 1 | 1 | 1 | 1 | 4 | 4 | 6 |
| 20–34 | 126 | 3.4 | 3 | 1 | 3 | 3 | 5 | 6 | 6 | 8 |
| 35–49 | 290 | 4.5 | 17 | 1 | 2 | 4 | 5 | 14 | 14 | 14 |
| 50–64 | 145 | 3.9 | 7 | 1 | 2 | 3 | 6 | 6 | 6 | 10 |
| 65+ | 109 | 4.6 | 9 | 1 | 2 | 4 | 7 | 9 | 10 | 14 |
| **2. MULTIPLE DX** | | | | | | | | | | |
| 0–19 Years | 101 | 5.9 | 107 | 1 | 4 | 4 | 6 | 13 | 22 | 81 |
| 20–34 | 268 | 4.2 | 25 | 1 | 3 | 3 | 4 | 8 | 9 | 24 |
| 35–49 | 854 | 4.6 | 23 | 2 | 2 | 3 | 5 | 8 | 12 | 19 |
| 50–64 | 1,083 | 4.9 | 15 | 2 | 2 | 4 | 6 | 10 | 11 | 18 |
| 65+ | 3,153 | 6.3 | 19 | 2 | 3 | 5 | 8 | 11 | 14 | 22 |
| **TOTAL SINGLE DX** | 698 | 4.0 | 11 | 1 | 2 | 3 | 5 | 7 | 11 | 14 |
| **TOTAL MULTIPLE DX** | 5,459 | 5.6 | 22 | 2 | 3 | 4 | 7 | 11 | 13 | 22 |
| **TOTAL** | | | | | | | | | | |
| 0–19 Years | 129 | 4.9 | 87 | 1 | 2 | 3 | 5 | 11 | 17 | 65 |
| 20–34 | 394 | 3.9 | 17 | 1 | 2 | 3 | 5 | 6 | 8 | 15 |
| 35–49 | 1,144 | 4.6 | 21 | 1 | 2 | 4 | 5 | 8 | 14 | 19 |
| 50–64 | 1,228 | 4.8 | 14 | 1 | 3 | 4 | 6 | 9 | 11 | 18 |
| 65+ | 3,262 | 6.3 | 19 | 2 | 3 | 5 | 8 | 11 | 14 | 22 |
| **GRAND TOTAL** | 6,157 | 5.4 | 20 | 2 | 3 | 4 | 7 | 10 | 13 | 21 |

## 03.93: INSERT SPINAL NEUROSTIM. Formerly included in operation group(s) 507.

| Type of Patients | Observed Patients | Avg. Stay | Variance | 10th | 25th | 50th | 75th | 90th | 95th | 99th |
|---|---|---|---|---|---|---|---|---|---|---|
| **1. SINGLE DX** | | | | | | | | | | |
| 0–19 Years | 3 | 4.2 | 7 | 1 | 1 | 6 | 6 | 6 | 6 | 6 |
| 20–34 | 45 | 2.8 | 2 | 1 | 1 | 3 | 3 | 4 | 4 | 5 |
| 35–49 | 166 | 1.7 | 1 | 1 | 1 | 2 | 2 | 3 | 4 | 5 |
| 50–64 | 72 | 1.7 | <1 | 1 | 1 | 2 | 2 | 3 | 4 | 5 |
| 65+ | 45 | 1.9 | 3 | 1 | 1 | 1 | 2 | 6 | 6 | 10 |
| **2. MULTIPLE DX** | | | | | | | | | | |
| 0–19 Years | 6 | 1.4 | <1 | 1 | 1 | 1 | 2 | 3 | 3 | 5 |
| 20–34 | 73 | 2.8 | 6 | 1 | 1 | 3 | 3 | 7 | 7 | 10 |
| 35–49 | 454 | 2.3 | 4 | 1 | 1 | 2 | 3 | 4 | 5 | 9 |
| 50–64 | 291 | 2.5 | 8 | 1 | 1 | 2 | 3 | 5 | 7 | 12 |
| 65+ | 199 | 3.7 | 30 | 1 | 1 | 2 | 3 | 9 | 17 | 22 |
| **TOTAL SINGLE DX** | 331 | 1.9 | 2 | 1 | 1 | 1 | 2 | 4 | 4 | 6 |
| **TOTAL MULTIPLE DX** | 1,023 | 2.6 | 10 | 1 | 1 | 2 | 3 | 5 | 7 | 18 |
| **TOTAL** | | | | | | | | | | |
| 0–19 Years | 9 | 2.3 | 4 | 1 | 1 | 1 | 3 | 6 | 6 | 6 |
| 20–34 | 118 | 2.8 | 4 | 1 | 1 | 2 | 4 | 7 | 7 | 10 |
| 35–49 | 620 | 2.1 | 3 | 1 | 1 | 2 | 3 | 4 | 5 | 8 |
| 50–64 | 363 | 2.3 | 6 | 1 | 1 | 2 | 3 | 5 | 6 | 10 |
| 65+ | 244 | 3.4 | 26 | 1 | 1 | 3 | 5 | 8 | 17 | 22 |
| **GRAND TOTAL** | 1,354 | 2.4 | 8 | 1 | 1 | 2 | 3 | 4 | 6 | 17 |

Length of Stay by Diagnosis and Operation, United States, 2000

## United States, October 1998–September 1999 Data, by Operation

### 03.95: SPINAL BLOOD PATCH. Formerly included in operation group(s) 507.

| Type of Patients | Observed Patients | Avg. Stay | Variance | Percentiles | | | | | | |
|---|---|---|---|---|---|---|---|---|---|---|
| | | | | 10th | 25th | 50th | 75th | 90th | 95th | 99th |
| **1. SINGLE DX** | | | | | | | | | | |
| 0–19 Years | 12 | 3.5 | 4 | 1 | 1 | 3 | 6 | 6 | 6 | 6 |
| 20–34 | 77 | 2.2 | 1 | 1 | 1 | 2 | 3 | 3 | 4 | 5 |
| 35–49 | 69 | 2.3 | 2 | 1 | 1 | 2 | 3 | 3 | 6 | 7 |
| 50–64 | 15 | 2.2 | 4 | 1 | 1 | 2 | 2 | 4 | 4 | 10 |
| 65+ | 3 | 3.9 | 4 | 2 | 2 | 4 | 4 | 7 | 7 | 7 |
| **2. MULTIPLE DX** | | | | | | | | | | |
| 0–19 Years | 58 | 3.2 | 3 | 1 | 2 | 3 | 5 | 5 | 6 | 8 |
| 20–34 | 333 | 2.7 | 4 | 1 | 1 | 2 | 3 | 5 | 7 | 10 |
| 35–49 | 227 | 3.5 | 13 | 1 | 2 | 2 | 4 | 6 | 9 | 25 |
| 50–64 | 60 | 3.3 | 8 | 1 | 1 | 3 | 5 | 7 | 7 | 19 |
| 65+ | 31 | 4.3 | 7 | 1 | 2 | 4 | 6 | 7 | 10 | 11 |
| **TOTAL SINGLE DX** | 176 | 2.4 | 2 | 1 | 1 | 2 | 3 | 4 | 6 | 7 |
| **TOTAL MULTIPLE DX** | 709 | 3.1 | 7 | 1 | 1 | 2 | 4 | 6 | 7 | 17 |
| **TOTAL** | | | | | | | | | | |
| 0–19 Years | 70 | 3.2 | 3 | 1 | 1 | 3 | 5 | 6 | 6 | 8 |
| 20–34 | 410 | 2.6 | 4 | 1 | 1 | 2 | 3 | 5 | 6 | 10 |
| 35–49 | 296 | 3.2 | 11 | 1 | 1 | 2 | 3 | 6 | 7 | 17 |
| 50–64 | 75 | 3.1 | 7 | 1 | 1 | 2 | 4 | 7 | 7 | 11 |
| 65+ | 34 | 4.3 | 7 | 2 | 2 | 4 | 6 | 7 | 10 | 11 |
| **GRAND TOTAL** | 885 | 3.0 | 7 | 1 | 1 | 2 | 4 | 6 | 7 | 17 |

### 04.01: EXC ACOUSTIC NEUROMA. Formerly included in operation group(s) 508.

| Type of Patients | Observed Patients | Avg. Stay | Variance | Percentiles | | | | | | |
|---|---|---|---|---|---|---|---|---|---|---|
| | | | | 10th | 25th | 50th | 75th | 90th | 95th | 99th |
| **1. SINGLE DX** | | | | | | | | | | |
| 0–19 Years | 4 | 4.2 | 4 | 2 | 2 | 3 | 6 | 6 | 6 | 6 |
| 20–34 | 25 | 4.7 | 2 | 3 | 4 | 4 | 5 | 6 | 7 | 9 |
| 35–49 | 91 | 4.2 | 2 | 2 | 3 | 4 | 5 | 6 | 7 | 8 |
| 50–64 | 71 | 4.3 | 2 | 3 | 3 | 4 | 5 | 6 | 7 | 10 |
| 65+ | 9 | 4.2 | 1 | 3 | 3 | 4 | 5 | 6 | 6 | 6 |
| **2. MULTIPLE DX** | | | | | | | | | | |
| 0–19 Years | 9 | 3.6 | 3 | 3 | 3 | 3 | 3 | 6 | 9 | 9 |
| 20–34 | 56 | 6.0 | 14 | 3 | 4 | 6 | 8 | 8 | 14 | 21 |
| 35–49 | 180 | 5.9 | 8 | 4 | 4 | 5 | 7 | 9 | 12 | 16 |
| 50–64 | 221 | 5.7 | 9 | 3 | 4 | 5 | 7 | 8 | 10 | 16 |
| 65+ | 104 | 6.7 | 37 | 3 | 4 | 5 | 7 | 10 | 15 | 33 |
| **TOTAL SINGLE DX** | 200 | 4.3 | 2 | 3 | 3 | 4 | 5 | 6 | 7 | 9 |
| **TOTAL MULTIPLE DX** | 570 | 5.9 | 15 | 3 | 4 | 5 | 7 | 8 | 12 | 20 |
| **TOTAL** | | | | | | | | | | |
| 0–19 Years | 13 | 3.7 | 3 | 3 | 3 | 3 | 3 | 6 | 7 | 9 |
| 20–34 | 81 | 5.8 | 12 | 3 | 4 | 5 | 7 | 8 | 8 | 21 |
| 35–49 | 271 | 5.4 | 7 | 4 | 4 | 5 | 6 | 8 | 12 | 14 |
| 50–64 | 292 | 5.4 | 8 | 3 | 4 | 5 | 6 | 8 | 10 | 15 |
| 65+ | 113 | 6.4 | 34 | 3 | 4 | 5 | 7 | 10 | 15 | 33 |
| **GRAND TOTAL** | 770 | 5.6 | 12 | 3 | 4 | 5 | 6 | 8 | 11 | 17 |

### 04.0: PERIPH NERVE INC/DIV/EXC. Formerly included in operation group(s) 508.

| Type of Patients | Observed Patients | Avg. Stay | Variance | Percentiles | | | | | | |
|---|---|---|---|---|---|---|---|---|---|---|
| | | | | 10th | 25th | 50th | 75th | 90th | 95th | 99th |
| **1. SINGLE DX** | | | | | | | | | | |
| 0–19 Years | 37 | 2.8 | 3 | 1 | 1 | 2 | 5 | 5 | 5 | 6 |
| 20–34 | 61 | 3.1 | 3 | 2 | 2 | 2 | 4 | 6 | 6 | 7 |
| 35–49 | 163 | 3.4 | 3 | 2 | 2 | 3 | 4 | 6 | 6 | 8 |
| 50–64 | 111 | 2.9 | 4 | 1 | 1 | 3 | 4 | 5 | 6 | 10 |
| 65+ | 58 | 2.6 | 4 | 1 | 1 | 2 | 4 | 6 | 8 | 8 |
| **2. MULTIPLE DX** | | | | | | | | | | |
| 0–19 Years | 67 | 3.7 | 9 | 1 | 2 | 3 | 4 | 6 | 9 | 30 |
| 20–34 | 156 | 4.9 | 14 | 1 | 3 | 4 | 7 | 8 | 8 | 20 |
| 35–49 | 350 | 4.8 | 13 | 1 | 2 | 4 | 6 | 8 | 12 | 21 |
| 50–64 | 366 | 5.1 | 12 | 1 | 3 | 5 | 6 | 8 | 12 | 16 |
| 65+ | 253 | 4.7 | 26 | 1 | 1 | 3 | 6 | 9 | 11 | 26 |
| **TOTAL SINGLE DX** | 430 | 3.1 | 3 | 1 | 2 | 3 | 4 | 5 | 6 | 8 |
| **TOTAL MULTIPLE DX** | 1,192 | 4.8 | 15 | 1 | 2 | 4 | 6 | 8 | 11 | 21 |
| **TOTAL** | | | | | | | | | | |
| 0–19 Years | 104 | 3.3 | 7 | 1 | 2 | 3 | 4 | 6 | 6 | 19 |
| 20–34 | 217 | 4.3 | 11 | 1 | 2 | 4 | 6 | 8 | 8 | 18 |
| 35–49 | 513 | 4.4 | 10 | 1 | 2 | 4 | 5 | 7 | 10 | 20 |
| 50–64 | 477 | 4.6 | 11 | 1 | 2 | 5 | 6 | 8 | 10 | 16 |
| 65+ | 311 | 4.3 | 22 | 1 | 1 | 3 | 6 | 8 | 11 | 24 |
| **GRAND TOTAL** | 1,622 | 4.3 | 13 | 1 | 2 | 4 | 6 | 8 | 10 | 18 |

### 04.07: PERIPH/CRAN NERV EXC NEC. Formerly included in operation group(s) 508.

| Type of Patients | Observed Patients | Avg. Stay | Variance | Percentiles | | | | | | |
|---|---|---|---|---|---|---|---|---|---|---|
| | | | | 10th | 25th | 50th | 75th | 90th | 95th | 99th |
| **1. SINGLE DX** | | | | | | | | | | |
| 0–19 Years | 20 | 3.2 | 2 | 1 | 2 | 3 | 5 | 5 | 5 | 5 |
| 20–34 | 23 | 2.6 | 2 | 2 | 2 | 2 | 3 | 6 | 6 | 6 |
| 35–49 | 52 | 2.6 | 2 | 1 | 1 | 3 | 3 | 5 | 5 | 6 |
| 50–64 | 22 | 1.3 | 1 | 1 | 1 | 1 | 1 | 2 | 3 | 10 |
| 65+ | 12 | 1.8 | 1 | 1 | 1 | 1 | 2 | 3 | 5 | 5 |
| **2. MULTIPLE DX** | | | | | | | | | | |
| 0–19 Years | 33 | 3.1 | 6 | 1 | 2 | 3 | 4 | 4 | 7 | 19 |
| 20–34 | 65 | 4.0 | 7 | 1 | 1 | 4 | 6 | 8 | 8 | 8 |
| 35–49 | 111 | 4.1 | 21 | 1 | 1 | 3 | 5 | 8 | 11 | 23 |
| 50–64 | 91 | 4.6 | 20 | 1 | 1 | 3 | 6 | 10 | 16 | 16 |
| 65+ | 65 | 3.0 | 8 | 1 | 1 | 2 | 3 | 7 | 10 | 11 |
| **TOTAL SINGLE DX** | 129 | 2.4 | 2 | 1 | 1 | 2 | 3 | 5 | 5 | 6 |
| **TOTAL MULTIPLE DX** | 365 | 3.9 | 15 | 1 | 1 | 3 | 5 | 8 | 11 | 21 |
| **TOTAL** | | | | | | | | | | |
| 0–19 Years | 53 | 3.1 | 4 | 1 | 2 | 3 | 4 | 5 | 5 | 10 |
| 20–34 | 88 | 3.4 | 6 | 1 | 2 | 2 | 5 | 8 | 8 | 8 |
| 35–49 | 163 | 3.6 | 15 | 1 | 1 | 3 | 4 | 7 | 9 | 23 |
| 50–64 | 113 | 3.7 | 17 | 1 | 1 | 2 | 5 | 9 | 15 | 16 |
| 65+ | 77 | 2.8 | 8 | 1 | 1 | 2 | 3 | 6 | 10 | 11 |
| **GRAND TOTAL** | 494 | 3.4 | 11 | 1 | 1 | 2 | 4 | 7 | 9 | 18 |

Length of Stay by Diagnosis and Operation, United States, 2000

# United States, October 1998–September 1999 Data, by Operation

## 04.1: DXTIC PX PERIPH NERV. Formerly included in operation group(s) 508, 512.

| Type of Patients | Observed Patients | Avg. Stay | Variance | 10th | 25th | 50th | 75th | 90th | 95th | 99th |
|---|---|---|---|---|---|---|---|---|---|---|
| **1. SINGLE DX** | | | | | | | | | | |
| 0–19 Years | 1 | 2.0 | 0 | 2 | 2 | 2 | 2 | 2 | 2 | 2 |
| 20–34 | 1 | 3.0 | 0 | 3 | 3 | 3 | 3 | 3 | 3 | 3 |
| 35–49 | 2 | 2.3 | 1 | 1 | 1 | 3 | 3 | 3 | 3 | 3 |
| 50–64 | 0 | | | | | | | | | |
| 65+ | 2 | 2.9 | 1 | 2 | 2 | 2 | 4 | 4 | 4 | 4 |
| **2. MULTIPLE DX** | | | | | | | | | | |
| 0–19 Years | 8 | 9.4 | 96 | 1 | 1 | 7 | 9 | 25 | 36 | 36 |
| 20–34 | 9 | 12.1 | 204 | 3 | 3 | 4 | 15 | 42 | 42 | 42 |
| 35–49 | 29 | 8.1 | 37 | 3 | 3 | 8 | 11 | 11 | 24 | 27 |
| 50–64 | 40 | 9.6 | 69 | 3 | 4 | 7 | 11 | 22 | 32 | 37 |
| 65+ | 73 | 13.1 | 87 | 3 | 6 | 11 | 18 | 28 | 28 | 37 |
| **TOTAL SINGLE DX** | 6 | 2.5 | <1 | 1 | 2 | 2 | 3 | 4 | 4 | 4 |
| **TOTAL MULTIPLE DX** | 159 | 10.7 | 80 | 3 | 4 | 8 | 14 | 26 | 28 | 42 |
| **TOTAL** | | | | | | | | | | |
| 0–19 Years | 9 | 8.2 | 87 | 1 | 1 | 5 | 9 | 25 | 36 | 36 |
| 20–34 | 10 | 11.7 | 198 | 3 | 3 | 4 | 15 | 42 | 42 | 42 |
| 35–49 | 31 | 7.9 | 37 | 2 | 3 | 8 | 11 | 11 | 24 | 27 |
| 50–64 | 40 | 9.6 | 69 | 3 | 4 | 7 | 11 | 22 | 32 | 37 |
| 65+ | 75 | 12.9 | 88 | 3 | 6 | 10 | 18 | 28 | 28 | 37 |
| **GRAND TOTAL** | 165 | 10.5 | 80 | 3 | 4 | 8 | 13 | 25 | 28 | 42 |

## 04.3: CRAN/PERIPH NERVE SUTURE. Formerly included in operation group(s) 509.

| Type of Patients | Observed Patients | Avg. Stay | Variance | 10th | 25th | 50th | 75th | 90th | 95th | 99th |
|---|---|---|---|---|---|---|---|---|---|---|
| **1. SINGLE DX** | | | | | | | | | | |
| 0–19 Years | 11 | 1.2 | <1 | 1 | 1 | 1 | 1 | 2 | 2 | 2 |
| 20–34 | 3 | 1.0 | 0 | 1 | 1 | 1 | 1 | 2 | 2 | 2 |
| 35–49 | 6 | 2.4 | 1 | 1 | 1 | 3 | 3 | 4 | 4 | 4 |
| 50–64 | 2 | 1.0 | 0 | 1 | 1 | 1 | 1 | 1 | 1 | 1 |
| 65+ | 0 | | | | | | | | | |
| **2. MULTIPLE DX** | | | | | | | | | | |
| 0–19 Years | 80 | 2.4 | 2 | 1 | 1 | 2 | 3 | 4 | 6 | 10 |
| 20–34 | 119 | 2.2 | 2 | 1 | 1 | 2 | 3 | 6 | 6 | 9 |
| 35–49 | 76 | 2.3 | 13 | 1 | 1 | 2 | 2 | 4 | 5 | 11 |
| 50–64 | 30 | 3.0 | 1 | 1 | 2 | 3 | 4 | 4 | 4 | 4 |
| 65+ | 18 | 4.5 | 10 | 2 | 2 | 3 | 7 | 7 | 8 | 17 |
| **TOTAL SINGLE DX** | 22 | 1.5 | <1 | 1 | 1 | 1 | 2 | 3 | 3 | 4 |
| **TOTAL MULTIPLE DX** | 323 | 2.6 | 6 | 1 | 1 | 2 | 3 | 4 | 7 | 10 |
| **TOTAL** | | | | | | | | | | |
| 0–19 Years | 91 | 2.4 | 2 | 1 | 1 | 2 | 3 | 4 | 6 | 10 |
| 20–34 | 122 | 2.2 | 2 | 1 | 1 | 2 | 3 | 4 | 4 | 8 |
| 35–49 | 82 | 2.3 | 12 | 1 | 1 | 2 | 2 | 4 | 5 | 11 |
| 50–64 | 32 | 3.0 | 1 | 1 | 2 | 3 | 4 | 4 | 4 | 4 |
| 65+ | 18 | 4.5 | 10 | 2 | 2 | 3 | 7 | 7 | 8 | 17 |
| **GRAND TOTAL** | 345 | 2.5 | 6 | 1 | 1 | 2 | 3 | 4 | 7 | 10 |

## 04.2: DESTR PERIPH/CRAN NERVES. Formerly included in operation group(s) 509.

| Type of Patients | Observed Patients | Avg. Stay | Variance | 10th | 25th | 50th | 75th | 90th | 95th | 99th |
|---|---|---|---|---|---|---|---|---|---|---|
| **1. SINGLE DX** | | | | | | | | | | |
| 0–19 Years | 1 | 1.0 | 0 | 1 | 1 | 1 | 1 | 1 | 1 | 1 |
| 20–34 | 1 | 6.0 | 0 | 6 | 6 | 6 | 6 | 6 | 6 | 6 |
| 35–49 | 4 | 3.6 | 11 | 1 | 1 | 4 | 4 | 9 | 9 | 9 |
| 50–64 | 3 | 1.4 | <1 | 1 | 1 | 1 | 1 | 2 | 2 | 2 |
| 65+ | 19 | 1.1 | <1 | 1 | 1 | 1 | 1 | 1 | 1 | 3 |
| **2. MULTIPLE DX** | | | | | | | | | | |
| 0–19 Years | 1 | 1.0 | 0 | 1 | 1 | 1 | 1 | 1 | 1 | 1 |
| 20–34 | 7 | 11.0 | 274 | 2 | 2 | 2 | 11 | 49 | 49 | 49 |
| 35–49 | 12 | 15.5 | 220 | 1 | 3 | 5 | 33 | 33 | 33 | 33 |
| 50–64 | 21 | 2.4 | 17 | 1 | 1 | 1 | 2 | 3 | 4 | 25 |
| 65+ | 63 | 4.5 | 31 | 1 | 1 | 3 | 6 | 14 | 15 | 26 |
| **TOTAL SINGLE DX** | 28 | 1.5 | 2 | 1 | 1 | 1 | 1 | 3 | 4 | 9 |
| **TOTAL MULTIPLE DX** | 104 | 5.5 | 76 | 1 | 1 | 2 | 4 | 14 | 33 | 49 |
| **TOTAL** | | | | | | | | | | |
| 0–19 Years | 2 | 1.0 | 0 | 1 | 1 | 1 | 1 | 1 | 1 | 1 |
| 20–34 | 8 | 10.7 | 260 | 2 | 2 | 2 | 11 | 49 | 49 | 49 |
| 35–49 | 16 | 13.9 | 207 | 1 | 2 | 4 | 33 | 33 | 33 | 33 |
| 50–64 | 24 | 2.3 | 15 | 1 | 1 | 1 | 2 | 3 | 4 | 25 |
| 65+ | 82 | 4.0 | 27 | 1 | 1 | 3 | 4 | 14 | 14 | 26 |
| **GRAND TOTAL** | 132 | 4.9 | 67 | 1 | 1 | 2 | 4 | 14 | 26 | 33 |

## 04.4: PERIPH NERV ADHESIOLYSIS. Formerly included in operation group(s) 509.

| Type of Patients | Observed Patients | Avg. Stay | Variance | 10th | 25th | 50th | 75th | 90th | 95th | 99th |
|---|---|---|---|---|---|---|---|---|---|---|
| **1. SINGLE DX** | | | | | | | | | | |
| 0–19 Years | 33 | 2.3 | <1 | 1 | 2 | 2 | 3 | 3 | 4 | 6 |
| 20–34 | 62 | 2.0 | 2 | 1 | 1 | 2 | 3 | 3 | 5 | 5 |
| 35–49 | 148 | 2.2 | 2 | 1 | 1 | 2 | 3 | 4 | 4 | 7 |
| 50–64 | 113 | 3.0 | 4 | 1 | 1 | 3 | 4 | 6 | 6 | 6 |
| 65+ | 60 | 2.6 | 4 | 1 | 1 | 2 | 3 | 5 | 5 | 15 |
| **2. MULTIPLE DX** | | | | | | | | | | |
| 0–19 Years | 79 | 5.0 | 35 | 1 | 2 | 3 | 5 | 12 | 12 | 32 |
| 20–34 | 146 | 3.7 | 30 | 1 | 2 | 3 | 6 | 10 | 10 | 29 |
| 35–49 | 329 | 3.2 | 14 | 1 | 1 | 2 | 4 | 7 | 10 | 17 |
| 50–64 | 317 | 3.3 | 13 | 1 | 1 | 3 | 4 | 7 | 9 | 21 |
| 65+ | 339 | 4.0 | 12 | 1 | 1 | 3 | 5 | 8 | 13 | 16 |
| **TOTAL SINGLE DX** | 416 | 2.5 | 3 | 1 | 1 | 2 | 3 | 5 | 6 | 6 |
| **TOTAL MULTIPLE DX** | 1,210 | 3.6 | 17 | 1 | 1 | 2 | 4 | 7 | 11 | 19 |
| **TOTAL** | | | | | | | | | | |
| 0–19 Years | 112 | 4.2 | 27 | 1 | 2 | 3 | 5 | 12 | 12 | 27 |
| 20–34 | 208 | 3.3 | 24 | 1 | 1 | 2 | 4 | 6 | 8 | 20 |
| 35–49 | 477 | 2.9 | 10 | 1 | 1 | 2 | 4 | 5 | 8 | 15 |
| 50–64 | 430 | 3.2 | 10 | 1 | 1 | 3 | 4 | 7 | 9 | 19 |
| 65+ | 399 | 3.8 | 11 | 1 | 1 | 3 | 5 | 8 | 12 | 16 |
| **GRAND TOTAL** | 1,626 | 3.3 | 13 | 1 | 1 | 2 | 4 | 6 | 10 | 18 |

Length of Stay by Diagnosis and Operation, United States, 2000

**United States, October 1998–September 1999 Data, by Operation**

**04.41: DECOMP TRIGEMINAL ROOT. Formerly included in operation group(s) 509.**

| Type of Patients | Observed Patients | Avg. Stay | Vari-ance | 10th | 25th | 50th | 75th | 90th | 95th | 99th |
|---|---|---|---|---|---|---|---|---|---|---|
| **1. SINGLE DX** | | | | | | | | | | |
| 0–19 Years | 1 | 3.0 | 0 | 3 | 3 | 3 | 3 | 3 | 3 | 3 |
| 20–34 | 12 | 2.8 | 1 | 2 | 2 | 3 | 3 | 5 | 5 | 5 |
| 35–49 | 39 | 3.3 | <1 | 2 | 3 | 3 | 4 | 4 | 4 | 5 |
| 50–64 | 50 | 3.2 | 4 | 2 | 3 | 3 | 3 | 4 | 5 | 7 |
| 65+ | 39 | 3.1 | 4 | 1 | 2 | 3 | 4 | 5 | 6 | 15 |
| **2. MULTIPLE DX** | | | | | | | | | | |
| 0–19 Years | 4 | 4.0 | 1 | 3 | 3 | 3 | 5 | 5 | 5 | 5 |
| 20–34 | 8 | 3.1 | 1 | 2 | 2 | 3 | 4 | 4 | 6 | 6 |
| 35–49 | 56 | 3.7 | 5 | 2 | 2 | 3 | 4 | 7 | 9 | 12 |
| 50–64 | 108 | 4.5 | 10 | 2 | 3 | 3 | 6 | 9 | 9 | 24 |
| 65+ | 93 | 4.3 | 9 | 2 | 3 | 4 | 5 | 6 | 7 | 13 |
| **TOTAL SINGLE DX** | 141 | 3.2 | 3 | 2 | 3 | 3 | 4 | 4 | 5 | 7 |
| **TOTAL MULTIPLE DX** | 269 | 4.3 | 8 | 2 | 3 | 3 | 5 | 7 | 9 | 14 |
| **TOTAL** | | | | | | | | | | |
| 0–19 Years | 5 | 3.7 | 1 | 3 | 3 | 3 | 5 | 5 | 5 | 5 |
| 20–34 | 20 | 2.9 | 1 | 2 | 2 | 2 | 3 | 5 | 5 | 6 |
| 35–49 | 95 | 3.5 | 3 | 2 | 2 | 3 | 4 | 4 | 7 | 12 |
| 50–64 | 158 | 4.1 | 8 | 2 | 3 | 3 | 4 | 7 | 9 | 17 |
| 65+ | 132 | 3.9 | 9 | 2 | 2 | 3 | 5 | 6 | 7 | 15 |
| **GRAND TOTAL** | 410 | 3.8 | 6 | 2 | 3 | 3 | 4 | 6 | 8 | 13 |

**04.49: PERIPH NERV ADHESIO NEC. Formerly included in operation group(s) 509.**

| Type of Patients | Observed Patients | Avg. Stay | Vari-ance | 10th | 25th | 50th | 75th | 90th | 95th | 99th |
|---|---|---|---|---|---|---|---|---|---|---|
| **1. SINGLE DX** | | | | | | | | | | |
| 0–19 Years | 26 | 2.0 | <1 | 1 | 1 | 2 | 2 | 3 | 3 | 6 |
| 20–34 | 26 | 1.4 | <1 | 1 | 1 | 1 | 2 | 2 | 3 | 6 |
| 35–49 | 49 | 1.6 | <1 | 1 | 1 | 1 | 2 | 3 | 3 | 5 |
| 50–64 | 26 | 1.1 | <1 | 1 | 1 | 1 | 1 | 1 | 2 | 3 |
| 65+ | 7 | 1.3 | <1 | 1 | 1 | 2 | 2 | 2 | 2 | 2 |
| **2. MULTIPLE DX** | | | | | | | | | | |
| 0–19 Years | 46 | 5.3 | 28 | 1 | 2 | 3 | 12 | 12 | 12 | 27 |
| 20–34 | 51 | 3.2 | 22 | 1 | 1 | 3 | 3 | 8 | 8 | 29 |
| 35–49 | 99 | 2.4 | 12 | 1 | 2 | 2 | 3 | 4 | 6 | 15 |
| 50–64 | 66 | 3.0 | 15 | 1 | 2 | 2 | 3 | 6 | 11 | 29 |
| 65+ | 52 | 3.8 | 17 | 1 | 2 | 4 | 4 | 13 | 13 | 13 |
| **TOTAL SINGLE DX** | 134 | 1.5 | <1 | 1 | 1 | 1 | 2 | 3 | 3 | 5 |
| **TOTAL MULTIPLE DX** | 314 | 3.3 | 18 | 1 | 1 | 2 | 3 | 8 | 12 | 27 |
| **TOTAL** | | | | | | | | | | |
| 0–19 Years | 72 | 4.2 | 21 | 1 | 2 | 2 | 4 | 12 | 12 | 27 |
| 20–34 | 77 | 2.5 | 15 | 1 | 1 | 1 | 2 | 5 | 8 | 29 |
| 35–49 | 148 | 2.1 | 8 | 1 | 1 | 2 | 2 | 5 | 6 | 15 |
| 50–64 | 92 | 2.5 | 12 | 1 | 1 | 2 | 3 | 5 | 8 | 14 |
| 65+ | 59 | 3.6 | 16 | 1 | 2 | 4 | 4 | 13 | 13 | 13 |
| **GRAND TOTAL** | 448 | 2.8 | 13 | 1 | 1 | 2 | 3 | 5 | 12 | 14 |

**04.43: CARPAL TUNNEL RELEASE. Formerly included in operation group(s) 509.**

| Type of Patients | Observed Patients | Avg. Stay | Vari-ance | 10th | 25th | 50th | 75th | 90th | 95th | 99th |
|---|---|---|---|---|---|---|---|---|---|---|
| **1. SINGLE DX** | | | | | | | | | | |
| 0–19 Years | 1 | 2.0 | 0 | 2 | 2 | 2 | 2 | 2 | 2 | 2 |
| 20–34 | 14 | 1.0 | 0 | 1 | 1 | 1 | 1 | 1 | 1 | 1 |
| 35–49 | 31 | 1.3 | <1 | 1 | 1 | 1 | 1 | 3 | 3 | 4 |
| 50–64 | 16 | 1.4 | <1 | 1 | 1 | 1 | 1 | 2 | 6 | 6 |
| 65+ | 9 | 1.1 | <1 | 1 | 1 | 1 | 1 | 1 | 1 | 3 |
| **2. MULTIPLE DX** | | | | | | | | | | |
| 0–19 Years | 17 | 5.1 | 77 | 1 | 1 | 2 | 6 | 7 | 16 | 51 |
| 20–34 | 63 | 3.5 | 29 | 1 | 2 | 3 | 4 | 5 | 8 | 13 |
| 35–49 | 129 | 3.5 | 14 | 1 | 1 | 2 | 4 | 8 | 10 | 17 |
| 50–64 | 96 | 2.2 | 6 | 1 | 1 | 2 | 2 | 5 | 6 | 13 |
| 65+ | 147 | 3.8 | 14 | 1 | 1 | 3 | 5 | 9 | 12 | 16 |
| **TOTAL SINGLE DX** | 71 | 1.2 | <1 | 1 | 1 | 1 | 1 | 2 | 3 | 6 |
| **TOTAL MULTIPLE DX** | 452 | 3.3 | 17 | 1 | 1 | 2 | 4 | 7 | 10 | 17 |
| **TOTAL** | | | | | | | | | | |
| 0–19 Years | 18 | 5.1 | 76 | 1 | 1 | 2 | 6 | 7 | 16 | 51 |
| 20–34 | 77 | 3.3 | 27 | 1 | 1 | 2 | 4 | 5 | 8 | 13 |
| 35–49 | 160 | 3.1 | 13 | 1 | 1 | 2 | 4 | 7 | 10 | 17 |
| 50–64 | 112 | 2.1 | 5 | 1 | 1 | 1 | 2 | 5 | 9 | 13 |
| 65+ | 156 | 3.6 | 13 | 1 | 1 | 2 | 5 | 8 | 11 | 16 |
| **GRAND TOTAL** | 523 | 3.1 | 15 | 1 | 2 | 2 | 4 | 7 | 10 | 16 |

**04.5: CRAN OR PERIPH NERV GRFT. Formerly included in operation group(s) 509.**

| Type of Patients | Observed Patients | Avg. Stay | Vari-ance | 10th | 25th | 50th | 75th | 90th | 95th | 99th |
|---|---|---|---|---|---|---|---|---|---|---|
| **1. SINGLE DX** | | | | | | | | | | |
| 0–19 Years | 29 | 1.9 | 2 | 1 | 1 | 2 | 2 | 3 | 3 | 7 |
| 20–34 | 10 | 2.0 | 2 | 1 | 1 | 1 | 4 | 4 | 4 | 4 |
| 35–49 | 8 | 2.2 | <1 | 2 | 2 | 2 | 3 | 3 | 3 | 3 |
| 50–64 | 0 | | | | | | | | | |
| 65+ | 0 | | | | | | | | | |
| **2. MULTIPLE DX** | | | | | | | | | | |
| 0–19 Years | 45 | 2.7 | 2 | 1 | 2 | 2 | 4 | 4 | 5 | 5 |
| 20–34 | 37 | 3.1 | 7 | 1 | 2 | 3 | 3 | 4 | 6 | 15 |
| 35–49 | 31 | 2.7 | 8 | 1 | 1 | 2 | 3 | 3 | 13 | 16 |
| 50–64 | 9 | 2.0 | <1 | 1 | 2 | 3 | 3 | 3 | 3 | 3 |
| 65+ | 4 | 3.2 | <1 | 2 | 2 | 3 | 4 | 4 | 4 | 4 |
| **TOTAL SINGLE DX** | 47 | 2.0 | 1 | 1 | 1 | 2 | 3 | 3 | 4 | 7 |
| **TOTAL MULTIPLE DX** | 126 | 2.8 | 4 | 1 | 2 | 2 | 3 | 4 | 5 | 13 |
| **TOTAL** | | | | | | | | | | |
| 0–19 Years | 74 | 2.4 | 2 | 1 | 1 | 2 | 3 | 4 | 5 | 7 |
| 20–34 | 47 | 2.8 | 6 | 1 | 1 | 3 | 3 | 4 | 6 | 15 |
| 35–49 | 39 | 2.6 | 7 | 1 | 1 | 2 | 3 | 3 | 13 | 16 |
| 50–64 | 9 | 2.0 | <1 | 1 | 2 | 3 | 3 | 3 | 3 | 3 |
| 65+ | 4 | 3.2 | <1 | 2 | 2 | 3 | 4 | 4 | 4 | 4 |
| **GRAND TOTAL** | 173 | 2.5 | 4 | 1 | 1 | 2 | 3 | 4 | 5 | 13 |

Length of Stay by Diagnosis and Operation, United States, 2000

# United States, October 1998–September 1999 Data, by Operation

## 04.6: PERIPH NERVES TRANSPOS. Formerly included in operation group(s) 509.

| Type of Patients | Observed Patients | Avg. Stay | Variance | 10th | 25th | 50th | 75th | 90th | 95th | 99th |
|---|---|---|---|---|---|---|---|---|---|---|
| **1. SINGLE DX** | | | | | | | | | | |
| 0–19 Years | 11 | 1.9 | 1 | 1 | 1 | 1 | 2 | 4 | 4 | 4 |
| 20–34 | 7 | 1.6 | <1 | 1 | 1 | 1 | 2 | 3 | 3 | 3 |
| 35–49 | 8 | 1.0 | <1 | 1 | 1 | 1 | 1 | 1 | 1 | 2 |
| 50–64 | 11 | 1.0 | <1 | 1 | 1 | 1 | 1 | 1 | 1 | 2 |
| 65+ | 6 | 1.2 | <1 | 1 | 1 | 1 | 1 | 2 | 2 | 2 |
| **2. MULTIPLE DX** | | | | | | | | | | |
| 0–19 Years | 16 | 4.7 | 45 | 1 | 1 | 1 | 3 | 18 | 18 | 23 |
| 20–34 | 16 | 2.2 | 5 | 1 | 1 | 2 | 3 | 3 | 4 | 6 |
| 35–49 | 54 | 3.6 | 8 | 1 | 1 | 2 | 7 | 7 | 8 | 9 |
| 50–64 | 36 | 1.5 | <1 | 1 | 1 | 1 | 2 | 3 | 3 | 3 |
| 65+ | 28 | 2.7 | 15 | 1 | 1 | 1 | 2 | 7 | 12 | 18 |
| **TOTAL SINGLE DX** | 43 | 1.2 | <1 | 1 | 1 | 1 | 1 | 2 | 2 | 4 |
| **TOTAL MULTIPLE DX** | 150 | 2.7 | 10 | 1 | 1 | 1 | 3 | 7 | 7 | 18 |
| **TOTAL** | | | | | | | | | | |
| 0–19 Years | 27 | 4.1 | 36 | 1 | 1 | 1 | 3 | 18 | 18 | 23 |
| 20–34 | 23 | 2.1 | 1 | 1 | 1 | 2 | 3 | 3 | 4 | 6 |
| 35–49 | 62 | 3.0 | 7 | 1 | 1 | 2 | 5 | 7 | 8 | 9 |
| 50–64 | 47 | 1.4 | <1 | 1 | 1 | 1 | 1 | 2 | 3 | 3 |
| 65+ | 34 | 2.6 | 14 | 1 | 1 | 1 | 2 | 7 | 9 | 18 |
| **GRAND TOTAL** | 193 | 2.4 | 8 | 1 | 1 | 1 | 3 | 7 | 7 | 18 |

## 04.8: PERIPHERAL NERVE INJECT. Formerly included in operation group(s) 512.

| Type of Patients | Observed Patients | Avg. Stay | Variance | 10th | 25th | 50th | 75th | 90th | 95th | 99th |
|---|---|---|---|---|---|---|---|---|---|---|
| **1. SINGLE DX** | | | | | | | | | | |
| 0–19 Years | 2 | 1.9 | <1 | 1 | 2 | 2 | 2 | 2 | 2 | 2 |
| 20–34 | 13 | 3.1 | 2 | 1 | 2 | 3 | 4 | 5 | 5 | 5 |
| 35–49 | 31 | 3.6 | 4 | 1 | 2 | 4 | 5 | 6 | 8 | 8 |
| 50–64 | 12 | 2.9 | 6 | 2 | 2 | 2 | 3 | 5 | 8 | 14 |
| 65+ | 19 | 2.2 | <1 | 1 | 2 | 2 | 3 | 3 | 4 | 4 |
| **2. MULTIPLE DX** | | | | | | | | | | |
| 0–19 Years | 13 | 11.8 | 329 | 1 | 3 | 4 | 8 | 28 | 64 | 64 |
| 20–34 | 125 | 4.7 | 15 | 1 | 2 | 4 | 6 | 8 | 12 | 24 |
| 35–49 | 328 | 5.4 | 34 | 2 | 3 | 4 | 6 | 9 | 13 | 35 |
| 50–64 | 270 | 5.4 | 18 | 2 | 3 | 4 | 7 | 10 | 15 | 20 |
| 65+ | 558 | 7.0 | 47 | 2 | 3 | 6 | 7 | 13 | 17 | 49 |
| **TOTAL SINGLE DX** | 77 | 3.2 | 4 | 1 | 2 | 3 | 5 | 6 | 6 | 8 |
| **TOTAL MULTIPLE DX** | 1,294 | 6.1 | 38 | 2 | 3 | 4 | 7 | 11 | 15 | 35 |
| **TOTAL** | | | | | | | | | | |
| 0–19 Years | 15 | 10.8 | 305 | 1 | 3 | 4 | 8 | 28 | 64 | 64 |
| 20–34 | 138 | 4.6 | 14 | 1 | 2 | 4 | 6 | 9 | 12 | 24 |
| 35–49 | 359 | 5.2 | 31 | 2 | 3 | 4 | 6 | 9 | 13 | 31 |
| 50–64 | 282 | 5.3 | 18 | 2 | 3 | 4 | 7 | 10 | 15 | 20 |
| 65+ | 577 | 6.9 | 47 | 2 | 3 | 6 | 7 | 13 | 17 | 49 |
| **GRAND TOTAL** | 1,371 | 5.9 | 36 | 2 | 3 | 4 | 7 | 11 | 15 | 32 |

## 04.7: OTHER PERIPH NEUROPLASTY. Formerly included in operation group(s) 509.

| Type of Patients | Observed Patients | Avg. Stay | Variance | 10th | 25th | 50th | 75th | 90th | 95th | 99th |
|---|---|---|---|---|---|---|---|---|---|---|
| **1. SINGLE DX** | | | | | | | | | | |
| 0–19 Years | 20 | 3.2 | 4 | 2 | 2 | 2 | 3 | 7 | 7 | 7 |
| 20–34 | 15 | 1.7 | <1 | 1 | 1 | 1 | 2 | 3 | 4 | 4 |
| 35–49 | 4 | 1.0 | 0 | 1 | 1 | 1 | 1 | 1 | 1 | 1 |
| 50–64 | 9 | 1.2 | <1 | 1 | 1 | 1 | 1 | 2 | 2 | 2 |
| 65+ | 1 | 10.0 | 0 | 10 | 10 | 10 | 10 | 10 | 10 | 10 |
| **2. MULTIPLE DX** | | | | | | | | | | |
| 0–19 Years | 42 | 2.3 | 3 | 1 | 1 | 2 | 3 | 3 | 4 | 11 |
| 20–34 | 68 | 2.3 | 5 | 1 | 1 | 2 | 3 | 4 | 5 | 12 |
| 35–49 | 46 | 2.0 | 4 | 2 | 1 | 2 | 2 | 3 | 5 | 14 |
| 50–64 | 20 | 2.2 | 1 | 1 | 1 | 2 | 2 | 3 | 3 | 7 |
| 65+ | 14 | 3.7 | 15 | 1 | 1 | 2 | 4 | 9 | 9 | 16 |
| **TOTAL SINGLE DX** | 49 | 2.3 | 3 | 1 | 1 | 2 | 3 | 4 | 7 | 10 |
| **TOTAL MULTIPLE DX** | 190 | 2.2 | 4 | 1 | 1 | 2 | 3 | 3 | 5 | 12 |
| **TOTAL** | | | | | | | | | | |
| 0–19 Years | 62 | 2.5 | 4 | 1 | 1 | 2 | 3 | 4 | 7 | 11 |
| 20–34 | 83 | 2.3 | 4 | 1 | 1 | 2 | 3 | 4 | 5 | 12 |
| 35–49 | 50 | 1.9 | 4 | 1 | 1 | 1 | 2 | 3 | 5 | 14 |
| 50–64 | 29 | 2.1 | 1 | 1 | 2 | 2 | 2 | 3 | 3 | 7 |
| 65+ | 15 | 4.0 | 16 | 1 | 1 | 2 | 9 | 9 | 10 | 16 |
| **GRAND TOTAL** | 239 | 2.2 | 4 | 1 | 1 | 2 | 3 | 3 | 5 | 11 |

## 04.81: ANES INJECT PERIPH NERVE. Formerly included in operation group(s) 512.

| Type of Patients | Observed Patients | Avg. Stay | Variance | 10th | 25th | 50th | 75th | 90th | 95th | 99th |
|---|---|---|---|---|---|---|---|---|---|---|
| **1. SINGLE DX** | | | | | | | | | | |
| 0–19 Years | 2 | 1.9 | <1 | 1 | 2 | 2 | 2 | 2 | 2 | 2 |
| 20–34 | 13 | 3.1 | 2 | 1 | 2 | 3 | 4 | 5 | 5 | 5 |
| 35–49 | 30 | 3.6 | 5 | 1 | 2 | 4 | 5 | 6 | 8 | 8 |
| 50–64 | 12 | 2.9 | 6 | 2 | 2 | 2 | 3 | 5 | 8 | 14 |
| 65+ | 16 | 2.3 | <1 | 1 | 2 | 2 | 3 | 3 | 4 | 4 |
| **2. MULTIPLE DX** | | | | | | | | | | |
| 0–19 Years | 13 | 11.8 | 329 | 1 | 3 | 4 | 8 | 28 | 64 | 64 |
| 20–34 | 125 | 4.7 | 15 | 1 | 2 | 4 | 6 | 9 | 12 | 24 |
| 35–49 | 318 | 5.3 | 34 | 2 | 3 | 4 | 6 | 9 | 13 | 35 |
| 50–64 | 256 | 5.3 | 17 | 2 | 3 | 4 | 7 | 10 | 13 | 20 |
| 65+ | 529 | 7.1 | 49 | 2 | 3 | 6 | 7 | 13 | 17 | 49 |
| **TOTAL SINGLE DX** | 73 | 3.2 | 4 | 1 | 2 | 3 | 5 | 6 | 6 | 8 |
| **TOTAL MULTIPLE DX** | 1,241 | 6.1 | 38 | 2 | 3 | 4 | 7 | 11 | 15 | 35 |
| **TOTAL** | | | | | | | | | | |
| 0–19 Years | 15 | 10.8 | 305 | 1 | 3 | 4 | 8 | 28 | 64 | 64 |
| 20–34 | 138 | 4.6 | 14 | 1 | 2 | 4 | 6 | 9 | 12 | 24 |
| 35–49 | 348 | 5.2 | 32 | 2 | 3 | 4 | 6 | 9 | 13 | 31 |
| 50–64 | 268 | 5.2 | 16 | 2 | 3 | 4 | 7 | 10 | 13 | 20 |
| 65+ | 545 | 7.0 | 48 | 2 | 3 | 6 | 7 | 13 | 17 | 49 |
| **GRAND TOTAL** | 1,314 | 5.9 | 37 | 2 | 3 | 4 | 7 | 10 | 15 | 32 |

Length of Stay by Diagnosis and Operation, United States, 2000

# United States, October 1998–September 1999 Data, by Operation

## 04.9: OTH PERIPH NERVE OPS. Formerly included in operation group(s) 509.

| Type of Patients | Observed Patients | Avg. Stay | Variance | 10th | 25th | 50th | 75th | 90th | 95th | 99th |
|---|---|---|---|---|---|---|---|---|---|---|
| **1. SINGLE DX** | | | | | | | | | | |
| 0–19 Years | 87 | 1.2 | 1 | 1 | 1 | 1 | 1 | 1 | 1 | 5 |
| 20–34 | 32 | 1.1 | <1 | 1 | 1 | 1 | 1 | 1 | 2 | 3 |
| 35–49 | 37 | 1.3 | <1 | 1 | 1 | 1 | 1 | 2 | 4 | 4 |
| 50–64 | 9 | 1.1 | <1 | 1 | 1 | 1 | 1 | 1 | 2 | 2 |
| 65+ | 0 | | | | | | | | | |
| **2. MULTIPLE DX** | | | | | | | | | | |
| 0–19 Years | 97 | 2.2 | 27 | 1 | 1 | 1 | 1 | 4 | 7 | 27 |
| 20–34 | 54 | 2.1 | 5 | 1 | 1 | 1 | 2 | 5 | 7 | 12 |
| 35–49 | 59 | 2.1 | 11 | 1 | 1 | 2 | 2 | 3 | 4 | 14 |
| 50–64 | 23 | 1.4 | <1 | 1 | 1 | 1 | 2 | 3 | 3 | 4 |
| 65+ | 17 | 4.1 | 27 | 1 | 1 | 2 | 4 | 11 | 13 | 24 |
| **TOTAL SINGLE DX** | 165 | 1.2 | <1 | 1 | 1 | 1 | 1 | 1 | 2 | 4 |
| **TOTAL MULTIPLE DX** | 250 | 2.2 | 18 | 1 | 1 | 1 | 2 | 4 | 7 | 27 |
| **TOTAL** | | | | | | | | | | |
| 0–19 Years | 184 | 1.7 | 15 | 1 | 1 | 1 | 1 | 3 | 4 | 26 |
| 20–34 | 86 | 1.4 | 2 | 1 | 1 | 1 | 1 | 2 | 4 | 9 |
| 35–49 | 96 | 1.7 | 5 | 1 | 1 | 1 | 2 | 3 | 4 | 13 |
| 50–64 | 32 | 1.2 | <1 | 1 | 1 | 1 | 2 | 2 | 2 | 4 |
| 65+ | 17 | 4.1 | 27 | 1 | 1 | 2 | 4 | 11 | 13 | 24 |
| **GRAND TOTAL** | 415 | 1.7 | 9 | 1 | 1 | 1 | 1 | 3 | 4 | 13 |

## 04.92: IMPL PERIPH NEUROSTIM. Formerly included in operation group(s) 509.

| Type of Patients | Observed Patients | Avg. Stay | Variance | 10th | 25th | 50th | 75th | 90th | 95th | 99th |
|---|---|---|---|---|---|---|---|---|---|---|
| **1. SINGLE DX** | | | | | | | | | | |
| 0–19 Years | 87 | 1.2 | 1 | 1 | 1 | 1 | 1 | 1 | 1 | 5 |
| 20–34 | 32 | 1.1 | <1 | 1 | 1 | 1 | 1 | 1 | 2 | 3 |
| 35–49 | 36 | 1.3 | <1 | 1 | 1 | 1 | 1 | 2 | 4 | 4 |
| 50–64 | 9 | 1.1 | <1 | 1 | 1 | 1 | 1 | 1 | 2 | 2 |
| 65+ | 0 | | | | | | | | | |
| **2. MULTIPLE DX** | | | | | | | | | | |
| 0–19 Years | 87 | 2.0 | 28 | 1 | 1 | 1 | 1 | 3 | 4 | 71 |
| 20–34 | 47 | 1.8 | 4 | 1 | 1 | 1 | 2 | 4 | 7 | 12 |
| 35–49 | 56 | 2.0 | 10 | 1 | 1 | 2 | 2 | 3 | 3 | 14 |
| 50–64 | 20 | 1.4 | <1 | 1 | 1 | 1 | 1 | 2 | 2 | 4 |
| 65+ | 11 | 3.2 | 35 | 1 | 1 | 2 | 2 | 7 | 24 | 24 |
| **TOTAL SINGLE DX** | 164 | 1.2 | <1 | 1 | 1 | 1 | 1 | 1 | 2 | 4 |
| **TOTAL MULTIPLE DX** | 221 | 2.0 | 18 | 1 | 1 | 1 | 2 | 3 | 4 | 27 |
| **TOTAL** | | | | | | | | | | |
| 0–19 Years | 174 | 1.6 | 14 | 1 | 1 | 1 | 1 | 2 | 3 | 26 |
| 20–34 | 79 | 1.3 | 1 | 1 | 1 | 1 | 1 | 2 | 3 | 7 |
| 35–49 | 92 | 1.6 | 4 | 1 | 1 | 1 | 2 | 2 | 3 | 7 |
| 50–64 | 29 | 1.2 | <1 | 1 | 1 | 1 | 1 | 2 | 2 | 4 |
| 65+ | 11 | 3.2 | 35 | 1 | 1 | 2 | 2 | 7 | 24 | 24 |
| **GRAND TOTAL** | 385 | 1.5 | 9 | 1 | 1 | 1 | 1 | 2 | 4 | 9 |

## 05.0: SYMPATH NERVE DIVISION. Formerly included in operation group(s) 511.

| Type of Patients | Observed Patients | Avg. Stay | Variance | 10th | 25th | 50th | 75th | 90th | 95th | 99th |
|---|---|---|---|---|---|---|---|---|---|---|
| **1. SINGLE DX** | | | | | | | | | | |
| 0–19 Years | 0 | | | | | | | | | |
| 20–34 | 0 | | | | | | | | | |
| 35–49 | 0 | | | | | | | | | |
| 50–64 | 0 | | | | | | | | | |
| 65+ | 0 | | | | | | | | | |
| **2. MULTIPLE DX** | | | | | | | | | | |
| 0–19 Years | 0 | | | | | | | | | |
| 20–34 | 1 | 3.0 | 0 | 3 | 3 | 3 | 3 | 3 | 3 | 3 |
| 35–49 | 1 | 2.0 | 0 | 2 | 2 | 2 | 2 | 2 | 2 | 2 |
| 50–64 | 3 | 2.4 | <1 | 2 | 2 | 2 | 3 | 3 | 3 | 3 |
| 65+ | 0 | | | | | | | | | |
| **TOTAL SINGLE DX** | 0 | | | | | | | | | |
| **TOTAL MULTIPLE DX** | 5 | 2.4 | <1 | 2 | 2 | 2 | 3 | 3 | 3 | 3 |
| **TOTAL** | | | | | | | | | | |
| 0–19 Years | 0 | | | | | | | | | |
| 20–34 | 1 | 3.0 | 0 | 3 | 3 | 3 | 3 | 3 | 3 | 3 |
| 35–49 | 1 | 2.0 | 0 | 2 | 2 | 2 | 2 | 2 | 2 | 2 |
| 50–64 | 3 | 2.4 | <1 | 2 | 2 | 2 | 3 | 3 | 3 | 3 |
| 65+ | 0 | | | | | | | | | |
| **GRAND TOTAL** | 5 | 2.4 | <1 | 2 | 2 | 2 | 3 | 3 | 3 | 3 |

## 05.1: SYMPATH NERVE DXTIC PX. Formerly included in operation group(s) 511, 512.

| Type of Patients | Observed Patients | Avg. Stay | Variance | 10th | 25th | 50th | 75th | 90th | 95th | 99th |
|---|---|---|---|---|---|---|---|---|---|---|
| **1. SINGLE DX** | | | | | | | | | | |
| 0–19 Years | 1 | 3.0 | 0 | 3 | 3 | 3 | 3 | 3 | 3 | 3 |
| 20–34 | 0 | | | | | | | | | |
| 35–49 | 0 | | | | | | | | | |
| 50–64 | 0 | | | | | | | | | |
| 65+ | 0 | | | | | | | | | |
| **2. MULTIPLE DX** | | | | | | | | | | |
| 0–19 Years | 0 | | | | | | | | | |
| 20–34 | 2 | 8.8 | <1 | 8 | 9 | 9 | 9 | 9 | 9 | 9 |
| 35–49 | 0 | | | | | | | | | |
| 50–64 | 0 | | | | | | | | | |
| 65+ | 0 | | | | | | | | | |
| **TOTAL SINGLE DX** | 1 | 3.0 | 0 | 3 | 3 | 3 | 3 | 3 | 3 | 3 |
| **TOTAL MULTIPLE DX** | 2 | 8.8 | <1 | 8 | 9 | 9 | 9 | 9 | 9 | 9 |
| **TOTAL** | | | | | | | | | | |
| 0–19 Years | 1 | 3.0 | 0 | 3 | 3 | 3 | 3 | 3 | 3 | 3 |
| 20–34 | 2 | 8.8 | <1 | 8 | 9 | 9 | 9 | 9 | 9 | 9 |
| 35–49 | 0 | | | | | | | | | |
| 50–64 | 0 | | | | | | | | | |
| 65+ | 0 | | | | | | | | | |
| **GRAND TOTAL** | 3 | 5.0 | 8 | 3 | 9 | 9 | 9 | 9 | 9 | 9 |

Length of Stay by Diagnosis and Operation, United States, 2000

**United States, October 1998–September 1999 Data, by Operation**

### 05.2: SYMPATHECTOMY. Formerly included in operation group(s) 510.

| Type of Patients | Observed Patients | Avg. Stay | Variance | Percentiles | | | | | | |
|---|---|---|---|---|---|---|---|---|---|---|
| | | | | 10th | 25th | 50th | 75th | 90th | 95th | 99th |
| **1. SINGLE DX** | | | | | | | | | | |
| 0–19 Years | 15 | 1.8 | 1 | 1 | 1 | 1 | 2 | 3 | 5 | 5 |
| 20–34 | 49 | 1.9 | 2 | 1 | 1 | 1 | 2 | 5 | 6 | 7 |
| 35–49 | 33 | 2.5 | 4 | 1 | 1 | 2 | 3 | 5 | 7 | 10 |
| 50–64 | 10 | 1.5 | <1 | 1 | 1 | 1 | 2 | 2 | 3 | 3 |
| 65+ | 8 | 2.7 | 2 | 1 | 2 | 2 | 4 | 4 | 6 | 6 |
| **2. MULTIPLE DX** | | | | | | | | | | |
| 0–19 Years | 15 | 2.7 | <1 | 1 | 3 | 3 | 3 | 3 | 3 | 5 |
| 20–34 | 61 | 3.3 | 12 | 1 | 1 | 2 | 3 | 6 | 12 | 19 |
| 35–49 | 136 | 3.9 | 33 | 1 | 1 | 2 | 4 | 7 | 11 | 22 |
| 50–64 | 74 | 6.1 | 22 | 1 | 2 | 5 | 9 | 12 | 14 | 23 |
| 65+ | 110 | 6.2 | 20 | 2 | 3 | 5 | 8 | 12 | 13 | 21 |
| **TOTAL SINGLE DX** | 115 | 2.2 | 3 | 1 | 1 | 2 | 3 | 4 | 6 | 7 |
| **TOTAL MULTIPLE DX** | 396 | 4.8 | 24 | 1 | 2 | 3 | 6 | 10 | 13 | 22 |
| **TOTAL** | | | | | | | | | | |
| 0–19 Years | 30 | 2.3 | 1 | 1 | 1 | 2 | 3 | 3 | 5 | 5 |
| 20–34 | 110 | 2.7 | 8 | 1 | 1 | 2 | 3 | 6 | 7 | 14 |
| 35–49 | 169 | 3.5 | 23 | 1 | 1 | 2 | 4 | 7 | 9 | 21 |
| 50–64 | 84 | 5.4 | 22 | 1 | 2 | 4 | 9 | 10 | 14 | 23 |
| 65+ | 118 | 5.9 | 19 | 2 | 3 | 5 | 8 | 12 | 13 | 21 |
| **GRAND TOTAL** | 511 | 4.0 | 19 | 1 | 1 | 3 | 5 | 9 | 12 | 21 |

### 05.3: SYMPATH NERVE INJECTION. Formerly included in operation group(s) 511.

| Type of Patients | Observed Patients | Avg. Stay | Variance | Percentiles | | | | | | |
|---|---|---|---|---|---|---|---|---|---|---|
| | | | | 10th | 25th | 50th | 75th | 90th | 95th | 99th |
| **1. SINGLE DX** | | | | | | | | | | |
| 0–19 Years | 1 | 9.0 | 0 | 9 | 9 | 9 | 9 | 9 | 9 | 9 |
| 20–34 | 16 | 3.4 | 13 | 1 | 1 | 3 | 4 | 9 | 9 | 14 |
| 35–49 | 28 | 3.6 | 16 | 1 | 1 | 3 | 4 | 7 | 8 | 24 |
| 50–64 | 14 | 2.6 | 2 | 1 | 2 | 2 | 3 | 4 | 4 | 6 |
| 65+ | 7 | 3.4 | 15 | 1 | 1 | 2 | 4 | 12 | 12 | 12 |
| **2. MULTIPLE DX** | | | | | | | | | | |
| 0–19 Years | 14 | 11.1 | 206 | 2 | 2 | 3 | 18 | 30 | 50 | 50 |
| 20–34 | 68 | 6.3 | 27 | 1 | 2 | 5 | 8 | 14 | 18 | 21 |
| 35–49 | 207 | 7.3 | 53 | 2 | 4 | 5 | 8 | 14 | 18 | 47 |
| 50–64 | 159 | 9.5 | 64 | 2 | 5 | 9 | 11 | 15 | 25 | 29 |
| 65+ | 218 | 8.0 | 46 | 2 | 4 | 7 | 10 | 14 | 18 | 40 |
| **TOTAL SINGLE DX** | 66 | 3.4 | 13 | 1 | 1 | 3 | 4 | 8 | 9 | 24 |
| **TOTAL MULTIPLE DX** | 666 | 8.1 | 56 | 2 | 4 | 6 | 10 | 14 | 22 | 47 |
| **TOTAL** | | | | | | | | | | |
| 0–19 Years | 15 | 11.0 | 201 | 2 | 2 | 3 | 18 | 30 | 50 | 50 |
| 20–34 | 84 | 5.6 | 25 | 1 | 1 | 4 | 8 | 14 | 18 | 21 |
| 35–49 | 235 | 6.8 | 49 | 2 | 3 | 5 | 8 | 14 | 18 | 47 |
| 50–64 | 173 | 9.2 | 63 | 2 | 4 | 8 | 11 | 15 | 25 | 29 |
| 65+ | 225 | 7.9 | 46 | 2 | 4 | 6 | 10 | 14 | 18 | 40 |
| **GRAND TOTAL** | 732 | 7.7 | 54 | 2 | 3 | 6 | 10 | 14 | 20 | 47 |

### 05.31: ANES INJECT SYMPATH NERV. Formerly included in operation group(s) 511.

| Type of Patients | Observed Patients | Avg. Stay | Variance | Percentiles | | | | | | |
|---|---|---|---|---|---|---|---|---|---|---|
| | | | | 10th | 25th | 50th | 75th | 90th | 95th | 99th |
| **1. SINGLE DX** | | | | | | | | | | |
| 0–19 Years | 1 | 9.0 | 0 | 9 | 9 | 9 | 9 | 9 | 9 | 9 |
| 20–34 | 15 | 3.3 | 13 | 1 | 1 | 3 | 4 | 9 | 9 | 14 |
| 35–49 | 28 | 3.6 | 16 | 1 | 1 | 3 | 4 | 7 | 8 | 24 |
| 50–64 | 13 | 2.6 | 2 | 1 | 1 | 3 | 3 | 4 | 4 | 6 |
| 65+ | 6 | 3.7 | 16 | 1 | 1 | 2 | 4 | 12 | 12 | 12 |
| **2. MULTIPLE DX** | | | | | | | | | | |
| 0–19 Years | 11 | 8.2 | 203 | 2 | 2 | 3 | 4 | 18 | 50 | 50 |
| 20–34 | 55 | 6.9 | 28 | 1 | 3 | 6 | 10 | 14 | 18 | 22 |
| 35–49 | 203 | 7.3 | 53 | 2 | 4 | 5 | 8 | 14 | 18 | 47 |
| 50–64 | 151 | 9.8 | 65 | 3 | 5 | 10 | 11 | 16 | 25 | 29 |
| 65+ | 205 | 8.2 | 47 | 2 | 4 | 7 | 10 | 14 | 18 | 48 |
| **TOTAL SINGLE DX** | 63 | 3.4 | 13 | 1 | 1 | 3 | 3 | 8 | 9 | 24 |
| **TOTAL MULTIPLE DX** | 625 | 8.3 | 56 | 2 | 4 | 7 | 10 | 14 | 20 | 47 |
| **TOTAL** | | | | | | | | | | |
| 0–19 Years | 12 | 8.2 | 194 | 2 | 2 | 3 | 8 | 18 | 50 | 50 |
| 20–34 | 70 | 5.9 | 26 | 1 | 1 | 4 | 8 | 14 | 18 | 21 |
| 35–49 | 231 | 6.8 | 49 | 2 | 3 | 5 | 8 | 14 | 18 | 47 |
| 50–64 | 164 | 9.4 | 65 | 2 | 4 | 9 | 11 | 15 | 25 | 29 |
| 65+ | 211 | 8.1 | 47 | 2 | 4 | 7 | 10 | 14 | 18 | 48 |
| **GRAND TOTAL** | 688 | 7.8 | 54 | 2 | 4 | 6 | 10 | 14 | 19 | 47 |

### 05.8: OTH SYMPATH NERVE OPS. Formerly included in operation group(s) 511.

| Type of Patients | Observed Patients | Avg. Stay | Variance | Percentiles | | | | | | |
|---|---|---|---|---|---|---|---|---|---|---|
| | | | | 10th | 25th | 50th | 75th | 90th | 95th | 99th |
| **1. SINGLE DX** | | | | | | | | | | |
| 0–19 Years | 0 | | | | | | | | | |
| 20–34 | 0 | | | | | | | | | |
| 35–49 | 0 | | | | | | | | | |
| 50–64 | 0 | | | | | | | | | |
| 65+ | 0 | | | | | | | | | |
| **2. MULTIPLE DX** | | | | | | | | | | |
| 0–19 Years | 0 | | | | | | | | | |
| 20–34 | 0 | | | | | | | | | |
| 35–49 | 3 | 5.2 | 17 | 1 | 3 | 3 | 3 | 10 | 10 | 10 |
| 50–64 | 1 | 28.0 | 0 | 28 | 28 | 28 | 28 | 28 | 28 | 28 |
| 65+ | 1 | 13.0 | 0 | 13 | 13 | 13 | 13 | 13 | 13 | 13 |
| **TOTAL SINGLE DX** | 0 | | | | | | | | | |
| **TOTAL MULTIPLE DX** | 5 | 20.7 | 108 | 3 | 13 | 28 | 28 | 28 | 28 | 28 |
| **TOTAL** | | | | | | | | | | |
| 0–19 Years | 0 | | | | | | | | | |
| 20–34 | 0 | | | | | | | | | |
| 35–49 | 3 | 5.2 | 17 | 1 | 3 | 3 | 3 | 10 | 10 | 10 |
| 50–64 | 1 | 28.0 | 0 | 28 | 28 | 28 | 28 | 28 | 28 | 28 |
| 65+ | 1 | 13.0 | 0 | 13 | 13 | 13 | 13 | 13 | 13 | 13 |
| **GRAND TOTAL** | 5 | 20.7 | 108 | 3 | 13 | 28 | 28 | 28 | 28 | 28 |

Length of Stay by Diagnosis and Operation, United States, 2000

## United States, October 1998–September 1999 Data, by Operation

### 05.9: OTHER NERVOUS SYSTEM OPS. Formerly included in operation group(s) 511.

| Type of Patients | Observed Patients | Avg. Stay | Vari-ance | Percentiles 10th | 25th | 50th | 75th | 90th | 95th | 99th |
|---|---|---|---|---|---|---|---|---|---|---|
| **1. SINGLE DX** | | | | | | | | | | |
| 0–19 Years | 0 | | | | | | | | | |
| 20–34 | 0 | | | | | | | | | |
| 35–49 | 0 | | | | | | | | | |
| 50–64 | 1 | 2.0 | 0 | 2 | 2 | 2 | 2 | 2 | 2 | 2 |
| 65+ | 0 | | | | | | | | | |
| **2. MULTIPLE DX** | | | | | | | | | | |
| 0–19 Years | 0 | | | | | | | | | |
| 20–34 | 0 | | | | | | | | | |
| 35–49 | 0 | | | | | | | | | |
| 50–64 | 0 | | | | | | | | | |
| 65+ | 0 | | | | | | | | | |
| **TOTAL SINGLE DX** | 1 | 2.0 | 0 | 2 | 2 | 2 | 2 | 2 | 2 | 2 |
| **TOTAL MULTIPLE DX** | 0 | | | | | | | | | |
| **TOTAL** | | | | | | | | | | |
| 0–19 Years | 0 | | | | | | | | | |
| 20–34 | 0 | | | | | | | | | |
| 35–49 | 0 | | | | | | | | | |
| 50–64 | 1 | 2.0 | 0 | 2 | 2 | 2 | 2 | 2 | 2 | 2 |
| 65+ | 0 | | | | | | | | | |
| **GRAND TOTAL** | 1 | 2.0 | 0 | 2 | 2 | 2 | 2 | 2 | 2 | 2 |

### 06.09: INC THYROID FIELD NEC. Formerly included in operation group(s) 514.

| Type of Patients | Observed Patients | Avg. Stay | Vari-ance | Percentiles 10th | 25th | 50th | 75th | 90th | 95th | 99th |
|---|---|---|---|---|---|---|---|---|---|---|
| **1. SINGLE DX** | | | | | | | | | | |
| 0–19 Years | 18 | 3.7 | 11 | 1 | 1 | 2 | 6 | 9 | 9 | 9 |
| 20–34 | 27 | 2.0 | 4 | 1 | 1 | 2 | 2 | 4 | 9 | 9 |
| 35–49 | 7 | 2.7 | 1 | 2 | 3 | 3 | 3 | 3 | 5 | 5 |
| 50–64 | 6 | 1.4 | <1 | 1 | 1 | 1 | 1 | 3 | 3 | 3 |
| 65+ | 2 | 1.0 | 0 | 1 | 1 | 1 | 1 | 1 | 1 | 1 |
| **2. MULTIPLE DX** | | | | | | | | | | |
| 0–19 Years | 38 | 4.3 | 9 | 1 | 2 | 3 | 7 | 9 | 9 | 10 |
| 20–34 | 77 | 4.9 | 28 | 1 | 2 | 4 | 8 | 8 | 10 | 48 |
| 35–49 | 62 | 4.2 | 28 | 1 | 3 | 3 | 5 | 8 | 9 | 24 |
| 50–64 | 45 | 5.5 | 25 | 2 | 4 | 4 | 8 | 12 | 18 | 23 |
| 65+ | 48 | 5.0 | 58 | 1 | 3 | 3 | 7 | 9 | 13 | 63 |
| **TOTAL SINGLE DX** | 60 | 2.7 | 7 | 1 | 1 | 1 | 3 | 8 | 9 | 9 |
| **TOTAL MULTIPLE DX** | 270 | 4.8 | 30 | 1 | 2 | 3 | 7 | 8 | 11 | 23 |
| **TOTAL** | | | | | | | | | | |
| 0–19 Years | 56 | 4.0 | 10 | 1 | 1 | 3 | 7 | 9 | 9 | 10 |
| 20–34 | 104 | 4.2 | 24 | 1 | 3 | 3 | 6 | 8 | 9 | 15 |
| 35–49 | 69 | 3.9 | 24 | 1 | 4 | 4 | 5 | 8 | 9 | 24 |
| 50–64 | 51 | 5.1 | 24 | 2 | 4 | 4 | 8 | 9 | 18 | 23 |
| 65+ | 50 | 4.7 | 55 | 1 | 3 | 3 | 7 | 9 | 11 | 63 |
| **GRAND TOTAL** | 330 | 4.3 | 25 | 1 | 3 | 3 | 6 | 8 | 9 | 23 |

### 06.0: THYROID FIELD INCISION. Formerly included in operation group(s) 514.

| Type of Patients | Observed Patients | Avg. Stay | Vari-ance | Percentiles 10th | 25th | 50th | 75th | 90th | 95th | 99th |
|---|---|---|---|---|---|---|---|---|---|---|
| **1. SINGLE DX** | | | | | | | | | | |
| 0–19 Years | 19 | 3.7 | 11 | 1 | 1 | 2 | 6 | 9 | 9 | 9 |
| 20–34 | 28 | 1.9 | 3 | 1 | 1 | 1 | 2 | 4 | 4 | 9 |
| 35–49 | 9 | 2.6 | 1 | 1 | 2 | 3 | 3 | 3 | 5 | 5 |
| 50–64 | 8 | 1.5 | <1 | 1 | 1 | 1 | 2 | 3 | 3 | 3 |
| 65+ | 4 | 1.8 | 2 | 1 | 1 | 1 | 4 | 4 | 4 | 4 |
| **2. MULTIPLE DX** | | | | | | | | | | |
| 0–19 Years | 42 | 4.2 | 9 | 1 | 2 | 3 | 7 | 9 | 9 | 10 |
| 20–34 | 81 | 4.9 | 28 | 1 | 2 | 3 | 8 | 8 | 10 | 15 |
| 35–49 | 77 | 3.8 | 17 | 1 | 2 | 3 | 4 | 8 | 8 | 18 |
| 50–64 | 73 | 4.8 | 19 | 1 | 2 | 3 | 6 | 8 | 15 | 23 |
| 65+ | 80 | 5.6 | 43 | 1 | 2 | 4 | 7 | 10 | 13 | 28 |
| **TOTAL SINGLE DX** | 68 | 2.6 | 6 | 1 | 1 | 1 | 3 | 6 | 9 | 9 |
| **TOTAL MULTIPLE DX** | 353 | 4.7 | 24 | 1 | 2 | 3 | 6 | 8 | 11 | 23 |
| **TOTAL** | | | | | | | | | | |
| 0–19 Years | 61 | 4.0 | 10 | 1 | 1 | 3 | 7 | 9 | 9 | 10 |
| 20–34 | 109 | 4.1 | 23 | 1 | 1 | 3 | 6 | 8 | 8 | 15 |
| 35–49 | 86 | 3.7 | 15 | 1 | 2 | 3 | 4 | 7 | 8 | 18 |
| 50–64 | 81 | 4.5 | 18 | 1 | 2 | 3 | 5 | 8 | 14 | 23 |
| 65+ | 84 | 5.4 | 41 | 1 | 2 | 4 | 7 | 10 | 12 | 28 |
| **GRAND TOTAL** | 421 | 4.3 | 22 | 1 | 2 | 3 | 5 | 8 | 10 | 23 |

### 06.1: THYROID/PARATHY DXTIC PX. Formerly included in operation group(s) 514, 516.

| Type of Patients | Observed Patients | Avg. Stay | Vari-ance | Percentiles 10th | 25th | 50th | 75th | 90th | 95th | 99th |
|---|---|---|---|---|---|---|---|---|---|---|
| **1. SINGLE DX** | | | | | | | | | | |
| 0–19 Years | 4 | 1.8 | <1 | 1 | 1 | 2 | 2 | 3 | 3 | 3 |
| 20–34 | 5 | 1.5 | <1 | 1 | 1 | 1 | 2 | 2 | 2 | 2 |
| 35–49 | 13 | 1.8 | 1 | 1 | 1 | 1 | 3 | 3 | 4 | 4 |
| 50–64 | 7 | 1.6 | <1 | 1 | 1 | 2 | 2 | 2 | 4 | 4 |
| 65+ | 4 | 1.5 | <1 | 1 | 1 | 1 | 2 | 2 | 2 | 2 |
| **2. MULTIPLE DX** | | | | | | | | | | |
| 0–19 Years | 1 | 2.0 | 0 | 2 | 2 | 2 | 2 | 2 | 2 | 2 |
| 20–34 | 18 | 6.3 | 25 | 1 | 2 | 6 | 6 | 14 | 20 | 20 |
| 35–49 | 50 | 4.2 | 14 | 1 | 2 | 2 | 6 | 10 | 14 | 14 |
| 50–64 | 79 | 3.9 | 12 | 1 | 1 | 2 | 5 | 10 | 13 | 13 |
| 65+ | 144 | 6.5 | 31 | 3 | 3 | 6 | 8 | 12 | 16 | 37 |
| **TOTAL SINGLE DX** | 33 | 1.7 | <1 | 1 | 1 | 1 | 2 | 3 | 4 | 4 |
| **TOTAL MULTIPLE DX** | 292 | 5.6 | 25 | 1 | 2 | 5 | 7 | 12 | 15 | 20 |
| **TOTAL** | | | | | | | | | | |
| 0–19 Years | 5 | 1.8 | <1 | 1 | 1 | 2 | 2 | 3 | 3 | 3 |
| 20–34 | 23 | 5.8 | 24 | 1 | 2 | 6 | 6 | 14 | 20 | 20 |
| 35–49 | 63 | 3.5 | 12 | 1 | 1 | 2 | 4 | 9 | 13 | 14 |
| 50–64 | 86 | 3.7 | 12 | 1 | 2 | 2 | 5 | 10 | 13 | 13 |
| 65+ | 148 | 6.5 | 31 | 3 | 3 | 6 | 8 | 12 | 16 | 37 |
| **GRAND TOTAL** | 325 | 5.2 | 24 | 1 | 2 | 4 | 7 | 11 | 14 | 20 |

Length of Stay by Diagnosis and Operation, United States, 2000

# United States, October 1998–September 1999 Data, by Operation

## 06.2: UNILAT THYROID LOBECTOMY. Formerly included in operation group(s) 513.

| Type of Patients | Observed Patients | Avg. Stay | Variance | Percentiles | | | | | | |
|---|---|---|---|---|---|---|---|---|---|---|
| | | | | 10th | 25th | 50th | 75th | 90th | 95th | 99th |
| **1. SINGLE DX** | | | | | | | | | | |
| 0–19 Years | 115 | 1.2 | <1 | 1 | 1 | 1 | 1 | 2 | 2 | 3 |
| 20–34 | 479 | 1.3 | <1 | 1 | 1 | 1 | 2 | 2 | 2 | 4 |
| 35–49 | 887 | 1.3 | <1 | 1 | 1 | 1 | 1 | 2 | 2 | 3 |
| 50–64 | 534 | 1.3 | <1 | 1 | 1 | 1 | 2 | 2 | 2 | 3 |
| 65+ | 231 | 1.4 | <1 | 1 | 1 | 1 | 2 | 2 | 3 | 4 |
| **2. MULTIPLE DX** | | | | | | | | | | |
| 0–19 Years | 39 | 1.8 | <1 | 1 | 1 | 2 | 2 | 2 | 2 | 3 |
| 20–34 | 315 | 1.5 | 2 | 1 | 1 | 1 | 2 | 2 | 3 | 5 |
| 35–49 | 1,028 | 1.5 | 1 | 1 | 1 | 1 | 2 | 3 | 3 | 6 |
| 50–64 | 980 | 1.6 | 2 | 1 | 1 | 1 | 2 | 2 | 3 | 7 |
| 65+ | 933 | 2.4 | 12 | 1 | 1 | 1 | 2 | 4 | 7 | 20 |
| **TOTAL SINGLE DX** | 2,246 | 1.3 | <1 | 1 | 1 | 1 | 1 | 2 | 2 | 4 |
| **TOTAL MULTIPLE DX** | 3,295 | 1.8 | 4 | 1 | 1 | 2 | 2 | 3 | 4 | 11 |
| **TOTAL** | | | | | | | | | | |
| 0–19 Years | 154 | 1.4 | <1 | 1 | 1 | 1 | 2 | 2 | 2 | 3 |
| 20–34 | 794 | 1.4 | 1 | 1 | 1 | 1 | 2 | 2 | 2 | 5 |
| 35–49 | 1,915 | 1.4 | <1 | 1 | 1 | 1 | 2 | 2 | 3 | 5 |
| 50–64 | 1,514 | 1.5 | 1 | 1 | 1 | 1 | 2 | 2 | 3 | 7 |
| 65+ | 1,164 | 2.1 | 9 | 1 | 1 | 1 | 2 | 4 | 6 | 15 |
| **GRAND TOTAL** | 5,541 | 1.6 | 3 | 1 | 1 | 1 | 2 | 2 | 3 | 7 |

## 06.39: PART THYROIDECTOMY NEC. Formerly included in operation group(s) 513.

| Type of Patients | Observed Patients | Avg. Stay | Variance | Percentiles | | | | | | |
|---|---|---|---|---|---|---|---|---|---|---|
| | | | | 10th | 25th | 50th | 75th | 90th | 95th | 99th |
| **1. SINGLE DX** | | | | | | | | | | |
| 0–19 Years | 63 | 1.9 | 4 | 1 | 1 | 1 | 2 | 4 | 4 | 15 |
| 20–34 | 272 | 1.4 | <1 | 1 | 1 | 1 | 2 | 2 | 3 | 5 |
| 35–49 | 441 | 1.4 | <1 | 1 | 1 | 1 | 2 | 2 | 3 | 5 |
| 50–64 | 247 | 1.5 | <1 | 1 | 1 | 1 | 2 | 2 | 3 | 4 |
| 65+ | 97 | 1.5 | <1 | 1 | 1 | 1 | 2 | 2 | 3 | 3 |
| **2. MULTIPLE DX** | | | | | | | | | | |
| 0–19 Years | 39 | 3.1 | 15 | 1 | 1 | 2 | 2 | 8 | 15 | 16 |
| 20–34 | 232 | 2.1 | 7 | 1 | 1 | 1 | 2 | 3 | 3 | 12 |
| 35–49 | 581 | 2.0 | 5 | 1 | 1 | 1 | 2 | 3 | 4 | 14 |
| 50–64 | 554 | 1.9 | 2 | 1 | 1 | 1 | 2 | 3 | 5 | 9 |
| 65+ | 450 | 3.5 | 29 | 1 | 1 | 2 | 3 | 8 | 15 | 21 |
| **TOTAL SINGLE DX** | 1,120 | 1.4 | <1 | 1 | 1 | 1 | 2 | 2 | 3 | 4 |
| **TOTAL MULTIPLE DX** | 1,856 | 2.3 | 10 | 1 | 1 | 2 | 2 | 4 | 6 | 19 |
| **TOTAL** | | | | | | | | | | |
| 0–19 Years | 102 | 2.4 | 8 | 1 | 1 | 1 | 2 | 4 | 8 | 16 |
| 20–34 | 504 | 1.7 | 4 | 1 | 1 | 1 | 2 | 3 | 3 | 14 |
| 35–49 | 1,022 | 1.8 | 3 | 1 | 1 | 1 | 2 | 3 | 4 | 14 |
| 50–64 | 801 | 1.8 | 2 | 1 | 1 | 1 | 2 | 3 | 4 | 7 |
| 65+ | 547 | 3.2 | 25 | 1 | 1 | 2 | 3 | 7 | 12 | 19 |
| **GRAND TOTAL** | 2,976 | 2.0 | 6 | 1 | 1 | 1 | 2 | 3 | 4 | 14 |

## 06.3: OTHER PART THYROIDECTOMY. Formerly included in operation group(s) 513.

| Type of Patients | Observed Patients | Avg. Stay | Variance | Percentiles | | | | | | |
|---|---|---|---|---|---|---|---|---|---|---|
| | | | | 10th | 25th | 50th | 75th | 90th | 95th | 99th |
| **1. SINGLE DX** | | | | | | | | | | |
| 0–19 Years | 76 | 1.8 | 3 | 1 | 1 | 1 | 2 | 3 | 4 | 15 |
| 20–34 | 289 | 1.4 | <1 | 1 | 1 | 1 | 2 | 2 | 3 | 3 |
| 35–49 | 474 | 1.4 | <1 | 1 | 1 | 1 | 2 | 2 | 3 | 5 |
| 50–64 | 267 | 1.5 | <1 | 1 | 1 | 1 | 2 | 2 | 3 | 4 |
| 65+ | 109 | 1.5 | <1 | 1 | 1 | 1 | 2 | 2 | 3 | 3 |
| **2. MULTIPLE DX** | | | | | | | | | | |
| 0–19 Years | 43 | 3.6 | 20 | 1 | 1 | 2 | 3 | 13 | 15 | 16 |
| 20–34 | 245 | 2.1 | 7 | 1 | 1 | 1 | 2 | 3 | 5 | 12 |
| 35–49 | 616 | 2.0 | 5 | 1 | 1 | 1 | 2 | 3 | 4 | 14 |
| 50–64 | 604 | 1.9 | 3 | 1 | 1 | 1 | 2 | 3 | 5 | 9 |
| 65+ | 498 | 3.5 | 30 | 1 | 1 | 2 | 3 | 8 | 15 | 33 |
| **TOTAL SINGLE DX** | 1,215 | 1.4 | <1 | 1 | 1 | 1 | 2 | 2 | 3 | 4 |
| **TOTAL MULTIPLE DX** | 2,006 | 2.3 | 10 | 1 | 1 | 2 | 2 | 4 | 6 | 19 |
| **TOTAL** | | | | | | | | | | |
| 0–19 Years | 119 | 2.5 | 10 | 1 | 1 | 1 | 2 | 4 | 13 | 15 |
| 20–34 | 534 | 1.7 | 3 | 1 | 1 | 1 | 2 | 3 | 4 | 8 |
| 35–49 | 1,090 | 1.7 | 3 | 1 | 1 | 1 | 2 | 3 | 4 | 14 |
| 50–64 | 871 | 1.8 | 2 | 1 | 1 | 1 | 2 | 3 | 5 | 8 |
| 65+ | 607 | 3.2 | 26 | 1 | 1 | 2 | 3 | 7 | 12 | 27 |
| **GRAND TOTAL** | 3,221 | 2.0 | 7 | 1 | 1 | 1 | 2 | 3 | 4 | 14 |

## 06.4: COMPLETE THYROIDECTOMY. Formerly included in operation group(s) 513.

| Type of Patients | Observed Patients | Avg. Stay | Variance | Percentiles | | | | | | |
|---|---|---|---|---|---|---|---|---|---|---|
| | | | | 10th | 25th | 50th | 75th | 90th | 95th | 99th |
| **1. SINGLE DX** | | | | | | | | | | |
| 0–19 Years | 47 | 1.5 | <1 | 1 | 1 | 1 | 2 | 2 | 3 | 4 |
| 20–34 | 285 | 1.6 | 1 | 1 | 1 | 1 | 2 | 3 | 3 | 5 |
| 35–49 | 450 | 1.7 | <1 | 1 | 2 | 2 | 3 | 3 | 3 | 5 |
| 50–64 | 216 | 1.5 | <1 | 1 | 1 | 1 | 2 | 2 | 3 | 4 |
| 65+ | 90 | 1.7 | <1 | 1 | 1 | 1 | 2 | 3 | 3 | 6 |
| **2. MULTIPLE DX** | | | | | | | | | | |
| 0–19 Years | 80 | 2.2 | 2 | 1 | 1 | 2 | 3 | 4 | 4 | 8 |
| 20–34 | 414 | 2.4 | 5 | 1 | 1 | 2 | 3 | 4 | 5 | 9 |
| 35–49 | 914 | 2.2 | 3 | 1 | 1 | 2 | 3 | 4 | 5 | 9 |
| 50–64 | 687 | 2.1 | 3 | 1 | 1 | 2 | 3 | 4 | 5 | 8 |
| 65+ | 571 | 2.9 | 13 | 1 | 1 | 2 | 3 | 5 | 9 | 21 |
| **TOTAL SINGLE DX** | 1,088 | 1.6 | <1 | 1 | 1 | 1 | 2 | 2 | 3 | 5 |
| **TOTAL MULTIPLE DX** | 2,666 | 2.3 | 5 | 1 | 1 | 2 | 3 | 4 | 6 | 11 |
| **TOTAL** | | | | | | | | | | |
| 0–19 Years | 127 | 1.9 | 1 | 1 | 1 | 2 | 2 | 3 | 4 | 7 |
| 20–34 | 699 | 2.1 | 4 | 1 | 1 | 1 | 3 | 3 | 5 | 8 |
| 35–49 | 1,364 | 2.0 | 2 | 1 | 1 | 1 | 3 | 3 | 4 | 7 |
| 50–64 | 903 | 2.0 | 3 | 1 | 1 | 2 | 3 | 3 | 5 | 7 |
| 65+ | 661 | 2.7 | 11 | 1 | 1 | 2 | 3 | 5 | 8 | 20 |
| **GRAND TOTAL** | 3,754 | 2.1 | 4 | 1 | 1 | 2 | 3 | 3 | 5 | 11 |

Length of Stay by Diagnosis and Operation, United States, 2000

23

# United States, October 1998–September 1999 Data, by Operation

## 06.5: SUBSTERNAL THYROIDECTOMY. Formerly included in operation group(s) 513.

| Type of Patients | Observed Patients | Avg. Stay | Variance | Percentiles | | | | | | |
|---|---|---|---|---|---|---|---|---|---|---|
| | | | | 10th | 25th | 50th | 75th | 90th | 95th | 99th |
| **1. SINGLE DX** | | | | | | | | | | |
| 0–19 Years | 6 | 1.2 | <1 | 1 | 1 | 1 | 1 | 2 | 2 | 2 |
| 20–34 | 15 | 1.2 | <1 | 1 | 1 | 1 | 1 | 2 | 2 | 3 |
| 35–49 | 55 | 1.6 | <1 | 1 | 1 | 1 | 2 | 4 | 4 | 4 |
| 50–64 | 26 | 1.9 | <1 | 1 | 1 | 2 | 2 | 3 | 3 | 5 |
| 65+ | 19 | 4.0 | 6 | 1 | 2 | 3 | 7 | 7 | 7 | 7 |
| **2. MULTIPLE DX** | | | | | | | | | | |
| 0–19 Years | 6 | 2.1 | 2 | 1 | 1 | 2 | 2 | 4 | 4 | 4 |
| 20–34 | 32 | 2.7 | 5 | 1 | 1 | 2 | 5 | 6 | 6 | 7 |
| 35–49 | 72 | 2.9 | 26 | 1 | 1 | 2 | 3 | 6 | 7 | 48 |
| 50–64 | 110 | 2.4 | 5 | 1 | 1 | 2 | 2 | 5 | 6 | 15 |
| 65+ | 139 | 3.9 | 28 | 1 | 1 | 2 | 4 | 9 | 12 | 19 |
| **TOTAL SINGLE DX** | 121 | 1.8 | 2 | 1 | 1 | 1 | 2 | 4 | 4 | 7 |
| **TOTAL MULTIPLE DX** | 359 | 3.2 | 19 | 1 | 1 | 2 | 3 | 6 | 9 | 19 |
| **TOTAL** | | | | | | | | | | |
| 0–19 Years | 12 | 1.5 | <1 | 1 | 1 | 1 | 2 | 2 | 4 | 4 |
| 20–34 | 47 | 2.1 | 3 | 1 | 1 | 1 | 2 | 6 | 6 | 7 |
| 35–49 | 127 | 2.1 | 10 | 1 | 1 | 1 | 2 | 4 | 4 | 7 |
| 50–64 | 136 | 2.3 | 4 | 1 | 1 | 2 | 2 | 4 | 6 | 8 |
| 65+ | 158 | 3.9 | 26 | 1 | 1 | 2 | 4 | 9 | 12 | 19 |
| **GRAND TOTAL** | 480 | 2.7 | 14 | 1 | 1 | 2 | 3 | 6 | 7 | 15 |

## 06.6: LINGUAL THYROID EXCISION. Formerly included in operation group(s) 513.

| Type of Patients | Observed Patients | Avg. Stay | Variance | Percentiles | | | | | | |
|---|---|---|---|---|---|---|---|---|---|---|
| | | | | 10th | 25th | 50th | 75th | 90th | 95th | 99th |
| **1. SINGLE DX** | | | | | | | | | | |
| 0–19 Years | 1 | 1.0 | 0 | 1 | 1 | 1 | 1 | 1 | 1 | 1 |
| 20–34 | 1 | 1.0 | 0 | 1 | 1 | 1 | 1 | 1 | 1 | 1 |
| 35–49 | 0 | | | | | | | | | |
| 50–64 | 1 | 3.0 | 0 | 3 | 3 | 3 | 3 | 3 | 3 | 3 |
| 65+ | 0 | | | | | | | | | |
| **2. MULTIPLE DX** | | | | | | | | | | |
| 0–19 Years | 0 | | | | | | | | | |
| 20–34 | 0 | | | | | | | | | |
| 35–49 | 2 | 1.9 | 1 | 1 | 1 | 1 | 3 | 3 | 3 | 3 |
| 50–64 | 2 | 2.0 | 0 | 2 | 2 | 2 | 2 | 2 | 2 | 2 |
| 65+ | 2 | 1.4 | <1 | 1 | 1 | 1 | 2 | 2 | 2 | 2 |
| **TOTAL SINGLE DX** | 3 | 1.4 | <1 | 1 | 1 | 1 | 1 | 3 | 3 | 3 |
| **TOTAL MULTIPLE DX** | 6 | 1.8 | <1 | 1 | 1 | 2 | 2 | 3 | 3 | 3 |
| **TOTAL** | | | | | | | | | | |
| 0–19 Years | 1 | 1.0 | 0 | 1 | 1 | 1 | 1 | 1 | 1 | 1 |
| 20–34 | 1 | 1.0 | 0 | 1 | 1 | 1 | 1 | 1 | 1 | 1 |
| 35–49 | 2 | 1.9 | 1 | 1 | 1 | 1 | 3 | 3 | 3 | 3 |
| 50–64 | 3 | 2.4 | <1 | 2 | 2 | 2 | 2 | 3 | 3 | 3 |
| 65+ | 2 | 1.4 | <1 | 1 | 1 | 1 | 2 | 2 | 2 | 2 |
| **GRAND TOTAL** | 9 | 1.5 | <1 | 1 | 1 | 1 | 2 | 3 | 3 | 3 |

## 06.7: THYROGLOSSAL DUCT EXC. Formerly included in operation group(s) 514.

| Type of Patients | Observed Patients | Avg. Stay | Variance | Percentiles | | | | | | |
|---|---|---|---|---|---|---|---|---|---|---|
| | | | | 10th | 25th | 50th | 75th | 90th | 95th | 99th |
| **1. SINGLE DX** | | | | | | | | | | |
| 0–19 Years | 150 | 1.3 | <1 | 1 | 1 | 1 | 1 | 2 | 3 | 4 |
| 20–34 | 24 | 1.6 | <1 | 1 | 1 | 1 | 2 | 3 | 3 | 7 |
| 35–49 | 33 | 1.3 | <1 | 1 | 1 | 1 | 1 | 2 | 3 | 5 |
| 50–64 | 13 | 1.1 | <1 | 1 | 1 | 1 | 1 | 2 | 2 | 2 |
| 65+ | 6 | 1.0 | <1 | 1 | 1 | 1 | 1 | 1 | 1 | 2 |
| **2. MULTIPLE DX** | | | | | | | | | | |
| 0–19 Years | 55 | 1.4 | <1 | 1 | 1 | 1 | 2 | 2 | 4 | 6 |
| 20–34 | 9 | 1.2 | <1 | 1 | 1 | 1 | 1 | 2 | 2 | 4 |
| 35–49 | 17 | 2.2 | 6 | 1 | 1 | 1 | 2 | 3 | 12 | 12 |
| 50–64 | 21 | 1.6 | <1 | 1 | 1 | 1 | 2 | 2 | 3 | 7 |
| 65+ | 10 | 1.9 | 2 | 1 | 1 | 1 | 2 | 6 | 6 | 6 |
| **TOTAL SINGLE DX** | 226 | 1.3 | <1 | 1 | 1 | 1 | 1 | 2 | 3 | 4 |
| **TOTAL MULTIPLE DX** | 112 | 1.6 | 1 | 1 | 1 | 1 | 2 | 2 | 4 | 6 |
| **TOTAL** | | | | | | | | | | |
| 0–19 Years | 205 | 1.3 | <1 | 1 | 1 | 1 | 1 | 2 | 3 | 4 |
| 20–34 | 33 | 1.4 | <1 | 1 | 1 | 1 | 1 | 2 | 3 | 4 |
| 35–49 | 50 | 1.4 | 2 | 1 | 1 | 1 | 1 | 2 | 3 | 8 |
| 50–64 | 34 | 1.4 | <1 | 1 | 1 | 1 | 2 | 2 | 2 | 7 |
| 65+ | 16 | 1.6 | 2 | 1 | 1 | 1 | 2 | 6 | 6 | 6 |
| **GRAND TOTAL** | 338 | 1.3 | <1 | 1 | 1 | 1 | 1 | 2 | 3 | 6 |

## 06.8: PARATHYROIDECTOMY. Formerly included in operation group(s) 514.

| Type of Patients | Observed Patients | Avg. Stay | Variance | Percentiles | | | | | | |
|---|---|---|---|---|---|---|---|---|---|---|
| | | | | 10th | 25th | 50th | 75th | 90th | 95th | 99th |
| **1. SINGLE DX** | | | | | | | | | | |
| 0–19 Years | 7 | 1.4 | <1 | 1 | 1 | 1 | 2 | 2 | 2 | 3 |
| 20–34 | 25 | 1.8 | 1 | 1 | 1 | 2 | 2 | 3 | 5 | 5 |
| 35–49 | 81 | 1.2 | <1 | 1 | 1 | 1 | 1 | 2 | 2 | 4 |
| 50–64 | 109 | 1.3 | <1 | 1 | 1 | 1 | 1 | 2 | 2 | 4 |
| 65+ | 71 | 1.4 | <1 | 1 | 1 | 1 | 2 | 2 | 2 | 3 |
| **2. MULTIPLE DX** | | | | | | | | | | |
| 0–19 Years | 34 | 3.7 | 9 | 1 | 1 | 3 | 7 | 8 | 8 | 16 |
| 20–34 | 187 | 4.3 | 30 | 1 | 1 | 2 | 6 | 9 | 13 | 25 |
| 35–49 | 691 | 3.1 | 14 | 1 | 1 | 2 | 3 | 8 | 12 | 17 |
| 50–64 | 1,079 | 2.6 | 11 | 1 | 1 | 2 | 3 | 6 | 9 | 16 |
| 65+ | 1,217 | 3.7 | 36 | 1 | 1 | 2 | 3 | 8 | 17 | 31 |
| **TOTAL SINGLE DX** | 293 | 1.3 | <1 | 1 | 1 | 1 | 2 | 2 | 2 | 4 |
| **TOTAL MULTIPLE DX** | 3,208 | 3.2 | 22 | 1 | 1 | 2 | 3 | 7 | 12 | 25 |
| **TOTAL** | | | | | | | | | | |
| 0–19 Years | 41 | 3.2 | 8 | 1 | 1 | 2 | 4 | 8 | 8 | 9 |
| 20–34 | 212 | 4.0 | 28 | 1 | 1 | 2 | 5 | 9 | 13 | 25 |
| 35–49 | 772 | 2.8 | 12 | 1 | 1 | 1 | 3 | 7 | 11 | 16 |
| 50–64 | 1,188 | 2.5 | 10 | 1 | 1 | 1 | 3 | 5 | 9 | 16 |
| 65+ | 1,288 | 3.6 | 34 | 1 | 1 | 2 | 3 | 8 | 17 | 31 |
| **GRAND TOTAL** | 3,501 | 3.0 | 20 | 1 | 1 | 2 | 3 | 7 | 11 | 24 |

Length of Stay by Diagnosis and Operation, United States, 2000

# United States, October 1998–September 1999 Data, by Operation

## 06.81: TOTAL PARATHYROIDECTOMY. Formerly included in operation group(s) 514.

| Type of Patients | Observed Patients | Avg. Stay | Vari- ance | Percentiles 10th | 25th | 50th | 75th | 90th | 95th | 99th |
|---|---|---|---|---|---|---|---|---|---|---|
| **1. SINGLE DX** | | | | | | | | | | |
| 0–19 Years | 0 | | | | | | | | | |
| 20–34 | 5 | 2.3 | 3 | 1 | 1 | 1 | 5 | 5 | 5 | 5 |
| 35–49 | 5 | 1.8 | 1 | 1 | 1 | 1 | 2 | 4 | 4 | 4 |
| 50–64 | 10 | 1.1 | <1 | 1 | 1 | 1 | 2 | 4 | 4 | 3 |
| 65+ | 10 | 1.3 | <1 | 1 | 1 | 1 | 2 | 2 | 2 | 2 |
| **2. MULTIPLE DX** | | | | | | | | | | |
| 0–19 Years | 5 | 3.7 | 3 | 2 | 2 | 4 | 4 | 4 | 8 | 8 |
| 20–34 | 40 | 6.2 | 14 | 2 | 4 | 6 | 8 | 13 | 15 | 15 |
| 35–49 | 119 | 5.0 | 26 | 1 | 2 | 2 | 7 | 14 | 14 | 21 |
| 50–64 | 126 | 3.9 | 17 | 1 | 1 | 2 | 2 | 10 | 12 | 22 |
| 65+ | 103 | 6.2 | 48 | 1 | 3 | 3 | 7 | 20 | 20 | 20 |
| **TOTAL SINGLE DX** | **30** | **1.4** | **<1** | **1** | **1** | **1** | **1** | **2** | **4** | **5** |
| **TOTAL MULTIPLE DX** | **393** | **5.1** | **28** | **1** | **1** | **3** | **6** | **14** | **18** | **20** |
| **TOTAL** | | | | | | | | | | |
| 0–19 Years | 5 | 3.7 | 3 | 2 | 2 | 4 | 4 | 4 | 8 | 8 |
| 20–34 | 45 | 5.8 | 15 | 3 | 3 | 5 | 7 | 13 | 15 | 15 |
| 35–49 | 124 | 4.9 | 26 | 1 | 1 | 2 | 7 | 14 | 14 | 21 |
| 50–64 | 136 | 3.5 | 16 | 1 | 1 | 2 | 2 | 9 | 11 | 22 |
| 65+ | 113 | 5.8 | 46 | 1 | 1 | 3 | 7 | 20 | 20 | 20 |
| **GRAND TOTAL** | **423** | **4.8** | **27** | **1** | **1** | **2** | **6** | **14** | **17** | **20** |

## 06.89: OTHER PARATHYROIDECTOMY. Formerly included in operation group(s) 514.

| Type of Patients | Observed Patients | Avg. Stay | Vari- ance | Percentiles 10th | 25th | 50th | 75th | 90th | 95th | 99th |
|---|---|---|---|---|---|---|---|---|---|---|
| **1. SINGLE DX** | | | | | | | | | | |
| 0–19 Years | 7 | 1.4 | <1 | 1 | 1 | 1 | 2 | 2 | 2 | 3 |
| 20–34 | 20 | 1.7 | <1 | 1 | 1 | 2 | 2 | 2 | 3 | 3 |
| 35–49 | 76 | 1.2 | <1 | 1 | 1 | 1 | 1 | 2 | 3 | 3 |
| 50–64 | 99 | 1.3 | <1 | 1 | 1 | 1 | 1 | 2 | 2 | 4 |
| 65+ | 61 | 1.4 | <1 | 1 | 1 | 1 | 2 | 2 | 2 | 3 |
| **2. MULTIPLE DX** | | | | | | | | | | |
| 0–19 Years | 29 | 3.7 | 10 | 1 | 1 | 2 | 7 | 8 | 9 | 16 |
| 20–34 | 147 | 3.8 | 33 | 1 | 1 | 2 | 5 | 8 | 12 | 35 |
| 35–49 | 572 | 2.6 | 9 | 1 | 1 | 2 | 3 | 5 | 9 | 15 |
| 50–64 | 953 | 2.5 | 10 | 1 | 1 | 1 | 2 | 5 | 9 | 15 |
| 65+ | 1,114 | 3.5 | 34 | 1 | 2 | 2 | 3 | 8 | 15 | 31 |
| **TOTAL SINGLE DX** | **263** | **1.3** | **<1** | **1** | **1** | **1** | **2** | **2** | **2** | **3** |
| **TOTAL MULTIPLE DX** | **2,815** | **2.9** | **21** | **1** | **1** | **2** | **3** | **6** | **11** | **28** |
| **TOTAL** | | | | | | | | | | |
| 0–19 Years | 36 | 3.1 | 8 | 1 | 1 | 2 | 2 | 6 | 8 | 9 |
| 20–34 | 167 | 3.6 | 30 | 1 | 1 | 2 | 3 | 9 | 12 | 25 |
| 35–49 | 648 | 2.3 | 9 | 1 | 1 | 1 | 2 | 4 | 8 | 14 |
| 50–64 | 1,052 | 2.4 | 10 | 1 | 1 | 1 | 2 | 4 | 8 | 14 |
| 65+ | 1,175 | 3.3 | 32 | 1 | 1 | 2 | 2 | 7 | 15 | 31 |
| **GRAND TOTAL** | **3,078** | **2.8** | **19** | **1** | **1** | **1** | **2** | **6** | **10** | **25** |

## 06.9: THYROID/PARATHY OPS NEC. Formerly included in operation group(s) 514.

| Type of Patients | Observed Patients | Avg. Stay | Vari- ance | Percentiles 10th | 25th | 50th | 75th | 90th | 95th | 99th |
|---|---|---|---|---|---|---|---|---|---|---|
| **1. SINGLE DX** | | | | | | | | | | |
| 0–19 Years | 0 | | | | | | | | | |
| 20–34 | 4 | 2.0 | 1 | 1 | 2 | 2 | 2 | 4 | 4 | 4 |
| 35–49 | 5 | 1.0 | 0 | 1 | 1 | 1 | 1 | 1 | 1 | 1 |
| 50–64 | 2 | 1.5 | <1 | 1 | 2 | 2 | 2 | 2 | 2 | 2 |
| 65+ | 2 | 2.9 | 9 | 1 | 1 | 1 | 7 | 7 | 7 | 7 |
| **2. MULTIPLE DX** | | | | | | | | | | |
| 0–19 Years | 13 | 4.5 | 10 | 1 | 2 | 4 | 6 | 12 | 12 | 12 |
| 20–34 | 12 | 2.8 | 7 | 1 | 1 | 1 | 2 | 7 | 7 | 11 |
| 35–49 | 26 | 4.6 | 19 | 1 | 1 | 3 | 7 | 9 | 14 | 22 |
| 50–64 | 22 | 3.2 | 8 | 1 | 1 | 1 | 5 | 8 | 8 | 9 |
| 65+ | 29 | 5.3 | 98 | 1 | 1 | 2 | 4 | 9 | 40 | 40 |
| **TOTAL SINGLE DX** | **13** | **1.7** | **3** | **1** | **1** | **1** | **2** | **4** | **7** | **7** |
| **TOTAL MULTIPLE DX** | **102** | **4.3** | **39** | **1** | **1** | **2** | **5** | **8** | **12** | **40** |
| **TOTAL** | | | | | | | | | | |
| 0–19 Years | 13 | 4.5 | 10 | 1 | 1 | 4 | 6 | 12 | 12 | 12 |
| 20–34 | 16 | 2.7 | 6 | 1 | 1 | 1 | 4 | 5 | 7 | 11 |
| 35–49 | 31 | 4.2 | 18 | 1 | 2 | 3 | 6 | 9 | 14 | 22 |
| 50–64 | 24 | 3.1 | 7 | 1 | 1 | 2 | 5 | 8 | 8 | 9 |
| 65+ | 31 | 5.2 | 93 | 1 | 1 | 2 | 4 | 8 | 40 | 40 |
| **GRAND TOTAL** | **115** | **4.1** | **36** | **1** | **1** | **2** | **5** | **8** | **12** | **40** |

## 07.0: ADRENAL FIELD EXPLOR. Formerly included in operation group(s) 515.

| Type of Patients | Observed Patients | Avg. Stay | Vari- ance | Percentiles 10th | 25th | 50th | 75th | 90th | 95th | 99th |
|---|---|---|---|---|---|---|---|---|---|---|
| **1. SINGLE DX** | | | | | | | | | | |
| 0–19 Years | 0 | | | | | | | | | |
| 20–34 | 0 | | | | | | | | | |
| 35–49 | 0 | | | | | | | | | |
| 50–64 | 0 | | | | | | | | | |
| 65+ | 0 | | | | | | | | | |
| **2. MULTIPLE DX** | | | | | | | | | | |
| 0–19 Years | 1 | 4.0 | 0 | 4 | 4 | 4 | 4 | 4 | 4 | 4 |
| 20–34 | 0 | | | | | | | | | |
| 35–49 | 1 | 18.0 | 0 | 18 | 18 | 18 | 18 | 18 | 18 | 18 |
| 50–64 | 0 | | | | | | | | | |
| 65+ | 0 | | | | | | | | | |
| **TOTAL SINGLE DX** | **0** | | | | | | | | | |
| **TOTAL MULTIPLE DX** | **2** | **8.7** | **52** | **4** | **4** | **4** | **18** | **18** | **18** | **18** |
| **TOTAL** | | | | | | | | | | |
| 0–19 Years | 1 | 4.0 | 0 | 4 | 4 | 4 | 4 | 4 | 4 | 4 |
| 20–34 | 0 | | | | | | | | | |
| 35–49 | 1 | 18.0 | 0 | 18 | 18 | 18 | 18 | 18 | 18 | 18 |
| 50–64 | 0 | | | | | | | | | |
| 65+ | 0 | | | | | | | | | |
| **GRAND TOTAL** | **2** | **8.7** | **52** | **4** | **4** | **4** | **18** | **18** | **18** | **18** |

Length of Stay by Diagnosis and Operation, United States, 2000

# United States, October 1998–September 1999 Data, by Operation

## 07.1: OTH ENDOCRINE DXTIC PX. Formerly included in operation group(s) 515, 516.

| Type of Patients | Observed Patients | Avg. Stay | Vari- ance | 10th | 25th | 50th | 75th | 90th | 95th | 99th |
|---|---|---|---|---|---|---|---|---|---|---|
| **1. SINGLE DX** | | | | | | | | | | |
| 0–19 Years | 4 | 3.2 | <1 | 3 | 3 | 3 | 3 | 4 | 4 | 4 |
| 20–34 | 3 | 2.0 | 3 | 1 | 1 | 1 | 4 | 4 | 4 | 4 |
| 35–49 | 4 | 3.3 | 10 | 1 | 1 | 4 | 4 | 10 | 10 | 10 |
| 50–64 | 2 | 13.4 | 16 | 15 | 15 | 15 | 15 | 15 | 15 | 15 |
| 65+ | 1 | 8.0 | 0 | 8 | 8 | 8 | 8 | 8 | 8 | 8 |
| **2. MULTIPLE DX** | | | | | | | | | | |
| 0–19 Years | 20 | 9.9 | 83 | 1 | 3 | 7 | 16 | 31 | 31 | 31 |
| 20–34 | 8 | 6.1 | 15 | 4 | 5 | 5 | 5 | 12 | 19 | 19 |
| 35–49 | 32 | 6.3 | 23 | 3 | 3 | 5 | 9 | 12 | 15 | 22 |
| 50–64 | 82 | 5.8 | 18 | 1 | 3 | 5 | 7 | 9 | 13 | 22 |
| 65+ | 129 | 7.1 | 26 | 2 | 4 | 7 | 9 | 12 | 16 | 24 |
| **TOTAL SINGLE DX** | 14 | 6.5 | 30 | 1 | 3 | 4 | 15 | 15 | 15 | 15 |
| **TOTAL MULTIPLE DX** | 271 | 6.9 | 29 | 1 | 3 | 6 | 9 | 12 | 17 | 31 |
| **TOTAL** | | | | | | | | | | |
| 0–19 Years | 24 | 7.7 | 66 | 1 | 3 | 4 | 10 | 17 | 31 | 31 |
| 20–34 | 11 | 5.5 | 15 | 3 | 4 | 5 | 5 | 7 | 19 | 19 |
| 35–49 | 36 | 5.9 | 22 | 1 | 3 | 4 | 9 | 12 | 15 | 22 |
| 50–64 | 84 | 6.6 | 23 | 2 | 3 | 6 | 9 | 15 | 15 | 22 |
| 65+ | 130 | 7.1 | 26 | 2 | 4 | 7 | 9 | 12 | 16 | 24 |
| **GRAND TOTAL** | 285 | 6.8 | 29 | 1 | 3 | 6 | 9 | 14 | 17 | 31 |

## 07.22: UNILATERAL ADRENALECTOMY. Formerly included in operation group(s) 515.

| Type of Patients | Observed Patients | Avg. Stay | Vari- ance | 10th | 25th | 50th | 75th | 90th | 95th | 99th |
|---|---|---|---|---|---|---|---|---|---|---|
| **1. SINGLE DX** | | | | | | | | | | |
| 0–19 Years | 18 | 3.4 | 1 | 3 | 3 | 3 | 4 | 4 | 6 | 7 |
| 20–34 | 13 | 4.9 | 6 | 2 | 2 | 3 | 7 | 7 | 7 | 10 |
| 35–49 | 28 | 3.6 | 1 | 1 | 4 | 4 | 4 | 5 | 5 | 7 |
| 50–64 | 25 | 3.7 | 2 | 2 | 2 | 4 | 5 | 5 | 6 | 8 |
| 65+ | 9 | 5.0 | 3 | 3 | 4 | 4 | 7 | 7 | 7 | 7 |
| **2. MULTIPLE DX** | | | | | | | | | | |
| 0–19 Years | 66 | 6.5 | 30 | 3 | 4 | 5 | 8 | 11 | 17 | 34 |
| 20–34 | 59 | 4.4 | 26 | 2 | 2 | 4 | 5 | 8 | 9 | 20 |
| 35–49 | 219 | 4.5 | 17 | 1 | 2 | 4 | 5 | 8 | 11 | 21 |
| 50–64 | 252 | 5.5 | 17 | 2 | 3 | 5 | 7 | 10 | 10 | 19 |
| 65+ | 164 | 8.5 | 52 | 3 | 4 | 6 | 10 | 17 | 27 | 35 |
| **TOTAL SINGLE DX** | 93 | 3.9 | 3 | 2 | 3 | 4 | 5 | 7 | 7 | 8 |
| **TOTAL MULTIPLE DX** | 760 | 5.7 | 28 | 2 | 3 | 4 | 7 | 10 | 16 | 31 |
| **TOTAL** | | | | | | | | | | |
| 0–19 Years | 84 | 5.5 | 23 | 3 | 3 | 4 | 6 | 10 | 15 | 34 |
| 20–34 | 72 | 4.5 | 22 | 2 | 2 | 3 | 6 | 7 | 9 | 20 |
| 35–49 | 247 | 4.4 | 15 | 1 | 2 | 4 | 5 | 7 | 10 | 19 |
| 50–64 | 277 | 5.3 | 16 | 2 | 3 | 5 | 6 | 10 | 10 | 19 |
| 65+ | 173 | 8.4 | 50 | 3 | 4 | 6 | 9 | 17 | 27 | 35 |
| **GRAND TOTAL** | 853 | 5.5 | 25 | 2 | 3 | 4 | 6 | 10 | 14 | 28 |

## 07.2: PARTIAL ADRENALECTOMY. Formerly included in operation group(s) 515.

| Type of Patients | Observed Patients | Avg. Stay | Vari- ance | 10th | 25th | 50th | 75th | 90th | 95th | 99th |
|---|---|---|---|---|---|---|---|---|---|---|
| **1. SINGLE DX** | | | | | | | | | | |
| 0–19 Years | 34 | 3.8 | 3 | 3 | 3 | 3 | 4 | 5 | 8 | 8 |
| 20–34 | 13 | 4.9 | 6 | 2 | 2 | 5 | 7 | 7 | 7 | 10 |
| 35–49 | 31 | 3.8 | 2 | 2 | 4 | 4 | 4 | 5 | 6 | 7 |
| 50–64 | 29 | 3.7 | 2 | 2 | 2 | 4 | 5 | 5 | 6 | 8 |
| 65+ | 9 | 5.0 | 3 | 3 | 4 | 4 | 7 | 7 | 7 | 7 |
| **2. MULTIPLE DX** | | | | | | | | | | |
| 0–19 Years | 104 | 11.8 | 199 | 3 | 4 | 6 | 11 | 50 | 50 | 50 |
| 20–34 | 75 | 4.6 | 27 | 2 | 2 | 3 | 5 | 8 | 12 | 23 |
| 35–49 | 247 | 4.5 | 15 | 2 | 2 | 4 | 5 | 8 | 10 | 21 |
| 50–64 | 279 | 5.5 | 16 | 2 | 3 | 5 | 7 | 10 | 10 | 19 |
| 65+ | 184 | 8.3 | 47 | 3 | 4 | 6 | 9 | 17 | 27 | 35 |
| **TOTAL SINGLE DX** | 116 | 4.0 | 3 | 2 | 3 | 4 | 5 | 7 | 7 | 8 |
| **TOTAL MULTIPLE DX** | 889 | 6.4 | 51 | 2 | 3 | 5 | 7 | 10 | 18 | 50 |
| **TOTAL** | | | | | | | | | | |
| 0–19 Years | 138 | 9.3 | 151 | 3 | 3 | 5 | 8 | 17 | 50 | 50 |
| 20–34 | 88 | 4.7 | 23 | 2 | 2 | 3 | 6 | 7 | 10 | 23 |
| 35–49 | 278 | 4.5 | 14 | 2 | 3 | 4 | 5 | 7 | 10 | 21 |
| 50–64 | 308 | 5.2 | 15 | 2 | 3 | 5 | 6 | 10 | 10 | 19 |
| 65+ | 193 | 8.2 | 46 | 3 | 4 | 6 | 9 | 16 | 27 | 35 |
| **GRAND TOTAL** | 1,005 | 6.0 | 45 | 2 | 3 | 4 | 7 | 10 | 16 | 50 |

## 07.3: BILATERAL ADRENALECTOMY. Formerly included in operation group(s) 515.

| Type of Patients | Observed Patients | Avg. Stay | Vari- ance | 10th | 25th | 50th | 75th | 90th | 95th | 99th |
|---|---|---|---|---|---|---|---|---|---|---|
| **1. SINGLE DX** | | | | | | | | | | |
| 0–19 Years | 2 | 2.0 | 0 | 2 | 2 | 2 | 2 | 2 | 2 | 2 |
| 20–34 | 1 | 2.0 | 0 | 2 | 2 | 2 | 2 | 2 | 2 | 2 |
| 35–49 | 0 | | | | | | | | | |
| 50–64 | 0 | | | | | | | | | |
| 65+ | 0 | | | | | | | | | |
| **2. MULTIPLE DX** | | | | | | | | | | |
| 0–19 Years | 6 | 5.2 | 7 | 4 | 4 | 4 | 5 | 13 | >99 | >99 |
| 20–34 | 2 | 3.4 | 4 | 2 | 2 | 2 | 5 | 5 | 5 | 5 |
| 35–49 | 10 | 6.2 | 9 | 3 | 4 | 6 | 7 | 11 | 11 | 11 |
| 50–64 | 13 | 7.2 | 28 | 2 | 3 | 6 | 7 | 17 | 22 | 22 |
| 65+ | 3 | 6.9 | 10 | 3 | 7 | 7 | 7 | 13 | 13 | 13 |
| **TOTAL SINGLE DX** | 3 | 2.0 | 0 | 2 | 2 | 2 | 2 | 2 | 2 | 2 |
| **TOTAL MULTIPLE DX** | 34 | 6.2 | 15 | 2 | 4 | 6 | 7 | 13 | 17 | >99 |
| **TOTAL** | | | | | | | | | | |
| 0–19 Years | 8 | 4.5 | 7 | 2 | 2 | 4 | 5 | 13 | >99 | >99 |
| 20–34 | 3 | 2.6 | 2 | 2 | 2 | 2 | 2 | 5 | 5 | 5 |
| 35–49 | 10 | 6.2 | 9 | 3 | 4 | 6 | 7 | 11 | 11 | 11 |
| 50–64 | 13 | 7.2 | 28 | 2 | 3 | 6 | 7 | 17 | 22 | 22 |
| 65+ | 3 | 6.9 | 10 | 3 | 7 | 7 | 7 | 13 | 13 | 13 |
| **GRAND TOTAL** | 37 | 5.7 | 15 | 2 | 3 | 5 | 7 | 13 | 17 | >99 |

Length of Stay by Diagnosis and Operation, United States, 2000

## United States, October 1998–September 1999 Data, by Operation

### 07.4: OTHER ADRENAL OPERATIONS. Formerly included in operation group(s) 515.

| Type of Patients | Observed Patients | Avg. Stay | Variance | 10th | 25th | 50th | 75th | 90th | 95th | 99th |
|---|---|---|---|---|---|---|---|---|---|---|
| **1. SINGLE DX** | | | | | | | | | | |
| 0–19 Years | 0 | | | | | | | | | |
| 20–34 | 0 | | | | | | | | | |
| 35–49 | 0 | | | | | | | | | |
| 50–64 | 0 | | | | | | | | | |
| 65+ | 0 | | | | | | | | | |
| **2. MULTIPLE DX** | | | | | | | | | | |
| 0–19 Years | 1 | 1.0 | 0 | 1 | 1 | | 1 | 1 | 1 | 1 |
| 20–34 | 2 | 8.9 | 64 | 1 | 1 | 14 | 14 | 14 | 14 | 14 |
| 35–49 | 0 | | | | | | | | | |
| 50–64 | 1 | 17.0 | 0 | 17 | 17 | 17 | 17 | 17 | 17 | 17 |
| 65+ | 0 | | | | | | | | | |
| **TOTAL SINGLE DX** | 0 | | | | | | | | | |
| **TOTAL MULTIPLE DX** | 4 | 10.6 | 61 | 1 | 1 | 14 | 17 | 17 | 17 | 17 |
| **TOTAL** | | | | | | | | | | |
| 0–19 Years | 1 | 1.0 | 0 | 1 | 1 | | 1 | 1 | 1 | 1 |
| 20–34 | 2 | 8.9 | 64 | 1 | 1 | 14 | 14 | 14 | 14 | 14 |
| 35–49 | 0 | | | | | | | | | |
| 50–64 | 1 | 17.0 | 0 | 17 | 17 | 17 | 17 | 17 | 17 | 17 |
| 65+ | 0 | | | | | | | | | |
| **GRAND TOTAL** | 4 | 10.6 | 61 | 1 | 1 | 14 | 17 | 17 | 17 | 17 |

### 07.5: PINEAL GLAND OPERATIONS. Formerly included in operation group(s) 515.

| Type of Patients | Observed Patients | Avg. Stay | Variance | 10th | 25th | 50th | 75th | 90th | 95th | 99th |
|---|---|---|---|---|---|---|---|---|---|---|
| **1. SINGLE DX** | | | | | | | | | | |
| 0–19 Years | 2 | 6.0 | 3 | 4 | 4 | 7 | 7 | 7 | 7 | 7 |
| 20–34 | 3 | 3.3 | <1 | 2 | 3 | 4 | 4 | 4 | 4 | 4 |
| 35–49 | 1 | 2.0 | 0 | 2 | 2 | 2 | 2 | 2 | 2 | 2 |
| 50–64 | 1 | 6.0 | 0 | 6 | 6 | 6 | 6 | 6 | 6 | 6 |
| 65+ | 0 | | | | | | | | | |
| **2. MULTIPLE DX** | | | | | | | | | | |
| 0–19 Years | 16 | 10.6 | 39 | 4 | 6 | 11 | 17 | 19 | 21 | 21 |
| 20–34 | 5 | 11.5 | 151 | 2 | 2 | 6 | 14 | 34 | 34 | 34 |
| 35–49 | 7 | 7.5 | 40 | 3 | 4 | 5 | 8 | 25 | 25 | 25 |
| 50–64 | 1 | 20.0 | 0 | 20 | 20 | 20 | 20 | 20 | 20 | 20 |
| 65+ | 1 | 5.0 | 0 | 5 | 5 | 5 | 5 | 5 | 5 | 5 |
| **TOTAL SINGLE DX** | 7 | 3.9 | 4 | 2 | 2 | 4 | 6 | 7 | 7 | 7 |
| **TOTAL MULTIPLE DX** | 30 | 9.6 | 52 | 3 | 4 | 7 | 14 | 20 | 25 | 34 |
| **TOTAL** | | | | | | | | | | |
| 0–19 Years | 18 | 10.2 | 37 | 4 | 5 | 7 | 17 | 19 | 21 | 21 |
| 20–34 | 8 | 7.8 | 95 | 2 | 2 | 4 | 6 | 14 | 34 | 34 |
| 35–49 | 8 | 6.6 | 38 | 2 | 3 | 5 | 8 | 8 | 25 | 25 |
| 50–64 | 2 | 12.4 | 77 | 6 | 6 | 6 | 20 | 20 | 20 | 20 |
| 65+ | 1 | 5.0 | | 5 | 5 | 5 | 5 | 5 | 5 | 5 |
| **GRAND TOTAL** | 37 | 8.5 | 48 | 2 | 4 | 6 | 11 | 19 | 21 | 34 |

### 07.6: HYPOPHYSECTOMY. Formerly included in operation group(s) 515.

| Type of Patients | Observed Patients | Avg. Stay | Variance | 10th | 25th | 50th | 75th | 90th | 95th | 99th |
|---|---|---|---|---|---|---|---|---|---|---|
| **1. SINGLE DX** | | | | | | | | | | |
| 0–19 Years | 23 | 3.4 | 4 | 2 | 2 | 3 | 4 | 5 | 9 | 12 |
| 20–34 | 110 | 3.6 | 2 | 2 | 4 | 4 | 4 | 5 | 6 | 8 |
| 35–49 | 124 | 4.4 | 6 | 2 | 3 | 4 | 5 | 10 | 10 | 10 |
| 50–64 | 107 | 3.3 | 2 | 2 | 2 | 3 | 4 | 5 | 6 | 9 |
| 65+ | 60 | 4.0 | 3 | 2 | 3 | 4 | 4 | 7 | 9 | 9 |
| **2. MULTIPLE DX** | | | | | | | | | | |
| 0–19 Years | 99 | 10.1 | 249 | 3 | 4 | 6 | 10 | 16 | 43 | >99 |
| 20–34 | 268 | 4.7 | 9 | 3 | 4 | 4 | 6 | 8 | 10 | 15 |
| 35–49 | 434 | 6.0 | 20 | 2 | 3 | 4 | 7 | 13 | 13 | 22 |
| 50–64 | 509 | 5.2 | 13 | 2 | 3 | 4 | 6 | 9 | 12 | 23 |
| 65+ | 415 | 6.3 | 39 | 3 | 3 | 4 | 7 | 11 | 17 | 41 |
| **TOTAL SINGLE DX** | 424 | 3.8 | 4 | 2 | 3 | 3 | 4 | 6 | 9 | 10 |
| **TOTAL MULTIPLE DX** | 1,725 | 5.8 | 33 | 2 | 3 | 4 | 6 | 11 | 13 | 30 |
| **TOTAL** | | | | | | | | | | |
| 0–19 Years | 122 | 8.6 | 202 | 2 | 3 | 5 | 9 | 15 | 36 | >99 |
| 20–34 | 378 | 4.4 | 7 | 2 | 3 | 4 | 5 | 7 | 10 | 15 |
| 35–49 | 558 | 5.6 | 17 | 2 | 3 | 4 | 7 | 13 | 13 | 21 |
| 50–64 | 616 | 4.9 | 12 | 2 | 3 | 4 | 6 | 8 | 11 | 23 |
| 65+ | 475 | 6.1 | 36 | 3 | 3 | 4 | 6 | 10 | 15 | 41 |
| **GRAND TOTAL** | 2,149 | 5.4 | 28 | 2 | 3 | 4 | 6 | 10 | 13 | 26 |

### 07.62: EXC PIT LES-TRANSSPHEN. Formerly included in operation group(s) 515.

| Type of Patients | Observed Patients | Avg. Stay | Variance | 10th | 25th | 50th | 75th | 90th | 95th | 99th |
|---|---|---|---|---|---|---|---|---|---|---|
| **1. SINGLE DX** | | | | | | | | | | |
| 0–19 Years | 17 | 3.2 | 4 | 2 | 2 | 3 | 3 | 5 | 9 | 9 |
| 20–34 | 78 | 3.4 | 2 | 3 | 3 | 3 | 5 | 5 | 5 | 8 |
| 35–49 | 79 | 4.6 | 7 | 2 | 3 | 3 | 5 | 10 | 10 | 10 |
| 50–64 | 65 | 3.2 | 2 | 2 | 3 | 3 | 4 | 5 | 6 | 9 |
| 65+ | 40 | 3.4 | 2 | 3 | 3 | 3 | 4 | 5 | 6 | 9 |
| **2. MULTIPLE DX** | | | | | | | | | | |
| 0–19 Years | 37 | 5.7 | 43 | 3 | 3 | 4 | 5 | 8 | 15 | 43 |
| 20–34 | 177 | 4.3 | 7 | 3 | 3 | 4 | 5 | 7 | 10 | 15 |
| 35–49 | 280 | 6.1 | 20 | 2 | 3 | 4 | 8 | 13 | 13 | 20 |
| 50–64 | 315 | 4.6 | 8 | 2 | 3 | 4 | 5 | 7 | 9 | 16 |
| 65+ | 268 | 6.2 | 39 | 3 | 3 | 4 | 6 | 11 | 17 | 42 |
| **TOTAL SINGLE DX** | 279 | 3.8 | 4 | 2 | 3 | 3 | 4 | 6 | 10 | 10 |
| **TOTAL MULTIPLE DX** | 1,077 | 5.4 | 20 | 2 | 3 | 4 | 6 | 11 | 13 | 24 |
| **TOTAL** | | | | | | | | | | |
| 0–19 Years | 54 | 4.8 | 29 | 2 | 3 | 3 | 5 | 8 | 9 | 43 |
| 20–34 | 255 | 4.0 | 6 | 2 | 3 | 3 | 4 | 6 | 8 | 15 |
| 35–49 | 359 | 5.8 | 18 | 2 | 3 | 4 | 7 | 13 | 13 | 18 |
| 50–64 | 380 | 4.4 | 7 | 3 | 3 | 4 | 6 | 7 | 9 | 16 |
| 65+ | 308 | 5.9 | 36 | 3 | 3 | 4 | 6 | 10 | 15 | 41 |
| **GRAND TOTAL** | 1,356 | 5.1 | 17 | 2 | 3 | 4 | 5 | 10 | 13 | 21 |

Length of Stay by Diagnosis and Operation, United States, 2000

# United States, October 1998–September 1999 Data, by Operation

## 07.65: TOT EXC PIT-TRANSSPHEN. Formerly included in operation group(s) 515.

| Type of Patients | Observed Patients | Avg. Stay | Variance | 10th | 25th | 50th | 75th | 90th | 95th | 99th |
|---|---|---|---|---|---|---|---|---|---|---|
| **1. SINGLE DX** | | | | | | | | | | |
| 0–19 Years | 2 | 2.3 | <1 | 2 | 2 | 2 | 3 | 3 | 3 | 3 |
| 20–34 | 23 | 3.8 | <1 | 2 | 4 | 4 | 4 | 4 | 5 | 6 |
| 35–49 | 37 | 3.9 | 2 | 2 | 3 | 4 | 4 | 7 | 7 | 8 |
| 50–64 | 33 | 3.4 | 2 | 2 | 3 | 3 | 4 | 5 | 7 | 8 |
| 65+ | 18 | 4.6 | 3 | 3 | 4 | 4 | 5 | 8 | 9 | 9 |
| **2. MULTIPLE DX** | | | | | | | | | | |
| 0–19 Years | 14 | 4.6 | 6 | 2 | 3 | 5 | 6 | 8 | 8 | 11 |
| 20–34 | 60 | 5.3 | 8 | 2 | 3 | 5 | 7 | 10 | 10 | 14 |
| 35–49 | 101 | 5.1 | 13 | 2 | 3 | 4 | 6 | 9 | 10 | 26 |
| 50–64 | 124 | 5.4 | 13 | 3 | 3 | 4 | 6 | 8 | 15 | 18 |
| 65+ | 112 | 4.9 | 8 | 2 | 3 | 4 | 6 | 8 | 10 | 17 |
| **TOTAL SINGLE DX** | 113 | 3.9 | 2 | 2 | 3 | 4 | 4 | 6 | 7 | 9 |
| **TOTAL MULTIPLE DX** | 411 | 5.2 | 11 | 2 | 3 | 4 | 6 | 9 | 11 | 18 |
| **TOTAL** | | | | | | | | | | |
| 0–19 Years | 16 | 4.1 | 5 | 2 | 2 | 3 | 6 | 7 | 8 | 11 |
| 20–34 | 83 | 4.7 | 6 | 2 | 3 | 4 | 5 | 7 | 10 | 14 |
| 35–49 | 138 | 4.7 | 10 | 2 | 3 | 4 | 5 | 7 | 9 | 26 |
| 50–64 | 157 | 5.0 | <1 | 3 | 3 | 4 | 5 | 8 | 11 | 18 |
| 65+ | 130 | 4.9 | 7 | 2 | 3 | 4 | 6 | 8 | 10 | 17 |
| **GRAND TOTAL** | 524 | 4.8 | 9 | 2 | 3 | 4 | 5 | 8 | 10 | 18 |

## 07.7: OTHER HYPOPHYSIS OPS. Formerly included in operation group(s) 515.

| Type of Patients | Observed Patients | Avg. Stay | Variance | 10th | 25th | 50th | 75th | 90th | 95th | 99th |
|---|---|---|---|---|---|---|---|---|---|---|
| **1. SINGLE DX** | | | | | | | | | | |
| 0–19 Years | 1 | 4.0 | 0 | 4 | 4 | 4 | 4 | 4 | 4 | 4 |
| 20–34 | 3 | 1.9 | <1 | 1 | 1 | 2 | 2 | 3 | 3 | 3 |
| 35–49 | 1 | 2.0 | 0 | 2 | 2 | 2 | 2 | 2 | 2 | 2 |
| 50–64 | 0 | | | | | | | | | |
| 65+ | 0 | | | | | | | | | |
| **2. MULTIPLE DX** | | | | | | | | | | |
| 0–19 Years | 3 | 3.9 | 6 | 1 | 1 | 5 | 5 | 6 | 6 | 6 |
| 20–34 | 0 | | | | | | | | | |
| 35–49 | 4 | 5.0 | 23 | 3 | 3 | 3 | 4 | 14 | 17 | 17 |
| 50–64 | 3 | 3.0 | <1 | 2 | 2 | 3 | 4 | 4 | 4 | 4 |
| 65+ | 11 | 6.4 | 134 | 1 | 2 | 2 | 3 | 15 | 42 | 42 |
| **TOTAL SINGLE DX** | 5 | 2.5 | 1 | 1 | 2 | 2 | 4 | 4 | 4 | 4 |
| **TOTAL MULTIPLE DX** | 21 | 5.2 | 67 | 1 | 2 | 3 | 4 | 14 | 17 | 42 |
| **TOTAL** | | | | | | | | | | |
| 0–19 Years | 4 | 4.0 | 2 | 1 | 4 | 4 | 5 | 6 | 6 | 6 |
| 20–34 | 3 | 1.9 | <1 | 1 | 1 | 2 | 2 | 3 | 3 | 3 |
| 35–49 | 5 | 4.6 | 21 | 2 | 3 | 3 | 4 | 14 | 17 | 17 |
| 50–64 | 3 | 3.0 | <1 | 2 | 2 | 3 | 4 | 4 | 4 | 4 |
| 65+ | 11 | 6.4 | 134 | 1 | 2 | 2 | 3 | 15 | 42 | 42 |
| **GRAND TOTAL** | 26 | 4.7 | 56 | 1 | 2 | 3 | 4 | 6 | 17 | 42 |

## 07.8: THYMECTOMY. Formerly included in operation group(s) 515.

| Type of Patients | Observed Patients | Avg. Stay | Variance | 10th | 25th | 50th | 75th | 90th | 95th | 99th |
|---|---|---|---|---|---|---|---|---|---|---|
| **1. SINGLE DX** | | | | | | | | | | |
| 0–19 Years | 25 | 3.4 | 4 | 1 | 2 | 3 | 4 | 5 | 6 | 12 |
| 20–34 | 30 | 4.1 | 6 | 2 | 3 | 3 | 4 | 5 | 12 | 12 |
| 35–49 | 31 | 3.3 | 1 | 2 | 2 | 3 | 4 | 4 | 5 | 8 |
| 50–64 | 24 | 3.6 | 5 | 2 | 3 | 3 | 4 | 5 | 5 | 15 |
| 65+ | 9 | 4.6 | 6 | 2 | 3 | 4 | 6 | 9 | 9 | 9 |
| **2. MULTIPLE DX** | | | | | | | | | | |
| 0–19 Years | 37 | 6.7 | 66 | 2 | 3 | 4 | 7 | 18 | 19 | 58 |
| 20–34 | 85 | 4.8 | 33 | 2 | 3 | 3 | 4 | 15 | 23 | 24 |
| 35–49 | 128 | 5.7 | 28 | 2 | 3 | 4 | 7 | 9 | 15 | 25 |
| 50–64 | 114 | 6.2 | 50 | 3 | 4 | 5 | 7 | 11 | 14 | 52 |
| 65+ | 88 | 6.4 | 45 | 2 | 3 | 5 | 6 | 11 | 16 | 43 |
| **TOTAL SINGLE DX** | 119 | 3.6 | 4 | 2 | 3 | 3 | 4 | 5 | 8 | 12 |
| **TOTAL MULTIPLE DX** | 452 | 5.9 | 41 | 2 | 3 | 4 | 7 | 10 | 16 | 28 |
| **TOTAL** | | | | | | | | | | |
| 0–19 Years | 62 | 5.4 | 45 | 2 | 3 | 4 | 5 | 10 | 19 | 58 |
| 20–34 | 115 | 4.7 | 29 | 2 | 3 | 3 | 4 | 10 | 19 | 23 |
| 35–49 | 159 | 5.3 | 24 | 2 | 3 | 4 | 7 | 8 | 12 | 24 |
| 50–64 | 138 | 5.9 | 46 | 3 | 4 | 5 | 6 | 8 | 14 | 23 |
| 65+ | 97 | 6.3 | 42 | 2 | 3 | 5 | 6 | 11 | 16 | 43 |
| **GRAND TOTAL** | 571 | 5.5 | 36 | 2 | 3 | 4 | 6 | 10 | 15 | 25 |

## 07.82: TOTAL EXCISION OF THYMUS. Formerly included in operation group(s) 515.

| Type of Patients | Observed Patients | Avg. Stay | Variance | 10th | 25th | 50th | 75th | 90th | 95th | 99th |
|---|---|---|---|---|---|---|---|---|---|---|
| **1. SINGLE DX** | | | | | | | | | | |
| 0–19 Years | 15 | 3.6 | 4 | 2 | 3 | 4 | 4 | 5 | 6 | 12 |
| 20–34 | 18 | 4.5 | 8 | 3 | 3 | 4 | 5 | 12 | 12 | 12 |
| 35–49 | 20 | 3.6 | <1 | 2 | 3 | 4 | 4 | 5 | 5 | 8 |
| 50–64 | 11 | 4.1 | 9 | 2 | 3 | 4 | 5 | 5 | 15 | 15 |
| 65+ | 3 | 4.1 | 1 | 3 | 3 | 4 | 4 | 6 | 6 | 6 |
| **2. MULTIPLE DX** | | | | | | | | | | |
| 0–19 Years | 22 | 7.8 | 87 | 3 | 4 | 4 | 7 | 19 | 19 | 58 |
| 20–34 | 60 | 6.6 | 51 | 2 | 3 | 3 | 6 | 23 | 23 | 28 |
| 35–49 | 89 | 5.9 | 32 | 3 | 3 | 4 | 7 | 9 | 15 | 37 |
| 50–64 | 68 | 5.7 | 32 | 3 | 4 | 5 | 6 | 7 | 14 | 23 |
| 65+ | 60 | 6.2 | 46 | 2 | 3 | 5 | 6 | 11 | 15 | 55 |
| **TOTAL SINGLE DX** | 67 | 3.9 | 4 | 2 | 3 | 4 | 4 | 5 | 6 | 12 |
| **TOTAL MULTIPLE DX** | 299 | 6.2 | 42 | 2 | 3 | 4 | 7 | 11 | 19 | 37 |
| **TOTAL** | | | | | | | | | | |
| 0–19 Years | 37 | 6.2 | 59 | 2 | 3 | 4 | 6 | 12 | 19 | 58 |
| 20–34 | 78 | 6.2 | 43 | 2 | 3 | 3 | 5 | 19 | 23 | 28 |
| 35–49 | 109 | 5.5 | 27 | 2 | 3 | 4 | 7 | 9 | 15 | 25 |
| 50–64 | 79 | 5.6 | 31 | 3 | 3 | 4 | 6 | 7 | 14 | 23 |
| 65+ | 63 | 6.1 | 45 | 2 | 3 | 5 | 6 | 11 | 15 | 43 |
| **GRAND TOTAL** | 366 | 5.8 | 37 | 2 | 3 | 4 | 6 | 10 | 16 | 28 |

Length of Stay by Diagnosis and Operation, United States, 2000

# United States, October 1998–September 1999 Data, by Operation

## 07.9: OTHER THYMUS OPERATIONS. Formerly included in operation group(s) 515.

| Type of Patients | Observed Patients | Avg. Stay | Variance | 10th | 25th | 50th | 75th | 90th | 95th | 99th |
|---|---|---|---|---|---|---|---|---|---|---|
| **1. SINGLE DX** | | | | | | | | | | |
| 0–19 Years | 0 | | | | | | | | | |
| 20–34 | 0 | | | | | | | | | |
| 35–49 | 1 | 1.0 | 0 | 1 | 1 | 1 | 1 | 1 | 1 | 1 |
| 50–64 | 0 | | | | | | | | | |
| 65+ | 0 | | | | | | | | | |
| **2. MULTIPLE DX** | | | | | | | | | | |
| 0–19 Years | 1 | 8.0 | 0 | 8 | 8 | 8 | 8 | 8 | 8 | 8 |
| 20–34 | 0 | | | | | | | | | |
| 35–49 | 0 | | | | | | | | | |
| 50–64 | 1 | 7.0 | 0 | 7 | 7 | 7 | 7 | 7 | 7 | 7 |
| 65+ | 0 | | | | | | | | | |
| **TOTAL SINGLE DX** | 1 | 1.0 | 0 | 1 | 1 | 1 | 1 | 1 | 1 | 1 |
| **TOTAL MULTIPLE DX** | 2 | 7.6 | <1 | 7 | 7 | 8 | 8 | 8 | 8 | 8 |
| **TOTAL** | | | | | | | | | | |
| 0–19 Years | 1 | 8.0 | 0 | 8 | 8 | 8 | 8 | 8 | 8 | 8 |
| 20–34 | 0 | | | | | | | | | |
| 35–49 | 1 | 1.0 | 0 | 1 | 1 | 1 | 1 | 1 | 1 | 1 |
| 50–64 | 1 | 7.0 | 0 | 7 | 7 | 7 | 7 | 7 | 7 | 7 |
| 65+ | 0 | | | | | | | | | |
| **GRAND TOTAL** | 3 | 4.5 | 14 | 1 | 1 | 7 | 8 | 8 | 8 | 8 |

## 08.1: DXTIC PX ON EYELID. Formerly included in operation group(s) 517, 532.

| Type of Patients | Observed Patients | Avg. Stay | Variance | 10th | 25th | 50th | 75th | 90th | 95th | 99th |
|---|---|---|---|---|---|---|---|---|---|---|
| **1. SINGLE DX** | | | | | | | | | | |
| 0–19 Years | 0 | | | | | | | | | |
| 20–34 | 0 | | | | | | | | | |
| 35–49 | 0 | | | | | | | | | |
| 50–64 | 0 | | | | | | | | | |
| 65+ | 0 | | | | | | | | | |
| **2. MULTIPLE DX** | | | | | | | | | | |
| 0–19 Years | 1 | 3.0 | 0 | 3 | 3 | 3 | 3 | 3 | 3 | 3 |
| 20–34 | 0 | | | | | | | | | |
| 35–49 | 4 | 4.1 | 9 | 2 | 2 | 2 | 5 | 11 | 11 | 11 |
| 50–64 | 3 | 8.0 | 18 | 7 | 7 | 7 | 7 | 7 | 25 | 27 |
| 65+ | 6 | 3.8 | 3 | 3 | 3 | 3 | 3 | 6 | 6 | 10 |
| **TOTAL SINGLE DX** | 0 | | | | | | | | | |
| **TOTAL MULTIPLE DX** | 14 | 5.3 | 13 | 3 | 3 | 5 | 7 | 7 | 7 | 25 |
| **TOTAL** | | | | | | | | | | |
| 0–19 Years | 1 | 3.0 | 0 | 3 | 3 | 3 | 3 | 3 | 3 | 3 |
| 20–34 | 0 | | | | | | | | | |
| 35–49 | 4 | 4.1 | 9 | 2 | 2 | 2 | 5 | 11 | 11 | 11 |
| 50–64 | 3 | 8.0 | 18 | 7 | 7 | 7 | 7 | 7 | 25 | 27 |
| 65+ | 6 | 3.8 | 3 | 3 | 3 | 3 | 3 | 6 | 6 | 10 |
| **GRAND TOTAL** | 14 | 5.3 | 13 | 3 | 3 | 5 | 7 | 7 | 7 | 25 |

## 08.0: EYELID INCISION. Formerly included in operation group(s) 518.

| Type of Patients | Observed Patients | Avg. Stay | Variance | 10th | 25th | 50th | 75th | 90th | 95th | 99th |
|---|---|---|---|---|---|---|---|---|---|---|
| **1. SINGLE DX** | | | | | | | | | | |
| 0–19 Years | 11 | 1.5 | <1 | 1 | 1 | 1 | 1 | 1 | 4 | 4 |
| 20–34 | 6 | 2.5 | <1 | 2 | 2 | 2 | 3 | 3 | 5 | 5 |
| 35–49 | 2 | 1.0 | 0 | 1 | 1 | 1 | 1 | 1 | 1 | 1 |
| 50–64 | 0 | | | | | | | | | |
| 65+ | 0 | | | | | | | | | |
| **2. MULTIPLE DX** | | | | | | | | | | |
| 0–19 Years | 24 | 3.3 | 3 | 1 | 3 | 3 | 4 | 6 | 7 | 7 |
| 20–34 | 11 | 3.6 | 5 | 1 | 3 | 3 | 6 | 7 | 7 | 7 |
| 35–49 | 14 | 4.6 | 9 | 2 | 2 | 4 | 6 | 7 | 12 | 14 |
| 50–64 | 10 | 3.8 | 7 | 2 | 2 | 3 | 4 | 9 | 9 | 9 |
| 65+ | 12 | 5.5 | 12 | 2 | 3 | 5 | 8 | 10 | 14 | 14 |
| **TOTAL SINGLE DX** | 19 | 1.7 | 1 | 1 | 1 | 1 | 2 | 3 | 4 | 5 |
| **TOTAL MULTIPLE DX** | 71 | 3.9 | 6 | 2 | 2 | 3 | 5 | 7 | 8 | 14 |
| **TOTAL** | | | | | | | | | | |
| 0–19 Years | 35 | 2.6 | 3 | 1 | 1 | 3 | 3 | 4 | 6 | 7 |
| 20–34 | 17 | 3.2 | 4 | 2 | 2 | 3 | 3 | 7 | 7 | 7 |
| 35–49 | 16 | 4.2 | 10 | 2 | 2 | 4 | 6 | 7 | 12 | 14 |
| 50–64 | 10 | 3.8 | 7 | 2 | 2 | 2 | 4 | 9 | 9 | 9 |
| 65+ | 12 | 5.5 | 12 | 2 | 3 | 5 | 8 | 10 | 14 | 14 |
| **GRAND TOTAL** | 90 | 3.3 | 6 | 1 | 2 | 3 | 4 | 7 | 8 | 14 |

## 08.2: EXC/DESTR EYELID LESION. Formerly included in operation group(s) 517.

| Type of Patients | Observed Patients | Avg. Stay | Variance | 10th | 25th | 50th | 75th | 90th | 95th | 99th |
|---|---|---|---|---|---|---|---|---|---|---|
| **1. SINGLE DX** | | | | | | | | | | |
| 0–19 Years | 67 | 1.1 | <1 | 1 | 1 | 1 | 1 | 1 | 1 | 6 |
| 20–34 | 3 | 4.2 | 5 | 1 | 2 | 6 | 6 | 6 | 6 | 6 |
| 35–49 | 2 | 3.4 | 13 | 1 | 1 | 1 | 2 | 8 | 8 | 8 |
| 50–64 | 2 | 1.8 | <1 | 1 | 1 | 1 | 2 | 2 | 2 | 2 |
| 65+ | 5 | 1.4 | <1 | 1 | 1 | 1 | 2 | 3 | 3 | 3 |
| **2. MULTIPLE DX** | | | | | | | | | | |
| 0–19 Years | 29 | 2.1 | 5 | 1 | 1 | 1 | 2 | 6 | 6 | 14 |
| 20–34 | 28 | 2.4 | 1 | 1 | 1 | 1 | 3 | 4 | 5 | 5 |
| 35–49 | 20 | 11.0 | 147 | 2 | 4 | 4 | 14 | 27 | 27 | 55 |
| 50–64 | 21 | 3.4 | 11 | 1 | 2 | 2 | 4 | 7 | 11 | 15 |
| 65+ | 64 | 5.6 | 20 | 3 | 4 | 4 | 6 | 10 | 18 | 19 |
| **TOTAL SINGLE DX** | 79 | 1.2 | 1 | 1 | 1 | 1 | 1 | 1 | 2 | 6 |
| **TOTAL MULTIPLE DX** | 162 | 4.0 | 25 | 1 | 1 | 2 | 5 | 8 | 13 | 27 |
| **TOTAL** | | | | | | | | | | |
| 0–19 Years | 96 | 1.4 | 2 | 1 | 1 | 1 | 1 | 1 | 6 | 6 |
| 20–34 | 31 | 2.5 | 1 | 1 | 2 | 2 | 3 | 4 | 5 | 6 |
| 35–49 | 22 | 10.3 | 139 | 2 | 4 | 4 | 12 | 27 | 27 | 55 |
| 50–64 | 23 | 3.3 | 11 | 1 | 1 | 2 | 4 | 7 | 11 | 15 |
| 65+ | 69 | 5.4 | 20 | 3 | 4 | 6 | 6 | 10 | 16 | 19 |
| **GRAND TOTAL** | 241 | 2.9 | 17 | 1 | 1 | 1 | 3 | 6 | 9 | 27 |

Length of Stay by Diagnosis and Operation, United States, 2000

# United States, October 1998–September 1999 Data, by Operation

## 08.3: PTOSIS/LID RETRACT REP. Formerly included in operation group(s) 518.

| Type of Patients | Observed Patients | Avg. Stay | Vari-ance | 10th | 25th | 50th | 75th | 90th | 95th | 99th |
|---|---|---|---|---|---|---|---|---|---|---|
| **1. SINGLE DX** | | | | | | | | | | |
| 0–19 Years | 15 | 1.0 | 0 | 1 | 1 | 1 | 1 | 1 | 1 | 1 |
| 20–34 | 1 | 1.0 | 0 | 1 | 1 | 1 | 1 | 1 | 1 | 1 |
| 35–49 | 0 | | | | | | | | | |
| 50–64 | 7 | 1.5 | <1 | 1 | 1 | 1 | 2 | 2 | 2 | 2 |
| 65+ | 1 | 1.0 | 0 | 1 | 1 | 1 | 1 | 1 | 1 | 1 |
| **2. MULTIPLE DX** | | | | | | | | | | |
| 0–19 Years | 16 | 1.3 | <1 | 1 | 1 | 1 | 1 | 2 | 3 | 5 |
| 20–34 | 2 | 1.6 | <1 | 1 | 1 | 2 | 2 | 2 | 2 | 2 |
| 35–49 | 8 | 1.1 | <1 | 1 | 1 | 1 | 1 | 1 | 2 | 2 |
| 50–64 | 27 | 1.2 | 1 | 1 | 1 | 1 | 1 | 2 | 2 | 2 |
| 65+ | 24 | 1.7 | 5 | 1 | 1 | 1 | 1 | 3 | 4 | 13 |
| **TOTAL SINGLE DX** | 24 | 1.1 | <1 | 1 | 1 | 1 | 1 | 2 | 2 | 2 |
| **TOTAL MULTIPLE DX** | 77 | 1.2 | 1 | 1 | 1 | 1 | 1 | 2 | 2 | 6 |
| **TOTAL** | | | | | | | | | | |
| 0–19 Years | 31 | 1.1 | <1 | 1 | 1 | 1 | 1 | 1 | 2 | 3 |
| 20–34 | 3 | 1.5 | <1 | 1 | 1 | 1 | 2 | 2 | 2 | 2 |
| 35–49 | 8 | 1.1 | <1 | 1 | 1 | 1 | 1 | 1 | 2 | 2 |
| 50–64 | 34 | 1.3 | <1 | 1 | 1 | 1 | 1 | 2 | 2 | 2 |
| 65+ | 25 | 1.7 | 5 | 1 | 1 | 1 | 1 | 3 | 4 | 13 |
| **GRAND TOTAL** | 101 | 1.2 | <1 | 1 | 1 | 1 | 1 | 2 | 2 | 5 |

## 08.4: ENTROPION/ECTROPION REP. Formerly included in operation group(s) 518.

| Type of Patients | Observed Patients | Avg. Stay | Vari-ance | 10th | 25th | 50th | 75th | 90th | 95th | 99th |
|---|---|---|---|---|---|---|---|---|---|---|
| **1. SINGLE DX** | | | | | | | | | | |
| 0–19 Years | 1 | 2.0 | 0 | 2 | 2 | 2 | 2 | 2 | 2 | 2 |
| 20–34 | 0 | | | | | | | | | |
| 35–49 | 1 | 1.0 | 0 | 1 | 1 | 1 | 1 | 1 | 1 | 1 |
| 50–64 | 0 | | | | | | | | | |
| 65+ | 1 | 1.0 | 0 | 1 | 1 | 1 | 1 | 1 | 1 | 1 |
| **2. MULTIPLE DX** | | | | | | | | | | |
| 0–19 Years | 8 | 1.7 | 2 | 1 | 1 | 1 | 1 | 3 | 3 | 5 |
| 20–34 | 7 | 2.7 | 3 | 1 | 2 | 2 | 3 | 7 | 7 | 7 |
| 35–49 | 4 | 4.5 | 2 | 2 | 2 | 5 | 6 | 6 | 6 | 6 |
| 50–64 | 5 | 14.8 | 86 | 2 | 2 | 21 | 21 | 21 | 21 | 21 |
| 65+ | 24 | 9.0 | 77 | 1 | 1 | 5 | 15 | 24 | 24 | 24 |
| **TOTAL SINGLE DX** | 3 | 1.8 | <1 | 1 | 2 | 2 | 2 | 2 | 2 | 2 |
| **TOTAL MULTIPLE DX** | 48 | 6.8 | 63 | 1 | 1 | 3 | 8 | 21 | 24 | 24 |
| **TOTAL** | | | | | | | | | | |
| 0–19 Years | 9 | 1.8 | 2 | 1 | 1 | 1 | 2 | 3 | 6 | 6 |
| 20–34 | 7 | 2.7 | 3 | 1 | 2 | 2 | 3 | 7 | 7 | 7 |
| 35–49 | 5 | 4.0 | 4 | 2 | 2 | 5 | 5 | 6 | 6 | 6 |
| 50–64 | 5 | 14.8 | 86 | 1 | 2 | 21 | 21 | 21 | 21 | 21 |
| 65+ | 25 | 8.8 | 76 | 1 | 1 | 4 | 15 | 24 | 24 | 24 |
| **GRAND TOTAL** | 51 | 6.3 | 59 | 1 | 1 | 2 | 6 | 21 | 24 | 24 |

## 08.5: OTH ADJUST LID POSITION. Formerly included in operation group(s) 518.

| Type of Patients | Observed Patients | Avg. Stay | Vari-ance | 10th | 25th | 50th | 75th | 90th | 95th | 99th |
|---|---|---|---|---|---|---|---|---|---|---|
| **1. SINGLE DX** | | | | | | | | | | |
| 0–19 Years | 8 | 1.7 | 1 | 1 | 1 | 1 | 3 | 3 | 4 | 4 |
| 20–34 | 2 | 1.0 | 0 | 1 | 1 | 1 | 1 | 1 | 1 | 1 |
| 35–49 | 3 | 1.0 | 0 | 1 | 1 | 1 | 1 | 1 | 1 | 1 |
| 50–64 | 1 | 3.0 | 0 | 3 | 3 | 3 | 3 | 3 | 3 | 3 |
| 65+ | 0 | | | | | | | | | |
| **2. MULTIPLE DX** | | | | | | | | | | |
| 0–19 Years | 31 | 2.8 | 13 | 1 | 1 | 2 | 3 | 6 | 8 | 11 |
| 20–34 | 28 | 3.7 | 3 | 1 | 3 | 3 | 5 | 5 | 6 | 12 |
| 35–49 | 34 | 5.6 | 40 | 1 | 2 | 3 | 7 | 11 | 23 | 27 |
| 50–64 | 40 | 7.8 | 74 | 1 | 3 | 4 | 6 | 25 | 25 | 37 |
| 65+ | 54 | 5.9 | 31 | 1 | 2 | 5 | 8 | 10 | 17 | 35 |
| **TOTAL SINGLE DX** | 14 | 1.5 | <1 | 1 | 1 | 1 | 1 | 3 | 4 | 4 |
| **TOTAL MULTIPLE DX** | 187 | 5.4 | 38 | 1 | 2 | 3 | 5 | 11 | 23 | 27 |
| **TOTAL** | | | | | | | | | | |
| 0–19 Years | 39 | 2.6 | 11 | 1 | 1 | 2 | 3 | 6 | 8 | 11 |
| 20–34 | 30 | 3.5 | 4 | 1 | 3 | 3 | 5 | 5 | 6 | 11 |
| 35–49 | 37 | 5.5 | 40 | 1 | 2 | 3 | 7 | 11 | 23 | 27 |
| 50–64 | 41 | 7.7 | 74 | 1 | 3 | 4 | 6 | 25 | 25 | 37 |
| 65+ | 54 | 5.9 | 31 | 1 | 2 | 5 | 8 | 10 | 17 | 35 |
| **GRAND TOTAL** | 201 | 5.1 | 37 | 1 | 1 | 3 | 5 | 11 | 22 | 27 |

## 08.6: EYELID RECONST W GRAFT. Formerly included in operation group(s) 518.

| Type of Patients | Observed Patients | Avg. Stay | Vari-ance | 10th | 25th | 50th | 75th | 90th | 95th | 99th |
|---|---|---|---|---|---|---|---|---|---|---|
| **1. SINGLE DX** | | | | | | | | | | |
| 0–19 Years | 1 | 1.0 | 0 | 1 | 1 | 1 | 1 | 1 | 1 | 1 |
| 20–34 | 1 | 1.0 | 0 | 1 | 1 | 1 | 1 | 1 | 1 | 1 |
| 35–49 | 2 | 1.4 | <1 | 1 | 1 | 1 | 2 | 2 | 2 | 2 |
| 50–64 | 3 | 1.0 | 0 | 1 | 1 | 1 | 1 | 1 | 1 | 1 |
| 65+ | 1 | 2.0 | 0 | 2 | 2 | 2 | 2 | 2 | 2 | 2 |
| **2. MULTIPLE DX** | | | | | | | | | | |
| 0–19 Years | 12 | 3.0 | 7 | 1 | 1 | 2 | 7 | 7 | 7 | 7 |
| 20–34 | 9 | 6.4 | 74 | 1 | 1 | 2 | 5 | 22 | 22 | 22 |
| 35–49 | 6 | 1.6 | <1 | 1 | 1 | 1 | 1 | 3 | 3 | 3 |
| 50–64 | 6 | 6.7 | 30 | 1 | 1 | 4 | 11 | 15 | 15 | 15 |
| 65+ | 18 | 6.1 | 39 | 2 | 2 | 5 | 9 | 9 | 27 | 27 |
| **TOTAL SINGLE DX** | 8 | 1.1 | <1 | 1 | 1 | 1 | 1 | 2 | 2 | 2 |
| **TOTAL MULTIPLE DX** | 51 | 4.5 | 34 | 1 | 1 | 2 | 5 | 11 | 22 | 27 |
| **TOTAL** | | | | | | | | | | |
| 0–19 Years | 13 | 2.7 | 6 | 1 | 1 | 2 | 5 | 7 | 7 | 7 |
| 20–34 | 10 | 4.6 | 56 | 1 | 1 | 1 | 2 | 22 | 22 | 22 |
| 35–49 | 8 | 1.5 | <1 | 1 | 1 | 1 | 4 | 3 | 3 | 3 |
| 50–64 | 9 | 3.1 | 19 | 1 | 2 | 4 | 4 | 11 | 15 | 15 |
| 65+ | 19 | 5.4 | 35 | 1 | 2 | 4 | 9 | 9 | 27 | 27 |
| **GRAND TOTAL** | 59 | 3.5 | 26 | 1 | 1 | 1 | 3 | 9 | 15 | 27 |

Length of Stay by Diagnosis and Operation, United States, 2000

# United States, October 1998–September 1999 Data, by Operation

## 08.7: OTHER EYELID RECONST. Formerly included in operation group(s) 518.

| Type of Patients | Observed Patients | Avg. Stay | Variance | 10th | 25th | 50th | 75th | 90th | 95th | 99th |
|---|---|---|---|---|---|---|---|---|---|---|
| **1. SINGLE DX** | | | | | | | | | | |
| 0–19 Years | 2 | 1.0 | 0 | 1 | 1 | 1 | 1 | 1 | 1 | 1 |
| 20–34 | 2 | | | | | | | | | |
| 35–49 | 1 | 2.0 | 0 | 2 | 2 | 2 | 2 | 2 | 2 | 2 |
| 50–64 | 3 | 1.3 | <1 | 1 | 1 | 1 | 1 | 2 | 2 | 2 |
| 65+ | 0 | | | | | | | | | |
| **2. MULTIPLE DX** | | | | | | | | | | |
| 0–19 Years | 12 | 1.5 | 1 | 1 | 1 | 1 | 1 | 4 | 4 | 5 |
| 20–34 | 7 | 2.3 | 5 | 1 | 2 | 2 | 2 | 5 | 5 | 5 |
| 35–49 | 13 | 3.9 | 29 | 1 | 1 | 1 | 2 | 13 | 18 | 18 |
| 50–64 | 21 | 2.3 | 15 | 1 | 1 | 1 | 2 | 3 | 4 | 24 |
| 65+ | 13 | 5.2 | 40 | 1 | 2 | 2 | 7 | 8 | 24 | 24 |
| **TOTAL SINGLE DX** | 6 | 1.5 | <1 | 1 | 1 | 2 | 2 | 2 | 2 | 2 |
| **TOTAL MULTIPLE DX** | 66 | 3.0 | 18 | 1 | 1 | 2 | 2 | 7 | 13 | 24 |
| **TOTAL** | | | | | | | | | | |
| 0–19 Years | 14 | 1.4 | 1 | 1 | 1 | 1 | 1 | 3 | 4 | 5 |
| 20–34 | 7 | 2.3 | 2 | 1 | 2 | 2 | 2 | 5 | 5 | 5 |
| 35–49 | 14 | 3.5 | 24 | 1 | 1 | 2 | 2 | 13 | 13 | 18 |
| 50–64 | 24 | 2.2 | 14 | 1 | 1 | 1 | 2 | 3 | 4 | 24 |
| 65+ | 13 | 5.2 | 40 | 1 | 2 | 2 | 7 | 8 | 24 | 24 |
| **GRAND TOTAL** | 72 | 2.8 | 17 | 1 | 1 | 2 | 2 | 5 | 13 | 24 |

## 08.8: OTHER REPAIR OF EYELID. Formerly included in operation group(s) 518.

| Type of Patients | Observed Patients | Avg. Stay | Variance | 10th | 25th | 50th | 75th | 90th | 95th | 99th |
|---|---|---|---|---|---|---|---|---|---|---|
| **1. SINGLE DX** | | | | | | | | | | |
| 0–19 Years | 112 | 1.1 | <1 | 1 | 1 | 1 | 1 | 1 | 2 | 3 |
| 20–34 | 14 | 1.2 | <1 | 1 | 1 | 1 | 1 | 1 | 2 | 6 |
| 35–49 | 11 | 1.1 | <1 | 1 | 1 | 1 | 1 | 1 | 2 | 2 |
| 50–64 | 7 | 1.0 | 0 | 1 | 1 | 1 | 1 | 1 | 1 | 1 |
| 65+ | 6 | 1.6 | <1 | 1 | 1 | 1 | 3 | 3 | 3 | 3 |
| **2. MULTIPLE DX** | | | | | | | | | | |
| 0–19 Years | 346 | 3.0 | 11 | 1 | 1 | 2 | 4 | 8 | 8 | 16 |
| 20–34 | 455 | 2.3 | 5 | 1 | 1 | 2 | 3 | 4 | 7 | 11 |
| 35–49 | 409 | 2.7 | 9 | 1 | 1 | 2 | 3 | 5 | 9 | 15 |
| 50–64 | 249 | 3.5 | 16 | 1 | 2 | 2 | 4 | 7 | 9 | 18 |
| 65+ | 688 | 5.2 | 24 | 2 | 2 | 4 | 6 | 10 | 14 | 22 |
| **TOTAL SINGLE DX** | 150 | 1.1 | <1 | 1 | 1 | 1 | 1 | 1 | 2 | 3 |
| **TOTAL MULTIPLE DX** | 2,147 | 3.3 | 14 | 1 | 1 | 2 | 4 | 7 | 10 | 18 |
| **TOTAL** | | | | | | | | | | |
| 0–19 Years | 458 | 2.7 | 10 | 1 | 1 | 1 | 3 | 6 | 8 | 16 |
| 20–34 | 469 | 2.3 | 5 | 1 | 1 | 2 | 3 | 4 | 6 | 11 |
| 35–49 | 409 | 2.7 | 9 | 1 | 1 | 2 | 3 | 5 | 9 | 15 |
| 50–64 | 256 | 3.5 | 16 | 1 | 2 | 2 | 4 | 7 | 8 | 18 |
| 65+ | 694 | 5.2 | 24 | 2 | 2 | 4 | 6 | 10 | 14 | 22 |
| **GRAND TOTAL** | 2,297 | 3.2 | 13 | 1 | 1 | 2 | 4 | 7 | 10 | 18 |

## 08.81: LINEAR REP EYELID LAC. Formerly included in operation group(s) 518.

| Type of Patients | Observed Patients | Avg. Stay | Variance | 10th | 25th | 50th | 75th | 90th | 95th | 99th |
|---|---|---|---|---|---|---|---|---|---|---|
| **1. SINGLE DX** | | | | | | | | | | |
| 0–19 Years | 96 | 1.1 | <1 | 1 | 1 | 1 | 1 | 1 | 2 | 3 |
| 20–34 | 10 | 1.1 | <1 | 1 | 1 | 1 | 1 | 1 | 2 | 3 |
| 35–49 | 4 | 1.0 | 0 | 1 | 1 | 1 | 1 | 1 | 1 | 1 |
| 50–64 | 2 | 1.0 | 0 | 1 | 1 | 1 | 1 | 1 | 1 | 1 |
| 65+ | 2 | 2.4 | 1 | 1 | 1 | 3 | 3 | 3 | 3 | 3 |
| **2. MULTIPLE DX** | | | | | | | | | | |
| 0–19 Years | 314 | 3.0 | 11 | 1 | 1 | 2 | 4 | 7 | 8 | 16 |
| 20–34 | 428 | 2.3 | 5 | 1 | 1 | 2 | 3 | 4 | 7 | 11 |
| 35–49 | 375 | 2.8 | 8 | 1 | 1 | 2 | 3 | 5 | 9 | 15 |
| 50–64 | 227 | 3.8 | 17 | 1 | 2 | 3 | 4 | 7 | 10 | 20 |
| 65+ | 669 | 5.2 | 24 | 1 | 2 | 4 | 6 | 10 | 15 | 22 |
| **TOTAL SINGLE DX** | 114 | 1.1 | <1 | 1 | 1 | 1 | 1 | 1 | 2 | 3 |
| **TOTAL MULTIPLE DX** | 2,013 | 3.4 | 14 | 1 | 1 | 2 | 4 | 7 | 10 | 19 |
| **TOTAL** | | | | | | | | | | |
| 0–19 Years | 410 | 2.8 | 10 | 1 | 1 | 1 | 3 | 6 | 8 | 16 |
| 20–34 | 438 | 2.3 | 5 | 1 | 1 | 2 | 3 | 4 | 7 | 11 |
| 35–49 | 379 | 2.7 | 8 | 1 | 1 | 2 | 3 | 5 | 9 | 15 |
| 50–64 | 229 | 3.8 | 17 | 1 | 2 | 3 | 4 | 7 | 10 | 20 |
| 65+ | 671 | 5.2 | 24 | 1 | 2 | 4 | 6 | 10 | 15 | 22 |
| **GRAND TOTAL** | 2,127 | 3.3 | 13 | 1 | 1 | 2 | 4 | 7 | 10 | 18 |

## 08.9: OTHER EYELID OPERATIONS. Formerly included in operation group(s) 518, 532.

| Type of Patients | Observed Patients | Avg. Stay | Variance | 10th | 25th | 50th | 75th | 90th | 95th | 99th |
|---|---|---|---|---|---|---|---|---|---|---|
| **1. SINGLE DX** | | | | | | | | | | |
| 0–19 Years | 3 | 3.1 | 1 | 1 | 3 | 3 | 4 | 4 | 4 | 4 |
| 20–34 | 1 | 2.0 | 0 | 2 | 2 | 2 | 2 | 2 | 2 | 2 |
| 35–49 | 0 | | | | | | | | | |
| 50–64 | 1 | 1.0 | 0 | 1 | 1 | 1 | 1 | 1 | 1 | 1 |
| 65+ | 0 | | | | | | | | | |
| **2. MULTIPLE DX** | | | | | | | | | | |
| 0–19 Years | 8 | 11.3 | 630 | 2 | 2 | 2 | 4 | 18 | 86 | 86 |
| 20–34 | 0 | | | | | | | | | |
| 35–49 | 3 | 22.5 | <1 | 22 | 22 | 22 | 22 | 24 | 24 | 24 |
| 50–64 | 1 | 6.0 | 0 | 6 | 6 | 6 | 6 | 6 | 6 | 6 |
| 65+ | 4 | 12.6 | 159 | 5 | 5 | 5 | 10 | 35 | 35 | 35 |
| **TOTAL SINGLE DX** | 5 | 2.7 | 1 | 1 | 2 | 3 | 4 | 4 | 4 | 4 |
| **TOTAL MULTIPLE DX** | 16 | 11.4 | 274 | 2 | 4 | 6 | 9 | 24 | 35 | 86 |
| **TOTAL** | | | | | | | | | | |
| 0–19 Years | 11 | 9.4 | 492 | 2 | 2 | 3 | 4 | 4 | 86 | 86 |
| 20–34 | 1 | 2.0 | 0 | 2 | 2 | 2 | 2 | 2 | 2 | 2 |
| 35–49 | 3 | 22.5 | <1 | 22 | 22 | 22 | 22 | 24 | 24 | 24 |
| 50–64 | 2 | 5.8 | 1 | 5 | 5 | 5 | 6 | 6 | 6 | 6 |
| 65+ | 4 | 12.6 | 159 | 5 | 5 | 5 | 10 | 35 | 35 | 35 |
| **GRAND TOTAL** | 21 | 10.2 | 246 | 2 | 3 | 6 | 6 | 22 | 35 | 86 |

# United States, October 1998–September 1999 Data, by Operation

## 09.0: LACRIMAL GLAND INCISION. Formerly included in operation group(s) 519.

| Type of Patients | Observed Patients | Avg. Stay | Vari-ance | 10th | 25th | 50th | 75th | 90th | 95th | 99th |
|---|---|---|---|---|---|---|---|---|---|---|
| **1. SINGLE DX** | | | | | | | | | | |
| 0–19 Years | 0 | | | | | | | | | |
| 20–34 | 0 | | | | | | | | | |
| 35–49 | 0 | | | | | | | | | |
| 50–64 | 0 | | | | | | | | | |
| 65+ | 0 | | | | | | | | | |
| **2. MULTIPLE DX** | | | | | | | | | | |
| 0–19 Years | 2 | 2.6 | <1 | 2 | 2 | 3 | 3 | 3 | 3 | 3 |
| 20–34 | 1 | 1.0 | 0 | 1 | 1 | 1 | 1 | 1 | 1 | 1 |
| 35–49 | 0 | | | | | | | | | |
| 50–64 | 0 | | | | | | | | | |
| 65+ | 1 | 2.0 | 0 | 2 | 2 | 2 | 2 | 2 | 2 | 2 |
| **TOTAL SINGLE DX** | 0 | | | | | | | | | |
| **TOTAL MULTIPLE DX** | 4 | 2.2 | <1 | 2 | 2 | 2 | 3 | 3 | 3 | 3 |
| **TOTAL** | | | | | | | | | | |
| 0–19 Years | 2 | 2.6 | <1 | 2 | 2 | 3 | 3 | 3 | 3 | 3 |
| 20–34 | 1 | 1.0 | 0 | 1 | 1 | 1 | 1 | 1 | 1 | 1 |
| 35–49 | 0 | | | | | | | | | |
| 50–64 | 0 | | | | | | | | | |
| 65+ | 1 | 2.0 | 0 | 2 | 2 | 2 | 2 | 2 | 2 | 2 |
| **GRAND TOTAL** | 4 | 2.2 | <1 | 2 | 2 | 2 | 3 | 3 | 3 | 3 |

## 09.1: LACRIMAL SYSTEM DXTIC PX. Formerly included in operation group(s) 519, 532.

| Type of Patients | Observed Patients | Avg. Stay | Vari-ance | 10th | 25th | 50th | 75th | 90th | 95th | 99th |
|---|---|---|---|---|---|---|---|---|---|---|
| **1. SINGLE DX** | | | | | | | | | | |
| 0–19 Years | 0 | | | | | | | | | |
| 20–34 | 0 | | | | | | | | | |
| 35–49 | 0 | | | | | | | | | |
| 50–64 | 0 | | | | | | | | | |
| 65+ | 0 | | | | | | | | | |
| **2. MULTIPLE DX** | | | | | | | | | | |
| 0–19 Years | 1 | 9.0 | 0 | 9 | 9 | 9 | 9 | 9 | 9 | 9 |
| 20–34 | 2 | 12.7 | 10 | 10 | 10 | 15 | 15 | 15 | 15 | 15 |
| 35–49 | 2 | 13.3 | 1 | 12 | 12 | 14 | 14 | 14 | 14 | 14 |
| 50–64 | 2 | 5.5 | <1 | 4 | 6 | 6 | 6 | 6 | 6 | 6 |
| 65+ | 2 | 1.4 | <1 | 1 | 1 | 1 | 2 | 2 | 2 | 2 |
| **TOTAL SINGLE DX** | 0 | | | | | | | | | |
| **TOTAL MULTIPLE DX** | 9 | 8.0 | 22 | 1 | 4 | 6 | 12 | 14 | 15 | 15 |
| **TOTAL** | | | | | | | | | | |
| 0–19 Years | 1 | 9.0 | 0 | 9 | 9 | 9 | 9 | 9 | 9 | 9 |
| 20–34 | 2 | 12.7 | 10 | 10 | 10 | 15 | 15 | 15 | 15 | 15 |
| 35–49 | 2 | 13.3 | 1 | 12 | 12 | 14 | 14 | 14 | 14 | 14 |
| 50–64 | 2 | 5.5 | <1 | 4 | 6 | 6 | 6 | 6 | 6 | 6 |
| 65+ | 2 | 1.4 | <1 | 1 | 1 | 1 | 2 | 2 | 2 | 2 |
| **GRAND TOTAL** | 9 | 8.0 | 22 | 1 | 4 | 6 | 12 | 14 | 15 | 15 |

## 09.2: LACRIMAL GLAND LES EXC. Formerly included in operation group(s) 519.

| Type of Patients | Observed Patients | Avg. Stay | Vari-ance | 10th | 25th | 50th | 75th | 90th | 95th | 99th |
|---|---|---|---|---|---|---|---|---|---|---|
| **1. SINGLE DX** | | | | | | | | | | |
| 0–19 Years | 2 | 2.2 | 0 | 1 | 1 | 3 | 3 | 3 | 3 | 3 |
| 20–34 | 1 | 1.0 | 0 | 1 | 1 | 1 | 1 | 1 | 1 | 1 |
| 35–49 | 2 | 1.0 | 0 | 1 | 1 | 1 | 1 | 1 | 1 | 1 |
| 50–64 | 1 | 1.0 | 0 | 1 | 1 | 1 | 1 | 1 | 1 | 1 |
| 65+ | 0 | | | | | | | | | |
| **2. MULTIPLE DX** | | | | | | | | | | |
| 0–19 Years | 2 | 1.3 | <1 | 1 | 1 | 1 | 1 | 2 | 2 | 2 |
| 20–34 | 0 | | | | | | | | | |
| 35–49 | 2 | 3.0 | 0 | 3 | 3 | 3 | 3 | 3 | 3 | 3 |
| 50–64 | 1 | 1.0 | 0 | 1 | 1 | 1 | 1 | 1 | 1 | 1 |
| 65+ | 1 | 2.0 | 0 | 2 | 2 | 2 | 2 | 2 | 2 | 2 |
| **TOTAL SINGLE DX** | 6 | 1.0 | <1 | 1 | 1 | 1 | 1 | 1 | 1 | 1 |
| **TOTAL MULTIPLE DX** | 6 | 2.2 | <1 | 1 | 1 | 2 | 3 | 3 | 3 | 3 |
| **TOTAL** | | | | | | | | | | |
| 0–19 Years | 4 | 1.5 | <1 | 1 | 1 | 1 | 2 | 3 | 3 | 3 |
| 20–34 | 1 | 1.0 | 0 | 1 | 1 | 1 | 1 | 1 | 1 | 1 |
| 35–49 | 4 | 1.3 | <1 | 1 | 3 | 3 | 3 | 3 | 3 | 3 |
| 50–64 | 2 | 1.0 | <1 | 1 | 1 | 1 | 1 | 1 | 1 | 1 |
| 65+ | 1 | 2.0 | 0 | 2 | 2 | 2 | 2 | 2 | 2 | 2 |
| **GRAND TOTAL** | 12 | 1.2 | <1 | 1 | 1 | 1 | 1 | 2 | 3 | 3 |

## 09.3: OTHER LACRIMAL GLAND OPS. Formerly included in operation group(s) 519.

| Type of Patients | Observed Patients | Avg. Stay | Vari-ance | 10th | 25th | 50th | 75th | 90th | 95th | 99th |
|---|---|---|---|---|---|---|---|---|---|---|
| **1. SINGLE DX** | | | | | | | | | | |
| 0–19 Years | 0 | | | | | | | | | |
| 20–34 | 0 | | | | | | | | | |
| 35–49 | 0 | | | | | | | | | |
| 50–64 | 0 | | | | | | | | | |
| 65+ | 0 | | | | | | | | | |
| **2. MULTIPLE DX** | | | | | | | | | | |
| 0–19 Years | 0 | | | | | | | | | |
| 20–34 | 0 | | | | | | | | | |
| 35–49 | 0 | | | | | | | | | |
| 50–64 | 0 | | | | | | | | | |
| 65+ | 0 | | | | | | | | | |
| **TOTAL SINGLE DX** | 0 | | | | | | | | | |
| **TOTAL MULTIPLE DX** | 0 | | | | | | | | | |
| **TOTAL** | | | | | | | | | | |
| 0–19 Years | 0 | | | | | | | | | |
| 20–34 | 0 | | | | | | | | | |
| 35–49 | 0 | | | | | | | | | |
| 50–64 | 0 | | | | | | | | | |
| 65+ | 0 | | | | | | | | | |
| **GRAND TOTAL** | 0 | | | | | | | | | |

Length of Stay by Diagnosis and Operation, United States, 2000

# United States, October 1998–September 1999 Data, by Operation

## 09.4: LACRIMAL PASSAGE MANIP. Formerly included in operation group(s) 532.

| Type of Patients | Observed Patients | Avg. Stay | Vari-ance | Percentiles | | | | | | |
|---|---|---|---|---|---|---|---|---|---|---|
| | | | | 10th | 25th | 50th | 75th | 90th | 95th | 99th |
| **1. SINGLE DX** | | | | | | | | | | |
| 0–19 Years | 87 | 1.0 | <1 | 1 | 1 | 1 | 1 | 1 | 1 | 1 |
| 20–34 | 0 | | | | | | | | | |
| 35–49 | 1 | 1.0 | 0 | 1 | 1 | 1 | 1 | 1 | 1 | 1 |
| 50–64 | 0 | | | | | | | | | |
| 65+ | 0 | | | | | | | | | |
| **2. MULTIPLE DX** | | | | | | | | | | |
| 0–19 Years | 86 | 4.0 | 26 | 1 | 1 | 2 | 5 | 7 | 16 | 23 |
| 20–34 | 1 | 10.0 | 0 | 10 | 10 | 10 | 10 | 10 | 10 | 10 |
| 35–49 | 6 | 1.7 | 3 | 1 | 1 | 1 | 1 | 5 | 5 | 5 |
| 50–64 | 1 | 8.0 | 0 | 8 | 8 | 8 | 8 | 8 | 8 | 8 |
| 65+ | 3 | 3.2 | <1 | 3 | 3 | 3 | 3 | 3 | 6 | 6 |
| **TOTAL SINGLE DX** | 88 | 1.0 | <1 | 1 | 1 | 1 | 1 | 1 | 1 | 1 |
| **TOTAL MULTIPLE DX** | 97 | 3.9 | 22 | 1 | 1 | 3 | 4 | 7 | 10 | 23 |
| **TOTAL** | | | | | | | | | | |
| 0–19 Years | 173 | 1.9 | 10 | 1 | 1 | 1 | 1 | 4 | 6 | 23 |
| 20–34 | 1 | 10.0 | 0 | 10 | 10 | 10 | 10 | 10 | 10 | 10 |
| 35–49 | 7 | 1.6 | 2 | 1 | 1 | 1 | 1 | 5 | 5 | 5 |
| 50–64 | 1 | 8.0 | 0 | 8 | 8 | 8 | 8 | 8 | 8 | 8 |
| 65+ | 3 | 3.2 | <1 | 3 | 3 | 3 | 3 | 3 | 6 | 6 |
| **GRAND TOTAL** | 185 | 2.0 | 9 | 1 | 1 | 1 | 1 | 4 | 6 | 23 |

## 09.5: INC LACRIMAL SAC/PASSG. Formerly included in operation group(s) 519.

| Type of Patients | Observed Patients | Avg. Stay | Vari-ance | Percentiles | | | | | | |
|---|---|---|---|---|---|---|---|---|---|---|
| | | | | 10th | 25th | 50th | 75th | 90th | 95th | 99th |
| **1. SINGLE DX** | | | | | | | | | | |
| 0–19 Years | 2 | 1.2 | <1 | 1 | 1 | 1 | 1 | 1 | 1 | 1 |
| 20–34 | 0 | | | | | | | | | |
| 35–49 | 3 | 1.9 | <1 | 1 | 1 | 2 | 3 | 3 | 3 | 3 |
| 50–64 | 1 | 1.0 | 0 | 1 | 1 | 1 | 1 | 1 | 1 | 1 |
| 65+ | 3 | 1.7 | 1 | 1 | 1 | 1 | 3 | 3 | 3 | 3 |
| **2. MULTIPLE DX** | | | | | | | | | | |
| 0–19 Years | 20 | 3.5 | 3 | 3 | 3 | 3 | 4 | 6 | 9 | 11 |
| 20–34 | 3 | 2.4 | 2 | 1 | 1 | 2 | 3 | 4 | 4 | 4 |
| 35–49 | 8 | 3.6 | 4 | 1 | 3 | 4 | 4 | 8 | 8 | 8 |
| 50–64 | 1 | 1.0 | 0 | 1 | 1 | 1 | 1 | 1 | 1 | 1 |
| 65+ | 7 | 4.1 | 15 | 2 | 3 | 3 | 3 | 6 | 18 | 18 |
| **TOTAL SINGLE DX** | 9 | 1.5 | <1 | 1 | 1 | 1 | 2 | 3 | 3 | 3 |
| **TOTAL MULTIPLE DX** | 39 | 3.5 | 4 | 2 | 3 | 3 | 3 | 6 | 9 | 11 |
| **TOTAL** | | | | | | | | | | |
| 0–19 Years | 22 | 3.3 | 3 | 1 | 1 | 3 | 3 | 3 | 9 | 9 |
| 20–34 | 3 | 2.4 | 2 | 1 | 1 | 2 | 2 | 4 | 4 | 4 |
| 35–49 | 11 | 3.1 | 4 | 1 | 2 | 3 | 3 | 6 | 8 | 8 |
| 50–64 | 2 | 1.0 | 0 | 1 | 1 | 1 | 1 | 1 | 1 | 1 |
| 65+ | 10 | 3.3 | 11 | 1 | 3 | 3 | 3 | 6 | 18 | 18 |
| **GRAND TOTAL** | 48 | 3.1 | 4 | 1 | 2 | 3 | 3 | 5 | 8 | 11 |

## 09.6: LACRIMAL SAC/PASSAGE EXC. Formerly included in operation group(s) 519.

| Type of Patients | Observed Patients | Avg. Stay | Vari-ance | Percentiles | | | | | | |
|---|---|---|---|---|---|---|---|---|---|---|
| | | | | 10th | 25th | 50th | 75th | 90th | 95th | 99th |
| **1. SINGLE DX** | | | | | | | | | | |
| 0–19 Years | 0 | | | | | | | | | |
| 20–34 | 0 | | | | | | | | | |
| 35–49 | 0 | | | | | | | | | |
| 50–64 | 0 | | | | | | | | | |
| 65+ | 0 | | | | | | | | | |
| **2. MULTIPLE DX** | | | | | | | | | | |
| 0–19 Years | 3 | 3.5 | 5 | 1 | 1 | 4 | 6 | 6 | 6 | 6 |
| 20–34 | 1 | 1.0 | 0 | 1 | 1 | 1 | 1 | 1 | 1 | 1 |
| 35–49 | 0 | | | | | | | | | |
| 50–64 | 0 | | | | | | | | | |
| 65+ | 4 | 2.7 | 1 | 2 | 2 | 2 | 4 | 4 | 5 | 5 |
| **TOTAL SINGLE DX** | 0 | | | | | | | | | |
| **TOTAL MULTIPLE DX** | 8 | 2.6 | 2 | 1 | 2 | 2 | 4 | 5 | 6 | 6 |
| **TOTAL** | | | | | | | | | | |
| 0–19 Years | 3 | 3.5 | 5 | 1 | 1 | 4 | 6 | 6 | 6 | 6 |
| 20–34 | 1 | 1.0 | 0 | 1 | 1 | 1 | 1 | 1 | 1 | 1 |
| 35–49 | 0 | | | | | | | | | |
| 50–64 | 0 | | | | | | | | | |
| 65+ | 4 | 2.7 | 1 | 2 | 2 | 2 | 4 | 4 | 5 | 5 |
| **GRAND TOTAL** | 8 | 2.6 | 2 | 1 | 2 | 2 | 4 | 5 | 6 | 6 |

## 09.7: CANALICULUS/PUNCTUM REP. Formerly included in operation group(s) 519.

| Type of Patients | Observed Patients | Avg. Stay | Vari-ance | Percentiles | | | | | | |
|---|---|---|---|---|---|---|---|---|---|---|
| | | | | 10th | 25th | 50th | 75th | 90th | 95th | 99th |
| **1. SINGLE DX** | | | | | | | | | | |
| 0–19 Years | 17 | 1.1 | <1 | 1 | 1 | 1 | 1 | 1 | 1 | 4 |
| 20–34 | 2 | 1.0 | 0 | 1 | 1 | 1 | 1 | 1 | 1 | 1 |
| 35–49 | 1 | 1.0 | 0 | 1 | 1 | 1 | 1 | 1 | 1 | 1 |
| 50–64 | 1 | 1.0 | 0 | 1 | 1 | 1 | 1 | 1 | 1 | 1 |
| 65+ | 0 | | | | | | | | | |
| **2. MULTIPLE DX** | | | | | | | | | | |
| 0–19 Years | 25 | 1.2 | <1 | 1 | 1 | 1 | 1 | 2 | 2 | 3 |
| 20–34 | 9 | 3.2 | 5 | 1 | 2 | 3 | 3 | 7 | 7 | 7 |
| 35–49 | 9 | 1.6 | <1 | 1 | 1 | 2 | 2 | 2 | 3 | 3 |
| 50–64 | 2 | 2.0 | 0 | 2 | 2 | 2 | 2 | 2 | 2 | 2 |
| 65+ | 1 | 3.0 | 0 | 3 | 3 | 3 | 3 | 3 | 3 | 3 |
| **TOTAL SINGLE DX** | 21 | 1.1 | <1 | 1 | 1 | 1 | 1 | 1 | 1 | 4 |
| **TOTAL MULTIPLE DX** | 46 | 2.0 | 3 | 1 | 1 | 1 | 3 | 3 | 7 | 7 |
| **TOTAL** | | | | | | | | | | |
| 0–19 Years | 42 | 1.2 | <1 | 1 | 1 | 1 | 1 | 2 | 2 | 4 |
| 20–34 | 11 | 3.1 | 5 | 1 | 3 | 3 | 3 | 7 | 7 | 7 |
| 35–49 | 10 | 1.5 | <1 | 1 | 1 | 1 | 2 | 3 | 3 | 3 |
| 50–64 | 3 | 1.4 | <1 | 1 | 1 | 2 | 3 | 3 | 3 | 3 |
| 65+ | 1 | 3.0 | 0 | 3 | 3 | 3 | 3 | 3 | 3 | 3 |
| **GRAND TOTAL** | 67 | 1.7 | 2 | 1 | 1 | 1 | 2 | 3 | 7 | 7 |

Length of Stay by Diagnosis and Operation, United States, 2000

# United States, October 1998–September 1999 Data, by Operation

## 09.8: NL FISTULIZATION. Formerly included in operation group(s) 519.

| Type of Patients | Observed Patients | Avg. Stay | Variance | 10th | 25th | 50th | 75th | 90th | 95th | 99th |
|---|---|---|---|---|---|---|---|---|---|---|
| **1. SINGLE DX** | | | | | | | | | | |
| 0–19 Years | 2 | 5.2 | 0 | 1 | 1 | 7 | 7 | 7 | 7 | 7 |
| 20–34 | 1 | 3.0 | 0 | 3 | 3 | 3 | 3 | 3 | 3 | 3 |
| 35–49 | 0 | | | | | | | | | |
| 50–64 | 1 | 1.0 | 0 | 1 | 1 | 1 | 1 | 1 | 1 | 1 |
| 65+ | 4 | 1.0 | 0 | 1 | 1 | 1 | 1 | 1 | 1 | 1 |
| **2. MULTIPLE DX** | | | | | | | | | | |
| 0–19 Years | 3 | 1.9 | <1 | 1 | 1 | 2 | 2 | 3 | 3 | 3 |
| 20–34 | 3 | 3.0 | 3 | 2 | 2 | 2 | 5 | 5 | 5 | 5 |
| 35–49 | 8 | 2.1 | 2 | 1 | 1 | 1 | 3 | 4 | 4 | 5 |
| 50–64 | 8 | 2.9 | 10 | 1 | 1 | 1 | 7 | 9 | 9 | 9 |
| 65+ | 31 | 2.3 | 13 | 1 | 1 | 3 | 3 | 4 | 4 | 33 |
| **TOTAL SINGLE DX** | 8 | 1.5 | 2 | 1 | 1 | 1 | 1 | 3 | 3 | 7 |
| **TOTAL MULTIPLE DX** | 53 | 2.3 | 9 | 1 | 1 | 1 | 3 | 4 | 7 | 9 |
| **TOTAL** | | | | | | | | | | |
| 0–19 Years | 5 | 2.6 | 4 | 1 | 1 | 2 | 3 | 7 | 7 | 7 |
| 20–34 | 4 | 3.0 | 1 | 2 | 2 | 3 | 3 | 5 | 5 | 5 |
| 35–49 | 8 | 2.1 | 2 | 1 | 1 | 1 | 3 | 4 | 4 | 5 |
| 50–64 | 9 | 2.7 | 9 | 1 | 1 | 1 | 2 | 9 | 9 | 9 |
| 65+ | 35 | 2.1 | 11 | 1 | 1 | 1 | 2 | 4 | 4 | 5 |
| **GRAND TOTAL** | 61 | 2.2 | 8 | 1 | 1 | 1 | 3 | 4 | 5 | 9 |

## 09.9: OTH LACRIMAL SYST OPS. Formerly included in operation group(s) 519.

| Type of Patients | Observed Patients | Avg. Stay | Variance | 10th | 25th | 50th | 75th | 90th | 95th | 99th |
|---|---|---|---|---|---|---|---|---|---|---|
| **1. SINGLE DX** | | | | | | | | | | |
| 0–19 Years | 3 | 1.0 | 0 | 1 | 1 | 1 | 1 | 1 | 1 | 1 |
| 20–34 | 0 | | | | | | | | | |
| 35–49 | 0 | | | | | | | | | |
| 50–64 | 0 | | | | | | | | | |
| 65+ | 0 | | | | | | | | | |
| **2. MULTIPLE DX** | | | | | | | | | | |
| 0–19 Years | 3 | 4.2 | 19 | 1 | 1 | 1 | 9 | 9 | 9 | 9 |
| 20–34 | 2 | 1.7 | <1 | 1 | 1 | 2 | 2 | 2 | 2 | 2 |
| 35–49 | 0 | | | | | | | | | |
| 50–64 | 0 | | | | | | | | | |
| 65+ | 1 | 1.0 | 0 | 1 | 1 | 1 | 1 | 1 | 1 | 1 |
| **TOTAL SINGLE DX** | 3 | 1.0 | 0 | 1 | 1 | 1 | 1 | 1 | 1 | 1 |
| **TOTAL MULTIPLE DX** | 6 | 2.8 | 10 | 1 | 1 | 1 | 2 | 9 | 9 | 9 |
| **TOTAL** | | | | | | | | | | |
| 0–19 Years | 6 | 1.4 | 3 | 1 | 1 | 1 | 1 | 2 | 2 | 9 |
| 20–34 | 2 | 1.7 | <1 | 1 | 1 | 2 | 2 | 2 | 2 | 2 |
| 35–49 | 0 | | | | | | | | | |
| 50–64 | 0 | | | | | | | | | |
| 65+ | 1 | 1.0 | 0 | 1 | 1 | 1 | 1 | 1 | 1 | 1 |
| **GRAND TOTAL** | 9 | 1.4 | 3 | 1 | 1 | 1 | 1 | 2 | 2 | 9 |

## 10.0: INC/RMVL FB-CONJUNCTIVA. Formerly included in operation group(s) 520.

| Type of Patients | Observed Patients | Avg. Stay | Variance | 10th | 25th | 50th | 75th | 90th | 95th | 99th |
|---|---|---|---|---|---|---|---|---|---|---|
| **1. SINGLE DX** | | | | | | | | | | |
| 0–19 Years | 0 | | | | | | | | | |
| 20–34 | 0 | | | | | | | | | |
| 35–49 | 0 | | | | | | | | | |
| 50–64 | 1 | 4.0 | 0 | 4 | 4 | 4 | 4 | 4 | 4 | 4 |
| 65+ | 0 | | | | | | | | | |
| **2. MULTIPLE DX** | | | | | | | | | | |
| 0–19 Years | 3 | 2.4 | <1 | 1 | 2 | 3 | 3 | 3 | 3 | 3 |
| 20–34 | 1 | 3.0 | 0 | 3 | 3 | 3 | 3 | 3 | 3 | 3 |
| 35–49 | 2 | 2.0 | 0 | 2 | 2 | 2 | 2 | 2 | 2 | 2 |
| 50–64 | 1 | 1.0 | 0 | 1 | 1 | 1 | 1 | 1 | 1 | 1 |
| 65+ | 0 | | | | | | | | | |
| **TOTAL SINGLE DX** | 1 | 4.0 | 0 | 4 | 4 | 4 | 4 | 4 | 4 | 4 |
| **TOTAL MULTIPLE DX** | 7 | 2.3 | <1 | 1 | 2 | 3 | 3 | 3 | 3 | 3 |
| **TOTAL** | | | | | | | | | | |
| 0–19 Years | 3 | 2.4 | <1 | 1 | 2 | 3 | 3 | 3 | 3 | 3 |
| 20–34 | 1 | 3.0 | 0 | 3 | 3 | 3 | 3 | 3 | 3 | 3 |
| 35–49 | 2 | 2.0 | 0 | 2 | 2 | 2 | 2 | 2 | 2 | 2 |
| 50–64 | 2 | 1.9 | 2 | 1 | 1 | 1 | 4 | 4 | 4 | 4 |
| 65+ | 0 | | | | | | | | | |
| **GRAND TOTAL** | 8 | 2.4 | <1 | 1 | 2 | 3 | 3 | 3 | 3 | 3 |

## 10.1: CONJUNCTIVA INCISION NEC. Formerly included in operation group(s) 520.

| Type of Patients | Observed Patients | Avg. Stay | Variance | 10th | 25th | 50th | 75th | 90th | 95th | 99th |
|---|---|---|---|---|---|---|---|---|---|---|
| **1. SINGLE DX** | | | | | | | | | | |
| 0–19 Years | 3 | 2.2 | 1 | 1 | 1 | 3 | 3 | 3 | 3 | 3 |
| 20–34 | 0 | | | | | | | | | |
| 35–49 | 2 | 4.0 | 0 | 4 | 4 | 4 | 4 | 4 | 4 | 4 |
| 50–64 | 2 | 4.0 | 0 | 4 | 4 | 4 | 4 | 4 | 4 | 4 |
| 65+ | 1 | 4.0 | 0 | 4 | 4 | 4 | 4 | 4 | 4 | 4 |
| **2. MULTIPLE DX** | | | | | | | | | | |
| 0–19 Years | 6 | 4.0 | 9 | 2 | 3 | 3 | 3 | 11 | 11 | 11 |
| 20–34 | 2 | 1.7 | <1 | 1 | 1 | 2 | 2 | 2 | 2 | 2 |
| 35–49 | 9 | 3.9 | 15 | 1 | 2 | 3 | 5 | 5 | 17 | 17 |
| 50–64 | 4 | 4.4 | <1 | 4 | 4 | 4 | 5 | 5 | 5 | 5 |
| 65+ | 5 | 2.9 | 3 | 1 | 1 | 4 | 4 | 4 | 5 | 5 |
| **TOTAL SINGLE DX** | 8 | 3.2 | 1 | 1 | 3 | 4 | 4 | 4 | 4 | 4 |
| **TOTAL MULTIPLE DX** | 26 | 3.6 | 7 | 1 | 2 | 3 | 4 | 5 | 11 | 17 |
| **TOTAL** | | | | | | | | | | |
| 0–19 Years | 9 | 3.5 | 7 | 1 | 3 | 3 | 3 | 11 | 11 | 11 |
| 20–34 | 2 | 1.7 | <1 | 1 | 1 | 2 | 2 | 2 | 2 | 2 |
| 35–49 | 11 | 3.9 | 13 | 1 | 2 | 4 | 5 | 5 | 17 | 17 |
| 50–64 | 6 | 4.3 | <1 | 4 | 4 | 4 | 5 | 5 | 5 | 5 |
| 65+ | 6 | 3.1 | 2 | 1 | 1 | 4 | 4 | 4 | 5 | 5 |
| **GRAND TOTAL** | 34 | 3.5 | 6 | 1 | 2 | 3 | 4 | 5 | 5 | 17 |

**United States, October 1998–September 1999 Data, by Operation**

## 10.2: CONJUNCTIVA DXTIC PX. Formerly included in operation group(s) 520, 532.

| Type of Patients | Observed Patients | Avg. Stay | Variance | 10th | 25th | 50th | 75th | 90th | 95th | 99th |
|---|---|---|---|---|---|---|---|---|---|---|
| **1. SINGLE DX** | | | | | | | | | | |
| 0–19 Years | 0 | | | | | | | | | |
| 20–34 | 0 | | | | | | | | | |
| 35–49 | 0 | | | | | | | | | |
| 50–64 | 0 | | | | | | | | | |
| 65+ | 0 | | | | | | | | | |
| **2. MULTIPLE DX** | | | | | | | | | | |
| 0–19 Years | 6 | 15.6 | 151 | 2 | 2 | 8 | 8 | 31 | 32 | 32 |
| 20–34 | 1 | 2.0 | 0 | 2 | 2 | 2 | 2 | 2 | 2 | 2 |
| 35–49 | 0 | | | | | | | | | |
| 50–64 | 1 | 15.0 | 0 | 15 | 15 | 15 | 15 | 15 | 15 | 15 |
| 65+ | 2 | 7.4 | 34 | 5 | 5 | 5 | 5 | 20 | 20 | 20 |
| **TOTAL SINGLE DX** | 0 | | | | | | | | | |
| **TOTAL MULTIPLE DX** | 10 | 13.1 | 122 | 2 | 5 | 8 | 22 | 31 | 32 | 32 |
| **TOTAL** | | | | | | | | | | |
| 0–19 Years | 6 | 15.6 | 151 | 2 | 2 | 8 | 8 | 31 | 32 | 32 |
| 20–34 | 1 | 2.0 | 0 | 2 | 2 | 2 | 2 | 2 | 2 | 2 |
| 35–49 | 0 | | | | | | | | | |
| 50–64 | 1 | 15.0 | 0 | 15 | 15 | 15 | 15 | 15 | 15 | 15 |
| 65+ | 2 | 7.4 | 34 | 5 | 5 | 5 | 5 | 20 | 20 | 20 |
| **GRAND TOTAL** | 10 | 13.1 | 122 | 2 | 5 | 8 | 22 | 31 | 32 | 32 |

## 10.3: EXC/DESTR CONJUNCT LES. Formerly included in operation group(s) 520.

| Type of Patients | Observed Patients | Avg. Stay | Variance | 10th | 25th | 50th | 75th | 90th | 95th | 99th |
|---|---|---|---|---|---|---|---|---|---|---|
| **1. SINGLE DX** | | | | | | | | | | |
| 0–19 Years | 3 | 1.4 | <1 | 1 | 1 | 1 | 1 | 2 | 2 | 2 |
| 20–34 | 1 | 1.0 | 0 | 1 | 1 | 1 | 1 | 1 | 1 | 1 |
| 35–49 | 0 | | | | | | | | | |
| 50–64 | 1 | 1.0 | 0 | 1 | 1 | 1 | 1 | 1 | 1 | 1 |
| 65+ | 0 | | | | | | | | | |
| **2. MULTIPLE DX** | | | | | | | | | | |
| 0–19 Years | 2 | 21.2 | 23 | 17 | 17 | 17 | 26 | 26 | 26 | 26 |
| 20–34 | 0 | | | | | | | | | |
| 35–49 | 1 | 1.0 | 0 | 1 | 1 | 1 | 1 | 1 | 1 | 1 |
| 50–64 | 1 | 3.0 | 0 | 3 | 3 | 3 | 3 | 3 | 3 | 3 |
| 65+ | 5 | 9.9 | 49 | 1 | 4 | 7 | 13 | 19 | 19 | 19 |
| **TOTAL SINGLE DX** | 5 | 1.2 | <1 | 1 | 1 | 1 | 1 | 2 | 2 | 2 |
| **TOTAL MULTIPLE DX** | 9 | 12.7 | 87 | 1 | 3 | 13 | 19 | 26 | 26 | 26 |
| **TOTAL** | | | | | | | | | | |
| 0–19 Years | 5 | 15.5 | 104 | 1 | 2 | 17 | 26 | 26 | 26 | 26 |
| 20–34 | 1 | 1.0 | 0 | 1 | 1 | 1 | 1 | 1 | 1 | 1 |
| 35–49 | 1 | 1.0 | 0 | 1 | 1 | 1 | 1 | 1 | 1 | 1 |
| 50–64 | 2 | 1.9 | 1 | 1 | 1 | 1 | 3 | 3 | 3 | 3 |
| 65+ | 5 | 9.9 | 49 | 1 | 4 | 7 | 13 | 19 | 19 | 19 |
| **GRAND TOTAL** | 14 | 10.0 | 90 | 1 | 1 | 7 | 17 | 26 | 26 | 26 |

## 10.4: CONJUNCTIVOPLASTY. Formerly included in operation group(s) 520.

| Type of Patients | Observed Patients | Avg. Stay | Variance | 10th | 25th | 50th | 75th | 90th | 95th | 99th |
|---|---|---|---|---|---|---|---|---|---|---|
| **1. SINGLE DX** | | | | | | | | | | |
| 0–19 Years | 1 | 1.0 | 0 | 1 | 1 | 1 | 1 | 1 | 1 | 1 |
| 20–34 | 1 | 1.0 | 0 | 1 | 1 | 1 | 1 | 1 | 1 | 1 |
| 35–49 | 1 | 2.0 | 0 | 2 | 2 | 2 | 2 | 2 | 2 | 2 |
| 50–64 | 0 | | | | | | | | | |
| 65+ | 1 | 1.0 | 0 | 1 | 1 | 1 | 1 | 1 | 1 | 1 |
| **2. MULTIPLE DX** | | | | | | | | | | |
| 0–19 Years | 1 | 4.0 | 0 | 4 | 4 | 4 | 4 | 4 | 4 | 4 |
| 20–34 | 6 | 22.3 | 66 | 6 | 24 | 26 | 26 | 26 | 26 | 26 |
| 35–49 | 0 | | | | | | | | | |
| 50–64 | 4 | 2.8 | 6 | 1 | 1 | 2 | 2 | 2 | 7 | 7 |
| 65+ | | | | | | | | | | |
| **TOTAL SINGLE DX** | 4 | 1.3 | <1 | 1 | 1 | 1 | 2 | 2 | 2 | 2 |
| **TOTAL MULTIPLE DX** | 11 | 18.8 | 111 | 2 | 6 | 26 | 26 | 26 | 26 | 26 |
| **TOTAL** | | | | | | | | | | |
| 0–19 Years | 2 | 2.3 | 4 | 1 | 1 | 1 | 1 | 4 | 4 | 4 |
| 20–34 | 1 | 1.0 | 0 | 1 | 1 | 1 | 1 | 1 | 1 | 1 |
| 35–49 | 7 | 21.3 | 81 | 2 | 24 | 26 | 26 | 26 | 26 | 26 |
| 50–64 | 0 | | | | | | | | | |
| 65+ | 5 | 2.6 | 6 | 1 | 1 | 2 | 2 | 2 | 7 | 7 |
| **GRAND TOTAL** | 15 | 16.8 | 130 | 1 | 2 | 26 | 26 | 26 | 26 | 26 |

## 10.5: CONJUNCT/LID ADHESIO. Formerly included in operation group(s) 520.

| Type of Patients | Observed Patients | Avg. Stay | Variance | 10th | 25th | 50th | 75th | 90th | 95th | 99th |
|---|---|---|---|---|---|---|---|---|---|---|
| **1. SINGLE DX** | | | | | | | | | | |
| 0–19 Years | 0 | | | | | | | | | |
| 20–34 | 0 | | | | | | | | | |
| 35–49 | 0 | | | | | | | | | |
| 50–64 | 0 | | | | | | | | | |
| 65+ | | | | | | | | | | |
| **2. MULTIPLE DX** | | | | | | | | | | |
| 0–19 Years | 2 | 11.3 | 42 | 5 | 5 | 17 | 17 | 17 | 17 | 17 |
| 20–34 | 0 | | | | | | | | | |
| 35–49 | 0 | | | | | | | | | |
| 50–64 | 0 | | | | | | | | | |
| 65+ | 1 | 1.0 | 0 | 1 | 1 | 1 | 1 | 1 | 1 | 1 |
| **TOTAL SINGLE DX** | 0 | | | | | | | | | |
| **TOTAL MULTIPLE DX** | 3 | 9.5 | 51 | 1 | 5 | 5 | 17 | 17 | 17 | 17 |
| **TOTAL** | | | | | | | | | | |
| 0–19 Years | 2 | 11.3 | 42 | 5 | 5 | 17 | 17 | 17 | 17 | 17 |
| 20–34 | 0 | | | | | | | | | |
| 35–49 | 0 | | | | | | | | | |
| 50–64 | 0 | | | | | | | | | |
| 65+ | 1 | 1.0 | 0 | 1 | 1 | 1 | 1 | 1 | 1 | 1 |
| **GRAND TOTAL** | 3 | 9.5 | 51 | 1 | 5 | 5 | 17 | 17 | 17 | 17 |

Length of Stay by Diagnosis and Operation, United States, 2000

# United States, October 1998–September 1999 Data, by Operation

## 10.6: REPAIR CONJUNCT LAC. Formerly included in operation group(s) 520.

| Type of Patients | Observed Patients | Avg. Stay | Variance | 10th | 25th | 50th | 75th | 90th | 95th | 99th |
|---|---|---|---|---|---|---|---|---|---|---|
| **1. SINGLE DX** | | | | | | | | | | |
| 0–19 Years | 5 | 1.1 | <1 | 1 | 1 | 1 | 1 | 1 | 2 | 2 |
| 20–34 | 0 | | | | | | | | | |
| 35–49 | 2 | 1.7 | <1 | 1 | 1 | 2 | 2 | 2 | 2 | 2 |
| 50–64 | 1 | 1.0 | 0 | 1 | 1 | 1 | 1 | 1 | 1 | 1 |
| 65+ | 0 | | | | | | | | | |
| **2. MULTIPLE DX** | | | | | | | | | | |
| 0–19 Years | 10 | 2.1 | 2 | 1 | 1 | 2 | 3 | 4 | 5 | 5 |
| 20–34 | 4 | 1.7 | <1 | 1 | 1 | 2 | 2 | 2 | 2 | 3 |
| 35–49 | 2 | 3.0 | <1 | 3 | 3 | 3 | 3 | 3 | 3 | 3 |
| 50–64 | 2 | 1.0 | 0 | 1 | 1 | 1 | 1 | 1 | 1 | 1 |
| 65+ | 3 | 3.5 | 4 | 2 | 2 | 3 | 6 | 6 | 6 | 6 |
| **TOTAL SINGLE DX** | 8 | 1.2 | <1 | 1 | 1 | 1 | 1 | 2 | 2 | 2 |
| **TOTAL MULTIPLE DX** | 21 | 2.4 | 1 | 1 | 1 | 3 | 3 | 3 | 3 | 6 |
| **TOTAL** | | | | | | | | | | |
| 0–19 Years | 15 | 1.5 | <1 | 1 | 1 | 1 | 1 | 3 | 3 | 5 |
| 20–34 | 4 | 1.7 | <1 | 1 | 1 | 2 | 2 | 2 | 2 | 2 |
| 35–49 | 4 | 2.7 | <1 | 2 | 3 | 3 | 3 | 3 | 3 | 3 |
| 50–64 | 3 | 1.0 | 0 | 1 | 1 | 1 | 1 | 1 | 1 | 1 |
| 65+ | 3 | 3.5 | 4 | 2 | 2 | 3 | 6 | 6 | 6 | 6 |
| **GRAND TOTAL** | 29 | 1.9 | 1 | 1 | 1 | 2 | 3 | 3 | 3 | 5 |

## 11.0: MAGNET REMOVAL CORNEA FB. Formerly included in operation group(s) 522.

| Type of Patients | Observed Patients | Avg. Stay | Variance | 10th | 25th | 50th | 75th | 90th | 95th | 99th |
|---|---|---|---|---|---|---|---|---|---|---|
| **1. SINGLE DX** | | | | | | | | | | |
| 0–19 Years | 0 | | | | | | | | | |
| 20–34 | 0 | | | | | | | | | |
| 35–49 | 0 | | | | | | | | | |
| 50–64 | 0 | | | | | | | | | |
| 65+ | 0 | | | | | | | | | |
| **2. MULTIPLE DX** | | | | | | | | | | |
| 0–19 Years | 1 | 3.0 | 0 | 3 | 3 | 3 | 3 | 3 | 3 | 3 |
| 20–34 | 0 | | | | | | | | | |
| 35–49 | 2 | 2.0 | 0 | 2 | 2 | 2 | 2 | 2 | 2 | 2 |
| 50–64 | 0 | | | | | | | | | |
| 65+ | 0 | | | | | | | | | |
| **TOTAL SINGLE DX** | 0 | | | | | | | | | |
| **TOTAL MULTIPLE DX** | 3 | 2.6 | <1 | 2 | 2 | 3 | 3 | 3 | 3 | 3 |
| **TOTAL** | | | | | | | | | | |
| 0–19 Years | 1 | 3.0 | 0 | 3 | 3 | 3 | 3 | 3 | 3 | 3 |
| 20–34 | 0 | | | | | | | | | |
| 35–49 | 2 | 2.0 | 0 | 2 | 2 | 2 | 2 | 2 | 2 | 2 |
| 50–64 | 0 | | | | | | | | | |
| 65+ | 0 | | | | | | | | | |
| **GRAND TOTAL** | 3 | 2.6 | <1 | 2 | 2 | 3 | 3 | 3 | 3 | 3 |

## 10.9: OTHER CONJUNCTIVAL OPS. Formerly included in operation group(s) 520.

| Type of Patients | Observed Patients | Avg. Stay | Variance | 10th | 25th | 50th | 75th | 90th | 95th | 99th |
|---|---|---|---|---|---|---|---|---|---|---|
| **1. SINGLE DX** | | | | | | | | | | |
| 0–19 Years | 4 | 3.0 | 2 | 1 | 2 | 4 | 4 | 4 | 4 | 4 |
| 20–34 | 0 | | | | | | | | | |
| 35–49 | 1 | 2.0 | 0 | 2 | 2 | 2 | 2 | 2 | 2 | 2 |
| 50–64 | 2 | 6.9 | <1 | 7 | 7 | 7 | 7 | 7 | 7 | 7 |
| 65+ | 3 | 1.2 | <1 | 1 | 1 | 1 | 1 | 2 | 2 | 2 |
| **2. MULTIPLE DX** | | | | | | | | | | |
| 0–19 Years | 7 | 4.3 | 2 | 1 | 3 | 5 | 5 | 6 | 6 | 6 |
| 20–34 | 2 | 1.3 | <1 | 1 | 1 | 1 | 2 | 2 | 2 | 2 |
| 35–49 | 8 | 3.2 | <1 | 2 | 3 | 3 | 4 | 4 | 4 | 4 |
| 50–64 | 6 | 4.0 | 20 | 1 | 1 | 1 | 11 | 11 | 11 | 11 |
| 65+ | 20 | 4.0 | 7 | 1 | 2 | 4 | 5 | 6 | 8 | 16 |
| **TOTAL SINGLE DX** | 10 | 5.1 | 6 | 1 | 2 | 7 | 7 | 7 | 7 | 7 |
| **TOTAL MULTIPLE DX** | 43 | 3.8 | 6 | 1 | 2 | 3 | 5 | 6 | 8 | 11 |
| **TOTAL** | | | | | | | | | | |
| 0–19 Years | 11 | 3.8 | 3 | 1 | 3 | 4 | 5 | 5 | 6 | 6 |
| 20–34 | 2 | 1.3 | <1 | 1 | 1 | 1 | 2 | 2 | 2 | 2 |
| 35–49 | 9 | 3.1 | <1 | 2 | 3 | 3 | 4 | 4 | 4 | 4 |
| 50–64 | 8 | 6.2 | 6 | 1 | 7 | 7 | 7 | 6 | 11 | 11 |
| 65+ | 23 | 3.7 | 7 | 1 | 2 | 3 | 5 | 6 | 8 | 16 |
| **GRAND TOTAL** | 53 | 4.2 | 6 | 1 | 2 | 4 | 6 | 7 | 7 | 11 |

## 11.1: CORNEAL INCISION. Formerly included in operation group(s) 522.

| Type of Patients | Observed Patients | Avg. Stay | Variance | 10th | 25th | 50th | 75th | 90th | 95th | 99th |
|---|---|---|---|---|---|---|---|---|---|---|
| **1. SINGLE DX** | | | | | | | | | | |
| 0–19 Years | 3 | 1.0 | <1 | 1 | 1 | 1 | 1 | 1 | 1 | 2 |
| 20–34 | 2 | 2.6 | <1 | 2 | 2 | 3 | 3 | 3 | 3 | 3 |
| 35–49 | 0 | | | | | | | | | |
| 50–64 | 0 | | | | | | | | | |
| 65+ | 0 | | | | | | | | | |
| **2. MULTIPLE DX** | | | | | | | | | | |
| 0–19 Years | 1 | 2.0 | 0 | 2 | 2 | 2 | 2 | 2 | 2 | 2 |
| 20–34 | 4 | 1.8 | <1 | 1 | 1 | 1 | 2 | 3 | 3 | 3 |
| 35–49 | 2 | 2.0 | 0 | 2 | 2 | 2 | 2 | 2 | 2 | 2 |
| 50–64 | 1 | 7.0 | 0 | 7 | 7 | 7 | 7 | 7 | 7 | 7 |
| 65+ | 2 | 3.0 | 6 | 1 | 1 | 5 | 5 | 5 | 5 | 5 |
| **TOTAL SINGLE DX** | 5 | 1.2 | <1 | 1 | 1 | 1 | 1 | 2 | 3 | 3 |
| **TOTAL MULTIPLE DX** | 10 | 2.5 | 3 | 1 | 2 | 2 | 2 | 5 | 7 | 7 |
| **TOTAL** | | | | | | | | | | |
| 0–19 Years | 4 | 1.1 | <1 | 1 | 1 | 1 | 1 | 2 | 2 | 2 |
| 20–34 | 6 | 2.0 | <1 | 1 | 2 | 2 | 3 | 3 | 3 | 3 |
| 35–49 | 2 | 2.0 | 0 | 2 | 2 | 2 | 2 | 2 | 2 | 2 |
| 50–64 | 1 | 7.0 | 0 | 7 | 7 | 7 | 7 | 7 | 7 | 7 |
| 65+ | 2 | 3.0 | 6 | 1 | 1 | 5 | 5 | 5 | 5 | 5 |
| **GRAND TOTAL** | 15 | 1.6 | 2 | 1 | 1 | 1 | 2 | 3 | 5 | 7 |

Length of Stay by Diagnosis and Operation, United States, 2000

# United States, October 1998–September 1999 Data, by Operation

## 11.2: DXTIC PX ON CORNEA. Formerly included in operation group(s) 522, 532.

| Type of Patients | Observed Patients | Avg. Stay | Variance | 10th | 25th | 50th | 75th | 90th | 95th | 99th |
|---|---|---|---|---|---|---|---|---|---|---|
| **1. SINGLE DX** | | | | | | | | | | |
| 0–19 Years | 1 | 4.0 | 0 | 4 | 4 | 4 | 4 | 4 | 4 | 4 |
| 20–34 | 2 | 3.3 | <1 | 3 | 3 | 3 | 4 | 4 | 4 | 4 |
| 35–49 | 0 | | | | | | | | | |
| 50–64 | 0 | | | | | | | | | |
| 65+ | 1 | 4.0 | 0 | 4 | 4 | 4 | 4 | 4 | 4 | 4 |
| **2. MULTIPLE DX** | | | | | | | | | | |
| 0–19 Years | 0 | | | | | | | | | |
| 20–34 | 0 | | | | | | | | | |
| 35–49 | 1 | 10.0 | 0 | 10 | 10 | 10 | 10 | 10 | 10 | 10 |
| 50–64 | 3 | 2.0 | 0 | 2 | 2 | 2 | 2 | 2 | 2 | 2 |
| 65+ | 4 | 11.8 | 52 | 4 | 4 | 15 | 10 | 20 | 20 | 20 |
| **TOTAL SINGLE DX** | 4 | 3.4 | <1 | 3 | 3 | 3 | 4 | 4 | 4 | 4 |
| **TOTAL MULTIPLE DX** | 8 | 7.3 | 40 | 2 | 2 | 4 | 10 | 20 | 20 | 20 |
| **TOTAL** | | | | | | | | | | |
| 0–19 Years | 1 | 4.0 | 0 | 4 | 4 | 4 | 4 | 4 | 4 | 4 |
| 20–34 | 2 | 3.3 | <1 | 3 | 3 | 3 | 4 | 4 | 4 | 4 |
| 35–49 | 1 | 10.0 | 0 | 10 | 10 | 10 | 10 | 10 | 10 | 10 |
| 50–64 | 3 | 2.0 | 0 | 2 | 2 | 2 | 2 | 2 | 2 | 2 |
| 65+ | 5 | 8.9 | 46 | 4 | 4 | 4 | 15 | 20 | 20 | 20 |
| **GRAND TOTAL** | 12 | 5.1 | 20 | 2 | 3 | 4 | 4 | 10 | 15 | 20 |

## 11.3: EXCISION OF PTERYGIUM. Formerly included in operation group(s) 522.

| Type of Patients | Observed Patients | Avg. Stay | Variance | 10th | 25th | 50th | 75th | 90th | 95th | 99th |
|---|---|---|---|---|---|---|---|---|---|---|
| **1. SINGLE DX** | | | | | | | | | | |
| 0–19 Years | 0 | | | | | | | | | |
| 20–34 | 1 | 1.0 | 0 | 1 | 1 | 1 | 1 | 1 | 1 | 1 |
| 35–49 | 2 | 1.0 | 0 | 1 | 1 | 1 | 1 | 1 | 1 | 1 |
| 50–64 | 0 | | | | | | | | | |
| 65+ | 0 | | | | | | | | | |
| **2. MULTIPLE DX** | | | | | | | | | | |
| 0–19 Years | 0 | | | | | | | | | |
| 20–34 | 0 | | | | | | | | | |
| 35–49 | 0 | | | | | | | | | |
| 50–64 | 3 | 1.8 | <1 | 1 | 2 | 2 | 2 | 2 | 2 | 2 |
| 65+ | 2 | 2.9 | 1 | 2 | 2 | 2 | 2 | 4 | 4 | 4 |
| **TOTAL SINGLE DX** | 3 | 1.0 | 0 | 1 | 1 | 1 | 1 | 1 | 1 | 1 |
| **TOTAL MULTIPLE DX** | 5 | 2.3 | <1 | 2 | 2 | 2 | 2 | 4 | 4 | 4 |
| **TOTAL** | | | | | | | | | | |
| 0–19 Years | 0 | | | | | | | | | |
| 20–34 | 1 | 1.0 | 0 | 1 | 1 | 1 | 1 | 1 | 1 | 1 |
| 35–49 | 2 | 1.0 | 0 | 1 | 1 | 1 | 1 | 1 | 1 | 1 |
| 50–64 | 3 | 1.8 | <1 | 1 | 2 | 2 | 2 | 2 | 2 | 2 |
| 65+ | 2 | 2.9 | 1 | 2 | 2 | 2 | 2 | 4 | 4 | 4 |
| **GRAND TOTAL** | 8 | 1.8 | <1 | 1 | 1 | 2 | 2 | 4 | 4 | 4 |

## 11.4: EXC/DESTR CORNEAL LESION. Formerly included in operation group(s) 522.

| Type of Patients | Observed Patients | Avg. Stay | Variance | 10th | 25th | 50th | 75th | 90th | 95th | 99th |
|---|---|---|---|---|---|---|---|---|---|---|
| **1. SINGLE DX** | | | | | | | | | | |
| 0–19 Years | 0 | | | | | | | | | |
| 20–34 | 1 | 1.0 | 0 | 1 | 1 | 1 | 1 | 1 | 1 | 1 |
| 35–49 | 0 | | | | | | | | | |
| 50–64 | 0 | | | | | | | | | |
| 65+ | 0 | | | | | | | | | |
| **2. MULTIPLE DX** | | | | | | | | | | |
| 0–19 Years | 8 | 2.1 | 4 | 1 | 1 | 1 | 1 | 7 | 7 | 7 |
| 20–34 | 0 | | | | | | | | | |
| 35–49 | 1 | 4.0 | 0 | 4 | 4 | 4 | 4 | 4 | 4 | 4 |
| 50–64 | 1 | 4.0 | 0 | 4 | 4 | 4 | 4 | 4 | 4 | 4 |
| 65+ | 5 | 5.4 | 64 | 1 | 1 | 1 | 1 | 20 | 20 | 20 |
| **TOTAL SINGLE DX** | 1 | 1.0 | 0 | 1 | 1 | 1 | 1 | 1 | 1 | 1 |
| **TOTAL MULTIPLE DX** | 15 | 3.2 | 20 | 1 | 1 | 1 | 4 | 7 | 17 | 20 |
| **TOTAL** | | | | | | | | | | |
| 0–19 Years | 8 | 2.1 | 4 | 1 | 1 | 1 | 1 | 7 | 7 | 7 |
| 20–34 | 1 | 1.0 | 0 | 1 | 1 | 1 | 1 | 1 | 1 | 1 |
| 35–49 | 1 | 4.0 | 0 | 4 | 4 | 4 | 4 | 4 | 4 | 4 |
| 50–64 | 1 | 4.0 | 0 | 4 | 4 | 4 | 4 | 4 | 4 | 4 |
| 65+ | 5 | 5.4 | 64 | 1 | 1 | 1 | 1 | 20 | 20 | 20 |
| **GRAND TOTAL** | 16 | 2.6 | 15 | 1 | 1 | 1 | 3 | 4 | 7 | 20 |

## 11.5: CORNEAL REPAIR. Formerly included in operation group(s) 522.

| Type of Patients | Observed Patients | Avg. Stay | Variance | 10th | 25th | 50th | 75th | 90th | 95th | 99th |
|---|---|---|---|---|---|---|---|---|---|---|
| **1. SINGLE DX** | | | | | | | | | | |
| 0–19 Years | 113 | 2.2 | 1 | 1 | 1 | 2 | 2 | 4 | 4 | 7 |
| 20–34 | 33 | 1.8 | <1 | 1 | 1 | 2 | 2 | 3 | 3 | 4 |
| 35–49 | 30 | 1.8 | <1 | 1 | 1 | 2 | 2 | 3 | 3 | 4 |
| 50–64 | 11 | 2.6 | 3 | 1 | 1 | 2 | 5 | 5 | 5 | 5 |
| 65+ | 9 | 1.3 | <1 | 1 | 1 | 1 | 1 | 1 | 4 | 4 |
| **2. MULTIPLE DX** | | | | | | | | | | |
| 0–19 Years | 145 | 3.2 | 6 | 1 | 2 | 3 | 3 | 5 | 9 | 13 |
| 20–34 | 87 | 2.6 | 3 | 1 | 1 | 2 | 3 | 4 | 6 | 8 |
| 35–49 | 70 | 2.3 | 4 | 1 | 2 | 2 | 3 | 4 | 6 | 11 |
| 50–64 | 35 | 3.1 | 10 | 1 | 2 | 3 | 3 | 4 | 6 | 16 |
| 65+ | 80 | 4.0 | 12 | 1 | 2 | 3 | 5 | 8 | 10 | 14 |
| **TOTAL SINGLE DX** | 196 | 2.1 | 1 | 1 | 1 | 2 | 3 | 4 | 5 | 5 |
| **TOTAL MULTIPLE DX** | 417 | 3.0 | 6 | 1 | 1 | 2 | 4 | 5 | 8 | 14 |
| **TOTAL** | | | | | | | | | | |
| 0–19 Years | 258 | 2.8 | 4 | 1 | 2 | 2 | 3 | 4 | 6 | 13 |
| 20–34 | 120 | 2.4 | 2 | 1 | 1 | 2 | 3 | 4 | 4 | 8 |
| 35–49 | 100 | 2.2 | 3 | 1 | 2 | 2 | 3 | 4 | 5 | 11 |
| 50–64 | 46 | 2.9 | 7 | 1 | 2 | 3 | 5 | 5 | 8 | 16 |
| 65+ | 89 | 3.7 | 11 | 1 | 3 | 3 | 5 | 8 | 8 | 14 |
| **GRAND TOTAL** | 613 | 2.7 | 5 | 1 | 2 | 3 | 3 | 5 | 6 | 13 |

Length of Stay by Diagnosis and Operation, United States, 2000

# United States, October 1998–September 1999 Data, by Operation

## 11.51: SUTURE OF CORNEAL LAC. Formerly included in operation group(s) 522.

| Type of Patients | Observed Patients | Avg. Stay | Variance | 10th | 25th | 50th | 75th | 90th | 95th | 99th |
|---|---|---|---|---|---|---|---|---|---|---|
| **1. SINGLE DX** | | | | | | | | | | |
| 0–19 Years | 99 | 2.1 | 1 | 1 | 1 | 2 | 3 | 4 | 4 | 5 |
| 20–34 | 32 | 1.8 | <1 | 1 | 1 | 2 | 2 | 3 | 3 | 3 |
| 35–49 | 26 | 1.8 | <1 | 1 | 1 | 2 | 2 | 3 | 3 | 4 |
| 50–64 | 9 | 2.6 | 3 | 1 | 1 | 2 | 5 | 5 | 5 | 5 |
| 65+ | 4 | 1.6 | 2 | 1 | 1 | 1 | 1 | 4 | 4 | 4 |
| **2. MULTIPLE DX** | | | | | | | | | | |
| 0–19 Years | 118 | 3.0 | 4 | 1 | 2 | 3 | 4 | 5 | 8 | 10 |
| 20–34 | 76 | 2.7 | 3 | 1 | 1 | 2 | 4 | 4 | 4 | 8 |
| 35–49 | 51 | 1.9 | 2 | 1 | 1 | 1 | 2 | 4 | 5 | 8 |
| 50–64 | 29 | 2.3 | 1 | 1 | 2 | 2 | 3 | 3 | 4 | 6 |
| 65+ | 40 | 4.0 | 9 | 1 | 1 | 4 | 5 | 8 | 8 | 13 |
| **TOTAL SINGLE DX** | 170 | 2.1 | 1 | 1 | 1 | 2 | 3 | 4 | 5 | 5 |
| **TOTAL MULTIPLE DX** | 314 | 2.7 | 4 | 1 | 1 | 2 | 3 | 4 | 6 | 10 |
| **TOTAL** | | | | | | | | | | |
| 0–19 Years | 217 | 2.6 | 3 | 1 | 2 | 2 | 3 | 4 | 5 | 9 |
| 20–34 | 108 | 2.4 | 2 | 1 | 1 | 2 | 2 | 3 | 4 | 8 |
| 35–49 | 77 | 1.9 | 2 | 1 | 1 | 1 | 2 | 3 | 4 | 6 |
| 50–64 | 38 | 2.4 | 2 | 1 | 2 | 2 | 3 | 5 | 5 | 6 |
| 65+ | 44 | 3.7 | 8 | 1 | 1 | 3 | 5 | 8 | 8 | 13 |
| **GRAND TOTAL** | 484 | 2.5 | 3 | 1 | 1 | 2 | 3 | 4 | 5 | 9 |

## 11.7: OTHER CORNEA RECONST. Formerly included in operation group(s) 522.

| Type of Patients | Observed Patients | Avg. Stay | Variance | 10th | 25th | 50th | 75th | 90th | 95th | 99th |
|---|---|---|---|---|---|---|---|---|---|---|
| **1. SINGLE DX** | | | | | | | | | | |
| 0–19 Years | 0 | | | | | | | | | |
| 20–34 | 1 | 40.0 | 0 | 40 | 40 | 40 | 40 | 40 | 40 | 40 |
| 35–49 | 1 | 2.0 | 0 | 2 | 2 | 2 | 2 | 2 | 2 | 2 |
| 50–64 | 0 | | | | | | | | | |
| 65+ | 1 | 4.0 | 0 | 4 | 4 | 4 | 4 | 4 | 4 | 4 |
| **2. MULTIPLE DX** | | | | | | | | | | |
| 0–19 Years | 0 | | | | | | | | | |
| 20–34 | 0 | | | | | | | | | |
| 35–49 | 0 | | | | | | | | | |
| 50–64 | 0 | | | | | | | | | |
| 65+ | 0 | | | | | | | | | |
| **TOTAL SINGLE DX** | 3 | 9.3 | 213 | 2 | 2 | 4 | 4 | 40 | 40 | 40 |
| **TOTAL MULTIPLE DX** | 0 | | | | | | | | | |
| **TOTAL** | | | | | | | | | | |
| 0–19 Years | 0 | | | | | | | | | |
| 20–34 | 1 | 40.0 | 0 | 40 | 40 | 40 | 40 | 40 | 40 | 40 |
| 35–49 | 1 | 2.0 | 0 | 2 | 2 | 2 | 2 | 2 | 2 | 2 |
| 50–64 | 0 | | | | | | | | | |
| 65+ | 1 | 4.0 | 0 | 4 | 4 | 4 | 4 | 4 | 4 | 4 |
| **GRAND TOTAL** | 3 | 9.3 | 213 | 2 | 2 | 4 | 4 | 40 | 40 | 40 |

## 11.6: CORNEAL TRANSPLANT. Formerly included in operation group(s) 521.

| Type of Patients | Observed Patients | Avg. Stay | Variance | 10th | 25th | 50th | 75th | 90th | 95th | 99th |
|---|---|---|---|---|---|---|---|---|---|---|
| **1. SINGLE DX** | | | | | | | | | | |
| 0–19 Years | 4 | 1.3 | <1 | 1 | 1 | 1 | 2 | 2 | 2 | 2 |
| 20–34 | 9 | 3.7 | 12 | 1 | 2 | 3 | 4 | 4 | 15 | 15 |
| 35–49 | 7 | 3.5 | 7 | 1 | 1 | 4 | 4 | 8 | 8 | 8 |
| 50–64 | 3 | 1.0 | 0 | 1 | 1 | 1 | 1 | 1 | 1 | 1 |
| 65+ | 20 | 2.3 | 2 | 1 | 1 | 2 | 3 | 4 | 5 | 6 |
| **2. MULTIPLE DX** | | | | | | | | | | |
| 0–19 Years | 8 | 2.4 | 3 | 1 | 1 | 2 | 3 | 6 | 6 | 6 |
| 20–34 | 21 | 3.1 | 8 | 1 | 1 | 2 | 3 | 8 | 9 | 10 |
| 35–49 | 35 | 4.3 | 30 | 1 | 2 | 2 | 3 | 11 | 17 | 28 |
| 50–64 | 40 | 4.5 | 31 | 1 | 1 | 2 | 7 | 9 | 13 | 36 |
| 65+ | 140 | 2.7 | 10 | 1 | 1 | 1 | 3 | 6 | 9 | 13 |
| **TOTAL SINGLE DX** | 43 | 3.0 | 7 | 1 | 1 | 2 | 4 | 5 | 8 | 15 |
| **TOTAL MULTIPLE DX** | 244 | 3.3 | 18 | 1 | 1 | 2 | 3 | 8 | 10 | 21 |
| **TOTAL** | | | | | | | | | | |
| 0–19 Years | 12 | 2.1 | 2 | 1 | 1 | 2 | 3 | 3 | 6 | 6 |
| 20–34 | 30 | 3.3 | 9 | 1 | 1 | 2 | 4 | 8 | 15 | 15 |
| 35–49 | 42 | 4.2 | 25 | 1 | 2 | 2 | 4 | 8 | 17 | 28 |
| 50–64 | 43 | 4.4 | 30 | 1 | 1 | 2 | 7 | 9 | 13 | 36 |
| 65+ | 160 | 2.7 | 9 | 1 | 1 | 1 | 3 | 6 | 9 | 13 |
| **GRAND TOTAL** | 287 | 3.3 | 16 | 1 | 1 | 2 | 4 | 8 | 10 | 21 |

## 11.9: OTHER CORNEAL OPERATIONS. Formerly included in operation group(s) 522.

| Type of Patients | Observed Patients | Avg. Stay | Variance | 10th | 25th | 50th | 75th | 90th | 95th | 99th |
|---|---|---|---|---|---|---|---|---|---|---|
| **1. SINGLE DX** | | | | | | | | | | |
| 0–19 Years | 0 | | | | | | | | | |
| 20–34 | 1 | 5.0 | 0 | 5 | 5 | 5 | 5 | 5 | 5 | 5 |
| 35–49 | 0 | | | | | | | | | |
| 50–64 | 0 | | | | | | | | | |
| 65+ | 0 | | | | | | | | | |
| **2. MULTIPLE DX** | | | | | | | | | | |
| 0–19 Years | 1 | 2.0 | 0 | 2 | 2 | 2 | 2 | 2 | 2 | 2 |
| 20–34 | 0 | | | | | | | | | |
| 35–49 | 0 | | | | | | | | | |
| 50–64 | 1 | 3.0 | 0 | 3 | 3 | 3 | 3 | 3 | 3 | 3 |
| 65+ | 2 | 3.7 | 4 | 1 | 1 | 5 | 5 | 5 | 5 | 5 |
| **TOTAL SINGLE DX** | 1 | 5.0 | 0 | 5 | 5 | 5 | 5 | 5 | 5 | 5 |
| **TOTAL MULTIPLE DX** | 4 | 3.1 | 1 | 2 | 3 | 3 | 3 | 5 | 5 | 5 |
| **TOTAL** | | | | | | | | | | |
| 0–19 Years | 1 | 2.0 | 0 | 2 | 2 | 2 | 2 | 2 | 2 | 2 |
| 20–34 | 1 | 5.0 | 0 | 5 | 5 | 5 | 5 | 5 | 5 | 5 |
| 35–49 | 0 | | | | | | | | | |
| 50–64 | 1 | 3.0 | 0 | 3 | 3 | 3 | 3 | 3 | 3 | 3 |
| 65+ | 2 | 3.7 | 4 | 1 | 1 | 5 | 5 | 5 | 5 | 5 |
| **GRAND TOTAL** | 5 | 3.4 | 1 | 2 | 3 | 3 | 5 | 5 | 5 | 5 |

Length of Stay by Diagnosis and Operation, United States, 2000

## United States, October 1998–September 1999 Data, by Operation

### 12.0: RMVL INOC FB ANT SEGMENT. Formerly included in operation group(s) 524.

| Type of Patients | Observed Patients | Avg. Stay | Variance | Percentiles | | | | | | |
|---|---|---|---|---|---|---|---|---|---|---|
| | | | | 10th | 25th | 50th | 75th | 90th | 95th | 99th |
| **1. SINGLE DX** | | | | | | | | | | |
| 0–19 Years | 3 | 1.1 | <1 | 1 | 1 | 1 | 1 | 2 | 2 | 2 |
| 20–34 | 5 | 2.0 | <1 | 2 | 2 | 2 | 2 | 2 | 3 | 3 |
| 35–49 | 1 | 1.0 | 0 | 1 | 1 | 1 | 1 | 1 | 1 | 1 |
| 50–64 | 0 | | | | | | | | | |
| 65+ | 0 | | | | | | | | | |
| **2. MULTIPLE DX** | | | | | | | | | | |
| 0–19 Years | 5 | 4.2 | 11 | 1 | 1 | 2 | 8 | 8 | 8 | 8 |
| 20–34 | 5 | 1.3 | 7 | 1 | 1 | 2 | 2 | 2 | 3 | 7 |
| 35–49 | 3 | 3.2 | 3 | 1 | 1 | 3 | 5 | 5 | 5 | 5 |
| 50–64 | 2 | 3.3 | <1 | 3 | 3 | 3 | 4 | 4 | 4 | 4 |
| 65+ | 2 | 2.3 | 1 | 1 | 1 | 3 | 3 | 3 | 3 | 3 |
| **TOTAL SINGLE DX** | 9 | 1.7 | <1 | 1 | 1 | 2 | 2 | 2 | 3 | 3 |
| **TOTAL MULTIPLE DX** | 17 | 2.5 | 5 | 1 | 1 | 1 | 3 | 8 | 8 | 8 |
| **TOTAL** | | | | | | | | | | |
| 0–19 Years | 8 | 3.3 | 10 | 1 | 1 | 1 | 8 | 8 | 8 | 8 |
| 20–34 | 10 | 1.6 | 7 | 1 | 2 | 2 | 2 | 2 | 3 | 7 |
| 35–49 | 4 | 2.6 | 3 | 1 | 1 | 3 | 5 | 5 | 5 | 5 |
| 50–64 | 2 | 3.3 | <1 | 3 | 3 | 3 | 4 | 4 | 4 | 4 |
| 65+ | 2 | 2.3 | 1 | 1 | 1 | 3 | 3 | 3 | 3 | 3 |
| **GRAND TOTAL** | 26 | 2.2 | 4 | 1 | 1 | 1 | 3 | 5 | 8 | 8 |

### 12.1: IRIDOTOMY/SMP IRIDECTOMY. Formerly included in operation group(s) 524.

| Type of Patients | Observed Patients | Avg. Stay | Variance | Percentiles | | | | | | |
|---|---|---|---|---|---|---|---|---|---|---|
| | | | | 10th | 25th | 50th | 75th | 90th | 95th | 99th |
| **1. SINGLE DX** | | | | | | | | | | |
| 0–19 Years | 0 | | | | | | | | | |
| 20–34 | 1 | 1.0 | 0 | 1 | 1 | 1 | 1 | 1 | 1 | 1 |
| 35–49 | 1 | 1.0 | 0 | 1 | 1 | 1 | 1 | 1 | 1 | 1 |
| 50–64 | 1 | 1.0 | 0 | 1 | 1 | 1 | 1 | 1 | 1 | 1 |
| 65+ | 5 | 1.7 | <1 | 2 | 2 | 2 | 2 | 2 | 2 | 2 |
| **2. MULTIPLE DX** | | | | | | | | | | |
| 0–19 Years | 3 | 1.0 | 0 | 1 | 1 | 1 | 1 | 1 | 1 | 1 |
| 20–34 | 2 | 3.8 | 7 | 1 | 1 | 6 | 6 | 6 | 6 | 6 |
| 35–49 | 3 | 2.0 | <1 | 1 | 2 | 2 | 3 | 3 | 3 | 3 |
| 50–64 | 16 | 5.5 | 28 | 2 | 4 | 4 | 5 | 16 | 16 | 26 |
| 65+ | 42 | 7.4 | 52 | 2 | 6 | 6 | 11 | 15 | 18 | 46 |
| **TOTAL SINGLE DX** | 8 | 1.5 | <1 | 1 | 1 | 1 | 2 | 2 | 2 | 2 |
| **TOTAL MULTIPLE DX** | 66 | 6.2 | 41 | 1 | 4 | 4 | 8 | 16 | 16 | 26 |
| **TOTAL** | | | | | | | | | | |
| 0–19 Years | 3 | 1.0 | 0 | 1 | 1 | 1 | 1 | 1 | 1 | 1 |
| 20–34 | 3 | 3.4 | 7 | 1 | 1 | 6 | 6 | 6 | 6 | 6 |
| 35–49 | 4 | 1.6 | <1 | 1 | 1 | 2 | 2 | 3 | 3 | 3 |
| 50–64 | 17 | 5.5 | 28 | 2 | 4 | 4 | 5 | 16 | 16 | 26 |
| 65+ | 47 | 6.8 | 50 | 1 | 2 | 5 | 11 | 15 | 18 | 46 |
| **GRAND TOTAL** | 74 | 5.8 | 39 | 1 | 1 | 4 | 7 | 16 | 16 | 26 |

### 12.2: ANTERIOR SEG DXTIC PX. Formerly included in operation group(s) 524, 532.

| Type of Patients | Observed Patients | Avg. Stay | Variance | Percentiles | | | | | | |
|---|---|---|---|---|---|---|---|---|---|---|
| | | | | 10th | 25th | 50th | 75th | 90th | 95th | 99th |
| **1. SINGLE DX** | | | | | | | | | | |
| 0–19 Years | 1 | 3.0 | 0 | 3 | 3 | 3 | 3 | 3 | 3 | 3 |
| 20–34 | 2 | 1.0 | 0 | 1 | 1 | 1 | 1 | 1 | 1 | 1 |
| 35–49 | 0 | | | | | | | | | |
| 50–64 | 1 | 1.0 | 0 | 1 | 1 | 1 | 1 | 1 | 1 | 1 |
| 65+ | 0 | | | | | | | | | |
| **2. MULTIPLE DX** | | | | | | | | | | |
| 0–19 Years | 5 | 7.4 | 8 | 6 | 6 | 7 | 10 | 10 | 10 | 10 |
| 20–34 | 0 | | | | | | | | | |
| 35–49 | 4 | 3.0 | 3 | 1 | 2 | 3 | 3 | 6 | 6 | 6 |
| 50–64 | 7 | 4.5 | 14 | 2 | 2 | 2 | 7 | 10 | 10 | 15 |
| 65+ | 16 | 3.5 | 2 | 2 | 3 | 3 | 4 | 5 | 7 | 8 |
| **TOTAL SINGLE DX** | 4 | 1.3 | <1 | 1 | 1 | 1 | 1 | 3 | 3 | 3 |
| **TOTAL MULTIPLE DX** | 32 | 4.2 | 8 | 1 | 3 | 3 | 6 | 8 | 10 | 10 |
| **TOTAL** | | | | | | | | | | |
| 0–19 Years | 6 | 7.1 | 8 | 3 | 6 | 7 | 10 | 10 | 10 | 10 |
| 20–34 | 2 | 1.0 | 0 | 1 | 1 | 1 | 1 | 1 | 1 | 1 |
| 35–49 | 4 | 3.0 | 3 | 1 | 2 | 3 | 3 | 6 | 6 | 6 |
| 50–64 | 8 | 4.2 | 13 | 2 | 2 | 3 | 7 | 10 | 10 | 15 |
| 65+ | 16 | 3.5 | 2 | 2 | 3 | 3 | 4 | 5 | 7 | 8 |
| **GRAND TOTAL** | 36 | 4.0 | 8 | 1 | 2 | 3 | 6 | 8 | 10 | 10 |

### 12.3: IRIDOPLASTY/COREOPLASTY. Formerly included in operation group(s) 524.

| Type of Patients | Observed Patients | Avg. Stay | Variance | Percentiles | | | | | | |
|---|---|---|---|---|---|---|---|---|---|---|
| | | | | 10th | 25th | 50th | 75th | 90th | 95th | 99th |
| **1. SINGLE DX** | | | | | | | | | | |
| 0–19 Years | 5 | 1.0 | 0 | 1 | 1 | 1 | 1 | 1 | 1 | 1 |
| 20–34 | 1 | 1.0 | 0 | 1 | 1 | 1 | 1 | 1 | 1 | 1 |
| 35–49 | 0 | | | | | | | | | |
| 50–64 | 0 | | | | | | | | | |
| 65+ | 1 | 1.0 | 0 | 1 | 1 | 1 | 1 | 1 | 1 | 1 |
| **2. MULTIPLE DX** | | | | | | | | | | |
| 0–19 Years | 6 | 2.6 | <1 | 1 | 2 | 3 | 3 | 3 | 4 | 4 |
| 20–34 | 4 | 1.7 | <1 | 1 | 1 | 1 | 3 | 3 | 3 | 3 |
| 35–49 | 1 | 1.0 | 0 | 1 | 1 | 1 | 1 | 1 | 1 | 1 |
| 50–64 | 3 | 8.7 | 38 | 1 | 6 | 6 | 15 | 15 | 15 | 15 |
| 65+ | 13 | 6.9 | 112 | 1 | 4 | 4 | 7 | 7 | 39 | 39 |
| **TOTAL SINGLE DX** | 7 | 1.0 | 0 | 1 | 1 | 1 | 1 | 1 | 1 | 1 |
| **TOTAL MULTIPLE DX** | 27 | 5.1 | 53 | 1 | 3 | 3 | 4 | 15 | 15 | 39 |
| **TOTAL** | | | | | | | | | | |
| 0–19 Years | 11 | 1.7 | 1 | 1 | 1 | 1 | 3 | 3 | 3 | 4 |
| 20–34 | 5 | 1.5 | <1 | 1 | 1 | 1 | 2 | 3 | 3 | 3 |
| 35–49 | 1 | 1.0 | 0 | 1 | 1 | 1 | 1 | 1 | 1 | 1 |
| 50–64 | 3 | 8.7 | 38 | 1 | 6 | 6 | 15 | 15 | 15 | 15 |
| 65+ | 14 | 6.3 | 105 | 1 | 1 | 4 | 7 | 15 | 39 | 39 |
| **GRAND TOTAL** | 34 | 3.7 | 39 | 1 | 1 | 1 | 4 | 7 | 15 | 39 |

Length of Stay by Diagnosis and Operation, United States, 2000

# United States, October 1998–September 1999 Data, by Operation

## 12.4: DESTR IRIS/CIL BODY LES. Formerly included in operation group(s) 524.

| Type of Patients | Observed Patients | Avg. Stay | Variance | Percentiles | | | | | | |
|---|---|---|---|---|---|---|---|---|---|---|
| | | | | 10th | 25th | 50th | 75th | 90th | 95th | 99th |
| **1. SINGLE DX** | | | | | | | | | | |
| 0–19 Years | 0 | | | | | | | | | |
| 20–34 | 0 | | | | | | | | | |
| 35–49 | 0 | | | | | | | | | |
| 50–64 | 0 | | | | | | | | | |
| 65+ | 2 | 2.6 | 4 | 1 | 1 | 4 | 4 | 4 | 4 | 4 |
| **2. MULTIPLE DX** | | | | | | | | | | |
| 0–19 Years | 2 | 4.8 | 2 | 4 | 4 | 4 | 7 | 7 | 7 | 7 |
| 20–34 | 0 | | | | | | | | | |
| 35–49 | 0 | | | | | | | | | |
| 50–64 | 0 | | | | | | | | | |
| 65+ | 2 | 9.8 | 1 | 9 | 9 | 9 | 11 | 11 | 11 | 11 |
| **TOTAL SINGLE DX** | 2 | 2.6 | 4 | 1 | 1 | 4 | 4 | 4 | 4 | 4 |
| **TOTAL MULTIPLE DX** | 4 | 7.5 | 9 | 4 | 4 | 9 | 9 | 11 | 11 | 11 |
| **TOTAL** | | | | | | | | | | |
| 0–19 Years | 2 | 4.8 | 2 | 4 | 4 | 4 | 7 | 7 | 7 | 7 |
| 20–34 | 0 | | | | | | | | | |
| 35–49 | 0 | | | | | | | | | |
| 50–64 | 0 | | | | | | | | | |
| 65+ | 4 | 7.4 | 15 | 1 | 4 | 9 | 11 | 11 | 11 | 11 |
| **GRAND TOTAL** | 6 | 6.5 | 11 | 4 | 4 | 7 | 9 | 11 | 11 | 11 |

## 12.5: INOC CIRCULAT FACILITAT. Formerly included in operation group(s) 523.

| Type of Patients | Observed Patients | Avg. Stay | Variance | Percentiles | | | | | | |
|---|---|---|---|---|---|---|---|---|---|---|
| | | | | 10th | 25th | 50th | 75th | 90th | 95th | 99th |
| **1. SINGLE DX** | | | | | | | | | | |
| 0–19 Years | 5 | 1.1 | <1 | 1 | 1 | 1 | 1 | 1 | 2 | 2 |
| 20–34 | 0 | | | | | | | | | |
| 35–49 | 0 | | | | | | | | | |
| 50–64 | 1 | 8.0 | 0 | 8 | 8 | 8 | 8 | 8 | 8 | 8 |
| 65+ | 2 | 2.4 | 1 | 1 | 1 | 3 | 3 | 3 | 3 | 3 |
| **2. MULTIPLE DX** | | | | | | | | | | |
| 0–19 Years | 19 | 2.7 | 6 | 1 | 1 | 2 | 3 | 6 | 10 | 10 |
| 20–34 | 2 | 4.6 | <1 | 4 | 4 | 5 | 5 | 5 | 5 | 5 |
| 35–49 | 0 | | | | | | | | | |
| 50–64 | 2 | 1.0 | 0 | 1 | 1 | 1 | 1 | 1 | 1 | 1 |
| 65+ | 7 | 5.8 | 46 | 1 | 1 | 3 | 9 | 9 | 24 | 24 |
| **TOTAL SINGLE DX** | 8 | 2.1 | 5 | 1 | 1 | 1 | 3 | 8 | 8 | 8 |
| **TOTAL MULTIPLE DX** | 30 | 3.3 | 14 | 1 | 1 | 2 | 4 | 9 | 10 | 24 |
| **TOTAL** | | | | | | | | | | |
| 0–19 Years | 24 | 2.4 | 6 | 1 | 1 | 1 | 3 | 6 | 10 | 10 |
| 20–34 | 2 | 4.6 | <1 | 4 | 4 | 5 | 5 | 5 | 5 | 5 |
| 35–49 | 0 | | | | | | | | | |
| 50–64 | 3 | 3.6 | 13 | 1 | 1 | 1 | 8 | 8 | 8 | 8 |
| 65+ | 9 | 5.0 | 37 | 1 | 1 | 3 | 9 | 9 | 24 | 24 |
| **GRAND TOTAL** | 38 | 3.0 | 12 | 1 | 1 | 1 | 3 | 8 | 10 | 24 |

## 12.6: SCLERAL FISTULIZATION. Formerly included in operation group(s) 523.

| Type of Patients | Observed Patients | Avg. Stay | Variance | Percentiles | | | | | | |
|---|---|---|---|---|---|---|---|---|---|---|
| | | | | 10th | 25th | 50th | 75th | 90th | 95th | 99th |
| **1. SINGLE DX** | | | | | | | | | | |
| 0–19 Years | 2 | 1.0 | 0 | 1 | 1 | 1 | 1 | 1 | 1 | 1 |
| 20–34 | 0 | | | | | | | | | |
| 35–49 | 5 | 2.4 | 2 | 1 | 2 | 2 | 4 | 4 | 4 | 4 |
| 50–64 | 12 | 2.5 | 4 | 1 | 2 | 2 | 4 | 5 | 5 | 9 |
| 65+ | 16 | 1.4 | <1 | 1 | 1 | 1 | 1 | 3 | 4 | 4 |
| **2. MULTIPLE DX** | | | | | | | | | | |
| 0–19 Years | 17 | 5.4 | 65 | 1 | 1 | 2 | 7 | 7 | 32 | 32 |
| 20–34 | 9 | 2.8 | 6 | 1 | 1 | 1 | 4 | 6 | 9 | 9 |
| 35–49 | 21 | 3.5 | 12 | 1 | 2 | 2 | 5 | 9 | 9 | 16 |
| 50–64 | 45 | 3.1 | 8 | 1 | 2 | 2 | 5 | 7 | 8 | 19 |
| 65+ | 169 | 2.3 | 11 | 1 | 1 | 1 | 2 | 5 | 7 | 23 |
| **TOTAL SINGLE DX** | 35 | 2.0 | 2 | 1 | 1 | 1 | 3 | 4 | 5 | 9 |
| **TOTAL MULTIPLE DX** | 261 | 3.1 | 19 | 1 | 1 | 1 | 4 | 7 | 9 | 32 |
| **TOTAL** | | | | | | | | | | |
| 0–19 Years | 19 | 5.1 | 63 | 1 | 1 | 2 | 7 | 7 | 32 | 32 |
| 20–34 | 9 | 2.8 | 6 | 1 | 1 | 1 | 4 | 6 | 9 | 9 |
| 35–49 | 26 | 3.3 | 10 | 1 | 1 | 2 | 5 | 6 | 8 | 16 |
| 50–64 | 57 | 3.0 | 7 | 1 | 1 | 2 | 4 | 7 | 6 | 12 |
| 65+ | 185 | 2.2 | 10 | 1 | 1 | 1 | 2 | 4 | 6 | 19 |
| **GRAND TOTAL** | 296 | 2.9 | 17 | 1 | 1 | 1 | 4 | 6 | 8 | 25 |

## 12.7: ELEVAT INOC PRESS RELIEF. Formerly included in operation group(s) 523.

| Type of Patients | Observed Patients | Avg. Stay | Variance | Percentiles | | | | | | |
|---|---|---|---|---|---|---|---|---|---|---|
| | | | | 10th | 25th | 50th | 75th | 90th | 95th | 99th |
| **1. SINGLE DX** | | | | | | | | | | |
| 0–19 Years | 0 | | | | | | | | | |
| 20–34 | 0 | | | | | | | | | |
| 35–49 | 2 | 1.0 | 0 | 1 | 1 | 1 | 1 | 1 | 1 | 1 |
| 50–64 | 2 | 1.0 | 0 | 1 | 1 | 1 | 1 | 1 | 1 | 1 |
| 65+ | 0 | | | | | | | | | |
| **2. MULTIPLE DX** | | | | | | | | | | |
| 0–19 Years | 5 | 1.4 | <1 | 1 | 1 | 1 | 2 | 2 | 2 | 2 |
| 20–34 | 1 | 1.0 | 0 | 1 | 1 | 1 | 1 | 1 | 1 | 1 |
| 35–49 | 6 | 6.1 | 7 | 4 | 4 | 4 | 9 | 9 | 9 | 9 |
| 50–64 | 5 | 5.3 | 11 | 1 | 3 | 3 | 10 | 10 | 10 | 10 |
| 65+ | 13 | 4.3 | 50 | 1 | 2 | 3 | 3 | 8 | 8 | 34 |
| **TOTAL SINGLE DX** | 4 | 1.0 | 0 | 1 | 1 | 1 | 1 | 1 | 1 | 1 |
| **TOTAL MULTIPLE DX** | 30 | 3.9 | 16 | 1 | 1 | 3 | 4 | 9 | 10 | 10 |
| **TOTAL** | | | | | | | | | | |
| 0–19 Years | 5 | 1.4 | <1 | 1 | 1 | 1 | 2 | 2 | 2 | 2 |
| 20–34 | 1 | 1.0 | 0 | 1 | 1 | 1 | 1 | 1 | 1 | 1 |
| 35–49 | 8 | 5.5 | 9 | 4 | 4 | 4 | 6 | 8 | 8 | 9 |
| 50–64 | 7 | 4.6 | 12 | 1 | 1 | 3 | 3 | 10 | 10 | 10 |
| 65+ | 13 | 4.3 | 50 | 1 | 2 | 3 | 3 | 8 | 8 | 34 |
| **GRAND TOTAL** | 34 | 3.7 | 15 | 1 | 1 | 3 | 4 | 9 | 10 | 10 |

Length of Stay by Diagnosis and Operation, United States, 2000

# United States, October 1998–September 1999 Data, by Operation

## 12.8: OPERATIONS ON SCLERA. Formerly included in operation group(s) 524.

| Type of Patients | Observed Patients | Avg. Stay | Variance | Percentiles | | | | | | |
|---|---|---|---|---|---|---|---|---|---|---|
| | | | | 10th | 25th | 50th | 75th | 90th | 95th | 99th |
| **1. SINGLE DX** | | | | | | | | | | |
| 0–19 Years | 13 | 2.4 | 2 | 1 | 2 | 2 | 2 | 5 | 6 | 6 |
| 20–34 | 15 | 2.1 | <1 | 1 | 1 | 2 | 2 | 3 | 6 | 4 |
| 35–49 | 3 | 2.7 | 2 | 1 | 3 | 2 | 4 | 3 | 4 | 4 |
| 50–64 | 1 | 3.0 | 0 | 3 | 3 | 3 | 3 | 3 | 3 | 3 |
| 65+ | 6 | 1.5 | <1 | 1 | 1 | 1 | 2 | 2 | 4 | 4 |
| **2. MULTIPLE DX** | | | | | | | | | | |
| 0–19 Years | 29 | 1.9 | 1 | 1 | 1 | 1 | 3 | 3 | 4 | 4 |
| 20–34 | 21 | 2.1 | 2 | 1 | 1 | 2 | 3 | 4 | 4 | 6 |
| 35–49 | 27 | 2.3 | 3 | 1 | 1 | 1 | 4 | 5 | 6 | 6 |
| 50–64 | 15 | 2.7 | 5 | 1 | 1 | 2 | 4 | 6 | 9 | 9 |
| 65+ | 53 | 4.1 | 24 | 1 | 2 | 3 | 4 | 13 | 13 | 37 |
| **TOTAL SINGLE DX** | 38 | 2.1 | 1 | 1 | 1 | 2 | 3 | 4 | 4 | 6 |
| **TOTAL MULTIPLE DX** | 145 | 2.9 | 11 | 1 | 1 | 2 | 3 | 6 | 7 | 13 |
| **TOTAL** | | | | | | | | | | |
| 0–19 Years | 42 | 2.1 | 1 | 1 | 1 | 2 | 3 | 4 | 4 | 6 |
| 20–34 | 36 | 2.1 | 1 | 1 | 1 | 2 | 3 | 4 | 4 | 5 |
| 35–49 | 30 | 2.3 | 3 | 1 | 1 | 1 | 3 | 5 | 6 | 6 |
| 50–64 | 16 | 2.7 | 5 | 1 | 1 | 2 | 3 | 6 | 9 | 9 |
| 65+ | 59 | 3.9 | 23 | 1 | 2 | 3 | 4 | 8 | 13 | 37 |
| **GRAND TOTAL** | 183 | 2.7 | 8 | 1 | 1 | 2 | 3 | 5 | 6 | 13 |

## 12.9: OTH ANTERIOR SEGMENT OPS. Formerly included in operation group(s) 524.

| Type of Patients | Observed Patients | Avg. Stay | Variance | Percentiles | | | | | | |
|---|---|---|---|---|---|---|---|---|---|---|
| | | | | 10th | 25th | 50th | 75th | 90th | 95th | 99th |
| **1. SINGLE DX** | | | | | | | | | | |
| 0–19 Years | 3 | 1.3 | <1 | 1 | 1 | 1 | 1 | 3 | 3 | 3 |
| 20–34 | 3 | 2.2 | 5 | 1 | 1 | 1 | 3 | 7 | 7 | 7 |
| 35–49 | 1 | 1.0 | 0 | 1 | 1 | 1 | 1 | 1 | 1 | 1 |
| 50–64 | 3 | 2.0 | 0 | 2 | 2 | 2 | 2 | 2 | 2 | 2 |
| 65+ | 4 | 4.3 | 6 | 1 | 3 | 3 | 7 | 7 | 7 | 7 |
| **2. MULTIPLE DX** | | | | | | | | | | |
| 0–19 Years | 26 | 6.8 | 11 | 3 | 5 | 6 | 10 | 10 | 12 | 16 |
| 20–34 | 9 | 5.7 | 35 | 2 | 2 | 2 | 7 | 17 | 17 | 17 |
| 35–49 | 12 | 5.9 | 61 | 2 | 2 | 2 | 5 | 23 | 23 | 23 |
| 50–64 | 29 | 4.1 | 17 | 1 | 2 | 3 | 5 | 11 | 13 | 23 |
| 65+ | 57 | 3.1 | 7 | 1 | 2 | 2 | 4 | 6 | 9 | 15 |
| **TOTAL SINGLE DX** | 14 | 2.3 | 4 | 1 | 1 | 1 | 3 | 7 | 7 | 7 |
| **TOTAL MULTIPLE DX** | 133 | 5.0 | 18 | 1 | 2 | 3 | 7 | 10 | 12 | 23 |
| **TOTAL** | | | | | | | | | | |
| 0–19 Years | 29 | 6.4 | 12 | 3 | 3 | 5 | 10 | 10 | 12 | 16 |
| 20–34 | 12 | 5.0 | 31 | 1 | 2 | 2 | 6 | 17 | 17 | 17 |
| 35–49 | 13 | 5.4 | 57 | 1 | 2 | 2 | 3 | 23 | 23 | 23 |
| 50–64 | 32 | 4.0 | 17 | 1 | 2 | 3 | 4 | 11 | 13 | 23 |
| 65+ | 61 | 3.2 | 7 | 1 | 2 | 2 | 4 | 7 | 9 | 15 |
| **GRAND TOTAL** | 147 | 4.8 | 17 | 2 | 2 | 3 | 6 | 10 | 12 | 23 |

## 13.0: REMOVAL FB FROM LENS. Formerly included in operation group(s) 527.

| Type of Patients | Observed Patients | Avg. Stay | Variance | Percentiles | | | | | | |
|---|---|---|---|---|---|---|---|---|---|---|
| | | | | 10th | 25th | 50th | 75th | 90th | 95th | 99th |
| **1. SINGLE DX** | | | | | | | | | | |
| 0–19 Years | 0 | | | | | | | | | |
| 20–34 | 0 | | | | | | | | | |
| 35–49 | 0 | | | | | | | | | |
| 50–64 | 0 | | | | | | | | | |
| 65+ | 0 | | | | | | | | | |
| **2. MULTIPLE DX** | | | | | | | | | | |
| 0–19 Years | 0 | | | | | | | | | |
| 20–34 | 0 | | | | | | | | | |
| 35–49 | 0 | | | | | | | | | |
| 50–64 | 0 | | | | | | | | | |
| 65+ | 0 | | | | | | | | | |
| **TOTAL SINGLE DX** | 0 | | | | | | | | | |
| **TOTAL MULTIPLE DX** | 0 | | | | | | | | | |
| **TOTAL** | | | | | | | | | | |
| 0–19 Years | 0 | | | | | | | | | |
| 20–34 | 0 | | | | | | | | | |
| 35–49 | 0 | | | | | | | | | |
| 50–64 | 0 | | | | | | | | | |
| 65+ | 0 | | | | | | | | | |
| **GRAND TOTAL** | 0 | | | | | | | | | |

## 13.1: INTRACAP LENS EXTRACTION. Formerly included in operation group(s) 525.

| Type of Patients | Observed Patients | Avg. Stay | Variance | Percentiles | | | | | | |
|---|---|---|---|---|---|---|---|---|---|---|
| | | | | 10th | 25th | 50th | 75th | 90th | 95th | 99th |
| **1. SINGLE DX** | | | | | | | | | | |
| 0–19 Years | 10 | 1.3 | <1 | 1 | 1 | 1 | 1 | 3 | 3 | 3 |
| 20–34 | 0 | | | | | | | | | |
| 35–49 | 0 | | | | | | | | | |
| 50–64 | 1 | 3.0 | 0 | 3 | 3 | 3 | 3 | 3 | 3 | 3 |
| 65+ | 3 | 1.5 | <1 | 1 | 1 | 1 | 3 | 3 | 3 | 3 |
| **2. MULTIPLE DX** | | | | | | | | | | |
| 0–19 Years | 23 | 1.7 | 2 | 1 | 1 | 1 | 2 | 4 | 6 | 7 |
| 20–34 | 0 | | | | | | | | | |
| 35–49 | 3 | 2.5 | 3 | 1 | 1 | 1 | 4 | 4 | 4 | 4 |
| 50–64 | 5 | 2.8 | 14 | 1 | 2 | 2 | 2 | 2 | 15 | 15 |
| 65+ | 13 | 3.4 | 2 | 2 | 2 | 4 | 4 | 5 | 5 | 7 |
| **TOTAL SINGLE DX** | 14 | 1.6 | <1 | 1 | 1 | 1 | 3 | 3 | 3 | 3 |
| **TOTAL MULTIPLE DX** | 44 | 2.2 | 3 | 1 | 1 | 1 | 3 | 4 | 6 | 7 |
| **TOTAL** | | | | | | | | | | |
| 0–19 Years | 33 | 1.7 | 2 | 1 | 1 | 1 | 2 | 4 | 6 | 7 |
| 20–34 | 0 | | | | | | | | | |
| 35–49 | 3 | 2.5 | 3 | 1 | 1 | 2 | 4 | 4 | 4 | 4 |
| 50–64 | 6 | 2.8 | 10 | 1 | 2 | 3 | 3 | 4 | 13 | 15 |
| 65+ | 16 | 2.7 | 2 | 1 | 3 | 3 | 4 | 7 | 5 | 7 |
| **GRAND TOTAL** | 58 | 2.1 | 3 | 1 | 1 | 1 | 3 | 4 | 5 | 7 |

Length of Stay by Diagnosis and Operation, United States, 2000

# United States, October 1998–September 1999 Data, by Operation

## 13.2: LIN EXTRACAPS LENS EXTR. Formerly included in operation group(s) 526.

| Type of Patients | Observed Patients | Avg. Stay | Variance | Percentiles | | | | | | |
|---|---|---|---|---|---|---|---|---|---|---|
| | | | | 10th | 25th | 50th | 75th | 90th | 95th | 99th |
| **1. SINGLE DX** | | | | | | | | | | |
| 0–19 Years | 0 | | | | | | | | | |
| 20–34 | 0 | | | | | | | | | |
| 35–49 | 0 | | | | | | | | | |
| 50–64 | 0 | | | | | | | | | |
| 65+ | 0 | | | | | | | | | |
| **2. MULTIPLE DX** | | | | | | | | | | |
| 0–19 Years | 2 | 2.9 | <1 | 3 | 3 | 3 | 3 | 3 | 3 | 3 |
| 20–34 | 0 | | | | | | | | | |
| 35–49 | 1 | 2.0 | 0 | 2 | 2 | 2 | 2 | 2 | 2 | 2 |
| 50–64 | 0 | | | | | | | | | |
| 65+ | 3 | 9.8 | 238 | 2 | 2 | 2 | 3 | 39 | 39 | 39 |
| **TOTAL SINGLE DX** | 0 | | | | | | | | | |
| **TOTAL MULTIPLE DX** | 6 | 5.5 | 102 | 2 | 2 | 3 | 3 | 3 | 39 | 39 |
| **TOTAL** | | | | | | | | | | |
| 0–19 Years | 2 | 2.9 | <1 | 3 | 3 | 3 | 3 | 3 | 3 | 3 |
| 20–34 | 0 | | | | | | | | | |
| 35–49 | 1 | 2.0 | 0 | 2 | 2 | 2 | 2 | 2 | 2 | 2 |
| 50–64 | 0 | | | | | | | | | |
| 65+ | 3 | 9.8 | 238 | 2 | 2 | 3 | 3 | 39 | 39 | 39 |
| **GRAND TOTAL** | 6 | 5.5 | 102 | 2 | 2 | 3 | 3 | 3 | 39 | 39 |

## 13.3: SIMP ASP LENS EXTRACTION. Formerly included in operation group(s) 526.

| Type of Patients | Observed Patients | Avg. Stay | Variance | Percentiles | | | | | | |
|---|---|---|---|---|---|---|---|---|---|---|
| | | | | 10th | 25th | 50th | 75th | 90th | 95th | 99th |
| **1. SINGLE DX** | | | | | | | | | | |
| 0–19 Years | 2 | 1.0 | 0 | 1 | 1 | 1 | 1 | 1 | 1 | 1 |
| 20–34 | 0 | | | | | | | | | |
| 35–49 | 0 | | | | | | | | | |
| 50–64 | 0 | | | | | | | | | |
| 65+ | 0 | | | | | | | | | |
| **2. MULTIPLE DX** | | | | | | | | | | |
| 0–19 Years | 1 | 8.0 | 0 | 8 | 8 | 8 | 8 | 8 | 8 | 8 |
| 20–34 | 1 | 2.0 | 0 | 2 | 2 | 2 | 2 | 2 | 2 | 2 |
| 35–49 | 1 | 1.0 | 0 | 1 | 1 | 1 | 1 | 1 | 1 | 1 |
| 50–64 | 2 | 7.8 | 56 | 1 | 1 | 14 | 14 | 14 | 14 | 14 |
| 65+ | 9 | 2.5 | 6 | 1 | 1 | 1 | 3 | 8 | 8 | 8 |
| **TOTAL SINGLE DX** | 2 | 1.0 | 0 | 1 | 1 | 1 | 1 | 1 | 1 | 1 |
| **TOTAL MULTIPLE DX** | 14 | 3.6 | 16 | 1 | 1 | 1 | 4 | 8 | 14 | 14 |
| **TOTAL** | | | | | | | | | | |
| 0–19 Years | 3 | 3.5 | 13 | 1 | 1 | 1 | 8 | 8 | 8 | 8 |
| 20–34 | 1 | 2.0 | 0 | 2 | 2 | 2 | 2 | 2 | 2 | 2 |
| 35–49 | 1 | 1.0 | 0 | 1 | 1 | 1 | 1 | 1 | 1 | 1 |
| 50–64 | 2 | 7.8 | 56 | 1 | 1 | 14 | 14 | 14 | 14 | 14 |
| 65+ | 9 | 2.5 | 6 | 1 | 1 | 1 | 3 | 8 | 8 | 8 |
| **GRAND TOTAL** | 16 | 3.2 | 14 | 1 | 1 | 1 | 4 | 8 | 14 | 14 |

## 13.4: FRAG-ASP EXTRACAPS LENS. Formerly included in operation group(s) 526.

| Type of Patients | Observed Patients | Avg. Stay | Variance | Percentiles | | | | | | |
|---|---|---|---|---|---|---|---|---|---|---|
| | | | | 10th | 25th | 50th | 75th | 90th | 95th | 99th |
| **1. SINGLE DX** | | | | | | | | | | |
| 0–19 Years | 2 | 1.0 | 0 | 1 | 1 | 1 | 1 | 1 | 1 | 1 |
| 20–34 | 5 | 1.3 | <1 | 1 | 1 | 1 | 1 | 3 | 3 | 3 |
| 35–49 | 17 | 1.2 | <1 | 1 | 1 | 1 | 1 | 2 | 3 | 4 |
| 50–64 | 22 | 1.5 | 2 | 1 | 1 | 1 | 1 | 5 | 5 | 5 |
| 65+ | 115 | 1.1 | <1 | 1 | 1 | 1 | 1 | 1 | 1 | 2 |
| **2. MULTIPLE DX** | | | | | | | | | | |
| 0–19 Years | 5 | 3.2 | 6 | 1 | 1 | 1 | 6 | 6 | 6 | 6 |
| 20–34 | 7 | 3.3 | 33 | 1 | 1 | 1 | 2 | 18 | 18 | 18 |
| 35–49 | 23 | 1.7 | 1 | 1 | 1 | 1 | 2 | 3 | 4 | 5 |
| 50–64 | 90 | 3.4 | 39 | 1 | 1 | 1 | 4 | 6 | 10 | 33 |
| 65+ | 521 | 3.7 | 43 | 1 | 1 | 1 | 4 | 7 | 18 | 34 |
| **TOTAL SINGLE DX** | 161 | 1.2 | <1 | 1 | 1 | 1 | 1 | 1 | 3 | 5 |
| **TOTAL MULTIPLE DX** | 646 | 3.5 | 39 | 1 | 1 | 1 | 4 | 6 | 16 | 33 |
| **TOTAL** | | | | | | | | | | |
| 0–19 Years | 7 | 2.9 | 6 | 1 | 1 | 1 | 6 | 6 | 6 | 6 |
| 20–34 | 12 | 2.4 | 19 | 1 | 1 | 1 | 2 | 3 | 18 | 18 |
| 35–49 | 40 | 1.5 | <1 | 1 | 1 | 1 | 2 | 3 | 4 | 5 |
| 50–64 | 112 | 3.2 | 35 | 1 | 1 | 1 | 4 | 5 | 8 | 33 |
| 65+ | 636 | 3.4 | 39 | 1 | 1 | 1 | 3 | 7 | 16 | 34 |
| **GRAND TOTAL** | 807 | 3.2 | 35 | 1 | 1 | 1 | 3 | 6 | 11 | 33 |

## 13.41: CATARACT PHACO & ASP. Formerly included in operation group(s) 526.

| Type of Patients | Observed Patients | Avg. Stay | Variance | Percentiles | | | | | | |
|---|---|---|---|---|---|---|---|---|---|---|
| | | | | 10th | 25th | 50th | 75th | 90th | 95th | 99th |
| **1. SINGLE DX** | | | | | | | | | | |
| 0–19 Years | 2 | 1.0 | 0 | 1 | 1 | 1 | 1 | 1 | 1 | 1 |
| 20–34 | 5 | 1.3 | <1 | 1 | 1 | 1 | 1 | 3 | 3 | 3 |
| 35–49 | 17 | 1.2 | <1 | 1 | 1 | 1 | 1 | 2 | 3 | 4 |
| 50–64 | 22 | 1.5 | 2 | 1 | 1 | 1 | 1 | 5 | 5 | 5 |
| 65+ | 115 | 1.1 | <1 | 1 | 1 | 1 | 1 | 1 | 1 | 2 |
| **2. MULTIPLE DX** | | | | | | | | | | |
| 0–19 Years | 3 | 1.3 | <1 | 1 | 1 | 1 | 1 | 3 | 3 | 3 |
| 20–34 | 7 | 3.3 | 33 | 1 | 1 | 1 | 2 | 18 | 18 | 18 |
| 35–49 | 22 | 1.6 | 1 | 1 | 1 | 1 | 2 | 3 | 4 | 5 |
| 50–64 | 85 | 3.6 | 41 | 1 | 1 | 1 | 4 | 6 | 13 | 33 |
| 65+ | 506 | 3.6 | 44 | 1 | 1 | 1 | 4 | 7 | 18 | 34 |
| **TOTAL SINGLE DX** | 161 | 1.2 | <1 | 1 | 1 | 1 | 1 | 1 | 3 | 5 |
| **TOTAL MULTIPLE DX** | 623 | 3.5 | 41 | 1 | 1 | 1 | 3 | 6 | 16 | 33 |
| **TOTAL** | | | | | | | | | | |
| 0–19 Years | 5 | 1.2 | <1 | 1 | 1 | 1 | 1 | 3 | 3 | 3 |
| 20–34 | 12 | 2.4 | 19 | 1 | 1 | 1 | 2 | 3 | 18 | 18 |
| 35–49 | 39 | 1.5 | <1 | 1 | 1 | 1 | 2 | 3 | 4 | 5 |
| 50–64 | 107 | 3.3 | 36 | 1 | 1 | 1 | 4 | 6 | 8 | 33 |
| 65+ | 621 | 3.4 | 40 | 1 | 1 | 1 | 3 | 7 | 18 | 34 |
| **GRAND TOTAL** | 784 | 3.1 | 35 | 1 | 1 | 1 | 3 | 6 | 12 | 33 |

Length of Stay by Diagnosis and Operation, United States, 2000

# United States, October 1998–September 1999 Data, by Operation

## 13.5: OTH EXTRACAPS LENS EXTR. Formerly included in operation group(s) 526.

| Type of Patients | Observed Patients | Avg. Stay | Variance | 10th | 25th | 50th | 75th | 90th | 95th | 99th |
|---|---|---|---|---|---|---|---|---|---|---|
| **1. SINGLE DX** | | | | | | | | | | |
| 0–19 Years | 1 | 1.0 | 0 | 1 | 1 | 1 | 1 | 1 | 1 | 1 |
| 20–34 | 3 | 2.8 | <1 | 1 | 3 | 3 | 3 | 3 | 3 | 3 |
| 35–49 | 0 | | | | | | | | | |
| 50–64 | 1 | 1.0 | 0 | 1 | 1 | 1 | 1 | 1 | 1 | 1 |
| 65+ | 3 | 1.0 | 0 | 1 | 1 | 1 | 1 | 1 | 1 | 1 |
| **2. MULTIPLE DX** | | | | | | | | | | |
| 0–19 Years | 10 | 4.3 | 38 | 1 | 1 | 2 | 2 | 20 | 20 | 20 |
| 20–34 | 3 | 1.2 | <1 | 1 | 1 | 1 | 1 | 3 | 3 | 3 |
| 35–49 | 6 | 2.8 | <1 | 1 | 3 | 3 | 3 | 4 | 4 | 4 |
| 50–64 | 15 | 4.0 | 25 | 1 | 1 | 1 | 4 | 14 | 14 | 14 |
| 65+ | 76 | 2.4 | 14 | 1 | 1 | 1 | 2 | 5 | 8 | 43 |
| **TOTAL SINGLE DX** | 8 | 2.2 | <1 | 1 | 1 | 3 | 3 | 3 | 3 | 3 |
| **TOTAL MULTIPLE DX** | 110 | 2.9 | 17 | 1 | 1 | 1 | 3 | 7 | 14 | 20 |
| **TOTAL** | | | | | | | | | | |
| 0–19 Years | 11 | 4.0 | 36 | 1 | 1 | 2 | 2 | 14 | 20 | 20 |
| 20–34 | 6 | 2.4 | <1 | 1 | 1 | 3 | 3 | 3 | 3 | 3 |
| 35–49 | 6 | 2.8 | <1 | 1 | 3 | 3 | 3 | 4 | 4 | 4 |
| 50–64 | 16 | 4.0 | 24 | 1 | 1 | 1 | 4 | 14 | 14 | 14 |
| 65+ | 79 | 2.3 | 13 | 1 | 1 | 1 | 2 | 5 | 7 | 21 |
| **GRAND TOTAL** | 118 | 2.8 | 15 | 1 | 1 | 1 | 3 | 5 | 14 | 20 |

## 13.6: OTH CATARACT EXTRACTION. Formerly included in operation group(s) 526.

| Type of Patients | Observed Patients | Avg. Stay | Variance | 10th | 25th | 50th | 75th | 90th | 95th | 99th |
|---|---|---|---|---|---|---|---|---|---|---|
| **1. SINGLE DX** | | | | | | | | | | |
| 0–19 Years | 5 | 1.0 | 0 | 1 | 1 | 1 | 1 | 1 | 1 | 1 |
| 20–34 | 0 | | | | | | | | | |
| 35–49 | 0 | | | | | | | | | |
| 50–64 | 0 | | | | | | | | | |
| 65+ | 1 | 4.0 | 0 | 4 | 4 | 4 | 4 | 4 | 4 | 4 |
| **2. MULTIPLE DX** | | | | | | | | | | |
| 0–19 Years | 5 | 4.6 | 88 | 1 | 1 | 1 | 4 | 4 | 32 | 32 |
| 20–34 | 1 | 1.0 | 0 | 1 | 1 | 1 | 1 | 1 | 1 | 1 |
| 35–49 | 0 | | | | | | | | | |
| 50–64 | 1 | 2.0 | 0 | 2 | 2 | 2 | 2 | 2 | 2 | 2 |
| 65+ | 27 | 7.8 | 75 | 1 | 3 | 7 | 9 | 16 | 17 | 64 |
| **TOTAL SINGLE DX** | 6 | 1.4 | 1 | 1 | 1 | 1 | 1 | 4 | 4 | 4 |
| **TOTAL MULTIPLE DX** | 34 | 6.5 | 73 | 1 | 1 | 4 | 7 | 14 | 17 | 64 |
| **TOTAL** | | | | | | | | | | |
| 0–19 Years | 10 | 3.4 | 61 | 1 | 1 | 1 | 1 | 4 | 32 | 32 |
| 20–34 | 1 | 1.0 | 0 | 1 | 1 | 1 | 1 | 1 | 1 | 1 |
| 35–49 | 0 | | | | | | | | | |
| 50–64 | 1 | 2.0 | 0 | 2 | 2 | 2 | 2 | 2 | 2 | 2 |
| 65+ | 28 | 7.7 | 74 | 1 | 3 | 7 | 7 | 16 | 17 | 64 |
| **GRAND TOTAL** | 40 | 6.1 | 69 | 1 | 1 | 4 | 7 | 14 | 17 | 64 |

## 13.7: INSERT PROSTHETIC LENS. Formerly included in operation group(s) 527.

| Type of Patients | Observed Patients | Avg. Stay | Variance | 10th | 25th | 50th | 75th | 90th | 95th | 99th |
|---|---|---|---|---|---|---|---|---|---|---|
| **1. SINGLE DX** | | | | | | | | | | |
| 0–19 Years | 1 | 1.0 | 0 | 1 | 1 | 1 | 1 | 1 | 1 | 1 |
| 20–34 | 0 | | | | | | | | | |
| 35–49 | 0 | | | | | | | | | |
| 50–64 | 0 | | | | | | | | | |
| 65+ | 2 | 1.0 | 0 | 1 | 1 | 1 | 1 | 1 | 1 | 1 |
| **2. MULTIPLE DX** | | | | | | | | | | |
| 0–19 Years | 2 | 1.0 | 0 | 1 | 1 | 1 | 1 | 1 | 1 | 1 |
| 20–34 | 3 | 2.4 | <1 | 1 | 1 | 3 | 3 | 3 | 3 | 3 |
| 35–49 | 3 | 1.0 | 0 | 1 | 1 | 1 | 1 | 1 | 1 | 1 |
| 50–64 | 7 | 3.5 | 13 | 1 | 1 | 2 | 4 | 10 | 10 | 10 |
| 65+ | 19 | 2.2 | 3 | 1 | 1 | 1 | 3 | 6 | 7 | 7 |
| **TOTAL SINGLE DX** | 3 | 1.0 | 0 | 1 | 1 | 1 | 1 | 1 | 1 | 1 |
| **TOTAL MULTIPLE DX** | 33 | 2.3 | 5 | 1 | 1 | 1 | 3 | 6 | 10 | 10 |
| **TOTAL** | | | | | | | | | | |
| 0–19 Years | 3 | 1.0 | 0 | 1 | 1 | 1 | 1 | 1 | 1 | 1 |
| 20–34 | 2 | 2.4 | <1 | 1 | 1 | 3 | 3 | 3 | 3 | 3 |
| 35–49 | 3 | 1.0 | 0 | 1 | 1 | 1 | 1 | 1 | 1 | 1 |
| 50–64 | 7 | 3.5 | 13 | 1 | 1 | 2 | 4 | 10 | 10 | 10 |
| 65+ | 21 | 2.1 | 3 | 1 | 1 | 1 | 3 | 4 | 7 | 7 |
| **GRAND TOTAL** | 36 | 2.2 | 5 | 1 | 1 | 1 | 3 | 4 | 10 | 10 |

## 13.8: IMPLANTED LENS REMOVAL. Formerly included in operation group(s) 527.

| Type of Patients | Observed Patients | Avg. Stay | Variance | 10th | 25th | 50th | 75th | 90th | 95th | 99th |
|---|---|---|---|---|---|---|---|---|---|---|
| **1. SINGLE DX** | | | | | | | | | | |
| 0–19 Years | 0 | | | | | | | | | |
| 20–34 | 0 | | | | | | | | | |
| 35–49 | 0 | | | | | | | | | |
| 50–64 | 0 | | | | | | | | | |
| 65+ | 0 | | | | | | | | | |
| **2. MULTIPLE DX** | | | | | | | | | | |
| 0–19 Years | 0 | | | | | | | | | |
| 20–34 | 0 | | | | | | | | | |
| 35–49 | 0 | | | | | | | | | |
| 50–64 | 1 | 1.0 | 0 | 1 | 1 | 1 | 1 | 1 | 1 | 1 |
| 65+ | 5 | 1.6 | 1 | 1 | 1 | 1 | 2 | 4 | 4 | 4 |
| **TOTAL SINGLE DX** | 0 | | | | | | | | | |
| **TOTAL MULTIPLE DX** | 6 | 1.4 | 1 | 1 | 1 | 1 | 1 | 1 | 4 | 4 |
| **TOTAL** | | | | | | | | | | |
| 0–19 Years | 0 | | | | | | | | | |
| 20–34 | 0 | | | | | | | | | |
| 35–49 | 0 | | | | | | | | | |
| 50–64 | 1 | 1.0 | 0 | 1 | 1 | 1 | 1 | 1 | 1 | 1 |
| 65+ | 5 | 1.6 | 1 | 1 | 1 | 1 | 2 | 4 | 4 | 4 |
| **GRAND TOTAL** | 6 | 1.4 | 1 | 1 | 1 | 1 | 1 | 1 | 4 | 4 |

Length of Stay by Diagnosis and Operation, United States, 2000

# United States, October 1998–September 1999 Data, by Operation

## 13.9: OTHER OPERATIONS ON LENS. Formerly included in operation group(s) 527.

| Type of Patients | Observed Patients | Avg. Stay | Variance | 10th | 25th | 50th | 75th | 90th | 95th | 99th |
|---|---|---|---|---|---|---|---|---|---|---|
| **1. SINGLE DX** | | | | | | | | | | |
| 0–19 Years | 0 | | | | | | | | | |
| 20–34 | 0 | | | | | | | | | |
| 35–49 | 0 | | | | | | | | | |
| 50–64 | 0 | | | | | | | | | |
| 65+ | 0 | | | | | | | | | |
| **2. MULTIPLE DX** | | | | | | | | | | |
| 0–19 Years | 1 | 3.0 | 0 | | | 3 | 3 | 3 | 3 | 3 |
| 20–34 | 0 | | | | | | | | | |
| 35–49 | 1 | 7.0 | 0 | 7 | 7 | 7 | 7 | 7 | 7 | 7 |
| 50–64 | 1 | 3.0 | 0 | 3 | 3 | 3 | 3 | 3 | 3 | 3 |
| 65+ | 2 | 6.4 | 30 | 2 | 2 | 2 | 11 | 11 | 11 | 11 |
| **TOTAL SINGLE DX** | 0 | | | | | | | | | |
| **TOTAL MULTIPLE DX** | 5 | 5.8 | 7 | 3 | 3 | 7 | 7 | 7 | 11 | 11 |
| **TOTAL** | | | | | | | | | | |
| 0–19 Years | 1 | 3.0 | 0 | 3 | 3 | 3 | 3 | 3 | 3 | 3 |
| 20–34 | 0 | | | | | | | | | |
| 35–49 | 1 | 7.0 | 0 | 7 | 7 | 7 | 7 | 7 | 7 | 7 |
| 50–64 | 1 | 3.0 | 0 | 3 | 3 | 3 | 3 | 3 | 3 | 3 |
| 65+ | 2 | 6.4 | 30 | 2 | 2 | 2 | 11 | 11 | 11 | 11 |
| **GRAND TOTAL** | 5 | 5.8 | 7 | 3 | 3 | 7 | 7 | 7 | 11 | 11 |

## 14.0: RMVL OF POST SEGMENT FB. Formerly included in operation group(s) 529.

| Type of Patients | Observed Patients | Avg. Stay | Variance | 10th | 25th | 50th | 75th | 90th | 95th | 99th |
|---|---|---|---|---|---|---|---|---|---|---|
| **1. SINGLE DX** | | | | | | | | | | |
| 0–19 Years | 1 | 1.0 | 0 | 1 | 1 | 1 | 1 | 1 | 1 | 1 |
| 20–34 | 0 | | | | | | | | | |
| 35–49 | 1 | 2.0 | 0 | 2 | 2 | 2 | 2 | 2 | 2 | 2 |
| 50–64 | 1 | 1.0 | 0 | 1 | 1 | 1 | 1 | 1 | 1 | 1 |
| 65+ | 0 | | | | | | | | | |
| **2. MULTIPLE DX** | | | | | | | | | | |
| 0–19 Years | 1 | 3.0 | 0 | 3 | 3 | 3 | 3 | 3 | 3 | 3 |
| 20–34 | 5 | 1.5 | <1 | 1 | 1 | 1 | 1 | 3 | 3 | 3 |
| 35–49 | 1 | 1.0 | 0 | 1 | 1 | 1 | 1 | 1 | 1 | 1 |
| 50–64 | 0 | | | | | | | | | |
| 65+ | 1 | 1.0 | 0 | 1 | 1 | 1 | 1 | 1 | 1 | 1 |
| **TOTAL SINGLE DX** | 3 | 1.3 | <1 | 1 | 1 | 1 | 2 | 2 | 2 | 2 |
| **TOTAL MULTIPLE DX** | 8 | 1.4 | <1 | 1 | 1 | 1 | 1 | 3 | 3 | 3 |
| **TOTAL** | | | | | | | | | | |
| 0–19 Years | 2 | 2.0 | 2 | 1 | 1 | 2 | 3 | 3 | 3 | 3 |
| 20–34 | 5 | 1.5 | <1 | 1 | 1 | 1 | 1 | 3 | 3 | 3 |
| 35–49 | 2 | 1.3 | <1 | 1 | 1 | 1 | 2 | 2 | 2 | 2 |
| 50–64 | 1 | 1.0 | 0 | 1 | 1 | 1 | 1 | 1 | 1 | 1 |
| 65+ | 1 | 1.0 | 0 | 1 | 1 | 1 | 1 | 1 | 1 | 1 |
| **GRAND TOTAL** | 11 | 1.4 | <1 | 1 | 1 | 1 | 2 | 3 | 3 | 3 |

## 14.1: DXTIC PX POSTERIOR SEG. Formerly included in operation group(s) 529, 532.

| Type of Patients | Observed Patients | Avg. Stay | Variance | 10th | 25th | 50th | 75th | 90th | 95th | 99th |
|---|---|---|---|---|---|---|---|---|---|---|
| **1. SINGLE DX** | | | | | | | | | | |
| 0–19 Years | 0 | | | | | | | | | |
| 20–34 | 1 | 4.0 | 0 | 4 | 4 | 4 | 4 | 4 | 4 | 4 |
| 35–49 | 0 | | | | | | | | | |
| 50–64 | 1 | 4.0 | 0 | 4 | 4 | 4 | 4 | 4 | 4 | 4 |
| 65+ | 6 | 2.4 | 1 | 1 | 2 | 2 | 3 | 4 | 4 | 4 |
| **2. MULTIPLE DX** | | | | | | | | | | |
| 0–19 Years | 3 | 3.0 | 10 | 1 | 1 | 1 | 8 | >99 | >99 | >99 |
| 20–34 | 0 | | | | | | | | | |
| 35–49 | 1 | 13.0 | 0 | 13 | 13 | 13 | 13 | 13 | 13 | 13 |
| 50–64 | 2 | 5.4 | <1 | 5 | 5 | 5 | 6 | 6 | 6 | 6 |
| 65+ | 12 | 3.8 | 7 | 2 | 2 | 2 | 5 | 6 | 12 | 12 |
| **TOTAL SINGLE DX** | 8 | 2.9 | 1 | 2 | 2 | 3 | 4 | 4 | 4 | 4 |
| **TOTAL MULTIPLE DX** | 18 | 4.5 | 14 | 1 | 2 | 3 | 8 | 13 | 13 | >99 |
| **TOTAL** | | | | | | | | | | |
| 0–19 Years | 3 | 3.0 | 10 | 1 | 1 | 1 | 8 | >99 | >99 | >99 |
| 20–34 | 1 | 4.0 | 0 | 4 | 4 | 4 | 4 | 4 | 4 | 4 |
| 35–49 | 1 | 13.0 | 0 | 13 | 13 | 13 | 13 | 13 | 13 | 13 |
| 50–64 | 3 | 5.0 | <1 | 4 | 4 | 5 | 6 | 6 | 6 | 7 |
| 65+ | 18 | 3.5 | 6 | 2 | 2 | 2 | 4 | 6 | 8 | 12 |
| **GRAND TOTAL** | 26 | 4.2 | 13 | 1 | 2 | 3 | 6 | 13 | 13 | >99 |

## 14.2: RETINA-CHOROID LES DESTR. Formerly included in operation group(s) 529.

| Type of Patients | Observed Patients | Avg. Stay | Variance | 10th | 25th | 50th | 75th | 90th | 95th | 99th |
|---|---|---|---|---|---|---|---|---|---|---|
| **1. SINGLE DX** | | | | | | | | | | |
| 0–19 Years | 28 | 1.4 | <1 | 1 | 1 | 1 | 2 | 2 | 3 | 3 |
| 20–34 | 4 | 4.4 | 6 | 1 | 1 | 6 | 6 | 7 | 7 | 7 |
| 35–49 | 7 | 6.2 | 2 | 3 | 7 | 7 | 7 | 7 | 8 | 8 |
| 50–64 | 10 | 6.9 | 3 | 1 | 7 | 7 | 8 | 8 | 8 | 8 |
| 65+ | 10 | 6.6 | 4 | 1 | 7 | 7 | 8 | 8 | 8 | 8 |
| **2. MULTIPLE DX** | | | | | | | | | | |
| 0–19 Years | 95 | 26.3 | >999 | 1 | 2 | 47 | >99 | >99 | >99 | >99 |
| 20–34 | 3 | 1.1 | <1 | 1 | 1 | 1 | 7 | 2 | 2 | 2 |
| 35–49 | 18 | 8.9 | 106 | 3 | 5 | 7 | 7 | 9 | 48 | 48 |
| 50–64 | 30 | 6.2 | 7 | 1 | 5 | 7 | 7 | 9 | 11 | 11 |
| 65+ | 53 | 5.5 | 18 | 1 | 3 | 5 | 7 | 9 | 13 | 26 |
| **TOTAL SINGLE DX** | 59 | 4.5 | 8 | 1 | 1 | 6 | 7 | 8 | 8 | 8 |
| **TOTAL MULTIPLE DX** | 199 | 15.1 | 753 | 1 | 2 | 7 | 73 | >99 | >99 | >99 |
| **TOTAL** | | | | | | | | | | |
| 0–19 Years | 123 | 20.5 | >999 | 1 | 1 | 3 | 97 | >99 | >99 | >99 |
| 20–34 | 7 | 2.8 | 6 | 1 | 1 | 1 | 6 | 7 | 7 | 7 |
| 35–49 | 25 | 7.9 | 70 | 2 | 5 | 7 | 7 | 9 | 17 | 48 |
| 50–64 | 40 | 6.4 | 17 | 1 | 6 | 7 | 8 | 9 | 11 | 11 |
| 65+ | 63 | 5.6 | 17 | 1 | 3 | 5 | 8 | 9 | 11 | 26 |
| **GRAND TOTAL** | 258 | 12.3 | 579 | 1 | 2 | 7 | 9 | 9 | >99 | >99 |

Length of Stay by Diagnosis and Operation, United States, 2000

# United States, October 1998–September 1999 Data, by Operation

## 14.3: REPAIR OF RETINAL TEAR. Formerly included in operation group(s) 528.

| Type of Patients | Observed Patients | Avg. Stay | Variance | 10th | 25th | 50th | 75th | 90th | 95th | 99th |
|---|---|---|---|---|---|---|---|---|---|---|
| **1. SINGLE DX** | | | | | | | | | | |
| 0–19 Years | 2 | 1.5 | <1 | 1 | 1 | 1 | 2 | 2 | 2 | 2 |
| 20–34 | 1 | 1.0 | 0 | 1 | 1 | 1 | 1 | 1 | 1 | 1 |
| 35–49 | 1 | 1.0 | 0 | 1 | 1 | 1 | 1 | 1 | 1 | 1 |
| 50–64 | 3 | 1.0 | 0 | 1 | 1 | 1 | 1 | 1 | 1 | 1 |
| 65+ | 0 | | | | | | | | | |
| **2. MULTIPLE DX** | | | | | | | | | | |
| 0–19 Years | 10 | 66.5 | >999 | 2 | 85 | 85 | 85 | 85 | 85 | 99 |
| 20–34 | 3 | 3.7 | 4 | 1 | 1 | 4 | 6 | 6 | 6 | 6 |
| 35–49 | 7 | 2.5 | 16 | 1 | 1 | 1 | 2 | 10 | 16 | 16 |
| 50–64 | 6 | 1.3 | <1 | 1 | 1 | 1 | 1 | 1 | 4 | 4 |
| 65+ | 18 | 1.8 | 6 | 1 | 1 | 1 | 3 | 3 | 5 | 15 |
| **TOTAL SINGLE DX** | 7 | 1.1 | <1 | 1 | 1 | 1 | 1 | 2 | 2 | 2 |
| **TOTAL MULTIPLE DX** | 44 | 27.2 | >999 | 1 | 85 | 85 | 85 | 85 | 85 | 99 |
| **TOTAL** | | | | | | | | | | |
| 0–19 Years | 12 | 62.4 | >999 | 85 | 85 | 85 | 85 | 85 | 85 | 99 |
| 20–34 | 4 | 3.3 | 5 | 1 | 4 | 4 | 4 | 6 | 6 | 6 |
| 35–49 | 8 | 2.4 | 15 | 1 | 1 | 1 | 1 | 10 | 16 | 16 |
| 50–64 | 9 | 1.2 | <1 | 1 | 1 | 1 | 1 | 1 | 4 | 4 |
| 65+ | 18 | 1.8 | 6 | 1 | 1 | 1 | 3 | 3 | 5 | 15 |
| **GRAND TOTAL** | 51 | 24.8 | >999 | 1 | 1 | 1 | 85 | 85 | 85 | 99 |

## 14.49: SCLERAL BUCKLING NEC. Formerly included in operation group(s) 528.

| Type of Patients | Observed Patients | Avg. Stay | Variance | 10th | 25th | 50th | 75th | 90th | 95th | 99th |
|---|---|---|---|---|---|---|---|---|---|---|
| **1. SINGLE DX** | | | | | | | | | | |
| 0–19 Years | 9 | 1.1 | <1 | 1 | 1 | 1 | 1 | 1 | 1 | 4 |
| 20–34 | 17 | 1.4 | <1 | 1 | 1 | 1 | 2 | 2 | 2 | 3 |
| 35–49 | 40 | 1.3 | <1 | 1 | 1 | 1 | 1 | 2 | 2 | 3 |
| 50–64 | 56 | 1.4 | <1 | 1 | 1 | 1 | 2 | 2 | 3 | 5 |
| 65+ | 75 | 1.2 | <1 | 1 | 1 | 1 | 1 | 2 | 2 | 2 |
| **2. MULTIPLE DX** | | | | | | | | | | |
| 0–19 Years | 46 | 2.2 | 26 | 1 | 1 | 1 | 2 | 3 | 24 | >99 |
| 20–34 | 49 | 1.5 | <1 | 1 | 1 | 1 | 2 | 2 | 3 | 3 |
| 35–49 | 83 | 1.5 | 3 | 1 | 1 | 1 | 1 | 2 | 4 | 8 |
| 50–64 | 153 | 2.1 | 7 | 1 | 1 | 1 | 2 | 4 | 7 | 16 |
| 65+ | 308 | 1.4 | 2 | 1 | 1 | 1 | 1 | 2 | 3 | 9 |
| **TOTAL SINGLE DX** | 197 | 1.3 | <1 | 1 | 1 | 1 | 1 | 2 | 2 | 4 |
| **TOTAL MULTIPLE DX** | 639 | 1.7 | 5 | 1 | 1 | 1 | 2 | 3 | 4 | 10 |
| **TOTAL** | | | | | | | | | | |
| 0–19 Years | 55 | 1.9 | 19 | 1 | 1 | 1 | 1 | 2 | 7 | >99 |
| 20–34 | 66 | 1.5 | <1 | 1 | 1 | 1 | 2 | 2 | 3 | 3 |
| 35–49 | 123 | 1.4 | 2 | 1 | 1 | 1 | 1 | 2 | 3 | 8 |
| 50–64 | 209 | 2.0 | 6 | 1 | 1 | 1 | 2 | 4 | 5 | 14 |
| 65+ | 383 | 1.3 | 1 | 1 | 1 | 1 | 1 | 2 | 3 | 6 |
| **GRAND TOTAL** | 836 | 1.6 | 4 | 1 | 1 | 1 | 2 | 2 | 3 | 9 |

## 14.4: REP RETINA DETACH/BUCKLE. Formerly included in operation group(s) 528.

| Type of Patients | Observed Patients | Avg. Stay | Variance | 10th | 25th | 50th | 75th | 90th | 95th | 99th |
|---|---|---|---|---|---|---|---|---|---|---|
| **1. SINGLE DX** | | | | | | | | | | |
| 0–19 Years | 11 | 1.0 | <1 | 1 | 1 | 1 | 1 | 1 | 1 | 4 |
| 20–34 | 22 | 1.4 | <1 | 1 | 1 | 1 | 1 | 2 | 2 | 4 |
| 35–49 | 54 | 1.4 | <1 | 1 | 1 | 1 | 1 | 2 | 3 | 3 |
| 50–64 | 71 | 1.3 | <1 | 1 | 1 | 1 | 1 | 2 | 3 | 5 |
| 65+ | 90 | 1.2 | <1 | 1 | 1 | 1 | 1 | 2 | 2 | 3 |
| **2. MULTIPLE DX** | | | | | | | | | | |
| 0–19 Years | 51 | 2.2 | 24 | 1 | 1 | 1 | 2 | 3 | 24 | >99 |
| 20–34 | 63 | 1.5 | <1 | 1 | 1 | 1 | 2 | 2 | 3 | 3 |
| 35–49 | 118 | 1.5 | 3 | 1 | 1 | 1 | 1 | 2 | 4 | 8 |
| 50–64 | 217 | 2.1 | 7 | 1 | 1 | 1 | 2 | 4 | 7 | 14 |
| 65+ | 421 | 1.3 | 1 | 1 | 1 | 1 | 1 | 2 | 2 | 6 |
| **TOTAL SINGLE DX** | 248 | 1.3 | <1 | 1 | 1 | 1 | 1 | 2 | 2 | 4 |
| **TOTAL MULTIPLE DX** | 870 | 1.7 | 4 | 1 | 1 | 2 | 2 | 3 | 4 | 14 |
| **TOTAL** | | | | | | | | | | |
| 0–19 Years | 62 | 1.9 | 18 | 1 | 1 | 1 | 1 | 2 | 7 | >99 |
| 20–34 | 85 | 1.5 | <1 | 1 | 1 | 1 | 2 | 2 | 3 | 3 |
| 35–49 | 172 | 1.5 | 2 | 1 | 1 | 1 | 1 | 2 | 4 | 7 |
| 50–64 | 288 | 1.9 | 5 | 1 | 1 | 1 | 2 | 4 | 5 | 14 |
| 65+ | 511 | 1.3 | 1 | 1 | 1 | 1 | 1 | 2 | 2 | 5 |
| **GRAND TOTAL** | 1,118 | 1.6 | 4 | 1 | 1 | 1 | 2 | 2 | 3 | 9 |

## 14.5: OTH REPAIR RETINA DETACH. Formerly included in operation group(s) 528.

| Type of Patients | Observed Patients | Avg. Stay | Variance | 10th | 25th | 50th | 75th | 90th | 95th | 99th |
|---|---|---|---|---|---|---|---|---|---|---|
| **1. SINGLE DX** | | | | | | | | | | |
| 0–19 Years | 6 | 1.1 | <1 | 1 | 1 | 1 | 1 | 1 | 2 | 2 |
| 20–34 | 4 | 1.0 | 0 | 1 | 1 | 1 | 1 | 1 | 1 | 1 |
| 35–49 | 6 | 1.0 | 0 | 1 | 1 | 1 | 1 | 1 | 1 | 1 |
| 50–64 | 18 | 1.5 | <1 | 1 | 1 | 1 | 2 | 2 | 2 | 3 |
| 65+ | 18 | 1.1 | <1 | 1 | 1 | 1 | 1 | 2 | 2 | 3 |
| **2. MULTIPLE DX** | | | | | | | | | | |
| 0–19 Years | 36 | 7.6 | 316 | 1 | 1 | 1 | 2 | 33 | 81 | >99 |
| 20–34 | 30 | 2.4 | 10 | 1 | 1 | 1 | 3 | 4 | 6 | 20 |
| 35–49 | 36 | 1.9 | 5 | 1 | 1 | 1 | 2 | 3 | 5 | 12 |
| 50–64 | 77 | 2.5 | 8 | 1 | 1 | 1 | 3 | 6 | 7 | 15 |
| 65+ | 128 | 1.4 | 1 | 1 | 1 | 1 | 1 | 2 | 4 | 8 |
| **TOTAL SINGLE DX** | 52 | 1.2 | <1 | 1 | 1 | 1 | 1 | 2 | 2 | 2 |
| **TOTAL MULTIPLE DX** | 307 | 2.4 | 33 | 1 | 1 | 1 | 2 | 4 | 7 | 30 |
| **TOTAL** | | | | | | | | | | |
| 0–19 Years | 42 | 5.7 | 232 | 1 | 1 | 1 | 2 | 23 | 75 | >99 |
| 20–34 | 34 | 2.2 | 9 | 1 | 1 | 1 | 2 | 4 | 5 | 20 |
| 35–49 | 42 | 1.7 | 4 | 1 | 1 | 1 | 1 | 3 | 5 | 12 |
| 50–64 | 95 | 2.3 | 6 | 1 | 1 | 1 | 2 | 6 | 7 | 15 |
| 65+ | 146 | 1.4 | 1 | 1 | 1 | 1 | 1 | 2 | 4 | 8 |
| **GRAND TOTAL** | 359 | 2.2 | 27 | 1 | 1 | 1 | 2 | 4 | 7 | 23 |

Length of Stay by Diagnosis and Operation, United States, 2000

**United States, October 1998–September 1999 Data, by Operation**

### 14.6: RMVL PROSTH MAT POST SEG. Formerly included in operation group(s) 529.

| Type of Patients | Observed Patients | Avg. Stay | Variance | 10th | 25th | 50th | 75th | 90th | 95th | 99th |
|---|---|---|---|---|---|---|---|---|---|---|
| **1. SINGLE DX** | | | | | | | | | | |
| 0–19 Years | 0 | | | | | | | | | |
| 20–34 | 0 | | | | | | | | | |
| 35–49 | 4 | 3.2 | 3 | | 1 | 4 | 4 | 5 | 5 | 5 |
| 50–64 | 4 | 2.3 | <1 | | 2 | 2 | 2 | 4 | 4 | 4 |
| 65+ | 3 | 2.5 | 8 | | 1 | 1 | 1 | 7 | 7 | 7 |
| **2. MULTIPLE DX** | | | | | | | | | | |
| 0–19 Years | 6 | 1.0 | 0 | 1 | 1 | 1 | 1 | 1 | 1 | 1 |
| 20–34 | 4 | 3.0 | 3 | 1 | 2 | 3 | 3 | 3 | 8 | 8 |
| 35–49 | 5 | 4.1 | 9 | 1 | 2 | 4 | 6 | 9 | 9 | 9 |
| 50–64 | 10 | 6.2 | 10 | 1 | 4 | 8 | 8 | 9 | 11 | 11 |
| 65+ | 17 | 3.6 | 10 | 1 | 1 | 3 | 5 | 7 | 11 | 11 |
| **TOTAL SINGLE DX** | 11 | 2.5 | 2 | 1 | 1 | 2 | 4 | 4 | 5 | 7 |
| **TOTAL MULTIPLE DX** | 42 | 4.0 | 10 | 1 | 1 | 3 | 7 | 8 | 11 | 11 |
| **TOTAL** | | | | | | | | | | |
| 0–19 Years | 6 | 1.0 | 0 | 1 | 1 | 1 | 1 | 1 | 1 | 1 |
| 20–34 | 4 | 3.0 | 3 | 1 | 2 | 3 | 3 | 3 | 8 | 8 |
| 35–49 | 9 | 3.8 | 7 | 1 | 2 | 4 | 5 | 9 | 9 | 9 |
| 50–64 | 14 | 4.8 | 11 | 1 | 4 | 4 | 8 | 8 | 11 | 11 |
| 65+ | 20 | 3.5 | 9 | 1 | 1 | 3 | 5 | 7 | 11 | 11 |
| **GRAND TOTAL** | 53 | 3.7 | 9 | 1 | 1 | 2 | 6 | 8 | 9 | 11 |

### 14.74: MECH VITRECTOMY NEC. Formerly included in operation group(s) 529.

| Type of Patients | Observed Patients | Avg. Stay | Variance | 10th | 25th | 50th | 75th | 90th | 95th | 99th |
|---|---|---|---|---|---|---|---|---|---|---|
| **1. SINGLE DX** | | | | | | | | | | |
| 0–19 Years | 14 | 1.5 | <1 | 1 | 1 | 1 | 1 | 2 | 2 | 3 |
| 20–34 | 7 | 2.5 | 3 | 1 | 1 | 1 | 4 | 4 | 4 | 8 |
| 35–49 | 9 | 2.1 | <1 | 1 | 2 | 2 | 2 | 3 | 3 | 4 |
| 50–64 | 22 | 1.5 | <1 | 1 | 1 | 1 | 2 | 2 | 3 | 3 |
| 65+ | 54 | 1.3 | <1 | 1 | 1 | 1 | 1 | 2 | 3 | 4 |
| **2. MULTIPLE DX** | | | | | | | | | | |
| 0–19 Years | 45 | 2.5 | 16 | 1 | 1 | 1 | 1 | 6 | 17 | 17 |
| 20–34 | 57 | 2.7 | 15 | 1 | 1 | 1 | 3 | 6 | 12 | 19 |
| 35–49 | 104 | 3.1 | 14 | 1 | 2 | 2 | 3 | 6 | 11 | 27 |
| 50–64 | 185 | 2.5 | 20 | 1 | 1 | 1 | 2 | 4 | 6 | 33 |
| 65+ | 538 | 2.0 | 9 | 1 | 1 | 1 | 2 | 4 | 5 | 14 |
| **TOTAL SINGLE DX** | 106 | 1.6 | <1 | 1 | 1 | 1 | 2 | 3 | 3 | 4 |
| **TOTAL MULTIPLE DX** | 929 | 2.4 | 14 | 1 | 1 | 1 | 2 | 5 | 7 | 21 |
| **TOTAL** | | | | | | | | | | |
| 0–19 Years | 59 | 2.3 | 12 | 1 | 1 | 1 | 2 | 4 | 9 | 17 |
| 20–34 | 64 | 2.7 | 13 | 1 | 1 | 1 | 3 | 6 | 12 | 19 |
| 35–49 | 113 | 3.0 | 13 | 1 | 2 | 2 | 3 | 5 | 10 | 27 |
| 50–64 | 207 | 2.4 | 19 | 1 | 1 | 1 | 2 | 4 | 6 | 33 |
| 65+ | 592 | 2.0 | 8 | 1 | 1 | 1 | 2 | 4 | 5 | 14 |
| **GRAND TOTAL** | 1,035 | 2.3 | 12 | 1 | 1 | 1 | 2 | 4 | 6 | 19 |

### 14.7: OPERATIONS ON VITREOUS. Formerly included in operation group(s) 529.

| Type of Patients | Observed Patients | Avg. Stay | Variance | 10th | 25th | 50th | 75th | 90th | 95th | 99th |
|---|---|---|---|---|---|---|---|---|---|---|
| **1. SINGLE DX** | | | | | | | | | | |
| 0–19 Years | 26 | 1.7 | 2 | 1 | 1 | 1 | 2 | 3 | 4 | 7 |
| 20–34 | 12 | 2.1 | 3 | 1 | 1 | 1 | 3 | 4 | 4 | 8 |
| 35–49 | 21 | 3.0 | 69 | 1 | 1 | 2 | 2 | 3 | 4 | 60 |
| 50–64 | 35 | 1.5 | <1 | 1 | 1 | 1 | 2 | 2 | 3 | 3 |
| 65+ | 81 | 1.8 | 2 | 1 | 1 | 1 | 2 | 4 | 7 | 7 |
| **2. MULTIPLE DX** | | | | | | | | | | |
| 0–19 Years | 75 | 3.0 | 12 | 1 | 1 | 1 | 4 | 5 | 11 | 17 |
| 20–34 | 98 | 3.9 | 59 | 1 | 1 | 1 | 3 | 7 | 19 | 24 |
| 35–49 | 152 | 3.3 | 17 | 1 | 2 | 2 | 3 | 8 | 10 | 27 |
| 50–64 | 267 | 2.6 | 20 | 1 | 1 | 1 | 2 | 5 | 7 | 33 |
| 65+ | 740 | 2.2 | 8 | 1 | 1 | 1 | 2 | 4 | 6 | 14 |
| **TOTAL SINGLE DX** | 175 | 2.0 | 17 | 1 | 1 | 1 | 2 | 3 | 4 | 7 |
| **TOTAL MULTIPLE DX** | 1,332 | 2.6 | 17 | 1 | 1 | 1 | 3 | 5 | 8 | 23 |
| **TOTAL** | | | | | | | | | | |
| 0–19 Years | 101 | 2.7 | 10 | 1 | 1 | 1 | 4 | 5 | 7 | 17 |
| 20–34 | 110 | 3.7 | 54 | 1 | 1 | 1 | 3 | 6 | 19 | 24 |
| 35–49 | 173 | 3.2 | 27 | 1 | 1 | 2 | 3 | 7 | 10 | 27 |
| 50–64 | 302 | 2.5 | 18 | 1 | 1 | 1 | 2 | 4 | 7 | 33 |
| 65+ | 821 | 2.1 | 8 | 1 | 1 | 1 | 2 | 4 | 6 | 13 |
| **GRAND TOTAL** | 1,507 | 2.5 | 17 | 1 | 1 | 1 | 3 | 5 | 7 | 23 |

### 14.9: OTHER POST SEGMENT OPS. Formerly included in operation group(s) 529.

| Type of Patients | Observed Patients | Avg. Stay | Variance | 10th | 25th | 50th | 75th | 90th | 95th | 99th |
|---|---|---|---|---|---|---|---|---|---|---|
| **1. SINGLE DX** | | | | | | | | | | |
| 0–19 Years | 6 | 1.1 | <1 | 1 | 1 | 1 | 1 | 2 | 2 | 2 |
| 20–34 | 2 | 1.0 | 0 | 1 | 1 | 1 | 1 | 1 | 1 | 1 |
| 35–49 | 6 | 1.0 | 0 | 1 | 1 | 1 | 1 | 1 | 1 | 1 |
| 50–64 | 13 | 1.2 | <1 | 1 | 1 | 1 | 1 | 2 | 2 | 2 |
| 65+ | 47 | 1.0 | <1 | 1 | 1 | 1 | 1 | 1 | 1 | 2 |
| **2. MULTIPLE DX** | | | | | | | | | | |
| 0–19 Years | 25 | 1.4 | 2 | 1 | 1 | 1 | 1 | 3 | 3 | 5 |
| 20–34 | 33 | 1.6 | <1 | 1 | 1 | 1 | 2 | 3 | 3 | 6 |
| 35–49 | 45 | 1.5 | <1 | 1 | 1 | 1 | 2 | 2 | 3 | 6 |
| 50–64 | 118 | 1.6 | 8 | 1 | 1 | 1 | 1 | 2 | 4 | 24 |
| 65+ | 309 | 1.3 | 1 | 1 | 1 | 1 | 1 | 2 | 2 | 8 |
| **TOTAL SINGLE DX** | 74 | 1.1 | <1 | 1 | 1 | 1 | 1 | 1 | 2 | 2 |
| **TOTAL MULTIPLE DX** | 530 | 1.4 | 3 | 1 | 1 | 1 | 1 | 2 | 3 | 8 |
| **TOTAL** | | | | | | | | | | |
| 0–19 Years | 31 | 1.4 | 1 | 1 | 1 | 1 | 1 | 2 | 3 | 5 |
| 20–34 | 35 | 1.6 | <1 | 1 | 1 | 1 | 2 | 3 | 3 | 6 |
| 35–49 | 51 | 1.5 | <1 | 1 | 1 | 1 | 2 | 2 | 3 | 6 |
| 50–64 | 131 | 1.6 | 8 | 1 | 1 | 1 | 1 | 2 | 3 | 24 |
| 65+ | 356 | 1.2 | 1 | 1 | 1 | 1 | 1 | 1 | 2 | 8 |
| **GRAND TOTAL** | 604 | 1.4 | 3 | 1 | 1 | 1 | 1 | 2 | 3 | 8 |

Length of Stay by Diagnosis and Operation, United States, 2000

## United States, October 1998–September 1999 Data, by Operation

### 15.0: EXOC MUSC-TEND DXTIC PX. Formerly included in operation group(s) 530, 532.

| Type of Patients | Observed Patients | Avg. Stay | Variance | 10th | 25th | 50th | 75th | 90th | 95th | 99th |
|---|---|---|---|---|---|---|---|---|---|---|
| **1. SINGLE DX** | | | | | | | | | | |
| 0–19 Years | 0 | | | | | | | | | |
| 20–34 | 0 | | | | | | | | | |
| 35–49 | 0 | | | | | | | | | |
| 50–64 | 0 | | | | | | | | | |
| 65+ | 0 | | | | | | | | | |
| **2. MULTIPLE DX** | | | | | | | | | | |
| 0–19 Years | 0 | | | | | | | | | |
| 20–34 | 0 | | | | | | | | | |
| 35–49 | 0 | | | | | | | | | |
| 50–64 | 1 | 6.0 | 0 | 6 | 6 | 6 | 6 | 6 | 6 | 6 |
| 65+ | 0 | | | | | | | | | |
| **TOTAL SINGLE DX** | 0 | | | | | | | | | |
| **TOTAL MULTIPLE DX** | 1 | 6.0 | 0 | 6 | 6 | 6 | 6 | 6 | 6 | 6 |
| **TOTAL** | | | | | | | | | | |
| 0–19 Years | 0 | | | | | | | | | |
| 20–34 | 0 | | | | | | | | | |
| 35–49 | 0 | | | | | | | | | |
| 50–64 | 1 | 6.0 | 0 | 6 | 6 | 6 | 6 | 6 | 6 | 6 |
| 65+ | 0 | | | | | | | | | |
| **GRAND TOTAL** | 1 | 6.0 | 0 | 6 | 6 | 6 | 6 | 6 | 6 | 6 |

### 15.1: 1 EXOC MUSC OPS W DETACH. Formerly included in operation group(s) 530.

| Type of Patients | Observed Patients | Avg. Stay | Variance | 10th | 25th | 50th | 75th | 90th | 95th | 99th |
|---|---|---|---|---|---|---|---|---|---|---|
| **1. SINGLE DX** | | | | | | | | | | |
| 0–19 Years | 209 | 1.0 | <1 | 1 | 1 | 1 | 1 | 1 | 1 | 2 |
| 20–34 | 0 | | | | | | | | | |
| 35–49 | 0 | | | | | | | | | |
| 50–64 | 0 | | | | | | | | | |
| 65+ | 1 | 5.0 | 0 | 5 | 5 | 5 | 5 | 5 | 5 | 5 |
| **2. MULTIPLE DX** | | | | | | | | | | |
| 0–19 Years | 62 | 1.3 | 11 | 1 | 1 | 1 | 1 | 1 | 1 | 3 |
| 20–34 | 3 | 2.6 | <1 | 2 | 2 | 3 | 3 | 3 | 3 | 3 |
| 35–49 | 4 | 2.7 | 2 | 2 | 2 | 2 | 2 | 5 | 5 | 5 |
| 50–64 | 2 | 1.8 | 3 | 1 | 1 | 1 | 1 | 5 | 5 | 5 |
| 65+ | 3 | 1.0 | 0 | 1 | 1 | 1 | 1 | 1 | 1 | 1 |
| **TOTAL SINGLE DX** | 210 | 1.0 | <1 | 1 | 1 | 1 | 1 | 1 | 1 | 2 |
| **TOTAL MULTIPLE DX** | 74 | 1.4 | 11 | 1 | 1 | 1 | 1 | 2 | 2 | 5 |
| **TOTAL** | | | | | | | | | | |
| 0–19 Years | 271 | 1.1 | 3 | 1 | 1 | 1 | 1 | 1 | 1 | 3 |
| 20–34 | 3 | 2.6 | <1 | 2 | 2 | 3 | 3 | 3 | 3 | 3 |
| 35–49 | 4 | 2.7 | 2 | 2 | 2 | 2 | 2 | 5 | 5 | 5 |
| 50–64 | 2 | 1.8 | 3 | 1 | 1 | 1 | 1 | 5 | 5 | 5 |
| 65+ | 4 | 2.2 | 4 | 1 | 1 | 1 | 1 | 5 | 5 | 5 |
| **GRAND TOTAL** | 284 | 1.1 | 3 | 1 | 1 | 1 | 1 | 1 | 1 | 3 |

### 15.2: OTH OPS ON 1 EXOC MUSCLE. Formerly included in operation group(s) 530.

| Type of Patients | Observed Patients | Avg. Stay | Variance | 10th | 25th | 50th | 75th | 90th | 95th | 99th |
|---|---|---|---|---|---|---|---|---|---|---|
| **1. SINGLE DX** | | | | | | | | | | |
| 0–19 Years | 1 | 1.0 | 0 | 1 | 1 | 1 | 1 | 1 | 1 | 1 |
| 20–34 | 0 | | | | | | | | | |
| 35–49 | 0 | | | | | | | | | |
| 50–64 | 0 | | | | | | | | | |
| 65+ | 0 | | | | | | | | | |
| **2. MULTIPLE DX** | | | | | | | | | | |
| 0–19 Years | 0 | | | | | | | | | |
| 20–34 | 0 | | | | | | | | | |
| 35–49 | 0 | | | | | | | | | |
| 50–64 | 0 | | | | | | | | | |
| 65+ | 0 | | | | | | | | | |
| **TOTAL SINGLE DX** | 1 | 1.0 | 0 | 1 | 1 | 1 | 1 | 1 | 1 | 1 |
| **TOTAL MULTIPLE DX** | 0 | | | | | | | | | |
| **TOTAL** | | | | | | | | | | |
| 0–19 Years | 1 | 1.0 | 0 | 1 | 1 | 1 | 1 | 1 | 1 | 1 |
| 20–34 | 0 | | | | | | | | | |
| 35–49 | 0 | | | | | | | | | |
| 50–64 | 0 | | | | | | | | | |
| 65+ | 0 | | | | | | | | | |
| **GRAND TOTAL** | 1 | 1.0 | 0 | 1 | 1 | 1 | 1 | 1 | 1 | 1 |

### 15.3: TEMP DETACH >1 EXOC MUSC. Formerly included in operation group(s) 530.

| Type of Patients | Observed Patients | Avg. Stay | Variance | 10th | 25th | 50th | 75th | 90th | 95th | 99th |
|---|---|---|---|---|---|---|---|---|---|---|
| **1. SINGLE DX** | | | | | | | | | | |
| 0–19 Years | 21 | 1.0 | 0 | 1 | 1 | 1 | 1 | 1 | 1 | 1 |
| 20–34 | 0 | | | | | | | | | |
| 35–49 | 1 | 4.0 | 0 | 4 | 4 | 4 | 4 | 4 | 4 | 4 |
| 50–64 | 0 | | | | | | | | | |
| 65+ | 0 | | | | | | | | | |
| **2. MULTIPLE DX** | | | | | | | | | | |
| 0–19 Years | 41 | 1.1 | <1 | 1 | 1 | 1 | 1 | 1 | 1 | 4 |
| 20–34 | 5 | 1.6 | 1 | 1 | 1 | 1 | 2 | 2 | 4 | 4 |
| 35–49 | 4 | 1.8 | 1 | 1 | 1 | 1 | 2 | 2 | 4 | 4 |
| 50–64 | 2 | 3.0 | 9 | 1 | 1 | 1 | 7 | 7 | 7 | 7 |
| 65+ | 1 | 27.0 | 0 | 27 | 27 | 27 | 27 | 27 | 27 | 27 |
| **TOTAL SINGLE DX** | 22 | 1.0 | <1 | 1 | 1 | 1 | 1 | 1 | 1 | 4 |
| **TOTAL MULTIPLE DX** | 53 | 1.3 | 3 | 1 | 1 | 1 | 1 | 2 | 2 | 7 |
| **TOTAL** | | | | | | | | | | |
| 0–19 Years | 62 | 1.1 | <1 | 1 | 1 | 1 | 1 | 1 | 1 | 4 |
| 20–34 | 5 | 1.6 | 1 | 1 | 1 | 2 | 2 | 4 | 4 | 4 |
| 35–49 | 5 | 2.3 | 2 | 1 | 1 | 2 | 4 | 4 | 4 | 4 |
| 50–64 | 2 | 3.0 | 9 | 1 | 1 | 7 | 7 | 7 | 7 | 7 |
| 65+ | 1 | 27.0 | 0 | 27 | 27 | 27 | 27 | 27 | 27 | 27 |
| **GRAND TOTAL** | 75 | 1.2 | 2 | 1 | 1 | 1 | 1 | 1 | 1 | 7 |

Length of Stay by Diagnosis and Operation, United States, 2000

# United States, October 1998–September 1999 Data, by Operation

## 15.4: OTH OPS ON >1 EXOC MUSC. Formerly included in operation group(s) 530.

| Type of Patients | Observed Patients | Avg. Stay | Vari-ance | Percentiles | | | | | | |
|---|---|---|---|---|---|---|---|---|---|---|
| | | | | 10th | 25th | 50th | 75th | 90th | 95th | 99th |
| **1. SINGLE DX** | | | | | | | | | | |
| 0–19 Years | 0 | | | | | | | | | |
| 20–34 | 0 | | | | | | | | | |
| 35–49 | 0 | | | | | | | | | |
| 50–64 | 0 | | | | | | | | | |
| 65+ | 0 | | | | | | | | | |
| **2. MULTIPLE DX** | | | | | | | | | | |
| 0–19 Years | 0 | | | | | | | | | |
| 20–34 | 0 | | | | | | | | | |
| 35–49 | 0 | | | | | | | | | |
| 50–64 | 0 | | | | | | | | | |
| 65+ | 0 | | | | | | | | | |
| **TOTAL SINGLE DX** | 0 | | | | | | | | | |
| **TOTAL MULTIPLE DX** | 0 | | | | | | | | | |
| **TOTAL** | | | | | | | | | | |
| 0–19 Years | 0 | | | | | | | | | |
| 20–34 | 0 | | | | | | | | | |
| 35–49 | 0 | | | | | | | | | |
| 50–64 | 0 | | | | | | | | | |
| 65+ | 0 | | | | | | | | | |
| **GRAND TOTAL** | 0 | | | | | | | | | |

## 15.5: EXOC MUSC TRANSPOSITION. Formerly included in operation group(s) 530.

| Type of Patients | Observed Patients | Avg. Stay | Vari-ance | Percentiles | | | | | | |
|---|---|---|---|---|---|---|---|---|---|---|
| | | | | 10th | 25th | 50th | 75th | 90th | 95th | 99th |
| **1. SINGLE DX** | | | | | | | | | | |
| 0–19 Years | 0 | | | | | | | | | |
| 20–34 | 0 | | | | | | | | | |
| 35–49 | 1 | 1.0 | 0 | 1 | 1 | 1 | 1 | 1 | 1 | 1 |
| 50–64 | 1 | 1.0 | 0 | 1 | 1 | 1 | 1 | 1 | 1 | 1 |
| 65+ | 0 | | | | | | | | | |
| **2. MULTIPLE DX** | | | | | | | | | | |
| 0–19 Years | 0 | | | | | | | | | |
| 20–34 | 0 | | | | | | | | | |
| 35–49 | 0 | | | | | | | | | |
| 50–64 | 0 | | | | | | | | | |
| 65+ | 1 | 1.0 | 0 | 1 | 1 | 1 | 1 | 1 | 1 | 1 |
| **TOTAL SINGLE DX** | 2 | 1.0 | 0 | 1 | 1 | 1 | 1 | 1 | 1 | 1 |
| **TOTAL MULTIPLE DX** | 1 | 1.0 | 0 | 1 | 1 | 1 | 1 | 1 | 1 | 1 |
| **TOTAL** | | | | | | | | | | |
| 0–19 Years | 0 | | | | | | | | | |
| 20–34 | 0 | | | | | | | | | |
| 35–49 | 1 | 1.0 | 0 | 1 | 1 | 1 | 1 | 1 | 1 | 1 |
| 50–64 | 1 | 1.0 | 0 | 1 | 1 | 1 | 1 | 1 | 1 | 1 |
| 65+ | 1 | 1.0 | 0 | 1 | 1 | 1 | 1 | 1 | 1 | 1 |
| **GRAND TOTAL** | 3 | 1.0 | 0 | 1 | 1 | 1 | 1 | 1 | 1 | 1 |

## 15.6: REV EXOC MUSCLE SURGERY. Formerly included in operation group(s) 530.

| Type of Patients | Observed Patients | Avg. Stay | Vari-ance | Percentiles | | | | | | |
|---|---|---|---|---|---|---|---|---|---|---|
| | | | | 10th | 25th | 50th | 75th | 90th | 95th | 99th |
| **1. SINGLE DX** | | | | | | | | | | |
| 0–19 Years | 6 | 1.0 | 0 | 1 | 1 | 1 | 1 | 1 | 1 | 1 |
| 20–34 | 0 | | | | | | | | | |
| 35–49 | 0 | | | | | | | | | |
| 50–64 | 0 | | | | | | | | | |
| 65+ | 0 | | | | | | | | | |
| **2. MULTIPLE DX** | | | | | | | | | | |
| 0–19 Years | 2 | 1.0 | 0 | 1 | 1 | 1 | 1 | 1 | 1 | 1 |
| 20–34 | 0 | | | | | | | | | |
| 35–49 | 1 | 2.0 | 0 | 2 | 2 | 2 | 2 | 2 | 2 | 2 |
| 50–64 | 0 | | | | | | | | | |
| 65+ | 0 | | | | | | | | | |
| **TOTAL SINGLE DX** | 6 | 1.0 | 0 | 1 | 1 | 1 | 1 | 1 | 1 | 1 |
| **TOTAL MULTIPLE DX** | 3 | 1.5 | <1 | 1 | 1 | 2 | 2 | 2 | 2 | 2 |
| **TOTAL** | | | | | | | | | | |
| 0–19 Years | 8 | 1.0 | 0 | 1 | 1 | 1 | 1 | 1 | 1 | 1 |
| 20–34 | 0 | | | | | | | | | |
| 35–49 | 1 | 2.0 | 0 | 2 | 2 | 2 | 2 | 2 | 2 | 2 |
| 50–64 | 0 | | | | | | | | | |
| 65+ | 0 | | | | | | | | | |
| **GRAND TOTAL** | 9 | 1.4 | <1 | 1 | 1 | 1 | 2 | 2 | 2 | 2 |

## 15.7: EXOC MUSCLE INJURY REP. Formerly included in operation group(s) 530.

| Type of Patients | Observed Patients | Avg. Stay | Vari-ance | Percentiles | | | | | | |
|---|---|---|---|---|---|---|---|---|---|---|
| | | | | 10th | 25th | 50th | 75th | 90th | 95th | 99th |
| **1. SINGLE DX** | | | | | | | | | | |
| 0–19 Years | 0 | | | | | | | | | |
| 20–34 | 0 | | | | | | | | | |
| 35–49 | 0 | | | | | | | | | |
| 50–64 | 0 | | | | | | | | | |
| 65+ | 1 | 2.0 | 0 | 2 | 2 | 2 | 2 | 2 | 2 | 2 |
| **2. MULTIPLE DX** | | | | | | | | | | |
| 0–19 Years | 5 | 1.6 | <1 | 1 | 1 | 1 | 2 | 3 | 3 | 3 |
| 20–34 | 7 | 2.9 | 3 | 1 | 1 | 3 | 4 | 5 | 5 | 5 |
| 35–49 | 2 | 2.0 | 0 | 2 | 2 | 2 | 2 | 2 | 2 | 2 |
| 50–64 | 2 | 5.6 | <1 | 4 | 6 | 6 | 6 | 6 | 6 | 6 |
| 65+ | 4 | 2.1 | 3 | 1 | 1 | 1 | 3 | 5 | 5 | 5 |
| **TOTAL SINGLE DX** | 1 | 2.0 | 0 | 2 | 2 | 2 | 2 | 2 | 2 | 2 |
| **TOTAL MULTIPLE DX** | 20 | 3.4 | 4 | 1 | 1 | 3 | 6 | 6 | 6 | 6 |
| **TOTAL** | | | | | | | | | | |
| 0–19 Years | 5 | 1.6 | <1 | 1 | 1 | 1 | 2 | 3 | 3 | 3 |
| 20–34 | 7 | 2.9 | 3 | 1 | 1 | 3 | 4 | 5 | 5 | 5 |
| 35–49 | 2 | 2.0 | 0 | 2 | 2 | 2 | 2 | 2 | 2 | 2 |
| 50–64 | 2 | 5.6 | <1 | 4 | 6 | 6 | 6 | 6 | 6 | 6 |
| 65+ | 5 | 2.0 | 2 | 1 | 1 | 1 | 3 | 5 | 5 | 5 |
| **GRAND TOTAL** | 21 | 3.4 | 4 | 1 | 2 | 3 | 6 | 6 | 6 | 6 |

Length of Stay by Diagnosis and Operation, United States, 2000

# United States, October 1998–September 1999 Data, by Operation

## 15.9: OTH EXOC MUSC-TEND OPS. Formerly included in operation group(s) 530.

| Type of Patients | Observed Patients | Avg. Stay | Variance | 10th | 25th | 50th | 75th | 90th | 95th | 99th |
|---|---|---|---|---|---|---|---|---|---|---|
| **1. SINGLE DX** | | | | | | | | | | |
| 0–19 Years | 0 | | | | | | | | | |
| 20–34 | 0 | | | | | | | | | |
| 35–49 | 1 | 1.0 | 0 | 1 | 1 | 1 | 1 | 1 | 1 | 1 |
| 50–64 | 0 | | | | | | | | | |
| 65+ | 0 | | | | | | | | | |
| **2. MULTIPLE DX** | | | | | | | | | | |
| 0–19 Years | 0 | | | | | | | | | |
| 20–34 | 0 | | | | | | | | | |
| 35–49 | 0 | | | | | | | | | |
| 50–64 | 1 | 6.0 | 0 | 6 | 6 | 6 | 6 | 6 | 6 | 6 |
| 65+ | 0 | | | | | | | | | |
| **TOTAL SINGLE DX** | 1 | 1.0 | 0 | 1 | 1 | 1 | 1 | 1 | 1 | 1 |
| **TOTAL MULTIPLE DX** | 1 | 6.0 | 0 | 6 | 6 | 6 | 6 | 6 | 6 | 6 |
| **TOTAL** | | | | | | | | | | |
| 0–19 Years | 0 | | | | | | | | | |
| 20–34 | 0 | | | | | | | | | |
| 35–49 | 1 | 1.0 | 0 | 1 | 1 | 1 | 1 | 1 | 1 | 1 |
| 50–64 | 1 | 6.0 | 0 | 6 | 6 | 6 | 6 | 6 | 6 | 6 |
| 65+ | 0 | | | | | | | | | |
| **GRAND TOTAL** | 2 | 4.6 | 6 | 1 | 1 | 6 | 6 | 6 | 6 | 6 |

## 16.09: ORBITOTOMY NEC. Formerly included in operation group(s) 531.

| Type of Patients | Observed Patients | Avg. Stay | Variance | 10th | 25th | 50th | 75th | 90th | 95th | 99th |
|---|---|---|---|---|---|---|---|---|---|---|
| **1. SINGLE DX** | | | | | | | | | | |
| 0–19 Years | 20 | 4.5 | 9 | 1 | 2 | 5 | 6 | 10 | 10 | 10 |
| 20–34 | 11 | 1.8 | <1 | 1 | 1 | 2 | 2 | 5 | 10 | 4 |
| 35–49 | 7 | 1.9 | 2 | 1 | 1 | 4 | 3 | 5 | 5 | 6 |
| 50–64 | 8 | 2.0 | <1 | 2 | 2 | 2 | 2 | 2 | 2 | 4 |
| 65+ | 0 | | | | | | | | | |
| **2. MULTIPLE DX** | | | | | | | | | | |
| 0–19 Years | 132 | 7.4 | 29 | 3 | 4 | 6 | 8 | 15 | 23 | 23 |
| 20–34 | 37 | 3.5 | 50 | 1 | 1 | 1 | 3 | 8 | 10 | 51 |
| 35–49 | 47 | 8.9 | 134 | 1 | 2 | 5 | 7 | 28 | 39 | 46 |
| 50–64 | 43 | 3.0 | 9 | 1 | 1 | 2 | 4 | 5 | 5 | 18 |
| 65+ | 41 | 3.5 | 11 | 1 | 1 | 2 | 6 | 10 | 10 | 12 |
| **TOTAL SINGLE DX** | 46 | 2.5 | 4 | 1 | 1 | 2 | 3 | 5 | 6 | 10 |
| **TOTAL MULTIPLE DX** | 300 | 5.8 | 47 | 1 | 2 | 4 | 7 | 12 | 23 | 39 |
| **TOTAL** | | | | | | | | | | |
| 0–19 Years | 152 | 7.1 | 28 | 2 | 4 | 6 | 8 | 14 | 23 | 23 |
| 20–34 | 48 | 3.1 | 41 | 1 | 1 | 1 | 2 | 6 | 10 | 51 |
| 35–49 | 54 | 6.7 | 103 | 1 | 1 | 3 | 7 | 28 | 39 | 46 |
| 50–64 | 51 | 2.8 | 8 | 1 | 1 | 2 | 4 | 4 | 5 | 18 |
| 65+ | 41 | 3.5 | 11 | 1 | 1 | 2 | 6 | 10 | 10 | 12 |
| **GRAND TOTAL** | 346 | 5.2 | 42 | 1 | 1 | 4 | 6 | 10 | 19 | 39 |

## 16.0: ORBITOTOMY. Formerly included in operation group(s) 531.

| Type of Patients | Observed Patients | Avg. Stay | Variance | 10th | 25th | 50th | 75th | 90th | 95th | 99th |
|---|---|---|---|---|---|---|---|---|---|---|
| **1. SINGLE DX** | | | | | | | | | | |
| 0–19 Years | 21 | 4.5 | 9 | 1 | 2 | 4 | 6 | 10 | 10 | 10 |
| 20–34 | 15 | 1.9 | <1 | 1 | 1 | 1 | 2 | 3 | 4 | 4 |
| 35–49 | 8 | 1.9 | 2 | 1 | 2 | 2 | 3 | 5 | 5 | 6 |
| 50–64 | 12 | 1.8 | <1 | 1 | 1 | 2 | 2 | 2 | 2 | 4 |
| 65+ | 1 | 1.0 | 0 | 1 | 1 | 1 | 1 | 1 | 1 | 1 |
| **2. MULTIPLE DX** | | | | | | | | | | |
| 0–19 Years | 136 | 7.4 | 29 | 3 | 4 | 6 | 8 | 15 | 23 | 23 |
| 20–34 | 50 | 3.3 | 42 | 1 | 1 | 1 | 3 | 8 | 9 | 51 |
| 35–49 | 53 | 8.9 | 136 | 1 | 2 | 5 | 7 | 28 | 39 | 46 |
| 50–64 | 46 | 3.0 | 9 | 1 | 1 | 2 | 4 | 5 | 5 | 18 |
| 65+ | 47 | 3.4 | 11 | 1 | 1 | 2 | 5 | 9 | 10 | 12 |
| **TOTAL SINGLE DX** | 57 | 2.4 | 4 | 1 | 1 | 2 | 3 | 5 | 6 | 10 |
| **TOTAL MULTIPLE DX** | 332 | 5.6 | 47 | 1 | 2 | 4 | 6 | 10 | 20 | 39 |
| **TOTAL** | | | | | | | | | | |
| 0–19 Years | 157 | 7.1 | 28 | 2 | 4 | 6 | 8 | 13 | 23 | 23 |
| 20–34 | 65 | 3.0 | 34 | 1 | 1 | 2 | 3 | 5 | 9 | 51 |
| 35–49 | 61 | 6.8 | 105 | 1 | 1 | 3 | 7 | 28 | 39 | 46 |
| 50–64 | 58 | 2.7 | 7 | 1 | 1 | 2 | 4 | 4 | 5 | 18 |
| 65+ | 48 | 3.4 | 11 | 1 | 1 | 2 | 5 | 9 | 10 | 12 |
| **GRAND TOTAL** | 389 | 5.1 | 41 | 1 | 1 | 3 | 6 | 10 | 19 | 39 |

## 16.1: RMVL PENETR FB EYE NOS. Formerly included in operation group(s) 531.

| Type of Patients | Observed Patients | Avg. Stay | Variance | 10th | 25th | 50th | 75th | 90th | 95th | 99th |
|---|---|---|---|---|---|---|---|---|---|---|
| **1. SINGLE DX** | | | | | | | | | | |
| 0–19 Years | 3 | 3.0 | 2 | 1 | 1 | 4 | 4 | 4 | 4 | 4 |
| 20–34 | 2 | 3.7 | <1 | 3 | 3 | 4 | 4 | 4 | 4 | 4 |
| 35–49 | 0 | | | | | | | | | |
| 50–64 | 0 | | | | | | | | | |
| 65+ | 0 | | | | | | | | | |
| **2. MULTIPLE DX** | | | | | | | | | | |
| 0–19 Years | 5 | 7.2 | 14 | 1 | 7 | 8 | 11 | 11 | 11 | 11 |
| 20–34 | 1 | 6.0 | | 6 | 6 | 6 | 6 | 6 | 6 | 6 |
| 35–49 | 3 | 1.8 | 2 | 1 | 1 | 1 | 3 | 4 | 4 | 4 |
| 50–64 | 1 | 4.0 | 0 | 4 | 4 | 4 | 4 | 4 | 4 | 4 |
| 65+ | 0 | | | | | | | | | |
| **TOTAL SINGLE DX** | 5 | 3.1 | 2 | 3 | 3 | 4 | 4 | 4 | 4 | 4 |
| **TOTAL MULTIPLE DX** | 10 | 5.0 | 9 | 1 | 2 | 6 | 6 | 8 | 11 | 11 |
| **TOTAL** | | | | | | | | | | |
| 0–19 Years | 8 | 4.4 | 10 | 1 | 2 | 4 | 7 | 8 | 11 | 11 |
| 20–34 | 3 | 5.2 | 1 | 3 | 4 | 6 | 6 | 6 | 6 | 6 |
| 35–49 | 3 | 1.8 | 2 | 1 | 1 | 1 | 3 | 4 | 4 | 4 |
| 50–64 | 1 | 4.0 | 0 | 4 | 4 | 4 | 4 | 4 | 4 | 4 |
| 65+ | 0 | | | | | | | | | |
| **GRAND TOTAL** | 15 | 4.2 | 7 | 1 | 3 | 4 | 6 | 8 | 11 | 11 |

Length of Stay by Diagnosis and Operation, United States, 2000

# United States, October 1998–September 1999 Data, by Operation

## 16.2: ORBIT & EYEBALL DXTIC PX. Formerly included in operation group(s) 531, 532.

| Type of Patients | Observed Patients | Avg. Stay | Variance | 10th | 25th | 50th | 75th | 90th | 95th | 99th |
|---|---|---|---|---|---|---|---|---|---|---|
| **1. SINGLE DX** | | | | | | | | | | |
| 0–19 Years | 12 | 2.1 | 4 | 1 | 1 | 1 | 2 | 6 | 6 | 6 |
| 20–34 | 0 | | | | | | | | | |
| 35–49 | 2 | 2.7 | 1 | 2 | 2 | 2 | 4 | 4 | 4 | 4 |
| 50–64 | 1 | 1.0 | 0 | 1 | 1 | 1 | 1 | 1 | 1 | 1 |
| 65+ | 1 | 2.0 | 0 | 2 | 2 | 2 | 2 | 2 | 2 | 2 |
| **2. MULTIPLE DX** | | | | | | | | | | |
| 0–19 Years | 15 | 7.1 | 50 | 1 | 1 | 3 | 11 | 20 | 20 | 24 |
| 20–34 | 3 | 5.2 | 22 | 1 | 1 | 1 | 10 | 10 | 10 | 10 |
| 35–49 | 10 | 6.5 | 77 | 2 | 2 | 3 | 7 | 27 | 27 | 36 |
| 50–64 | 12 | 5.4 | 11 | 1 | 1 | 8 | 8 | 8 | 8 | 9 |
| 65+ | 24 | 4.9 | 15 | 1 | 1 | 6 | 7 | 7 | 14 | 16 |
| **TOTAL SINGLE DX** | 16 | 2.2 | 3 | 1 | 1 | 1 | 2 | 5 | 6 | 6 |
| **TOTAL MULTIPLE DX** | 64 | 5.7 | 30 | 1 | 1 | 4 | 8 | 11 | 16 | 27 |
| **TOTAL** | | | | | | | | | | |
| 0–19 Years | 27 | 4.9 | 35 | 1 | 1 | 2 | 6 | 15 | 20 | 24 |
| 20–34 | 3 | 5.2 | 22 | 1 | 1 | 1 | 10 | 10 | 10 | 10 |
| 35–49 | 12 | 5.7 | 63 | 2 | 2 | 3 | 4 | 13 | 27 | 36 |
| 50–64 | 13 | 5.2 | 11 | 1 | 1 | 8 | 8 | 8 | 8 | 9 |
| 65+ | 25 | 4.9 | 14 | 1 | 1 | 6 | 7 | 7 | 14 | 16 |
| **GRAND TOTAL** | 80 | 5.1 | 27 | 1 | 1 | 3 | 7 | 11 | 15 | 27 |

## 16.3: EVISCERATION OF EYEBALL. Formerly included in operation group(s) 531.

| Type of Patients | Observed Patients | Avg. Stay | Variance | 10th | 25th | 50th | 75th | 90th | 95th | 99th |
|---|---|---|---|---|---|---|---|---|---|---|
| **1. SINGLE DX** | | | | | | | | | | |
| 0–19 Years | 2 | 2.6 | <1 | 2 | 2 | 3 | 3 | 3 | 3 | 3 |
| 20–34 | 0 | | | | | | | | | |
| 35–49 | 2 | 5.1 | 3 | 2 | 6 | 6 | 6 | 6 | 6 | 6 |
| 50–64 | 1 | 3.0 | 0 | 3 | 3 | 3 | 3 | 3 | 3 | 3 |
| 65+ | 3 | 2.1 | <1 | 1 | 2 | 2 | 2 | 4 | 4 | 4 |
| **2. MULTIPLE DX** | | | | | | | | | | |
| 0–19 Years | 6 | 4.7 | 5 | 2 | 2 | 6 | 6 | 6 | 8 | 8 |
| 20–34 | 16 | 6.3 | 70 | 1 | 2 | 3 | 8 | 10 | 33 | 33 |
| 35–49 | 21 | 5.1 | 23 | 1 | 3 | 4 | 5 | 9 | 11 | 31 |
| 50–64 | 12 | 4.4 | 49 | 1 | 1 | 1 | 2 | 22 | 22 | 22 |
| 65+ | 44 | 5.4 | 49 | 1 | 2 | 3 | 7 | 12 | 20 | 42 |
| **TOTAL SINGLE DX** | 8 | 4.2 | 4 | 2 | 2 | 6 | 6 | 6 | 6 | 6 |
| **TOTAL MULTIPLE DX** | 99 | 5.2 | 41 | 1 | 2 | 3 | 6 | 11 | 22 | 33 |
| **TOTAL** | | | | | | | | | | |
| 0–19 Years | 8 | 4.3 | 5 | 2 | 2 | 6 | 6 | 6 | 8 | 8 |
| 20–34 | 16 | 6.3 | 70 | 1 | 2 | 3 | 8 | 10 | 33 | 33 |
| 35–49 | 23 | 5.1 | 19 | 2 | 3 | 4 | 6 | 9 | 11 | 31 |
| 50–64 | 13 | 4.3 | 48 | 1 | 2 | 1 | 2 | 22 | 22 | 22 |
| 65+ | 47 | 5.1 | 46 | 1 | 2 | 3 | 7 | 12 | 20 | 42 |
| **GRAND TOTAL** | 107 | 5.1 | 37 | 1 | 2 | 3 | 6 | 10 | 20 | 33 |

## 16.4: ENUCLEATION OF EYEBALL. Formerly included in operation group(s) 531.

| Type of Patients | Observed Patients | Avg. Stay | Variance | 10th | 25th | 50th | 75th | 90th | 95th | 99th |
|---|---|---|---|---|---|---|---|---|---|---|
| **1. SINGLE DX** | | | | | | | | | | |
| 0–19 Years | 14 | 1.5 | 1 | 1 | 1 | 1 | 1 | 3 | 5 | 5 |
| 20–34 | 7 | 4.9 | 102 | 1 | 1 | 1 | 1 | 30 | 30 | 30 |
| 35–49 | 7 | 1.9 | <1 | 1 | 2 | 2 | 2 | 2 | 3 | 3 |
| 50–64 | 5 | 1.1 | <1 | 1 | 1 | 1 | 1 | 1 | 2 | 2 |
| 65+ | 9 | 1.3 | <1 | 1 | 1 | 1 | 1 | 2 | 2 | 5 |
| **2. MULTIPLE DX** | | | | | | | | | | |
| 0–19 Years | 40 | 3.3 | 9 | 1 | 1 | 2 | 4 | 6 | 11 | 14 |
| 20–34 | 35 | 4.6 | 28 | 1 | 1 | 2 | 7 | 13 | 21 | 21 |
| 35–49 | 58 | 2.9 | 7 | 1 | 1 | 2 | 3 | 5 | 11 | 12 |
| 50–64 | 43 | 3.3 | 11 | 1 | 1 | 2 | 4 | 7 | 8 | 22 |
| 65+ | 105 | 3.6 | 12 | 1 | 1 | 2 | 5 | 8 | 11 | 15 |
| **TOTAL SINGLE DX** | 42 | 2.1 | 20 | 1 | 1 | 1 | 2 | 2 | 3 | 30 |
| **TOTAL MULTIPLE DX** | 281 | 3.4 | 12 | 1 | 1 | 2 | 4 | 7 | 11 | 21 |
| **TOTAL** | | | | | | | | | | |
| 0–19 Years | 54 | 3.0 | 8 | 1 | 1 | 2 | 4 | 6 | 9 | 14 |
| 20–34 | 42 | 4.7 | 42 | 1 | 1 | 2 | 6 | 13 | 21 | 30 |
| 35–49 | 65 | 2.8 | 6 | 1 | 1 | 2 | 3 | 5 | 9 | 12 |
| 50–64 | 48 | 3.1 | 10 | 1 | 1 | 2 | 4 | 6 | 8 | 22 |
| 65+ | 114 | 3.3 | 11 | 1 | 1 | 2 | 5 | 8 | 11 | 15 |
| **GRAND TOTAL** | 323 | 3.2 | 13 | 1 | 1 | 2 | 4 | 7 | 11 | 21 |

## 16.5: EXENTERATION OF ORBIT. Formerly included in operation group(s) 531.

| Type of Patients | Observed Patients | Avg. Stay | Variance | 10th | 25th | 50th | 75th | 90th | 95th | 99th |
|---|---|---|---|---|---|---|---|---|---|---|
| **1. SINGLE DX** | | | | | | | | | | |
| 0–19 Years | 1 | 2.0 | 0 | 2 | 2 | 2 | 2 | 2 | 2 | 2 |
| 20–34 | 0 | | | | | | | | | |
| 35–49 | 3 | 3.4 | <1 | 2 | 2 | 4 | 4 | 4 | 4 | 4 |
| 50–64 | 1 | 2.0 | 0 | 2 | 2 | 2 | 2 | 2 | 2 | 2 |
| 65+ | 1 | 7.0 | 0 | 7 | 7 | 7 | 7 | 7 | 7 | 7 |
| **2. MULTIPLE DX** | | | | | | | | | | |
| 0–19 Years | 4 | 8.7 | 32 | 1 | 1 | 13 | 13 | 13 | 13 | 13 |
| 20–34 | 3 | 11.2 | 170 | 5 | 5 | 5 | 7 | 37 | 37 | 37 |
| 35–49 | 5 | 4.7 | 6 | 3 | 4 | 4 | 5 | 10 | 10 | 10 |
| 50–64 | 9 | 8.0 | 51 | 1 | 2 | 7 | 7 | 15 | 28 | 28 |
| 65+ | 21 | 4.7 | 18 | 1 | 2 | 3 | 6 | 12 | 18 | 18 |
| **TOTAL SINGLE DX** | 6 | 3.0 | 2 | 2 | 2 | 2 | 4 | 4 | 7 | 7 |
| **TOTAL MULTIPLE DX** | 42 | 6.4 | 36 | 1 | 3 | 4 | 7 | 13 | 15 | 37 |
| **TOTAL** | | | | | | | | | | |
| 0–19 Years | 5 | 7.6 | 33 | 1 | 2 | 13 | 13 | 13 | 13 | 13 |
| 20–34 | 3 | 11.2 | 170 | 5 | 5 | 5 | 7 | 37 | 37 | 37 |
| 35–49 | 8 | 4.4 | 5 | 2 | 4 | 4 | 4 | 10 | 10 | 10 |
| 50–64 | 10 | 7.4 | 49 | 1 | 3 | 7 | 7 | 15 | 28 | 28 |
| 65+ | 22 | 4.7 | 18 | 1 | 2 | 3 | 6 | 12 | 18 | 18 |
| **GRAND TOTAL** | 48 | 6.0 | 33 | 1 | 3 | 4 | 7 | 13 | 15 | 28 |

## United States, October 1998–September 1999 Data, by Operation

### 16.6: 2ND PX POST RMVL EYEBALL. Formerly included in operation group(s) 531.

| Type of Patients | Observed Patients | Avg. Stay | Variance | 10th | 25th | 50th | 75th | 90th | 95th | 99th |
|---|---|---|---|---|---|---|---|---|---|---|
| **1. SINGLE DX** | | | | | | | | | | |
| 0–19 Years | 2 | 1.0 | 0 | 1 | 1 | 1 | 1 | 1 | 1 | 1 |
| 20–34 | 1 | 1.0 | 0 | 1 | 1 | 1 | 1 | 1 | 1 | 1 |
| 35–49 | 1 | 1.0 | 0 | 1 | 1 | 1 | 1 | 1 | 1 | 1 |
| 50–64 | 0 | | | | | | | | | |
| 65+ | 0 | | | | | | | | | |
| **2. MULTIPLE DX** | | | | | | | | | | |
| 0–19 Years | 6 | 2.2 | <1 | 1 | 2 | 2 | 3 | 3 | 3 | 3 |
| 20–34 | 7 | 3.4 | 3 | 1 | 3 | 3 | 3 | 7 | 7 | 7 |
| 35–49 | 4 | 3.0 | 2 | 2 | 2 | 3 | 5 | 5 | 5 | 5 |
| 50–64 | 7 | 4.9 | 5 | 1 | 4 | 6 | 6 | 6 | 6 | 9 |
| 65+ | 11 | 10.7 | 148 | 1 | 2 | 4 | 19 | 19 | 19 | 56 |
| **TOTAL SINGLE DX** | 4 | 1.0 | 0 | 1 | 1 | 1 | 1 | 1 | 1 | 1 |
| **TOTAL MULTIPLE DX** | 35 | 5.3 | 42 | 1 | 2 | 3 | 6 | 7 | 19 | 19 |
| **TOTAL** | | | | | | | | | | |
| 0–19 Years | 8 | 2.1 | <1 | 1 | 1 | 2 | 3 | 3 | 3 | 3 |
| 20–34 | 8 | 3.1 | 4 | 1 | 1 | 3 | 3 | 7 | 7 | 7 |
| 35–49 | 5 | 2.2 | 2 | 1 | 1 | 2 | 2 | 5 | 5 | 5 |
| 50–64 | 7 | 4.9 | 5 | 1 | 4 | 6 | 6 | 6 | 6 | 9 |
| 65+ | 11 | 10.7 | 148 | 1 | 2 | 4 | 19 | 19 | 19 | 56 |
| **GRAND TOTAL** | 39 | 4.8 | 39 | 1 | 2 | 3 | 6 | 7 | 19 | 19 |

### 16.7: OCULAR/ORBITAL IMPL RMVL. Formerly included in operation group(s) 531.

| Type of Patients | Observed Patients | Avg. Stay | Variance | 10th | 25th | 50th | 75th | 90th | 95th | 99th |
|---|---|---|---|---|---|---|---|---|---|---|
| **1. SINGLE DX** | | | | | | | | | | |
| 0–19 Years | 1 | 1.0 | 0 | 1 | 1 | 1 | 1 | 1 | 1 | 1 |
| 20–34 | 0 | | | | | | | | | |
| 35–49 | 0 | | | | | | | | | |
| 50–64 | 0 | | | | | | | | | |
| 65+ | 0 | | | | | | | | | |
| **2. MULTIPLE DX** | | | | | | | | | | |
| 0–19 Years | 8 | 5.5 | 9 | 1 | 4 | 5 | 9 | 9 | 9 | 9 |
| 20–34 | 5 | 2.5 | 4 | 1 | 2 | 2 | 2 | 8 | 8 | 8 |
| 35–49 | 2 | 3.4 | 6 | 2 | 2 | 2 | 7 | 7 | 7 | 7 |
| 50–64 | 4 | 3.3 | <1 | 3 | 3 | 3 | 4 | 4 | 6 | 6 |
| 65+ | 8 | 5.0 | 23 | 1 | 1 | 4 | 10 | 14 | 14 | 14 |
| **TOTAL SINGLE DX** | 1 | 1.0 | 0 | 1 | 1 | 1 | 1 | 1 | 1 | 1 |
| **TOTAL MULTIPLE DX** | 27 | 3.8 | 6 | 2 | 2 | 3 | 4 | 8 | 9 | 14 |
| **TOTAL** | | | | | | | | | | |
| 0–19 Years | 9 | 4.7 | 10 | 1 | 4 | 4 | 8 | 9 | 9 | 9 |
| 20–34 | 5 | 2.5 | 4 | 1 | 2 | 2 | 2 | 8 | 8 | 8 |
| 35–49 | 4 | 3.4 | 6 | 1 | 2 | 2 | 7 | 7 | 7 | 7 |
| 50–64 | 4 | 3.3 | <1 | 3 | 3 | 3 | 4 | 4 | 6 | 6 |
| 65+ | 8 | 5.0 | 23 | 1 | 1 | 4 | 10 | 14 | 14 | 14 |
| **GRAND TOTAL** | 28 | 3.7 | 6 | 1 | 2 | 3 | 4 | 8 | 9 | 14 |

### 16.8: EYEBALL/ORBIT INJ REPAIR. Formerly included in operation group(s) 531.

| Type of Patients | Observed Patients | Avg. Stay | Variance | 10th | 25th | 50th | 75th | 90th | 95th | 99th |
|---|---|---|---|---|---|---|---|---|---|---|
| **1. SINGLE DX** | | | | | | | | | | |
| 0–19 Years | 41 | 2.5 | 1 | 1 | 1 | 3 | 3 | 3 | 5 | 6 |
| 20–34 | 29 | 2.0 | 1 | 1 | 1 | 1 | 2 | 3 | 4 | 7 |
| 35–49 | 23 | 1.7 | <1 | 1 | 1 | 2 | 2 | 3 | 3 | 5 |
| 50–64 | 3 | 4.3 | <1 | 3 | 4 | 4 | 5 | 5 | 5 | 5 |
| 65+ | 6 | 2.0 | 1 | 1 | 1 | 2 | 2 | 4 | 4 | 4 |
| **2. MULTIPLE DX** | | | | | | | | | | |
| 0–19 Years | 75 | 3.2 | 5 | 1 | 2 | 3 | 4 | 6 | 7 | 8 |
| 20–34 | 84 | 2.8 | 2 | 1 | 2 | 2 | 3 | 4 | 7 | 8 |
| 35–49 | 80 | 3.1 | 8 | 1 | 1 | 2 | 4 | 6 | 10 | 17 |
| 50–64 | 31 | 2.5 | 2 | 1 | 2 | 3 | 3 | 3 | 6 | 9 |
| 65+ | 106 | 3.8 | 10 | 1 | 2 | 3 | 5 | 6 | 8 | 13 |
| **TOTAL SINGLE DX** | 102 | 2.3 | 2 | 1 | 1 | 2 | 3 | 4 | 5 | 6 |
| **TOTAL MULTIPLE DX** | 376 | 3.2 | 6 | 1 | 2 | 3 | 4 | 5 | 7 | 12 |
| **TOTAL** | | | | | | | | | | |
| 0–19 Years | 116 | 2.9 | 3 | 1 | 2 | 3 | 3 | 5 | 6 | 7 |
| 20–34 | 113 | 2.6 | 2 | 1 | 2 | 2 | 3 | 4 | 6 | 7 |
| 35–49 | 103 | 2.7 | 6 | 1 | 1 | 2 | 3 | 5 | 9 | 11 |
| 50–64 | 34 | 2.8 | 6 | 2 | 2 | 3 | 3 | 6 | 8 | 9 |
| 65+ | 112 | 3.7 | 10 | 1 | 2 | 3 | 5 | 6 | 8 | 13 |
| **GRAND TOTAL** | 478 | 2.9 | 5 | 1 | 2 | 3 | 3 | 5 | 6 | 11 |

### 16.82: REPAIR EYEBALL RUPTURE. Formerly included in operation group(s) 531.

| Type of Patients | Observed Patients | Avg. Stay | Variance | 10th | 25th | 50th | 75th | 90th | 95th | 99th |
|---|---|---|---|---|---|---|---|---|---|---|
| **1. SINGLE DX** | | | | | | | | | | |
| 0–19 Years | 27 | 2.8 | <1 | 2 | 3 | 3 | 3 | 3 | 4 | 6 |
| 20–34 | 19 | 2.0 | 2 | 1 | 1 | 1 | 3 | 3 | 6 | 7 |
| 35–49 | 15 | 1.6 | <1 | 1 | 1 | 1 | 2 | 3 | 3 | 4 |
| 50–64 | 2 | 3.8 | <1 | 3 | 4 | 4 | 4 | 4 | 4 | 4 |
| 65+ | 4 | 1.7 | <1 | 1 | 1 | 2 | 2 | 2 | 2 | 2 |
| **2. MULTIPLE DX** | | | | | | | | | | |
| 0–19 Years | 50 | 3.1 | 3 | 1 | 2 | 3 | 4 | 6 | 7 | 8 |
| 20–34 | 54 | 3.0 | 4 | 1 | 1 | 3 | 4 | 6 | 6 | 12 |
| 35–49 | 46 | 3.3 | 10 | 1 | 1 | 2 | 4 | 5 | 10 | 17 |
| 50–64 | 24 | 2.4 | 2 | 1 | 2 | 2 | 3 | 3 | 7 | 9 |
| 65+ | 80 | 3.8 | 10 | 1 | 2 | 3 | 5 | 5 | 7 | 16 |
| **TOTAL SINGLE DX** | 67 | 2.4 | 1 | 2 | 2 | 3 | 3 | 3 | 4 | 6 |
| **TOTAL MULTIPLE DX** | 254 | 3.3 | 7 | 1 | 2 | 3 | 4 | 5 | 7 | 13 |
| **TOTAL** | | | | | | | | | | |
| 0–19 Years | 77 | 3.0 | 2 | 2 | 2 | 3 | 3 | 4 | 6 | 7 |
| 20–34 | 73 | 2.6 | 3 | 1 | 1 | 2 | 3 | 6 | 6 | 8 |
| 35–49 | 61 | 2.6 | 6 | 1 | 1 | 2 | 3 | 4 | 4 | 17 |
| 50–64 | 26 | 2.6 | 2 | 2 | 2 | 3 | 3 | 4 | 4 | 9 |
| 65+ | 84 | 3.7 | 10 | 1 | 2 | 3 | 4 | 5 | 7 | 13 |
| **GRAND TOTAL** | 321 | 3.0 | 5 | 1 | 2 | 3 | 4 | 5 | 6 | 10 |

Length of Stay by Diagnosis and Operation, United States, 2000

# United States, October 1998–September 1999 Data, by Operation

## 16.9: OTHER EYE & ORBIT OPS. Formerly included in operation group(s) 531.

| Type of Patients | Observed Patients | Avg. Stay | Variance | 10th | 25th | 50th | 75th | 90th | 95th | 99th |
|---|---|---|---|---|---|---|---|---|---|---|
| **1. SINGLE DX** | | | | | | | | | | |
| 0–19 Years | 28 | 3.4 | 1 | 1 | 2 | 4 | 4 | 5 | 5 | 5 |
| 20–34 | 4 | 1.9 | 2 | 1 | 1 | 1 | 3 | 5 | 5 | 5 |
| 35–49 | 9 | 2.1 | 2 | 1 | 1 | 1 | 2 | 5 | 5 | 5 |
| 50–64 | 1 | 1.0 | 0 | 1 | 1 | 1 | 1 | 1 | 1 | 1 |
| 65+ | 2 | 2.4 | <1 | 2 | 2 | 2 | 3 | 3 | 3 | 3 |
| **2. MULTIPLE DX** | | | | | | | | | | |
| 0–19 Years | 35 | 6.4 | 75 | 1 | 3 | 5 | 6 | 16 | 16 | 74 |
| 20–34 | 22 | 3.3 | 12 | 1 | 1 | 4 | 4 | 9 | 12 | 12 |
| 35–49 | 30 | 3.4 | 5 | 1 | 1 | 4 | 4 | 6 | 7 | 11 |
| 50–64 | 22 | 4.7 | 12 | 1 | 2 | 4 | 7 | 12 | 12 | 14 |
| 65+ | 45 | 3.8 | 42 | 1 | 1 | 2 | 3 | 6 | 9 | 35 |
| **TOTAL SINGLE DX** | 44 | 3.1 | 2 | 1 | 2 | 4 | 4 | 5 | 5 | 5 |
| **TOTAL MULTIPLE DX** | 154 | 4.5 | 36 | 1 | 1 | 3 | 5 | 9 | 12 | 29 |
| **TOTAL** | | | | | | | | | | |
| 0–19 Years | 63 | 4.8 | 38 | 1 | 3 | 4 | 5 | 6 | 16 | 26 |
| 20–34 | 26 | 3.1 | 11 | 1 | 1 | 1 | 4 | 9 | 12 | 12 |
| 35–49 | 39 | 3.0 | 4 | 1 | 1 | 2 | 4 | 6 | 7 | 10 |
| 50–64 | 23 | 4.7 | 12 | 1 | 2 | 4 | 7 | 12 | 12 | 14 |
| 65+ | 47 | 3.8 | 41 | 1 | 1 | 2 | 3 | 6 | 9 | 35 |
| **GRAND TOTAL** | 198 | 4.1 | 26 | 1 | 1 | 3 | 5 | 7 | 12 | 26 |

## 18.1: EXTERNAL EAR DXTIC PX. Formerly included in operation group(s) 533, 539.

| Type of Patients | Observed Patients | Avg. Stay | Variance | 10th | 25th | 50th | 75th | 90th | 95th | 99th |
|---|---|---|---|---|---|---|---|---|---|---|
| **1. SINGLE DX** | | | | | | | | | | |
| 0–19 Years | 6 | 1.9 | 2 | 1 | 1 | 1 | 2 | 4 | 6 | 6 |
| 20–34 | 0 | | | | | | | | | |
| 35–49 | 1 | 1.0 | 0 | 1 | 1 | 1 | 1 | 1 | 1 | 1 |
| 50–64 | 1 | 3.0 | 0 | 3 | 3 | 3 | 3 | 3 | 3 | 3 |
| 65+ | 0 | | | | | | | | | |
| **2. MULTIPLE DX** | | | | | | | | | | |
| 0–19 Years | 22 | 5.1 | 63 | 1 | 1 | 3 | 4 | 9 | 9 | 42 |
| 20–34 | 5 | 5.2 | 9 | 4 | 4 | 4 | 4 | 7 | 14 | 14 |
| 35–49 | 6 | 5.6 | 9 | 3 | 6 | 6 | 6 | 6 | 6 | 9 |
| 50–64 | 8 | 6.7 | 12 | 3 | 5 | 6 | 9 | 12 | 16 | 16 |
| 65+ | 34 | 8.0 | 78 | 1 | 3 | 6 | 8 | 13 | 13 | 47 |
| **TOTAL SINGLE DX** | 8 | 2.0 | 2 | 1 | 1 | 1 | 2 | 4 | 6 | 6 |
| **TOTAL MULTIPLE DX** | 75 | 6.3 | 54 | 1 | 3 | 5 | 7 | 12 | 13 | 47 |
| **TOTAL** | | | | | | | | | | |
| 0–19 Years | 28 | 4.6 | 54 | 1 | 1 | 3 | 4 | 9 | 9 | 42 |
| 20–34 | 5 | 5.2 | 9 | 4 | 4 | 4 | 4 | 7 | 14 | 14 |
| 35–49 | 7 | 5.3 | 3 | 3 | 6 | 6 | 6 | 6 | 6 | 9 |
| 50–64 | 9 | 6.4 | 12 | 3 | 5 | 6 | 9 | 12 | 16 | 16 |
| 65+ | 34 | 8.0 | 78 | 1 | 3 | 6 | 8 | 13 | 13 | 47 |
| **GRAND TOTAL** | 83 | 6.0 | 51 | 1 | 2 | 4 | 6 | 9 | 13 | 47 |

## 18.0: EXTERNAL EAR INCISION. Formerly included in operation group(s) 533, 539.

| Type of Patients | Observed Patients | Avg. Stay | Variance | 10th | 25th | 50th | 75th | 90th | 95th | 99th |
|---|---|---|---|---|---|---|---|---|---|---|
| **1. SINGLE DX** | | | | | | | | | | |
| 0–19 Years | 78 | 3.3 | 5 | 1 | 1 | 2 | 6 | 7 | 7 | 7 |
| 20–34 | 14 | 2.6 | 2 | 1 | 1 | 2 | 4 | 4 | 4 | 7 |
| 35–49 | 11 | 2.5 | 2 | 2 | 2 | 2 | 3 | 3 | 5 | 8 |
| 50–64 | 2 | 4.2 | 1 | 3 | 3 | 5 | 5 | 5 | 5 | 5 |
| 65+ | 0 | | | | | | | | | |
| **2. MULTIPLE DX** | | | | | | | | | | |
| 0–19 Years | 99 | 4.2 | 6 | 2 | 2 | 3 | 5 | 7 | 8 | 13 |
| 20–34 | 36 | 3.6 | 4 | 1 | 2 | 4 | 5 | 6 | 7 | 9 |
| 35–49 | 41 | 3.8 | 6 | 1 | 2 | 3 | 5 | 7 | 9 | 11 |
| 50–64 | 19 | 6.6 | 16 | 2 | 3 | 6 | 10 | 12 | 15 | 15 |
| 65+ | 18 | 4.7 | 10 | 3 | 3 | 3 | 5 | 9 | 11 | 14 |
| **TOTAL SINGLE DX** | 105 | 3.2 | 4 | 1 | 1 | 2 | 4 | 7 | 7 | 8 |
| **TOTAL MULTIPLE DX** | 213 | 4.3 | 8 | 1 | 2 | 4 | 5 | 7 | 11 | 13 |
| **TOTAL** | | | | | | | | | | |
| 0–19 Years | 177 | 3.7 | 6 | 2 | 2 | 3 | 5 | 7 | 7 | 13 |
| 20–34 | 50 | 3.3 | 3 | 1 | 2 | 4 | 5 | 5 | 7 | 9 |
| 35–49 | 52 | 3.5 | 5 | 2 | 2 | 3 | 5 | 7 | 8 | 11 |
| 50–64 | 21 | 6.5 | 16 | 3 | 3 | 6 | 9 | 12 | 12 | 15 |
| 65+ | 18 | 4.7 | 10 | 3 | 3 | 3 | 5 | 9 | 11 | 14 |
| **GRAND TOTAL** | 318 | 3.9 | 7 | 1 | 2 | 3 | 5 | 7 | 9 | 13 |

## 18.2: EXC/DESTR EXT EAR LESION. Formerly included in operation group(s) 533.

| Type of Patients | Observed Patients | Avg. Stay | Variance | 10th | 25th | 50th | 75th | 90th | 95th | 99th |
|---|---|---|---|---|---|---|---|---|---|---|
| **1. SINGLE DX** | | | | | | | | | | |
| 0–19 Years | 35 | 1.4 | 2 | 1 | 1 | 1 | 1 | 2 | 6 | 6 |
| 20–34 | 4 | 3.2 | 8 | 1 | 1 | 1 | 7 | 7 | 7 | 7 |
| 35–49 | 4 | 1.5 | <1 | 1 | 1 | 1 | 2 | 2 | 2 | 2 |
| 50–64 | 1 | 3.0 | 0 | 3 | 3 | 3 | 3 | 3 | 3 | 3 |
| 65+ | 4 | 2.6 | <1 | 1 | 3 | 3 | 3 | 3 | 3 | 3 |
| **2. MULTIPLE DX** | | | | | | | | | | |
| 0–19 Years | 272 | 2.7 | 10 | 1 | 1 | 2 | 3 | 5 | 7 | 16 |
| 20–34 | 18 | 3.3 | 5 | 1 | 2 | 2 | 5 | 6 | 8 | 9 |
| 35–49 | 17 | 7.4 | 36 | 2 | 2 | 6 | 11 | 14 | 14 | 27 |
| 50–64 | 16 | 4.5 | 18 | 1 | 3 | 3 | 5 | 13 | 14 | 14 |
| 65+ | 70 | 6.1 | 24 | 3 | 5 | 5 | 5 | 8 | 12 | 29 |
| **TOTAL SINGLE DX** | 48 | 1.6 | 2 | 1 | 1 | 1 | 1 | 3 | 6 | 6 |
| **TOTAL MULTIPLE DX** | 393 | 3.8 | 17 | 1 | 2 | 2 | 5 | 8 | 10 | 27 |
| **TOTAL** | | | | | | | | | | |
| 0–19 Years | 307 | 2.4 | 8 | 1 | 2 | 2 | 3 | 4 | 6 | 16 |
| 20–34 | 22 | 3.3 | 5 | 1 | 2 | 2 | 5 | 6 | 8 | 9 |
| 35–49 | 21 | 6.0 | 34 | 2 | 2 | 3 | 10 | 14 | 14 | 27 |
| 50–64 | 17 | 4.1 | 14 | 1 | 2 | 5 | 5 | 13 | 14 | 14 |
| 65+ | 74 | 6.0 | 23 | 2 | 5 | 5 | 5 | 8 | 12 | 29 |
| **GRAND TOTAL** | 441 | 3.4 | 15 | 1 | 2 | 2 | 5 | 7 | 8 | 23 |

Length of Stay by Diagnosis and Operation, United States, 2000

## United States, October 1998–September 1999 Data, by Operation

### 18.29: DESTR EXT EAR LES NEC. Formerly included in operation group(s) 533.

| Type of Patients | Observed Patients | Avg. Stay | Variance | 10th | 25th | 50th | 75th | 90th | 95th | 99th |
|---|---|---|---|---|---|---|---|---|---|---|
| **1. SINGLE DX** | | | | | | | | | | |
| 0-19 Years | 23 | 1.5 | 2 | 1 | 1 | 1 | 1 | 2 | 6 | 6 |
| 20-34 | 3 | 3.9 | 9 | 1 | 1 | 3 | 7 | 7 | 7 | 7 |
| 35-49 | 3 | 3.0 | 0 | 1 | 1 | 3 | 3 | 3 | 3 | 3 |
| 50-64 | 1 | 3.0 | 0 | 3 | 3 | 3 | 3 | 3 | 3 | 3 |
| 65+ | 4 | 2.6 | <1 | 1 | 3 | 3 | 3 | 3 | 3 | 3 |
| **2. MULTIPLE DX** | | | | | | | | | | |
| 0-19 Years | 264 | 2.7 | 10 | 1 | 1 | 2 | 3 | 5 | 7 | 16 |
| 20-34 | 18 | 3.3 | 5 | 1 | 2 | 2 | 5 | 6 | 7 | 9 |
| 35-49 | 17 | 7.4 | 36 | 2 | 2 | 6 | 11 | 14 | 14 | 27 |
| 50-64 | 16 | 4.5 | 18 | 1 | 2 | 3 | 5 | 13 | 14 | 14 |
| 65+ | 70 | 6.1 | 24 | 3 | 5 | 5 | 5 | 8 | 12 | 29 |
| **TOTAL SINGLE DX** | 34 | 1.8 | 2 | 1 | 1 | 1 | 2 | 3 | 6 | 7 |
| **TOTAL MULTIPLE DX** | 385 | 3.9 | 17 | 1 | 2 | 2 | 5 | 8 | 10 | 27 |
| **TOTAL** | | | | | | | | | | |
| 0-19 Years | 287 | 2.5 | 9 | 1 | 1 | 2 | 3 | 4 | 7 | 16 |
| 20-34 | 21 | 3.3 | 5 | 1 | 2 | 2 | 5 | 6 | 8 | 9 |
| 35-49 | 20 | 6.5 | 36 | 2 | 2 | 5 | 10 | 14 | 14 | 27 |
| 50-64 | 17 | 4.1 | 14 | 1 | 2 | 3 | 3 | 13 | 14 | 14 |
| 65+ | 74 | 6.0 | 23 | 2 | 5 | 5 | 5 | 8 | 12 | 29 |
| **GRAND TOTAL** | 419 | 3.6 | 16 | 1 | 1 | 2 | 5 | 7 | 9 | 24 |

### 18.4: SUTURE EXT EAR LAC. Formerly included in operation group(s) 533.

| Type of Patients | Observed Patients | Avg. Stay | Variance | 10th | 25th | 50th | 75th | 90th | 95th | 99th |
|---|---|---|---|---|---|---|---|---|---|---|
| **1. SINGLE DX** | | | | | | | | | | |
| 0-19 Years | 20 | 2.1 | 2 | 1 | 1 | 1 | 3 | 3 | 6 | 6 |
| 20-34 | 10 | 2.0 | <1 | 1 | 2 | 2 | 2 | 2 | 5 | 5 |
| 35-49 | 1 | 1.0 | 0 | 1 | 1 | 1 | 1 | 1 | 1 | 1 |
| 50-64 | 1 | 1.0 | 0 | 1 | 1 | 1 | 1 | 1 | 1 | 1 |
| 65+ | 1 | 1.0 | 0 | 1 | 1 | 1 | 1 | 1 | 1 | 1 |
| **2. MULTIPLE DX** | | | | | | | | | | |
| 0-19 Years | 114 | 2.4 | 4 | 1 | 1 | 2 | 3 | 5 | 6 | 12 |
| 20-34 | 138 | 4.8 | 78 | 1 | 2 | 2 | 4 | 10 | 24 | 57 |
| 35-49 | 119 | 2.7 | 9 | 1 | 1 | 2 | 3 | 4 | 9 | 17 |
| 50-64 | 63 | 3.7 | 10 | 1 | 1 | 2 | 6 | 8 | 9 | 17 |
| 65+ | 100 | 4.8 | 9 | 1 | 2 | 5 | 7 | 8 | 10 | 13 |
| **TOTAL SINGLE DX** | 33 | 2.0 | 2 | 1 | 1 | 2 | 2 | 3 | 5 | 6 |
| **TOTAL MULTIPLE DX** | 534 | 3.6 | 26 | 1 | 1 | 2 | 4 | 7 | 9 | 24 |
| **TOTAL** | | | | | | | | | | |
| 0-19 Years | 134 | 2.4 | 4 | 1 | 1 | 2 | 3 | 5 | 6 | 12 |
| 20-34 | 148 | 4.6 | 73 | 1 | 2 | 2 | 4 | 9 | 24 | 57 |
| 35-49 | 120 | 2.6 | 9 | 1 | 2 | 2 | 3 | 4 | 9 | 17 |
| 50-64 | 64 | 3.7 | 10 | 1 | 2 | 5 | 6 | 8 | 9 | 17 |
| 65+ | 101 | 4.8 | 9 | 1 | 2 | 5 | 7 | 8 | 10 | 13 |
| **GRAND TOTAL** | 567 | 3.5 | 25 | 1 | 1 | 2 | 4 | 7 | 9 | 24 |

### 18.3: OTHER EXTERNAL EAR EXC. Formerly included in operation group(s) 533.

| Type of Patients | Observed Patients | Avg. Stay | Variance | 10th | 25th | 50th | 75th | 90th | 95th | 99th |
|---|---|---|---|---|---|---|---|---|---|---|
| **1. SINGLE DX** | | | | | | | | | | |
| 0-19 Years | 1 | 1.0 | 0 | 1 | 1 | 1 | 1 | 1 | 1 | 1 |
| 20-34 | 1 | 1.0 | 0 | 1 | 1 | 1 | 1 | 1 | 1 | 1 |
| 35-49 | 2 | 1.1 | <1 | 1 | 1 | 1 | 1 | 1 | 2 | 2 |
| 50-64 | 2 | 1.0 | 0 | 1 | 1 | 1 | 1 | 1 | 1 | 1 |
| 65+ | 3 | 1.5 | <1 | 1 | 1 | 2 | 2 | 2 | 2 | 2 |
| **2. MULTIPLE DX** | | | | | | | | | | |
| 0-19 Years | 2 | 3.6 | 1 | 1 | 4 | 4 | 4 | 4 | 4 | 4 |
| 20-34 | 1 | 3.0 | 0 | 3 | 3 | 3 | 3 | 3 | 3 | 3 |
| 35-49 | 2 | 4.0 | 0 | 4 | 4 | 4 | 4 | 4 | 4 | 4 |
| 50-64 | 10 | 5.6 | 8 | 2 | 4 | 5 | 8 | 11 | 11 | 11 |
| 65+ | 49 | 4.9 | 21 | 1 | 2 | 3 | 7 | 13 | 17 | 17 |
| **TOTAL SINGLE DX** | 9 | 1.2 | <1 | 1 | 1 | 1 | 1 | 2 | 2 | 2 |
| **TOTAL MULTIPLE DX** | 64 | 5.0 | 17 | 1 | 2 | 4 | 7 | 11 | 14 | 17 |
| **TOTAL** | | | | | | | | | | |
| 0-19 Years | 3 | 3.4 | 2 | 1 | 4 | 4 | 4 | 4 | 4 | 4 |
| 20-34 | 2 | 2.1 | 2 | 1 | 1 | 3 | 3 | 3 | 3 | 3 |
| 35-49 | 4 | 1.4 | 1 | 1 | 1 | 1 | 1 | 4 | 4 | 4 |
| 50-64 | 12 | 4.7 | 10 | 1 | 2 | 4 | 8 | 8 | 11 | 11 |
| 65+ | 52 | 4.6 | 20 | 1 | 1 | 3 | 7 | 13 | 17 | 17 |
| **GRAND TOTAL** | 73 | 4.2 | 16 | 1 | 1 | 3 | 5 | 9 | 13 | 17 |

### 18.5: CORRECTION PROMINENT EAR. Formerly included in operation group(s) 533.

| Type of Patients | Observed Patients | Avg. Stay | Variance | 10th | 25th | 50th | 75th | 90th | 95th | 99th |
|---|---|---|---|---|---|---|---|---|---|---|
| **1. SINGLE DX** | | | | | | | | | | |
| 0-19 Years | 6 | 1.0 | 0 | 1 | 1 | 1 | 1 | 1 | 1 | 1 |
| 20-34 | 1 | 1.0 | 0 | 1 | 1 | 1 | 1 | 1 | 1 | 1 |
| 35-49 | 0 | | | | | | | | | |
| 50-64 | 0 | | | | | | | | | |
| **2. MULTIPLE DX** | | | | | | | | | | |
| 0-19 Years | 11 | 1.0 | 0 | 1 | 1 | 1 | 1 | 1 | 1 | 1 |
| 20-34 | 1 | 1.0 | 0 | 1 | 1 | 1 | 1 | 1 | 1 | 1 |
| 35-49 | 1 | 1.0 | 0 | 1 | 1 | 1 | 1 | 1 | 1 | 1 |
| 50-64 | 2 | 1.0 | 0 | 1 | 1 | 1 | 1 | 1 | 1 | 1 |
| 65+ | 0 | | | | | | | | | |
| **TOTAL SINGLE DX** | 8 | 1.0 | 0 | 1 | 1 | 1 | 1 | 1 | 1 | 1 |
| **TOTAL MULTIPLE DX** | 15 | 1.0 | 0 | 1 | 1 | 1 | 1 | 1 | 1 | 1 |
| **TOTAL** | | | | | | | | | | |
| 0-19 Years | 17 | 1.0 | 0 | 1 | 1 | 1 | 1 | 1 | 1 | 1 |
| 20-34 | 2 | 1.0 | 0 | 1 | 1 | 1 | 1 | 1 | 1 | 1 |
| 35-49 | 2 | 1.0 | 0 | 1 | 1 | 1 | 1 | 1 | 1 | 1 |
| 50-64 | 2 | 1.0 | 0 | 1 | 1 | 1 | 1 | 1 | 1 | 1 |
| 65+ | 0 | | | | | | | | | |
| **GRAND TOTAL** | 23 | 1.0 | 0 | 1 | 1 | 1 | 1 | 1 | 1 | 1 |

Length of Stay by Diagnosis and Operation, United States, 2000

## United States, October 1998–September 1999 Data, by Operation

### 18.6: EXT AUDIT CANAL RECONST. Formerly included in operation group(s) 533.

| Type of Patients | Observed Patients | Avg. Stay | Variance | 10th | 25th | 50th | 75th | 90th | 95th | 99th |
|---|---|---|---|---|---|---|---|---|---|---|
| **1. SINGLE DX** | | | | | | | | | | |
| 0–19 Years | 37 | 1.6 | 1 | 1 | 1 | 1 | 2 | 4 | 4 | 4 |
| 20–34 | 2 | 1.5 | <1 | 1 | 1 | 1 | 2 | 2 | 2 | 2 |
| 35–49 | 1 | 3.0 | 0 | 3 | 3 | 3 | 3 | 3 | 3 | 3 |
| 50–64 | 1 | 1.0 | 0 | 1 | 1 | 1 | 1 | 1 | 1 | 1 |
| 65+ | 2 | 4.9 | 15 | 1 | 1 | 8 | 8 | 8 | 8 | 8 |
| **2. MULTIPLE DX** | | | | | | | | | | |
| 0–19 Years | 61 | 1.8 | 1 | 1 | 1 | 1 | 3 | 3 | 3 | 5 |
| 20–34 | 5 | 3.9 | 18 | 2 | 2 | 2 | 4 | 5 | 17 | 17 |
| 35–49 | 6 | 2.8 | 12 | 1 | 1 | 2 | 3 | 11 | 11 | 11 |
| 50–64 | 4 | 2.7 | 2 | 1 | 2 | 2 | 4 | 5 | 5 | 5 |
| 65+ | 12 | 2.0 | 1 | 1 | 1 | 3 | 3 | 3 | 4 | 5 |
| **TOTAL SINGLE DX** | 43 | 1.7 | 2 | 1 | 1 | 1 | 2 | 4 | 4 | 8 |
| **TOTAL MULTIPLE DX** | 88 | 2.1 | 3 | 1 | 1 | 1 | 3 | 3 | 4 | 11 |
| **TOTAL** | | | | | | | | | | |
| 0–19 Years | 98 | 1.7 | 1 | 1 | 1 | 1 | 3 | 3 | 4 | 5 |
| 20–34 | 7 | 3.5 | 16 | 1 | 2 | 2 | 4 | 5 | 17 | 17 |
| 35–49 | 7 | 2.8 | 11 | 1 | 1 | 2 | 3 | 11 | 11 | 11 |
| 50–64 | 5 | 2.4 | 2 | 1 | 1 | 2 | 4 | 5 | 5 | 5 |
| 65+ | 14 | 2.2 | 3 | 1 | 1 | 1 | 3 | 4 | 5 | 8 |
| **GRAND TOTAL** | 131 | 1.9 | 3 | 1 | 1 | 1 | 3 | 3 | 4 | 8 |

### 18.7: OTH PLASTIC REP EXT EAR. Formerly included in operation group(s) 533.

| Type of Patients | Observed Patients | Avg. Stay | Variance | 10th | 25th | 50th | 75th | 90th | 95th | 99th |
|---|---|---|---|---|---|---|---|---|---|---|
| **1. SINGLE DX** | | | | | | | | | | |
| 0–19 Years | 151 | 1.8 | <1 | 1 | 1 | 1 | 2 | 3 | 4 | 4 |
| 20–34 | 14 | 3.4 | 10 | 1 | 1 | 1 | 8 | 8 | 8 | 8 |
| 35–49 | 6 | 1.2 | <1 | 1 | 1 | 1 | 1 | 2 | 2 | 2 |
| 50–64 | 6 | 1.3 | <1 | 1 | 1 | 1 | 2 | 2 | 2 | 2 |
| 65+ | 2 | 1.0 | 0 | 1 | 1 | 1 | 1 | 1 | 1 | 1 |
| **2. MULTIPLE DX** | | | | | | | | | | |
| 0–19 Years | 146 | 1.9 | 2 | 1 | 1 | 1 | 2 | 4 | 5 | 6 |
| 20–34 | 50 | 2.9 | 6 | 1 | 2 | 2 | 3 | 6 | 9 | 13 |
| 35–49 | 23 | 3.2 | 9 | 1 | 2 | 3 | 4 | 6 | 11 | 14 |
| 50–64 | 27 | 2.6 | 4 | 1 | 1 | 3 | 3 | 6 | 6 | 6 |
| 65+ | 47 | 3.4 | 6 | 1 | 3 | 3 | 3 | 5 | 7 | 16 |
| **TOTAL SINGLE DX** | 179 | 1.8 | 2 | 1 | 1 | 1 | 2 | 3 | 4 | 8 |
| **TOTAL MULTIPLE DX** | 293 | 2.5 | 4 | 1 | 1 | 2 | 3 | 5 | 6 | 10 |
| **TOTAL** | | | | | | | | | | |
| 0–19 Years | 297 | 1.8 | 1 | 1 | 1 | 1 | 2 | 4 | 4 | 6 |
| 20–34 | 64 | 3.1 | 7 | 1 | 1 | 2 | 3 | 8 | 8 | 10 |
| 35–49 | 29 | 2.7 | 3 | 1 | 1 | 2 | 3 | 3 | 4 | 14 |
| 50–64 | 33 | 2.5 | 4 | 1 | 1 | 2 | 3 | 6 | 6 | 16 |
| 65+ | 49 | 3.4 | 6 | 1 | 3 | 3 | 3 | 5 | 7 | 16 |
| **GRAND TOTAL** | 472 | 2.2 | 3 | 1 | 1 | 1 | 3 | 4 | 6 | 9 |

### 18.9: OTHER EXT EAR OPERATIONS. Formerly included in operation group(s) 533.

| Type of Patients | Observed Patients | Avg. Stay | Variance | 10th | 25th | 50th | 75th | 90th | 95th | 99th |
|---|---|---|---|---|---|---|---|---|---|---|
| **1. SINGLE DX** | | | | | | | | | | |
| 0–19 Years | 0 | | | | | | | | | |
| 20–34 | 0 | | | | | | | | | |
| 35–49 | 0 | | | | | | | | | |
| 50–64 | 0 | | | | | | | | | |
| 65+ | 0 | | | | | | | | | |
| **2. MULTIPLE DX** | | | | | | | | | | |
| 0–19 Years | 0 | | | | | | | | | |
| 20–34 | 0 | | | | | | | | | |
| 35–49 | 1 | 3.0 | 0 | 3 | 3 | 3 | 3 | 3 | 3 | 3 |
| 50–64 | 1 | 8.0 | 0 | 8 | 8 | 8 | 8 | 8 | 8 | 8 |
| 65+ | 0 | | | | | | | | | |
| **TOTAL SINGLE DX** | 0 | | | | | | | | | |
| **TOTAL MULTIPLE DX** | 2 | 4.2 | 5 | 3 | 3 | 3 | 3 | 8 | 8 | 8 |
| **TOTAL** | | | | | | | | | | |
| 0–19 Years | 0 | | | | | | | | | |
| 20–34 | 0 | | | | | | | | | |
| 35–49 | 1 | 3.0 | 0 | 3 | 3 | 3 | 3 | 3 | 3 | 3 |
| 50–64 | 1 | 8.0 | 0 | 8 | 8 | 8 | 8 | 8 | 8 | 8 |
| 65+ | 0 | | | | | | | | | |
| **GRAND TOTAL** | 2 | 4.2 | 5 | 3 | 3 | 3 | 3 | 8 | 8 | 8 |

### 19.0: STAPES MOBILIZATION. Formerly included in operation group(s) 534.

| Type of Patients | Observed Patients | Avg. Stay | Variance | 10th | 25th | 50th | 75th | 90th | 95th | 99th |
|---|---|---|---|---|---|---|---|---|---|---|
| **1. SINGLE DX** | | | | | | | | | | |
| 0–19 Years | 0 | | | | | | | | | |
| 20–34 | 0 | | | | | | | | | |
| 35–49 | 0 | | | | | | | | | |
| 50–64 | 1 | 1.0 | 0 | 1 | 1 | 1 | 1 | 1 | 1 | 1 |
| 65+ | 0 | | | | | | | | | |
| **2. MULTIPLE DX** | | | | | | | | | | |
| 0–19 Years | 2 | 1.0 | 0 | 1 | 1 | 1 | 1 | 1 | 1 | 1 |
| 20–34 | 1 | 1.0 | 0 | 1 | 1 | 1 | 1 | 1 | 1 | 1 |
| 35–49 | 3 | 1.5 | <1 | 1 | 1 | 1 | 2 | 2 | 2 | 2 |
| 50–64 | 0 | | | | | | | | | |
| 65+ | 1 | 1.0 | 0 | 1 | 1 | 1 | 1 | 1 | 1 | 1 |
| **TOTAL SINGLE DX** | 1 | 1.0 | 0 | 1 | 1 | 1 | 1 | 1 | 1 | 1 |
| **TOTAL MULTIPLE DX** | 7 | 1.2 | <1 | 1 | 1 | 1 | 1 | 2 | 2 | 2 |
| **TOTAL** | | | | | | | | | | |
| 0–19 Years | 2 | 1.0 | 0 | 1 | 1 | 1 | 1 | 1 | 1 | 1 |
| 20–34 | 1 | 1.0 | 0 | 1 | 1 | 1 | 1 | 1 | 1 | 1 |
| 35–49 | 3 | 1.5 | <1 | 1 | 1 | 1 | 2 | 2 | 2 | 2 |
| 50–64 | 1 | 1.0 | 0 | 1 | 1 | 1 | 1 | 1 | 1 | 1 |
| 65+ | 1 | 1.0 | 0 | 1 | 1 | 1 | 1 | 1 | 1 | 1 |
| **GRAND TOTAL** | 8 | 1.2 | <1 | 1 | 1 | 1 | 1 | 2 | 2 | 2 |

Length of Stay by Diagnosis and Operation, United States, 2000

# United States, October 1998–September 1999 Data, by Operation

## 19.1: STAPEDECTOMY. Formerly included in operation group(s) 534.

| Type of Patients | Observed Patients | Avg. Stay | Variance | 10th | 25th | 50th | 75th | 90th | 95th | 99th |
|---|---|---|---|---|---|---|---|---|---|---|
| **1. SINGLE DX** | | | | | | | | | | |
| 0–19 Years | 2 | 1.0 | 0 | | | | | | | |
| 20–34 | 7 | 1.0 | 0 | 1 | 1 | 1 | 1 | 1 | 1 | 1 |
| 35–49 | 18 | 1.0 | <1 | 1 | 1 | 1 | 1 | 1 | 1 | 1 |
| 50–64 | 10 | 1.3 | <1 | 1 | 1 | 1 | 2 | 2 | 2 | 3 |
| 65+ | 4 | 1.0 | 0 | 1 | 1 | 1 | 1 | 1 | 1 | 1 |
| **2. MULTIPLE DX** | | | | | | | | | | |
| 0–19 Years | 3 | 1.1 | <1 | 1 | 1 | 1 | 1 | 2 | 2 | 2 |
| 20–34 | 9 | 1.2 | <1 | 1 | 1 | 1 | 1 | 1 | 2 | 6 |
| 35–49 | 32 | 1.4 | <1 | 1 | 1 | 2 | 2 | 2 | 3 | 4 |
| 50–64 | 25 | 1.6 | 1 | 1 | 1 | 2 | 2 | 3 | 5 | 6 |
| 65+ | 15 | 2.4 | 1 | 1 | 1 | 3 | 3 | 3 | 5 | 5 |
| **TOTAL SINGLE DX** | 41 | 1.1 | <1 | 1 | 1 | 1 | 1 | 2 | 2 | 2 |
| **TOTAL MULTIPLE DX** | 84 | 1.6 | 1 | 1 | 1 | 2 | 2 | 3 | 4 | 6 |
| **TOTAL** | | | | | | | | | | |
| 0–19 Years | 5 | 1.1 | <1 | 1 | 1 | 1 | 1 | 2 | 2 | 2 |
| 20–34 | 16 | 1.1 | <1 | 1 | 1 | 1 | 1 | 1 | 1 | 6 |
| 35–49 | 50 | 1.2 | <1 | 1 | 1 | 1 | 2 | 2 | 2 | 4 |
| 50–64 | 35 | 1.4 | <1 | 1 | 1 | 2 | 3 | 3 | 5 | 6 |
| 65+ | 19 | 2.1 | 1 | 1 | 1 | 2 | 3 | 3 | 5 | 5 |
| **GRAND TOTAL** | 125 | 1.4 | <1 | 1 | 1 | 1 | 1 | 2 | 3 | 5 |

## 19.2: STAPEDECTOMY REVISION. Formerly included in operation group(s) 534.

| Type of Patients | Observed Patients | Avg. Stay | Variance | 10th | 25th | 50th | 75th | 90th | 95th | 99th |
|---|---|---|---|---|---|---|---|---|---|---|
| **1. SINGLE DX** | | | | | | | | | | |
| 0–19 Years | 0 | | | | | | | | | |
| 20–34 | 2 | 1.0 | 0 | 1 | 1 | 1 | 1 | 1 | 1 | 1 |
| 35–49 | 1 | 1.0 | 0 | 1 | 1 | 1 | 1 | 1 | 1 | 1 |
| 50–64 | 0 | | | | | | | | | |
| 65+ | 4 | 1.3 | <1 | 1 | 1 | 1 | 2 | 2 | 2 | 2 |
| **2. MULTIPLE DX** | | | | | | | | | | |
| 0–19 Years | 1 | 1.0 | 0 | 1 | 1 | 1 | 1 | 1 | 1 | 1 |
| 20–34 | 1 | 1.0 | 0 | 1 | 1 | 1 | 1 | 1 | 1 | 1 |
| 35–49 | 8 | 1.2 | <1 | 1 | 1 | 1 | 1 | 1 | 3 | 3 |
| 50–64 | 4 | 1.0 | 0 | 1 | 1 | 1 | 1 | 1 | 1 | 1 |
| 65+ | 4 | 1.4 | <1 | 1 | 1 | 1 | 1 | 4 | 4 | 4 |
| **TOTAL SINGLE DX** | 7 | 1.1 | <1 | 1 | 1 | 1 | 1 | 1 | 2 | 2 |
| **TOTAL MULTIPLE DX** | 18 | 1.2 | <1 | 1 | 1 | 1 | 1 | 1 | 3 | 4 |
| **TOTAL** | | | | | | | | | | |
| 0–19 Years | 1 | 1.0 | 0 | 1 | 1 | 1 | 1 | 1 | 1 | 1 |
| 20–34 | 3 | 1.0 | 0 | 1 | 1 | 1 | 1 | 1 | 1 | 1 |
| 35–49 | 9 | 1.2 | <1 | 1 | 1 | 1 | 1 | 1 | 3 | 3 |
| 50–64 | 4 | 1.0 | <1 | 1 | 1 | 1 | 1 | 1 | 1 | 1 |
| 65+ | 8 | 1.4 | <1 | 1 | 1 | 1 | 1 | 4 | 4 | 4 |
| **GRAND TOTAL** | 25 | 1.1 | <1 | 1 | 1 | 1 | 1 | 1 | 3 | 4 |

## 19.3: OSSICULAR CHAIN OPS NEC. Formerly included in operation group(s) 534.

| Type of Patients | Observed Patients | Avg. Stay | Variance | 10th | 25th | 50th | 75th | 90th | 95th | 99th |
|---|---|---|---|---|---|---|---|---|---|---|
| **1. SINGLE DX** | | | | | | | | | | |
| 0–19 Years | 0 | | | | | | | | | |
| 20–34 | 1 | 1.0 | 0 | 1 | 1 | 1 | 1 | 1 | 1 | 1 |
| 35–49 | 0 | | | | | | | | | |
| 50–64 | 0 | | | | | | | | | |
| 65+ | 2 | 2.0 | 0 | 2 | 2 | 2 | 2 | 2 | 2 | 2 |
| **2. MULTIPLE DX** | | | | | | | | | | |
| 0–19 Years | 4 | 1.0 | 0 | 1 | 1 | 1 | 1 | 1 | 1 | 1 |
| 20–34 | 1 | 1.0 | 0 | 1 | 1 | 1 | 1 | 1 | 1 | 1 |
| 35–49 | 4 | 1.0 | 0 | 1 | 1 | 1 | 1 | 1 | 1 | 1 |
| 50–64 | 5 | 1.1 | <1 | 1 | 1 | 2 | 2 | 2 | 3 | 3 |
| 65+ | 1 | 1.0 | 0 | 1 | 1 | 1 | 1 | 1 | 1 | 1 |
| **TOTAL SINGLE DX** | 3 | 1.7 | <1 | 1 | 1 | 2 | 2 | 2 | 2 | 2 |
| **TOTAL MULTIPLE DX** | 15 | 1.0 | <1 | 1 | 1 | 1 | 1 | 1 | 1 | 3 |
| **TOTAL** | | | | | | | | | | |
| 0–19 Years | 4 | 1.0 | 0 | 1 | 1 | 1 | 1 | 1 | 1 | 1 |
| 20–34 | 2 | 1.0 | 0 | 1 | 1 | 1 | 1 | 1 | 1 | 1 |
| 35–49 | 4 | 1.0 | 0 | 1 | 1 | 1 | 1 | 1 | 1 | 1 |
| 50–64 | 5 | 1.1 | <1 | 1 | 1 | 2 | 2 | 2 | 2 | 3 |
| 65+ | 3 | 1.6 | <1 | 1 | 1 | 2 | 2 | 2 | 2 | 2 |
| **GRAND TOTAL** | 18 | 1.1 | <1 | 1 | 1 | 1 | 1 | 1 | 2 | 3 |

## 19.4: MYRINGOPLASTY. Formerly included in operation group(s) 535.

| Type of Patients | Observed Patients | Avg. Stay | Variance | 10th | 25th | 50th | 75th | 90th | 95th | 99th |
|---|---|---|---|---|---|---|---|---|---|---|
| **1. SINGLE DX** | | | | | | | | | | |
| 0–19 Years | 70 | 1.0 | <1 | 1 | 1 | 1 | 1 | 1 | 1 | 2 |
| 20–34 | 6 | 1.2 | <1 | 1 | 1 | 1 | 2 | 2 | 2 | 2 |
| 35–49 | 2 | 1.7 | <1 | 1 | 1 | 2 | 2 | 2 | 2 | 2 |
| 50–64 | 2 | 1.0 | 0 | 1 | 1 | 1 | 1 | 1 | 1 | 1 |
| 65+ | 3 | 1.0 | 0 | 1 | 1 | 1 | 1 | 1 | 1 | 1 |
| **2. MULTIPLE DX** | | | | | | | | | | |
| 0–19 Years | 101 | 1.4 | 2 | 1 | 1 | 1 | 1 | 2 | 3 | 8 |
| 20–34 | 10 | 1.5 | <1 | 1 | 1 | 1 | 2 | 3 | 3 | 8 |
| 35–49 | 11 | 2.7 | 6 | 1 | 2 | 2 | 4 | 7 | 7 | 7 |
| 50–64 | 18 | 1.5 | <1 | 1 | 1 | 1 | 2 | 2 | 3 | 6 |
| 65+ | 11 | 1.0 | <1 | 1 | 1 | 1 | 1 | 1 | 1 | 2 |
| **TOTAL SINGLE DX** | 83 | 1.0 | <1 | 1 | 1 | 1 | 1 | 1 | 1 | 2 |
| **TOTAL MULTIPLE DX** | 151 | 1.5 | 2 | 1 | 1 | 1 | 1 | 2 | 3 | 8 |
| **TOTAL** | | | | | | | | | | |
| 0–19 Years | 171 | 1.3 | 2 | 1 | 1 | 1 | 1 | 2 | 3 | 8 |
| 20–34 | 16 | 1.4 | <1 | 1 | 1 | 1 | 2 | 3 | 3 | 3 |
| 35–49 | 13 | 2.6 | 6 | 1 | 1 | 1 | 3 | 7 | 7 | 7 |
| 50–64 | 20 | 1.5 | <1 | 1 | 1 | 1 | 2 | 2 | 3 | 6 |
| 65+ | 14 | 1.0 | <1 | 1 | 1 | 1 | 1 | 1 | 1 | 2 |
| **GRAND TOTAL** | 234 | 1.4 | 2 | 1 | 1 | 1 | 1 | 2 | 3 | 8 |

Length of Stay by Diagnosis and Operation, United States, 2000

# United States, October 1998–September 1999 Data, by Operation

## 19.5: OTHER TYMPANOPLASTY. Formerly included in operation group(s) 535.

| Type of Patients | Observed Patients | Avg. Stay | Variance | 10th | 25th | 50th | 75th | 90th | 95th | 99th |
|---|---|---|---|---|---|---|---|---|---|---|
| **1. SINGLE DX** | | | | | | | | | | |
| 0–19 Years | 9 | 1.4 | <1 | 1 | 1 | 1 | 1 | 3 | 3 | 3 |
| 20–34 | 3 | 1.0 | 0 | 1 | 1 | 1 | 1 | 1 | 1 | 1 |
| 35–49 | 5 | 1.0 | 0 | 1 | 1 | 1 | 1 | 1 | 1 | 1 |
| 50–64 | 3 | 1.4 | <1 | 1 | 1 | 1 | 2 | 2 | 2 | 2 |
| 65+ | 1 | 1.0 | 0 | 1 | 1 | 1 | 1 | 1 | 1 | 1 |
| **2. MULTIPLE DX** | | | | | | | | | | |
| 0–19 Years | 26 | 1.0 | <1 | 1 | 1 | 1 | 1 | 1 | 1 | 1 |
| 20–34 | 4 | 1.4 | <1 | 1 | 1 | 1 | 2 | 2 | 2 | 2 |
| 35–49 | 9 | 1.3 | <1 | 1 | 1 | 1 | 1 | 2 | 4 | 4 |
| 50–64 | 8 | 1.4 | <1 | 1 | 1 | 1 | 2 | 2 | 2 | 2 |
| 65+ | 8 | 2.0 | 4 | 1 | 1 | 1 | 1 | 6 | 6 | 6 |
| **TOTAL SINGLE DX** | 21 | 1.2 | <1 | 1 | 1 | 1 | 1 | 2 | 3 | 3 |
| **TOTAL MULTIPLE DX** | 55 | 1.2 | <1 | 1 | 1 | 1 | 1 | 2 | 2 | 4 |
| **TOTAL** | | | | | | | | | | |
| 0–19 Years | 35 | 1.1 | <1 | 1 | 1 | 1 | 1 | 1 | 2 | 3 |
| 20–34 | 7 | 1.2 | <1 | 1 | 1 | 1 | 1 | 2 | 2 | 2 |
| 35–49 | 14 | 1.3 | <1 | 1 | 1 | 1 | 1 | 2 | 4 | 4 |
| 50–64 | 11 | 1.4 | <1 | 1 | 1 | 1 | 2 | 2 | 2 | 2 |
| 65+ | 9 | 1.8 | 3 | 1 | 1 | 1 | 1 | 6 | 6 | 6 |
| **GRAND TOTAL** | 76 | 1.2 | <1 | 1 | 1 | 1 | 1 | 2 | 2 | 4 |

## 19.6: TYMPANOPLASTY REVISION. Formerly included in operation group(s) 538.

| Type of Patients | Observed Patients | Avg. Stay | Variance | 10th | 25th | 50th | 75th | 90th | 95th | 99th |
|---|---|---|---|---|---|---|---|---|---|---|
| **1. SINGLE DX** | | | | | | | | | | |
| 0–19 Years | 3 | 1.0 | 0 | 1 | 1 | 1 | 1 | 1 | 1 | 1 |
| 20–34 | 1 | 1.0 | 0 | 1 | 1 | 1 | 1 | 1 | 1 | 1 |
| 35–49 | 0 | | | | | | | | | |
| 50–64 | 0 | | | | | | | | | |
| 65+ | 0 | | | | | | | | | |
| **2. MULTIPLE DX** | | | | | | | | | | |
| 0–19 Years | 13 | 1.0 | 0 | 1 | 1 | 1 | 1 | 1 | 1 | 1 |
| 20–34 | 3 | 1.3 | <1 | 1 | 1 | 1 | 2 | 2 | 2 | 2 |
| 35–49 | 10 | 1.2 | <1 | 1 | 1 | 1 | 1 | 3 | 3 | 3 |
| 50–64 | 4 | 1.3 | <1 | 1 | 1 | 1 | 1 | 2 | 2 | 2 |
| 65+ | 4 | 2.0 | 2 | 1 | 1 | 1 | 4 | 4 | 4 | 4 |
| **TOTAL SINGLE DX** | 4 | 1.0 | 0 | 1 | 1 | 1 | 1 | 1 | 1 | 1 |
| **TOTAL MULTIPLE DX** | 34 | 1.1 | <1 | 1 | 1 | 1 | 1 | 1 | 3 | 4 |
| **TOTAL** | | | | | | | | | | |
| 0–19 Years | 16 | 1.0 | 0 | 1 | 1 | 1 | 1 | 1 | 1 | 1 |
| 20–34 | 4 | 1.2 | <1 | 1 | 1 | 1 | 1 | 2 | 2 | 2 |
| 35–49 | 10 | 1.2 | <1 | 1 | 1 | 1 | 1 | 2 | 3 | 3 |
| 50–64 | 4 | 1.3 | <1 | 1 | 1 | 1 | 1 | 2 | 2 | 2 |
| 65+ | 4 | 2.0 | 2 | 1 | 1 | 1 | 4 | 4 | 4 | 4 |
| **GRAND TOTAL** | 38 | 1.1 | <1 | 1 | 1 | 1 | 1 | 1 | 3 | 4 |

## 19.9: MIDDLE EAR REPAIR NEC. Formerly included in operation group(s) 538.

| Type of Patients | Observed Patients | Avg. Stay | Variance | 10th | 25th | 50th | 75th | 90th | 95th | 99th |
|---|---|---|---|---|---|---|---|---|---|---|
| **1. SINGLE DX** | | | | | | | | | | |
| 0–19 Years | 0 | | | | | | | | | |
| 20–34 | 1 | 1.0 | 0 | 1 | 1 | 1 | 1 | 1 | 1 | 1 |
| 35–49 | 1 | 1.0 | 0 | 1 | 1 | 1 | 1 | 1 | 1 | 1 |
| 50–64 | 1 | 4.0 | 0 | 4 | 4 | 4 | 4 | 4 | 4 | 4 |
| 65+ | 1 | 2.0 | 0 | 2 | 2 | 2 | 2 | 2 | 2 | 2 |
| **2. MULTIPLE DX** | | | | | | | | | | |
| 0–19 Years | 5 | 5.5 | 85 | 1 | 1 | 1 | 4 | 25 | 25 | 25 |
| 20–34 | 0 | | | | | | | | | |
| 35–49 | 5 | 4.9 | 18 | 1 | 2 | 2 | 11 | 11 | 11 | 11 |
| 50–64 | 2 | 2.9 | 1 | 2 | 2 | 2 | 4 | 4 | 4 | 4 |
| 65+ | 4 | 7.0 | 5 | 6 | 6 | 6 | 9 | 9 | 9 | 9 |
| **TOTAL SINGLE DX** | 4 | 2.0 | 2 | 1 | 1 | 1 | 4 | 4 | 4 | 4 |
| **TOTAL MULTIPLE DX** | 16 | 6.0 | 26 | 1 | 2 | 6 | 9 | 11 | 11 | 25 |
| **TOTAL** | | | | | | | | | | |
| 0–19 Years | 5 | 5.5 | 85 | 1 | 1 | 1 | 4 | 25 | 25 | 25 |
| 20–34 | 1 | 1.0 | 0 | 1 | 1 | 1 | 1 | 1 | 1 | 1 |
| 35–49 | 6 | 4.6 | 18 | 1 | 2 | 2 | 11 | 11 | 11 | 11 |
| 50–64 | 3 | 3.3 | 1 | 2 | 2 | 4 | 4 | 4 | 4 | 4 |
| 65+ | 5 | 6.8 | 5 | 4 | 6 | 6 | 9 | 9 | 9 | 9 |
| **GRAND TOTAL** | 20 | 5.6 | 25 | 1 | 2 | 6 | 9 | 9 | 11 | 25 |

## 20.0: MYRINGOTOMY. Formerly included in operation group(s) 536.

| Type of Patients | Observed Patients | Avg. Stay | Variance | 10th | 25th | 50th | 75th | 90th | 95th | 99th |
|---|---|---|---|---|---|---|---|---|---|---|
| **1. SINGLE DX** | | | | | | | | | | |
| 0–19 Years | 340 | 1.2 | <1 | 1 | 1 | 1 | 1 | 2 | 3 | 4 |
| 20–34 | 1 | 1.0 | 0 | 1 | 1 | 1 | 1 | 1 | 1 | 1 |
| 35–49 | 4 | 4.7 | 4 | 3 | 3 | 3 | 7 | 7 | 7 | 7 |
| 50–64 | 2 | 1.5 | <1 | 1 | 1 | 1 | 2 | 2 | 2 | 2 |
| 65+ | 3 | 1.3 | <1 | 1 | 1 | 1 | 1 | 3 | 3 | 3 |
| **2. MULTIPLE DX** | | | | | | | | | | |
| 0–19 Years | 1,973 | 2.8 | 14 | 1 | 1 | 1 | 3 | 6 | 9 | 17 |
| 20–34 | 52 | 5.2 | 19 | 2 | 2 | 3 | 6 | 10 | 15 | 22 |
| 35–49 | 80 | 5.7 | 25 | 1 | 1 | 4 | 9 | 11 | 14 | 21 |
| 50–64 | 90 | 6.2 | 64 | 2 | 4 | 5 | 8 | 11 | 19 | 32 |
| 65+ | 133 | 9.0 | 78 | 2 | 4 | 7 | 11 | 18 | 22 | 36 |
| **TOTAL SINGLE DX** | 350 | 1.2 | <1 | 1 | 1 | 1 | 1 | 2 | 3 | 4 |
| **TOTAL MULTIPLE DX** | 2,328 | 3.3 | 21 | 1 | 1 | 2 | 4 | 7 | 11 | 21 |
| **TOTAL** | | | | | | | | | | |
| 0–19 Years | 2,313 | 2.5 | 12 | 1 | 1 | 1 | 3 | 5 | 8 | 16 |
| 20–34 | 53 | 5.1 | 19 | 2 | 2 | 3 | 6 | 10 | 15 | 22 |
| 35–49 | 84 | 5.7 | 25 | 1 | 1 | 4 | 9 | 11 | 14 | 21 |
| 50–64 | 92 | 6.1 | 64 | 1 | 1 | 5 | 8 | 11 | 15 | 32 |
| 65+ | 136 | 8.7 | 78 | 2 | 3 | 7 | 11 | 18 | 22 | 36 |
| **GRAND TOTAL** | 2,678 | 2.9 | 18 | 1 | 1 | 1 | 3 | 7 | 10 | 21 |

Length of Stay by Diagnosis and Operation, United States, 2000

# United States, October 1998–September 1999 Data, by Operation

## 20.01: MYRINGOTOMY W INTUBATION. Formerly included in operation group(s) 536.

| Type of Patients | Observed Patients | Avg. Stay | Vari-ance | 10th | 25th | 50th | 75th | 90th | 95th | 99th |
|---|---|---|---|---|---|---|---|---|---|---|
| **1. SINGLE DX** | | | | | | | | | | |
| 0–19 Years | 325 | 1.2 | <1 | 1 | 1 | 1 | 1 | 1 | 3 | 4 |
| 20–34 | 0 | | | | | | | | | |
| 35–49 | 3 | 6.0 | 3 | 3 | 6 | 7 | 7 | 7 | 7 | 7 |
| 50–64 | 1 | 1.0 | 0 | 1 | 1 | 1 | 1 | 1 | 1 | 1 |
| 65+ | 1 | 1.0 | 0 | 1 | 1 | 1 | 1 | 1 | 1 | 1 |
| **2. MULTIPLE DX** | | | | | | | | | | |
| 0–19 Years | 1,878 | 2.8 | 14 | 1 | 1 | 1 | 3 | 6 | 9 | 17 |
| 20–34 | 43 | 5.4 | 22 | 1 | 2 | 3 | 8 | 13 | 15 | 22 |
| 35–49 | 72 | 5.7 | 27 | 2 | 2 | 4 | 7 | 11 | 16 | 21 |
| 50–64 | 81 | 6.0 | 70 | 1 | 2 | 5 | 7 | 11 | 15 | 32 |
| 65+ | 115 | 8.6 | 46 | 2 | 3 | 7 | 12 | 18 | 22 | 29 |
| **TOTAL SINGLE DX** | 330 | 1.2 | <1 | 1 | 1 | 1 | 1 | 1 | 3 | 4 |
| **TOTAL MULTIPLE DX** | 2,185 | 3.2 | 20 | 1 | 1 | 2 | 4 | 7 | 11 | 21 |
| **TOTAL** | | | | | | | | | | |
| 0–19 Years | 2,203 | 2.5 | 12 | 1 | 1 | 3 | 3 | 5 | 8 | 16 |
| 20–34 | 43 | 5.4 | 22 | 1 | 2 | 3 | 8 | 13 | 15 | 22 |
| 35–49 | 72 | 5.7 | 27 | 1 | 2 | 4 | 7 | 11 | 16 | 21 |
| 50–64 | 81 | 6.0 | 69 | 1 | 1 | 5 | 7 | 11 | 15 | 32 |
| 65+ | 116 | 8.4 | 46 | 2 | 3 | 7 | 12 | 18 | 22 | 29 |
| **GRAND TOTAL** | 2,515 | 2.9 | 17 | 1 | 1 | 1 | 3 | 7 | 10 | 21 |

## 20.1: TYMPANOSTOMY TUBE RMVL. Formerly included in operation group(s) 538.

| Type of Patients | Observed Patients | Avg. Stay | Vari-ance | 10th | 25th | 50th | 75th | 90th | 95th | 99th |
|---|---|---|---|---|---|---|---|---|---|---|
| **1. SINGLE DX** | | | | | | | | | | |
| 0–19 Years | 11 | 1.2 | <1 | 1 | 1 | 1 | 1 | 1 | 3 | 5 |
| 20–34 | 0 | | | | | | | | | |
| 35–49 | 0 | | | | | | | | | |
| 50–64 | 0 | | | | | | | | | |
| 65+ | 0 | | | | | | | | | |
| **2. MULTIPLE DX** | | | | | | | | | | |
| 0–19 Years | 39 | 3.3 | 8 | 1 | 1 | 3 | 5 | 6 | 8 | 13 |
| 20–34 | 1 | 3.0 | 0 | 3 | 3 | 3 | 3 | 3 | 3 | 3 |
| 35–49 | 1 | | | | | | | | | |
| 50–64 | 0 | | | | | | | | | |
| 65+ | 1 | 6.0 | 0 | 6 | 6 | 6 | 6 | 6 | 6 | 6 |
| **TOTAL SINGLE DX** | 11 | 1.2 | <1 | 1 | 1 | 1 | 1 | 1 | 3 | 5 |
| **TOTAL MULTIPLE DX** | 41 | 3.4 | 7 | 1 | 1 | 3 | 5 | 6 | 8 | 13 |
| **TOTAL** | | | | | | | | | | |
| 0–19 Years | 50 | 2.8 | 7 | 1 | 1 | 3 | 4 | 6 | 8 | 13 |
| 20–34 | 0 | | | | | | | | | |
| 35–49 | 1 | 3.0 | 0 | 3 | 3 | 3 | 3 | 3 | 3 | 3 |
| 50–64 | 0 | | | | | | | | | |
| 65+ | 1 | 6.0 | 0 | 6 | 6 | 6 | 6 | 6 | 6 | 6 |
| **GRAND TOTAL** | 52 | 2.8 | 6 | 1 | 1 | 1 | 4 | 6 | 8 | 13 |

## 20.2: MASTOID & MID EAR INC. Formerly included in operation group(s) 538.

| Type of Patients | Observed Patients | Avg. Stay | Vari-ance | 10th | 25th | 50th | 75th | 90th | 95th | 99th |
|---|---|---|---|---|---|---|---|---|---|---|
| **1. SINGLE DX** | | | | | | | | | | |
| 0–19 Years | 10 | 2.6 | 2 | 1 | 2 | 2 | 4 | 5 | 5 | 5 |
| 20–34 | 4 | 1.6 | <1 | 1 | 1 | 1 | 2 | 2 | 2 | 2 |
| 35–49 | 3 | 3.3 | 20 | 1 | 1 | 1 | 1 | 12 | 12 | 12 |
| 50–64 | 1 | 1.0 | 0 | 1 | 1 | 1 | 1 | 1 | 1 | 1 |
| 65+ | 1 | 2.0 | 0 | 2 | 2 | 2 | 2 | 2 | 2 | 2 |
| **2. MULTIPLE DX** | | | | | | | | | | |
| 0–19 Years | 19 | 5.0 | 36 | 1 | 4 | 4 | 5 | 5 | 24 | 24 |
| 20–34 | 3 | 5.6 | 3 | 4 | 7 | 7 | 7 | 7 | 7 | 7 |
| 35–49 | 5 | 2.4 | 2 | 1 | 1 | 3 | 3 | 5 | 5 | 5 |
| 50–64 | 3 | 5.2 | 3 | 3 | 6 | 6 | 6 | 6 | 6 | 6 |
| 65+ | 3 | 6.8 | 9 | 4 | 4 | 6 | 10 | 10 | 10 | 10 |
| **TOTAL SINGLE DX** | 19 | 2.4 | 3 | 1 | 1 | 2 | 2 | 5 | 5 | 12 |
| **TOTAL MULTIPLE DX** | 33 | 4.7 | 26 | 1 | 2 | 4 | 5 | 7 | 24 | 24 |
| **TOTAL** | | | | | | | | | | |
| 0–19 Years | 29 | 4.1 | 25 | 1 | 1 | 4 | 5 | 5 | 24 | 24 |
| 20–34 | 7 | 3.2 | 5 | 1 | 1 | 2 | 4 | 7 | 7 | 7 |
| 35–49 | 8 | 2.6 | 6 | 1 | 1 | 2 | 3 | 5 | 5 | 12 |
| 50–64 | 4 | 4.0 | 6 | 1 | 6 | 6 | 6 | 6 | 6 | 6 |
| 65+ | 4 | 4.8 | 11 | 2 | 4 | 4 | 6 | 10 | 10 | 10 |
| **GRAND TOTAL** | 52 | 3.9 | 19 | 1 | 1 | 3 | 5 | 6 | 7 | 24 |

## 20.3: MID & INNER EAR DXTIC PX. Formerly included in operation group(s) 538, 539.

| Type of Patients | Observed Patients | Avg. Stay | Vari-ance | 10th | 25th | 50th | 75th | 90th | 95th | 99th |
|---|---|---|---|---|---|---|---|---|---|---|
| **1. SINGLE DX** | | | | | | | | | | |
| 0–19 Years | 1 | 2.0 | 0 | 2 | 2 | 2 | 2 | 2 | 2 | 2 |
| 20–34 | 0 | | | | | | | | | |
| 35–49 | 0 | | | | | | | | | |
| 50–64 | 0 | | | | | | | | | |
| 65+ | 0 | | | | | | | | | |
| **2. MULTIPLE DX** | | | | | | | | | | |
| 0–19 Years | 7 | 3.2 | 6 | 1 | 3 | 3 | 3 | 7 | 7 | 14 |
| 20–34 | 1 | 6.0 | 0 | 6 | 6 | 6 | 6 | 6 | 6 | 6 |
| 35–49 | 2 | 14.0 | 0 | 14 | 14 | 14 | 14 | 14 | 14 | 14 |
| 50–64 | 0 | | | | | | | | | |
| 65+ | 4 | 12.2 | 168 | 6 | 6 | 8 | 8 | 40 | 40 | 40 |
| **TOTAL SINGLE DX** | 1 | 2.0 | 0 | 2 | 2 | 2 | 2 | 2 | 2 | 2 |
| **TOTAL MULTIPLE DX** | 14 | 5.3 | 39 | 1 | 3 | 3 | 7 | 14 | 14 | 40 |
| **TOTAL** | | | | | | | | | | |
| 0–19 Years | 8 | 3.2 | 6 | 1 | 3 | 3 | 3 | 7 | 7 | 14 |
| 20–34 | 1 | 6.0 | 0 | 6 | 6 | 6 | 6 | 6 | 6 | 6 |
| 35–49 | 2 | 14.0 | 0 | 14 | 14 | 14 | 14 | 14 | 14 | 14 |
| 50–64 | 0 | | | | | | | | | |
| 65+ | 4 | 12.2 | 168 | 6 | 6 | 8 | 8 | 40 | 40 | 40 |
| **GRAND TOTAL** | 15 | 5.2 | 38 | 1 | 3 | 3 | 6 | 14 | 14 | 40 |

Length of Stay by Diagnosis and Operation, United States, 2000

**United States, October 1998–September 1999 Data, by Operation**

## 20.4: MASTOIDECTOMY. Formerly included in operation group(s) 537.

| Type of Patients | Observed Patients | Avg. Stay | Variance | 10th | 25th | 50th | 75th | 90th | 95th | 99th |
|---|---|---|---|---|---|---|---|---|---|---|
| **1. SINGLE DX** | | | | | | | | | | |
| 0–19 Years | 67 | 1.7 | 3 | 1 | 1 | 1 | 1 | 6 | 6 | 7 |
| 20–34 | 27 | 1.5 | 2 | 1 | 1 | 1 | 2 | 3 | 3 | 12 |
| 35–49 | 39 | 1.6 | 2 | 1 | 1 | 1 | 2 | 4 | 4 | 6 |
| 50–64 | 18 | 1.3 | <1 | 1 | 1 | 1 | 1 | 1 | 3 | 5 |
| 65+ | 10 | 1.5 | 1 | 1 | 1 | 2 | 2 | 2 | 5 | 5 |
| **2. MULTIPLE DX** | | | | | | | | | | |
| 0–19 Years | 253 | 3.2 | 26 | 1 | 1 | 1 | 4 | 8 | 9 | 16 |
| 20–34 | 67 | 2.7 | 5 | 1 | 1 | 1 | 4 | 6 | 8 | 11 |
| 35–49 | 111 | 4.4 | 39 | 1 | 1 | 1 | 4 | 16 | 16 | 29 |
| 50–64 | 88 | 2.6 | 9 | 1 | 1 | 1 | 3 | 6 | 9 | 15 |
| 65+ | 137 | 6.4 | 79 | 1 | 1 | 2 | 7 | 15 | 21 | 37 |
| **TOTAL SINGLE DX** | 161 | 1.6 | 2 | 1 | 1 | 1 | 1 | 3 | 5 | 6 |
| **TOTAL MULTIPLE DX** | 656 | 3.9 | 34 | 1 | 1 | 1 | 4 | 9 | 15 | 29 |
| **TOTAL** | | | | | | | | | | |
| 0–19 Years | 320 | 3.0 | 22 | 1 | 1 | 1 | 4 | 7 | 9 | 16 |
| 20–34 | 94 | 2.2 | 4 | 1 | 1 | 1 | 3 | 5 | 6 | 11 |
| 35–49 | 150 | 3.9 | 33 | 1 | 1 | 1 | 4 | 16 | 16 | 29 |
| 50–64 | 106 | 2.4 | 8 | 1 | 1 | 1 | 2 | 6 | 8 | 15 |
| 65+ | 147 | 6.1 | 76 | 1 | 1 | 2 | 7 | 15 | 21 | 37 |
| **GRAND TOTAL** | 817 | 3.4 | 29 | 1 | 1 | 1 | 4 | 8 | 15 | 25 |

## 20.49: MASTOIDECTOMY NEC. Formerly included in operation group(s) 537.

| Type of Patients | Observed Patients | Avg. Stay | Variance | 10th | 25th | 50th | 75th | 90th | 95th | 99th |
|---|---|---|---|---|---|---|---|---|---|---|
| **1. SINGLE DX** | | | | | | | | | | |
| 0–19 Years | 26 | 2.0 | 4 | 1 | 1 | 1 | 1 | 6 | 6 | 7 |
| 20–34 | 10 | 1.2 | <1 | 1 | 1 | 1 | 1 | 2 | 3 | 4 |
| 35–49 | 16 | 1.5 | <1 | 1 | 1 | 1 | 2 | 3 | 4 | 4 |
| 50–64 | 5 | 1.3 | <1 | 1 | 1 | 1 | 1 | 3 | 3 | 3 |
| 65+ | 6 | 1.8 | 2 | 1 | 1 | 1 | 2 | 5 | 5 | 5 |
| **2. MULTIPLE DX** | | | | | | | | | | |
| 0–19 Years | 93 | 3.1 | 10 | 1 | 1 | 2 | 4 | 7 | 8 | 16 |
| 20–34 | 28 | 3.0 | 6 | 1 | 1 | 2 | 3 | 8 | 9 | 11 |
| 35–49 | 52 | 6.0 | 49 | 1 | 1 | 2 | 12 | 16 | 16 | 29 |
| 50–64 | 45 | 2.5 | 8 | 1 | 1 | 1 | 2 | 6 | 9 | 12 |
| 65+ | 53 | 8.5 | 80 | 1 | 1 | 4 | 15 | 16 | 31 | 37 |
| **TOTAL SINGLE DX** | 63 | 1.6 | 2 | 1 | 1 | 1 | 1 | 4 | 6 | 6 |
| **TOTAL MULTIPLE DX** | 271 | 4.5 | 33 | 1 | 1 | 2 | 5 | 15 | 16 | 29 |
| **TOTAL** | | | | | | | | | | |
| 0–19 Years | 119 | 2.9 | 9 | 1 | 1 | 1 | 4 | 7 | 8 | 16 |
| 20–34 | 38 | 2.1 | 4 | 1 | 1 | 1 | 3 | 5 | 8 | 9 |
| 35–49 | 68 | 5.1 | 42 | 1 | 1 | 1 | 7 | 16 | 16 | 29 |
| 50–64 | 50 | 2.4 | 7 | 1 | 1 | 1 | 2 | 6 | 9 | 12 |
| 65+ | 59 | 8.0 | 77 | 1 | 1 | 3 | 15 | 16 | 31 | 37 |
| **GRAND TOTAL** | 334 | 3.9 | 28 | 1 | 1 | 1 | 4 | 12 | 16 | 29 |

## 20.42: RADICAL MASTOIDECTOMY. Formerly included in operation group(s) 537.

| Type of Patients | Observed Patients | Avg. Stay | Variance | 10th | 25th | 50th | 75th | 90th | 95th | 99th |
|---|---|---|---|---|---|---|---|---|---|---|
| **1. SINGLE DX** | | | | | | | | | | |
| 0–19 Years | 35 | 1.1 | <1 | 1 | 1 | 1 | 1 | 1 | 1 | 4 |
| 20–34 | 15 | 1.7 | 3 | 1 | 1 | 1 | 1 | 2 | 3 | 12 |
| 35–49 | 17 | 1.8 | 3 | 1 | 1 | 1 | 1 | 2 | 6 | 9 |
| 50–64 | 10 | 1.0 | 0 | 1 | 1 | 1 | 1 | 1 | 1 | 1 |
| 65+ | 4 | 1.0 | 0 | 1 | 1 | 1 | 1 | 1 | 1 | 1 |
| **2. MULTIPLE DX** | | | | | | | | | | |
| 0–19 Years | 117 | 2.9 | 45 | 1 | 1 | 1 | 2 | 7 | 9 | 9 |
| 20–34 | 28 | 2.4 | 2 | 1 | 1 | 2 | 4 | 4 | 6 | 6 |
| 35–49 | 44 | 2.2 | 5 | 1 | 1 | 1 | 2 | 4 | 6 | 12 |
| 50–64 | 31 | 2.2 | 4 | 1 | 1 | 1 | 3 | 4 | 6 | 8 |
| 65+ | 58 | 5.2 | 122 | 1 | 1 | 1 | 4 | 17 | 25 | 79 |
| **TOTAL SINGLE DX** | 81 | 1.4 | 2 | 1 | 1 | 1 | 1 | 2 | 3 | 9 |
| **TOTAL MULTIPLE DX** | 278 | 3.0 | 42 | 1 | 1 | 1 | 3 | 6 | 9 | 30 |
| **TOTAL** | | | | | | | | | | |
| 0–19 Years | 152 | 2.5 | 37 | 1 | 1 | 1 | 2 | 6 | 9 | 9 |
| 20–34 | 43 | 2.1 | 3 | 1 | 1 | 1 | 3 | 4 | 5 | 12 |
| 35–49 | 61 | 2.1 | 5 | 1 | 1 | 1 | 2 | 4 | 6 | 12 |
| 50–64 | 41 | 1.9 | 3 | 1 | 1 | 1 | 2 | 4 | 8 | 8 |
| 65+ | 62 | 5.0 | 116 | 1 | 1 | 2 | 4 | 17 | 25 | 79 |
| **GRAND TOTAL** | 359 | 2.7 | 34 | 1 | 1 | 1 | 2 | 5 | 9 | 25 |

## 20.5: OTH MIDDLE EAR EXCISION. Formerly included in operation group(s) 538.

| Type of Patients | Observed Patients | Avg. Stay | Variance | 10th | 25th | 50th | 75th | 90th | 95th | 99th |
|---|---|---|---|---|---|---|---|---|---|---|
| **1. SINGLE DX** | | | | | | | | | | |
| 0–19 Years | 12 | 1.4 | <1 | 1 | 1 | 1 | 2 | 2 | 2 | 7 |
| 20–34 | 5 | 3.8 | 2 | 2 | 3 | 4 | 5 | 5 | 5 | 5 |
| 35–49 | 2 | 2.3 | 3 | 1 | 1 | 1 | 4 | 4 | 4 | 4 |
| 50–64 | 3 | 1.1 | <1 | 1 | 1 | 1 | 1 | 1 | 2 | 2 |
| 65+ | 0 | | | | | | | | | |
| **2. MULTIPLE DX** | | | | | | | | | | |
| 0–19 Years | 29 | 2.3 | 8 | 1 | 1 | 1 | 2 | 2 | 10 | 10 |
| 20–34 | 2 | 2.9 | 2 | 2 | 2 | 2 | 5 | 5 | 5 | 5 |
| 35–49 | 6 | 5.1 | 7 | 4 | 4 | 4 | 9 | 9 | 8 | 9 |
| 50–64 | 13 | 4.4 | 3 | 4 | 3 | 4 | 6 | 7 | 8 | 8 |
| 65+ | 12 | 3.1 | 18 | 1 | 2 | 2 | 2 | 3 | 14 | 26 |
| **TOTAL SINGLE DX** | 22 | 1.6 | 1 | 1 | 1 | 1 | 2 | 3 | 4 | 7 |
| **TOTAL MULTIPLE DX** | 62 | 2.8 | 10 | 1 | 1 | 1 | 3 | 9 | 10 | 10 |
| **TOTAL** | | | | | | | | | | |
| 0–19 Years | 41 | 2.1 | 7 | 1 | 1 | 1 | 2 | 3 | 10 | 10 |
| 20–34 | 7 | 3.5 | 2 | 2 | 2 | 4 | 5 | 5 | 5 | 5 |
| 35–49 | 8 | 4.4 | 7 | 4 | 4 | 4 | 4 | 9 | 9 | 12 |
| 50–64 | 16 | 2.8 | 4 | 1 | 1 | 3 | 4 | 6 | 7 | 8 |
| 65+ | 12 | 3.1 | 18 | 1 | 2 | 2 | 2 | 3 | 14 | 26 |
| **GRAND TOTAL** | 84 | 2.5 | 8 | 1 | 1 | 1 | 3 | 6 | 10 | 10 |

Length of Stay by Diagnosis and Operation, United States, 2000

# United States, October 1998–September 1999 Data, by Operation

## 20.6: FENESTRATION INNER EAR. Formerly included in operation group(s) 538.

| Type of Patients | Observed Patients | Avg. Stay | Variance | Percentiles | | | | | | |
|---|---|---|---|---|---|---|---|---|---|---|
| | | | | 10th | 25th | 50th | 75th | 90th | 95th | 99th |
| **1. SINGLE DX** | | | | | | | | | | |
| 0–19 Years | 0 | | | | | | | | | |
| 20–34 | 1 | 1.0 | 0 | 1 | 1 | 1 | 1 | 1 | 1 | 1 |
| 35–49 | 0 | | | | | | | | | |
| 50–64 | 1 | 4.0 | 0 | 4 | 4 | 4 | 4 | 4 | 4 | 4 |
| 65+ | 0 | | | | | | | | | |
| **2. MULTIPLE DX** | | | | | | | | | | |
| 0–19 Years | 0 | | | | | | | | | |
| 20–34 | 1 | 1.0 | 0 | 1 | 1 | 1 | 1 | 1 | 1 | 1 |
| 35–49 | 1 | 7.0 | 0 | 7 | 7 | 7 | 7 | 7 | 7 | 7 |
| 50–64 | 0 | | | | | | | | | |
| 65+ | 0 | | | | | | | | | |
| **TOTAL SINGLE DX** | 2 | 2.8 | 3 | 1 | 1 | 4 | 4 | 4 | 4 | 4 |
| **TOTAL MULTIPLE DX** | 2 | 2.8 | 10 | 1 | 1 | 7 | 7 | 7 | 7 | 7 |
| **TOTAL** | | | | | | | | | | |
| 0–19 Years | 0 | | | | | | | | | |
| 20–34 | 1 | 1.0 | 0 | 1 | 1 | 1 | 1 | 1 | 1 | 1 |
| 35–49 | 1 | 1.0 | 0 | 1 | 1 | 1 | 1 | 1 | 1 | 1 |
| 50–64 | 2 | 5.4 | 3 | 4 | 4 | 4 | 4 | 4 | 4 | 4 |
| 65+ | 0 | | | | | | | | | |
| **GRAND TOTAL** | 4 | 2.8 | 6 | 1 | 1 | 1 | 4 | 7 | 7 | 7 |

## 20.7: INC/EXC/DESTR INNER EAR. Formerly included in operation group(s) 538.

| Type of Patients | Observed Patients | Avg. Stay | Variance | Percentiles | | | | | | |
|---|---|---|---|---|---|---|---|---|---|---|
| | | | | 10th | 25th | 50th | 75th | 90th | 95th | 99th |
| **1. SINGLE DX** | | | | | | | | | | |
| 0–19 Years | 3 | 3.1 | 2 | 1 | 3 | 3 | 4 | 4 | 4 | 4 |
| 20–34 | 3 | 2.2 | 1 | 1 | 1 | 3 | 1 | 3 | 3 | 3 |
| 35–49 | 12 | 2.7 | 3 | 1 | 1 | 2 | 5 | 5 | 5 | 5 |
| 50–64 | 7 | 1.2 | <1 | 1 | 1 | 1 | 1 | 2 | 2 | 2 |
| 65+ | 5 | 2.5 | 1 | 2 | 2 | 2 | 4 | 4 | 4 | 4 |
| **2. MULTIPLE DX** | | | | | | | | | | |
| 0–19 Years | 5 | 2.2 | 6 | 1 | 1 | 1 | 2 | 4 | 11 | 11 |
| 20–34 | 5 | 1.6 | <1 | 1 | 1 | 2 | 2 | 2 | 3 | 3 |
| 35–49 | 23 | 2.3 | <1 | 1 | 2 | 2 | 3 | 3 | 3 | 3 |
| 50–64 | 35 | 2.1 | 1 | 1 | 1 | 2 | 3 | 4 | 4 | 7 |
| 65+ | 34 | 4.2 | 6 | 1 | 2 | 4 | 6 | 6 | 6 | 13 |
| **TOTAL SINGLE DX** | 30 | 2.0 | 2 | 1 | 1 | 1 | 3 | 5 | 5 | 5 |
| **TOTAL MULTIPLE DX** | 102 | 2.7 | 3 | 1 | 2 | 2 | 3 | 6 | 6 | 11 |
| **TOTAL** | | | | | | | | | | |
| 0–19 Years | 8 | 2.3 | 6 | 1 | 1 | 1 | 3 | 4 | 11 | 11 |
| 20–34 | 8 | 1.9 | <1 | 1 | 1 | 2 | 3 | 3 | 3 | 3 |
| 35–49 | 35 | 2.3 | <1 | 1 | 2 | 2 | 3 | 3 | 4 | 5 |
| 50–64 | 42 | 1.8 | 1 | 1 | 1 | 2 | 3 | 3 | 4 | 5 |
| 65+ | 39 | 4.1 | 6 | 1 | 2 | 4 | 6 | 6 | 6 | 13 |
| **GRAND TOTAL** | 132 | 2.6 | 3 | 1 | 1 | 2 | 3 | 5 | 6 | 7 |

## 20.8: EUSTACHIAN TUBE OPS. Formerly included in operation group(s) 538.

| Type of Patients | Observed Patients | Avg. Stay | Variance | Percentiles | | | | | | |
|---|---|---|---|---|---|---|---|---|---|---|
| | | | | 10th | 25th | 50th | 75th | 90th | 95th | 99th |
| **1. SINGLE DX** | | | | | | | | | | |
| 0–19 Years | 1 | 1.0 | 0 | 1 | 1 | 1 | 1 | 1 | 1 | 1 |
| 20–34 | 0 | | | | | | | | | |
| 35–49 | 1 | 3.0 | 0 | 3 | 3 | 3 | 3 | 3 | 3 | 3 |
| 50–64 | 0 | | | | | | | | | |
| 65+ | 0 | | | | | | | | | |
| **2. MULTIPLE DX** | | | | | | | | | | |
| 0–19 Years | 2 | 1.8 | <1 | 1 | 2 | 2 | 2 | 2 | 2 | 2 |
| 20–34 | 0 | | | | | | | | | |
| 35–49 | 0 | | | | | | | | | |
| 50–64 | 1 | 8.0 | 0 | 8 | 8 | 8 | 8 | 8 | 8 | 8 |
| 65+ | 0 | | | | | | | | | |
| **TOTAL SINGLE DX** | 2 | 2.2 | 1 | 1 | 1 | 3 | 3 | 3 | 3 | 3 |
| **TOTAL MULTIPLE DX** | 3 | 4.9 | 10 | 2 | 2 | 2 | 8 | 8 | 8 | 8 |
| **TOTAL** | | | | | | | | | | |
| 0–19 Years | 3 | 1.6 | <1 | 1 | 1 | 2 | 2 | 2 | 2 | 2 |
| 20–34 | 0 | | | | | | | | | |
| 35–49 | 1 | 3.0 | 0 | 3 | 3 | 3 | 3 | 3 | 3 | 3 |
| 50–64 | 1 | 8.0 | 0 | 8 | 8 | 8 | 8 | 8 | 8 | 8 |
| 65+ | 0 | | | | | | | | | |
| **GRAND TOTAL** | 5 | 4.2 | 9 | 1 | 2 | 3 | 8 | 8 | 8 | 8 |

## 20.9: OTHER ME & IE OPS. Formerly included in operation group(s) 538.

| Type of Patients | Observed Patients | Avg. Stay | Variance | Percentiles | | | | | | |
|---|---|---|---|---|---|---|---|---|---|---|
| | | | | 10th | 25th | 50th | 75th | 90th | 95th | 99th |
| **1. SINGLE DX** | | | | | | | | | | |
| 0–19 Years | 139 | 1.1 | <1 | 1 | 1 | 1 | 1 | 1 | 2 | 3 |
| 20–34 | 15 | 1.2 | <1 | 1 | 1 | 1 | 1 | 2 | 3 | 3 |
| 35–49 | 15 | 1.3 | <1 | 1 | 1 | 1 | 1 | 3 | 3 | 3 |
| 50–64 | 8 | 1.1 | <1 | 1 | 1 | 1 | 1 | 1 | 2 | 2 |
| 65+ | 14 | 1.1 | <1 | 1 | 1 | 1 | 1 | 1 | 1 | 2 |
| **2. MULTIPLE DX** | | | | | | | | | | |
| 0–19 Years | 91 | 1.8 | 10 | 1 | 1 | 1 | 1 | 3 | 5 | 8 |
| 20–34 | 16 | 1.4 | 3 | 1 | 1 | 1 | 1 | 3 | 5 | 13 |
| 35–49 | 42 | 2.8 | 5 | 1 | 2 | 2 | 4 | 5 | 8 | 11 |
| 50–64 | 35 | 2.6 | 3 | 1 | 1 | 2 | 4 | 5 | 5 | 6 |
| 65+ | 35 | 1.7 | 2 | 1 | 1 | 1 | 2 | 3 | 5 | 9 |
| **TOTAL SINGLE DX** | 191 | 1.1 | <1 | 1 | 1 | 1 | 1 | 1 | 2 | 3 |
| **TOTAL MULTIPLE DX** | 219 | 2.0 | 7 | 1 | 1 | 1 | 2 | 5 | 5 | 9 |
| **TOTAL** | | | | | | | | | | |
| 0–19 Years | 230 | 1.4 | 4 | 1 | 1 | 1 | 1 | 2 | 3 | 5 |
| 20–34 | 31 | 1.3 | 2 | 1 | 1 | 1 | 1 | 2 | 3 | 13 |
| 35–49 | 57 | 2.5 | 5 | 1 | 2 | 2 | 3 | 5 | 5 | 11 |
| 50–64 | 43 | 2.4 | 3 | 1 | 1 | 2 | 4 | 5 | 5 | 6 |
| 65+ | 49 | 1.6 | 2 | 1 | 1 | 1 | 1 | 3 | 5 | 9 |
| **GRAND TOTAL** | 410 | 1.6 | 4 | 1 | 1 | 1 | 1 | 3 | 5 | 8 |

Length of Stay by Diagnosis and Operation, United States, 2000

# United States, October 1998–September 1999 Data, by Operation

## 21.0: CONTROL OF EPISTAXIS. Formerly included in operation group(s) 543, 556.

| Type of Patients | Observed Patients | Avg. Stay | Variance | 10th | 25th | 50th | 75th | 90th | 95th | 99th |
|---|---|---|---|---|---|---|---|---|---|---|
| **1. SINGLE DX** | | | | | | | | | | |
| 0–19 Years | 24 | 2.7 | 9 | 1 | 1 | 2 | 3 | 10 | 11 | 11 |
| 20–34 | 58 | 2.4 | 1 | 1 | 1 | 3 | 3 | 4 | 4 | 6 |
| 35–49 | 95 | 2.1 | 1 | 1 | 1 | 2 | 3 | 4 | 5 | 5 |
| 50–64 | 98 | 2.6 | 2 | 1 | 1 | 2 | 3 | 5 | 6 | 6 |
| 65+ | 89 | 2.6 | 3 | 1 | 1 | 2 | 3 | 5 | 7 | 7 |
| **2. MULTIPLE DX** | | | | | | | | | | |
| 0–19 Years | 102 | 4.4 | 24 | 2 | 3 | 3 | 4 | 7 | 12 | 31 |
| 20–34 | 211 | 3.3 | 8 | 1 | 1 | 3 | 4 | 7 | 9 | 15 |
| 35–49 | 600 | 3.7 | 12 | 1 | 2 | 3 | 4 | 7 | 10 | 18 |
| 50–64 | 1,003 | 3.9 | 12 | 1 | 2 | 3 | 5 | 8 | 9 | 19 |
| 65+ | 2,549 | 4.3 | 16 | 1 | 2 | 3 | 5 | 9 | 12 | 21 |
| **TOTAL SINGLE DX** | 364 | 2.4 | 2 | 1 | 1 | 2 | 3 | 4 | 5 | 7 |
| **TOTAL MULTIPLE DX** | 4,465 | 4.1 | 15 | 1 | 2 | 3 | 5 | 8 | 10 | 20 |
| **TOTAL** | | | | | | | | | | |
| 0–19 Years | 126 | 4.2 | 23 | 2 | 2 | 3 | 4 | 7 | 12 | 30 |
| 20–34 | 269 | 3.1 | 6 | 1 | 1 | 3 | 4 | 6 | 7 | 13 |
| 35–49 | 695 | 3.5 | 11 | 1 | 2 | 3 | 4 | 7 | 10 | 17 |
| 50–64 | 1,101 | 3.8 | 12 | 1 | 2 | 3 | 5 | 8 | 9 | 19 |
| 65+ | 2,638 | 4.2 | 16 | 1 | 2 | 3 | 5 | 8 | 11 | 20 |
| **GRAND TOTAL** | 4,829 | 4.0 | 14 | 1 | 2 | 3 | 5 | 8 | 10 | 19 |

## 21.01: ANT NAS PACK FOR EPISTX. Formerly included in operation group(s) 556.

| Type of Patients | Observed Patients | Avg. Stay | Variance | 10th | 25th | 50th | 75th | 90th | 95th | 99th |
|---|---|---|---|---|---|---|---|---|---|---|
| **1. SINGLE DX** | | | | | | | | | | |
| 0–19 Years | 4 | 1.2 | <1 | 1 | 1 | 1 | 1 | 2 | 2 | 2 |
| 20–34 | 12 | 2.3 | 1 | 1 | 1 | 3 | 3 | 4 | 4 | 4 |
| 35–49 | 15 | 1.8 | <1 | 1 | 1 | 2 | 2 | 3 | 4 | 4 |
| 50–64 | 13 | 1.9 | <1 | 1 | 1 | 1 | 2 | 3 | 3 | 3 |
| 65+ | 22 | 1.7 | 1 | 1 | 2 | 2 | 2 | 3 | 4 | 5 |
| **2. MULTIPLE DX** | | | | | | | | | | |
| 0–19 Years | 45 | 4.1 | 20 | 2 | 3 | 3 | 3 | 7 | 12 | 31 |
| 20–34 | 76 | 2.5 | 6 | 1 | 1 | 2 | 3 | 5 | 7 | 12 |
| 35–49 | 190 | 4.0 | 13 | 1 | 2 | 3 | 4 | 10 | 12 | 16 |
| 50–64 | 285 | 4.1 | 18 | 1 | 2 | 3 | 5 | 8 | 13 | 19 |
| 65+ | 884 | 4.3 | 18 | 1 | 2 | 3 | 5 | 8 | 11 | 22 |
| **TOTAL SINGLE DX** | 66 | 1.8 | 1 | 1 | 1 | 1 | 2 | 3 | 4 | 5 |
| **TOTAL MULTIPLE DX** | 1,480 | 4.1 | 17 | 1 | 2 | 3 | 5 | 8 | 12 | 21 |
| **TOTAL** | | | | | | | | | | |
| 0–19 Years | 49 | 4.1 | 19 | 1 | 3 | 3 | 3 | 7 | 12 | 31 |
| 20–34 | 88 | 2.5 | 6 | 1 | 1 | 2 | 3 | 5 | 7 | 12 |
| 35–49 | 205 | 3.9 | 13 | 1 | 2 | 2 | 4 | 10 | 11 | 16 |
| 50–64 | 298 | 4.0 | 17 | 1 | 1 | 3 | 5 | 8 | 13 | 19 |
| 65+ | 906 | 4.2 | 17 | 1 | 2 | 3 | 5 | 7 | 11 | 22 |
| **GRAND TOTAL** | 1,546 | 4.0 | 16 | 1 | 2 | 3 | 5 | 8 | 11 | 21 |

## 21.02: POST NAS PACK FOR EPISTX. Formerly included in operation group(s) 543.

| Type of Patients | Observed Patients | Avg. Stay | Variance | 10th | 25th | 50th | 75th | 90th | 95th | 99th |
|---|---|---|---|---|---|---|---|---|---|---|
| **1. SINGLE DX** | | | | | | | | | | |
| 0–19 Years | 5 | 4.0 | 12 | 1 | 1 | 3 | 3 | 10 | 10 | 10 |
| 20–34 | 15 | 2.5 | 1 | 1 | 1 | 3 | 3 | 3 | 4 | 6 |
| 35–49 | 33 | 2.7 | 2 | 2 | 2 | 3 | 3 | 5 | 5 | 5 |
| 50–64 | 36 | 3.0 | 3 | 1 | 2 | 3 | 4 | 6 | 6 | 6 |
| 65+ | 30 | 2.3 | <1 | 1 | 2 | 2 | 3 | 3 | 5 | 5 |
| **2. MULTIPLE DX** | | | | | | | | | | |
| 0–19 Years | 9 | 2.3 | 3 | 1 | 1 | 2 | 3 | 5 | 6 | 7 |
| 20–34 | 53 | 3.5 | 6 | 1 | 2 | 3 | 5 | 7 | 7 | 17 |
| 35–49 | 181 | 3.8 | 10 | 1 | 2 | 3 | 5 | 6 | 7 | 21 |
| 50–64 | 319 | 3.7 | 7 | 1 | 2 | 3 | 4 | 6 | 8 | 12 |
| 65+ | 707 | 3.7 | 9 | 1 | 2 | 3 | 4 | 6 | 8 | 14 |
| **TOTAL SINGLE DX** | 119 | 2.6 | 2 | 1 | 2 | 3 | 3 | 5 | 5 | 6 |
| **TOTAL MULTIPLE DX** | 1,269 | 3.7 | 8 | 1 | 2 | 3 | 4 | 6 | 8 | 15 |
| **TOTAL** | | | | | | | | | | |
| 0–19 Years | 14 | 2.9 | 7 | 1 | 1 | 2 | 3 | 7 | 10 | 10 |
| 20–34 | 68 | 3.2 | 5 | 1 | 2 | 3 | 3 | 6 | 7 | 17 |
| 35–49 | 214 | 3.6 | 9 | 1 | 2 | 3 | 4 | 6 | 7 | 16 |
| 50–64 | 355 | 3.6 | 6 | 1 | 2 | 3 | 4 | 6 | 8 | 11 |
| 65+ | 737 | 3.6 | 8 | 1 | 2 | 3 | 4 | 6 | 8 | 14 |
| **GRAND TOTAL** | 1,388 | 3.6 | 8 | 1 | 2 | 3 | 4 | 6 | 8 | 14 |

## 21.03: CAUT TO CNTRL EPISTAXIS. Formerly included in operation group(s) 543.

| Type of Patients | Observed Patients | Avg. Stay | Variance | 10th | 25th | 50th | 75th | 90th | 95th | 99th |
|---|---|---|---|---|---|---|---|---|---|---|
| **1. SINGLE DX** | | | | | | | | | | |
| 0–19 Years | 13 | 2.5 | 8 | 1 | 1 | 1 | 2 | 8 | 11 | 11 |
| 20–34 | 23 | 2.3 | 2 | 1 | 1 | 2 | 4 | 4 | 5 | 6 |
| 35–49 | 32 | 1.7 | <1 | 1 | 1 | 1 | 2 | 3 | 3 | 6 |
| 50–64 | 27 | 2.2 | <1 | 1 | 1 | 2 | 2 | 3 | 3 | 5 |
| 65+ | 27 | 3.6 | 6 | 1 | 2 | 3 | 7 | 7 | 7 | 7 |
| **2. MULTIPLE DX** | | | | | | | | | | |
| 0–19 Years | 39 | 5.5 | 37 | 2 | 2 | 4 | 5 | 8 | 21 | 30 |
| 20–34 | 58 | 3.7 | 9 | 1 | 2 | 3 | 5 | 7 | 9 | 15 |
| 35–49 | 162 | 3.4 | 12 | 1 | 2 | 3 | 4 | 7 | 8 | 21 |
| 50–64 | 291 | 3.9 | 15 | 1 | 2 | 3 | 5 | 8 | 9 | 15 |
| 65+ | 753 | 4.7 | 21 | 1 | 3 | 3 | 6 | 10 | 15 | 21 |
| **TOTAL SINGLE DX** | 122 | 2.4 | 4 | 1 | 1 | 2 | 3 | 5 | 7 | 11 |
| **TOTAL MULTIPLE DX** | 1,303 | 4.3 | 18 | 1 | 2 | 3 | 5 | 9 | 13 | 21 |
| **TOTAL** | | | | | | | | | | |
| 0–19 Years | 52 | 4.7 | 31 | 1 | 2 | 3 | 5 | 8 | 17 | 30 |
| 20–34 | 81 | 3.3 | 8 | 1 | 1 | 3 | 4 | 7 | 9 | 15 |
| 35–49 | 194 | 3.1 | 10 | 1 | 2 | 2 | 5 | 8 | 9 | 18 |
| 50–64 | 318 | 3.8 | 14 | 1 | 2 | 3 | 5 | 8 | 9 | 15 |
| 65+ | 780 | 4.7 | 20 | 1 | 2 | 3 | 6 | 10 | 15 | 21 |
| **GRAND TOTAL** | 1,425 | 4.2 | 17 | 1 | 2 | 3 | 5 | 9 | 12 | 20 |

Length of Stay by Diagnosis and Operation, United States, 2000

# United States, October 1998–September 1999 Data, by Operation

## 21.1: INCISION OF NOSE. Formerly included in operation group(s) 542.

| Type of Patients | Observed Patients | Avg. Stay | Variance | 10th | 25th | 50th | 75th | 90th | 95th | 99th |
|---|---|---|---|---|---|---|---|---|---|---|
| **1. SINGLE DX** | | | | | | | | | | |
| 0–19 Years | 7 | 1.8 | <1 | 1 | 1 | 2 | 2 | 2 | 2 | 2 |
| 20–34 | 4 | 1.6 | <1 | 1 | 1 | 1 | 2 | 3 | 3 | 3 |
| 35–49 | 4 | 2.2 | <1 | 1 | 1 | 3 | 3 | 3 | 3 | 3 |
| 50–64 | 2 | 1.6 | <1 | 1 | 1 | 2 | 2 | 2 | 2 | 2 |
| 65+ | 0 | | | | | | | | | |
| **2. MULTIPLE DX** | | | | | | | | | | |
| 0–19 Years | 20 | 2.5 | 2 | 1 | 2 | 2 | 3 | 5 | 5 | 9 |
| 20–34 | 6 | 4.1 | 4 | 3 | 3 | 3 | 6 | 6 | 10 | 10 |
| 35–49 | 21 | 3.8 | 15 | 2 | 2 | 3 | 3 | 9 | 9 | 23 |
| 50–64 | 12 | 8.4 | 297 | 1 | 1 | 2 | 5 | 36 | 67 | 67 |
| 65+ | 13 | 4.0 | 3 | 2 | 2 | 4 | 6 | 7 | 7 | 7 |
| **TOTAL SINGLE DX** | 17 | 1.9 | <1 | 1 | 1 | 2 | 3 | 3 | 3 | 3 |
| **TOTAL MULTIPLE DX** | 72 | 4.0 | 40 | 1 | 2 | 3 | 4 | 6 | 9 | 36 |
| **TOTAL** | | | | | | | | | | |
| 0–19 Years | 27 | 2.3 | 2 | 1 | 2 | 2 | 4 | 5 | 5 | 9 |
| 20–34 | 10 | 3.7 | 4 | 2 | 3 | 3 | 6 | 6 | 6 | 10 |
| 35–49 | 25 | 3.3 | 11 | 1 | 2 | 3 | 3 | 5 | 9 | 23 |
| 50–64 | 14 | 7.8 | 273 | 1 | 1 | 2 | 4 | 36 | 67 | 67 |
| 65+ | 13 | 4.0 | 3 | 2 | 2 | 4 | 6 | 7 | 7 | 7 |
| **GRAND TOTAL** | 89 | 3.7 | 34 | 1 | 2 | 3 | 4 | 6 | 7 | 36 |

## 21.2: NASAL DIAGNOSTIC PX. Formerly included in operation group(s) 542, 556.

| Type of Patients | Observed Patients | Avg. Stay | Variance | 10th | 25th | 50th | 75th | 90th | 95th | 99th |
|---|---|---|---|---|---|---|---|---|---|---|
| **1. SINGLE DX** | | | | | | | | | | |
| 0–19 Years | 9 | 2.8 | 11 | 1 | 1 | 1 | 2 | 2 | 10 | 10 |
| 20–34 | 2 | 3.5 | <1 | 2 | 2 | 4 | 4 | 4 | 4 | 4 |
| 35–49 | 3 | 1.1 | <1 | 1 | 1 | 1 | 1 | 2 | 2 | 2 |
| 50–64 | 0 | | | | | | | | | |
| 65+ | 1 | 2.0 | 0 | 2 | 2 | 2 | 2 | 2 | 2 | 2 |
| **2. MULTIPLE DX** | | | | | | | | | | |
| 0–19 Years | 48 | 5.6 | 89 | 1 | 2 | 3 | 6 | 10 | 12 | 62 |
| 20–34 | 15 | 7.3 | 150 | 1 | 1 | 3 | 4 | 42 | 42 | 42 |
| 35–49 | 37 | 5.4 | 21 | 2 | 2 | 4 | 6 | 10 | 12 | 25 |
| 50–64 | 47 | 5.6 | 18 | 2 | 4 | 5 | 6 | 9 | 11 | 24 |
| 65+ | 107 | 7.0 | 34 | 2 | 3 | 5 | 9 | 13 | 18 | 27 |
| **TOTAL SINGLE DX** | 15 | 2.4 | 6 | 1 | 1 | 2 | 2 | 4 | 10 | 10 |
| **TOTAL MULTIPLE DX** | 254 | 6.2 | 48 | 1 | 2 | 4 | 7 | 13 | 17 | 42 |
| **TOTAL** | | | | | | | | | | |
| 0–19 Years | 57 | 5.1 | 75 | 1 | 2 | 2 | 6 | 10 | 12 | 62 |
| 20–34 | 17 | 7.0 | 139 | 1 | 2 | 3 | 4 | 12 | 42 | 42 |
| 35–49 | 40 | 5.1 | 21 | 1 | 2 | 3 | 6 | 10 | 12 | 25 |
| 50–64 | 47 | 5.6 | 18 | 2 | 4 | 5 | 6 | 9 | 11 | 24 |
| 65+ | 108 | 6.9 | 34 | 2 | 3 | 5 | 9 | 13 | 18 | 27 |
| **GRAND TOTAL** | 269 | 6.0 | 46 | 1 | 2 | 4 | 7 | 13 | 17 | 42 |

## 21.3: NASAL LESION DESTR/EXC. Formerly included in operation group(s) 542.

| Type of Patients | Observed Patients | Avg. Stay | Variance | 10th | 25th | 50th | 75th | 90th | 95th | 99th |
|---|---|---|---|---|---|---|---|---|---|---|
| **1. SINGLE DX** | | | | | | | | | | |
| 0–19 Years | 19 | 1.8 | 1 | 1 | 1 | 1 | 1 | 4 | 4 | 4 |
| 20–34 | 4 | 3.1 | 11 | 1 | 2 | 2 | 2 | 11 | 11 | 11 |
| 35–49 | 2 | 1.0 | 0 | 1 | 1 | 1 | 1 | 1 | 1 | 1 |
| 50–64 | 0 | | | | | | | | | |
| 65+ | 9 | 2.1 | 2 | 1 | 1 | 2 | 3 | 3 | 6 | 6 |
| **2. MULTIPLE DX** | | | | | | | | | | |
| 0–19 Years | 36 | 3.1 | 15 | 1 | 1 | 2 | 2 | 7 | 7 | 23 |
| 20–34 | 22 | 3.6 | 6 | 1 | 1 | 2 | 6 | 7 | 7 | 7 |
| 35–49 | 31 | 3.4 | 17 | 1 | 2 | 4 | 4 | 8 | 8 | 32 |
| 50–64 | 33 | 4.5 | 14 | 1 | 2 | 4 | 6 | 7 | 16 | 19 |
| 65+ | 94 | 4.5 | 18 | 1 | 4 | 6 | 6 | 10 | 11 | 19 |
| **TOTAL SINGLE DX** | 34 | 1.9 | 2 | 1 | 1 | 2 | 2 | 4 | 4 | 11 |
| **TOTAL MULTIPLE DX** | 216 | 3.8 | 16 | 1 | 2 | 2 | 5 | 7 | 10 | 20 |
| **TOTAL** | | | | | | | | | | |
| 0–19 Years | 55 | 2.8 | 13 | 1 | 1 | 2 | 2 | 6 | 7 | 23 |
| 20–34 | 26 | 3.5 | 6 | 2 | 2 | 6 | 6 | 7 | 7 | 11 |
| 35–49 | 33 | 3.3 | 16 | 1 | 1 | 2 | 4 | 8 | 8 | 32 |
| 50–64 | 33 | 4.5 | 14 | 1 | 2 | 4 | 6 | 7 | 16 | 19 |
| 65+ | 103 | 4.3 | 17 | 1 | 3 | 6 | 6 | 10 | 11 | 19 |
| **GRAND TOTAL** | 250 | 3.6 | 15 | 1 | 1 | 2 | 5 | 7 | 10 | 19 |

## 21.4: RESECTION OF NOSE. Formerly included in operation group(s) 542.

| Type of Patients | Observed Patients | Avg. Stay | Variance | 10th | 25th | 50th | 75th | 90th | 95th | 99th |
|---|---|---|---|---|---|---|---|---|---|---|
| **1. SINGLE DX** | | | | | | | | | | |
| 0–19 Years | 0 | | | | | | | | | |
| 20–34 | 0 | | | | | | | | | |
| 35–49 | 1 | 3.0 | 0 | 3 | 3 | 3 | 3 | 3 | 3 | 3 |
| 50–64 | 0 | | | | | | | | | |
| 65+ | 1 | 1.0 | 0 | 1 | 1 | 1 | 1 | 1 | 1 | 1 |
| **2. MULTIPLE DX** | | | | | | | | | | |
| 0–19 Years | 0 | | | | | | | | | |
| 20–34 | 0 | | | | | | | | | |
| 35–49 | 1 | 1.0 | 0 | 1 | 1 | 1 | 1 | 1 | 1 | 1 |
| 50–64 | 3 | 1.6 | <1 | 1 | 1 | 2 | 2 | 2 | 2 | 2 |
| 65+ | 24 | 5.7 | 48 | 1 | 1 | 3 | 6 | 15 | 16 | 31 |
| **TOTAL SINGLE DX** | 2 | 2.0 | 2 | 1 | 1 | 3 | 3 | 3 | 3 | 3 |
| **TOTAL MULTIPLE DX** | 28 | 5.4 | 46 | 1 | 1 | 3 | 6 | 14 | 16 | 31 |
| **TOTAL** | | | | | | | | | | |
| 0–19 Years | 0 | | | | | | | | | |
| 20–34 | 0 | | | | | | | | | |
| 35–49 | 2 | 1.7 | 1 | 1 | 1 | 1 | 3 | 3 | 3 | 3 |
| 50–64 | 3 | 1.6 | <1 | 1 | 1 | 2 | 3 | 3 | 3 | 3 |
| 65+ | 25 | 5.6 | 48 | 1 | 1 | 3 | 6 | 15 | 16 | 31 |
| **GRAND TOTAL** | 30 | 5.3 | 45 | 1 | 1 | 3 | 6 | 14 | 16 | 31 |

Length of Stay by Diagnosis and Operation, United States, 2000

# United States, October 1998–September 1999 Data, by Operation

## 21.5: SUBMUC NAS SEPTUM RESECT. Formerly included in operation group(s) 540.

| Type of Patients | Observed Patients | Avg. Stay | Variance | 10th | 25th | 50th | 75th | 90th | 95th | 99th |
|---|---|---|---|---|---|---|---|---|---|---|
| **1. SINGLE DX** | | | | | | | | | | |
| 0–19 Years | 3 | 1.6 | <1 | 1 | 1 | 2 | 2 | 2 | 2 | 2 |
| 20–34 | 2 | 1.2 | <1 | 1 | 1 | 1 | 1 | 2 | 2 | 2 |
| 35–49 | 5 | 1.2 | <1 | 1 | 1 | 1 | 1 | 2 | 2 | 2 |
| 50–64 | 2 | 1.4 | <1 | 1 | 1 | 1 | 1 | 3 | 3 | 3 |
| 65+ | 1 | 2.0 | 0 | 2 | 2 | 2 | 2 | 2 | 2 | 2 |
| **2. MULTIPLE DX** | | | | | | | | | | |
| 0–19 Years | 30 | 1.5 | 3 | 1 | 1 | 1 | 1 | 2 | 3 | >99 |
| 20–34 | 49 | 2.8 | 18 | 1 | 1 | 1 | 2 | 9 | 9 | 23 |
| 35–49 | 108 | 1.6 | 2 | 1 | 1 | 1 | 2 | 2 | 3 | 9 |
| 50–64 | 76 | 1.9 | 4 | 1 | 1 | 1 | 2 | 4 | 8 | 8 |
| 65+ | 44 | 2.5 | 8 | 2 | 1 | 1 | 3 | 5 | 9 | 15 |
| **TOTAL SINGLE DX** | 13 | 1.4 | <1 | 1 | 1 | 1 | 2 | 2 | 2 | 3 |
| **TOTAL MULTIPLE DX** | 307 | 1.9 | 6 | 1 | 1 | 1 | 2 | 3 | 7 | 15 |
| **TOTAL** | | | | | | | | | | |
| 0–19 Years | 33 | 1.5 | 3 | 1 | 1 | 1 | 2 | 2 | 3 | >99 |
| 20–34 | 51 | 2.8 | 17 | 1 | 1 | 1 | 2 | 9 | 9 | 23 |
| 35–49 | 113 | 1.6 | 2 | 1 | 1 | 1 | 2 | 2 | 3 | 9 |
| 50–64 | 78 | 1.9 | 4 | 1 | 1 | 1 | 2 | 4 | 8 | 8 |
| 65+ | 45 | 2.5 | 8 | 1 | 1 | 1 | 3 | 5 | 9 | 15 |
| **GRAND TOTAL** | 320 | 1.9 | 6 | 1 | 1 | 1 | 2 | 3 | 7 | 15 |

## 21.6: TURBINECTOMY. Formerly included in operation group(s) 542.

| Type of Patients | Observed Patients | Avg. Stay | Variance | 10th | 25th | 50th | 75th | 90th | 95th | 99th |
|---|---|---|---|---|---|---|---|---|---|---|
| **1. SINGLE DX** | | | | | | | | | | |
| 0–19 Years | 5 | 2.1 | 2 | 1 | 1 | 2 | 4 | 4 | 4 | 4 |
| 20–34 | 3 | 1.4 | 1 | 1 | 1 | 1 | 1 | 4 | 4 | 4 |
| 35–49 | 1 | 1.0 | 0 | 1 | 1 | 1 | 1 | 1 | 1 | 1 |
| 50–64 | 5 | 1.7 | 2 | 1 | 1 | 1 | 3 | 3 | 4 | 5 |
| 65+ | 0 | | | | | | | | | |
| **2. MULTIPLE DX** | | | | | | | | | | |
| 0–19 Years | 41 | 3.1 | 7 | 1 | 1 | 2 | 4 | 7 | 9 | 17 |
| 20–34 | 19 | 2.0 | 2 | 1 | 1 | 1 | 3 | 4 | 4 | 4 |
| 35–49 | 34 | 5.4 | 137 | 1 | 2 | 3 | 4 | 9 | 50 | 50 |
| 50–64 | 37 | 3.3 | 7 | 1 | 1 | 1 | 4 | 6 | 7 | 16 |
| 65+ | 21 | 2.2 | 8 | 1 | 1 | 1 | 2 | 5 | 7 | 16 |
| **TOTAL SINGLE DX** | 14 | 1.7 | 2 | 1 | 1 | 1 | 3 | 4 | 4 | 5 |
| **TOTAL MULTIPLE DX** | 152 | 3.2 | 33 | 1 | 1 | 2 | 4 | 5 | 9 | 50 |
| **TOTAL** | | | | | | | | | | |
| 0–19 Years | 46 | 3.0 | 7 | 1 | 1 | 2 | 4 | 7 | 9 | 17 |
| 20–34 | 22 | 1.9 | 2 | 1 | 1 | 1 | 3 | 4 | 4 | 4 |
| 35–49 | 35 | 5.3 | 135 | 1 | 1 | 3 | 4 | 5 | 50 | 50 |
| 50–64 | 42 | 3.0 | 6 | 1 | 1 | 3 | 4 | 5 | 5 | 16 |
| 65+ | 21 | 2.2 | 8 | 1 | 1 | 1 | 2 | 5 | 7 | 16 |
| **GRAND TOTAL** | 166 | 3.1 | 31 | 1 | 1 | 2 | 4 | 5 | 8 | 50 |

## 21.7: NASAL FRACTURE REDUCTION. Formerly included in operation group(s) 543.

| Type of Patients | Observed Patients | Avg. Stay | Variance | 10th | 25th | 50th | 75th | 90th | 95th | 99th |
|---|---|---|---|---|---|---|---|---|---|---|
| **1. SINGLE DX** | | | | | | | | | | |
| 0–19 Years | 20 | 1.1 | <1 | 1 | 1 | 1 | 1 | 1 | 1 | 5 |
| 20–34 | 15 | 1.6 | 1 | 1 | 1 | 1 | 2 | 2 | 2 | 9 |
| 35–49 | 5 | 1.8 | 1 | 1 | 1 | 1 | 3 | 3 | 3 | 3 |
| 50–64 | 2 | 6.2 | 4 | 2 | 7 | 7 | 7 | 7 | 7 | 7 |
| 65+ | 3 | 1.2 | <1 | 1 | 1 | 1 | 1 | 2 | 2 | 2 |
| **2. MULTIPLE DX** | | | | | | | | | | |
| 0–19 Years | 119 | 4.1 | 17 | 1 | 2 | 3 | 4 | 9 | 18 | 18 |
| 20–34 | 136 | 3.8 | 13 | 1 | 1 | 3 | 5 | 8 | 8 | 14 |
| 35–49 | 111 | 3.5 | 11 | 1 | 1 | 2 | 4 | 8 | 9 | 15 |
| 50–64 | 65 | 3.6 | 9 | 1 | 1 | 3 | 5 | 7 | 10 | 13 |
| 65+ | 65 | 4.8 | 12 | 1 | 2 | 4 | 6 | 9 | 10 | 15 |
| **TOTAL SINGLE DX** | 45 | 1.5 | 2 | 1 | 1 | 1 | 1 | 2 | 3 | 7 |
| **TOTAL MULTIPLE DX** | 496 | 3.9 | 13 | 1 | 1 | 3 | 5 | 9 | 10 | 18 |
| **TOTAL** | | | | | | | | | | |
| 0–19 Years | 139 | 3.7 | 16 | 1 | 1 | 2 | 4 | 9 | 12 | 18 |
| 20–34 | 151 | 3.6 | 12 | 1 | 1 | 2 | 5 | 8 | 8 | 14 |
| 35–49 | 116 | 3.5 | 11 | 1 | 1 | 3 | 4 | 8 | 9 | 15 |
| 50–64 | 67 | 3.7 | 9 | 1 | 1 | 3 | 6 | 7 | 10 | 13 |
| 65+ | 68 | 4.6 | 12 | 1 | 2 | 4 | 6 | 9 | 10 | 15 |
| **GRAND TOTAL** | 541 | 3.7 | 13 | 1 | 1 | 2 | 5 | 8 | 9 | 18 |

## 21.71: CLSD REDUCTION NASAL FX. Formerly included in operation group(s) 543.

| Type of Patients | Observed Patients | Avg. Stay | Variance | 10th | 25th | 50th | 75th | 90th | 95th | 99th |
|---|---|---|---|---|---|---|---|---|---|---|
| **1. SINGLE DX** | | | | | | | | | | |
| 0–19 Years | 16 | 1.1 | <1 | 1 | 1 | 1 | 1 | 1 | 1 | 5 |
| 20–34 | 11 | 1.6 | <1 | 1 | 1 | 1 | 2 | 2 | 2 | 6 |
| 35–49 | 1 | 1.0 | 0 | 1 | 1 | 1 | 1 | 1 | 1 | 1 |
| 50–64 | 0 | | | | | | | | | |
| 65+ | 2 | 1.0 | 0 | 1 | 1 | 1 | 1 | 1 | 1 | 1 |
| **2. MULTIPLE DX** | | | | | | | | | | |
| 0–19 Years | 75 | 4.6 | 23 | 1 | 1 | 3 | 5 | 9 | 18 | 18 |
| 20–34 | 64 | 3.5 | 22 | 1 | 1 | 2 | 4 | 8 | 10 | 19 |
| 35–49 | 59 | 3.5 | 12 | 1 | 2 | 2 | 4 | 9 | 10 | 15 |
| 50–64 | 31 | 5.2 | 13 | 2 | 2 | 4 | 7 | 12 | 13 | 13 |
| 65+ | 42 | 5.2 | 16 | 1 | 2 | 4 | 9 | 10 | 12 | 13 |
| **TOTAL SINGLE DX** | 30 | 1.3 | <1 | 1 | 1 | 1 | 1 | 2 | 2 | 5 |
| **TOTAL MULTIPLE DX** | 271 | 4.2 | 19 | 1 | 1 | 3 | 5 | 9 | 14 | 18 |
| **TOTAL** | | | | | | | | | | |
| 0–19 Years | 91 | 3.9 | 20 | 1 | 1 | 2 | 4 | 9 | 18 | 18 |
| 20–34 | 75 | 3.1 | 18 | 1 | 1 | 2 | 4 | 6 | 9 | 19 |
| 35–49 | 60 | 3.5 | 12 | 1 | 2 | 2 | 4 | 9 | 10 | 15 |
| 50–64 | 31 | 5.2 | 13 | 2 | 2 | 4 | 7 | 12 | 13 | 13 |
| 65+ | 44 | 5.0 | 16 | 1 | 1 | 4 | 9 | 9 | 12 | 15 |
| **GRAND TOTAL** | 301 | 3.8 | 17 | 1 | 1 | 2 | 4 | 9 | 13 | 18 |

Length of Stay by Diagnosis and Operation

# United States, October 1998–September 1999 Data, by Operation

## 21.88: SEPTOPLASTY NEC. Formerly included in operation group(s) 541.

| Type of Patients | Observed Patients | Avg. Stay | Variance | 10th | 25th | 50th | 75th | 90th | 95th | 99th |
|---|---|---|---|---|---|---|---|---|---|---|
| **1. SINGLE DX** | | | | | | | | | | |
| 0–19 Years | 11 | 1.4 | <1 | 1 | 1 | 1 | 2 | 2 | 2 | 6 |
| 20–34 | 6 | 1.5 | <1 | 1 | 1 | 1 | 2 | 2 | 2 | 4 |
| 35–49 | 5 | 1.5 | <1 | 1 | 1 | 1 | 1 | 2 | 4 | 4 |
| 50–64 | 8 | 2.0 | 4 | 1 | 1 | 2 | 2 | 4 | 4 | 8 |
| 65+ | 4 | 1.4 | <1 | 1 | 1 | 1 | 2 | 2 | 2 | 2 |
| **2. MULTIPLE DX** | | | | | | | | | | |
| 0–19 Years | 85 | 2.1 | 11 | 1 | 1 | 1 | 2 | 3 | 4 | 29 |
| 20–34 | 145 | 2.0 | 3 | 1 | 1 | 1 | 2 | 4 | 5 | 10 |
| 35–49 | 229 | 1.8 | 2 | 1 | 1 | 1 | 2 | 3 | 5 | 10 |
| 50–64 | 176 | 2.6 | 6 | 1 | 2 | 2 | 3 | 5 | 7 | 18 |
| 65+ | 139 | 2.6 | 6 | 1 | 2 | 2 | 3 | 4 | 7 | 12 |
| **TOTAL SINGLE DX** | 34 | 1.6 | 1 | 1 | 1 | 1 | 2 | 2 | 4 | 8 |
| **TOTAL MULTIPLE DX** | 774 | 2.1 | 5 | 1 | 1 | 1 | 2 | 4 | 6 | 12 |
| **TOTAL** | | | | | | | | | | |
| 0–19 Years | 96 | 2.0 | 10 | 1 | 1 | 1 | 2 | 3 | 4 | 29 |
| 20–34 | 151 | 2.0 | 3 | 1 | 1 | 1 | 2 | 3 | 5 | 10 |
| 35–49 | 234 | 1.7 | 2 | 1 | 1 | 1 | 2 | 3 | 5 | 10 |
| 50–64 | 184 | 2.6 | 6 | 1 | 2 | 2 | 3 | 5 | 7 | 18 |
| 65+ | 143 | 2.6 | 6 | 1 | 2 | 2 | 3 | 4 | 7 | 12 |
| **GRAND TOTAL** | 808 | 2.1 | 5 | 1 | 1 | 1 | 2 | 4 | 6 | 10 |

## 21.9: OTHER NASAL OPERATIONS. Formerly included in operation group(s) 543.

| Type of Patients | Observed Patients | Avg. Stay | Variance | 10th | 25th | 50th | 75th | 90th | 95th | 99th |
|---|---|---|---|---|---|---|---|---|---|---|
| **1. SINGLE DX** | | | | | | | | | | |
| 0–19 Years | 9 | 1.8 | 2 | 1 | 1 | 1 | 2 | 3 | 3 | 8 |
| 20–34 | 0 | | | | | | | | | |
| 35–49 | 0 | | | | | | | | | |
| 50–64 | 0 | | | | | | | | | |
| 65+ | | | | | | | | | | |
| **2. MULTIPLE DX** | | | | | | | | | | |
| 0–19 Years | 28 | 10.3 | 163 | 1 | 1 | 3 | 11 | 34 | 34 | 34 |
| 20–34 | 3 | 1.3 | <1 | 1 | 1 | 1 | 3 | 3 | 3 | 3 |
| 35–49 | 4 | 2.5 | <1 | 1 | 1 | 3 | 3 | 3 | 3 | 3 |
| 50–64 | 3 | 1.5 | <1 | 1 | 1 | 1 | 2 | 2 | 3 | 3 |
| 65+ | 1 | 3.0 | 0 | 3 | 3 | 3 | 3 | 3 | 3 | 3 |
| **TOTAL SINGLE DX** | 9 | 1.8 | 2 | 1 | 1 | 1 | 2 | 3 | 3 | 8 |
| **TOTAL MULTIPLE DX** | 39 | 6.6 | 108 | 1 | 1 | 3 | 4 | 34 | 34 | 34 |
| **TOTAL** | | | | | | | | | | |
| 0–19 Years | 37 | 7.8 | 130 | 1 | 1 | 3 | 6 | 34 | 34 | 34 |
| 20–34 | 3 | 1.3 | <1 | 1 | 1 | 1 | 2 | 2 | 2 | 2 |
| 35–49 | 4 | 2.5 | <1 | 1 | 1 | 3 | 3 | 3 | 3 | 3 |
| 50–64 | 3 | 1.5 | <1 | 1 | 1 | 1 | 3 | 3 | 3 | 3 |
| 65+ | 1 | 3.0 | 0 | 3 | 3 | 3 | 3 | 3 | 3 | 3 |
| **GRAND TOTAL** | 48 | 5.7 | 92 | 1 | 1 | 2 | 3 | 21 | 34 | 34 |

## 21.8: NASAL REP & PLASTIC OPS. Formerly included in operation group(s) 541.

| Type of Patients | Observed Patients | Avg. Stay | Variance | 10th | 25th | 50th | 75th | 90th | 95th | 99th |
|---|---|---|---|---|---|---|---|---|---|---|
| **1. SINGLE DX** | | | | | | | | | | |
| 0–19 Years | 105 | 2.0 | 11 | 1 | 1 | 1 | 2 | 3 | 4 | 30 |
| 20–34 | 34 | 1.6 | <1 | 1 | 1 | 2 | 2 | 2 | 4 | 4 |
| 35–49 | 18 | 1.6 | <1 | 1 | 1 | 2 | 2 | 2 | 3 | 5 |
| 50–64 | 14 | 1.8 | <1 | 1 | 1 | 2 | 2 | 2 | 2 | 8 |
| 65+ | 16 | 1.4 | <1 | 1 | 1 | 1 | 2 | 2 | 2 | 4 |
| **2. MULTIPLE DX** | | | | | | | | | | |
| 0–19 Years | 386 | 2.0 | 6 | 1 | 1 | 1 | 2 | 3 | 6 | 13 |
| 20–34 | 322 | 2.1 | 3 | 1 | 1 | 2 | 2 | 4 | 6 | 9 |
| 35–49 | 405 | 2.1 | 5 | 1 | 1 | 2 | 2 | 5 | 6 | 10 |
| 50–64 | 282 | 3.2 | 54 | 2 | 2 | 3 | 3 | 5 | 7 | 19 |
| 65+ | 407 | 3.1 | 10 | 1 | 1 | 4 | 4 | 6 | 9 | 16 |
| **TOTAL SINGLE DX** | 187 | 1.8 | 6 | 1 | 1 | 1 | 2 | 3 | 4 | 12 |
| **TOTAL MULTIPLE DX** | 1,802 | 2.4 | 14 | 1 | 1 | 1 | 3 | 5 | 6 | 14 |
| **TOTAL** | | | | | | | | | | |
| 0–19 Years | 491 | 2.0 | 8 | 1 | 1 | 1 | 2 | 3 | 5 | 14 |
| 20–34 | 356 | 2.0 | 3 | 1 | 1 | 1 | 2 | 4 | 5 | 9 |
| 35–49 | 423 | 2.1 | 5 | 1 | 1 | 2 | 2 | 4 | 6 | 10 |
| 50–64 | 296 | 3.1 | 50 | 1 | 2 | 2 | 3 | 5 | 7 | 18 |
| 65+ | 423 | 3.1 | 9 | 1 | 1 | 2 | 4 | 6 | 9 | 16 |
| **GRAND TOTAL** | 1,989 | 2.3 | 13 | 1 | 1 | 1 | 2 | 4 | 6 | 14 |

## 21.81: NASAL LACERATION SUTURE. Formerly included in operation group(s) 541.

| Type of Patients | Observed Patients | Avg. Stay | Variance | 10th | 25th | 50th | 75th | 90th | 95th | 99th |
|---|---|---|---|---|---|---|---|---|---|---|
| **1. SINGLE DX** | | | | | | | | | | |
| 0–19 Years | 18 | 2.2 | 2 | 1 | 1 | 2 | 4 | 4 | 4 | 4 |
| 20–34 | 1 | 2.0 | 0 | 2 | 2 | 2 | 2 | 2 | 2 | 2 |
| 35–49 | 1 | 1.0 | 0 | 1 | 1 | 1 | 1 | 1 | 1 | 1 |
| 50–64 | 1 | 2.0 | 0 | 2 | 2 | 2 | 2 | 2 | 2 | 2 |
| 65+ | 0 | | | | | | | | | |
| **2. MULTIPLE DX** | | | | | | | | | | |
| 0–19 Years | 74 | 1.8 | 3 | 1 | 1 | 1 | 2 | 4 | 6 | 7 |
| 20–34 | 91 | 2.0 | 2 | 1 | 1 | 1 | 2 | 4 | 5 | 9 |
| 35–49 | 84 | 2.5 | 6 | 1 | 1 | 2 | 3 | 5 | 5 | 9 |
| 50–64 | 38 | 3.1 | 10 | 2 | 2 | 2 | 3 | 5 | 15 | 16 |
| 65+ | 125 | 4.0 | 12 | 1 | 1 | 3 | 5 | 8 | 12 | 16 |
| **TOTAL SINGLE DX** | 21 | 2.2 | 2 | 1 | 1 | 1 | 4 | 4 | 4 | 4 |
| **TOTAL MULTIPLE DX** | 412 | 2.7 | 7 | 1 | 1 | 2 | 3 | 5 | 7 | 15 |
| **TOTAL** | | | | | | | | | | |
| 0–19 Years | 92 | 1.9 | 2 | 1 | 1 | 1 | 2 | 4 | 6 | 7 |
| 20–34 | 92 | 2.0 | 2 | 1 | 1 | 1 | 2 | 4 | 5 | 9 |
| 35–49 | 85 | 2.5 | 6 | 1 | 1 | 2 | 3 | 5 | 5 | 9 |
| 50–64 | 39 | 3.0 | 10 | 2 | 2 | 2 | 3 | 5 | 15 | 16 |
| 65+ | 125 | 4.0 | 12 | 1 | 2 | 3 | 5 | 8 | 12 | 16 |
| **GRAND TOTAL** | 433 | 2.7 | 7 | 1 | 1 | 2 | 3 | 5 | 7 | 15 |

Length of Stay by Diagnosis and Operation, United States, 2000

# United States, October 1998–September 1999 Data, by Operation

## 22.0: NASAL SINUS ASP & LAVAGE. Formerly included in operation group(s) 545.

| Type of Patients | Observed Patients | Avg. Stay | Variance | Percentiles 10th | 25th | 50th | 75th | 90th | 95th | 99th |
|---|---|---|---|---|---|---|---|---|---|---|
| **1. SINGLE DX** | | | | | | | | | | |
| 0–19 Years | 3 | 1.7 | <1 | 1 | 1 | 2 | 2 | 2 | 2 | 2 |
| 20–34 | 3 | 1.2 | <1 | 1 | 1 | 2 | 4 | 1 | 3 | 3 |
| 35–49 | 2 | 3.4 | <1 | 3 | 3 | 3 | 4 | 4 | 4 | 4 |
| 50–64 | 1 | 2.0 | 0 | 2 | 2 | 2 | 2 | 2 | 2 | 2 |
| 65+ | 0 | | | | | | | | | |
| **2. MULTIPLE DX** | | | | | | | | | | |
| 0–19 Years | 53 | 7.0 | 80 | 1 | 2 | 4 | 5 | 12 | 23 | 42 |
| 20–34 | 26 | 5.8 | 28 | 2 | 2 | 4 | 6 | 14 | 18 | 28 |
| 35–49 | 20 | 7.5 | 38 | 2 | 3 | 4 | 14 | 14 | 22 | 25 |
| 50–64 | 19 | 6.5 | 14 | 3 | 4 | 5 | 8 | 11 | 13 | 20 |
| 65+ | 28 | 8.7 | 30 | 3 | 5 | 7 | 11 | 17 | 22 | 23 |
| **TOTAL SINGLE DX** | 9 | 1.7 | <1 | 1 | 1 | 2 | 2 | 3 | 3 | 4 |
| **TOTAL MULTIPLE DX** | 146 | 7.0 | 46 | 2 | 3 | 5 | 10 | 14 | 19 | 42 |
| **TOTAL** | | | | | | | | | | |
| 0–19 Years | 56 | 6.1 | 71 | 1 | 2 | 3 | 7 | 12 | 23 | 42 |
| 20–34 | 29 | 4.9 | 26 | 1 | 2 | 3 | 6 | 14 | 18 | 28 |
| 35–49 | 22 | 7.1 | 36 | 2 | 3 | 4 | 14 | 14 | 15 | 25 |
| 50–64 | 20 | 6.4 | 14 | 3 | 4 | 5 | 8 | 11 | 13 | 20 |
| 65+ | 28 | 8.7 | 30 | 3 | 5 | 7 | 11 | 17 | 22 | 23 |
| **GRAND TOTAL** | 155 | 6.4 | 43 | 1 | 2 | 4 | 8 | 14 | 18 | 42 |

## 22.1: NASAL SINUS DXTIC PX. Formerly included in operation group(s) 545, 556.

| Type of Patients | Observed Patients | Avg. Stay | Variance | Percentiles 10th | 25th | 50th | 75th | 90th | 95th | 99th |
|---|---|---|---|---|---|---|---|---|---|---|
| **1. SINGLE DX** | | | | | | | | | | |
| 0–19 Years | 6 | 11.8 | 52 | 2 | 2 | 17 | 17 | 17 | 17 | 17 |
| 20–34 | 4 | 3.6 | 8 | 1 | 2 | 2 | 4 | 8 | 8 | 8 |
| 35–49 | 8 | 2.2 | 14 | 1 | 1 | 1 | 1 | 4 | 12 | 18 |
| 50–64 | 4 | 1.7 | <1 | 1 | 1 | 1 | 3 | 3 | 3 | 3 |
| 65+ | 1 | 1.0 | 0 | 1 | 1 | 1 | 1 | 1 | 1 | 1 |
| **2. MULTIPLE DX** | | | | | | | | | | |
| 0–19 Years | 43 | 3.8 | 20 | 1 | 2 | 2 | 5 | 7 | 11 | 14 |
| 20–34 | 31 | 6.1 | 117 | 1 | 2 | 4 | 7 | 7 | 13 | 79 |
| 35–49 | 41 | 5.8 | 43 | 2 | 3 | 4 | 7 | 10 | 15 | 41 |
| 50–64 | 41 | 3.5 | 16 | 1 | 2 | 2 | 4 | 8 | 10 | 10 |
| 65+ | 82 | 6.5 | 30 | 1 | 3 | 5 | 9 | 17 | 19 | 26 |
| **TOTAL SINGLE DX** | 23 | 5.0 | 42 | 1 | 1 | 1 | 4 | 17 | 17 | 18 |
| **TOTAL MULTIPLE DX** | 238 | 5.2 | 42 | 1 | 2 | 3 | 7 | 10 | 14 | 26 |
| **TOTAL** | | | | | | | | | | |
| 0–19 Years | 49 | 5.0 | 33 | 1 | 2 | 2 | 6 | 7 | 17 | 17 |
| 20–34 | 35 | 6.0 | 110 | 1 | 2 | 4 | 7 | 7 | 9 | 79 |
| 35–49 | 49 | 4.7 | 37 | 1 | 1 | 2 | 6 | 9 | 15 | 41 |
| 50–64 | 45 | 3.4 | 16 | 1 | 3 | 3 | 4 | 8 | 10 | 10 |
| 65+ | 83 | 6.5 | 30 | 1 | 3 | 5 | 9 | 15 | 19 | 26 |
| **GRAND TOTAL** | 261 | 5.2 | 42 | 1 | 2 | 3 | 7 | 10 | 17 | 26 |

## 22.2: INTRANASAL ANTROTOMY. Formerly included in operation group(s) 545.

| Type of Patients | Observed Patients | Avg. Stay | Variance | Percentiles 10th | 25th | 50th | 75th | 90th | 95th | 99th |
|---|---|---|---|---|---|---|---|---|---|---|
| **1. SINGLE DX** | | | | | | | | | | |
| 0–19 Years | 11 | 1.4 | <1 | 1 | 1 | 1 | 1 | 3 | 3 | 3 |
| 20–34 | 2 | 1.5 | <1 | 1 | 1 | 2 | 2 | 3 | 3 | 3 |
| 35–49 | 6 | 1.5 | <1 | 1 | 1 | 1 | 1 | 4 | 4 | 4 |
| 50–64 | 2 | 1.3 | <1 | 1 | 1 | 1 | 2 | 2 | 2 | 2 |
| 65+ | 2 | 1.6 | <1 | 1 | 1 | 1 | 2 | 2 | 2 | 2 |
| **2. MULTIPLE DX** | | | | | | | | | | |
| 0–19 Years | 59 | 4.9 | 22 | 1 | 1 | 3 | 8 | 14 | 15 | 17 |
| 20–34 | 19 | 3.3 | 18 | 1 | 1 | 2 | 3 | 4 | 10 | 28 |
| 35–49 | 26 | 12.1 | 357 | 1 | 1 | 2 | 11 | 49 | 49 | 49 |
| 50–64 | 18 | 4.8 | 154 | 1 | 1 | 2 | 5 | 8 | 10 | 86 |
| 65+ | 21 | 6.8 | 33 | 1 | 6 | 6 | 9 | 17 | 17 | 21 |
| **TOTAL SINGLE DX** | 23 | 1.4 | <1 | 1 | 1 | 1 | 1 | 3 | 3 | 4 |
| **TOTAL MULTIPLE DX** | 143 | 6.1 | 125 | 1 | 1 | 3 | 5 | 14 | 21 | 49 |
| **TOTAL** | | | | | | | | | | |
| 0–19 Years | 70 | 3.4 | 16 | 1 | 1 | 2 | 3 | 9 | 14 | 17 |
| 20–34 | 21 | 3.3 | 17 | 1 | 1 | 3 | 3 | 4 | 10 | 28 |
| 35–49 | 32 | 10.2 | 309 | 1 | 1 | 1 | 4 | 49 | 49 | 49 |
| 50–64 | 20 | 4.7 | 149 | 1 | 2 | 2 | 5 | 8 | 10 | 86 |
| 65+ | 23 | 6.5 | 33 | 1 | 6 | 6 | 9 | 17 | 17 | 21 |
| **GRAND TOTAL** | 166 | 5.1 | 101 | 1 | 1 | 2 | 4 | 11 | 17 | 49 |

## 22.3: EXT MAXILLARY ANTROTOMY. Formerly included in operation group(s) 544.

| Type of Patients | Observed Patients | Avg. Stay | Variance | Percentiles 10th | 25th | 50th | 75th | 90th | 95th | 99th |
|---|---|---|---|---|---|---|---|---|---|---|
| **1. SINGLE DX** | | | | | | | | | | |
| 0–19 Years | 8 | 2.3 | <1 | 1 | 2 | 2 | 3 | 3 | 4 | 4 |
| 20–34 | 4 | 1.0 | 0 | 1 | 1 | 1 | 1 | 1 | 1 | 1 |
| 35–49 | 5 | 1.7 | <1 | 1 | 1 | 1 | 2 | 2 | 2 | 2 |
| 50–64 | 2 | 1.0 | 0 | 1 | 1 | 1 | 1 | 1 | 1 | 1 |
| 65+ | 3 | 1.7 | 2 | 1 | 1 | 1 | 1 | 4 | 4 | 4 |
| **2. MULTIPLE DX** | | | | | | | | | | |
| 0–19 Years | 33 | 7.2 | 82 | 1 | 3 | 5 | 9 | 14 | 17 | 54 |
| 20–34 | 33 | 3.7 | 21 | 1 | 1 | 1 | 5 | 9 | 13 | 25 |
| 35–49 | 61 | 4.0 | 25 | 2 | 2 | 2 | 4 | 9 | 12 | 35 |
| 50–64 | 43 | 3.7 | 8 | 1 | 1 | 2 | 5 | 7 | 10 | 17 |
| 65+ | 51 | 4.8 | 43 | 1 | 1 | 2 | 7 | 12 | 19 | 36 |
| **TOTAL SINGLE DX** | 22 | 1.7 | <1 | 1 | 1 | 2 | 2 | 3 | 3 | 4 |
| **TOTAL MULTIPLE DX** | 221 | 4.4 | 29 | 1 | 2 | 2 | 5 | 10 | 14 | 25 |
| **TOTAL** | | | | | | | | | | |
| 0–19 Years | 41 | 6.6 | 75 | 1 | 2 | 4 | 9 | 14 | 14 | 54 |
| 20–34 | 37 | 3.5 | 20 | 1 | 1 | 1 | 4 | 8 | 13 | 25 |
| 35–49 | 66 | 3.8 | 22 | 1 | 2 | 2 | 4 | 7 | 12 | 25 |
| 50–64 | 45 | 3.7 | 8 | 1 | 1 | 2 | 5 | 7 | 10 | 17 |
| 65+ | 54 | 4.6 | 41 | 1 | 2 | 2 | 4 | 12 | 19 | 36 |
| **GRAND TOTAL** | 243 | 4.2 | 28 | 1 | 2 | 2 | 5 | 9 | 13 | 25 |

Length of Stay by Diagnosis and Operation, United States, 2000

**United States, October 1998–September 1999 Data, by Operation**

## 22.4: FRONT SINUSOT & SINUSECT. Formerly included in operation group(s) 545.

| Type of Patients | Observed Patients | Avg. Stay | Variance | 10th | 25th | 50th | 75th | 90th | 95th | 99th |
|---|---|---|---|---|---|---|---|---|---|---|
| **1. SINGLE DX** | | | | | | | | | | |
| 0–19 Years | 9 | 2.0 | <1 | 1 | 1 | 2 | 3 | 3 | 3 | 3 |
| 20–34 | 10 | 2.2 | <1 | 1 | 2 | 2 | 3 | 3 | 3 | 4 |
| 35–49 | 26 | 2.1 | <1 | 1 | 2 | 2 | 3 | 4 | 4 | 4 |
| 50–64 | 11 | 1.8 | <1 | 1 | 1 | 1 | 2 | 3 | 4 | 4 |
| 65+ | 6 | 2.7 | 2 | 2 | 2 | 2 | 3 | 5 | 5 | 5 |
| **2. MULTIPLE DX** | | | | | | | | | | |
| 0–19 Years | 35 | 6.3 | 19 | 1 | 3 | 5 | 9 | 11 | 15 | 20 |
| 20–34 | 70 | 4.3 | 20 | 1 | 3 | 3 | 5 | 8 | 14 | 25 |
| 35–49 | 82 | 3.8 | 15 | 1 | 2 | 3 | 4 | 7 | 11 | 11 |
| 50–64 | 86 | 4.0 | 19 | 1 | 2 | 3 | 4 | 7 | 13 | 23 |
| 65+ | 52 | 5.4 | 18 | 2 | 2 | 4 | 8 | 10 | 11 | 17 |
| **TOTAL SINGLE DX** | 62 | 2.1 | 1 | 1 | 1 | 2 | 3 | 4 | 4 | 5 |
| **TOTAL MULTIPLE DX** | 325 | 4.4 | 18 | 1 | 2 | 3 | 5 | 9 | 12 | 25 |
| **TOTAL** | | | | | | | | | | |
| 0–19 Years | 44 | 5.5 | 19 | 1 | 2 | 5 | 8 | 11 | 15 | 20 |
| 20–34 | 80 | 4.1 | 18 | 1 | 2 | 3 | 5 | 8 | 11 | 25 |
| 35–49 | 108 | 3.3 | 12 | 1 | 2 | 2 | 4 | 5 | 9 | 25 |
| 50–64 | 97 | 3.9 | 18 | 1 | 2 | 3 | 4 | 6 | 13 | 23 |
| 65+ | 58 | 5.0 | 16 | 2 | 2 | 4 | 7 | 10 | 10 | 17 |
| **GRAND TOTAL** | 387 | 4.1 | 17 | 1 | 2 | 3 | 5 | 8 | 11 | 23 |

## 22.6: OTHER NASAL SINUSECTOMY. Formerly included in operation group(s) 545.

| Type of Patients | Observed Patients | Avg. Stay | Variance | 10th | 25th | 50th | 75th | 90th | 95th | 99th |
|---|---|---|---|---|---|---|---|---|---|---|
| **1. SINGLE DX** | | | | | | | | | | |
| 0–19 Years | 48 | 2.6 | 5 | 1 | 1 | 1 | 5 | 5 | 6 | 9 |
| 20–34 | 21 | 2.3 | 1 | 1 | 2 | 2 | 3 | 3 | 5 | 9 |
| 35–49 | 39 | 2.7 | 4 | 1 | 1 | 2 | 2 | 5 | 6 | 10 |
| 50–64 | 19 | 2.0 | 3 | 1 | 1 | 1 | 3 | 4 | 7 | 8 |
| 65+ | 23 | 1.6 | 1 | 1 | 1 | 1 | 2 | 3 | 3 | 6 |
| **2. MULTIPLE DX** | | | | | | | | | | |
| 0–19 Years | 566 | 5.5 | 45 | 1 | 3 | 3 | 7 | 13 | 15 | 36 |
| 20–34 | 266 | 4.1 | 26 | 1 | 2 | 2 | 4 | 10 | 15 | 27 |
| 35–49 | 465 | 4.2 | 33 | 1 | 2 | 2 | 5 | 10 | 12 | 27 |
| 50–64 | 399 | 4.9 | 55 | 1 | 2 | 4 | 5 | 12 | 18 | 34 |
| 65+ | 411 | 4.8 | 27 | 1 | 2 | 4 | 4 | 10 | 16 | 27 |
| **TOTAL SINGLE DX** | 150 | 2.4 | 4 | 1 | 1 | 1 | 4 | 5 | 6 | 9 |
| **TOTAL MULTIPLE DX** | 2,107 | 4.7 | 39 | 1 | 1 | 2 | 5 | 11 | 15 | 34 |
| **TOTAL** | | | | | | | | | | |
| 0–19 Years | 614 | 5.1 | 41 | 1 | 1 | 3 | 6 | 12 | 14 | 35 |
| 20–34 | 287 | 4.0 | 24 | 1 | 1 | 2 | 4 | 9 | 15 | 27 |
| 35–49 | 504 | 4.1 | 31 | 1 | 2 | 2 | 5 | 10 | 12 | 27 |
| 50–64 | 418 | 4.8 | 53 | 1 | 2 | 4 | 5 | 12 | 18 | 34 |
| 65+ | 434 | 4.7 | 27 | 1 | 2 | 4 | 4 | 10 | 16 | 27 |
| **GRAND TOTAL** | 2,257 | 4.6 | 37 | 1 | 1 | 2 | 5 | 10 | 15 | 34 |

## 22.5: OTHER NASAL SINUSOTOMY. Formerly included in operation group(s) 545.

| Type of Patients | Observed Patients | Avg. Stay | Variance | 10th | 25th | 50th | 75th | 90th | 95th | 99th |
|---|---|---|---|---|---|---|---|---|---|---|
| **1. SINGLE DX** | | | | | | | | | | |
| 0–19 Years | 5 | 2.6 | 1 | 1 | 1 | 3 | 3 | 4 | 4 | 4 |
| 20–34 | 3 | 3.7 | 1 | 2 | 2 | 3 | 5 | 5 | 5 | 5 |
| 35–49 | 1 | 4.0 | 0 | 4 | 4 | 4 | 4 | 4 | 4 | 4 |
| 50–64 | 3 | 2.9 | 1 | 2 | 2 | 3 | 3 | 5 | 5 | 5 |
| 65+ | 2 | 2.5 | 4 | 1 | 1 | 1 | 4 | 4 | 4 | 4 |
| **2. MULTIPLE DX** | | | | | | | | | | |
| 0–19 Years | 30 | 7.7 | 45 | 1 | 3 | 6 | 12 | 13 | 26 | 30 |
| 20–34 | 32 | 7.6 | 56 | 3 | 3 | 6 | 9 | 15 | 33 | 33 |
| 35–49 | 44 | 5.5 | 26 | 1 | 2 | 4 | 7 | 12 | 18 | 21 |
| 50–64 | 28 | 5.5 | 44 | 1 | 2 | 2 | 8 | 15 | 23 | 23 |
| 65+ | 34 | 6.1 | 51 | 1 | 1 | 3 | 6 | 20 | 21 | 35 |
| **TOTAL SINGLE DX** | 14 | 3.1 | 1 | 1 | 2 | 3 | 4 | 5 | 5 | 5 |
| **TOTAL MULTIPLE DX** | 168 | 6.5 | 44 | 1 | 2 | 4 | 9 | 15 | 21 | 33 |
| **TOTAL** | | | | | | | | | | |
| 0–19 Years | 35 | 7.0 | 42 | 1 | 3 | 5 | 12 | 13 | 26 | 30 |
| 20–34 | 35 | 7.2 | 52 | 2 | 3 | 6 | 9 | 15 | 21 | 33 |
| 35–49 | 45 | 5.4 | 25 | 1 | 2 | 4 | 7 | 12 | 18 | 21 |
| 50–64 | 31 | 5.2 | 40 | 1 | 2 | 2 | 8 | 15 | 23 | 23 |
| 65+ | 36 | 6.0 | 50 | 1 | 1 | 3 | 6 | 20 | 21 | 35 |
| **GRAND TOTAL** | 182 | 6.2 | 42 | 1 | 2 | 4 | 8 | 15 | 21 | 33 |

## 22.62: EXC MAX SINUS LESION NEC. Formerly included in operation group(s) 545.

| Type of Patients | Observed Patients | Avg. Stay | Variance | 10th | 25th | 50th | 75th | 90th | 95th | 99th |
|---|---|---|---|---|---|---|---|---|---|---|
| **1. SINGLE DX** | | | | | | | | | | |
| 0–19 Years | 7 | 1.8 | <1 | 1 | 1 | 1 | 2 | 3 | 3 | 4 |
| 20–34 | 2 | 3.1 | 1 | 2 | 2 | 2 | 2 | 3 | 3 | 4 |
| 35–49 | 17 | 2.6 | 3 | 1 | 1 | 2 | 5 | 5 | 5 | 6 |
| 50–64 | 5 | 2.6 | <1 | 1 | 3 | 3 | 3 | 3 | 3 | 3 |
| 65+ | 10 | 1.1 | <1 | 1 | 1 | 1 | 1 | 1 | 2 | 2 |
| **2. MULTIPLE DX** | | | | | | | | | | |
| 0–19 Years | 81 | 9.3 | 112 | 1 | 3 | 5 | 11 | 21 | 34 | 43 |
| 20–34 | 52 | 4.3 | 33 | 1 | 1 | 2 | 5 | 12 | 18 | 23 |
| 35–49 | 88 | 4.4 | 16 | 1 | 2 | 3 | 5 | 12 | 12 | 19 |
| 50–64 | 99 | 6.4 | 46 | 1 | 3 | 3 | 10 | 15 | 19 | 31 |
| 65+ | 90 | 4.4 | 15 | 1 | 2 | 4 | 4 | 8 | 12 | 24 |
| **TOTAL SINGLE DX** | 41 | 2.2 | 2 | 1 | 1 | 2 | 3 | 5 | 5 | 6 |
| **TOTAL MULTIPLE DX** | 410 | 5.6 | 44 | 1 | 2 | 4 | 6 | 12 | 18 | 34 |
| **TOTAL** | | | | | | | | | | |
| 0–19 Years | 88 | 8.5 | 106 | 1 | 2 | 4 | 11 | 21 | 34 | 43 |
| 20–34 | 54 | 4.3 | 32 | 1 | 1 | 3 | 5 | 12 | 18 | 23 |
| 35–49 | 105 | 4.0 | 14 | 1 | 3 | 3 | 5 | 8 | 12 | 17 |
| 50–64 | 104 | 6.2 | 45 | 2 | 3 | 4 | 10 | 15 | 19 | 31 |
| 65+ | 100 | 4.2 | 15 | 1 | 2 | 4 | 4 | 7 | 12 | 24 |
| **GRAND TOTAL** | 451 | 5.3 | 42 | 1 | 2 | 3 | 6 | 12 | 17 | 34 |

Length of Stay by Diagnosis and Operation, United States, 2000

# United States, October 1998–September 1999 Data, by Operation

## 22.63: ETHMOIDECTOMY. Formerly included in operation group(s) 545.

| Type of Patients | Observed Patients | Avg. Stay | Variance | 10th | 25th | 50th | 75th | 90th | 95th | 99th |
|---|---|---|---|---|---|---|---|---|---|---|
| **1. SINGLE DX** | | | | | | | | | | |
| 0–19 Years | 36 | 3.4 | 5 | 1 | 1 | 4 | 6 | 6 | 6 | 9 |
| 20–34 | 11 | 2.2 | 1 | 2 | 2 | 2 | 3 | 3 | 5 | 5 |
| 35–49 | 15 | 2.9 | 6 | 1 | 1 | 2 | 4 | 6 | 10 | 10 |
| 50–64 | 12 | 1.4 | 2 | 1 | 1 | 1 | 1 | 2 | 4 | 7 |
| 65+ | 10 | 2.1 | 3 | 1 | 1 | 3 | 3 | 6 | 6 | 6 |
| **2. MULTIPLE DX** | | | | | | | | | | |
| 0–19 Years | 461 | 4.8 | 32 | 1 | 1 | 3 | 7 | 11 | 14 | 28 |
| 20–34 | 190 | 3.8 | 18 | 1 | 1 | 2 | 4 | 8 | 12 | 24 |
| 35–49 | 312 | 4.1 | 34 | 1 | 1 | 2 | 5 | 10 | 11 | 37 |
| 50–64 | 259 | 3.2 | 20 | 1 | 1 | 2 | 4 | 7 | 10 | 24 |
| 65+ | 257 | 4.6 | 27 | 1 | 1 | 4 | 4 | 10 | 16 | 24 |
| **TOTAL SINGLE DX** | 84 | 2.8 | 5 | 1 | 1 | 1 | 5 | 6 | 6 | 10 |
| **TOTAL MULTIPLE DX** | 1,479 | 4.1 | 27 | 1 | 1 | 2 | 5 | 10 | 13 | 24 |
| **TOTAL** | | | | | | | | | | |
| 0–19 Years | 497 | 4.7 | 29 | 1 | 1 | 3 | 6 | 11 | 14 | 25 |
| 20–34 | 201 | 3.8 | 17 | 1 | 1 | 2 | 4 | 8 | 12 | 24 |
| 35–49 | 327 | 4.0 | 33 | 1 | 1 | 2 | 5 | 10 | 11 | 37 |
| 50–64 | 271 | 3.1 | 19 | 1 | 1 | 2 | 4 | 7 | 10 | 24 |
| 65+ | 267 | 4.5 | 26 | 1 | 1 | 4 | 4 | 10 | 16 | 24 |
| **GRAND TOTAL** | 1,563 | 4.0 | 26 | 1 | 1 | 2 | 5 | 10 | 13 | 24 |

## 22.9: OTHER NASAL SINUS OPS. Formerly included in operation group(s) 545.

| Type of Patients | Observed Patients | Avg. Stay | Variance | 10th | 25th | 50th | 75th | 90th | 95th | 99th |
|---|---|---|---|---|---|---|---|---|---|---|
| **1. SINGLE DX** | | | | | | | | | | |
| 0–19 Years | 0 | | | | | | | | | |
| 20–34 | 0 | | | | | | | | | |
| 35–49 | 0 | | | | | | | | | |
| 50–64 | 0 | | | | | | | | | |
| 65+ | 0 | | | | | | | | | |
| **2. MULTIPLE DX** | | | | | | | | | | |
| 0–19 Years | 14 | 8.8 | 146 | 1 | 3 | 3 | 12 | 20 | 52 | 52 |
| 20–34 | 2 | 5.6 | 4 | 4 | 4 | 7 | 7 | 7 | 7 | 7 |
| 35–49 | 7 | 2.5 | 3 | 1 | 1 | 2 | 4 | 5 | 5 | 6 |
| 50–64 | 5 | 2.1 | 2 | 1 | 1 | 1 | 4 | 4 | 4 | 4 |
| 65+ | 6 | 8.2 | 34 | 1 | 2 | 7 | 10 | 21 | 21 | 21 |
| **TOTAL SINGLE DX** | 0 | | | | | | | | | |
| **TOTAL MULTIPLE DX** | 34 | 6.2 | 80 | 1 | 1 | 3 | 7 | 14 | 20 | 52 |
| **TOTAL** | | | | | | | | | | |
| 0–19 Years | 14 | 8.8 | 146 | 1 | 3 | 3 | 12 | 20 | 52 | 52 |
| 20–34 | 2 | 5.6 | 4 | 4 | 4 | 7 | 7 | 7 | 7 | 7 |
| 35–49 | 7 | 2.5 | 3 | 1 | 1 | 2 | 4 | 5 | 5 | 6 |
| 50–64 | 5 | 2.1 | 2 | 1 | 1 | 1 | 4 | 4 | 4 | 4 |
| 65+ | 6 | 8.2 | 34 | 1 | 2 | 7 | 10 | 21 | 21 | 21 |
| **GRAND TOTAL** | 34 | 6.2 | 80 | 1 | 1 | 3 | 7 | 14 | 20 | 52 |

## 22.7: NASAL SINUS REPAIR. Formerly included in operation group(s) 545.

| Type of Patients | Observed Patients | Avg. Stay | Variance | 10th | 25th | 50th | 75th | 90th | 95th | 99th |
|---|---|---|---|---|---|---|---|---|---|---|
| **1. SINGLE DX** | | | | | | | | | | |
| 0–19 Years | 1 | 2.0 | 0 | 2 | 2 | 2 | 2 | 2 | 2 | 2 |
| 20–34 | 1 | 3.0 | 0 | 3 | 3 | 3 | 3 | 3 | 3 | 3 |
| 35–49 | 2 | 1.0 | 0 | 1 | 1 | 1 | 1 | 1 | 1 | 1 |
| 50–64 | 2 | 5.1 | 3 | 6 | 6 | 6 | 6 | 6 | 6 | 6 |
| 65+ | 1 | 2.0 | 0 | 2 | 2 | 2 | 2 | 2 | 2 | 2 |
| **2. MULTIPLE DX** | | | | | | | | | | |
| 0–19 Years | 13 | 5.3 | 114 | 1 | 1 | 1 | 2 | 5 | 37 | 37 |
| 20–34 | 16 | 6.8 | 38 | 1 | 1 | 3 | 14 | 14 | 14 | 19 |
| 35–49 | 28 | 2.3 | 3 | 1 | 1 | 2 | 3 | 4 | 5 | 8 |
| 50–64 | 10 | 1.7 | 1 | 1 | 1 | 1 | 2 | 4 | 5 | 5 |
| 65+ | 5 | 2.8 | <1 | 2 | 2 | 3 | 3 | 4 | 4 | 4 |
| **TOTAL SINGLE DX** | 7 | 2.7 | 3 | 2 | 2 | 2 | 3 | 6 | 6 | 6 |
| **TOTAL MULTIPLE DX** | 72 | 4.0 | 29 | 1 | 1 | 2 | 4 | 14 | 14 | 37 |
| **TOTAL** | | | | | | | | | | |
| 0–19 Years | 14 | 4.8 | 97 | 1 | 1 | 2 | 2 | 5 | 37 | 37 |
| 20–34 | 17 | 6.7 | 37 | 1 | 1 | 3 | 14 | 14 | 14 | 19 |
| 35–49 | 30 | 2.3 | 3 | 1 | 1 | 2 | 3 | 4 | 5 | 8 |
| 50–64 | 12 | 2.1 | 3 | 1 | 1 | 1 | 2 | 5 | 6 | 6 |
| 65+ | 6 | 2.7 | <1 | 2 | 2 | 3 | 3 | 4 | 4 | 4 |
| **GRAND TOTAL** | 79 | 3.9 | 28 | 1 | 1 | 2 | 4 | 14 | 14 | 19 |

## 23.0: FORCEPS TOOTH EXTRACTION. Formerly included in operation group(s) 546.

| Type of Patients | Observed Patients | Avg. Stay | Variance | 10th | 25th | 50th | 75th | 90th | 95th | 99th |
|---|---|---|---|---|---|---|---|---|---|---|
| **1. SINGLE DX** | | | | | | | | | | |
| 0–19 Years | 31 | 1.4 | 2 | 1 | 1 | 1 | 1 | 3 | 6 | 6 |
| 20–34 | 10 | 5.8 | 50 | 1 | 1 | 2 | 6 | 22 | 22 | 22 |
| 35–49 | 4 | 2.0 | <1 | 2 | 2 | 2 | 2 | 2 | 3 | 3 |
| 50–64 | 3 | 2.0 | 2 | 1 | 1 | 1 | 4 | 4 | 4 | 4 |
| 65+ | 4 | 1.7 | <1 | 1 | 1 | 2 | 2 | 2 | 2 | 2 |
| **2. MULTIPLE DX** | | | | | | | | | | |
| 0–19 Years | 365 | 2.1 | 8 | 1 | 1 | 1 | 2 | 4 | 7 | 14 |
| 20–34 | 166 | 5.8 | 30 | 1 | 2 | 3 | 8 | 16 | 25 | >99 |
| 35–49 | 215 | 5.5 | 40 | 1 | 2 | 3 | 7 | 13 | 21 | 35 |
| 50–64 | 135 | 8.1 | 37 | 2 | 3 | 6 | 12 | 17 | 23 | 24 |
| 65+ | 159 | 7.0 | 72 | 1 | 3 | 6 | 8 | 12 | 19 | 42 |
| **TOTAL SINGLE DX** | 52 | 1.9 | 6 | 1 | 1 | 1 | 2 | 4 | 6 | 13 |
| **TOTAL MULTIPLE DX** | 1,040 | 4.7 | 33 | 1 | 1 | 3 | 6 | 12 | 16 | 48 |
| **TOTAL** | | | | | | | | | | |
| 0–19 Years | 396 | 2.1 | 7 | 1 | 1 | 1 | 2 | 4 | 6 | 14 |
| 20–34 | 176 | 5.8 | 31 | 1 | 2 | 3 | 8 | 16 | 25 | >99 |
| 35–49 | 219 | 5.2 | 38 | 1 | 2 | 3 | 7 | 11 | 20 | 35 |
| 50–64 | 138 | 7.8 | 37 | 2 | 3 | 5 | 12 | 17 | 21 | 24 |
| 65+ | 163 | 6.9 | 71 | 2 | 3 | 6 | 8 | 12 | 19 | 42 |
| **GRAND TOTAL** | 1,092 | 4.4 | 32 | 1 | 1 | 2 | 6 | 12 | 16 | 36 |

# United States, October 1998–September 1999 Data, by Operation

## 23.09: TOOTH EXTRACTION NEC. Formerly included in operation group(s) 546.

| Type of Patients | Observed Patients | Avg. Stay | Variance | 10th | 25th | 50th | 75th | 90th | 95th | 99th |
|---|---|---|---|---|---|---|---|---|---|---|
| **1. SINGLE DX** | | | | | | | | | | |
| 0–19 Years | 28 | 1.4 | <1 | 1 | 1 | 1 | 1 | 3 | 6 | 6 |
| 20–34 | 10 | 5.8 | 50 | 1 | 1 | 2 | 6 | 22 | 22 | 22 |
| 35–49 | 6 | 4.0 | <1 | 2 | 2 | 2 | 4 | 4 | 4 | 4 |
| 50–64 | 3 | 2.0 | 2 | 1 | 2 | 1 | 2 | 4 | 4 | 4 |
| 65+ | 4 | 1.7 | <1 | 1 | 1 | 2 | 2 | 2 | 2 | 2 |
| **2. MULTIPLE DX** | | | | | | | | | | |
| 0–19 Years | 299 | 2.0 | 8 | 1 | 1 | 1 | 2 | 4 | 6 | 14 |
| 20–34 | 164 | 5.8 | 31 | 1 | 2 | 3 | 9 | 16 | 27 | >99 |
| 35–49 | 211 | 5.6 | 41 | 2 | 2 | 3 | 7 | 13 | 21 | 35 |
| 50–64 | 133 | 8.1 | 38 | 2 | 3 | 6 | 12 | 17 | 23 | 24 |
| 65+ | 156 | 7.0 | 72 | 3 | 3 | 6 | 7 | 12 | 19 | 42 |
| **TOTAL SINGLE DX** | 49 | 1.9 | 6 | 1 | 1 | 1 | 2 | 4 | 6 | 13 |
| **TOTAL MULTIPLE DX** | 963 | 4.8 | 35 | 1 | 1 | 3 | 6 | 12 | 16 | 49 |
| **TOTAL** | | | | | | | | | | |
| 0–19 Years | 327 | 2.0 | 8 | 1 | 1 | 2 | 2 | 4 | 6 | 12 |
| 20–34 | 174 | 5.8 | 31 | 1 | 2 | 3 | 9 | 16 | 25 | >99 |
| 35–49 | 215 | 5.3 | 38 | 1 | 2 | 3 | 7 | 11 | 20 | 35 |
| 50–64 | 136 | 7.8 | 38 | 2 | 3 | 5 | 12 | 17 | 23 | 24 |
| 65+ | 160 | 6.9 | 72 | 3 | 3 | 5 | 7 | 12 | 19 | 42 |
| **GRAND TOTAL** | 1,012 | 4.5 | 33 | 1 | 1 | 2 | 6 | 12 | 16 | 48 |

## 23.19: SURG TOOTH EXTRACT NEC. Formerly included in operation group(s) 546.

| Type of Patients | Observed Patients | Avg. Stay | Variance | 10th | 25th | 50th | 75th | 90th | 95th | 99th |
|---|---|---|---|---|---|---|---|---|---|---|
| **1. SINGLE DX** | | | | | | | | | | |
| 0–19 Years | 34 | 1.5 | <1 | 1 | 1 | 1 | 2 | 3 | 4 | 4 |
| 20–34 | 10 | 2.5 | 2 | 2 | 2 | 2 | 3 | 3 | 5 | 6 |
| 35–49 | 5 | 3.9 | 2 | 1 | 2 | 5 | 5 | 5 | 5 | 5 |
| 50–64 | 2 | 2.1 | 4 | 1 | 1 | 1 | 5 | 5 | 5 | 5 |
| 65+ | 1 | 1.0 | 0 | 1 | 1 | 1 | 1 | 1 | 1 | 1 |
| **2. MULTIPLE DX** | | | | | | | | | | |
| 0–19 Years | 262 | 2.9 | 17 | 1 | 1 | 2 | 3 | 5 | 10 | 33 |
| 20–34 | 207 | 4.2 | 30 | 1 | 1 | 3 | 5 | 9 | 12 | 30 |
| 35–49 | 237 | 6.4 | 54 | 2 | 2 | 4 | 7 | 15 | 18 | 35 |
| 50–64 | 170 | 5.1 | 31 | 1 | 2 | 3 | 6 | 9 | 12 | 35 |
| 65+ | 242 | 4.5 | 22 | 1 | 3 | 3 | 7 | 11 | 15 | 20 |
| **TOTAL SINGLE DX** | 52 | 1.8 | 2 | 1 | 1 | 1 | 2 | 4 | 5 | 6 |
| **TOTAL MULTIPLE DX** | 1,118 | 4.5 | 32 | 1 | 1 | 3 | 5 | 10 | 15 | 34 |
| **TOTAL** | | | | | | | | | | |
| 0–19 Years | 296 | 2.7 | 15 | 1 | 1 | 3 | 3 | 5 | 10 | 33 |
| 20–34 | 217 | 4.1 | 29 | 1 | 1 | 5 | 5 | 8 | 11 | 28 |
| 35–49 | 242 | 6.3 | 53 | 2 | 2 | 4 | 7 | 15 | 18 | 35 |
| 50–64 | 172 | 5.1 | 31 | 1 | 2 | 3 | 6 | 9 | 11 | 35 |
| 65+ | 243 | 4.5 | 22 | 1 | 3 | 3 | 7 | 11 | 15 | 20 |
| **GRAND TOTAL** | 1,170 | 4.3 | 30 | 1 | 1 | 3 | 5 | 9 | 15 | 33 |

## 23.1: SURG REMOVAL OF TOOTH. Formerly included in operation group(s) 546.

| Type of Patients | Observed Patients | Avg. Stay | Variance | 10th | 25th | 50th | 75th | 90th | 95th | 99th |
|---|---|---|---|---|---|---|---|---|---|---|
| **1. SINGLE DX** | | | | | | | | | | |
| 0–19 Years | 34 | 1.5 | <1 | 1 | 1 | 1 | 2 | 3 | 4 | 4 |
| 20–34 | 11 | 2.5 | 2 | 1 | 2 | 2 | 3 | 3 | 5 | 6 |
| 35–49 | 6 | 3.7 | 3 | 1 | 2 | 5 | 5 | 5 | 5 | 5 |
| 50–64 | 2 | 2.1 | 4 | 1 | 1 | 1 | 5 | 5 | 5 | 5 |
| 65+ | 1 | 1.0 | 0 | 1 | 1 | 1 | 1 | 1 | 1 | 1 |
| **2. MULTIPLE DX** | | | | | | | | | | |
| 0–19 Years | 262 | 2.9 | 17 | 1 | 1 | 2 | 3 | 5 | 10 | 33 |
| 20–34 | 213 | 4.2 | 29 | 1 | 1 | 3 | 5 | 9 | 12 | 30 |
| 35–49 | 245 | 6.4 | 54 | 2 | 2 | 4 | 7 | 15 | 18 | 35 |
| 50–64 | 174 | 5.4 | 47 | 2 | 2 | 3 | 6 | 9 | 13 | 35 |
| 65+ | 246 | 4.5 | 22 | 1 | 1 | 3 | 7 | 11 | 15 | 20 |
| **TOTAL SINGLE DX** | 54 | 1.8 | 2 | 1 | 1 | 1 | 2 | 4 | 5 | 6 |
| **TOTAL MULTIPLE DX** | 1,140 | 4.5 | 34 | 1 | 1 | 3 | 5 | 10 | 15 | 34 |
| **TOTAL** | | | | | | | | | | |
| 0–19 Years | 296 | 2.7 | 15 | 1 | 1 | 3 | 3 | 5 | 10 | 33 |
| 20–34 | 224 | 4.1 | 28 | 1 | 1 | 3 | 5 | 8 | 11 | 28 |
| 35–49 | 251 | 6.3 | 53 | 2 | 2 | 4 | 7 | 15 | 18 | 35 |
| 50–64 | 176 | 5.4 | 47 | 1 | 2 | 3 | 6 | 9 | 13 | 35 |
| 65+ | 247 | 4.5 | 22 | 1 | 1 | 3 | 7 | 11 | 15 | 20 |
| **GRAND TOTAL** | 1,194 | 4.3 | 32 | 1 | 1 | 3 | 5 | 9 | 15 | 33 |

## 23.2: TOOTH RESTOR BY FILLING. Formerly included in operation group(s) 547.

| Type of Patients | Observed Patients | Avg. Stay | Variance | 10th | 25th | 50th | 75th | 90th | 95th | 99th |
|---|---|---|---|---|---|---|---|---|---|---|
| **1. SINGLE DX** | | | | | | | | | | |
| 0–19 Years | 18 | 1.0 | 0 | 1 | 1 | 1 | 1 | 1 | 1 | 1 |
| 20–34 | 0 | | | | | | | | | |
| 35–49 | 0 | | | | | | | | | |
| 50–64 | 0 | | | | | | | | | |
| **2. MULTIPLE DX** | | | | | | | | | | |
| 0–19 Years | 111 | 1.2 | 2 | 1 | 1 | 1 | 1 | 1 | 2 | 7 |
| 20–34 | 19 | 4.7 | 92 | 1 | 1 | 1 | 3 | 32 | 32 | 32 |
| 35–49 | 10 | 1.2 | <1 | 1 | 1 | 1 | 1 | 1 | 1 | 5 |
| 50–64 | 3 | 1.0 | 0 | 1 | 1 | 1 | 1 | 1 | 1 | 1 |
| 65+ | 0 | | | | | | | | | |
| **TOTAL SINGLE DX** | 18 | 1.0 | 0 | 1 | 1 | 1 | 1 | 1 | 1 | 1 |
| **TOTAL MULTIPLE DX** | 143 | 1.4 | 7 | 1 | 1 | 1 | 1 | 1 | 3 | 11 |
| **TOTAL** | | | | | | | | | | |
| 0–19 Years | 129 | 1.2 | 1 | 1 | 1 | 1 | 1 | 1 | 1 | 7 |
| 20–34 | 19 | 4.7 | 92 | 1 | 1 | 1 | 3 | 32 | 32 | 32 |
| 35–49 | 10 | 1.2 | <1 | 1 | 1 | 1 | 1 | 1 | 1 | 5 |
| 50–64 | 3 | 1.0 | 0 | 1 | 1 | 1 | 1 | 1 | 1 | 1 |
| 65+ | 0 | | | | | | | | | |
| **GRAND TOTAL** | 161 | 1.3 | 5 | 1 | 1 | 1 | 1 | 1 | 2 | 11 |

Length of Stay by Diagnosis and Operation, United States, 2000

# United States, October 1998–September 1999 Data, by Operation

## 23.3: TOOTH RESTOR BY INLAY. Formerly included in operation group(s) 547.

| Type of Patients | Observed Patients | Avg. Stay | Variance | 10th | 25th | 50th | 75th | 90th | 95th | 99th |
|---|---|---|---|---|---|---|---|---|---|---|
| **1. SINGLE DX** | | | | | | | | | | |
| 0–19 Years | 0 | | | | | | | | | |
| 20–34 | 0 | | | | | | | | | |
| 35–49 | 0 | | | | | | | | | |
| 50–64 | 0 | | | | | | | | | |
| 65+ | 0 | | | | | | | | | |
| **2. MULTIPLE DX** | | | | | | | | | | |
| 0–19 Years | 1 | 1.0 | 0 | 1 | 1 | 1 | 1 | 1 | 1 | 1 |
| 20–34 | 0 | | | | | | | | | |
| 35–49 | 0 | | | | | | | | | |
| 50–64 | 0 | | | | | | | | | |
| 65+ | 0 | | | | | | | | | |
| **TOTAL SINGLE DX** | 0 | | | | | | | | | |
| **TOTAL MULTIPLE DX** | 1 | 1.0 | 0 | 1 | 1 | 1 | 1 | 1 | 1 | 1 |
| **TOTAL** | | | | | | | | | | |
| 0–19 Years | 1 | 1.0 | 0 | 1 | 1 | 1 | 1 | 1 | 1 | 1 |
| 20–34 | 0 | | | | | | | | | |
| 35–49 | 0 | | | | | | | | | |
| 50–64 | 0 | | | | | | | | | |
| 65+ | 0 | | | | | | | | | |
| **GRAND TOTAL** | 1 | 1.0 | 0 | 1 | 1 | 1 | 1 | 1 | 1 | 1 |

## 23.4: OTHER DENTAL RESTORATION. Formerly included in operation group(s) 547.

| Type of Patients | Observed Patients | Avg. Stay | Variance | 10th | 25th | 50th | 75th | 90th | 95th | 99th |
|---|---|---|---|---|---|---|---|---|---|---|
| **1. SINGLE DX** | | | | | | | | | | |
| 0–19 Years | 165 | 1.0 | 0 | 1 | 1 | 1 | 1 | 1 | 1 | 1 |
| 20–34 | 0 | | | | | | | | | |
| 35–49 | 0 | | | | | | | | | |
| 50–64 | 0 | | | | | | | | | |
| 65+ | 0 | | | | | | | | | |
| **2. MULTIPLE DX** | | | | | | | | | | |
| 0–19 Years | 139 | 2.0 | 13 | 1 | 1 | 1 | 1 | 3 | 6 | 23 |
| 20–34 | 4 | 1.2 | <1 | 1 | 1 | 1 | 1 | 2 | 2 | 2 |
| 35–49 | 7 | 4.0 | 12 | 1 | 1 | 2 | 9 | 9 | 9 | 9 |
| 50–64 | 0 | | | | | | | | | |
| 65+ | 0 | | | | | | | | | |
| **TOTAL SINGLE DX** | 165 | 1.0 | 0 | 1 | 1 | 1 | 1 | 1 | 1 | 1 |
| **TOTAL MULTIPLE DX** | 150 | 2.1 | 13 | 1 | 1 | 1 | 2 | 3 | 7 | 23 |
| **TOTAL** | | | | | | | | | | |
| 0–19 Years | 304 | 1.7 | 10 | 1 | 1 | 1 | 1 | 3 | 4 | 23 |
| 20–34 | 4 | 1.2 | <1 | 1 | 1 | 1 | 1 | 2 | 2 | 2 |
| 35–49 | 7 | 4.0 | 12 | 1 | 1 | 2 | 9 | 9 | 9 | 9 |
| 50–64 | 0 | | | | | | | | | |
| 65+ | 0 | | | | | | | | | |
| **GRAND TOTAL** | 315 | 1.8 | 10 | 1 | 1 | 1 | 1 | 3 | 6 | 23 |

## 23.5: TOOTH IMPLANTATION. Formerly included in operation group(s) 547.

| Type of Patients | Observed Patients | Avg. Stay | Variance | 10th | 25th | 50th | 75th | 90th | 95th | 99th |
|---|---|---|---|---|---|---|---|---|---|---|
| **1. SINGLE DX** | | | | | | | | | | |
| 0–19 Years | 0 | | | | | | | | | |
| 20–34 | 0 | | | | | | | | | |
| 35–49 | 0 | | | | | | | | | |
| 50–64 | 0 | | | | | | | | | |
| 65+ | 1 | 1.0 | 0 | 1 | 1 | 1 | 1 | 1 | 1 | 1 |
| **2. MULTIPLE DX** | | | | | | | | | | |
| 0–19 Years | 5 | 1.7 | 1 | 1 | 1 | 1 | 2 | 4 | 4 | 4 |
| 20–34 | 1 | 1.0 | 0 | 1 | 1 | 1 | 1 | 1 | 1 | 1 |
| 35–49 | 0 | | | | | | | | | |
| 50–64 | 0 | | | | | | | | | |
| 65+ | 0 | | | | | | | | | |
| **TOTAL SINGLE DX** | 1 | 1.0 | 0 | 1 | 1 | 1 | 1 | 1 | 1 | 1 |
| **TOTAL MULTIPLE DX** | 6 | 1.6 | 1 | 1 | 1 | 1 | 2 | 4 | 4 | 4 |
| **TOTAL** | | | | | | | | | | |
| 0–19 Years | 5 | 1.7 | 1 | 1 | 1 | 1 | 2 | 4 | 4 | 4 |
| 20–34 | 1 | 1.0 | 0 | 1 | 1 | 1 | 1 | 1 | 1 | 1 |
| 35–49 | 0 | | | | | | | | | |
| 50–64 | 0 | | | | | | | | | |
| 65+ | 1 | 1.0 | 0 | 1 | 1 | 1 | 1 | 1 | 1 | 1 |
| **GRAND TOTAL** | 7 | 1.5 | 1 | 1 | 1 | 1 | 2 | 4 | 4 | 4 |

## 23.6: PROSTHETIC DENTAL IMPL. Formerly included in operation group(s) 547.

| Type of Patients | Observed Patients | Avg. Stay | Variance | 10th | 25th | 50th | 75th | 90th | 95th | 99th |
|---|---|---|---|---|---|---|---|---|---|---|
| **1. SINGLE DX** | | | | | | | | | | |
| 0–19 Years | 0 | | | | | | | | | |
| 20–34 | 1 | 1.0 | 0 | 1 | 1 | 1 | 1 | 1 | 1 | 1 |
| 35–49 | 1 | 2.0 | 0 | 2 | 2 | 2 | 2 | 2 | 2 | 2 |
| 50–64 | 0 | | | | | | | | | |
| 65+ | 0 | | | | | | | | | |
| **2. MULTIPLE DX** | | | | | | | | | | |
| 0–19 Years | 1 | 1.0 | 0 | 1 | 1 | 1 | 1 | 1 | 1 | 1 |
| 20–34 | 2 | 1.9 | <1 | 2 | 2 | 2 | 2 | 2 | 2 | 2 |
| 35–49 | 1 | 1.0 | 0 | 1 | 1 | 1 | 1 | 1 | 1 | 1 |
| 50–64 | 1 | 1.0 | 0 | 1 | 1 | 1 | 1 | 1 | 1 | 1 |
| 65+ | 2 | 1.0 | 0 | 1 | 1 | 1 | 1 | 1 | 1 | 1 |
| **TOTAL SINGLE DX** | 2 | 1.2 | <1 | 1 | 1 | 1 | 1 | 1 | 2 | 2 |
| **TOTAL MULTIPLE DX** | 7 | 1.8 | <1 | 1 | 2 | 2 | 2 | 2 | 2 | 2 |
| **TOTAL** | | | | | | | | | | |
| 0–19 Years | 1 | 1.0 | 0 | 1 | 1 | 1 | 1 | 1 | 1 | 1 |
| 20–34 | 3 | 1.9 | <1 | 1 | 1 | 2 | 2 | 2 | 2 | 2 |
| 35–49 | 2 | 1.4 | <1 | 1 | 1 | 1 | 1 | 2 | 2 | 2 |
| 50–64 | 1 | 1.0 | <1 | 1 | 1 | 1 | 1 | 1 | 1 | 1 |
| 65+ | 2 | 1.0 | 0 | 1 | 1 | 1 | 1 | 1 | 1 | 1 |
| **GRAND TOTAL** | 9 | 1.8 | <1 | 1 | 2 | 2 | 2 | 2 | 2 | 2 |

Length of Stay by Diagnosis and Operation, United States, 2000

# United States, October 1998–September 1999 Data, by Operation

## 23.7: ROOT CANAL TX & APICOECT. Formerly included in operation group(s) 548.

| Type of Patients | Observed Patients | Avg. Stay | Variance | 10th | 25th | 50th | 75th | 90th | 95th | 99th |
|---|---|---|---|---|---|---|---|---|---|---|
| **1. SINGLE DX** | | | | | | | | | | |
| 0–19 Years | 3 | 1.2 | <1 | 1 | 1 | 1 | 1 | 2 | 2 | 2 |
| 20–34 | 0 | | | | | | | | | |
| 35–49 | 0 | | | | | | | | | |
| 50–64 | 0 | | | | | | | | | |
| 65+ | 0 | | | | | | | | | |
| **2. MULTIPLE DX** | | | | | | | | | | |
| 0–19 Years | 13 | 1.9 | 2 | 1 | 1 | 2 | 2 | 4 | 4 | 7 |
| 20–34 | 4 | 5.8 | 56 | 1 | 1 | 1 | 18 | 18 | 18 | 18 |
| 35–49 | 3 | 2.8 | <1 | 2 | 2 | 3 | 3 | 4 | 4 | 4 |
| 50–64 | 1 | 6.0 | 0 | 6 | 6 | 6 | 6 | 6 | 6 | 6 |
| 65+ | 2 | 10.1 | 39 | 4 | 4 | 15 | 15 | 15 | 15 | 15 |
| **TOTAL SINGLE DX** | 3 | 1.2 | <1 | 1 | 1 | 1 | 1 | 2 | 2 | 2 |
| **TOTAL MULTIPLE DX** | 23 | 3.2 | 19 | 1 | 1 | 2 | 3 | 7 | 18 | 18 |
| **TOTAL** | | | | | | | | | | |
| 0–19 Years | 16 | 1.9 | 2 | 1 | 1 | 1 | 2 | 4 | 4 | 7 |
| 20–34 | 4 | 5.8 | 56 | 1 | 1 | 1 | 18 | 18 | 18 | 18 |
| 35–49 | 3 | 2.8 | <1 | 2 | 2 | 3 | 3 | 4 | 4 | 4 |
| 50–64 | 1 | 6.0 | 0 | 6 | 6 | 6 | 6 | 6 | 6 | 6 |
| 65+ | 2 | 10.1 | 39 | 4 | 4 | 15 | 15 | 15 | 15 | 15 |
| **GRAND TOTAL** | 26 | 3.1 | 18 | 1 | 1 | 2 | 3 | 7 | 15 | 18 |

## 24.1: TOOTH & GUM DXTIC PX. Formerly included in operation group(s) 548, 556.

| Type of Patients | Observed Patients | Avg. Stay | Variance | 10th | 25th | 50th | 75th | 90th | 95th | 99th |
|---|---|---|---|---|---|---|---|---|---|---|
| **1. SINGLE DX** | | | | | | | | | | |
| 0–19 Years | 0 | | | | | | | | | |
| 20–34 | 0 | | | | | | | | | |
| 35–49 | 0 | | | | | | | | | |
| 50–64 | 0 | | | | | | | | | |
| 65+ | 0 | | | | | | | | | |
| **2. MULTIPLE DX** | | | | | | | | | | |
| 0–19 Years | 2 | 4.9 | 35 | 1 | 1 | 1 | 12 | 12 | 12 | 12 |
| 20–34 | 3 | 7.5 | 10 | 6 | 6 | 6 | 6 | 13 | 13 | 13 |
| 35–49 | 2 | 4.9 | 26 | 1 | 1 | 1 | 9 | 9 | 9 | 9 |
| 50–64 | 1 | 10.0 | 0 | 10 | 10 | 10 | 10 | 10 | 10 | 10 |
| 65+ | 8 | 4.2 | 8 | 2 | 2 | 4 | 5 | 9 | 11 | 11 |
| **TOTAL SINGLE DX** | 0 | | | | | | | | | |
| **TOTAL MULTIPLE DX** | 16 | 4.9 | 12 | 2 | 2 | 5 | 6 | 10 | 12 | 13 |
| **TOTAL** | | | | | | | | | | |
| 0–19 Years | 2 | 4.9 | 35 | 1 | 1 | 1 | 12 | 12 | 12 | 12 |
| 20–34 | 3 | 7.5 | 10 | 6 | 6 | 6 | 6 | 13 | 13 | 13 |
| 35–49 | 2 | 4.9 | 26 | 1 | 1 | 1 | 9 | 9 | 9 | 9 |
| 50–64 | 1 | 10.0 | 0 | 10 | 10 | 10 | 10 | 10 | 10 | 10 |
| 65+ | 8 | 4.2 | 8 | 2 | 2 | 4 | 5 | 9 | 11 | 11 |
| **GRAND TOTAL** | 16 | 4.9 | 12 | 2 | 2 | 5 | 6 | 10 | 12 | 13 |

## 24.0: GUM OR ALVEOLAR INCISION. Formerly included in operation group(s) 548.

| Type of Patients | Observed Patients | Avg. Stay | Variance | 10th | 25th | 50th | 75th | 90th | 95th | 99th |
|---|---|---|---|---|---|---|---|---|---|---|
| **1. SINGLE DX** | | | | | | | | | | |
| 0–19 Years | 10 | 2.6 | 4 | 2 | 2 | 2 | 2 | 4 | 6 | 11 |
| 20–34 | 11 | 2.7 | 2 | 2 | 2 | 2 | 3 | 6 | 6 | 6 |
| 35–49 | 12 | 4.1 | 3 | 2 | 3 | 3 | 5 | 7 | 7 | 7 |
| 50–64 | 0 | | | | | | | | | |
| 65+ | 0 | | | | | | | | | |
| **2. MULTIPLE DX** | | | | | | | | | | |
| 0–19 Years | 58 | 3.0 | 2 | 1 | 2 | 3 | 3 | 5 | 5 | 5 |
| 20–34 | 46 | 2.7 | 2 | 1 | 2 | 2 | 3 | 4 | 6 | 6 |
| 35–49 | 50 | 3.8 | 13 | 2 | 2 | 4 | 4 | 5 | 7 | 30 |
| 50–64 | 23 | 3.4 | 2 | 2 | 2 | 3 | 4 | 5 | 7 | 7 |
| 65+ | 15 | 6.5 | 11 | 3 | 4 | 6 | 8 | 13 | 13 | 13 |
| **TOTAL SINGLE DX** | 33 | 3.3 | 4 | 2 | 2 | 2 | 5 | 7 | 7 | 11 |
| **TOTAL MULTIPLE DX** | 192 | 3.3 | 5 | 1 | 2 | 3 | 4 | 5 | 6 | 12 |
| **TOTAL** | | | | | | | | | | |
| 0–19 Years | 68 | 3.0 | 2 | 1 | 2 | 3 | 3 | 5 | 5 | 6 |
| 20–34 | 57 | 2.7 | 2 | 1 | 2 | 2 | 3 | 4 | 6 | 6 |
| 35–49 | 62 | 3.9 | 10 | 2 | 2 | 3 | 5 | 6 | 7 | 30 |
| 50–64 | 23 | 3.4 | 2 | 2 | 2 | 3 | 4 | 5 | 7 | 7 |
| 65+ | 15 | 6.5 | 11 | 3 | 4 | 6 | 8 | 13 | 13 | 13 |
| **GRAND TOTAL** | 225 | 3.3 | 5 | 2 | 2 | 3 | 4 | 5 | 6 | 11 |

## 24.2: GINGIVOPLASTY. Formerly included in operation group(s) 548.

| Type of Patients | Observed Patients | Avg. Stay | Variance | 10th | 25th | 50th | 75th | 90th | 95th | 99th |
|---|---|---|---|---|---|---|---|---|---|---|
| **1. SINGLE DX** | | | | | | | | | | |
| 0–19 Years | 2 | 1.0 | 0 | 1 | 1 | 1 | 1 | 1 | 1 | 1 |
| 20–34 | 0 | | | | | | | | | |
| 35–49 | 0 | | | | | | | | | |
| 50–64 | 0 | | | | | | | | | |
| 65+ | 0 | | | | | | | | | |
| **2. MULTIPLE DX** | | | | | | | | | | |
| 0–19 Years | 5 | 4.5 | 8 | 1 | 2 | 7 | 7 | 7 | 7 | 7 |
| 20–34 | 1 | 2.0 | 0 | 2 | 2 | 2 | 2 | 2 | 2 | 2 |
| 35–49 | 2 | 1.4 | <1 | 1 | 1 | 1 | 2 | 2 | 2 | 2 |
| 50–64 | 2 | 1.5 | <1 | 1 | 1 | 2 | 2 | 2 | 2 | 2 |
| 65+ | 2 | 2.8 | 6 | 1 | 1 | 1 | 5 | 5 | 5 | 5 |
| **TOTAL SINGLE DX** | 2 | 1.0 | 0 | 1 | 1 | 1 | 1 | 1 | 1 | 1 |
| **TOTAL MULTIPLE DX** | 12 | 3.4 | 7 | 1 | 1 | 2 | 7 | 7 | 7 | 7 |
| **TOTAL** | | | | | | | | | | |
| 0–19 Years | 7 | 4.2 | 8 | 1 | 1 | 2 | 7 | 7 | 7 | 7 |
| 20–34 | 1 | 2.0 | 0 | 2 | 2 | 2 | 2 | 2 | 2 | 2 |
| 35–49 | 2 | 1.4 | <1 | 1 | 1 | 1 | 2 | 2 | 2 | 2 |
| 50–64 | 2 | 1.5 | <1 | 1 | 1 | 1 | 5 | 5 | 5 | 5 |
| 65+ | 2 | 2.8 | 6 | 1 | 1 | 1 | 5 | 5 | 5 | 5 |
| **GRAND TOTAL** | 14 | 3.2 | 6 | 1 | 1 | 2 | 7 | 7 | 7 | 7 |

Length of Stay by Diagnosis and Operation, United States, 2000

# United States, October 1998–September 1999 Data, by Operation

## 24.3: OTHER OPERATIONS ON GUMS. Formerly included in operation group(s) 548.

| Type of Patients | Observed Patients | Avg. Stay | Variance | 10th | 25th | 50th | 75th | 90th | 95th | 99th |
|---|---|---|---|---|---|---|---|---|---|---|
| **1. SINGLE DX** | | | | | | | | | | |
| 0–19 Years | 6 | 1.7 | 1 | 1 | 1 | 1 | 2 | 3 | 5 | 5 |
| 20–34 | 0 | | | | | | | | | |
| 35–49 | 0 | | | | | | | | | |
| 50–64 | 1 | 1.0 | 0 | 1 | 1 | 1 | 1 | 1 | 1 | 1 |
| 65+ | 3 | 1.4 | <1 | 1 | 1 | 1 | 2 | 2 | 2 | 2 |
| **2. MULTIPLE DX** | | | | | | | | | | |
| 0–19 Years | 38 | 3.1 | 8 | 1 | 1 | 2 | 6 | 6 | 9 | 11 |
| 20–34 | 14 | 2.2 | 2 | 1 | 1 | 2 | 2 | 3 | 5 | 8 |
| 35–49 | 10 | 2.6 | 3 | 1 | 1 | 2 | 4 | 6 | 6 | 6 |
| 50–64 | 7 | 5.5 | 57 | 1 | 2 | 3 | 8 | 8 | 28 | 28 |
| 65+ | 19 | 5.4 | 17 | 1 | 2 | 4 | 8 | 12 | 13 | 13 |
| **TOTAL SINGLE DX** | 10 | 1.6 | 1 | 1 | 1 | 1 | 2 | 2 | 4 | 5 |
| **TOTAL MULTIPLE DX** | 88 | 3.4 | 11 | 1 | 1 | 2 | 5 | 8 | 10 | 13 |
| **TOTAL** | | | | | | | | | | |
| 0–19 Years | 44 | 2.9 | 7 | 1 | 1 | 2 | 4 | 6 | 9 | 11 |
| 20–34 | 14 | 2.2 | 2 | 1 | 1 | 2 | 2 | 3 | 5 | 8 |
| 35–49 | 10 | 2.6 | 3 | 1 | 1 | 2 | 4 | 6 | 6 | 6 |
| 50–64 | 8 | 5.1 | 53 | 1 | 1 | 3 | 8 | 8 | 28 | 28 |
| 65+ | 22 | 5.0 | 17 | 1 | 2 | 3 | 8 | 12 | 13 | 13 |
| **GRAND TOTAL** | 98 | 3.2 | 11 | 1 | 1 | 2 | 4 | 7 | 10 | 13 |

## 24.4: EXC OF DENTAL LES OF JAW. Formerly included in operation group(s) 548.

| Type of Patients | Observed Patients | Avg. Stay | Variance | 10th | 25th | 50th | 75th | 90th | 95th | 99th |
|---|---|---|---|---|---|---|---|---|---|---|
| **1. SINGLE DX** | | | | | | | | | | |
| 0–19 Years | 18 | 1.0 | <1 | 1 | 1 | 1 | 1 | 1 | 1 | 2 |
| 20–34 | 5 | 1.9 | <1 | 2 | 2 | 2 | 2 | 2 | 2 | 2 |
| 35–49 | 6 | 1.6 | <1 | 1 | 1 | 2 | 2 | 2 | 2 | 2 |
| 50–64 | 1 | 2.0 | 0 | 2 | 2 | 2 | 2 | 2 | 2 | 2 |
| 65+ | 1 | 3.0 | 0 | 3 | 3 | 3 | 3 | 3 | 3 | 3 |
| **2. MULTIPLE DX** | | | | | | | | | | |
| 0–19 Years | 32 | 2.4 | 7 | 1 | 1 | 1 | 3 | 9 | 9 | 9 |
| 20–34 | 11 | 3.8 | 23 | 1 | 1 | 1 | 3 | 15 | 15 | 15 |
| 35–49 | 30 | 7.0 | 99 | 1 | 2 | 2 | 10 | 17 | 37 | 37 |
| 50–64 | 17 | 4.4 | 32 | 2 | 3 | 3 | 3 | 5 | 23 | 31 |
| 65+ | 31 | 3.1 | 10 | 1 | 1 | 2 | 3 | 10 | 11 | 12 |
| **TOTAL SINGLE DX** | 31 | 1.3 | <1 | 1 | 1 | 1 | 2 | 2 | 2 | 2 |
| **TOTAL MULTIPLE DX** | 121 | 4.3 | 41 | 1 | 1 | 3 | 3 | 10 | 15 | 37 |
| **TOTAL** | | | | | | | | | | |
| 0–19 Years | 50 | 1.8 | 4 | 1 | 1 | 1 | 1 | 3 | 9 | 9 |
| 20–34 | 16 | 2.7 | 10 | 1 | 2 | 2 | 2 | 3 | 12 | 15 |
| 35–49 | 36 | 6.5 | 92 | 2 | 3 | 3 | 9 | 17 | 37 | 37 |
| 50–64 | 18 | 4.3 | 32 | 2 | 3 | 3 | 3 | 5 | 23 | 31 |
| 65+ | 32 | 3.1 | 10 | 1 | 1 | 2 | 3 | 10 | 11 | 12 |
| **GRAND TOTAL** | 152 | 3.6 | 33 | 1 | 2 | 2 | 3 | 9 | 11 | 37 |

## 24.5: ALVEOLOPLASTY. Formerly included in operation group(s) 548.

| Type of Patients | Observed Patients | Avg. Stay | Variance | 10th | 25th | 50th | 75th | 90th | 95th | 99th |
|---|---|---|---|---|---|---|---|---|---|---|
| **1. SINGLE DX** | | | | | | | | | | |
| 0–19 Years | 60 | 1.2 | <1 | 1 | 1 | 1 | 1 | 2 | 2 | 4 |
| 20–34 | 0 | | | | | | | | | |
| 35–49 | 1 | 1.0 | 0 | 1 | 1 | 1 | 1 | 1 | 1 | 1 |
| 50–64 | 0 | | | | | | | | | |
| 65+ | 2 | 1.7 | <1 | 1 | 1 | 2 | 2 | 2 | 2 | 2 |
| **2. MULTIPLE DX** | | | | | | | | | | |
| 0–19 Years | 150 | 1.3 | 1 | 1 | 1 | 1 | 1 | 2 | 2 | 4 |
| 20–34 | 24 | 11.8 | 80 | 4 | 6 | 8 | 26 | 26 | 26 | 26 |
| 35–49 | 99 | 6.8 | 42 | 1 | 2 | 5 | 9 | 13 | 23 | 34 |
| 50–64 | 110 | 6.3 | 42 | 1 | 2 | 4 | 8 | 14 | 17 | 31 |
| 65+ | 122 | 11.7 | 239 | 1 | 2 | 5 | 14 | 48 | 48 | 48 |
| **TOTAL SINGLE DX** | 63 | 1.2 | <1 | 1 | 1 | 1 | 1 | 2 | 2 | 4 |
| **TOTAL MULTIPLE DX** | 505 | 6.0 | 81 | 1 | 1 | 2 | 8 | 15 | 26 | 48 |
| **TOTAL** | | | | | | | | | | |
| 0–19 Years | 210 | 1.3 | 1 | 1 | 1 | 1 | 1 | 2 | 2 | 4 |
| 20–34 | 24 | 11.8 | 80 | 4 | 6 | 8 | 26 | 26 | 26 | 26 |
| 35–49 | 100 | 6.8 | 42 | 1 | 2 | 5 | 9 | 13 | 23 | 34 |
| 50–64 | 110 | 6.3 | 42 | 1 | 2 | 4 | 8 | 14 | 17 | 31 |
| 65+ | 124 | 11.4 | 235 | 1 | 2 | 5 | 14 | 48 | 48 | 48 |
| **GRAND TOTAL** | 568 | 5.4 | 73 | 1 | 1 | 2 | 6 | 13 | 26 | 48 |

## 24.6: EXPOSURE OF TOOTH. Formerly included in operation group(s) 547.

| Type of Patients | Observed Patients | Avg. Stay | Variance | 10th | 25th | 50th | 75th | 90th | 95th | 99th |
|---|---|---|---|---|---|---|---|---|---|---|
| **1. SINGLE DX** | | | | | | | | | | |
| 0–19 Years | 0 | | | | | | | | | |
| 20–34 | 0 | | | | | | | | | |
| 35–49 | 0 | | | | | | | | | |
| 50–64 | 0 | | | | | | | | | |
| 65+ | 0 | | | | | | | | | |
| **2. MULTIPLE DX** | | | | | | | | | | |
| 0–19 Years | 0 | | | | | | | | | |
| 20–34 | 0 | | | | | | | | | |
| 35–49 | 1 | 1.0 | 0 | 1 | 1 | 1 | 1 | 1 | 1 | 1 |
| 50–64 | 0 | | | | | | | | | |
| 65+ | 0 | | | | | | | | | |
| **TOTAL SINGLE DX** | 0 | | | | | | | | | |
| **TOTAL MULTIPLE DX** | 1 | 1.0 | 0 | 1 | 1 | 1 | 1 | 1 | 1 | 1 |
| **TOTAL** | | | | | | | | | | |
| 0–19 Years | 0 | | | | | | | | | |
| 20–34 | 0 | | | | | | | | | |
| 35–49 | 1 | 1.0 | 0 | 1 | 1 | 1 | 1 | 1 | 1 | 1 |
| 50–64 | 0 | | | | | | | | | |
| 65+ | 0 | | | | | | | | | |
| **GRAND TOTAL** | 1 | 1.0 | 0 | 1 | 1 | 1 | 1 | 1 | 1 | 1 |

## United States, October 1998–September 1999 Data, by Operation

### 24.7: APPL ORTHODONT APPLIANCE. Formerly included in operation group(s) 547.

| Type of Patients | Observed Patients | Avg. Stay | Variance | Percentiles | | | | | | |
|---|---|---|---|---|---|---|---|---|---|---|
| | | | | 10th | 25th | 50th | 75th | 90th | 95th | 99th |
| **1. SINGLE DX** | | | | | | | | | | |
| 0–19 Years | 12 | 1.3 | <1 | 1 | 1 | 1 | 1 | 2 | 3 | 3 |
| 20–34 | 1 | 2.0 | 0 | 2 | 2 | 2 | 2 | 2 | 2 | 2 |
| 35–49 | 0 | | | | | | | | | |
| 50–64 | 0 | | | | | | | | | |
| 65+ | 0 | | | | | | | | | |
| **2. MULTIPLE DX** | | | | | | | | | | |
| 0–19 Years | 7 | 1.8 | 4 | 1 | 1 | 2 | 2 | 3 | 3 | 10 |
| 20–34 | 5 | 3.3 | 4 | 2 | 2 | 3 | 3 | 3 | 9 | 9 |
| 35–49 | 2 | 4.6 | 17 | 1 | 1 | 8 | 8 | 8 | 8 | 8 |
| 50–64 | 2 | 2.5 | <1 | 2 | 2 | 3 | 3 | 3 | 3 | 3 |
| 65+ | 0 | | | | | | | | | |
| **TOTAL SINGLE DX** | 13 | 1.3 | <1 | 1 | 1 | 1 | 1 | 2 | 3 | 3 |
| **TOTAL MULTIPLE DX** | 16 | 2.5 | 5 | 1 | 2 | 2 | 3 | 3 | 9 | 10 |
| **TOTAL** | | | | | | | | | | |
| 0–19 Years | 19 | 1.4 | 1 | 1 | 1 | 1 | 1 | 2 | 3 | 10 |
| 20–34 | 6 | 3.2 | 4 | 2 | 2 | 3 | 3 | 3 | 9 | 9 |
| 35–49 | 2 | 4.6 | 17 | 1 | 1 | 8 | 8 | 8 | 8 | 8 |
| 50–64 | 2 | 2.5 | <1 | 2 | 2 | 3 | 3 | 3 | 3 | 3 |
| 65+ | 0 | | | | | | | | | |
| **GRAND TOTAL** | 29 | 1.8 | 2 | 1 | 1 | 1 | 2 | 3 | 3 | 9 |

### 24.8: OTHER ORTHODONTIC OP. Formerly included in operation group(s) 547.

| Type of Patients | Observed Patients | Avg. Stay | Variance | Percentiles | | | | | | |
|---|---|---|---|---|---|---|---|---|---|---|
| | | | | 10th | 25th | 50th | 75th | 90th | 95th | 99th |
| **1. SINGLE DX** | | | | | | | | | | |
| 0–19 Years | 0 | | | | | | | | | |
| 20–34 | 2 | 2.9 | 3 | 2 | 2 | 2 | 5 | 5 | 5 | 5 |
| 35–49 | 1 | 1.0 | 0 | 1 | 1 | 1 | 1 | 1 | 1 | 1 |
| 50–64 | 0 | | | | | | | | | |
| 65+ | 0 | | | | | | | | | |
| **2. MULTIPLE DX** | | | | | | | | | | |
| 0–19 Years | 3 | 1.4 | <1 | 1 | 1 | 1 | 2 | 2 | 2 | 2 |
| 20–34 | 1 | 1.0 | 0 | 1 | 1 | 1 | 1 | 1 | 1 | 1 |
| 35–49 | 1 | 7.0 | 0 | 7 | 7 | 7 | 7 | 7 | 7 | 7 |
| 50–64 | 0 | | | | | | | | | |
| 65+ | 1 | 2.0 | | 2 | 2 | 2 | 2 | 2 | 2 | 2 |
| **TOTAL SINGLE DX** | 3 | 2.4 | 3 | 1 | 2 | 2 | 2 | 5 | 5 | 5 |
| **TOTAL MULTIPLE DX** | 6 | 2.0 | 4 | 1 | 1 | 1 | 2 | 2 | 7 | 7 |
| **TOTAL** | | | | | | | | | | |
| 0–19 Years | 3 | 1.4 | <1 | 1 | 1 | 1 | 2 | 2 | 2 | 2 |
| 20–34 | 3 | 1.6 | 2 | 1 | 1 | 1 | 2 | 2 | 5 | 5 |
| 35–49 | 2 | 5.4 | 9 | 1 | 1 | 7 | 7 | 7 | 7 | 7 |
| 50–64 | 0 | | | | | | | | | |
| 65+ | 1 | 2.0 | | 2 | 2 | 2 | 2 | 2 | 2 | 2 |
| **GRAND TOTAL** | 9 | 2.1 | 3 | 1 | 1 | 1 | 2 | 5 | 7 | 7 |

### 24.9: OTHER DENTAL OPERATION. Formerly included in operation group(s) 548.

| Type of Patients | Observed Patients | Avg. Stay | Variance | Percentiles | | | | | | |
|---|---|---|---|---|---|---|---|---|---|---|
| | | | | 10th | 25th | 50th | 75th | 90th | 95th | 99th |
| **1. SINGLE DX** | | | | | | | | | | |
| 0–19 Years | 1 | 1.0 | 0 | 1 | 1 | 1 | 1 | 1 | 1 | 1 |
| 20–34 | 0 | | | | | | | | | |
| 35–49 | 0 | | | | | | | | | |
| 50–64 | 1 | 3.0 | 0 | 3 | 3 | 3 | 3 | 3 | 3 | 3 |
| 65+ | 0 | | | | | | | | | |
| **2. MULTIPLE DX** | | | | | | | | | | |
| 0–19 Years | 3 | 2.3 | 1 | 1 | 1 | 3 | 3 | 3 | 3 | 3 |
| 20–34 | 1 | 2.0 | 0 | 2 | 2 | 2 | 3 | 3 | 2 | 2 |
| 35–49 | 4 | 21.7 | 738 | 1 | 2 | 2 | 55 | 55 | 55 | 55 |
| 50–64 | 2 | 2.4 | <1 | 1 | 1 | 3 | 3 | 3 | 3 | 3 |
| 65+ | 3 | 2.4 | 3 | 1 | 2 | 2 | 2 | 7 | 7 | 7 |
| **TOTAL SINGLE DX** | 2 | 2.3 | 1 | 1 | 1 | 3 | 3 | 3 | 3 | 3 |
| **TOTAL MULTIPLE DX** | 13 | 7.2 | 245 | 1 | 2 | 2 | 3 | 7 | 55 | 55 |
| **TOTAL** | | | | | | | | | | |
| 0–19 Years | 4 | 2.1 | 1 | 1 | 1 | 3 | 3 | 3 | 3 | 3 |
| 20–34 | 1 | 2.0 | 0 | 2 | 2 | 2 | 2 | 2 | 2 | 2 |
| 35–49 | 4 | 21.7 | 738 | 1 | 2 | 2 | 55 | 55 | 55 | 55 |
| 50–64 | 3 | 2.6 | <1 | 1 | 3 | 3 | 3 | 3 | 3 | 3 |
| 65+ | 3 | 2.4 | 3 | 1 | 2 | 2 | 2 | 7 | 7 | 7 |
| **GRAND TOTAL** | 15 | 6.8 | 226 | 1 | 2 | 2 | 3 | 7 | 55 | 55 |

### 25.0: DXTIC PX ON TONGUE. Formerly included in operation group(s) 551, 556.

| Type of Patients | Observed Patients | Avg. Stay | Variance | Percentiles | | | | | | |
|---|---|---|---|---|---|---|---|---|---|---|
| | | | | 10th | 25th | 50th | 75th | 90th | 95th | 99th |
| **1. SINGLE DX** | | | | | | | | | | |
| 0–19 Years | 1 | 1.0 | 0 | 1 | 1 | 1 | 1 | 1 | 1 | 1 |
| 20–34 | 0 | | | | | | | | | |
| 35–49 | 3 | 1.8 | 2 | 1 | 1 | 1 | 4 | 4 | 4 | 4 |
| 50–64 | 2 | 9.8 | 46 | 4 | 4 | 15 | 15 | 15 | 15 | 15 |
| 65+ | 3 | 1.0 | 0 | 1 | 1 | 1 | 1 | 1 | 1 | 1 |
| **2. MULTIPLE DX** | | | | | | | | | | |
| 0–19 Years | 4 | 3.6 | 7 | 1 | 3 | 5 | 5 | 8 | 8 | 8 |
| 20–34 | 8 | 5.8 | 14 | 1 | 3 | 6 | 6 | 13 | 13 | 13 |
| 35–49 | 27 | 11.1 | 110 | 2 | 4 | 8 | 12 | 35 | 35 | 35 |
| 50–64 | 46 | 7.7 | 52 | 1 | 3 | 6 | 11 | 15 | 20 | 43 |
| 65+ | 58 | 8.1 | 81 | 1 | 6 | 6 | 11 | 18 | 37 | 37 |
| **TOTAL SINGLE DX** | 9 | 2.9 | 18 | 1 | 1 | 1 | 4 | 4 | 15 | 15 |
| **TOTAL MULTIPLE DX** | 143 | 8.1 | 68 | 1 | 2 | 6 | 11 | 17 | 29 | 37 |
| **TOTAL** | | | | | | | | | | |
| 0–19 Years | 5 | 3.1 | 6 | 1 | 3 | 5 | 5 | 5 | 8 | 8 |
| 20–34 | 8 | 5.8 | 14 | 1 | 3 | 6 | 6 | 13 | 13 | 13 |
| 35–49 | 30 | 10.4 | 107 | 1 | 4 | 8 | 12 | 35 | 35 | 35 |
| 50–64 | 48 | 7.8 | 52 | 1 | 3 | 6 | 11 | 15 | 20 | 43 |
| 65+ | 61 | 7.9 | 80 | 1 | 6 | 6 | 10 | 17 | 37 | 37 |
| **GRAND TOTAL** | 152 | 7.9 | 67 | 1 | 2 | 6 | 11 | 17 | 29 | 37 |

Length of Stay by Diagnosis and Operation

# United States, October 1998–September 1999 Data, by Operation

## 25.1: EXC/DESTR TONGUE LES. Formerly included in operation group(s) 551.

| Type of Patients | Observed Patients | Avg. Stay | Variance | 10th | 25th | 50th | 75th | 90th | 95th | 99th |
|---|---|---|---|---|---|---|---|---|---|---|
| **1. SINGLE DX** | | | | | | | | | | |
| 0–19 Years | 13 | 1.2 | <1 | 1 | 1 | 1 | 1 | 1 | 2 | 7 |
| 20–34 | 3 | 2.8 | 3 | 1 | 1 | 4 | 4 | 4 | 4 | 4 |
| 35–49 | 8 | 3.1 | 8 | 1 | 1 | 1 | 4 | 8 | 9 | 9 |
| 50–64 | 5 | 2.0 | <1 | 1 | 1 | 2 | 3 | 3 | 3 | 3 |
| 65+ | 4 | 1.1 | <1 | 1 | 1 | 1 | 1 | 2 | 2 | 2 |
| **2. MULTIPLE DX** | | | | | | | | | | |
| 0–19 Years | 15 | 1.7 | 1 | 1 | 1 | 1 | 3 | 3 | 3 | 5 |
| 20–34 | 11 | 3.7 | 4 | 1 | 1 | 5 | 5 | 5 | 6 | 9 |
| 35–49 | 28 | 5.0 | 35 | 1 | 1 | 3 | 7 | 10 | 12 | 37 |
| 50–64 | 56 | 6.3 | 119 | 1 | 2 | 4 | 6 | 8 | 14 | 48 |
| 65+ | 80 | 5.4 | 39 | 1 | 2 | 3 | 7 | 15 | 17 | 37 |
| **TOTAL SINGLE DX** | 33 | 1.7 | 3 | 1 | 1 | 1 | 2 | 4 | 4 | 9 |
| **TOTAL MULTIPLE DX** | 190 | 5.1 | 54 | 1 | 1 | 3 | 5 | 10 | 16 | 45 |
| **TOTAL** | | | | | | | | | | |
| 0–19 Years | 28 | 1.5 | 1 | 1 | 1 | 1 | 1 | 3 | 3 | 7 |
| 20–34 | 14 | 3.6 | 4 | 1 | 1 | 4 | 5 | 5 | 6 | 9 |
| 35–49 | 36 | 4.6 | 31 | 1 | 1 | 3 | 7 | 9 | 11 | 37 |
| 50–64 | 61 | 6.0 | 112 | 1 | 2 | 4 | 6 | 7 | 14 | 48 |
| 65+ | 84 | 5.2 | 38 | 1 | 2 | 3 | 7 | 13 | 17 | 37 |
| **GRAND TOTAL** | 223 | 4.6 | 48 | 1 | 1 | 3 | 5 | 9 | 15 | 45 |

## 25.2: PARTIAL GLOSSECTOMY. Formerly included in operation group(s) 551.

| Type of Patients | Observed Patients | Avg. Stay | Variance | 10th | 25th | 50th | 75th | 90th | 95th | 99th |
|---|---|---|---|---|---|---|---|---|---|---|
| **1. SINGLE DX** | | | | | | | | | | |
| 0–19 Years | 7 | 4.6 | 25 | 1 | 2 | 3 | 3 | 16 | 16 | 16 |
| 20–34 | 4 | 3.0 | 7 | 1 | 1 | 2 | 3 | 7 | 7 | 7 |
| 35–49 | 21 | 2.8 | 5 | 1 | 1 | 2 | 4 | 7 | 7 | 9 |
| 50–64 | 23 | 2.6 | 6 | 1 | 1 | 1 | 3 | 6 | 6 | 14 |
| 65+ | 15 | 2.1 | 2 | 1 | 1 | 2 | 2 | 5 | 5 | 5 |
| **2. MULTIPLE DX** | | | | | | | | | | |
| 0–19 Years | 33 | 4.3 | 24 | 2 | 2 | 5 | 5 | 7 | 11 | 37 |
| 20–34 | 11 | 7.9 | 16 | 2 | 4 | 9 | 10 | 12 | 16 | 16 |
| 35–49 | 61 | 5.4 | 17 | 1 | 2 | 5 | 7 | 8 | 12 | 31 |
| 50–64 | 121 | 5.1 | 34 | 1 | 1 | 3 | 7 | 11 | 13 | 37 |
| 65+ | 187 | 5.3 | 21 | 1 | 2 | 4 | 7 | 10 | 13 | 22 |
| **TOTAL SINGLE DX** | 70 | 2.7 | 7 | 1 | 1 | 2 | 3 | 6 | 7 | 14 |
| **TOTAL MULTIPLE DX** | 413 | 5.2 | 24 | 1 | 2 | 4 | 7 | 10 | 13 | 25 |
| **TOTAL** | | | | | | | | | | |
| 0–19 Years | 40 | 4.4 | 24 | 2 | 2 | 3 | 5 | 7 | 13 | 37 |
| 20–34 | 15 | 7.0 | 17 | 2 | 3 | 7 | 10 | 12 | 12 | 16 |
| 35–49 | 82 | 4.9 | 16 | 1 | 2 | 5 | 7 | 8 | 9 | 14 |
| 50–64 | 144 | 4.5 | 28 | 1 | 1 | 3 | 6 | 10 | 11 | 37 |
| 65+ | 202 | 5.0 | 20 | 1 | 2 | 4 | 7 | 10 | 13 | 22 |
| **GRAND TOTAL** | 483 | 4.8 | 22 | 1 | 2 | 3 | 7 | 10 | 13 | 22 |

## 25.3: COMPLETE GLOSSECTOMY. Formerly included in operation group(s) 551.

| Type of Patients | Observed Patients | Avg. Stay | Variance | 10th | 25th | 50th | 75th | 90th | 95th | 99th |
|---|---|---|---|---|---|---|---|---|---|---|
| **1. SINGLE DX** | | | | | | | | | | |
| 0–19 Years | 0 | | | | | | | | | |
| 20–34 | 0 | | | | | | | | | |
| 35–49 | 0 | | | | | | | | | |
| 50–64 | 0 | | | | | | | | | |
| 65+ | 0 | | | | | | | | | |
| **2. MULTIPLE DX** | | | | | | | | | | |
| 0–19 Years | 0 | | | | | | | | | |
| 20–34 | 1 | 7.0 | 0 | 7 | 7 | 7 | 7 | 7 | 7 | 7 |
| 35–49 | 5 | 11.8 | 44 | 7 | 7 | 11 | 13 | 24 | 24 | 24 |
| 50–64 | 4 | 10.3 | 13 | 8 | 8 | 9 | 11 | 17 | 17 | 17 |
| 65+ | 4 | 14.2 | 35 | 12 | 12 | 12 | 12 | 27 | 27 | 27 |
| **TOTAL SINGLE DX** | 0 | | | | | | | | | |
| **TOTAL MULTIPLE DX** | 14 | 11.7 | 27 | 7 | 8 | 11 | 12 | 17 | 24 | 27 |
| **TOTAL** | | | | | | | | | | |
| 0–19 Years | 0 | | | | | | | | | |
| 20–34 | 1 | 7.0 | 0 | 7 | 7 | 7 | 7 | 7 | 7 | 7 |
| 35–49 | 5 | 11.8 | 44 | 7 | 7 | 11 | 13 | 24 | 24 | 24 |
| 50–64 | 4 | 10.3 | 13 | 8 | 8 | 9 | 11 | 17 | 17 | 17 |
| 65+ | 4 | 14.2 | 35 | 12 | 12 | 12 | 12 | 27 | 27 | 27 |
| **GRAND TOTAL** | 14 | 11.7 | 27 | 7 | 8 | 11 | 12 | 17 | 24 | 27 |

## 25.4: RADICAL GLOSSECTOMY. Formerly included in operation group(s) 551.

| Type of Patients | Observed Patients | Avg. Stay | Variance | 10th | 25th | 50th | 75th | 90th | 95th | 99th |
|---|---|---|---|---|---|---|---|---|---|---|
| **1. SINGLE DX** | | | | | | | | | | |
| 0–19 Years | 0 | | | | | | | | | |
| 20–34 | 0 | | | | | | | | | |
| 35–49 | 0 | | | | | | | | | |
| 50–64 | 0 | | | | | | | | | |
| 65+ | 0 | | | | | | | | | |
| **2. MULTIPLE DX** | | | | | | | | | | |
| 0–19 Years | 0 | | | | | | | | | |
| 20–34 | 0 | | | | | | | | | |
| 35–49 | 2 | 17.5 | <1 | 17 | 17 | 17 | 18 | 18 | 18 | 18 |
| 50–64 | 5 | 12.5 | 76 | 7 | 8 | 9 | 15 | 31 | 31 | 31 |
| 65+ | 8 | 9.2 | 53 | 2 | 2 | 7 | 18 | 21 | 21 | 21 |
| **TOTAL SINGLE DX** | 0 | | | | | | | | | |
| **TOTAL MULTIPLE DX** | 15 | 10.5 | 57 | 2 | 6 | 8 | 18 | 21 | 21 | 31 |
| **TOTAL** | | | | | | | | | | |
| 0–19 Years | 0 | | | | | | | | | |
| 20–34 | 0 | | | | | | | | | |
| 35–49 | 2 | 17.5 | <1 | 17 | 17 | 17 | 18 | 18 | 18 | 18 |
| 50–64 | 5 | 12.5 | 76 | 7 | 8 | 9 | 15 | 31 | 31 | 31 |
| 65+ | 8 | 9.2 | 53 | 2 | 2 | 7 | 18 | 21 | 21 | 21 |
| **GRAND TOTAL** | 15 | 10.5 | 57 | 2 | 6 | 8 | 18 | 21 | 21 | 31 |

# United States, October 1998–September 1999 Data, by Operation

## 25.5: REPAIR OF TONGUE. Formerly included in operation group(s) 551.

| Type of Patients | Observed Patients | Avg. Stay | Variance | Percentiles | | | | | | |
|---|---|---|---|---|---|---|---|---|---|---|
| | | | | 10th | 25th | 50th | 75th | 90th | 95th | 99th |
| **1. SINGLE DX** | | | | | | | | | | |
| 0–19 Years | 19 | 1.1 | <1 | 1 | 1 | 1 | 1 | 1 | 3 | 3 |
| 20–34 | 0 | | | | | | | | | |
| 35–49 | 2 | 1.0 | 0 | 1 | 1 | 1 | 1 | 1 | 1 | 1 |
| 50–64 | 1 | 2.0 | 0 | 2 | 2 | 2 | 2 | 2 | 2 | 2 |
| 65+ | 0 | | | | | | | | | |
| **2. MULTIPLE DX** | | | | | | | | | | |
| 0–19 Years | 65 | 5.3 | 53 | 1 | 1 | 2 | 5 | 18 | 24 | 32 |
| 20–34 | 36 | 2.9 | 6 | 1 | 2 | 4 | 4 | 7 | 9 | 9 |
| 35–49 | 38 | 5.0 | 13 | 2 | 2 | 4 | 7 | 7 | 12 | 17 |
| 50–64 | 31 | 3.5 | 9 | 1 | 2 | 3 | 5 | 6 | 7 | 16 |
| 65+ | 31 | 4.9 | 19 | 1 | 2 | 4 | 6 | 9 | 18 | 18 |
| **TOTAL SINGLE DX** | 22 | 1.1 | <1 | 1 | 1 | 1 | 1 | 1 | 2 | 3 |
| **TOTAL MULTIPLE DX** | 201 | 4.7 | 24 | 1 | 1 | 2 | 7 | 10 | 17 | 24 |
| **TOTAL** | | | | | | | | | | |
| 0–19 Years | 84 | 4.5 | 46 | 1 | 1 | 1 | 4 | 17 | 18 | 24 |
| 20–34 | 36 | 2.9 | 6 | 1 | 1 | 2 | 4 | 7 | 9 | 9 |
| 35–49 | 40 | 4.9 | 13 | 2 | 2 | 4 | 7 | 7 | 12 | 17 |
| 50–64 | 32 | 3.5 | 8 | 1 | 2 | 3 | 5 | 6 | 7 | 16 |
| 65+ | 31 | 4.9 | 19 | 1 | 2 | 4 | 6 | 9 | 18 | 18 |
| **GRAND TOTAL** | 223 | 4.5 | 23 | 1 | 1 | 2 | 7 | 9 | 17 | 24 |

## 25.9: OTHER TONGUE OPERATIONS. Formerly included in operation group(s) 551, 556.

| Type of Patients | Observed Patients | Avg. Stay | Variance | Percentiles | | | | | | |
|---|---|---|---|---|---|---|---|---|---|---|
| | | | | 10th | 25th | 50th | 75th | 90th | 95th | 99th |
| **1. SINGLE DX** | | | | | | | | | | |
| 0–19 Years | 22 | 1.2 | <1 | 1 | 1 | 1 | 1 | 1 | 2 | 2 |
| 20–34 | 1 | 2.0 | 0 | 2 | 2 | 2 | 2 | 2 | 2 | 2 |
| 35–49 | 1 | 3.0 | 0 | 3 | 3 | 3 | 3 | 3 | 3 | 3 |
| 50–64 | 1 | 1.0 | 0 | 1 | 1 | 1 | 1 | 1 | 1 | 1 |
| 65+ | 1 | 4.0 | 0 | 4 | 4 | 4 | 4 | 4 | 4 | 4 |
| **2. MULTIPLE DX** | | | | | | | | | | |
| 0–19 Years | 279 | 2.7 | 9 | 1 | 2 | 2 | 3 | 4 | 6 | 21 |
| 20–34 | 6 | 2.1 | 1 | 1 | 2 | 2 | 2 | 4 | 4 | 4 |
| 35–49 | 5 | 2.5 | 4 | 1 | 1 | 3 | 3 | 6 | 6 | 6 |
| 50–64 | 3 | 1.0 | 0 | 1 | 1 | 1 | 1 | 1 | 1 | 1 |
| 65+ | 7 | 5.0 | 2 | 3 | 4 | 6 | 6 | 6 | 8 | 8 |
| **TOTAL SINGLE DX** | 26 | 1.3 | <1 | 1 | 1 | 1 | 1 | 2 | 2 | 2 |
| **TOTAL MULTIPLE DX** | 300 | 2.8 | 9 | 1 | 2 | 2 | 3 | 4 | 6 | 21 |
| **TOTAL** | | | | | | | | | | |
| 0–19 Years | 301 | 2.5 | 8 | 1 | 1 | 2 | 3 | 4 | 5 | 21 |
| 20–34 | 7 | 2.1 | 1 | 1 | 2 | 3 | 4 | 4 | 4 | 4 |
| 35–49 | 6 | 2.7 | 2 | 1 | 1 | 3 | 3 | 6 | 6 | 6 |
| 50–64 | 4 | 1.0 | 0 | 1 | 1 | 1 | 1 | 1 | 1 | 1 |
| 65+ | 8 | 4.9 | 2 | 3 | 4 | 5 | 6 | 6 | 8 | 8 |
| **GRAND TOTAL** | 326 | 2.5 | 8 | 1 | 1 | 2 | 3 | 4 | 6 | 21 |

## 26.0: INC SALIVARY GLAND/DUCT. Formerly included in operation group(s) 549.

| Type of Patients | Observed Patients | Avg. Stay | Variance | Percentiles | | | | | | |
|---|---|---|---|---|---|---|---|---|---|---|
| | | | | 10th | 25th | 50th | 75th | 90th | 95th | 99th |
| **1. SINGLE DX** | | | | | | | | | | |
| 0–19 Years | 9 | 3.7 | 5 | 1 | 1 | 4 | 6 | 6 | 8 | 8 |
| 20–34 | 6 | 2.8 | <1 | 2 | 2 | 3 | 3 | 4 | 4 | 4 |
| 35–49 | 7 | 4.2 | 10 | 1 | 3 | 4 | 4 | 5 | 13 | 13 |
| 50–64 | 5 | 3.1 | <1 | 2 | 2 | 3 | 3 | 4 | 6 | 6 |
| 65+ | 3 | 3.7 | 4 | 2 | 2 | 3 | 6 | 6 | 6 | 6 |
| **2. MULTIPLE DX** | | | | | | | | | | |
| 0–19 Years | 15 | 3.9 | 15 | 1 | 1 | 2 | 8 | 10 | 10 | 12 |
| 20–34 | 11 | 2.2 | <1 | 2 | 2 | 2 | 3 | 4 | 4 | 7 |
| 35–49 | 21 | 6.2 | 5 | 3 | 4 | 8 | 8 | 8 | 8 | 10 |
| 50–64 | 25 | 4.8 | 15 | 2 | 2 | 4 | 6 | 7 | 17 | 18 |
| 65+ | 56 | 5.9 | 15 | 2 | 4 | 4 | 7 | 11 | 13 | 22 |
| **TOTAL SINGLE DX** | 30 | 3.5 | 4 | 1 | 2 | 3 | 4 | 6 | 6 | 13 |
| **TOTAL MULTIPLE DX** | 128 | 4.4 | 11 | 2 | 2 | 3 | 6 | 8 | 10 | 17 |
| **TOTAL** | | | | | | | | | | |
| 0–19 Years | 24 | 3.8 | 10 | 1 | 1 | 3 | 6 | 10 | 10 | 12 |
| 20–34 | 17 | 2.3 | <1 | 2 | 2 | 2 | 2 | 3 | 4 | 7 |
| 35–49 | 28 | 5.8 | 7 | 2 | 4 | 5 | 8 | 8 | 8 | 13 |
| 50–64 | 30 | 4.5 | 12 | 2 | 2 | 3 | 5 | 7 | 17 | 18 |
| 65+ | 59 | 5.8 | 15 | 2 | 4 | 4 | 7 | 11 | 13 | 22 |
| **GRAND TOTAL** | 158 | 4.2 | 10 | 2 | 2 | 3 | 6 | 8 | 10 | 17 |

## 26.1: SALIVARY GLAND DXTIC PX. Formerly included in operation group(s) 549, 556.

| Type of Patients | Observed Patients | Avg. Stay | Variance | Percentiles | | | | | | |
|---|---|---|---|---|---|---|---|---|---|---|
| | | | | 10th | 25th | 50th | 75th | 90th | 95th | 99th |
| **1. SINGLE DX** | | | | | | | | | | |
| 0–19 Years | 3 | 2.2 | 7 | 1 | 1 | 1 | 1 | 7 | 7 | 7 |
| 20–34 | 0 | | | | | | | | | |
| 35–49 | 3 | 1.0 | 0 | 1 | 1 | 1 | 1 | 1 | 1 | 1 |
| 50–64 | 5 | 1.7 | <1 | 1 | 1 | 2 | 2 | 3 | 3 | 5 |
| 65+ | 1 | 4.0 | 0 | 4 | 4 | 4 | 4 | 4 | 4 | 4 |
| **2. MULTIPLE DX** | | | | | | | | | | |
| 0–19 Years | 10 | 6.9 | 247 | 1 | 1 | 3 | 7 | 7 | 8 | 76 |
| 20–34 | 9 | 10.7 | 71 | 7 | 8 | 9 | 10 | 10 | 43 | 43 |
| 35–49 | 23 | 3.5 | 17 | 1 | 1 | 1 | 4 | 8 | 8 | 27 |
| 50–64 | 30 | 6.8 | 40 | 2 | 2 | 7 | 10 | 10 | 16 | 39 |
| 65+ | 82 | 7.2 | 26 | 1 | 3 | 7 | 9 | 15 | 19 | 19 |
| **TOTAL SINGLE DX** | 12 | 1.8 | 2 | 1 | 1 | 1 | 2 | 3 | 5 | 7 |
| **TOTAL MULTIPLE DX** | 154 | 6.5 | 44 | 1 | 2 | 6 | 9 | 10 | 17 | 27 |
| **TOTAL** | | | | | | | | | | |
| 0–19 Years | 13 | 5.8 | 194 | 1 | 1 | 1 | 7 | 7 | 8 | 76 |
| 20–34 | 9 | 10.7 | 71 | 7 | 8 | 9 | 10 | 10 | 43 | 43 |
| 35–49 | 26 | 3.4 | 16 | 1 | 1 | 1 | 4 | 8 | 8 | 19 |
| 50–64 | 35 | 5.8 | 36 | 1 | 3 | 4 | 6 | 10 | 11 | 39 |
| 65+ | 83 | 7.1 | 26 | 1 | 3 | 5 | 9 | 15 | 19 | 19 |
| **GRAND TOTAL** | 166 | 6.0 | 42 | 1 | 2 | 5 | 8 | 10 | 17 | 27 |

Length of Stay by Diagnosis and Operation, United States, 2000

# United States, October 1998–September 1999 Data, by Operation

## 26.2: EXC OF SG LESION. Formerly included in operation group(s) 549.

| Type of Patients | Observed Patients | Avg. Stay | Vari-ance | 10th | 25th | 50th | 75th | 90th | 95th | 99th |
|---|---|---|---|---|---|---|---|---|---|---|
| **1. SINGLE DX** | | | | | | | | | | |
| 0–19 Years | 25 | 1.3 | 1 | 1 | 1 | 1 | 2 | 3 | 3 | 7 |
| 20–34 | 14 | 1.6 | <1 | 1 | 1 | 1 | 2 | 3 | 3 | 3 |
| 35–49 | 15 | 1.2 | <1 | 1 | 1 | 1 | 1 | 2 | 2 | 2 |
| 50–64 | 19 | 1.4 | 1 | 1 | 1 | 1 | 1 | 2 | 2 | 7 |
| 65+ | 10 | 1.3 | <1 | 1 | 1 | 1 | 2 | 2 | 3 | 2 |
| **2. MULTIPLE DX** | | | | | | | | | | |
| 0–19 Years | 19 | 6.0 | 39 | 1 | 2 | 4 | 7 | 17 | 17 | 17 |
| 20–34 | 8 | 1.4 | <1 | 1 | 1 | 1 | 2 | 3 | 3 | 3 |
| 35–49 | 18 | 2.2 | 8 | 1 | 1 | 1 | 3 | 6 | 6 | 16 |
| 50–64 | 26 | 4.0 | 50 | 1 | 1 | 2 | 6 | 7 | 14 | 48 |
| 65+ | 54 | 2.2 | 9 | 1 | 1 | 1 | 2 | 5 | 6 | 18 |
| **TOTAL SINGLE DX** | 83 | 1.4 | <1 | 1 | 1 | 1 | 1 | 2 | 2 | 7 |
| **TOTAL MULTIPLE DX** | 125 | 3.1 | 21 | 1 | 1 | 1 | 4 | 6 | 16 | 17 |
| **TOTAL** | | | | | | | | | | |
| 0–19 Years | 44 | 3.5 | 24 | 1 | 1 | 1 | 4 | 17 | 17 | 17 |
| 20–34 | 22 | 1.5 | <1 | 1 | 1 | 1 | 2 | 2 | 3 | 3 |
| 35–49 | 33 | 1.8 | 5 | 1 | 1 | 1 | 2 | 3 | 6 | 16 |
| 50–64 | 45 | 2.2 | 17 | 1 | 1 | 1 | 2 | 3 | 7 | 14 |
| 65+ | 64 | 2.2 | 8 | 1 | 1 | 1 | 2 | 5 | 5 | 18 |
| **GRAND TOTAL** | 208 | 2.4 | 13 | 1 | 1 | 1 | 2 | 5 | 7 | 17 |

## 26.3: SIALOADENECTOMY. Formerly included in operation group(s) 549.

| Type of Patients | Observed Patients | Avg. Stay | Vari-ance | 10th | 25th | 50th | 75th | 90th | 95th | 99th |
|---|---|---|---|---|---|---|---|---|---|---|
| **1. SINGLE DX** | | | | | | | | | | |
| 0–19 Years | 65 | 1.7 | 2 | 1 | 1 | 1 | 2 | 2 | 3 | 7 |
| 20–34 | 143 | 1.3 | <1 | 1 | 1 | 1 | 1 | 2 | 2 | 4 |
| 35–49 | 258 | 1.4 | <1 | 1 | 1 | 1 | 2 | 2 | 3 | 5 |
| 50–64 | 224 | 1.3 | <1 | 1 | 1 | 1 | 1 | 2 | 2 | 4 |
| 65+ | 178 | 1.6 | 2 | 1 | 1 | 1 | 2 | 2 | 3 | 13 |
| **2. MULTIPLE DX** | | | | | | | | | | |
| 0–19 Years | 93 | 3.8 | 23 | 1 | 1 | 2 | 4 | 7 | 22 | 22 |
| 20–34 | 96 | 1.7 | 2 | 1 | 1 | 1 | 2 | 3 | 4 | 9 |
| 35–49 | 316 | 2.0 | 5 | 1 | 1 | 1 | 2 | 3 | 4 | 13 |
| 50–64 | 467 | 2.1 | 6 | 1 | 1 | 1 | 2 | 4 | 6 | 12 |
| 65+ | 799 | 2.2 | 5 | 1 | 1 | 2 | 2 | 4 | 6 | 10 |
| **TOTAL SINGLE DX** | 868 | 1.4 | <1 | 1 | 1 | 1 | 2 | 2 | 3 | 5 |
| **TOTAL MULTIPLE DX** | 1,771 | 2.2 | 6 | 1 | 1 | 1 | 2 | 4 | 6 | 14 |
| **TOTAL** | | | | | | | | | | |
| 0–19 Years | 158 | 3.0 | 16 | 1 | 1 | 2 | 3 | 5 | 8 | 22 |
| 20–34 | 239 | 1.4 | 1 | 1 | 1 | 1 | 1 | 2 | 3 | 6 |
| 35–49 | 574 | 1.7 | 3 | 1 | 1 | 1 | 2 | 3 | 4 | 13 |
| 50–64 | 691 | 1.8 | 4 | 1 | 1 | 1 | 2 | 3 | 4 | 10 |
| 65+ | 977 | 2.1 | 5 | 1 | 1 | 1 | 2 | 4 | 5 | 11 |
| **GRAND TOTAL** | 2,639 | 1.9 | 5 | 1 | 1 | 1 | 2 | 3 | 5 | 12 |

## 26.30: SIALOADENECTOMY NOS. Formerly included in operation group(s) 549.

| Type of Patients | Observed Patients | Avg. Stay | Vari-ance | 10th | 25th | 50th | 75th | 90th | 95th | 99th |
|---|---|---|---|---|---|---|---|---|---|---|
| **1. SINGLE DX** | | | | | | | | | | |
| 0–19 Years | 16 | 1.5 | <1 | 1 | 1 | 1 | 2 | 3 | 3 | 3 |
| 20–34 | 25 | 1.1 | <1 | 1 | 1 | 1 | 1 | 2 | 2 | 3 |
| 35–49 | 40 | 1.3 | <1 | 1 | 1 | 1 | 1 | 2 | 2 | 3 |
| 50–64 | 28 | 1.2 | <1 | 1 | 1 | 1 | 1 | 2 | 3 | 4 |
| 65+ | 28 | 1.7 | <1 | 1 | 1 | 2 | 2 | 2 | 3 | 4 |
| **2. MULTIPLE DX** | | | | | | | | | | |
| 0–19 Years | 21 | 2.5 | 3 | 1 | 1 | 2 | 3 | 7 | 7 | 7 |
| 20–34 | 15 | 1.8 | 2 | 1 | 1 | 1 | 2 | 4 | 5 | 5 |
| 35–49 | 38 | 3.1 | 16 | 1 | 1 | 1 | 2 | 13 | 13 | 16 |
| 50–64 | 61 | 3.0 | 17 | 1 | 1 | 2 | 3 | 6 | 12 | 20 |
| 65+ | 103 | 2.6 | 8 | 1 | 1 | 2 | 3 | 5 | 7 | 17 |
| **TOTAL SINGLE DX** | 137 | 1.3 | <1 | 1 | 1 | 1 | 1 | 2 | 2 | 4 |
| **TOTAL MULTIPLE DX** | 238 | 2.7 | 11 | 1 | 1 | 2 | 3 | 5 | 9 | 20 |
| **TOTAL** | | | | | | | | | | |
| 0–19 Years | 37 | 2.2 | 3 | 1 | 1 | 2 | 3 | 3 | 7 | 7 |
| 20–34 | 40 | 1.2 | <1 | 1 | 1 | 1 | 1 | 2 | 2 | 4 |
| 35–49 | 78 | 2.2 | 9 | 1 | 1 | 1 | 2 | 3 | 13 | 13 |
| 50–64 | 89 | 2.3 | 11 | 1 | 1 | 2 | 3 | 5 | 5 | 20 |
| 65+ | 131 | 2.5 | 7 | 1 | 1 | 2 | 3 | 5 | 7 | 17 |
| **GRAND TOTAL** | 375 | 2.1 | 7 | 1 | 1 | 1 | 2 | 4 | 6 | 17 |

## 26.31: PARTIAL SIALOADENECTOMY. Formerly included in operation group(s) 549.

| Type of Patients | Observed Patients | Avg. Stay | Vari-ance | 10th | 25th | 50th | 75th | 90th | 95th | 99th |
|---|---|---|---|---|---|---|---|---|---|---|
| **1. SINGLE DX** | | | | | | | | | | |
| 0–19 Years | 22 | 1.4 | <1 | 1 | 1 | 1 | 2 | 2 | 2 | 3 |
| 20–34 | 76 | 1.2 | <1 | 1 | 1 | 1 | 1 | 2 | 2 | 3 |
| 35–49 | 126 | 1.4 | <1 | 1 | 1 | 1 | 2 | 2 | 2 | 5 |
| 50–64 | 125 | 1.2 | <1 | 1 | 1 | 1 | 1 | 2 | 3 | 4 |
| 65+ | 89 | 1.3 | <1 | 1 | 1 | 1 | 2 | 2 | 3 | 4 |
| **2. MULTIPLE DX** | | | | | | | | | | |
| 0–19 Years | 25 | 2.8 | 3 | 1 | 2 | 2 | 4 | 4 | 4 | 10 |
| 20–34 | 53 | 1.5 | 2 | 1 | 1 | 1 | 1 | 3 | 4 | 9 |
| 35–49 | 150 | 1.8 | 2 | 1 | 1 | 1 | 2 | 3 | 4 | 11 |
| 50–64 | 241 | 1.8 | 5 | 1 | 1 | 1 | 2 | 3 | 4 | 10 |
| 65+ | 365 | 1.7 | 5 | 1 | 1 | 2 | 2 | 3 | 3 | 9 |
| **TOTAL SINGLE DX** | 438 | 1.3 | <1 | 1 | 1 | 1 | 1 | 2 | 2 | 4 |
| **TOTAL MULTIPLE DX** | 834 | 1.8 | 3 | 1 | 1 | 1 | 2 | 3 | 4 | 10 |
| **TOTAL** | | | | | | | | | | |
| 0–19 Years | 47 | 2.2 | 3 | 1 | 1 | 2 | 3 | 4 | 4 | 10 |
| 20–34 | 129 | 1.4 | <1 | 1 | 1 | 1 | 1 | 2 | 3 | 6 |
| 35–49 | 276 | 1.6 | 2 | 1 | 1 | 1 | 2 | 3 | 4 | 7 |
| 50–64 | 366 | 1.6 | 3 | 1 | 1 | 1 | 2 | 3 | 4 | 10 |
| 65+ | 454 | 1.6 | 2 | 1 | 1 | 1 | 2 | 3 | 3 | 7 |
| **GRAND TOTAL** | 1,272 | 1.6 | 2 | 1 | 1 | 1 | 2 | 3 | 4 | 9 |

Length of Stay by Diagnosis and Operation, United States, 2000

# United States, October 1998–September 1999 Data, by Operation

## 26.32: COMPLETE SIALOADENECTOMY. Formerly included in operation group(s) 549.

| Type of Patients | Observed Patients | Avg. Stay | Variance | 10th | 25th | 50th | 75th | 90th | 95th | 99th |
|---|---|---|---|---|---|---|---|---|---|---|
| **1. SINGLE DX** | | | | | | | | | | |
| 0–19 Years | 27 | 2.1 | 4 | 1 | 1 | 2 | 2 | 3 | 7 | 14 |
| 20–34 | 42 | 1.6 | <1 | 1 | 1 | 1 | 2 | 3 | 3 | 6 |
| 35–49 | 92 | 1.5 | <1 | 1 | 1 | 1 | 2 | 2 | 3 | 5 |
| 50–64 | 71 | 1.4 | <1 | 1 | 1 | 1 | 2 | 2 | 3 | 3 |
| 65+ | 61 | 2.0 | 5 | 1 | 1 | 1 | 2 | 3 | 4 | 13 |
| **2. MULTIPLE DX** | | | | | | | | | | |
| 0–19 Years | 47 | 5.7 | 51 | 2 | 2 | 3 | 5 | 22 | 22 | 22 |
| 20–34 | 28 | 1.9 | 4 | 1 | 1 | 1 | 2 | 2 | 3 | 12 |
| 35–49 | 128 | 1.9 | 5 | 1 | 1 | 2 | 2 | 3 | 4 | 15 |
| 50–64 | 165 | 2.1 | 4 | 1 | 1 | 2 | 2 | 3 | 6 | 10 |
| 65+ | 331 | 2.7 | 7 | 1 | 1 | 2 | 3 | 5 | 8 | 13 |
| **TOTAL SINGLE DX** | 293 | 1.7 | 2 | 1 | 1 | 1 | 2 | 2 | 3 | 7 |
| **TOTAL MULTIPLE DX** | 699 | 2.5 | 9 | 1 | 1 | 2 | 3 | 5 | 8 | 21 |
| **TOTAL** | | | | | | | | | | |
| 0–19 Years | 74 | 4.1 | 33 | 1 | 1 | 2 | 3 | 9 | 22 | 22 |
| 20–34 | 70 | 1.8 | 2 | 1 | 1 | 1 | 2 | 3 | 3 | 11 |
| 35–49 | 220 | 1.8 | 3 | 1 | 1 | 1 | 2 | 3 | 3 | 9 |
| 50–64 | 236 | 1.9 | 3 | 1 | 1 | 2 | 2 | 3 | 4 | 10 |
| 65+ | 392 | 2.6 | 7 | 1 | 1 | 2 | 3 | 5 | 8 | 13 |
| **GRAND TOTAL** | 992 | 2.3 | 7 | 1 | 1 | 2 | 2 | 4 | 6 | 15 |

## 26.9: OTH SALIVARY OPERATIONS. Formerly included in operation group(s) 549.

| Type of Patients | Observed Patients | Avg. Stay | Variance | 10th | 25th | 50th | 75th | 90th | 95th | 99th |
|---|---|---|---|---|---|---|---|---|---|---|
| **1. SINGLE DX** | | | | | | | | | | |
| 0–19 Years | 1 | 1.0 | 0 | 1 | 1 | 1 | 1 | 1 | 1 | 1 |
| 20–34 | 1 | 3.0 | 0 | 3 | 3 | 3 | 3 | 3 | 3 | 3 |
| 35–49 | 1 | 2.0 | 0 | 2 | 2 | 2 | 2 | 2 | 2 | 2 |
| 50–64 | 0 | | | | | | | | | |
| 65+ | 0 | | | | | | | | | |
| **2. MULTIPLE DX** | | | | | | | | | | |
| 0–19 Years | 3 | 2.2 | <1 | 2 | 2 | 2 | 2 | 3 | 3 | 3 |
| 20–34 | 3 | 2.9 | 1 | 2 | 3 | 3 | 4 | 4 | 4 | 4 |
| 35–49 | 1 | 2.0 | 0 | 2 | 2 | 2 | 2 | 2 | 2 | 2 |
| 50–64 | 3 | 3.3 | <1 | 3 | 3 | 3 | 4 | 4 | 4 | 4 |
| 65+ | 18 | 5.9 | 21 | 2 | 2 | 4 | 8 | 14 | 18 | 18 |
| **TOTAL SINGLE DX** | 3 | 2.2 | <1 | 1 | 2 | 2 | 3 | 3 | 3 | 3 |
| **TOTAL MULTIPLE DX** | 28 | 4.6 | 15 | 2 | 2 | 3 | 4 | 9 | 15 | 18 |
| **TOTAL** | | | | | | | | | | |
| 0–19 Years | 4 | 2.1 | <1 | 2 | 2 | 2 | 2 | 3 | 3 | 3 |
| 20–34 | 4 | 2.9 | 1 | 2 | 3 | 3 | 3 | 3 | 4 | 4 |
| 35–49 | 2 | 2.0 | 0 | 2 | 2 | 2 | 2 | 2 | 2 | 2 |
| 50–64 | 3 | 3.3 | <1 | 3 | 3 | 3 | 4 | 4 | 4 | 4 |
| 65+ | 18 | 5.9 | 21 | 2 | 2 | 4 | 8 | 14 | 18 | 18 |
| **GRAND TOTAL** | 31 | 4.4 | 14 | 2 | 2 | 3 | 4 | 8 | 15 | 18 |

## 26.4: SG & DUCT REPAIR. Formerly included in operation group(s) 549.

| Type of Patients | Observed Patients | Avg. Stay | Variance | 10th | 25th | 50th | 75th | 90th | 95th | 99th |
|---|---|---|---|---|---|---|---|---|---|---|
| **1. SINGLE DX** | | | | | | | | | | |
| 0–19 Years | 2 | 1.4 | <1 | 1 | 1 | 1 | 1 | 3 | 3 | 3 |
| 20–34 | 2 | 2.0 | 0 | 2 | 2 | 2 | 2 | 2 | 2 | 2 |
| 35–49 | 0 | | | | | | | | | |
| 50–64 | 0 | | | | | | | | | |
| 65+ | 0 | | | | | | | | | |
| **2. MULTIPLE DX** | | | | | | | | | | |
| 0–19 Years | 10 | 2.9 | 5 | 1 | 1 | 2 | 3 | 7 | 7 | 7 |
| 20–34 | 5 | 3.3 | 13 | 1 | 1 | 2 | 4 | 4 | 14 | 14 |
| 35–49 | 4 | 5.2 | 64 | 1 | 2 | 2 | 3 | 23 | 23 | 23 |
| 50–64 | 1 | 4.0 | 0 | 4 | 4 | 4 | 4 | 4 | 4 | 4 |
| 65+ | 3 | 4.7 | 35 | 2 | 2 | 2 | 2 | 18 | 18 | 18 |
| **TOTAL SINGLE DX** | 4 | 1.6 | <1 | 1 | 1 | 2 | 2 | 3 | 3 | 3 |
| **TOTAL MULTIPLE DX** | 23 | 3.8 | 22 | 1 | 2 | 2 | 3 | 7 | 18 | 23 |
| **TOTAL** | | | | | | | | | | |
| 0–19 Years | 12 | 2.7 | 4 | 1 | 1 | 2 | 3 | 7 | 7 | 7 |
| 20–34 | 7 | 3.1 | 11 | 1 | 2 | 2 | 3 | 4 | 14 | 14 |
| 35–49 | 4 | 5.2 | 64 | 1 | 2 | 2 | 3 | 23 | 23 | 23 |
| 50–64 | 1 | 4.0 | 0 | 4 | 4 | 4 | 4 | 4 | 4 | 4 |
| 65+ | 3 | 4.7 | 35 | 2 | 2 | 2 | 2 | 18 | 18 | 18 |
| **GRAND TOTAL** | 27 | 3.6 | 21 | 1 | 2 | 2 | 3 | 7 | 18 | 23 |

## 27.0: DRAIN FACE & MOUTH FLOOR. Formerly included in operation group(s) 551.

| Type of Patients | Observed Patients | Avg. Stay | Variance | 10th | 25th | 50th | 75th | 90th | 95th | 99th |
|---|---|---|---|---|---|---|---|---|---|---|
| **1. SINGLE DX** | | | | | | | | | | |
| 0–19 Years | 113 | 3.1 | 3 | 1 | 2 | 3 | 4 | 6 | 6 | 7 |
| 20–34 | 91 | 2.8 | 1 | 2 | 2 | 3 | 3 | 5 | 5 | 7 |
| 35–49 | 71 | 3.1 | 3 | 1 | 2 | 3 | 3 | 6 | 6 | 8 |
| 50–64 | 12 | 2.7 | <1 | 2 | 2 | 3 | 3 | 4 | 4 | 4 |
| 65+ | 4 | 4.2 | 2 | 2 | 3 | 5 | 5 | 5 | 5 | 5 |
| **2. MULTIPLE DX** | | | | | | | | | | |
| 0–19 Years | 318 | 3.6 | 11 | 2 | 2 | 3 | 4 | 6 | 7 | 10 |
| 20–34 | 581 | 3.7 | 6 | 2 | 3 | 3 | 5 | 6 | 8 | 12 |
| 35–49 | 521 | 4.3 | 12 | 1 | 2 | 3 | 5 | 8 | 12 | 17 |
| 50–64 | 222 | 4.9 | 25 | 2 | 3 | 3 | 6 | 9 | 11 | 24 |
| 65+ | 177 | 5.4 | 12 | 2 | 3 | 5 | 7 | 9 | 12 | 19 |
| **TOTAL SINGLE DX** | 291 | 3.0 | 2 | 2 | 2 | 3 | 4 | 5 | 6 | 7 |
| **TOTAL MULTIPLE DX** | 1,819 | 4.2 | 12 | 2 | 2 | 3 | 5 | 7 | 10 | 17 |
| **TOTAL** | | | | | | | | | | |
| 0–19 Years | 431 | 3.5 | 9 | 1 | 2 | 3 | 4 | 6 | 7 | 10 |
| 20–34 | 672 | 3.6 | 5 | 2 | 2 | 3 | 4 | 6 | 7 | 12 |
| 35–49 | 592 | 4.2 | 11 | 1 | 2 | 3 | 5 | 7 | 12 | 17 |
| 50–64 | 234 | 4.8 | 25 | 2 | 3 | 3 | 6 | 9 | 11 | 24 |
| 65+ | 181 | 5.4 | 11 | 2 | 3 | 5 | 7 | 9 | 12 | 19 |
| **GRAND TOTAL** | 2,110 | 4.0 | 11 | 2 | 3 | 3 | 5 | 7 | 9 | 17 |

Length of Stay by Diagnosis and Operation, United States, 2000

# United States, October 1998–September 1999 Data, by Operation

## 27.1: INCISION OF PALATE. Formerly included in operation group(s) 551.

| Type of Patients | Observed Patients | Avg. Stay | Variance | 10th | 25th | 50th | 75th | 90th | 95th | 99th |
|---|---|---|---|---|---|---|---|---|---|---|
| **1. SINGLE DX** | | | | | | | | | | |
| 0–19 Years | 1 | 1.0 | 0 | 1 | 1 | 1 | 1 | 1 | 1 | 1 |
| 20–34 | 3 | 1.6 | <1 | 1 | 1 | 2 | 2 | 2 | 2 | 2 |
| 35–49 | 0 | | | | | | | | | |
| 50–64 | 0 | | | | | | | | | |
| 65+ | 0 | | | | | | | | | |
| **2. MULTIPLE DX** | | | | | | | | | | |
| 0–19 Years | 5 | 5.8 | 79 | 2 | 3 | 3 | 3 | 7 | 37 | 37 |
| 20–34 | 2 | 4.5 | 3 | 3 | 3 | 6 | 6 | 6 | 6 | 6 |
| 35–49 | 3 | 3.3 | 1 | 2 | 2 | 4 | 4 | 4 | 4 | 4 |
| 50–64 | 2 | 6.7 | 33 | 3 | 3 | 3 | 12 | 12 | 12 | 12 |
| 65+ | 2 | 4.8 | <1 | 5 | 5 | 5 | 5 | 5 | 5 | 5 |
| **TOTAL SINGLE DX** | 4 | 1.4 | <1 | 1 | 1 | 1 | 2 | 2 | 2 | 2 |
| **TOTAL MULTIPLE DX** | 14 | 4.9 | 21 | 2 | 3 | 5 | 5 | 6 | 7 | 37 |
| **TOTAL** | | | | | | | | | | |
| 0–19 Years | 6 | 5.1 | 70 | 1 | 2 | 3 | 3 | 7 | 37 | 37 |
| 20–34 | 5 | 3.0 | 4 | 1 | 2 | 2 | 3 | 6 | 6 | 6 |
| 35–49 | 3 | 3.3 | 1 | 2 | 2 | 4 | 4 | 4 | 4 | 4 |
| 50–64 | 2 | 6.7 | 33 | 3 | 3 | 3 | 12 | 12 | 12 | 12 |
| 65+ | 2 | 4.8 | <1 | 5 | 5 | 5 | 5 | 5 | 5 | 5 |
| **GRAND TOTAL** | 18 | 4.5 | 20 | 2 | 3 | 4 | 5 | 6 | 7 | 37 |

## 27.2: ORAL CAVITY DXTIC PX. Formerly included in operation group(s) 551, 556.

| Type of Patients | Observed Patients | Avg. Stay | Variance | 10th | 25th | 50th | 75th | 90th | 95th | 99th |
|---|---|---|---|---|---|---|---|---|---|---|
| **1. SINGLE DX** | | | | | | | | | | |
| 0–19 Years | 5 | 2.4 | <1 | 1 | 2 | 3 | 3 | 3 | 3 | 3 |
| 20–34 | 1 | 1.0 | 0 | 1 | 1 | 1 | 1 | 1 | 1 | 1 |
| 35–49 | 0 | | | | | | | | | |
| 50–64 | 2 | 2.8 | 7 | 1 | 1 | 1 | 5 | 5 | 5 | 5 |
| 65+ | 1 | 1.0 | 0 | 1 | 1 | 1 | 1 | 1 | 1 | 1 |
| **2. MULTIPLE DX** | | | | | | | | | | |
| 0–19 Years | 20 | 9.0 | 110 | 1 | 1 | 6 | 10 | 25 | 25 | 58 |
| 20–34 | 13 | 5.8 | 29 | 1 | 1 | 5 | 7 | 13 | 13 | 24 |
| 35–49 | 44 | 7.3 | 78 | 1 | 2 | 5 | 7 | 16 | 37 | 37 |
| 50–64 | 51 | 6.4 | 52 | 1 | 2 | 4 | 8 | 14 | 25 | 31 |
| 65+ | 66 | 8.6 | 57 | 2 | 3 | 6 | 13 | 18 | 18 | 26 |
| **TOTAL SINGLE DX** | 9 | 2.3 | 1 | 1 | 1 | 2 | 3 | 3 | 5 | 5 |
| **TOTAL MULTIPLE DX** | 194 | 7.7 | 65 | 1 | 2 | 6 | 8 | 18 | 25 | 37 |
| **TOTAL** | | | | | | | | | | |
| 0–19 Years | 25 | 8.0 | 98 | 1 | 1 | 5 | 8 | 25 | 25 | 58 |
| 20–34 | 14 | 5.6 | 29 | 1 | 1 | 5 | 7 | 13 | 13 | 24 |
| 35–49 | 44 | 7.3 | 78 | 1 | 2 | 5 | 7 | 16 | 37 | 37 |
| 50–64 | 53 | 6.4 | 51 | 1 | 2 | 4 | 8 | 14 | 25 | 31 |
| 65+ | 67 | 8.6 | 57 | 2 | 3 | 6 | 13 | 18 | 18 | 26 |
| **GRAND TOTAL** | 203 | 7.5 | 64 | 1 | 2 | 5 | 8 | 18 | 25 | 37 |

## 27.3: EXC BONY PALATE LES/TISS. Formerly included in operation group(s) 551.

| Type of Patients | Observed Patients | Avg. Stay | Variance | 10th | 25th | 50th | 75th | 90th | 95th | 99th |
|---|---|---|---|---|---|---|---|---|---|---|
| **1. SINGLE DX** | | | | | | | | | | |
| 0–19 Years | 2 | 1.0 | 0 | 1 | 1 | 1 | 1 | 1 | 1 | 1 |
| 20–34 | 5 | 2.0 | <1 | 1 | 1 | 2 | 3 | 3 | 3 | 3 |
| 35–49 | 5 | 2.0 | <1 | 1 | 2 | 2 | 3 | 3 | 3 | 3 |
| 50–64 | 6 | 1.8 | <1 | 1 | 2 | 2 | 2 | 3 | 3 | 3 |
| 65+ | 2 | 2.5 | <1 | 2 | 2 | 3 | 3 | 3 | 3 | 3 |
| **2. MULTIPLE DX** | | | | | | | | | | |
| 0–19 Years | 5 | 6.2 | 56 | 2 | 2 | 4 | 4 | 22 | 22 | 22 |
| 20–34 | 2 | 1.7 | <1 | 1 | 1 | 2 | 2 | 2 | 2 | 2 |
| 35–49 | 10 | 6.3 | 57 | 1 | 1 | 2 | 10 | 18 | 24 | 24 |
| 50–64 | 18 | 2.8 | 4 | 1 | 1 | 2 | 3 | 5 | 9 | 9 |
| 65+ | 46 | 4.6 | 18 | 1 | 2 | 3 | 6 | 11 | 13 | 21 |
| **TOTAL SINGLE DX** | 20 | 1.7 | <1 | 1 | 1 | 1 | 2 | 3 | 3 | 3 |
| **TOTAL MULTIPLE DX** | 81 | 4.5 | 22 | 1 | 2 | 3 | 5 | 10 | 16 | 24 |
| **TOTAL** | | | | | | | | | | |
| 0–19 Years | 7 | 2.5 | 21 | 1 | 1 | 2 | 2 | 4 | 4 | 22 |
| 20–34 | 7 | 1.9 | <1 | 1 | 1 | 2 | 3 | 3 | 3 | 3 |
| 35–49 | 15 | 5.2 | 46 | 1 | 1 | 2 | 10 | 18 | 24 | 24 |
| 50–64 | 24 | 2.5 | 3 | 1 | 2 | 3 | 3 | 4 | 9 | 9 |
| 65+ | 48 | 4.5 | 17 | 1 | 2 | 3 | 6 | 11 | 13 | 21 |
| **GRAND TOTAL** | 101 | 3.8 | 18 | 1 | 1 | 2 | 4 | 9 | 13 | 22 |

## 27.4: OTHER EXCISION OF MOUTH. Formerly included in operation group(s) 551.

| Type of Patients | Observed Patients | Avg. Stay | Variance | 10th | 25th | 50th | 75th | 90th | 95th | 99th |
|---|---|---|---|---|---|---|---|---|---|---|
| **1. SINGLE DX** | | | | | | | | | | |
| 0–19 Years | 35 | 1.8 | 2 | 1 | 1 | 1 | 3 | 3 | 7 | 7 |
| 20–34 | 8 | 1.3 | <1 | 1 | 1 | 1 | 2 | 2 | 2 | 2 |
| 35–49 | 7 | 2.9 | 7 | 1 | 1 | 1 | 6 | 6 | 7 | 7 |
| 50–64 | 17 | 2.8 | 5 | 1 | 1 | 1 | 5 | 5 | 8 | 8 |
| 65+ | 20 | 2.4 | 5 | 1 | 1 | 2 | 2 | 5 | 5 | 12 |
| **2. MULTIPLE DX** | | | | | | | | | | |
| 0–19 Years | 63 | 3.1 | 14 | 1 | 1 | 2 | 4 | 7 | 9 | 23 |
| 20–34 | 30 | 3.6 | 7 | 1 | 1 | 4 | 6 | 6 | 7 | 14 |
| 35–49 | 55 | 9.1 | 72 | 1 | 2 | 9 | 12 | 17 | 22 | 48 |
| 50–64 | 132 | 6.6 | 49 | 1 | 2 | 5 | 10 | 13 | 20 | 40 |
| 65+ | 267 | 6.2 | 60 | 1 | 2 | 4 | 8 | 13 | 18 | 39 |
| **TOTAL SINGLE DX** | 87 | 2.2 | 4 | 1 | 1 | 1 | 3 | 5 | 7 | 8 |
| **TOTAL MULTIPLE DX** | 547 | 6.0 | 52 | 1 | 2 | 4 | 8 | 12 | 18 | 39 |
| **TOTAL** | | | | | | | | | | |
| 0–19 Years | 98 | 2.6 | 10 | 1 | 1 | 1 | 3 | 5 | 7 | 23 |
| 20–34 | 38 | 3.3 | 7 | 1 | 1 | 3 | 4 | 6 | 7 | 14 |
| 35–49 | 62 | 8.3 | 68 | 1 | 2 | 8 | 11 | 14 | 22 | 48 |
| 50–64 | 149 | 6.1 | 45 | 1 | 2 | 4 | 9 | 12 | 17 | 40 |
| 65+ | 287 | 6.0 | 57 | 1 | 2 | 4 | 8 | 12 | 18 | 39 |
| **GRAND TOTAL** | 634 | 5.5 | 47 | 1 | 1 | 3 | 7 | 11 | 17 | 37 |

Length of Stay by Diagnosis and Operation, United States, 2000

## United States, October 1998–September 1999 Data, by Operation

### 27.49: EXCISION OF MOUTH NEC. Formerly included in operation group(s) 551.

| Type of Patients | Observed Patients | Avg. Stay | Variance | 10th | 25th | 50th | 75th | 90th | 95th | 99th |
|---|---|---|---|---|---|---|---|---|---|---|
| **1. SINGLE DX** | | | | | | | | | | |
| 0–19 Years | 14 | 1.6 | <1 | 1 | 1 | 1 | 3 | 3 | 3 | 3 |
| 20–34 | 4 | 1.3 | <1 | 1 | 1 | 1 | 2 | 3 | 3 | 2 |
| 35–49 | 4 | 4.5 | 7 | 1 | 1 | 6 | 6 | 7 | 7 | 7 |
| 50–64 | 12 | 2.0 | 5 | 1 | 1 | 1 | 1 | 8 | 8 | 8 |
| 65+ | 15 | 2.8 | 6 | 1 | 2 | 2 | 2 | 5 | 12 | 12 |
| **2. MULTIPLE DX** | | | | | | | | | | |
| 0–19 Years | 27 | 4.9 | 26 | 1 | 2 | 3 | 6 | 9 | 23 | 23 |
| 20–34 | 13 | 3.0 | 10 | 1 | 1 | 1 | 3 | 7 | 9 | 12 |
| 35–49 | 34 | 10.5 | 85 | 1 | 4 | 10 | 12 | 21 | 22 | 48 |
| 50–64 | 101 | 7.4 | 58 | 1 | 2 | 5 | 10 | 16 | 20 | 42 |
| 65+ | 179 | 6.0 | 33 | 1 | 2 | 5 | 9 | 12 | 18 | 29 |
| **TOTAL SINGLE DX** | 49 | 2.2 | 4 | 1 | 1 | 1 | 3 | 5 | 6 | 12 |
| **TOTAL MULTIPLE DX** | 354 | 6.7 | 46 | 1 | 2 | 5 | 9 | 14 | 20 | 37 |
| **TOTAL** | | | | | | | | | | |
| 0–19 Years | 41 | 3.2 | 16 | 1 | 1 | 2 | 3 | 7 | 9 | 23 |
| 20–34 | 17 | 2.7 | 8 | 1 | 1 | 1 | 3 | 7 | 9 | 12 |
| 35–49 | 38 | 9.9 | 80 | 1 | 3 | 9 | 12 | 21 | 22 | 48 |
| 50–64 | 113 | 6.8 | 55 | 1 | 2 | 5 | 10 | 15 | 20 | 42 |
| 65+ | 194 | 5.8 | 32 | 1 | 2 | 4 | 9 | 12 | 15 | 29 |
| **GRAND TOTAL** | 403 | 6.1 | 43 | 1 | 1 | 4 | 9 | 12 | 18 | 37 |

### 27.51: SUTURE OF LIP LACERATION. Formerly included in operation group(s) 551.

| Type of Patients | Observed Patients | Avg. Stay | Variance | 10th | 25th | 50th | 75th | 90th | 95th | 99th |
|---|---|---|---|---|---|---|---|---|---|---|
| **1. SINGLE DX** | | | | | | | | | | |
| 0–19 Years | 68 | 1.2 | <1 | 1 | 1 | 1 | 1 | 2 | 2 | 2 |
| 20–34 | 2 | 1.0 | 0 | 1 | 1 | 1 | 1 | | | 1 |
| 35–49 | 5 | 1.2 | <1 | 1 | 1 | 1 | 1 | 2 | 2 | 2 |
| 50–64 | 0 | | | | | | | | | |
| 65+ | 0 | | | | | | | | | |
| **2. MULTIPLE DX** | | | | | | | | | | |
| 0–19 Years | 229 | 2.2 | 18 | 1 | 1 | 1 | 2 | 3 | 4 | 10 |
| 20–34 | 282 | 2.0 | 4 | 1 | 1 | 1 | 2 | 4 | 6 | 11 |
| 35–49 | 222 | 2.6 | 5 | 1 | 1 | 2 | 3 | 5 | 7 | 12 |
| 50–64 | 119 | 3.4 | 13 | 1 | 1 | 2 | 4 | 8 | 10 | 19 |
| 65+ | 261 | 4.4 | 32 | 1 | 2 | 3 | 5 | 9 | 10 | 46 |
| **TOTAL SINGLE DX** | 75 | 1.2 | <1 | 1 | 1 | 1 | 1 | 2 | 2 | 2 |
| **TOTAL MULTIPLE DX** | 1,113 | 2.8 | 15 | 1 | 1 | 2 | 3 | 6 | 9 | 15 |
| **TOTAL** | | | | | | | | | | |
| 0–19 Years | 297 | 2.1 | 16 | 1 | 1 | 1 | 2 | 3 | 4 | 9 |
| 20–34 | 284 | 2.0 | 4 | 1 | 1 | 1 | 2 | 4 | 6 | 11 |
| 35–49 | 227 | 2.6 | 5 | 1 | 1 | 2 | 3 | 5 | 7 | 12 |
| 50–64 | 119 | 3.4 | 13 | 1 | 1 | 2 | 4 | 8 | 10 | 19 |
| 65+ | 261 | 4.4 | 32 | 1 | 2 | 3 | 5 | 9 | 10 | 46 |
| **GRAND TOTAL** | 1,188 | 2.8 | 14 | 1 | 1 | 2 | 3 | 5 | 9 | 15 |

### 27.5: PLASTIC REPAIR OF MOUTH. Formerly included in operation group(s) 551.

| Type of Patients | Observed Patients | Avg. Stay | Variance | 10th | 25th | 50th | 75th | 90th | 95th | 99th |
|---|---|---|---|---|---|---|---|---|---|---|
| **1. SINGLE DX** | | | | | | | | | | |
| 0–19 Years | 433 | 1.4 | 1 | 1 | 1 | 1 | 1 | 2 | 3 | 8 |
| 20–34 | 6 | 1.2 | <1 | 1 | 1 | 1 | 1 | 2 | 2 | 2 |
| 35–49 | 7 | 1.2 | <1 | 1 | 1 | 1 | 1 | 2 | 2 | 2 |
| 50–64 | 4 | 3.2 | 4 | 2 | 2 | 2 | 5 | 5 | 5 | 5 |
| 65+ | 3 | 1.2 | <1 | 1 | 1 | 1 | 1 | 3 | 3 | 3 |
| **2. MULTIPLE DX** | | | | | | | | | | |
| 0–19 Years | 849 | 1.7 | 6 | 1 | 1 | 1 | 2 | 3 | 4 | 8 |
| 20–34 | 366 | 2.0 | 4 | 1 | 1 | 1 | 2 | 4 | 6 | 11 |
| 35–49 | 309 | 3.0 | 12 | 1 | 1 | 2 | 3 | 5 | 9 | 23 |
| 50–64 | 163 | 3.5 | 11 | 1 | 1 | 2 | 5 | 7 | 10 | 19 |
| 65+ | 321 | 4.3 | 31 | 1 | 2 | 3 | 5 | 9 | 10 | 45 |
| **TOTAL SINGLE DX** | 453 | 1.4 | 1 | 1 | 1 | 1 | 1 | 2 | 3 | 8 |
| **TOTAL MULTIPLE DX** | 2,008 | 2.5 | 11 | 1 | 1 | 2 | 3 | 5 | 7 | 14 |
| **TOTAL** | | | | | | | | | | |
| 0–19 Years | 1,282 | 1.6 | 4 | 1 | 1 | 1 | 2 | 3 | 4 | 8 |
| 20–34 | 372 | 2.0 | 4 | 1 | 1 | 1 | 2 | 4 | 6 | 11 |
| 35–49 | 316 | 2.9 | 11 | 1 | 1 | 2 | 3 | 5 | 8 | 23 |
| 50–64 | 167 | 3.5 | 11 | 1 | 1 | 2 | 5 | 7 | 10 | 19 |
| 65+ | 324 | 4.2 | 30 | 1 | 2 | 3 | 4 | 9 | 10 | 45 |
| **GRAND TOTAL** | 2,461 | 2.3 | 9 | 1 | 1 | 1 | 2 | 4 | 6 | 12 |

### 27.54: REPAIR OF CLEFT LIP. Formerly included in operation group(s) 551.

| Type of Patients | Observed Patients | Avg. Stay | Variance | 10th | 25th | 50th | 75th | 90th | 95th | 99th |
|---|---|---|---|---|---|---|---|---|---|---|
| **1. SINGLE DX** | | | | | | | | | | |
| 0–19 Years | 319 | 1.3 | <1 | 1 | 1 | 1 | 1 | 2 | 3 | 4 |
| 20–34 | 0 | | | | | | | | | |
| 35–49 | 0 | 1.0 | 0 | 1 | 1 | 1 | 1 | 1 | 1 | 1 |
| 50–64 | 0 | | | | | | | | | |
| 65+ | 0 | | | | | | | | | |
| **2. MULTIPLE DX** | | | | | | | | | | |
| 0–19 Years | 483 | 1.5 | 2 | 1 | 1 | 1 | 2 | 2 | 3 | 8 |
| 20–34 | 9 | 1.6 | 2 | 1 | 1 | 1 | 1 | 2 | 6 | 6 |
| 35–49 | 3 | 1.2 | <1 | 1 | 1 | 1 | 1 | 2 | 2 | 2 |
| 50–64 | 1 | 2.0 | 0 | 2 | 2 | 2 | 2 | 2 | 2 | 2 |
| 65+ | 0 | | | | | | | | | |
| **TOTAL SINGLE DX** | 320 | 1.3 | <1 | 1 | 1 | 1 | 1 | 2 | 3 | 4 |
| **TOTAL MULTIPLE DX** | 496 | 1.5 | 2 | 1 | 1 | 1 | 2 | 2 | 3 | 8 |
| **TOTAL** | | | | | | | | | | |
| 0–19 Years | 802 | 1.4 | 1 | 1 | 1 | 1 | 1 | 2 | 3 | 8 |
| 20–34 | 9 | 1.6 | 2 | 1 | 1 | 1 | 1 | 2 | 6 | 6 |
| 35–49 | 4 | 1.1 | <1 | 1 | 1 | 1 | 1 | 2 | 2 | 2 |
| 50–64 | 1 | 2.0 | 0 | 2 | 2 | 2 | 2 | 2 | 2 | 2 |
| 65+ | 0 | | | | | | | | | |
| **GRAND TOTAL** | 816 | 1.4 | 1 | 1 | 1 | 1 | 1 | 2 | 3 | 8 |

Length of Stay by Diagnosis and Operation, United States, 2000

# United States, October 1998–September 1999 Data, by Operation

## 27.6: PALATOPLASTY. Formerly included in operation group(s) 550.

| Type of Patients | Observed Patients | Avg. Stay | Vari-ance | Percentiles | | | | | | |
|---|---|---|---|---|---|---|---|---|---|---|
| | | | | 10th | 25th | 50th | 75th | 90th | 95th | 99th |
| **1. SINGLE DX** | | | | | | | | | | |
| 0–19 Years | 619 | 1.5 | <1 | 1 | 1 | 1 | 2 | 2 | 3 | 4 |
| 20–34 | 10 | 3.0 | 3 | 1 | 1 | 2 | 5 | 5 | 5 | 5 |
| 35–49 | 28 | 2.3 | 3 | 1 | 1 | 2 | 3 | 3 | 3 | 9 |
| 50–64 | 6 | 1.7 | <1 | 1 | 1 | 2 | 2 | 2 | 2 | 3 |
| 65+ | 4 | 3.5 | 5 | 1 | 1 | 3 | 6 | 6 | 6 | 6 |
| **2. MULTIPLE DX** | | | | | | | | | | |
| 0–19 Years | 1,499 | 1.8 | 4 | 1 | 1 | 1 | 2 | 3 | 4 | 6 |
| 20–34 | 164 | 1.9 | 2 | 1 | 1 | 1 | 2 | 3 | 4 | 10 |
| 35–49 | 450 | 1.7 | 2 | 1 | 1 | 1 | 2 | 3 | 4 | 8 |
| 50–64 | 304 | 1.9 | 3 | 1 | 1 | 1 | 2 | 3 | 4 | 10 |
| 65+ | 86 | 1.8 | 2 | 1 | 1 | 1 | 2 | 3 | 5 | 7 |
| **TOTAL SINGLE DX** | 667 | 1.6 | <1 | 1 | 1 | 1 | 2 | 3 | 3 | 5 |
| **TOTAL MULTIPLE DX** | 2,503 | 1.8 | 4 | 1 | 1 | 1 | 2 | 3 | 4 | 7 |
| **TOTAL** | | | | | | | | | | |
| 0–19 Years | 2,118 | 1.8 | 3 | 1 | 1 | 1 | 2 | 3 | 3 | 6 |
| 20–34 | 174 | 1.9 | 3 | 1 | 1 | 1 | 2 | 4 | 5 | 10 |
| 35–49 | 478 | 1.7 | 2 | 1 | 1 | 1 | 2 | 3 | 4 | 9 |
| 50–64 | 310 | 1.8 | 3 | 1 | 1 | 1 | 2 | 3 | 4 | 10 |
| 65+ | 90 | 1.8 | 3 | 1 | 1 | 1 | 2 | 4 | 5 | 7 |
| **GRAND TOTAL** | 3,170 | 1.8 | 3 | 1 | 1 | 1 | 2 | 3 | 4 | 6 |

## 27.62: CLEFT PALATE CORRECTION. Formerly included in operation group(s) 550.

| Type of Patients | Observed Patients | Avg. Stay | Vari-ance | Percentiles | | | | | | |
|---|---|---|---|---|---|---|---|---|---|---|
| | | | | 10th | 25th | 50th | 75th | 90th | 95th | 99th |
| **1. SINGLE DX** | | | | | | | | | | |
| 0–19 Years | 410 | 1.6 | <1 | 1 | 1 | 1 | 2 | 3 | 3 | 4 |
| 20–34 | 3 | 1.3 | <1 | 1 | 1 | 1 | 2 | 2 | 2 | 2 |
| 35–49 | 1 | 3.0 | 0 | 3 | 3 | 3 | 3 | 3 | 3 | 3 |
| 50–64 | 0 | | | | | | | | | |
| 65+ | 0 | | | | | | | | | |
| **2. MULTIPLE DX** | | | | | | | | | | |
| 0–19 Years | 927 | 1.8 | 2 | 1 | 1 | 1 | 2 | 3 | 3 | 6 |
| 20–34 | 3 | 1.7 | <1 | 1 | 1 | 2 | 2 | 2 | 2 | 2 |
| 35–49 | 6 | 1.3 | <1 | 1 | 1 | 1 | 2 | 2 | 2 | 2 |
| 50–64 | 1 | 1.0 | 0 | 1 | 1 | 1 | 1 | 1 | 1 | 1 |
| 65+ | 3 | 1.8 | <1 | 1 | 2 | 2 | 2 | 2 | 2 | 2 |
| **TOTAL SINGLE DX** | 414 | 1.6 | <1 | 1 | 1 | 1 | 2 | 3 | 3 | 4 |
| **TOTAL MULTIPLE DX** | 940 | 1.8 | 2 | 1 | 1 | 1 | 2 | 3 | 3 | 6 |
| **TOTAL** | | | | | | | | | | |
| 0–19 Years | 1,337 | 1.7 | 2 | 1 | 1 | 1 | 2 | 3 | 3 | 5 |
| 20–34 | 6 | 1.5 | <1 | 1 | 1 | 1 | 2 | 2 | 2 | 2 |
| 35–49 | 7 | 2.7 | <1 | 1 | 3 | 3 | 3 | 3 | 3 | 3 |
| 50–64 | 1 | 1.0 | 0 | 1 | 1 | 1 | 1 | 1 | 1 | 1 |
| 65+ | 3 | 1.8 | <1 | 1 | 2 | 2 | 2 | 2 | 2 | 2 |
| **GRAND TOTAL** | 1,354 | 1.7 | 2 | 1 | 1 | 1 | 2 | 3 | 3 | 5 |

## 27.63: REV CLEFT PALATE REPAIR. Formerly included in operation group(s) 550.

| Type of Patients | Observed Patients | Avg. Stay | Vari-ance | Percentiles | | | | | | |
|---|---|---|---|---|---|---|---|---|---|---|
| | | | | 10th | 25th | 50th | 75th | 90th | 95th | 99th |
| **1. SINGLE DX** | | | | | | | | | | |
| 0–19 Years | 159 | 1.5 | <1 | 1 | 1 | | 2 | 2 | 3 | 6 |
| 20–34 | 0 | | | | | | | | | |
| 35–49 | 0 | 2.0 | 0 | 2 | 2 | 2 | 2 | 2 | 2 | 2 |
| 50–64 | 0 | | | | | | | | | |
| 65+ | 0 | | | | | | | | | |
| **2. MULTIPLE DX** | | | | | | | | | | |
| 0–19 Years | 406 | 1.8 | 1 | 1 | 1 | 1 | 2 | 3 | 4 | 5 |
| 20–34 | 5 | 1.2 | <1 | 1 | 1 | 1 | 1 | 2 | 2 | 2 |
| 35–49 | 5 | 2.5 | 2 | 1 | 2 | 2 | 4 | 4 | 4 | 4 |
| 50–64 | 1 | 1.0 | 0 | 1 | 1 | 1 | 1 | 1 | 1 | 1 |
| 65+ | 1 | 4.0 | 0 | 4 | 4 | 4 | 4 | 4 | 4 | 4 |
| **TOTAL SINGLE DX** | 160 | 1.5 | <1 | 1 | 1 | 1 | 2 | 2 | 3 | 6 |
| **TOTAL MULTIPLE DX** | 418 | 1.8 | 1 | 1 | 1 | 1 | 2 | 3 | 4 | 5 |
| **TOTAL** | | | | | | | | | | |
| 0–19 Years | 565 | 1.7 | 1 | 1 | 1 | 1 | 2 | 3 | 4 | 6 |
| 20–34 | 5 | 1.2 | <1 | 1 | 1 | 1 | 1 | 2 | 2 | 2 |
| 35–49 | 6 | 2.2 | <1 | 1 | 2 | 2 | 4 | 4 | 4 | 4 |
| 50–64 | 1 | 1.0 | 0 | 1 | 1 | 1 | 1 | 1 | 1 | 1 |
| 65+ | 1 | 4.0 | 0 | 4 | 4 | 4 | 4 | 4 | 4 | 4 |
| **GRAND TOTAL** | 578 | 1.7 | 1 | 1 | 1 | 1 | 2 | 3 | 4 | 6 |

## 27.69: OTHER PLASTIC REP PALATE. Formerly included in operation group(s) 550.

| Type of Patients | Observed Patients | Avg. Stay | Vari-ance | Percentiles | | | | | | |
|---|---|---|---|---|---|---|---|---|---|---|
| | | | | 10th | 25th | 50th | 75th | 90th | 95th | 99th |
| **1. SINGLE DX** | | | | | | | | | | |
| 0–19 Years | 25 | 1.3 | <1 | 1 | 1 | 1 | 1 | 2 | 3 | 3 |
| 20–34 | 7 | 3.6 | 3 | 1 | 1 | 5 | 5 | 5 | 5 | 5 |
| 35–49 | 26 | 1.8 | 3 | 1 | 1 | 1 | 2 | 3 | 3 | 9 |
| 50–64 | 6 | 1.7 | <1 | 1 | 1 | 2 | 2 | 2 | 2 | 3 |
| 65+ | 4 | 3.5 | 5 | 1 | 1 | 3 | 6 | 6 | 6 | 6 |
| **2. MULTIPLE DX** | | | | | | | | | | |
| 0–19 Years | 156 | 2.8 | 30 | 1 | 1 | 1 | 3 | 4 | 6 | 39 |
| 20–34 | 154 | 1.8 | 3 | 1 | 1 | 1 | 2 | 3 | 4 | 11 |
| 35–49 | 433 | 1.7 | 2 | 1 | 1 | 1 | 2 | 3 | 3 | 8 |
| 50–64 | 300 | 1.8 | 2 | 1 | 1 | 1 | 2 | 3 | 3 | 8 |
| 65+ | 79 | 1.7 | 3 | 1 | 1 | 1 | 2 | 3 | 5 | 7 |
| **TOTAL SINGLE DX** | 68 | 1.8 | 2 | 1 | 1 | 1 | 2 | 3 | 5 | 9 |
| **TOTAL MULTIPLE DX** | 1,122 | 1.9 | 6 | 1 | 1 | 1 | 2 | 3 | 4 | 10 |
| **TOTAL** | | | | | | | | | | |
| 0–19 Years | 181 | 2.5 | 25 | 1 | 1 | 1 | 2 | 4 | 6 | 39 |
| 20–34 | 161 | 1.9 | 3 | 1 | 1 | 1 | 2 | 4 | 5 | 11 |
| 35–49 | 459 | 1.7 | 2 | 1 | 1 | 1 | 2 | 3 | 3 | 9 |
| 50–64 | 306 | 1.8 | 2 | 1 | 1 | 1 | 2 | 3 | 4 | 8 |
| 65+ | 83 | 1.8 | 3 | 1 | 1 | 1 | 2 | 3 | 5 | 7 |
| **GRAND TOTAL** | 1,190 | 1.9 | 6 | 1 | 1 | 1 | 2 | 3 | 4 | 10 |

Length of Stay by Diagnosis and Operation, United States, 2000

# United States, October 1998–September 1999 Data, by Operation

## 27.7: OPERATIONS ON UVULA. Formerly included in operation group(s) 551.

| Type of Patients | Observed Patients | Avg. Stay | Variance | 10th | 25th | 50th | 75th | 90th | 95th | 99th |
|---|---|---|---|---|---|---|---|---|---|---|
| **1. SINGLE DX** | | | | | | | | | | |
| 0–19 Years | 2 | 1.0 | 0 | 1 | 1 | 1 | 1 | 1 | 1 | 1 |
| 20–34 | 1 | 4.0 | 0 | 4 | 4 | 4 | 4 | 4 | 4 | 4 |
| 35–49 | 5 | 1.0 | 0 | 1 | 1 | 1 | 1 | 1 | 1 | 1 |
| 50–64 | 1 | 1.0 | 0 | 1 | 1 | 1 | 1 | 1 | 1 | 1 |
| 65+ | 1 | 1.0 | 0 | 1 | 1 | 1 | 1 | 1 | 1 | 1 |
| **2. MULTIPLE DX** | | | | | | | | | | |
| 0–19 Years | 21 | 1.9 | 10 | 1 | 1 | 1 | 1 | 3 | 4 | 17 |
| 20–34 | 16 | 2.1 | 6 | 1 | 1 | 1 | 2 | 7 | 9 | 9 |
| 35–49 | 32 | 3.8 | 29 | 1 | 1 | 1 | 2 | 16 | 16 | 16 |
| 50–64 | 9 | 2.0 | 1 | 1 | 1 | 2 | 2 | 4 | 4 | 4 |
| 65+ | 8 | 2.9 | 3 | 1 | 1 | 3 | 4 | 5 | 5 | 5 |
| **TOTAL SINGLE DX** | 10 | 1.2 | <1 | 1 | 1 | 1 | 1 | 1 | 4 | 4 |
| **TOTAL MULTIPLE DX** | 86 | 2.7 | 16 | 1 | 2 | 1 | 2 | 7 | 16 | 17 |
| **TOTAL** | | | | | | | | | | |
| 0–19 Years | 23 | 1.9 | 9 | 1 | 1 | 1 | 1 | 3 | 4 | 17 |
| 20–34 | 17 | 2.2 | 6 | 1 | 1 | 1 | 2 | 7 | 9 | 9 |
| 35–49 | 37 | 3.4 | 27 | 1 | 1 | 1 | 2 | 16 | 16 | 16 |
| 50–64 | 10 | 1.9 | 1 | 1 | 1 | 1 | 2 | 4 | 4 | 4 |
| 65+ | 9 | 2.7 | 3 | 1 | 1 | 3 | 4 | 5 | 5 | 5 |
| **GRAND TOTAL** | 96 | 2.6 | 15 | 1 | 1 | 1 | 2 | 7 | 16 | 17 |

## 28.0: TONSIL/PERITONSILLAR I&D. Formerly included in operation group(s) 555.

| Type of Patients | Observed Patients | Avg. Stay | Variance | 10th | 25th | 50th | 75th | 90th | 95th | 99th |
|---|---|---|---|---|---|---|---|---|---|---|
| **1. SINGLE DX** | | | | | | | | | | |
| 0–19 Years | 413 | 2.5 | 4 | 1 | 1 | 2 | 3 | 6 | 7 | 9 |
| 20–34 | 243 | 1.9 | 1 | 1 | 1 | 2 | 2 | 3 | 4 | 5 |
| 35–49 | 110 | 1.7 | 1 | 1 | 1 | 2 | 2 | 3 | 4 | 5 |
| 50–64 | 24 | 1.8 | <1 | 1 | 1 | 2 | 2 | 3 | 3 | 4 |
| 65+ | 6 | 2.1 | | 1 | 2 | 2 | 3 | 4 | 4 | 4 |
| **2. MULTIPLE DX** | | | | | | | | | | |
| 0–19 Years | 484 | 3.1 | 5 | 1 | 2 | 2 | 4 | 6 | 7 | 11 |
| 20–34 | 289 | 2.7 | 7 | 1 | 1 | 2 | 3 | 5 | 7 | 10 |
| 35–49 | 195 | 3.6 | 17 | 1 | 1 | 3 | 5 | 7 | 9 | 17 |
| 50–64 | 81 | 4.0 | 18 | 2 | 2 | 3 | 4 | 6 | 10 | 30 |
| 65+ | 58 | 10.6 | 157 | 2 | 2 | 6 | 13 | 41 | 41 | 43 |
| **TOTAL SINGLE DX** | 796 | 2.2 | 3 | 1 | 1 | 2 | 2 | 4 | 6 | 9 |
| **TOTAL MULTIPLE DX** | 1,107 | 3.4 | 16 | 1 | 1 | 2 | 4 | 6 | 9 | 18 |
| **TOTAL** | | | | | | | | | | |
| 0–19 Years | 897 | 2.8 | 4 | 1 | 1 | 2 | 3 | 6 | 7 | 11 |
| 20–34 | 532 | 2.3 | 4 | 1 | 1 | 2 | 3 | 4 | 5 | 10 |
| 35–49 | 305 | 2.9 | 12 | 1 | 1 | 2 | 4 | 6 | 8 | 12 |
| 50–64 | 105 | 3.6 | 16 | 2 | 2 | 3 | 3 | 6 | 10 | 30 |
| 65+ | 64 | 9.8 | 149 | 2 | 2 | 6 | 10 | 41 | 41 | 43 |
| **GRAND TOTAL** | 1,903 | 2.9 | 11 | 1 | 1 | 2 | 3 | 5 | 7 | 12 |

## 27.9: OTH OPS ON MOUTH & FACE. Formerly included in operation group(s) 551, 556.

| Type of Patients | Observed Patients | Avg. Stay | Variance | 10th | 25th | 50th | 75th | 90th | 95th | 99th |
|---|---|---|---|---|---|---|---|---|---|---|
| **1. SINGLE DX** | | | | | | | | | | |
| 0–19 Years | 10 | 3.8 | 8 | 1 | 1 | 4 | 7 | 7 | 7 | 7 |
| 20–34 | 6 | 2.1 | 1 | 1 | 1 | 2 | 3 | 3 | 5 | 5 |
| 35–49 | 5 | 3.4 | 3 | 1 | 1 | 4 | 5 | 5 | 5 | 5 |
| 50–64 | 1 | 1.0 | 0 | 1 | 1 | 1 | 1 | 1 | 1 | 1 |
| 65+ | 0 | | | | | | | | | |
| **2. MULTIPLE DX** | | | | | | | | | | |
| 0–19 Years | 31 | 3.6 | 3 | 1 | 2 | 3 | 5 | 5 | 6 | 9 |
| 20–34 | 40 | 4.4 | 14 | 2 | 2 | 3 | 5 | 9 | 10 | 29 |
| 35–49 | 41 | 3.2 | 12 | 2 | 2 | 3 | 3 | 6 | 7 | 16 |
| 50–64 | 16 | 6.7 | 31 | 2 | 2 | 3 | 11 | 15 | 15 | 19 |
| 65+ | 13 | 5.0 | 15 | 2 | 3 | 3 | 10 | 12 | 12 | 12 |
| **TOTAL SINGLE DX** | 22 | 2.9 | 5 | 1 | 1 | 2 | 4 | 4 | 7 | 7 |
| **TOTAL MULTIPLE DX** | 141 | 4.0 | 10 | 2 | 2 | 3 | 5 | 5 | 6 | 16 |
| **TOTAL** | | | | | | | | | | |
| 0–19 Years | 41 | 3.6 | 4 | 1 | 2 | 3 | 5 | 5 | 6 | 9 |
| 20–34 | 46 | 3.9 | 12 | 1 | 2 | 3 | 5 | 5 | 10 | 16 |
| 35–49 | 46 | 3.2 | 5 | 2 | 2 | 3 | 4 | 5 | 6 | 16 |
| 50–64 | 17 | 6.4 | 31 | 2 | 2 | 3 | 11 | 15 | 15 | 19 |
| 65+ | 13 | 5.0 | 15 | 2 | 3 | 3 | 10 | 12 | 12 | 12 |
| **GRAND TOTAL** | 163 | 3.8 | 10 | 1 | 2 | 3 | 5 | 5 | 7 | 16 |

## 28.1: TONSIL ADENOID DXTIC PX. Formerly included in operation group(s) 555, 556.

| Type of Patients | Observed Patients | Avg. Stay | Variance | 10th | 25th | 50th | 75th | 90th | 95th | 99th |
|---|---|---|---|---|---|---|---|---|---|---|
| **1. SINGLE DX** | | | | | | | | | | |
| 0–19 Years | 5 | 1.4 | <1 | 1 | 1 | 1 | 2 | 2 | 2 | 2 |
| 20–34 | 5 | 1.2 | <1 | 1 | 1 | 1 | 2 | 2 | 2 | 2 |
| 35–49 | 1 | 2.0 | 0 | 2 | 2 | 3 | 3 | 3 | 3 | 3 |
| 50–64 | 1 | 2.0 | 0 | 2 | 2 | 2 | 2 | 2 | 2 | 2 |
| 65+ | 1 | 1.0 | 0 | 1 | 1 | 1 | 1 | 1 | 1 | 1 |
| **2. MULTIPLE DX** | | | | | | | | | | |
| 0–19 Years | 5 | 3.0 | 1 | 2 | 2 | 2 | 3 | 3 | 6 | 6 |
| 20–34 | 11 | 3.7 | 2 | 2 | 2 | 5 | 5 | 5 | 5 | 5 |
| 35–49 | 22 | 3.9 | 57 | 2 | 2 | 2 | 2 | 6 | 15 | 27 |
| 50–64 | 23 | 5.7 | 36 | 1 | 1 | 3 | 8 | 19 | 19 | 21 |
| 65+ | 31 | 7.8 | 58 | 3 | 3 | 5 | 13 | 16 | 22 | 44 |
| **TOTAL SINGLE DX** | 14 | 1.4 | <1 | 1 | 1 | 1 | 2 | 2 | 2 | 3 |
| **TOTAL MULTIPLE DX** | 92 | 4.7 | 47 | 1 | 2 | 2 | 5 | 12 | 16 | 27 |
| **TOTAL** | | | | | | | | | | |
| 0–19 Years | 10 | 2.1 | 1 | 1 | 1 | 3 | 3 | 3 | 3 | 6 |
| 20–34 | 16 | 3.3 | 3 | 1 | 1 | 2 | 2 | 5 | 5 | 5 |
| 35–49 | 24 | 3.8 | 56 | 2 | 2 | 2 | 2 | 6 | 15 | 27 |
| 50–64 | 24 | 5.4 | 35 | 1 | 1 | 5 | 8 | 12 | 19 | 21 |
| 65+ | 32 | 7.5 | 57 | 2 | 3 | 5 | 13 | 16 | 22 | 44 |
| **GRAND TOTAL** | 106 | 4.5 | 44 | 1 | 2 | 2 | 5 | 12 | 16 | 27 |

Length of Stay by Diagnosis and Operation, United States, 2000

# United States, October 1998–September 1999 Data, by Operation

## 28.2: TONSILLECTOMY. Formerly included in operation group(s) 552.

| Type of Patients | Observed Patients | Avg. Stay | Variance | 10th | 25th | 50th | 75th | 90th | 95th | 99th |
|---|---|---|---|---|---|---|---|---|---|---|
| **1. SINGLE DX** | | | | | | | | | | |
| 0–19 Years | 362 | 1.5 | <1 | 1 | 1 | 1 | 2 | 3 | 4 | 5 |
| 20–34 | 108 | 1.6 | <1 | 1 | 1 | 1 | 2 | 3 | 3 | 4 |
| 35–49 | 40 | 1.7 | <1 | 1 | 1 | 1 | 2 | 3 | 3 | 4 |
| 50–64 | 9 | 1.7 | 1 | 1 | 1 | 1 | 2 | 4 | 4 | 4 |
| 65+ | 7 | 1.6 | <1 | 1 | 1 | 2 | 2 | 2 | 2 | 2 |
| **2. MULTIPLE DX** | | | | | | | | | | |
| 0–19 Years | 523 | 1.9 | 4 | 1 | 1 | 1 | 2 | 4 | 5 | 8 |
| 20–34 | 242 | 2.2 | 3 | 1 | 1 | 1 | 3 | 4 | 6 | 9 |
| 35–49 | 174 | 2.6 | 9 | 1 | 1 | 2 | 3 | 4 | 7 | 13 |
| 50–64 | 76 | 4.0 | 24 | 1 | 1 | 2 | 4 | 9 | 13 | 27 |
| 65+ | 48 | 4.1 | 13 | 1 | 1 | 3 | 6 | 10 | 11 | 13 |
| **TOTAL SINGLE DX** | 526 | 1.5 | <1 | 1 | 1 | 1 | 2 | 3 | 3 | 4 |
| **TOTAL MULTIPLE DX** | 1,063 | 2.3 | 6 | 1 | 1 | 1 | 3 | 4 | 6 | 12 |
| **TOTAL** | | | | | | | | | | |
| 0–19 Years | 885 | 1.7 | 3 | 1 | 1 | 1 | 2 | 3 | 4 | 8 |
| 20–34 | 350 | 2.0 | 3 | 1 | 1 | 1 | 3 | 4 | 5 | 9 |
| 35–49 | 214 | 2.3 | 7 | 1 | 1 | 2 | 3 | 4 | 6 | 12 |
| 50–64 | 85 | 3.8 | 23 | 1 | 1 | 2 | 4 | 8 | 12 | 27 |
| 65+ | 55 | 3.9 | 12 | 1 | 1 | 3 | 5 | 10 | 11 | 13 |
| **GRAND TOTAL** | 1,589 | 2.1 | 5 | 1 | 1 | 1 | 2 | 4 | 5 | 10 |

## 28.3: T&A. Formerly included in operation group(s) 553.

| Type of Patients | Observed Patients | Avg. Stay | Variance | 10th | 25th | 50th | 75th | 90th | 95th | 99th |
|---|---|---|---|---|---|---|---|---|---|---|
| **1. SINGLE DX** | | | | | | | | | | |
| 0–19 Years | 792 | 1.3 | <1 | 1 | 1 | 1 | 1 | 2 | 3 | 4 |
| 20–34 | 12 | 1.1 | <1 | 1 | 1 | 1 | 1 | 1 | 1 | 4 |
| 35–49 | 2 | 1.0 | 0 | 1 | 1 | 1 | 1 | 1 | 1 | 1 |
| 50–64 | 0 | | | | | | | | | |
| 65+ | 0 | | | | | | | | | |
| **2. MULTIPLE DX** | | | | | | | | | | |
| 0–19 Years | 3,437 | 2.0 | 9 | 1 | 1 | 1 | 2 | 4 | 5 | 15 |
| 20–34 | 42 | 2.6 | 4 | 1 | 2 | 2 | 3 | 5 | 6 | 7 |
| 35–49 | 22 | 3.3 | 5 | 1 | 2 | 3 | 5 | 5 | 5 | 15 |
| 50–64 | 2 | 2.4 | <1 | 2 | 2 | 2 | 3 | 3 | 3 | 3 |
| 65+ | 0 | | | | | | | | | |
| **TOTAL SINGLE DX** | 806 | 1.3 | <1 | 1 | 1 | 1 | 1 | 2 | 3 | 4 |
| **TOTAL MULTIPLE DX** | 3,503 | 2.0 | 9 | 1 | 1 | 1 | 2 | 4 | 5 | 15 |
| **TOTAL** | | | | | | | | | | |
| 0–19 Years | 4,229 | 1.9 | 7 | 1 | 1 | 1 | 2 | 3 | 5 | 14 |
| 20–34 | 54 | 2.0 | 3 | 1 | 1 | 1 | 2 | 4 | 6 | 7 |
| 35–49 | 24 | 3.2 | 5 | 1 | 2 | 3 | 5 | 5 | 5 | 15 |
| 50–64 | 2 | 2.4 | <1 | 2 | 2 | 2 | 3 | 3 | 3 | 3 |
| 65+ | 0 | | | | | | | | | |
| **GRAND TOTAL** | 4,309 | 1.9 | 7 | 1 | 1 | 1 | 2 | 3 | 5 | 14 |

## 28.4: EXCISION OF TONSIL TAG. Formerly included in operation group(s) 555.

| Type of Patients | Observed Patients | Avg. Stay | Variance | 10th | 25th | 50th | 75th | 90th | 95th | 99th |
|---|---|---|---|---|---|---|---|---|---|---|
| **1. SINGLE DX** | | | | | | | | | | |
| 0–19 Years | 0 | | | | | | | | | |
| 20–34 | 0 | | | | | | | | | |
| 35–49 | 0 | | | | | | | | | |
| 50–64 | 0 | | | | | | | | | |
| 65+ | 0 | | | | | | | | | |
| **2. MULTIPLE DX** | | | | | | | | | | |
| 0–19 Years | 0 | | | | | | | | | |
| 20–34 | 0 | | | | | | | | | |
| 35–49 | 0 | | | | | | | | | |
| 50–64 | 0 | | | | | | | | | |
| 65+ | 1 | 1.0 | 0 | 1 | 1 | 1 | 1 | 1 | 1 | 1 |
| **TOTAL SINGLE DX** | 0 | | | | | | | | | |
| **TOTAL MULTIPLE DX** | 1 | 1.0 | 0 | 1 | 1 | 1 | 1 | 1 | 1 | 1 |
| **TOTAL** | | | | | | | | | | |
| 0–19 Years | 0 | | | | | | | | | |
| 20–34 | 0 | | | | | | | | | |
| 35–49 | 0 | | | | | | | | | |
| 50–64 | 0 | | | | | | | | | |
| 65+ | 1 | 1.0 | 0 | 1 | 1 | 1 | 1 | 1 | 1 | 1 |
| **GRAND TOTAL** | 1 | 1.0 | 0 | 1 | 1 | 1 | 1 | 1 | 1 | 1 |

## 28.5: EXCISION LINGUAL TONSIL. Formerly included in operation group(s) 555.

| Type of Patients | Observed Patients | Avg. Stay | Variance | 10th | 25th | 50th | 75th | 90th | 95th | 99th |
|---|---|---|---|---|---|---|---|---|---|---|
| **1. SINGLE DX** | | | | | | | | | | |
| 0–19 Years | 0 | | | | | | | | | |
| 20–34 | 1 | 3.0 | 0 | 3 | 3 | 3 | 3 | 3 | 3 | 3 |
| 35–49 | 1 | 2.0 | 0 | 2 | 2 | 2 | 2 | 2 | 2 | 2 |
| 50–64 | 0 | | | | | | | | | |
| 65+ | 0 | | | | | | | | | |
| **2. MULTIPLE DX** | | | | | | | | | | |
| 0–19 Years | 1 | 3.0 | 0 | 3 | 3 | 3 | 3 | 3 | 3 | 3 |
| 20–34 | 1 | 5.0 | 0 | 5 | 5 | 5 | 5 | 5 | 5 | 5 |
| 35–49 | 2 | 1.1 | <1 | 1 | 1 | 1 | 1 | 1 | 2 | 2 |
| 50–64 | 2 | 1.0 | 0 | 1 | 1 | 1 | 1 | 1 | 1 | 1 |
| 65+ | 0 | | | | | | | | | |
| **TOTAL SINGLE DX** | 2 | 2.6 | <1 | 2 | 2 | 3 | 3 | 3 | 3 | 3 |
| **TOTAL MULTIPLE DX** | 6 | 1.7 | 2 | 1 | 1 | 1 | 2 | 4 | 5 | 5 |
| **TOTAL** | | | | | | | | | | |
| 0–19 Years | 1 | 3.0 | 0 | 3 | 3 | 3 | 3 | 3 | 3 | 3 |
| 20–34 | 2 | 4.5 | <1 | 3 | 3 | 5 | 5 | 5 | 5 | 5 |
| 35–49 | 3 | 1.2 | <1 | 1 | 1 | 1 | 1 | 2 | 2 | 2 |
| 50–64 | 2 | 1.0 | 0 | 1 | 1 | 1 | 1 | 1 | 1 | 1 |
| 65+ | 0 | | | | | | | | | |
| **GRAND TOTAL** | 8 | 1.8 | 2 | 1 | 1 | 1 | 2 | 5 | 5 | 5 |

Length of Stay by Diagnosis and Operation, United States, 2000

# United States, October 1998–September 1999 Data, by Operation

## 28.6: ADENOIDECTOMY. Formerly included in operation group(s) 554.

| Type of Patients | Observed Patients | Avg. Stay | Variance | 10th | 25th | 50th | 75th | 90th | 95th | 99th |
|---|---|---|---|---|---|---|---|---|---|---|
| **1. SINGLE DX** | | | | | | | | | | |
| 0–19 Years | 37 | 1.1 | <1 | 1 | 1 | 1 | 1 | 1 | 2 | 3 |
| 20–34 | 1 | 1.0 | 0 | 1 | 1 | 1 | 1 | 1 | 1 | 1 |
| 35–49 | 0 | | | | | | | | | |
| 50–64 | 0 | | | | | | | | | |
| 65+ | 0 | | | | | | | | | |
| **2. MULTIPLE DX** | | | | | | | | | | |
| 0–19 Years | 254 | 2.9 | 28 | 1 | 1 | 1 | 2 | 7 | 15 | 26 |
| 20–34 | 2 | 10.2 | 87 | 1 | 1 | 18 | 18 | 18 | 18 | 18 |
| 35–49 | 5 | 1.2 | <1 | 1 | 1 | 1 | 1 | 2 | 2 | 2 |
| 50–64 | 1 | 13.0 | 0 | 13 | 13 | 13 | 13 | 13 | 13 | 13 |
| 65+ | 1 | 7.0 | 0 | 7 | 7 | 7 | 7 | 7 | 7 | 7 |
| **TOTAL SINGLE DX** | 38 | 1.1 | <1 | 1 | 1 | 1 | 1 | 1 | 2 | 3 |
| **TOTAL MULTIPLE DX** | 263 | 2.8 | 26 | 1 | 1 | 1 | 2 | 6 | 15 | 26 |
| **TOTAL** | | | | | | | | | | |
| 0–19 Years | 291 | 2.7 | 25 | 1 | 1 | 1 | 2 | 5 | 15 | 26 |
| 20–34 | 3 | 7.3 | 77 | 1 | 1 | 18 | 18 | 18 | 18 | 18 |
| 35–49 | 5 | 1.2 | <1 | 1 | 1 | 1 | 1 | 2 | 2 | 2 |
| 50–64 | 1 | 13.0 | 0 | 13 | 13 | 13 | 13 | 13 | 13 | 13 |
| 65+ | 1 | 7.0 | 0 | 7 | 7 | 7 | 7 | 7 | 7 | 7 |
| **GRAND TOTAL** | 301 | 2.6 | 24 | 1 | 1 | 1 | 2 | 5 | 14 | 25 |

## 28.7: HEMOR CONTROL POST T&A. Formerly included in operation group(s) 555.

| Type of Patients | Observed Patients | Avg. Stay | Variance | 10th | 25th | 50th | 75th | 90th | 95th | 99th |
|---|---|---|---|---|---|---|---|---|---|---|
| **1. SINGLE DX** | | | | | | | | | | |
| 0–19 Years | 430 | 1.3 | <1 | 1 | 1 | 1 | 2 | 2 | 2 | 3 |
| 20–34 | 117 | 1.3 | <1 | 1 | 1 | 1 | 1 | 2 | 3 | 3 |
| 35–49 | 26 | 1.3 | <1 | 1 | 1 | 1 | 2 | 2 | 2 | 4 |
| 50–64 | 4 | 6.2 | 50 | 1 | 16 | 16 | 16 | 16 | 16 | 16 |
| 65+ | 1 | 1.0 | 0 | 1 | 1 | 1 | 1 | 1 | 1 | 1 |
| **2. MULTIPLE DX** | | | | | | | | | | |
| 0–19 Years | 231 | 1.8 | 2 | 1 | 1 | 1 | 2 | 3 | 4 | 9 |
| 20–34 | 61 | 2.0 | 2 | 1 | 1 | 2 | 2 | 3 | 6 | 8 |
| 35–49 | 29 | 2.0 | 5 | 1 | 1 | 1 | 2 | 3 | 3 | 13 |
| 50–64 | 13 | 1.4 | <1 | 1 | 1 | 1 | 2 | 2 | 3 | 4 |
| 65+ | 3 | 10.1 | 72 | 2 | 2 | 14 | 19 | 19 | 19 | 19 |
| **TOTAL SINGLE DX** | 578 | 1.4 | <1 | 1 | 1 | 1 | 2 | 2 | 3 | 3 |
| **TOTAL MULTIPLE DX** | 337 | 1.9 | 3 | 1 | 1 | 1 | 2 | 3 | 4 | 9 |
| **TOTAL** | | | | | | | | | | |
| 0–19 Years | 661 | 1.5 | <1 | 1 | 1 | 1 | 2 | 2 | 3 | 5 |
| 20–34 | 178 | 1.5 | 1 | 1 | 1 | 1 | 2 | 3 | 3 | 8 |
| 35–49 | 55 | 1.7 | 3 | 1 | 1 | 1 | 2 | 3 | 4 | 13 |
| 50–64 | 17 | 2.8 | 20 | 1 | 1 | 2 | 2 | 16 | 16 | 16 |
| 65+ | 4 | 8.3 | 71 | 2 | 2 | 14 | 19 | 19 | 19 | 19 |
| **GRAND TOTAL** | 915 | 1.5 | 2 | 1 | 1 | 1 | 2 | 2 | 3 | 7 |

## 28.9: OTHER TONSIL/ADENOID OPS. Formerly included in operation group(s) 555.

| Type of Patients | Observed Patients | Avg. Stay | Variance | 10th | 25th | 50th | 75th | 90th | 95th | 99th |
|---|---|---|---|---|---|---|---|---|---|---|
| **1. SINGLE DX** | | | | | | | | | | |
| 0–19 Years | 11 | 1.4 | <1 | 1 | 1 | 1 | 2 | 2 | 4 | 4 |
| 20–34 | 5 | 1.1 | <1 | 1 | 1 | 1 | 1 | 2 | 2 | 2 |
| 35–49 | 2 | 2.0 | 0 | 2 | 2 | 2 | 2 | 2 | 2 | 2 |
| 50–64 | 1 | 1.0 | 0 | 1 | 1 | 1 | 1 | 1 | 1 | 1 |
| 65+ | 0 | | | | | | | | | |
| **2. MULTIPLE DX** | | | | | | | | | | |
| 0–19 Years | 13 | 1.4 | <1 | 1 | 1 | 1 | 2 | 2 | 2 | 5 |
| 20–34 | 5 | 2.9 | 18 | 1 | 1 | 1 | 3 | 3 | 16 | 16 |
| 35–49 | 10 | 7.4 | 36 | 1 | 3 | 5 | 15 | 15 | 15 | 15 |
| 50–64 | 6 | 7.0 | 49 | 3 | 3 | 6 | 6 | 7 | 29 | 29 |
| 65+ | 9 | 4.6 | 16 | 1 | 2 | 4 | 5 | 6 | 6 | 21 |
| **TOTAL SINGLE DX** | 19 | 1.4 | <1 | 1 | 1 | 1 | 2 | 2 | 2 | 4 |
| **TOTAL MULTIPLE DX** | 43 | 4.9 | 33 | 1 | 1 | 3 | 6 | 12 | 15 | 29 |
| **TOTAL** | | | | | | | | | | |
| 0–19 Years | 24 | 1.4 | <1 | 1 | 1 | 1 | 2 | 2 | 2 | 5 |
| 20–34 | 10 | 1.8 | 8 | 1 | 1 | 1 | 1 | 3 | 3 | 16 |
| 35–49 | 12 | 6.6 | 34 | 1 | 3 | 3 | 12 | 15 | 15 | 15 |
| 50–64 | 7 | 6.8 | 49 | 3 | 3 | 6 | 6 | 7 | 29 | 29 |
| 65+ | 9 | 4.6 | 16 | 1 | 2 | 4 | 5 | 6 | 6 | 21 |
| **GRAND TOTAL** | 62 | 3.8 | 26 | 1 | 1 | 2 | 5 | 6 | 15 | 29 |

## 29.0: PHARYNGOTOMY. Formerly included in operation group(s) 555.

| Type of Patients | Observed Patients | Avg. Stay | Variance | 10th | 25th | 50th | 75th | 90th | 95th | 99th |
|---|---|---|---|---|---|---|---|---|---|---|
| **1. SINGLE DX** | | | | | | | | | | |
| 0–19 Years | 11 | 2.8 | 2 | 2 | 2 | 2 | 3 | 5 | 5 | 5 |
| 20–34 | 2 | 3.1 | 2 | 2 | 2 | 2 | 5 | 5 | 5 | 5 |
| 35–49 | 0 | | | | | | | | | |
| 50–64 | 2 | 2.9 | <1 | 2 | 3 | 3 | 3 | 3 | 3 | 3 |
| 65+ | 0 | | | | | | | | | |
| **2. MULTIPLE DX** | | | | | | | | | | |
| 0–19 Years | 14 | 4.8 | 6 | 2 | 2 | 5 | 7 | 7 | 10 | 10 |
| 20–34 | 3 | 2.0 | 3 | 1 | 1 | 1 | 2 | 5 | 5 | 5 |
| 35–49 | 10 | 9.1 | 47 | 2 | 3 | 6 | 15 | 15 | 15 | 29 |
| 50–64 | 8 | 5.9 | 7 | 2 | 4 | 6 | 8 | 8 | 8 | 8 |
| 65+ | 10 | 6.7 | 14 | 1 | 6 | 8 | 8 | 8 | 11 | 20 |
| **TOTAL SINGLE DX** | 15 | 2.9 | 1 | 2 | 2 | 3 | 3 | 5 | 5 | 5 |
| **TOTAL MULTIPLE DX** | 45 | 6.4 | 20 | 2 | 3 | 6 | 8 | 11 | 15 | 29 |
| **TOTAL** | | | | | | | | | | |
| 0–19 Years | 25 | 4.1 | 6 | 2 | 2 | 3 | 5 | 7 | 10 | 10 |
| 20–34 | 5 | 2.6 | 3 | 2 | 2 | 2 | 2 | 5 | 5 | 5 |
| 35–49 | 10 | 9.1 | 47 | 2 | 3 | 6 | 15 | 15 | 15 | 29 |
| 50–64 | 10 | 4.7 | 6 | 2 | 3 | 3 | 8 | 8 | 8 | 9 |
| 65+ | 10 | 6.7 | 14 | 1 | 6 | 8 | 8 | 8 | 11 | 20 |
| **GRAND TOTAL** | 60 | 5.4 | 17 | 2 | 2 | 4 | 8 | 9 | 15 | 20 |

Length of Stay by Diagnosis and Operation, United States, 2000

## United States, October 1998–September 1999 Data, by Operation

### 29.1: PHARYNGEAL DXTIC PX. Formerly included in operation group(s) 555, 556.

| Type of Patients | Observed Patients | Avg. Stay | Vari-ance | Percentiles | | | | | | |
|---|---|---|---|---|---|---|---|---|---|---|
| | | | | 10th | 25th | 50th | 75th | 90th | 95th | 99th |
| **1. SINGLE DX** | | | | | | | | | | |
| 0–19 Years | 41 | 1.9 | <1 | 1 | 1 | 2 | 2 | 3 | 3 | 6 |
| 20–34 | 17 | 2.3 | 2 | 1 | 1 | 2 | 2 | 4 | 7 | 7 |
| 35–49 | 15 | 2.3 | <1 | 1 | 2 | 2 | 3 | 3 | 3 | 4 |
| 50–64 | 7 | 1.9 | 1 | 1 | 1 | 2 | 2 | 4 | 4 | 4 |
| 65+ | 3 | 1.9 | 3 | 1 | 1 | 1 | 1 | 5 | 5 | 5 |
| **2. MULTIPLE DX** | | | | | | | | | | |
| 0–19 Years | 142 | 5.7 | 88 | 1 | 2 | 3 | 8 | 11 | 13 | 90 |
| 20–34 | 44 | 3.1 | 13 | 1 | 1 | 2 | 4 | 5 | 9 | 26 |
| 35–49 | 107 | 4.0 | 25 | 1 | 1 | 2 | 5 | 8 | 16 | 21 |
| 50–64 | 139 | 5.8 | 35 | 1 | 2 | 4 | 7 | 15 | 19 | 32 |
| 65+ | 272 | 6.4 | 28 | 2 | 3 | 6 | 8 | 13 | 15 | 31 |
| **TOTAL SINGLE DX** | 83 | 2.1 | 1 | 1 | 1 | 2 | 3 | 3 | 3 | 6 |
| **TOTAL MULTIPLE DX** | 704 | 5.4 | 42 | 1 | 2 | 4 | 7 | 11 | 15 | 35 |
| **TOTAL** | | | | | | | | | | |
| 0–19 Years | 183 | 4.8 | 70 | 1 | 1 | 2 | 6 | 9 | 12 | 73 |
| 20–34 | 61 | 2.9 | 10 | 1 | 1 | 2 | 3 | 5 | 8 | 15 |
| 35–49 | 122 | 3.7 | 21 | 1 | 1 | 2 | 5 | 6 | 15 | 21 |
| 50–64 | 146 | 5.6 | 34 | 1 | 1 | 4 | 7 | 15 | 17 | 32 |
| 65+ | 275 | 6.3 | 28 | 2 | 3 | 5 | 8 | 13 | 15 | 31 |
| **GRAND TOTAL** | 787 | 5.0 | 38 | 1 | 2 | 3 | 6 | 11 | 15 | 31 |

### 29.2: EXC BRANCHIAL CLEFT CYST. Formerly included in operation group(s) 555.

| Type of Patients | Observed Patients | Avg. Stay | Vari-ance | Percentiles | | | | | | |
|---|---|---|---|---|---|---|---|---|---|---|
| | | | | 10th | 25th | 50th | 75th | 90th | 95th | 99th |
| **1. SINGLE DX** | | | | | | | | | | |
| 0–19 Years | 39 | 2.0 | 1 | 1 | 1 | 2 | 2 | 3 | 3 | 5 |
| 20–34 | 21 | 1.3 | <1 | 1 | 1 | 1 | 2 | 2 | 2 | 3 |
| 35–49 | 16 | 1.8 | 4 | 1 | 1 | 1 | 2 | 2 | 7 | 9 |
| 50–64 | 8 | 1.9 | <1 | 1 | 2 | 2 | 2 | 2 | 3 | 3 |
| 65+ | 3 | 1.3 | <1 | 1 | 2 | 2 | 2 | 2 | 2 | 2 |
| **2. MULTIPLE DX** | | | | | | | | | | |
| 0–19 Years | 30 | 2.8 | 6 | 1 | 1 | 2 | 4 | 5 | 5 | 15 |
| 20–34 | 10 | 3.1 | 17 | 1 | 1 | 2 | 3 | 12 | 12 | 12 |
| 35–49 | 15 | 2.3 | 4 | 1 | 1 | 1 | 3 | 5 | 5 | 8 |
| 50–64 | 7 | 2.0 | <1 | 1 | 2 | 2 | 2 | 3 | 4 | 4 |
| 65+ | 6 | 1.8 | 1 | 1 | 1 | 2 | 2 | 3 | 4 | 4 |
| **TOTAL SINGLE DX** | 87 | 1.7 | 1 | 1 | 1 | 1 | 2 | 3 | 3 | 7 |
| **TOTAL MULTIPLE DX** | 68 | 2.6 | 6 | 1 | 1 | 2 | 3 | 5 | 7 | 14 |
| **TOTAL** | | | | | | | | | | |
| 0–19 Years | 69 | 2.3 | 3 | 1 | 1 | 2 | 3 | 4 | 5 | 11 |
| 20–34 | 31 | 1.7 | 4 | 1 | 1 | 1 | 1 | 2 | 3 | 12 |
| 35–49 | 31 | 2.0 | 4 | 1 | 1 | 1 | 2 | 5 | 7 | 9 |
| 50–64 | 15 | 2.0 | <1 | 1 | 2 | 2 | 2 | 3 | 4 | 4 |
| 65+ | 9 | 1.6 | 1 | 1 | 1 | 2 | 2 | 3 | 4 | 4 |
| **GRAND TOTAL** | 155 | 2.0 | 3 | 1 | 1 | 2 | 2 | 3 | 5 | 12 |

### 29.11: PHARYNGOSCOPY. Formerly included in operation group(s) 556.

| Type of Patients | Observed Patients | Avg. Stay | Vari-ance | Percentiles | | | | | | |
|---|---|---|---|---|---|---|---|---|---|---|
| | | | | 10th | 25th | 50th | 75th | 90th | 95th | 99th |
| **1. SINGLE DX** | | | | | | | | | | |
| 0–19 Years | 38 | 1.9 | 1 | 1 | 1 | 2 | 2 | 3 | 3 | 6 |
| 20–34 | 15 | 2.3 | 2 | 1 | 1 | 2 | 2 | 4 | 7 | 7 |
| 35–49 | 10 | 2.3 | <1 | 2 | 2 | 2 | 3 | 3 | 3 | 4 |
| 50–64 | 5 | 2.2 | 1 | 1 | 1 | 2 | 2 | 4 | 4 | 4 |
| 65+ | 2 | 1.0 | 0 | 1 | 1 | 1 | 1 | 1 | 1 | 1 |
| **2. MULTIPLE DX** | | | | | | | | | | |
| 0–19 Years | 134 | 5.4 | 91 | 1 | 2 | 3 | 7 | 11 | 13 | 90 |
| 20–34 | 38 | 2.7 | 6 | 1 | 1 | 2 | 3 | 4 | 8 | 15 |
| 35–49 | 77 | 4.5 | 18 | 1 | 2 | 4 | 5 | 9 | 15 | 26 |
| 50–64 | 89 | 6.3 | 29 | 2 | 2 | 5 | 8 | 14 | 15 | 36 |
| 65+ | 196 | 6.3 | 25 | 2 | 3 | 5 | 7 | 13 | 15 | 24 |
| **TOTAL SINGLE DX** | 70 | 2.0 | 1 | 1 | 1 | 2 | 2 | 3 | 4 | 7 |
| **TOTAL MULTIPLE DX** | 534 | 5.5 | 43 | 1 | 2 | 4 | 7 | 11 | 15 | 36 |
| **TOTAL** | | | | | | | | | | |
| 0–19 Years | 172 | 4.5 | 71 | 1 | 1 | 2 | 5 | 9 | 12 | 73 |
| 20–34 | 53 | 2.6 | 5 | 1 | 1 | 2 | 3 | 4 | 7 | 15 |
| 35–49 | 87 | 4.1 | 15 | 1 | 2 | 3 | 5 | 7 | 13 | 21 |
| 50–64 | 94 | 6.0 | 28 | 1 | 2 | 5 | 7 | 14 | 15 | 36 |
| 65+ | 198 | 6.2 | 25 | 2 | 3 | 5 | 7 | 12 | 15 | 24 |
| **GRAND TOTAL** | 604 | 5.0 | 38 | 1 | 2 | 3 | 6 | 10 | 14 | 26 |

### 29.3: EXC/DESTR PHARYNGEAL LES. Formerly included in operation group(s) 555.

| Type of Patients | Observed Patients | Avg. Stay | Vari-ance | Percentiles | | | | | | |
|---|---|---|---|---|---|---|---|---|---|---|
| | | | | 10th | 25th | 50th | 75th | 90th | 95th | 99th |
| **1. SINGLE DX** | | | | | | | | | | |
| 0–19 Years | 20 | 3.6 | 6 | 1 | 2 | 3 | 5 | 7 | 8 | 10 |
| 20–34 | 6 | 3.1 | 4 | 1 | 1 | 3 | 6 | 6 | 6 | 6 |
| 35–49 | 20 | 2.9 | 2 | 1 | 1 | 3 | 4 | 4 | 6 | 6 |
| 50–64 | 15 | 1.9 | 1 | 1 | 1 | 1 | 2 | 6 | 6 | 7 |
| 65+ | 27 | 3.3 | 7 | 1 | 2 | 3 | 4 | 5 | 6 | 14 |
| **2. MULTIPLE DX** | | | | | | | | | | |
| 0–19 Years | 37 | 7.8 | 95 | 2 | 3 | 3 | 9 | 15 | 29 | 45 |
| 20–34 | 6 | 4.2 | 6 | 2 | 2 | 2 | 7 | 8 | 8 | 8 |
| 35–49 | 34 | 3.8 | 13 | 1 | 2 | 4 | 5 | 9 | 8 | 21 |
| 50–64 | 123 | 6.7 | 40 | 1 | 2 | 5 | 8 | 12 | 15 | 38 |
| 65+ | 327 | 5.3 | 30 | 1 | 2 | 3 | 7 | 10 | 16 | 25 |
| **TOTAL SINGLE DX** | 88 | 2.9 | 5 | 1 | 1 | 2 | 4 | 6 | 7 | 10 |
| **TOTAL MULTIPLE DX** | 527 | 5.7 | 36 | 1 | 2 | 4 | 7 | 12 | 16 | 34 |
| **TOTAL** | | | | | | | | | | |
| 0–19 Years | 57 | 6.0 | 60 | 2 | 2 | 3 | 7 | 12 | 22 | 45 |
| 20–34 | 12 | 3.9 | 6 | 1 | 2 | 3 | 6 | 7 | 4 | 8 |
| 35–49 | 54 | 3.6 | 10 | 1 | 2 | 4 | 4 | 7 | 4 | 21 |
| 50–64 | 138 | 6.2 | 37 | 1 | 2 | 5 | 8 | 12 | 15 | 38 |
| 65+ | 354 | 5.2 | 29 | 1 | 2 | 3 | 6 | 10 | 16 | 25 |
| **GRAND TOTAL** | 615 | 5.3 | 32 | 1 | 2 | 4 | 7 | 11 | 15 | 29 |

Length of Stay by Diagnosis and Operation, United States, 2000

# United States, October 1998–September 1999 Data, by Operation

## 29.4: PLASTIC OP ON PHARYNX. Formerly included in operation group(s) 555.

| Type of Patients | Observed Patients | Avg. Stay | Vari-ance | 10th | 25th | 50th | 75th | 90th | 95th | 99th |
|---|---|---|---|---|---|---|---|---|---|---|
| **1. SINGLE DX** | | | | | | | | | | |
| 0-19 Years | 92 | 1.9 | 2 | 1 | 1 | 2 | 2 | 3 | 3 | 10 |
| 20-34 | 21 | 1.2 | <1 | 1 | 1 | 1 | 1 | 2 | 3 | 4 |
| 35-49 | 74 | 1.8 | <1 | 1 | 1 | 2 | 2 | 2 | 4 | 4 |
| 50-64 | 32 | 1.7 | <1 | 1 | 1 | 2 | 2 | 3 | 3 | 6 |
| 65+ | 4 | 2.5 | 1 | 1 | 2 | 2 | 4 | 4 | 4 | 4 |
| **2. MULTIPLE DX** | | | | | | | | | | |
| 0-19 Years | 186 | 3.1 | 59 | 1 | 2 | 2 | 3 | 4 | 5 | 42 |
| 20-34 | 149 | 1.6 | 1 | 1 | 1 | 1 | 2 | 3 | 3 | 5 |
| 35-49 | 484 | 1.7 | 3 | 1 | 1 | 1 | 2 | 3 | 4 | 7 |
| 50-64 | 264 | 1.7 | 1 | 1 | 1 | 1 | 2 | 3 | 4 | 6 |
| 65+ | 92 | 2.2 | 7 | 1 | 2 | 2 | 3 | 3 | 6 | 18 |
| **TOTAL SINGLE DX** | 223 | 1.8 | 1 | 1 | 1 | 2 | 2 | 3 | 3 | 6 |
| **TOTAL MULTIPLE DX** | 1,175 | 1.9 | 11 | 1 | 1 | 1 | 2 | 3 | 4 | 8 |
| **TOTAL** | | | | | | | | | | |
| 0-19 Years | 278 | 2.8 | 42 | 1 | 1 | 2 | 3 | 4 | 5 | 42 |
| 20-34 | 170 | 1.6 | 1 | 1 | 1 | 1 | 2 | 3 | 3 | 5 |
| 35-49 | 558 | 1.7 | 3 | 1 | 1 | 1 | 2 | 3 | 4 | 7 |
| 50-64 | 296 | 1.7 | 1 | 1 | 1 | 2 | 2 | 3 | 4 | 6 |
| 65+ | 96 | 2.2 | 7 | 1 | 2 | 2 | 3 | 3 | 6 | 18 |
| **GRAND TOTAL** | 1,398 | 1.9 | 10 | 1 | 1 | 1 | 2 | 3 | 4 | 8 |

## 29.9: OTHER PHARYNGEAL OPS. Formerly included in operation group(s) 555.

| Type of Patients | Observed Patients | Avg. Stay | Vari-ance | 10th | 25th | 50th | 75th | 90th | 95th | 99th |
|---|---|---|---|---|---|---|---|---|---|---|
| **1. SINGLE DX** | | | | | | | | | | |
| 0-19 Years | 7 | 2.3 | <1 | 2 | 2 | 2 | 2 | 4 | 4 | 4 |
| 20-34 | 2 | 3.0 | 0 | 3 | 3 | 3 | 3 | 3 | 3 | 3 |
| 35-49 | 3 | 4.9 | <1 | 4 | 5 | 5 | 5 | 5 | 5 | 5 |
| 50-64 | 0 | | | | | | | | | |
| 65+ | 0 | | | | | | | | | |
| **2. MULTIPLE DX** | | | | | | | | | | |
| 0-19 Years | 13 | 29.6 | 878 | 1 | 2 | 6 | 64 | 64 | 64 | 64 |
| 20-34 | 2 | 6.7 | <1 | 5 | 7 | 7 | 7 | 7 | 7 | 7 |
| 35-49 | 1 | 21.0 | 0 | 21 | 21 | 21 | 21 | 21 | 21 | 21 |
| 50-64 | 2 | 3.0 | 0 | 2 | 3 | 3 | 3 | 3 | 3 | 3 |
| 65+ | 1 | 2.0 | 0 | 2 | 2 | 2 | 2 | 2 | 2 | 2 |
| **TOTAL SINGLE DX** | 12 | 2.9 | 2 | 2 | 2 | 2 | 4 | 5 | 5 | 5 |
| **TOTAL MULTIPLE DX** | 19 | 12.8 | 426 | 2 | 3 | 3 | 7 | 64 | 64 | 64 |
| **TOTAL** | | | | | | | | | | |
| 0-19 Years | 20 | 15.2 | 596 | 2 | 2 | 7 | 64 | 64 | 64 | 64 |
| 20-34 | 4 | 5.8 | 3 | 3 | 5 | 7 | 7 | 7 | 7 | 7 |
| 35-49 | 4 | 10.4 | 62 | 5 | 5 | 5 | 21 | 21 | 21 | 21 |
| 50-64 | 2 | 3.0 | 0 | 3 | 3 | 3 | 3 | 3 | 3 | 3 |
| 65+ | 1 | 2.0 | 0 | 2 | 2 | 2 | 2 | 2 | 2 | 2 |
| **GRAND TOTAL** | 31 | 9.5 | 308 | 2 | 2 | 3 | 5 | 36 | 64 | 64 |

## 29.5: OTHER PHARYNGEAL REPAIR. Formerly included in operation group(s) 555.

| Type of Patients | Observed Patients | Avg. Stay | Vari-ance | 10th | 25th | 50th | 75th | 90th | 95th | 99th |
|---|---|---|---|---|---|---|---|---|---|---|
| **1. SINGLE DX** | | | | | | | | | | |
| 0-19 Years | 9 | 1.8 | 1 | 1 | 1 | 1 | 2 | 3 | 3 | 3 |
| 20-34 | 1 | 3.0 | 0 | 3 | 3 | 3 | 3 | 3 | 3 | 3 |
| 35-49 | 2 | 3.0 | 1 | 2 | 2 | 2 | 4 | 4 | 4 | 4 |
| 50-64 | 0 | | | | | | | | | |
| 65+ | 0 | | | | | | | | | |
| **2. MULTIPLE DX** | | | | | | | | | | |
| 0-19 Years | 10 | 1.8 | 2 | 1 | 1 | 1 | 2 | 3 | 4 | 10 |
| 20-34 | 11 | 3.9 | 5 | 2 | 2 | 4 | 4 | 4 | 10 | 10 |
| 35-49 | 3 | 5.3 | 3 | 3 | 4 | 4 | 7 | 7 | 7 | 7 |
| 50-64 | 16 | 7.9 | 36 | 2 | 7 | 7 | 10 | 15 | 15 | 28 |
| 65+ | 14 | 9.5 | 124 | 3 | 3 | 4 | 13 | 19 | 44 | 44 |
| **TOTAL SINGLE DX** | 12 | 2.1 | 1 | 1 | 1 | 2 | 3 | 3 | 4 | 6 |
| **TOTAL MULTIPLE DX** | 54 | 5.9 | 47 | 1 | 2 | 4 | 7 | 13 | 15 | 44 |
| **TOTAL** | | | | | | | | | | |
| 0-19 Years | 19 | 1.8 | 2 | 1 | 1 | 1 | 2 | 3 | 4 | 10 |
| 20-34 | 12 | 3.7 | 4 | 1 | 3 | 4 | 4 | 4 | 10 | 10 |
| 35-49 | 5 | 4.7 | 4 | 2 | 3 | 4 | 7 | 7 | 7 | 7 |
| 50-64 | 16 | 7.9 | 36 | 1 | 3 | 7 | 10 | 15 | 15 | 28 |
| 65+ | 14 | 9.5 | 124 | 2 | 3 | 4 | 13 | 19 | 44 | 44 |
| **GRAND TOTAL** | 66 | 5.3 | 42 | 1 | 2 | 3 | 6 | 12 | 15 | 44 |

## 30.0: EXC/DESTR LES LARYNX. Formerly included in operation group(s) 557.

| Type of Patients | Observed Patients | Avg. Stay | Vari-ance | 10th | 25th | 50th | 75th | 90th | 95th | 99th |
|---|---|---|---|---|---|---|---|---|---|---|
| **1. SINGLE DX** | | | | | | | | | | |
| 0-19 Years | 83 | 1.6 | <1 | 1 | 1 | 1 | 2 | 3 | 3 | 4 |
| 20-34 | 8 | 1.6 | <1 | 1 | 1 | 2 | 2 | 3 | 3 | 3 |
| 35-49 | 12 | 1.5 | <1 | 1 | 1 | 1 | 2 | 3 | 3 | 3 |
| 50-64 | 11 | 1.1 | <1 | 1 | 1 | 1 | 1 | 1 | 2 | 2 |
| 65+ | 10 | 1.1 | <1 | 1 | 1 | 2 | 2 | 2 | 2 | 2 |
| **2. MULTIPLE DX** | | | | | | | | | | |
| 0-19 Years | 218 | 4.6 | 42 | 1 | 1 | 2 | 6 | 11 | 17 | 30 |
| 20-34 | 22 | 2.8 | 12 | 1 | 1 | 2 | 4 | 4 | 4 | 31 |
| 35-49 | 67 | 2.7 | 13 | 1 | 1 | 2 | 3 | 6 | 8 | 36 |
| 50-64 | 109 | 5.2 | 56 | 1 | 1 | 3 | 6 | 11 | 14 | 42 |
| 65+ | 124 | 4.9 | 33 | 1 | 1 | 3 | 6 | 11 | 17 | 28 |
| **TOTAL SINGLE DX** | 124 | 1.5 | <1 | 1 | 1 | 1 | 2 | 3 | 3 | 4 |
| **TOTAL MULTIPLE DX** | 540 | 4.3 | 37 | 1 | 1 | 2 | 5 | 10 | 15 | 42 |
| **TOTAL** | | | | | | | | | | |
| 0-19 Years | 301 | 3.7 | 32 | 1 | 1 | 2 | 3 | 9 | 15 | 30 |
| 20-34 | 30 | 2.6 | 10 | 1 | 1 | 2 | 3 | 4 | 4 | 11 |
| 35-49 | 79 | 2.6 | 12 | 1 | 1 | 2 | 3 | 6 | 8 | 36 |
| 50-64 | 120 | 5.0 | 54 | 1 | 1 | 3 | 5 | 11 | 13 | 42 |
| 65+ | 134 | 4.6 | 31 | 1 | 1 | 3 | 6 | 9 | 17 | 28 |
| **GRAND TOTAL** | 664 | 3.8 | 32 | 1 | 2 | 2 | 4 | 9 | 12 | 36 |

Length of Stay by Diagnosis and Operation, United States, 2000

# United States, October 1998–September 1999 Data, by Operation

## 30.09: EXC/DESTR LARYNX LES NEC. Formerly included in operation group(s) 557.

| Type of Patients | Observed Patients | Avg. Stay | Vari-ance | Percentiles 10th | 25th | 50th | 75th | 90th | 95th | 99th |
|---|---|---|---|---|---|---|---|---|---|---|
| **1. SINGLE DX** | | | | | | | | | | |
| 0–19 Years | 83 | 1.6 | <1 | 1 | 1 | 1 | 2 | 3 | 3 | 4 |
| 20–34 | 8 | 1.6 | <1 | 1 | 1 | 1 | 2 | 2 | 2 | 2 |
| 35–49 | 11 | 1.6 | <1 | 1 | 1 | 1 | 2 | 3 | 3 | 3 |
| 50–64 | 11 | 1.1 | <1 | 1 | 1 | 1 | 1 | 1 | 2 | 2 |
| 65+ | 10 | 1.1 | <1 | 1 | 1 | 1 | 1 | 2 | 2 | 2 |
| **2. MULTIPLE DX** | | | | | | | | | | |
| 0–19 Years | 208 | 4.6 | 43 | 1 | 1 | 2 | 6 | 11 | 17 | 30 |
| 20–34 | 21 | 2.8 | 12 | 1 | 1 | 2 | 4 | 4 | 4 | 31 |
| 35–49 | 67 | 2.7 | 13 | 1 | 1 | 2 | 3 | 6 | 8 | 36 |
| 50–64 | 108 | 5.2 | 56 | 1 | 1 | 3 | 6 | 11 | 14 | 42 |
| 65+ | 124 | 4.9 | 33 | 1 | 1 | 3 | 6 | 11 | 17 | 28 |
| **TOTAL SINGLE DX** | 123 | 1.6 | <1 | 1 | 1 | 1 | 2 | 3 | 3 | 4 |
| **TOTAL MULTIPLE DX** | 528 | 4.3 | 38 | 1 | 1 | 2 | 5 | 10 | 15 | 42 |
| **TOTAL** | | | | | | | | | | |
| 0–19 Years | 291 | 3.7 | 33 | 1 | 1 | 2 | 3 | 9 | 16 | 30 |
| 20–34 | 29 | 2.6 | 10 | 1 | 1 | 2 | 3 | 4 | 4 | 11 |
| 35–49 | 78 | 2.6 | 12 | 1 | 1 | 2 | 3 | 6 | 8 | 36 |
| 50–64 | 119 | 5.0 | 54 | 1 | 1 | 2 | 5 | 11 | 12 | 42 |
| 65+ | 134 | 4.6 | 31 | 1 | 1 | 3 | 6 | 9 | 17 | 28 |
| **GRAND TOTAL** | 651 | 3.8 | 32 | 1 | 1 | 2 | 4 | 9 | 12 | 36 |

## 30.1: HEMILARYNGECTOMY. Formerly included in operation group(s) 558.

| Type of Patients | Observed Patients | Avg. Stay | Vari-ance | Percentiles 10th | 25th | 50th | 75th | 90th | 95th | 99th |
|---|---|---|---|---|---|---|---|---|---|---|
| **1. SINGLE DX** | | | | | | | | | | |
| 0–19 Years | 0 | | | | | | | | | |
| 20–34 | 0 | | | | | | | | | |
| 35–49 | 0 | | | | | | | | | |
| 50–64 | 6 | 8.4 | 4 | 5 | 7 | 10 | 10 | 10 | 10 | 10 |
| 65+ | 4 | 8.4 | 5 | 5 | 5 | 9 | 9 | 11 | 11 | 11 |
| **2. MULTIPLE DX** | | | | | | | | | | |
| 0–19 Years | 0 | | | | | | | | | |
| 20–34 | 1 | 9.0 | 0 | 9 | 9 | 9 | 9 | 9 | 9 | 9 |
| 35–49 | 2 | 16.0 | 40 | 8 | 8 | 20 | 20 | 20 | 20 | 20 |
| 50–64 | 10 | 10.2 | 85 | 5 | 5 | 6 | 8 | 19 | 38 | 38 |
| 65+ | 15 | 9.3 | 18 | 7 | 7 | 7 | 11 | 13 | 21 | 24 |
| **TOTAL SINGLE DX** | 10 | 8.4 | 5 | 5 | 7 | 9 | 10 | 10 | 11 | 11 |
| **TOTAL MULTIPLE DX** | 28 | 10.0 | 49 | 5 | 6 | 7 | 11 | 20 | 24 | 38 |
| **TOTAL** | | | | | | | | | | |
| 0–19 Years | 0 | | | | | | | | | |
| 20–34 | 1 | 9.0 | 0 | 9 | 9 | 9 | 9 | 9 | 9 | 9 |
| 35–49 | 2 | 16.0 | 40 | 9 | 9 | 20 | 20 | 20 | 20 | 20 |
| 50–64 | 16 | 9.5 | 59 | 8 | 8 | 8 | 10 | 18 | 38 | 38 |
| 65+ | 19 | 9.1 | 16 | 7 | 7 | 8 | 11 | 12 | 21 | 24 |
| **GRAND TOTAL** | 38 | 9.6 | 39 | 5 | 7 | 8 | 10 | 18 | 21 | 38 |

## 30.2: PARTIAL LARYNGECTOMY NEC. Formerly included in operation group(s) 558.

| Type of Patients | Observed Patients | Avg. Stay | Vari-ance | Percentiles 10th | 25th | 50th | 75th | 90th | 95th | 99th |
|---|---|---|---|---|---|---|---|---|---|---|
| **1. SINGLE DX** | | | | | | | | | | |
| 0–19 Years | 6 | 3.0 | 2 | 1 | 2 | 3 | 3 | 5 | 5 | 5 |
| 20–34 | 1 | 5.0 | 0 | 5 | 5 | 5 | 5 | 5 | 5 | 5 |
| 35–49 | 1 | 9.0 | 0 | 9 | 9 | 9 | 9 | 9 | 9 | 9 |
| 50–64 | 8 | 7.6 | 38 | 3 | 3 | 6 | 11 | 19 | 19 | 19 |
| 65+ | 9 | 4.0 | 8 | 1 | 1 | 4 | 6 | 8 | 9 | 9 |
| **2. MULTIPLE DX** | | | | | | | | | | |
| 0–19 Years | 39 | 8.9 | 349 | 2 | 2 | 3 | 8 | 14 | 73 | 95 |
| 20–34 | 5 | 7.1 | 105 | 2 | 2 | 3 | 5 | 32 | 32 | 32 |
| 35–49 | 9 | 5.6 | 184 | 1 | 1 | 1 | 3 | 20 | 20 | 88 |
| 50–64 | 42 | 8.2 | 27 | 1 | 4 | 8 | 12 | 14 | 17 | 24 |
| 65+ | 51 | 5.3 | 27 | 1 | 2 | 3 | 8 | 12 | 14 | 24 |
| **TOTAL SINGLE DX** | 25 | 5.7 | 21 | 1 | 3 | 5 | 6 | 11 | 19 | 19 |
| **TOTAL MULTIPLE DX** | 146 | 7.1 | 127 | 1 | 2 | 3 | 9 | 12 | 20 | 73 |
| **TOTAL** | | | | | | | | | | |
| 0–19 Years | 45 | 8.1 | 304 | 2 | 2 | 3 | 5 | 14 | 24 | 95 |
| 20–34 | 6 | 6.6 | 81 | 2 | 2 | 5 | 5 | 32 | 32 | 32 |
| 35–49 | 10 | 6.0 | 163 | 1 | 1 | 1 | 8 | 20 | 20 | 88 |
| 50–64 | 50 | 8.1 | 29 | 1 | 4 | 6 | 12 | 16 | 19 | 24 |
| 65+ | 60 | 5.1 | 25 | 1 | 2 | 3 | 8 | 10 | 12 | 24 |
| **GRAND TOTAL** | 171 | 6.9 | 112 | 1 | 2 | 3 | 9 | 12 | 19 | 73 |

## 30.3: COMPLETE LARYNGECTOMY. Formerly included in operation group(s) 559.

| Type of Patients | Observed Patients | Avg. Stay | Vari-ance | Percentiles 10th | 25th | 50th | 75th | 90th | 95th | 99th |
|---|---|---|---|---|---|---|---|---|---|---|
| **1. SINGLE DX** | | | | | | | | | | |
| 0–19 Years | 0 | | | | | | | | | |
| 20–34 | 0 | | | | | | | | | |
| 35–49 | 4 | 11.9 | 21 | 4 | 7 | 15 | 15 | 15 | 15 | 15 |
| 50–64 | 23 | 8.2 | 6 | 5 | 6 | 9 | 9 | 12 | 12 | 14 |
| 65+ | 18 | 10.3 | 3 | 8 | 11 | 11 | 11 | 11 | 11 | 12 |
| **2. MULTIPLE DX** | | | | | | | | | | |
| 0–19 Years | 1 | 25.0 | 0 | 25 | 25 | 25 | 25 | 25 | 25 | 25 |
| 20–34 | 3 | 16.9 | 177 | 9 | 9 | 14 | >99 | >99 | >99 | >99 |
| 35–49 | 44 | 13.3 | 90 | 5 | 7 | 9 | 16 | 23 | 36 | 44 |
| 50–64 | 185 | 10.5 | 42 | 5 | 7 | 9 | 12 | 17 | 23 | 38 |
| 65+ | 260 | 11.0 | 47 | 6 | 7 | 9 | 12 | 21 | 27 | 37 |
| **TOTAL SINGLE DX** | 45 | 9.9 | 5 | 6 | 9 | 11 | 11 | 11 | 12 | 15 |
| **TOTAL MULTIPLE DX** | 493 | 11.0 | 50 | 5 | 7 | 9 | 12 | 20 | 27 | 44 |
| **TOTAL** | | | | | | | | | | |
| 0–19 Years | 1 | 25.0 | 0 | 25 | 25 | 25 | 25 | 25 | 25 | 25 |
| 20–34 | 3 | 16.9 | 177 | 9 | 9 | 14 | >99 | >99 | >99 | >99 |
| 35–49 | 48 | 13.2 | 85 | 5 | 7 | 9 | 16 | 23 | 36 | 44 |
| 50–64 | 208 | 10.2 | 38 | 5 | 7 | 9 | 11 | 16 | 22 | 38 |
| 65+ | 278 | 10.8 | 36 | 6 | 7 | 10 | 11 | 19 | 25 | 37 |
| **GRAND TOTAL** | 538 | 10.8 | 42 | 5 | 7 | 9 | 12 | 18 | 24 | 44 |

Length of Stay by Diagnosis and Operation, United States, 2000

# United States, October 1998–September 1999 Data, by Operation

## 30.4: RADICAL LARYNGECTOMY. Formerly included in operation group(s) 559.

| Type of Patients | Observed Patients | Avg. Stay | Vari-ance | 10th | 25th | 50th | 75th | 90th | 95th | 99th |
|---|---|---|---|---|---|---|---|---|---|---|
| **1. SINGLE DX** | | | | | | | | | | |
| 0–19 Years | 0 | | | | | | | | | |
| 20–34 | 0 | | | | | | | | | |
| 35–49 | 7 | 8.6 | 8 | 3 | 7 | 9 | 11 | 11 | 11 | 11 |
| 50–64 | 14 | 8.8 | 18 | 1 | 8 | 9 | 11 | 15 | 15 | 15 |
| 65+ | 8 | 12.6 | 81 | 5 | 7 | 13 | 14 | 14 | 39 | 39 |
| **2. MULTIPLE DX** | | | | | | | | | | |
| 0–19 Years | 0 | | | | | | | | | |
| 20–34 | 4 | 11.9 | 16 | 6 | 11 | 11 | 13 | 19 | 19 | 19 |
| 35–49 | 90 | 13.6 | 75 | 6 | 7 | 9 | 20 | 28 | 28 | 40 |
| 50–64 | 329 | 13.7 | 103 | 7 | 8 | 10 | 16 | 22 | 36 | 64 |
| 65+ | 281 | 12.7 | 72 | 6 | 8 | 10 | 16 | 21 | 25 | 56 |
| **TOTAL SINGLE DX** | 29 | 9.4 | 28 | 3 | 7 | 9 | 11 | 15 | 15 | 39 |
| **TOTAL MULTIPLE DX** | 704 | 13.3 | 87 | 6 | 8 | 10 | 16 | 22 | 30 | 58 |
| **TOTAL** | | | | | | | | | | |
| 0–19 Years | 0 | | | | | | | | | |
| 20–34 | 4 | 11.9 | 16 | 6 | 11 | 11 | 13 | 19 | 19 | 19 |
| 35–49 | 97 | 13.4 | 73 | 6 | 7 | 9 | 20 | 28 | 28 | 40 |
| 50–64 | 343 | 13.4 | 100 | 6 | 8 | 10 | 15 | 22 | 36 | 64 |
| 65+ | 289 | 12.7 | 72 | 6 | 8 | 10 | 16 | 21 | 25 | 56 |
| **GRAND TOTAL** | 733 | 13.2 | 86 | 6 | 8 | 10 | 16 | 22 | 30 | 57 |

## 31.0: INJECTION OF LARYNX. Formerly included in operation group(s) 561.

| Type of Patients | Observed Patients | Avg. Stay | Vari-ance | 10th | 25th | 50th | 75th | 90th | 95th | 99th |
|---|---|---|---|---|---|---|---|---|---|---|
| **1. SINGLE DX** | | | | | | | | | | |
| 0–19 Years | 1 | 1.0 | 0 | 1 | 1 | 1 | 1 | 1 | 1 | 1 |
| 20–34 | 0 | | | | | | | | | |
| 35–49 | 0 | | | | | | | | | |
| 50–64 | 1 | 1.0 | 0 | 1 | 1 | 1 | 1 | 1 | 1 | 1 |
| 65+ | 1 | 1.0 | 0 | 1 | 1 | 1 | 1 | 1 | 1 | 1 |
| **2. MULTIPLE DX** | | | | | | | | | | |
| 0–19 Years | 3 | 3.0 | 47 | 1 | 1 | 1 | 1 | 2 | 27 | 27 |
| 20–34 | 0 | | | | | | | | | |
| 35–49 | 1 | 3.0 | 0 | 3 | 3 | 3 | 3 | 3 | 3 | 3 |
| 50–64 | 10 | 11.6 | 179 | 1 | 2 | 6 | 10 | 32 | 43 | 43 |
| 65+ | 23 | 6.8 | 133 | 1 | 1 | 4 | 5 | 16 | 44 | 58 |
| **TOTAL SINGLE DX** | 3 | 1.0 | 0 | 1 | 1 | 1 | 1 | 1 | 1 | 1 |
| **TOTAL MULTIPLE DX** | 37 | 6.9 | 128 | 1 | 1 | 2 | 6 | 16 | 32 | 58 |
| **TOTAL** | | | | | | | | | | |
| 0–19 Years | 4 | 2.9 | 44 | 1 | 1 | 1 | 1 | 2 | 27 | 27 |
| 20–34 | 0 | | | | | | | | | |
| 35–49 | 1 | 3.0 | 0 | 3 | 3 | 3 | 3 | 3 | 3 | 3 |
| 50–64 | 11 | 11.0 | 175 | 1 | 3 | 6 | 10 | 32 | 43 | 43 |
| 65+ | 24 | 6.3 | 124 | 1 | 1 | 2 | 5 | 16 | 44 | 58 |
| **GRAND TOTAL** | 40 | 6.5 | 121 | 1 | 1 | 2 | 6 | 16 | 32 | 58 |

## 31.1: TEMPORARY TRACHEOSTOMY. Formerly included in operation group(s) 560.

| Type of Patients | Observed Patients | Avg. Stay | Vari-ance | 10th | 25th | 50th | 75th | 90th | 95th | 99th |
|---|---|---|---|---|---|---|---|---|---|---|
| **1. SINGLE DX** | | | | | | | | | | |
| 0–19 Years | 22 | 11.2 | 48 | 4 | 7 | 11 | 13 | 16 | 33 | 33 |
| 20–34 | 16 | 10.4 | 187 | 3 | 6 | 8 | 8 | 14 | 41 | 94 |
| 35–49 | 40 | 10.8 | 78 | 3 | 4 | 6 | 14 | 25 | 25 | 31 |
| 50–64 | 45 | 5.5 | 12 | 2 | 3 | 5 | 7 | 9 | 12 | 19 |
| 65+ | 34 | 7.8 | 32 | 2 | 5 | 6 | 7 | 17 | 24 | 25 |
| **2. MULTIPLE DX** | | | | | | | | | | |
| 0–19 Years | 887 | 28.6 | 445 | 9 | 14 | 25 | 44 | 82 | >99 | >99 |
| 20–34 | 1,160 | 29.6 | 438 | 7 | 14 | 26 | 43 | 66 | 86 | >99 |
| 35–49 | 2,110 | 29.1 | 439 | 6 | 13 | 25 | 43 | 63 | 81 | >99 |
| 50–64 | 3,233 | 28.3 | 407 | 6 | 11 | 25 | 42 | 59 | 72 | >99 |
| 65+ | 5,325 | 31.2 | 409 | 8 | 16 | 28 | 45 | 63 | 79 | >99 |
| **TOTAL SINGLE DX** | 157 | 8.9 | 65 | 3 | 5 | 7 | 11 | 19 | 25 | 33 |
| **TOTAL MULTIPLE DX** | 12,715 | 29.8 | 420 | 7 | 14 | 27 | 43 | 64 | 82 | >99 |
| **TOTAL** | | | | | | | | | | |
| 0–19 Years | 909 | 28.1 | 443 | 8 | 13 | 24 | 43 | 80 | >99 | >99 |
| 20–34 | 1,176 | 29.3 | 440 | 7 | 13 | 25 | 42 | 66 | 86 | >99 |
| 35–49 | 2,150 | 28.6 | 438 | 6 | 12 | 24 | 43 | 63 | 81 | >99 |
| 50–64 | 3,278 | 28.0 | 409 | 6 | 11 | 25 | 42 | 58 | 72 | >99 |
| 65+ | 5,359 | 31.1 | 410 | 8 | 16 | 28 | 44 | 63 | 78 | >99 |
| **GRAND TOTAL** | 12,872 | 29.5 | 422 | 7 | 14 | 26 | 43 | 63 | 81 | >99 |

## 31.2: PERMANENT TRACHEOSTOMY. Formerly included in operation group(s) 560.

| Type of Patients | Observed Patients | Avg. Stay | Vari-ance | 10th | 25th | 50th | 75th | 90th | 95th | 99th |
|---|---|---|---|---|---|---|---|---|---|---|
| **1. SINGLE DX** | | | | | | | | | | |
| 0–19 Years | 3 | 8.6 | 2 | 8 | 8 | 8 | 8 | 11 | 11 | 11 |
| 20–34 | 5 | 7.4 | 11 | 3 | 4 | 10 | 10 | 10 | 10 | 10 |
| 35–49 | 12 | 8.3 | 23 | 2 | 5 | 8 | 12 | 15 | 17 | 17 |
| 50–64 | 13 | 12.8 | 407 | 1 | 2 | 4 | 11 | 65 | 65 | 65 |
| 65+ | 11 | 7.3 | 29 | 2 | 2 | 7 | 12 | 13 | 20 | 20 |
| **2. MULTIPLE DX** | | | | | | | | | | |
| 0–19 Years | 216 | 27.7 | 394 | 9 | 14 | 24 | 44 | >99 | >99 | >99 |
| 20–34 | 153 | 25.6 | 301 | 6 | 12 | 23 | 40 | 55 | 86 | >99 |
| 35–49 | 389 | 23.9 | 372 | 4 | 10 | 20 | 34 | 52 | 75 | >99 |
| 50–64 | 733 | 25.1 | 548 | 8 | 8 | 19 | 35 | 61 | 90 | >99 |
| 65+ | 1,384 | 29.7 | 394 | 8 | 15 | 27 | 42 | 67 | 84 | >99 |
| **TOTAL SINGLE DX** | 44 | 9.2 | 116 | 2 | 4 | 8 | 11 | 15 | 20 | 65 |
| **TOTAL MULTIPLE DX** | 2,875 | 27.5 | 429 | 6 | 12 | 23 | 40 | 65 | 90 | >99 |
| **TOTAL** | | | | | | | | | | |
| 0–19 Years | 219 | 27.5 | 394 | 9 | 14 | 24 | 44 | 93 | >99 | >99 |
| 20–34 | 158 | 24.9 | 302 | 5 | 11 | 22 | 38 | 55 | 68 | >99 |
| 35–49 | 401 | 23.3 | 367 | 4 | 9 | 19 | 33 | 52 | 70 | >99 |
| 50–64 | 746 | 24.9 | 548 | 4 | 8 | 18 | 35 | 61 | 90 | >99 |
| 65+ | 1,395 | 29.6 | 394 | 8 | 15 | 27 | 42 | 67 | 84 | >99 |
| **GRAND TOTAL** | 2,919 | 27.2 | 429 | 6 | 12 | 23 | 39 | 65 | 90 | >99 |

Length of Stay by Diagnosis and Operation, United States, 2000

# United States, October 1998–September 1999 Data, by Operation

## 31.29: OTHER PERM TRACHEOSTOMY. Formerly included in operation group(s) 560.

| Type of Patients | Observed Patients | Avg. Stay | Vari-ance | 10th | 25th | 50th | 75th | 90th | 95th | 99th |
|---|---|---|---|---|---|---|---|---|---|---|
| **1. SINGLE DX** | | | | | | | | | | |
| 0-19 Years | 3 | 8.6 | 2 | 8 | 8 | 8 | 8 | 11 | 11 | 11 |
| 20-34 | 4 | 6.8 | 12 | 3 | 4 | 10 | 10 | 10 | 10 | 10 |
| 35-49 | 12 | 8.3 | 23 | 2 | 5 | 8 | 12 | 15 | 17 | 17 |
| 50-64 | 13 | 12.8 | 407 | 1 | 2 | 4 | 11 | 65 | 65 | 65 |
| 65+ | 11 | 7.3 | 29 | 2 | 2 | 7 | 12 | 13 | 20 | 20 |
| **2. MULTIPLE DX** | | | | | | | | | | |
| 0-19 Years | 216 | 27.7 | 394 | 9 | 14 | 24 | 44 | >99 | >99 | >99 |
| 20-34 | 153 | 25.6 | 301 | 6 | 12 | 23 | 40 | 55 | 70 | >99 |
| 35-49 | 389 | 23.9 | 372 | 4 | 10 | 20 | 34 | 52 | 75 | >99 |
| 50-64 | 728 | 25.1 | 547 | 4 | 8 | 19 | 35 | 61 | 90 | >99 |
| 65+ | 1,381 | 29.7 | 393 | 8 | 15 | 27 | 42 | 67 | 84 | >99 |
| **TOTAL SINGLE DX** | 43 | 9.1 | 119 | 2 | 4 | 7 | 12 | 15 | 20 | 65 |
| **TOTAL MULTIPLE DX** | 2,867 | 27.5 | 428 | 6 | 12 | 23 | 40 | 65 | 90 | >99 |
| **TOTAL** | | | | | | | | | | |
| 0-19 Years | 219 | 27.5 | 394 | 9 | 14 | 24 | 44 | 93 | >99 | >99 |
| 20-34 | 157 | 25.0 | 303 | 5 | 11 | 22 | 38 | 55 | 68 | >99 |
| 35-49 | 401 | 23.3 | 367 | 4 | 9 | 19 | 33 | 52 | 70 | >99 |
| 50-64 | 741 | 24.9 | 547 | 4 | 8 | 18 | 35 | 61 | 90 | >99 |
| 65+ | 1,392 | 29.6 | 393 | 8 | 15 | 27 | 42 | 67 | 84 | >99 |
| **GRAND TOTAL** | 2,910 | 27.2 | 428 | 6 | 12 | 23 | 39 | 65 | 90 | >99 |

## 31.3: INC LARYNX/TRACHEA NEC. Formerly included in operation group(s) 561.

| Type of Patients | Observed Patients | Avg. Stay | Vari-ance | 10th | 25th | 50th | 75th | 90th | 95th | 99th |
|---|---|---|---|---|---|---|---|---|---|---|
| **1. SINGLE DX** | | | | | | | | | | |
| 0-19 Years | 1 | 2.0 | 0 | 2 | 2 | 2 | 2 | 2 | 2 | 2 |
| 20-34 | 1 | 1.0 | 0 | 1 | 1 | 1 | 1 | 1 | 1 | 1 |
| 35-49 | 3 | 1.2 | <1 | 1 | 1 | 1 | 1 | 2 | 2 | 2 |
| 50-64 | 2 | 3.2 | 9 | 1 | 1 | 1 | 6 | 6 | 6 | 6 |
| 65+ | 2 | 1.1 | <1 | 1 | 1 | 1 | 1 | 2 | 2 | 2 |
| **2. MULTIPLE DX** | | | | | | | | | | |
| 0-19 Years | 14 | 8.1 | 116 | 1 | 1 | 1 | 17 | 29 | 29 | 33 |
| 20-34 | 3 | 2.9 | 4 | 1 | 1 | 3 | 5 | 5 | 5 | 5 |
| 35-49 | 4 | 4.1 | 5 | 2 | 2 | 4 | 7 | 7 | 7 | 7 |
| 50-64 | 7 | 6.2 | 6 | 2 | 4 | 7 | 8 | 8 | 8 | 8 |
| 65+ | 8 | 6.7 | 39 | 1 | 3 | 5 | 8 | 22 | 22 | 22 |
| **TOTAL SINGLE DX** | 9 | 1.3 | <1 | 1 | 1 | 1 | 1 | 2 | 2 | 6 |
| **TOTAL MULTIPLE DX** | 36 | 6.9 | 68 | 1 | 1 | 4 | 8 | 17 | 29 | 33 |
| **TOTAL** | | | | | | | | | | |
| 0-19 Years | 15 | 7.9 | 114 | 1 | 1 | 1 | 17 | 29 | 29 | 33 |
| 20-34 | 4 | 2.7 | 4 | 1 | 1 | 1 | 5 | 5 | 5 | 5 |
| 35-49 | 7 | 1.6 | 1 | 1 | 1 | 7 | 2 | 2 | 4 | 7 |
| 50-64 | 9 | 5.9 | 7 | 1 | 4 | 3 | 8 | 8 | 8 | 8 |
| 65+ | 10 | 4.7 | 32 | 1 | 1 | 3 | 5 | 8 | 22 | 22 |
| **GRAND TOTAL** | 45 | 5.2 | 54 | 1 | 1 | 2 | 7 | 17 | 29 | 33 |

## 31.4: LARYNX/TRACHEA DXTIC PX. Formerly included in operation group(s) 557, 558, 581.

| Type of Patients | Observed Patients | Avg. Stay | Vari-ance | 10th | 25th | 50th | 75th | 90th | 95th | 99th |
|---|---|---|---|---|---|---|---|---|---|---|
| **1. SINGLE DX** | | | | | | | | | | |
| 0-19 Years | 864 | 1.7 | 2 | 1 | 1 | 1 | 2 | 3 | 4 | 7 |
| 20-34 | 60 | 1.7 | 1 | 1 | 1 | 1 | 2 | 3 | 4 | 5 |
| 35-49 | 66 | 2.5 | 7 | 1 | 1 | 2 | 3 | 4 | 4 | 10 |
| 50-64 | 46 | 2.3 | 7 | 1 | 1 | 2 | 2 | 4 | 5 | 6 |
| 65+ | 25 | 3.3 | 17 | 1 | 1 | 2 | 5 | 9 | 11 | 22 |
| **2. MULTIPLE DX** | | | | | | | | | | |
| 0-19 Years | 2,686 | 4.7 | 61 | 1 | 2 | 2 | 4 | 9 | 16 | 47 |
| 20-34 | 207 | 4.0 | 37 | 1 | 1 | 2 | 4 | 8 | 15 | 25 |
| 35-49 | 546 | 4.8 | 20 | 1 | 2 | 3 | 6 | 10 | 14 | 19 |
| 50-64 | 723 | 6.0 | 60 | 1 | 3 | 4 | 7 | 12 | 16 | 44 |
| 65+ | 1,233 | 6.5 | 32 | 1 | 3 | 5 | 9 | 13 | 18 | 28 |
| **TOTAL SINGLE DX** | 1,061 | 1.9 | 3 | 1 | 1 | 1 | 2 | 3 | 4 | 9 |
| **TOTAL MULTIPLE DX** | 5,395 | 5.2 | 50 | 1 | 2 | 3 | 6 | 11 | 16 | 42 |
| **TOTAL** | | | | | | | | | | |
| 0-19 Years | 3,550 | 3.9 | 47 | 1 | 1 | 2 | 3 | 8 | 13 | 43 |
| 20-34 | 267 | 3.4 | 29 | 1 | 2 | 2 | 3 | 6 | 13 | 25 |
| 35-49 | 612 | 4.5 | 19 | 1 | 2 | 3 | 6 | 10 | 14 | 19 |
| 50-64 | 769 | 5.7 | 57 | 1 | 2 | 3 | 7 | 12 | 16 | 44 |
| 65+ | 1,258 | 6.3 | 32 | 1 | 3 | 5 | 8 | 13 | 17 | 28 |
| **GRAND TOTAL** | 6,456 | 4.6 | 43 | 1 | 1 | 2 | 5 | 10 | 14 | 34 |

## 31.42: LARYNGOSCOPY/TRACHEOSCPY. Formerly included in operation group(s) 581.

| Type of Patients | Observed Patients | Avg. Stay | Vari-ance | 10th | 25th | 50th | 75th | 90th | 95th | 99th |
|---|---|---|---|---|---|---|---|---|---|---|
| **1. SINGLE DX** | | | | | | | | | | |
| 0-19 Years | 857 | 1.7 | 2 | 1 | 1 | 1 | 2 | 3 | 4 | 7 |
| 20-34 | 56 | 1.7 | 1 | 1 | 1 | 1 | 2 | 3 | 4 | 5 |
| 35-49 | 64 | 2.6 | 7 | 1 | 1 | 2 | 3 | 4 | 4 | 10 |
| 50-64 | 33 | 2.5 | 9 | 1 | 1 | 2 | 3 | 4 | 5 | 30 |
| 65+ | 17 | 2.6 | 10 | 1 | 1 | 2 | 2 | 9 | 9 | 11 |
| **2. MULTIPLE DX** | | | | | | | | | | |
| 0-19 Years | 2,660 | 4.7 | 61 | 1 | 2 | 2 | 4 | 9 | 16 | 47 |
| 20-34 | 196 | 4.0 | 38 | 1 | 1 | 2 | 4 | 8 | 18 | 25 |
| 35-49 | 474 | 4.6 | 19 | 1 | 2 | 3 | 6 | 10 | 14 | 19 |
| 50-64 | 569 | 5.7 | 49 | 1 | 2 | 4 | 7 | 11 | 15 | 36 |
| 65+ | 1,024 | 6.5 | 33 | 2 | 3 | 5 | 8 | 13 | 18 | 29 |
| **TOTAL SINGLE DX** | 1,027 | 1.9 | 2 | 1 | 1 | 1 | 2 | 3 | 4 | 9 |
| **TOTAL MULTIPLE DX** | 4,923 | 5.1 | 50 | 1 | 2 | 3 | 6 | 11 | 16 | 42 |
| **TOTAL** | | | | | | | | | | |
| 0-19 Years | 3,517 | 3.9 | 47 | 1 | 1 | 2 | 3 | 8 | 13 | 43 |
| 20-34 | 252 | 3.5 | 30 | 1 | 2 | 2 | 3 | 6 | 13 | 25 |
| 35-49 | 538 | 4.3 | 18 | 1 | 2 | 3 | 5 | 10 | 14 | 19 |
| 50-64 | 602 | 5.5 | 47 | 1 | 2 | 4 | 6 | 10 | 15 | 34 |
| 65+ | 1,041 | 6.3 | 33 | 1 | 3 | 4 | 8 | 13 | 17 | 29 |
| **GRAND TOTAL** | 5,950 | 4.5 | 42 | 1 | 1 | 2 | 5 | 9 | 14 | 35 |

## United States, October 1998–September 1999 Data, by Operation

### 31.43: CLSD (ENDO) BX LARYNX. Formerly included in operation group(s) 557.

| Type of Patients | Observed Patients | Avg. Stay | Variance | 10th | 25th | 50th | 75th | 90th | 95th | 99th |
|---|---|---|---|---|---|---|---|---|---|---|
| **1. SINGLE DX** | | | | | | | | | | |
| 0–19 Years | 2 | 2.3 | 6 | 1 | 1 | 1 | 6 | 6 | 6 | 6 |
| 20–34 | 3 | 1.0 | 0 | 1 | 1 | 1 | 1 | 1 | 1 | 1 |
| 35–49 | 1 | 1.0 | 0 | 1 | 1 | 1 | 1 | 1 | 1 | 1 |
| 50–64 | 11 | 1.7 | <1 | 1 | 1 | 2 | 2 | 2 | 2 | 3 |
| 65+ | 7 | 6.3 | 11 | 1 | 3 | 7 | 9 | 10 | 10 | 10 |
| **2. MULTIPLE DX** | | | | | | | | | | |
| 0–19 Years | 11 | 6.1 | 51 | 2 | 2 | 4 | 5 | 23 | 23 | 23 |
| 20–34 | 7 | 2.1 | 1 | 1 | 1 | 1 | 4 | 4 | 4 | 5 |
| 35–49 | 59 | 6.3 | 24 | 1 | 2 | 5 | 9 | 12 | 16 | 19 |
| 50–64 | 132 | 6.3 | 65 | 2 | 2 | 5 | 10 | 12 | 15 | 44 |
| 65+ | 164 | 6.4 | 26 | 1 | 3 | 5 | 10 | 11 | 17 | 24 |
| **TOTAL SINGLE DX** | 24 | 2.5 | 6 | 1 | 1 | 2 | 2 | 7 | 9 | 10 |
| **TOTAL MULTIPLE DX** | 373 | 6.2 | 39 | 1 | 2 | 4 | 10 | 12 | 16 | 27 |
| **TOTAL** | | | | | | | | | | |
| 0–19 Years | 13 | 5.3 | 43 | 1 | 2 | 2 | 5 | 14 | 23 | 23 |
| 20–34 | 10 | 2.0 | 1 | 1 | 1 | 2 | 2 | 4 | 4 | 5 |
| 35–49 | 60 | 6.2 | 24 | 1 | 1 | 5 | 9 | 11 | 16 | 19 |
| 50–64 | 143 | 5.9 | 61 | 1 | 2 | 3 | 10 | 12 | 15 | 31 |
| 65+ | 171 | 6.4 | 26 | 1 | 3 | 5 | 10 | 11 | 17 | 24 |
| **GRAND TOTAL** | 397 | 6.0 | 38 | 1 | 2 | 4 | 10 | 12 | 15 | 27 |

### 31.5: LOC EXC/DESTR LARYNX LES. Formerly included in operation group(s) 558.

| Type of Patients | Observed Patients | Avg. Stay | Variance | 10th | 25th | 50th | 75th | 90th | 95th | 99th |
|---|---|---|---|---|---|---|---|---|---|---|
| **1. SINGLE DX** | | | | | | | | | | |
| 0–19 Years | 14 | 4.4 | 19 | 1 | 1 | 2 | 7 | 9 | 9 | 19 |
| 20–34 | 2 | 1.9 | <1 | 1 | 2 | 2 | 2 | 2 | 2 | 2 |
| 35–49 | 5 | 3.6 | 3 | 2 | 2 | 5 | 5 | 5 | 5 | 5 |
| 50–64 | 5 | 2.5 | 7 | 1 | 1 | 1 | 7 | 7 | 7 | 7 |
| 65+ | 3 | 1.7 | <1 | 1 | 1 | 2 | 2 | 2 | 2 | 2 |
| **2. MULTIPLE DX** | | | | | | | | | | |
| 0–19 Years | 180 | 6.4 | 72 | 1 | 1 | 4 | 8 | 14 | 21 | 28 |
| 20–34 | 22 | 7.3 | 91 | 1 | 1 | 5 | 8 | 9 | 17 | 52 |
| 35–49 | 31 | 7.4 | 44 | 2 | 2 | 6 | 9 | 11 | 19 | 35 |
| 50–64 | 69 | 6.9 | 71 | 1 | 3 | 5 | 7 | 17 | 17 | 70 |
| 65+ | 56 | 10.6 | 80 | 1 | 3 | 7 | 21 | 21 | 21 | 38 |
| **TOTAL SINGLE DX** | 29 | 3.3 | 9 | 1 | 1 | 2 | 5 | 7 | 7 | 19 |
| **TOTAL MULTIPLE DX** | 358 | 7.1 | 72 | 1 | 2 | 5 | 8 | 17 | 21 | 35 |
| **TOTAL** | | | | | | | | | | |
| 0–19 Years | 194 | 6.3 | 70 | 1 | 1 | 4 | 8 | 13 | 21 | 28 |
| 20–34 | 24 | 6.6 | 84 | 1 | 1 | 5 | 8 | 9 | 17 | 52 |
| 35–49 | 36 | 6.8 | 40 | 2 | 2 | 5 | 9 | 9 | 17 | 35 |
| 50–64 | 74 | 6.6 | 68 | 1 | 2 | 4 | 7 | 14 | 17 | 70 |
| 65+ | 59 | 10.4 | 80 | 1 | 2 | 7 | 21 | 21 | 21 | 38 |
| **GRAND TOTAL** | 387 | 6.9 | 70 | 1 | 2 | 5 | 8 | 17 | 21 | 35 |

### 31.6: REPAIR OF LARYNX. Formerly included in operation group(s) 561.

| Type of Patients | Observed Patients | Avg. Stay | Variance | 10th | 25th | 50th | 75th | 90th | 95th | 99th |
|---|---|---|---|---|---|---|---|---|---|---|
| **1. SINGLE DX** | | | | | | | | | | |
| 0–19 Years | 33 | 3.2 | 5 | 1 | 1 | 4 | 4 | 5 | 7 | 13 |
| 20–34 | 3 | 3.1 | <1 | 1 | 3 | 3 | 3 | 4 | 4 | 4 |
| 35–49 | 1 | 1.8 | <1 | 1 | 1 | 1 | 3 | 3 | 3 | 3 |
| 50–64 | 5 | 1.0 | 0 | 1 | 1 | 1 | 1 | 1 | 1 | 1 |
| 65+ | 3 | 1.0 | 0 | 1 | 1 | 1 | 1 | 1 | 1 | 1 |
| **2. MULTIPLE DX** | | | | | | | | | | |
| 0–19 Years | 187 | 10.4 | 129 | 4 | 4 | 7 | 13 | 22 | 40 | 65 |
| 20–34 | 18 | 9.3 | 367 | 1 | 1 | 2 | 3 | 29 | 80 | 80 |
| 35–49 | 34 | 4.5 | 33 | 1 | 1 | 3 | 5 | 9 | 21 | 24 |
| 50–64 | 53 | 5.1 | 121 | 1 | 1 | 2 | 4 | 8 | 19 | 55 |
| 65+ | 74 | 2.6 | 13 | 1 | 1 | 1 | 2 | 6 | 11 | 20 |
| **TOTAL SINGLE DX** | 55 | 2.7 | 4 | 1 | 1 | 2 | 4 | 5 | 6 | 10 |
| **TOTAL MULTIPLE DX** | 366 | 7.5 | 117 | 1 | 1 | 4 | 9 | 18 | 25 | 65 |
| **TOTAL** | | | | | | | | | | |
| 0–19 Years | 220 | 9.3 | 116 | 1 | 3 | 6 | 12 | 19 | 29 | 65 |
| 20–34 | 21 | 7.9 | 294 | 1 | 1 | 2 | 4 | 12 | 29 | 80 |
| 35–49 | 45 | 3.9 | 27 | 1 | 1 | 2 | 4 | 6 | 21 | 24 |
| 50–64 | 58 | 4.9 | 115 | 1 | 1 | 1 | 4 | 8 | 15 | 55 |
| 65+ | 77 | 2.5 | 13 | 1 | 1 | 1 | 2 | 6 | 11 | 20 |
| **GRAND TOTAL** | 421 | 6.9 | 105 | 1 | 1 | 4 | 8 | 16 | 22 | 65 |

### 31.69: OTHER LARYNGEAL REPAIR. Formerly included in operation group(s) 561.

| Type of Patients | Observed Patients | Avg. Stay | Variance | 10th | 25th | 50th | 75th | 90th | 95th | 99th |
|---|---|---|---|---|---|---|---|---|---|---|
| **1. SINGLE DX** | | | | | | | | | | |
| 0–19 Years | 32 | 3.1 | 6 | 1 | 1 | 3 | 4 | 5 | 7 | 13 |
| 20–34 | 9 | 1.0 | 0 | 1 | 1 | 1 | 1 | 1 | 1 | 1 |
| 35–49 | 5 | 1.1 | <1 | 1 | 1 | 1 | 1 | 1 | 2 | 2 |
| 50–64 | 5 | 1.0 | 0 | 1 | 1 | 1 | 1 | 1 | 1 | 1 |
| 65+ | 3 | 1.0 | 0 | 1 | 1 | 1 | 1 | 1 | 1 | 1 |
| **2. MULTIPLE DX** | | | | | | | | | | |
| 0–19 Years | 184 | 10.5 | 129 | 4 | 4 | 7 | 13 | 22 | 40 | 65 |
| 20–34 | 15 | 9.6 | 438 | 1 | 1 | 2 | 3 | 29 | 80 | 80 |
| 35–49 | 28 | 3.7 | 24 | 1 | 1 | 3 | 4 | 6 | 19 | 21 |
| 50–64 | 49 | 4.9 | 116 | 1 | 2 | 2 | 4 | 8 | 11 | 55 |
| 65+ | 71 | 2.6 | 14 | 1 | 1 | 2 | 2 | 6 | 11 | 20 |
| **TOTAL SINGLE DX** | 50 | 2.6 | 5 | 1 | 1 | 2 | 4 | 5 | 7 | 13 |
| **TOTAL MULTIPLE DX** | 347 | 7.5 | 119 | 1 | 1 | 4 | 9 | 18 | 25 | 65 |
| **TOTAL** | | | | | | | | | | |
| 0–19 Years | 216 | 9.3 | 117 | 1 | 3 | 6 | 12 | 19 | 29 | 65 |
| 20–34 | 16 | 9.3 | 425 | 1 | 1 | 2 | 3 | 29 | 80 | 80 |
| 35–49 | 37 | 3.2 | 20 | 1 | 1 | 1 | 3 | 6 | 19 | 21 |
| 50–64 | 54 | 4.7 | 110 | 1 | 1 | 1 | 4 | 8 | 11 | 55 |
| 65+ | 74 | 2.5 | 13 | 1 | 1 | 2 | 2 | 6 | 11 | 20 |
| **GRAND TOTAL** | 397 | 6.9 | 108 | 1 | 1 | 4 | 8 | 16 | 22 | 65 |

Length of Stay by Diagnosis and Operation

# United States, October 1998–September 1999 Data, by Operation

## 31.7: REPAIR OF TRACHEA. Formerly included in operation group(s) 561.

| Type of Patients | Observed Patients | Avg. Stay | Variance | Percentiles | | | | | | |
|---|---|---|---|---|---|---|---|---|---|---|
| | | | | 10th | 25th | 50th | 75th | 90th | 95th | 99th |
| **1. SINGLE DX** | | | | | | | | | | |
| 0–19 Years | 50 | 5.9 | 47 | 1 | 1 | 3 | 10 | 12 | 21 | 28 |
| 20–34 | 6 | 2.4 | 2 | 2 | 2 | 2 | 2 | 2 | 7 | 7 |
| 35–49 | 1 | 1.0 | 0 | 1 | 1 | 1 | 1 | 1 | 1 | 1 |
| 50–64 | 6 | 4.9 | 47 | 1 | 1 | 1 | 4 | 15 | 24 | 24 |
| 65+ | 3 | 1.3 | <1 | 1 | 1 | 1 | 2 | 2 | 2 | 2 |
| **2. MULTIPLE DX** | | | | | | | | | | |
| 0–19 Years | 336 | 12.3 | 177 | 1 | 3 | 8 | 16 | 30 | 46 | 70 |
| 20–34 | 41 | 8.3 | 106 | 3 | 4 | 4 | 8 | 20 | 26 | 61 |
| 35–49 | 82 | 6.3 | 68 | 1 | 1 | 3 | 8 | 20 | 24 | >99 |
| 50–64 | 144 | 8.3 | 227 | 1 | 1 | 3 | 8 | 26 | 47 | >99 |
| 65+ | 167 | 8.3 | 92 | 1 | 2 | 5 | 12 | 17 | 27 | 48 |
| **TOTAL SINGLE DX** | 66 | 5.2 | 41 | 1 | 1 | 2 | 6 | 12 | 21 | 28 |
| **TOTAL MULTIPLE DX** | 770 | 9.7 | 166 | 1 | 2 | 5 | 12 | 25 | 42 | 83 |
| **TOTAL** | | | | | | | | | | |
| 0–19 Years | 386 | 11.1 | 159 | 1 | 2 | 7 | 15 | 28 | 44 | 61 |
| 20–34 | 47 | 7.0 | 89 | 2 | 2 | 4 | 8 | 13 | 26 | 61 |
| 35–49 | 83 | 6.3 | 68 | 1 | 1 | 3 | 8 | 20 | 24 | >99 |
| 50–64 | 150 | 8.1 | 218 | 1 | 1 | 3 | 8 | 26 | 43 | >99 |
| 65+ | 170 | 8.2 | 92 | 1 | 2 | 5 | 12 | 17 | 27 | 48 |
| **GRAND TOTAL** | 836 | 9.2 | 154 | 1 | 2 | 5 | 11 | 23 | 39 | 83 |

## 31.74: REVISION OF TRACHEOSTOMY. Formerly included in operation group(s) 561.

| Type of Patients | Observed Patients | Avg. Stay | Variance | Percentiles | | | | | | |
|---|---|---|---|---|---|---|---|---|---|---|
| | | | | 10th | 25th | 50th | 75th | 90th | 95th | 99th |
| **1. SINGLE DX** | | | | | | | | | | |
| 0–19 Years | 3 | 4.3 | 3 | 1 | 5 | 5 | 5 | 5 | 5 | 5 |
| 20–34 | 0 | | | | | | | | | |
| 35–49 | 0 | | | | | | | | | |
| 50–64 | 1 | 24.0 | 0 | 24 | 24 | 24 | 24 | 24 | 24 | 24 |
| 65+ | 1 | 1.0 | 0 | 1 | 1 | 1 | 1 | 1 | 1 | 1 |
| **2. MULTIPLE DX** | | | | | | | | | | |
| 0–19 Years | 53 | 7.2 | 117 | 1 | 1 | 2 | 8 | 18 | 36 | 44 |
| 20–34 | 13 | 11.1 | 157 | 1 | 4 | 4 | 22 | 26 | 26 | 67 |
| 35–49 | 47 | 6.8 | 74 | 1 | 1 | 3 | 12 | 21 | 28 | >99 |
| 50–64 | 93 | 8.9 | 274 | 1 | 1 | 2 | 8 | 26 | 83 | >99 |
| 65+ | 106 | 10.2 | 119 | 1 | 2 | 6 | 15 | 19 | 28 | 61 |
| **TOTAL SINGLE DX** | 5 | 6.6 | 52 | 1 | 5 | 5 | 5 | 24 | 24 | 24 |
| **TOTAL MULTIPLE DX** | 312 | 8.8 | 187 | 1 | 1 | 4 | 11 | 26 | 37 | >99 |
| **TOTAL** | | | | | | | | | | |
| 0–19 Years | 56 | 6.9 | 106 | 1 | 1 | 3 | 5 | 17 | 36 | 44 |
| 20–34 | 13 | 11.1 | 157 | 1 | 4 | 4 | 22 | 26 | 26 | 67 |
| 35–49 | 47 | 6.8 | 74 | 1 | 1 | 2 | 12 | 21 | 28 | >99 |
| 50–64 | 94 | 9.0 | 274 | 1 | 2 | 2 | 8 | 26 | 83 | >99 |
| 65+ | 107 | 10.2 | 119 | 1 | 2 | 6 | 15 | 19 | 28 | 61 |
| **GRAND TOTAL** | 317 | 8.8 | 184 | 1 | 1 | 4 | 11 | 26 | 37 | >99 |

## 31.9: OTHER LARYNX/TRACHEA OPS. Formerly included in operation group(s) 561.

| Type of Patients | Observed Patients | Avg. Stay | Variance | Percentiles | | | | | | |
|---|---|---|---|---|---|---|---|---|---|---|
| | | | | 10th | 25th | 50th | 75th | 90th | 95th | 99th |
| **1. SINGLE DX** | | | | | | | | | | |
| 0–19 Years | 15 | 2.9 | 3 | 1 | 2 | 2 | 5 | 5 | 5 | 5 |
| 20–34 | 3 | 2.8 | <1 | 2 | 2 | 3 | 4 | 4 | 4 | 4 |
| 35–49 | 5 | 1.2 | <1 | 1 | 1 | 1 | 1 | 2 | 2 | 2 |
| 50–64 | 4 | 1.5 | <1 | 1 | 1 | 1 | 2 | 3 | 3 | 3 |
| 65+ | 5 | 1.0 | 0 | 1 | 1 | 1 | 1 | 1 | 1 | 1 |
| **2. MULTIPLE DX** | | | | | | | | | | |
| 0–19 Years | 105 | 8.9 | 108 | 1 | 1 | 4 | 16 | 19 | 27 | 47 |
| 20–34 | 23 | 5.8 | 55 | 1 | 1 | 3 | 7 | 17 | 26 | 26 |
| 35–49 | 51 | 3.3 | 9 | 1 | 1 | 3 | 4 | 5 | 9 | 15 |
| 50–64 | 72 | 6.8 | 56 | 1 | 1 | 5 | 10 | 16 | 18 | 43 |
| 65+ | 93 | 6.6 | 48 | 1 | 2 | 3 | 8 | 18 | 23 | 25 |
| **TOTAL SINGLE DX** | 32 | 2.0 | 2 | 1 | 1 | 1 | 2 | 5 | 5 | 5 |
| **TOTAL MULTIPLE DX** | 344 | 6.6 | 63 | 1 | 1 | 3 | 8 | 17 | 23 | 40 |
| **TOTAL** | | | | | | | | | | |
| 0–19 Years | 120 | 8.4 | 101 | 1 | 1 | 4 | 15 | 18 | 27 | 47 |
| 20–34 | 26 | 5.6 | 52 | 1 | 1 | 2 | 7 | 17 | 26 | 26 |
| 35–49 | 56 | 3.2 | 9 | 1 | 1 | 3 | 4 | 5 | 7 | 15 |
| 50–64 | 76 | 6.7 | 55 | 1 | 1 | 3 | 9 | 16 | 18 | 43 |
| 65+ | 98 | 6.3 | 47 | 1 | 2 | 3 | 8 | 18 | 23 | 25 |
| **GRAND TOTAL** | 376 | 6.3 | 60 | 1 | 1 | 3 | 8 | 16 | 22 | 40 |

## 32.0: LOC EXC/DESTR BRONCH LES. Formerly included in operation group(s) 562.

| Type of Patients | Observed Patients | Avg. Stay | Variance | Percentiles | | | | | | |
|---|---|---|---|---|---|---|---|---|---|---|
| | | | | 10th | 25th | 50th | 75th | 90th | 95th | 99th |
| **1. SINGLE DX** | | | | | | | | | | |
| 0–19 Years | 14 | 3.6 | 3 | 2 | 3 | 3 | 5 | 6 | 6 | 6 |
| 20–34 | 4 | 4.7 | 2 | 4 | 4 | 4 | 4 | 7 | 7 | 7 |
| 35–49 | 6 | 3.9 | 6 | 2 | 2 | 2 | 4 | 8 | 8 | 8 |
| 50–64 | 6 | 2.9 | 4 | 1 | 2 | 2 | 5 | 6 | 6 | 6 |
| 65+ | 1 | 6.0 | 0 | 6 | 6 | 6 | 6 | 6 | 6 | 6 |
| **2. MULTIPLE DX** | | | | | | | | | | |
| 0–19 Years | 29 | 5.7 | 17 | 1 | 3 | 5 | 6 | 10 | 16 | 19 |
| 20–34 | 9 | 9.3 | 228 | 2 | 4 | 5 | 5 | 52 | 52 | 52 |
| 35–49 | 29 | 4.2 | 15 | 1 | 3 | 3 | 5 | 7 | 9 | 25 |
| 50–64 | 49 | 5.3 | 16 | 2 | 3 | 4 | 6 | 13 | 16 | 16 |
| 65+ | 60 | 5.0 | 31 | 1 | 2 | 3 | 7 | 11 | 12 | 21 |
| **TOTAL SINGLE DX** | 31 | 3.7 | 4 | 2 | 2 | 4 | 6 | 6 | 7 | 8 |
| **TOTAL MULTIPLE DX** | 176 | 5.3 | 32 | 1 | 2 | 4 | 6 | 11 | 13 | 25 |
| **TOTAL** | | | | | | | | | | |
| 0–19 Years | 43 | 4.7 | 11 | 2 | 2 | 4 | 6 | 8 | 10 | 19 |
| 20–34 | 13 | 7.8 | 156 | 3 | 4 | 5 | 5 | 7 | 52 | 52 |
| 35–49 | 35 | 4.2 | 13 | 1 | 2 | 3 | 5 | 8 | 9 | 25 |
| 50–64 | 55 | 5.1 | 16 | 1 | 2 | 4 | 6 | 13 | 16 | 16 |
| 65+ | 61 | 5.0 | 31 | 1 | 2 | 3 | 7 | 11 | 12 | 21 |
| **GRAND TOTAL** | 207 | 5.0 | 27 | 1 | 2 | 4 | 6 | 10 | 13 | 21 |

## United States, October 1998–September 1999 Data, by Operation

### 32.1: OTHER BRONCHIAL EXCISION. Formerly included in operation group(s) 563.

| Type of Patients | Observed Patients | Avg. Stay | Variance | 10th | 25th | 50th | 75th | 90th | 95th | 99th |
|---|---|---|---|---|---|---|---|---|---|---|
| **1. SINGLE DX** | | | | | | | | | | |
| 0-19 Years | 0 | | | | | | | | | |
| 20-34 | 2 | 4.1 | 4 | | 5 | 5 | 5 | 5 | 5 | 5 |
| 35-49 | 2 | 5.8 | 1 | | 5 | 5 | 7 | 7 | 7 | 7 |
| 50-64 | 0 | | | | | | | | | |
| 65+ | 0 | | | | | | | | | |
| **2. MULTIPLE DX** | | | | | | | | | | |
| 0-19 Years | 2 | 12.7 | 7 | 8 | 14 | 14 | 14 | 14 | 14 | 14 |
| 20-34 | 1 | 13.0 | 0 | 13 | 13 | 13 | 13 | 13 | 13 | 13 |
| 35-49 | 2 | 5.8 | 1 | 5 | 5 | 5 | 7 | 7 | 7 | 7 |
| 50-64 | 10 | 5.9 | 5 | 2 | 5 | 5 | 7 | 9 | 9 | 11 |
| 65+ | 2 | 13.0 | 0 | 13 | 13 | 13 | 13 | 13 | 13 | 13 |
| **TOTAL SINGLE DX** | 4 | 5.0 | 3 | 1 | 5 | 5 | 5 | 7 | 7 | 7 |
| **TOTAL MULTIPLE DX** | 17 | 8.3 | 15 | 5 | 5 | 7 | 13 | 13 | 14 | 14 |
| **TOTAL** | | | | | | | | | | |
| 0-19 Years | 2 | 12.7 | 7 | 8 | 14 | 14 | 14 | 14 | 14 | 14 |
| 20-34 | 3 | 7.7 | 24 | 1 | 5 | 5 | 13 | 13 | 13 | 13 |
| 35-49 | 4 | 5.8 | 1 | 5 | 5 | 5 | 7 | 7 | 7 | 7 |
| 50-64 | 10 | 5.9 | 5 | 2 | 5 | 5 | 7 | 9 | 9 | 11 |
| 65+ | 2 | 13.0 | 0 | 13 | 13 | 13 | 13 | 13 | 13 | 13 |
| **GRAND TOTAL** | 21 | 7.7 | 14 | 5 | 5 | 7 | 13 | 13 | 14 | 14 |

### 32.2: LOC EXC/DESTR LUNG LES. Formerly included in operation group(s) 564.

| Type of Patients | Observed Patients | Avg. Stay | Variance | 10th | 25th | 50th | 75th | 90th | 95th | 99th |
|---|---|---|---|---|---|---|---|---|---|---|
| **1. SINGLE DX** | | | | | | | | | | |
| 0-19 Years | 75 | 4.7 | 9 | 2 | 3 | 4 | 6 | 9 | 11 | 16 |
| 20-34 | 110 | 4.5 | 7 | 2 | 3 | 4 | 5 | 9 | 9 | 15 |
| 35-49 | 128 | 4.3 | 15 | 2 | 3 | 4 | 4 | 7 | 10 | 30 |
| 50-64 | 123 | 3.7 | 5 | 2 | 2 | 3 | 4 | 6 | 9 | 12 |
| 65+ | 79 | 3.8 | 4 | 2 | 2 | 3 | 5 | 7 | 7 | 12 |
| **2. MULTIPLE DX** | | | | | | | | | | |
| 0-19 Years | 341 | 8.1 | 90 | 3 | 4 | 6 | 10 | 14 | 18 | 56 |
| 20-34 | 589 | 8.7 | 39 | 3 | 4 | 7 | 11 | 16 | 21 | 29 |
| 35-49 | 1,040 | 7.4 | 45 | 2 | 3 | 5 | 9 | 14 | 24 | 32 |
| 50-64 | 1,774 | 7.2 | 56 | 2 | 3 | 5 | 8 | 15 | 22 | 33 |
| 65+ | 2,269 | 8.0 | 46 | 2 | 4 | 6 | 10 | 16 | 23 | 31 |
| **TOTAL SINGLE DX** | 515 | 4.2 | 10 | 2 | 3 | 4 | 5 | 7 | 9 | 15 |
| **TOTAL MULTIPLE DX** | 6,013 | 7.8 | 51 | 2 | 4 | 6 | 10 | 15 | 22 | 32 |
| **TOTAL** | | | | | | | | | | |
| 0-19 Years | 416 | 7.5 | 78 | 2 | 4 | 5 | 9 | 13 | 16 | 54 |
| 20-34 | 699 | 8.0 | 36 | 2 | 4 | 6 | 11 | 16 | 21 | 27 |
| 35-49 | 1,168 | 6.9 | 42 | 2 | 3 | 5 | 8 | 14 | 21 | 32 |
| 50-64 | 1,897 | 7.0 | 54 | 2 | 3 | 5 | 8 | 14 | 20 | 33 |
| 65+ | 2,348 | 7.9 | 46 | 2 | 4 | 6 | 10 | 16 | 23 | 31 |
| **GRAND TOTAL** | 6,528 | 7.5 | 48 | 2 | 3 | 5 | 9 | 15 | 21 | 32 |

### 32.21: EMPHYSEM BLEB PLICATION. Formerly included in operation group(s) 564.

| Type of Patients | Observed Patients | Avg. Stay | Variance | 10th | 25th | 50th | 75th | 90th | 95th | 99th |
|---|---|---|---|---|---|---|---|---|---|---|
| **1. SINGLE DX** | | | | | | | | | | |
| 0-19 Years | 7 | 6.6 | 14 | 4 | 5 | 5 | 6 | 6 | 16 | 16 |
| 20-34 | 10 | 3.4 | 4 | 2 | 2 | 2 | 2 | 4 | 6 | 7 |
| 35-49 | 6 | 3.8 | 2 | 3 | 3 | 4 | 4 | 4 | 4 | 12 |
| 50-64 | 0 | | | | | | | | | |
| 65+ | 0 | | | | | | | | | |
| **2. MULTIPLE DX** | | | | | | | | | | |
| 0-19 Years | 40 | 9.1 | 130 | 3 | 5 | 7 | 11 | 14 | 14 | 96 |
| 20-34 | 74 | 8.5 | 26 | 4 | 5 | 8 | 11 | 14 | 15 | 25 |
| 35-49 | 61 | 7.8 | 39 | 2 | 5 | 5 | 9 | 16 | 18 | 35 |
| 50-64 | 54 | 13.7 | 125 | 5 | 6 | 12 | 15 | 29 | 30 | 89 |
| 65+ | 51 | 11.5 | 64 | 3 | 4 | 11 | 17 | 23 | 29 | 34 |
| **TOTAL SINGLE DX** | 23 | 3.9 | 3 | 3 | 3 | 4 | 4 | 5 | 6 | 12 |
| **TOTAL MULTIPLE DX** | 280 | 9.8 | 77 | 3 | 5 | 8 | 12 | 17 | 25 | 35 |
| **TOTAL** | | | | | | | | | | |
| 0-19 Years | 47 | 8.9 | 122 | 3 | 5 | 6 | 11 | 14 | 14 | 96 |
| 20-34 | 84 | 7.9 | 26 | 2 | 4 | 7 | 10 | 14 | 15 | 25 |
| 35-49 | 67 | 5.9 | 26 | 5 | 5 | 4 | 6 | 12 | 16 | 29 |
| 50-64 | 54 | 13.7 | 125 | 5 | 6 | 12 | 15 | 29 | 30 | 89 |
| 65+ | 51 | 11.5 | 64 | 3 | 4 | 11 | 17 | 23 | 29 | 34 |
| **GRAND TOTAL** | 303 | 8.6 | 67 | 3 | 4 | 6 | 11 | 15 | 19 | 34 |

### 32.28: ENDO EXC/DESTR LUNG LES. Formerly included in operation group(s) 564.

| Type of Patients | Observed Patients | Avg. Stay | Variance | 10th | 25th | 50th | 75th | 90th | 95th | 99th |
|---|---|---|---|---|---|---|---|---|---|---|
| **1. SINGLE DX** | | | | | | | | | | |
| 0-19 Years | 10 | 3.3 | 5 | 2 | 2 | 3 | 3 | 6 | 7 | 14 |
| 20-34 | 12 | 5.0 | 19 | 1 | 3 | 3 | 6 | 9 | 9 | 22 |
| 35-49 | 9 | 3.2 | 27 | 1 | 1 | 1 | 2 | 6 | 20 | 20 |
| 50-64 | 4 | 2.2 | <1 | 2 | 2 | 2 | 2 | 3 | 3 | 3 |
| 65+ | 8 | 2.1 | <1 | 2 | 2 | 2 | 2 | 3 | 3 | 4 |
| **2. MULTIPLE DX** | | | | | | | | | | |
| 0-19 Years | 24 | 7.1 | 14 | 2 | 4 | 7 | 9 | 12 | 14 | 15 |
| 20-34 | 52 | 7.1 | 18 | 3 | 3 | 7 | 11 | 11 | 11 | 20 |
| 35-49 | 70 | 5.8 | 24 | 1 | 1 | 5 | 8 | 10 | 12 | 27 |
| 50-64 | 89 | 4.4 | 19 | 2 | 3 | 3 | 4 | 10 | 14 | 22 |
| 65+ | 103 | 7.0 | 31 | 3 | 3 | 5 | 9 | 16 | 16 | 22 |
| **TOTAL SINGLE DX** | 43 | 3.4 | 12 | 1 | 2 | 2 | 3 | 6 | 9 | 20 |
| **TOTAL MULTIPLE DX** | 338 | 6.1 | 24 | 1 | 2 | 4 | 9 | 12 | 16 | 22 |
| **TOTAL** | | | | | | | | | | |
| 0-19 Years | 34 | 6.0 | 15 | 2 | 3 | 5 | 9 | 12 | 12 | 15 |
| 20-34 | 64 | 6.8 | 18 | 3 | 3 | 6 | 10 | 11 | 11 | 22 |
| 35-49 | 79 | 5.5 | 25 | 1 | 1 | 5 | 8 | 10 | 12 | 27 |
| 50-64 | 93 | 4.3 | 19 | 2 | 2 | 3 | 4 | 10 | 14 | 22 |
| 65+ | 111 | 6.7 | 31 | 2 | 3 | 6 | 9 | 16 | 16 | 22 |
| **GRAND TOTAL** | 381 | 5.9 | 24 | 1 | 2 | 4 | 9 | 11 | 16 | 22 |

Length of Stay by Diagnosis and Operation, United States, 2000

# United States, October 1998–September 1999 Data, by Operation

## 32.29: LOC EXC LUNG LES NEC. Formerly included in operation group(s) 564.

| Type of Patients | Observed Patients | Avg. Stay | Variance | 10th | 25th | 50th | 75th | 90th | 95th | 99th |
|---|---|---|---|---|---|---|---|---|---|---|
| **1. SINGLE DX** | | | | | | | | | | |
| 0–19 Years | 58 | 4.8 | 9 | 2 | 3 | 4 | 7 | 9 | 11 | 15 |
| 20–34 | 88 | 4.5 | 7 | 2 | 3 | 4 | 5 | 9 | 9 | 15 |
| 35–49 | 111 | 4.7 | 22 | 2 | 2 | 4 | 5 | 9 | 12 | 30 |
| 50–64 | 117 | 3.5 | 4 | 2 | 2 | 3 | 4 | 6 | 7 | 12 |
| 65+ | 71 | 4.0 | 4 | 2 | 3 | 4 | 5 | 7 | 7 | 12 |
| **2. MULTIPLE DX** | | | | | | | | | | |
| 0–19 Years | 275 | 7.8 | 80 | 3 | 4 | 5 | 10 | 14 | 18 | 56 |
| 20–34 | 463 | 8.9 | 43 | 3 | 4 | 7 | 12 | 18 | 22 | 29 |
| 35–49 | 902 | 7.5 | 47 | 2 | 3 | 5 | 9 | 14 | 24 | 32 |
| 50–64 | 1,568 | 6.8 | 48 | 2 | 3 | 5 | 7 | 13 | 20 | 34 |
| 65+ | 2,058 | 7.9 | 44 | 2 | 4 | 6 | 10 | 16 | 23 | 29 |
| **TOTAL SINGLE DX** | 445 | 4.3 | 10 | 2 | 3 | 4 | 5 | 7 | 9 | 14 |
| **TOTAL MULTIPLE DX** | 5,266 | 7.6 | 48 | 2 | 4 | 6 | 9 | 15 | 21 | 32 |
| **TOTAL** | | | | | | | | | | |
| 0–19 Years | 333 | 7.3 | 69 | 2 | 3 | 5 | 8 | 13 | 17 | 56 |
| 20–34 | 551 | 8.1 | 39 | 2 | 4 | 6 | 11 | 16 | 21 | 28 |
| 35–49 | 1,013 | 7.2 | 45 | 2 | 3 | 5 | 8 | 14 | 24 | 32 |
| 50–64 | 1,685 | 6.6 | 46 | 2 | 3 | 5 | 7 | 13 | 19 | 31 |
| 65+ | 2,129 | 7.8 | 43 | 2 | 4 | 6 | 10 | 16 | 22 | 29 |
| **GRAND TOTAL** | 5,711 | 7.3 | 46 | 2 | 3 | 5 | 9 | 14 | 21 | 32 |

## 32.4: LOBECTOMY OF LUNG. Formerly included in operation group(s) 565.

| Type of Patients | Observed Patients | Avg. Stay | Variance | 10th | 25th | 50th | 75th | 90th | 95th | 99th |
|---|---|---|---|---|---|---|---|---|---|---|
| **1. SINGLE DX** | | | | | | | | | | |
| 0–19 Years | 42 | 8.9 | 199 | 3 | 4 | 4 | 8 | 9 | 58 | 58 |
| 20–34 | 9 | 6.0 | 2 | 5 | 5 | 5 | 7 | 8 | 8 | 8 |
| 35–49 | 59 | 5.1 | 2 | 4 | 5 | 5 | 6 | 7 | 7 | 8 |
| 50–64 | 120 | 5.8 | 7 | 3 | 5 | 5 | 7 | 9 | 11 | 15 |
| 65+ | 117 | 5.8 | 14 | 3 | 4 | 5 | 6 | 8 | 10 | 23 |
| **2. MULTIPLE DX** | | | | | | | | | | |
| 0–19 Years | 137 | 13.5 | 173 | 5 | 7 | 11 | 15 | 23 | 28 | 98 |
| 20–34 | 109 | 9.0 | 57 | 4 | 5 | 5 | 10 | 13 | 20 | 47 |
| 35–49 | 662 | 8.7 | 65 | 4 | 5 | 7 | 9 | 16 | 22 | 45 |
| 50–64 | 2,747 | 8.4 | 38 | 4 | 5 | 7 | 9 | 14 | 20 | 41 |
| 65+ | 4,529 | 9.1 | 40 | 4 | 6 | 7 | 11 | 15 | 20 | 37 |
| **TOTAL SINGLE DX** | 347 | 6.2 | 43 | 3 | 4 | 5 | 6 | 8 | 10 | 58 |
| **TOTAL MULTIPLE DX** | 8,184 | 8.9 | 45 | 4 | 5 | 7 | 10 | 15 | 20 | 41 |
| **TOTAL** | | | | | | | | | | |
| 0–19 Years | 179 | 12.4 | 183 | 4 | 5 | 8 | 14 | 22 | 29 | 91 |
| 20–34 | 118 | 8.9 | 55 | 4 | 5 | 7 | 10 | 13 | 19 | 47 |
| 35–49 | 721 | 8.5 | 62 | 4 | 5 | 6 | 9 | 15 | 22 | 45 |
| 50–64 | 2,867 | 8.3 | 37 | 4 | 5 | 7 | 9 | 14 | 20 | 41 |
| 65+ | 4,646 | 9.0 | 39 | 4 | 6 | 7 | 10 | 15 | 20 | 37 |
| **GRAND TOTAL** | 8,531 | 8.8 | 45 | 4 | 5 | 7 | 10 | 15 | 20 | 41 |

## 32.3: SEGMENTAL LUNG RESECTION. Formerly included in operation group(s) 564.

| Type of Patients | Observed Patients | Avg. Stay | Variance | 10th | 25th | 50th | 75th | 90th | 95th | 99th |
|---|---|---|---|---|---|---|---|---|---|---|
| **1. SINGLE DX** | | | | | | | | | | |
| 0–19 Years | 20 | 5.1 | 15 | 2 | 3 | 4 | 7 | 9 | 18 | 18 |
| 20–34 | 13 | 4.4 | 5 | 3 | 3 | 4 | 5 | 5 | 5 | 12 |
| 35–49 | 27 | 6.8 | 47 | 2 | 4 | 5 | 6 | 17 | 17 | 48 |
| 50–64 | 31 | 4.9 | 2 | 3 | 4 | 5 | 6 | 7 | 8 | 8 |
| 65+ | 29 | 5.1 | 5 | 3 | 4 | 5 | 6 | 9 | 10 | 10 |
| **2. MULTIPLE DX** | | | | | | | | | | |
| 0–19 Years | 68 | 11.7 | 140 | 3 | 5 | 7 | 21 | 29 | 84 | >99 |
| 20–34 | 52 | 8.1 | 46 | 3 | 5 | 7 | 9 | 17 | 19 | >99 |
| 35–49 | 183 | 9.4 | 43 | 3 | 5 | 7 | 13 | 15 | 18 | 38 |
| 50–64 | 587 | 8.1 | 38 | 3 | 6 | 6 | 9 | 14 | 19 | 34 |
| 65+ | 902 | 9.8 | 53 | 4 | 6 | 8 | 11 | 17 | 24 | 36 |
| **TOTAL SINGLE DX** | 120 | 5.3 | 15 | 3 | 4 | 4 | 6 | 8 | 10 | 18 |
| **TOTAL MULTIPLE DX** | 1,792 | 9.3 | 53 | 4 | 5 | 7 | 11 | 17 | 23 | 46 |
| **TOTAL** | | | | | | | | | | |
| 0–19 Years | 88 | 10.4 | 121 | 3 | 4 | 7 | 14 | 28 | 47 | >99 |
| 20–34 | 65 | 7.3 | 39 | 3 | 4 | 6 | 8 | 17 | 19 | >99 |
| 35–49 | 210 | 9.1 | 44 | 3 | 5 | 7 | 13 | 15 | 18 | 38 |
| 50–64 | 618 | 7.9 | 37 | 4 | 5 | 6 | 9 | 14 | 18 | 34 |
| 65+ | 931 | 9.7 | 53 | 4 | 6 | 8 | 11 | 17 | 24 | 36 |
| **GRAND TOTAL** | 1,912 | 9.1 | 51 | 4 | 5 | 7 | 11 | 17 | 23 | 46 |

## 32.5: COMPLETE PNEUMONECTOMY. Formerly included in operation group(s) 565.

| Type of Patients | Observed Patients | Avg. Stay | Variance | 10th | 25th | 50th | 75th | 90th | 95th | 99th |
|---|---|---|---|---|---|---|---|---|---|---|
| **1. SINGLE DX** | | | | | | | | | | |
| 0–19 Years | 1 | 1.0 | 0 | 1 | 1 | 1 | 1 | 1 | 1 | 1 |
| 20–34 | 4 | 12.5 | 61 | 4 | 5 | 6 | 20 | 20 | 20 | 20 |
| 35–49 | 8 | 6.3 | 120 | 4 | 4 | 4 | 4 | 8 | 18 | 78 |
| 50–64 | 8 | 8.1 | 7 | 4 | 6 | 8 | 11 | 11 | 11 | 11 |
| 65+ | 6 | 6.0 | 2 | 4 | 5 | 6 | 7 | 9 | 9 | 9 |
| **2. MULTIPLE DX** | | | | | | | | | | |
| 0–19 Years | 21 | 10.1 | 42 | 4 | 4 | 8 | 14 | 22 | 25 | 25 |
| 20–34 | 19 | 11.0 | 120 | 3 | 5 | 6 | 11 | 24 | 48 | 48 |
| 35–49 | 125 | 17.2 | 597 | 4 | 5 | 7 | 13 | 82 | 82 | 82 |
| 50–64 | 455 | 8.2 | 43 | 4 | 5 | 6 | 9 | 13 | 17 | 33 |
| 65+ | 505 | 8.9 | 35 | 4 | 5 | 7 | 10 | 14 | 20 | 36 |
| **TOTAL SINGLE DX** | 27 | 7.8 | 76 | 4 | 4 | 5 | 8 | 20 | 20 | 78 |
| **TOTAL MULTIPLE DX** | 1,125 | 9.5 | 103 | 4 | 5 | 7 | 10 | 15 | 21 | 82 |
| **TOTAL** | | | | | | | | | | |
| 0–19 Years | 22 | 9.8 | 43 | 4 | 4 | 6 | 14 | 20 | 25 | 25 |
| 20–34 | 23 | 11.5 | 101 | 4 | 5 | 6 | 20 | 20 | 35 | 48 |
| 35–49 | 133 | 15.9 | 551 | 4 | 4 | 7 | 12 | 82 | 82 | 82 |
| 50–64 | 463 | 8.2 | 42 | 4 | 5 | 6 | 10 | 13 | 17 | 33 |
| 65+ | 511 | 8.9 | 35 | 4 | 5 | 7 | 10 | 14 | 20 | 36 |
| **GRAND TOTAL** | 1,152 | 9.5 | 102 | 4 | 5 | 7 | 10 | 15 | 21 | 82 |

Length of Stay by Diagnosis and Operation

# United States, October 1998–September 1999 Data, by Operation

## 32.6: RAD DISSECT THOR STRUCT. Formerly included in operation group(s) 567.

| Type of Patients | Observed Patients | Avg. Stay | Vari-ance | 10th | 25th | 50th | 75th | 90th | 95th | 99th |
|---|---|---|---|---|---|---|---|---|---|---|
| **1. SINGLE DX** | | | | | | | | | | |
| 0–19 Years | 0 | | | | | | | | | |
| 20–34 | 0 | | | | | | | | | |
| 35–49 | 1 | 10.0 | 0 | 10 | 10 | 10 | 10 | 10 | 10 | 10 |
| 50–64 | 1 | 7.0 | 0 | 7 | 7 | 7 | 7 | 7 | 7 | 7 |
| 65+ | 1 | 4.0 | 0 | 4 | 4 | 4 | 4 | 4 | 4 | 4 |
| **2. MULTIPLE DX** | | | | | | | | | | |
| 0–19 Years | 3 | 6.2 | 26 | 1 | 1 | 4 | 11 | 11 | 11 | 11 |
| 20–34 | 1 | 8.0 | 0 | 8 | 8 | 8 | 8 | 8 | 8 | 8 |
| 35–49 | 5 | 9.0 | 41 | 4 | 4 | 9 | 11 | 20 | 20 | 20 |
| 50–64 | 31 | 8.1 | 46 | 4 | 4 | 5 | 10 | 14 | 19 | 39 |
| 65+ | 30 | 13.1 | 94 | 6 | 7 | 11 | 15 | 24 | 29 | 59 |
| **TOTAL SINGLE DX** | 3 | 6.5 | 9 | 4 | 4 | 7 | 10 | 10 | 10 | 10 |
| **TOTAL MULTIPLE DX** | 70 | 9.9 | 68 | 4 | 5 | 8 | 12 | 17 | 24 | 39 |
| **TOTAL** | | | | | | | | | | |
| 0–19 Years | 3 | 6.2 | 26 | 1 | 1 | 4 | 11 | 11 | 11 | 11 |
| 20–34 | 1 | 8.0 | 0 | 8 | 8 | 8 | 8 | 8 | 8 | 8 |
| 35–49 | 6 | 9.2 | 36 | 4 | 4 | 9 | 11 | 20 | 20 | 20 |
| 50–64 | 32 | 8.1 | 46 | 4 | 4 | 5 | 10 | 14 | 19 | 39 |
| 65+ | 31 | 12.9 | 94 | 6 | 7 | 10 | 15 | 24 | 29 | 59 |
| **GRAND TOTAL** | 73 | 9.9 | 67 | 4 | 5 | 7 | 12 | 17 | 24 | 39 |

## 33.0: INCISION OF BRONCHUS. Formerly included in operation group(s) 562.

| Type of Patients | Observed Patients | Avg. Stay | Vari-ance | 10th | 25th | 50th | 75th | 90th | 95th | 99th |
|---|---|---|---|---|---|---|---|---|---|---|
| **1. SINGLE DX** | | | | | | | | | | |
| 0–19 Years | 0 | | | | | | | | | |
| 20–34 | 0 | | | | | | | | | |
| 35–49 | 0 | | | | | | | | | |
| 50–64 | 0 | | | | | | | | | |
| 65+ | 0 | | | | | | | | | |
| **2. MULTIPLE DX** | | | | | | | | | | |
| 0–19 Years | 0 | | | | | | | | | |
| 20–34 | 0 | | | | | | | | | |
| 35–49 | 1 | 4.0 | 0 | 4 | 4 | 4 | 4 | 4 | 4 | 4 |
| 50–64 | 0 | | | | | | | | | |
| 65+ | 3 | 6.9 | 6 | 3 | 7 | 7 | 7 | 9 | 9 | 9 |
| **TOTAL SINGLE DX** | 0 | | | | | | | | | |
| **TOTAL MULTIPLE DX** | 4 | 6.0 | 6 | 3 | 4 | 7 | 7 | 9 | 9 | 9 |
| **TOTAL** | | | | | | | | | | |
| 0–19 Years | 0 | | | | | | | | | |
| 20–34 | 0 | | | | | | | | | |
| 35–49 | 1 | 4.0 | 0 | 4 | 4 | 4 | 4 | 4 | 4 | 4 |
| 50–64 | 0 | | | | | | | | | |
| 65+ | 3 | 6.9 | 6 | 3 | 7 | 7 | 7 | 9 | 9 | 9 |
| **GRAND TOTAL** | 4 | 6.0 | 6 | 3 | 4 | 7 | 7 | 9 | 9 | 9 |

## 32.9: OTHER EXCISION OF LUNG. Formerly included in operation group(s) 567.

| Type of Patients | Observed Patients | Avg. Stay | Vari-ance | 10th | 25th | 50th | 75th | 90th | 95th | 99th |
|---|---|---|---|---|---|---|---|---|---|---|
| **1. SINGLE DX** | | | | | | | | | | |
| 0–19 Years | 2 | 2.6 | 2 | 2 | 2 | 2 | 4 | 4 | 4 | 4 |
| 20–34 | 0 | | | | | | | | | |
| 35–49 | 1 | 2.0 | 0 | 2 | 2 | 2 | 2 | 2 | 2 | 2 |
| 50–64 | 1 | 6.0 | 0 | 6 | 6 | 6 | 6 | 6 | 6 | 6 |
| 65+ | 1 | 8.0 | 0 | 8 | 8 | 8 | 8 | 8 | 8 | 8 |
| **2. MULTIPLE DX** | | | | | | | | | | |
| 0–19 Years | 3 | 11.8 | <1 | 11 | 11 | 12 | 12 | 13 | 13 | 13 |
| 20–34 | 4 | 9.0 | 16 | 4 | 4 | 10 | 11 | 13 | 13 | 13 |
| 35–49 | 3 | 6.7 | 14 | 6 | 6 | 6 | 8 | 8 | 8 | 8 |
| 50–64 | 11 | 8.9 | 14 | 5 | 6 | 8 | 11 | 13 | 18 | 18 |
| 65+ | 16 | 6.3 | 15 | 1 | 4 | 5 | 8 | 13 | 13 | 16 |
| **TOTAL SINGLE DX** | 5 | 4.4 | 6 | 2 | 2 | 4 | 6 | 8 | 8 | 8 |
| **TOTAL MULTIPLE DX** | 37 | 7.7 | 15 | 4 | 4 | 7 | 11 | 13 | 13 | 18 |
| **TOTAL** | | | | | | | | | | |
| 0–19 Years | 5 | 9.8 | 16 | 2 | 11 | 11 | 12 | 13 | 13 | 13 |
| 20–34 | 4 | 9.0 | 16 | 4 | 4 | 10 | 11 | 13 | 13 | 13 |
| 35–49 | 4 | 5.2 | 6 | 2 | 2 | 6 | 6 | 8 | 8 | 8 |
| 50–64 | 12 | 8.4 | 12 | 5 | 6 | 8 | 10 | 13 | 18 | 18 |
| 65+ | 17 | 6.3 | 14 | 1 | 4 | 5 | 8 | 12 | 13 | 16 |
| **GRAND TOTAL** | 42 | 7.2 | 15 | 2 | 4 | 7 | 11 | 13 | 13 | 18 |

## 33.1: INCISION OF LUNG. Formerly included in operation group(s) 567.

| Type of Patients | Observed Patients | Avg. Stay | Vari-ance | 10th | 25th | 50th | 75th | 90th | 95th | 99th |
|---|---|---|---|---|---|---|---|---|---|---|
| **1. SINGLE DX** | | | | | | | | | | |
| 0–19 Years | 1 | 4.0 | 0 | 4 | 4 | 4 | 4 | 4 | 4 | 4 |
| 20–34 | 2 | | | | | | | | | |
| 35–49 | 2 | 6.4 | 3 | 5 | 5 | 5 | 8 | 8 | 8 | 8 |
| 50–64 | 0 | | | | | | | | | |
| 65+ | 1 | 5.0 | 0 | 5 | 5 | 5 | 5 | 5 | 5 | 5 |
| **2. MULTIPLE DX** | | | | | | | | | | |
| 0–19 Years | 10 | 8.9 | 55 | 2 | 2 | 6 | 15 | 23 | 24 | 24 |
| 20–34 | 9 | 14.0 | 110 | 4 | 4 | 10 | 28 | 28 | 28 | 28 |
| 35–49 | 23 | 8.4 | 17 | 3 | 4 | 9 | 11 | 12 | 17 | 17 |
| 50–64 | 32 | 12.7 | 59 | 4 | 7 | 12 | 16 | 23 | 30 | 35 |
| 65+ | 36 | 13.3 | 63 | 5 | 10 | 11 | 17 | 22 | 30 | 30 |
| **TOTAL SINGLE DX** | 4 | 5.2 | 2 | 4 | 4 | 5 | 5 | 8 | 8 | 8 |
| **TOTAL MULTIPLE DX** | 110 | 11.5 | 57 | 3 | 6 | 10 | 15 | 22 | 29 | 30 |
| **TOTAL** | | | | | | | | | | |
| 0–19 Years | 11 | 8.2 | 50 | 2 | 2 | 6 | 13 | 15 | 24 | 24 |
| 20–34 | 9 | 14.0 | 110 | 4 | 4 | 10 | 28 | 28 | 28 | 28 |
| 35–49 | 25 | 8.3 | 16 | 3 | 5 | 9 | 11 | 12 | 17 | 17 |
| 50–64 | 32 | 12.7 | 59 | 4 | 7 | 12 | 16 | 23 | 30 | 35 |
| 65+ | 37 | 13.2 | 63 | 5 | 9 | 11 | 17 | 22 | 30 | 30 |
| **GRAND TOTAL** | 114 | 11.3 | 57 | 3 | 6 | 10 | 15 | 22 | 28 | 30 |

Length of Stay by Diagnosis and Operation, United States, 2000

# United States, October 1998–September 1999 Data, by Operation

## 33.2: BRONCHIAL/LUNG DXTIC PX. Formerly included in operation group(s) 562, 564, 566, 581.

| Type of Patients | Observed Patients | Avg. Stay | Vari-ance | Percentiles | | | | | | |
|---|---|---|---|---|---|---|---|---|---|---|
| | | | | 10th | 25th | 50th | 75th | 90th | 95th | 99th |
| **1. SINGLE DX** | | | | | | | | | | |
| 0–19 Years | 400 | 2.9 | 11 | 1 | 1 | 1 | 3 | 6 | 12 | 15 |
| 20–34 | 132 | 5.2 | 11 | 1 | 3 | 4 | 7 | 11 | 12 | 15 |
| 35–49 | 256 | 4.3 | 9 | 1 | 2 | 4 | 5 | 7 | 10 | 14 |
| 50–64 | 227 | 4.3 | 13 | 1 | 2 | 3 | 5 | 7 | 10 | 16 |
| 65+ | 199 | 4.2 | 13 | 1 | 2 | 3 | 6 | 9 | 11 | 19 |
| **2. MULTIPLE DX** | | | | | | | | | | |
| 0–19 Years | 2,285 | 8.0 | 92 | 1 | 2 | 5 | 10 | 18 | 25 | 48 |
| 20–34 | 2,130 | 9.8 | 80 | 3 | 4 | 7 | 12 | 20 | 33 | 39 |
| 35–49 | 6,118 | 8.9 | 65 | 2 | 4 | 7 | 11 | 17 | 22 | 45 |
| 50–64 | 10,966 | 8.8 | 62 | 2 | 4 | 7 | 11 | 17 | 25 | 40 |
| 65+ | 22,533 | 9.3 | 53 | 3 | 5 | 8 | 12 | 17 | 23 | 37 |
| **TOTAL SINGLE DX** | 1,214 | 3.8 | 12 | 1 | 1 | 3 | 5 | 8 | 11 | 15 |
| **TOTAL MULTIPLE DX** | 44,032 | 9.1 | 61 | 2 | 4 | 7 | 11 | 17 | 23 | 39 |
| **TOTAL** | | | | | | | | | | |
| 0–19 Years | 2,685 | 7.2 | 82 | 1 | 2 | 4 | 9 | 16 | 22 | 44 |
| 20–34 | 2,262 | 9.5 | 77 | 3 | 4 | 7 | 12 | 19 | 32 | 38 |
| 35–49 | 6,374 | 8.7 | 63 | 2 | 4 | 7 | 11 | 17 | 22 | 43 |
| 50–64 | 11,193 | 8.7 | 61 | 2 | 4 | 7 | 11 | 17 | 24 | 40 |
| 65+ | 22,732 | 9.3 | 53 | 3 | 5 | 8 | 12 | 17 | 23 | 37 |
| **GRAND TOTAL** | 45,246 | 8.9 | 60 | 2 | 4 | 7 | 11 | 17 | 23 | 39 |

## 33.23: OTHER BRONCHOSCOPY. Formerly included in operation group(s) 566.

| Type of Patients | Observed Patients | Avg. Stay | Vari-ance | Percentiles | | | | | | |
|---|---|---|---|---|---|---|---|---|---|---|
| | | | | 10th | 25th | 50th | 75th | 90th | 95th | 99th |
| **1. SINGLE DX** | | | | | | | | | | |
| 0–19 Years | 232 | 2.2 | 9 | 1 | 1 | 1 | 2 | 4 | 6 | 16 |
| 20–34 | 8 | 2.0 | <1 | 1 | 1 | 1 | 2 | 4 | 4 | 4 |
| 35–49 | 15 | 4.0 | 8 | 1 | 2 | 4 | 5 | 7 | 7 | 13 |
| 50–64 | 14 | 2.6 | 9 | 1 | 1 | 1 | 2 | 9 | 9 | 12 |
| 65+ | 12 | 4.0 | 6 | 1 | 2 | 4 | 6 | 6 | 9 | 9 |
| **2. MULTIPLE DX** | | | | | | | | | | |
| 0–19 Years | 828 | 6.4 | 63 | 1 | 2 | 4 | 8 | 15 | 20 | 40 |
| 20–34 | 182 | 9.2 | 79 | 2 | 4 | 6 | 11 | 19 | 28 | 46 |
| 35–49 | 394 | 7.8 | 70 | 2 | 4 | 6 | 9 | 15 | 19 | 38 |
| 50–64 | 445 | 10.2 | 88 | 3 | 4 | 7 | 13 | 25 | 25 | 44 |
| 65+ | 819 | 10.0 | 73 | 3 | 4 | 7 | 12 | 20 | 29 | 47 |
| **TOTAL SINGLE DX** | 281 | 2.3 | 8 | 1 | 1 | 1 | 2 | 5 | 7 | 15 |
| **TOTAL MULTIPLE DX** | 2,668 | 8.4 | 74 | 1 | 3 | 6 | 11 | 18 | 25 | 44 |
| **TOTAL** | | | | | | | | | | |
| 0–19 Years | 1,060 | 5.5 | 54 | 1 | 1 | 3 | 7 | 14 | 18 | 36 |
| 20–34 | 190 | 9.0 | 77 | 2 | 4 | 6 | 11 | 19 | 26 | 46 |
| 35–49 | 409 | 7.7 | 69 | 1 | 3 | 5 | 9 | 15 | 19 | 37 |
| 50–64 | 459 | 9.9 | 87 | 1 | 3 | 7 | 13 | 25 | 25 | 44 |
| 65+ | 831 | 10.0 | 73 | 3 | 4 | 7 | 12 | 20 | 29 | 47 |
| **GRAND TOTAL** | 2,949 | 7.8 | 71 | 1 | 2 | 5 | 10 | 17 | 25 | 43 |

## 33.22: FIBER-OPTIC BRONCHOSCOPY. Formerly included in operation group(s) 566.

| Type of Patients | Observed Patients | Avg. Stay | Vari-ance | Percentiles | | | | | | |
|---|---|---|---|---|---|---|---|---|---|---|
| | | | | 10th | 25th | 50th | 75th | 90th | 95th | 99th |
| **1. SINGLE DX** | | | | | | | | | | |
| 0–19 Years | 75 | 2.2 | 4 | 1 | 1 | 1 | 3 | 6 | 7 | 12 |
| 20–34 | 18 | 3.2 | 2 | 1 | 2 | 4 | 4 | 4 | 4 | 6 |
| 35–49 | 19 | 4.3 | 6 | 1 | 2 | 5 | 5 | 7 | 10 | 10 |
| 50–64 | 16 | 3.5 | 5 | 1 | 2 | 3 | 5 | 7 | 7 | 7 |
| 65+ | 15 | 4.2 | 15 | 1 | 1 | 2 | 8 | 9 | 14 | 14 |
| **2. MULTIPLE DX** | | | | | | | | | | |
| 0–19 Years | 495 | 7.7 | 69 | 1 | 2 | 5 | 10 | 17 | 25 | 48 |
| 20–34 | 233 | 7.1 | 32 | 2 | 4 | 6 | 9 | 13 | 16 | 29 |
| 35–49 | 496 | 8.4 | 39 | 3 | 4 | 7 | 11 | 16 | 18 | 34 |
| 50–64 | 758 | 8.4 | 115 | 3 | 4 | 6 | 10 | 15 | 23 | 92 |
| 65+ | 1,377 | 9.6 | 46 | 3 | 5 | 8 | 12 | 17 | 21 | 33 |
| **TOTAL SINGLE DX** | 143 | 2.9 | 6 | 1 | 1 | 2 | 4 | 7 | 7 | 12 |
| **TOTAL MULTIPLE DX** | 3,359 | 8.6 | 64 | 2 | 4 | 7 | 12 | 16 | 21 | 39 |
| **TOTAL** | | | | | | | | | | |
| 0–19 Years | 570 | 6.9 | 64 | 1 | 2 | 4 | 9 | 16 | 23 | 48 |
| 20–34 | 251 | 6.8 | 31 | 2 | 4 | 5 | 9 | 13 | 16 | 28 |
| 35–49 | 515 | 8.2 | 38 | 2 | 4 | 7 | 11 | 16 | 18 | 34 |
| 50–64 | 774 | 8.3 | 113 | 3 | 3 | 6 | 10 | 15 | 22 | 92 |
| 65+ | 1,392 | 9.5 | 46 | 3 | 5 | 8 | 12 | 17 | 21 | 33 |
| **GRAND TOTAL** | 3,502 | 8.4 | 63 | 2 | 4 | 7 | 11 | 16 | 21 | 38 |

## 33.24: CLSD (ENDO) BRONCHUS BX. Formerly included in operation group(s) 562.

| Type of Patients | Observed Patients | Avg. Stay | Vari-ance | Percentiles | | | | | | |
|---|---|---|---|---|---|---|---|---|---|---|
| | | | | 10th | 25th | 50th | 75th | 90th | 95th | 99th |
| **1. SINGLE DX** | | | | | | | | | | |
| 0–19 Years | 47 | 5.2 | 19 | 1 | 2 | 3 | 7 | 14 | 15 | 15 |
| 20–34 | 38 | 6.8 | 13 | 1 | 4 | 8 | 11 | 11 | 11 | 16 |
| 35–49 | 68 | 4.2 | 6 | 2 | 2 | 5 | 5 | 7 | 8 | 14 |
| 50–64 | 45 | 5.0 | 13 | 2 | 2 | 4 | 7 | 8 | 11 | 23 |
| 65+ | 51 | 5.5 | 18 | 1 | 2 | 4 | 7 | 10 | 13 | 19 |
| **2. MULTIPLE DX** | | | | | | | | | | |
| 0–19 Years | 498 | 8.4 | 87 | 1 | 3 | 6 | 11 | 17 | 22 | 37 |
| 20–34 | 866 | 9.4 | 56 | 3 | 5 | 7 | 13 | 17 | 24 | 36 |
| 35–49 | 2,485 | 9.0 | 62 | 3 | 4 | 7 | 11 | 17 | 23 | 47 |
| 50–64 | 4,307 | 8.4 | 37 | 3 | 4 | 7 | 11 | 15 | 20 | 29 |
| 65+ | 9,252 | 9.6 | 51 | 3 | 5 | 8 | 12 | 18 | 23 | 36 |
| **TOTAL SINGLE DX** | 249 | 5.3 | 14 | 1 | 2 | 4 | 7 | 11 | 13 | 19 |
| **TOTAL MULTIPLE DX** | 17,408 | 9.1 | 51 | 3 | 5 | 7 | 11 | 17 | 22 | 35 |
| **TOTAL** | | | | | | | | | | |
| 0–19 Years | 545 | 8.1 | 82 | 1 | 3 | 6 | 10 | 16 | 21 | 37 |
| 20–34 | 904 | 9.3 | 54 | 3 | 5 | 8 | 12 | 17 | 23 | 36 |
| 35–49 | 2,553 | 8.8 | 61 | 3 | 4 | 7 | 11 | 17 | 22 | 43 |
| 50–64 | 4,352 | 8.3 | 37 | 3 | 4 | 7 | 10 | 15 | 20 | 29 |
| 65+ | 9,303 | 9.5 | 51 | 3 | 5 | 8 | 12 | 18 | 23 | 36 |
| **GRAND TOTAL** | 17,657 | 9.1 | 51 | 3 | 5 | 7 | 11 | 17 | 22 | 35 |

Length of Stay by Diagnosis and Operation, United States, 2000

## United States, October 1998–September 1999 Data, by Operation

### 33.26: CLSD (NEEDLE) LUNG BX. Formerly included in operation group(s) 564.

| Type of Patients | Observed Patients | Avg. Stay | Variance | Percentiles | | | | | | |
|---|---|---|---|---|---|---|---|---|---|---|
| | | | | 10th | 25th | 50th | 75th | 90th | 95th | 99th |
| **1. SINGLE DX** | | | | | | | | | | |
| 0–19 Years | 3 | 1.9 | 3 | 1 | 1 | 1 | 1 | 6 | 6 | 6 |
| 20–34 | 3 | 2.6 | 4 | 1 | 1 | 1 | 5 | 5 | 5 | 5 |
| 35–49 | 12 | 3.2 | 6 | 1 | 1 | 1 | 5 | 5 | 5 | 11 |
| 50–64 | 17 | 6.0 | 33 | 1 | 1 | 3 | 9 | 16 | 16 | 16 |
| 65+ | 27 | 3.0 | 7 | 1 | 1 | 2 | 4 | 7 | 9 | 10 |
| **2. MULTIPLE DX** | | | | | | | | | | |
| 0–19 Years | 30 | 9.1 | 71 | 1 | 2 | 8 | 15 | 19 | 35 | 36 |
| 20–34 | 50 | 13.1 | 148 | 2 | 3 | 6 | 26 | 32 | 32 | 40 |
| 35–49 | 326 | 8.2 | 83 | 2 | 4 | 6 | 10 | 15 | 18 | 74 |
| 50–64 | 1,085 | 6.6 | 37 | 2 | 3 | 5 | 8 | 13 | 19 | 27 |
| 65+ | 3,030 | 7.7 | 39 | 2 | 3 | 6 | 10 | 15 | 20 | 29 |
| **TOTAL SINGLE DX** | 62 | 3.6 | 14 | 1 | 1 | 2 | 5 | 9 | 13 | 16 |
| **TOTAL MULTIPLE DX** | 4,521 | 7.5 | 43 | 2 | 3 | 6 | 10 | 15 | 20 | 32 |
| **TOTAL** | | | | | | | | | | |
| 0–19 Years | 33 | 7.2 | 63 | 1 | 3 | 5 | 11 | 15 | 19 | 35 |
| 20–34 | 53 | 12.5 | 146 | 2 | 3 | 6 | 26 | 32 | 32 | 40 |
| 35–49 | 338 | 8.0 | 81 | 2 | 3 | 6 | 10 | 14 | 17 | 74 |
| 50–64 | 1,102 | 6.6 | 37 | 2 | 3 | 5 | 8 | 13 | 19 | 27 |
| 65+ | 3,057 | 7.6 | 39 | 2 | 3 | 6 | 10 | 15 | 20 | 29 |
| **GRAND TOTAL** | 4,583 | 7.4 | 43 | 2 | 3 | 6 | 10 | 14 | 20 | 32 |

### 33.27: ENDO LUNG BX (CLOSED). Formerly included in operation group(s) 564.

| Type of Patients | Observed Patients | Avg. Stay | Variance | Percentiles | | | | | | |
|---|---|---|---|---|---|---|---|---|---|---|
| | | | | 10th | 25th | 50th | 75th | 90th | 95th | 99th |
| **1. SINGLE DX** | | | | | | | | | | |
| 0–19 Years | 12 | 5.6 | 17 | 2 | 3 | 6 | 6 | 12 | 15 | 15 |
| 20–34 | 36 | 5.1 | 6 | 2 | 3 | 5 | 7 | 7 | 9 | 13 |
| 35–49 | 59 | 6.4 | 14 | 2 | 4 | 6 | 7 | 13 | 14 | 19 |
| 50–64 | 46 | 4.7 | 22 | 3 | 3 | 4 | 6 | 7 | 9 | 37 |
| 65+ | 42 | 5.1 | 17 | 1 | 2 | 4 | 7 | 11 | 14 | 17 |
| **2. MULTIPLE DX** | | | | | | | | | | |
| 0–19 Years | 122 | 10.3 | 102 | 1 | 4 | 7 | 14 | 24 | 31 | 44 |
| 20–34 | 619 | 11.2 | 96 | 4 | 5 | 8 | 12 | 31 | 36 | 37 |
| 35–49 | 1,755 | 9.5 | 69 | 3 | 5 | 8 | 11 | 17 | 23 | 50 |
| 50–64 | 3,180 | 10.4 | 75 | 3 | 5 | 8 | 12 | 24 | 27 | 43 |
| 65+ | 6,590 | 9.8 | 56 | 3 | 5 | 8 | 13 | 18 | 23 | 39 |
| **TOTAL SINGLE DX** | 195 | 5.4 | 15 | 1 | 3 | 5 | 7 | 10 | 13 | 17 |
| **TOTAL MULTIPLE DX** | 12,266 | 10.0 | 66 | 3 | 5 | 8 | 12 | 19 | 26 | 43 |
| **TOTAL** | | | | | | | | | | |
| 0–19 Years | 134 | 9.8 | 95 | 1 | 3 | 6 | 13 | 23 | 31 | 44 |
| 20–34 | 655 | 10.8 | 92 | 3 | 5 | 7 | 12 | 26 | 36 | 37 |
| 35–49 | 1,814 | 9.3 | 67 | 3 | 5 | 8 | 11 | 16 | 23 | 50 |
| 50–64 | 3,226 | 10.3 | 75 | 3 | 5 | 8 | 12 | 24 | 27 | 43 |
| 65+ | 6,632 | 9.8 | 56 | 3 | 5 | 8 | 13 | 18 | 23 | 38 |
| **GRAND TOTAL** | 12,461 | 9.9 | 65 | 3 | 5 | 8 | 12 | 19 | 25 | 42 |

### 33.28: OPEN BIOPSY OF LUNG. Formerly included in operation group(s) 564.

| Type of Patients | Observed Patients | Avg. Stay | Variance | Percentiles | | | | | | |
|---|---|---|---|---|---|---|---|---|---|---|
| | | | | 10th | 25th | 50th | 75th | 90th | 95th | 99th |
| **1. SINGLE DX** | | | | | | | | | | |
| 0–19 Years | 28 | 4.8 | 15 | 1 | 2 | 3 | 8 | 11 | 13 | 13 |
| 20–34 | 27 | 5.3 | 19 | 2 | 4 | 4 | 6 | 15 | 15 | 20 |
| 35–49 | 83 | 3.0 | 4 | 1 | 2 | 3 | 3 | 5 | 7 | 10 |
| 50–64 | 87 | 3.7 | 4 | 1 | 2 | 3 | 5 | 6 | 7 | 10 |
| 65+ | 51 | 2.9 | 5 | 1 | 2 | 2 | 3 | 6 | 7 | 15 |
| **2. MULTIPLE DX** | | | | | | | | | | |
| 0–19 Years | 223 | 13.8 | 248 | 2 | 3 | 7 | 18 | 36 | 45 | 89 |
| 20–34 | 166 | 10.3 | 173 | 2 | 3 | 6 | 14 | 21 | 32 | 91 |
| 35–49 | 622 | 8.0 | 67 | 2 | 3 | 4 | 10 | 18 | 23 | 42 |
| 50–64 | 1,128 | 8.0 | 74 | 2 | 3 | 5 | 10 | 16 | 27 | 40 |
| 65+ | 1,340 | 8.5 | 68 | 2 | 3 | 6 | 11 | 19 | 25 | 40 |
| **TOTAL SINGLE DX** | 276 | 3.6 | 8 | 1 | 2 | 3 | 5 | 7 | 9 | 15 |
| **TOTAL MULTIPLE DX** | 3,479 | 8.7 | 88 | 2 | 3 | 5 | 11 | 19 | 27 | 44 |
| **TOTAL** | | | | | | | | | | |
| 0–19 Years | 251 | 12.6 | 227 | 2 | 3 | 6 | 17 | 34 | 42 | 89 |
| 20–34 | 193 | 9.6 | 154 | 2 | 3 | 6 | 12 | 20 | 30 | 91 |
| 35–49 | 705 | 7.4 | 62 | 2 | 3 | 4 | 10 | 18 | 21 | 37 |
| 50–64 | 1,215 | 7.8 | 71 | 2 | 3 | 5 | 10 | 16 | 26 | 40 |
| 65+ | 1,391 | 8.2 | 66 | 2 | 3 | 5 | 10 | 19 | 25 | 40 |
| **GRAND TOTAL** | 3,755 | 8.3 | 84 | 2 | 3 | 5 | 10 | 19 | 26 | 43 |

### 33.3: SURG COLLAPSE OF LUNG. Formerly included in operation group(s) 567.

| Type of Patients | Observed Patients | Avg. Stay | Variance | Percentiles | | | | | | |
|---|---|---|---|---|---|---|---|---|---|---|
| | | | | 10th | 25th | 50th | 75th | 90th | 95th | 99th |
| **1. SINGLE DX** | | | | | | | | | | |
| 0–19 Years | 13 | 4.0 | 7 | 2 | 3 | 3 | 6 | 6 | 11 | 11 |
| 20–34 | 20 | 4.3 | 3 | 2 | 4 | 5 | 6 | 6 | 6 | 6 |
| 35–49 | 11 | 4.4 | 2 | 2 | 5 | 5 | 5 | 5 | 5 | 7 |
| 50–64 | 3 | 3.3 | 1 | 4 | 4 | 4 | 4 | 4 | 4 | 4 |
| 65+ | 1 | 4.0 | 0 | 4 | 4 | 4 | 4 | 4 | 4 | 4 |
| **2. MULTIPLE DX** | | | | | | | | | | |
| 0–19 Years | 23 | 5.4 | 10 | 3 | 3 | 6 | 8 | 8 | 10 | 14 |
| 20–34 | 42 | 6.4 | 41 | 2 | 4 | 5 | 6 | 11 | 21 | 35 |
| 35–49 | 45 | 7.7 | 68 | 2 | 3 | 4 | 8 | 21 | 21 | 37 |
| 50–64 | 68 | 12.0 | 334 | 4 | 8 | 8 | 10 | 18 | 34 | 90 |
| 65+ | 77 | 11.0 | 73 | 3 | 5 | 8 | 13 | 21 | 32 | 42 |
| **TOTAL SINGLE DX** | 48 | 4.2 | 3 | 2 | 3 | 4 | 5 | 5 | 7 | 11 |
| **TOTAL MULTIPLE DX** | 255 | 9.4 | 139 | 2 | 4 | 6 | 10 | 19 | 28 | 90 |
| **TOTAL** | | | | | | | | | | |
| 0–19 Years | 36 | 5.0 | 10 | 2 | 3 | 4 | 7 | 9 | 10 | 14 |
| 20–34 | 62 | 5.6 | 28 | 4 | 4 | 4 | 5 | 8 | 14 | 35 |
| 35–49 | 56 | 7.0 | 57 | 3 | 3 | 5 | 7 | 21 | 21 | 37 |
| 50–64 | 71 | 11.8 | 327 | 2 | 4 | 8 | 13 | 18 | 34 | 90 |
| 65+ | 78 | 10.9 | 73 | 3 | 5 | 8 | 13 | 21 | 32 | 42 |
| **GRAND TOTAL** | 303 | 8.5 | 121 | 2 | 4 | 5 | 9 | 16 | 22 | 90 |

Length of Stay by Diagnosis and Operation, United States, 2000

# United States, October 1998–September 1999 Data, by Operation

## 33.4: LUNG AND BRONCHUS REPAIR. Formerly included in operation group(s) 563, 567.

| Type of Patients | Observed Patients | Avg. Stay | Variance | 10th | 25th | 50th | 75th | 90th | 95th | 99th |
|---|---|---|---|---|---|---|---|---|---|---|
| **1. SINGLE DX** | | | | | | | | | | |
| 0–19 Years | 0 | | | | | | | | | |
| 20–34 | 0 | | | | | | | | | |
| 35–49 | 2 | 4.7 | 3 | 3 | 3 | 6 | 6 | 6 | 6 | 6 |
| 50–64 | 0 | | | | | | | | | |
| 65+ | 0 | | | | | | | | | |
| **2. MULTIPLE DX** | | | | | | | | | | |
| 0–19 Years | 15 | 6.8 | 38 | 3 | 4 | 4 | 6 | 8 | 26 | 26 |
| 20–34 | 27 | 11.3 | 25 | 5 | 7 | 11 | 15 | 15 | 15 | 27 |
| 35–49 | 24 | 12.9 | 84 | 4 | 9 | 9 | 17 | 20 | 24 | 55 |
| 50–64 | 13 | 10.6 | 34 | 3 | 6 | 11 | 13 | 20 | 20 | 20 |
| 65+ | 15 | 18.3 | 215 | 3 | 4 | 15 | 20 | 51 | 51 | 51 |
| **TOTAL SINGLE DX** | 2 | 4.7 | 3 | 3 | 3 | 6 | 6 | 6 | 6 | 6 |
| **TOTAL MULTIPLE DX** | 94 | 10.9 | 78 | 4 | 4 | 8 | 15 | 20 | 26 | 51 |
| **TOTAL** | | | | | | | | | | |
| 0–19 Years | 15 | 6.8 | 38 | 3 | 4 | 4 | 6 | 8 | 26 | 26 |
| 20–34 | 27 | 11.3 | 25 | 5 | 7 | 11 | 15 | 15 | 15 | 27 |
| 35–49 | 26 | 12.3 | 83 | 3 | 6 | 9 | 17 | 20 | 24 | 55 |
| 50–64 | 13 | 10.6 | 34 | 3 | 6 | 11 | 13 | 20 | 20 | 20 |
| 65+ | 15 | 18.3 | 215 | 3 | 4 | 15 | 20 | 51 | 51 | 51 |
| **GRAND TOTAL** | 96 | 10.8 | 77 | 4 | 4 | 8 | 15 | 20 | 26 | 51 |

## 33.6: HEART-LUNG TRANSPLANT. Formerly included in operation group(s) 572.

| Type of Patients | Observed Patients | Avg. Stay | Variance | 10th | 25th | 50th | 75th | 90th | 95th | 99th |
|---|---|---|---|---|---|---|---|---|---|---|
| **1. SINGLE DX** | | | | | | | | | | |
| 0–19 Years | 0 | | | | | | | | | |
| 20–34 | 0 | | | | | | | | | |
| 35–49 | 0 | | | | | | | | | |
| 50–64 | 0 | | | | | | | | | |
| 65+ | 0 | | | | | | | | | |
| **2. MULTIPLE DX** | | | | | | | | | | |
| 0–19 Years | 3 | 28.4 | 492 | 15 | 15 | >99 | >99 | >99 | >99 | >99 |
| 20–34 | 3 | 17.4 | 44 | 14 | 14 | 15 | 15 | 30 | 30 | 30 |
| 35–49 | 1 | 15.0 | 0 | 15 | 15 | 15 | 15 | 15 | 15 | 15 |
| 50–64 | 2 | 15.1 | 22 | 9 | 9 | 18 | 18 | 18 | 18 | 18 |
| 65+ | 0 | | | | | | | | | |
| **TOTAL SINGLE DX** | 0 | | | | | | | | | |
| **TOTAL MULTIPLE DX** | 9 | 23.7 | 344 | 15 | 15 | 64 | >99 | >99 | >99 | >99 |
| **TOTAL** | | | | | | | | | | |
| 0–19 Years | 3 | 28.4 | 492 | 15 | 15 | >99 | >99 | >99 | >99 | >99 |
| 20–34 | 3 | 17.4 | 44 | 14 | 14 | 15 | 15 | 30 | 30 | 30 |
| 35–49 | 1 | 15.0 | 0 | 15 | 15 | 15 | 15 | 15 | 15 | 15 |
| 50–64 | 2 | 15.1 | 22 | 9 | 9 | 18 | 18 | 18 | 18 | 18 |
| 65+ | 0 | | | | | | | | | |
| **GRAND TOTAL** | 9 | 23.7 | 344 | 15 | 15 | 64 | >99 | >99 | >99 | >99 |

## 33.5: LUNG TRANSPLANTATION. Formerly included in operation group(s) 567.

| Type of Patients | Observed Patients | Avg. Stay | Variance | 10th | 25th | 50th | 75th | 90th | 95th | 99th |
|---|---|---|---|---|---|---|---|---|---|---|
| **1. SINGLE DX** | | | | | | | | | | |
| 0–19 Years | 1 | 8.0 | 0 | 8 | 8 | 8 | 8 | 8 | 8 | 8 |
| 20–34 | 2 | 8.6 | 1 | 8 | 8 | 8 | 10 | 10 | 10 | 10 |
| 35–49 | 1 | 22.0 | 0 | 22 | 22 | 22 | 22 | 22 | 22 | 22 |
| 50–64 | 5 | 5.4 | 2 | 4 | 4 | 6 | 7 | 7 | 7 | 7 |
| 65+ | 1 | 14.0 | 0 | 14 | 14 | 14 | 14 | 14 | 14 | 14 |
| **2. MULTIPLE DX** | | | | | | | | | | |
| 0–19 Years | 20 | 32.5 | 373 | 14 | 25 | 31 | 48 | >99 | >99 | >99 |
| 20–34 | 31 | 22.3 | 121 | 11 | 14 | 19 | 29 | 32 | 50 | 52 |
| 35–49 | 56 | 18.5 | 185 | 7 | 11 | 15 | 22 | 37 | 46 | >99 |
| 50–64 | 124 | 16.5 | 131 | 7 | 9 | 13 | 22 | 31 | 40 | >99 |
| 65+ | 8 | 28.8 | 489 | 9 | 12 | 15 | 51 | 61 | 61 | 61 |
| **TOTAL SINGLE DX** | 10 | 7.8 | 21 | 4 | 5 | 7 | 8 | 14 | 22 | 22 |
| **TOTAL MULTIPLE DX** | 239 | 20.6 | 223 | 8 | 11 | 16 | 27 | 46 | 78 | >99 |
| **TOTAL** | | | | | | | | | | |
| 0–19 Years | 21 | 32.1 | 376 | 14 | 25 | 31 | 48 | >99 | >99 | >99 |
| 20–34 | 33 | 21.3 | 125 | 11 | 13 | 19 | 27 | 32 | 50 | 52 |
| 35–49 | 57 | 18.5 | 183 | 7 | 11 | 15 | 22 | 37 | 46 | >99 |
| 50–64 | 129 | 15.9 | 130 | 6 | 8 | 12 | 22 | 30 | 39 | >99 |
| 65+ | 9 | 27.7 | 465 | 9 | 12 | 15 | 51 | 61 | 61 | 61 |
| **GRAND TOTAL** | 249 | 20.1 | 221 | 8 | 10 | 15 | 27 | 46 | 78 | >99 |

## 33.9: OTHER BRONCHIAL LUNG OPS. Formerly included in operation group(s) 563, 567.

| Type of Patients | Observed Patients | Avg. Stay | Variance | 10th | 25th | 50th | 75th | 90th | 95th | 99th |
|---|---|---|---|---|---|---|---|---|---|---|
| **1. SINGLE DX** | | | | | | | | | | |
| 0–19 Years | 2 | 7.0 | 34 | 3 | 3 | 3 | 13 | 13 | 13 | 13 |
| 20–34 | 2 | 1.0 | 0 | 1 | 1 | 1 | 1 | 1 | 1 | 1 |
| 35–49 | 0 | | | | | | | | | |
| 50–64 | 4 | 1.4 | <1 | 1 | 1 | 1 | 1 | 3 | 3 | 3 |
| 65+ | 1 | 1.0 | 0 | 1 | 1 | 1 | 1 | 1 | 1 | 1 |
| **2. MULTIPLE DX** | | | | | | | | | | |
| 0–19 Years | 45 | 9.1 | 88 | 2 | 4 | 6 | 11 | 20 | 26 | 30 |
| 20–34 | 18 | 4.7 | 18 | 1 | 2 | 2 | 7 | 10 | 17 | 17 |
| 35–49 | 34 | 10.1 | 76 | 1 | 2 | 7 | 18 | 22 | 27 | 36 |
| 50–64 | 54 | 11.4 | 105 | 1 | 4 | 8 | 14 | 25 | 36 | 48 |
| 65+ | 63 | 10.1 | 76 | 3 | 4 | 8 | 14 | 20 | 21 | 28 |
| **TOTAL SINGLE DX** | 9 | 2.6 | 13 | 1 | 1 | 1 | 3 | 3 | 13 | 13 |
| **TOTAL MULTIPLE DX** | 214 | 9.8 | 82 | 1 | 4 | 7 | 14 | 20 | 25 | 42 |
| **TOTAL** | | | | | | | | | | |
| 0–19 Years | 47 | 9.1 | 87 | 2 | 4 | 6 | 11 | 20 | 26 | 30 |
| 20–34 | 20 | 4.5 | 17 | 1 | 1 | 2 | 7 | 10 | 17 | 17 |
| 35–49 | 34 | 10.1 | 76 | 1 | 2 | 7 | 18 | 22 | 27 | 36 |
| 50–64 | 58 | 11.0 | 105 | 1 | 3 | 8 | 14 | 24 | 26 | 48 |
| 65+ | 64 | 10.1 | 76 | 3 | 4 | 8 | 14 | 20 | 21 | 28 |
| **GRAND TOTAL** | 223 | 9.6 | 81 | 1 | 3 | 7 | 14 | 20 | 25 | 42 |

Length of Stay by Diagnosis and Operation, United States, 2000

# United States, October 1998–September 1999 Data, by Operation

## 34.0: INC CHEST WALL & PLEURA. Formerly included in operation group(s) 568.

| Type of Patients | Observed Patients | Avg. Stay | Variance | 10th | 25th | 50th | 75th | 90th | 95th | 99th |
|---|---|---|---|---|---|---|---|---|---|---|
| **1. SINGLE DX** | | | | | | | | | | |
| 0–19 Years | 514 | 3.6 | 6 | 1 | 2 | 3 | 4 | 6 | 8 | 11 |
| 20–34 | 892 | 3.7 | 5 | 2 | 2 | 3 | 5 | 7 | 8 | 11 |
| 35–49 | 503 | 3.2 | 5 | 1 | 2 | 3 | 4 | 7 | 8 | 11 |
| 50–64 | 168 | 4.0 | 6 | 2 | 3 | 3 | 4 | 7 | 9 | 12 |
| 65+ | 75 | 3.8 | 8 | 1 | 2 | 3 | 5 | 7 | 10 | 14 |
| **2. MULTIPLE DX** | | | | | | | | | | |
| 0–19 Years | 1,628 | 9.0 | 122 | 2 | 4 | 7 | 10 | 15 | 22 | 75 |
| 20–34 | 2,362 | 6.0 | 38 | 2 | 3 | 4 | 8 | 11 | 17 | 28 |
| 35–49 | 3,138 | 6.6 | 28 | 2 | 3 | 5 | 7 | 13 | 17 | 26 |
| 50–64 | 3,466 | 7.5 | 44 | 2 | 3 | 6 | 9 | 15 | 19 | 35 |
| 65+ | 6,075 | 8.5 | 43 | 3 | 4 | 7 | 11 | 16 | 21 | 35 |
| **TOTAL SINGLE DX** | 2,152 | 3.6 | 5 | 1 | 2 | 3 | 4 | 7 | 8 | 11 |
| **TOTAL MULTIPLE DX** | 16,669 | 7.6 | 49 | 2 | 3 | 6 | 10 | 15 | 20 | 35 |
| **TOTAL** | | | | | | | | | | |
| 0–19 Years | 2,142 | 7.8 | 101 | 2 | 3 | 5 | 9 | 14 | 20 | 70 |
| 20–34 | 3,254 | 5.3 | 29 | 2 | 3 | 4 | 6 | 10 | 13 | 24 |
| 35–49 | 3,641 | 6.1 | 26 | 2 | 3 | 5 | 8 | 12 | 16 | 25 |
| 50–64 | 3,634 | 7.4 | 43 | 2 | 3 | 5 | 9 | 15 | 19 | 35 |
| 65+ | 6,150 | 8.5 | 43 | 3 | 4 | 7 | 11 | 16 | 21 | 35 |
| **GRAND TOTAL** | 18,821 | 7.1 | 46 | 2 | 3 | 5 | 9 | 14 | 19 | 35 |

## 34.02: EXPLORATORY THORACOTOMY. Formerly included in operation group(s) 568.

| Type of Patients | Observed Patients | Avg. Stay | Variance | 10th | 25th | 50th | 75th | 90th | 95th | 99th |
|---|---|---|---|---|---|---|---|---|---|---|
| **1. SINGLE DX** | | | | | | | | | | |
| 0–19 Years | 4 | 4.4 | 1 | 3 | 4 | 4 | 5 | 6 | 6 | 6 |
| 20–34 | 1 | 3.0 | 0 | 3 | 3 | 3 | 3 | 3 | 3 | 3 |
| 35–49 | 4 | 5.4 | 6 | 2 | 2 | 7 | 7 | 7 | 7 | 7 |
| 50–64 | 6 | 5.1 | 9 | 4 | 4 | 4 | 4 | 7 | 15 | 15 |
| 65+ | 9 | 3.9 | 9 | 1 | 1 | 4 | 7 | 7 | 10 | 10 |
| **2. MULTIPLE DX** | | | | | | | | | | |
| 0–19 Years | 20 | 18.6 | 693 | 3 | 5 | 7 | 21 | 99 | 99 | >99 |
| 20–34 | 36 | 6.5 | 67 | 1 | 3 | 4 | 6 | 20 | 20 | 36 |
| 35–49 | 59 | 6.5 | 39 | 4 | 4 | 5 | 6 | 11 | 21 | 31 |
| 50–64 | 128 | 8.3 | 64 | 3 | 4 | 6 | 9 | 17 | 23 | 39 |
| 65+ | 185 | 7.4 | 31 | 3 | 4 | 6 | 9 | 14 | 18 | 27 |
| **TOTAL SINGLE DX** | 24 | 4.5 | 7 | 1 | 3 | 4 | 6 | 7 | 10 | 15 |
| **TOTAL MULTIPLE DX** | 428 | 7.9 | 84 | 3 | 4 | 5 | 8 | 16 | 21 | 42 |
| **TOTAL** | | | | | | | | | | |
| 0–19 Years | 24 | 16.9 | 633 | 3 | 5 | 7 | 19 | 26 | 99 | >99 |
| 20–34 | 37 | 6.5 | 66 | 1 | 3 | 4 | 6 | 20 | 20 | 36 |
| 35–49 | 63 | 6.5 | 38 | 4 | 4 | 4 | 6 | 11 | 21 | 31 |
| 50–64 | 134 | 8.1 | 62 | 3 | 4 | 5 | 9 | 17 | 23 | 39 |
| 65+ | 194 | 7.2 | 30 | 3 | 4 | 5 | 9 | 14 | 17 | 27 |
| **GRAND TOTAL** | 452 | 7.8 | 81 | 3 | 4 | 5 | 8 | 16 | 21 | 42 |

## 34.01: INCISION OF CHEST WALL. Formerly included in operation group(s) 568.

| Type of Patients | Observed Patients | Avg. Stay | Variance | 10th | 25th | 50th | 75th | 90th | 95th | 99th |
|---|---|---|---|---|---|---|---|---|---|---|
| **1. SINGLE DX** | | | | | | | | | | |
| 0–19 Years | 15 | 3.1 | 5 | 1 | 1 | 4 | 4 | 7 | 7 | 7 |
| 20–34 | 7 | 3.5 | 6 | 1 | 1 | 4 | 5 | 6 | 8 | 8 |
| 35–49 | 7 | 2.5 | 5 | 1 | 1 | 2 | 3 | 7 | 7 | 7 |
| 50–64 | 6 | 3.6 | 11 | 1 | 1 | 2 | 5 | 10 | 10 | 10 |
| 65+ | 4 | 5.3 | 11 | 1 | 4 | 5 | 5 | 11 | 11 | 11 |
| **2. MULTIPLE DX** | | | | | | | | | | |
| 0–19 Years | 30 | 3.4 | 15 | 1 | 1 | 2 | 4 | 8 | 12 | 21 |
| 20–34 | 20 | 6.2 | 73 | 2 | 3 | 4 | 6 | 7 | 16 | 54 |
| 35–49 | 86 | 6.1 | 29 | 1 | 2 | 4 | 11 | 12 | 14 | 26 |
| 50–64 | 133 | 4.4 | 22 | 1 | 1 | 2 | 5 | 11 | 16 | 18 |
| 65+ | 160 | 7.4 | 76 | 1 | 2 | 5 | 9 | 15 | 20 | 54 |
| **TOTAL SINGLE DX** | 39 | 3.3 | 6 | 1 | 1 | 3 | 5 | 7 | 7 | 11 |
| **TOTAL MULTIPLE DX** | 429 | 5.7 | 43 | 1 | 2 | 3 | 8 | 12 | 17 | 30 |
| **TOTAL** | | | | | | | | | | |
| 0–19 Years | 45 | 3.3 | 10 | 1 | 2 | 2 | 4 | 7 | 8 | 21 |
| 20–34 | 27 | 5.8 | 63 | 2 | 3 | 4 | 6 | 7 | 16 | 54 |
| 35–49 | 93 | 5.9 | 28 | 1 | 2 | 3 | 11 | 12 | 14 | 26 |
| 50–64 | 139 | 4.4 | 22 | 1 | 1 | 2 | 5 | 11 | 16 | 18 |
| 65+ | 164 | 7.3 | 74 | 1 | 2 | 5 | 9 | 15 | 20 | 54 |
| **GRAND TOTAL** | 468 | 5.5 | 40 | 1 | 2 | 3 | 7 | 12 | 16 | 28 |

## 34.04: INSERT INTERCOSTAL CATH. Formerly included in operation group(s) 568.

| Type of Patients | Observed Patients | Avg. Stay | Variance | 10th | 25th | 50th | 75th | 90th | 95th | 99th |
|---|---|---|---|---|---|---|---|---|---|---|
| **1. SINGLE DX** | | | | | | | | | | |
| 0–19 Years | 421 | 3.6 | 6 | 1 | 2 | 3 | 4 | 6 | 8 | 12 |
| 20–34 | 717 | 3.7 | 5 | 2 | 2 | 3 | 5 | 7 | 8 | 10 |
| 35–49 | 405 | 3.1 | 5 | 1 | 2 | 3 | 3 | 6 | 7 | 10 |
| 50–64 | 122 | 3.6 | 4 | 2 | 2 | 3 | 4 | 6 | 7 | 11 |
| 65+ | 48 | 3.6 | 5 | 2 | 2 | 3 | 5 | 6 | 7 | 13 |
| **2. MULTIPLE DX** | | | | | | | | | | |
| 0–19 Years | 1,316 | 9.1 | 124 | 3 | 4 | 7 | 10 | 15 | 22 | 75 |
| 20–34 | 1,930 | 5.8 | 33 | 2 | 3 | 4 | 7 | 11 | 15 | 24 |
| 35–49 | 2,465 | 6.5 | 26 | 2 | 3 | 4 | 8 | 13 | 17 | 24 |
| 50–64 | 2,535 | 7.2 | 40 | 2 | 3 | 5 | 9 | 14 | 18 | 35 |
| 65+ | 4,685 | 8.5 | 42 | 3 | 4 | 7 | 11 | 16 | 21 | 35 |
| **TOTAL SINGLE DX** | 1,713 | 3.5 | 5 | 1 | 2 | 3 | 4 | 7 | 8 | 11 |
| **TOTAL MULTIPLE DX** | 12,931 | 7.5 | 48 | 2 | 3 | 6 | 9 | 14 | 19 | 35 |
| **TOTAL** | | | | | | | | | | |
| 0–19 Years | 1,737 | 7.9 | 104 | 2 | 3 | 5 | 9 | 14 | 20 | 70 |
| 20–34 | 2,647 | 5.2 | 25 | 2 | 3 | 4 | 6 | 9 | 12 | 22 |
| 35–49 | 2,870 | 6.0 | 24 | 2 | 3 | 5 | 7 | 12 | 15 | 24 |
| 50–64 | 2,657 | 7.1 | 39 | 2 | 3 | 5 | 9 | 14 | 18 | 35 |
| 65+ | 4,733 | 8.4 | 42 | 3 | 4 | 7 | 11 | 16 | 21 | 35 |
| **GRAND TOTAL** | 14,644 | 7.1 | 44 | 2 | 3 | 5 | 9 | 14 | 18 | 35 |

Length of Stay by Diagnosis and Operation, United States, 2000

# United States, October 1998–September 1999 Data, by Operation

## 34.09: OTHER PLEURAL INCISION. Formerly included in operation group(s) 568.

| Type of Patients | Observed Patients | Avg. Stay | Vari- ance | Percentiles | | | | | | |
|---|---|---|---|---|---|---|---|---|---|---|
| | | | | 10th | 25th | 50th | 75th | 90th | 95th | 99th |
| **1. SINGLE DX** | | | | | | | | | | |
| 0–19 Years | 74 | 3.8 | 4 | 2 | 3 | 5 | 5 | 6 | 8 | 11 |
| 20–34 | 167 | 3.5 | 5 | 1 | 2 | 3 | 4 | 6 | 8 | 12 |
| 35–49 | 87 | 3.8 | 9 | 1 | 2 | 3 | 4 | 9 | 11 | 11 |
| 50–64 | 33 | 4.8 | 11 | 2 | 3 | 3 | 6 | 9 | 12 | 12 |
| 65+ | 10 | 5.9 | 26 | 2 | 2 | 3 | 8 | 14 | 15 | 15 |
| **2. MULTIPLE DX** | | | | | | | | | | |
| 0–19 Years | 252 | 7.9 | 50 | 2 | 4 | 6 | 10 | 15 | 20 | 44 |
| 20–34 | 372 | 6.3 | 56 | 2 | 3 | 6 | 7 | 11 | 17 | 29 |
| 35–49 | 502 | 6.8 | 35 | 2 | 3 | 5 | 8 | 14 | 20 | 27 |
| 50–64 | 602 | 8.8 | 46 | 3 | 4 | 6 | 12 | 18 | 22 | 36 |
| 65+ | 955 | 8.8 | 46 | 3 | 4 | 7 | 12 | 16 | 22 | 32 |
| **TOTAL SINGLE DX** | 371 | 3.8 | 7 | 1 | 2 | 3 | 4 | 8 | 10 | 12 |
| **TOTAL MULTIPLE DX** | 2,683 | 8.0 | 47 | 2 | 4 | 6 | 10 | 16 | 21 | 32 |
| **TOTAL** | | | | | | | | | | |
| 0–19 Years | 326 | 6.9 | 42 | 2 | 3 | 5 | 9 | 13 | 19 | 31 |
| 20–34 | 539 | 5.5 | 42 | 2 | 3 | 4 | 6 | 10 | 13 | 27 |
| 35–49 | 589 | 6.4 | 33 | 2 | 3 | 5 | 8 | 13 | 18 | 27 |
| 50–64 | 635 | 8.6 | 45 | 3 | 4 | 6 | 11 | 18 | 22 | 36 |
| 65+ | 965 | 8.8 | 46 | 3 | 4 | 7 | 12 | 16 | 22 | 32 |
| **GRAND TOTAL** | 3,054 | 7.5 | 44 | 2 | 3 | 5 | 9 | 16 | 20 | 32 |

## 34.1: INCISION OF MEDIASTINUM. Formerly included in operation group(s) 569.

| Type of Patients | Observed Patients | Avg. Stay | Vari- ance | Percentiles | | | | | | |
|---|---|---|---|---|---|---|---|---|---|---|
| | | | | 10th | 25th | 50th | 75th | 90th | 95th | 99th |
| **1. SINGLE DX** | | | | | | | | | | |
| 0–19 Years | 1 | 1.0 | 0 | 1 | 1 | 1 | 1 | 1 | 1 | 1 |
| 20–34 | 4 | 1.9 | <1 | 1 | 2 | 2 | 2 | 3 | 3 | 3 |
| 35–49 | 6 | 1.0 | 0 | 1 | 1 | 1 | 1 | 1 | 1 | 1 |
| 50–64 | 3 | 2.4 | 3 | 1 | 1 | 1 | 4 | 4 | 4 | 4 |
| 65+ | 1 | 1.0 | 0 | 1 | 1 | 1 | 1 | 1 | 1 | 1 |
| **2. MULTIPLE DX** | | | | | | | | | | |
| 0–19 Years | 13 | 25.3 | 393 | 7 | 17 | 55 | >99 | >99 | >99 | >99 |
| 20–34 | 17 | 8.4 | 74 | 4 | 4 | 4 | 9 | 27 | 27 | 36 |
| 35–49 | 35 | 9.2 | 71 | 1 | 3 | 7 | 14 | 19 | 30 | 32 |
| 50–64 | 66 | 15.0 | 374 | 2 | 5 | 7 | 17 | 65 | 65 | 75 |
| 65+ | 85 | 9.4 | 66 | 1 | 3 | 9 | 11 | 19 | 26 | 38 |
| **TOTAL SINGLE DX** | 15 | 1.5 | <1 | 1 | 1 | 1 | 2 | 3 | 4 | 4 |
| **TOTAL MULTIPLE DX** | 216 | 11.6 | 185 | 1 | 4 | 8 | 14 | 30 | 65 | >99 |
| **TOTAL** | | | | | | | | | | |
| 0–19 Years | 14 | 23.2 | 406 | 2 | 16 | 55 | >99 | >99 | >99 | >99 |
| 20–34 | 21 | 7.6 | 69 | 2 | 4 | 4 | 9 | 25 | 27 | 36 |
| 35–49 | 41 | 8.3 | 70 | 1 | 2 | 4 | 13 | 19 | 30 | 32 |
| 50–64 | 69 | 14.7 | 369 | 1 | 4 | 6 | 17 | 48 | 65 | 75 |
| 65+ | 86 | 9.3 | 66 | 1 | 3 | 9 | 11 | 19 | 26 | 38 |
| **GRAND TOTAL** | 231 | 11.2 | 181 | 1 | 3 | 7 | 13 | 29 | 65 | >99 |

## 34.2: THORAX DXTIC PROCEDURES. Formerly included in operation group(s) 569, 581.

| Type of Patients | Observed Patients | Avg. Stay | Vari- ance | Percentiles | | | | | | |
|---|---|---|---|---|---|---|---|---|---|---|
| | | | | 10th | 25th | 50th | 75th | 90th | 95th | 99th |
| **1. SINGLE DX** | | | | | | | | | | |
| 0–19 Years | 39 | 6.8 | 21 | 2 | 3 | 6 | 9 | 16 | 16 | 16 |
| 20–34 | 84 | 3.3 | 3 | 1 | 2 | 3 | 4 | 5 | 7 | 9 |
| 35–49 | 106 | 2.1 | 4 | 1 | 1 | 1 | 2 | 4 | 7 | 9 |
| 50–64 | 66 | 2.4 | 4 | 1 | 1 | 2 | 3 | 5 | 5 | 14 |
| 65+ | 65 | 2.5 | 5 | 1 | 1 | 1 | 3 | 7 | 7 | 8 |
| **2. MULTIPLE DX** | | | | | | | | | | |
| 0–19 Years | 146 | 11.5 | 127 | 2 | 4 | 9 | 14 | 23 | 35 | 65 |
| 20–34 | 272 | 6.7 | 31 | 1 | 3 | 6 | 8 | 13 | 19 | 27 |
| 35–49 | 669 | 8.1 | 50 | 1 | 2 | 7 | 11 | 17 | 22 | 31 |
| 50–64 | 1,233 | 7.1 | 43 | 1 | 3 | 5 | 11 | 15 | 18 | 28 |
| 65+ | 2,280 | 7.4 | 42 | 1 | 3 | 6 | 10 | 15 | 19 | 32 |
| **TOTAL SINGLE DX** | 360 | 3.3 | 9 | 1 | 1 | 2 | 4 | 7 | 9 | 16 |
| **TOTAL MULTIPLE DX** | 4,600 | 7.5 | 47 | 1 | 2 | 6 | 11 | 15 | 20 | 33 |
| **TOTAL** | | | | | | | | | | |
| 0–19 Years | 185 | 10.3 | 103 | 2 | 4 | 7 | 14 | 21 | 35 | 65 |
| 20–34 | 356 | 5.7 | 25 | 1 | 2 | 4 | 7 | 11 | 15 | 25 |
| 35–49 | 775 | 7.5 | 49 | 1 | 2 | 6 | 10 | 16 | 22 | 31 |
| 50–64 | 1,299 | 6.9 | 42 | 1 | 2 | 5 | 11 | 15 | 18 | 28 |
| 65+ | 2,345 | 7.3 | 42 | 1 | 2 | 6 | 10 | 15 | 19 | 32 |
| **GRAND TOTAL** | 4,960 | 7.2 | 45 | 1 | 2 | 5 | 10 | 15 | 19 | 32 |

## 34.21: TRANSPLEURA THORACOSCOPY. Formerly included in operation group(s) 569.

| Type of Patients | Observed Patients | Avg. Stay | Vari- ance | Percentiles | | | | | | |
|---|---|---|---|---|---|---|---|---|---|---|
| | | | | 10th | 25th | 50th | 75th | 90th | 95th | 99th |
| **1. SINGLE DX** | | | | | | | | | | |
| 0–19 Years | 13 | 3.7 | 13 | 1 | 2 | 2 | 3 | 9 | 14 | 14 |
| 20–34 | 24 | 3.9 | 2 | 3 | 3 | 4 | 4 | 4 | 7 | 8 |
| 35–49 | 22 | 2.2 | 3 | 1 | 2 | 2 | 2 | 3 | 4 | 11 |
| 50–64 | 7 | 1.8 | <1 | 1 | 1 | 1 | 2 | 3 | 3 | 3 |
| 65+ | 17 | 2.6 | 5 | 1 | 1 | 1 | 3 | 7 | 7 | 8 |
| **2. MULTIPLE DX** | | | | | | | | | | |
| 0–19 Years | 57 | 10.8 | 37 | 3 | 6 | 10 | 14 | 21 | 23 | 23 |
| 20–34 | 68 | 7.5 | 27 | 3 | 6 | 6 | 7 | 14 | 19 | 35 |
| 35–49 | 172 | 11.5 | 80 | 1 | 5 | 8 | 17 | 24 | 31 | 31 |
| 50–64 | 282 | 8.6 | 61 | 2 | 3 | 7 | 13 | 16 | 20 | 38 |
| 65+ | 556 | 9.0 | 55 | 2 | 4 | 7 | 13 | 19 | 22 | 38 |
| **TOTAL SINGLE DX** | 83 | 3.3 | 4 | 1 | 2 | 3 | 4 | 5 | 7 | 11 |
| **TOTAL MULTIPLE DX** | 1,135 | 9.2 | 58 | 2 | 4 | 7 | 13 | 19 | 22 | 36 |
| **TOTAL** | | | | | | | | | | |
| 0–19 Years | 70 | 9.5 | 40 | 2 | 4 | 9 | 14 | 20 | 22 | 23 |
| 20–34 | 92 | 6.1 | 20 | 3 | 4 | 8 | 7 | 10 | 15 | 24 |
| 35–49 | 194 | 10.2 | 79 | 1 | 3 | 6 | 16 | 22 | 31 | 31 |
| 50–64 | 289 | 8.5 | 60 | 1 | 4 | 7 | 13 | 16 | 19 | 38 |
| 65+ | 573 | 8.7 | 54 | 2 | 4 | 7 | 12 | 18 | 22 | 38 |
| **GRAND TOTAL** | 1,218 | 8.6 | 55 | 2 | 4 | 6 | 12 | 18 | 22 | 35 |

Length of Stay by Diagnosis and Operation, United States, 2000

# United States, October 1998–September 1999 Data, by Operation

## 34.22: MEDIASTINOSCOPY. Formerly included in operation group(s) 569.

| Type of Patients | Observed Patients | Avg. Stay | Variance | 10th | 25th | 50th | 75th | 90th | 95th | 99th |
|---|---|---|---|---|---|---|---|---|---|---|
| **1. SINGLE DX** | | | | | | | | | | |
| 0–19 Years | 3 | 4.2 | 3 | 3 | 3 | 3 | 6 | 6 | 6 | 6 |
| 20–34 | 31 | 2.1 | 4 | 1 | 1 | 1 | 2 | 5 | 7 | 12 |
| 35–49 | 44 | 1.5 | 1 | 1 | 1 | 1 | 1 | 2 | 4 | 4 |
| 50–64 | 32 | 2.0 | 2 | 1 | 1 | 1 | 3 | 3 | 5 | 9 |
| 65+ | 28 | 1.7 | 3 | 1 | 1 | 1 | 1 | 3 | 8 | 8 |
| **2. MULTIPLE DX** | | | | | | | | | | |
| 0–19 Years | 8 | 5.0 | 12 | 6 | 7 | 7 | 9 | 9 | 9 | 9 |
| 20–34 | 84 | 5.9 | 40 | 1 | 1 | 4 | 8 | 16 | 22 | 25 |
| 35–49 | 235 | 6.5 | 43 | 1 | 1 | 5 | 9 | 13 | 17 | 32 |
| 50–64 | 501 | 5.4 | 38 | 1 | 1 | 2 | 8 | 14 | 21 | 25 |
| 65+ | 724 | 5.7 | 34 | 1 | 1 | 4 | 8 | 14 | 18 | 28 |
| **TOTAL SINGLE DX** | 138 | 1.9 | 3 | 1 | 1 | 1 | 2 | 4 | 6 | 9 |
| **TOTAL MULTIPLE DX** | 1,552 | 5.8 | 37 | 1 | 1 | 4 | 9 | 14 | 18 | 28 |
| **TOTAL** | | | | | | | | | | |
| 0–19 Years | 11 | 4.7 | 9 | 3 | 5 | 5 | 7 | 9 | 9 | 9 |
| 20–34 | 115 | 4.9 | 33 | 1 | 2 | 2 | 6 | 12 | 19 | 25 |
| 35–49 | 279 | 5.9 | 41 | 1 | 1 | 5 | 9 | 13 | 16 | 32 |
| 50–64 | 533 | 5.2 | 37 | 1 | 1 | 2 | 8 | 13 | 20 | 25 |
| 65+ | 752 | 5.6 | 33 | 1 | 1 | 4 | 8 | 14 | 18 | 28 |
| **GRAND TOTAL** | 1,690 | 5.5 | 35 | 1 | 1 | 3 | 9 | 13 | 18 | 26 |

## 34.25: CLSD MEDIASTINAL BX. Formerly included in operation group(s) 569.

| Type of Patients | Observed Patients | Avg. Stay | Variance | 10th | 25th | 50th | 75th | 90th | 95th | 99th |
|---|---|---|---|---|---|---|---|---|---|---|
| **1. SINGLE DX** | | | | | | | | | | |
| 0–19 Years | 4 | 11.5 | 25 | 3 | 9 | 16 | 16 | 16 | 16 | 16 |
| 20–34 | 8 | 1.8 | 2 | 1 | 1 | 1 | 1 | 3 | 6 | 6 |
| 35–49 | 13 | 2.5 | 6 | 1 | 1 | 2 | 3 | 5 | 9 | 9 |
| 50–64 | 5 | 2.3 | 2 | 1 | 1 | 2 | 3 | 5 | 5 | 5 |
| 65+ | 2 | 4.1 | 5 | 3 | 3 | 3 | 3 | 8 | 8 | 8 |
| **2. MULTIPLE DX** | | | | | | | | | | |
| 0–19 Years | 11 | 11.6 | 74 | 3 | 5 | 12 | 14 | 14 | 36 | 36 |
| 20–34 | 41 | 6.9 | 42 | 2 | 3 | 7 | 8 | 11 | 16 | 38 |
| 35–49 | 62 | 6.8 | 25 | 1 | 1 | 7 | 12 | 12 | 12 | 20 |
| 50–64 | 81 | 7.5 | 28 | 1 | 3 | 6 | 13 | 13 | 15 | 23 |
| 65+ | 165 | 7.0 | 38 | 1 | 3 | 6 | 9 | 14 | 16 | 27 |
| **TOTAL SINGLE DX** | 32 | 5.7 | 31 | 1 | 1 | 3 | 9 | 16 | 16 | 16 |
| **TOTAL MULTIPLE DX** | 360 | 7.2 | 34 | 1 | 3 | 6 | 11 | 13 | 16 | 27 |
| **TOTAL** | | | | | | | | | | |
| 0–19 Years | 15 | 11.6 | 49 | 3 | 8 | 12 | 16 | 16 | 16 | 36 |
| 20–34 | 49 | 5.9 | 39 | 1 | 2 | 4 | 7 | 10 | 16 | 38 |
| 35–49 | 75 | 6.5 | 25 | 1 | 1 | 5 | 12 | 12 | 12 | 20 |
| 50–64 | 86 | 7.2 | 28 | 1 | 3 | 6 | 13 | 13 | 14 | 23 |
| 65+ | 167 | 7.0 | 38 | 1 | 3 | 6 | 9 | 14 | 16 | 27 |
| **GRAND TOTAL** | 392 | 7.1 | 34 | 1 | 3 | 6 | 11 | 13 | 16 | 25 |

## 34.24: PLEURAL BIOPSY. Formerly included in operation group(s) 569.

| Type of Patients | Observed Patients | Avg. Stay | Variance | 10th | 25th | 50th | 75th | 90th | 95th | 99th |
|---|---|---|---|---|---|---|---|---|---|---|
| **1. SINGLE DX** | | | | | | | | | | |
| 0–19 Years | 3 | 10.9 | 48 | 3 | 3 | 11 | 17 | 17 | 17 | 17 |
| 20–34 | 1 | 2.0 | 0 | 2 | 2 | 2 | 2 | 2 | 2 | 2 |
| 35–49 | 7 | 3.2 | 5 | 1 | 1 | 3 | 5 | 8 | 8 | 8 |
| 50–64 | 15 | 3.9 | 9 | 2 | 2 | 3 | 5 | 5 | 14 | 14 |
| 65+ | 12 | 2.6 | 4 | 1 | 2 | 2 | 4 | 4 | 7 | 7 |
| **2. MULTIPLE DX** | | | | | | | | | | |
| 0–19 Years | 7 | 8.8 | 10 | 6 | 7 | 9 | 11 | 14 | 14 | 14 |
| 20–34 | 24 | 7.7 | 22 | 3 | 3 | 6 | 11 | 15 | 15 | 19 |
| 35–49 | 106 | 8.9 | 28 | 2 | 6 | 10 | 10 | 17 | 19 | 25 |
| 50–64 | 211 | 8.5 | 36 | 2 | 3 | 7 | 15 | 15 | 18 | 26 |
| 65+ | 516 | 8.2 | 37 | 2 | 4 | 7 | 11 | 16 | 19 | 29 |
| **TOTAL SINGLE DX** | 38 | 3.3 | 8 | 1 | 2 | 2 | 4 | 5 | 8 | 17 |
| **TOTAL MULTIPLE DX** | 864 | 8.4 | 35 | 2 | 4 | 7 | 11 | 15 | 19 | 29 |
| **TOTAL** | | | | | | | | | | |
| 0–19 Years | 10 | 9.3 | 17 | 3 | 7 | 9 | 12 | 14 | 17 | 17 |
| 20–34 | 25 | 6.7 | 23 | 2 | 3 | 6 | 11 | 15 | 15 | 19 |
| 35–49 | 113 | 8.7 | 29 | 2 | 5 | 9 | 10 | 16 | 19 | 25 |
| 50–64 | 226 | 8.4 | 36 | 2 | 3 | 7 | 15 | 15 | 18 | 26 |
| 65+ | 528 | 8.1 | 37 | 2 | 4 | 7 | 11 | 16 | 19 | 29 |
| **GRAND TOTAL** | 902 | 8.2 | 35 | 2 | 3 | 7 | 11 | 15 | 19 | 29 |

## 34.26: OPEN MEDIASTINAL BIOPSY. Formerly included in operation group(s) 569.

| Type of Patients | Observed Patients | Avg. Stay | Variance | 10th | 25th | 50th | 75th | 90th | 95th | 99th |
|---|---|---|---|---|---|---|---|---|---|---|
| **1. SINGLE DX** | | | | | | | | | | |
| 0–19 Years | 10 | 6.1 | 7 | 3 | 5 | 7 | 7 | 7 | 14 | 14 |
| 20–34 | 19 | 3.2 | 3 | 1 | 2 | 2 | 4 | 5 | 7 | 8 |
| 35–49 | 16 | 2.6 | 7 | 1 | 1 | 1 | 2 | 8 | 8 | 8 |
| 50–64 | 4 | 3.1 | 7 | 1 | 1 | 1 | 7 | 7 | 7 | 7 |
| 65+ | 3 | 2.7 | 2 | 1 | 3 | 3 | 3 | 4 | 4 | 4 |
| **2. MULTIPLE DX** | | | | | | | | | | |
| 0–19 Years | 45 | 14.3 | 257 | 2 | 2 | 6 | 17 | 17 | 47 | 65 |
| 20–34 | 51 | 5.2 | 21 | 1 | 2 | 2 | 7 | 11 | 13 | 26 |
| 35–49 | 59 | 5.4 | 38 | 1 | 1 | 4 | 6 | 13 | 16 | 26 |
| 50–64 | 106 | 5.9 | 27 | 1 | 2 | 4 | 8 | 14 | 15 | 22 |
| 65+ | 140 | 6.1 | 35 | 1 | 2 | 4 | 8 | 15 | 15 | 23 |
| **TOTAL SINGLE DX** | 52 | 4.2 | 8 | 1 | 2 | 4 | 7 | 7 | 8 | 14 |
| **TOTAL MULTIPLE DX** | 401 | 7.0 | 72 | 1 | 2 | 4 | 9 | 15 | 21 | 42 |
| **TOTAL** | | | | | | | | | | |
| 0–19 Years | 55 | 11.9 | 199 | 2 | 4 | 6 | 15 | 15 | 35 | 65 |
| 20–34 | 70 | 4.7 | 17 | 1 | 2 | 3 | 6 | 11 | 11 | 26 |
| 35–49 | 75 | 4.9 | 34 | 1 | 1 | 3 | 6 | 12 | 15 | 26 |
| 50–64 | 110 | 5.9 | 27 | 1 | 2 | 4 | 8 | 14 | 15 | 22 |
| 65+ | 143 | 6.0 | 35 | 1 | 2 | 4 | 8 | 14 | 15 | 23 |
| **GRAND TOTAL** | 453 | 6.7 | 65 | 1 | 2 | 4 | 8 | 15 | 19 | 39 |

Length of Stay by Diagnosis and Operation, United States, 2000

# United States, October 1998–September 1999 Data, by Operation

## 34.5: PLEURECTOMY. Formerly included in operation group(s) 569.

| Type of Patients | Observed Patients | Avg. Stay | Vari-ance | 10th | 25th | 50th | 75th | 90th | 95th | 99th |
|---|---|---|---|---|---|---|---|---|---|---|
| **1. SINGLE DX** | | | | | | | | | | |
| 0–19 Years | 21 | 6.2 | 11 | 2 | 3 | 6 | 9 | 11 | 13 | 18 |
| 20–34 | 17 | 5.1 | 10 | 3 | 3 | 6 | 7 | 9 | 10 | 15 |
| 35–49 | 37 | 5.3 | 10 | 3 | 4 | 4 | 6 | 8 | 9 | 16 |
| 50–64 | 20 | 5.4 | 11 | 2 | 2 | 5 | 6 | 6 | 9 | 28 |
| 65+ | 10 | 3.9 | 7 | 2 | 2 | 3 | 5 | 7 | 13 | 13 |
| **2. MULTIPLE DX** | | | | | | | | | | |
| 0–19 Years | 388 | 12.4 | 58 | 6 | 8 | 11 | 15 | 19 | 24 | 35 |
| 20–34 | 310 | 12.5 | 88 | 4 | 7 | 11 | 15 | 23 | 27 | 62 |
| 35–49 | 725 | 14.4 | 103 | 5 | 7 | 13 | 18 | 24 | 37 | 52 |
| 50–64 | 812 | 14.6 | 121 | 5 | 8 | 12 | 18 | 26 | 35 | 69 |
| 65+ | 922 | 14.3 | 82 | 5 | 8 | 13 | 18 | 27 | 34 | >99 |
| **TOTAL SINGLE DX** | 105 | 5.4 | 11 | 2 | 3 | 5 | 6 | 9 | 11 | 16 |
| **TOTAL MULTIPLE DX** | 3,157 | 14.0 | 95 | 5 | 8 | 12 | 17 | 24 | 33 | 55 |
| **TOTAL** | | | | | | | | | | |
| 0–19 Years | 409 | 11.9 | 57 | 6 | 8 | 11 | 14 | 19 | 24 | 34 |
| 20–34 | 327 | 12.1 | 87 | 3 | 6 | 10 | 15 | 22 | 27 | 62 |
| 35–49 | 762 | 13.9 | 102 | 5 | 7 | 12 | 18 | 24 | 36 | 52 |
| 50–64 | 832 | 14.3 | 120 | 5 | 8 | 11 | 18 | 26 | 35 | 69 |
| 65+ | 932 | 14.2 | 82 | 5 | 8 | 13 | 18 | 27 | 34 | >99 |
| **GRAND TOTAL** | 3,262 | 13.6 | 94 | 5 | 7 | 11 | 17 | 24 | 32 | 54 |

## 34.51: DECORTICATION OF LUNG. Formerly included in operation group(s) 569.

| Type of Patients | Observed Patients | Avg. Stay | Vari-ance | 10th | 25th | 50th | 75th | 90th | 95th | 99th |
|---|---|---|---|---|---|---|---|---|---|---|
| **1. SINGLE DX** | | | | | | | | | | |
| 0–19 Years | 14 | 6.9 | 7 | 4 | 6 | 6 | 9 | 11 | 11 | 18 |
| 20–34 | 9 | 5.3 | 11 | 3 | 3 | 3 | 7 | 9 | 15 | 15 |
| 35–49 | 32 | 5.7 | 10 | 4 | 4 | 5 | 7 | 8 | 10 | 16 |
| 50–64 | 10 | 6.5 | 16 | 5 | 5 | 6 | 6 | 7 | 9 | 28 |
| 65+ | 4 | 5.0 | 14 | 3 | 3 | 4 | 4 | 13 | 13 | 13 |
| **2. MULTIPLE DX** | | | | | | | | | | |
| 0–19 Years | 358 | 12.8 | 60 | 6 | 8 | 11 | 15 | 19 | 25 | 39 |
| 20–34 | 261 | 14.2 | 92 | 6 | 8 | 12 | 17 | 24 | 28 | 63 |
| 35–49 | 667 | 14.9 | 108 | 5 | 8 | 13 | 18 | 25 | 38 | 52 |
| 50–64 | 726 | 15.4 | 127 | 5 | 8 | 13 | 19 | 27 | 38 | 69 |
| 65+ | 789 | 14.9 | 83 | 6 | 9 | 13 | 19 | 28 | 34 | >99 |
| **TOTAL SINGLE DX** | 69 | 6.0 | 10 | 3 | 4 | 6 | 7 | 9 | 11 | 18 |
| **TOTAL MULTIPLE DX** | 2,801 | 14.7 | 98 | 6 | 8 | 13 | 18 | 25 | 34 | 63 |
| **TOTAL** | | | | | | | | | | |
| 0–19 Years | 372 | 12.5 | 59 | 6 | 8 | 11 | 15 | 19 | 25 | 35 |
| 20–34 | 270 | 13.9 | 92 | 6 | 8 | 12 | 17 | 24 | 27 | 63 |
| 35–49 | 699 | 14.4 | 107 | 5 | 7 | 12 | 18 | 25 | 37 | 52 |
| 50–64 | 736 | 15.3 | 126 | 5 | 8 | 12 | 18 | 27 | 37 | 69 |
| 65+ | 793 | 14.9 | 83 | 6 | 9 | 13 | 19 | 28 | 34 | >99 |
| **GRAND TOTAL** | 2,870 | 14.5 | 98 | 6 | 8 | 12 | 18 | 25 | 34 | 62 |

## 34.3: DESTR MEDIASTINUM LES. Formerly included in operation group(s) 569.

| Type of Patients | Observed Patients | Avg. Stay | Vari-ance | 10th | 25th | 50th | 75th | 90th | 95th | 99th |
|---|---|---|---|---|---|---|---|---|---|---|
| **1. SINGLE DX** | | | | | | | | | | |
| 0–19 Years | 49 | 4.7 | 4 | 2 | 3 | 4 | 6 | 8 | 9 | 9 |
| 20–34 | 30 | 3.9 | 4 | 2 | 3 | 4 | 5 | 6 | 9 | 10 |
| 35–49 | 46 | 3.5 | 3 | 1 | 2 | 4 | 4 | 6 | 6 | 8 |
| 50–64 | 22 | 3.5 | <1 | 3 | 3 | 4 | 4 | 4 | 5 | 5 |
| 65+ | 4 | 6.7 | 11 | 3 | 4 | 4 | 10 | 10 | 10 | 10 |
| **2. MULTIPLE DX** | | | | | | | | | | |
| 0–19 Years | 79 | 7.1 | 37 | 2 | 4 | 6 | 8 | 13 | 15 | 39 |
| 20–34 | 61 | 5.2 | 20 | 1 | 3 | 4 | 6 | 10 | 14 | 32 |
| 35–49 | 98 | 5.6 | 32 | 2 | 3 | 4 | 6 | 10 | 16 | 31 |
| 50–64 | 89 | 4.6 | 38 | 1 | 3 | 4 | 6 | 7 | 10 | 21 |
| 65+ | 113 | 6.6 | 42 | 2 | 3 | 4 | 8 | 16 | 22 | 31 |
| **TOTAL SINGLE DX** | 151 | 4.1 | 4 | 2 | 3 | 4 | 5 | 7 | 8 | 10 |
| **TOTAL MULTIPLE DX** | 440 | 5.7 | 36 | 1 | 3 | 4 | 6 | 10 | 15 | 31 |
| **TOTAL** | | | | | | | | | | |
| 0–19 Years | 128 | 6.1 | 25 | 2 | 4 | 5 | 7 | 9 | 15 | 26 |
| 20–34 | 91 | 4.9 | 17 | 1 | 3 | 4 | 5 | 10 | 14 | 17 |
| 35–49 | 144 | 4.8 | 22 | 1 | 3 | 4 | 6 | 8 | 13 | 23 |
| 50–64 | 111 | 4.5 | 33 | 1 | 3 | 4 | 6 | 6 | 10 | 21 |
| 65+ | 117 | 6.6 | 41 | 2 | 3 | 4 | 8 | 12 | 22 | 31 |
| **GRAND TOTAL** | 591 | 5.3 | 29 | 2 | 3 | 4 | 6 | 9 | 14 | 26 |

## 34.4: EXC/DESTR CHEST WALL LES. Formerly included in operation group(s) 569.

| Type of Patients | Observed Patients | Avg. Stay | Vari-ance | 10th | 25th | 50th | 75th | 90th | 95th | 99th |
|---|---|---|---|---|---|---|---|---|---|---|
| **1. SINGLE DX** | | | | | | | | | | |
| 0–19 Years | 34 | 2.9 | 3 | 1 | 1 | 3 | 4 | 6 | 6 | 7 |
| 20–34 | 12 | 2.7 | 3 | 1 | 2 | 2 | 3 | 6 | 6 | 6 |
| 35–49 | 28 | 3.5 | 4 | 1 | 2 | 3 | 5 | 6 | 7 | 7 |
| 50–64 | 11 | 3.7 | 2 | 1 | 3 | 4 | 4 | 6 | 6 | 8 |
| 65+ | 9 | 2.5 | 2 | 1 | 2 | 2 | 3 | 6 | 6 | 6 |
| **2. MULTIPLE DX** | | | | | | | | | | |
| 0–19 Years | 38 | 7.4 | 27 | 2 | 3 | 5 | 13 | 14 | 15 | 26 |
| 20–34 | 43 | 5.4 | 25 | 1 | 1 | 3 | 7 | 13 | 18 | 21 |
| 35–49 | 67 | 6.3 | 35 | 2 | 3 | 4 | 8 | 12 | 18 | 29 |
| 50–64 | 120 | 7.5 | 36 | 2 | 3 | 6 | 11 | 13 | 17 | 30 |
| 65+ | 163 | 7.0 | 76 | 1 | 3 | 5 | 8 | 14 | 20 | 30 |
| **TOTAL SINGLE DX** | 94 | 3.1 | 3 | 1 | 2 | 3 | 4 | 6 | 6 | 7 |
| **TOTAL MULTIPLE DX** | 431 | 6.9 | 51 | 1 | 3 | 5 | 8 | 13 | 18 | 30 |
| **TOTAL** | | | | | | | | | | |
| 0–19 Years | 72 | 5.0 | 19 | 1 | 3 | 4 | 6 | 13 | 14 | 22 |
| 20–34 | 55 | 4.8 | 21 | 1 | 2 | 3 | 6 | 9 | 15 | 21 |
| 35–49 | 95 | 5.6 | 28 | 1 | 3 | 4 | 7 | 11 | 16 | 29 |
| 50–64 | 131 | 7.1 | 34 | 2 | 3 | 5 | 10 | 13 | 16 | 30 |
| 65+ | 172 | 6.8 | 73 | 1 | 3 | 5 | 8 | 12 | 19 | 30 |
| **GRAND TOTAL** | 525 | 6.2 | 45 | 1 | 3 | 4 | 8 | 13 | 16 | 30 |

Length of Stay by Diagnosis and Operation, United States, 2000

## United States, October 1998–September 1999 Data, by Operation

### 34.59: OTHER PLEURAL EXCISION. Formerly included in operation group(s) 569.

| Type of Patients | Observed Patients | Avg. Stay | Vari-ance | 10th | 25th | 50th | 75th | 90th | 95th | 99th |
|---|---|---|---|---|---|---|---|---|---|---|
| **1. SINGLE DX** | | | | | | | | | | |
| 0–19 Years | 7 | 4.9 | 17 | 2 | 2 | 3 | 6 | 13 | 13 | 13 |
| 20–34 | 8 | 4.8 | 8 | 1 | 3 | 4 | 3 | 7 | 10 | 10 |
| 35–49 | 5 | 2.6 | 4 | 1 | 1 | 3 | 3 | 5 | 7 | 7 |
| 50–64 | 10 | 4.4 | 6 | 2 | 2 | 4 | 6 | 6 | 11 | 11 |
| 65+ | 6 | 3.3 | 3 | 2 | 2 | 2 | 5 | 6 | 7 | 7 |
| **2. MULTIPLE DX** | | | | | | | | | | |
| 0–19 Years | 30 | 7.9 | 14 | 4 | 4 | 8 | 10 | 11 | 13 | 21 |
| 20–34 | 49 | 6.9 | 36 | 3 | 4 | 5 | 8 | 11 | 24 | 28 |
| 35–49 | 58 | 10.2 | 49 | 3 | 5 | 7 | 16 | 20 | 22 | 27 |
| 50–64 | 86 | 8.6 | 38 | 3 | 4 | 7 | 9 | 16 | 20 | 40 |
| 65+ | 133 | 9.7 | 50 | 4 | 5 | 7 | 12 | 20 | 23 | 39 |
| **TOTAL SINGLE DX** | 36 | 4.1 | 9 | 2 | 2 | 3 | 6 | 7 | 11 | 13 |
| **TOTAL MULTIPLE DX** | 356 | 8.9 | 43 | 3 | 5 | 7 | 11 | 17 | 22 | 32 |
| **TOTAL** | | | | | | | | | | |
| 0–19 Years | 37 | 7.2 | 16 | 3 | 4 | 7 | 10 | 11 | 13 | 21 |
| 20–34 | 57 | 6.7 | 34 | 3 | 3 | 5 | 8 | 11 | 21 | 28 |
| 35–49 | 63 | 9.7 | 49 | 3 | 5 | 7 | 15 | 20 | 22 | 27 |
| 50–64 | 96 | 8.1 | 36 | 3 | 4 | 7 | 9 | 16 | 20 | 32 |
| 65+ | 139 | 9.4 | 50 | 3 | 5 | 7 | 11 | 19 | 23 | 39 |
| **GRAND TOTAL** | 392 | 8.4 | 41 | 3 | 4 | 7 | 10 | 16 | 22 | 32 |

### 34.6: SCARIFICATION OF PLEURA. Formerly included in operation group(s) 569.

| Type of Patients | Observed Patients | Avg. Stay | Vari-ance | 10th | 25th | 50th | 75th | 90th | 95th | 99th |
|---|---|---|---|---|---|---|---|---|---|---|
| **1. SINGLE DX** | | | | | | | | | | |
| 0–19 Years | 29 | 9.6 | 75 | 3 | 4 | 7 | 11 | 31 | 31 | 31 |
| 20–34 | 38 | 4.3 | 8 | 2 | 3 | 4 | 5 | 7 | 8 | 10 |
| 35–49 | 10 | 3.4 | 2 | 3 | 3 | 3 | 3 | 4 | 7 | 11 |
| 50–64 | 3 | 2.4 | 1 | 1 | 1 | 3 | 3 | 4 | 4 | 4 |
| 65+ | 3 | 11.9 | 28 | 4 | 7 | 16 | 16 | 16 | 16 | 16 |
| **2. MULTIPLE DX** | | | | | | | | | | |
| 0–19 Years | 73 | 9.7 | 87 | 4 | 5 | 8 | 11 | 18 | 20 | 54 |
| 20–34 | 121 | 7.6 | 54 | 2 | 4 | 6 | 9 | 13 | 17 | 39 |
| 35–49 | 154 | 10.2 | 58 | 3 | 4 | 7 | 15 | 21 | 21 | 29 |
| 50–64 | 246 | 8.9 | 51 | 3 | 5 | 7 | 11 | 18 | 24 | 33 |
| 65+ | 448 | 10.4 | 48 | 4 | 5 | 9 | 14 | 19 | 23 | 35 |
| **TOTAL SINGLE DX** | 83 | 6.1 | 36 | 2 | 3 | 4 | 7 | 11 | 16 | 31 |
| **TOTAL MULTIPLE DX** | 1,042 | 9.7 | 54 | 3 | 5 | 8 | 12 | 20 | 22 | 35 |
| **TOTAL** | | | | | | | | | | |
| 0–19 Years | 102 | 9.7 | 83 | 4 | 5 | 7 | 11 | 18 | 31 | 52 |
| 20–34 | 159 | 6.6 | 41 | 2 | 3 | 5 | 8 | 11 | 14 | 23 |
| 35–49 | 164 | 9.5 | 56 | 3 | 4 | 7 | 14 | 21 | 21 | 29 |
| 50–64 | 249 | 8.7 | 51 | 3 | 4 | 6 | 11 | 17 | 23 | 33 |
| 65+ | 451 | 10.4 | 48 | 4 | 5 | 9 | 14 | 19 | 23 | 35 |
| **GRAND TOTAL** | 1,125 | 9.3 | 54 | 3 | 4 | 7 | 12 | 19 | 22 | 35 |

### 34.7: REPAIR OF CHEST WALL. Formerly included in operation group(s) 569.

| Type of Patients | Observed Patients | Avg. Stay | Vari-ance | 10th | 25th | 50th | 75th | 90th | 95th | 99th |
|---|---|---|---|---|---|---|---|---|---|---|
| **1. SINGLE DX** | | | | | | | | | | |
| 0–19 Years | 413 | 4.4 | 2 | 3 | 3 | 4 | 6 | 6 | 7 | 8 |
| 20–34 | 17 | 4.1 | 4 | 3 | 3 | 4 | 7 | 6 | 7 | 7 |
| 35–49 | 5 | 3.5 | 11 | 1 | 2 | 2 | 3 | 11 | 11 | 11 |
| 50–64 | 6 | 2.8 | 3 | 1 | 2 | 2 | 3 | 7 | 7 | 7 |
| 65+ | 2 | 3.2 | 5 | 1 | 1 | 5 | 5 | 5 | 5 | 5 |
| **2. MULTIPLE DX** | | | | | | | | | | |
| 0–19 Years | 351 | 5.5 | 19 | 3 | 4 | 5 | 6 | 9 | 11 | 24 |
| 20–34 | 50 | 9.6 | 149 | 2 | 4 | 5 | 8 | 25 | 60 | >99 |
| 35–49 | 79 | 8.1 | 99 | 1 | 2 | 5 | 9 | 18 | 29 | 83 |
| 50–64 | 226 | 8.7 | 100 | 2 | 3 | 6 | 10 | 18 | 24 | 46 |
| 65+ | 249 | 8.5 | 113 | 2 | 2 | 5 | 11 | 19 | 27 | 97 |
| **TOTAL SINGLE DX** | 447 | 4.3 | 2 | 3 | 3 | 4 | 6 | 6 | 7 | 10 |
| **TOTAL MULTIPLE DX** | 955 | 7.4 | 76 | 2 | 3 | 5 | 9 | 15 | 23 | 60 |
| **TOTAL** | | | | | | | | | | |
| 0–19 Years | 764 | 4.8 | 9 | 3 | 3 | 4 | 6 | 7 | 9 | 15 |
| 20–34 | 67 | 7.6 | 102 | 1 | 3 | 5 | 7 | 25 | 30 | >99 |
| 35–49 | 88 | 7.8 | 94 | 1 | 2 | 4 | 9 | 18 | 29 | 83 |
| 50–64 | 232 | 8.6 | 99 | 2 | 3 | 6 | 10 | 18 | 24 | 46 |
| 65+ | 251 | 8.5 | 113 | 2 | 2 | 5 | 11 | 19 | 27 | 97 |
| **GRAND TOTAL** | 1,402 | 6.2 | 48 | 2 | 3 | 4 | 6 | 11 | 17 | 39 |

### 34.74: PECTUS DEFORMITY REPAIR. Formerly included in operation group(s) 569.

| Type of Patients | Observed Patients | Avg. Stay | Vari-ance | 10th | 25th | 50th | 75th | 90th | 95th | 99th |
|---|---|---|---|---|---|---|---|---|---|---|
| **1. SINGLE DX** | | | | | | | | | | |
| 0–19 Years | 405 | 4.4 | 2 | 3 | 3 | 4 | 6 | 6 | 7 | 10 |
| 20–34 | 9 | 4.8 | 3 | 3 | 3 | 5 | 7 | 7 | 7 | 7 |
| 35–49 | 2 | 2.2 | 1 | 1 | 1 | 3 | 3 | 3 | 3 | 3 |
| 50–64 | 0 | | | | | | | | | |
| 65+ | 0 | | | | | | | | | |
| **2. MULTIPLE DX** | | | | | | | | | | |
| 0–19 Years | 323 | 5.0 | 6 | 3 | 4 | 5 | 6 | 9 | 11 | 11 |
| 20–34 | 16 | 5.4 | 11 | 4 | 4 | 5 | 5 | 6 | 9 | 21 |
| 35–49 | 2 | 6.7 | 4 | 5 | 5 | 8 | 8 | 8 | 8 | 8 |
| 50–64 | 0 | | | | | | | | | |
| 65+ | 1 | 1.0 | 0 | 1 | 1 | 1 | 1 | 1 | 1 | 1 |
| **TOTAL SINGLE DX** | 416 | 4.4 | 2 | 3 | 3 | 4 | 6 | 6 | 7 | 8 |
| **TOTAL MULTIPLE DX** | 342 | 5.0 | 6 | 3 | 4 | 5 | 6 | 8 | 11 | 11 |
| **TOTAL** | | | | | | | | | | |
| 0–19 Years | 728 | 4.6 | 4 | 3 | 3 | 4 | 6 | 7 | 8 | 11 |
| 20–34 | 25 | 5.1 | 7 | 3 | 4 | 5 | 6 | 7 | 7 | 21 |
| 35–49 | 4 | 4.0 | 8 | 1 | 3 | 3 | 5 | 8 | 8 | 8 |
| 50–64 | 0 | | | | | | | | | |
| 65+ | 1 | 1.0 | 0 | 1 | 1 | 1 | 1 | 1 | 1 | 1 |
| **GRAND TOTAL** | 758 | 4.6 | 4 | 3 | 3 | 4 | 6 | 7 | 7 | 11 |

Length of Stay by Diagnosis and Operation, United States, 2000

# Length of Stay by Diagnosis and Operation, United States, October 1998–September 1999 Data, by Operation

## 34.79: OTHER CHEST WALL REPAIR. Formerly included in operation group(s) 569.

| Type of Patients | Observed Patients | Avg. Stay | Variance | 10th | 25th | 50th | 75th | 90th | 95th | 99th |
|---|---|---|---|---|---|---|---|---|---|---|
| **1. SINGLE DX** | | | | | | | | | | |
| 0–19 Years | 1 | 3.0 | 0 | 3 | 3 | 3 | 3 | 3 | 3 | 3 |
| 20–34 | 1 | 1.0 | 0 | 1 | 1 | 1 | 1 | 1 | 1 | 1 |
| 35–49 | 3 | 6.6 | 20 | 2 | 4 | 4 | 11 | 11 | 11 | 11 |
| 50–64 | 5 | 3.4 | 5 | 1 | 2 | 3 | 4 | 7 | 7 | 7 |
| 65+ | 1 | 5.0 | 0 | 5 | 5 | 5 | 5 | 5 | 5 | 5 |
| **2. MULTIPLE DX** | | | | | | | | | | |
| 0–19 Years | 15 | 12.2 | 232 | 3 | 5 | 7 | 15 | 27 | 27 | 88 |
| 20–34 | 8 | 5.3 | 2 | 3 | 5 | 5 | 7 | 7 | 7 | 7 |
| 35–49 | 54 | 6.6 | 35 | 2 | 2 | 5 | 9 | 13 | 17 | 36 |
| 50–64 | 194 | 7.3 | 57 | 2 | 3 | 4 | 9 | 18 | 20 | 39 |
| 65+ | 209 | 7.6 | 75 | 2 | 2 | 5 | 10 | 16 | 21 | 46 |
| **TOTAL SINGLE DX** | 11 | 4.1 | 10 | 1 | 2 | 3 | 5 | 11 | 11 | 11 |
| **TOTAL MULTIPLE DX** | 480 | 7.5 | 68 | 2 | 3 | 5 | 9 | 16 | 21 | 46 |
| **TOTAL** | | | | | | | | | | |
| 0–19 Years | 16 | 11.9 | 227 | 3 | 5 | 7 | 15 | 27 | 27 | 88 |
| 20–34 | 9 | 4.8 | 4 | 1 | 4 | 5 | 7 | 7 | 7 | 7 |
| 35–49 | 57 | 6.6 | 35 | 2 | 2 | 5 | 9 | 13 | 17 | 36 |
| 50–64 | 199 | 7.3 | 56 | 2 | 3 | 4 | 9 | 18 | 20 | 39 |
| 65+ | 210 | 7.6 | 75 | 2 | 2 | 5 | 10 | 16 | 21 | 46 |
| **GRAND TOTAL** | 491 | 7.4 | 68 | 2 | 3 | 5 | 9 | 16 | 20 | 46 |

## 34.9: OTHER OPS ON THORAX. Formerly included in operation group(s) 569, 580, 581.

| Type of Patients | Observed Patients | Avg. Stay | Variance | 10th | 25th | 50th | 75th | 90th | 95th | 99th |
|---|---|---|---|---|---|---|---|---|---|---|
| **1. SINGLE DX** | | | | | | | | | | |
| 0–19 Years | 26 | 3.2 | 4 | 2 | 2 | 3 | 4 | 4 | 7 | 14 |
| 20–34 | 56 | 4.7 | 12 | 1 | 2 | 4 | 6 | 8 | 10 | 18 |
| 35–49 | 47 | 3.7 | 5 | 1 | 2 | 4 | 4 | 7 | 8 | 10 |
| 50–64 | 32 | 5.0 | 7 | 2 | 2 | 6 | 7 | 7 | 7 | 12 |
| 65+ | 52 | 6.3 | 17 | 2 | 3 | 6 | 8 | 12 | 12 | 16 |
| **2. MULTIPLE DX** | | | | | | | | | | |
| 0–19 Years | 671 | 8.8 | 75 | 2 | 4 | 7 | 11 | 16 | 26 | 64 |
| 20–34 | 765 | 8.1 | 40 | 2 | 4 | 7 | 10 | 16 | 19 | 27 |
| 35–49 | 2,750 | 7.1 | 37 | 2 | 3 | 5 | 9 | 14 | 17 | 35 |
| 50–64 | 5,420 | 7.0 | 32 | 2 | 3 | 6 | 9 | 14 | 18 | 27 |
| 65+ | 18,001 | 8.0 | 36 | 2 | 4 | 7 | 10 | 15 | 19 | 30 |
| **TOTAL SINGLE DX** | 213 | 4.5 | 10 | 1 | 2 | 4 | 6 | 8 | 12 | 16 |
| **TOTAL MULTIPLE DX** | 27,607 | 7.7 | 37 | 2 | 4 | 6 | 10 | 15 | 19 | 30 |
| **TOTAL** | | | | | | | | | | |
| 0–19 Years | 697 | 8.3 | 71 | 2 | 3 | 7 | 10 | 15 | 26 | 58 |
| 20–34 | 821 | 7.9 | 39 | 2 | 4 | 6 | 10 | 16 | 19 | 27 |
| 35–49 | 2,797 | 7.0 | 37 | 2 | 3 | 5 | 9 | 14 | 17 | 35 |
| 50–64 | 5,452 | 7.0 | 32 | 2 | 3 | 6 | 9 | 14 | 17 | 27 |
| 65+ | 18,053 | 8.0 | 36 | 2 | 4 | 7 | 10 | 15 | 19 | 30 |
| **GRAND TOTAL** | 27,820 | 7.7 | 36 | 2 | 4 | 6 | 10 | 15 | 19 | 30 |

## 34.8: OPERATIONS ON DIAPHRAGM. Formerly included in operation group(s) 569.

| Type of Patients | Observed Patients | Avg. Stay | Variance | 10th | 25th | 50th | 75th | 90th | 95th | 99th |
|---|---|---|---|---|---|---|---|---|---|---|
| **1. SINGLE DX** | | | | | | | | | | |
| 0–19 Years | 9 | 6.4 | 9 | 3 | 4 | 6 | 10 | 10 | 10 | 10 |
| 20–34 | 3 | 4.8 | 5 | 3 | 3 | 4 | 7 | 7 | 8 | 8 |
| 35–49 | 5 | 4.1 | 1 | 4 | 4 | 4 | 4 | 4 | 7 | 7 |
| 50–64 | 1 | 1.0 | 0 | 1 | 1 | 1 | 1 | 1 | 1 | 1 |
| 65+ | 0 | | | | | | | | | |
| **2. MULTIPLE DX** | | | | | | | | | | |
| 0–19 Years | 90 | 9.8 | 102 | 3 | 5 | 7 | 12 | 18 | 22 | 90 |
| 20–34 | 150 | 9.5 | 103 | 3 | 4 | 6 | 11 | 20 | 29 | 44 |
| 35–49 | 97 | 10.8 | 70 | 3 | 4 | 9 | 18 | 18 | 24 | 45 |
| 50–64 | 33 | 13.7 | 257 | 3 | 4 | 9 | 19 | 19 | 48 | 90 |
| 65+ | 28 | 15.8 | 109 | 5 | 7 | 20 | 20 | 23 | 24 | 71 |
| **TOTAL SINGLE DX** | 18 | 5.2 | 7 | 3 | 3 | 4 | 7 | 10 | 10 | 10 |
| **TOTAL MULTIPLE DX** | 398 | 10.8 | 113 | 3 | 4 | 7 | 14 | 20 | 26 | 53 |
| **TOTAL** | | | | | | | | | | |
| 0–19 Years | 99 | 9.5 | 94 | 3 | 5 | 7 | 11 | 17 | 22 | 31 |
| 20–34 | 153 | 9.2 | 99 | 3 | 4 | 6 | 10 | 18 | 29 | 44 |
| 35–49 | 102 | 10.3 | 68 | 3 | 4 | 8 | 16 | 18 | 24 | 45 |
| 50–64 | 34 | 13.6 | 256 | 3 | 4 | 9 | 19 | 19 | 48 | 90 |
| 65+ | 28 | 15.8 | 109 | 5 | 7 | 20 | 20 | 23 | 24 | 71 |
| **GRAND TOTAL** | 416 | 10.5 | 109 | 3 | 4 | 7 | 14 | 20 | 24 | 53 |

## 34.91: THORACENTESIS. Formerly included in operation group(s) 580.

| Type of Patients | Observed Patients | Avg. Stay | Variance | 10th | 25th | 50th | 75th | 90th | 95th | 99th |
|---|---|---|---|---|---|---|---|---|---|---|
| **1. SINGLE DX** | | | | | | | | | | |
| 0–19 Years | 21 | 3.0 | 3 | 2 | 2 | 2 | 4 | 4 | 7 | 7 |
| 20–34 | 47 | 4.5 | 13 | 1 | 2 | 4 | 6 | 8 | 12 | 18 |
| 35–49 | 41 | 3.6 | 5 | 1 | 2 | 4 | 4 | 6 | 8 | 10 |
| 50–64 | 30 | 4.9 | 8 | 2 | 2 | 7 | 7 | 7 | 7 | 12 |
| 65+ | 47 | 4.8 | 16 | 1 | 3 | 4 | 7 | 10 | 14 | 23 |
| **2. MULTIPLE DX** | | | | | | | | | | |
| 0–19 Years | 648 | 8.8 | 76 | 2 | 4 | 7 | 10 | 16 | 26 | 66 |
| 20–34 | 720 | 8.2 | 40 | 2 | 4 | 7 | 10 | 16 | 19 | 27 |
| 35–49 | 2,625 | 7.0 | 37 | 2 | 3 | 5 | 9 | 14 | 17 | 35 |
| 50–64 | 5,115 | 6.9 | 32 | 2 | 3 | 6 | 9 | 14 | 17 | 27 |
| 65+ | 17,406 | 8.0 | 36 | 2 | 4 | 7 | 10 | 15 | 19 | 30 |
| **TOTAL SINGLE DX** | 186 | 4.0 | 9 | 1 | 2 | 4 | 6 | 7 | 8 | 16 |
| **TOTAL MULTIPLE DX** | 26,514 | 7.7 | 37 | 2 | 4 | 6 | 10 | 15 | 19 | 30 |
| **TOTAL** | | | | | | | | | | |
| 0–19 Years | 669 | 8.3 | 72 | 2 | 3 | 7 | 10 | 15 | 26 | 58 |
| 20–34 | 767 | 8.0 | 39 | 2 | 4 | 6 | 10 | 16 | 19 | 27 |
| 35–49 | 2,666 | 7.0 | 37 | 2 | 3 | 5 | 9 | 14 | 17 | 35 |
| 50–64 | 5,145 | 6.9 | 32 | 2 | 3 | 6 | 9 | 14 | 17 | 27 |
| 65+ | 17,453 | 7.9 | 36 | 2 | 4 | 7 | 10 | 15 | 19 | 30 |
| **GRAND TOTAL** | 26,700 | 7.7 | 36 | 2 | 4 | 6 | 10 | 15 | 19 | 30 |

Length of Stay by Diagnosis and Operation, United States, 2000

# United States, October 1998–September 1999 Data, by Operation

## 34.92: INJECT INTO THOR CAVIT. Formerly included in operation group(s) 581.

| Type of Patients | Observed Patients | Avg. Stay | Variance | 10th | 25th | 50th | 75th | 90th | 95th | 99th |
|---|---|---|---|---|---|---|---|---|---|---|
| **1. SINGLE DX** | | | | | | | | | | |
| 0–19 Years | 5 | 4.1 | 11 | 3 | 3 | 3 | 5 | 4 | 10 | 20 |
| 20–34 | 9 | 5.6 | 4 | 3 | 4 | 5 | 8 | 4 | 8 | 8 |
| 35–49 | 5 | 5.0 | 3 | 3 | 3 | 5 | 7 | 7 | 7 | 7 |
| 50–64 | 2 | 5.5 | 1 | 3 | 6 | 6 | 6 | 6 | 6 | 6 |
| 65+ | 5 | 9.0 | 8 | 6 | 6 | 8 | 12 | 12 | 12 | 12 |
| **2. MULTIPLE DX** | | | | | | | | | | |
| 0–19 Years | 14 | 6.9 | 42 | 2 | 4 | 5 | 6 | 15 | 27 | 27 |
| 20–34 | 39 | 7.1 | 48 | 3 | 3 | 6 | 8 | 14 | 27 | 60 |
| 35–49 | 115 | 7.3 | 26 | 3 | 4 | 6 | 9 | 14 | 19 | 26 |
| 50–64 | 295 | 8.0 | 34 | 3 | 4 | 7 | 9 | 15 | 22 | 27 |
| 65+ | 573 | 8.7 | 31 | 6 | 5 | 7 | 11 | 16 | 20 | 28 |
| **TOTAL SINGLE DX** | 26 | 6.7 | 12 | 3 | 3 | 6 | 8 | 12 | 12 | 12 |
| **TOTAL MULTIPLE DX** | 1,036 | 8.3 | 32 | 5 | 5 | 7 | 10 | 16 | 19 | 28 |
| **TOTAL** | | | | | | | | | | |
| 0–19 Years | 19 | 5.5 | 28 | 3 | 3 | 5 | 7 | 10 | 20 | 27 |
| 20–34 | 48 | 6.9 | 43 | 3 | 4 | 6 | 8 | 9 | 10 | 27 |
| 35–49 | 120 | 7.3 | 25 | 3 | 4 | 6 | 9 | 14 | 19 | 26 |
| 50–64 | 297 | 7.9 | 33 | 3 | 4 | 7 | 9 | 15 | 22 | 27 |
| 65+ | 578 | 8.7 | 30 | 6 | 5 | 7 | 11 | 16 | 20 | 28 |
| **GRAND TOTAL** | 1,062 | 8.2 | 31 | 3 | 5 | 7 | 10 | 15 | 19 | 28 |

## 35.1: OPEN HEART VALVULOPLASTY. Formerly included in operation group(s) 572.

| Type of Patients | Observed Patients | Avg. Stay | Variance | 10th | 25th | 50th | 75th | 90th | 95th | 99th |
|---|---|---|---|---|---|---|---|---|---|---|
| **1. SINGLE DX** | | | | | | | | | | |
| 0–19 Years | 69 | 4.6 | 7 | 2 | 3 | 4 | 5 | 11 | 11 | 11 |
| 20–34 | 14 | 3.7 | <1 | 3 | 3 | 4 | 5 | 4 | 5 | 5 |
| 35–49 | 14 | 4.7 | <1 | 4 | 4 | 5 | 5 | 5 | 6 | 7 |
| 50–64 | 11 | 4.7 | <1 | 4 | 4 | 5 | 5 | 5 | 6 | 9 |
| 65+ | 5 | 3.7 | <1 | 3 | 3 | 3 | 4 | 5 | 5 | 5 |
| **2. MULTIPLE DX** | | | | | | | | | | |
| 0–19 Years | 655 | 7.5 | 104 | 3 | 3 | 4 | 7 | 15 | 26 | 42 |
| 20–34 | 79 | 7.9 | 76 | 3 | 4 | 5 | 8 | 14 | 26 | 46 |
| 35–49 | 307 | 6.9 | 32 | 3 | 4 | 5 | 8 | 11 | 17 | 33 |
| 50–64 | 571 | 7.9 | 27 | 4 | 5 | 6 | 9 | 13 | 17 | 29 |
| 65+ | 832 | 11.9 | 78 | 5 | 6 | 8 | 13 | 28 | 34 | 34 |
| **TOTAL SINGLE DX** | 113 | 4.5 | 4 | 3 | 3 | 4 | 5 | 7 | 11 | 11 |
| **TOTAL MULTIPLE DX** | 2,444 | 9.3 | 74 | 3 | 5 | 7 | 10 | 19 | 32 | 38 |
| **TOTAL** | | | | | | | | | | |
| 0–19 Years | 724 | 7.1 | 93 | 3 | 3 | 4 | 7 | 14 | 22 | 42 |
| 20–34 | 93 | 7.3 | 68 | 3 | 4 | 5 | 7 | 12 | 26 | 46 |
| 35–49 | 321 | 6.7 | 30 | 3 | 4 | 5 | 7 | 11 | 16 | 33 |
| 50–64 | 582 | 7.8 | 26 | 4 | 5 | 6 | 9 | 13 | 17 | 29 |
| 65+ | 837 | 11.8 | 78 | 5 | 6 | 8 | 13 | 28 | 34 | 34 |
| **GRAND TOTAL** | 2,557 | 9.0 | 71 | 3 | 4 | 6 | 10 | 17 | 30 | 38 |

## 35.0: CLOSED HEART VALVOTOMY. Formerly included in operation group(s) 579.

| Type of Patients | Observed Patients | Avg. Stay | Variance | 10th | 25th | 50th | 75th | 90th | 95th | 99th |
|---|---|---|---|---|---|---|---|---|---|---|
| **1. SINGLE DX** | | | | | | | | | | |
| 0–19 Years | 4 | 2.9 | 4 | 1 | 1 | 1 | 1 | 5 | 5 | 5 |
| 20–34 | 0 | | | | | | | | | |
| 35–49 | 0 | | | | | | | | | |
| 50–64 | 0 | | | | | | | | | |
| **2. MULTIPLE DX** | | | | | | | | | | |
| 0–19 Years | 23 | 6.2 | 50 | 1 | 1 | 3 | 10 | 18 | 18 | 33 |
| 20–34 | 3 | 6.4 | 87 | 1 | 1 | 2 | 20 | 20 | 20 | 60 |
| 35–49 | 5 | 2.2 | 9 | 1 | 1 | 1 | 1 | 10 | 10 | 10 |
| 50–64 | 6 | 1.4 | <1 | 1 | 1 | 1 | 2 | 2 | 3 | 3 |
| 65+ | 2 | 3.6 | <1 | 3 | 3 | 3 | 5 | 5 | 5 | 5 |
| **TOTAL SINGLE DX** | 4 | 2.9 | 4 | 1 | 1 | 1 | 1 | 5 | 5 | 5 |
| **TOTAL MULTIPLE DX** | 39 | 4.8 | 38 | 1 | 1 | 2 | 5 | 18 | 18 | 33 |
| **TOTAL** | | | | | | | | | | |
| 0–19 Years | 27 | 5.2 | 38 | 1 | 1 | 3 | 5 | 18 | 18 | 33 |
| 20–34 | 3 | 6.4 | 87 | 1 | 1 | 2 | 20 | 20 | 20 | 60 |
| 35–49 | 5 | 2.2 | 9 | 1 | 1 | 1 | 1 | 10 | 10 | 10 |
| 50–64 | 6 | 1.4 | <1 | 1 | 1 | 1 | 2 | 2 | 3 | 3 |
| 65+ | 2 | 3.6 | <1 | 3 | 3 | 3 | 5 | 5 | 5 | 5 |
| **GRAND TOTAL** | 43 | 4.4 | 31 | 1 | 1 | 2 | 5 | 13 | 18 | 20 |

## 35.11: OPN AORTIC VALVULOPLASTY. Formerly included in operation group(s) 572.

| Type of Patients | Observed Patients | Avg. Stay | Variance | 10th | 25th | 50th | 75th | 90th | 95th | 99th |
|---|---|---|---|---|---|---|---|---|---|---|
| **1. SINGLE DX** | | | | | | | | | | |
| 0–19 Years | 46 | 3.8 | 2 | 2 | 3 | 4 | 4 | 7 | 7 | 7 |
| 20–34 | 0 | | | | | | | | | |
| 35–49 | 1 | 4.0 | 0 | 4 | 4 | 4 | 4 | 4 | 4 | 4 |
| 50–64 | 1 | 5.0 | 0 | 5 | 5 | 5 | 5 | 5 | 5 | 5 |
| 65+ | 0 | | | | | | | | | |
| **2. MULTIPLE DX** | | | | | | | | | | |
| 0–19 Years | 241 | 5.8 | 32 | 3 | 3 | 4 | 7 | 9 | 16 | 27 |
| 20–34 | 13 | 8.8 | 165 | 3 | 3 | 6 | 12 | 12 | 12 | 75 |
| 35–49 | 29 | 5.3 | 11 | 3 | 3 | 4 | 6 | 8 | 11 | 19 |
| 50–64 | 39 | 9.1 | 19 | 5 | 5 | 8 | 12 | 13 | 19 | 21 |
| 65+ | 57 | 11.7 | 82 | 4 | 7 | 10 | 12 | 19 | 24 | 56 |
| **TOTAL SINGLE DX** | 48 | 3.8 | 2 | 2 | 3 | 4 | 4 | 7 | 7 | 7 |
| **TOTAL MULTIPLE DX** | 379 | 7.2 | 48 | 3 | 3 | 5 | 8 | 13 | 19 | 33 |
| **TOTAL** | | | | | | | | | | |
| 0–19 Years | 287 | 5.5 | 28 | 2 | 3 | 4 | 6 | 8 | 16 | 27 |
| 20–34 | 13 | 8.8 | 165 | 3 | 3 | 6 | 12 | 12 | 12 | 75 |
| 35–49 | 30 | 5.1 | 9 | 3 | 3 | 4 | 6 | 8 | 11 | 19 |
| 50–64 | 40 | 9.0 | 18 | 4 | 5 | 8 | 12 | 13 | 19 | 21 |
| 65+ | 57 | 11.7 | 82 | 4 | 7 | 10 | 12 | 19 | 24 | 56 |
| **GRAND TOTAL** | 427 | 6.7 | 43 | 3 | 3 | 4 | 8 | 12 | 17 | 27 |

Length of Stay by Diagnosis and Operation, United States, 2000

# United States, October 1998–September 1999 Data, by Operation

## 35.21: REPL AORTIC VALVE-TISSUE. Formerly included in operation group(s) 570.

| Type of Patients | Observed Patients | Avg. Stay | Variance | Percentiles | | | | | | |
|---|---|---|---|---|---|---|---|---|---|---|
| | | | | 10th | 25th | 50th | 75th | 90th | 95th | 99th |
| **1. SINGLE DX** | | | | | | | | | | |
| 0–19 Years | 28 | 3.6 | <1 | 3 | 3 | 3 | 4 | 5 | 5 | 6 |
| 20–34 | 11 | 4.2 | <1 | 3 | 4 | 4 | 5 | 5 | 5 | 5 |
| 35–49 | 22 | 4.2 | 4 | 2 | 3 | 4 | 5 | 7 | 9 | 9 |
| 50–64 | 5 | 4.2 | <1 | 4 | 4 | 4 | 4 | 5 | 5 | 5 |
| 65+ | 7 | 5.6 | 3 | 3 | 4 | 6 | 6 | 8 | 8 | 8 |
| **2. MULTIPLE DX** | | | | | | | | | | |
| 0–19 Years | 190 | 7.5 | 71 | 3 | 4 | 5 | 6 | 12 | 25 | 56 |
| 20–34 | 118 | 7.5 | 26 | 3 | 4 | 5 | 10 | 15 | 16 | 25 |
| 35–49 | 235 | 8.2 | 54 | 3 | 4 | 5 | 9 | 19 | 25 | 42 |
| 50–64 | 422 | 8.6 | 52 | 4 | 5 | 6 | 10 | 15 | 21 | 33 |
| 65+ | 2,877 | 10.4 | 61 | 5 | 6 | 8 | 12 | 18 | 25 | 44 |
| **TOTAL SINGLE DX** | 73 | 4.0 | 2 | 3 | 3 | 4 | 4 | 5 | 6 | 9 |
| **TOTAL MULTIPLE DX** | 3,842 | 9.9 | 60 | 4 | 5 | 8 | 11 | 18 | 24 | 44 |
| **TOTAL** | | | | | | | | | | |
| 0–19 Years | 218 | 6.9 | 62 | 3 | 4 | 5 | 6 | 12 | 25 | 56 |
| 20–34 | 129 | 7.1 | 24 | 3 | 4 | 5 | 9 | 15 | 16 | 25 |
| 35–49 | 257 | 7.9 | 51 | 4 | 4 | 5 | 9 | 18 | 23 | 42 |
| 50–64 | 427 | 8.6 | 51 | 4 | 5 | 6 | 9 | 15 | 21 | 33 |
| 65+ | 2,884 | 10.4 | 61 | 5 | 6 | 8 | 12 | 18 | 25 | 44 |
| **GRAND TOTAL** | 3,915 | 9.8 | 60 | 4 | 5 | 8 | 11 | 17 | 24 | 44 |

## 35.22: REPL AORTIC VALVE NEC. Formerly included in operation group(s) 570.

| Type of Patients | Observed Patients | Avg. Stay | Variance | Percentiles | | | | | | |
|---|---|---|---|---|---|---|---|---|---|---|
| | | | | 10th | 25th | 50th | 75th | 90th | 95th | 99th |
| **1. SINGLE DX** | | | | | | | | | | |
| 0–19 Years | 5 | 4.5 | 1 | 4 | 4 | 4 | 4 | 6 | 7 | 7 |
| 20–34 | 16 | 5.2 | 4 | 4 | 4 | 5 | 6 | 7 | 7 | 13 |
| 35–49 | 40 | 4.6 | 2 | 3 | 3 | 5 | 5 | 7 | 7 | 8 |
| 50–64 | 48 | 4.9 | 3 | 3 | 3 | 5 | 6 | 8 | 8 | 9 |
| 65+ | 35 | 5.2 | 2 | 4 | 4 | 5 | 5 | 7 | 8 | 11 |
| **2. MULTIPLE DX** | | | | | | | | | | |
| 0–19 Years | 72 | 8.8 | 143 | 3 | 4 | 5 | 8 | 15 | 21 | 66 |
| 20–34 | 200 | 9.1 | 54 | 4 | 5 | 6 | 11 | 17 | 19 | 48 |
| 35–49 | 874 | 8.9 | 66 | 4 | 5 | 6 | 9 | 17 | 26 | 57 |
| 50–64 | 2,043 | 8.8 | 41 | 4 | 5 | 7 | 10 | 15 | 20 | 34 |
| 65+ | 4,158 | 10.8 | 61 | 5 | 6 | 8 | 13 | 19 | 25 | 50 |
| **TOTAL SINGLE DX** | 144 | 4.9 | 3 | 3 | 4 | 5 | 6 | 7 | 8 | 10 |
| **TOTAL MULTIPLE DX** | 7,347 | 10.0 | 57 | 4 | 6 | 8 | 12 | 17 | 24 | 47 |
| **TOTAL** | | | | | | | | | | |
| 0–19 Years | 77 | 6.9 | 114 | 3 | 4 | 5 | 7 | 11 | 19 | 66 |
| 20–34 | 216 | 8.6 | 53 | 4 | 5 | 6 | 10 | 17 | 18 | 48 |
| 35–49 | 914 | 8.6 | 64 | 4 | 5 | 6 | 9 | 16 | 26 | 45 |
| 50–64 | 2,091 | 8.7 | 40 | 4 | 5 | 7 | 10 | 15 | 20 | 34 |
| 65+ | 4,193 | 10.8 | 61 | 5 | 6 | 8 | 13 | 19 | 25 | 50 |
| **GRAND TOTAL** | 7,491 | 9.8 | 57 | 4 | 5 | 7 | 12 | 17 | 23 | 45 |

## 35.12: OPN MITRAL VALVULOPLASTY. Formerly included in operation group(s) 572.

| Type of Patients | Observed Patients | Avg. Stay | Variance | Percentiles | | | | | | |
|---|---|---|---|---|---|---|---|---|---|---|
| | | | | 10th | 25th | 50th | 75th | 90th | 95th | 99th |
| **1. SINGLE DX** | | | | | | | | | | |
| 0–19 Years | 15 | 4.1 | 1 | 3 | 3 | 4 | 5 | 5 | 6 | 6 |
| 20–34 | 13 | 3.7 | <1 | 3 | 3 | 4 | 4 | 5 | 6 | 5 |
| 35–49 | 12 | 4.9 | <1 | 4 | 5 | 5 | 5 | 4 | 6 | 7 |
| 50–64 | 10 | 4.7 | <1 | 4 | 4 | 5 | 5 | 5 | 6 | 9 |
| 65+ | 5 | 3.7 | <1 | 3 | 3 | 3 | 4 | 5 | 5 | 5 |
| **2. MULTIPLE DX** | | | | | | | | | | |
| 0–19 Years | 236 | 8.6 | 186 | 3 | 3 | 4 | 8 | 16 | 35 | 99 |
| 20–34 | 60 | 6.9 | 44 | 3 | 3 | 5 | 6 | 11 | 26 | 46 |
| 35–49 | 265 | 6.8 | 27 | 3 | 4 | 5 | 8 | 11 | 16 | 32 |
| 50–64 | 521 | 7.7 | 25 | 4 | 5 | 6 | 9 | 13 | 16 | 29 |
| 65+ | 758 | 11.9 | 78 | 5 | 6 | 8 | 13 | 32 | 34 | 34 |
| **TOTAL SINGLE DX** | 55 | 4.4 | <1 | 3 | 4 | 5 | 5 | 5 | 6 | 7 |
| **TOTAL MULTIPLE DX** | 1,840 | 9.7 | 77 | 4 | 5 | 7 | 11 | 20 | 34 | 38 |
| **TOTAL** | | | | | | | | | | |
| 0–19 Years | 251 | 8.4 | 179 | 3 | 3 | 4 | 7 | 14 | 31 | 99 |
| 20–34 | 73 | 6.4 | 38 | 3 | 4 | 5 | 6 | 10 | 19 | 26 |
| 35–49 | 277 | 6.6 | 25 | 3 | 4 | 5 | 7 | 11 | 15 | 29 |
| 50–64 | 531 | 7.6 | 25 | 4 | 5 | 6 | 8 | 13 | 15 | 29 |
| 65+ | 763 | 11.8 | 78 | 5 | 6 | 8 | 13 | 32 | 34 | 34 |
| **GRAND TOTAL** | 1,895 | 9.5 | 75 | 4 | 5 | 7 | 10 | 20 | 34 | 38 |

## 35.2: HEART VALVE REPLACEMENT. Formerly included in operation group(s) 570.

| Type of Patients | Observed Patients | Avg. Stay | Variance | Percentiles | | | | | | |
|---|---|---|---|---|---|---|---|---|---|---|
| | | | | 10th | 25th | 50th | 75th | 90th | 95th | 99th |
| **1. SINGLE DX** | | | | | | | | | | |
| 0–19 Years | 55 | 3.9 | 1 | 3 | 3 | 4 | 5 | 5 | 6 | 7 |
| 20–34 | 35 | 4.9 | 3 | 3 | 4 | 5 | 5 | 6 | 7 | 14 |
| 35–49 | 82 | 4.6 | 3 | 3 | 3 | 4 | 5 | 7 | 8 | 9 |
| 50–64 | 70 | 4.9 | 3 | 3 | 3 | 4 | 6 | 8 | 8 | 9 |
| 65+ | 50 | 5.3 | 2 | 4 | 4 | 5 | 6 | 7 | 8 | 11 |
| **2. MULTIPLE DX** | | | | | | | | | | |
| 0–19 Years | 591 | 9.3 | 122 | 3 | 4 | 5 | 8 | 18 | 36 | 60 |
| 20–34 | 483 | 8.9 | 51 | 4 | 5 | 6 | 10 | 17 | 20 | 42 |
| 35–49 | 1,784 | 8.8 | 62 | 4 | 5 | 6 | 9 | 17 | 25 | 47 |
| 50–64 | 3,883 | 9.3 | 49 | 4 | 5 | 7 | 11 | 16 | 22 | 36 |
| 65+ | 9,542 | 11.1 | 67 | 5 | 6 | 8 | 13 | 20 | 27 | 50 |
| **TOTAL SINGLE DX** | 292 | 4.6 | 3 | 3 | 4 | 4 | 5 | 7 | 8 | 9 |
| **TOTAL MULTIPLE DX** | 16,283 | 10.3 | 65 | 4 | 6 | 8 | 12 | 19 | 26 | 49 |
| **TOTAL** | | | | | | | | | | |
| 0–19 Years | 646 | 8.7 | 112 | 3 | 4 | 5 | 8 | 16 | 32 | 57 |
| 20–34 | 518 | 8.6 | 48 | 4 | 5 | 6 | 10 | 17 | 19 | 38 |
| 35–49 | 1,866 | 8.6 | 60 | 4 | 5 | 6 | 9 | 16 | 25 | 45 |
| 50–64 | 3,953 | 9.2 | 48 | 4 | 5 | 7 | 11 | 16 | 22 | 36 |
| 65+ | 9,592 | 11.0 | 67 | 5 | 6 | 8 | 13 | 20 | 27 | 50 |
| **GRAND TOTAL** | 16,575 | 10.2 | 65 | 4 | 6 | 8 | 12 | 18 | 25 | 49 |

Length of Stay by Diagnosis and Operation, United States, 2000

# United States, October 1998–September 1999 Data, by Operation

## 35.23: REPL MITRAL VALVE W TISS. Formerly included in operation group(s) 570.

| Type of Patients | Observed Patients | Avg. Stay | Variance | 10th | 25th | 50th | 75th | 90th | 95th | 99th |
|---|---|---|---|---|---|---|---|---|---|---|
| **1. SINGLE DX** | | | | | | | | | | |
| 0–19 Years | 1 | 4.0 | 0 | 4 | 4 | 4 | 4 | 4 | 4 | 4 |
| 20–34 | 0 | | | | | | | | | |
| 35–49 | 1 | 5.0 | 0 | 5 | 5 | 5 | 5 | 5 | 5 | 5 |
| 50–64 | 1 | 6.0 | 0 | 6 | 6 | 6 | 6 | 6 | 6 | 6 |
| 65+ | 0 | | | | | | | | | |
| **2. MULTIPLE DX** | | | | | | | | | | |
| 0–19 Years | 10 | 7.0 | 16 | 4 | 5 | 6 | 6 | 16 | 16 | 16 |
| 20–34 | 10 | 19.8 | 394 | 5 | 6 | 9 | 20 | 59 | 59 | 59 |
| 35–49 | 39 | 10.3 | 49 | 4 | 6 | 8 | 12 | 24 | 25 | 38 |
| 50–64 | 93 | 16.3 | 160 | 6 | 7 | 10 | 27 | 36 | 36 | 51 |
| 65+ | 689 | 12.6 | 87 | 6 | 7 | 9 | 15 | 23 | 30 | 53 |
| **TOTAL SINGLE DX** | 3 | 4.5 | <1 | 4 | 4 | 4 | 5 | 5 | 6 | 6 |
| **TOTAL MULTIPLE DX** | 841 | 12.9 | 95 | 6 | 7 | 9 | 15 | 25 | 35 | 52 |
| **TOTAL** | | | | | | | | | | |
| 0–19 Years | 11 | 6.5 | 14 | 4 | 6 | 6 | 6 | 16 | 16 | 16 |
| 20–34 | 10 | 19.8 | 394 | 5 | 6 | 9 | 20 | 59 | 59 | 59 |
| 35–49 | 40 | 10.2 | 49 | 4 | 6 | 8 | 12 | 24 | 25 | 38 |
| 50–64 | 94 | 16.2 | 159 | 6 | 7 | 10 | 27 | 36 | 36 | 51 |
| 65+ | 689 | 12.6 | 87 | 6 | 7 | 9 | 15 | 23 | 30 | 53 |
| **GRAND TOTAL** | 844 | 12.8 | 95 | 6 | 7 | 9 | 15 | 25 | 35 | 52 |

## 35.3: TISS ADJ TO HRT VALV OPS. Formerly included in operation group(s) 572.

| Type of Patients | Observed Patients | Avg. Stay | Variance | 10th | 25th | 50th | 75th | 90th | 95th | 99th |
|---|---|---|---|---|---|---|---|---|---|---|
| **1. SINGLE DX** | | | | | | | | | | |
| 0–19 Years | 15 | 4.1 | 2 | 3 | 3 | 4 | 6 | 6 | 6 | 6 |
| 20–34 | 4 | 5.1 | 5 | 4 | 4 | 4 | 5 | 10 | 10 | 10 |
| 35–49 | 8 | 4.5 | <1 | 3 | 4 | 5 | 5 | 6 | 6 | 6 |
| 50–64 | 3 | 4.0 | <1 | 3 | 3 | 4 | 5 | 5 | 5 | 5 |
| 65+ | 1 | 10.0 | 0 | 10 | 10 | 10 | 10 | 10 | 10 | 10 |
| **2. MULTIPLE DX** | | | | | | | | | | |
| 0–19 Years | 132 | 5.8 | 41 | 2 | 3 | 4 | 6 | 10 | 16 | 50 |
| 20–34 | 21 | 13.2 | 245 | 3 | 4 | 6 | 22 | 31 | 31 | 83 |
| 35–49 | 71 | 10.2 | 82 | 3 | 5 | 7 | 11 | 15 | 31 | 32 |
| 50–64 | 193 | 8.7 | 38 | 4 | 5 | 7 | 10 | 16 | 20 | 41 |
| 65+ | 370 | 12.0 | 72 | 5 | 6 | 9 | 14 | 23 | 30 | 38 |
| **TOTAL SINGLE DX** | 31 | 4.4 | 2 | 3 | 3 | 4 | 5 | 5 | 6 | 10 |
| **TOTAL MULTIPLE DX** | 787 | 10.2 | 70 | 4 | 5 | 7 | 12 | 21 | 29 | 41 |
| **TOTAL** | | | | | | | | | | |
| 0–19 Years | 147 | 5.6 | 37 | 3 | 3 | 4 | 6 | 8 | 13 | 50 |
| 20–34 | 25 | 12.4 | 225 | 3 | 4 | 5 | 20 | 22 | 31 | 83 |
| 35–49 | 79 | 9.6 | 77 | 4 | 5 | 6 | 10 | 28 | 31 | 32 |
| 50–64 | 196 | 8.6 | 38 | 4 | 5 | 6 | 10 | 16 | 20 | 41 |
| 65+ | 371 | 12.0 | 72 | 5 | 6 | 9 | 14 | 23 | 30 | 38 |
| **GRAND TOTAL** | 818 | 10.0 | 69 | 4 | 5 | 7 | 12 | 21 | 28 | 41 |

## 35.24: REPL MITRAL VALVE NEC. Formerly included in operation group(s) 570.

| Type of Patients | Observed Patients | Avg. Stay | Variance | 10th | 25th | 50th | 75th | 90th | 95th | 99th |
|---|---|---|---|---|---|---|---|---|---|---|
| **1. SINGLE DX** | | | | | | | | | | |
| 0–19 Years | 4 | 5.0 | 2 | 2 | 5 | 5 | 5 | 7 | 7 | 9 |
| 20–34 | 7 | 6.0 | 7 | 5 | 5 | 5 | 5 | 8 | 14 | 14 |
| 35–49 | 18 | 5.2 | 3 | 4 | 4 | 5 | 6 | 7 | 8 | 10 |
| 50–64 | 16 | 4.8 | 2 | 3 | 4 | 4 | 5 | 6 | 8 | 9 |
| 65+ | 8 | 6.6 | 3 | 5 | 5 | 6 | 8 | 9 | 9 | 9 |
| **2. MULTIPLE DX** | | | | | | | | | | |
| 0–19 Years | 99 | 16.8 | 254 | 5 | 7 | 10 | 19 | 50 | 50 | 61 |
| 20–34 | 111 | 9.7 | 49 | 5 | 5 | 8 | 11 | 16 | 22 | 51 |
| 35–49 | 596 | 8.6 | 57 | 4 | 5 | 6 | 11 | 16 | 20 | 47 |
| 50–64 | 1,292 | 9.7 | 48 | 5 | 6 | 8 | 11 | 17 | 22 | 42 |
| 65+ | 1,800 | 12.1 | 81 | 5 | 7 | 9 | 15 | 22 | 29 | 62 |
| **TOTAL SINGLE DX** | 53 | 5.3 | 3 | 4 | 4 | 5 | 6 | 7 | 9 | 14 |
| **TOTAL MULTIPLE DX** | 3,898 | 10.9 | 74 | 5 | 6 | 8 | 13 | 20 | 27 | 53 |
| **TOTAL** | | | | | | | | | | |
| 0–19 Years | 103 | 16.2 | 249 | 5 | 7 | 10 | 17 | 50 | 50 | 61 |
| 20–34 | 118 | 9.5 | 48 | 5 | 5 | 8 | 11 | 16 | 22 | 51 |
| 35–49 | 614 | 8.6 | 56 | 4 | 5 | 6 | 9 | 15 | 20 | 47 |
| 50–64 | 1,308 | 9.7 | 48 | 5 | 6 | 7 | 11 | 17 | 22 | 42 |
| 65+ | 1,808 | 12.1 | 81 | 5 | 7 | 9 | 15 | 22 | 29 | 62 |
| **GRAND TOTAL** | 3,951 | 10.8 | 74 | 6 | 6 | 8 | 13 | 20 | 27 | 53 |

## 35.33: ANNULOPLASTY. Formerly included in operation group(s) 572.

| Type of Patients | Observed Patients | Avg. Stay | Variance | 10th | 25th | 50th | 75th | 90th | 95th | 99th |
|---|---|---|---|---|---|---|---|---|---|---|
| **1. SINGLE DX** | | | | | | | | | | |
| 0–19 Years | 0 | | | | | | | | | |
| 20–34 | 2 | 5.4 | 8 | 3 | 3 | 4 | 4 | 10 | 10 | 10 |
| 35–49 | 6 | 4.2 | 1 | 3 | 3 | 4 | 5 | 5 | 5 | 6 |
| 50–64 | 3 | 4.0 | <1 | 3 | 3 | 4 | 5 | 5 | 5 | 5 |
| 65+ | 1 | 10.0 | 0 | 10 | 10 | 10 | 10 | 10 | 10 | 10 |
| **2. MULTIPLE DX** | | | | | | | | | | |
| 0–19 Years | 32 | 11.1 | 159 | 4 | 4 | 6 | 17 | 35 | 50 | >99 |
| 20–34 | 18 | 12.3 | 249 | 3 | 3 | 5 | 20 | 22 | 22 | 83 |
| 35–49 | 59 | 8.8 | 58 | 4 | 4 | 7 | 10 | 15 | 28 | 32 |
| 50–64 | 190 | 8.8 | 38 | 4 | 5 | 7 | 10 | 16 | 20 | 41 |
| 65+ | 367 | 12.0 | 72 | 5 | 6 | 9 | 14 | 23 | 30 | 38 |
| **TOTAL SINGLE DX** | 12 | 4.7 | 4 | 3 | 3 | 4 | 5 | 10 | 10 | 10 |
| **TOTAL MULTIPLE DX** | 666 | 10.9 | 72 | 4 | 6 | 8 | 13 | 21 | 29 | 43 |
| **TOTAL** | | | | | | | | | | |
| 0–19 Years | 32 | 11.1 | 159 | 4 | 4 | 6 | 17 | 35 | 50 | >99 |
| 20–34 | 20 | 11.7 | 232 | 3 | 3 | 6 | 15 | 22 | 22 | 83 |
| 35–49 | 65 | 8.5 | 56 | 4 | 4 | 6 | 10 | 15 | 28 | 32 |
| 50–64 | 193 | 8.7 | 38 | 4 | 5 | 7 | 10 | 16 | 20 | 41 |
| 65+ | 368 | 12.0 | 72 | 5 | 6 | 9 | 14 | 23 | 30 | 38 |
| **GRAND TOTAL** | 678 | 10.8 | 71 | 4 | 6 | 8 | 13 | 21 | 29 | 43 |

Length of Stay by Diagnosis and Operation, United States, 2000

# United States, October 1998–September 1999 Data, by Operation

## 35.4: SEPTAL DEFECT PRODUCTION. Formerly included in operation group(s) 572.

| Type of Patients | Observed Patients | Avg. Stay | Variance | 10th | 25th | 50th | 75th | 90th | 95th | 99th |
|---|---|---|---|---|---|---|---|---|---|---|
| **1. SINGLE DX** | | | | | | | | | | |
| 0–19 Years | 1 | 3.0 | 0 | 3 | 3 | 3 | 3 | 3 | 3 | 3 |
| 20–34 | 0 | | | | | | | | | |
| 35–49 | 0 | | | | | | | | | |
| 50–64 | 0 | | | | | | | | | |
| 65+ | 0 | | | | | | | | | |
| **2. MULTIPLE DX** | | | | | | | | | | |
| 0–19 Years | 102 | 12.0 | 104 | 3 | 5 | 9 | 14 | 29 | 35 | 43 |
| 20–34 | 1 | 16.0 | 0 | 16 | 16 | 16 | 16 | 16 | 16 | 16 |
| 35–49 | 0 | | | | | | | | | |
| 50–64 | 1 | 2.0 | 0 | 2 | 2 | 2 | 2 | 2 | 2 | 2 |
| 65+ | 2 | 8.5 | 12 | 6 | 6 | 6 | 12 | 12 | 12 | 12 |
| **TOTAL SINGLE DX** | 1 | 3.0 | 0 | 3 | 3 | 3 | 3 | 3 | 3 | 3 |
| **TOTAL MULTIPLE DX** | 106 | 11.9 | 102 | 3 | 5 | 9 | 14 | 25 | 35 | 43 |
| **TOTAL** | | | | | | | | | | |
| 0–19 Years | 103 | 11.9 | 103 | 3 | 5 | 9 | 14 | 25 | 35 | 43 |
| 20–34 | 1 | 16.0 | 0 | 16 | 16 | 16 | 16 | 16 | 16 | 16 |
| 35–49 | 0 | | | | | | | | | |
| 50–64 | 1 | 2.0 | 0 | 2 | 2 | 2 | 2 | 2 | 2 | 2 |
| 65+ | 2 | 8.5 | 12 | 6 | 6 | 6 | 12 | 12 | 12 | 12 |
| **GRAND TOTAL** | 107 | 11.8 | 102 | 3 | 5 | 9 | 14 | 25 | 35 | 43 |

## 35.5: PROSTH REP HEART SEPTA. Formerly included in operation group(s) 572, 579.

| Type of Patients | Observed Patients | Avg. Stay | Variance | 10th | 25th | 50th | 75th | 90th | 95th | 99th |
|---|---|---|---|---|---|---|---|---|---|---|
| **1. SINGLE DX** | | | | | | | | | | |
| 0–19 Years | 163 | 2.6 | 2 | 1 | 2 | 2 | 3 | 4 | 5 | 7 |
| 20–34 | 7 | 4.5 | <1 | 3 | 5 | 5 | 5 | 5 | 5 | 5 |
| 35–49 | 12 | 1.7 | 2 | 1 | 1 | 1 | 1 | 4 | 5 | 5 |
| 50–64 | 2 | 3.5 | <1 | 3 | 3 | 3 | 3 | 5 | 5 | 5 |
| 65+ | 1 | 1.0 | 0 | 1 | 1 | 1 | 1 | 1 | 1 | 1 |
| **2. MULTIPLE DX** | | | | | | | | | | |
| 0–19 Years | 976 | 7.8 | 72 | 3 | 3 | 5 | 8 | 15 | 23 | 50 |
| 20–34 | 41 | 5.4 | 24 | 2 | 4 | 4 | 5 | 10 | 10 | 42 |
| 35–49 | 58 | 4.5 | 12 | 2 | 2 | 4 | 5 | 9 | 11 | 20 |
| 50–64 | 38 | 7.3 | 15 | 4 | 4 | 6 | 10 | 13 | 15 | 20 |
| 65+ | 39 | 11.3 | 58 | 3 | 5 | 9 | 17 | 23 | 27 | 27 |
| **TOTAL SINGLE DX** | 185 | 2.7 | 2 | 1 | 1 | 2 | 3 | 5 | 5 | 7 |
| **TOTAL MULTIPLE DX** | 1,152 | 7.6 | 66 | 3 | 3 | 5 | 8 | 15 | 22 | 50 |
| **TOTAL** | | | | | | | | | | |
| 0–19 Years | 1,139 | 6.9 | 64 | 2 | 3 | 4 | 7 | 14 | 21 | 50 |
| 20–34 | 48 | 5.1 | 16 | 3 | 4 | 4 | 5 | 9 | 10 | 16 |
| 35–49 | 70 | 3.7 | 11 | 1 | 1 | 3 | 5 | 7 | 11 | 20 |
| 50–64 | 40 | 7.1 | 15 | 3 | 4 | 6 | 10 | 13 | 15 | 20 |
| 65+ | 40 | 11.1 | 59 | 3 | 5 | 9 | 17 | 23 | 27 | 27 |
| **GRAND TOTAL** | 1,337 | 6.7 | 58 | 2 | 3 | 4 | 7 | 14 | 20 | 48 |

## 35.53: PROSTH REP VSD. Formerly included in operation group(s) 572.

| Type of Patients | Observed Patients | Avg. Stay | Variance | 10th | 25th | 50th | 75th | 90th | 95th | 99th |
|---|---|---|---|---|---|---|---|---|---|---|
| **1. SINGLE DX** | | | | | | | | | | |
| 0–19 Years | 59 | 3.0 | 1 | 2 | 2 | 3 | 4 | 5 | 5 | 7 |
| 20–34 | 0 | | | | | | | | | |
| 35–49 | 1 | 4.0 | 0 | 4 | 4 | 4 | 4 | 4 | 4 | 4 |
| 50–64 | 1 | 5.0 | 0 | 5 | 5 | 5 | 5 | 5 | 5 | 5 |
| 65+ | 0 | | | | | | | | | |
| **2. MULTIPLE DX** | | | | | | | | | | |
| 0–19 Years | 623 | 7.4 | 64 | 3 | 4 | 5 | 7 | 15 | 21 | 50 |
| 20–34 | 10 | 5.6 | 10 | 4 | 4 | 4 | 6 | 10 | 10 | 16 |
| 35–49 | 3 | 5.7 | 3 | 3 | 5 | 7 | 7 | 7 | 7 | 7 |
| 50–64 | 5 | 11.1 | 18 | 5 | 7 | 14 | 15 | 15 | 15 | 15 |
| 65+ | 9 | 17.6 | 23 | 8 | 17 | 19 | 22 | 23 | 23 | 23 |
| **TOTAL SINGLE DX** | 61 | 3.1 | 1 | 2 | 2 | 3 | 4 | 5 | 5 | 7 |
| **TOTAL MULTIPLE DX** | 650 | 7.5 | 63 | 3 | 4 | 5 | 8 | 15 | 21 | 50 |
| **TOTAL** | | | | | | | | | | |
| 0–19 Years | 682 | 7.0 | 60 | 3 | 3 | 5 | 7 | 14 | 20 | 50 |
| 20–34 | 10 | 5.6 | 10 | 4 | 4 | 4 | 6 | 10 | 10 | 16 |
| 35–49 | 4 | 5.3 | 2 | 4 | 5 | 5 | 7 | 7 | 7 | 7 |
| 50–64 | 6 | 10.6 | 20 | 5 | 7 | 14 | 15 | 15 | 15 | 15 |
| 65+ | 9 | 17.6 | 23 | 8 | 17 | 19 | 22 | 23 | 23 | 23 |
| **GRAND TOTAL** | 711 | 7.1 | 59 | 3 | 3 | 5 | 7 | 15 | 21 | 50 |

## 35.6: TISS GRFT REP HRT SEPTA. Formerly included in operation group(s) 572.

| Type of Patients | Observed Patients | Avg. Stay | Variance | 10th | 25th | 50th | 75th | 90th | 95th | 99th |
|---|---|---|---|---|---|---|---|---|---|---|
| **1. SINGLE DX** | | | | | | | | | | |
| 0–19 Years | 163 | 3.0 | <1 | 2 | 2 | 3 | 4 | 4 | 4 | 6 |
| 20–34 | 17 | 3.3 | <1 | 3 | 3 | 3 | 4 | 4 | 6 | 6 |
| 35–49 | 25 | 3.8 | <1 | 2 | 3 | 4 | 4 | 5 | 6 | 7 |
| 50–64 | 2 | 2.8 | 1 | 2 | 2 | 2 | 4 | 4 | 4 | 4 |
| 65+ | 0 | | | | | | | | | |
| **2. MULTIPLE DX** | | | | | | | | | | |
| 0–19 Years | 745 | 6.8 | 71 | 2 | 3 | 4 | 7 | 16 | 18 | >99 |
| 20–34 | 58 | 4.2 | 5 | 3 | 3 | 3 | 5 | 6 | 7 | 12 |
| 35–49 | 106 | 5.3 | 14 | 3 | 4 | 4 | 6 | 8 | 12 | 21 |
| 50–64 | 89 | 9.4 | 75 | 3 | 4 | 5 | 14 | 18 | 30 | 30 |
| 65+ | 53 | 12.5 | 363 | 4 | 5 | 7 | 10 | 27 | 81 | >99 |
| **TOTAL SINGLE DX** | 207 | 3.1 | 1 | 2 | 2 | 3 | 4 | 4 | 5 | 6 |
| **TOTAL MULTIPLE DX** | 1,051 | 7.1 | 79 | 3 | 3 | 5 | 7 | 17 | 18 | 99 |
| **TOTAL** | | | | | | | | | | |
| 0–19 Years | 908 | 6.2 | 60 | 2 | 3 | 4 | 6 | 13 | 18 | >99 |
| 20–34 | 75 | 4.1 | 4 | 3 | 3 | 3 | 5 | 8 | 7 | 12 |
| 35–49 | 131 | 5.0 | 11 | 3 | 3 | 5 | 5 | 8 | 10 | 21 |
| 50–64 | 91 | 9.3 | 75 | 4 | 4 | 5 | 13 | 18 | 30 | 30 |
| 65+ | 53 | 12.5 | 363 | 4 | 5 | 7 | 10 | 27 | 81 | >99 |
| **GRAND TOTAL** | 1,258 | 6.5 | 69 | 2 | 3 | 4 | 7 | 14 | 18 | 98 |

Length of Stay by Diagnosis and Operation, United States, 2000

## United States, October 1998–September 1999 Data, by Operation

### 35.61: REPAIR ASD W TISS GRAFT. Formerly included in operation group(s) 572.

| Type of Patients | Observed Patients | Avg. Stay | Variance | 10th | 25th | 50th | 75th | 90th | 95th | 99th |
|---|---|---|---|---|---|---|---|---|---|---|
| **1. SINGLE DX** | | | | | | | | | | |
| 0–19 Years | 128 | 2.9 | <1 | 2 | 2 | 3 | 4 | 4 | 4 | 5 |
| 20–34 | 17 | 3.3 | <1 | 3 | 3 | 3 | 4 | 4 | 6 | 6 |
| 35–49 | 25 | 3.8 | <1 | 3 | 3 | 4 | 4 | 5 | 6 | 7 |
| 50–64 | 2 | 2.8 | 1 | 2 | 3 | 2 | 4 | 4 | 4 | 4 |
| 65+ | 0 | | | | | | | | | |
| **2. MULTIPLE DX** | | | | | | | | | | |
| 0–19 Years | 330 | 4.1 | 17 | 2 | 3 | 3 | 4 | 7 | 11 | >99 |
| 20–34 | 51 | 3.7 | 2 | 3 | 3 | 4 | 4 | 5 | 6 | 9 |
| 35–49 | 102 | 5.5 | 15 | 3 | 4 | 4 | 6 | 8 | 12 | 21 |
| 50–64 | 80 | 9.0 | 52 | 3 | 4 | 5 | 14 | 18 | 30 | 30 |
| 65+ | 37 | 6.9 | 9 | 4 | 5 | 7 | 9 | 11 | 13 | >99 |
| **TOTAL SINGLE DX** | 172 | 3.1 | <1 | 2 | 2 | 3 | 4 | 4 | 4 | 6 |
| **TOTAL MULTIPLE DX** | 600 | 5.4 | 25 | 2 | 3 | 4 | 5 | 10 | 17 | >99 |
| **TOTAL** | | | | | | | | | | |
| 0–19 Years | 458 | 3.8 | 13 | 2 | 3 | 3 | 4 | 5 | 9 | >99 |
| 20–34 | 68 | 3.6 | 2 | 3 | 3 | 4 | 4 | 5 | 6 | 9 |
| 35–49 | 127 | 5.1 | 12 | 3 | 3 | 4 | 5 | 8 | 11 | 21 |
| 50–64 | 82 | 9.0 | 52 | 3 | 4 | 5 | 14 | 18 | 30 | 30 |
| 65+ | 37 | 6.9 | 9 | 4 | 5 | 7 | 9 | 11 | 13 | >99 |
| **GRAND TOTAL** | 772 | 4.9 | 21 | 2 | 3 | 4 | 5 | 9 | 17 | 62 |

### 35.62: REPAIR VSD W TISS GRAFT. Formerly included in operation group(s) 572.

| Type of Patients | Observed Patients | Avg. Stay | Variance | 10th | 25th | 50th | 75th | 90th | 95th | 99th |
|---|---|---|---|---|---|---|---|---|---|---|
| **1. SINGLE DX** | | | | | | | | | | |
| 0–19 Years | 27 | 3.1 | <1 | 2 | 3 | 3 | 3 | 4 | 6 | 6 |
| 20–34 | 0 | | | | | | | | | |
| 35–49 | 0 | | | | | | | | | |
| 50–64 | 0 | | | | | | | | | |
| 65+ | 0 | | | | | | | | | |
| **2. MULTIPLE DX** | | | | | | | | | | |
| 0–19 Years | 258 | 7.8 | 44 | 3 | 4 | 6 | 9 | 18 | 18 | 32 |
| 20–34 | 6 | 5.9 | 4 | 2 | 6 | 6 | 6 | 7 | 12 | 12 |
| 35–49 | 3 | 4.0 | <1 | 3 | 4 | 4 | 4 | 4 | 4 | 8 |
| 50–64 | 8 | 18.0 | 519 | 8 | 9 | 12 | 13 | 17 | 90 | 90 |
| 65+ | 12 | 34.4 | >999 | 9 | 9 | 15 | 41 | 99 | 99 | 99 |
| **TOTAL SINGLE DX** | 27 | 3.1 | <1 | 2 | 3 | 3 | 3 | 4 | 6 | 6 |
| **TOTAL MULTIPLE DX** | 287 | 8.6 | 110 | 3 | 4 | 6 | 9 | 18 | 20 | 81 |
| **TOTAL** | | | | | | | | | | |
| 0–19 Years | 285 | 7.3 | 41 | 3 | 3 | 5 | 8 | 16 | 18 | 32 |
| 20–34 | 6 | 5.9 | 4 | 2 | 6 | 6 | 6 | 7 | 12 | 12 |
| 35–49 | 3 | 4.0 | <1 | 3 | 4 | 4 | 4 | 4 | 4 | 8 |
| 50–64 | 8 | 18.0 | 519 | 8 | 9 | 12 | 13 | 17 | 90 | 90 |
| 65+ | 12 | 34.4 | >999 | 9 | 9 | 15 | 41 | 99 | 99 | 99 |
| **GRAND TOTAL** | 314 | 8.1 | 103 | 3 | 4 | 5 | 9 | 18 | 20 | 79 |

### 35.7: HEART SEPTA REP NEC/NOS. Formerly included in operation group(s) 572.

| Type of Patients | Observed Patients | Avg. Stay | Variance | 10th | 25th | 50th | 75th | 90th | 95th | 99th |
|---|---|---|---|---|---|---|---|---|---|---|
| **1. SINGLE DX** | | | | | | | | | | |
| 0–19 Years | 338 | 2.8 | 1 | 1 | 2 | 3 | 3 | 4 | 5 | 5 |
| 20–34 | 31 | 3.7 | <1 | 3 | 3 | 3 | 4 | 5 | 5 | 6 |
| 35–49 | 26 | 3.2 | 1 | 2 | 3 | 4 | 4 | 5 | 5 | 7 |
| 50–64 | 4 | 5.7 | 3 | 4 | 4 | 7 | 7 | 7 | 7 | 7 |
| 65+ | 0 | | | | | | | | | |
| **2. MULTIPLE DX** | | | | | | | | | | |
| 0–19 Years | 895 | 5.7 | 33 | 2 | 3 | 4 | 6 | 11 | 14 | 42 |
| 20–34 | 89 | 4.4 | 5 | 3 | 3 | 4 | 5 | 6 | 7 | 16 |
| 35–49 | 159 | 4.2 | 5 | 3 | 3 | 4 | 5 | 6 | 8 | 15 |
| 50–64 | 115 | 5.8 | 16 | 3 | 4 | 4 | 6 | 10 | 15 | 24 |
| 65+ | 86 | 11.4 | 99 | 4 | 5 | 8 | 11 | 33 | 33 | 37 |
| **TOTAL SINGLE DX** | 399 | 2.8 | 2 | 2 | 2 | 3 | 4 | 4 | 5 | 6 |
| **TOTAL MULTIPLE DX** | 1,344 | 5.8 | 33 | 3 | 3 | 4 | 6 | 10 | 14 | 34 |
| **TOTAL** | | | | | | | | | | |
| 0–19 Years | 1,233 | 4.7 | 25 | 2 | 3 | 4 | 5 | 9 | 13 | 30 |
| 20–34 | 120 | 4.2 | 4 | 3 | 3 | 4 | 5 | 6 | 7 | 16 |
| 35–49 | 185 | 4.0 | 4 | 3 | 3 | 4 | 4 | 6 | 7 | 15 |
| 50–64 | 119 | 5.8 | 16 | 3 | 4 | 4 | 6 | 9 | 15 | 24 |
| 65+ | 86 | 11.4 | 99 | 4 | 5 | 8 | 11 | 33 | 33 | 37 |
| **GRAND TOTAL** | 1,743 | 5.0 | 27 | 2 | 3 | 4 | 5 | 9 | 13 | 33 |

### 35.71: REPAIR ASD NEC. Formerly included in operation group(s) 572.

| Type of Patients | Observed Patients | Avg. Stay | Variance | 10th | 25th | 50th | 75th | 90th | 95th | 99th |
|---|---|---|---|---|---|---|---|---|---|---|
| **1. SINGLE DX** | | | | | | | | | | |
| 0–19 Years | 290 | 2.6 | 1 | 1 | 2 | 3 | 3 | 4 | 4 | 5 |
| 20–34 | 31 | 3.7 | <1 | 3 | 3 | 3 | 4 | 5 | 5 | 6 |
| 35–49 | 25 | 3.2 | 1 | 2 | 3 | 3 | 3 | 5 | 5 | 7 |
| 50–64 | 4 | 5.7 | 3 | 4 | 4 | 7 | 7 | 7 | 7 | 7 |
| 65+ | 0 | | | | | | | | | |
| **2. MULTIPLE DX** | | | | | | | | | | |
| 0–19 Years | 501 | 4.6 | 20 | 2 | 3 | 4 | 5 | 7 | 13 | 43 |
| 20–34 | 71 | 4.1 | 3 | 3 | 3 | 4 | 5 | 6 | 7 | 10 |
| 35–49 | 144 | 4.0 | 3 | 3 | 3 | 4 | 4 | 6 | 7 | 10 |
| 50–64 | 107 | 5.5 | 15 | 3 | 4 | 4 | 5 | 9 | 13 | 24 |
| 65+ | 67 | 7.7 | 25 | 4 | 5 | 7 | 8 | 11 | 18 | 34 |
| **TOTAL SINGLE DX** | 350 | 2.7 | 1 | 1 | 2 | 3 | 3 | 4 | 5 | 5 |
| **TOTAL MULTIPLE DX** | 890 | 4.8 | 16 | 2 | 3 | 5 | 5 | 8 | 11 | 34 |
| **TOTAL** | | | | | | | | | | |
| 0–19 Years | 791 | 3.8 | 13 | 2 | 3 | 4 | 5 | 5 | 7 | 29 |
| 20–34 | 102 | 4.0 | 2 | 3 | 3 | 4 | 5 | 5 | 7 | 10 |
| 35–49 | 169 | 3.9 | 3 | 3 | 3 | 4 | 4 | 6 | 6 | 10 |
| 50–64 | 111 | 5.5 | 15 | 3 | 4 | 4 | 5 | 9 | 12 | 24 |
| 65+ | 67 | 7.7 | 25 | 4 | 5 | 7 | 8 | 11 | 18 | 34 |
| **GRAND TOTAL** | 1,240 | 4.2 | 13 | 2 | 3 | 5 | 5 | 6 | 9 | 24 |

Length of Stay by Diagnosis and Operation, United States, 2000

## United States, October 1998–September 1999 Data, by Operation

### 35.72: REPAIR VSD NEC. Formerly included in operation group(s) 572.

| Type of Patients | Observed Patients | Avg. Stay | Variance | 10th | 25th | 50th | 75th | 90th | 95th | 99th |
|---|---|---|---|---|---|---|---|---|---|---|
| **1. SINGLE DX** | | | | | | | | | | |
| 0–19 Years | 39 | 3.5 | 3 | 2 | 3 | 4 | 4 | 4 | 5 | 17 |
| 20–34 | 0 | | | | | | | | | |
| 35–49 | 1 | 4.0 | 0 | 4 | 4 | 4 | 4 | 4 | 4 | 4 |
| 50–64 | 0 | | | | | | | | | |
| 65+ | 0 | | | | | | | | | |
| **2. MULTIPLE DX** | | | | | | | | | | |
| 0–19 Years | 273 | 6.3 | 22 | 3 | 3 | 5 | 8 | 12 | 14 | 22 |
| 20–34 | 15 | 5.0 | 8 | 3 | 3 | 5 | 5 | 6 | 6 | 19 |
| 35–49 | 15 | 5.2 | 16 | 3 | 3 | 3 | 6 | 11 | 15 | 20 |
| 50–64 | 3 | 13.6 | 13 | 6 | 15 | 15 | 15 | 16 | 16 | 16 |
| 65+ | 18 | 24.4 | 133 | 7 | 11 | 33 | 33 | 33 | 33 | 48 |
| **TOTAL SINGLE DX** | 40 | 3.5 | 3 | 2 | 3 | 4 | 4 | 4 | 5 | 17 |
| **TOTAL MULTIPLE DX** | 324 | 7.3 | 46 | 3 | 3 | 5 | 9 | 13 | 20 | 33 |
| **TOTAL** | | | | | | | | | | |
| 0–19 Years | 312 | 5.9 | 21 | 3 | 3 | 4 | 7 | 12 | 13 | 21 |
| 20–34 | 15 | 5.0 | 8 | 3 | 3 | 5 | 5 | 6 | 6 | 19 |
| 35–49 | 16 | 5.2 | 16 | 3 | 3 | 3 | 6 | 11 | 15 | 20 |
| 50–64 | 3 | 13.6 | 13 | 6 | 15 | 15 | 15 | 16 | 16 | 16 |
| 65+ | 18 | 24.4 | 133 | 7 | 11 | 33 | 33 | 33 | 33 | 48 |
| **GRAND TOTAL** | 364 | 6.8 | 42 | 3 | 3 | 4 | 8 | 13 | 17 | 33 |

### 35.8: TOT REP CONG CARD ANOM. Formerly included in operation group(s) 572.

| Type of Patients | Observed Patients | Avg. Stay | Variance | 10th | 25th | 50th | 75th | 90th | 95th | 99th |
|---|---|---|---|---|---|---|---|---|---|---|
| **1. SINGLE DX** | | | | | | | | | | |
| 0–19 Years | 63 | 5.0 | 3 | 3 | 4 | 5 | 6 | 7 | 8 | 11 |
| 20–34 | 2 | 5.8 | 1 | 5 | 5 | 5 | 7 | 7 | 7 | 7 |
| 35–49 | 0 | | | | | | | | | |
| 50–64 | 1 | 20.0 | 0 | 20 | 20 | 20 | 20 | 20 | 20 | 20 |
| 65+ | 1 | 7.0 | 0 | 7 | 7 | 7 | 7 | 7 | 7 | 7 |
| **2. MULTIPLE DX** | | | | | | | | | | |
| 0–19 Years | 958 | 11.9 | 118 | 4 | 6 | 8 | 14 | 21 | 32 | 60 |
| 20–34 | 10 | 8.1 | 79 | 3 | 4 | 5 | 9 | 14 | 42 | 42 |
| 35–49 | 3 | 6.3 | 4 | 4 | 4 | 7 | 8 | 8 | 8 | 8 |
| 50–64 | 7 | 9.1 | 27 | 4 | 4 | 6 | 16 | 16 | 16 | 16 |
| 65+ | 1 | 8.0 | 0 | 8 | 8 | 8 | 8 | 8 | 8 | 8 |
| **TOTAL SINGLE DX** | 67 | 5.6 | 11 | 3 | 4 | 5 | 6 | 8 | 11 | 20 |
| **TOTAL MULTIPLE DX** | 979 | 11.8 | 117 | 4 | 6 | 8 | 14 | 21 | 32 | 60 |
| **TOTAL** | | | | | | | | | | |
| 0–19 Years | 1,021 | 11.2 | 111 | 4 | 6 | 8 | 13 | 20 | 31 | 57 |
| 20–34 | 12 | 7.5 | 60 | 3 | 4 | 5 | 7 | 14 | 17 | 42 |
| 35–49 | 3 | 6.3 | 4 | 4 | 4 | 7 | 8 | 8 | 8 | 8 |
| 50–64 | 8 | 13.8 | 45 | 4 | 5 | 16 | 20 | 20 | 20 | 20 |
| 65+ | 2 | 7.6 | <1 | 7 | 7 | 8 | 8 | 8 | 8 | 8 |
| **GRAND TOTAL** | 1,046 | 11.2 | 110 | 4 | 5 | 8 | 13 | 20 | 31 | 57 |

### 35.81: TOT REP TETRALOGY FALLOT. Formerly included in operation group(s) 572.

| Type of Patients | Observed Patients | Avg. Stay | Variance | 10th | 25th | 50th | 75th | 90th | 95th | 99th |
|---|---|---|---|---|---|---|---|---|---|---|
| **1. SINGLE DX** | | | | | | | | | | |
| 0–19 Years | 57 | 4.8 | 3 | 3 | 4 | 4 | 6 | 7 | 7 | 11 |
| 20–34 | 1 | 7.0 | 0 | 7 | 7 | 7 | 7 | 7 | 7 | 7 |
| 35–49 | 0 | | | | | | | | | |
| 50–64 | 1 | 20.0 | 0 | 20 | 20 | 20 | 20 | 20 | 20 | 20 |
| 65+ | 0 | | | | | | | | | |
| **2. MULTIPLE DX** | | | | | | | | | | |
| 0–19 Years | 577 | 10.2 | 107 | 4 | 6 | 7 | 11 | 17 | 25 | 83 |
| 20–34 | 7 | 12.2 | 127 | 5 | 6 | 9 | 14 | 42 | 42 | 42 |
| 35–49 | 2 | 7.5 | <1 | 7 | 7 | 7 | 8 | 8 | 8 | 8 |
| 50–64 | 3 | 13.6 | 16 | 6 | 10 | 16 | 16 | 16 | 16 | 16 |
| 65+ | 0 | | | | | | | | | |
| **TOTAL SINGLE DX** | 59 | 5.6 | 14 | 3 | 4 | 4 | 6 | 7 | 13 | 20 |
| **TOTAL MULTIPLE DX** | 589 | 10.2 | 107 | 4 | 6 | 7 | 11 | 17 | 25 | 83 |
| **TOTAL** | | | | | | | | | | |
| 0–19 Years | 634 | 9.5 | 98 | 4 | 5 | 7 | 10 | 16 | 23 | 54 |
| 20–34 | 8 | 11.2 | 104 | 5 | 6 | 7 | 9 | 17 | 42 | 42 |
| 35–49 | 2 | 7.5 | <1 | 7 | 7 | 7 | 8 | 8 | 8 | 8 |
| 50–64 | 4 | 17.6 | 16 | 10 | 16 | 20 | 20 | 20 | 20 | 20 |
| 65+ | 0 | | | | | | | | | |
| **GRAND TOTAL** | 648 | 9.6 | 97 | 4 | 5 | 7 | 10 | 17 | 23 | 54 |

### 35.9: VALVES & SEPTA OPS NEC. Formerly included in operation group(s) 572.

| Type of Patients | Observed Patients | Avg. Stay | Variance | 10th | 25th | 50th | 75th | 90th | 95th | 99th |
|---|---|---|---|---|---|---|---|---|---|---|
| **1. SINGLE DX** | | | | | | | | | | |
| 0–19 Years | 140 | 2.6 | 5 | 1 | 1 | 1 | 4 | 6 | 6 | 10 |
| 20–34 | 5 | 1.4 | <1 | 1 | 1 | 1 | 2 | 2 | 2 | 2 |
| 35–49 | 8 | 1.3 | <1 | 1 | 1 | 1 | 2 | 2 | 2 | 2 |
| 50–64 | 3 | 1.3 | <1 | 1 | 1 | 1 | 2 | 2 | 2 | 2 |
| 65+ | 6 | 1.2 | <1 | 1 | 1 | 1 | 1 | 2 | 2 | 2 |
| **2. MULTIPLE DX** | | | | | | | | | | |
| 0–19 Years | 1,015 | 8.5 | 71 | 1 | 4 | 6 | 10 | 18 | 25 | 47 |
| 20–34 | 37 | 5.5 | 38 | 1 | 1 | 4 | 7 | 11 | 24 | 32 |
| 35–49 | 48 | 4.8 | 15 | 1 | 2 | 4 | 6 | 7 | 10 | 15 |
| 50–64 | 62 | 8.0 | 102 | 1 | 2 | 4 | 10 | 13 | 16 | 35 |
| 65+ | 112 | 5.7 | 36 | 1 | 2 | 3 | 7 | 14 | 19 | 27 |
| **TOTAL SINGLE DX** | 162 | 2.5 | 4 | 1 | 1 | 1 | 4 | 6 | 6 | 8 |
| **TOTAL MULTIPLE DX** | 1,274 | 7.9 | 67 | 1 | 3 | 6 | 9 | 17 | 24 | 45 |
| **TOTAL** | | | | | | | | | | |
| 0–19 Years | 1,155 | 7.8 | 68 | 1 | 3 | 6 | 9 | 17 | 24 | 47 |
| 20–34 | 42 | 5.4 | 37 | 1 | 1 | 4 | 7 | 11 | 24 | 32 |
| 35–49 | 56 | 4.5 | 15 | 1 | 2 | 4 | 6 | 7 | 10 | 15 |
| 50–64 | 65 | 7.8 | 100 | 1 | 2 | 7 | 10 | 13 | 16 | 35 |
| 65+ | 118 | 5.5 | 35 | 1 | 3 | 3 | 7 | 13 | 19 | 27 |
| **GRAND TOTAL** | 1,436 | 7.4 | 64 | 1 | 3 | 6 | 9 | 15 | 23 | 43 |

Length of Stay by Diagnosis and Operation, United States, 2000

# United States, October 1998–September 1999 Data, by Operation

## 35.94: CREAT CONDUIT ATRIUM-PA. Formerly included in operation group(s) 572.

| Type of Patients | Observed Patients | Avg. Stay | Variance | 10th | 25th | 50th | 75th | 90th | 95th | 99th |
|---|---|---|---|---|---|---|---|---|---|---|
| **1. SINGLE DX** | | | | | | | | | | |
| 0–19 Years | 21 | 5.4 | 3 | 3 | 4 | 5 | 6 | 7 | 8 | 14 |
| 20–34 | 0 | | | | | | | | | |
| 35–49 | 0 | | | | | | | | | |
| 50–64 | 0 | | | | | | | | | |
| 65+ | 0 | | | | | | | | | |
| **2. MULTIPLE DX** | | | | | | | | | | |
| 0–19 Years | 480 | 9.9 | 58 | 4 | 5 | 7 | 11 | 19 | 24 | 43 |
| 20–34 | 6 | 14.0 | 55 | 4 | 9 | 11 | 24 | 24 | 24 | 24 |
| 35–49 | 1 | 15.0 | 0 | 15 | 15 | 15 | 15 | 15 | 15 | 15 |
| 50–64 | 0 | | | | | | | | | |
| 65+ | 0 | | | | | | | | | |
| **TOTAL SINGLE DX** | 21 | 5.4 | 3 | 3 | 4 | 5 | 6 | 7 | 8 | 14 |
| **TOTAL MULTIPLE DX** | 487 | 9.9 | 58 | 4 | 5 | 7 | 11 | 20 | 24 | 43 |
| **TOTAL** | | | | | | | | | | |
| 0–19 Years | 501 | 9.6 | 56 | 4 | 5 | 7 | 11 | 19 | 24 | 43 |
| 20–34 | 6 | 14.0 | 55 | 4 | 9 | 11 | 24 | 24 | 24 | 24 |
| 35–49 | 1 | 15.0 | 0 | 15 | 15 | 15 | 15 | 15 | 15 | 15 |
| 50–64 | 0 | | | | | | | | | |
| 65+ | 0 | | | | | | | | | |
| **GRAND TOTAL** | 508 | 9.6 | 56 | 4 | 5 | 7 | 11 | 19 | 24 | 43 |

## 35.96: PERC VALVULOPLASTY. Formerly included in operation group(s) 572.

| Type of Patients | Observed Patients | Avg. Stay | Variance | 10th | 25th | 50th | 75th | 90th | 95th | 99th |
|---|---|---|---|---|---|---|---|---|---|---|
| **1. SINGLE DX** | | | | | | | | | | |
| 0–19 Years | 111 | 1.5 | 1 | 1 | 1 | 1 | 1 | 3 | 5 | 5 |
| 20–34 | 5 | 1.4 | <1 | 1 | 1 | 1 | 2 | 2 | 2 | 2 |
| 35–49 | 8 | 1.3 | <1 | 1 | 1 | 1 | 2 | 2 | 2 | 2 |
| 50–64 | 3 | 1.3 | <1 | 1 | 1 | 1 | 2 | 2 | 2 | 2 |
| 65+ | 6 | 1.2 | <1 | 1 | 1 | 1 | 1 | 2 | 2 | 2 |
| **2. MULTIPLE DX** | | | | | | | | | | |
| 0–19 Years | 237 | 4.3 | 66 | 1 | 1 | 1 | 3 | 12 | 19 | 36 |
| 20–34 | 14 | 2.4 | 7 | 1 | 2 | 3 | 6 | 6 | 6 | 15 |
| 35–49 | 32 | 3.7 | 6 | 1 | 1 | 3 | 6 | 6 | 13 | 10 |
| 50–64 | 41 | 6.2 | 124 | 1 | 1 | 2 | 10 | 13 | 13 | 99 |
| 65+ | 93 | 5.0 | 32 | 1 | 1 | 3 | 6 | 11 | 19 | 27 |
| **TOTAL SINGLE DX** | 133 | 1.5 | <1 | 1 | 1 | 1 | 2 | 3 | 4 | 5 |
| **TOTAL MULTIPLE DX** | 417 | 4.4 | 53 | 1 | 1 | 2 | 5 | 10 | 16 | 30 |
| **TOTAL** | | | | | | | | | | |
| 0–19 Years | 348 | 3.5 | 49 | 1 | 1 | 1 | 2 | 7 | 16 | 33 |
| 20–34 | 19 | 2.4 | 6 | 1 | 1 | 2 | 6 | 6 | 6 | 15 |
| 35–49 | 40 | 3.4 | 6 | 1 | 2 | 2 | 6 | 6 | 13 | 10 |
| 50–64 | 44 | 6.0 | 119 | 1 | 1 | 2 | 10 | 13 | 13 | 99 |
| 65+ | 99 | 4.8 | 31 | 1 | 1 | 3 | 5 | 11 | 19 | 27 |
| **GRAND TOTAL** | 550 | 3.8 | 44 | 1 | 1 | 1 | 4 | 9 | 14 | 30 |

## 36.0: RMVL COR ART OBSTR/STENT. Formerly included in operation group(s) 573, 579.

| Type of Patients | Observed Patients | Avg. Stay | Variance | 10th | 25th | 50th | 75th | 90th | 95th | 99th |
|---|---|---|---|---|---|---|---|---|---|---|
| **1. SINGLE DX** | | | | | | | | | | |
| 0–19 Years | 11 | 1.1 | <1 | 1 | 1 | 1 | 1 | 1 | 2 | 2 |
| 20–34 | 15 | 1.6 | <1 | 1 | 1 | 1 | 2 | 3 | 4 | 4 |
| 35–49 | 540 | 1.8 | 1 | 1 | 1 | 1 | 2 | 3 | 5 | 6 |
| 50–64 | 1,393 | 1.6 | 1 | 1 | 1 | 1 | 2 | 3 | 4 | 6 |
| 65+ | 1,460 | 1.5 | 1 | 1 | 1 | 1 | 2 | 3 | 3 | 5 |
| **2. MULTIPLE DX** | | | | | | | | | | |
| 0–19 Years | 72 | 4.1 | 49 | 1 | 1 | 3 | 5 | 13 | 13 | 55 |
| 20–34 | 685 | 3.2 | 9 | 1 | 2 | 3 | 4 | 5 | 7 | 15 |
| 35–49 | 18,116 | 2.9 | 5 | 1 | 1 | 2 | 4 | 5 | 7 | 11 |
| 50–64 | 51,644 | 2.8 | 6 | 1 | 1 | 2 | 4 | 5 | 7 | 12 |
| 65+ | 66,397 | 3.6 | 13 | 1 | 1 | 2 | 4 | 7 | 10 | 18 |
| **TOTAL SINGLE DX** | 3,419 | 1.6 | 1 | 1 | 1 | 1 | 2 | 3 | 3 | 6 |
| **TOTAL MULTIPLE DX** | 136,914 | 3.2 | 10 | 1 | 1 | 2 | 4 | 6 | 8 | 15 |
| **TOTAL** | | | | | | | | | | |
| 0–19 Years | 83 | 3.9 | 46 | 1 | 1 | 1 | 4 | 12 | 13 | 55 |
| 20–34 | 700 | 3.2 | 9 | 1 | 2 | 3 | 4 | 5 | 6 | 14 |
| 35–49 | 18,656 | 2.8 | 5 | 1 | 1 | 2 | 4 | 5 | 7 | 11 |
| 50–64 | 53,037 | 2.7 | 6 | 1 | 1 | 2 | 4 | 5 | 7 | 11 |
| 65+ | 67,857 | 3.5 | 13 | 1 | 1 | 2 | 4 | 7 | 10 | 18 |
| **GRAND TOTAL** | 140,333 | 3.1 | 9 | 1 | 1 | 2 | 4 | 6 | 8 | 15 |

## 36.01: 1 PTCA/ATHERECT W/O TL. Formerly included in operation group(s) 573.

| Type of Patients | Observed Patients | Avg. Stay | Variance | 10th | 25th | 50th | 75th | 90th | 95th | 99th |
|---|---|---|---|---|---|---|---|---|---|---|
| **1. SINGLE DX** | | | | | | | | | | |
| 0–19 Years | 7 | 1.0 | 0 | 1 | 1 | 1 | 1 | 1 | 1 | 1 |
| 20–34 | 14 | 1.5 | <1 | 1 | 1 | 1 | 2 | 3 | 3 | 4 |
| 35–49 | 454 | 1.8 | 1 | 1 | 1 | 1 | 2 | 3 | 5 | 6 |
| 50–64 | 1,126 | 1.6 | 1 | 1 | 1 | 1 | 2 | 3 | 3 | 6 |
| 65+ | 1,191 | 1.5 | 1 | 1 | 1 | 1 | 2 | 3 | 3 | 5 |
| **2. MULTIPLE DX** | | | | | | | | | | |
| 0–19 Years | 54 | 3.5 | 56 | 1 | 1 | 2 | 2 | 9 | 12 | 55 |
| 20–34 | 549 | 3.2 | 9 | 1 | 2 | 3 | 4 | 5 | 6 | 17 |
| 35–49 | 14,356 | 2.8 | 5 | 1 | 1 | 2 | 4 | 5 | 7 | 11 |
| 50–64 | 40,451 | 2.8 | 6 | 1 | 1 | 2 | 4 | 5 | 7 | 11 |
| 65+ | 51,711 | 3.5 | 13 | 1 | 1 | 2 | 4 | 7 | 10 | 18 |
| **TOTAL SINGLE DX** | 2,792 | 1.6 | 1 | 1 | 1 | 1 | 2 | 3 | 4 | 6 |
| **TOTAL MULTIPLE DX** | 107,121 | 3.1 | 9 | 1 | 1 | 2 | 4 | 6 | 8 | 15 |
| **TOTAL** | | | | | | | | | | |
| 0–19 Years | 61 | 3.3 | 52 | 1 | 1 | 1 | 2 | 9 | 12 | 55 |
| 20–34 | 563 | 3.2 | 9 | 1 | 2 | 3 | 4 | 5 | 6 | 17 |
| 35–49 | 14,810 | 2.8 | 5 | 1 | 1 | 2 | 4 | 5 | 7 | 11 |
| 50–64 | 41,577 | 2.7 | 6 | 1 | 1 | 2 | 4 | 5 | 7 | 11 |
| 65+ | 52,902 | 3.5 | 13 | 1 | 1 | 2 | 4 | 7 | 10 | 18 |
| **GRAND TOTAL** | 109,913 | 3.1 | 9 | 1 | 1 | 2 | 4 | 6 | 8 | 15 |

Length of Stay by Diagnosis and Operation, United States, 2000

# United States, October 1998–September 1999 Data, by Operation

## 36.02: 1 PTCA/ATHERECT W TL. Formerly included in operation group(s) 573.

| Type of Patients | Observed Patients | Avg. Stay | Vari-ance | Percentiles 10th | 25th | 50th | 75th | 90th | 95th | 99th |
|---|---|---|---|---|---|---|---|---|---|---|
| **1. SINGLE DX** | | | | | | | | | | |
| 0–19 Years | 0 | | | | | | | | | |
| 20–34 | 0 | | | | | | | | | |
| 35–49 | 25 | 2.2 | 1 | 1 | 1 | 2 | 3 | 4 | 5 | 5 |
| 50–64 | 52 | 2.0 | 2 | 1 | 1 | 2 | 2 | 4 | 5 | 5 |
| 65+ | 49 | 1.5 | <1 | 1 | 1 | 1 | 2 | 2 | 4 | 4 |
| **2. MULTIPLE DX** | | | | | | | | | | |
| 0–19 Years | 3 | 5.0 | 10 | 1 | 3 | 3 | 8 | 8 | 8 | 8 |
| 20–34 | 34 | 3.7 | 3 | 2 | 3 | 3 | 4 | 5 | 7 | 12 |
| 35–49 | 943 | 3.4 | 5 | 1 | 2 | 3 | 4 | 6 | 8 | 10 |
| 50–64 | 2,444 | 3.0 | 5 | 1 | 1 | 3 | 4 | 5 | 7 | 12 |
| 65+ | 2,597 | 3.8 | 12 | 1 | 1 | 3 | 5 | 8 | 10 | 16 |
| **TOTAL SINGLE DX** | 126 | 1.8 | 1 | 1 | 1 | 1 | 2 | 4 | 4 | 5 |
| **TOTAL MULTIPLE DX** | 6,021 | 3.4 | 8 | 1 | 1 | 3 | 4 | 6 | 8 | 14 |
| **TOTAL** | | | | | | | | | | |
| 0–19 Years | 3 | 5.0 | 10 | 1 | 3 | 3 | 8 | 8 | 8 | 8 |
| 20–34 | 34 | 3.7 | 3 | 2 | 3 | 3 | 4 | 5 | 7 | 12 |
| 35–49 | 968 | 3.4 | 5 | 1 | 2 | 3 | 4 | 6 | 8 | 10 |
| 50–64 | 2,496 | 2.9 | 5 | 1 | 1 | 3 | 4 | 5 | 7 | 12 |
| 65+ | 2,646 | 3.7 | 12 | 1 | 1 | 3 | 5 | 8 | 10 | 16 |
| **GRAND TOTAL** | 6,147 | 3.3 | 8 | 1 | 1 | 3 | 4 | 6 | 8 | 14 |

## 36.06: INSERT CORONARY STENT. Formerly included in operation group(s) 573.

| Type of Patients | Observed Patients | Avg. Stay | Vari-ance | Percentiles 10th | 25th | 50th | 75th | 90th | 95th | 99th |
|---|---|---|---|---|---|---|---|---|---|---|
| **1. SINGLE DX** | | | | | | | | | | |
| 0–19 Years | 1 | 1.0 | 0 | 1 | 1 | 1 | 1 | 1 | 1 | 1 |
| 20–34 | 0 | | | | | | | | | |
| 35–49 | 10 | 1.6 | <1 | 1 | 1 | 1 | 2 | 3 | 3 | 3 |
| 50–64 | 28 | 1.2 | <1 | 1 | 1 | 1 | 1 | 2 | 2 | 5 |
| 65+ | 23 | 1.5 | <1 | 1 | 1 | 1 | 2 | 4 | 4 | 4 |
| **2. MULTIPLE DX** | | | | | | | | | | |
| 0–19 Years | 8 | 1.4 | 1 | 1 | 1 | 1 | 1 | 2 | 4 | 5 |
| 20–34 | 25 | 2.7 | 6 | 1 | 1 | 2 | 4 | 6 | 6 | 15 |
| 35–49 | 590 | 3.2 | 18 | 1 | 1 | 2 | 4 | 5 | 6 | 20 |
| 50–64 | 1,648 | 3.0 | 8 | 1 | 1 | 2 | 4 | 6 | 7 | 14 |
| 65+ | 2,028 | 4.5 | 22 | 1 | 1 | 3 | 6 | 10 | 14 | 23 |
| **TOTAL SINGLE DX** | 62 | 1.4 | <1 | 1 | 1 | 1 | 1 | 2 | 4 | 5 |
| **TOTAL MULTIPLE DX** | 4,299 | 3.7 | 16 | 1 | 1 | 3 | 4 | 7 | 11 | 22 |
| **TOTAL** | | | | | | | | | | |
| 0–19 Years | 9 | 1.4 | <1 | 1 | 1 | 1 | 1 | 2 | 4 | 5 |
| 20–34 | 25 | 2.7 | 6 | 1 | 1 | 2 | 4 | 6 | 6 | 15 |
| 35–49 | 600 | 3.1 | 17 | 1 | 1 | 2 | 4 | 5 | 6 | 20 |
| 50–64 | 1,676 | 2.9 | 8 | 1 | 1 | 2 | 4 | 6 | 7 | 14 |
| 65+ | 2,051 | 4.4 | 22 | 1 | 1 | 3 | 6 | 10 | 14 | 23 |
| **GRAND TOTAL** | 4,361 | 3.7 | 16 | 1 | 1 | 2 | 4 | 7 | 11 | 21 |

## 36.05: PTCA/ATHERECT-MULT VESS. Formerly included in operation group(s) 573.

| Type of Patients | Observed Patients | Avg. Stay | Vari-ance | Percentiles 10th | 25th | 50th | 75th | 90th | 95th | 99th |
|---|---|---|---|---|---|---|---|---|---|---|
| **1. SINGLE DX** | | | | | | | | | | |
| 0–19 Years | 2 | 1.5 | <1 | 1 | 1 | 1 | 2 | 2 | 2 | 2 |
| 20–34 | 1 | 4.0 | 0 | 4 | 4 | 4 | 4 | 4 | 4 | 4 |
| 35–49 | 51 | 1.5 | <1 | 1 | 1 | 1 | 2 | 3 | 3 | 5 |
| 50–64 | 186 | 1.5 | <1 | 1 | 1 | 1 | 2 | 3 | 3 | 5 |
| 65+ | 196 | 1.3 | <1 | 1 | 1 | 1 | 1 | 2 | 2 | 4 |
| **2. MULTIPLE DX** | | | | | | | | | | |
| 0–19 Years | 5 | 1.6 | <1 | 1 | 1 | 1 | 2 | 3 | 3 | 3 |
| 20–34 | 74 | 2.4 | 5 | 1 | 1 | 2 | 3 | 4 | 6 | 14 |
| 35–49 | 2,206 | 2.8 | 5 | 1 | 1 | 2 | 4 | 5 | 7 | 11 |
| 50–64 | 7,037 | 2.7 | 7 | 1 | 1 | 2 | 3 | 5 | 7 | 13 |
| 65+ | 9,967 | 3.5 | 12 | 1 | 1 | 2 | 4 | 7 | 10 | 17 |
| **TOTAL SINGLE DX** | 436 | 1.4 | <1 | 1 | 1 | 1 | 1 | 2 | 3 | 4 |
| **TOTAL MULTIPLE DX** | 19,289 | 3.1 | 10 | 1 | 1 | 2 | 4 | 6 | 9 | 16 |
| **TOTAL** | | | | | | | | | | |
| 0–19 Years | 7 | 1.6 | <1 | 1 | 1 | 1 | 2 | 3 | 3 | 3 |
| 20–34 | 75 | 2.4 | 5 | 1 | 1 | 2 | 3 | 4 | 6 | 14 |
| 35–49 | 2,257 | 2.7 | 5 | 1 | 1 | 2 | 4 | 5 | 7 | 11 |
| 50–64 | 7,223 | 2.7 | 7 | 1 | 1 | 2 | 3 | 5 | 7 | 13 |
| 65+ | 10,163 | 3.4 | 12 | 1 | 1 | 2 | 4 | 7 | 10 | 17 |
| **GRAND TOTAL** | 19,725 | 3.1 | 9 | 1 | 1 | 2 | 4 | 6 | 8 | 15 |

## 36.1: HRT REVASC BYPASS ANAST. Formerly included in operation group(s) 574.

| Type of Patients | Observed Patients | Avg. Stay | Vari-ance | Percentiles 10th | 25th | 50th | 75th | 90th | 95th | 99th |
|---|---|---|---|---|---|---|---|---|---|---|
| **1. SINGLE DX** | | | | | | | | | | |
| 0–19 Years | 2 | 9.0 | 37 | 3 | 3 | 13 | 13 | 13 | 13 | 13 |
| 20–34 | 1 | 7.0 | 0 | 7 | 7 | 7 | 7 | 7 | 7 | 7 |
| 35–49 | 57 | 5.0 | 2 | 3 | 4 | 5 | 6 | 6 | 7 | 8 |
| 50–64 | 229 | 5.3 | 2 | 4 | 4 | 5 | 6 | 7 | 9 | 10 |
| 65+ | 205 | 6.1 | 4 | 4 | 5 | 5 | 8 | 9 | 9 | 9 |
| **2. MULTIPLE DX** | | | | | | | | | | |
| 0–19 Years | 9 | 5.9 | 36 | 1 | 1 | 5 | 6 | 13 | 25 | 25 |
| 20–34 | 199 | 7.0 | 13 | 3 | 5 | 6 | 8 | 10 | 15 | 21 |
| 35–49 | 7,449 | 7.0 | 17 | 4 | 5 | 6 | 8 | 11 | 13 | 22 |
| 50–64 | 31,238 | 7.6 | 22 | 4 | 5 | 6 | 9 | 12 | 15 | 27 |
| 65+ | 44,014 | 9.3 | 38 | 5 | 6 | 8 | 11 | 16 | 20 | 34 |
| **TOTAL SINGLE DX** | 494 | 5.7 | 3 | 4 | 5 | 5 | 7 | 9 | 9 | 10 |
| **TOTAL MULTIPLE DX** | 82,909 | 8.5 | 31 | 4 | 5 | 7 | 10 | 14 | 18 | 30 |
| **TOTAL** | | | | | | | | | | |
| 0–19 Years | 11 | 6.3 | 35 | 1 | 3 | 5 | 6 | 13 | 25 | 25 |
| 20–34 | 200 | 7.0 | 13 | 3 | 5 | 6 | 8 | 10 | 15 | 21 |
| 35–49 | 7,506 | 7.0 | 17 | 4 | 5 | 6 | 8 | 11 | 13 | 22 |
| 50–64 | 31,467 | 7.5 | 22 | 4 | 5 | 6 | 9 | 12 | 15 | 26 |
| 65+ | 44,219 | 9.3 | 38 | 5 | 6 | 8 | 11 | 16 | 20 | 34 |
| **GRAND TOTAL** | 83,403 | 8.4 | 31 | 4 | 5 | 7 | 10 | 14 | 18 | 30 |

Length of Stay by Diagnosis and Operation, United States, 2000

# United States, October 1998–September 1999 Data, by Operation

## 36.11: AO-COR BYPASS-1 COR ART. Formerly included in operation group(s) 574.

| Type of Patients | Observed Patients | Avg. Stay | Variance | 10th | 25th | 50th | 75th | 90th | 95th | 99th |
|---|---|---|---|---|---|---|---|---|---|---|
| **1. SINGLE DX** | | | | | | | | | | |
| 0–19 Years | 1 | 13.0 | 0 | 13 | 13 | 13 | 13 | 13 | 13 | 13 |
| 20–34 | 0 | | | | | | | | | |
| 35–49 | 10 | 4.7 | 2 | 3 | 4 | 6 | 6 | 7 | 7 | 7 |
| 50–64 | 21 | 4.8 | 3 | 3 | 4 | 5 | 5 | 8 | 8 | 10 |
| 65+ | 27 | 5.7 | 2 | 4 | 5 | 7 | 7 | 8 | 9 | 9 |
| **2. MULTIPLE DX** | | | | | | | | | | |
| 0–19 Years | 2 | 11.4 | 116 | 5 | 5 | 5 | 25 | 25 | 25 | 25 |
| 20–34 | 43 | 7.0 | 14 | 4 | 4 | 7 | 9 | 11 | 14 | 21 |
| 35–49 | 1,088 | 6.8 | 15 | 4 | 5 | 6 | 8 | 11 | 12 | 22 |
| 50–64 | 3,653 | 7.0 | 26 | 4 | 5 | 6 | 8 | 11 | 14 | 22 |
| 65+ | 4,053 | 9.1 | 52 | 4 | 5 | 7 | 10 | 15 | 19 | 36 |
| **TOTAL SINGLE DX** | 59 | 5.3 | 4 | 4 | 4 | 5 | 7 | 8 | 9 | 13 |
| **TOTAL MULTIPLE DX** | 8,839 | 8.0 | 37 | 4 | 5 | 7 | 9 | 13 | 16 | 31 |
| **TOTAL** | | | | | | | | | | |
| 0–19 Years | 3 | 11.9 | 75 | 5 | 5 | 13 | 13 | 25 | 25 | 25 |
| 20–34 | 43 | 7.0 | 14 | 4 | 4 | 7 | 9 | 11 | 14 | 21 |
| 35–49 | 1,098 | 6.8 | 14 | 4 | 5 | 6 | 8 | 11 | 12 | 22 |
| 50–64 | 3,674 | 7.0 | 26 | 4 | 5 | 6 | 8 | 11 | 14 | 22 |
| 65+ | 4,080 | 9.1 | 52 | 4 | 5 | 7 | 10 | 15 | 19 | 36 |
| **GRAND TOTAL** | 8,898 | 7.9 | 37 | 4 | 5 | 7 | 9 | 13 | 16 | 31 |

## 36.13: AO-COR BYPASS-3 COR ART. Formerly included in operation group(s) 574.

| Type of Patients | Observed Patients | Avg. Stay | Variance | 10th | 25th | 50th | 75th | 90th | 95th | 99th |
|---|---|---|---|---|---|---|---|---|---|---|
| **1. SINGLE DX** | | | | | | | | | | |
| 0–19 Years | 0 | | | | | | | | | |
| 20–34 | 0 | | | | | | | | | |
| 35–49 | 11 | 5.9 | 2 | 5 | 6 | 6 | 6 | 7 | 8 | 13 |
| 50–64 | 58 | 5.2 | 2 | 4 | 4 | 5 | 6 | 7 | 7 | 10 |
| 65+ | 51 | 5.6 | 6 | 4 | 4 | 5 | 7 | 8 | 9 | 20 |
| **2. MULTIPLE DX** | | | | | | | | | | |
| 0–19 Years | 1 | 13.0 | 0 | 13 | 13 | 13 | 13 | 13 | 13 | 13 |
| 20–34 | 47 | 7.3 | 18 | 4 | 6 | 6 | 7 | 11 | 17 | 26 |
| 35–49 | 1,890 | 7.4 | 21 | 4 | 5 | 6 | 9 | 11 | 14 | 22 |
| 50–64 | 8,849 | 7.9 | 26 | 5 | 6 | 7 | 9 | 13 | 16 | 30 |
| 65+ | 13,445 | 9.7 | 37 | 5 | 6 | 8 | 11 | 16 | 21 | 34 |
| **TOTAL SINGLE DX** | 120 | 5.5 | 3 | 4 | 4 | 5 | 6 | 7 | 8 | 10 |
| **TOTAL MULTIPLE DX** | 24,232 | 8.9 | 33 | 4 | 6 | 7 | 10 | 15 | 19 | 31 |
| **TOTAL** | | | | | | | | | | |
| 0–19 Years | 1 | 13.0 | 0 | 13 | 13 | 13 | 13 | 13 | 13 | 13 |
| 20–34 | 47 | 7.3 | 18 | 4 | 6 | 6 | 7 | 11 | 17 | 26 |
| 35–49 | 1,901 | 7.4 | 21 | 4 | 5 | 6 | 9 | 11 | 14 | 22 |
| 50–64 | 8,907 | 7.9 | 26 | 5 | 6 | 7 | 9 | 13 | 16 | 30 |
| 65+ | 13,496 | 9.6 | 37 | 5 | 6 | 8 | 11 | 16 | 21 | 34 |
| **GRAND TOTAL** | 24,352 | 8.9 | 33 | 4 | 6 | 7 | 10 | 15 | 19 | 30 |

## 36.12: AO-COR BYPASS-2 COR ART. Formerly included in operation group(s) 574.

| Type of Patients | Observed Patients | Avg. Stay | Variance | 10th | 25th | 50th | 75th | 90th | 95th | 99th |
|---|---|---|---|---|---|---|---|---|---|---|
| **1. SINGLE DX** | | | | | | | | | | |
| 0–19 Years | 0 | | | | | | | | | |
| 20–34 | 0 | | | | | | | | | |
| 35–49 | 12 | 4.3 | 1 | 3 | 3 | 4 | 6 | 6 | 6 | 6 |
| 50–64 | 78 | 5.4 | 2 | 4 | 4 | 5 | 7 | 7 | 8 | 11 |
| 65+ | 57 | 5.9 | 3 | 4 | 5 | 6 | 6 | 8 | 9 | 13 |
| **2. MULTIPLE DX** | | | | | | | | | | |
| 0–19 Years | 2 | 3.3 | 7 | 1 | 1 | 1 | 6 | 6 | 6 | 6 |
| 20–34 | 38 | 6.7 | 8 | 3 | 4 | 6 | 10 | 10 | 10 | 11 |
| 35–49 | 1,925 | 7.0 | 14 | 4 | 5 | 7 | 8 | 11 | 14 | 21 |
| 50–64 | 8,375 | 7.4 | 18 | 4 | 5 | 7 | 9 | 12 | 14 | 24 |
| 65+ | 11,497 | 9.2 | 32 | 5 | 6 | 8 | 11 | 15 | 19 | 34 |
| **TOTAL SINGLE DX** | 147 | 5.6 | 3 | 4 | 5 | 6 | 6 | 8 | 8 | 11 |
| **TOTAL MULTIPLE DX** | 21,837 | 8.3 | 26 | 4 | 5 | 7 | 10 | 14 | 17 | 29 |
| **TOTAL** | | | | | | | | | | |
| 0–19 Years | 2 | 3.3 | 7 | 1 | 1 | 1 | 6 | 6 | 6 | 6 |
| 20–34 | 38 | 6.7 | 8 | 3 | 4 | 6 | 10 | 10 | 10 | 11 |
| 35–49 | 1,937 | 6.9 | 14 | 4 | 5 | 7 | 8 | 11 | 14 | 21 |
| 50–64 | 8,453 | 7.4 | 18 | 4 | 5 | 7 | 9 | 12 | 14 | 24 |
| 65+ | 11,554 | 9.2 | 32 | 5 | 6 | 8 | 11 | 15 | 19 | 33 |
| **GRAND TOTAL** | 21,984 | 8.3 | 26 | 4 | 5 | 7 | 10 | 14 | 17 | 29 |

## 36.14: AO-COR BYPASS-4+ COR ART. Formerly included in operation group(s) 574.

| Type of Patients | Observed Patients | Avg. Stay | Variance | 10th | 25th | 50th | 75th | 90th | 95th | 99th |
|---|---|---|---|---|---|---|---|---|---|---|
| **1. SINGLE DX** | | | | | | | | | | |
| 0–19 Years | 0 | | | | | | | | | |
| 20–34 | 0 | | | | | | | | | |
| 35–49 | 8 | 5.3 | 2 | 4 | 5 | 5 | 6 | 8 | 8 | 8 |
| 50–64 | 35 | 5.6 | 1 | 5 | 5 | 5 | 7 | 7 | 7 | 7 |
| 65+ | 43 | 6.4 | 4 | 5 | 5 | 5 | 9 | 9 | 9 | 9 |
| **2. MULTIPLE DX** | | | | | | | | | | |
| 0–19 Years | 0 | | | | | | | | | |
| 20–34 | 28 | 8.1 | 14 | 5 | 6 | 6 | 10 | 15 | 15 | 15 |
| 35–49 | 1,140 | 7.5 | 18 | 4 | 5 | 7 | 9 | 10 | 14 | 26 |
| 50–64 | 5,415 | 8.0 | 19 | 4 | 5 | 7 | 9 | 13 | 16 | 25 |
| 65+ | 8,843 | 9.7 | 43 | 5 | 6 | 8 | 11 | 16 | 21 | 36 |
| **TOTAL SINGLE DX** | 86 | 6.2 | 3 | 5 | 5 | 5 | 9 | 9 | 9 | 9 |
| **TOTAL MULTIPLE DX** | 15,426 | 9.0 | 34 | 4 | 6 | 7 | 10 | 15 | 19 | 32 |
| **TOTAL** | | | | | | | | | | |
| 0–19 Years | 0 | | | | | | | | | |
| 20–34 | 28 | 8.1 | 14 | 5 | 6 | 6 | 10 | 15 | 15 | 15 |
| 35–49 | 1,148 | 7.5 | 18 | 4 | 5 | 7 | 9 | 10 | 14 | 26 |
| 50–64 | 5,450 | 8.0 | 19 | 4 | 5 | 7 | 9 | 13 | 16 | 25 |
| 65+ | 8,886 | 9.6 | 42 | 5 | 6 | 8 | 11 | 16 | 21 | 36 |
| **GRAND TOTAL** | 15,512 | 8.9 | 33 | 4 | 6 | 7 | 10 | 15 | 18 | 32 |

Length of Stay by Diagnosis and Operation, United States, 2000

# United States, October 1998–September 1999 Data, by Operation

## 36.15: 1 INT MAM-COR ART BYPASS. Formerly included in operation group(s) 574.

| Type of Patients | Observed Patients | Avg. Stay | Vari-ance | Percentiles | | | | | | |
|---|---|---|---|---|---|---|---|---|---|---|
| | | | | 10th | 25th | 50th | 75th | 90th | 95th | 99th |
| **1. SINGLE DX** | | | | | | | | | | |
| 0–19 Years | 1 | 3.0 | 0 | 3 | 3 | 3 | 3 | 3 | 3 | 3 |
| 20–34 | 1 | 7.0 | 0 | 7 | 7 | 7 | 7 | 7 | 7 | 7 |
| 35–49 | 12 | 4.3 | <1 | 3 | 4 | 4 | 5 | 5 | 5 | 5 |
| 50–64 | 33 | 5.0 | 4 | 3 | 3 | 4 | 7 | 7 | 8 | 13 |
| 65+ | 26 | 5.0 | 4 | 2 | 4 | 5 | 6 | 7 | 9 | 11 |
| **2. MULTIPLE DX** | | | | | | | | | | |
| 0–19 Years | 3 | 5.0 | 4 | 3 | 3 | 5 | 7 | 7 | 7 | 7 |
| 20–34 | 32 | 6.4 | 14 | 3 | 4 | 6 | 7 | 11 | 16 | 19 |
| 35–49 | 1,177 | 6.4 | 17 | 3 | 4 | 5 | 7 | 10 | 12 | 22 |
| 50–64 | 4,341 | 7.1 | 21 | 4 | 5 | 6 | 8 | 11 | 15 | 25 |
| 65+ | 5,762 | 8.5 | 35 | 4 | 5 | 7 | 10 | 15 | 20 | 34 |
| **TOTAL SINGLE DX** | 73 | 4.9 | 4 | 3 | 4 | 4 | 6 | 7 | 8 | 11 |
| **TOTAL MULTIPLE DX** | 11,315 | 7.8 | 29 | 4 | 5 | 6 | 9 | 13 | 17 | 29 |
| **TOTAL** | | | | | | | | | | |
| 0–19 Years | 4 | 4.5 | 3 | 3 | 3 | 3 | 5 | 7 | 7 | 7 |
| 20–34 | 33 | 6.4 | 14 | 3 | 4 | 6 | 7 | 11 | 16 | 19 |
| 35–49 | 1,189 | 6.4 | 17 | 3 | 4 | 5 | 7 | 10 | 12 | 22 |
| 50–64 | 4,374 | 7.1 | 21 | 4 | 4 | 6 | 8 | 11 | 15 | 25 |
| 65+ | 5,788 | 8.5 | 35 | 4 | 5 | 7 | 10 | 15 | 20 | 34 |
| **GRAND TOTAL** | 11,388 | 7.8 | 28 | 4 | 5 | 6 | 9 | 13 | 17 | 29 |

## 36.16: 2 INT MAM-COR ART BYPASS. Formerly included in operation group(s) 574.

| Type of Patients | Observed Patients | Avg. Stay | Vari-ance | Percentiles | | | | | | |
|---|---|---|---|---|---|---|---|---|---|---|
| | | | | 10th | 25th | 50th | 75th | 90th | 95th | 99th |
| **1. SINGLE DX** | | | | | | | | | | |
| 0–19 Years | 0 | | | | | | | | | |
| 20–34 | 0 | | | | | | | | | |
| 35–49 | 4 | 3.3 | 3 | 2 | 2 | 3 | 3 | 6 | 6 | 6 |
| 50–64 | 4 | 4.7 | <1 | 4 | 4 | 5 | 5 | 5 | 5 | 7 |
| 65+ | 1 | 4.0 | 0 | 4 | 4 | 4 | 4 | 4 | 4 | 4 |
| **2. MULTIPLE DX** | | | | | | | | | | |
| 0–19 Years | 1 | 5.0 | 0 | 5 | 5 | 5 | 5 | 5 | 5 | 5 |
| 20–34 | 9 | 5.7 | <1 | 4 | 6 | 6 | 6 | 6 | 7 | 7 |
| 35–49 | 198 | 6.7 | 11 | 4 | 5 | 6 | 8 | 10 | 12 | 16 |
| 50–64 | 507 | 7.1 | 28 | 4 | 5 | 6 | 8 | 11 | 13 | 24 |
| 65+ | 336 | 7.7 | 17 | 4 | 5 | 7 | 9 | 12 | 15 | 28 |
| **TOTAL SINGLE DX** | 9 | 4.4 | <1 | 3 | 4 | 5 | 5 | 5 | 5 | 6 |
| **TOTAL MULTIPLE DX** | 1,051 | 7.2 | 21 | 4 | 5 | 6 | 8 | 11 | 13 | 24 |
| **TOTAL** | | | | | | | | | | |
| 0–19 Years | 1 | 5.0 | 0 | 5 | 5 | 5 | 5 | 5 | 5 | 5 |
| 20–34 | 9 | 5.7 | <1 | 4 | 6 | 6 | 6 | 6 | 7 | 7 |
| 35–49 | 202 | 6.7 | 11 | 4 | 6 | 6 | 8 | 10 | 12 | 16 |
| 50–64 | 511 | 7.1 | 27 | 4 | 5 | 6 | 8 | 11 | 13 | 24 |
| 65+ | 337 | 7.7 | 17 | 4 | 5 | 7 | 9 | 12 | 15 | 28 |
| **GRAND TOTAL** | 1,060 | 7.2 | 21 | 4 | 5 | 6 | 8 | 11 | 13 | 24 |

## 36.2: ARTERIAL IMPLANT REVASC. Formerly included in operation group(s) 579.

| Type of Patients | Observed Patients | Avg. Stay | Vari-ance | Percentiles | | | | | | |
|---|---|---|---|---|---|---|---|---|---|---|
| | | | | 10th | 25th | 50th | 75th | 90th | 95th | 99th |
| **1. SINGLE DX** | | | | | | | | | | |
| 0–19 Years | 0 | | | | | | | | | |
| 20–34 | 0 | | | | | | | | | |
| 35–49 | 0 | | | | | | | | | |
| 50–64 | 0 | | | | | | | | | |
| 65+ | 0 | | | | | | | | | |
| **2. MULTIPLE DX** | | | | | | | | | | |
| 0–19 Years | 1 | 17.0 | 0 | 17 | 17 | 17 | 17 | 17 | 17 | 17 |
| 20–34 | 0 | | | | | | | | | |
| 35–49 | 1 | 6.0 | 0 | 6 | 6 | 6 | 6 | 6 | 6 | 6 |
| 50–64 | 1 | 9.0 | 0 | 9 | 9 | 9 | 9 | 9 | 9 | 9 |
| 65+ | 3 | 12.2 | 80 | 5 | 5 | 9 | 25 | 25 | 25 | 25 |
| **TOTAL SINGLE DX** | 0 | | | | | | | | | |
| **TOTAL MULTIPLE DX** | 6 | 11.6 | 63 | 5 | 5 | 9 | 17 | 25 | 25 | 25 |
| **TOTAL** | | | | | | | | | | |
| 0–19 Years | 1 | 17.0 | 0 | 17 | 17 | 17 | 17 | 17 | 17 | 17 |
| 20–34 | 0 | | | | | | | | | |
| 35–49 | 1 | 6.0 | 0 | 6 | 6 | 6 | 6 | 6 | 6 | 6 |
| 50–64 | 1 | 9.0 | 0 | 9 | 9 | 9 | 9 | 9 | 9 | 9 |
| 65+ | 3 | 12.2 | 80 | 5 | 5 | 9 | 25 | 25 | 25 | 25 |
| **GRAND TOTAL** | 6 | 11.6 | 63 | 5 | 5 | 9 | 17 | 25 | 25 | 25 |

## 36.3: HEART REVASC NEC. Formerly included in operation group(s) 579.

| Type of Patients | Observed Patients | Avg. Stay | Vari-ance | Percentiles | | | | | | |
|---|---|---|---|---|---|---|---|---|---|---|
| | | | | 10th | 25th | 50th | 75th | 90th | 95th | 99th |
| **1. SINGLE DX** | | | | | | | | | | |
| 0–19 Years | 0 | | | | | | | | | |
| 20–34 | 0 | | | | | | | | | |
| 35–49 | 0 | | | | | | | | | |
| 50–64 | 2 | 1.0 | 0 | 1 | 1 | 1 | 1 | 1 | 1 | 1 |
| 65+ | 1 | 1.0 | 0 | 1 | 1 | 1 | 1 | 1 | 1 | 1 |
| **2. MULTIPLE DX** | | | | | | | | | | |
| 0–19 Years | 1 | 10.0 | 0 | 10 | 10 | 10 | 10 | 10 | 10 | 10 |
| 20–34 | 2 | 4.0 | 0 | 4 | 4 | 4 | 4 | 4 | 4 | 4 |
| 35–49 | 26 | 4.9 | 3 | 3 | 4 | 5 | 6 | 7 | 8 | 9 |
| 50–64 | 165 | 5.7 | 34 | 1 | 3 | 5 | 6 | 9 | 13 | 26 |
| 65+ | 136 | 5.6 | 17 | 1 | 3 | 4 | 7 | 12 | 14 | 17 |
| **TOTAL SINGLE DX** | 3 | 1.0 | 0 | 1 | 1 | 1 | 1 | 1 | 1 | 1 |
| **TOTAL MULTIPLE DX** | 330 | 5.6 | 24 | 1 | 3 | 5 | 6 | 10 | 14 | 26 |
| **TOTAL** | | | | | | | | | | |
| 0–19 Years | 1 | 10.0 | 0 | 10 | 10 | 10 | 10 | 10 | 10 | 10 |
| 20–34 | 2 | 4.0 | 0 | 4 | 4 | 5 | 6 | 7 | 8 | 9 |
| 35–49 | 26 | 4.9 | 3 | 3 | 4 | 5 | 6 | 7 | 8 | 9 |
| 50–64 | 167 | 5.7 | 34 | 1 | 3 | 5 | 6 | 9 | 13 | 26 |
| 65+ | 137 | 5.6 | 17 | 1 | 3 | 4 | 7 | 12 | 14 | 17 |
| **GRAND TOTAL** | 333 | 5.6 | 24 | 1 | 3 | 5 | 6 | 10 | 14 | 26 |

Length of Stay by Diagnosis and Operation, United States, 2000

# United States, October 1998–September 1999 Data, by Operation

## 36.9: OTHER HEART VESSEL OPS. Formerly included in operation group(s) 579.

| Type of Patients | Observed Patients | Avg. Stay | Variance | Percentiles 10th | 25th | 50th | 75th | 90th | 95th | 99th |
|---|---|---|---|---|---|---|---|---|---|---|
| **1. SINGLE DX** | | | | | | | | | | |
| 0–19 Years | 9 | 4.6 | 10 | 1 | 3 | 3 | 9 | 9 | 9 | 9 |
| 20–34 | 1 | 3.0 | 0 | 3 | 3 | 3 | 3 | 3 | 3 | 3 |
| 35–49 | 1 | 4.0 | 0 | 4 | 4 | 4 | 4 | 4 | 4 | 4 |
| 50–64 | 0 | | | | | | | | | |
| 65+ | 0 | | | | | | | | | |
| **2. MULTIPLE DX** | | | | | | | | | | |
| 0–19 Years | 33 | 16.7 | 214 | 4 | 6 | 11 | 34 | 37 | 61 | >99 |
| 20–34 | 4 | 18.8 | 17 | 20 | 20 | 20 | 20 | 20 | 20 | 20 |
| 35–49 | 15 | 8.8 | 38 | 4 | 5 | 7 | 9 | 17 | 24 | 24 |
| 50–64 | 43 | 8.8 | 31 | 4 | 5 | 7 | 10 | 19 | 22 | 30 |
| 65+ | 66 | 9.4 | 26 | 5 | 7 | 8 | 12 | 16 | 20 | 28 |
| **TOTAL SINGLE DX** | 11 | 4.5 | 9 | 3 | 3 | 3 | 9 | 9 | 9 | 9 |
| **TOTAL MULTIPLE DX** | 161 | 11.6 | 80 | 4 | 6 | 8 | 15 | 22 | 37 | 61 |
| **TOTAL** | | | | | | | | | | |
| 0–19 Years | 42 | 12.2 | 172 | 3 | 3 | 9 | 14 | 37 | 37 | >99 |
| 20–34 | 5 | 18.0 | 27 | 20 | 20 | 20 | 20 | 20 | 20 | 20 |
| 35–49 | 16 | 8.5 | 37 | 4 | 5 | 7 | 8 | 17 | 24 | 24 |
| 50–64 | 43 | 8.8 | 31 | 4 | 5 | 7 | 10 | 19 | 22 | 30 |
| 65+ | 66 | 9.4 | 26 | 5 | 7 | 8 | 12 | 16 | 20 | 28 |
| **GRAND TOTAL** | 172 | 10.8 | 77 | 3 | 5 | 8 | 14 | 20 | 31 | 61 |

## 37.1: CARDIOTOMY & PERICARDIOT. Formerly included in operation group(s) 579.

| Type of Patients | Observed Patients | Avg. Stay | Variance | Percentiles 10th | 25th | 50th | 75th | 90th | 95th | 99th |
|---|---|---|---|---|---|---|---|---|---|---|
| **1. SINGLE DX** | | | | | | | | | | |
| 0–19 Years | 9 | 5.2 | 5 | 2 | 3 | 7 | 7 | 7 | 7 | 7 |
| 20–34 | 7 | 5.3 | 39 | 2 | 3 | 3 | 5 | 9 | 26 | 26 |
| 35–49 | 8 | 3.3 | 2 | 1 | 2 | 4 | 4 | 5 | 5 | 5 |
| 50–64 | 16 | 4.5 | 2 | 2 | 5 | 5 | 5 | 5 | 7 | 8 |
| 65+ | 8 | 4.5 | 7 | 2 | 3 | 3 | 8 | 9 | 9 | 9 |
| **2. MULTIPLE DX** | | | | | | | | | | |
| 0–19 Years | 99 | 11.2 | 134 | 3 | 4 | 7 | 13 | 29 | 33 | 66 |
| 20–34 | 182 | 8.7 | 50 | 3 | 4 | 8 | 8 | 17 | 24 | 36 |
| 35–49 | 458 | 9.3 | 49 | 3 | 4 | 7 | 13 | 20 | 22 | 31 |
| 50–64 | 730 | 9.6 | 57 | 3 | 5 | 7 | 12 | 18 | 22 | 41 |
| 65+ | 991 | 11.6 | 78 | 4 | 6 | 10 | 14 | 22 | 29 | 52 |
| **TOTAL SINGLE DX** | 48 | 4.7 | 11 | 2 | 3 | 5 | 5 | 7 | 8 | 26 |
| **TOTAL MULTIPLE DX** | 2,460 | 10.4 | 68 | 3 | 5 | 8 | 13 | 20 | 27 | 46 |
| **TOTAL** | | | | | | | | | | |
| 0–19 Years | 108 | 10.9 | 129 | 3 | 4 | 7 | 12 | 29 | 33 | 66 |
| 20–34 | 189 | 8.5 | 50 | 3 | 4 | 7 | 8 | 17 | 24 | 36 |
| 35–49 | 466 | 9.2 | 49 | 3 | 4 | 7 | 12 | 20 | 22 | 31 |
| 50–64 | 746 | 9.4 | 55 | 3 | 5 | 7 | 11 | 18 | 22 | 40 |
| 65+ | 999 | 11.6 | 78 | 4 | 6 | 10 | 14 | 21 | 29 | 52 |
| **GRAND TOTAL** | 2,508 | 10.2 | 68 | 3 | 5 | 8 | 13 | 20 | 26 | 46 |

## 37.0: PERICARDIOCENTESIS. Formerly included in operation group(s) 579.

| Type of Patients | Observed Patients | Avg. Stay | Variance | Percentiles 10th | 25th | 50th | 75th | 90th | 95th | 99th |
|---|---|---|---|---|---|---|---|---|---|---|
| **1. SINGLE DX** | | | | | | | | | | |
| 0–19 Years | 19 | 2.8 | 1 | 1 | 2 | 3 | 3 | 5 | 5 | 5 |
| 20–34 | 6 | 2.8 | 1 | 1 | 2 | 3 | 4 | 4 | 5 | 5 |
| 35–49 | 7 | 2.1 | 1 | 1 | 2 | 2 | 2 | 2 | 6 | 6 |
| 50–64 | 4 | 1.4 | <1 | 1 | 1 | 1 | 2 | 2 | 2 | 2 |
| 65+ | 6 | 3.2 | 13 | 1 | 1 | 2 | 9 | 9 | 9 | 9 |
| **2. MULTIPLE DX** | | | | | | | | | | |
| 0–19 Years | 118 | 6.0 | 44 | 1 | 2 | 4 | 9 | 11 | 14 | 40 |
| 20–34 | 82 | 7.4 | 134 | 2 | 4 | 5 | 7 | 11 | 14 | 95 |
| 35–49 | 209 | 5.9 | 19 | 2 | 3 | 5 | 8 | 11 | 15 | 21 |
| 50–64 | 292 | 6.5 | 66 | 2 | 3 | 5 | 8 | 12 | 16 | 33 |
| 65+ | 406 | 6.8 | 26 | 2 | 4 | 6 | 9 | 13 | 17 | 25 |
| **TOTAL SINGLE DX** | 42 | 2.7 | 3 | 1 | 2 | 2 | 3 | 5 | 5 | 9 |
| **TOTAL MULTIPLE DX** | 1,107 | 6.5 | 44 | 2 | 3 | 5 | 8 | 12 | 16 | 27 |
| **TOTAL** | | | | | | | | | | |
| 0–19 Years | 137 | 5.6 | 40 | 1 | 2 | 4 | 7 | 11 | 14 | 40 |
| 20–34 | 88 | 6.9 | 120 | 2 | 3 | 5 | 7 | 9 | 14 | 95 |
| 35–49 | 216 | 5.7 | 19 | 2 | 3 | 5 | 8 | 11 | 13 | 21 |
| 50–64 | 296 | 6.5 | 65 | 2 | 3 | 5 | 8 | 12 | 16 | 33 |
| 65+ | 412 | 6.8 | 26 | 2 | 4 | 6 | 9 | 13 | 17 | 25 |
| **GRAND TOTAL** | 1,149 | 6.3 | 43 | 2 | 3 | 5 | 8 | 12 | 16 | 27 |

## 37.12: PERICARDIOTOMY. Formerly included in operation group(s) 579.

| Type of Patients | Observed Patients | Avg. Stay | Variance | Percentiles 10th | 25th | 50th | 75th | 90th | 95th | 99th |
|---|---|---|---|---|---|---|---|---|---|---|
| **1. SINGLE DX** | | | | | | | | | | |
| 0–19 Years | 8 | 5.3 | 5 | 2 | 3 | 7 | 7 | 7 | 7 | 7 |
| 20–34 | 6 | 8.2 | 76 | 1 | 2 | 5 | 9 | 26 | 26 | 26 |
| 35–49 | 8 | 3.3 | 2 | 1 | 2 | 4 | 4 | 5 | 5 | 5 |
| 50–64 | 16 | 4.5 | 2 | 2 | 5 | 5 | 5 | 5 | 7 | 8 |
| 65+ | 8 | 4.5 | 7 | 2 | 3 | 3 | 8 | 9 | 9 | 9 |
| **2. MULTIPLE DX** | | | | | | | | | | |
| 0–19 Years | 91 | 11.5 | 138 | 3 | 4 | 7 | 13 | 29 | 33 | 66 |
| 20–34 | 179 | 8.7 | 50 | 3 | 4 | 8 | 8 | 18 | 24 | 36 |
| 35–49 | 446 | 9.4 | 49 | 3 | 4 | 7 | 13 | 20 | 22 | 31 |
| 50–64 | 692 | 9.5 | 58 | 3 | 5 | 7 | 12 | 18 | 22 | 42 |
| 65+ | 935 | 11.6 | 80 | 4 | 6 | 10 | 14 | 21 | 30 | 52 |
| **TOTAL SINGLE DX** | 46 | 4.9 | 13 | 2 | 3 | 5 | 5 | 7 | 9 | 26 |
| **TOTAL MULTIPLE DX** | 2,343 | 10.4 | 70 | 3 | 5 | 8 | 13 | 20 | 27 | 46 |
| **TOTAL** | | | | | | | | | | |
| 0–19 Years | 99 | 11.2 | 133 | 3 | 4 | 7 | 13 | 29 | 33 | 66 |
| 20–34 | 185 | 8.7 | 51 | 3 | 4 | 7 | 8 | 18 | 24 | 36 |
| 35–49 | 454 | 9.3 | 49 | 3 | 4 | 7 | 13 | 20 | 22 | 31 |
| 50–64 | 708 | 9.3 | 57 | 3 | 5 | 7 | 11 | 18 | 22 | 41 |
| 65+ | 943 | 11.6 | 80 | 4 | 6 | 10 | 14 | 21 | 30 | 52 |
| **GRAND TOTAL** | 2,389 | 10.2 | 69 | 3 | 5 | 8 | 13 | 20 | 27 | 46 |

Length of Stay by Diagnosis and Operation, United States, 2000

## United States, October 1998–September 1999 Data, by Operation

### 37.2: DXTIC PX HRT/PERICARDIUM. Formerly included in operation group(s) 575, 579, 581.

| Type of Patients | Observed Patients | Avg. Stay | Vari-ance | Percentiles | | | | | | |
|---|---|---|---|---|---|---|---|---|---|---|
| | | | | 10th | 25th | 50th | 75th | 90th | 95th | 99th |
| **1. SINGLE DX** | | | | | | | | | | |
| 0–19 Years | 366 | 2.2 | 12 | 1 | 1 | 1 | 2 | 4 | 7 | 20 |
| 20–34 | 380 | 2.3 | 5 | 1 | 1 | 2 | 3 | 4 | 5 | 13 |
| 35–49 | 1,814 | 2.2 | 4 | 1 | 1 | 2 | 3 | 4 | 5 | 11 |
| 50–64 | 1,647 | 1.9 | 2 | 1 | 1 | 1 | 2 | 3 | 4 | 7 |
| 65+ | 954 | 2.6 | 4 | 1 | 1 | 2 | 4 | 6 | 6 | 8 |
| **2. MULTIPLE DX** | | | | | | | | | | |
| 0–19 Years | 1,697 | 4.7 | 62 | 1 | 1 | 2 | 5 | 12 | 18 | 36 |
| 20–34 | 2,652 | 3.5 | 11 | 1 | 1 | 3 | 4 | 7 | 9 | 16 |
| 35–49 | 27,317 | 3.2 | 7 | 1 | 1 | 2 | 4 | 6 | 8 | 13 |
| 50–64 | 56,137 | 3.6 | 10 | 1 | 2 | 3 | 4 | 7 | 9 | 16 |
| 65+ | 76,847 | 4.6 | 16 | 1 | 2 | 4 | 6 | 9 | 12 | 19 |
| **TOTAL SINGLE DX** | 5,161 | 2.2 | 4 | 1 | 1 | 1 | 3 | 5 | 5 | 11 |
| **TOTAL MULTIPLE DX** | 164,650 | 4.0 | 13 | 1 | 2 | 3 | 5 | 8 | 10 | 17 |
| **TOTAL** | | | | | | | | | | |
| 0–19 Years | 2,063 | 4.2 | 53 | 1 | 1 | 1 | 4 | 10 | 17 | 33 |
| 20–34 | 3,032 | 3.3 | 10 | 1 | 1 | 2 | 4 | 6 | 9 | 15 |
| 35–49 | 29,131 | 3.1 | 7 | 1 | 1 | 2 | 4 | 6 | 8 | 13 |
| 50–64 | 57,784 | 3.5 | 10 | 1 | 2 | 3 | 4 | 7 | 9 | 15 |
| 65+ | 77,801 | 4.5 | 16 | 1 | 2 | 4 | 6 | 9 | 12 | 19 |
| **GRAND TOTAL** | 169,811 | 3.9 | 13 | 1 | 2 | 3 | 5 | 8 | 10 | 17 |

### 37.21: RT HEART CARDIAC CATH. Formerly included in operation group(s) 575.

| Type of Patients | Observed Patients | Avg. Stay | Vari-ance | Percentiles | | | | | | |
|---|---|---|---|---|---|---|---|---|---|---|
| | | | | 10th | 25th | 50th | 75th | 90th | 95th | 99th |
| **1. SINGLE DX** | | | | | | | | | | |
| 0–19 Years | 44 | 2.8 | 5 | 1 | 1 | 2 | 5 | 6 | 6 | 9 |
| 20–34 | 13 | 2.6 | 2 | 1 | 1 | 3 | 4 | 4 | 5 | 5 |
| 35–49 | 17 | 1.9 | 1 | 1 | 1 | 2 | 2 | 3 | 4 | 5 |
| 50–64 | 17 | 2.1 | 3 | 1 | 1 | 1 | 3 | 4 | 7 | 8 |
| 65+ | 9 | 4.1 | 4 | 2 | 3 | 3 | 5 | 6 | 9 | 9 |
| **2. MULTIPLE DX** | | | | | | | | | | |
| 0–19 Years | 182 | 6.8 | 138 | 1 | 1 | 2 | 8 | 17 | 25 | 84 |
| 20–34 | 136 | 6.4 | 46 | 1 | 2 | 5 | 8 | 11 | 16 | 45 |
| 35–49 | 427 | 5.3 | 32 | 1 | 2 | 4 | 7 | 10 | 13 | 28 |
| 50–64 | 838 | 6.7 | 51 | 2 | 3 | 6 | 9 | 14 | 18 | 41 |
| 65+ | 947 | 7.2 | 39 | 1 | 3 | 6 | 10 | 16 | 20 | 28 |
| **TOTAL SINGLE DX** | 100 | 2.8 | 4 | 1 | 1 | 2 | 4 | 5 | 6 | 9 |
| **TOTAL MULTIPLE DX** | 2,530 | 6.7 | 51 | 1 | 2 | 5 | 9 | 14 | 18 | 34 |
| **TOTAL** | | | | | | | | | | |
| 0–19 Years | 226 | 6.2 | 120 | 1 | 1 | 2 | 6 | 14 | 21 | 84 |
| 20–34 | 149 | 6.1 | 43 | 1 | 2 | 5 | 8 | 11 | 16 | 45 |
| 35–49 | 444 | 5.2 | 31 | 1 | 1 | 4 | 7 | 10 | 13 | 28 |
| 50–64 | 855 | 6.6 | 50 | 1 | 3 | 4 | 9 | 14 | 18 | 41 |
| 65+ | 956 | 7.2 | 39 | 1 | 3 | 6 | 9 | 16 | 19 | 28 |
| **GRAND TOTAL** | 2,630 | 6.5 | 50 | 1 | 2 | 4 | 8 | 14 | 18 | 33 |

### 37.22: LEFT HEART CARDIAC CATH. Formerly included in operation group(s) 575.

| Type of Patients | Observed Patients | Avg. Stay | Vari-ance | Percentiles | | | | | | |
|---|---|---|---|---|---|---|---|---|---|---|
| | | | | 10th | 25th | 50th | 75th | 90th | 95th | 99th |
| **1. SINGLE DX** | | | | | | | | | | |
| 0–19 Years | 19 | 1.6 | <1 | 1 | 1 | 1 | 2 | 3 | 3 | 5 |
| 20–34 | 203 | 2.2 | 1 | 1 | 1 | 2 | 3 | 4 | 5 | 5 |
| 35–49 | 1,504 | 2.2 | 4 | 1 | 2 | 2 | 2 | 4 | 5 | 11 |
| 50–64 | 1,350 | 1.9 | 2 | 1 | 1 | 2 | 2 | 3 | 4 | 7 |
| 65+ | 724 | 2.6 | 3 | 1 | 2 | 2 | 4 | 5 | 6 | 7 |
| **2. MULTIPLE DX** | | | | | | | | | | |
| 0–19 Years | 93 | 4.6 | 35 | 1 | 1 | 2 | 4 | 15 | 23 | 23 |
| 20–34 | 1,659 | 2.8 | 5 | 1 | 1 | 2 | 4 | 5 | 7 | 11 |
| 35–49 | 22,441 | 2.9 | 5 | 1 | 2 | 2 | 4 | 6 | 7 | 11 |
| 50–64 | 45,151 | 3.3 | 7 | 1 | 2 | 3 | 4 | 6 | 8 | 13 |
| 65+ | 57,300 | 4.1 | 13 | 1 | 2 | 3 | 5 | 8 | 10 | 18 |
| **TOTAL SINGLE DX** | 3,800 | 2.2 | 3 | 1 | 1 | 2 | 3 | 4 | 5 | 11 |
| **TOTAL MULTIPLE DX** | 126,644 | 3.6 | 10 | 1 | 2 | 3 | 5 | 7 | 9 | 15 |
| **TOTAL** | | | | | | | | | | |
| 0–19 Years | 112 | 3.9 | 28 | 1 | 1 | 1 | 4 | 11 | 15 | 23 |
| 20–34 | 1,862 | 2.7 | 4 | 1 | 1 | 2 | 4 | 5 | 7 | 11 |
| 35–49 | 23,945 | 2.8 | 5 | 1 | 1 | 2 | 4 | 5 | 7 | 11 |
| 50–64 | 46,501 | 3.2 | 7 | 1 | 2 | 3 | 4 | 6 | 8 | 13 |
| 65+ | 58,024 | 4.1 | 13 | 1 | 2 | 3 | 5 | 8 | 10 | 17 |
| **GRAND TOTAL** | 130,444 | 3.5 | 10 | 1 | 2 | 3 | 4 | 7 | 9 | 15 |

### 37.23: RT/LEFT HEART CARD CATH. Formerly included in operation group(s) 575.

| Type of Patients | Observed Patients | Avg. Stay | Vari-ance | Percentiles | | | | | | |
|---|---|---|---|---|---|---|---|---|---|---|
| | | | | 10th | 25th | 50th | 75th | 90th | 95th | 99th |
| **1. SINGLE DX** | | | | | | | | | | |
| 0–19 Years | 148 | 2.2 | 11 | 1 | 1 | 1 | 2 | 4 | 7 | 20 |
| 20–34 | 27 | 2.3 | 4 | 1 | 2 | 1 | 3 | 7 | 7 | 7 |
| 35–49 | 87 | 2.0 | 3 | 1 | 1 | 1 | 2 | 5 | 6 | 8 |
| 50–64 | 112 | 1.8 | 2 | 1 | 1 | 1 | 2 | 3 | 5 | 7 |
| 65+ | 78 | 1.6 | 2 | 1 | 1 | 1 | 2 | 2 | 3 | 6 |
| **2. MULTIPLE DX** | | | | | | | | | | |
| 0–19 Years | 1,033 | 4.4 | 59 | 1 | 1 | 1 | 4 | 10 | 17 | 37 |
| 20–34 | 470 | 4.5 | 14 | 1 | 2 | 3 | 6 | 10 | 11 | 16 |
| 35–49 | 3,372 | 4.2 | 12 | 1 | 2 | 3 | 6 | 8 | 10 | 16 |
| 50–64 | 8,008 | 4.7 | 15 | 1 | 2 | 3 | 6 | 9 | 11 | 20 |
| 65+ | 14,606 | 5.6 | 19 | 1 | 3 | 5 | 7 | 11 | 14 | 21 |
| **TOTAL SINGLE DX** | 452 | 1.9 | 5 | 1 | 1 | 1 | 2 | 3 | 5 | 10 |
| **TOTAL MULTIPLE DX** | 27,489 | 5.1 | 19 | 1 | 2 | 4 | 7 | 10 | 13 | 21 |
| **TOTAL** | | | | | | | | | | |
| 0–19 Years | 1,181 | 4.0 | 53 | 1 | 1 | 1 | 4 | 9 | 16 | 36 |
| 20–34 | 497 | 4.4 | 14 | 1 | 2 | 3 | 6 | 10 | 11 | 16 |
| 35–49 | 3,459 | 4.2 | 12 | 1 | 2 | 3 | 5 | 8 | 10 | 16 |
| 50–64 | 8,120 | 4.7 | 12 | 1 | 2 | 3 | 6 | 9 | 11 | 20 |
| 65+ | 14,684 | 5.5 | 19 | 1 | 2 | 5 | 7 | 11 | 13 | 21 |
| **GRAND TOTAL** | 27,941 | 5.0 | 19 | 1 | 2 | 4 | 7 | 10 | 13 | 21 |

Length of Stay by Diagnosis and Operation, United States, 2000

# United States, October 1998–September 1999 Data, by Operation

## 37.25: CARDIAC BIOPSY. Formerly included in operation group(s) 579.

| Type of Patients | Observed Patients | Avg. Stay | Variance | 10th | 25th | 50th | 75th | 90th | 95th | 99th |
|---|---|---|---|---|---|---|---|---|---|---|
| **1. SINGLE DX** | | | | | | | | | | |
| 0–19 Years | 24 | 2.9 | 8 | 1 | 1 | 2 | 3 | 7 | 12 | 12 |
| 20–34 | 4 | 2.2 | 2 | 1 | 1 | 1 | 3 | 7 | 12 | 12 |
| 35–49 | 1 | 1.0 | 0 | 1 | 1 | 1 | 1 | 1 | 1 | 1 |
| 50–64 | 8 | 2.1 | 6 | 1 | 1 | 1 | 1 | 6 | 9 | 9 |
| 65+ | 2 | 2.7 | <1 | 2 | 1 | 3 | 3 | 3 | 3 | 3 |
| **2. MULTIPLE DX** | | | | | | | | | | |
| 0–19 Years | 143 | 5.6 | 47 | 1 | 1 | 2 | 7 | 16 | 19 | 29 |
| 20–34 | 46 | 6.9 | 46 | 1 | 2 | 5 | 8 | 15 | 21 | 33 |
| 35–49 | 118 | 6.2 | 39 | 1 | 2 | 4 | 7 | 14 | 19 | 29 |
| 50–64 | 229 | 6.2 | 40 | 2 | 3 | 4 | 7 | 12 | 16 | 33 |
| 65+ | 62 | 6.6 | 41 | 1 | 2 | 4 | 8 | 17 | 21 | 21 |
| **TOTAL SINGLE DX** | 39 | 2.7 | 7 | 1 | 1 | 2 | 3 | 6 | 12 | 12 |
| **TOTAL MULTIPLE DX** | 598 | 6.0 | 43 | 1 | 2 | 4 | 8 | 15 | 20 | 29 |
| **TOTAL** | | | | | | | | | | |
| 0–19 Years | 167 | 5.1 | 41 | 1 | 1 | 2 | 7 | 15 | 19 | 24 |
| 20–34 | 50 | 6.6 | 45 | 1 | 2 | 5 | 8 | 15 | 21 | 33 |
| 35–49 | 119 | 6.1 | 39 | 1 | 2 | 4 | 7 | 14 | 19 | 29 |
| 50–64 | 237 | 6.0 | 39 | 1 | 2 | 4 | 7 | 11 | 16 | 33 |
| 65+ | 64 | 6.5 | 41 | 1 | 2 | 4 | 8 | 17 | 21 | 21 |
| **GRAND TOTAL** | 637 | 5.8 | 41 | 1 | 1 | 3 | 7 | 15 | 19 | 29 |

## 37.26: CARD EPS/RECORD STUDIES. Formerly included in operation group(s) 581.

| Type of Patients | Observed Patients | Avg. Stay | Variance | 10th | 25th | 50th | 75th | 90th | 95th | 99th |
|---|---|---|---|---|---|---|---|---|---|---|
| **1. SINGLE DX** | | | | | | | | | | |
| 0–19 Years | 128 | 2.0 | 17 | 1 | 1 | 1 | 1 | 4 | 4 | 32 |
| 20–34 | 125 | 2.5 | 11 | 1 | 1 | 1 | 2 | 5 | 13 | 13 |
| 35–49 | 194 | 2.1 | 2 | 1 | 1 | 1 | 3 | 5 | 5 | 5 |
| 50–64 | 156 | 1.8 | 2 | 1 | 1 | 1 | 2 | 4 | 5 | 7 |
| 65+ | 137 | 4.0 | 7 | 1 | 1 | 4 | 5 | 8 | 8 | 8 |
| **2. MULTIPLE DX** | | | | | | | | | | |
| 0–19 Years | 236 | 3.4 | 16 | 1 | 1 | 2 | 5 | 8 | 9 | 25 |
| 20–34 | 320 | 3.1 | 6 | 1 | 1 | 3 | 4 | 6 | 6 | 11 |
| 35–49 | 903 | 3.9 | 13 | 1 | 2 | 3 | 5 | 8 | 11 | 16 |
| 50–64 | 1,805 | 4.8 | 20 | 1 | 2 | 4 | 7 | 10 | 12 | 21 |
| 65+ | 3,763 | 5.9 | 23 | 1 | 2 | 5 | 8 | 11 | 15 | 23 |
| **TOTAL SINGLE DX** | 740 | 2.4 | 7 | 1 | 1 | 1 | 3 | 5 | 8 | 13 |
| **TOTAL MULTIPLE DX** | 7,027 | 5.2 | 21 | 1 | 2 | 4 | 7 | 11 | 13 | 21 |
| **TOTAL** | | | | | | | | | | |
| 0–19 Years | 364 | 2.8 | 17 | 1 | 1 | 1 | 4 | 6 | 8 | 31 |
| 20–34 | 445 | 3.0 | 7 | 1 | 1 | 2 | 4 | 6 | 7 | 13 |
| 35–49 | 1,097 | 3.4 | 11 | 1 | 1 | 2 | 4 | 7 | 9 | 16 |
| 50–64 | 1,961 | 4.5 | 19 | 1 | 1 | 3 | 6 | 9 | 12 | 21 |
| 65+ | 3,900 | 5.8 | 23 | 1 | 2 | 5 | 8 | 11 | 15 | 22 |
| **GRAND TOTAL** | 7,767 | 4.8 | 20 | 1 | 2 | 4 | 7 | 10 | 13 | 21 |

## 37.3: PERICARDIECT/EXC HRT LES. Formerly included in operation group(s) 578, 579.

| Type of Patients | Observed Patients | Avg. Stay | Variance | 10th | 25th | 50th | 75th | 90th | 95th | 99th |
|---|---|---|---|---|---|---|---|---|---|---|
| **1. SINGLE DX** | | | | | | | | | | |
| 0–19 Years | 145 | 1.6 | 1 | 1 | 1 | 1 | 2 | 3 | 4 | 6 |
| 20–34 | 85 | 1.7 | 2 | 1 | 1 | 1 | 2 | 4 | 5 | 7 |
| 35–49 | 124 | 1.3 | <1 | 1 | 1 | 1 | 1 | 2 | 3 | 5 |
| 50–64 | 74 | 1.6 | 1 | 1 | 1 | 1 | 1 | 4 | 5 | 6 |
| 65+ | 60 | 1.6 | 2 | 1 | 1 | 1 | 2 | 3 | 4 | 11 |
| **2. MULTIPLE DX** | | | | | | | | | | |
| 0–19 Years | 316 | 4.6 | 84 | 1 | 1 | 3 | 5 | 9 | 12 | 86 |
| 20–34 | 214 | 3.5 | 40 | 1 | 1 | 2 | 5 | 7 | 10 | 32 |
| 35–49 | 506 | 5.7 | 42 | 1 | 1 | 3 | 7 | 20 | 20 | 21 |
| 50–64 | 824 | 5.2 | 39 | 1 | 1 | 3 | 6 | 11 | 15 | 31 |
| 65+ | 1,384 | 6.5 | 45 | 1 | 2 | 4 | 8 | 15 | 19 | 38 |
| **TOTAL SINGLE DX** | 488 | 1.5 | 1 | 1 | 1 | 1 | 1 | 3 | 4 | 6 |
| **TOTAL MULTIPLE DX** | 3,244 | 5.6 | 48 | 1 | 1 | 3 | 7 | 13 | 19 | 35 |
| **TOTAL** | | | | | | | | | | |
| 0–19 Years | 461 | 3.8 | 63 | 1 | 1 | 2 | 4 | 7 | 10 | 45 |
| 20–34 | 299 | 3.0 | 31 | 1 | 1 | 1 | 3 | 6 | 9 | 23 |
| 35–49 | 630 | 4.6 | 35 | 1 | 1 | 2 | 5 | 14 | 20 | 20 |
| 50–64 | 898 | 4.9 | 37 | 1 | 1 | 3 | 6 | 11 | 14 | 29 |
| 65+ | 1,444 | 6.3 | 44 | 1 | 2 | 4 | 8 | 15 | 18 | 38 |
| **GRAND TOTAL** | 3,732 | 5.1 | 44 | 1 | 1 | 3 | 6 | 12 | 17 | 29 |

## 37.31: PERICARDIECTOMY. Formerly included in operation group(s) 579.

| Type of Patients | Observed Patients | Avg. Stay | Variance | 10th | 25th | 50th | 75th | 90th | 95th | 99th |
|---|---|---|---|---|---|---|---|---|---|---|
| **1. SINGLE DX** | | | | | | | | | | |
| 0–19 Years | 5 | 5.4 | 4 | 3 | 4 | 5 | 8 | 8 | 8 | 8 |
| 20–34 | 9 | 3.8 | 2 | 2 | 2 | 4 | 5 | 6 | 6 | 6 |
| 35–49 | 9 | 2.7 | <1 | 1 | 3 | 3 | 3 | 3 | 3 | 4 |
| 50–64 | 3 | 4.6 | <1 | 4 | 4 | 5 | 5 | 5 | 5 | 5 |
| 65+ | 1 | 11.0 | 0 | 11 | 11 | 11 | 11 | 11 | 11 | 11 |
| **2. MULTIPLE DX** | | | | | | | | | | |
| 0–19 Years | 12 | 7.1 | 34 | 2 | 4 | 5 | 7 | 17 | 21 | 23 |
| 20–34 | 23 | 11.3 | 76 | 5 | 6 | 8 | 15 | 23 | 32 | 37 |
| 35–49 | 74 | 12.8 | 54 | 3 | 5 | 15 | 20 | 20 | 20 | 20 |
| 50–64 | 105 | 9.6 | 117 | 4 | 5 | 6 | 13 | 18 | 28 | 48 |
| 65+ | 98 | 12.9 | 49 | 4 | 6 | 13 | 17 | 19 | 25 | 29 |
| **TOTAL SINGLE DX** | 27 | 4.0 | 4 | 2 | 3 | 4 | 5 | 6 | 8 | 11 |
| **TOTAL MULTIPLE DX** | 312 | 11.6 | 75 | 3 | 5 | 10 | 17 | 20 | 22 | 38 |
| **TOTAL** | | | | | | | | | | |
| 0–19 Years | 17 | 6.7 | 26 | 3 | 4 | 5 | 7 | 17 | 21 | 23 |
| 20–34 | 32 | 9.7 | 69 | 2 | 5 | 6 | 13 | 18 | 32 | 37 |
| 35–49 | 83 | 12.1 | 57 | 3 | 4 | 11 | 20 | 20 | 20 | 20 |
| 50–64 | 108 | 9.3 | 113 | 2 | 3 | 6 | 12 | 18 | 28 | 48 |
| 65+ | 99 | 12.9 | 49 | 4 | 6 | 13 | 17 | 19 | 25 | 29 |
| **GRAND TOTAL** | 339 | 11.2 | 74 | 3 | 5 | 9 | 17 | 20 | 21 | 38 |

Length of Stay by Diagnosis and Operation, United States, 2000

# United States, October 1998–September 1999 Data, by Operation

## 37.33: HEART LES EXC/DESTR NEC. Formerly included in operation group(s) 579.

| Type of Patients | Observed Patients | Avg. Stay | Vari-ance | 10th | 25th | 50th | 75th | 90th | 95th | 99th |
|---|---|---|---|---|---|---|---|---|---|---|
| **1. SINGLE DX** | | | | | | | | | | |
| 0–19 Years | 27 | 2.5 | 2 | 1 | 1 | 3 | 3 | 4 | 4 | 5 |
| 20–34 | 3 | 3.9 | 1 | 3 | 3 | 3 | 5 | 5 | 5 | 5 |
| 35–49 | 2 | 6.8 | 6 | 5 | 5 | 5 | 9 | 9 | 9 | 9 |
| 50–64 | 4 | 2.4 | 1 | 1 | 1 | 3 | 3 | 4 | 4 | 4 |
| 65+ | 1 | 4.0 | 0 | 4 | 4 | 4 | 4 | 4 | 4 | 4 |
| **2. MULTIPLE DX** | | | | | | | | | | |
| 0–19 Years | 98 | 7.9 | 235 | 3 | 3 | 4 | 5 | 12 | 22 | 86 |
| 20–34 | 25 | 4.2 | 5 | 3 | 3 | 3 | 5 | 7 | 10 | 11 |
| 35–49 | 84 | 8.6 | 35 | 3 | 5 | 8 | 11 | 16 | 21 | 24 |
| 50–64 | 113 | 7.2 | 20 | 3 | 4 | 6 | 9 | 13 | 17 | 23 |
| 65+ | 157 | 11.0 | 119 | 2 | 4 | 7 | 14 | 29 | 38 | 38 |
| **TOTAL SINGLE DX** | 37 | 2.8 | 2 | 1 | 1 | 3 | 4 | 4 | 5 | 9 |
| **TOTAL MULTIPLE DX** | 477 | 8.7 | 111 | 2 | 3 | 6 | 10 | 18 | 25 | 55 |
| **TOTAL** | | | | | | | | | | |
| 0–19 Years | 125 | 6.8 | 194 | 2 | 3 | 3 | 5 | 10 | 14 | 86 |
| 20–34 | 28 | 4.2 | 5 | 3 | 3 | 3 | 5 | 7 | 9 | 11 |
| 35–49 | 86 | 8.6 | 35 | 3 | 5 | 8 | 11 | 16 | 21 | 24 |
| 50–64 | 117 | 7.1 | 20 | 3 | 4 | 6 | 9 | 12 | 17 | 23 |
| 65+ | 158 | 11.0 | 119 | 2 | 4 | 7 | 14 | 29 | 38 | 38 |
| **GRAND TOTAL** | 514 | 8.3 | 106 | 2 | 3 | 5 | 9 | 17 | 23 | 55 |

## 37.34: CATH ABLATION HEART LES. Formerly included in operation group(s) 578.

| Type of Patients | Observed Patients | Avg. Stay | Vari-ance | 10th | 25th | 50th | 75th | 90th | 95th | 99th |
|---|---|---|---|---|---|---|---|---|---|---|
| **1. SINGLE DX** | | | | | | | | | | |
| 0–19 Years | 113 | 1.3 | <1 | 1 | 1 | 1 | 1 | 2 | 2 | 4 |
| 20–34 | 73 | 1.4 | 1 | 1 | 1 | 1 | 1 | 2 | 3 | 7 |
| 35–49 | 113 | 1.2 | <1 | 1 | 1 | 1 | 1 | 2 | 3 | 5 |
| 50–64 | 67 | 1.3 | <1 | 1 | 1 | 1 | 1 | 2 | 3 | 6 |
| 65+ | 57 | 1.4 | <1 | 1 | 1 | 1 | 1 | 3 | 3 | 4 |
| **2. MULTIPLE DX** | | | | | | | | | | |
| 0–19 Years | 189 | 2.4 | 7 | 1 | 1 | 1 | 3 | 6 | 7 | 11 |
| 20–34 | 164 | 2.1 | 6 | 1 | 1 | 1 | 3 | 4 | 6 | 13 |
| 35–49 | 337 | 2.6 | 12 | 1 | 1 | 2 | 5 | 5 | 8 | 13 |
| 50–64 | 537 | 3.1 | 9 | 1 | 1 | 2 | 5 | 6 | 8 | 12 |
| 65+ | 1,037 | 4.4 | 17 | 1 | 1 | 3 | 6 | 9 | 12 | 22 |
| **TOTAL SINGLE DX** | 423 | 1.3 | <1 | 1 | 1 | 1 | 1 | 2 | 3 | 5 |
| **TOTAL MULTIPLE DX** | 2,264 | 3.4 | 13 | 1 | 1 | 2 | 4 | 7 | 10 | 19 |
| **TOTAL** | | | | | | | | | | |
| 0–19 Years | 302 | 2.0 | 5 | 1 | 1 | 1 | 2 | 6 | 6 | 11 |
| 20–34 | 237 | 1.9 | 5 | 1 | 1 | 1 | 2 | 4 | 6 | 13 |
| 35–49 | 450 | 2.1 | 9 | 1 | 1 | 1 | 2 | 4 | 6 | 11 |
| 50–64 | 604 | 2.9 | 9 | 1 | 1 | 2 | 4 | 6 | 8 | 12 |
| 65+ | 1,094 | 4.2 | 17 | 1 | 1 | 3 | 6 | 9 | 12 | 22 |
| **GRAND TOTAL** | 2,687 | 3.0 | 12 | 1 | 1 | 2 | 4 | 7 | 9 | 17 |

## 37.4: REP HEART & PERICARDIUM. Formerly included in operation group(s) 579.

| Type of Patients | Observed Patients | Avg. Stay | Vari-ance | 10th | 25th | 50th | 75th | 90th | 95th | 99th |
|---|---|---|---|---|---|---|---|---|---|---|
| **1. SINGLE DX** | | | | | | | | | | |
| 0–19 Years | 1 | 6.0 | 0 | 6 | 6 | 6 | 6 | 6 | 6 | 6 |
| 20–34 | 0 | | | | | | | | | |
| 35–49 | 1 | 4.0 | 0 | 4 | 4 | 4 | 4 | 4 | 4 | 4 |
| 50–64 | 0 | | | | | | | | | |
| 65+ | 0 | | | | | | | | | |
| **2. MULTIPLE DX** | | | | | | | | | | |
| 0–19 Years | 20 | 11.9 | 149 | 3 | 4 | 6 | 13 | 41 | 41 | 41 |
| 20–34 | 55 | 8.1 | 42 | 4 | 5 | 5 | 11 | 11 | 18 | 37 |
| 35–49 | 46 | 6.5 | 42 | 4 | 4 | 4 | 8 | 9 | 11 | 23 |
| 50–64 | 21 | 8.1 | 23 | 3 | 4 | 6 | 12 | 16 | 16 | 17 |
| 65+ | 22 | 7.9 | 12 | 4 | 6 | 7 | 9 | 12 | 14 | 19 |
| **TOTAL SINGLE DX** | 2 | 4.8 | 2 | 4 | 4 | 4 | 6 | 6 | 6 | 6 |
| **TOTAL MULTIPLE DX** | 164 | 7.9 | 47 | 4 | 4 | 6 | 9 | 13 | 18 | 41 |
| **TOTAL** | | | | | | | | | | |
| 0–19 Years | 21 | 11.8 | 147 | 3 | 4 | 6 | 13 | 41 | 41 | 41 |
| 20–34 | 55 | 8.1 | 42 | 4 | 5 | 5 | 11 | 11 | 18 | 37 |
| 35–49 | 47 | 6.5 | 42 | 4 | 4 | 4 | 8 | 9 | 11 | 23 |
| 50–64 | 21 | 8.1 | 23 | 3 | 4 | 6 | 12 | 16 | 16 | 17 |
| 65+ | 22 | 7.9 | 12 | 4 | 6 | 7 | 9 | 12 | 14 | 19 |
| **GRAND TOTAL** | 166 | 7.9 | 47 | 4 | 4 | 6 | 9 | 13 | 18 | 41 |

## 37.5: HEART TRANSPLANTATION. Formerly included in operation group(s) 572.

| Type of Patients | Observed Patients | Avg. Stay | Vari-ance | 10th | 25th | 50th | 75th | 90th | 95th | 99th |
|---|---|---|---|---|---|---|---|---|---|---|
| **1. SINGLE DX** | | | | | | | | | | |
| 0–19 Years | 1 | 7.0 | 0 | 7 | 7 | 7 | 7 | 7 | 7 | 7 |
| 20–34 | 0 | | | | | | | | | |
| 35–49 | 1 | 13.0 | 0 | 13 | 13 | 13 | 13 | 13 | 13 | 13 |
| 50–64 | 0 | | | | | | | | | |
| 65+ | 0 | | | | | | | | | |
| **2. MULTIPLE DX** | | | | | | | | | | |
| 0–19 Years | 95 | 39.0 | 630 | 9 | 21 | 53 | >99 | >99 | >99 | >99 |
| 20–34 | 33 | 31.4 | 717 | 9 | 16 | 36 | >99 | >99 | >99 | >99 |
| 35–49 | 65 | 31.7 | 709 | 9 | 12 | 29 | 94 | >99 | >99 | >99 |
| 50–64 | 192 | 33.4 | 705 | 9 | 14 | 38 | >99 | >99 | >99 | >99 |
| 65+ | 38 | 28.9 | 395 | 8 | 12 | 35 | 61 | >99 | >99 | >99 |
| **TOTAL SINGLE DX** | 2 | 12.0 | 7 | 7 | 13 | 13 | 13 | 13 | 13 | 13 |
| **TOTAL MULTIPLE DX** | 423 | 34.3 | 661 | 9 | 15 | 42 | 99 | >99 | >99 | >99 |
| **TOTAL** | | | | | | | | | | |
| 0–19 Years | 96 | 38.9 | 631 | 9 | 21 | 53 | >99 | >99 | >99 | >99 |
| 20–34 | 33 | 31.4 | 717 | 9 | 16 | 36 | >99 | >99 | >99 | >99 |
| 35–49 | 66 | 31.2 | 701 | 9 | 13 | 27 | 94 | >99 | >99 | >99 |
| 50–64 | 192 | 33.4 | 705 | 9 | 14 | 38 | >99 | >99 | >99 | >99 |
| 65+ | 38 | 28.9 | 395 | 8 | 12 | 35 | 61 | >99 | >99 | >99 |
| **GRAND TOTAL** | 425 | 34.2 | 661 | 9 | 15 | 42 | 99 | >99 | >99 | >99 |

Length of Stay by Diagnosis and Operation, United States, 2000

## 37.6: IMPL HEART ASSIST SYST. Formerly included in operation group(s) 571.

| Type of Patients | Observed Patients | Avg. Stay | Variance | Percentiles | | | | | | |
|---|---|---|---|---|---|---|---|---|---|---|
| | | | | 10th | 25th | 50th | 75th | 90th | 95th | 99th |
| **1. SINGLE DX** | | | | | | | | | | |
| 0–19 Years | 1 | 3.0 | 0 | 3 | 3 | 3 | 3 | 3 | 3 | 3 |
| 20–34 | 0 | | | | | | | | | |
| 35–49 | 3 | 4.0 | 2 | 1 | 4 | 4 | 4 | 6 | 6 | 6 |
| 50–64 | 4 | 2.6 | 4 | 1 | 1 | 2 | 2 | 6 | 6 | 6 |
| 65+ | 4 | 2.1 | 5 | 1 | 1 | 1 | 2 | 8 | 8 | 8 |
| **2. MULTIPLE DX** | | | | | | | | | | |
| 0–19 Years | 4 | 42.6 | 906 | 9 | 10 | 64 | 65 | 65 | 65 | 65 |
| 20–34 | 21 | 9.0 | 115 | 3 | 3 | 8 | 10 | 15 | 16 | 67 |
| 35–49 | 340 | 7.2 | 48 | 3 | 4 | 5 | 8 | 13 | 19 | 36 |
| 50–64 | 986 | 8.5 | 75 | 3 | 4 | 6 | 10 | 17 | 24 | 60 |
| 65+ | 1,394 | 9.8 | 60 | 3 | 5 | 8 | 12 | 18 | 24 | 37 |
| **TOTAL SINGLE DX** | 12 | 2.7 | 4 | 1 | 1 | 2 | 4 | 6 | 8 | 8 |
| **TOTAL MULTIPLE DX** | 2,745 | 9.0 | 66 | 3 | 5 | 7 | 11 | 17 | 23 | 53 |
| **TOTAL** | | | | | | | | | | |
| 0–19 Years | 5 | 29.1 | 955 | 3 | 3 | 10 | 64 | 65 | 65 | 65 |
| 20–34 | 21 | 9.0 | 115 | 3 | 3 | 8 | 10 | 15 | 16 | 67 |
| 35–49 | 343 | 7.1 | 47 | 3 | 4 | 5 | 8 | 13 | 19 | 36 |
| 50–64 | 990 | 8.5 | 75 | 3 | 4 | 6 | 10 | 17 | 24 | 60 |
| 65+ | 1,398 | 9.7 | 60 | 3 | 5 | 8 | 12 | 18 | 24 | 37 |
| **GRAND TOTAL** | 2,757 | 9.0 | 66 | 3 | 4 | 7 | 11 | 17 | 23 | 53 |

## 37.61: PULSATION BALLOON IMPL. Formerly included in operation group(s) 571.

| Type of Patients | Observed Patients | Avg. Stay | Variance | Percentiles | | | | | | |
|---|---|---|---|---|---|---|---|---|---|---|
| | | | | 10th | 25th | 50th | 75th | 90th | 95th | 99th |
| **1. SINGLE DX** | | | | | | | | | | |
| 0–19 Years | 0 | | | | | | | | | |
| 20–34 | 0 | | | | | | | | | |
| 35–49 | 3 | 4.0 | 2 | 1 | 4 | 4 | 4 | 6 | 6 | 6 |
| 50–64 | 3 | 1.7 | <1 | 1 | 1 | 2 | 2 | 2 | 2 | 2 |
| 65+ | 4 | 2.1 | 5 | 1 | 1 | 1 | 2 | 8 | 8 | 8 |
| **2. MULTIPLE DX** | | | | | | | | | | |
| 0–19 Years | 1 | 9.0 | 0 | 9 | 9 | 9 | 9 | 9 | 9 | 9 |
| 20–34 | 18 | 7.7 | 33 | 3 | 3 | 8 | 10 | 15 | 15 | 38 |
| 35–49 | 329 | 6.8 | 31 | 3 | 4 | 5 | 8 | 12 | 17 | 26 |
| 50–64 | 947 | 8.0 | 52 | 3 | 4 | 6 | 9 | 15 | 20 | 34 |
| 65+ | 1,371 | 9.7 | 53 | 3 | 5 | 8 | 12 | 18 | 24 | 35 |
| **TOTAL SINGLE DX** | 10 | 2.5 | 4 | 1 | 1 | 2 | 4 | 6 | 8 | 8 |
| **TOTAL MULTIPLE DX** | 2,666 | 8.7 | 51 | 3 | 4 | 7 | 11 | 16 | 21 | 34 |
| **TOTAL** | | | | | | | | | | |
| 0–19 Years | 1 | 9.0 | 0 | 9 | 9 | 9 | 9 | 9 | 9 | 9 |
| 20–34 | 18 | 7.7 | 33 | 3 | 4 | 8 | 10 | 15 | 15 | 38 |
| 35–49 | 332 | 6.8 | 30 | 3 | 4 | 5 | 8 | 12 | 16 | 25 |
| 50–64 | 950 | 8.0 | 52 | 3 | 4 | 6 | 9 | 15 | 20 | 34 |
| 65+ | 1,375 | 9.6 | 54 | 3 | 5 | 8 | 12 | 18 | 24 | 35 |
| **GRAND TOTAL** | 2,676 | 8.7 | 51 | 3 | 4 | 7 | 11 | 16 | 21 | 34 |

## 37.7: CARDIAC PACER LEAD OP. Formerly included in operation group(s) 577, 581.

| Type of Patients | Observed Patients | Avg. Stay | Variance | Percentiles | | | | | | |
|---|---|---|---|---|---|---|---|---|---|---|
| | | | | 10th | 25th | 50th | 75th | 90th | 95th | 99th |
| **1. SINGLE DX** | | | | | | | | | | |
| 0–19 Years | 36 | 1.7 | <1 | 1 | 1 | 1 | 1 | 3 | 4 | 4 |
| 20–34 | 26 | 1.9 | 2 | 1 | 1 | 1 | 2 | 4 | 4 | 6 |
| 35–49 | 53 | 1.8 | 2 | 1 | 1 | 1 | 2 | 4 | 6 | 6 |
| 50–64 | 117 | 1.7 | 3 | 1 | 1 | 1 | 2 | 3 | 5 | 10 |
| 65+ | 581 | 1.7 | 2 | 1 | 1 | 1 | 2 | 3 | 4 | 7 |
| **2. MULTIPLE DX** | | | | | | | | | | |
| 0–19 Years | 125 | 3.6 | 18 | 1 | 1 | 2 | 4 | 6 | 13 | 21 |
| 20–34 | 127 | 3.0 | 7 | 1 | 1 | 2 | 4 | 6 | 8 | 17 |
| 35–49 | 530 | 4.1 | 14 | 2 | 2 | 3 | 6 | 8 | 11 | 18 |
| 50–64 | 2,245 | 4.9 | 32 | 2 | 2 | 4 | 6 | 9 | 13 | 26 |
| 65+ | 17,291 | 5.1 | 21 | 1 | 2 | 4 | 7 | 10 | 14 | 21 |
| **TOTAL SINGLE DX** | 813 | 1.7 | 2 | 1 | 1 | 1 | 2 | 3 | 4 | 7 |
| **TOTAL MULTIPLE DX** | 20,318 | 5.1 | 22 | 1 | 2 | 4 | 7 | 10 | 13 | 21 |
| **TOTAL** | | | | | | | | | | |
| 0–19 Years | 161 | 3.2 | 15 | 1 | 1 | 2 | 4 | 5 | 8 | 21 |
| 20–34 | 153 | 2.8 | 7 | 1 | 1 | 2 | 3 | 6 | 7 | 17 |
| 35–49 | 583 | 3.9 | 13 | 1 | 2 | 3 | 5 | 8 | 11 | 18 |
| 50–64 | 2,362 | 4.8 | 31 | 1 | 2 | 4 | 6 | 9 | 13 | 26 |
| 65+ | 17,872 | 5.0 | 20 | 1 | 2 | 4 | 7 | 10 | 14 | 21 |
| **GRAND TOTAL** | 21,131 | 4.9 | 21 | 2 | 2 | 4 | 7 | 10 | 13 | 21 |

## 37.71: INSERT TV LEAD-VENTRICLE. Formerly included in operation group(s) 577.

| Type of Patients | Observed Patients | Avg. Stay | Variance | Percentiles | | | | | | |
|---|---|---|---|---|---|---|---|---|---|---|
| | | | | 10th | 25th | 50th | 75th | 90th | 95th | 99th |
| **1. SINGLE DX** | | | | | | | | | | |
| 0–19 Years | 0 | | | | | | | | | |
| 20–34 | 1 | 1.0 | 0 | 1 | 1 | 1 | 1 | 1 | 1 | 1 |
| 35–49 | 2 | 2.0 | 0 | 2 | 2 | 2 | 2 | 2 | 2 | 2 |
| 50–64 | 1 | 1.6 | <1 | 2 | 2 | 2 | 3 | 8 | 16 | 16 |
| 65+ | 19 | 3.0 | 12 | 1 | 1 | 2 | 3 | 8 | 16 | 16 |
| **2. MULTIPLE DX** | | | | | | | | | | |
| 0–19 Years | 3 | 3.2 | 6 | 1 | 1 | 1 | 6 | 6 | 6 | 6 |
| 20–34 | 3 | 3.3 | 1 | 2 | 2 | 4 | 4 | 4 | 4 | 4 |
| 35–49 | 14 | 7.9 | 49 | 5 | 6 | 6 | 7 | 13 | 15 | 49 |
| 50–64 | 64 | 3.3 | 12 | 1 | 1 | 2 | 4 | 7 | 10 | 14 |
| 65+ | 940 | 6.4 | 29 | 1 | 3 | 5 | 9 | 12 | 16 | 25 |
| **TOTAL SINGLE DX** | 23 | 2.7 | 10 | 1 | 1 | 2 | 2 | 5 | 8 | 16 |
| **TOTAL MULTIPLE DX** | 1,024 | 6.2 | 29 | 1 | 3 | 5 | 9 | 12 | 16 | 25 |
| **TOTAL** | | | | | | | | | | |
| 0–19 Years | 3 | 3.2 | 6 | 1 | 1 | 2 | 6 | 6 | 6 | 6 |
| 20–34 | 4 | 2.2 | 2 | 1 | 1 | 2 | 4 | 4 | 4 | 4 |
| 35–49 | 15 | 7.8 | 49 | 4 | 6 | 6 | 7 | 13 | 15 | 49 |
| 50–64 | 66 | 3.2 | 11 | 1 | 1 | 2 | 4 | 7 | 10 | 14 |
| 65+ | 959 | 6.4 | 29 | 1 | 3 | 5 | 9 | 12 | 16 | 25 |
| **GRAND TOTAL** | 1,047 | 6.2 | 28 | 1 | 2 | 5 | 8 | 12 | 15 | 25 |

Length of Stay by Diagnosis and Operation, United States, 2000

# United States, October 1998–September 1999 Data, by Operation

## 37.76: REPL TRANSVENOUS LEAD(S). Formerly included in operation group(s) 577.

| Type of Patients | Observed Patients | Avg. Stay | Variance | Percentiles | | | | | | |
|---|---|---|---|---|---|---|---|---|---|---|
| | | | | 10th | 25th | 50th | 75th | 90th | 95th | 99th |
| **1. SINGLE DX** | | | | | | | | | | |
| 0–19 Years | 2 | 2.2 | <1 | 2 | 2 | 2 | 2 | 3 | 3 | 3 |
| 20–34 | 1 | 2.0 | 0 | 2 | 2 | 2 | 2 | 3 | 3 | 3 |
| 35–49 | 2 | 3.0 | 3 | 4 | 4 | 4 | 4 | 4 | 4 | 4 |
| 50–64 | 5 | 1.2 | <1 | 1 | 1 | 1 | 1 | 2 | 2 | 2 |
| 65+ | 36 | 1.2 | <1 | 1 | 1 | 1 | 1 | 2 | 3 | 3 |
| **2. MULTIPLE DX** | | | | | | | | | | |
| 0–19 Years | 25 | 2.1 | 2 | 1 | 1 | 2 | 3 | 3 | 5 | 9 |
| 20–34 | 11 | 1.8 | 1 | 1 | 1 | 1 | 2 | 4 | 4 | 4 |
| 35–49 | 26 | 3.2 | 8 | 1 | 2 | 2 | 3 | 8 | 10 | 12 |
| 50–64 | 63 | 3.0 | 10 | 1 | 2 | 2 | 4 | 4 | 5 | 21 |
| 65+ | 415 | 3.8 | 18 | 1 | 2 | 2 | 4 | 10 | 13 | 18 |
| **TOTAL SINGLE DX** | 46 | 1.3 | <1 | 1 | 1 | 1 | 1 | 2 | 3 | 4 |
| **TOTAL MULTIPLE DX** | 540 | 3.5 | 16 | 1 | 1 | 2 | 4 | 9 | 13 | 18 |
| **TOTAL** | | | | | | | | | | |
| 0–19 Years | 27 | 2.1 | 2 | 1 | 1 | 2 | 3 | 3 | 5 | 9 |
| 20–34 | 12 | 1.8 | 1 | 1 | 2 | 1 | 2 | 4 | 4 | 4 |
| 35–49 | 28 | 3.2 | 8 | 1 | 2 | 2 | 4 | 8 | 10 | 12 |
| 50–64 | 68 | 2.9 | 9 | 1 | 2 | 2 | 4 | 4 | 5 | 21 |
| 65+ | 451 | 3.6 | 18 | 1 | 2 | 2 | 4 | 10 | 13 | 18 |
| **GRAND TOTAL** | 586 | 3.4 | 15 | 1 | 1 | 2 | 4 | 8 | 13 | 18 |

## 37.78: INSERT TEMP TV PACER. Formerly included in operation group(s) 577.

| Type of Patients | Observed Patients | Avg. Stay | Variance | Percentiles | | | | | | |
|---|---|---|---|---|---|---|---|---|---|---|
| | | | | 10th | 25th | 50th | 75th | 90th | 95th | 99th |
| **1. SINGLE DX** | | | | | | | | | | |
| 0–19 Years | 1 | 4.0 | 0 | 4 | 4 | 4 | 4 | 4 | 4 | 4 |
| 20–34 | 0 | | | | | | | | | |
| 35–49 | 0 | | | | | | | | | |
| 50–64 | 2 | 1.6 | <1 | 1 | 1 | 2 | 2 | 2 | 2 | 2 |
| 65+ | 4 | 3.5 | 3 | 2 | 2 | 3 | 6 | 6 | 6 | 6 |
| **2. MULTIPLE DX** | | | | | | | | | | |
| 0–19 Years | 6 | 7.5 | 24 | 5 | 5 | 5 | 8 | 13 | 24 | 24 |
| 20–34 | 8 | 4.4 | 32 | 1 | 1 | 1 | 6 | 12 | 17 | 21 |
| 35–49 | 30 | 6.3 | 12 | 2 | 3 | 5 | 8 | 12 | 12 | 14 |
| 50–64 | 172 | 6.4 | 67 | 3 | 3 | 4 | 7 | 11 | 16 | 56 |
| 65+ | 834 | 6.9 | 22 | 3 | 4 | 6 | 9 | 12 | 16 | 24 |
| **TOTAL SINGLE DX** | 7 | 3.2 | 2 | 1 | 2 | 3 | 4 | 6 | 6 | 6 |
| **TOTAL MULTIPLE DX** | 1,050 | 6.8 | 29 | 2 | 4 | 5 | 9 | 12 | 16 | 24 |
| **TOTAL** | | | | | | | | | | |
| 0–19 Years | 7 | 6.7 | 20 | 4 | 5 | 5 | 8 | 13 | 13 | 24 |
| 20–34 | 8 | 4.4 | 32 | 1 | 1 | 1 | 6 | 12 | 17 | 21 |
| 35–49 | 30 | 6.3 | 12 | 2 | 3 | 5 | 8 | 12 | 12 | 14 |
| 50–64 | 174 | 6.3 | 67 | 2 | 3 | 4 | 7 | 11 | 16 | 56 |
| 65+ | 838 | 6.9 | 22 | 2 | 4 | 6 | 9 | 12 | 16 | 24 |
| **GRAND TOTAL** | 1,057 | 6.8 | 29 | 2 | 4 | 5 | 9 | 12 | 16 | 24 |

## 37.72: INSERT TV LEAD-ATR&VENT. Formerly included in operation group(s) 577.

| Type of Patients | Observed Patients | Avg. Stay | Variance | Percentiles | | | | | | |
|---|---|---|---|---|---|---|---|---|---|---|
| | | | | 10th | 25th | 50th | 75th | 90th | 95th | 99th |
| **1. SINGLE DX** | | | | | | | | | | |
| 0–19 Years | 28 | 1.4 | <1 | 1 | 1 | 1 | 2 | 2 | 3 | 3 |
| 20–34 | 22 | 1.8 | 1 | 1 | 1 | 2 | 2 | 4 | 5 | 6 |
| 35–49 | 45 | 2.1 | 3 | 1 | 1 | 2 | 2 | 5 | 6 | 6 |
| 50–64 | 98 | 1.8 | 3 | 1 | 1 | 2 | 2 | 3 | 6 | 10 |
| 65+ | 472 | 1.8 | 2 | 1 | 1 | 2 | 2 | 3 | 4 | 7 |
| **2. MULTIPLE DX** | | | | | | | | | | |
| 0–19 Years | 48 | 2.6 | 3 | 1 | 1 | 2 | 4 | 4 | 5 | 9 |
| 20–34 | 86 | 3.1 | 5 | 1 | 1 | 2 | 4 | 7 | 7 | 9 |
| 35–49 | 423 | 3.9 | 12 | 1 | 2 | 3 | 5 | 8 | 10 | 18 |
| 50–64 | 1,840 | 5.0 | 30 | 1 | 2 | 4 | 6 | 9 | 13 | 26 |
| 65+ | 14,459 | 5.0 | 19 | 1 | 2 | 4 | 7 | 10 | 13 | 21 |
| **TOTAL SINGLE DX** | 665 | 1.8 | 2 | 1 | 1 | 1 | 2 | 3 | 4 | 7 |
| **TOTAL MULTIPLE DX** | 16,856 | 4.9 | 20 | 1 | 2 | 4 | 6 | 10 | 13 | 21 |
| **TOTAL** | | | | | | | | | | |
| 0–19 Years | 76 | 2.2 | 3 | 1 | 2 | 2 | 3 | 4 | 5 | 8 |
| 20–34 | 108 | 2.8 | 5 | 1 | 2 | 2 | 4 | 6 | 7 | 9 |
| 35–49 | 468 | 3.8 | 11 | 1 | 2 | 3 | 5 | 7 | 9 | 18 |
| 50–64 | 1,938 | 4.8 | 29 | 1 | 2 | 4 | 6 | 9 | 13 | 25 |
| 65+ | 14,931 | 4.9 | 19 | 1 | 2 | 4 | 6 | 10 | 13 | 21 |
| **GRAND TOTAL** | 17,521 | 4.8 | 20 | 1 | 2 | 4 | 6 | 9 | 13 | 21 |

## 37.75: REVISION PACEMAKER LEAD. Formerly included in operation group(s) 577.

| Type of Patients | Observed Patients | Avg. Stay | Variance | Percentiles | | | | | | |
|---|---|---|---|---|---|---|---|---|---|---|
| | | | | 10th | 25th | 50th | 75th | 90th | 95th | 99th |
| **1. SINGLE DX** | | | | | | | | | | |
| 0–19 Years | 1 | 4.0 | 0 | 4 | 4 | 4 | 4 | 4 | 4 | 4 |
| 20–34 | 1 | 4.0 | 0 | 4 | 4 | 4 | 4 | 4 | 4 | 4 |
| 35–49 | 3 | 1.2 | <1 | 1 | 1 | 1 | 1 | 2 | 2 | 3 |
| 50–64 | 8 | 1.4 | <1 | 1 | 1 | 1 | 2 | 2 | 3 | 3 |
| 65+ | 34 | 1.5 | <1 | 1 | 1 | 1 | 2 | 2 | 3 | 3 |
| **2. MULTIPLE DX** | | | | | | | | | | |
| 0–19 Years | 12 | 3.2 | 13 | 1 | 1 | 2 | 3 | 6 | 6 | 18 |
| 20–34 | 8 | 3.7 | 7 | 2 | 2 | 2 | 4 | 7 | 10 | 10 |
| 35–49 | 24 | 2.1 | 2 | 1 | 1 | 1 | 3 | 4 | 6 | 6 |
| 50–64 | 61 | 3.2 | 8 | 1 | 1 | 3 | 3 | 6 | 12 | 14 |
| 65+ | 383 | 3.7 | 14 | 1 | 1 | 3 | 5 | 7 | 10 | 23 |
| **TOTAL SINGLE DX** | 47 | 1.5 | <1 | 1 | 1 | 1 | 2 | 2 | 3 | 4 |
| **TOTAL MULTIPLE DX** | 488 | 3.6 | 13 | 1 | 1 | 3 | 5 | 7 | 10 | 20 |
| **TOTAL** | | | | | | | | | | |
| 0–19 Years | 13 | 3.2 | 12 | 1 | 2 | 2 | 3 | 6 | 6 | 18 |
| 20–34 | 9 | 3.7 | 6 | 2 | 2 | 3 | 4 | 7 | 10 | 10 |
| 35–49 | 27 | 2.0 | 2 | 1 | 1 | 1 | 3 | 4 | 6 | 6 |
| 50–64 | 69 | 3.0 | 8 | 1 | 1 | 3 | 3 | 6 | 12 | 14 |
| 65+ | 417 | 3.4 | 13 | 1 | 1 | 2 | 5 | 7 | 9 | 20 |
| **GRAND TOTAL** | 535 | 3.3 | 12 | 1 | 1 | 2 | 4 | 7 | 9 | 18 |

# United States, October 1998–September 1999 Data, by Operation

## 37.8: CARDIAC PACEMAKER DEV OP. Formerly included in operation group(s) 577.

| Type of Patients | Observed Patients | Vari-ance | Avg. Stay | 10th | 25th | 50th | 75th | 90th | 95th | 99th |
|---|---|---|---|---|---|---|---|---|---|---|
| **1. SINGLE DX** | | | | | | | | | | |
| 0-19 Years | 51 | 6 | 2.0 | 1 | 1 | 1 | 2 | 3 | 3 | 8 |
| 20-34 | 22 | <1 | 1.4 | 1 | 1 | 1 | 1 | 2 | 3 | 7 |
| 35-49 | 46 | <1 | 1.8 | 1 | 1 | 2 | 2 | 2 | 3 | 5 |
| 50-64 | 127 | <1 | 1.8 | 1 | 1 | 1 | 2 | 3 | 4 | 6 |
| 65+ | 653 | 2 | 1.9 | 1 | 1 | 1 | 2 | 4 | 5 | 8 |
| **2. MULTIPLE DX** | | | | | | | | | | |
| 0-19 Years | 302 | 45 | 4.2 | 1 | 1 | 2 | 3 | 11 | 18 | 32 |
| 20-34 | 154 | 14 | 3.8 | 1 | 1 | 3 | 4 | 8 | 9 | 21 |
| 35-49 | 445 | 24 | 4.5 | 1 | 2 | 3 | 6 | 10 | 11 | 25 |
| 50-64 | 1,979 | 36 | 5.3 | 1 | 2 | 4 | 7 | 11 | 15 | 32 |
| 65+ | 18,497 | 34 | 5.6 | 1 | 2 | 4 | 7 | 12 | 16 | 30 |
| **TOTAL SINGLE DX** | 899 | 2 | 1.9 | 1 | 1 | 1 | 2 | 3 | 5 | 8 |
| **TOTAL MULTIPLE DX** | 21,377 | 34 | 5.6 | 1 | 2 | 4 | 7 | 12 | 16 | 30 |
| **TOTAL** | | | | | | | | | | |
| 0-19 Years | 353 | 39 | 3.8 | 1 | 1 | 2 | 3 | 8 | 18 | 31 |
| 20-34 | 176 | 13 | 3.5 | 1 | 2 | 2 | 4 | 7 | 9 | 18 |
| 35-49 | 491 | 21 | 4.0 | 1 | 2 | 3 | 5 | 8 | 10 | 25 |
| 50-64 | 2,106 | 35 | 5.1 | 1 | 2 | 3 | 6 | 11 | 15 | 29 |
| 65+ | 19,150 | 33 | 5.5 | 1 | 2 | 4 | 7 | 12 | 15 | 29 |
| **GRAND TOTAL** | 22,276 | 33 | 5.4 | 1 | 2 | 4 | 7 | 11 | 15 | 29 |

## 37.80: INSERT PACEMAKER DEV NOS. Formerly included in operation group(s) 577.

| Type of Patients | Observed Patients | Vari-ance | Avg. Stay | 10th | 25th | 50th | 75th | 90th | 95th | 99th |
|---|---|---|---|---|---|---|---|---|---|---|
| **1. SINGLE DX** | | | | | | | | | | |
| 0-19 Years | 5 | 78 | 7.4 | 1 | 1 | 3 | 8 | 25 | 25 | 25 |
| 20-34 | 1 | 0 | 1.0 | 1 | 1 | 1 | 1 | 1 | 1 | 1 |
| 35-49 | 2 | 0 | 1.0 | 1 | 1 | 1 | 1 | 1 | 1 | 1 |
| 50-64 | 2 | 0 | 1.0 | 1 | 1 | 1 | 1 | 1 | 1 | 1 |
| 65+ | 23 | 1 | 2.0 | 1 | 1 | 1 | 3 | 4 | 4 | 4 |
| **2. MULTIPLE DX** | | | | | | | | | | |
| 0-19 Years | 5 | 19 | 4.1 | 1 | 2 | 3 | 5 | 5 | 17 | 17 |
| 20-34 | 4 | 7 | 3.2 | 1 | 2 | 2 | 2 | 9 | 9 | 9 |
| 35-49 | 10 | 41 | 5.8 | 1 | 2 | 4 | 6 | 12 | 25 | 25 |
| 50-64 | 42 | 18 | 4.4 | 1 | 2 | 3 | 6 | 8 | 13 | 29 |
| 65+ | 549 | 29 | 5.3 | 1 | 2 | 4 | 6 | 11 | 15 | 25 |
| **TOTAL SINGLE DX** | 33 | 17 | 2.7 | 1 | 1 | 1 | 3 | 4 | 8 | 25 |
| **TOTAL MULTIPLE DX** | 610 | 28 | 5.2 | 1 | 2 | 4 | 6 | 11 | 14 | 25 |
| **TOTAL** | | | | | | | | | | |
| 0-19 Years | 10 | 54 | 6.0 | 1 | 1 | 3 | 8 | 17 | 25 | 25 |
| 20-34 | 5 | 6 | 2.8 | 1 | 2 | 2 | 2 | 9 | 9 | 9 |
| 35-49 | 12 | 38 | 5.2 | 1 | 1 | 4 | 4 | 12 | 25 | 25 |
| 50-64 | 44 | 18 | 4.3 | 1 | 2 | 3 | 6 | 8 | 13 | 29 |
| 65+ | 572 | 28 | 5.2 | 1 | 2 | 4 | 6 | 11 | 14 | 25 |
| **GRAND TOTAL** | 643 | 28 | 5.1 | 1 | 2 | 4 | 6 | 11 | 14 | 25 |

## 37.81: INSERT SINGLE CHAMB DEV. Formerly included in operation group(s) 577.

| Type of Patients | Observed Patients | Vari-ance | Avg. Stay | 10th | 25th | 50th | 75th | 90th | 95th | 99th |
|---|---|---|---|---|---|---|---|---|---|---|
| **1. SINGLE DX** | | | | | | | | | | |
| 0-19 Years | 7 | 6 | 2.8 | 1 | 1 | 2 | 3 | 7 | 7 | 7 |
| 20-34 | 0 | | | | | | | | | |
| 35-49 | 2 | 2 | 3.2 | 2 | 2 | 4 | 4 | 4 | 4 | 4 |
| 50-64 | 10 | 6 | 2.7 | 1 | 1 | 1 | 6 | 6 | 7 | 7 |
| 65+ | 57 | 2 | 2.1 | 1 | 1 | 1 | 3 | 5 | 5 | 6 |
| **2. MULTIPLE DX** | | | | | | | | | | |
| 0-19 Years | 20 | 82 | 6.0 | 1 | 1 | 2 | 5 | 18 | 32 | 36 |
| 20-34 | 8 | 27 | 5.1 | 2 | 3 | 3 | 4 | 15 | 18 | 18 |
| 35-49 | 35 | 15 | 4.8 | 1 | 2 | 4 | 6 | 10 | 13 | 20 |
| 50-64 | 203 | 41 | 6.1 | 1 | 2 | 4 | 7 | 15 | 19 | 28 |
| 65+ | 2,934 | 32 | 6.4 | 1 | 3 | 5 | 8 | 13 | 17 | 26 |
| **TOTAL SINGLE DX** | 76 | 3 | 2.2 | 1 | 1 | 1 | 3 | 5 | 6 | 7 |
| **TOTAL MULTIPLE DX** | 3,200 | 33 | 6.3 | 1 | 3 | 5 | 8 | 13 | 17 | 27 |
| **TOTAL** | | | | | | | | | | |
| 0-19 Years | 27 | 69 | 5.4 | 1 | 1 | 3 | 5 | 18 | 32 | 36 |
| 20-34 | 8 | 27 | 5.1 | 2 | 3 | 3 | 5 | 15 | 18 | 18 |
| 35-49 | 37 | 15 | 4.7 | 1 | 2 | 4 | 6 | 10 | 13 | 20 |
| 50-64 | 213 | 41 | 6.0 | 1 | 2 | 5 | 7 | 15 | 19 | 28 |
| 65+ | 2,991 | 32 | 6.3 | 1 | 3 | 5 | 8 | 13 | 16 | 26 |
| **GRAND TOTAL** | 3,276 | 33 | 6.3 | 1 | 3 | 5 | 8 | 13 | 17 | 27 |

## 37.82: INSERT RATE-RESPON DEV. Formerly included in operation group(s) 577.

| Type of Patients | Observed Patients | Vari-ance | Avg. Stay | 10th | 25th | 50th | 75th | 90th | 95th | 99th |
|---|---|---|---|---|---|---|---|---|---|---|
| **1. SINGLE DX** | | | | | | | | | | |
| 0-19 Years | 6 | <1 | 2.1 | 2 | 2 | 2 | 2 | 3 | 3 | 3 |
| 20-34 | 0 | | | | | | | | | |
| 35-49 | 8 | <1 | 1.2 | 1 | 1 | 1 | 1 | 2 | 2 | 2 |
| 50-64 | 14 | <1 | 2.2 | 1 | 1 | 3 | 3 | 3 | 3 | 3 |
| 65+ | 79 | 3 | 1.9 | 1 | 1 | 2 | 2 | 4 | 5 | 11 |
| **2. MULTIPLE DX** | | | | | | | | | | |
| 0-19 Years | 12 | 44 | 8.4 | 1 | 2 | 7 | 14 | 14 | 18 | 18 |
| 20-34 | 6 | 86 | 7.5 | 3 | 3 | 3 | 6 | 9 | 34 | 34 |
| 35-49 | 53 | 9 | 4.0 | 1 | 2 | 3 | 6 | 8 | 10 | 13 |
| 50-64 | 290 | 37 | 6.8 | 1 | 2 | 5 | 11 | 15 | 19 | 26 |
| 65+ | 3,965 | 41 | 6.5 | 1 | 2 | 5 | 8 | 13 | 20 | 29 |
| **TOTAL SINGLE DX** | 107 | 2 | 2.0 | 1 | 1 | 2 | 3 | 4 | 5 | 11 |
| **TOTAL MULTIPLE DX** | 4,326 | 40 | 6.5 | 1 | 2 | 5 | 8 | 14 | 19 | 29 |
| **TOTAL** | | | | | | | | | | |
| 0-19 Years | 18 | 34 | 5.6 | 1 | 2 | 3 | 7 | 18 | 18 | 18 |
| 20-34 | 6 | 86 | 7.5 | 3 | 3 | 3 | 8 | 14 | 34 | 34 |
| 35-49 | 61 | 9 | 3.8 | 1 | 1 | 3 | 5 | 8 | 10 | 13 |
| 50-64 | 304 | 36 | 6.5 | 1 | 2 | 4 | 9 | 15 | 17 | 26 |
| 65+ | 4,044 | 40 | 6.4 | 1 | 2 | 5 | 8 | 13 | 19 | 29 |
| **GRAND TOTAL** | 4,433 | 40 | 6.4 | 1 | 2 | 5 | 8 | 14 | 19 | 29 |

Length of Stay by Diagnosis and Operation, United States, 2000

# United States, October 1998–September 1999 Data, by Operation

## 37.83: INSERT DUAL-CHAMBER DEV. Formerly included in operation group(s) 577.

| Type of Patients | Observed Patients | Avg. Stay | Variance | 10th | 25th | 50th | 75th | 90th | 95th | 99th |
|---|---|---|---|---|---|---|---|---|---|---|
| **1. SINGLE DX** | | | | | | | | | | |
| 0–19 Years | 22 | 1.3 | <1 | 1 | 1 | 1 | 1 | 2 | 2 | 4 |
| 20–34 | 11 | 1.8 | 2 | 1 | 1 | 1 | 2 | 3 | 3 | 7 |
| 35–49 | 19 | 1.8 | <1 | 1 | 1 | 2 | 2 | 2 | 2 | 5 |
| 50–64 | 58 | 1.6 | 1 | 1 | 1 | 1 | 2 | 3 | 4 | 8 |
| 65+ | 236 | 2.2 | 3 | 1 | 1 | 2 | 3 | 4 | 7 | 8 |
| **2. MULTIPLE DX** | | | | | | | | | | |
| 0–19 Years | 77 | 4.6 | 51 | 1 | 1 | 2 | 5 | 9 | 18 | 32 |
| 20–34 | 53 | 4.8 | 16 | 1 | 2 | 4 | 7 | 9 | 13 | 21 |
| 35–49 | 204 | 4.4 | 16 | 1 | 2 | 3 | 6 | 9 | 12 | 21 |
| 50–64 | 1,050 | 4.8 | 16 | 1 | 2 | 4 | 6 | 9 | 12 | 19 |
| 65+ | 7,772 | 5.8 | 37 | 1 | 2 | 4 | 7 | 12 | 16 | 37 |
| **TOTAL SINGLE DX** | 346 | 2.0 | 2 | 1 | 1 | 2 | 2 | 4 | 5 | 8 |
| **TOTAL MULTIPLE DX** | 9,156 | 5.7 | 34 | 1 | 2 | 4 | 7 | 12 | 15 | 35 |
| **TOTAL** | | | | | | | | | | |
| 0–19 Years | 99 | 3.5 | 37 | 1 | 1 | 1 | 3 | 8 | 11 | 31 |
| 20–34 | 64 | 4.4 | 15 | 1 | 2 | 4 | 6 | 9 | 12 | 21 |
| 35–49 | 223 | 3.7 | 13 | 1 | 2 | 2 | 5 | 8 | 10 | 21 |
| 50–64 | 1,108 | 4.6 | 15 | 1 | 2 | 4 | 6 | 9 | 11 | 18 |
| 65+ | 8,008 | 5.7 | 36 | 1 | 2 | 4 | 7 | 12 | 16 | 37 |
| **GRAND TOTAL** | 9,502 | 5.5 | 33 | 1 | 2 | 4 | 7 | 11 | 15 | 34 |

## 37.85: REPL W 1-CHAMBER DEVICE. Formerly included in operation group(s) 577.

| Type of Patients | Observed Patients | Avg. Stay | Variance | 10th | 25th | 50th | 75th | 90th | 95th | 99th |
|---|---|---|---|---|---|---|---|---|---|---|
| **1. SINGLE DX** | | | | | | | | | | |
| 0–19 Years | 6 | 1.8 | <1 | 1 | 2 | 2 | 2 | 2 | 2 | 2 |
| 20–34 | 1 | 1.0 | 0 | 1 | 1 | 1 | 1 | 1 | 1 | 1 |
| 35–49 | 0 | | | | | | | | | |
| 50–64 | 2 | 1.6 | <1 | 1 | 1 | 2 | 2 | 2 | 2 | 2 |
| 65+ | 63 | 1.2 | <1 | 1 | 1 | 1 | 1 | 2 | 2 | 4 |
| **2. MULTIPLE DX** | | | | | | | | | | |
| 0–19 Years | 32 | 2.3 | 8 | 1 | 1 | 1 | 2 | 5 | 11 | 11 |
| 20–34 | 11 | 1.7 | 3 | 1 | 1 | 1 | 2 | 4 | 7 | 7 |
| 35–49 | 18 | 4.7 | 25 | 1 | 2 | 3 | 5 | 8 | 18 | 22 |
| 50–64 | 36 | 3.1 | 8 | 1 | 1 | 2 | 4 | 8 | 9 | 11 |
| 65+ | 589 | 3.3 | 11 | 1 | 1 | 2 | 4 | 8 | 11 | 16 |
| **TOTAL SINGLE DX** | 72 | 1.2 | <1 | 1 | 1 | 1 | 1 | 2 | 2 | 4 |
| **TOTAL MULTIPLE DX** | 686 | 3.3 | 11 | 1 | 1 | 2 | 4 | 8 | 11 | 16 |
| **TOTAL** | | | | | | | | | | |
| 0–19 Years | 38 | 2.3 | 7 | 1 | 1 | 1 | 2 | 5 | 11 | 11 |
| 20–34 | 12 | 1.7 | 3 | 1 | 1 | 1 | 2 | 4 | 7 | 7 |
| 35–49 | 18 | 4.7 | 25 | 1 | 2 | 3 | 5 | 8 | 18 | 22 |
| 50–64 | 38 | 3.1 | 8 | 1 | 1 | 2 | 4 | 8 | 9 | 11 |
| 65+ | 652 | 3.2 | 11 | 1 | 1 | 2 | 4 | 7 | 10 | 16 |
| **GRAND TOTAL** | 758 | 3.1 | 11 | 1 | 1 | 2 | 4 | 7 | 10 | 16 |

## 37.86: REPL W RATE-RESPON DEV. Formerly included in operation group(s) 577.

| Type of Patients | Observed Patients | Avg. Stay | Variance | 10th | 25th | 50th | 75th | 90th | 95th | 99th |
|---|---|---|---|---|---|---|---|---|---|---|
| **1. SINGLE DX** | | | | | | | | | | |
| 0–19 Years | 2 | 1.5 | <1 | | 1 | | 2 | 2 | 2 | 2 |
| 20–34 | 0 | | | | | | | | | |
| 35–49 | 3 | 1.7 | 1 | 1 | 1 | 1 | 3 | 3 | 3 | 3 |
| 50–64 | 7 | 2.2 | 1 | 1 | 1 | 2 | 2 | 4 | 4 | 4 |
| 65+ | 51 | 1.9 | 4 | 1 | 1 | 1 | 2 | 3 | 4 | 14 |
| **2. MULTIPLE DX** | | | | | | | | | | |
| 0–19 Years | 22 | 6.3 | 99 | | 1 | 2 | 2 | 29 | 29 | 29 |
| 20–34 | 11 | 1.7 | <1 | 1 | 1 | 1 | 3 | 3 | 3 | 3 |
| 35–49 | 23 | 4.1 | 34 | 1 | 2 | 3 | 4 | 5 | 12 | 34 |
| 50–64 | 59 | 3.4 | 9 | 1 | 1 | 2 | 6 | 8 | 9 | 13 |
| 65+ | 728 | 3.2 | 11 | 1 | 1 | 2 | 4 | 7 | 9 | 16 |
| **TOTAL SINGLE DX** | 63 | 1.9 | 4 | 1 | 1 | 1 | 2 | 3 | 4 | 14 |
| **TOTAL MULTIPLE DX** | 843 | 3.4 | 15 | 1 | 1 | 2 | 4 | 7 | 9 | 24 |
| **TOTAL** | | | | | | | | | | |
| 0–19 Years | 24 | 6.2 | 98 | | 1 | 2 | 2 | 29 | 29 | 29 |
| 20–34 | 11 | 1.7 | <1 | 1 | 1 | 1 | 3 | 3 | 3 | 3 |
| 35–49 | 26 | 3.8 | 31 | 1 | 2 | 3 | 4 | 5 | 12 | 34 |
| 50–64 | 66 | 3.2 | 8 | 1 | 1 | 2 | 5 | 8 | 9 | 13 |
| 65+ | 779 | 3.2 | 11 | 1 | 1 | 2 | 4 | 7 | 9 | 16 |
| **GRAND TOTAL** | 906 | 3.3 | 15 | 1 | 1 | 2 | 4 | 7 | 9 | 24 |

## 37.87: REPL W DUAL-CHAMB DEVICE. Formerly included in operation group(s) 577.

| Type of Patients | Observed Patients | Avg. Stay | Variance | 10th | 25th | 50th | 75th | 90th | 95th | 99th |
|---|---|---|---|---|---|---|---|---|---|---|
| **1. SINGLE DX** | | | | | | | | | | |
| 0–19 Years | 1 | 2.0 | 0 | 2 | 2 | 2 | 2 | 2 | 2 | 2 |
| 20–34 | 8 | 1.3 | <1 | 1 | 1 | 1 | 2 | 2 | 2 | 2 |
| 35–49 | 12 | 2.0 | 2 | 1 | 1 | 2 | 2 | 4 | 7 | 7 |
| 50–64 | 31 | 1.2 | <1 | 1 | 1 | 1 | 1 | 2 | 4 | 4 |
| 65+ | 137 | 1.5 | <1 | 1 | 1 | 1 | 2 | 2 | 2 | 6 |
| **2. MULTIPLE DX** | | | | | | | | | | |
| 0–19 Years | 118 | 2.2 | 3 | 1 | 1 | 2 | 3 | 4 | 5 | 8 |
| 20–34 | 51 | 2.9 | 4 | 1 | 2 | 2 | 4 | 4 | 7 | 10 |
| 35–49 | 85 | 3.7 | 45 | 1 | 2 | 2 | 5 | 6 | 6 | 53 |
| 50–64 | 248 | 2.8 | 12 | 1 | 2 | 2 | 3 | 7 | 9 | 18 |
| 65+ | 1,759 | 3.2 | 13 | 1 | 2 | 2 | 4 | 7 | 10 | 19 |
| **TOTAL SINGLE DX** | 189 | 1.5 | <1 | 1 | 1 | 1 | 2 | 2 | 2 | 6 |
| **TOTAL MULTIPLE DX** | 2,261 | 3.2 | 14 | 1 | 1 | 2 | 4 | 7 | 9 | 19 |
| **TOTAL** | | | | | | | | | | |
| 0–19 Years | 119 | 2.2 | 3 | 1 | 1 | 2 | 3 | 4 | 5 | 8 |
| 20–34 | 59 | 2.7 | 4 | 1 | 1 | 2 | 4 | 4 | 7 | 10 |
| 35–49 | 97 | 3.5 | 41 | 1 | 1 | 2 | 4 | 6 | 6 | 53 |
| 50–64 | 279 | 2.7 | 11 | 1 | 1 | 2 | 3 | 7 | 8 | 18 |
| 65+ | 1,896 | 3.1 | 12 | 1 | 1 | 2 | 4 | 7 | 10 | 18 |
| **GRAND TOTAL** | 2,450 | 3.0 | 13 | 1 | 1 | 2 | 4 | 7 | 9 | 18 |

Length of Stay by Diagnosis and Operation, United States, 2000

## United States, October 1998–September 1999 Data, by Operation

### 37.89: REV/RMVL PACEMAKER DEV. Formerly included in operation group(s) 577.

| Type of Patients | Observed Patients | Avg. Stay | Variance | 10th | 25th | 50th | 75th | 90th | 95th | 99th |
|---|---|---|---|---|---|---|---|---|---|---|
| **1. SINGLE DX** | | | | | | | | | | |
| 0–19 Years | 2 | 1.8 | <1 | 1 | 2 | 2 | 2 | 2 | 2 | 2 |
| 20–34 | 1 | 1.0 | 0 | 1 | 1 | 1 | 1 | 1 | 1 | 1 |
| 35–49 | 0 | | | | | | | | | |
| 50–64 | 3 | 2.5 | <1 | 1 | 1 | 3 | 3 | 3 | 3 | 3 |
| 65+ | 7 | 2.4 | 22 | 1 | 1 | 1 | 1 | 1 | 17 | 17 |
| **2. MULTIPLE DX** | | | | | | | | | | |
| 0–19 Years | 16 | 7.4 | 124 | 1 | 1 | 1 | 13 | 20 | 44 | 44 |
| 20–34 | 10 | 4.1 | 18 | 1 | 1 | 1 | 8 | 9 | 15 | 15 |
| 35–49 | 17 | 8.0 | 31 | 1 | 4 | 10 | 10 | 10 | 15 | 26 |
| 50–64 | 51 | 20.6 | 350 | 2 | 4 | 12 | 46 | 46 | 46 | 46 |
| 65+ | 201 | 6.3 | 35 | 1 | 2 | 5 | 8 | 13 | 15 | 35 |
| **TOTAL SINGLE DX** | 13 | 2.0 | 7 | 1 | 1 | 1 | 3 | 3 | 3 | 17 |
| **TOTAL MULTIPLE DX** | 295 | 8.9 | 122 | 1 | 2 | 5 | 10 | 20 | 46 | 46 |
| **TOTAL** | | | | | | | | | | |
| 0–19 Years | 18 | 7.0 | 118 | 1 | 1 | 1 | 9 | 20 | 20 | 44 |
| 20–34 | 11 | 2.9 | 13 | 1 | 1 | 1 | 2 | 8 | 9 | 15 |
| 35–49 | 17 | 8.0 | 31 | 1 | 4 | 10 | 10 | 10 | 15 | 26 |
| 50–64 | 54 | 18.3 | 342 | 2 | 3 | 9 | 46 | 46 | 46 | 46 |
| 65+ | 208 | 6.2 | 35 | 1 | 2 | 5 | 8 | 13 | 16 | 35 |
| **GRAND TOTAL** | 308 | 8.5 | 118 | 1 | 2 | 5 | 10 | 20 | 46 | 46 |

### 37.9: HRT/PERICARDIUM OPS NEC. Formerly included in operation group(s) 576, 579, 584.

| Type of Patients | Observed Patients | Avg. Stay | Variance | 10th | 25th | 50th | 75th | 90th | 95th | 99th |
|---|---|---|---|---|---|---|---|---|---|---|
| **1. SINGLE DX** | | | | | | | | | | |
| 0–19 Years | 21 | 2.5 | 7 | 1 | 1 | 2 | 2 | 2 | 2 | 9 |
| 20–34 | 28 | 2.0 | 3 | 1 | 1 | 1 | 1 | 1 | 6 | 7 |
| 35–49 | 29 | 2.5 | 4 | 1 | 1 | 2 | 3 | 5 | 7 | 9 |
| 50–64 | 44 | 2.2 | 3 | 1 | 1 | 2 | 3 | 4 | 5 | 9 |
| 65+ | 83 | 1.7 | 1 | 1 | 1 | 2 | 2 | 2 | 3 | 8 |
| **2. MULTIPLE DX** | | | | | | | | | | |
| 0–19 Years | 76 | 5.5 | 52 | 1 | 2 | 2 | 6 | 13 | 17 | 37 |
| 20–34 | 143 | 6.6 | 36 | 1 | 2 | 5 | 10 | 13 | 18 | 24 |
| 35–49 | 771 | 6.2 | 37 | 1 | 2 | 5 | 8 | 14 | 17 | 30 |
| 50–64 | 2,378 | 6.7 | 45 | 1 | 2 | 5 | 9 | 14 | 19 | 36 |
| 65+ | 4,721 | 6.8 | 40 | 1 | 2 | 5 | 9 | 15 | 18 | 30 |
| **TOTAL SINGLE DX** | 205 | 2.0 | 3 | 1 | 1 | 2 | 2 | 4 | 7 | 9 |
| **TOTAL MULTIPLE DX** | 8,089 | 6.7 | 41 | 1 | 2 | 5 | 9 | 14 | 18 | 30 |
| **TOTAL** | | | | | | | | | | |
| 0–19 Years | 97 | 4.9 | 45 | 1 | 1 | 2 | 6 | 13 | 17 | 37 |
| 20–34 | 171 | 5.7 | 33 | 1 | 2 | 4 | 7 | 13 | 17 | 24 |
| 35–49 | 800 | 6.1 | 36 | 1 | 2 | 5 | 8 | 14 | 17 | 30 |
| 50–64 | 2,422 | 6.7 | 44 | 1 | 2 | 5 | 9 | 13 | 19 | 36 |
| 65+ | 4,804 | 6.7 | 39 | 1 | 2 | 5 | 9 | 14 | 18 | 30 |
| **GRAND TOTAL** | 8,294 | 6.6 | 40 | 1 | 2 | 5 | 9 | 14 | 18 | 30 |

### 37.94: IMPL/REPL AICD TOT SYST. Formerly included in operation group(s) 576.

| Type of Patients | Observed Patients | Avg. Stay | Variance | 10th | 25th | 50th | 75th | 90th | 95th | 99th |
|---|---|---|---|---|---|---|---|---|---|---|
| **1. SINGLE DX** | | | | | | | | | | |
| 0–19 Years | 18 | 2.5 | 7 | 1 | 1 | 1 | 1 | 7 | 9 | 9 |
| 20–34 | 19 | 3.0 | 7 | 1 | 1 | 2 | 6 | 7 | 9 | 11 |
| 35–49 | 19 | 2.8 | 4 | 1 | 1 | 2 | 4 | 7 | 7 | 9 |
| 50–64 | 32 | 2.3 | 3 | 1 | 1 | 2 | 3 | 4 | 5 | 9 |
| 65+ | 46 | 1.9 | 2 | 1 | 1 | 2 | 2 | 2 | 4 | 8 |
| **2. MULTIPLE DX** | | | | | | | | | | |
| 0–19 Years | 50 | 6.1 | 60 | 2 | 2 | 4 | 8 | 17 | 17 | 28 |
| 20–34 | 105 | 7.4 | 32 | 1 | 3 | 6 | 11 | 15 | 18 | 24 |
| 35–49 | 667 | 6.8 | 42 | 1 | 2 | 5 | 9 | 14 | 18 | 30 |
| 50–64 | 2,035 | 7.2 | 46 | 1 | 3 | 6 | 9 | 14 | 20 | 36 |
| 65+ | 3,817 | 7.6 | 41 | 2 | 3 | 6 | 10 | 16 | 19 | 30 |
| **TOTAL SINGLE DX** | 134 | 2.3 | 4 | 1 | 1 | 2 | 2 | 5 | 7 | 9 |
| **TOTAL MULTIPLE DX** | 6,674 | 7.4 | 43 | 1 | 3 | 6 | 10 | 15 | 19 | 32 |
| **TOTAL** | | | | | | | | | | |
| 0–19 Years | 68 | 5.1 | 48 | 1 | 1 | 2 | 6 | 14 | 17 | 28 |
| 20–34 | 124 | 6.9 | 31 | 1 | 3 | 5 | 10 | 13 | 18 | 24 |
| 35–49 | 686 | 6.7 | 41 | 1 | 2 | 5 | 9 | 14 | 18 | 30 |
| 50–64 | 2,067 | 7.1 | 46 | 1 | 3 | 6 | 9 | 14 | 19 | 36 |
| 65+ | 3,863 | 7.5 | 41 | 2 | 3 | 6 | 10 | 16 | 19 | 30 |
| **GRAND TOTAL** | 6,808 | 7.3 | 42 | 1 | 3 | 6 | 10 | 15 | 19 | 31 |

### 37.98: REPL AICD GENERATOR ONLY. Formerly included in operation group(s) 584.

| Type of Patients | Observed Patients | Avg. Stay | Variance | 10th | 25th | 50th | 75th | 90th | 95th | 99th |
|---|---|---|---|---|---|---|---|---|---|---|
| **1. SINGLE DX** | | | | | | | | | | |
| 0–19 Years | 0 | | | | | | | | | |
| 20–34 | 3 | 1.1 | <1 | 1 | 1 | 1 | 1 | 2 | 2 | 2 |
| 35–49 | 3 | 1.3 | <1 | 1 | 1 | 1 | 2 | 2 | 2 | 2 |
| 50–64 | 6 | 1.0 | 0 | 1 | 1 | 1 | 1 | 1 | 1 | 1 |
| 65+ | 28 | 1.1 | <1 | 1 | 1 | 1 | 1 | 2 | 2 | 2 |
| **2. MULTIPLE DX** | | | | | | | | | | |
| 0–19 Years | 13 | 3.5 | 15 | 1 | 1 | 2 | 4 | 13 | 13 | 13 |
| 20–34 | 19 | 2.5 | 18 | 1 | 1 | 1 | 2 | 3 | 3 | 21 |
| 35–49 | 37 | 1.7 | 2 | 1 | 1 | 1 | 2 | 3 | 4 | 7 |
| 50–64 | 191 | 2.4 | 6 | 1 | 1 | 1 | 3 | 6 | 7 | 13 |
| 65+ | 580 | 2.6 | 9 | 1 | 1 | 1 | 3 | 7 | 8 | 14 |
| **TOTAL SINGLE DX** | 40 | 1.1 | <1 | 1 | 1 | 1 | 1 | 2 | 2 | 2 |
| **TOTAL MULTIPLE DX** | 840 | 2.6 | 8 | 1 | 1 | 1 | 3 | 6 | 8 | 13 |
| **TOTAL** | | | | | | | | | | |
| 0–19 Years | 13 | 3.5 | 15 | 1 | 1 | 1 | 4 | 13 | 13 | 13 |
| 20–34 | 22 | 2.2 | 14 | 1 | 1 | 1 | 2 | 2 | 7 | 21 |
| 35–49 | 40 | 1.6 | 2 | 1 | 1 | 1 | 3 | 3 | 4 | 7 |
| 50–64 | 197 | 2.4 | 6 | 1 | 1 | 1 | 3 | 6 | 6 | 13 |
| 65+ | 608 | 2.6 | 8 | 1 | 1 | 1 | 3 | 7 | 8 | 14 |
| **GRAND TOTAL** | 880 | 2.5 | 8 | 1 | 1 | 1 | 3 | 6 | 8 | 13 |

Length of Stay by Diagnosis and Operation, United States, 2000

# United States, October 1998–September 1999 Data, by Operation

## 38.03: UPPER LIMB VESSEL INC. Formerly included in operation group(s) 590.

| Type of Patients | Observed Patients | Avg. Stay | Vari- ance | Percentiles | | | | | | |
|---|---|---|---|---|---|---|---|---|---|---|
| | | | | 10th | 25th | 50th | 75th | 90th | 95th | 99th |
| 1. SINGLE DX | | | | | | | | | | |
| 0–19 Years | 3 | 2.8 | 2 | 1 | 1 | 3 | 4 | 4 | 4 | 4 |
| 20–34 | 5 | 3.6 | 3 | 1 | 2 | 4 | 4 | 7 | 7 | 7 |
| 35–49 | 6 | 1.8 | 2 | 1 | 1 | 1 | 4 | 4 | 4 | 4 |
| 50–64 | 6 | 4.3 | 13 | 1 | 2 | 3 | 5 | 11 | 11 | 11 |
| 65+ | 5 | 2.7 | 3 | 1 | 1 | 2 | 4 | 5 | 5 | 5 |
| 2. MULTIPLE DX | | | | | | | | | | |
| 0–19 Years | 15 | 3.6 | 14 | 1 | 1 | 3 | 3 | 6 | 9 | 20 |
| 20–34 | 62 | 7.1 | 16 | 2 | 4 | 8 | 10 | 10 | 10 | 19 |
| 35–49 | 159 | 5.4 | 26 | 1 | 2 | 3 | 7 | 12 | 15 | 29 |
| 50–64 | 261 | 5.7 | 27 | 1 | 2 | 4 | 9 | 12 | 15 | 29 |
| 65+ | 730 | 8.1 | 46 | 2 | 3 | 6 | 12 | 18 | 18 | 27 |
| TOTAL SINGLE DX | 25 | 3.0 | 5 | 1 | 1 | 3 | 4 | 5 | 7 | 11 |
| TOTAL MULTIPLE DX | 1,227 | 7.1 | 39 | 1 | 3 | 5 | 10 | 18 | 18 | 27 |
| TOTAL | | | | | | | | | | |
| 0–19 Years | 18 | 3.5 | 13 | 1 | 1 | 3 | 3 | 6 | 9 | 20 |
| 20–34 | 67 | 6.9 | 16 | 1 | 3 | 8 | 10 | 10 | 10 | 19 |
| 35–49 | 165 | 5.2 | 25 | 1 | 2 | 3 | 6 | 12 | 15 | 29 |
| 50–64 | 267 | 5.7 | 27 | 2 | 2 | 4 | 8 | 12 | 15 | 29 |
| 65+ | 735 | 8.1 | 46 | 2 | 3 | 6 | 12 | 18 | 18 | 27 |
| GRAND TOTAL | 1,252 | 7.1 | 39 | 1 | 3 | 5 | 10 | 18 | 18 | 27 |

## 38.08: LOWER LIMB ARTERY INC. Formerly included in operation group(s) 590.

| Type of Patients | Observed Patients | Avg. Stay | Vari- ance | Percentiles | | | | | | |
|---|---|---|---|---|---|---|---|---|---|---|
| | | | | 10th | 25th | 50th | 75th | 90th | 95th | 99th |
| 1. SINGLE DX | | | | | | | | | | |
| 0–19 Years | 3 | 4.6 | 6 | 2 | 2 | 3 | 7 | 7 | 7 | 7 |
| 20–34 | 2 | 8.2 | 15 | 2 | 10 | 10 | 10 | 10 | 10 | 10 |
| 35–49 | 7 | 2.4 | 15 | 1 | 1 | 1 | 2 | 3 | 12 | 17 |
| 50–64 | 17 | 2.5 | 2 | 1 | 1 | 2 | 3 | 5 | 6 | 8 |
| 65+ | 16 | 4.0 | 8 | 1 | 2 | 3 | 5 | 7 | 13 | 13 |
| 2. MULTIPLE DX | | | | | | | | | | |
| 0–19 Years | 20 | 8.0 | 51 | 1 | 1 | 7 | 12 | 18 | 22 | 26 |
| 20–34 | 39 | 9.4 | 91 | 3 | 5 | 5 | 10 | 22 | 28 | 61 |
| 35–49 | 212 | 10.2 | 81 | 2 | 4 | 8 | 16 | 17 | 25 | 53 |
| 50–64 | 521 | 6.7 | 37 | 2 | 3 | 5 | 8 | 14 | 17 | 27 |
| 65+ | 1,586 | 8.1 | 41 | 3 | 4 | 7 | 10 | 15 | 20 | 40 |
| TOTAL SINGLE DX | 45 | 3.1 | 8 | 1 | 1 | 2 | 3 | 7 | 10 | 13 |
| TOTAL MULTIPLE DX | 2,378 | 8.0 | 45 | 2 | 4 | 6 | 10 | 16 | 20 | 40 |
| TOTAL | | | | | | | | | | |
| 0–19 Years | 23 | 7.6 | 46 | 1 | 2 | 7 | 12 | 17 | 22 | 26 |
| 20–34 | 41 | 9.3 | 87 | 3 | 5 | 5 | 10 | 16 | 28 | 61 |
| 35–49 | 219 | 9.9 | 81 | 1 | 4 | 8 | 16 | 16 | 25 | 53 |
| 50–64 | 538 | 6.5 | 36 | 2 | 3 | 5 | 8 | 14 | 17 | 27 |
| 65+ | 1,602 | 8.0 | 41 | 3 | 4 | 7 | 10 | 15 | 20 | 40 |
| GRAND TOTAL | 2,423 | 7.9 | 45 | 2 | 4 | 6 | 10 | 16 | 20 | 40 |

## 37.99: OTH OPS HRT/PERICARDIUM. Formerly included in operation group(s) 579.

| Type of Patients | Observed Patients | Avg. Stay | Vari- ance | Percentiles | | | | | | |
|---|---|---|---|---|---|---|---|---|---|---|
| | | | | 10th | 25th | 50th | 75th | 90th | 95th | 99th |
| 1. SINGLE DX | | | | | | | | | | |
| 0–19 Years | 3 | 1.8 | 3 | 1 | 1 | 1 | 1 | 5 | 5 | 5 |
| 20–34 | 4 | 1.4 | <1 | 1 | 1 | 1 | 2 | 2 | 2 | 2 |
| 35–49 | 2 | 2.1 | 5 | 1 | 1 | 1 | 1 | 6 | 6 | 6 |
| 50–64 | 2 | 1.7 | <1 | 1 | 1 | 2 | 2 | 2 | 2 | 2 |
| 65+ | 2 | 1.9 | 2 | 1 | 1 | 1 | 3 | 3 | 3 | 3 |
| 2. MULTIPLE DX | | | | | | | | | | |
| 0–19 Years | 9 | 9.0 | 175 | 1 | 1 | 1 | 7 | 37 | 37 | 37 |
| 20–34 | 11 | 6.7 | 11 | 1 | 6 | 6 | 7 | 11 | 11 | 18 |
| 35–49 | 45 | 5.0 | 9 | 2 | 3 | 5 | 7 | 8 | 10 | 16 |
| 50–64 | 99 | 6.2 | 45 | 1 | 2 | 6 | 7 | 10 | 15 | 37 |
| 65+ | 185 | 5.4 | 28 | 1 | 2 | 4 | 7 | 13 | 18 | 26 |
| TOTAL SINGLE DX | 13 | 1.6 | 1 | 1 | 1 | 1 | 2 | 2 | 5 | 6 |
| TOTAL MULTIPLE DX | 349 | 5.6 | 30 | 1 | 2 | 4 | 7 | 10 | 17 | 28 |
| TOTAL | | | | | | | | | | |
| 0–19 Years | 12 | 7.1 | 139 | 1 | 1 | 1 | 6 | 37 | 37 | 37 |
| 20–34 | 15 | 5.1 | 14 | 1 | 1 | 6 | 5 | 11 | 11 | 18 |
| 35–49 | 47 | 4.9 | 9 | 1 | 3 | 5 | 7 | 8 | 10 | 16 |
| 50–64 | 101 | 6.1 | 44 | 1 | 2 | 5 | 7 | 10 | 15 | 37 |
| 65+ | 187 | 5.4 | 28 | 1 | 2 | 4 | 7 | 13 | 18 | 26 |
| GRAND TOTAL | 362 | 5.5 | 30 | 1 | 2 | 4 | 7 | 10 | 16 | 28 |

## 38.0: INCISION OF VESSEL. Formerly included in operation group(s) 590.

| Type of Patients | Observed Patients | Avg. Stay | Vari- ance | Percentiles | | | | | | |
|---|---|---|---|---|---|---|---|---|---|---|
| | | | | 10th | 25th | 50th | 75th | 90th | 95th | 99th |
| 1. SINGLE DX | | | | | | | | | | |
| 0–19 Years | 7 | 3.8 | 3 | 2 | 3 | 4 | 4 | 7 | 7 | 7 |
| 20–34 | 14 | 4.8 | 12 | 1 | 2 | 4 | 6 | 10 | 11 | 14 |
| 35–49 | 18 | 3.0 | 17 | 1 | 1 | 1 | 3 | 12 | 12 | 17 |
| 50–64 | 30 | 2.7 | 4 | 1 | 1 | 2 | 3 | 5 | 8 | 11 |
| 65+ | 25 | 3.3 | 6 | 1 | 2 | 3 | 4 | 6 | 7 | 13 |
| 2. MULTIPLE DX | | | | | | | | | | |
| 0–19 Years | 54 | 7.5 | 103 | 1 | 2 | 3 | 11 | 17 | 20 | 70 |
| 20–34 | 138 | 8.5 | 41 | 2 | 4 | 8 | 10 | 14 | 18 | 32 |
| 35–49 | 484 | 8.4 | 65 | 2 | 3 | 6 | 12 | 16 | 24 | 36 |
| 50–64 | 970 | 6.7 | 48 | 2 | 3 | 5 | 9 | 14 | 17 | 34 |
| 65+ | 2,644 | 8.2 | 44 | 2 | 4 | 7 | 10 | 17 | 20 | 37 |
| TOTAL SINGLE DX | 94 | 3.2 | 8 | 1 | 1 | 2 | 4 | 7 | 11 | 13 |
| TOTAL MULTIPLE DX | 4,290 | 7.9 | 48 | 2 | 3 | 6 | 10 | 16 | 20 | 36 |
| TOTAL | | | | | | | | | | |
| 0–19 Years | 61 | 7.1 | 93 | 1 | 2 | 3 | 9 | 15 | 20 | 70 |
| 20–34 | 152 | 8.2 | 40 | 2 | 4 | 8 | 10 | 14 | 17 | 32 |
| 35–49 | 502 | 8.2 | 64 | 1 | 3 | 6 | 12 | 16 | 23 | 36 |
| 50–64 | 1,000 | 6.6 | 47 | 2 | 2 | 5 | 9 | 14 | 17 | 31 |
| 65+ | 2,669 | 8.1 | 44 | 2 | 4 | 7 | 10 | 17 | 20 | 37 |
| GRAND TOTAL | 4,384 | 7.8 | 48 | 2 | 3 | 6 | 10 | 16 | 19 | 36 |

Length of Stay by Diagnosis and Operation, United States, 2000

# United States, October 1998–September 1999 Data, by Operation

## 38.1: ENDARTERECTOMY. Formerly included in operation group(s) 586, 590.

| Type of Patients | Observed Patients | Avg. Stay | Vari-ance | Percentiles 10th | 25th | 50th | 75th | 90th | 95th | 99th |
|---|---|---|---|---|---|---|---|---|---|---|
| **1. SINGLE DX** | | | | | | | | | | |
| 0–19 Years | 0 | | | | | | | | | |
| 20–34 | 1 | 6.0 | 0 | 6 | 6 | 6 | 6 | 6 | 6 | 6 |
| 35–49 | 91 | 2.1 | 1 | 1 | 1 | 2 | 2 | 3 | 4 | 6 |
| 50–64 | 717 | 1.8 | <1 | 1 | 1 | 2 | 2 | 3 | 4 | 6 |
| 65+ | 2,049 | 1.9 | 2 | 1 | 1 | 2 | 2 | 3 | 4 | 7 |
| **2. MULTIPLE DX** | | | | | | | | | | |
| 0–19 Years | 2 | 7.4 | 7 | 4 | 4 | 9 | 9 | 9 | 9 | 9 |
| 20–34 | 32 | 5.7 | 18 | 2 | 3 | 5 | 6 | 11 | 14 | 21 |
| 35–49 | 973 | 3.9 | 20 | 1 | 1 | 2 | 4 | 9 | 12 | 21 |
| 50–64 | 9,761 | 3.1 | 14 | 1 | 1 | 2 | 3 | 6 | 10 | 20 |
| 65+ | 31,033 | 3.4 | 15 | 1 | 1 | 2 | 4 | 8 | 10 | 19 |
| **TOTAL SINGLE DX** | 2,858 | 1.9 | 1 | 1 | 1 | 2 | 2 | 3 | 4 | 6 |
| **TOTAL MULTIPLE DX** | 41,801 | 3.4 | 15 | 1 | 1 | 2 | 4 | 7 | 10 | 19 |
| **TOTAL** | | | | | | | | | | |
| 0–19 Years | 2 | 7.4 | 7 | 4 | 4 | 9 | 9 | 9 | 9 | 9 |
| 20–34 | 33 | 5.8 | 13 | 2 | 4 | 6 | 6 | 8 | 14 | 21 |
| 35–49 | 1,064 | 3.7 | 18 | 1 | 1 | 2 | 4 | 8 | 12 | 21 |
| 50–64 | 10,478 | 3.0 | 13 | 1 | 1 | 2 | 3 | 6 | 9 | 19 |
| 65+ | 33,082 | 3.4 | 14 | 1 | 1 | 2 | 4 | 7 | 10 | 18 |
| **GRAND TOTAL** | 44,659 | 3.3 | 14 | 1 | 1 | 2 | 4 | 7 | 10 | 19 |

## 38.16: ABDOMINAL ENDARTERECTOMY. Formerly included in operation group(s) 590.

| Type of Patients | Observed Patients | Avg. Stay | Vari-ance | Percentiles 10th | 25th | 50th | 75th | 90th | 95th | 99th |
|---|---|---|---|---|---|---|---|---|---|---|
| **1. SINGLE DX** | | | | | | | | | | |
| 0–19 Years | 0 | | | | | | | | | |
| 20–34 | 0 | | | | | | | | | |
| 35–49 | 1 | 7.0 | 0 | 7 | 7 | 7 | 7 | 7 | 7 | 7 |
| 50–64 | 2 | 2.4 | <1 | 2 | 2 | 2 | 3 | 3 | 3 | 3 |
| 65+ | 1 | 7.0 | 0 | 7 | 7 | 7 | 7 | 7 | 7 | 7 |
| **2. MULTIPLE DX** | | | | | | | | | | |
| 0–19 Years | 0 | | | | | | | | | |
| 20–34 | 0 | | | | | | | | | |
| 35–49 | 47 | 6.7 | 38 | 2 | 4 | 4 | 8 | 16 | 21 | 31 |
| 50–64 | 137 | 7.3 | 60 | 1 | 3 | 5 | 9 | 16 | 22 | 38 |
| 65+ | 227 | 9.1 | 58 | 3 | 4 | 8 | 10 | 18 | 22 | 36 |
| **TOTAL SINGLE DX** | 4 | 3.9 | 6 | 2 | 2 | 3 | 7 | 7 | 7 | 7 |
| **TOTAL MULTIPLE DX** | 411 | 8.3 | 57 | 2 | 3 | 7 | 10 | 18 | 22 | 36 |
| **TOTAL** | | | | | | | | | | |
| 0–19 Years | 0 | | | | | | | | | |
| 20–34 | 0 | | | | | | | | | |
| 35–49 | 48 | 6.7 | 37 | 2 | 4 | 4 | 8 | 16 | 21 | 31 |
| 50–64 | 139 | 7.2 | 59 | 1 | 3 | 5 | 9 | 15 | 22 | 38 |
| 65+ | 228 | 9.1 | 58 | 3 | 4 | 8 | 10 | 18 | 22 | 36 |
| **GRAND TOTAL** | 415 | 8.3 | 57 | 2 | 3 | 7 | 10 | 17 | 22 | 36 |

## 38.12: HEAD/NK ENDARTERECT NEC. Formerly included in operation group(s) 586.

| Type of Patients | Observed Patients | Avg. Stay | Vari-ance | Percentiles 10th | 25th | 50th | 75th | 90th | 95th | 99th |
|---|---|---|---|---|---|---|---|---|---|---|
| **1. SINGLE DX** | | | | | | | | | | |
| 0–19 Years | 0 | | | | | | | | | |
| 20–34 | 1 | 6.0 | 0 | 6 | 6 | 6 | 6 | 6 | 6 | 6 |
| 35–49 | 75 | 2.0 | 1 | 1 | 1 | 2 | 2 | 3 | 4 | 6 |
| 50–64 | 681 | 1.7 | 1 | 1 | 1 | 2 | 2 | 3 | 4 | 6 |
| 65+ | 2,019 | 1.9 | 1 | 1 | 1 | 2 | 2 | 3 | 4 | 7 |
| **2. MULTIPLE DX** | | | | | | | | | | |
| 0–19 Years | 0 | | | | | | | | | |
| 20–34 | 10 | 4.1 | 22 | 1 | 2 | 2 | 4 | 14 | 14 | 14 |
| 35–49 | 688 | 2.9 | 12 | 1 | 1 | 2 | 3 | 6 | 8 | 18 |
| 50–64 | 8,893 | 2.9 | 11 | 1 | 1 | 2 | 3 | 6 | 8 | 17 |
| 65+ | 29,508 | 3.3 | 13 | 1 | 1 | 2 | 4 | 7 | 10 | 18 |
| **TOTAL SINGLE DX** | 2,776 | 1.9 | 1 | 1 | 1 | 2 | 2 | 3 | 4 | 6 |
| **TOTAL MULTIPLE DX** | 39,099 | 3.2 | 13 | 1 | 1 | 2 | 3 | 7 | 9 | 18 |
| **TOTAL** | | | | | | | | | | |
| 0–19 Years | 0 | | | | | | | | | |
| 20–34 | 11 | 5.3 | 9 | 2 | 2 | 6 | 6 | 6 | 14 | 14 |
| 35–49 | 763 | 2.8 | 11 | 1 | 2 | 2 | 3 | 5 | 8 | 18 |
| 50–64 | 9,574 | 2.8 | 10 | 1 | 1 | 2 | 3 | 6 | 8 | 16 |
| 65+ | 31,527 | 3.2 | 12 | 1 | 1 | 2 | 4 | 7 | 9 | 17 |
| **GRAND TOTAL** | 41,875 | 3.1 | 12 | 1 | 1 | 2 | 3 | 7 | 9 | 17 |

## 38.18: LOWER LIMB ENDARTERECT. Formerly included in operation group(s) 590.

| Type of Patients | Observed Patients | Avg. Stay | Vari-ance | Percentiles 10th | 25th | 50th | 75th | 90th | 95th | 99th |
|---|---|---|---|---|---|---|---|---|---|---|
| **1. SINGLE DX** | | | | | | | | | | |
| 0–19 Years | 0 | | | | | | | | | |
| 20–34 | 0 | | | | | | | | | |
| 35–49 | 13 | 2.2 | <1 | 2 | 2 | 2 | 2 | 3 | 4 | 4 |
| 50–64 | 27 | 2.6 | 1 | 2 | 2 | 2 | 4 | 4 | 4 | 4 |
| 65+ | 28 | 2.8 | 3 | 2 | 2 | 2 | 4 | 5 | 5 | 9 |
| **2. MULTIPLE DX** | | | | | | | | | | |
| 0–19 Years | 0 | | | | | | | | | |
| 20–34 | 14 | 5.2 | 3 | 3 | 5 | 5 | 6 | 6 | 10 | 11 |
| 35–49 | 171 | 5.8 | 31 | 1 | 2 | 3 | 8 | 14 | 18 | 25 |
| 50–64 | 611 | 5.0 | 32 | 1 | 2 | 3 | 6 | 11 | 15 | 26 |
| 65+ | 1,165 | 5.9 | 32 | 2 | 2 | 4 | 8 | 13 | 17 | 29 |
| **TOTAL SINGLE DX** | 68 | 2.5 | 1 | 1 | 2 | 2 | 3 | 4 | 5 | 6 |
| **TOTAL MULTIPLE DX** | 1,961 | 5.6 | 32 | 2 | 2 | 4 | 7 | 13 | 15 | 28 |
| **TOTAL** | | | | | | | | | | |
| 0–19 Years | 0 | | | | | | | | | |
| 20–34 | 14 | 5.2 | 3 | 3 | 5 | 5 | 6 | 6 | 10 | 11 |
| 35–49 | 184 | 5.2 | 27 | 1 | 2 | 3 | 6 | 14 | 18 | 25 |
| 50–64 | 638 | 4.9 | 31 | 1 | 2 | 3 | 6 | 11 | 15 | 25 |
| 65+ | 1,193 | 5.9 | 31 | 2 | 2 | 4 | 7 | 13 | 17 | 29 |
| **GRAND TOTAL** | 2,029 | 5.5 | 31 | 2 | 2 | 4 | 7 | 12 | 15 | 28 |

Length of Stay by Diagnosis and Operation, United States, 2000

# United States, October 1998–September 1999 Data, by Operation

## 38.2: DXTIC BLOOD VESSELS PX. Formerly included in operation group(s) 590, 596.

| Type of Patients | Observed Patients | Avg. Stay | Variance | Percentiles | | | | | | |
|---|---|---|---|---|---|---|---|---|---|---|
| | | | | 10th | 25th | 50th | 75th | 90th | 95th | 99th |
| **1. SINGLE DX** | | | | | | | | | | |
| 0–19 Years | 1 | 1.0 | 0 | 1 | 1 | 1 | 1 | 1 | 1 | 1 |
| 20–34 | 1 | 2.0 | 0 | 2 | 2 | 2 | 2 | 2 | 2 | 2 |
| 35–49 | 3 | 3.4 | 2 | 1 | 4 | 4 | 4 | 4 | 4 | 4 |
| 50–64 | 8 | 6.8 | 18 | 1 | 3 | 4 | 11 | 11 | 13 | 13 |
| 65+ | 18 | 2.9 | 4 | 1 | 2 | 2 | 3 | 7 | 8 | 9 |
| **2. MULTIPLE DX** | | | | | | | | | | |
| 0–19 Years | 4 | 23.8 | 190 | 7 | 7 | 34 | 34 | 34 | 34 | 34 |
| 20–34 | 4 | 2.9 | 3 | 1 | 1 | 3 | 4 | 5 | 5 | 5 |
| 35–49 | 71 | 7.0 | 22 | 2 | 4 | 7 | 8 | 12 | 14 | 26 |
| 50–64 | 343 | 7.4 | 28 | 3 | 4 | 6 | 9 | 16 | 19 | 24 |
| 65+ | 1,495 | 7.6 | 33 | 3 | 4 | 6 | 10 | 14 | 18 | 29 |
| **TOTAL SINGLE DX** | 31 | 3.8 | 11 | 1 | 2 | 2 | 4 | 11 | 11 | 13 |
| **TOTAL MULTIPLE DX** | 1,917 | 7.6 | 33 | 3 | 4 | 6 | 9 | 14 | 19 | 29 |
| **TOTAL** | | | | | | | | | | |
| 0–19 Years | 5 | 13.6 | 235 | 1 | 1 | 7 | 34 | 34 | 34 | 34 |
| 20–34 | 5 | 2.7 | 3 | 1 | 1 | 3 | 4 | 5 | 5 | 5 |
| 35–49 | 74 | 6.9 | 22 | 2 | 4 | 6 | 8 | 11 | 14 | 26 |
| 50–64 | 351 | 7.4 | 28 | 3 | 4 | 6 | 9 | 15 | 19 | 24 |
| 65+ | 1,513 | 7.5 | 33 | 2 | 4 | 6 | 9 | 14 | 18 | 24 |
| **GRAND TOTAL** | 1,948 | 7.5 | 33 | 2 | 4 | 6 | 9 | 14 | 19 | 29 |

## 38.3: VESSEL RESECT W ANAST. Formerly included in operation group(s) 590.

| Type of Patients | Observed Patients | Avg. Stay | Variance | Percentiles | | | | | | |
|---|---|---|---|---|---|---|---|---|---|---|
| | | | | 10th | 25th | 50th | 75th | 90th | 95th | 99th |
| **1. SINGLE DX** | | | | | | | | | | |
| 0–19 Years | 31 | 3.0 | <1 | 2 | 2 | 3 | 4 | 4 | 4 | 7 |
| 20–34 | 3 | 2.8 | <1 | 2 | 3 | 3 | 3 | 3 | 3 | 3 |
| 35–49 | 4 | 3.2 | 6 | 1 | 1 | 2 | 6 | 6 | 6 | 6 |
| 50–64 | 5 | 2.0 | <1 | 1 | 1 | 2 | 2 | 2 | 2 | 5 |
| 65+ | 3 | 4.1 | 2 | 3 | 3 | 4 | 4 | 6 | 6 | 6 |
| **2. MULTIPLE DX** | | | | | | | | | | |
| 0–19 Years | 313 | 8.7 | 88 | 3 | 4 | 5 | 10 | 18 | 32 | 56 |
| 20–34 | 41 | 6.3 | 89 | 1 | 1 | 4 | 8 | 18 | 19 | 73 |
| 35–49 | 49 | 7.5 | 38 | 2 | 3 | 6 | 11 | 17 | 17 | 22 |
| 50–64 | 94 | 8.2 | 45 | 2 | 4 | 6 | 10 | 18 | 25 | 29 |
| 65+ | 268 | 8.0 | 51 | 2 | 4 | 7 | 9 | 15 | 23 | 48 |
| **TOTAL SINGLE DX** | 46 | 2.9 | 1 | 2 | 2 | 3 | 3 | 4 | 4 | 6 |
| **TOTAL MULTIPLE DX** | 765 | 8.2 | 68 | 2 | 4 | 6 | 9 | 17 | 25 | 48 |
| **TOTAL** | | | | | | | | | | |
| 0–19 Years | 344 | 7.8 | 78 | 2 | 3 | 5 | 8 | 17 | 30 | 49 |
| 20–34 | 44 | 6.1 | 83 | 1 | 2 | 3 | 8 | 18 | 19 | 73 |
| 35–49 | 53 | 7.2 | 37 | 2 | 3 | 6 | 11 | 17 | 17 | 22 |
| 50–64 | 99 | 7.5 | 44 | 2 | 3 | 5 | 9 | 18 | 25 | 29 |
| 65+ | 271 | 8.0 | 51 | 2 | 4 | 7 | 9 | 15 | 23 | 48 |
| **GRAND TOTAL** | 811 | 7.7 | 64 | 2 | 3 | 5 | 8 | 16 | 25 | 48 |

## 38.21: BLOOD VESSEL BIOPSY. Formerly included in operation group(s) 590.

| Type of Patients | Observed Patients | Avg. Stay | Variance | Percentiles | | | | | | |
|---|---|---|---|---|---|---|---|---|---|---|
| | | | | 10th | 25th | 50th | 75th | 90th | 95th | 99th |
| **1. SINGLE DX** | | | | | | | | | | |
| 0–19 Years | 0 | | | | | | | | | |
| 20–34 | 1 | 2.0 | 0 | 2 | 2 | 2 | 2 | 2 | 2 | 2 |
| 35–49 | 3 | 3.4 | 2 | 1 | 4 | 4 | 4 | 4 | 4 | 4 |
| 50–64 | 8 | 6.8 | 18 | 1 | 3 | 4 | 11 | 11 | 13 | 13 |
| 65+ | 18 | 2.9 | 4 | 1 | 2 | 2 | 3 | 7 | 8 | 9 |
| **2. MULTIPLE DX** | | | | | | | | | | |
| 0–19 Years | 2 | 34.0 | 0 | 34 | 34 | 34 | 34 | 34 | 34 | 34 |
| 20–34 | 4 | 2.9 | 3 | 1 | 1 | 3 | 4 | 5 | 5 | 5 |
| 35–49 | 64 | 7.4 | 21 | 3 | 5 | 7 | 8 | 12 | 14 | 26 |
| 50–64 | 337 | 7.4 | 28 | 3 | 4 | 6 | 9 | 16 | 19 | 24 |
| 65+ | 1,480 | 7.6 | 33 | 3 | 4 | 6 | 9 | 14 | 18 | 29 |
| **TOTAL SINGLE DX** | 30 | 4.1 | 11 | 1 | 2 | 2 | 6 | 11 | 11 | 13 |
| **TOTAL MULTIPLE DX** | 1,887 | 7.6 | 33 | 3 | 4 | 6 | 9 | 14 | 19 | 29 |
| **TOTAL** | | | | | | | | | | |
| 0–19 Years | 2 | 34.0 | 0 | 34 | 34 | 34 | 34 | 34 | 34 | 34 |
| 20–34 | 5 | 2.7 | 3 | 1 | 1 | 3 | 4 | 5 | 5 | 5 |
| 35–49 | 67 | 7.3 | 21 | 3 | 4 | 6 | 8 | 12 | 14 | 26 |
| 50–64 | 345 | 7.4 | 28 | 3 | 4 | 6 | 9 | 15 | 19 | 24 |
| 65+ | 1,498 | 7.5 | 33 | 2 | 4 | 6 | 9 | 14 | 18 | 24 |
| **GRAND TOTAL** | 1,917 | 7.5 | 33 | 3 | 4 | 6 | 9 | 14 | 19 | 29 |

## 38.34: AORTA RESECTION & ANAST. Formerly included in operation group(s) 590.

| Type of Patients | Observed Patients | Avg. Stay | Variance | Percentiles | | | | | | |
|---|---|---|---|---|---|---|---|---|---|---|
| | | | | 10th | 25th | 50th | 75th | 90th | 95th | 99th |
| **1. SINGLE DX** | | | | | | | | | | |
| 0–19 Years | 25 | 3.1 | <1 | 2 | 2 | 3 | 4 | 4 | 4 | 7 |
| 20–34 | 0 | | | | | | | | | |
| 35–49 | 0 | | | | | | | | | |
| 50–64 | 1 | 5.0 | 0 | 5 | 5 | 5 | 5 | 5 | 5 | 5 |
| 65+ | 1 | 4.0 | 0 | 4 | 4 | 4 | 4 | 4 | 4 | 4 |
| **2. MULTIPLE DX** | | | | | | | | | | |
| 0–19 Years | 295 | 8.8 | 89 | 3 | 4 | 5 | 10 | 19 | 32 | 56 |
| 20–34 | 4 | 14.6 | 98 | 8 | 8 | 8 | 27 | 27 | 27 | 27 |
| 35–49 | 3 | 6.9 | 9 | 4 | 4 | 7 | 10 | 10 | 10 | 10 |
| 50–64 | 31 | 7.8 | 28 | 4 | 4 | 7 | 8 | 16 | 21 | 29 |
| 65+ | 97 | 9.4 | 64 | 5 | 6 | 7 | 9 | 15 | 21 | 48 |
| **TOTAL SINGLE DX** | 27 | 3.1 | <1 | 2 | 2 | 3 | 4 | 4 | 4 | 7 |
| **TOTAL MULTIPLE DX** | 430 | 8.9 | 79 | 3 | 4 | 6 | 10 | 17 | 30 | 50 |
| **TOTAL** | | | | | | | | | | |
| 0–19 Years | 320 | 7.9 | 80 | 2 | 3 | 5 | 8 | 17 | 30 | 52 |
| 20–34 | 4 | 14.6 | 98 | 8 | 8 | 8 | 27 | 27 | 27 | 27 |
| 35–49 | 3 | 6.9 | 9 | 4 | 4 | 7 | 10 | 10 | 10 | 10 |
| 50–64 | 32 | 7.8 | 28 | 4 | 4 | 7 | 8 | 16 | 21 | 29 |
| 65+ | 98 | 9.4 | 63 | 5 | 6 | 7 | 9 | 15 | 21 | 48 |
| **GRAND TOTAL** | 457 | 8.2 | 73 | 3 | 4 | 5 | 9 | 16 | 30 | 49 |

Length of Stay by Diagnosis and Operation, United States, 2000

## 38.4: VESSEL RESECT W REPL. Formerly included in operation group(s) 587, 590.

| Type of Patients | Observed Patients | Avg. Stay | Variance | 10th | 25th | 50th | 75th | 90th | 95th | 99th |
|---|---|---|---|---|---|---|---|---|---|---|
| **1. SINGLE DX** | | | | | | | | | | |
| 0–19 Years | 20 | 3.8 | <1 | 3 | 3 | 4 | 4 | 5 | 5 | 5 |
| 20–34 | 9 | 3.6 | <1 | 3 | 3 | 4 | 4 | 4 | 4 | 6 |
| 35–49 | 23 | 4.5 | <1 | 2 | 3 | 4 | 6 | 7 | 8 | 11 |
| 50–64 | 63 | 4.7 | 4 | 3 | 4 | 5 | 5 | 7 | 8 | 12 |
| 65+ | 124 | 5.9 | 6 | 3 | 5 | 6 | 7 | 8 | 9 | 16 |
| **2. MULTIPLE DX** | | | | | | | | | | |
| 0–19 Years | 207 | 9.4 | 73 | 3 | 4 | 7 | 11 | 20 | 23 | 54 |
| 20–34 | 142 | 11.3 | 155 | 3 | 4 | 8 | 13 | 23 | 24 | 75 |
| 35–49 | 386 | 8.4 | 67 | 2 | 4 | 6 | 9 | 15 | 23 | 45 |
| 50–64 | 2,292 | 8.4 | 58 | 5 | 5 | 6 | 9 | 15 | 20 | 42 |
| 65+ | 9,152 | 9.9 | 64 | 5 | 6 | 8 | 11 | 17 | 24 | 45 |
| **TOTAL SINGLE DX** | 239 | 5.2 | 5 | 3 | 4 | 5 | 6 | 8 | 9 | 11 |
| **TOTAL MULTIPLE DX** | 12,179 | 9.5 | 64 | 4 | 6 | 7 | 10 | 17 | 23 | 45 |
| **TOTAL** | | | | | | | | | | |
| 0–19 Years | 227 | 8.9 | 69 | 3 | 4 | 6 | 11 | 20 | 23 | 54 |
| 20–34 | 151 | 10.6 | 145 | 3 | 4 | 7 | 12 | 23 | 23 | 75 |
| 35–49 | 409 | 8.1 | 64 | 2 | 4 | 6 | 9 | 14 | 22 | 45 |
| 50–64 | 2,355 | 8.3 | 57 | 4 | 5 | 6 | 9 | 14 | 20 | 42 |
| 65+ | 9,276 | 9.8 | 63 | 5 | 6 | 8 | 11 | 17 | 24 | 45 |
| **GRAND TOTAL** | 12,418 | 9.5 | 63 | 4 | 5 | 7 | 10 | 17 | 23 | 44 |

## 38.45: THOR VESS RESECT W REPL. Formerly included in operation group(s) 587.

| Type of Patients | Observed Patients | Avg. Stay | Variance | 10th | 25th | 50th | 75th | 90th | 95th | 99th |
|---|---|---|---|---|---|---|---|---|---|---|
| **1. SINGLE DX** | | | | | | | | | | |
| 0–19 Years | 16 | 4.0 | <1 | 3 | 4 | 4 | 4 | 5 | 5 | 5 |
| 20–34 | 3 | 3.9 | <1 | 3 | 4 | 4 | 4 | 5 | 4 | 5 |
| 35–49 | 3 | 6.3 | 9 | 4 | 4 | 4 | 8 | 11 | 11 | 11 |
| 50–64 | 4 | 6.1 | 6 | 4 | 6 | 7 | 9 | 9 | 9 | 9 |
| 65+ | 5 | 6.6 | 4 | 3 | 6 | 7 | 8 | 8 | 8 | 8 |
| **2. MULTIPLE DX** | | | | | | | | | | |
| 0–19 Years | 160 | 9.6 | 61 | 4 | 5 | 7 | 11 | 22 | 23 | 42 |
| 20–34 | 74 | 12.6 | 85 | 4 | 6 | 10 | 23 | 23 | 23 | 47 |
| 35–49 | 131 | 10.6 | 81 | 5 | 6 | 7 | 13 | 19 | 23 | 52 |
| 50–64 | 243 | 13.1 | 115 | 6 | 7 | 9 | 15 | 30 | 38 | 49 |
| 65+ | 477 | 16.3 | 203 | 6 | 8 | 11 | 18 | 34 | 46 | 77 |
| **TOTAL SINGLE DX** | 32 | 4.4 | 2 | 3 | 4 | 4 | 4 | 7 | 8 | 11 |
| **TOTAL MULTIPLE DX** | 1,085 | 13.7 | 147 | 5 | 7 | 9 | 16 | 28 | 38 | 62 |
| **TOTAL** | | | | | | | | | | |
| 0–19 Years | 176 | 9.1 | 58 | 4 | 4 | 7 | 11 | 20 | 23 | 42 |
| 20–34 | 78 | 11.4 | 82 | 3 | 5 | 8 | 18 | 23 | 23 | 47 |
| 35–49 | 134 | 10.5 | 79 | 5 | 6 | 7 | 13 | 18 | 23 | 52 |
| 50–64 | 247 | 13.1 | 114 | 5 | 7 | 9 | 15 | 27 | 38 | 49 |
| 65+ | 482 | 16.2 | 202 | 6 | 8 | 11 | 18 | 34 | 46 | 77 |
| **GRAND TOTAL** | 1,117 | 13.3 | 145 | 4 | 6 | 9 | 16 | 27 | 37 | 61 |

## 38.44: ABD AORTA RESECT W REPL. Formerly included in operation group(s) 587.

| Type of Patients | Observed Patients | Avg. Stay | Variance | 10th | 25th | 50th | 75th | 90th | 95th | 99th |
|---|---|---|---|---|---|---|---|---|---|---|
| **1. SINGLE DX** | | | | | | | | | | |
| 0–19 Years | 1 | 2.0 | 0 | 2 | 2 | 2 | 2 | 2 | 2 | 2 |
| 20–34 | 0 | | | | | | | | | |
| 35–49 | 6 | 6.2 | 6 | 3 | 4 | 6 | 7 | 10 | 10 | 10 |
| 50–64 | 42 | 5.2 | 3 | 4 | 5 | 5 | 5 | 7 | 8 | 12 |
| 65+ | 98 | 6.3 | 5 | 4 | 5 | 6 | 7 | 8 | 9 | 16 |
| **2. MULTIPLE DX** | | | | | | | | | | |
| 0–19 Years | 15 | 7.2 | 75 | 3 | 4 | 5 | 8 | 12 | 18 | >99 |
| 20–34 | 14 | 22.1 | 927 | 3 | 4 | 8 | 17 | 75 | 95 | 95 |
| 35–49 | 112 | 9.0 | 76 | 4 | 5 | 6 | 9 | 15 | 24 | 48 |
| 50–64 | 1,725 | 8.4 | 52 | 5 | 5 | 6 | 9 | 14 | 20 | 41 |
| 65+ | 7,831 | 9.8 | 54 | 5 | 6 | 8 | 11 | 17 | 23 | 42 |
| **TOTAL SINGLE DX** | 147 | 6.0 | 5 | 4 | 5 | 6 | 7 | 8 | 9 | 16 |
| **TOTAL MULTIPLE DX** | 9,697 | 9.6 | 55 | 5 | 6 | 7 | 10 | 16 | 22 | 42 |
| **TOTAL** | | | | | | | | | | |
| 0–19 Years | 16 | 6.8 | 70 | 3 | 4 | 5 | 7 | 12 | 18 | >99 |
| 20–34 | 14 | 22.1 | 927 | 3 | 4 | 8 | 17 | 75 | 95 | 95 |
| 35–49 | 118 | 8.9 | 74 | 4 | 5 | 6 | 8 | 14 | 24 | 48 |
| 50–64 | 1,767 | 8.4 | 51 | 5 | 5 | 6 | 9 | 14 | 20 | 41 |
| 65+ | 7,929 | 9.8 | 54 | 5 | 6 | 8 | 11 | 17 | 23 | 42 |
| **GRAND TOTAL** | 9,844 | 9.5 | 55 | 5 | 6 | 7 | 10 | 16 | 22 | 42 |

## 38.48: LEG ARTERY RESECT W REPL. Formerly included in operation group(s) 590.

| Type of Patients | Observed Patients | Avg. Stay | Variance | 10th | 25th | 50th | 75th | 90th | 95th | 99th |
|---|---|---|---|---|---|---|---|---|---|---|
| **1. SINGLE DX** | | | | | | | | | | |
| 0–19 Years | 1 | 3.0 | 0 | 3 | 3 | 3 | 3 | 3 | 3 | 3 |
| 20–34 | 1 | 4.0 | 0 | 3 | 4 | 4 | 4 | 4 | 4 | 4 |
| 35–49 | 6 | 4.7 | 5 | 2 | 3 | 3 | 7 | 7 | 7 | 7 |
| 50–64 | 13 | 3.0 | 2 | 1 | 1 | 3 | 4 | 4 | 6 | 6 |
| 65+ | 16 | 2.1 | 3 | 1 | 1 | 2 | 2 | 6 | 6 | 6 |
| **2. MULTIPLE DX** | | | | | | | | | | |
| 0–19 Years | 15 | 5.8 | 27 | 3 | 3 | 3 | 10 | 12 | 16 | 29 |
| 20–34 | 24 | 10.4 | 150 | 2 | 4 | 8 | 9 | 17 | 32 | 65 |
| 35–49 | 52 | 7.2 | 55 | 1 | 2 | 6 | 8 | 12 | 19 | 39 |
| 50–64 | 174 | 4.3 | 14 | 2 | 3 | 4 | 7 | 8 | 10 | 18 |
| 65+ | 539 | 6.1 | 42 | 2 | 3 | 6 | 7 | 12 | 16 | 40 |
| **TOTAL SINGLE DX** | 37 | 3.0 | 4 | 1 | 1 | 3 | 4 | 6 | 7 | 7 |
| **TOTAL MULTIPLE DX** | 804 | 5.9 | 40 | 2 | 2 | 4 | 7 | 11 | 15 | 39 |
| **TOTAL** | | | | | | | | | | |
| 0–19 Years | 16 | 5.7 | 27 | 3 | 3 | 3 | 5 | 12 | 16 | 29 |
| 20–34 | 25 | 10.2 | 146 | 3 | 4 | 8 | 9 | 17 | 32 | 65 |
| 35–49 | 58 | 6.8 | 49 | 2 | 3 | 6 | 7 | 12 | 19 | 39 |
| 50–64 | 187 | 4.2 | 13 | 1 | 2 | 4 | 5 | 8 | 10 | 18 |
| 65+ | 555 | 6.0 | 42 | 2 | 3 | 4 | 7 | 12 | 16 | 40 |
| **GRAND TOTAL** | 841 | 5.7 | 39 | 2 | 2 | 4 | 7 | 11 | 15 | 38 |

Length of Stay by Diagnosis and Operation, United States, 2000

# United States, October 1998–September 1999 Data, by Operation

## 38.5: LIG&STRIP VARICOSE VEINS. Formerly included in operation group(s) 582.

| Type of Patients | Observed Patients | Avg. Stay | Vari- ance | Percentiles | | | | | | |
|---|---|---|---|---|---|---|---|---|---|---|
| | | | | 10th | 25th | 50th | 75th | 90th | 95th | 99th |
| **1. SINGLE DX** | | | | | | | | | | |
| 0-19 Years | 3 | 4.7 | 7 | 2 | 2 | 7 | 7 | 7 | 7 | 7 |
| 20-34 | 50 | 1.4 | 2 | 1 | 1 | 1 | 1 | 2 | 3 | 14 |
| 35-49 | 89 | 2.1 | 4 | 1 | 1 | 1 | 2 | 7 | 7 | 7 |
| 50-64 | 65 | 1.2 | <1 | 1 | 1 | 1 | 1 | 2 | 2 | 3 |
| 65+ | 60 | 1.9 | 2 | 1 | 1 | 2 | 2 | 3 | 5 | 8 |
| **2. MULTIPLE DX** | | | | | | | | | | |
| 0-19 Years | 5 | 17.1 | 97 | 5 | 5 | 20 | 26 | 26 | 26 | 26 |
| 20-34 | 36 | 3.3 | 10 | 1 | 1 | 2 | 5 | 8 | 11 | 18 |
| 35-49 | 153 | 3.9 | 19 | 1 | 1 | 2 | 5 | 11 | 11 | 16 |
| 50-64 | 165 | 3.9 | 14 | 1 | 1 | 2 | 7 | 9 | 9 | 17 |
| 65+ | 207 | 4.3 | 24 | 1 | 2 | 3 | 5 | 8 | 14 | 24 |
| **TOTAL SINGLE DX** | 267 | 1.7 | 2 | 1 | 1 | 1 | 2 | 3 | 5 | 7 |
| **TOTAL MULTIPLE DX** | 566 | 4.1 | 20 | 1 | 1 | 2 | 5 | 11 | 11 | 24 |
| **TOTAL** | | | | | | | | | | |
| 0-19 Years | 8 | 10.3 | 85 | 2 | 2 | 7 | 20 | 26 | 26 | 26 |
| 20-34 | 86 | 2.0 | 6 | 1 | 1 | 1 | 2 | 5 | 7 | 14 |
| 35-49 | 242 | 3.5 | 16 | 1 | 1 | 2 | 4 | 11 | 11 | 11 |
| 50-64 | 230 | 3.1 | 11 | 1 | 1 | 2 | 3 | 9 | 9 | 16 |
| 65+ | 267 | 3.9 | 21 | 1 | 2 | 3 | 4 | 7 | 14 | 24 |
| **GRAND TOTAL** | 833 | 3.4 | 16 | 1 | 1 | 2 | 4 | 9 | 11 | 22 |

## 38.6: OTHER VESSEL EXCISION. Formerly included in operation group(s) 590.

| Type of Patients | Observed Patients | Avg. Stay | Vari- ance | Percentiles | | | | | | |
|---|---|---|---|---|---|---|---|---|---|---|
| | | | | 10th | 25th | 50th | 75th | 90th | 95th | 99th |
| **1. SINGLE DX** | | | | | | | | | | |
| 0-19 Years | 59 | 3.0 | 6 | 1 | 1 | 2 | 3 | 6 | 10 | 10 |
| 20-34 | 26 | 4.2 | 5 | 1 | 3 | 3 | 5 | 7 | 9 | 11 |
| 35-49 | 19 | 4.2 | 5 | 2 | 2 | 4 | 6 | 8 | 8 | 8 |
| 50-64 | 17 | 9.9 | 126 | 1 | 2 | 3 | 26 | 26 | 26 | 26 |
| 65+ | 13 | 3.1 | 4 | 1 | 3 | 3 | 5 | 6 | 7 | 7 |
| **2. MULTIPLE DX** | | | | | | | | | | |
| 0-19 Years | 252 | 9.6 | 99 | 3 | 4 | 7 | 10 | 17 | 26 | 55 |
| 20-34 | 83 | 7.3 | 96 | 1 | 2 | 5 | 8 | 16 | 19 | 51 |
| 35-49 | 195 | 9.2 | 108 | 2 | 2 | 6 | 13 | 19 | 29 | 49 |
| 50-64 | 250 | 6.7 | 49 | 2 | 3 | 5 | 8 | 12 | 17 | 39 |
| 65+ | 460 | 8.4 | 62 | 2 | 4 | 6 | 10 | 16 | 25 | 36 |
| **TOTAL SINGLE DX** | 134 | 3.9 | 21 | 1 | 1 | 3 | 5 | 7 | 10 | 26 |
| **TOTAL MULTIPLE DX** | 1,240 | 8.4 | 76 | 2 | 3 | 6 | 10 | 17 | 24 | 50 |
| **TOTAL** | | | | | | | | | | |
| 0-19 Years | 311 | 8.1 | 85 | 2 | 3 | 6 | 10 | 13 | 23 | 55 |
| 20-34 | 109 | 6.4 | 72 | 1 | 2 | 4 | 7 | 11 | 19 | 40 |
| 35-49 | 214 | 8.7 | 100 | 2 | 2 | 5 | 12 | 18 | 26 | 49 |
| 50-64 | 267 | 6.8 | 54 | 2 | 3 | 5 | 8 | 13 | 19 | 39 |
| 65+ | 473 | 8.3 | 61 | 2 | 3 | 6 | 10 | 16 | 25 | 36 |
| **GRAND TOTAL** | 1,374 | 7.9 | 72 | 2 | 3 | 5 | 9 | 16 | 23 | 45 |

## 38.59: LOWER LIMB VV LIG&STRIP. Formerly included in operation group(s) 582.

| Type of Patients | Observed Patients | Avg. Stay | Vari- ance | Percentiles | | | | | | |
|---|---|---|---|---|---|---|---|---|---|---|
| | | | | 10th | 25th | 50th | 75th | 90th | 95th | 99th |
| **1. SINGLE DX** | | | | | | | | | | |
| 0-19 Years | 1 | 7.0 | 0 | 7 | 7 | 7 | 7 | 7 | 7 | 7 |
| 20-34 | 49 | 1.4 | 2 | 1 | 1 | 1 | 1 | 2 | 3 | 14 |
| 35-49 | 86 | 2.2 | 4 | 1 | 1 | 1 | 2 | 7 | 7 | 7 |
| 50-64 | 65 | 1.2 | <1 | 1 | 1 | 1 | 1 | 2 | 2 | 3 |
| 65+ | 60 | 1.9 | 2 | 1 | 1 | 2 | 2 | 3 | 5 | 8 |
| **2. MULTIPLE DX** | | | | | | | | | | |
| 0-19 Years | 0 | | | | | | | | | |
| 20-34 | 32 | 2.8 | 7 | 1 | 1 | 2 | 3 | 7 | 8 | 11 |
| 35-49 | 147 | 3.9 | 18 | 1 | 1 | 2 | 5 | 11 | 11 | 11 |
| 50-64 | 161 | 3.9 | 14 | 1 | 1 | 2 | 7 | 9 | 9 | 17 |
| 65+ | 198 | 4.2 | 19 | 1 | 2 | 3 | 4 | 8 | 14 | 24 |
| **TOTAL SINGLE DX** | 261 | 1.7 | 2 | 1 | 1 | 1 | 2 | 3 | 5 | 7 |
| **TOTAL MULTIPLE DX** | 538 | 4.0 | 17 | 1 | 1 | 2 | 5 | 9 | 11 | 22 |
| **TOTAL** | | | | | | | | | | |
| 0-19 Years | 1 | 7.0 | 0 | 7 | 7 | 7 | 7 | 7 | 7 | 7 |
| 20-34 | 81 | 1.8 | 4 | 1 | 1 | 1 | 2 | 3 | 5 | 11 |
| 35-49 | 233 | 3.5 | 15 | 1 | 1 | 2 | 4 | 9 | 11 | 11 |
| 50-64 | 226 | 3.1 | 11 | 1 | 1 | 2 | 3 | 9 | 9 | 16 |
| 65+ | 258 | 3.8 | 17 | 1 | 2 | 3 | 4 | 6 | 13 | 24 |
| **GRAND TOTAL** | 799 | 3.3 | 14 | 1 | 2 | 2 | 4 | 9 | 11 | 19 |

## 38.64: EXCISION OF AORTA. Formerly included in operation group(s) 590.

| Type of Patients | Observed Patients | Avg. Stay | Vari- ance | Percentiles | | | | | | |
|---|---|---|---|---|---|---|---|---|---|---|
| | | | | 10th | 25th | 50th | 75th | 90th | 95th | 99th |
| **1. SINGLE DX** | | | | | | | | | | |
| 0-19 Years | 35 | 3.2 | 2 | 2 | 2 | 3 | 4 | 6 | 6 | 8 |
| 20-34 | 0 | | | | | | | | | |
| 35-49 | 1 | 4.0 | 0 | 4 | 4 | 4 | 4 | 4 | 4 | 4 |
| 50-64 | 1 | 8.0 | 0 | 8 | 8 | 8 | 8 | 8 | 8 | 8 |
| 65+ | 0 | | | | | | | | | |
| **2. MULTIPLE DX** | | | | | | | | | | |
| 0-19 Years | 203 | 9.2 | 88 | 3 | 4 | 6 | 11 | 17 | 25 | 55 |
| 20-34 | 4 | 1.9 | 4 | 1 | 1 | 1 | 1 | 4 | 8 | 8 |
| 35-49 | 2 | 25.1 | 186 | 4 | 4 | 33 | 33 | 33 | 33 | 33 |
| 50-64 | 17 | 10.1 | 168 | 4 | 6 | 6 | 8 | 10 | 32 | 74 |
| 65+ | 52 | 16.4 | 161 | 6 | 7 | 9 | 36 | 36 | 36 | 36 |
| **TOTAL SINGLE DX** | 37 | 3.3 | 2 | 2 | 2 | 3 | 4 | 6 | 6 | 8 |
| **TOTAL MULTIPLE DX** | 278 | 10.6 | 116 | 3 | 5 | 7 | 11 | 27 | 36 | 55 |
| **TOTAL** | | | | | | | | | | |
| 0-19 Years | 238 | 8.3 | 79 | 3 | 3 | 6 | 10 | 13 | 21 | 55 |
| 20-34 | 4 | 1.9 | 4 | 1 | 1 | 1 | 1 | 4 | 8 | 8 |
| 35-49 | 3 | 19.3 | 227 | 4 | 4 | 33 | 33 | 33 | 33 | 33 |
| 50-64 | 18 | 10.0 | 164 | 4 | 6 | 6 | 8 | 10 | 32 | 74 |
| 65+ | 52 | 16.4 | 161 | 6 | 7 | 9 | 36 | 36 | 36 | 36 |
| **GRAND TOTAL** | 315 | 9.8 | 108 | 3 | 4 | 6 | 10 | 22 | 36 | 55 |

Length of Stay by Diagnosis and Operation, United States, 2000

# United States, October 1998–September 1999 Data, by Operation

## 38.68: LOWER LIMB ARTERY EXC. Formerly included in operation group(s) 590.

| Type of Patients | Observed Patients | Avg. Stay | Variance | 10th | 25th | 50th | 75th | 90th | 95th | 99th |
|---|---|---|---|---|---|---|---|---|---|---|
| **1. SINGLE DX** | | | | | | | | | | |
| 0–19 Years | 3 | 1.3 | <1 | 1 | 1 | 1 | 2 | 2 | 2 | 2 |
| 20–34 | 4 | 3.0 | 4 | 1 | 1 | 4 | 5 | 5 | 5 | 5 |
| 35–49 | 0 | | | | | | | | | |
| 50–64 | 4 | 1.7 | <1 | 1 | 1 | 1 | 3 | 3 | 3 | 3 |
| 65+ | 3 | 2.3 | 1 | 1 | 1 | 3 | 3 | 3 | 3 | 3 |
| **2. MULTIPLE DX** | | | | | | | | | | |
| 0–19 Years | 0 | | | | | | | | | |
| 20–34 | 8 | 10.4 | 147 | 4 | 4 | 4 | 14 | 38 | 38 | 38 |
| 35–49 | 35 | 4.7 | 15 | 1 | 2 | 3 | 6 | 11 | 15 | 15 |
| 50–64 | 80 | 4.9 | 8 | 2 | 3 | 4 | 7 | 9 | 9 | 12 |
| 65+ | 213 | 5.4 | 21 | 1 | 3 | 5 | 7 | 10 | 12 | 17 |
| **TOTAL SINGLE DX** | 14 | 2.0 | 2 | 1 | 1 | 1 | 3 | 4 | 5 | 5 |
| **TOTAL MULTIPLE DX** | 336 | 5.3 | 20 | 2 | 3 | 5 | 7 | 9 | 12 | 17 |
| **TOTAL** | | | | | | | | | | |
| 0–19 Years | 3 | 1.3 | <1 | 1 | 1 | 1 | 2 | 2 | 2 | 2 |
| 20–34 | 12 | 8.3 | 117 | 1 | 4 | 4 | 7 | 38 | 38 | 38 |
| 35–49 | 35 | 4.7 | 15 | 1 | 2 | 3 | 6 | 11 | 15 | 15 |
| 50–64 | 84 | 4.8 | 8 | 2 | 3 | 4 | 7 | 9 | 9 | 12 |
| 65+ | 216 | 5.4 | 21 | 1 | 3 | 5 | 7 | 10 | 12 | 17 |
| **GRAND TOTAL** | 350 | 5.2 | 20 | 1 | 3 | 4 | 7 | 9 | 12 | 17 |

## 38.8: OTHER SURG VESSEL OCCL. Formerly included in operation group(s) 590.

| Type of Patients | Observed Patients | Avg. Stay | Variance | 10th | 25th | 50th | 75th | 90th | 95th | 99th |
|---|---|---|---|---|---|---|---|---|---|---|
| **1. SINGLE DX** | | | | | | | | | | |
| 0–19 Years | 362 | 2.1 | 8 | 1 | 1 | 1 | 2 | 3 | 5 | 19 |
| 20–34 | 100 | 2.3 | 3 | 1 | 1 | 1 | 2 | 3 | 5 | 10 |
| 35–49 | 146 | 2.0 | 3 | 1 | 1 | 1 | 2 | 4 | 5 | 11 |
| 50–64 | 88 | 2.3 | 4 | 1 | 1 | 2 | 2 | 4 | 6 | 10 |
| 65+ | 42 | 2.2 | 5 | 1 | 1 | 1 | 3 | 5 | 6 | 12 |
| **2. MULTIPLE DX** | | | | | | | | | | |
| 0–19 Years | 990 | 16.6 | 630 | 1 | 2 | 6 | 26 | 93 | >99 | >99 |
| 20–34 | 422 | 5.3 | 44 | 1 | 2 | 3 | 6 | 10 | 17 | 36 |
| 35–49 | 710 | 5.0 | 52 | 1 | 1 | 3 | 5 | 11 | 16 | 43 |
| 50–64 | 614 | 8.6 | 204 | 1 | 2 | 4 | 9 | 18 | 28 | 83 |
| 65+ | 897 | 7.6 | 65 | 1 | 2 | 5 | 9 | 17 | 21 | 40 |
| **TOTAL SINGLE DX** | 738 | 2.1 | 6 | 1 | 1 | 1 | 2 | 4 | 5 | 14 |
| **TOTAL MULTIPLE DX** | 3,633 | 9.6 | 267 | 1 | 2 | 4 | 10 | 27 | 74 | >99 |
| **TOTAL** | | | | | | | | | | |
| 0–19 Years | 1,352 | 12.6 | 503 | 1 | 1 | 3 | 14 | 81 | >99 | >99 |
| 20–34 | 522 | 4.6 | 37 | 1 | 1 | 3 | 5 | 10 | 14 | 33 |
| 35–49 | 856 | 4.5 | 45 | 1 | 1 | 2 | 5 | 10 | 15 | 36 |
| 50–64 | 702 | 7.7 | 180 | 1 | 2 | 4 | 8 | 16 | 26 | 83 |
| 65+ | 939 | 7.4 | 64 | 1 | 2 | 5 | 9 | 17 | 21 | 40 |
| **GRAND TOTAL** | 4,371 | 8.3 | 230 | 1 | 2 | 3 | 8 | 21 | 63 | >99 |

## 38.7: INTERRUPTION VENA CAVA. Formerly included in operation group(s) 588.

| Type of Patients | Observed Patients | Avg. Stay | Variance | 10th | 25th | 50th | 75th | 90th | 95th | 99th |
|---|---|---|---|---|---|---|---|---|---|---|
| **1. SINGLE DX** | | | | | | | | | | |
| 0–19 Years | 2 | 4.6 | <1 | 4 | 4 | 5 | 5 | 5 | 5 | 5 |
| 20–34 | 14 | 9.5 | 53 | 3 | 5 | 6 | 21 | 21 | 21 | 21 |
| 35–49 | 22 | 5.4 | 7 | 2 | 4 | 5 | 8 | 8 | 8 | 11 |
| 50–64 | 21 | 3.5 | 5 | 1 | 2 | 3 | 5 | 6 | 9 | 9 |
| 65+ | 20 | 3.5 | 6 | 2 | 2 | 3 | 4 | 8 | 9 | 13 |
| **2. MULTIPLE DX** | | | | | | | | | | |
| 0–19 Years | 23 | 8.9 | 151 | 2 | 5 | 5 | 8 | 14 | 41 | 68 |
| 20–34 | 279 | 10.9 | 105 | 2 | 5 | 9 | 14 | 20 | 29 | 69 |
| 35–49 | 905 | 10.2 | 87 | 3 | 5 | 8 | 12 | 20 | 26 | 54 |
| 50–64 | 1,847 | 10.4 | 68 | 3 | 5 | 8 | 13 | 21 | 27 | 41 |
| 65+ | 5,631 | 10.4 | 74 | 3 | 5 | 8 | 13 | 20 | 27 | 43 |
| **TOTAL SINGLE DX** | 79 | 5.1 | 18 | 1 | 3 | 4 | 6 | 9 | 11 | 21 |
| **TOTAL MULTIPLE DX** | 8,685 | 10.4 | 75 | 3 | 5 | 8 | 13 | 20 | 27 | 45 |
| **TOTAL** | | | | | | | | | | |
| 0–19 Years | 25 | 8.7 | 146 | 3 | 5 | 5 | 8 | 14 | 41 | 68 |
| 20–34 | 293 | 10.9 | 103 | 3 | 5 | 9 | 14 | 20 | 28 | 69 |
| 35–49 | 927 | 10.1 | 86 | 3 | 5 | 8 | 12 | 20 | 26 | 54 |
| 50–64 | 1,868 | 10.3 | 68 | 3 | 5 | 8 | 13 | 21 | 27 | 41 |
| 65+ | 5,651 | 10.4 | 74 | 3 | 5 | 8 | 13 | 20 | 27 | 43 |
| **GRAND TOTAL** | 8,764 | 10.3 | 75 | 3 | 5 | 8 | 13 | 20 | 27 | 45 |

## 38.81: OCCLUSION IC VESSELS NEC. Formerly included in operation group(s) 590.

| Type of Patients | Observed Patients | Avg. Stay | Variance | 10th | 25th | 50th | 75th | 90th | 95th | 99th |
|---|---|---|---|---|---|---|---|---|---|---|
| **1. SINGLE DX** | | | | | | | | | | |
| 0–19 Years | 17 | 2.6 | 6 | 1 | 1 | 2 | 2 | 7 | 8 | 9 |
| 20–34 | 26 | 2.7 | 4 | 1 | 1 | 1 | 4 | 4 | 5 | 10 |
| 35–49 | 55 | 2.0 | 3 | 1 | 1 | 1 | 2 | 4 | 5 | 14 |
| 50–64 | 31 | 2.8 | 10 | 1 | 2 | 2 | 3 | 8 | 8 | 16 |
| 65+ | 10 | 2.7 | 10 | 1 | 1 | 1 | 3 | 6 | 12 | 12 |
| **2. MULTIPLE DX** | | | | | | | | | | |
| 0–19 Years | 28 | 11.0 | 98 | 1 | 4 | 7 | 16 | 22 | 32 | 41 |
| 20–34 | 55 | 4.6 | 63 | 1 | 1 | 2 | 5 | 9 | 16 | 62 |
| 35–49 | 136 | 5.1 | 46 | 1 | 2 | 2 | 6 | 13 | 16 | 36 |
| 50–64 | 111 | 6.4 | 47 | 1 | 2 | 3 | 10 | 16 | 25 | 28 |
| 65+ | 72 | 6.9 | 65 | 1 | 2 | 3 | 9 | 21 | 26 | 30 |
| **TOTAL SINGLE DX** | 139 | 2.4 | 5 | 1 | 1 | 2 | 3 | 5 | 7 | 14 |
| **TOTAL MULTIPLE DX** | 402 | 6.2 | 58 | 1 | 2 | 3 | 8 | 16 | 23 | 36 |
| **TOTAL** | | | | | | | | | | |
| 0–19 Years | 45 | 8.0 | 81 | 1 | 1 | 5 | 13 | 22 | 32 | 41 |
| 20–34 | 81 | 3.8 | 39 | 1 | 1 | 2 | 4 | 8 | 10 | 40 |
| 35–49 | 191 | 4.0 | 33 | 1 | 1 | 2 | 4 | 10 | 14 | 36 |
| 50–64 | 142 | 5.7 | 41 | 1 | 2 | 3 | 8 | 14 | 22 | 28 |
| 65+ | 82 | 6.6 | 61 | 2 | 2 | 3 | 8 | 21 | 25 | 30 |
| **GRAND TOTAL** | 541 | 5.1 | 46 | 1 | 1 | 2 | 6 | 14 | 19 | 32 |

## United States, October 1998–September 1999 Data, by Operation

### 38.82: OCCL HEAD/NECK VESS NEC. Formerly included in operation group(s) 590.

| Type of Patients | Observed Patients | Avg. Stay | Vari-ance | Percentiles | | | | | | |
|---|---|---|---|---|---|---|---|---|---|---|
| | | | | 10th | 25th | 50th | 75th | 90th | 95th | 99th |
| **1. SINGLE DX** | | | | | | | | | | |
| 0–19 Years | 21 | 1.9 | 1 | 1 | 1 | 2 | 2 | 2 | 5 | 5 |
| 20–34 | 28 | 2.5 | 3 | 1 | 1 | 2 | 5 | 5 | 5 | 5 |
| 35–49 | 34 | 2.2 | 2 | 1 | 1 | 2 | 3 | 4 | 4 | 5 |
| 50–64 | 27 | 2.2 | 4 | 1 | 1 | 1 | 3 | 5 | 5 | 10 |
| 65+ | 15 | 1.4 | <1 | 1 | 1 | 2 | 2 | 3 | 3 | 3 |
| **2. MULTIPLE DX** | | | | | | | | | | |
| 0–19 Years | 29 | 5.5 | 29 | 1 | 2 | 2 | 11 | 12 | 18 | 19 |
| 20–34 | 66 | 3.9 | 41 | 1 | 1 | 2 | 4 | 8 | 14 | 23 |
| 35–49 | 124 | 3.3 | 9 | 1 | 2 | 2 | 4 | 6 | 10 | 17 |
| 50–64 | 117 | 5.4 | 41 | 1 | 2 | 3 | 6 | 10 | 17 | 34 |
| 65+ | 168 | 5.5 | 38 | 1 | 2 | 4 | 7 | 13 | 17 | 30 |
| **TOTAL SINGLE DX** | 125 | 2.1 | 2 | 1 | 1 | 2 | 3 | 5 | 5 | 10 |
| **TOTAL MULTIPLE DX** | 504 | 4.7 | 32 | 1 | 2 | 3 | 6 | 11 | 15 | 26 |
| **TOTAL** | | | | | | | | | | |
| 0–19 Years | 50 | 4.3 | 23 | 2 | 2 | 2 | 4 | 12 | 18 | 19 |
| 20–34 | 94 | 3.5 | 30 | 1 | 1 | 2 | 4 | 7 | 11 | 22 |
| 35–49 | 158 | 3.1 | 7 | 1 | 2 | 2 | 4 | 6 | 9 | 17 |
| 50–64 | 144 | 4.6 | 34 | 1 | 2 | 3 | 6 | 10 | 12 | 31 |
| 65+ | 183 | 5.3 | 36 | 1 | 2 | 3 | 7 | 12 | 17 | 30 |
| **GRAND TOTAL** | 629 | 4.2 | 27 | 1 | 1 | 2 | 5 | 10 | 14 | 24 |

### 38.86: SURG OCCL ABD ARTERY NEC. Formerly included in operation group(s) 590.

| Type of Patients | Observed Patients | Avg. Stay | Vari-ance | Percentiles | | | | | | |
|---|---|---|---|---|---|---|---|---|---|---|
| | | | | 10th | 25th | 50th | 75th | 90th | 95th | 99th |
| **1. SINGLE DX** | | | | | | | | | | |
| 0–19 Years | 7 | 3.8 | 3 | 1 | 2 | 5 | 5 | 5 | 5 | 6 |
| 20–34 | 13 | 1.7 | 4 | 1 | 1 | 1 | 1 | 5 | 5 | 14 |
| 35–49 | 30 | 2.1 | 7 | 1 | 2 | 1 | 2 | 7 | 11 | 11 |
| 50–64 | 10 | 2.9 | 2 | 1 | 2 | 3 | 4 | 4 | 6 | 6 |
| 65+ | 3 | 4.2 | 3 | 1 | 5 | 5 | 5 | 5 | 5 | 5 |
| **2. MULTIPLE DX** | | | | | | | | | | |
| 0–19 Years | 39 | 9.8 | 34 | 4 | 7 | 10 | 10 | 17 | 17 | 30 |
| 20–34 | 105 | 5.5 | 37 | 1 | 1 | 4 | 6 | 10 | 18 | 32 |
| 35–49 | 214 | 4.7 | 49 | 1 | 2 | 2 | 5 | 10 | 16 | 36 |
| 50–64 | 179 | 6.7 | 55 | 1 | 3 | 4 | 9 | 13 | 20 | 38 |
| 65+ | 323 | 8.9 | 85 | 2 | 3 | 6 | 10 | 20 | 26 | 50 |
| **TOTAL SINGLE DX** | 63 | 2.4 | 5 | 1 | 1 | 1 | 3 | 5 | 6 | 11 |
| **TOTAL MULTIPLE DX** | 860 | 7.0 | 64 | 1 | 2 | 5 | 9 | 16 | 20 | 41 |
| **TOTAL** | | | | | | | | | | |
| 0–19 Years | 46 | 9.2 | 34 | 3 | 5 | 10 | 10 | 17 | 17 | 30 |
| 20–34 | 118 | 4.8 | 33 | 1 | 1 | 3 | 6 | 9 | 18 | 32 |
| 35–49 | 244 | 4.4 | 45 | 1 | 2 | 4 | 5 | 10 | 16 | 36 |
| 50–64 | 189 | 6.5 | 53 | 1 | 3 | 6 | 8 | 13 | 19 | 38 |
| 65+ | 326 | 8.8 | 85 | 2 | 3 | 6 | 10 | 20 | 26 | 50 |
| **GRAND TOTAL** | 923 | 6.7 | 61 | 1 | 2 | 4 | 9 | 15 | 20 | 41 |

### 38.85: OCCL THORACIC VESS NEC. Formerly included in operation group(s) 590.

| Type of Patients | Observed Patients | Avg. Stay | Vari-ance | Percentiles | | | | | | |
|---|---|---|---|---|---|---|---|---|---|---|
| | | | | 10th | 25th | 50th | 75th | 90th | 95th | 99th |
| **1. SINGLE DX** | | | | | | | | | | |
| 0–19 Years | 291 | 2.0 | 9 | 1 | 1 | 1 | 2 | 3 | 4 | 19 |
| 20–34 | 9 | 3.5 | 7 | 1 | 3 | 3 | 4 | 6 | 11 | 11 |
| 35–49 | 6 | 1.6 | <1 | 1 | 1 | 1 | 2 | 3 | 3 | 3 |
| 50–64 | 2 | 1.4 | <1 | 2 | 1 | 1 | 2 | 2 | 3 | 3 |
| 65+ | 2 | 3.1 | 1 | 2 | 2 | 4 | 4 | 4 | 4 | 4 |
| **2. MULTIPLE DX** | | | | | | | | | | |
| 0–19 Years | 771 | 19.4 | 767 | 1 | 2 | 7 | 52 | >99 | >99 | >99 |
| 20–34 | 76 | 7.6 | 49 | 1 | 4 | 6 | 10 | 11 | 17 | 55 |
| 35–49 | 47 | 6.3 | 29 | 2 | 3 | 5 | 7 | 15 | 18 | 28 |
| 50–64 | 73 | 7.2 | 44 | 2 | 2 | 6 | 9 | 16 | 18 | 33 |
| 65+ | 73 | 10.1 | 101 | 1 | 3 | 7 | 13 | 22 | 22 | 40 |
| **TOTAL SINGLE DX** | 310 | 2.1 | 8 | 1 | 1 | 1 | 2 | 3 | 4 | 19 |
| **TOTAL MULTIPLE DX** | 1,040 | 16.6 | 616 | 1 | 3 | 6 | 26 | 93 | >99 | >99 |
| **TOTAL** | | | | | | | | | | |
| 0–19 Years | 1,062 | 14.4 | 609 | 1 | 1 | 3 | 21 | 89 | >99 | >99 |
| 20–34 | 85 | 7.3 | 47 | 1 | 3 | 6 | 10 | 11 | 14 | 55 |
| 35–49 | 53 | 5.9 | 28 | 3 | 3 | 5 | 7 | 15 | 16 | 23 |
| 50–64 | 75 | 7.1 | 43 | 2 | 2 | 6 | 8 | 16 | 18 | 33 |
| 65+ | 75 | 9.9 | 100 | 1 | 3 | 7 | 13 | 22 | 22 | 40 |
| **GRAND TOTAL** | 1,350 | 13.1 | 508 | 1 | 1 | 4 | 14 | 81 | >99 | >99 |

### 38.9: PUNCTURE OF VESSEL. Formerly included in operation group(s) 590, 595, 596.

| Type of Patients | Observed Patients | Avg. Stay | Vari-ance | Percentiles | | | | | | |
|---|---|---|---|---|---|---|---|---|---|---|
| | | | | 10th | 25th | 50th | 75th | 90th | 95th | 99th |
| **1. SINGLE DX** | | | | | | | | | | |
| 0–19 Years | 985 | 5.5 | 20 | 2 | 3 | 4 | 7 | 13 | 14 | 22 |
| 20–34 | 482 | 5.0 | 19 | 1 | 2 | 4 | 6 | 10 | 13 | 21 |
| 35–49 | 422 | 5.0 | 14 | 1 | 3 | 4 | 6 | 9 | 14 | 19 |
| 50–64 | 259 | 4.3 | 13 | 1 | 2 | 3 | 6 | 9 | 10 | 17 |
| 65+ | 159 | 5.6 | 23 | 1 | 2 | 4 | 8 | 10 | 15 | 21 |
| **2. MULTIPLE DX** | | | | | | | | | | |
| 0–19 Years | 13,896 | 13.3 | 251 | 2 | 4 | 8 | 15 | 34 | 52 | 88 |
| 20–34 | 6,974 | 8.1 | 58 | 2 | 3 | 6 | 10 | 16 | 22 | 36 |
| 35–49 | 14,589 | 7.9 | 53 | 2 | 4 | 6 | 10 | 15 | 21 | 38 |
| 50–64 | 15,995 | 8.3 | 53 | 2 | 4 | 6 | 10 | 16 | 22 | 37 |
| 65+ | 30,056 | 9.6 | 61 | 3 | 5 | 8 | 12 | 18 | 24 | 39 |
| **TOTAL SINGLE DX** | 2,307 | 5.2 | 18 | 1 | 2 | 4 | 7 | 11 | 14 | 21 |
| **TOTAL MULTIPLE DX** | 81,510 | 9.5 | 94 | 2 | 4 | 7 | 11 | 19 | 26 | 55 |
| **TOTAL** | | | | | | | | | | |
| 0–19 Years | 14,881 | 12.6 | 235 | 2 | 4 | 7 | 14 | 32 | 49 | 87 |
| 20–34 | 7,456 | 7.9 | 56 | 2 | 3 | 6 | 10 | 16 | 22 | 35 |
| 35–49 | 15,011 | 7.8 | 52 | 2 | 4 | 6 | 10 | 15 | 21 | 37 |
| 50–64 | 16,254 | 8.2 | 52 | 2 | 4 | 6 | 10 | 16 | 22 | 36 |
| 65+ | 30,215 | 9.6 | 60 | 3 | 5 | 8 | 12 | 18 | 24 | 39 |
| **GRAND TOTAL** | 83,817 | 9.4 | 92 | 2 | 4 | 7 | 11 | 19 | 26 | 54 |

Length of Stay by Diagnosis and Operation, United States, 2000

## United States, October 1998–September 1999 Data, by Operation

### 38.91: ARTERIAL CATHETERIZATION. Formerly included in operation group(s) 590.

| Type of Patients | Observed Patients | Avg. Stay | Variance | Percentiles | | | | | | |
|---|---|---|---|---|---|---|---|---|---|---|
| | | | | 10th | 25th | 50th | 75th | 90th | 95th | 99th |
| **1. SINGLE DX** | | | | | | | | | | |
| 0–19 Years | 74 | 4.3 | 6 | 1 | 2 | 4 | 6 | 9 | 9 | 9 |
| 20–34 | 11 | 2.4 | 5 | 1 | 1 | 4 | 7 | 7 | 7 | 7 |
| 35–49 | 19 | 5.3 | 30 | 2 | 2 | 4 | 5 | 10 | 21 | 21 |
| 50–64 | 16 | 3.7 | 4 | 2 | 2 | 4 | 4 | 7 | 7 | 8 |
| 65+ | 10 | 2.8 | 5 | 1 | 1 | 2 | 3 | 7 | 8 | 8 |
| **2. MULTIPLE DX** | | | | | | | | | | |
| 0–19 Years | 4,780 | 18.7 | 420 | 3 | 6 | 10 | 25 | 53 | 71 | 99 |
| 20–34 | 189 | 5.9 | 30 | 2 | 3 | 5 | 8 | 12 | 16 | 33 |
| 35–49 | 372 | 6.5 | 28 | 2 | 3 | 5 | 8 | 13 | 16 | 28 |
| 50–64 | 561 | 6.9 | 36 | 2 | 3 | 6 | 8 | 13 | 17 | 34 |
| 65+ | 924 | 7.7 | 34 | 2 | 4 | 6 | 10 | 16 | 19 | 29 |
| **TOTAL SINGLE DX** | 130 | 4.1 | 9 | 1 | 2 | 3 | 5 | 8 | 9 | 21 |
| **TOTAL MULTIPLE DX** | 6,826 | 14.9 | 323 | 2 | 5 | 8 | 17 | 40 | 61 | 95 |
| **TOTAL** | | | | | | | | | | |
| 0–19 Years | 4,854 | 18.5 | 416 | 3 | 6 | 10 | 24 | 52 | 71 | 99 |
| 20–34 | 200 | 5.7 | 29 | 2 | 3 | 4 | 7 | 12 | 16 | 33 |
| 35–49 | 391 | 6.4 | 28 | 2 | 3 | 5 | 8 | 13 | 16 | 27 |
| 50–64 | 577 | 6.8 | 35 | 2 | 3 | 6 | 8 | 13 | 17 | 34 |
| 65+ | 934 | 7.6 | 34 | 2 | 4 | 6 | 10 | 16 | 19 | 29 |
| **GRAND TOTAL** | 6,956 | 14.7 | 320 | 2 | 5 | 8 | 17 | 40 | 60 | 95 |

### 38.92: UMBILICAL VEIN CATH. Formerly included in operation group(s) 590.

| Type of Patients | Observed Patients | Avg. Stay | Variance | Percentiles | | | | | | |
|---|---|---|---|---|---|---|---|---|---|---|
| | | | | 10th | 25th | 50th | 75th | 90th | 95th | 99th |
| **1. SINGLE DX** | | | | | | | | | | |
| 0–19 Years | 11 | 4.5 | 6 | 2 | 3 | 4 | 8 | 8 | 8 | 9 |
| 20–34 | 0 | | | | | | | | | |
| 35–49 | 0 | | | | | | | | | |
| 50–64 | 0 | | | | | | | | | |
| 65+ | | | | | | | | | | |
| **2. MULTIPLE DX** | | | | | | | | | | |
| 0–19 Years | 1,737 | 14.7 | 273 | 3 | 5 | 8 | 17 | 40 | 56 | 86 |
| 20–34 | 0 | | | | | | | | | |
| 35–49 | 3 | 13.9 | 35 | 7 | 7 | 17 | 17 | 20 | 20 | 20 |
| 50–64 | 0 | | | | | | | | | |
| 65+ | 5 | 21.2 | 116 | 7 | 12 | 22 | 34 | 34 | 34 | 34 |
| **TOTAL SINGLE DX** | 11 | 4.5 | 6 | 2 | 3 | 4 | 8 | 8 | 8 | 9 |
| **TOTAL MULTIPLE DX** | 1,745 | 14.7 | 272 | 3 | 5 | 8 | 17 | 40 | 56 | 86 |
| **TOTAL** | | | | | | | | | | |
| 0–19 Years | 1,748 | 14.6 | 272 | 3 | 5 | 8 | 17 | 39 | 56 | 86 |
| 20–34 | 0 | | | | | | | | | |
| 35–49 | 3 | 13.9 | 35 | 7 | 7 | 17 | 17 | 20 | 20 | 20 |
| 50–64 | 0 | | | | | | | | | |
| 65+ | 5 | 21.2 | 116 | 7 | 12 | 22 | 34 | 34 | 34 | 34 |
| **GRAND TOTAL** | 1,756 | 14.6 | 271 | 3 | 5 | 8 | 17 | 39 | 55 | 86 |

### 38.93: VENOUS CATHETER NEC. Formerly included in operation group(s) 595.

| Type of Patients | Observed Patients | Avg. Stay | Variance | Percentiles | | | | | | |
|---|---|---|---|---|---|---|---|---|---|---|
| | | | | 10th | 25th | 50th | 75th | 90th | 95th | 99th |
| **1. SINGLE DX** | | | | | | | | | | |
| 0–19 Years | 801 | 5.9 | 21 | 2 | 3 | 4 | 7 | 13 | 15 | 22 |
| 20–34 | 430 | 5.2 | 20 | 1 | 2 | 4 | 7 | 11 | 14 | 22 |
| 35–49 | 354 | 5.1 | 13 | 2 | 3 | 4 | 6 | 11 | 14 | 16 |
| 50–64 | 204 | 4.4 | 12 | 1 | 2 | 3 | 6 | 9 | 10 | 14 |
| 65+ | 104 | 6.4 | 22 | 1 | 3 | 5 | 10 | 11 | 15 | 21 |
| **2. MULTIPLE DX** | | | | | | | | | | |
| 0–19 Years | 6,500 | 10.8 | 139 | 3 | 4 | 7 | 13 | 24 | 36 | 70 |
| 20–34 | 5,685 | 8.5 | 62 | 2 | 4 | 6 | 10 | 17 | 23 | 37 |
| 35–49 | 11,601 | 8.2 | 56 | 2 | 4 | 6 | 10 | 16 | 22 | 38 |
| 50–64 | 11,457 | 8.9 | 56 | 3 | 4 | 7 | 11 | 17 | 23 | 39 |
| 65+ | 21,779 | 10.2 | 63 | 3 | 5 | 8 | 13 | 19 | 25 | 41 |
| **TOTAL SINGLE DX** | 1,893 | 5.5 | 19 | 2 | 3 | 4 | 7 | 12 | 14 | 21 |
| **TOTAL MULTIPLE DX** | 57,022 | 9.4 | 70 | 3 | 4 | 7 | 12 | 18 | 25 | 44 |
| **TOTAL** | | | | | | | | | | |
| 0–19 Years | 7,301 | 10.0 | 124 | 3 | 4 | 7 | 12 | 21 | 33 | 68 |
| 20–34 | 6,115 | 8.3 | 60 | 2 | 4 | 6 | 10 | 17 | 23 | 37 |
| 35–49 | 11,955 | 8.1 | 54 | 2 | 4 | 6 | 10 | 16 | 22 | 38 |
| 50–64 | 11,661 | 8.8 | 56 | 3 | 4 | 7 | 11 | 17 | 23 | 39 |
| 65+ | 21,883 | 10.1 | 63 | 3 | 5 | 8 | 13 | 19 | 24 | 40 |
| **GRAND TOTAL** | 58,915 | 9.2 | 69 | 3 | 4 | 7 | 11 | 18 | 24 | 43 |

### 38.94: VENOUS CUTDOWN. Formerly included in operation group(s) 590.

| Type of Patients | Observed Patients | Avg. Stay | Variance | Percentiles | | | | | | |
|---|---|---|---|---|---|---|---|---|---|---|
| | | | | 10th | 25th | 50th | 75th | 90th | 95th | 99th |
| **1. SINGLE DX** | | | | | | | | | | |
| 0–19 Years | 12 | 1.5 | <1 | 1 | 1 | 1 | 2 | 3 | 3 | 5 |
| 20–34 | 0 | | | | | | | | | |
| 35–49 | 3 | 4.2 | 4 | 2 | 2 | 5 | 6 | 6 | 6 | 6 |
| 50–64 | 2 | 2.6 | 3 | 2 | 2 | 2 | 2 | 2 | 8 | 8 |
| 65+ | 1 | 4.0 | 0 | 4 | 4 | 4 | 4 | 4 | 4 | 4 |
| **2. MULTIPLE DX** | | | | | | | | | | |
| 0–19 Years | 163 | 17.5 | 452 | 3 | 4 | 9 | 22 | 47 | 75 | 99 |
| 20–34 | 37 | 9.6 | 111 | 3 | 4 | 8 | 10 | 14 | 40 | 47 |
| 35–49 | 74 | 8.9 | 35 | 1 | 4 | 8 | 14 | 16 | 16 | 26 |
| 50–64 | 79 | 9.4 | 81 | 2 | 4 | 7 | 11 | 26 | 27 | 36 |
| 65+ | 142 | 10.9 | 65 | 2 | 5 | 9 | 14 | 25 | 26 | 42 |
| **TOTAL SINGLE DX** | 18 | 1.8 | 2 | 1 | 1 | 1 | 2 | 3 | 5 | 8 |
| **TOTAL MULTIPLE DX** | 495 | 12.7 | 221 | 2 | 4 | 8 | 16 | 26 | 41 | 98 |
| **TOTAL** | | | | | | | | | | |
| 0–19 Years | 175 | 15.8 | 427 | 1 | 3 | 8 | 20 | 47 | 75 | 99 |
| 20–34 | 37 | 9.6 | 111 | 3 | 4 | 8 | 10 | 14 | 40 | 47 |
| 35–49 | 77 | 8.8 | 35 | 1 | 3 | 8 | 14 | 16 | 16 | 26 |
| 50–64 | 81 | 9.0 | 79 | 1 | 2 | 7 | 11 | 24 | 27 | 36 |
| 65+ | 143 | 10.9 | 65 | 2 | 5 | 9 | 14 | 25 | 26 | 42 |
| **GRAND TOTAL** | 513 | 12.1 | 215 | 1 | 4 | 8 | 14 | 26 | 39 | 86 |

Length of Stay by Diagnosis and Operation, United States, 2000

# United States, October 1998–September 1999 Data, by Operation

## 38.95: VENOUS CATH FOR RD. Formerly included in operation group(s) 595.

| Type of Patients | Observed Patients | Avg. Stay | Variance | 10th | 25th | 50th | 75th | 90th | 95th | 99th |
|---|---|---|---|---|---|---|---|---|---|---|
| **1. SINGLE DX** | | | | | | | | | | |
| 0–19 Years | 13 | 3.2 | 2 | 1 | 2 | 4 | 4 | 4 | 4 | 5 |
| 20–34 | 26 | 3.2 | 8 | 1 | 2 | 2 | 3 | 5 | 10 | 15 |
| 35–49 | 35 | 4.0 | 35 | 1 | 1 | 2 | 4 | 8 | 27 | 27 |
| 50–64 | 24 | 4.6 | 30 | 2 | 2 | 2 | 5 | 17 | 17 | 23 |
| 65+ | 28 | 3.2 | 25 | 1 | 1 | 2 | 2 | 7 | 16 | 27 |
| **2. MULTIPLE DX** | | | | | | | | | | |
| 0–19 Years | 284 | 6.0 | 34 | 1 | 2 | 4 | 8 | 12 | 16 | 29 |
| 20–34 | 917 | 6.4 | 32 | 1 | 3 | 5 | 8 | 13 | 16 | 26 |
| 35–49 | 2,212 | 7.2 | 48 | 1 | 3 | 5 | 9 | 14 | 19 | 40 |
| 50–64 | 3,283 | 7.1 | 42 | 1 | 3 | 6 | 9 | 14 | 19 | 31 |
| 65+ | 5,509 | 8.8 | 60 | 1 | 3 | 7 | 12 | 19 | 23 | 36 |
| **TOTAL SINGLE DX** | 126 | 3.6 | 21 | 1 | 1 | 2 | 4 | 6 | 16 | 27 |
| **TOTAL MULTIPLE DX** | 12,205 | 7.8 | 51 | 1 | 3 | 6 | 10 | 16 | 22 | 34 |
| **TOTAL** | | | | | | | | | | |
| 0–19 Years | 297 | 5.9 | 33 | 2 | 2 | 4 | 8 | 11 | 16 | 29 |
| 20–34 | 943 | 6.3 | 31 | 1 | 3 | 5 | 8 | 13 | 16 | 26 |
| 35–49 | 2,247 | 7.2 | 48 | 1 | 3 | 5 | 9 | 14 | 19 | 40 |
| 50–64 | 3,307 | 7.1 | 42 | 1 | 3 | 6 | 9 | 14 | 19 | 31 |
| 65+ | 5,537 | 8.7 | 60 | 1 | 3 | 7 | 12 | 19 | 23 | 36 |
| **GRAND TOTAL** | 12,331 | 7.8 | 51 | 1 | 3 | 6 | 10 | 16 | 22 | 34 |

## 38.99: VENOUS PUNCTURE NEC. Formerly included in operation group(s) 596.

| Type of Patients | Observed Patients | Avg. Stay | Variance | 10th | 25th | 50th | 75th | 90th | 95th | 99th |
|---|---|---|---|---|---|---|---|---|---|---|
| **1. SINGLE DX** | | | | | | | | | | |
| 0–19 Years | 45 | 3.1 | 2 | 2 | 2 | 3 | 4 | 5 | 5 | 7 |
| 20–34 | 5 | 3.5 | 2 | 2 | 2 | 3 | 4 | 6 | 6 | 6 |
| 35–49 | 3 | 2.3 | 2 | 1 | 2 | 2 | 2 | 5 | 5 | 5 |
| 50–64 | 1 | 1.0 | 0 | 1 | 1 | 1 | 1 | 1 | 1 | 1 |
| 65+ | 3 | 3.9 | 8 | 1 | 1 | 4 | 4 | 8 | 8 | 8 |
| **2. MULTIPLE DX** | | | | | | | | | | |
| 0–19 Years | 251 | 4.8 | 36 | 1 | 2 | 3 | 6 | 9 | 14 | 22 |
| 20–34 | 29 | 5.5 | 16 | 2 | 3 | 4 | 8 | 9 | 11 | 21 |
| 35–49 | 84 | 5.7 | 28 | 1 | 3 | 3 | 7 | 16 | 16 | 16 |
| 50–64 | 140 | 5.6 | 23 | 2 | 3 | 4 | 7 | 14 | 14 | 25 |
| 65+ | 170 | 5.5 | 33 | 2 | 3 | 4 | 6 | 9 | 13 | 22 |
| **TOTAL SINGLE DX** | 57 | 3.1 | 2 | 2 | 2 | 3 | 4 | 5 | 5 | 7 |
| **TOTAL MULTIPLE DX** | 674 | 5.3 | 31 | 1 | 2 | 4 | 6 | 11 | 16 | 22 |
| **TOTAL** | | | | | | | | | | |
| 0–19 Years | 296 | 4.6 | 31 | 1 | 2 | 3 | 5 | 9 | 11 | 22 |
| 20–34 | 34 | 5.3 | 15 | 2 | 3 | 4 | 7 | 9 | 11 | 21 |
| 35–49 | 87 | 5.6 | 27 | 1 | 3 | 3 | 7 | 16 | 16 | 16 |
| 50–64 | 141 | 5.6 | 23 | 2 | 3 | 4 | 7 | 14 | 14 | 25 |
| 65+ | 173 | 5.5 | 33 | 2 | 3 | 4 | 6 | 9 | 13 | 22 |
| **GRAND TOTAL** | 731 | 5.2 | 29 | 1 | 2 | 3 | 6 | 10 | 15 | 22 |

## 38.98: ARTERIAL PUNCTURE NEC. Formerly included in operation group(s) 590.

| Type of Patients | Observed Patients | Avg. Stay | Variance | 10th | 25th | 50th | 75th | 90th | 95th | 99th |
|---|---|---|---|---|---|---|---|---|---|---|
| **1. SINGLE DX** | | | | | | | | | | |
| 0–19 Years | 29 | 2.6 | 1 | 2 | 2 | 2 | 3 | 5 | 5 | 5 |
| 20–34 | 10 | 1.9 | <1 | 1 | 1 | 2 | 2 | 3 | 4 | 4 |
| 35–49 | 8 | 4.1 | 3 | 3 | 3 | 3 | 6 | 6 | 6 | 6 |
| 50–64 | 12 | 4.2 | 8 | 2 | 2 | 3 | 5 | 10 | 11 | 11 |
| 65+ | 13 | 4.4 | 3 | 2 | 3 | 4 | 5 | 6 | 8 | 8 |
| **2. MULTIPLE DX** | | | | | | | | | | |
| 0–19 Years | 181 | 5.3 | 19 | 1 | 3 | 4 | 7 | 10 | 13 | 24 |
| 20–34 | 117 | 3.9 | 12 | 1 | 2 | 3 | 5 | 8 | 11 | 12 |
| 35–49 | 243 | 3.8 | 10 | 1 | 2 | 4 | 5 | 7 | 8 | 24 |
| 50–64 | 475 | 4.7 | 13 | 2 | 3 | 4 | 6 | 8 | 10 | 17 |
| 65+ | 1,527 | 5.5 | 16 | 2 | 3 | 5 | 7 | 9 | 12 | 22 |
| **TOTAL SINGLE DX** | 72 | 3.3 | 3 | 2 | 2 | 3 | 4 | 6 | 6 | 11 |
| **TOTAL MULTIPLE DX** | 2,543 | 5.1 | 15 | 2 | 3 | 4 | 6 | 9 | 11 | 21 |
| **TOTAL** | | | | | | | | | | |
| 0–19 Years | 210 | 5.0 | 18 | 1 | 2 | 4 | 7 | 10 | 13 | 24 |
| 20–34 | 127 | 3.8 | 11 | 1 | 2 | 3 | 4 | 8 | 11 | 12 |
| 35–49 | 251 | 3.8 | 10 | 1 | 2 | 4 | 5 | 7 | 8 | 24 |
| 50–64 | 487 | 4.7 | 13 | 2 | 3 | 4 | 6 | 8 | 10 | 17 |
| 65+ | 1,540 | 5.5 | 16 | 2 | 3 | 5 | 7 | 9 | 12 | 22 |
| **GRAND TOTAL** | 2,615 | 5.0 | 15 | 2 | 3 | 4 | 6 | 9 | 11 | 20 |

## 39.0: SYSTEMIC TO PA SHUNT. Formerly included in operation group(s) 583.

| Type of Patients | Observed Patients | Avg. Stay | Variance | 10th | 25th | 50th | 75th | 90th | 95th | 99th |
|---|---|---|---|---|---|---|---|---|---|---|
| **1. SINGLE DX** | | | | | | | | | | |
| 0–19 Years | 6 | 14.5 | 37 | 5 | 8 | 17 | 19 | 19 | 19 | 19 |
| 20–34 | 0 | | | | | | | | | |
| 35–49 | 0 | | | | | | | | | |
| 50–64 | 0 | | | | | | | | | |
| **2. MULTIPLE DX** | | | | | | | | | | |
| 0–19 Years | 418 | 17.5 | 295 | 4 | 6 | 11 | 22 | 42 | 66 | >99 |
| 20–34 | 1 | 7.0 | 0 | 7 | 7 | 7 | 7 | 7 | 7 | 7 |
| 35–49 | 1 | 4.0 | 0 | 4 | 4 | 4 | 4 | 4 | 4 | 4 |
| 50–64 | 2 | 25.0 | 551 | 1 | 1 | 40 | 40 | 40 | 40 | 40 |
| 65+ | 1 | 2.0 | 0 | 2 | 2 | 2 | 2 | 2 | 2 | 2 |
| **TOTAL SINGLE DX** | 6 | 14.5 | 37 | 5 | 8 | 17 | 19 | 19 | 19 | 19 |
| **TOTAL MULTIPLE DX** | 423 | 17.4 | 295 | 4 | 6 | 11 | 22 | 42 | 65 | >99 |
| **TOTAL** | | | | | | | | | | |
| 0–19 Years | 424 | 17.4 | 293 | 4 | 6 | 12 | 22 | 42 | 65 | >99 |
| 20–34 | 1 | 7.0 | 0 | 7 | 7 | 7 | 7 | 7 | 7 | 7 |
| 35–49 | 1 | 4.0 | 0 | 4 | 4 | 4 | 4 | 4 | 4 | 4 |
| 50–64 | 2 | 25.0 | 551 | 1 | 1 | 40 | 40 | 40 | 40 | 40 |
| 65+ | 1 | 2.0 | 0 | 2 | 2 | 2 | 2 | 2 | 2 | 2 |
| **GRAND TOTAL** | 429 | 17.4 | 292 | 4 | 6 | 11 | 22 | 41 | 65 | >99 |

Length of Stay by Diagnosis and Operation, United States, 2000

# United States, October 1998–September 1999 Data, by Operation

## 39.1: INTRA-ABD VENOUS SHUNT. Formerly included in operation group(s) 583.

| Type of Patients | Observed Patients | Avg. Stay | Variance | 10th | 25th | 50th | 75th | 90th | 95th | 99th |
|---|---|---|---|---|---|---|---|---|---|---|
| **1. SINGLE DX** | | | | | | | | | | |
| 0–19 Years | 0 | | | | | | | | | |
| 20–34 | 0 | | | | | | | | | |
| 35–49 | 2 | 9.0 | 0 | 9 | 9 | 9 | 9 | 9 | 9 | 9 |
| 50–64 | 3 | 2.1 | 2 | 1 | 1 | 1 | 4 | 4 | 4 | 4 |
| 65+ | 2 | 8.6 | 54 | 4 | 4 | 4 | 16 | 16 | 16 | 16 |
| **2. MULTIPLE DX** | | | | | | | | | | |
| 0–19 Years | 24 | 14.0 | 133 | 5 | 7 | 8 | 31 | 31 | 43 | >99 |
| 20–34 | 33 | 6.8 | 23 | 2 | 2 | 6 | 9 | 13 | 16 | 27 |
| 35–49 | 433 | 7.7 | 51 | 2 | 3 | 6 | 9 | 16 | 21 | 35 |
| 50–64 | 380 | 8.8 | 66 | 2 | 4 | 6 | 11 | 19 | 26 | 35 |
| 65+ | 287 | 10.5 | 88 | 2 | 4 | 8 | 14 | 22 | 28 | 44 |
| **TOTAL SINGLE DX** | 7 | 5.5 | 21 | 1 | 1 | 4 | 9 | 9 | 16 | 16 |
| **TOTAL MULTIPLE DX** | 1,157 | 8.9 | 68 | 2 | 4 | 7 | 11 | 19 | 26 | 38 |
| **TOTAL** | | | | | | | | | | |
| 0–19 Years | 24 | 14.0 | 133 | 5 | 7 | 8 | 31 | 31 | 43 | >99 |
| 20–34 | 33 | 6.8 | 23 | 2 | 3 | 6 | 9 | 13 | 16 | 27 |
| 35–49 | 435 | 7.7 | 51 | 2 | 3 | 6 | 9 | 16 | 21 | 35 |
| 50–64 | 383 | 8.7 | 66 | 2 | 4 | 6 | 11 | 19 | 26 | 35 |
| 65+ | 289 | 10.5 | 87 | 2 | 4 | 8 | 14 | 22 | 28 | 44 |
| **GRAND TOTAL** | 1,164 | 8.9 | 68 | 2 | 4 | 7 | 11 | 19 | 26 | 38 |

## 39.21: CAVAL-PA ANASTOMOSIS. Formerly included in operation group(s) 583.

| Type of Patients | Observed Patients | Avg. Stay | Variance | 10th | 25th | 50th | 75th | 90th | 95th | 99th |
|---|---|---|---|---|---|---|---|---|---|---|
| **1. SINGLE DX** | | | | | | | | | | |
| 0–19 Years | 8 | 3.8 | 1 | 2 | 4 | 4 | 4 | 5 | 5 | 8 |
| 20–34 | 0 | | | | | | | | | |
| 35–49 | 0 | | | | | | | | | |
| 50–64 | 0 | | | | | | | | | |
| 65+ | 0 | | | | | | | | | |
| **2. MULTIPLE DX** | | | | | | | | | | |
| 0–19 Years | 391 | 10.3 | 193 | 4 | 5 | 8 | 9 | 16 | 32 | 84 |
| 20–34 | 4 | 6.8 | 4 | 5 | 5 | 6 | 8 | 10 | 10 | 10 |
| 35–49 | 2 | 3.0 | 6 | 1 | 1 | 1 | 5 | 5 | 5 | 5 |
| 50–64 | 1 | 4.0 | 0 | 4 | 4 | 4 | 4 | 4 | 4 | 4 |
| 65+ | 2 | 9.8 | <1 | 9 | 10 | 10 | 10 | 10 | 10 | 10 |
| **TOTAL SINGLE DX** | 8 | 3.8 | 1 | 4 | 4 | 4 | 4 | 5 | 5 | 8 |
| **TOTAL MULTIPLE DX** | 400 | 10.2 | 189 | 4 | 5 | 7 | 9 | 16 | 32 | 84 |
| **TOTAL** | | | | | | | | | | |
| 0–19 Years | 399 | 10.1 | 187 | 4 | 5 | 8 | 9 | 16 | 32 | 84 |
| 20–34 | 4 | 6.8 | 4 | 5 | 5 | 6 | 8 | 10 | 10 | 10 |
| 35–49 | 2 | 3.0 | 6 | 1 | 1 | 1 | 5 | 5 | 5 | 5 |
| 50–64 | 1 | 4.0 | 0 | 4 | 4 | 4 | 4 | 4 | 4 | 4 |
| 65+ | 2 | 9.8 | <1 | 9 | 10 | 10 | 10 | 10 | 10 | 10 |
| **GRAND TOTAL** | 408 | 10.0 | 184 | 4 | 5 | 6 | 9 | 16 | 32 | 84 |

## 39.2: OTHER SHUNT/VASC BYPASS. Formerly included in operation group(s) 583, 585.

| Type of Patients | Observed Patients | Avg. Stay | Variance | 10th | 25th | 50th | 75th | 90th | 95th | 99th |
|---|---|---|---|---|---|---|---|---|---|---|
| **1. SINGLE DX** | | | | | | | | | | |
| 0–19 Years | 32 | 3.0 | 3 | 1 | 2 | 2 | 4 | 6 | 7 | 7 |
| 20–34 | 50 | 2.9 | 12 | 1 | 1 | 2 | 3 | 6 | 10 | 27 |
| 35–49 | 199 | 3.1 | 5 | 1 | 1 | 3 | 5 | 5 | 6 | 16 |
| 50–64 | 424 | 3.5 | 6 | 1 | 2 | 3 | 5 | 6 | 7 | 15 |
| 65+ | 465 | 3.7 | 5 | 1 | 2 | 3 | 5 | 6 | 7 | 13 |
| **2. MULTIPLE DX** | | | | | | | | | | |
| 0–19 Years | 570 | 8.8 | 141 | 2 | 4 | 6 | 9 | 15 | 25 | 84 |
| 20–34 | 910 | 7.4 | 54 | 1 | 3 | 6 | 9 | 16 | 22 | 33 |
| 35–49 | 4,438 | 6.7 | 40 | 2 | 3 | 5 | 8 | 13 | 18 | 34 |
| 50–64 | 13,222 | 7.4 | 48 | 2 | 3 | 6 | 10 | 15 | 21 | 35 |
| 65+ | 23,851 | 8.3 | 54 | 2 | 4 | 6 | 10 | 16 | 22 | 37 |
| **TOTAL SINGLE DX** | 1,170 | 3.5 | 6 | 1 | 2 | 3 | 5 | 6 | 7 | 13 |
| **TOTAL MULTIPLE DX** | 42,991 | 7.8 | 52 | 2 | 3 | 6 | 10 | 16 | 21 | 36 |
| **TOTAL** | | | | | | | | | | |
| 0–19 Years | 602 | 8.4 | 133 | 2 | 4 | 6 | 8 | 15 | 23 | 84 |
| 20–34 | 960 | 7.3 | 54 | 1 | 3 | 6 | 9 | 15 | 21 | 33 |
| 35–49 | 4,637 | 6.5 | 39 | 1 | 3 | 5 | 8 | 13 | 17 | 33 |
| 50–64 | 13,646 | 7.2 | 47 | 2 | 4 | 6 | 10 | 15 | 20 | 35 |
| 65+ | 24,316 | 8.2 | 53 | 2 | 4 | 6 | 10 | 16 | 22 | 37 |
| **GRAND TOTAL** | 44,161 | 7.7 | 51 | 2 | 3 | 6 | 9 | 16 | 21 | 36 |

## 39.22: AORTA-SCL-CAROTID BYPASS. Formerly included in operation group(s) 583.

| Type of Patients | Observed Patients | Avg. Stay | Variance | 10th | 25th | 50th | 75th | 90th | 95th | 99th |
|---|---|---|---|---|---|---|---|---|---|---|
| **1. SINGLE DX** | | | | | | | | | | |
| 0–19 Years | 0 | | | | | | | | | |
| 20–34 | 1 | 5.0 | 0 | 5 | 5 | 5 | 5 | 5 | 5 | 5 |
| 35–49 | 4 | 3.0 | 2 | 1 | 3 | 3 | 3 | 5 | 5 | 5 |
| 50–64 | 18 | 2.6 | 6 | 1 | 1 | 2 | 3 | 4 | 9 | 16 |
| 65+ | 22 | 2.3 | 1 | 1 | 1 | 2 | 3 | 4 | 5 | 5 |
| **2. MULTIPLE DX** | | | | | | | | | | |
| 0–19 Years | 5 | 8.0 | 39 | 2 | 2 | 6 | 6 | 15 | 16 | 16 |
| 20–34 | 10 | 9.9 | 162 | 2 | 2 | 2 | 14 | 35 | 35 | 35 |
| 35–49 | 70 | 3.6 | 7 | 1 | 2 | 3 | 4 | 7 | 9 | 13 |
| 50–64 | 296 | 4.5 | 19 | 2 | 2 | 3 | 5 | 10 | 16 | 21 |
| 65+ | 362 | 5.3 | 39 | 2 | 2 | 3 | 7 | 12 | 15 | 33 |
| **TOTAL SINGLE DX** | 45 | 2.6 | 3 | 1 | 1 | 2 | 3 | 5 | 5 | 13 |
| **TOTAL MULTIPLE DX** | 743 | 4.9 | 30 | 1 | 2 | 3 | 6 | 10 | 15 | 30 |
| **TOTAL** | | | | | | | | | | |
| 0–19 Years | 5 | 8.0 | 39 | 2 | 2 | 6 | 6 | 15 | 16 | 16 |
| 20–34 | 11 | 9.3 | 144 | 2 | 2 | 4 | 14 | 35 | 35 | 35 |
| 35–49 | 74 | 3.6 | 7 | 1 | 3 | 3 | 4 | 7 | 9 | 13 |
| 50–64 | 314 | 4.4 | 19 | 1 | 2 | 3 | 5 | 10 | 15 | 21 |
| 65+ | 384 | 5.2 | 38 | 2 | 2 | 3 | 7 | 11 | 15 | 33 |
| **GRAND TOTAL** | 788 | 4.8 | 29 | 1 | 2 | 3 | 6 | 10 | 15 | 30 |

Length of Stay by Diagnosis and Operation, United States, 2000

# United States, October 1998–September 1999 Data, by Operation

## 39.25: AORTA-ILIAC-FEMORAL BYP. Formerly included in operation group(s) 583.

| Type of Patients | Observed Patients | Avg. Stay | Vari-ance | 10th | 25th | 50th | 75th | 90th | 95th | 99th |
|---|---|---|---|---|---|---|---|---|---|---|
| **1. SINGLE DX** | | | | | | | | | | |
| 0–19 Years | 0 | | | | | | | | | |
| 20–34 | 0 | | | | | | | | | |
| 35–49 | 27 | 5.4 | 12 | 2 | 4 | 4 | 6 | 7 | 16 | 16 |
| 50–64 | 66 | 5.5 | 2 | 4 | 5 | 5 | 6 | 8 | 8 | 9 |
| 65+ | 29 | 4.9 | 9 | 2 | 3 | 4 | 6 | 7 | 8 | 22 |
| **2. MULTIPLE DX** | | | | | | | | | | |
| 0–19 Years | 11 | 9.1 | 63 | 4 | 5 | 7 | 8 | 16 | 16 | 39 |
| 20–34 | 18 | 13.0 | 151 | 4 | 6 | 11 | 13 | 27 | 35 | 58 |
| 35–49 | 728 | 6.9 | 22 | 4 | 5 | 6 | 7 | 10 | 14 | 25 |
| 50–64 | 2,465 | 7.9 | 32 | 4 | 5 | 6 | 8 | 13 | 18 | 31 |
| 65+ | 2,634 | 9.6 | 53 | 4 | 6 | 7 | 11 | 19 | 22 | 44 |
| **TOTAL SINGLE DX** | 122 | 5.3 | 6 | 3 | 4 | 5 | 6 | 7 | 8 | 16 |
| **TOTAL MULTIPLE DX** | 5,856 | 8.5 | 41 | 4 | 5 | 7 | 9 | 15 | 22 | 35 |
| **TOTAL** | | | | | | | | | | |
| 0–19 Years | 11 | 9.1 | 63 | 4 | 5 | 7 | 8 | 16 | 16 | 39 |
| 20–34 | 18 | 13.0 | 151 | 4 | 6 | 11 | 13 | 27 | 35 | 58 |
| 35–49 | 755 | 6.9 | 22 | 4 | 5 | 6 | 7 | 10 | 15 | 25 |
| 50–64 | 2,531 | 7.8 | 31 | 4 | 5 | 6 | 8 | 13 | 18 | 31 |
| 65+ | 2,663 | 9.5 | 53 | 4 | 6 | 7 | 11 | 19 | 22 | 44 |
| **GRAND TOTAL** | 5,978 | 8.4 | 40 | 4 | 5 | 7 | 9 | 15 | 22 | 35 |

## 39.27: ARTERIOVENOSTOMY FOR RD. Formerly included in operation group(s) 585.

| Type of Patients | Observed Patients | Avg. Stay | Vari-ance | 10th | 25th | 50th | 75th | 90th | 95th | 99th |
|---|---|---|---|---|---|---|---|---|---|---|
| **1. SINGLE DX** | | | | | | | | | | |
| 0–19 Years | 8 | 1.7 | <1 | 1 | 1 | 2 | 2 | 2 | 2 | 2 |
| 20–34 | 37 | 2.5 | 17 | 1 | 1 | 1 | 2 | 5 | 10 | 27 |
| 35–49 | 91 | 2.0 | 5 | 1 | 1 | 1 | 2 | 3 | 7 | 10 |
| 50–64 | 66 | 1.6 | 2 | 1 | 1 | 1 | 2 | 2 | 5 | 10 |
| 65+ | 116 | 2.7 | 14 | 1 | 1 | 1 | 2 | 8 | 13 | 19 |
| **2. MULTIPLE DX** | | | | | | | | | | |
| 0–19 Years | 119 | 5.8 | 33 | 1 | 1 | 3 | 10 | 12 | 17 | 27 |
| 20–34 | 750 | 6.6 | 36 | 1 | 2 | 6 | 9 | 13 | 16 | 29 |
| 35–49 | 2,185 | 6.7 | 44 | 1 | 2 | 5 | 9 | 13 | 18 | 31 |
| 50–64 | 3,722 | 8.1 | 65 | 3 | 3 | 6 | 10 | 18 | 23 | 35 |
| 65+ | 5,560 | 9.0 | 72 | 1 | 3 | 7 | 13 | 19 | 25 | 41 |
| **TOTAL SINGLE DX** | 318 | 2.1 | 8 | 1 | 1 | 1 | 2 | 4 | 8 | 17 |
| **TOTAL MULTIPLE DX** | 12,336 | 8.1 | 63 | 1 | 3 | 6 | 11 | 17 | 23 | 38 |
| **TOTAL** | | | | | | | | | | |
| 0–19 Years | 127 | 5.2 | 30 | 1 | 1 | 3 | 8 | 12 | 14 | 21 |
| 20–34 | 787 | 6.5 | 36 | 1 | 2 | 6 | 9 | 13 | 16 | 29 |
| 35–49 | 2,276 | 6.6 | 44 | 1 | 2 | 5 | 9 | 13 | 18 | 31 |
| 50–64 | 3,788 | 8.0 | 65 | 1 | 3 | 6 | 10 | 18 | 23 | 35 |
| 65+ | 5,676 | 8.9 | 72 | 1 | 3 | 7 | 13 | 19 | 25 | 40 |
| **GRAND TOTAL** | 12,654 | 8.0 | 63 | 1 | 2 | 6 | 11 | 17 | 23 | 38 |

## 39.29: VASC SHUNT & BYPASS NEC. Formerly included in operation group(s) 583.

| Type of Patients | Observed Patients | Avg. Stay | Vari-ance | 10th | 25th | 50th | 75th | 90th | 95th | 99th |
|---|---|---|---|---|---|---|---|---|---|---|
| **1. SINGLE DX** | | | | | | | | | | |
| 0–19 Years | 4 | 3.1 | <1 | 1 | 3 | 3 | 4 | 4 | 4 | 4 |
| 20–34 | 11 | 3.5 | 2 | 2 | 3 | 3 | 3 | 7 | 7 | 7 |
| 35–49 | 73 | 3.6 | 3 | 2 | 2 | 4 | 5 | 5 | 5 | 8 |
| 50–64 | 273 | 3.6 | 6 | 2 | 2 | 3 | 5 | 6 | 7 | 19 |
| 65+ | 295 | 3.9 | 2 | 2 | 3 | 4 | 5 | 5 | 6 | 9 |
| **2. MULTIPLE DX** | | | | | | | | | | |
| 0–19 Years | 22 | 6.2 | 35 | 2 | 5 | 5 | 5 | 12 | 16 | 42 |
| 20–34 | 111 | 7.9 | 59 | 2 | 3 | 5 | 12 | 18 | 19 | 36 |
| 35–49 | 1,365 | 6.6 | 43 | 2 | 3 | 4 | 8 | 14 | 19 | 30 |
| 50–64 | 6,522 | 6.8 | 44 | 2 | 3 | 5 | 8 | 15 | 18 | 35 |
| 65+ | 15,022 | 7.8 | 47 | 3 | 4 | 6 | 10 | 15 | 21 | 36 |
| **TOTAL SINGLE DX** | 656 | 3.7 | 4 | 2 | 2 | 3 | 5 | 5 | 7 | 10 |
| **TOTAL MULTIPLE DX** | 23,042 | 7.5 | 46 | 2 | 3 | 5 | 9 | 15 | 20 | 35 |
| **TOTAL** | | | | | | | | | | |
| 0–19 Years | 26 | 5.9 | 33 | 2 | 4 | 5 | 5 | 10 | 16 | 42 |
| 20–34 | 122 | 7.7 | 57 | 2 | 3 | 5 | 10 | 18 | 18 | 36 |
| 35–49 | 1,438 | 6.3 | 41 | 2 | 3 | 4 | 8 | 14 | 18 | 30 |
| 50–64 | 6,795 | 6.6 | 43 | 2 | 3 | 5 | 8 | 14 | 18 | 35 |
| 65+ | 15,317 | 7.7 | 46 | 3 | 4 | 6 | 9 | 15 | 20 | 35 |
| **GRAND TOTAL** | 23,698 | 7.3 | 45 | 2 | 3 | 5 | 9 | 15 | 20 | 35 |

## 39.3: SUTURE OF VESSEL. Formerly included in operation group(s) 590.

| Type of Patients | Observed Patients | Avg. Stay | Vari-ance | 10th | 25th | 50th | 75th | 90th | 95th | 99th |
|---|---|---|---|---|---|---|---|---|---|---|
| **1. SINGLE DX** | | | | | | | | | | |
| 0–19 Years | 9 | 1.3 | <1 | 1 | 1 | 1 | 1 | 2 | 3 | 3 |
| 20–34 | 20 | 1.2 | <1 | 1 | 1 | 1 | 1 | 2 | 3 | 6 |
| 35–49 | 25 | 1.9 | 1 | 1 | 1 | 1 | 3 | 4 | 4 | 5 |
| 50–64 | 8 | 1.9 | 1 | 1 | 1 | 1 | 3 | 3 | 4 | 5 |
| 65+ | 8 | 2.4 | 3 | 1 | 1 | 1 | 5 | 5 | 5 | 5 |
| **2. MULTIPLE DX** | | | | | | | | | | |
| 0–19 Years | 145 | 5.1 | 35 | 1 | 1 | 3 | 6 | 15 | 21 | 29 |
| 20–34 | 329 | 3.4 | 16 | 1 | 1 | 2 | 4 | 6 | 9 | 18 |
| 35–49 | 296 | 5.2 | 44 | 1 | 1 | 3 | 6 | 12 | 26 | 26 |
| 50–64 | 233 | 6.7 | 37 | 3 | 3 | 5 | 9 | 12 | 17 | 28 |
| 65+ | 407 | 7.1 | 50 | 1 | 2 | 4 | 9 | 16 | 22 | 30 |
| **TOTAL SINGLE DX** | 70 | 1.6 | 1 | 1 | 1 | 1 | 2 | 3 | 4 | 5 |
| **TOTAL MULTIPLE DX** | 1,410 | 5.5 | 39 | 1 | 2 | 3 | 7 | 12 | 20 | 28 |
| **TOTAL** | | | | | | | | | | |
| 0–19 Years | 154 | 4.9 | 33 | 1 | 1 | 3 | 6 | 13 | 21 | 29 |
| 20–34 | 349 | 3.2 | 15 | 1 | 1 | 2 | 4 | 6 | 8 | 18 |
| 35–49 | 321 | 5.0 | 42 | 1 | 1 | 3 | 5 | 12 | 26 | 26 |
| 50–64 | 241 | 6.4 | 36 | 2 | 2 | 5 | 9 | 12 | 17 | 28 |
| 65+ | 415 | 7.0 | 49 | 1 | 2 | 4 | 9 | 16 | 22 | 30 |
| **GRAND TOTAL** | 1,480 | 5.2 | 37 | 1 | 1 | 3 | 6 | 12 | 18 | 28 |

Length of Stay by Diagnosis and Operation, United States, 2000

# United States, October 1998–September 1999 Data, by Operation

## 39.31: SUTURE OF ARTERY. Formerly included in operation group(s) 590.

| Type of Patients | Observed Patients | Avg. Stay | Vari-ance | 10th | 25th | 50th | 75th | 90th | 95th | 99th |
|---|---|---|---|---|---|---|---|---|---|---|
| **1. SINGLE DX** | | | | | | | | | | |
| 0–19 Years | 8 | 1.3 | <1 | 1 | 1 | 1 | 1 | 3 | 3 | 3 |
| 20–34 | 17 | 1.2 | <1 | 1 | 1 | 1 | 1 | 1 | 3 | 6 |
| 35–49 | 21 | 1.8 | 1 | 1 | 1 | 1 | 3 | 4 | 4 | 5 |
| 50–64 | 5 | 2.1 | 2 | 1 | 1 | 1 | 3 | 3 | 5 | 5 |
| 65+ | 7 | 2.7 | 4 | 1 | 1 | 1 | 5 | 5 | 5 | 5 |
| **2. MULTIPLE DX** | | | | | | | | | | |
| 0–19 Years | 122 | 5.1 | 39 | 1 | 1 | 3 | 6 | 16 | 21 | 29 |
| 20–34 | 246 | 3.0 | 7 | 1 | 1 | 2 | 4 | 6 | 7 | 13 |
| 35–49 | 226 | 5.3 | 49 | 1 | 1 | 3 | 6 | 14 | 26 | 26 |
| 50–64 | 182 | 6.6 | 37 | 1 | 3 | 5 | 9 | 12 | 17 | 28 |
| 65+ | 318 | 6.9 | 43 | 1 | 2 | 4 | 9 | 17 | 22 | 30 |
| **TOTAL SINGLE DX** | 58 | 1.7 | 1 | 1 | 1 | 1 | 2 | 3 | 4 | 5 |
| **TOTAL MULTIPLE DX** | 1,094 | 5.3 | 36 | 1 | 1 | 3 | 6 | 12 | 20 | 27 |
| **TOTAL** | | | | | | | | | | |
| 0–19 Years | 130 | 4.8 | 37 | 1 | 1 | 2 | 5 | 15 | 21 | 29 |
| 20–34 | 263 | 2.9 | 7 | 1 | 1 | 2 | 4 | 5 | 7 | 13 |
| 35–49 | 247 | 5.0 | 46 | 1 | 1 | 4 | 5 | 14 | 26 | 26 |
| 50–64 | 187 | 6.3 | 36 | 1 | 2 | 4 | 9 | 12 | 17 | 28 |
| 65+ | 325 | 6.8 | 43 | 1 | 2 | 4 | 9 | 16 | 22 | 30 |
| **GRAND TOTAL** | 1,152 | 5.1 | 35 | 1 | 1 | 3 | 6 | 11 | 20 | 27 |

## 39.42: REV AV SHUNT FOR RD. Formerly included in operation group(s) 585.

| Type of Patients | Observed Patients | Avg. Stay | Vari-ance | 10th | 25th | 50th | 75th | 90th | 95th | 99th |
|---|---|---|---|---|---|---|---|---|---|---|
| **1. SINGLE DX** | | | | | | | | | | |
| 0–19 Years | 3 | 3.1 | 8 | 1 | 1 | 3 | 3 | 9 | 9 | 9 |
| 20–34 | 4 | 1.6 | <1 | 1 | 1 | 2 | 3 | 9 | 9 | 9 |
| 35–49 | 3 | 1.2 | <1 | 1 | 1 | 1 | 1 | 2 | 2 | 2 |
| 50–64 | 11 | 1.2 | <1 | 1 | 1 | 1 | 1 | 2 | 2 | 2 |
| 65+ | 10 | 1.4 | 2 | 1 | 1 | 1 | 1 | 1 | 3 | 6 |
| **2. MULTIPLE DX** | | | | | | | | | | |
| 0–19 Years | 33 | 5.1 | 61 | 1 | 1 | 2 | 3 | 12 | 19 | 36 |
| 20–34 | 371 | 4.1 | 32 | 1 | 1 | 2 | 4 | 10 | 16 | 31 |
| 35–49 | 1,130 | 4.5 | 32 | 1 | 1 | 3 | 6 | 10 | 14 | 31 |
| 50–64 | 1,883 | 4.4 | 28 | 1 | 1 | 3 | 6 | 10 | 13 | 29 |
| 65+ | 2,596 | 4.7 | 39 | 1 | 1 | 2 | 5 | 11 | 17 | 30 |
| **TOTAL SINGLE DX** | 31 | 1.5 | 2 | 1 | 1 | 1 | 1 | 3 | 3 | 9 |
| **TOTAL MULTIPLE DX** | 6,013 | 4.5 | 34 | 1 | 1 | 2 | 6 | 10 | 15 | 31 |
| **TOTAL** | | | | | | | | | | |
| 0–19 Years | 36 | 4.9 | 55 | 1 | 1 | 2 | 3 | 12 | 12 | 36 |
| 20–34 | 375 | 4.1 | 32 | 1 | 1 | 2 | 4 | 10 | 16 | 31 |
| 35–49 | 1,133 | 4.5 | 32 | 1 | 1 | 3 | 6 | 10 | 14 | 31 |
| 50–64 | 1,894 | 4.4 | 28 | 1 | 1 | 3 | 6 | 10 | 13 | 29 |
| 65+ | 2,606 | 4.7 | 38 | 1 | 1 | 2 | 5 | 11 | 17 | 30 |
| **GRAND TOTAL** | 6,044 | 4.5 | 34 | 1 | 1 | 2 | 6 | 10 | 15 | 31 |

## 39.4: VASCULAR PX REVISION. Formerly included in operation group(s) 585, 590.

| Type of Patients | Observed Patients | Avg. Stay | Vari-ance | 10th | 25th | 50th | 75th | 90th | 95th | 99th |
|---|---|---|---|---|---|---|---|---|---|---|
| **1. SINGLE DX** | | | | | | | | | | |
| 0–19 Years | 5 | 2.5 | 7 | 1 | 1 | 1 | 3 | 9 | 9 | 9 |
| 20–34 | 9 | 1.9 | 1 | 1 | 1 | 2 | 2 | 4 | 4 | 4 |
| 35–49 | 26 | 1.8 | 2 | 1 | 1 | 2 | 2 | 2 | 3 | 14 |
| 50–64 | 50 | 1.8 | 4 | 1 | 1 | 1 | 2 | 4 | 7 | 10 |
| 65+ | 61 | 3.6 | 8 | 1 | 3 | 3 | 5 | 7 | 9 | 17 |
| **2. MULTIPLE DX** | | | | | | | | | | |
| 0–19 Years | 157 | 6.5 | 67 | 1 | 2 | 3 | 8 | 14 | 19 | 37 |
| 20–34 | 1,069 | 5.6 | 41 | 1 | 1 | 3 | 7 | 16 | 16 | 33 |
| 35–49 | 3,374 | 5.3 | 38 | 1 | 2 | 3 | 7 | 12 | 16 | 31 |
| 50–64 | 6,425 | 5.6 | 44 | 1 | 2 | 3 | 7 | 12 | 17 | 33 |
| 65+ | 9,186 | 5.6 | 40 | 1 | 2 | 4 | 7 | 12 | 18 | 33 |
| **TOTAL SINGLE DX** | 151 | 2.3 | 5 | 1 | 1 | 1 | 2 | 5 | 7 | 13 |
| **TOTAL MULTIPLE DX** | 20,211 | 5.6 | 41 | 1 | 2 | 3 | 7 | 12 | 17 | 32 |
| **TOTAL** | | | | | | | | | | |
| 0–19 Years | 162 | 6.4 | 65 | 1 | 2 | 3 | 8 | 14 | 18 | 37 |
| 20–34 | 1,078 | 5.6 | 41 | 1 | 1 | 3 | 7 | 16 | 16 | 33 |
| 35–49 | 3,400 | 5.3 | 38 | 1 | 2 | 3 | 7 | 12 | 16 | 31 |
| 50–64 | 6,475 | 5.5 | 44 | 1 | 2 | 3 | 7 | 12 | 17 | 30 |
| 65+ | 9,247 | 5.6 | 39 | 1 | 2 | 4 | 7 | 12 | 18 | 31 |
| **GRAND TOTAL** | 20,362 | 5.5 | 41 | 1 | 2 | 3 | 7 | 12 | 17 | 32 |

## 39.43: RMVL AV SHUNT FOR RD. Formerly included in operation group(s) 585.

| Type of Patients | Observed Patients | Avg. Stay | Vari-ance | 10th | 25th | 50th | 75th | 90th | 95th | 99th |
|---|---|---|---|---|---|---|---|---|---|---|
| **1. SINGLE DX** | | | | | | | | | | |
| 0–19 Years | 0 | | | | | | | | | |
| 20–34 | 0 | | | | | | | | | |
| 35–49 | 2 | 1.0 | 0 | 1 | 1 | 1 | 1 | 1 | 1 | 1 |
| 50–64 | 0 | | | | | | | | | |
| 65+ | 0 | | | | | | | | | |
| **2. MULTIPLE DX** | | | | | | | | | | |
| 0–19 Years | 8 | 8.7 | 244 | 4 | 5 | 5 | 5 | 6 | 71 | 71 |
| 20–34 | 152 | 7.1 | 43 | 2 | 3 | 5 | 9 | 15 | 19 | 46 |
| 35–49 | 424 | 7.2 | 51 | 1 | 3 | 5 | 10 | 15 | 19 | 38 |
| 50–64 | 474 | 8.6 | 77 | 2 | 3 | 6 | 11 | 20 | 28 | 37 |
| 65+ | 511 | 8.6 | 65 | 2 | 3 | 6 | 12 | 20 | 25 | 35 |
| **TOTAL SINGLE DX** | 2 | 1.0 | 0 | 1 | 1 | 1 | 1 | 1 | 1 | 1 |
| **TOTAL MULTIPLE DX** | 1,569 | 8.1 | 64 | 2 | 3 | 5 | 11 | 17 | 25 | 37 |
| **TOTAL** | | | | | | | | | | |
| 0–19 Years | 8 | 8.7 | 244 | 4 | 5 | 5 | 5 | 6 | 71 | 71 |
| 20–34 | 152 | 7.1 | 43 | 2 | 3 | 5 | 9 | 15 | 19 | 46 |
| 35–49 | 426 | 7.2 | 51 | 2 | 3 | 5 | 10 | 15 | 19 | 38 |
| 50–64 | 474 | 8.6 | 77 | 2 | 3 | 6 | 11 | 20 | 28 | 37 |
| 65+ | 511 | 8.6 | 65 | 2 | 3 | 6 | 12 | 20 | 25 | 35 |
| **GRAND TOTAL** | 1,571 | 8.1 | 64 | 2 | 3 | 5 | 11 | 17 | 25 | 37 |

# United States, October 1998–September 1999 Data, by Operation

## 39.49: VASCULAR PX REVISION NEC. Formerly included in operation group(s) 590.

| Type of Patients | Observed Patients | Avg. Stay | Variance | Percentiles | | | | | | |
|---|---|---|---|---|---|---|---|---|---|---|
| | | | | 10th | 25th | 50th | 75th | 90th | 95th | 99th |
| **1. SINGLE DX** | | | | | | | | | | |
| 0–19 Years | 2 | 1.0 | 0 | 1 | 1 | 1 | | 1 | 1 | 1 |
| 20–34 | 4 | 2.2 | 2 | 1 | 1 | 2 | 4 | 4 | 4 | 4 |
| 35–49 | 21 | 1.9 | 3 | 1 | 1 | 2 | 2 | 2 | 3 | 14 |
| 50–64 | 39 | 1.9 | 5 | 1 | 1 | 1 | 1 | 4 | 7 | 10 |
| 65+ | 50 | 3.9 | 8 | 1 | 2 | 3 | 5 | 7 | 9 | 17 |
| **2. MULTIPLE DX** | | | | | | | | | | |
| 0–19 Years | 116 | 6.7 | 55 | 1 | 2 | 4 | 10 | 14 | 18 | 37 |
| 20–34 | 541 | 6.4 | 46 | 1 | 2 | 4 | 9 | 16 | 16 | 30 |
| 35–49 | 1,812 | 5.4 | 37 | 1 | 2 | 4 | 7 | 11 | 16 | 29 |
| 50–64 | 4,047 | 5.7 | 47 | 1 | 2 | 4 | 7 | 12 | 17 | 34 |
| 65+ | 6,046 | 5.8 | 37 | 1 | 2 | 4 | 7 | 12 | 17 | 31 |
| **TOTAL SINGLE DX** | 116 | 2.3 | 6 | 1 | 1 | 1 | 3 | 5 | 7 | 13 |
| **TOTAL MULTIPLE DX** | 12,562 | 5.8 | 41 | 1 | 2 | 4 | 7 | 12 | 17 | 32 |
| **TOTAL** | | | | | | | | | | |
| 0–19 Years | 118 | 6.6 | 54 | 1 | 2 | 4 | 10 | 14 | 18 | 37 |
| 20–34 | 545 | 6.4 | 46 | 1 | 2 | 4 | 9 | 16 | 16 | 30 |
| 35–49 | 1,833 | 5.3 | 37 | 1 | 2 | 3 | 7 | 11 | 16 | 29 |
| 50–64 | 4,086 | 5.6 | 46 | 1 | 2 | 4 | 7 | 12 | 17 | 33 |
| 65+ | 6,096 | 5.8 | 37 | 1 | 2 | 4 | 7 | 12 | 17 | 31 |
| **GRAND TOTAL** | 12,678 | 5.7 | 41 | 1 | 2 | 4 | 7 | 12 | 17 | 32 |

## 39.5: OTHER VESSEL REPAIR. Formerly included in operation group(s) 589, 590.

| Type of Patients | Observed Patients | Avg. Stay | Variance | Percentiles | | | | | | |
|---|---|---|---|---|---|---|---|---|---|---|
| | | | | 10th | 25th | 50th | 75th | 90th | 95th | 99th |
| **1. SINGLE DX** | | | | | | | | | | |
| 0–19 Years | 81 | 2.6 | 4 | 1 | 1 | 2 | 3 | 5 | 6 | 11 |
| 20–34 | 97 | 6.7 | 11 | 2 | 5 | 6 | 9 | 10 | 11 | 20 |
| 35–49 | 281 | 5.7 | 20 | 1 | 2 | 4 | 9 | 12 | 15 | 15 |
| 50–64 | 413 | 3.2 | 8 | 1 | 1 | 2 | 5 | 7 | 8 | 13 |
| 65+ | 417 | 2.4 | 12 | 1 | 1 | 1 | 2 | 6 | 7 | 19 |
| **2. MULTIPLE DX** | | | | | | | | | | |
| 0–19 Years | 684 | 5.9 | 79 | 1 | 1 | 4 | 7 | 13 | 19 | 89 |
| 20–34 | 809 | 7.1 | 50 | 1 | 2 | 5 | 9 | 15 | 20 | 34 |
| 35–49 | 3,037 | 7.9 | 73 | 1 | 2 | 5 | 11 | 18 | 24 | 39 |
| 50–64 | 6,927 | 6.3 | 65 | 1 | 1 | 3 | 8 | 16 | 22 | 41 |
| 65+ | 13,239 | 5.4 | 43 | 1 | 1 | 3 | 7 | 13 | 18 | 33 |
| **TOTAL SINGLE DX** | 1,289 | 3.9 | 14 | 1 | 1 | 2 | 6 | 9 | 12 | 19 |
| **TOTAL MULTIPLE DX** | 24,696 | 6.0 | 55 | 1 | 1 | 3 | 8 | 14 | 21 | 38 |
| **TOTAL** | | | | | | | | | | |
| 0–19 Years | 765 | 5.6 | 73 | 1 | 1 | 3 | 7 | 13 | 19 | 75 |
| 20–34 | 906 | 7.0 | 44 | 1 | 2 | 6 | 9 | 14 | 19 | 29 |
| 35–49 | 3,318 | 7.7 | 68 | 1 | 2 | 5 | 11 | 17 | 23 | 39 |
| 50–64 | 7,340 | 6.2 | 62 | 1 | 1 | 3 | 7 | 15 | 22 | 41 |
| 65+ | 13,656 | 5.3 | 43 | 1 | 1 | 3 | 7 | 12 | 17 | 33 |
| **GRAND TOTAL** | 25,985 | 5.9 | 53 | 1 | 1 | 3 | 8 | 14 | 20 | 37 |

## 39.50: PTA/ATHERECT OTH VESSEL. Formerly included in operation group(s) 590.

| Type of Patients | Observed Patients | Avg. Stay | Variance | Percentiles | | | | | | |
|---|---|---|---|---|---|---|---|---|---|---|
| | | | | 10th | 25th | 50th | 75th | 90th | 95th | 99th |
| **1. SINGLE DX** | | | | | | | | | | |
| 0–19 Years | 43 | 1.5 | 2 | 1 | 1 | | 1 | 3 | 6 | 7 |
| 20–34 | 19 | 5.1 | 3 | 1 | 5 | 6 | 6 | 6 | 7 | 8 |
| 35–49 | 93 | 1.7 | 2 | 1 | 1 | 1 | 2 | 3 | 4 | 8 |
| 50–64 | 265 | 2.0 | 4 | 1 | 1 | 1 | 2 | 5 | 6 | 11 |
| 65+ | 344 | 1.6 | 4 | 1 | 1 | 1 | 1 | 2 | 4 | 6 |
| **2. MULTIPLE DX** | | | | | | | | | | |
| 0–19 Years | 396 | 3.5 | 54 | 1 | 1 | 1 | 5 | 8 | 12 | 75 |
| 20–34 | 395 | 5.2 | 31 | 1 | 1 | 4 | 6 | 11 | 15 | 25 |
| 35–49 | 1,726 | 4.5 | 33 | 1 | 1 | 2 | 5 | 10 | 14 | 29 |
| 50–64 | 4,923 | 4.2 | 29 | 1 | 1 | 2 | 5 | 10 | 15 | 26 |
| 65+ | 10,394 | 4.6 | 33 | 1 | 1 | 2 | 6 | 11 | 16 | 28 |
| **TOTAL SINGLE DX** | 764 | 1.9 | 4 | 1 | 1 | 1 | 2 | 4 | 6 | 9 |
| **TOTAL MULTIPLE DX** | 17,834 | 4.5 | 32 | 1 | 1 | 2 | 6 | 10 | 15 | 28 |
| **TOTAL** | | | | | | | | | | |
| 0–19 Years | 439 | 3.4 | 50 | 1 | 1 | 1 | 3 | 8 | 12 | 75 |
| 20–34 | 414 | 5.2 | 29 | 1 | 1 | 4 | 6 | 10 | 15 | 24 |
| 35–49 | 1,819 | 4.3 | 31 | 1 | 1 | 2 | 5 | 10 | 14 | 28 |
| 50–64 | 5,188 | 4.1 | 28 | 1 | 1 | 2 | 5 | 9 | 14 | 25 |
| 65+ | 10,738 | 4.5 | 32 | 1 | 1 | 2 | 6 | 11 | 16 | 28 |
| **GRAND TOTAL** | 18,598 | 4.4 | 31 | 1 | 1 | 2 | 6 | 10 | 15 | 27 |

## 39.51: CLIPPING OF ANEURYSM. Formerly included in operation group(s) 589.

| Type of Patients | Observed Patients | Avg. Stay | Variance | Percentiles | | | | | | |
|---|---|---|---|---|---|---|---|---|---|---|
| | | | | 10th | 25th | 50th | 75th | 90th | 95th | 99th |
| **1. SINGLE DX** | | | | | | | | | | |
| 0–19 Years | 4 | 7.5 | 9 | 5 | 5 | 8 | 11 | 11 | 11 | 11 |
| 20–34 | 44 | 8.2 | 9 | 5 | 6 | 7 | 10 | 10 | 13 | 20 |
| 35–49 | 130 | 8.0 | 18 | 3 | 4 | 9 | 11 | 15 | 15 | 15 |
| 50–64 | 93 | 6.2 | 6 | 3 | 4 | 7 | 7 | 8 | 10 | 15 |
| 65+ | 18 | 11.3 | 42 | 3 | 4 | 10 | 19 | 19 | 19 | 19 |
| **2. MULTIPLE DX** | | | | | | | | | | |
| 0–19 Years | 11 | 15.2 | 81 | 6 | 10 | 13 | 19 | 19 | 27 | 52 |
| 20–34 | 133 | 12.3 | 46 | 3 | 9 | 12 | 14 | 20 | 24 | 35 |
| 35–49 | 795 | 14.1 | 82 | 4 | 8 | 13 | 18 | 26 | 32 | 41 |
| 50–64 | 894 | 14.7 | 144 | 4 | 6 | 11 | 20 | 34 | 38 | 50 |
| 65+ | 440 | 15.2 | 126 | 4 | 7 | 13 | 19 | 31 | 41 | 52 |
| **TOTAL SINGLE DX** | 289 | 7.7 | 16 | 3 | 5 | 7 | 10 | 13 | 15 | 19 |
| **TOTAL MULTIPLE DX** | 2,273 | 14.4 | 114 | 4 | 7 | 12 | 19 | 28 | 37 | 50 |
| **TOTAL** | | | | | | | | | | |
| 0–19 Years | 15 | 13.2 | 73 | 5 | 7 | 13 | 19 | 19 | 19 | 52 |
| 20–34 | 177 | 10.8 | 36 | 4 | 7 | 10 | 14 | 17 | 21 | 34 |
| 35–49 | 925 | 13.2 | 77 | 4 | 7 | 12 | 17 | 25 | 31 | 39 |
| 50–64 | 987 | 13.9 | 138 | 4 | 6 | 9 | 19 | 31 | 38 | 50 |
| 65+ | 458 | 15.0 | 123 | 4 | 7 | 13 | 19 | 30 | 41 | 51 |
| **GRAND TOTAL** | 2,562 | 13.6 | 106 | 4 | 6 | 11 | 17 | 27 | 36 | 50 |

© 2000 by HCIA-Sachs, L.L.C.

Length of Stay by Diagnosis and Operation, United States, 2000

# United States, October 1998–September 1999 Data, by Operation

## 39.56: REP VESS W TISS PATCH. Formerly included in operation group(s) 590.

| Type of Patients | Observed Patients | Avg. Stay | Variance | Percentiles | | | | | | |
|---|---|---|---|---|---|---|---|---|---|---|
| | | | | 10th | 25th | 50th | 75th | 90th | 95th | 99th |
| **1. SINGLE DX** | | | | | | | | | | |
| 0–19 Years | 7 | 3.7 | <1 | 3 | 3 | 3 | 3 | 4 | 5 | 7 |
| 20–34 | 4 | 3.8 | <1 | 3 | 4 | 4 | 4 | 4 | 5 | 4 |
| 35–49 | 11 | 3.7 | 7 | 1 | 1 | 3 | 7 | 7 | 8 | 8 |
| 50–64 | 2 | 3.0 | 2 | 2 | 2 | 4 | 4 | 4 | 4 | 4 |
| 65+ | 9 | 2.3 | 2 | 1 | 2 | 2 | 2 | 2 | 6 | 6 |
| **2. MULTIPLE DX** | | | | | | | | | | |
| 0–19 Years | 110 | 7.4 | 56 | 3 | 4 | 5 | 9 | 13 | 15 | 35 |
| 20–34 | 94 | 6.7 | 58 | 2 | 3 | 4 | 8 | 16 | 23 | 44 |
| 35–49 | 92 | 6.6 | 98 | 1 | 2 | 4 | 7 | 11 | 19 | 65 |
| 50–64 | 101 | 8.8 | 85 | 2 | 3 | 6 | 12 | 16 | 21 | 46 |
| 65+ | 126 | 5.5 | 34 | 1 | 2 | 3 | 6 | 14 | 20 | 25 |
| **TOTAL SINGLE DX** | 33 | 3.4 | 3 | 1 | 2 | 3 | 4 | 7 | 7 | 8 |
| **TOTAL MULTIPLE DX** | 523 | 6.9 | 63 | 2 | 2 | 4 | 8 | 15 | 21 | 46 |
| **TOTAL** | | | | | | | | | | |
| 0–19 Years | 117 | 7.0 | 52 | 2 | 3 | 4 | 9 | 13 | 15 | 35 |
| 20–34 | 98 | 6.5 | 55 | 2 | 3 | 4 | 7 | 15 | 23 | 44 |
| 35–49 | 103 | 6.3 | 89 | 1 | 2 | 4 | 7 | 10 | 19 | 65 |
| 50–64 | 103 | 8.7 | 84 | 2 | 3 | 6 | 12 | 16 | 21 | 46 |
| 65+ | 135 | 5.4 | 33 | 1 | 2 | 3 | 6 | 13 | 20 | 25 |
| **GRAND TOTAL** | 556 | 6.7 | 60 | 2 | 2 | 4 | 8 | 14 | 20 | 46 |

## 39.57: REP VESS W SYNTH PATCH. Formerly included in operation group(s) 590.

| Type of Patients | Observed Patients | Avg. Stay | Variance | Percentiles | | | | | | |
|---|---|---|---|---|---|---|---|---|---|---|
| | | | | 10th | 25th | 50th | 75th | 90th | 95th | 99th |
| **1. SINGLE DX** | | | | | | | | | | |
| 0–19 Years | 4 | 3.7 | 1 | 3 | 3 | 3 | 5 | 5 | 5 | 5 |
| 20–34 | 3 | 3.3 | 5 | 2 | 2 | 2 | 3 | 3 | 7 | 7 |
| 35–49 | 0 | | | | | | | | | |
| 50–64 | 4 | 3.7 | 13 | 2 | 2 | 2 | 2 | 2 | 12 | 12 |
| 65+ | 6 | 3.8 | 6 | 2 | 2 | 2 | 7 | 7 | 7 | 7 |
| **2. MULTIPLE DX** | | | | | | | | | | |
| 0–19 Years | 59 | 8.2 | 163 | 3 | 5 | 5 | 8 | 37 | >99 | >99 |
| 20–34 | 50 | 9.8 | 54 | 2 | 7 | 7 | 17 | 20 | 21 | >99 |
| 35–49 | 68 | 7.5 | 44 | 2 | 6 | 6 | 10 | 10 | 15 | 33 |
| 50–64 | 131 | 6.8 | 74 | 1 | 4 | 4 | 6 | 14 | 18 | 52 |
| 65+ | 222 | 5.5 | 41 | 1 | 4 | 4 | 6 | 11 | 17 | 26 |
| **TOTAL SINGLE DX** | 17 | 3.7 | 8 | 2 | 3 | 5 | 7 | 7 | 12 | 12 |
| **TOTAL MULTIPLE DX** | 530 | 6.8 | 66 | 1 | 3 | 5 | 9 | 14 | 20 | >99 |
| **TOTAL** | | | | | | | | | | |
| 0–19 Years | 63 | 8.1 | 159 | 3 | 4 | 5 | 8 | 23 | >99 | >99 |
| 20–34 | 53 | 9.5 | 54 | 2 | 3 | 7 | 17 | 20 | 21 | >99 |
| 35–49 | 68 | 7.5 | 44 | 1 | 2 | 6 | 10 | 10 | 15 | 33 |
| 50–64 | 135 | 6.7 | 71 | 1 | 2 | 4 | 8 | 14 | 17 | 52 |
| 65+ | 228 | 5.5 | 40 | 1 | 2 | 4 | 6 | 11 | 17 | 26 |
| **GRAND TOTAL** | 547 | 6.7 | 65 | 1 | 3 | 4 | 8 | 14 | 20 | >99 |

## 39.52: ANEURYSM REPAIR NEC. Formerly included in operation group(s) 590.

| Type of Patients | Observed Patients | Avg. Stay | Variance | Percentiles | | | | | | |
|---|---|---|---|---|---|---|---|---|---|---|
| | | | | 10th | 25th | 50th | 75th | 90th | 95th | 99th |
| **1. SINGLE DX** | | | | | | | | | | |
| 0–19 Years | 4 | 2.6 | 4 | 1 | 1 | 2 | 2 | 6 | 6 | 6 |
| 20–34 | 8 | 5.0 | 9 | 2 | 2 | 4 | 4 | 6 | 9 | 9 |
| 35–49 | 20 | 3.6 | 16 | 1 | 1 | 2 | 5 | 7 | 15 | 17 |
| 50–64 | 26 | 2.9 | 2 | 1 | 1 | 3 | 3 | 4 | 7 | 7 |
| 65+ | 19 | 2.9 | 5 | 1 | 1 | 2 | 5 | 6 | 8 | 8 |
| **2. MULTIPLE DX** | | | | | | | | | | |
| 0–19 Years | 5 | 4.2 | 12 | 1 | 1 | 5 | 5 | 12 | 12 | 12 |
| 20–34 | 32 | 5.4 | 24 | 1 | 2 | 4 | 8 | 12 | 16 | 24 |
| 35–49 | 125 | 8.6 | 118 | 2 | 2 | 6 | 12 | 14 | 20 | 72 |
| 50–64 | 488 | 6.0 | 30 | 1 | 3 | 5 | 7 | 10 | 17 | 30 |
| 65+ | 1,410 | 7.0 | 54 | 2 | 3 | 5 | 9 | 13 | 19 | 37 |
| **TOTAL SINGLE DX** | 77 | 3.2 | 6 | 1 | 2 | 3 | 4 | 6 | 8 | 15 |
| **TOTAL MULTIPLE DX** | 2,060 | 6.8 | 52 | 2 | 3 | 5 | 9 | 13 | 19 | 34 |
| **TOTAL** | | | | | | | | | | |
| 0–19 Years | 9 | 3.7 | 10 | 1 | 1 | 2 | 5 | 6 | 12 | 12 |
| 20–34 | 40 | 5.3 | 21 | 1 | 2 | 4 | 8 | 9 | 16 | 24 |
| 35–49 | 145 | 8.0 | 109 | 2 | 2 | 5 | 12 | 13 | 20 | 72 |
| 50–64 | 514 | 5.8 | 29 | 1 | 3 | 5 | 7 | 10 | 16 | 28 |
| 65+ | 1,429 | 6.9 | 54 | 2 | 3 | 5 | 9 | 13 | 19 | 37 |
| **GRAND TOTAL** | 2,137 | 6.7 | 51 | 2 | 3 | 5 | 9 | 13 | 18 | 34 |

## 39.53: AV FISTULA REPAIR. Formerly included in operation group(s) 590.

| Type of Patients | Observed Patients | Avg. Stay | Variance | Percentiles | | | | | | |
|---|---|---|---|---|---|---|---|---|---|---|
| | | | | 10th | 25th | 50th | 75th | 90th | 95th | 99th |
| **1. SINGLE DX** | | | | | | | | | | |
| 0–19 Years | 8 | 2.2 | <1 | 2 | 2 | 2 | 2 | 3 | 4 | 5 |
| 20–34 | 7 | 2.9 | 2 | 1 | 1 | 3 | 4 | 5 | 5 | 5 |
| 35–49 | 15 | 2.2 | 3 | 1 | 1 | 2 | 2 | 6 | 6 | 7 |
| 50–64 | 10 | 1.8 | 1 | 1 | 1 | 1 | 2 | 3 | 5 | 5 |
| 65+ | 12 | 4.8 | 6 | 1 | 2 | 7 | 7 | 7 | 7 | 7 |
| **2. MULTIPLE DX** | | | | | | | | | | |
| 0–19 Years | 19 | 13.8 | 297 | 1 | 3 | 3 | 39 | 39 | 39 | 51 |
| 20–34 | 37 | 3.4 | 8 | 1 | 2 | 2 | 4 | 9 | 9 | 11 |
| 35–49 | 112 | 4.8 | 20 | 1 | 1 | 3 | 7 | 11 | 11 | 22 |
| 50–64 | 181 | 6.0 | 32 | 1 | 2 | 4 | 8 | 13 | 14 | 28 |
| 65+ | 262 | 6.9 | 46 | 1 | 2 | 5 | 10 | 15 | 17 | 33 |
| **TOTAL SINGLE DX** | 52 | 3.3 | 5 | 1 | 1 | 2 | 5 | 7 | 7 | 7 |
| **TOTAL MULTIPLE DX** | 611 | 6.4 | 49 | 1 | 2 | 4 | 8 | 14 | 18 | 39 |
| **TOTAL** | | | | | | | | | | |
| 0–19 Years | 27 | 11.4 | 258 | 1 | 1 | 3 | 5 | 39 | 39 | 51 |
| 20–34 | 44 | 3.3 | 7 | 1 | 1 | 2 | 4 | 9 | 9 | 11 |
| 35–49 | 127 | 4.6 | 19 | 1 | 1 | 3 | 7 | 11 | 11 | 18 |
| 50–64 | 191 | 5.9 | 32 | 1 | 2 | 4 | 7 | 13 | 14 | 28 |
| 65+ | 274 | 6.7 | 44 | 1 | 2 | 5 | 9 | 15 | 17 | 31 |
| **GRAND TOTAL** | 663 | 6.2 | 47 | 2 | 2 | 4 | 8 | 14 | 17 | 39 |

133

Length of Stay by Diagnosis and Operation, United States, 2000

# United States, October 1998–September 1999 Data, by Operation

## 39.59: REPAIR OF VESSEL NEC. Formerly included in operation group(s) 590.

| Type of Patients | Observed Patients | Avg. Stay | Vari-ance | 10th | 25th | 50th | 75th | 90th | 95th | 99th |
|---|---|---|---|---|---|---|---|---|---|---|
| **1. SINGLE DX** | | | | | | | | | | |
| 0–19 Years | 6 | 2.5 | <1 | 2 | 2 | 3 | 3 | 3 | 3 | 3 |
| 20–34 | 9 | 2.5 | <1 | 2 | 2 | 3 | 3 | 4 | 4 | 4 |
| 35–49 | 10 | 7.0 | 11 | 1 | 2 | 9 | 9 | 9 | 9 | 9 |
| 50–64 | 9 | 1.5 | <1 | 1 | 1 | 1 | 2 | 2 | 4 | 4 |
| 65+ | 8 | 1.4 | <1 | 1 | 1 | 1 | 2 | 3 | 4 | 4 |
| **2. MULTIPLE DX** | | | | | | | | | | |
| 0–19 Years | 60 | 8.3 | 71 | 2 | 3 | 5 | 11 | 24 | 31 | 38 |
| 20–34 | 58 | 7.8 | 94 | 2 | 3 | 8 | 8 | 15 | 15 | 75 |
| 35–49 | 98 | 3.4 | 25 | 1 | 1 | 2 | 4 | 8 | 11 | 28 |
| 50–64 | 175 | 6.3 | 46 | 1 | 2 | 4 | 8 | 17 | 21 | 29 |
| 65+ | 310 | 5.7 | 45 | 1 | 2 | 3 | 7 | 13 | 17 | 35 |
| **TOTAL SINGLE DX** | 42 | 4.1 | 11 | 1 | 2 | 2 | 9 | 9 | 9 | 9 |
| **TOTAL MULTIPLE DX** | 701 | 6.0 | 52 | 1 | 2 | 4 | 8 | 13 | 21 | 32 |
| **TOTAL** | | | | | | | | | | |
| 0–19 Years | 66 | 7.5 | 66 | 2 | 3 | 4 | 10 | 22 | 24 | 38 |
| 20–34 | 67 | 7.3 | 88 | 2 | 2 | 7 | 8 | 12 | 15 | 73 |
| 35–49 | 108 | 4.0 | 24 | 1 | 1 | 2 | 5 | 9 | 11 | 28 |
| 50–64 | 184 | 6.2 | 45 | 1 | 2 | 4 | 8 | 17 | 21 | 29 |
| 65+ | 318 | 5.6 | 44 | 1 | 2 | 3 | 7 | 12 | 17 | 35 |
| **GRAND TOTAL** | 743 | 5.9 | 50 | 1 | 2 | 3 | 8 | 12 | 21 | 32 |

## 39.8: VASCULAR BODY OPERATIONS. Formerly included in operation group(s) 590.

| Type of Patients | Observed Patients | Avg. Stay | Vari-ance | 10th | 25th | 50th | 75th | 90th | 95th | 99th |
|---|---|---|---|---|---|---|---|---|---|---|
| **1. SINGLE DX** | | | | | | | | | | |
| 0–19 Years | 0 | | | | | | | | | |
| 20–34 | 3 | 2.2 | 1 | | | | 2 | 4 | 4 | 4 |
| 35–49 | 8 | 2.0 | 3 | 1 | 1 | 1 | 3 | 3 | 7 | 7 |
| 50–64 | 5 | 1.0 | 0 | 1 | 1 | 1 | 1 | 1 | 1 | 1 |
| 65+ | 3 | 2.2 | <1 | 1 | 1 | 2 | 3 | 3 | 3 | 3 |
| **2. MULTIPLE DX** | | | | | | | | | | |
| 0–19 Years | 1 | 11.0 | 0 | 11 | 11 | 11 | 11 | 11 | 11 | 11 |
| 20–34 | 3 | 5.0 | 3 | 4 | 4 | 4 | 5 | 8 | 8 | 8 |
| 35–49 | 18 | 2.5 | 3 | 1 | 1 | 2 | 4 | 5 | 5 | 6 |
| 50–64 | 17 | 2.6 | 2 | 1 | 2 | 3 | 3 | 4 | 5 | 8 |
| 65+ | 30 | 4.6 | 24 | 1 | 2 | 3 | 4 | 11 | 19 | 20 |
| **TOTAL SINGLE DX** | 19 | 1.7 | 1 | 1 | 1 | 1 | 2 | 3 | 4 | 7 |
| **TOTAL MULTIPLE DX** | 69 | 3.8 | 15 | 1 | 2 | 2 | 4 | 11 | 11 | 20 |
| **TOTAL** | | | | | | | | | | |
| 0–19 Years | 1 | 11.0 | 0 | 11 | 11 | 11 | 11 | 11 | 11 | 11 |
| 20–34 | 6 | 3.6 | 4 | 1 | 2 | 4 | 4 | 5 | 8 | 8 |
| 35–49 | 26 | 2.3 | 2 | 1 | 1 | 2 | 3 | 5 | 6 | 7 |
| 50–64 | 22 | 2.1 | 2 | 1 | 2 | 3 | 3 | 4 | 5 | 8 |
| 65+ | 33 | 4.5 | 23 | 1 | 2 | 3 | 4 | 11 | 19 | 20 |
| **GRAND TOTAL** | 88 | 3.4 | 13 | 1 | 1 | 2 | 4 | 7 | 11 | 20 |

## 39.6: OPEN HEART AUXILIARY PX. Formerly included in operation group(s) 590.

| Type of Patients | Observed Patients | Avg. Stay | Vari-ance | 10th | 25th | 50th | 75th | 90th | 95th | 99th |
|---|---|---|---|---|---|---|---|---|---|---|
| **1. SINGLE DX** | | | | | | | | | | |
| 0–19 Years | 1 | 27.0 | 0 | 27 | 27 | 27 | 27 | 27 | 27 | 27 |
| 20–34 | 0 | | | | | | | | | |
| 35–49 | 0 | | | | | | | | | |
| 50–64 | 0 | | | | | | | | | |
| 65+ | 0 | | | | | | | | | |
| **2. MULTIPLE DX** | | | | | | | | | | |
| 0–19 Years | 95 | 28.8 | 344 | 6 | 17 | 26 | 39 | 54 | 80 | >99 |
| 20–34 | 3 | 10.5 | 15 | 6 | 6 | 12 | 14 | 14 | 14 | 14 |
| 35–49 | 11 | 5.8 | 20 | 3 | 3 | 4 | 7 | 9 | 20 | 20 |
| 50–64 | 23 | 6.7 | 6 | 4 | 5 | 6 | 8 | 11 | 11 | 12 |
| 65+ | 53 | 8.1 | 19 | 4 | 5 | 7 | 10 | 15 | 15 | 17 |
| **TOTAL SINGLE DX** | 1 | 27.0 | 0 | 27 | 27 | 27 | 27 | 27 | 27 | 27 |
| **TOTAL MULTIPLE DX** | 185 | 21.0 | 329 | 4 | 7 | 17 | 29 | 47 | 69 | >99 |
| **TOTAL** | | | | | | | | | | |
| 0–19 Years | 96 | 28.7 | 335 | 6 | 17 | 26 | 39 | 54 | 80 | >99 |
| 20–34 | 3 | 10.5 | 15 | 6 | 6 | 12 | 14 | 14 | 14 | 14 |
| 35–49 | 11 | 5.8 | 20 | 3 | 3 | 4 | 7 | 9 | 20 | 20 |
| 50–64 | 23 | 6.7 | 6 | 4 | 5 | 6 | 8 | 11 | 11 | 12 |
| 65+ | 53 | 8.1 | 19 | 4 | 5 | 7 | 10 | 15 | 15 | 17 |
| **GRAND TOTAL** | 186 | 21.1 | 324 | 4 | 7 | 17 | 29 | 46 | 69 | >99 |

## 39.9: OTHER VESSEL OPERATIONS. Formerly included in operation group(s) 584, 585, 590, 596.

| Type of Patients | Observed Patients | Avg. Stay | Vari-ance | 10th | 25th | 50th | 75th | 90th | 95th | 99th |
|---|---|---|---|---|---|---|---|---|---|---|
| **1. SINGLE DX** | | | | | | | | | | |
| 0–19 Years | 39 | 2.4 | 5 | 1 | 1 | 2 | 2 | 5 | 5 | 13 |
| 20–34 | 61 | 2.5 | 5 | 1 | 1 | 2 | 2 | 5 | 8 | 9 |
| 35–49 | 101 | 2.3 | 2 | 1 | 1 | 2 | 3 | 4 | 5 | 8 |
| 50–64 | 70 | 3.4 | 72 | 1 | 1 | 2 | 4 | 6 | 8 | 10 |
| 65+ | 107 | 3.2 | 11 | 1 | 2 | 2 | 5 | 6 | 8 | 18 |
| **2. MULTIPLE DX** | | | | | | | | | | |
| 0–19 Years | 647 | 3.9 | 25 | 1 | 1 | 2 | 5 | 9 | 12 | 24 |
| 20–34 | 4,141 | 4.1 | 18 | 1 | 2 | 3 | 5 | 8 | 11 | 20 |
| 35–49 | 11,406 | 4.6 | 21 | 1 | 2 | 3 | 6 | 9 | 12 | 23 |
| 50–64 | 16,994 | 5.5 | 33 | 2 | 2 | 4 | 7 | 11 | 16 | 35 |
| 65+ | 27,037 | 5.9 | 33 | 1 | 2 | 4 | 7 | 12 | 16 | 30 |
| **TOTAL SINGLE DX** | 378 | 2.8 | 14 | 1 | 1 | 2 | 3 | 6 | 7 | 14 |
| **TOTAL MULTIPLE DX** | 60,225 | 5.4 | 30 | 1 | 2 | 4 | 7 | 11 | 15 | 29 |
| **TOTAL** | | | | | | | | | | |
| 0–19 Years | 686 | 3.8 | 24 | 1 | 2 | 3 | 4 | 9 | 12 | 24 |
| 20–34 | 4,202 | 4.1 | 18 | 1 | 2 | 3 | 5 | 8 | 11 | 20 |
| 35–49 | 11,507 | 4.6 | 21 | 1 | 2 | 4 | 6 | 9 | 12 | 23 |
| 50–64 | 17,064 | 5.5 | 33 | 2 | 2 | 4 | 7 | 11 | 16 | 35 |
| 65+ | 27,144 | 5.8 | 33 | 1 | 2 | 4 | 7 | 12 | 16 | 30 |
| **GRAND TOTAL** | 60,603 | 5.4 | 30 | 1 | 2 | 4 | 7 | 11 | 15 | 29 |

Length of Stay by Diagnosis and Operation, United States, 2000

# United States, October 1998–September 1999 Data, by Operation

## 39.93: INSERT VESS-VESS CANNULA. Formerly included in operation group(s) 585.

| Type of Patients | Observed Patients | Avg. Stay | Variance | 10th | 25th | 50th | 75th | 90th | 95th | 99th |
|---|---|---|---|---|---|---|---|---|---|---|
| **1. SINGLE DX** | | | | | | | | | | |
| 0–19 Years | 2 | 5.0 | 0 | 5 | 5 | 5 | 5 | 5 | 5 | 5 |
| 20–34 | 4 | 6.7 | 10 | 8 | 8 | 8 | 9 | 9 | 9 | 9 |
| 35–49 | 4 | 2.3 | <1 | 2 | 2 | 2 | 2 | 4 | 4 | 4 |
| 50–64 | 8 | 2.6 | 9 | 1 | 1 | 1 | 1 | 8 | 8 | 8 |
| 65+ | 7 | 1.0 | 0 | 1 | 1 | 1 | 1 | 1 | 1 | 1 |
| **2. MULTIPLE DX** | | | | | | | | | | |
| 0–19 Years | 22 | 6.6 | 58 | 1 | 3 | 4 | 8 | 18 | 26 | 34 |
| 20–34 | 73 | 5.9 | 33 | 1 | 2 | 4 | 8 | 14 | 16 | 24 |
| 35–49 | 179 | 8.6 | 62 | 2 | 4 | 6 | 11 | 15 | 20 | 43 |
| 50–64 | 359 | 7.5 | 46 | 3 | 3 | 6 | 9 | 15 | 22 | >99 |
| 65+ | 504 | 14.8 | 211 | 2 | 4 | 9 | 19 | 43 | 43 | 46 |
| **TOTAL SINGLE DX** | 25 | 3.0 | 8 | 1 | 1 | 1 | 5 | 8 | 9 | 9 |
| **TOTAL MULTIPLE DX** | 1,137 | 10.9 | 137 | 1 | 3 | 7 | 12 | 31 | 43 | 43 |
| **TOTAL** | | | | | | | | | | |
| 0–19 Years | 24 | 6.5 | 54 | 1 | 3 | 4 | 7 | 18 | 26 | 34 |
| 20–34 | 77 | 5.9 | 32 | 1 | 2 | 4 | 8 | 14 | 16 | 24 |
| 35–49 | 183 | 8.5 | 62 | 2 | 4 | 6 | 11 | 15 | 20 | 43 |
| 50–64 | 367 | 7.5 | 46 | 3 | 3 | 6 | 9 | 15 | 22 | >99 |
| 65+ | 511 | 14.6 | 211 | 2 | 4 | 9 | 18 | 43 | 43 | 46 |
| **GRAND TOTAL** | 1,162 | 10.8 | 136 | 1 | 3 | 7 | 12 | 31 | 43 | 43 |

## 39.95: HEMODIALYSIS. Formerly included in operation group(s) 584.

| Type of Patients | Observed Patients | Avg. Stay | Variance | 10th | 25th | 50th | 75th | 90th | 95th | 99th |
|---|---|---|---|---|---|---|---|---|---|---|
| **1. SINGLE DX** | | | | | | | | | | |
| 0–19 Years | 14 | 3.2 | 9 | 1 | 1 | 2 | 3 | 5 | 13 | 13 |
| 20–34 | 32 | 2.4 | 5 | 1 | 1 | 2 | 2 | 7 | 8 | 13 |
| 35–49 | 65 | 2.6 | 5 | 1 | 1 | 2 | 3 | 4 | 5 | 8 |
| 50–64 | 40 | 2.9 | 5 | 1 | 1 | 2 | 4 | 6 | 9 | 10 |
| 65+ | 80 | 3.5 | 12 | 1 | 2 | 2 | 6 | 6 | 8 | 18 |
| **2. MULTIPLE DX** | | | | | | | | | | |
| 0–19 Years | 531 | 3.8 | 22 | 1 | 1 | 2 | 5 | 9 | 11 | 24 |
| 20–34 | 3,984 | 4.1 | 18 | 1 | 2 | 3 | 5 | 8 | 11 | 20 |
| 35–49 | 11,067 | 4.6 | 20 | 1 | 2 | 3 | 5 | 11 | 12 | 23 |
| 50–64 | 16,410 | 5.5 | 33 | 1 | 2 | 4 | 7 | 11 | 15 | 35 |
| 65+ | 26,123 | 5.7 | 27 | 2 | 2 | 4 | 7 | 12 | 15 | 26 |
| **TOTAL SINGLE DX** | 231 | 3.0 | 7 | 1 | 1 | 2 | 4 | 6 | 8 | 18 |
| **TOTAL MULTIPLE DX** | 58,115 | 5.3 | 27 | 1 | 2 | 4 | 6 | 11 | 14 | 27 |
| **TOTAL** | | | | | | | | | | |
| 0–19 Years | 545 | 3.8 | 22 | 1 | 2 | 2 | 5 | 9 | 11 | 24 |
| 20–34 | 4,016 | 4.1 | 18 | 1 | 2 | 3 | 5 | 8 | 11 | 20 |
| 35–49 | 11,132 | 4.6 | 20 | 1 | 2 | 3 | 5 | 11 | 12 | 23 |
| 50–64 | 16,450 | 5.5 | 33 | 1 | 2 | 4 | 7 | 11 | 15 | 35 |
| 65+ | 26,203 | 5.6 | 27 | 2 | 2 | 4 | 7 | 12 | 15 | 26 |
| **GRAND TOTAL** | 58,346 | 5.3 | 27 | 1 | 2 | 4 | 6 | 11 | 14 | 27 |

## 39.98: HEMORRHAGE CONTROL NOS. Formerly included in operation group(s) 590.

| Type of Patients | Observed Patients | Avg. Stay | Variance | 10th | 25th | 50th | 75th | 90th | 95th | 99th |
|---|---|---|---|---|---|---|---|---|---|---|
| **1. SINGLE DX** | | | | | | | | | | |
| 0–19 Years | 12 | 1.2 | <1 | 1 | 1 | 1 | 1 | 2 | 2 | 3 |
| 20–34 | 19 | 1.7 | 2 | 1 | 1 | 1 | 1 | 4 | 2 | 7 |
| 35–49 | 23 | 1.4 | <1 | 1 | 1 | 1 | 1 | 4 | 3 | 8 |
| 50–64 | 7 | 11.0 | 739 | 1 | 1 | 2 | 4 | 85 | 85 | 85 |
| 65+ | 4 | 1.6 | <1 | 1 | 1 | 1 | 2 | 2 | 2 | 2 |
| **2. MULTIPLE DX** | | | | | | | | | | |
| 0–19 Years | 38 | 5.2 | 50 | 1 | 2 | 2 | 5 | 14 | 16 | 34 |
| 20–34 | 61 | 3.2 | 5 | 1 | 2 | 2 | 4 | 6 | 7 | 9 |
| 35–49 | 100 | 3.4 | 11 | 1 | 2 | 2 | 4 | 7 | 9 | 14 |
| 50–64 | 98 | 4.2 | 27 | 1 | 2 | 2 | 4 | 12 | 17 | 25 |
| 65+ | 165 | 7.6 | 81 | 2 | 2 | 3 | 9 | 25 | 25 | 42 |
| **TOTAL SINGLE DX** | 65 | 2.2 | 59 | 1 | 1 | 1 | 2 | 3 | 4 | 8 |
| **TOTAL MULTIPLE DX** | 462 | 5.2 | 45 | 1 | 2 | 3 | 5 | 12 | 23 | 30 |
| **TOTAL** | | | | | | | | | | |
| 0–19 Years | 50 | 4.5 | 43 | 1 | 1 | 2 | 4 | 14 | 16 | 34 |
| 20–34 | 80 | 2.8 | 4 | 1 | 1 | 2 | 4 | 6 | 6 | 9 |
| 35–49 | 123 | 3.1 | 10 | 1 | 2 | 2 | 4 | 5 | 9 | 12 |
| 50–64 | 105 | 4.5 | 54 | 1 | 2 | 2 | 4 | 12 | 17 | 30 |
| 65+ | 169 | 7.5 | 80 | 2 | 2 | 3 | 9 | 25 | 25 | 42 |
| **GRAND TOTAL** | 527 | 4.9 | 47 | 1 | 2 | 2 | 5 | 11 | 20 | 30 |

## 40.0: INC LYMPHATIC STRUCTURE. Formerly included in operation group(s) 591.

| Type of Patients | Observed Patients | Avg. Stay | Variance | 10th | 25th | 50th | 75th | 90th | 95th | 99th |
|---|---|---|---|---|---|---|---|---|---|---|
| **1. SINGLE DX** | | | | | | | | | | |
| 0–19 Years | 69 | 3.7 | 4 | 1 | 2 | 2 | 4 | 6 | 6 | 8 |
| 20–34 | 1 | 6.0 | 0 | 6 | 6 | 6 | 6 | 6 | 6 | 6 |
| 35–49 | 3 | 2.8 | 7 | 1 | 1 | 1 | 1 | 7 | 7 | 7 |
| 50–64 | 3 | 3.0 | 1 | 2 | 2 | 3 | 3 | 5 | 5 | 5 |
| 65+ | 0 | | | | | | | | | |
| **2. MULTIPLE DX** | | | | | | | | | | |
| 0–19 Years | 84 | 5.9 | 18 | 2 | 3 | 5 | 5 | 10 | 12 | 29 |
| 20–34 | 15 | 5.2 | 6 | 3 | 5 | 5 | 5 | 9 | 10 | 12 |
| 35–49 | 13 | 6.8 | 22 | 3 | 4 | 4 | 13 | 13 | 13 | 21 |
| 50–64 | 28 | 3.4 | 7 | 1 | 1 | 4 | 5 | 15 | 15 | 35 |
| 65+ | 34 | 7.6 | 56 | 2 | 3 | 5 | 9 | 15 | 31 | 31 |
| **TOTAL SINGLE DX** | 76 | 3.7 | 4 | 1 | 2 | 4 | 4 | 6 | 6 | 8 |
| **TOTAL MULTIPLE DX** | 174 | 6.0 | 24 | 2 | 3 | 5 | 7 | 12 | 15 | 31 |
| **TOTAL** | | | | | | | | | | |
| 0–19 Years | 153 | 4.8 | 13 | 1 | 3 | 4 | 5 | 9 | 11 | 17 |
| 20–34 | 16 | 5.2 | 5 | 2 | 5 | 5 | 5 | 8 | 10 | 12 |
| 35–49 | 16 | 6.6 | 22 | 2 | 4 | 4 | 13 | 13 | 13 | 21 |
| 50–64 | 31 | 3.4 | 6 | 2 | 3 | 4 | 7 | 15 | 15 | 35 |
| 65+ | 34 | 7.6 | 56 | 2 | 3 | 5 | 9 | 15 | 31 | 31 |
| **GRAND TOTAL** | 250 | 5.2 | 19 | 1 | 3 | 5 | 6 | 9 | 13 | 29 |

Length of Stay by Diagnosis and Operation, United States, 2000

# United States, October 1998–September 1999 Data, by Operation

## 40.1: LYMPHATIC DXTIC PX. Formerly included in operation group(s) 591, 596.

| Type of Patients | Observed Patients | Avg. Stay | Vari-ance | Percentiles | | | | | | |
|---|---|---|---|---|---|---|---|---|---|---|
| | | | | 10th | 25th | 50th | 75th | 90th | 95th | 99th |
| **1. SINGLE DX** | | | | | | | | | | |
| 0–19 Years | 120 | 3.8 | 7 | 1 | 2 | 3 | 5 | 8 | 8 | 13 |
| 20–34 | 61 | 2.6 | 5 | 1 | 1 | 2 | 3 | 4 | 6 | 10 |
| 35–49 | 74 | 3.4 | 7 | 1 | 1 | 2 | 5 | 7 | 9 | 10 |
| 50–64 | 52 | 3.4 | 8 | 1 | 1 | 3 | 5 | 7 | 8 | 14 |
| 65+ | 46 | 3.0 | 7 | 1 | 1 | 2 | 4 | 9 | 9 | 9 |
| **2. MULTIPLE DX** | | | | | | | | | | |
| 0–19 Years | 295 | 9.2 | 89 | 1 | 3 | 7 | 11 | 18 | 34 | 48 |
| 20–34 | 321 | 8.8 | 61 | 2 | 4 | 7 | 10 | 18 | 21 | 42 |
| 35–49 | 749 | 9.6 | 97 | 2 | 4 | 7 | 12 | 25 | 25 | 56 |
| 50–64 | 1,061 | 8.0 | 51 | 1 | 3 | 6 | 10 | 16 | 21 | 36 |
| 65+ | 1,738 | 8.7 | 49 | 2 | 4 | 7 | 11 | 16 | 22 | 36 |
| **TOTAL SINGLE DX** | 353 | 3.4 | 7 | 1 | 1 | 2 | 5 | 7 | 9 | 13 |
| **TOTAL MULTIPLE DX** | 4,164 | 8.7 | 63 | 2 | 4 | 7 | 11 | 17 | 24 | 42 |
| **TOTAL** | | | | | | | | | | |
| 0–19 Years | 415 | 7.5 | 70 | 1 | 2 | 5 | 9 | 15 | 25 | 42 |
| 20–34 | 382 | 7.8 | 57 | 1 | 3 | 6 | 10 | 17 | 21 | 42 |
| 35–49 | 823 | 9.1 | 92 | 2 | 3 | 6 | 11 | 23 | 25 | 56 |
| 50–64 | 1,113 | 7.8 | 50 | 2 | 3 | 6 | 10 | 16 | 21 | 36 |
| 65+ | 1,784 | 8.6 | 49 | 2 | 4 | 7 | 11 | 16 | 22 | 36 |
| **GRAND TOTAL** | 4,517 | 8.3 | 60 | 2 | 3 | 6 | 11 | 16 | 23 | 41 |

## 40.11: LYMPHATIC STRUCT BIOPSY. Formerly included in operation group(s) 591.

| Type of Patients | Observed Patients | Avg. Stay | Vari-ance | Percentiles | | | | | | |
|---|---|---|---|---|---|---|---|---|---|---|
| | | | | 10th | 25th | 50th | 75th | 90th | 95th | 99th |
| **1. SINGLE DX** | | | | | | | | | | |
| 0–19 Years | 117 | 3.9 | 7 | 1 | 2 | 3 | 5 | 8 | 8 | 13 |
| 20–34 | 61 | 2.6 | 5 | 1 | 1 | 2 | 3 | 4 | 6 | 10 |
| 35–49 | 73 | 3.3 | 7 | 1 | 1 | 2 | 5 | 7 | 9 | 10 |
| 50–64 | 52 | 3.4 | 8 | 1 | 1 | 3 | 5 | 7 | 8 | 14 |
| 65+ | 44 | 2.8 | 6 | 1 | 1 | 2 | 3 | 8 | 9 | 9 |
| **2. MULTIPLE DX** | | | | | | | | | | |
| 0–19 Years | 291 | 9.3 | 90 | 1 | 3 | 7 | 11 | 18 | 34 | 48 |
| 20–34 | 318 | 8.8 | 59 | 2 | 4 | 7 | 10 | 18 | 21 | 42 |
| 35–49 | 747 | 9.6 | 97 | 2 | 4 | 7 | 12 | 25 | 25 | 56 |
| 50–64 | 1,052 | 8.0 | 51 | 1 | 3 | 6 | 11 | 16 | 21 | 36 |
| 65+ | 1,727 | 8.7 | 47 | 2 | 4 | 7 | 11 | 16 | 22 | 36 |
| **TOTAL SINGLE DX** | 347 | 3.4 | 7 | 1 | 1 | 2 | 5 | 7 | 9 | 13 |
| **TOTAL MULTIPLE DX** | 4,135 | 8.7 | 62 | 2 | 4 | 7 | 11 | 17 | 24 | 42 |
| **TOTAL** | | | | | | | | | | |
| 0–19 Years | 408 | 7.6 | 70 | 1 | 2 | 5 | 9 | 15 | 25 | 42 |
| 20–34 | 379 | 7.8 | 55 | 1 | 3 | 6 | 10 | 17 | 21 | 36 |
| 35–49 | 820 | 9.1 | 92 | 2 | 3 | 6 | 11 | 23 | 25 | 56 |
| 50–64 | 1,104 | 7.8 | 50 | 1 | 3 | 6 | 10 | 16 | 21 | 36 |
| 65+ | 1,771 | 8.6 | 47 | 2 | 4 | 7 | 11 | 16 | 21 | 36 |
| **GRAND TOTAL** | 4,482 | 8.3 | 60 | 2 | 3 | 6 | 11 | 16 | 23 | 41 |

## 40.2: SMP EXC LYMPHATIC STRUCT. Formerly included in operation group(s) 591.

| Type of Patients | Observed Patients | Avg. Stay | Vari-ance | Percentiles | | | | | | |
|---|---|---|---|---|---|---|---|---|---|---|
| | | | | 10th | 25th | 50th | 75th | 90th | 95th | 99th |
| **1. SINGLE DX** | | | | | | | | | | |
| 0–19 Years | 157 | 2.3 | 3 | 1 | 1 | 2 | 3 | 5 | 5 | 6 |
| 20–34 | 53 | 2.1 | 2 | 1 | 1 | 2 | 2 | 4 | 5 | 6 |
| 35–49 | 80 | 1.9 | 2 | 1 | 1 | 1 | 2 | 4 | 5 | 7 |
| 50–64 | 85 | 2.7 | 7 | 1 | 1 | 2 | 3 | 4 | 5 | 9 |
| 65+ | 68 | 1.8 | 1 | 1 | 1 | 1 | 2 | 4 | 4 | 5 |
| **2. MULTIPLE DX** | | | | | | | | | | |
| 0–19 Years | 185 | 5.7 | 64 | 1 | 2 | 4 | 7 | 11 | 18 | 34 |
| 20–34 | 160 | 9.8 | 257 | 1 | 2 | 4 | 9 | 21 | 71 | 71 |
| 35–49 | 360 | 6.1 | 31 | 1 | 2 | 5 | 8 | 15 | 16 | 22 |
| 50–64 | 485 | 4.7 | 40 | 1 | 3 | 3 | 5 | 14 | 16 | 23 |
| 65+ | 805 | 5.8 | 56 | 1 | 2 | 3 | 8 | 12 | 17 | 34 |
| **TOTAL SINGLE DX** | 443 | 2.2 | 3 | 1 | 1 | 1 | 3 | 4 | 5 | 9 |
| **TOTAL MULTIPLE DX** | 1,995 | 5.8 | 63 | 1 | 2 | 3 | 7 | 13 | 16 | 37 |
| **TOTAL** | | | | | | | | | | |
| 0–19 Years | 342 | 4.2 | 39 | 1 | 1 | 3 | 5 | 8 | 12 | 33 |
| 20–34 | 213 | 8.0 | 208 | 1 | 2 | 4 | 6 | 16 | 26 | 71 |
| 35–49 | 440 | 5.3 | 28 | 1 | 1 | 3 | 7 | 14 | 15 | 22 |
| 50–64 | 570 | 4.5 | 36 | 1 | 1 | 3 | 5 | 11 | 16 | 20 |
| 65+ | 873 | 5.5 | 53 | 1 | 2 | 3 | 7 | 12 | 17 | 34 |
| **GRAND TOTAL** | 2,438 | 5.1 | 54 | 1 | 1 | 3 | 6 | 12 | 16 | 34 |

## 40.21: EXC DEEP CERVICAL NODE. Formerly included in operation group(s) 591.

| Type of Patients | Observed Patients | Avg. Stay | Vari-ance | Percentiles | | | | | | |
|---|---|---|---|---|---|---|---|---|---|---|
| | | | | 10th | 25th | 50th | 75th | 90th | 95th | 99th |
| **1. SINGLE DX** | | | | | | | | | | |
| 0–19 Years | 39 | 2.9 | 2 | 1 | 2 | 2 | 4 | 5 | 5 | 6 |
| 20–34 | 5 | 2.6 | 7 | 1 | 1 | 2 | 2 | 8 | 8 | 8 |
| 35–49 | 10 | 2.0 | 2 | 1 | 1 | 1 | 4 | 4 | 4 | 4 |
| 50–64 | 7 | 7.2 | 11 | 1 | 9 | 9 | 9 | 9 | 9 | 9 |
| 65+ | 5 | 1.0 | 0 | 1 | 1 | 1 | 1 | 1 | 1 | 1 |
| **2. MULTIPLE DX** | | | | | | | | | | |
| 0–19 Years | 52 | 6.7 | 48 | 1 | 2 | 4 | 10 | 13 | 21 | 34 |
| 20–34 | 34 | 7.6 | 27 | 1 | 3 | 7 | 11 | 15 | 20 | 21 |
| 35–49 | 63 | 6.7 | 32 | 2 | 3 | 5 | 8 | 9 | 18 | 28 |
| 50–64 | 69 | 5.3 | 103 | 1 | 1 | 2 | 7 | 9 | 16 | 90 |
| 65+ | 123 | 6.8 | 68 | 1 | 3 | 4 | 8 | 15 | 18 | 28 |
| **TOTAL SINGLE DX** | 66 | 3.5 | 7 | 1 | 1 | 2 | 4 | 9 | 9 | 9 |
| **TOTAL MULTIPLE DX** | 341 | 6.5 | 62 | 1 | 2 | 4 | 8 | 13 | 18 | 34 |
| **TOTAL** | | | | | | | | | | |
| 0–19 Years | 91 | 5.2 | 33 | 1 | 2 | 4 | 5 | 11 | 15 | 34 |
| 20–34 | 39 | 7.1 | 27 | 1 | 3 | 6 | 11 | 14 | 20 | 21 |
| 35–49 | 73 | 6.2 | 31 | 1 | 2 | 5 | 8 | 11 | 18 | 28 |
| 50–64 | 76 | 5.6 | 89 | 1 | 1 | 3 | 8 | 11 | 15 | 24 |
| 65+ | 128 | 6.7 | 68 | 1 | 2 | 4 | 8 | 15 | 18 | 23 |
| **GRAND TOTAL** | 407 | 5.9 | 53 | 1 | 2 | 4 | 8 | 12 | 18 | 28 |

Length of Stay by Diagnosis and Operation, United States, 2000

## United States, October 1998–September 1999 Data, by Operation

### 40.23: EXC AXILLARY LYMPH NODE. Formerly included in operation group(s) 591.

| Type of Patients | Observed Patients | Avg. Stay | Variance | 10th | 25th | 50th | 75th | 90th | 95th | 99th |
|---|---|---|---|---|---|---|---|---|---|---|
| **1. SINGLE DX** | | | | | | | | | | |
| 0–19 Years | 4 | 1.0 | <1 | 1 | 1 | 1 | 1 | 1 | 1 | 2 |
| 20–34 | 9 | 1.4 | <1 | 1 | 1 | 1 | 2 | 2 | 2 | 3 |
| 35–49 | 37 | 1.4 | <1 | 1 | 1 | 1 | 1 | 3 | 3 | 4 |
| 50–64 | 39 | 1.7 | 1 | 1 | 1 | 1 | 2 | 4 | 4 | 4 |
| 65+ | 25 | 1.2 | <1 | 1 | 1 | 1 | 1 | 2 | 2 | 4 |
| **2. MULTIPLE DX** | | | | | | | | | | |
| 0–19 Years | 11 | 8.3 | 121 | 1 | 2 | 3 | 5 | 33 | 33 | 33 |
| 20–34 | 25 | 7.1 | 80 | 2 | 2 | 2 | 11 | 16 | 26 | 42 |
| 35–49 | 83 | 3.5 | 11 | 1 | 1 | 2 | 5 | 8 | 10 | 14 |
| 50–64 | 114 | 2.6 | 14 | 1 | 1 | 1 | 3 | 4 | 10 | 20 |
| 65+ | 216 | 5.0 | 63 | 1 | 1 | 2 | 7 | 11 | 17 | 35 |
| **TOTAL SINGLE DX** | 114 | 1.5 | <1 | 1 | 1 | 1 | 2 | 3 | 4 | 4 |
| **TOTAL MULTIPLE DX** | 449 | 4.2 | 44 | 1 | 1 | 2 | 5 | 10 | 15 | 34 |
| **TOTAL** | | | | | | | | | | |
| 0–19 Years | 15 | 6.3 | 97 | 2 | 2 | 2 | 5 | 33 | 33 | 33 |
| 20–34 | 34 | 5.8 | 68 | 1 | 2 | 2 | 5 | 16 | 21 | 42 |
| 35–49 | 120 | 2.7 | 8 | 1 | 1 | 1 | 3 | 6 | 8 | 13 |
| 50–64 | 153 | 2.3 | 11 | 1 | 1 | 1 | 2 | 4 | 10 | 15 |
| 65+ | 241 | 4.6 | 58 | 1 | 1 | 2 | 6 | 10 | 17 | 35 |
| **GRAND TOTAL** | 563 | 3.6 | 36 | 1 | 1 | 2 | 3 | 8 | 13 | 33 |

### 40.29: SMP EXC LYMPHATIC NEC. Formerly included in operation group(s) 591.

| Type of Patients | Observed Patients | Avg. Stay | Variance | 10th | 25th | 50th | 75th | 90th | 95th | 99th |
|---|---|---|---|---|---|---|---|---|---|---|
| **1. SINGLE DX** | | | | | | | | | | |
| 0–19 Years | 95 | 2.1 | 2 | 1 | 1 | 1 | 1 | 5 | 5 | 5 |
| 20–34 | 24 | 2.2 | 2 | 1 | 1 | 2 | 3 | 5 | 5 | 5 |
| 35–49 | 18 | 2.0 | 2 | 1 | 1 | 2 | 2 | 4 | 6 | 6 |
| 50–64 | 23 | 2.0 | 1 | 1 | 1 | 2 | 3 | 4 | 4 | 4 |
| 65+ | 23 | 2.6 | 1 | 2 | 2 | 2 | 4 | 4 | 4 | 5 |
| **2. MULTIPLE DX** | | | | | | | | | | |
| 0–19 Years | 96 | 4.9 | 75 | 1 | 3 | 3 | 5 | 8 | 10 | 46 |
| 20–34 | 71 | 13.5 | 475 | 2 | 3 | 6 | 7 | 71 | 71 | 71 |
| 35–49 | 129 | 7.2 | 36 | 2 | 2 | 6 | 11 | 15 | 16 | 21 |
| 50–64 | 196 | 5.5 | 36 | 1 | 2 | 3 | 6 | 16 | 16 | 23 |
| 65+ | 306 | 5.8 | 52 | 1 | 2 | 3 | 8 | 11 | 18 | 40 |
| **TOTAL SINGLE DX** | 183 | 2.1 | 2 | 1 | 1 | 2 | 3 | 4 | 5 | 6 |
| **TOTAL MULTIPLE DX** | 798 | 6.4 | 81 | 1 | 2 | 4 | 7 | 15 | 16 | 66 |
| **TOTAL** | | | | | | | | | | |
| 0–19 Years | 191 | 3.5 | 40 | 1 | 1 | 2 | 4 | 6 | 8 | 28 |
| 20–34 | 95 | 10.5 | 374 | 2 | 2 | 4 | 6 | 26 | 71 | 71 |
| 35–49 | 147 | 6.4 | 34 | 1 | 2 | 4 | 8 | 15 | 15 | 21 |
| 50–64 | 219 | 5.4 | 34 | 1 | 2 | 3 | 5 | 16 | 16 | 21 |
| 65+ | 329 | 5.6 | 49 | 1 | 2 | 3 | 7 | 11 | 17 | 40 |
| **GRAND TOTAL** | 981 | 5.7 | 70 | 1 | 2 | 3 | 6 | 15 | 16 | 49 |

### 40.24: EXC INGUINAL LYMPH NODE. Formerly included in operation group(s) 591.

| Type of Patients | Observed Patients | Avg. Stay | Variance | 10th | 25th | 50th | 75th | 90th | 95th | 99th |
|---|---|---|---|---|---|---|---|---|---|---|
| **1. SINGLE DX** | | | | | | | | | | |
| 0–19 Years | 19 | 2.6 | 8 | 1 | 1 | 2 | 3 | 4 | 5 | 15 |
| 20–34 | 15 | 2.1 | 2 | 1 | 1 | 2 | 2 | 4 | 6 | 6 |
| 35–49 | 14 | 3.1 | 4 | 1 | 1 | 3 | 5 | 7 | 7 | 7 |
| 50–64 | 16 | 2.1 | 1 | 1 | 1 | 2 | 3 | 3 | 4 | 5 |
| 65+ | 15 | 2.0 | 1 | 1 | 1 | 2 | 3 | 3 | 4 | 5 |
| **2. MULTIPLE DX** | | | | | | | | | | |
| 0–19 Years | 26 | 5.1 | 39 | 1 | 2 | 2 | 7 | 12 | 22 | 26 |
| 20–34 | 29 | 4.8 | 20 | 1 | 4 | 4 | 6 | 12 | 12 | 23 |
| 35–49 | 84 | 5.6 | 30 | 1 | 4 | 4 | 9 | 14 | 17 | 22 |
| 50–64 | 103 | 4.4 | 10 | 2 | 4 | 4 | 5 | 7 | 10 | 17 |
| 65+ | 157 | 6.1 | 39 | 3 | 4 | 4 | 8 | 12 | 16 | 29 |
| **TOTAL SINGLE DX** | 79 | 2.4 | 4 | 1 | 1 | 2 | 3 | 4 | 5 | 15 |
| **TOTAL MULTIPLE DX** | 399 | 5.4 | 28 | 1 | 2 | 4 | 7 | 12 | 15 | 26 |
| **TOTAL** | | | | | | | | | | |
| 0–19 Years | 45 | 4.0 | 26 | 1 | 1 | 2 | 4 | 11 | 15 | 26 |
| 20–34 | 44 | 4.1 | 16 | 1 | 1 | 2 | 5 | 12 | 12 | 23 |
| 35–49 | 98 | 5.3 | 27 | 1 | 2 | 4 | 5 | 12 | 17 | 22 |
| 50–64 | 119 | 4.1 | 9 | 2 | 2 | 3 | 5 | 7 | 10 | 17 |
| 65+ | 172 | 5.7 | 37 | 2 | 2 | 4 | 7 | 12 | 15 | 27 |
| **GRAND TOTAL** | 478 | 4.9 | 26 | 1 | 2 | 3 | 6 | 11 | 14 | 26 |

### 40.3: REGIONAL LYMPH NODE EXC. Formerly included in operation group(s) 592.

| Type of Patients | Observed Patients | Avg. Stay | Variance | 10th | 25th | 50th | 75th | 90th | 95th | 99th |
|---|---|---|---|---|---|---|---|---|---|---|
| **1. SINGLE DX** | | | | | | | | | | |
| 0–19 Years | 20 | 4.2 | 10 | 1 | 3 | 3 | 8 | 9 | 9 | 9 |
| 20–34 | 24 | 3.9 | 3 | 1 | 2 | 5 | 5 | 5 | 6 | 9 |
| 35–49 | 34 | 1.8 | 2 | 1 | 1 | 1 | 2 | 5 | 5 | 7 |
| 50–64 | 57 | 2.4 | 4 | 1 | 1 | 1 | 3 | 6 | 6 | 6 |
| 65+ | 54 | 1.4 | 1 | 1 | 1 | 1 | 1 | 2 | 3 | 6 |
| **2. MULTIPLE DX** | | | | | | | | | | |
| 0–19 Years | 38 | 4.8 | 10 | 3 | 3 | 4 | 7 | 7 | 7 | 13 |
| 20–34 | 99 | 4.6 | 13 | 1 | 2 | 4 | 6 | 8 | 13 | 14 |
| 35–49 | 201 | 4.5 | 16 | 1 | 2 | 4 | 6 | 10 | 11 | 16 |
| 50–64 | 375 | 3.2 | 16 | 1 | 1 | 2 | 4 | 5 | 8 | 17 |
| 65+ | 537 | 3.4 | 17 | 1 | 1 | 2 | 3 | 8 | 13 | 21 |
| **TOTAL SINGLE DX** | 189 | 2.3 | 4 | 1 | 1 | 1 | 3 | 5 | 6 | 9 |
| **TOTAL MULTIPLE DX** | 1,250 | 3.6 | 16 | 1 | 1 | 2 | 4 | 7 | 11 | 20 |
| **TOTAL** | | | | | | | | | | |
| 0–19 Years | 58 | 4.7 | 10 | 2 | 3 | 3 | 7 | 7 | 9 | 10 |
| 20–34 | 123 | 4.4 | 11 | 1 | 2 | 4 | 6 | 7 | 10 | 14 |
| 35–49 | 235 | 4.1 | 15 | 1 | 1 | 3 | 6 | 9 | 11 | 16 |
| 50–64 | 432 | 3.1 | 15 | 1 | 1 | 2 | 4 | 6 | 8 | 17 |
| 65+ | 591 | 3.2 | 16 | 1 | 2 | 2 | 3 | 8 | 12 | 21 |
| **GRAND TOTAL** | 1,439 | 3.5 | 15 | 1 | 2 | 2 | 4 | 7 | 10 | 19 |

Length of Stay by Diagnosis and Operation, United States, 2000

# United States, October 1998–September 1999 Data, by Operation

## 40.4: RAD EXC CERV LYMPH NODE. Formerly included in operation group(s) 592.

| Type of Patients | Observed Patients | Avg. Stay | Variance | 10th | 25th | 50th | 75th | 90th | 95th | 99th |
|---|---|---|---|---|---|---|---|---|---|---|
| **1. SINGLE DX** | | | | | | | | | | |
| 0–19 Years | 15 | 2.2 | 2 | 1 | 1 | 2 | 2 | 3 | 8 | 8 |
| 20–34 | 14 | 2.7 | 3 | 1 | 2 | 3 | 3 | 5 | 5 | 7 |
| 35–49 | 58 | 2.8 | 3 | 1 | 2 | 2 | 4 | 5 | 6 | 10 |
| 50–64 | 67 | 2.5 | 2 | 1 | 2 | 2 | 3 | 4 | 4 | 8 |
| 65+ | 42 | 2.9 | 3 | 1 | 2 | 2 | 4 | 6 | 6 | 10 |
| **2. MULTIPLE DX** | | | | | | | | | | |
| 0–19 Years | 35 | 4.9 | 125 | 1 | 1 | 2 | 5 | 8 | 11 | 72 |
| 20–34 | 64 | 2.8 | 1 | 1 | 2 | 3 | 3 | 4 | 4 | 7 |
| 35–49 | 387 | 3.9 | 19 | 1 | 2 | 3 | 4 | 8 | 14 | 18 |
| 50–64 | 767 | 4.7 | 18 | 2 | 2 | 3 | 5 | 11 | 15 | 15 |
| 65+ | 973 | 4.9 | 24 | 2 | 2 | 3 | 5 | 10 | 14 | 22 |
| **TOTAL SINGLE DX** | 196 | 2.7 | 3 | 1 | 2 | 2 | 3 | 5 | 6 | 10 |
| **TOTAL MULTIPLE DX** | 2,226 | 4.5 | 21 | 1 | 2 | 3 | 5 | 10 | 14 | 20 |
| **TOTAL** | | | | | | | | | | |
| 0–19 Years | 50 | 4.3 | 96 | 1 | 1 | 2 | 3 | 8 | 9 | 72 |
| 20–34 | 78 | 2.8 | 1 | 1 | 2 | 3 | 3 | 4 | 5 | 7 |
| 35–49 | 445 | 3.8 | 18 | 2 | 2 | 3 | 4 | 8 | 11 | 15 |
| 50–64 | 834 | 4.5 | 17 | 2 | 2 | 3 | 5 | 11 | 15 | 15 |
| 65+ | 1,015 | 4.8 | 23 | 2 | 2 | 3 | 5 | 10 | 14 | 22 |
| **GRAND TOTAL** | 2,422 | 4.4 | 20 | 1 | 2 | 3 | 5 | 9 | 14 | 20 |

## 40.41: UNILAT RAD NECK DISSECT. Formerly included in operation group(s) 592.

| Type of Patients | Observed Patients | Avg. Stay | Variance | 10th | 25th | 50th | 75th | 90th | 95th | 99th |
|---|---|---|---|---|---|---|---|---|---|---|
| **1. SINGLE DX** | | | | | | | | | | |
| 0–19 Years | 13 | 1.8 | <1 | 1 | 1 | 2 | 2 | 3 | 3 | 3 |
| 20–34 | 12 | 2.6 | 2 | 1 | 2 | 2 | 3 | 5 | 5 | 5 |
| 35–49 | 45 | 2.7 | 2 | 1 | 2 | 2 | 4 | 5 | 5 | 7 |
| 50–64 | 60 | 2.5 | 2 | 1 | 1 | 2 | 3 | 4 | 4 | 8 |
| 65+ | 39 | 2.9 | 4 | 1 | 2 | 2 | 4 | 6 | 6 | 10 |
| **2. MULTIPLE DX** | | | | | | | | | | |
| 0–19 Years | 31 | 5.1 | 134 | 1 | 1 | 2 | 5 | 8 | 11 | 72 |
| 20–34 | 51 | 2.8 | <1 | 2 | 2 | 3 | 3 | 4 | 4 | 6 |
| 35–49 | 343 | 3.8 | 19 | 1 | 2 | 3 | 4 | 8 | 14 | 14 |
| 50–64 | 677 | 4.7 | 19 | 2 | 2 | 3 | 5 | 11 | 15 | 15 |
| 65+ | 882 | 4.8 | 24 | 2 | 2 | 3 | 5 | 10 | 15 | 22 |
| **TOTAL SINGLE DX** | 169 | 2.7 | 2 | 1 | 2 | 2 | 3 | 5 | 6 | 7 |
| **TOTAL MULTIPLE DX** | 1,984 | 4.5 | 22 | 1 | 2 | 3 | 5 | 10 | 15 | 19 |
| **TOTAL** | | | | | | | | | | |
| 0–19 Years | 44 | 4.4 | 105 | 1 | 2 | 2 | 3 | 8 | 9 | 72 |
| 20–34 | 63 | 2.8 | <1 | 2 | 2 | 3 | 3 | 4 | 4 | 6 |
| 35–49 | 388 | 3.7 | 17 | 1 | 2 | 3 | 4 | 7 | 11 | 14 |
| 50–64 | 737 | 4.6 | 18 | 1 | 2 | 3 | 5 | 11 | 15 | 15 |
| 65+ | 921 | 4.7 | 23 | 2 | 2 | 3 | 5 | 10 | 14 | 22 |
| **GRAND TOTAL** | 2,153 | 4.4 | 21 | 1 | 2 | 3 | 5 | 9 | 14 | 18 |

## 40.5: OTH RAD NODE DISSECTION. Formerly included in operation group(s) 592.

| Type of Patients | Observed Patients | Avg. Stay | Variance | 10th | 25th | 50th | 75th | 90th | 95th | 99th |
|---|---|---|---|---|---|---|---|---|---|---|
| **1. SINGLE DX** | | | | | | | | | | |
| 0–19 Years | 3 | 1.2 | <1 | 1 | 1 | 1 | 1 | 2 | 2 | 2 |
| 20–34 | 17 | 4.3 | 1 | 3 | 3 | 5 | 5 | 6 | 6 | 6 |
| 35–49 | 13 | 3.3 | <1 | 2 | 2 | 4 | 4 | 4 | 4 | 4 |
| 50–64 | 22 | 2.4 | 5 | 1 | 1 | 1 | 3 | 5 | 7 | 9 |
| 65+ | 35 | 2.7 | 5 | 1 | 1 | 1 | 4 | 7 | 7 | 7 |
| **2. MULTIPLE DX** | | | | | | | | | | |
| 0–19 Years | 14 | 6.4 | 9 | 2 | 4 | 5 | 9 | 11 | 11 | 12 |
| 20–34 | 70 | 4.7 | 8 | 2 | 3 | 5 | 6 | 7 | 7 | 20 |
| 35–49 | 124 | 5.3 | 13 | 1 | 2 | 5 | 8 | 8 | 9 | 15 |
| 50–64 | 215 | 4.1 | 12 | 1 | 2 | 3 | 5 | 8 | 10 | 14 |
| 65+ | 231 | 4.8 | 18 | 1 | 2 | 4 | 6 | 11 | 13 | 21 |
| **TOTAL SINGLE DX** | 90 | 3.0 | 4 | 1 | 1 | 3 | 4 | 6 | 7 | 9 |
| **TOTAL MULTIPLE DX** | 654 | 4.7 | 14 | 1 | 2 | 4 | 6 | 8 | 11 | 19 |
| **TOTAL** | | | | | | | | | | |
| 0–19 Years | 17 | 5.7 | 11 | 1 | 4 | 5 | 9 | 11 | 11 | 12 |
| 20–34 | 87 | 4.7 | 7 | 2 | 3 | 5 | 6 | 7 | 7 | 20 |
| 35–49 | 137 | 5.1 | 12 | 1 | 2 | 4 | 8 | 8 | 10 | 15 |
| 50–64 | 237 | 4.0 | 12 | 1 | 2 | 3 | 5 | 8 | 10 | 14 |
| 65+ | 266 | 4.5 | 17 | 1 | 2 | 3 | 6 | 9 | 13 | 19 |
| **GRAND TOTAL** | 744 | 4.5 | 13 | 1 | 2 | 4 | 6 | 8 | 11 | 19 |

## 40.6: THORACIC DUCT OPERATIONS. Formerly included in operation group(s) 596.

| Type of Patients | Observed Patients | Avg. Stay | Variance | 10th | 25th | 50th | 75th | 90th | 95th | 99th |
|---|---|---|---|---|---|---|---|---|---|---|
| **1. SINGLE DX** | | | | | | | | | | |
| 0–19 Years | 0 | | | | | | | | | |
| 20–34 | 0 | | | | | | | | | |
| 35–49 | 0 | | | | | | | | | |
| 50–64 | 0 | | | | | | | | | |
| 65+ | | | | | | | | | | |
| **2. MULTIPLE DX** | | | | | | | | | | |
| 0–19 Years | 10 | 42.9 | 419 | 12 | 17 | 49 | 49 | 58 | 74 | 95 |
| 20–34 | 2 | 7.3 | 12 | 5 | 5 | 5 | 11 | 11 | 11 | 11 |
| 35–49 | 4 | 11.7 | 27 | 3 | 7 | 15 | 15 | 15 | 15 | 15 |
| 50–64 | 8 | 13.4 | 167 | 7 | 7 | 9 | 16 | 30 | 49 | 49 |
| 65+ | 7 | 20.6 | 119 | 3 | 17 | 20 | 30 | 37 | 38 | 38 |
| **TOTAL SINGLE DX** | 0 | | | | | | | | | |
| **TOTAL MULTIPLE DX** | 31 | 25.5 | 412 | 5 | 11 | 15 | 49 | 49 | 58 | 95 |
| **TOTAL** | | | | | | | | | | |
| 0–19 Years | 10 | 42.9 | 419 | 12 | 17 | 49 | 49 | 58 | 74 | 95 |
| 20–34 | 2 | 7.3 | 12 | 5 | 5 | 5 | 11 | 11 | 11 | 11 |
| 35–49 | 4 | 11.7 | 27 | 3 | 7 | 15 | 15 | 15 | 15 | 15 |
| 50–64 | 8 | 13.4 | 167 | 7 | 7 | 9 | 16 | 30 | 49 | 49 |
| 65+ | 7 | 20.6 | 119 | 3 | 17 | 20 | 30 | 37 | 38 | 38 |
| **GRAND TOTAL** | 31 | 25.5 | 412 | 5 | 11 | 15 | 49 | 49 | 58 | 95 |

Length of Stay by Diagnosis and Operation, United States, 2000

# United States, October 1998–September 1999 Data, by Operation

## 40.9: LYMPHATIC STRUCT OPS NEC. Formerly included in operation group(s) 596.

| Type of Patients | Observed Patients | Avg. Stay | Variance | Percentiles | | | | | | |
|---|---|---|---|---|---|---|---|---|---|---|
| | | | | 10th | 25th | 50th | 75th | 90th | 95th | 99th |
| **1. SINGLE DX** | | | | | | | | | | |
| 0–19 Years | 8 | 1.4 | <1 | 1 | 1 | 1 | 1 | 3 | 4 | 4 |
| 20–34 | 0 | | | | | | | | | |
| 35–49 | 1 | 1.0 | 0 | 1 | 1 | 1 | 1 | 1 | 1 | 1 |
| 50–64 | 2 | 4.0 | 0 | 4 | 4 | 4 | 4 | 4 | 4 | 4 |
| 65+ | 4 | 2.3 | 1 | 2 | 2 | 2 | 3 | 4 | 4 | 4 |
| **2. MULTIPLE DX** | | | | | | | | | | |
| 0–19 Years | 11 | 23.4 | >999 | 1 | 4 | 4 | 77 | 77 | 77 | 77 |
| 20–34 | 3 | 6.5 | 4 | 7 | 7 | 7 | 7 | 7 | 8 | 8 |
| 35–49 | 7 | 3.6 | 16 | 1 | 1 | 1 | 8 | 10 | 10 | 12 |
| 50–64 | 16 | 8.6 | 85 | 2 | 3 | 6 | 11 | 29 | 29 | 37 |
| 65+ | 23 | 5.8 | 22 | 1 | 3 | 5 | 7 | 11 | 19 | 23 |
| **TOTAL SINGLE DX** | 15 | 1.8 | 1 | 1 | 1 | 1 | 3 | 4 | 4 | 4 |
| **TOTAL MULTIPLE DX** | 60 | 9.8 | 309 | 1 | 2 | 5 | 7 | 19 | 77 | 77 |
| **TOTAL** | | | | | | | | | | |
| 0–19 Years | 19 | 14.7 | 792 | 1 | 1 | 2 | 5 | 77 | 77 | 77 |
| 20–34 | 3 | 6.5 | 4 | 7 | 7 | 7 | 7 | 7 | 8 | 8 |
| 35–49 | 8 | 3.4 | 15 | 1 | 1 | 1 | 8 | 10 | 10 | 12 |
| 50–64 | 18 | 8.2 | 80 | 2 | 3 | 6 | 11 | 29 | 29 | 37 |
| 65+ | 27 | 5.4 | 21 | 1 | 1 | 5 | 7 | 9 | 19 | 23 |
| **GRAND TOTAL** | 75 | 8.4 | 265 | 1 | 1 | 4 | 7 | 12 | 37 | 77 |

## 41.0: BONE MARROW TRANSPLANT. Formerly included in operation group(s) 593.

| Type of Patients | Observed Patients | Avg. Stay | Variance | Percentiles | | | | | | |
|---|---|---|---|---|---|---|---|---|---|---|
| | | | | 10th | 25th | 50th | 75th | 90th | 95th | 99th |
| **1. SINGLE DX** | | | | | | | | | | |
| 0–19 Years | 24 | 23.5 | 90 | 5 | 20 | 26 | 29 | 30 | 30 | 39 |
| 20–34 | 5 | 21.8 | 329 | 9 | 9 | 9 | 30 | 54 | 54 | 54 |
| 35–49 | 13 | 12.4 | 78 | 1 | 2 | 16 | 20 | 23 | 24 | 24 |
| 50–64 | 15 | 7.8 | 54 | 1 | 1 | 4 | 17 | 18 | 20 | 20 |
| 65+ | 0 | | | | | | | | | |
| **2. MULTIPLE DX** | | | | | | | | | | |
| 0–19 Years | 650 | 34.0 | 235 | 21 | 24 | 31 | 40 | 61 | 85 | >99 |
| 20–34 | 377 | 24.4 | 132 | 13 | 18 | 22 | 30 | 38 | 46 | 69 |
| 35–49 | 910 | 22.7 | 111 | 10 | 17 | 21 | 27 | 36 | 42 | 61 |
| 50–64 | 818 | 21.0 | 97 | 10 | 17 | 20 | 25 | 32 | 39 | 59 |
| 65+ | 62 | 20.2 | 102 | 7 | 17 | 19 | 23 | 27 | 31 | 74 |
| **TOTAL SINGLE DX** | 57 | 17.5 | 174 | 1 | 9 | 17 | 27 | 30 | 39 | 54 |
| **TOTAL MULTIPLE DX** | 2,817 | 26.0 | 180 | 14 | 18 | 23 | 32 | 43 | 56 | >99 |
| **TOTAL** | | | | | | | | | | |
| 0–19 Years | 674 | 33.7 | 233 | 21 | 24 | 31 | 39 | 61 | 84 | >99 |
| 20–34 | 382 | 24.3 | 140 | 9 | 17 | 22 | 30 | 38 | 47 | 69 |
| 35–49 | 923 | 22.6 | 112 | 10 | 17 | 21 | 27 | 36 | 42 | 61 |
| 50–64 | 833 | 20.7 | 100 | 8 | 16 | 20 | 25 | 32 | 39 | 59 |
| 65+ | 62 | 20.2 | 102 | 7 | 17 | 19 | 23 | 27 | 31 | 74 |
| **GRAND TOTAL** | 2,874 | 25.8 | 182 | 13 | 18 | 23 | 32 | 43 | 56 | >99 |

## 41.03: ALLO MARROW TRANSPL NEC. Formerly included in operation group(s) 593.

| Type of Patients | Observed Patients | Avg. Stay | Variance | Percentiles | | | | | | |
|---|---|---|---|---|---|---|---|---|---|---|
| | | | | 10th | 25th | 50th | 75th | 90th | 95th | 99th |
| **1. SINGLE DX** | | | | | | | | | | |
| 0–19 Years | 5 | 29.2 | 58 | 20 | 20 | 30 | 39 | 39 | 39 | 39 |
| 20–34 | 2 | 46.2 | 139 | 30 | 30 | 54 | 54 | 54 | 54 | 54 |
| 35–49 | 0 | | | | | | | | | |
| 50–64 | 1 | 1.0 | 0 | 1 | 1 | 1 | 1 | 1 | 1 | 1 |
| 65+ | 0 | | | | | | | | | |
| **2. MULTIPLE DX** | | | | | | | | | | |
| 0–19 Years | 198 | 42.2 | 254 | 26 | 33 | 39 | 54 | 76 | >99 | >99 |
| 20–34 | 113 | 31.7 | 95 | 22 | 27 | 31 | 37 | 45 | 47 | 70 |
| 35–49 | 174 | 31.0 | 85 | 22 | 26 | 30 | 36 | 41 | 46 | 57 |
| 50–64 | 84 | 30.2 | 103 | 19 | 24 | 29 | 35 | 45 | 57 | >99 |
| 65+ | 2 | 53.4 | 831 | 22 | 22 | 74 | 74 | 74 | 74 | 74 |
| **TOTAL SINGLE DX** | 8 | 21.9 | 451 | 1 | 1 | 20 | 39 | 54 | 54 | 54 |
| **TOTAL MULTIPLE DX** | 571 | 36.1 | 199 | 23 | 28 | 33 | 44 | 58 | 76 | >99 |
| **TOTAL** | | | | | | | | | | |
| 0–19 Years | 203 | 42.0 | 253 | 26 | 32 | 39 | 54 | 76 | >99 | >99 |
| 20–34 | 115 | 32.4 | 106 | 22 | 27 | 31 | 38 | 47 | 54 | 70 |
| 35–49 | 174 | 31.0 | 85 | 22 | 26 | 30 | 36 | 41 | 46 | 57 |
| 50–64 | 85 | 27.8 | 159 | 16 | 23 | 28 | 34 | 45 | 57 | >99 |
| 65+ | 2 | 53.4 | 831 | 22 | 22 | 74 | 74 | 74 | 74 | 74 |
| **GRAND TOTAL** | 579 | 35.7 | 211 | 22 | 28 | 33 | 43 | 58 | 75 | >99 |

## 41.04: AUTLOG STEM CELL TRANSPL. Formerly included in operation group(s) 593.

| Type of Patients | Observed Patients | Avg. Stay | Variance | Percentiles | | | | | | |
|---|---|---|---|---|---|---|---|---|---|---|
| | | | | 10th | 25th | 50th | 75th | 90th | 95th | 99th |
| **1. SINGLE DX** | | | | | | | | | | |
| 0–19 Years | 9 | 21.6 | 89 | 4 | 22 | 26 | 26 | 30 | 30 | 30 |
| 20–34 | 2 | 10.5 | 18 | 9 | 9 | 9 | 9 | 22 | 22 | 22 |
| 35–49 | 7 | 11.5 | 69 | 1 | 1 | 14 | 20 | 21 | 21 | 21 |
| 50–64 | 13 | 10.9 | 46 | 1 | 4 | 10 | 17 | 20 | 20 | 20 |
| 65+ | 0 | | | | | | | | | |
| **2. MULTIPLE DX** | | | | | | | | | | |
| 0–19 Years | 198 | 24.5 | 52 | 20 | 21 | 24 | 26 | 31 | 35 | 49 |
| 20–34 | 178 | 18.8 | 51 | 9 | 16 | 19 | 21 | 26 | 31 | 45 |
| 35–49 | 565 | 19.2 | 67 | 8 | 16 | 19 | 22 | 28 | 33 | 48 |
| 50–64 | 619 | 19.6 | 73 | 9 | 16 | 19 | 23 | 28 | 34 | 50 |
| 65+ | 54 | 19.0 | 53 | 7 | 17 | 19 | 23 | 27 | 31 | 38 |
| **TOTAL SINGLE DX** | 31 | 14.1 | 77 | 3 | 9 | 10 | 22 | 26 | 27 | 30 |
| **TOTAL MULTIPLE DX** | 1,614 | 20.3 | 68 | 10 | 17 | 20 | 24 | 28 | 33 | 48 |
| **TOTAL** | | | | | | | | | | |
| 0–19 Years | 207 | 24.4 | 54 | 19 | 22 | 24 | 26 | 31 | 35 | 48 |
| 20–34 | 180 | 18.4 | 52 | 8 | 16 | 18 | 21 | 26 | 31 | 45 |
| 35–49 | 572 | 19.1 | 67 | 8 | 16 | 19 | 22 | 28 | 33 | 48 |
| 50–64 | 632 | 19.4 | 74 | 8 | 16 | 19 | 23 | 28 | 34 | 50 |
| 65+ | 54 | 19.0 | 53 | 7 | 17 | 19 | 23 | 27 | 31 | 38 |
| **GRAND TOTAL** | 1,645 | 20.2 | 69 | 9 | 17 | 20 | 24 | 28 | 33 | 48 |

Length of Stay by Diagnosis and Operation, United States, 2000

# United States, October 1998–September 1999 Data, by Operation

## 41.1: PUNCTURE OF SPLEEN. Formerly included in operation group(s) 594.

| Type of Patients | Observed Patients | Avg. Stay | Vari-ance | Percentiles | | | | | | |
|---|---|---|---|---|---|---|---|---|---|---|
| | | | | 10th | 25th | 50th | 75th | 90th | 95th | 99th |
| **1. SINGLE DX** | | | | | | | | | | |
| 0–19 Years | 0 | | | | | | | | | |
| 20–34 | 0 | | | | | | | | | |
| 35–49 | 0 | | | | | | | | | |
| 50–64 | 0 | | | | | | | | | |
| 65+ | 0 | | | | | | | | | |
| **2. MULTIPLE DX** | | | | | | | | | | |
| 0–19 Years | 3 | 3.2 | 10 | 2 | 2 | 3 | 3 | 3 | 16 | 16 |
| 20–34 | 3 | 5.7 | 6 | 3 | 3 | 6 | 8 | 8 | 8 | 8 |
| 35–49 | 7 | 13.0 | 55 | 2 | 4 | 14 | 19 | 23 | 23 | 23 |
| 50–64 | 7 | 11.5 | 79 | 2 | 5 | 13 | 13 | 19 | 39 | 39 |
| 65+ | 6 | 10.9 | 41 | 4 | 5 | 8 | 14 | 22 | 22 | 22 |
| **TOTAL SINGLE DX** | 0 | | | | | | | | | |
| **TOTAL MULTIPLE DX** | 26 | 9.4 | 58 | 2 | 3 | 8 | 14 | 19 | 23 | 39 |
| **TOTAL** | | | | | | | | | | |
| 0–19 Years | 3 | 3.2 | 10 | 2 | 2 | 3 | 3 | 3 | 16 | 16 |
| 20–34 | 3 | 5.7 | 6 | 3 | 3 | 6 | 8 | 8 | 8 | 8 |
| 35–49 | 7 | 13.0 | 55 | 2 | 4 | 14 | 19 | 23 | 23 | 23 |
| 50–64 | 7 | 11.5 | 79 | 2 | 5 | 13 | 13 | 19 | 39 | 39 |
| 65+ | 6 | 10.9 | 41 | 4 | 5 | 8 | 14 | 22 | 22 | 22 |
| **GRAND TOTAL** | 26 | 9.4 | 58 | 2 | 3 | 8 | 14 | 19 | 23 | 39 |

## 41.2: SPLENOTOMY. Formerly included in operation group(s) 594.

| Type of Patients | Observed Patients | Avg. Stay | Vari-ance | Percentiles | | | | | | |
|---|---|---|---|---|---|---|---|---|---|---|
| | | | | 10th | 25th | 50th | 75th | 90th | 95th | 99th |
| **1. SINGLE DX** | | | | | | | | | | |
| 0–19 Years | 0 | | | | | | | | | |
| 20–34 | 0 | | | | | | | | | |
| 35–49 | 0 | | | | | | | | | |
| 50–64 | 0 | | | | | | | | | |
| 65+ | | | | | | | | | | |
| **2. MULTIPLE DX** | | | | | | | | | | |
| 0–19 Years | 6 | 10.8 | 84 | 4 | 4 | 5 | 23 | 23 | 23 | 23 |
| 20–34 | 1 | 8.0 | 0 | 8 | 8 | 8 | 8 | 8 | 8 | 8 |
| 35–49 | 4 | 9.7 | 18 | 4 | 4 | 10 | 10 | 16 | 16 | 16 |
| 50–64 | 1 | 1.0 | 0 | 1 | 1 | 1 | 1 | 1 | 1 | 1 |
| 65+ | 4 | 9.6 | 61 | 2 | 2 | 5 | 13 | 21 | 21 | 21 |
| **TOTAL SINGLE DX** | 0 | | | | | | | | | |
| **TOTAL MULTIPLE DX** | 16 | 9.6 | 55 | 2 | 4 | 8 | 13 | 23 | 23 | 23 |
| **TOTAL** | | | | | | | | | | |
| 0–19 Years | 6 | 10.8 | 84 | 4 | 4 | 5 | 23 | 23 | 23 | 23 |
| 20–34 | 1 | 8.0 | 0 | 8 | 8 | 8 | 8 | 8 | 8 | 8 |
| 35–49 | 4 | 9.7 | 18 | 4 | 4 | 10 | 10 | 16 | 16 | 16 |
| 50–64 | 1 | 1.0 | 0 | 1 | 1 | 1 | 1 | 1 | 1 | 1 |
| 65+ | 4 | 9.6 | 61 | 2 | 2 | 5 | 13 | 21 | 21 | 21 |
| **GRAND TOTAL** | 16 | 9.6 | 55 | 2 | 4 | 8 | 13 | 23 | 23 | 23 |

## 41.3: MARROW & SPLEEN DXTIC PX. Formerly included in operation group(s) 594, 596.

| Type of Patients | Observed Patients | Avg. Stay | Vari-ance | Percentiles | | | | | | |
|---|---|---|---|---|---|---|---|---|---|---|
| | | | | 10th | 25th | 50th | 75th | 90th | 95th | 99th |
| **1. SINGLE DX** | | | | | | | | | | |
| 0–19 Years | 427 | 4.3 | 16 | 1 | 1 | 3 | 6 | 9 | 10 | 21 |
| 20–34 | 80 | 4.5 | 11 | 2 | 2 | 4 | 6 | 7 | 13 | 17 |
| 35–49 | 80 | 3.6 | 7 | 2 | 2 | 2 | 4 | 8 | 9 | 13 |
| 50–64 | 56 | 4.1 | 20 | 1 | 2 | 3 | 4 | 7 | 15 | 30 |
| 65+ | 65 | 3.5 | 12 | 1 | 1 | 2 | 6 | 7 | 8 | 21 |
| **2. MULTIPLE DX** | | | | | | | | | | |
| 0–19 Years | 1,539 | 9.6 | 111 | 2 | 4 | 6 | 11 | 21 | 31 | 63 |
| 20–34 | 946 | 9.4 | 87 | 2 | 4 | 6 | 11 | 22 | 30 | 42 |
| 35–49 | 1,789 | 9.1 | 76 | 2 | 4 | 7 | 12 | 18 | 27 | 43 |
| 50–64 | 2,612 | 9.1 | 74 | 3 | 4 | 7 | 10 | 19 | 27 | 42 |
| 65+ | 7,088 | 8.6 | 53 | 3 | 4 | 7 | 10 | 17 | 24 | 36 |
| **TOTAL SINGLE DX** | 708 | 4.2 | 14 | 1 | 2 | 3 | 6 | 8 | 10 | 21 |
| **TOTAL MULTIPLE DX** | 13,974 | 8.9 | 69 | 2 | 4 | 7 | 11 | 18 | 26 | 42 |
| **TOTAL** | | | | | | | | | | |
| 0–19 Years | 1,966 | 8.4 | 94 | 1 | 3 | 6 | 9 | 17 | 27 | 60 |
| 20–34 | 1,026 | 8.8 | 81 | 2 | 3 | 6 | 11 | 21 | 28 | 42 |
| 35–49 | 1,869 | 8.9 | 74 | 2 | 4 | 6 | 11 | 18 | 27 | 43 |
| 50–64 | 2,668 | 9.0 | 73 | 3 | 4 | 7 | 10 | 19 | 27 | 42 |
| 65+ | 7,153 | 8.6 | 53 | 2 | 4 | 7 | 10 | 17 | 23 | 36 |
| **GRAND TOTAL** | 14,682 | 8.7 | 67 | 2 | 4 | 6 | 10 | 18 | 26 | 41 |

## 41.31: BONE MARROW BIOPSY. Formerly included in operation group(s) 594.

| Type of Patients | Observed Patients | Avg. Stay | Vari-ance | Percentiles | | | | | | |
|---|---|---|---|---|---|---|---|---|---|---|
| | | | | 10th | 25th | 50th | 75th | 90th | 95th | 99th |
| **1. SINGLE DX** | | | | | | | | | | |
| 0–19 Years | 426 | 4.3 | 16 | 1 | 1 | 3 | 6 | 9 | 10 | 21 |
| 20–34 | 80 | 4.5 | 11 | 2 | 2 | 4 | 6 | 7 | 13 | 17 |
| 35–49 | 80 | 3.6 | 7 | 2 | 2 | 2 | 4 | 8 | 9 | 13 |
| 50–64 | 55 | 4.1 | 20 | 1 | 2 | 3 | 4 | 7 | 15 | 30 |
| 65+ | 65 | 3.5 | 12 | 1 | 1 | 2 | 6 | 7 | 8 | 21 |
| **2. MULTIPLE DX** | | | | | | | | | | |
| 0–19 Years | 1,537 | 9.6 | 111 | 2 | 4 | 6 | 11 | 21 | 31 | 63 |
| 20–34 | 943 | 9.4 | 87 | 2 | 4 | 6 | 11 | 22 | 30 | 42 |
| 35–49 | 1,779 | 9.1 | 76 | 2 | 4 | 7 | 12 | 18 | 27 | 43 |
| 50–64 | 2,606 | 9.0 | 74 | 3 | 4 | 7 | 10 | 19 | 27 | 42 |
| 65+ | 7,059 | 8.6 | 53 | 3 | 4 | 7 | 10 | 17 | 24 | 36 |
| **TOTAL SINGLE DX** | 706 | 4.2 | 14 | 1 | 2 | 3 | 6 | 8 | 10 | 21 |
| **TOTAL MULTIPLE DX** | 13,924 | 8.9 | 69 | 2 | 4 | 7 | 11 | 18 | 26 | 42 |
| **TOTAL** | | | | | | | | | | |
| 0–19 Years | 1,963 | 8.4 | 94 | 1 | 3 | 6 | 9 | 17 | 27 | 60 |
| 20–34 | 1,023 | 8.9 | 81 | 2 | 3 | 6 | 11 | 21 | 28 | 42 |
| 35–49 | 1,859 | 8.9 | 74 | 2 | 4 | 6 | 11 | 18 | 27 | 43 |
| 50–64 | 2,661 | 9.0 | 73 | 3 | 4 | 7 | 10 | 19 | 27 | 42 |
| 65+ | 7,124 | 8.6 | 53 | 2 | 4 | 7 | 10 | 17 | 24 | 36 |
| **GRAND TOTAL** | 14,630 | 8.7 | 67 | 2 | 4 | 6 | 10 | 18 | 26 | 41 |

Length of Stay by Diagnosis and Operation, United States, 2000

# United States, October 1998–September 1999 Data, by Operation

## 41.4: EXC/DESTR SPLENIC TISSUE. Formerly included in operation group(s) 594.

| Type of Patients | Observed Patients | Variance | Avg. Stay | Percentiles |||||||
|---|---|---|---|---|---|---|---|---|---|---|
| | | | | 10th | 25th | 50th | 75th | 90th | 95th | 99th |
| **1. SINGLE DX** | | | | | | | | | | |
| 0–19 Years | 31 | 2 | 3.8 | 2 | 3 | 3 | 4 | 7 | 7 | 7 |
| 20–34 | 13 | 1 | 2.1 | 1 | 1 | 2 | 3 | 3 | 4 | 5 |
| 35–49 | 1 | 0 | 3.0 | 3 | 3 | 3 | 3 | 3 | 3 | 3 |
| 50–64 | 1 | 0 | 2.0 | 2 | 2 | 2 | 2 | 2 | 2 | 2 |
| 65+ | 1 | 0 | 2.0 | 2 | 2 | 2 | 2 | 2 | 2 | 2 |
| **2. MULTIPLE DX** | | | | | | | | | | |
| 0–19 Years | 38 | 11 | 6.9 | 3 | 4 | 7 | 9 | 10 | 12 | 15 |
| 20–34 | 16 | 14 | 6.0 | 2 | 4 | 6 | 8 | 8 | 10 | 25 |
| 35–49 | 13 | 295 | 11.5 | 5 | 6 | 6 | 9 | 14 | 83 | 83 |
| 50–64 | 4 | 11 | 8.4 | 5 | 7 | 7 | 13 | 13 | 13 | 13 |
| 65+ | 6 | 40 | 11.3 | 2 | 2 | 15 | 15 | 15 | 20 | 20 |
| **TOTAL SINGLE DX** | 47 | 2 | 3.5 | 2 | 2 | 3 | 4 | 6 | 7 | 7 |
| **TOTAL MULTIPLE DX** | 77 | 89 | 8.3 | 3 | 5 | 6 | 9 | 13 | 15 | 83 |
| **TOTAL** | | | | | | | | | | |
| 0–19 Years | 69 | 8 | 5.1 | 2 | 3 | 4 | 7 | 9 | 10 | 13 |
| 20–34 | 29 | 13 | 4.8 | 1 | 2 | 5 | 6 | 8 | 8 | 25 |
| 35–49 | 14 | 289 | 11.3 | 5 | 6 | 6 | 8 | 14 | 83 | 83 |
| 50–64 | 5 | 15 | 7.2 | 2 | 5 | 7 | 8 | 13 | 13 | 13 |
| 65+ | 7 | 46 | 9.5 | 2 | 2 | 13 | 15 | 15 | 20 | 20 |
| **GRAND TOTAL** | 124 | 59 | 6.3 | 2 | 3 | 5 | 7 | 10 | 14 | 25 |

## 41.5: TOTAL SPLENECTOMY. Formerly included in operation group(s) 594.

| Type of Patients | Observed Patients | Variance | Avg. Stay | Percentiles |||||||
|---|---|---|---|---|---|---|---|---|---|---|
| | | | | 10th | 25th | 50th | 75th | 90th | 95th | 99th |
| **1. SINGLE DX** | | | | | | | | | | |
| 0–19 Years | 247 | 2 | 3.1 | 2 | 3 | 3 | 4 | 5 | 6 | 8 |
| 20–34 | 168 | 5 | 3.6 | 2 | 2 | 4 | 4 | 5 | 6 | 14 |
| 35–49 | 120 | 8 | 4.0 | 2 | 2 | 3 | 5 | 7 | 11 | 11 |
| 50–64 | 65 | 4 | 3.0 | 1 | 2 | 2 | 4 | 5 | 6 | 15 |
| 65+ | 38 | 13 | 5.7 | 2 | 3 | 5 | 8 | 11 | 11 | 15 |
| **2. MULTIPLE DX** | | | | | | | | | | |
| 0–19 Years | 610 | 63 | 7.2 | 3 | 3 | 5 | 7 | 14 | 23 | 54 |
| 20–34 | 763 | 87 | 8.0 | 3 | 4 | 6 | 9 | 15 | 20 | 73 |
| 35–49 | 1,045 | 114 | 10.0 | 3 | 4 | 6 | 11 | 19 | 33 | 53 |
| 50–64 | 868 | 52 | 8.4 | 3 | 4 | 6 | 10 | 16 | 22 | 38 |
| 65+ | 1,062 | 84 | 9.8 | 3 | 5 | 7 | 11 | 20 | 26 | 48 |
| **TOTAL SINGLE DX** | 638 | 5 | 3.6 | 1 | 2 | 3 | 4 | 6 | 7 | 12 |
| **TOTAL MULTIPLE DX** | 4,348 | 84 | 8.9 | 3 | 4 | 6 | 10 | 17 | 26 | 52 |
| **TOTAL** | | | | | | | | | | |
| 0–19 Years | 857 | 49 | 6.0 | 2 | 3 | 4 | 6 | 10 | 17 | 35 |
| 20–34 | 931 | 73 | 7.1 | 2 | 4 | 5 | 8 | 12 | 18 | 73 |
| 35–49 | 1,165 | 105 | 9.3 | 3 | 4 | 6 | 10 | 17 | 33 | 52 |
| 50–64 | 933 | 50 | 8.0 | 3 | 4 | 6 | 9 | 15 | 21 | 37 |
| 65+ | 1,100 | 82 | 9.7 | 3 | 5 | 7 | 11 | 19 | 26 | 48 |
| **GRAND TOTAL** | 4,986 | 76 | 8.1 | 3 | 4 | 5 | 9 | 15 | 22 | 52 |

## 41.9: OTH SPLEEN & MARROW OPS. Formerly included in operation group(s) 594.

| Type of Patients | Observed Patients | Variance | Avg. Stay | Percentiles |||||||
|---|---|---|---|---|---|---|---|---|---|---|
| | | | | 10th | 25th | 50th | 75th | 90th | 95th | 99th |
| **1. SINGLE DX** | | | | | | | | | | |
| 0–19 Years | 64 | 9 | 2.2 | 1 | 1 | 1 | 3 | 4 | 6 | 23 |
| 20–34 | 53 | 5 | 3.0 | 1 | 1 | 1 | 6 | 6 | 6 | 6 |
| 35–49 | 36 | <1 | 1.0 | 1 | 1 | 1 | 1 | 1 | 1 | 1 |
| 50–64 | 12 | 12 | 2.5 | 1 | 1 | 1 | 1 | 11 | 11 | 11 |
| 65+ | 1 | 0 | 1.0 | 1 | 1 | 1 | 1 | 1 | 1 | 1 |
| **2. MULTIPLE DX** | | | | | | | | | | |
| 0–19 Years | 128 | 7 | 5.0 | 1 | 4 | 5 | 6 | 8 | 9 | 13 |
| 20–34 | 102 | 37 | 7.5 | 2 | 5 | 6 | 8 | 13 | 19 | 32 |
| 35–49 | 63 | 21 | 6.8 | 1 | 5 | 6 | 8 | 12 | 15 | 21 |
| 50–64 | 33 | 42 | 5.9 | 1 | 3 | 4 | 6 | 16 | 22 | 31 |
| 65+ | 12 | 124 | 15.2 | 3 | 4 | 15 | 29 | 29 | 29 | 31 |
| **TOTAL SINGLE DX** | 166 | 7 | 2.2 | 1 | 1 | 1 | 3 | 6 | 6 | 11 |
| **TOTAL MULTIPLE DX** | 338 | 27 | 6.4 | 1 | 4 | 6 | 7 | 10 | 16 | 31 |
| **TOTAL** | | | | | | | | | | |
| 0–19 Years | 192 | 10 | 3.9 | 1 | 1 | 4 | 6 | 7 | 9 | 13 |
| 20–34 | 155 | 31 | 5.9 | 1 | 2 | 5 | 7 | 10 | 17 | 32 |
| 35–49 | 99 | 22 | 5.0 | 1 | 1 | 5 | 7 | 10 | 13 | 21 |
| 50–64 | 45 | 38 | 5.3 | 1 | 1 | 4 | 5 | 11 | 16 | 31 |
| 65+ | 13 | 127 | 14.5 | 3 | 4 | 14 | 29 | 29 | 29 | 31 |
| **GRAND TOTAL** | 504 | 24 | 4.9 | 1 | 1 | 4 | 6 | 9 | 12 | 29 |

## 42.0: ESOPHAGOTOMY. Formerly included in operation group(s) 597.

| Type of Patients | Observed Patients | Variance | Avg. Stay | Percentiles |||||||
|---|---|---|---|---|---|---|---|---|---|---|
| | | | | 10th | 25th | 50th | 75th | 90th | 95th | 99th |
| **1. SINGLE DX** | | | | | | | | | | |
| 0–19 Years | 3 | <1 | 1.9 | 1 | 1 | 2 | 3 | 3 | 3 | 3 |
| 20–34 | 1 | 0 | 6.0 | 6 | 6 | 6 | 6 | 6 | 6 | 6 |
| 35–49 | 0 | | | | | | | | | |
| 50–64 | 0 | | | | | | | | | |
| 65+ | 0 | | | | | | | | | |
| **2. MULTIPLE DX** | | | | | | | | | | |
| 0–19 Years | 3 | 66 | 17.7 | 9 | 9 | 17 | 26 | 26 | 26 | 26 |
| 20–34 | 2 | 21 | 6.5 | 2 | 2 | 10 | 10 | 10 | 10 | 10 |
| 35–49 | 2 | 11 | 8.1 | 4 | 4 | 10 | 10 | 10 | 10 | 10 |
| 50–64 | 11 | 95 | 17.1 | 5 | 13 | 18 | 25 | 32 | 32 | 32 |
| 65+ | 8 | 82 | 8.0 | 2 | 2 | 6 | 11 | 13 | 35 | 35 |
| **TOTAL SINGLE DX** | 4 | 5 | 3.0 | 1 | 1 | 3 | 6 | 6 | 6 | 6 |
| **TOTAL MULTIPLE DX** | 26 | 94 | 13.3 | 2 | 5 | 10 | 20 | 26 | 32 | 35 |
| **TOTAL** | | | | | | | | | | |
| 0–19 Years | 6 | 94 | 14.6 | 2 | 9 | 9 | 26 | 26 | 26 | 26 |
| 20–34 | 3 | 14 | 6.4 | 2 | 2 | 6 | 10 | 12 | 10 | 10 |
| 35–49 | 2 | 11 | 8.1 | 4 | 4 | 10 | 10 | 17 | 10 | 10 |
| 50–64 | 11 | 95 | 17.1 | 5 | 13 | 18 | 25 | 32 | 32 | 32 |
| 65+ | 8 | 82 | 8.0 | 2 | 2 | 6 | 11 | 13 | 35 | 35 |
| **GRAND TOTAL** | 30 | 94 | 12.5 | 2 | 5 | 10 | 18 | 26 | 32 | 35 |

Length of Stay by Diagnosis and Operation, United States, 2000

# United States, October 1998–September 1999 Data, by Operation

## 42.1: ESOPHAGOSTOMY. Formerly included in operation group(s) 597.

| Type of Patients | Observed Patients | Avg. Stay | Variance | Percentiles 10th | 25th | 50th | 75th | 90th | 95th | 99th |
|---|---|---|---|---|---|---|---|---|---|---|
| **1. SINGLE DX** | | | | | | | | | | |
| 0–19 Years | 1 | 10.0 | 0 | 10 | 10 | 10 | 10 | 10 | 10 | 10 |
| 20–34 | 0 | | | | | | | | | |
| 35–49 | 0 | | | | | | | | | |
| 50–64 | 0 | | | | | | | | | |
| 65+ | 0 | | | | | | | | | |
| **2. MULTIPLE DX** | | | | | | | | | | |
| 0–19 Years | 6 | 18.0 | 411 | 2 | 5 | 29 | >99 | >99 | >99 | >99 |
| 20–34 | 0 | | | | | | | | | |
| 35–49 | 3 | 13.6 | 21 | 4 | 12 | 16 | 16 | 16 | 16 | 16 |
| 50–64 | 3 | 32.2 | >999 | 7 | 7 | 20 | 20 | 89 | 89 | 89 |
| 65+ | 6 | 22.2 | 73 | 12 | 15 | 27 | 28 | 35 | 35 | 35 |
| **TOTAL SINGLE DX** | 1 | 10.0 | 0 | 10 | 10 | 10 | 10 | 10 | 10 | 10 |
| **TOTAL MULTIPLE DX** | 18 | 19.9 | 270 | 4 | 12 | 16 | 28 | 89 | >99 | >99 |
| **TOTAL** | | | | | | | | | | |
| 0–19 Years | 7 | 16.4 | 330 | 2 | 5 | 18 | 52 | >99 | >99 | >99 |
| 20–34 | 0 | | | | | | | | | |
| 35–49 | 3 | 13.6 | 21 | 4 | 12 | 16 | 16 | 16 | 16 | 16 |
| 50–64 | 3 | 32.2 | >999 | 7 | 7 | 20 | 20 | 89 | 89 | 89 |
| 65+ | 6 | 22.2 | 73 | 12 | 15 | 27 | 28 | 35 | 35 | 35 |
| **GRAND TOTAL** | 19 | 19.4 | 261 | 4 | 12 | 16 | 28 | 89 | >99 | >99 |

## 42.2: ESOPHAGEAL DXTIC PX. Formerly included in operation group(s) 597, 598, 631.

| Type of Patients | Observed Patients | Avg. Stay | Variance | Percentiles 10th | 25th | 50th | 75th | 90th | 95th | 99th |
|---|---|---|---|---|---|---|---|---|---|---|
| **1. SINGLE DX** | | | | | | | | | | |
| 0–19 Years | 456 | 1.3 | 1 | 1 | 1 | 1 | 1 | 2 | 2 | 7 |
| 20–34 | 17 | 5.3 | 3 | 1 | 6 | 6 | 6 | 6 | 6 | 7 |
| 35–49 | 30 | 2.1 | 3 | 1 | 1 | 1 | 3 | 4 | 6 | 7 |
| 50–64 | 19 | 1.4 | <1 | 1 | 1 | 1 | 2 | 2 | 2 | 3 |
| 65+ | 11 | 1.9 | 3 | 1 | 1 | 1 | 2 | 3 | 7 | 7 |
| **2. MULTIPLE DX** | | | | | | | | | | |
| 0–19 Years | 362 | 4.2 | 61 | 1 | 1 | 2 | 4 | 9 | 14 | 37 |
| 20–34 | 79 | 6.3 | 32 | 1 | 3 | 5 | 7 | 20 | 20 | 20 |
| 35–49 | 265 | 4.9 | 23 | 1 | 2 | 4 | 7 | 9 | 12 | 25 |
| 50–64 | 408 | 6.1 | 23 | 1 | 3 | 5 | 8 | 13 | 15 | 24 |
| 65+ | 987 | 6.4 | 30 | 2 | 3 | 5 | 8 | 13 | 17 | 28 |
| **TOTAL SINGLE DX** | 533 | 1.6 | 3 | 1 | 1 | 1 | 1 | 3 | 6 | 7 |
| **TOTAL MULTIPLE DX** | 2,101 | 5.7 | 34 | 1 | 2 | 4 | 7 | 12 | 15 | 26 |
| **TOTAL** | | | | | | | | | | |
| 0–19 Years | 818 | 2.6 | 30 | 1 | 1 | 1 | 2 | 5 | 9 | 19 |
| 20–34 | 96 | 5.9 | 20 | 1 | 3 | 6 | 6 | 11 | 20 | 20 |
| 35–49 | 295 | 4.7 | 22 | 1 | 2 | 3 | 7 | 9 | 12 | 25 |
| 50–64 | 427 | 5.8 | 23 | 1 | 2 | 5 | 8 | 12 | 14 | 24 |
| 65+ | 998 | 6.3 | 30 | 2 | 3 | 5 | 8 | 13 | 17 | 28 |
| **GRAND TOTAL** | 2,634 | 4.8 | 30 | 1 | 1 | 3 | 6 | 10 | 14 | 24 |

## 42.23: ESOPHAGOSCOPY NEC. Formerly included in operation group(s) 598.

| Type of Patients | Observed Patients | Avg. Stay | Variance | Percentiles 10th | 25th | 50th | 75th | 90th | 95th | 99th |
|---|---|---|---|---|---|---|---|---|---|---|
| **1. SINGLE DX** | | | | | | | | | | |
| 0–19 Years | 427 | 1.3 | 1 | 1 | 1 | 1 | 1 | 2 | 2 | 8 |
| 20–34 | 16 | 5.3 | 3 | 1 | 6 | 6 | 6 | 6 | 6 | 7 |
| 35–49 | 25 | 1.9 | 4 | 1 | 1 | 1 | 2 | 4 | 6 | 9 |
| 50–64 | 18 | 1.4 | <1 | 1 | 1 | 1 | 2 | 2 | 2 | 3 |
| 65+ | 11 | 1.9 | 3 | 1 | 1 | 1 | 2 | 3 | 7 | 7 |
| **2. MULTIPLE DX** | | | | | | | | | | |
| 0–19 Years | 252 | 2.8 | 50 | 1 | 1 | 1 | 2 | 5 | 7 | 17 |
| 20–34 | 64 | 4.7 | 9 | 1 | 2 | 4 | 6 | 8 | 11 | 13 |
| 35–49 | 226 | 4.9 | 25 | 1 | 2 | 3 | 7 | 9 | 12 | 25 |
| 50–64 | 328 | 6.2 | 23 | 1 | 3 | 5 | 8 | 13 | 15 | 25 |
| 65+ | 804 | 6.1 | 26 | 2 | 3 | 5 | 7 | 12 | 15 | 28 |
| **TOTAL SINGLE DX** | 497 | 1.6 | 3 | 1 | 1 | 1 | 1 | 3 | 6 | 8 |
| **TOTAL MULTIPLE DX** | 1,674 | 5.4 | 30 | 1 | 2 | 4 | 7 | 10 | 14 | 25 |
| **TOTAL** | | | | | | | | | | |
| 0–19 Years | 679 | 1.8 | 19 | 1 | 1 | 1 | 1 | 3 | 5 | 14 |
| 20–34 | 80 | 5.0 | 6 | 1 | 3 | 6 | 6 | 7 | 8 | 13 |
| 35–49 | 251 | 4.7 | 24 | 1 | 2 | 3 | 7 | 9 | 12 | 25 |
| 50–64 | 346 | 5.9 | 23 | 1 | 2 | 5 | 8 | 11 | 15 | 22 |
| 65+ | 815 | 6.1 | 26 | 2 | 3 | 5 | 7 | 12 | 15 | 28 |
| **GRAND TOTAL** | 2,171 | 4.5 | 26 | 1 | 1 | 3 | 6 | 9 | 13 | 22 |

## 42.24: CLSD (ENDO) ESOPH BX. Formerly included in operation group(s) 597.

| Type of Patients | Observed Patients | Avg. Stay | Variance | Percentiles 10th | 25th | 50th | 75th | 90th | 95th | 99th |
|---|---|---|---|---|---|---|---|---|---|---|
| **1. SINGLE DX** | | | | | | | | | | |
| 0–19 Years | 4 | 1.8 | 1 | 1 | 1 | 2 | 2 | 4 | 4 | 4 |
| 20–34 | 1 | 3.0 | 0 | 3 | 3 | 3 | 3 | 3 | 3 | 3 |
| 35–49 | 3 | 2.9 | 3 | 1 | 1 | 3 | 3 | 6 | 6 | 6 |
| 50–64 | 1 | 2.0 | 0 | 2 | 2 | 2 | 2 | 2 | 2 | 2 |
| 65+ | 0 | | | | | | | | | |
| **2. MULTIPLE DX** | | | | | | | | | | |
| 0–19 Years | 19 | 6.9 | 135 | 2 | 2 | 4 | 5 | 12 | 14 | 71 |
| 20–34 | 13 | 5.6 | 25 | 2 | 2 | 4 | 5 | 15 | 16 | 16 |
| 35–49 | 35 | 4.7 | 15 | 2 | 3 | 4 | 5 | 10 | 14 | 16 |
| 50–64 | 69 | 5.4 | 24 | 1 | 3 | 4 | 7 | 13 | 15 | 24 |
| 65+ | 162 | 7.8 | 45 | 2 | 3 | 6 | 10 | 17 | 19 | 28 |
| **TOTAL SINGLE DX** | 9 | 2.3 | 2 | 1 | 1 | 2 | 3 | 4 | 4 | 6 |
| **TOTAL MULTIPLE DX** | 298 | 6.7 | 48 | 2 | 3 | 5 | 8 | 14 | 18 | 32 |
| **TOTAL** | | | | | | | | | | |
| 0–19 Years | 23 | 6.3 | 123 | 1 | 2 | 3 | 5 | 12 | 14 | 71 |
| 20–34 | 14 | 5.4 | 23 | 2 | 2 | 3 | 5 | 15 | 16 | 16 |
| 35–49 | 38 | 4.6 | 14 | 2 | 3 | 4 | 5 | 10 | 14 | 16 |
| 50–64 | 70 | 5.4 | 24 | 1 | 3 | 4 | 7 | 13 | 15 | 24 |
| 65+ | 162 | 7.8 | 45 | 2 | 3 | 6 | 10 | 17 | 19 | 28 |
| **GRAND TOTAL** | 307 | 6.6 | 47 | 1 | 3 | 5 | 8 | 14 | 18 | 32 |

Length of Stay by Diagnosis and Operation, United States, 2000

# United States, October 1998–September 1999 Data, by Operation

## 42.3: EXC/DESTR ESOPH LES/TISS. Formerly included in operation group(s) 597.

| Type of Patients | Observed Patients | Avg. Stay | Variance | 10th | 25th | 50th | 75th | 90th | 95th | 99th |
|---|---|---|---|---|---|---|---|---|---|---|
| **1. SINGLE DX** | | | | | | | | | | |
| 0-19 Years | 12 | 2.7 | 1 | 1 | 2 | 3 | 3 | 5 | 5 | 5 |
| 20-34 | 10 | 2.6 | 8 | 1 | 1 | 1 | 4 | 10 | 5 | 5 |
| 35-49 | 28 | 2.7 | 2 | 1 | 2 | 2 | 3 | 5 | 6 | 6 |
| 50-64 | 34 | 2.7 | <1 | 1 | 2 | 3 | 3 | 3 | 4 | 5 |
| 65+ | 25 | 3.5 | 2 | 1 | 2 | 4 | 4 | 5 | 6 | 6 |
| **2. MULTIPLE DX** | | | | | | | | | | |
| 0-19 Years | 99 | 4.1 | 23 | 1 | 1 | 3 | 5 | 9 | 11 | 26 |
| 20-34 | 261 | 4.0 | 9 | 1 | 2 | 3 | 5 | 7 | 11 | 18 |
| 35-49 | 1,788 | 5.7 | 28 | 2 | 3 | 4 | 6 | 11 | 16 | 28 |
| 50-64 | 1,574 | 5.2 | 25 | 2 | 3 | 4 | 6 | 9 | 12 | 24 |
| 65+ | 1,822 | 5.8 | 21 | 2 | 3 | 5 | 7 | 11 | 14 | 24 |
| **TOTAL SINGLE DX** | **109** | **2.8** | **2** | **1** | **2** | **3** | **3** | **4** | **5** | **7** |
| **TOTAL MULTIPLE DX** | **5,544** | **5.5** | **24** | **2** | **3** | **4** | **6** | **10** | **14** | **24** |
| **TOTAL** | | | | | | | | | | |
| 0-19 Years | 111 | 4.0 | 21 | 1 | 1 | 3 | 4 | 9 | 11 | 26 |
| 20-34 | 271 | 4.0 | 9 | 1 | 2 | 3 | 5 | 7 | 11 | 15 |
| 35-49 | 1,816 | 5.7 | 28 | 2 | 3 | 4 | 6 | 11 | 16 | 28 |
| 50-64 | 1,608 | 5.1 | 24 | 2 | 3 | 4 | 6 | 8 | 11 | 24 |
| 65+ | 1,847 | 5.8 | 21 | 2 | 3 | 5 | 7 | 11 | 14 | 23 |
| **GRAND TOTAL** | **5,653** | **5.4** | **24** | **2** | **3** | **4** | **6** | **10** | **14** | **24** |

## 42.4: EXCISION OF ESOPHAGUS. Formerly included in operation group(s) 597.

| Type of Patients | Observed Patients | Avg. Stay | Variance | 10th | 25th | 50th | 75th | 90th | 95th | 99th |
|---|---|---|---|---|---|---|---|---|---|---|
| **1. SINGLE DX** | | | | | | | | | | |
| 0-19 Years | 4 | 14.6 | 18 | 7 | 13 | 15 | 18 | 18 | 18 | 18 |
| 20-34 | 1 | 11.0 | 0 | 11 | 11 | 11 | 11 | 11 | 11 | 11 |
| 35-49 | 5 | 8.1 | 1 | 6 | 8 | 8 | 8 | 10 | 10 | 10 |
| 50-64 | 10 | 11.0 | 13 | 7 | 9 | 10 | 14 | 18 | 18 | 18 |
| 65+ | 2 | 8.9 | 3 | 7 | 7 | 10 | 10 | 10 | 10 | 10 |
| **2. MULTIPLE DX** | | | | | | | | | | |
| 0-19 Years | 25 | 20.8 | 181 | 6 | 10 | 18 | 34 | 34 | 37 | >99 |
| 20-34 | 19 | 18.8 | 144 | 7 | 8 | 15 | 29 | 39 | 40 | 40 |
| 35-49 | 102 | 13.9 | 84 | 7 | 8 | 10 | 15 | 30 | 31 | 49 |
| 50-64 | 299 | 15.9 | 123 | 8 | 9 | 12 | 19 | 39 | 40 | 49 |
| 65+ | 306 | 15.1 | 111 | 8 | 10 | 12 | 17 | 25 | 33 | 85 |
| **TOTAL SINGLE DX** | **22** | **10.8** | **14** | **7** | **8** | **10** | **13** | **18** | **18** | **18** |
| **TOTAL MULTIPLE DX** | **751** | **15.4** | **116** | **8** | **9** | **12** | **17** | **30** | **40** | **59** |
| **TOTAL** | | | | | | | | | | |
| 0-19 Years | 29 | 19.5 | 151 | 6 | 9 | 18 | 29 | 34 | 37 | >99 |
| 20-34 | 20 | 18.4 | 139 | 7 | 9 | 15 | 29 | 39 | 40 | 40 |
| 35-49 | 107 | 13.6 | 81 | 7 | 8 | 10 | 15 | 30 | 30 | 49 |
| 50-64 | 309 | 15.7 | 121 | 7 | 9 | 12 | 19 | 39 | 40 | 49 |
| 65+ | 308 | 15.0 | 111 | 8 | 10 | 12 | 17 | 25 | 33 | 85 |
| **GRAND TOTAL** | **773** | **15.3** | **113** | **8** | **9** | **12** | **17** | **30** | **40** | **58** |

## 42.33: ENDO EXC/DESTR ESOPH LES. Formerly included in operation group(s) 597.

| Type of Patients | Observed Patients | Avg. Stay | Variance | 10th | 25th | 50th | 75th | 90th | 95th | 99th |
|---|---|---|---|---|---|---|---|---|---|---|
| **1. SINGLE DX** | | | | | | | | | | |
| 0-19 Years | 8 | 2.2 | <1 | 1 | 1 | 3 | 3 | 3 | 3 | 3 |
| 20-34 | 7 | 2.2 | 9 | 1 | 1 | 1 | 1 | 10 | 10 | 10 |
| 35-49 | 24 | 2.6 | 9 | 2 | 2 | 2 | 3 | 4 | 7 | 7 |
| 50-64 | 19 | 2.8 | <1 | 2 | 2 | 3 | 3 | 3 | 4 | 4 |
| 65+ | 3 | 4.8 | 2 | 3 | 4 | 6 | 6 | 6 | 6 | 6 |
| **2. MULTIPLE DX** | | | | | | | | | | |
| 0-19 Years | 86 | 3.7 | 15 | 1 | 1 | 3 | 4 | 7 | 10 | 26 |
| 20-34 | 249 | 3.9 | 9 | 1 | 2 | 3 | 4 | 7 | 11 | 15 |
| 35-49 | 1,758 | 5.7 | 28 | 2 | 3 | 4 | 6 | 11 | 16 | 28 |
| 50-64 | 1,511 | 5.2 | 25 | 2 | 3 | 4 | 6 | 8 | 12 | 24 |
| 65+ | 1,630 | 5.8 | 20 | 2 | 3 | 5 | 7 | 10 | 14 | 23 |
| **TOTAL SINGLE DX** | **61** | **2.7** | **2** | **1** | **2** | **3** | **3** | **4** | **6** | **10** |
| **TOTAL MULTIPLE DX** | **5,234** | **5.5** | **24** | **2** | **3** | **4** | **6** | **10** | **14** | **24** |
| **TOTAL** | | | | | | | | | | |
| 0-19 Years | 94 | 3.7 | 14 | 1 | 1 | 3 | 4 | 7 | 10 | 19 |
| 20-34 | 256 | 3.9 | 9 | 1 | 2 | 3 | 4 | 7 | 11 | 15 |
| 35-49 | 1,782 | 5.7 | 28 | 2 | 3 | 4 | 6 | 11 | 16 | 28 |
| 50-64 | 1,530 | 5.2 | 25 | 2 | 3 | 4 | 6 | 8 | 12 | 24 |
| 65+ | 1,633 | 5.8 | 20 | 2 | 3 | 5 | 7 | 10 | 14 | 23 |
| **GRAND TOTAL** | **5,295** | **5.4** | **24** | **2** | **3** | **4** | **6** | **10** | **14** | **24** |

## 42.41: PARTIAL ESOPHAGECTOMY. Formerly included in operation group(s) 597.

| Type of Patients | Observed Patients | Avg. Stay | Variance | 10th | 25th | 50th | 75th | 90th | 95th | 99th |
|---|---|---|---|---|---|---|---|---|---|---|
| **1. SINGLE DX** | | | | | | | | | | |
| 0-19 Years | 3 | 11.4 | 13 | 7 | 7 | 13 | 15 | 15 | 15 | 15 |
| 20-34 | 0 | | | | | | | | | |
| 35-49 | 4 | 8.3 | <1 | 8 | 8 | 8 | 8 | 10 | 10 | 10 |
| 50-64 | 5 | 10.8 | 10 | 8 | 13 | 13 | 14 | 14 | 14 | 14 |
| 65+ | 1 | 7.0 | 0 | 7 | 7 | 7 | 7 | 7 | 7 | 7 |
| **2. MULTIPLE DX** | | | | | | | | | | |
| 0-19 Years | 17 | 22.1 | 234 | 6 | 10 | 18 | 34 | 34 | 37 | 80 |
| 20-34 | 12 | 23.6 | 168 | 7 | 11 | 23 | 37 | 40 | 40 | 40 |
| 35-49 | 62 | 13.5 | 71 | 8 | 8 | 10 | 14 | 30 | 30 | 33 |
| 50-64 | 178 | 15.3 | 104 | 8 | 9 | 11 | 19 | 29 | 40 | 46 |
| 65+ | 207 | 15.3 | 120 | 8 | 10 | 12 | 17 | 25 | 36 | 85 |
| **TOTAL SINGLE DX** | **13** | **9.5** | **7** | **7** | **8** | **8** | **13** | **14** | **14** | **15** |
| **TOTAL MULTIPLE DX** | **476** | **15.4** | **114** | **8** | **9** | **11** | **18** | **30** | **40** | **58** |
| **TOTAL** | | | | | | | | | | |
| 0-19 Years | 20 | 20.4 | 213 | 6 | 10 | 15 | 34 | 34 | 37 | 80 |
| 20-34 | 12 | 23.6 | 168 | 7 | 11 | 23 | 37 | 40 | 40 | 40 |
| 35-49 | 66 | 13.0 | 66 | 8 | 8 | 10 | 12 | 30 | 30 | 33 |
| 50-64 | 183 | 15.3 | 103 | 8 | 9 | 11 | 19 | 29 | 40 | 46 |
| 65+ | 208 | 15.3 | 120 | 8 | 10 | 12 | 17 | 25 | 36 | 85 |
| **GRAND TOTAL** | **489** | **15.2** | **112** | **8** | **9** | **11** | **17** | **29** | **40** | **58** |

Length of Stay by Diagnosis and Operation, United States, 2000

# United States, October 1998–September 1999 Data, by Operation

## 42.5: INTRATHOR ESOPH ANAST. Formerly included in operation group(s) 597.

| Type of Patients | Observed Patients | Avg. Stay | Variance | 10th | 25th | 50th | 75th | 90th | 95th | 99th |
|---|---|---|---|---|---|---|---|---|---|---|
| **1. SINGLE DX** | | | | | | | | | | |
| 0–19 Years | 1 | 20.0 | 0 | 20 | 20 | 20 | 20 | 20 | 20 | 20 |
| 20–34 | 1 | 3.0 | 0 | 3 | 3 | 3 | 3 | 3 | 3 | 3 |
| 35–49 | 1 | 2.0 | 0 | 2 | 2 | 2 | 2 | 2 | 2 | 2 |
| 50–64 | 1 | 8.0 | 0 | 8 | 8 | 8 | 8 | 8 | 8 | 8 |
| 65+ | 0 | | | | | | | | | |
| **2. MULTIPLE DX** | | | | | | | | | | |
| 0–19 Years | 35 | 44.0 | >999 | 8 | 13 | 22 | 91 | 91 | 91 | >99 |
| 20–34 | 4 | 10.0 | 98 | 5 | 5 | 5 | 10 | 24 | 40 | 40 |
| 35–49 | 9 | 10.1 | 26 | 6 | 6 | 10 | 12 | 22 | >99 | >99 |
| 50–64 | 19 | 17.0 | 118 | 9 | 10 | 16 | 23 | 30 | 31 | 62 |
| 65+ | 18 | 23.4 | 170 | 9 | 19 | 27 | 27 | 27 | 29 | 84 |
| **TOTAL SINGLE DX** | 4 | 11.3 | 74 | 2 | 3 | 8 | 20 | 20 | 20 | 20 |
| **TOTAL MULTIPLE DX** | 85 | 28.9 | 805 | 6 | 10 | 19 | 28 | 91 | 91 | >99 |
| **TOTAL** | | | | | | | | | | |
| 0–19 Years | 36 | 43.5 | >999 | 8 | 13 | 21 | 91 | 91 | 91 | >99 |
| 20–34 | 5 | 9.7 | 96 | 5 | 5 | 5 | 5 | 24 | 24 | 40 |
| 35–49 | 10 | 9.6 | 28 | 6 | 6 | 7 | 12 | 22 | >99 | >99 |
| 50–64 | 20 | 16.8 | 117 | 9 | 10 | 16 | 23 | 30 | 31 | 62 |
| 65+ | 18 | 23.4 | 170 | 9 | 19 | 27 | 27 | 27 | 29 | 84 |
| **GRAND TOTAL** | 89 | 28.6 | 795 | 6 | 10 | 19 | 28 | 91 | 91 | >99 |

## 42.6: ANTESTERNAL ESOPH ANAST. Formerly included in operation group(s) 597.

| Type of Patients | Observed Patients | Avg. Stay | Variance | 10th | 25th | 50th | 75th | 90th | 95th | 99th |
|---|---|---|---|---|---|---|---|---|---|---|
| **1. SINGLE DX** | | | | | | | | | | |
| 0–19 Years | 0 | | | | | | | | | |
| 20–34 | 0 | | | | | | | | | |
| 35–49 | 0 | | | | | | | | | |
| 50–64 | 0 | | | | | | | | | |
| 65+ | 0 | | | | | | | | | |
| **2. MULTIPLE DX** | | | | | | | | | | |
| 0–19 Years | 1 | 9.0 | 0 | 9 | 9 | 9 | 9 | 9 | 9 | 9 |
| 20–34 | 0 | | | | | | | | | |
| 35–49 | 1 | 62.0 | 0 | 62 | 62 | 62 | 62 | 62 | 62 | 62 |
| 50–64 | 3 | 20.6 | 84 | 7 | 23 | 23 | 23 | 34 | 34 | 34 |
| 65+ | 5 | 8.7 | 16 | 5 | 6 | 6 | 12 | 15 | 15 | 15 |
| **TOTAL SINGLE DX** | 0 | | | | | | | | | |
| **TOTAL MULTIPLE DX** | 10 | 21.6 | 377 | 6 | 7 | 15 | 23 | 62 | 62 | 62 |
| **TOTAL** | | | | | | | | | | |
| 0–19 Years | 1 | 9.0 | 0 | 9 | 9 | 9 | 9 | 9 | 9 | 9 |
| 20–34 | 0 | | | | | | | | | |
| 35–49 | 1 | 62.0 | 0 | 62 | 62 | 62 | 62 | 62 | 62 | 62 |
| 50–64 | 3 | 20.6 | 84 | 7 | 23 | 23 | 23 | 34 | 34 | 34 |
| 65+ | 5 | 8.7 | 16 | 5 | 6 | 6 | 12 | 15 | 15 | 15 |
| **GRAND TOTAL** | 10 | 21.6 | 377 | 6 | 7 | 15 | 23 | 62 | 62 | 62 |

## 42.7: ESOPHAGOMYOTOMY. Formerly included in operation group(s) 597.

| Type of Patients | Observed Patients | Avg. Stay | Variance | 10th | 25th | 50th | 75th | 90th | 95th | 99th |
|---|---|---|---|---|---|---|---|---|---|---|
| **1. SINGLE DX** | | | | | | | | | | |
| 0–19 Years | 18 | 2.8 | 2 | 1 | 2 | 3 | 4 | 5 | 5 | 6 |
| 20–34 | 40 | 2.8 | 1 | 1 | 2 | 3 | 3 | 5 | 5 | 7 |
| 35–49 | 30 | 2.6 | 3 | 1 | 2 | 2 | 3 | 4 | 8 | 9 |
| 50–64 | 14 | 2.2 | 2 | 1 | 1 | 2 | 4 | 4 | 5 | 7 |
| 65+ | 4 | 2.1 | <1 | 2 | 2 | 2 | 2 | 2 | 3 | 3 |
| **2. MULTIPLE DX** | | | | | | | | | | |
| 0–19 Years | 21 | 5.0 | 17 | 2 | 3 | 5 | 5 | 8 | 8 | 28 |
| 20–34 | 52 | 4.9 | 5 | 2 | 3 | 4 | 6 | 6 | 7 | 18 |
| 35–49 | 90 | 4.5 | 15 | 2 | 3 | 4 | 6 | 7 | 10 | 22 |
| 50–64 | 94 | 9.0 | 69 | 2 | 3 | 5 | 13 | 23 | 23 | 23 |
| 65+ | 90 | 6.8 | 52 | 1 | 2 | 4 | 8 | 18 | 24 | 30 |
| **TOTAL SINGLE DX** | 106 | 2.6 | 2 | 1 | 2 | 2 | 3 | 4 | 5 | 8 |
| **TOTAL MULTIPLE DX** | 347 | 6.5 | 40 | 2 | 2 | 5 | 6 | 18 | 23 | 27 |
| **TOTAL** | | | | | | | | | | |
| 0–19 Years | 39 | 3.9 | 11 | 1 | 2 | 3 | 5 | 6 | 8 | 28 |
| 20–34 | 92 | 4.3 | 5 | 2 | 3 | 4 | 6 | 6 | 6 | 11 |
| 35–49 | 120 | 4.0 | 13 | 2 | 2 | 3 | 6 | 7 | 9 | 20 |
| 50–64 | 108 | 8.3 | 66 | 2 | 3 | 5 | 11 | 23 | 23 | 23 |
| 65+ | 94 | 6.4 | 50 | 1 | 2 | 3 | 8 | 18 | 24 | 30 |
| **GRAND TOTAL** | 453 | 5.7 | 35 | 2 | 2 | 4 | 6 | 11 | 23 | 24 |

## 42.8: OTHER ESOPHAGEAL REPAIR. Formerly included in operation group(s) 597.

| Type of Patients | Observed Patients | Avg. Stay | Variance | 10th | 25th | 50th | 75th | 90th | 95th | 99th |
|---|---|---|---|---|---|---|---|---|---|---|
| **1. SINGLE DX** | | | | | | | | | | |
| 0–19 Years | 12 | 7.6 | 15 | 3 | 6 | 7 | 7 | 15 | 15 | 16 |
| 20–34 | 4 | 6.2 | 3 | 6 | 6 | 6 | 6 | 15 | 15 | 15 |
| 35–49 | 3 | 6.1 | 9 | 2 | 5 | 5 | 9 | 9 | 9 | 9 |
| 50–64 | 3 | 4.0 | <1 | 3 | 3 | 4 | 5 | 5 | 5 | 5 |
| 65+ | 2 | 1.5 | <1 | 1 | 1 | 2 | 2 | 2 | 2 | 2 |
| **2. MULTIPLE DX** | | | | | | | | | | |
| 0–19 Years | 57 | 21.6 | 707 | 4 | 5 | 13 | 27 | 68 | 99 | >99 |
| 20–34 | 25 | 11.1 | 53 | 5 | 7 | 10 | 13 | 16 | 22 | 37 |
| 35–49 | 78 | 13.1 | 186 | 2 | 5 | 9 | 16 | 29 | 30 | 97 |
| 50–64 | 123 | 8.9 | 99 | 1 | 3 | 5 | 10 | 18 | 30 | 56 |
| 65+ | 228 | 11.3 | 109 | 3 | 5 | 9 | 13 | 24 | 33 | 53 |
| **TOTAL SINGLE DX** | 24 | 6.4 | 9 | 3 | 6 | 6 | 7 | 9 | 15 | 15 |
| **TOTAL MULTIPLE DX** | 511 | 12.2 | 202 | 2 | 4 | 9 | 13 | 27 | 37 | 99 |
| **TOTAL** | | | | | | | | | | |
| 0–19 Years | 69 | 19.4 | 625 | 3 | 5 | 10 | 20 | 68 | 99 | >99 |
| 20–34 | 29 | 8.7 | 34 | 6 | 6 | 6 | 10 | 15 | 21 | 37 |
| 35–49 | 81 | 12.9 | 183 | 2 | 5 | 9 | 16 | 29 | 30 | 97 |
| 50–64 | 126 | 8.8 | 98 | 1 | 3 | 5 | 10 | 18 | 30 | 56 |
| 65+ | 230 | 11.3 | 109 | 3 | 5 | 9 | 13 | 24 | 33 | 53 |
| **GRAND TOTAL** | 535 | 11.9 | 193 | 2 | 4 | 8 | 13 | 27 | 35 | 99 |

Length of Stay by Diagnosis and Operation, United States, 2000

# United States, October 1998–September 1999 Data, by Operation

## 42.9: OTHER ESOPHAGEAL OPS. Formerly included in operation group(s) 597.

| Type of Patients | Observed Patients | Avg. Stay | Variance | Percentiles 10th | 25th | 50th | 75th | 90th | 95th | 99th |
|---|---|---|---|---|---|---|---|---|---|---|
| **1. SINGLE DX** | | | | | | | | | | |
| 0–19 Years | 37 | 2.2 | 4 | 1 | 1 | 1 | 2 | 6 | 6 | 6 |
| 20–34 | 7 | 1.1 | <1 | 1 | 1 | 1 | 1 | 2 | 2 | 2 |
| 35–49 | 6 | 5.4 | 15 | 1 | 1 | 9 | 9 | 9 | 9 | 9 |
| 50–64 | 5 | 3.2 | 2 | 1 | 1 | 4 | 4 | 5 | 5 | 5 |
| 65+ | 9 | 2.9 | 19 | 1 | 1 | 2 | 2 | 4 | 18 | 18 |
| **2. MULTIPLE DX** | | | | | | | | | | |
| 0–19 Years | 153 | 5.6 | 97 | 1 | 1 | 2 | 7 | 13 | 17 | 76 |
| 20–34 | 92 | 3.2 | 8 | 1 | 2 | 3 | 3 | 6 | 6 | 14 |
| 35–49 | 390 | 5.1 | 23 | 2 | 2 | 4 | 7 | 11 | 14 | 31 |
| 50–64 | 733 | 4.8 | 22 | 2 | 2 | 3 | 6 | 10 | 13 | 26 |
| 65+ | 2,865 | 5.8 | 29 | 1 | 3 | 4 | 7 | 11 | 15 | 25 |
| **TOTAL SINGLE DX** | 64 | 2.7 | 8 | 1 | 1 | 1 | 4 | 6 | 9 | 9 |
| **TOTAL MULTIPLE DX** | 4,233 | 5.5 | 31 | 1 | 2 | 4 | 7 | 11 | 14 | 26 |
| **TOTAL** | | | | | | | | | | |
| 0–19 Years | 190 | 4.9 | 79 | 1 | 1 | 2 | 6 | 11 | 17 | 76 |
| 20–34 | 99 | 3.1 | 8 | 1 | 2 | 2 | 3 | 6 | 9 | 14 |
| 35–49 | 396 | 5.2 | 23 | 1 | 2 | 4 | 7 | 11 | 14 | 31 |
| 50–64 | 738 | 4.7 | 22 | 1 | 2 | 3 | 6 | 10 | 13 | 26 |
| 65+ | 2,874 | 5.8 | 29 | 1 | 3 | 4 | 7 | 11 | 15 | 25 |
| **GRAND TOTAL** | 4,297 | 5.4 | 31 | 1 | 2 | 4 | 7 | 11 | 14 | 26 |

## 42.92: ESOPHAGEAL DILATION. Formerly included in operation group(s) 597.

| Type of Patients | Observed Patients | Avg. Stay | Variance | Percentiles 10th | 25th | 50th | 75th | 90th | 95th | 99th |
|---|---|---|---|---|---|---|---|---|---|---|
| **1. SINGLE DX** | | | | | | | | | | |
| 0–19 Years | 35 | 2.3 | 4 | 1 | 1 | 1 | 2 | 6 | 6 | 6 |
| 20–34 | 7 | 1.1 | <1 | 1 | 1 | 1 | 1 | 2 | 2 | 2 |
| 35–49 | 6 | 5.4 | 15 | 1 | 1 | 9 | 9 | 9 | 9 | 9 |
| 50–64 | 5 | 3.2 | 2 | 1 | 1 | 4 | 4 | 5 | 5 | 5 |
| 65+ | 8 | 3.0 | 22 | 1 | 1 | 2 | 4 | 4 | 18 | 18 |
| **2. MULTIPLE DX** | | | | | | | | | | |
| 0–19 Years | 150 | 5.5 | 95 | 1 | 1 | 2 | 7 | 13 | 17 | 76 |
| 20–34 | 88 | 3.1 | 9 | 1 | 2 | 2 | 3 | 6 | 6 | 14 |
| 35–49 | 356 | 5.1 | 24 | 2 | 2 | 4 | 6 | 11 | 14 | 31 |
| 50–64 | 713 | 4.7 | 22 | 2 | 2 | 3 | 6 | 10 | 13 | 26 |
| 65+ | 2,842 | 5.8 | 30 | 1 | 3 | 4 | 7 | 11 | 15 | 25 |
| **TOTAL SINGLE DX** | 61 | 2.7 | 8 | 1 | 1 | 1 | 4 | 6 | 9 | 9 |
| **TOTAL MULTIPLE DX** | 4,149 | 5.5 | 31 | 1 | 2 | 4 | 7 | 11 | 14 | 26 |
| **TOTAL** | | | | | | | | | | |
| 0–19 Years | 185 | 4.8 | 77 | 1 | 1 | 2 | 6 | 11 | 17 | 76 |
| 20–34 | 95 | 3.0 | 8 | 1 | 2 | 2 | 3 | 6 | 9 | 14 |
| 35–49 | 362 | 5.1 | 24 | 1 | 2 | 4 | 6 | 11 | 14 | 31 |
| 50–64 | 718 | 4.7 | 22 | 1 | 2 | 3 | 6 | 10 | 13 | 26 |
| 65+ | 2,850 | 5.8 | 30 | 1 | 3 | 4 | 7 | 11 | 15 | 25 |
| **GRAND TOTAL** | 4,210 | 5.4 | 31 | 1 | 2 | 4 | 7 | 11 | 14 | 25 |

## 43.0: GASTROTOMY. Formerly included in operation group(s) 599.

| Type of Patients | Observed Patients | Avg. Stay | Variance | Percentiles 10th | 25th | 50th | 75th | 90th | 95th | 99th |
|---|---|---|---|---|---|---|---|---|---|---|
| **1. SINGLE DX** | | | | | | | | | | |
| 0–19 Years | 9 | 3.5 | 5 | 1 | 1 | 4 | 5 | 7 | 7 | 7 |
| 20–34 | 1 | 3.0 | 0 | 3 | 3 | 3 | 3 | 3 | 3 | 3 |
| 35–49 | 1 | 7.0 | 0 | 7 | 7 | 7 | 7 | 7 | 7 | 7 |
| 50–64 | 1 | 1.0 | 0 | 1 | 1 | 1 | 1 | 1 | 1 | 1 |
| 65+ | 0 | | | | | | | | | |
| **2. MULTIPLE DX** | | | | | | | | | | |
| 0–19 Years | 20 | 9.2 | 58 | 2 | 4 | 6 | 13 | 22 | 22 | 22 |
| 20–34 | 25 | 6.3 | 14 | 3 | 4 | 5 | 5 | 14 | 14 | >99 |
| 35–49 | 53 | 9.6 | 124 | 4 | 4 | 5 | 8 | 22 | 31 | 76 |
| 50–64 | 32 | 19.4 | 427 | 4 | 6 | 12 | 18 | 65 | 65 | 65 |
| 65+ | 50 | 13.3 | 110 | 4 | 6 | 10 | 22 | 28 | 28 | 45 |
| **TOTAL SINGLE DX** | 12 | 3.5 | 5 | 1 | 1 | 4 | 5 | 7 | 7 | 7 |
| **TOTAL MULTIPLE DX** | 180 | 11.5 | 159 | 4 | 4 | 6 | 14 | 24 | 31 | 65 |
| **TOTAL** | | | | | | | | | | |
| 0–19 Years | 29 | 7.8 | 50 | 1 | 4 | 5 | 10 | 22 | 22 | 22 |
| 20–34 | 26 | 6.3 | 14 | 3 | 4 | 5 | 9 | 14 | 14 | >99 |
| 35–49 | 54 | 9.6 | 123 | 4 | 4 | 5 | 8 | 22 | 31 | 76 |
| 50–64 | 33 | 19.1 | 425 | 4 | 6 | 12 | 18 | 65 | 65 | 65 |
| 65+ | 50 | 13.3 | 110 | 4 | 6 | 10 | 22 | 28 | 28 | 45 |
| **GRAND TOTAL** | 192 | 11.2 | 156 | 4 | 4 | 6 | 13 | 23 | 31 | 65 |

## 43.1: GASTROSTOMY. Formerly included in operation group(s) 600.

| Type of Patients | Observed Patients | Avg. Stay | Variance | Percentiles 10th | 25th | 50th | 75th | 90th | 95th | 99th |
|---|---|---|---|---|---|---|---|---|---|---|
| **1. SINGLE DX** | | | | | | | | | | |
| 0–19 Years | 86 | 2.3 | 29 | 1 | 1 | 1 | 2 | 3 | 4 | 11 |
| 20–34 | 5 | 2.8 | 10 | 1 | 1 | 2 | 3 | 10 | 10 | 10 |
| 35–49 | 7 | 4.8 | 10 | 1 | 2 | 7 | 7 | 9 | 10 | 10 |
| 50–64 | 27 | 1.7 | 3 | 1 | 1 | 1 | 2 | 3 | 7 | 9 |
| 65+ | 69 | 6.3 | 21 | 1 | 2 | 5 | 9 | 11 | 15 | 18 |
| **2. MULTIPLE DX** | | | | | | | | | | |
| 0–19 Years | 1,495 | 8.1 | 155 | 1 | 2 | 3 | 10 | 21 | 34 | 88 |
| 20–34 | 318 | 12.0 | 129 | 2 | 6 | 15 | 15 | 26 | 33 | 75 |
| 35–49 | 927 | 11.3 | 96 | 3 | 5 | 10 | 15 | 22 | 31 | 65 |
| 50–64 | 2,651 | 12.0 | 111 | 2 | 5 | 9 | 16 | 25 | 32 | 59 |
| 65+ | 21,879 | 11.5 | 75 | 3 | 6 | 9 | 14 | 21 | 27 | 43 |
| **TOTAL SINGLE DX** | 194 | 3.4 | 26 | 1 | 1 | 2 | 4 | 9 | 10 | 18 |
| **TOTAL MULTIPLE DX** | 27,270 | 11.3 | 86 | 3 | 6 | 9 | 14 | 22 | 28 | 47 |
| **TOTAL** | | | | | | | | | | |
| 0–19 Years | 1,581 | 7.7 | 148 | 1 | 2 | 3 | 9 | 20 | 31 | 85 |
| 20–34 | 323 | 11.9 | 128 | 2 | 5 | 8 | 15 | 26 | 33 | 75 |
| 35–49 | 934 | 11.2 | 95 | 3 | 5 | 10 | 15 | 22 | 31 | 65 |
| 50–64 | 2,678 | 11.9 | 111 | 2 | 5 | 9 | 16 | 25 | 32 | 59 |
| 65+ | 21,948 | 11.5 | 75 | 3 | 6 | 9 | 14 | 21 | 27 | 43 |
| **GRAND TOTAL** | 27,464 | 11.3 | 86 | 3 | 5 | 9 | 14 | 22 | 28 | 47 |

Length of Stay by Diagnosis and Operation, United States, 2000

# United States, October 1998–September 1999 Data, by Operation

## 43.11: PERC (ENDO) GASTROSTOMY. Formerly included in operation group(s) 600.

| Type of Patients | Observed Patients | Avg. Stay | Variance | 10th | 25th | 50th | 75th | 90th | 95th | 99th |
|---|---|---|---|---|---|---|---|---|---|---|
| **1. SINGLE DX** | | | | | | | | | | |
| 0–19 Years | 51 | 2.4 | 45 | 1 | 1 | 1 | 2 | 3 | 4 | 57 |
| 20–34 | 4 | 1.7 | <1 | 1 | 1 | 1 | 3 | 3 | 3 | 3 |
| 35–49 | 4 | 5.5 | 9 | 1 | 3 | 7 | 7 | 9 | 9 | 9 |
| 50–64 | 24 | 1.6 | 3 | 1 | 1 | 1 | 1 | 3 | 3 | 9 |
| 65+ | 51 | 6.2 | 17 | 2 | 2 | 6 | 9 | 11 | 12 | 18 |
| **2. MULTIPLE DX** | | | | | | | | | | |
| 0–19 Years | 981 | 7.0 | 104 | 1 | 2 | 3 | 9 | 20 | 27 | 67 |
| 20–34 | 272 | 12.1 | 137 | 2 | 5 | 9 | 15 | 26 | 34 | 75 |
| 35–49 | 802 | 11.2 | 97 | 3 | 4 | 8 | 15 | 22 | 32 | 65 |
| 50–64 | 2,410 | 12.0 | 115 | 2 | 5 | 9 | 15 | 26 | 33 | 59 |
| 65+ | 20,685 | 11.5 | 76 | 4 | 6 | 9 | 15 | 22 | 27 | 43 |
| **TOTAL SINGLE DX** | 134 | 3.5 | 32 | 1 | 1 | 2 | 4 | 9 | 10 | 18 |
| **TOTAL MULTIPLE DX** | 25,150 | 11.4 | 83 | 3 | 6 | 9 | 15 | 22 | 28 | 46 |
| **TOTAL** | | | | | | | | | | |
| 0–19 Years | 1,032 | 6.7 | 101 | 1 | 1 | 2 | 8 | 18 | 26 | 63 |
| 20–34 | 276 | 12.0 | 137 | 2 | 5 | 9 | 15 | 26 | 33 | 75 |
| 35–49 | 806 | 11.2 | 97 | 3 | 4 | 8 | 15 | 22 | 32 | 65 |
| 50–64 | 2,434 | 11.8 | 115 | 2 | 5 | 9 | 15 | 25 | 33 | 59 |
| 65+ | 20,736 | 11.5 | 76 | 4 | 6 | 9 | 14 | 22 | 27 | 43 |
| **GRAND TOTAL** | 25,284 | 11.3 | 83 | 2 | 6 | 9 | 14 | 22 | 28 | 46 |

## 43.19: GASTROSTOMY NEC. Formerly included in operation group(s) 600.

| Type of Patients | Observed Patients | Avg. Stay | Variance | 10th | 25th | 50th | 75th | 90th | 95th | 99th |
|---|---|---|---|---|---|---|---|---|---|---|
| **1. SINGLE DX** | | | | | | | | | | |
| 0–19 Years | 35 | 2.1 | <1 | 1 | 1 | 2 | 3 | 3 | 4 | 4 |
| 20–34 | 1 | 10.0 | | 10 | 10 | 10 | 10 | 10 | 10 | 10 |
| 35–49 | 3 | 3.2 | 9 | 1 | 1 | 2 | 7 | 7 | 7 | 7 |
| 50–64 | 3 | 3.6 | 5 | 2 | 2 | 2 | 4 | 7 | 7 | 7 |
| 65+ | 18 | 6.7 | 42 | 1 | 3 | 5 | 9 | 13 | 27 | 27 |
| **2. MULTIPLE DX** | | | | | | | | | | |
| 0–19 Years | 514 | 10.2 | 244 | 2 | 2 | 4 | 11 | 24 | 54 | 96 |
| 20–34 | 46 | 11.5 | 84 | 4 | 6 | 7 | 14 | 23 | 27 | 54 |
| 35–49 | 125 | 11.5 | 87 | 3 | 7 | 10 | 12 | 21 | 28 | 55 |
| 50–64 | 241 | 12.5 | 84 | 3 | 5 | 12 | 17 | 22 | 28 | 51 |
| 65+ | 1,194 | 10.7 | 70 | 3 | 5 | 9 | 14 | 20 | 26 | 42 |
| **TOTAL SINGLE DX** | 60 | 3.0 | 11 | 1 | 2 | 2 | 3 | 5 | 9 | 15 |
| **TOTAL MULTIPLE DX** | 2,120 | 10.9 | 113 | 2 | 4 | 8 | 14 | 22 | 28 | 64 |
| **TOTAL** | | | | | | | | | | |
| 0–19 Years | 549 | 9.5 | 229 | 2 | 2 | 4 | 11 | 24 | 52 | 96 |
| 20–34 | 47 | 11.5 | 83 | 4 | 6 | 7 | 14 | 23 | 27 | 54 |
| 35–49 | 128 | 11.5 | 87 | 3 | 5 | 10 | 12 | 21 | 28 | 55 |
| 50–64 | 244 | 12.4 | 84 | 3 | 5 | 11 | 17 | 22 | 28 | 51 |
| 65+ | 1,212 | 10.7 | 70 | 3 | 5 | 9 | 14 | 20 | 26 | 42 |
| **GRAND TOTAL** | 2,180 | 10.7 | 112 | 2 | 4 | 8 | 14 | 21 | 28 | 64 |

## 43.3: PYLOROMYOTOMY. Formerly included in operation group(s) 599.

| Type of Patients | Observed Patients | Avg. Stay | Variance | 10th | 25th | 50th | 75th | 90th | 95th | 99th |
|---|---|---|---|---|---|---|---|---|---|---|
| **1. SINGLE DX** | | | | | | | | | | |
| 0–19 Years | 2,210 | 2.2 | 1 | 1 | 2 | 2 | 3 | 3 | 4 | 6 |
| 20–34 | 0 | | | | | | | | | |
| 35–49 | 0 | | | | | | | | | |
| 50–64 | 0 | | | | | | | | | |
| 65+ | 0 | | | | | | | | | |
| **2. MULTIPLE DX** | | | | | | | | | | |
| 0–19 Years | 1,390 | 3.5 | 19 | 2 | 2 | 3 | 4 | 5 | 7 | 17 |
| 20–34 | 1 | 9.0 | 0 | 9 | 9 | 9 | 9 | 9 | 9 | 9 |
| 35–49 | 2 | 21.3 | 251 | 4 | 4 | 32 | 32 | 32 | 32 | 32 |
| 50–64 | 5 | 13.6 | 203 | 2 | 2 | 12 | 20 | 38 | 38 | 38 |
| 65+ | 6 | 25.7 | 211 | 8 | 8 | 38 | 38 | 38 | 38 | 38 |
| **TOTAL SINGLE DX** | 2,210 | 2.2 | 1 | 1 | 2 | 2 | 3 | 3 | 4 | 6 |
| **TOTAL MULTIPLE DX** | 1,404 | 3.6 | 22 | 2 | 2 | 3 | 4 | 5 | 8 | 25 |
| **TOTAL** | | | | | | | | | | |
| 0–19 Years | 3,600 | 2.7 | 8 | 1 | 2 | 2 | 3 | 4 | 5 | 11 |
| 20–34 | 1 | 9.0 | 0 | 9 | 9 | 9 | 9 | 9 | 9 | 9 |
| 35–49 | 2 | 21.3 | 251 | 4 | 4 | 32 | 32 | 32 | 32 | 32 |
| 50–64 | 5 | 13.6 | 203 | 2 | 2 | 12 | 20 | 38 | 38 | 38 |
| 65+ | 6 | 25.7 | 211 | 8 | 8 | 38 | 38 | 38 | 38 | 38 |
| **GRAND TOTAL** | 3,614 | 2.7 | 9 | 1 | 2 | 2 | 3 | 4 | 5 | 11 |

## 43.4: LOC EXC GASTRIC LES. Formerly included in operation group(s) 601.

| Type of Patients | Observed Patients | Avg. Stay | Variance | 10th | 25th | 50th | 75th | 90th | 95th | 99th |
|---|---|---|---|---|---|---|---|---|---|---|
| **1. SINGLE DX** | | | | | | | | | | |
| 0–19 Years | 8 | 1.9 | 3 | 1 | 1 | 1 | 1 | 5 | 6 | 6 |
| 20–34 | 4 | 5.1 | <1 | 4 | 5 | 5 | 6 | 6 | 6 | 6 |
| 35–49 | 16 | 4.0 | 4 | 2 | 2 | 5 | 5 | 5 | 8 | 8 |
| 50–64 | 12 | 5.3 | 3 | 3 | 4 | 5 | 6 | 8 | 8 | 8 |
| 65+ | 8 | 3.3 | 6 | 1 | 1 | 2 | 4 | 8 | 8 | 10 |
| **2. MULTIPLE DX** | | | | | | | | | | |
| 0–19 Years | 21 | 6.5 | 21 | 2 | 4 | 5 | 9 | 9 | 9 | 31 |
| 20–34 | 67 | 5.6 | 22 | 2 | 3 | 4 | 8 | 9 | 10 | 41 |
| 35–49 | 229 | 4.6 | 22 | 1 | 3 | 4 | 6 | 8 | 10 | 20 |
| 50–64 | 499 | 5.6 | 22 | 2 | 3 | 5 | 7 | 11 | 15 | 24 |
| 65+ | 1,390 | 7.2 | 35 | 2 | 3 | 6 | 9 | 13 | 18 | 29 |
| **TOTAL SINGLE DX** | 48 | 3.6 | 5 | 1 | 1 | 4 | 5 | 6 | 8 | 10 |
| **TOTAL MULTIPLE DX** | 2,206 | 6.5 | 30 | 2 | 3 | 5 | 8 | 12 | 16 | 29 |
| **TOTAL** | | | | | | | | | | |
| 0–19 Years | 29 | 4.3 | 18 | 1 | 1 | 4 | 6 | 9 | 9 | 31 |
| 20–34 | 71 | 5.6 | 22 | 2 | 3 | 5 | 8 | 9 | 10 | 16 |
| 35–49 | 245 | 4.6 | 21 | 2 | 3 | 5 | 6 | 8 | 10 | 20 |
| 50–64 | 511 | 5.6 | 21 | 2 | 3 | 5 | 7 | 11 | 15 | 24 |
| 65+ | 1,398 | 7.2 | 35 | 2 | 3 | 6 | 9 | 13 | 18 | 29 |
| **GRAND TOTAL** | 2,254 | 6.4 | 30 | 2 | 3 | 5 | 8 | 11 | 16 | 29 |

## United States, October 1998–September 1999 Data, by Operation

### 43.41: ENDO EXC GASTRIC LES. Formerly included in operation group(s) 601.

| Type of Patients | Observed Patients | Avg. Stay | Vari-ance | Percentiles | | | | | | |
|---|---|---|---|---|---|---|---|---|---|---|
| | | | | 10th | 25th | 50th | 75th | 90th | 95th | 99th |
| **1. SINGLE DX** | | | | | | | | | | |
| 0–19 Years | 0 | | | | | | | | | |
| 20–34 | 1 | 4.0 | 0 | 4 | 4 | 4 | 4 | 4 | 4 | 4 |
| 35–49 | 4 | 1.6 | <1 | 1 | 1 | 2 | 2 | 2 | 2 | 2 |
| 50–64 | 1 | 6.0 | 0 | 6 | 6 | 6 | 6 | 6 | 6 | 6 |
| 65+ | 3 | 1.3 | <1 | 1 | 1 | 1 | 2 | 2 | 2 | 2 |
| **2. MULTIPLE DX** | | | | | | | | | | |
| 0–19 Years | 7 | 5.3 | 8 | 2 | 4 | 4 | 9 | 9 | 9 | 9 |
| 20–34 | 41 | 5.1 | 25 | 2 | 2 | 4 | 7 | 9 | 9 | 41 |
| 35–49 | 144 | 3.7 | 8 | 1 | 2 | 3 | 4 | 7 | 8 | 18 |
| 50–64 | 322 | 5.0 | 21 | 1 | 2 | 4 | 6 | 10 | 15 | 23 |
| 65+ | 1,044 | 6.3 | 23 | 2 | 3 | 5 | 8 | 11 | 15 | 25 |
| **TOTAL SINGLE DX** | 9 | 3.6 | 5 | 1 | 1 | 2 | 6 | 6 | 6 | 6 |
| **TOTAL MULTIPLE DX** | 1,558 | 5.7 | 22 | 2 | 3 | 4 | 7 | 10 | 14 | 23 |
| **TOTAL** | | | | | | | | | | |
| 0–19 Years | 7 | 5.3 | 8 | 2 | 4 | 4 | 9 | 9 | 9 | 9 |
| 20–34 | 42 | 5.1 | 25 | 2 | 2 | 4 | 7 | 9 | 9 | 41 |
| 35–49 | 148 | 3.7 | 8 | 1 | 2 | 3 | 4 | 7 | 8 | 18 |
| 50–64 | 323 | 5.0 | 21 | 1 | 2 | 4 | 6 | 10 | 15 | 23 |
| 65+ | 1,047 | 6.3 | 23 | 2 | 3 | 5 | 8 | 11 | 15 | 25 |
| **GRAND TOTAL** | 1,567 | 5.7 | 22 | 2 | 3 | 4 | 7 | 10 | 14 | 23 |

### 43.42: LOC GASTRIC LES EXC NEC. Formerly included in operation group(s) 601.

| Type of Patients | Observed Patients | Avg. Stay | Vari-ance | Percentiles | | | | | | |
|---|---|---|---|---|---|---|---|---|---|---|
| | | | | 10th | 25th | 50th | 75th | 90th | 95th | 99th |
| **1. SINGLE DX** | | | | | | | | | | |
| 0–19 Years | 7 | 3.9 | 3 | 1 | 3 | 4 | 5 | 6 | 6 | 6 |
| 20–34 | 3 | 5.4 | <1 | 5 | 5 | 5 | 6 | 6 | 6 | 6 |
| 35–49 | 12 | 4.6 | 3 | 5 | 5 | 5 | 5 | 8 | 8 | 8 |
| 50–64 | 10 | 5.4 | 4 | 2 | 3 | 5 | 6 | 8 | 10 | 10 |
| 65+ | 5 | 4.6 | 5 | 2 | 4 | 4 | 6 | 8 | 8 | 8 |
| **2. MULTIPLE DX** | | | | | | | | | | |
| 0–19 Years | 12 | 8.3 | 40 | 4 | 5 | 8 | 9 | 9 | 31 | 31 |
| 20–34 | 23 | 7.6 | 10 | 4 | 5 | 7 | 9 | 13 | 13 | 16 |
| 35–49 | 81 | 6.8 | 48 | 3 | 4 | 6 | 8 | 10 | 14 | >99 |
| 50–64 | 165 | 7.0 | 21 | 3 | 4 | 6 | 8 | 11 | 17 | 30 |
| 65+ | 316 | 10.9 | 65 | 4 | 6 | 8 | 13 | 21 | 27 | 47 |
| **TOTAL SINGLE DX** | 37 | 4.7 | 4 | 2 | 3 | 5 | 5 | 8 | 8 | 10 |
| **TOTAL MULTIPLE DX** | 597 | 9.0 | 50 | 3 | 5 | 7 | 10 | 16 | 23 | 45 |
| **TOTAL** | | | | | | | | | | |
| 0–19 Years | 19 | 6.4 | 29 | 2 | 4 | 5 | 8 | 9 | 9 | 31 |
| 20–34 | 26 | 7.4 | 9 | 4 | 5 | 6 | 9 | 11 | 13 | 16 |
| 35–49 | 93 | 6.6 | 45 | 3 | 4 | 6 | 8 | 10 | 13 | >99 |
| 50–64 | 175 | 7.0 | 21 | 3 | 4 | 6 | 8 | 11 | 17 | 30 |
| 65+ | 321 | 10.9 | 65 | 4 | 6 | 8 | 13 | 21 | 27 | 47 |
| **GRAND TOTAL** | 634 | 8.8 | 49 | 3 | 5 | 7 | 10 | 15 | 23 | 45 |

### 43.5: PROXIMAL GASTRECTOMY. Formerly included in operation group(s) 602.

| Type of Patients | Observed Patients | Avg. Stay | Vari-ance | Percentiles | | | | | | |
|---|---|---|---|---|---|---|---|---|---|---|
| | | | | 10th | 25th | 50th | 75th | 90th | 95th | 99th |
| **1. SINGLE DX** | | | | | | | | | | |
| 0–19 Years | 0 | | | | | | | | | |
| 20–34 | 0 | | | | | | | | | |
| 35–49 | 2 | 6.0 | 0 | 6 | 6 | 6 | 6 | 6 | 6 | 6 |
| 50–64 | 5 | 7.2 | 2 | 5 | 7 | 7 | 9 | 9 | 9 | 9 |
| 65+ | 1 | 9.0 | 0 | 9 | 9 | 9 | 9 | 9 | 9 | 9 |
| **2. MULTIPLE DX** | | | | | | | | | | |
| 0–19 Years | 0 | | | | | | | | | |
| 20–34 | 3 | 23.9 | 274 | 8 | 8 | 22 | 41 | 41 | 41 | 41 |
| 35–49 | 45 | 14.8 | 106 | 7 | 9 | 12 | 17 | 27 | 31 | 58 |
| 50–64 | 97 | 13.6 | 120 | 6 | 8 | 11 | 15 | 29 | 50 | >99 |
| 65+ | 159 | 15.8 | 176 | 7 | 9 | 11 | 17 | 30 | 43 | 74 |
| **TOTAL SINGLE DX** | 8 | 7.2 | 2 | 6 | 6 | 7 | 9 | 9 | 9 | 9 |
| **TOTAL MULTIPLE DX** | 304 | 15.1 | 153 | 7 | 9 | 11 | 16 | 29 | 43 | 74 |
| **TOTAL** | | | | | | | | | | |
| 0–19 Years | 0 | | | | | | | | | |
| 20–34 | 3 | 23.9 | 274 | 8 | 8 | 22 | 41 | 41 | 41 | 41 |
| 35–49 | 47 | 14.5 | 105 | 6 | 9 | 12 | 17 | 27 | 31 | 58 |
| 50–64 | 102 | 13.4 | 117 | 6 | 8 | 11 | 15 | 29 | 44 | >99 |
| 65+ | 160 | 15.8 | 176 | 7 | 9 | 10 | 17 | 30 | 43 | 74 |
| **GRAND TOTAL** | 312 | 14.9 | 151 | 7 | 9 | 11 | 16 | 29 | 43 | 74 |

### 43.6: DISTAL GASTRECTOMY. Formerly included in operation group(s) 602.

| Type of Patients | Observed Patients | Avg. Stay | Vari-ance | Percentiles | | | | | | |
|---|---|---|---|---|---|---|---|---|---|---|
| | | | | 10th | 25th | 50th | 75th | 90th | 95th | 99th |
| **1. SINGLE DX** | | | | | | | | | | |
| 0–19 Years | 2 | 6.3 | <1 | 6 | 6 | 6 | 7 | 7 | 7 | 7 |
| 20–34 | 3 | 3.8 | 3 | 2 | 3 | 3 | 6 | 6 | 6 | 6 |
| 35–49 | 14 | 7.1 | 6 | 4 | 7 | 7 | 7 | 8 | 14 | 14 |
| 50–64 | 10 | 7.0 | 18 | 4 | 6 | 6 | 7 | 16 | 16 | 16 |
| 65+ | 3 | 8.0 | 2 | 6 | 6 | 9 | 9 | 9 | 9 | 9 |
| **2. MULTIPLE DX** | | | | | | | | | | |
| 0–19 Years | 7 | 16.5 | 95 | 9 | 9 | 9 | 31 | 31 | 31 | 35 |
| 20–34 | 27 | 10.4 | 39 | 5 | 7 | 8 | 14 | 18 | 24 | 35 |
| 35–49 | 146 | 8.4 | 22 | 5 | 6 | 7 | 9 | 12 | 15 | 33 |
| 50–64 | 189 | 11.0 | 48 | 6 | 7 | 9 | 13 | 19 | 25 | 38 |
| 65+ | 320 | 12.0 | 72 | 6 | 7 | 10 | 15 | 19 | 25 | 60 |
| **TOTAL SINGLE DX** | 32 | 7.0 | 10 | 4 | 6 | 7 | 7 | 9 | 16 | 16 |
| **TOTAL MULTIPLE DX** | 689 | 11.0 | 57 | 6 | 6 | 9 | 13 | 19 | 25 | 39 |
| **TOTAL** | | | | | | | | | | |
| 0–19 Years | 9 | 15.2 | 94 | 7 | 9 | 9 | 23 | 31 | 31 | 35 |
| 20–34 | 30 | 10.0 | 40 | 4 | 6 | 8 | 14 | 18 | 24 | 35 |
| 35–49 | 160 | 8.2 | 20 | 5 | 6 | 7 | 9 | 12 | 14 | 33 |
| 50–64 | 199 | 10.6 | 47 | 6 | 6 | 8 | 12 | 19 | 23 | 38 |
| 65+ | 323 | 11.9 | 71 | 6 | 7 | 9 | 15 | 19 | 25 | 45 |
| **GRAND TOTAL** | 721 | 10.7 | 55 | 5 | 6 | 8 | 12 | 19 | 25 | 39 |

Length of Stay by Diagnosis and Operation, United States, 2000

# United States, October 1998–September 1999 Data, by Operation

## 43.7: PART GASTRECTOMY W ANAST. Formerly included in operation group(s) 602.

| Type of Patients | Observed Patients | Avg. Stay | Vari-ance | Percentiles | | | | | | |
|---|---|---|---|---|---|---|---|---|---|---|
| | | | | 10th | 25th | 50th | 75th | 90th | 95th | 99th |
| **1. SINGLE DX** | | | | | | | | | | |
| 0–19 Years | 0 | | | | | | | | | |
| 20–34 | 5 | 3.8 | 2 | 3 | 3 | 3 | 4 | 7 | 7 | 7 |
| 35–49 | 16 | 6.4 | 3 | 4 | 6 | 7 | 7 | 7 | 8 | 12 |
| 50–64 | 15 | 6.2 | 1 | 5 | 5 | 6 | 7 | 8 | 9 | >99 |
| 65+ | 8 | 8.3 | 3 | 7 | 7 | 8 | 9 | 10 | 12 | 12 |
| **2. MULTIPLE DX** | | | | | | | | | | |
| 0–19 Years | 6 | 11.1 | 26 | 9 | 9 | 9 | 9 | 22 | 26 | 26 |
| 20–34 | 60 | 10.7 | 130 | 5 | 7 | 7 | 11 | 21 | 26 | 90 |
| 35–49 | 386 | 13.0 | 84 | 5 | 7 | 10 | 16 | 25 | 33 | 45 |
| 50–64 | 583 | 12.8 | 84 | 6 | 8 | 9 | 15 | 23 | 29 | 53 |
| 65+ | 1,131 | 15.0 | 95 | 7 | 8 | 12 | 18 | 27 | 32 | 52 |
| **TOTAL SINGLE DX** | 44 | 6.0 | 4 | 3 | 5 | 6 | 7 | 8 | 9 | >99 |
| **TOTAL MULTIPLE DX** | 2,166 | 13.8 | 93 | 6 | 8 | 11 | 17 | 26 | 32 | 51 |
| **TOTAL** | | | | | | | | | | |
| 0–19 Years | 6 | 11.1 | 26 | 9 | 9 | 9 | 9 | 22 | 26 | 26 |
| 20–34 | 65 | 10.2 | 123 | 5 | 7 | 7 | 11 | 21 | 24 | 90 |
| 35–49 | 402 | 12.7 | 82 | 5 | 7 | 10 | 16 | 25 | 33 | 45 |
| 50–64 | 598 | 12.6 | 83 | 6 | 8 | 9 | 15 | 22 | 29 | 53 |
| 65+ | 1,139 | 15.0 | 95 | 7 | 8 | 12 | 18 | 27 | 32 | 52 |
| **GRAND TOTAL** | 2,210 | 13.7 | 92 | 6 | 8 | 11 | 17 | 26 | 32 | 51 |

## 43.8: OTH PARTIAL GASTRECTOMY. Formerly included in operation group(s) 602.

| Type of Patients | Observed Patients | Avg. Stay | Vari-ance | Percentiles | | | | | | |
|---|---|---|---|---|---|---|---|---|---|---|
| | | | | 10th | 25th | 50th | 75th | 90th | 95th | 99th |
| **1. SINGLE DX** | | | | | | | | | | |
| 0–19 Years | 3 | 11.8 | 50 | 5 | 6 | 6 | 19 | 19 | 19 | 19 |
| 20–34 | 6 | 4.4 | <1 | 4 | 4 | 4 | 5 | 5 | 6 | 6 |
| 35–49 | 8 | 6.4 | 15 | 4 | 5 | 5 | 5 | 11 | 11 | 22 |
| 50–64 | 11 | 6.7 | 13 | 5 | 5 | 6 | 6 | 7 | 18 | 18 |
| 65+ | 11 | 8.4 | 12 | 4 | 5 | 8 | 12 | 13 | 13 | 13 |
| **2. MULTIPLE DX** | | | | | | | | | | |
| 0–19 Years | 10 | 7.8 | 9 | 6 | 6 | 6 | 3 | 15 | 15 | 15 |
| 20–34 | 31 | 10.6 | 145 | 5 | 5 | 6 | 9 | 33 | 39 | 73 |
| 35–49 | 118 | 8.7 | 20 | 4 | 6 | 7 | 10 | 14 | 18 | 27 |
| 50–64 | 203 | 10.0 | 36 | 5 | 6 | 8 | 11 | 16 | 19 | 32 |
| 65+ | 408 | 12.8 | 80 | 6 | 7 | 10 | 15 | 22 | 27 | 63 |
| **TOTAL SINGLE DX** | 39 | 6.9 | 16 | 4 | 5 | 5 | 7 | 13 | 18 | 19 |
| **TOTAL MULTIPLE DX** | 770 | 11.2 | 63 | 5 | 6 | 9 | 14 | 19 | 24 | 40 |
| **TOTAL** | | | | | | | | | | |
| 0–19 Years | 13 | 8.5 | 18 | 6 | 6 | 6 | 8 | 15 | 19 | 19 |
| 20–34 | 37 | 9.1 | 116 | 4 | 5 | 5 | 8 | 14 | 24 | 90 |
| 35–49 | 126 | 8.5 | 20 | 4 | 6 | 7 | 10 | 14 | 18 | 27 |
| 50–64 | 214 | 9.8 | 36 | 5 | 6 | 8 | 11 | 16 | 19 | 32 |
| 65+ | 419 | 12.7 | 79 | 6 | 7 | 10 | 15 | 22 | 27 | 63 |
| **GRAND TOTAL** | 809 | 11.0 | 61 | 5 | 6 | 9 | 13 | 18 | 24 | 40 |

## 43.89: PARTIAL GASTRECTOMY NEC. Formerly included in operation group(s) 602.

| Type of Patients | Observed Patients | Avg. Stay | Vari-ance | Percentiles | | | | | | |
|---|---|---|---|---|---|---|---|---|---|---|
| | | | | 10th | 25th | 50th | 75th | 90th | 95th | 99th |
| **1. SINGLE DX** | | | | | | | | | | |
| 0–19 Years | 3 | 11.8 | 50 | 5 | 6 | 6 | 19 | 19 | 19 | 19 |
| 20–34 | 6 | 4.4 | <1 | 4 | 4 | 4 | 5 | 5 | 6 | 6 |
| 35–49 | 8 | 6.4 | 15 | 4 | 5 | 5 | 5 | 11 | 11 | 22 |
| 50–64 | 11 | 6.7 | 13 | 5 | 6 | 6 | 6 | 7 | 18 | 18 |
| 65+ | 11 | 8.4 | 12 | 4 | 5 | 5 | 12 | 13 | 13 | 13 |
| **2. MULTIPLE DX** | | | | | | | | | | |
| 0–19 Years | 10 | 7.8 | 9 | 6 | 6 | 6 | 8 | 15 | 15 | 15 |
| 20–34 | 30 | 10.7 | 147 | 5 | 5 | 6 | 9 | 33 | 39 | 73 |
| 35–49 | 117 | 8.6 | 20 | 4 | 6 | 7 | 10 | 14 | 18 | 27 |
| 50–64 | 203 | 10.0 | 36 | 5 | 6 | 8 | 11 | 16 | 19 | 32 |
| 65+ | 403 | 12.6 | 73 | 6 | 7 | 10 | 15 | 22 | 27 | 59 |
| **TOTAL SINGLE DX** | 39 | 6.9 | 16 | 4 | 5 | 6 | 7 | 13 | 18 | 19 |
| **TOTAL MULTIPLE DX** | 763 | 11.1 | 58 | 5 | 6 | 9 | 14 | 18 | 24 | 39 |
| **TOTAL** | | | | | | | | | | |
| 0–19 Years | 13 | 8.5 | 18 | 6 | 6 | 6 | 8 | 15 | 19 | 19 |
| 20–34 | 36 | 9.1 | 117 | 4 | 5 | 6 | 8 | 14 | 39 | 73 |
| 35–49 | 125 | 8.5 | 20 | 4 | 6 | 7 | 10 | 14 | 18 | 27 |
| 50–64 | 214 | 9.8 | 36 | 5 | 6 | 8 | 11 | 16 | 19 | 32 |
| 65+ | 414 | 12.5 | 72 | 6 | 7 | 10 | 15 | 22 | 27 | 59 |
| **GRAND TOTAL** | 802 | 10.9 | 57 | 5 | 6 | 9 | 13 | 18 | 24 | 39 |

## 43.9: TOTAL GASTRECTOMY. Formerly included in operation group(s) 603.

| Type of Patients | Observed Patients | Avg. Stay | Vari-ance | Percentiles | | | | | | |
|---|---|---|---|---|---|---|---|---|---|---|
| | | | | 10th | 25th | 50th | 75th | 90th | 95th | 99th |
| **1. SINGLE DX** | | | | | | | | | | |
| 0–19 Years | 0 | | | | | | | | | |
| 20–34 | 4 | 9.8 | 3 | 9 | 9 | 9 | 9 | 13 | 13 | 13 |
| 35–49 | 5 | 8.8 | <1 | 8 | 9 | 9 | 9 | 10 | 10 | 10 |
| 50–64 | 9 | 14.4 | 159 | 6 | 8 | 10 | 16 | 46 | 46 | 46 |
| 65+ | 6 | 12.0 | 6 | 10 | 10 | 10 | 14 | 15 | 17 | 17 |
| **2. MULTIPLE DX** | | | | | | | | | | |
| 0–19 Years | 2 | 13.7 | <1 | 13 | 13 | 14 | 14 | 14 | 14 | 14 |
| 20–34 | 20 | 15.0 | 16 | 8 | 15 | 15 | 15 | 22 | 22 | 22 |
| 35–49 | 174 | 15.6 | 74 | 8 | 11 | 11 | 15 | 24 | 39 | 51 |
| 50–64 | 396 | 14.1 | 86 | 8 | 9 | 12 | 16 | 22 | 29 | 58 |
| 65+ | 538 | 15.5 | 87 | 8 | 10 | 12 | 18 | 28 | 35 | 49 |
| **TOTAL SINGLE DX** | 24 | 11.0 | 42 | 8 | 9 | 9 | 10 | 15 | 17 | 46 |
| **TOTAL MULTIPLE DX** | 1,130 | 14.9 | 82 | 8 | 10 | 12 | 16 | 24 | 34 | 53 |
| **TOTAL** | | | | | | | | | | |
| 0–19 Years | 2 | 13.7 | <1 | 13 | 13 | 14 | 14 | 14 | 14 | 14 |
| 20–34 | 24 | 14.8 | 16 | 9 | 10 | 15 | 15 | 22 | 22 | 22 |
| 35–49 | 179 | 15.2 | 72 | 8 | 9 | 11 | 15 | 24 | 39 | 51 |
| 50–64 | 405 | 14.1 | 87 | 8 | 10 | 12 | 16 | 22 | 29 | 58 |
| 65+ | 544 | 15.4 | 86 | 8 | 10 | 12 | 18 | 28 | 35 | 49 |
| **GRAND TOTAL** | 1,154 | 14.8 | 82 | 8 | 10 | 12 | 16 | 24 | 34 | 53 |

Length of Stay by Diagnosis and Operation, United States, 2000

# United States, October 1998–September 1999 Data, by Operation

## 43.99: TOTAL GASTRECTOMY NEC. Formerly included in operation group(s) 603.

| Type of Patients | Observed Patients | Avg. Stay | Variance | 10th | 25th | 50th | 75th | 90th | 95th | 99th |
|---|---|---|---|---|---|---|---|---|---|---|
| **1. SINGLE DX** | | | | | | | | | | |
| 0–19 Years | 0 | | | | | | | | | |
| 20–34 | 4 | 9.8 | 3 | 9 | 9 | 9 | 9 | 13 | 13 | 13 |
| 35–49 | 5 | 8.8 | 4 | 8 | 9 | 9 | 16 | 9 | 10 | 10 |
| 50–64 | 9 | 14.4 | <1 | 6 | 9 | 10 | 16 | 46 | 46 | 46 |
| 65+ | 6 | 12.0 | 6 | 10 | 10 | 10 | 14 | 15 | 17 | 17 |
| **2. MULTIPLE DX** | | | | | | | | | | |
| 0–19 Years | 2 | 13.7 | <1 | 13 | 13 | 14 | 14 | 14 | 14 | 14 |
| 20–34 | 19 | 15.1 | 15 | 9 | 15 | 15 | 15 | 22 | 22 | 22 |
| 35–49 | 168 | 15.2 | 59 | 8 | 10 | 15 | 15 | 22 | 35 | 45 |
| 50–64 | 381 | 14.1 | 88 | 8 | 10 | 11 | 16 | 22 | 29 | 58 |
| 65+ | 530 | 15.4 | 86 | 8 | 10 | 12 | 18 | 28 | 35 | 49 |
| **TOTAL SINGLE DX** | 24 | 11.0 | 42 | 8 | 9 | 9 | 10 | 15 | 17 | 46 |
| **TOTAL MULTIPLE DX** | 1,100 | 14.9 | 80 | 8 | 10 | 12 | 16 | 24 | 33 | 54 |
| **TOTAL** | | | | | | | | | | |
| 0–19 Years | 2 | 13.7 | <1 | 13 | 13 | 14 | 14 | 14 | 14 | 14 |
| 20–34 | 23 | 14.9 | 15 | 9 | 15 | 15 | 15 | 22 | 22 | 22 |
| 35–49 | 173 | 14.8 | 58 | 8 | 10 | 15 | 15 | 21 | 35 | 45 |
| 50–64 | 390 | 14.1 | 88 | 8 | 10 | 11 | 16 | 22 | 30 | 58 |
| 65+ | 536 | 15.4 | 85 | 8 | 10 | 12 | 18 | 27 | 35 | 49 |
| **GRAND TOTAL** | 1,124 | 14.8 | 79 | 8 | 10 | 12 | 16 | 24 | 33 | 53 |

## 44.01: TRUNCAL VAGOTOMY. Formerly included in operation group(s) 604.

| Type of Patients | Observed Patients | Avg. Stay | Variance | 10th | 25th | 50th | 75th | 90th | 95th | 99th |
|---|---|---|---|---|---|---|---|---|---|---|
| **1. SINGLE DX** | | | | | | | | | | |
| 0–19 Years | 3 | 5.5 | 2 | 4 | 4 | 5 | 7 | 7 | 7 | 7 |
| 20–34 | 1 | 4.0 | 0 | 4 | 4 | 4 | 4 | 4 | 4 | 4 |
| 35–49 | 3 | 5.2 | 7 | 3 | 3 | 5 | 5 | 10 | 10 | 10 |
| 50–64 | 2 | 5.7 | <1 | 5 | 5 | 6 | 6 | 6 | 6 | 6 |
| 65+ | 2 | 5.5 | <1 | 5 | 5 | 6 | 6 | 6 | 6 | 6 |
| **2. MULTIPLE DX** | | | | | | | | | | |
| 0–19 Years | 0 | | | | | | | | | |
| 20–34 | 19 | 7.5 | 11 | 4 | 5 | 7 | 7 | 13 | 14 | 15 |
| 35–49 | 76 | 9.6 | 62 | 5 | 5 | 8 | 11 | 14 | 21 | 53 |
| 50–64 | 96 | 9.3 | 36 | 6 | 6 | 7 | 12 | 17 | 22 | 32 |
| 65+ | 127 | 13.8 | 119 | 6 | 8 | 11 | 16 | 24 | 30 | 80 |
| **TOTAL SINGLE DX** | 11 | 5.2 | 3 | 3 | 4 | 5 | 6 | 7 | 10 | 10 |
| **TOTAL MULTIPLE DX** | 318 | 11.0 | 78 | 5 | 7 | 9 | 13 | 18 | 26 | 53 |
| **TOTAL** | | | | | | | | | | |
| 0–19 Years | 3 | 5.5 | 2 | 4 | 5 | 5 | 7 | 7 | 7 | 7 |
| 20–34 | 20 | 7.2 | 11 | 4 | 5 | 7 | 7 | 13 | 14 | 15 |
| 35–49 | 79 | 9.5 | 61 | 5 | 6 | 8 | 11 | 14 | 21 | 53 |
| 50–64 | 98 | 9.3 | 36 | 4 | 6 | 7 | 12 | 17 | 22 | 32 |
| 65+ | 129 | 13.7 | 119 | 6 | 8 | 11 | 16 | 24 | 30 | 80 |
| **GRAND TOTAL** | 329 | 10.9 | 77 | 5 | 6 | 8 | 13 | 18 | 25 | 53 |

## 44.0: VAGOTOMY. Formerly included in operation group(s) 604.

| Type of Patients | Observed Patients | Avg. Stay | Variance | 10th | 25th | 50th | 75th | 90th | 95th | 99th |
|---|---|---|---|---|---|---|---|---|---|---|
| **1. SINGLE DX** | | | | | | | | | | |
| 0–19 Years | 4 | 6.0 | 3 | 4 | 5 | 5 | 7 | 8 | 8 | 8 |
| 20–34 | 4 | 5.8 | 4 | 2 | 4 | 7 | 7 | 7 | 7 | 7 |
| 35–49 | 11 | 4.4 | 2 | 2 | 4 | 5 | 5 | 5 | 6 | 6 |
| 50–64 | 5 | 5.6 | 2 | 2 | 5 | 6 | 7 | 5 | 6 | 7 |
| 65+ | 2 | 5.5 | <1 | 5 | 5 | 6 | 6 | 6 | 6 | 6 |
| **2. MULTIPLE DX** | | | | | | | | | | |
| 0–19 Years | 3 | 4.3 | 2 | 4 | 4 | 4 | 4 | 4 | 4 | 10 |
| 20–34 | 42 | 7.2 | 13 | 4 | 5 | 6 | 7 | 14 | 15 | 21 |
| 35–49 | 147 | 11.0 | 74 | 5 | 6 | 9 | 9 | 15 | 21 | 53 |
| 50–64 | 155 | 9.5 | 35 | 4 | 6 | 7 | 12 | 17 | 22 | 30 |
| 65+ | 195 | 14.2 | 103 | 6 | 9 | 11 | 17 | 25 | 35 | 58 |
| **TOTAL SINGLE DX** | 26 | 5.0 | 3 | 2 | 4 | 5 | 6 | 7 | 7 | 10 |
| **TOTAL MULTIPLE DX** | 542 | 11.4 | 74 | 5 | 6 | 9 | 14 | 19 | 25 | 48 |
| **TOTAL** | | | | | | | | | | |
| 0–19 Years | 7 | 4.6 | 2 | 4 | 4 | 4 | 4 | 7 | 8 | 10 |
| 20–34 | 46 | 7.0 | 12 | 4 | 5 | 6 | 13 | 13 | 15 | 21 |
| 35–49 | 158 | 10.5 | 71 | 5 | 5 | 7 | 15 | 15 | 21 | 53 |
| 50–64 | 160 | 9.4 | 35 | 4 | 6 | 7 | 12 | 17 | 22 | 30 |
| 65+ | 197 | 14.2 | 103 | 6 | 9 | 11 | 17 | 25 | 35 | 58 |
| **GRAND TOTAL** | 568 | 11.1 | 72 | 5 | 6 | 9 | 14 | 19 | 25 | 48 |

## 44.1: GASTRIC DXTIC PX. Formerly included in operation group(s) 598, 601, 606, 631.

| Type of Patients | Observed Patients | Avg. Stay | Variance | 10th | 25th | 50th | 75th | 90th | 95th | 99th |
|---|---|---|---|---|---|---|---|---|---|---|
| **1. SINGLE DX** | | | | | | | | | | |
| 0–19 Years | 27 | 1.3 | <1 | 1 | 1 | 1 | 2 | 2 | 3 | 3 |
| 20–34 | 5 | 2.4 | <1 | 2 | 2 | 2 | 4 | 4 | 5 | 5 |
| 35–49 | 12 | 4.9 | 44 | 1 | 2 | 2 | 6 | 8 | 27 | 27 |
| 50–64 | 4 | 2.1 | <1 | 1 | 2 | 2 | 3 | 3 | 3 | 3 |
| 65+ | 5 | 5.3 | 6 | 1 | 4 | 7 | 7 | 7 | 7 | 7 |
| **2. MULTIPLE DX** | | | | | | | | | | |
| 0–19 Years | 57 | 3.0 | 11 | 1 | 2 | 3 | 3 | 8 | 9 | 16 |
| 20–34 | 92 | 5.5 | 23 | 1 | 2 | 4 | 7 | 11 | 21 | 21 |
| 35–49 | 245 | 5.3 | 22 | 1 | 2 | 4 | 6 | 10 | 14 | 25 |
| 50–64 | 327 | 6.2 | 68 | 2 | 3 | 4 | 8 | 14 | 17 | 43 |
| 65+ | 890 | 7.2 | 42 | 2 | 3 | 6 | 8 | 14 | 19 | 32 |
| **TOTAL SINGLE DX** | 53 | 2.3 | 8 | 1 | 1 | 1 | 2 | 5 | 7 | 8 |
| **TOTAL MULTIPLE DX** | 1,611 | 6.4 | 43 | 1 | 3 | 5 | 7 | 13 | 18 | 31 |
| **TOTAL** | | | | | | | | | | |
| 0–19 Years | 84 | 2.5 | 9 | 1 | 1 | 2 | 2 | 6 | 8 | 14 |
| 20–34 | 97 | 5.3 | 22 | 2 | 2 | 4 | 7 | 10 | 17 | 21 |
| 35–49 | 257 | 5.3 | 22 | 1 | 2 | 4 | 6 | 10 | 14 | 25 |
| 50–64 | 331 | 6.2 | 68 | 2 | 3 | 4 | 7 | 14 | 17 | 43 |
| 65+ | 895 | 7.2 | 42 | 2 | 3 | 6 | 8 | 14 | 19 | 32 |
| **GRAND TOTAL** | 1,664 | 6.2 | 43 | 1 | 2 | 5 | 7 | 12 | 18 | 31 |

Length of Stay by Diagnosis and Operation, United States, 2000

## United States, October 1998–September 1999 Data, by Operation

### 44.13: GASTROSCOPY NEC. Formerly included in operation group(s) 598.

| Type of Patients | Observed Patients | Avg. Stay | Variance | Percentiles | | | | | | |
|---|---|---|---|---|---|---|---|---|---|---|
| | | | | 10th | 25th | 50th | 75th | 90th | 95th | 99th |
| **1. SINGLE DX** | | | | | | | | | | |
| 0–19 Years | 23 | 1.4 | <1 | 1 | 1 | 1 | 1 | 3 | 3 | 3 |
| 20–34 | 3 | 3.7 | 2 | 2 | 2 | 4 | 5 | 5 | 5 | 5 |
| 35–49 | 7 | 5.4 | 73 | 1 | 1 | 2 | 5 | 27 | 27 | 27 |
| 50–64 | 3 | 2.0 | <1 | 1 | 2 | 2 | 2 | 3 | 3 | 3 |
| 65+ | 3 | 6.2 | 3 | 2 | 6 | 7 | 7 | 7 | 7 | 7 |
| **2. MULTIPLE DX** | | | | | | | | | | |
| 0–19 Years | 42 | 2.9 | 12 | 1 | 1 | 2 | 3 | 8 | 9 | 9 |
| 20–34 | 47 | 5.3 | 27 | 1 | 2 | 7 | 7 | 10 | 21 | 21 |
| 35–49 | 116 | 4.8 | 16 | 1 | 2 | 4 | 6 | 9 | 14 | 19 |
| 50–64 | 149 | 6.8 | 72 | 2 | 3 | 4 | 7 | 15 | 18 | 58 |
| 65+ | 444 | 7.3 | 34 | 2 | 4 | 7 | 8 | 13 | 19 | 29 |
| **TOTAL SINGLE DX** | 39 | 2.3 | 10 | 1 | 1 | 2 | 2 | 6 | 7 | 27 |
| **TOTAL MULTIPLE DX** | 798 | 6.5 | 37 | 2 | 3 | 5 | 8 | 12 | 18 | 29 |
| **TOTAL** | | | | | | | | | | |
| 0–19 Years | 65 | 2.4 | 9 | 1 | 1 | 1 | 3 | 6 | 8 | 9 |
| 20–34 | 50 | 5.2 | 26 | 1 | 2 | 3 | 7 | 10 | 21 | 21 |
| 35–49 | 123 | 4.8 | 18 | 1 | 2 | 4 | 6 | 9 | 14 | 19 |
| 50–64 | 152 | 6.6 | 70 | 2 | 3 | 4 | 7 | 15 | 18 | 58 |
| 65+ | 447 | 7.3 | 34 | 2 | 4 | 7 | 8 | 13 | 19 | 29 |
| **GRAND TOTAL** | 837 | 6.3 | 37 | 1 | 3 | 5 | 7 | 12 | 18 | 29 |

### 44.2: PYLOROPLASTY. Formerly included in operation group(s) 604.

| Type of Patients | Observed Patients | Avg. Stay | Variance | Percentiles | | | | | | |
|---|---|---|---|---|---|---|---|---|---|---|
| | | | | 10th | 25th | 50th | 75th | 90th | 95th | 99th |
| **1. SINGLE DX** | | | | | | | | | | |
| 0–19 Years | 40 | 3.7 | 3 | 2 | 2 | 3 | 5 | 6 | 6 | 6 |
| 20–34 | 9 | 4.8 | <1 | 4 | 4 | 4 | 5 | 6 | 6 | 6 |
| 35–49 | 15 | 4.5 | 2 | 4 | 4 | 4 | 4 | 6 | 9 | 10 |
| 50–64 | 7 | 5.6 | 13 | 5 | 5 | 5 | 5 | 6 | 17 | 17 |
| 65+ | 6 | 4.9 | 13 | 1 | 2 | 3 | 8 | 10 | 10 | 10 |
| **2. MULTIPLE DX** | | | | | | | | | | |
| 0–19 Years | 61 | 6.4 | 29 | 3 | 4 | 4 | 6 | 14 | 21 | 24 |
| 20–34 | 46 | 4.5 | 27 | 1 | 1 | 2 | 7 | 8 | 17 | 29 |
| 35–49 | 216 | 7.4 | 38 | 2 | 4 | 6 | 8 | 16 | 20 | 29 |
| 50–64 | 248 | 8.6 | 52 | 3 | 4 | 7 | 11 | 18 | 25 | 36 |
| 65+ | 436 | 10.2 | 58 | 3 | 5 | 8 | 12 | 20 | 23 | 38 |
| **TOTAL SINGLE DX** | 77 | 4.2 | 5 | 2 | 2 | 4 | 5 | 6 | 6 | 10 |
| **TOTAL MULTIPLE DX** | 1,007 | 8.6 | 51 | 2 | 4 | 7 | 11 | 18 | 22 | 35 |
| **TOTAL** | | | | | | | | | | |
| 0–19 Years | 101 | 5.4 | 22 | 2 | 3 | 4 | 6 | 9 | 17 | 24 |
| 20–34 | 55 | 4.5 | 24 | 1 | 1 | 2 | 6 | 8 | 17 | 29 |
| 35–49 | 231 | 7.1 | 36 | 1 | 4 | 6 | 8 | 15 | 19 | 27 |
| 50–64 | 255 | 8.5 | 51 | 4 | 4 | 7 | 11 | 17 | 25 | 36 |
| 65+ | 442 | 10.1 | 58 | 3 | 5 | 8 | 12 | 20 | 23 | 38 |
| **GRAND TOTAL** | 1,084 | 8.3 | 49 | 2 | 4 | 6 | 10 | 17 | 21 | 34 |

### 44.14: CLSD (ENDO) GASTRIC BX. Formerly included in operation group(s) 601.

| Type of Patients | Observed Patients | Avg. Stay | Variance | Percentiles | | | | | | |
|---|---|---|---|---|---|---|---|---|---|---|
| | | | | 10th | 25th | 50th | 75th | 90th | 95th | 99th |
| **1. SINGLE DX** | | | | | | | | | | |
| 0–19 Years | 3 | 1.3 | <1 | 1 | 1 | 1 | 2 | 2 | 2 | 2 |
| 20–34 | 2 | 2.1 | <1 | 2 | 2 | 2 | 2 | 2 | 3 | 3 |
| 35–49 | 5 | 4.3 | 8 | 2 | 2 | 3 | 8 | 8 | 8 | 8 |
| 50–64 | 0 | | | | | | | | | |
| 65+ | 2 | 2.3 | 3 | 1 | 1 | 1 | 4 | 4 | 4 | 4 |
| **2. MULTIPLE DX** | | | | | | | | | | |
| 0–19 Years | 7 | 9.9 | 20 | 4 | 6 | 7 | 14 | 16 | 16 | 16 |
| 20–34 | 38 | 5.2 | 16 | 2 | 3 | 4 | 6 | 9 | 15 | 21 |
| 35–49 | 101 | 4.3 | 7 | 2 | 2 | 4 | 5 | 8 | 10 | 14 |
| 50–64 | 140 | 4.4 | 21 | 1 | 1 | 3 | 6 | 8 | 14 | 19 |
| 65+ | 389 | 6.1 | 35 | 2 | 3 | 5 | 7 | 12 | 16 | 26 |
| **TOTAL SINGLE DX** | 12 | 2.5 | 4 | 1 | 2 | 2 | 2 | 4 | 8 | 8 |
| **TOTAL MULTIPLE DX** | 675 | 5.4 | 27 | 1 | 2 | 4 | 6 | 11 | 15 | 22 |
| **TOTAL** | | | | | | | | | | |
| 0–19 Years | 10 | 7.3 | 30 | 1 | 2 | 7 | 13 | 14 | 16 | 16 |
| 20–34 | 40 | 4.7 | 15 | 2 | 2 | 3 | 5 | 9 | 10 | 21 |
| 35–49 | 106 | 4.3 | 7 | 2 | 2 | 4 | 5 | 8 | 10 | 14 |
| 50–64 | 140 | 4.4 | 21 | 1 | 1 | 3 | 6 | 9 | 14 | 19 |
| 65+ | 391 | 6.1 | 35 | 2 | 3 | 5 | 7 | 12 | 16 | 26 |
| **GRAND TOTAL** | 687 | 5.3 | 26 | 1 | 2 | 4 | 6 | 11 | 15 | 22 |

### 44.22: ENDO DILATION PYLORUS. Formerly included in operation group(s) 604.

| Type of Patients | Observed Patients | Avg. Stay | Variance | Percentiles | | | | | | |
|---|---|---|---|---|---|---|---|---|---|---|
| | | | | 10th | 25th | 50th | 75th | 90th | 95th | 99th |
| **1. SINGLE DX** | | | | | | | | | | |
| 0–19 Years | 0 | | | | | | | | | |
| 20–34 | 1 | 4.0 | 0 | 4 | 4 | 4 | 4 | 4 | 4 | 4 |
| 35–49 | 3 | 3.2 | 2 | 1 | 1 | 1 | 4 | 4 | 4 | 4 |
| 50–64 | 1 | 1.0 | 0 | 1 | 1 | 1 | 1 | 1 | 1 | 1 |
| 65+ | 3 | 1.9 | <1 | 1 | 1 | 2 | 3 | 3 | 3 | 3 |
| **2. MULTIPLE DX** | | | | | | | | | | |
| 0–19 Years | 5 | 2.5 | 3 | 1 | 1 | 2 | 3 | 6 | 6 | 6 |
| 20–34 | 28 | 3.5 | 24 | 1 | 1 | 3 | 3 | 8 | 9 | 29 |
| 35–49 | 95 | 5.6 | 37 | 1 | 2 | 4 | 6 | 15 | 20 | 29 |
| 50–64 | 122 | 4.4 | 15 | 1 | 2 | 3 | 6 | 9 | 14 | 20 |
| 65+ | 221 | 6.7 | 32 | 2 | 3 | 6 | 8 | 13 | 15 | 23 |
| **TOTAL SINGLE DX** | 8 | 2.5 | 2 | 1 | 1 | 2 | 4 | 4 | 4 | 4 |
| **TOTAL MULTIPLE DX** | 471 | 5.6 | 29 | 1 | 2 | 4 | 7 | 12 | 15 | 24 |
| **TOTAL** | | | | | | | | | | |
| 0–19 Years | 5 | 2.5 | 3 | 1 | 1 | 2 | 3 | 6 | 6 | 6 |
| 20–34 | 29 | 3.6 | 24 | 1 | 2 | 4 | 4 | 7 | 9 | 29 |
| 35–49 | 98 | 5.6 | 36 | 1 | 2 | 4 | 6 | 15 | 20 | 29 |
| 50–64 | 123 | 4.4 | 14 | 1 | 1 | 3 | 6 | 9 | 14 | 20 |
| 65+ | 224 | 6.7 | 32 | 2 | 3 | 6 | 8 | 13 | 15 | 23 |
| **GRAND TOTAL** | 479 | 5.6 | 29 | 1 | 2 | 4 | 7 | 11 | 15 | 24 |

Length of Stay by Diagnosis and Operation, United States, 2000

# United States, October 1998–September 1999 Data, by Operation

## 44.31: HIGH GASTRIC BYPASS. Formerly included in operation group(s) 606.

| Type of Patients | Observed Patients | Avg. Stay | Variance | Percentiles | | | | | | |
|---|---|---|---|---|---|---|---|---|---|---|
| | | | | 10th | 25th | 50th | 75th | 90th | 95th | 99th |
| **1. SINGLE DX** | | | | | | | | | | |
| 0–19 Years | 6 | 3.6 | <1 | 3 | 3 | 3 | 4 | 4 | 5 | 7 |
| 20–34 | 88 | 3.3 | <1 | 2 | 3 | 3 | 3 | 4 | 5 | 8 |
| 35–49 | 79 | 3.5 | 1 | 2 | 3 | 4 | 4 | 5 | 5 | 7 |
| 50–64 | 13 | 3.9 | 13 | 3 | 3 | 3 | 4 | 5 | 5 | 21 |
| 65+ | 1 | 3.0 | 0 | 3 | 3 | 3 | 3 | 3 | 3 | 3 |
| **2. MULTIPLE DX** | | | | | | | | | | |
| 0–19 Years | 42 | 4.1 | 4 | 3 | 3 | 3 | 5 | 5 | 7 | 12 |
| 20–34 | 1,006 | 3.8 | 3 | 3 | 3 | 3 | 4 | 5 | 6 | 10 |
| 35–49 | 1,798 | 4.0 | 3 | 3 | 3 | 4 | 4 | 6 | 7 | 13 |
| 50–64 | 647 | 4.7 | 13 | 3 | 4 | 4 | 5 | 7 | 11 | 20 |
| 65+ | 25 | 5.2 | 12 | 3 | 4 | 4 | 5 | 7 | 15 | 19 |
| **TOTAL SINGLE DX** | 187 | 3.4 | 2 | 2 | 3 | 3 | 4 | 4 | 5 | 7 |
| **TOTAL MULTIPLE DX** | 3,518 | 4.1 | 7 | 3 | 3 | 3 | 4 | 6 | 7 | 15 |
| **TOTAL** | | | | | | | | | | |
| 0–19 Years | 48 | 3.9 | 3 | 3 | 3 | 3 | 5 | 5 | 6 | 12 |
| 20–34 | 1,094 | 3.7 | 3 | 3 | 3 | 3 | 4 | 5 | 6 | 9 |
| 35–49 | 1,877 | 4.0 | 7 | 3 | 3 | 4 | 4 | 6 | 7 | 12 |
| 50–64 | 660 | 4.7 | 13 | 3 | 3 | 4 | 5 | 7 | 11 | 20 |
| 65+ | 26 | 5.1 | 11 | 3 | 4 | 4 | 5 | 7 | 15 | 19 |
| **GRAND TOTAL** | 3,705 | 4.0 | 7 | 3 | 3 | 3 | 4 | 6 | 7 | 14 |

## 44.39: GASTROENTEROSTOMY NEC. Formerly included in operation group(s) 606.

| Type of Patients | Observed Patients | Avg. Stay | Variance | Percentiles | | | | | | |
|---|---|---|---|---|---|---|---|---|---|---|
| | | | | 10th | 25th | 50th | 75th | 90th | 95th | 99th |
| **1. SINGLE DX** | | | | | | | | | | |
| 0–19 Years | 8 | 4.9 | 3 | 3 | 3 | 5 | 7 | 7 | 7 | 7 |
| 20–34 | 58 | 4.3 | 1 | 3 | 4 | 4 | 5 | 6 | 6 | 7 |
| 35–49 | 58 | 4.1 | 2 | 4 | 4 | 4 | 4 | 5 | 5 | 8 |
| 50–64 | 20 | 4.8 | 11 | 4 | 4 | 4 | 4 | 7 | 9 | 26 |
| 65+ | 1 | 7.0 | 0 | 7 | 7 | 7 | 7 | 7 | 7 | 7 |
| **2. MULTIPLE DX** | | | | | | | | | | |
| 0–19 Years | 36 | 13.4 | 136 | 3 | 4 | 10 | 19 | 23 | 35 | 58 |
| 20–34 | 361 | 4.9 | 27 | 2 | 3 | 4 | 5 | 8 | 10 | 39 |
| 35–49 | 710 | 5.7 | 38 | 2 | 3 | 4 | 6 | 11 | 17 | 33 |
| 50–64 | 592 | 9.9 | 81 | 2 | 4 | 7 | 14 | 25 | 33 | >99 |
| 65+ | 680 | 17.0 | 129 | 7 | 10 | 14 | 20 | 34 | 42 | 53 |
| **TOTAL SINGLE DX** | 145 | 4.3 | 3 | 3 | 4 | 4 | 5 | 6 | 7 | 9 |
| **TOTAL MULTIPLE DX** | 2,379 | 9.8 | 97 | 2 | 3 | 6 | 13 | 22 | 31 | 53 |
| **TOTAL** | | | | | | | | | | |
| 0–19 Years | 44 | 12.1 | 125 | 3 | 4 | 7 | 7 | 19 | 23 | 58 |
| 20–34 | 419 | 4.8 | 23 | 2 | 3 | 4 | 5 | 7 | 9 | 27 |
| 35–49 | 768 | 5.5 | 35 | 2 | 3 | 4 | 5 | 11 | 16 | 33 |
| 50–64 | 612 | 9.6 | 78 | 2 | 4 | 6 | 13 | 23 | 32 | >99 |
| 65+ | 681 | 17.0 | 129 | 7 | 10 | 14 | 20 | 34 | 42 | 53 |
| **GRAND TOTAL** | 2,524 | 9.4 | 92 | 2 | 3 | 5 | 12 | 22 | 30 | 52 |

## 44.29: OTHER PYLOROPLASTY. Formerly included in operation group(s) 604.

| Type of Patients | Observed Patients | Avg. Stay | Variance | Percentiles | | | | | | |
|---|---|---|---|---|---|---|---|---|---|---|
| | | | | 10th | 25th | 50th | 75th | 90th | 95th | 99th |
| **1. SINGLE DX** | | | | | | | | | | |
| 0–19 Years | 37 | 3.7 | 4 | 2 | 2 | 3 | 6 | 6 | 6 | 6 |
| 20–34 | 8 | 4.9 | <1 | 4 | 4 | 5 | 5 | 6 | 6 | 6 |
| 35–49 | 12 | 4.6 | 2 | 4 | 4 | 5 | 4 | 6 | 9 | 10 |
| 50–64 | 6 | 6.0 | 12 | 5 | 5 | 5 | 5 | 6 | 17 | 17 |
| 65+ | 3 | 8.0 | 5 | 5 | 5 | 8 | 10 | 10 | 10 | 10 |
| **2. MULTIPLE DX** | | | | | | | | | | |
| 0–19 Years | 54 | 6.3 | 28 | 3 | 4 | 4 | 6 | 14 | 22 | 24 |
| 20–34 | 18 | 7.9 | 21 | 4 | 5 | 7 | 8 | 16 | 20 | 20 |
| 35–49 | 119 | 8.8 | 35 | 4 | 6 | 7 | 10 | 16 | 16 | 27 |
| 50–64 | 123 | 11.7 | 59 | 5 | 7 | 8 | 14 | 23 | 29 | 41 |
| 65+ | 211 | 13.0 | 62 | 6 | 8 | 11 | 16 | 21 | 29 | 45 |
| **TOTAL SINGLE DX** | 66 | 4.4 | 5 | 2 | 3 | 4 | 5 | 6 | 6 | 17 |
| **TOTAL MULTIPLE DX** | 525 | 10.9 | 56 | 4 | 6 | 8 | 13 | 20 | 26 | 43 |
| **TOTAL** | | | | | | | | | | |
| 0–19 Years | 91 | 5.3 | 21 | 2 | 3 | 4 | 6 | 9 | 18 | 24 |
| 20–34 | 26 | 7.1 | 17 | 4 | 5 | 6 | 7 | 10 | 20 | 20 |
| 35–49 | 131 | 8.1 | 33 | 4 | 5 | 6 | 9 | 16 | 16 | 27 |
| 50–64 | 129 | 11.3 | 57 | 5 | 6 | 8 | 14 | 21 | 26 | 41 |
| 65+ | 214 | 13.0 | 62 | 6 | 8 | 11 | 16 | 21 | 29 | 45 |
| **GRAND TOTAL** | 591 | 10.1 | 55 | 4 | 5 | 8 | 12 | 20 | 25 | 41 |

## 44.3: GASTROENTEROSTOMY. Formerly included in operation group(s) 606.

| Type of Patients | Observed Patients | Avg. Stay | Variance | Percentiles | | | | | | |
|---|---|---|---|---|---|---|---|---|---|---|
| | | | | 10th | 25th | 50th | 75th | 90th | 95th | 99th |
| **1. SINGLE DX** | | | | | | | | | | |
| 0–19 Years | 14 | 4.0 | 2 | 3 | 3 | 4 | 4 | 7 | 7 | 7 |
| 20–34 | 146 | 3.6 | 1 | 3 | 3 | 3 | 4 | 5 | 6 | 7 |
| 35–49 | 137 | 3.8 | 2 | 2 | 3 | 4 | 4 | 5 | 5 | 7 |
| 50–64 | 33 | 4.6 | 11 | 3 | 3 | 4 | 4 | 5 | 7 | 26 |
| 65+ | 2 | 5.8 | 4 | 3 | 3 | 7 | 7 | 7 | 7 | 7 |
| **2. MULTIPLE DX** | | | | | | | | | | |
| 0–19 Years | 78 | 8.4 | 87 | 3 | 3 | 5 | 11 | 21 | 23 | 58 |
| 20–34 | 1,367 | 4.0 | 9 | 3 | 3 | 3 | 5 | 5 | 7 | 13 |
| 35–49 | 2,508 | 4.5 | 18 | 2 | 3 | 3 | 5 | 8 | 10 | 23 |
| 50–64 | 1,239 | 7.4 | 55 | 3 | 3 | 4 | 8 | 18 | 26 | 51 |
| 65+ | 705 | 16.7 | 130 | 6 | 9 | 13 | 20 | 33 | 42 | 53 |
| **TOTAL SINGLE DX** | 332 | 3.8 | 3 | 2 | 3 | 4 | 4 | 5 | 6 | 8 |
| **TOTAL MULTIPLE DX** | 5,897 | 6.5 | 52 | 3 | 3 | 4 | 6 | 14 | 21 | 42 |
| **TOTAL** | | | | | | | | | | |
| 0–19 Years | 92 | 7.4 | 70 | 3 | 3 | 4 | 7 | 19 | 23 | 35 |
| 20–34 | 1,513 | 4.0 | 8 | 3 | 3 | 3 | 4 | 5 | 7 | 13 |
| 35–49 | 2,645 | 4.5 | 17 | 2 | 3 | 4 | 5 | 9 | 10 | 22 |
| 50–64 | 1,272 | 7.3 | 54 | 3 | 3 | 4 | 8 | 17 | 26 | 50 |
| 65+ | 707 | 16.6 | 130 | 6 | 9 | 13 | 20 | 33 | 42 | 53 |
| **GRAND TOTAL** | 6,229 | 6.3 | 49 | 3 | 4 | 6 | 13 | 20 | 20 | 40 |

Length of Stay by Diagnosis and Operation, United States, 2000

# United States, October 1998–September 1999 Data, by Operation

## 44.42: SUT DUODENAL ULCER SITE. Formerly included in operation group(s) 606.

| Type of Patients | Observed Patients | Avg. Stay | Vari-ance | 10th | 25th | 50th | 75th | 90th | 95th | 99th |
|---|---|---|---|---|---|---|---|---|---|---|
| **1. SINGLE DX** | | | | | | | | | | |
| 0–19 Years | 11 | 6.7 | 3 | 5 | 6 | 6 | 9 | 9 | 9 | 9 |
| 20–34 | 35 | 5.2 | 2 | 4 | 4 | 5 | 6 | 7 | 7 | 8 |
| 35–49 | 57 | 5.6 | 2 | 5 | 5 | 5 | 6 | 7 | 8 | 10 |
| 50–64 | 16 | 6.0 | 2 | 6 | 6 | 6 | 7 | 7 | 7 | 11 |
| 65+ | 19 | 7.7 | 6 | 4 | 5 | 8 | 10 | 11 | 11 | 11 |
| **2. MULTIPLE DX** | | | | | | | | | | |
| 0–19 Years | 17 | 8.4 | 6 | 6 | 7 | 7 | 11 | 11 | 11 | 13 |
| 20–34 | 95 | 7.0 | 15 | 4 | 5 | 6 | 7 | 12 | 14 | 28 |
| 35–49 | 379 | 8.5 | 35 | 5 | 6 | 7 | 10 | 15 | 20 | 35 |
| 50–64 | 356 | 10.1 | 57 | 6 | 6 | 8 | 11 | 17 | 27 | 42 |
| 65+ | 875 | 13.4 | 67 | 6 | 8 | 11 | 18 | 22 | 28 | 43 |
| **TOTAL SINGLE DX** | 138 | 6.0 | 3 | 4 | 5 | 6 | 7 | 9 | 9 | 11 |
| **TOTAL MULTIPLE DX** | 1,722 | 11.3 | 60 | 5 | 6 | 9 | 14 | 22 | 25 | 40 |
| **TOTAL** | | | | | | | | | | |
| 0–19 Years | 28 | 7.6 | 5 | 5 | 6 | 7 | 9 | 11 | 11 | 11 |
| 20–34 | 130 | 6.6 | 13 | 4 | 5 | 6 | 7 | 11 | 14 | 21 |
| 35–49 | 436 | 8.1 | 32 | 5 | 6 | 7 | 9 | 13 | 19 | 34 |
| 50–64 | 372 | 9.9 | 56 | 5 | 6 | 8 | 10 | 17 | 26 | 42 |
| 65+ | 894 | 13.3 | 67 | 6 | 8 | 11 | 18 | 22 | 28 | 43 |
| **GRAND TOTAL** | 1,860 | 11.0 | 58 | 5 | 6 | 8 | 13 | 22 | 24 | 40 |

## 44.43: ENDO CNTRL GASTRIC BLEED. Formerly included in operation group(s) 605.

| Type of Patients | Observed Patients | Avg. Stay | Vari-ance | 10th | 25th | 50th | 75th | 90th | 95th | 99th |
|---|---|---|---|---|---|---|---|---|---|---|
| **1. SINGLE DX** | | | | | | | | | | |
| 0–19 Years | 1 | 2.0 | 0 | 2 | 2 | 2 | 2 | 2 | 2 | 2 |
| 20–34 | 23 | 3.1 | 1 | 2 | 2 | 4 | 4 | 4 | 4 | 4 |
| 35–49 | 29 | 2.7 | 4 | 1 | 2 | 2 | 3 | 3 | 4 | 14 |
| 50–64 | 33 | 2.5 | <1 | 1 | 2 | 3 | 3 | 5 | 4 | 14 |
| 65+ | 29 | 3.1 | 3 | 2 | 2 | 3 | 3 | 5 | 8 | 11 |
| **2. MULTIPLE DX** | | | | | | | | | | |
| 0–19 Years | 49 | 2.8 | 2 | 1 | 2 | 3 | 3 | 4 | 4 | 7 |
| 20–34 | 334 | 3.3 | 9 | 2 | 2 | 3 | 4 | 5 | 7 | 16 |
| 35–49 | 1,250 | 3.8 | 9 | 2 | 2 | 3 | 4 | 6 | 8 | 15 |
| 50–64 | 2,101 | 4.6 | 17 | 2 | 2 | 3 | 5 | 8 | 13 | 22 |
| 65+ | 6,643 | 5.6 | 22 | 2 | 3 | 4 | 6 | 11 | 15 | 24 |
| **TOTAL SINGLE DX** | 115 | 2.8 | 2 | 1 | 2 | 3 | 3 | 4 | 4 | 11 |
| **TOTAL MULTIPLE DX** | 10,377 | 5.0 | 19 | 2 | 3 | 4 | 6 | 9 | 14 | 22 |
| **TOTAL** | | | | | | | | | | |
| 0–19 Years | 50 | 2.8 | 2 | 1 | 2 | 3 | 3 | 4 | 4 | 7 |
| 20–34 | 357 | 3.3 | 8 | 2 | 2 | 3 | 4 | 5 | 7 | 16 |
| 35–49 | 1,279 | 3.8 | 9 | 2 | 2 | 3 | 4 | 6 | 8 | 15 |
| 50–64 | 2,134 | 4.5 | 17 | 2 | 2 | 3 | 5 | 8 | 13 | 22 |
| 65+ | 6,672 | 5.5 | 22 | 2 | 3 | 4 | 6 | 10 | 15 | 24 |
| **GRAND TOTAL** | 10,492 | 5.0 | 19 | 2 | 3 | 4 | 6 | 9 | 14 | 22 |

## 44.4: CNTRL PEPTIC ULCER HEMOR. Formerly included in operation group(s) 605, 606.

| Type of Patients | Observed Patients | Avg. Stay | Vari-ance | 10th | 25th | 50th | 75th | 90th | 95th | 99th |
|---|---|---|---|---|---|---|---|---|---|---|
| **1. SINGLE DX** | | | | | | | | | | |
| 0–19 Years | 13 | 6.6 | 3 | 5 | 6 | 6 | 9 | 9 | 9 | 9 |
| 20–34 | 70 | 4.2 | 3 | 2 | 4 | 4 | 5 | 7 | 7 | 8 |
| 35–49 | 119 | 4.9 | 5 | 2 | 3 | 5 | 6 | 8 | 8 | 10 |
| 50–64 | 68 | 3.8 | 4 | 1 | 3 | 3 | 5 | 6 | 7 | 10 |
| 65+ | 54 | 4.6 | 9 | 2 | 2 | 3 | 8 | 9 | 10 | 11 |
| **2. MULTIPLE DX** | | | | | | | | | | |
| 0–19 Years | 79 | 5.8 | 27 | 2 | 3 | 4 | 7 | 11 | 15 | 25 |
| 20–34 | 499 | 4.3 | 13 | 2 | 2 | 4 | 5 | 7 | 9 | 20 |
| 35–49 | 1,853 | 5.4 | 25 | 2 | 3 | 4 | 6 | 10 | 14 | 25 |
| 50–64 | 2,672 | 5.9 | 35 | 2 | 3 | 4 | 7 | 11 | 16 | 34 |
| 65+ | 8,021 | 6.9 | 40 | 2 | 3 | 5 | 9 | 15 | 19 | 29 |
| **TOTAL SINGLE DX** | 324 | 4.6 | 5 | 2 | 3 | 4 | 6 | 8 | 9 | 11 |
| **TOTAL MULTIPLE DX** | 13,124 | 6.4 | 36 | 2 | 3 | 4 | 8 | 13 | 18 | 29 |
| **TOTAL** | | | | | | | | | | |
| 0–19 Years | 92 | 6.0 | 22 | 2 | 3 | 5 | 7 | 11 | 15 | 25 |
| 20–34 | 569 | 4.3 | 12 | 2 | 2 | 4 | 5 | 7 | 8 | 18 |
| 35–49 | 1,972 | 5.3 | 24 | 2 | 3 | 4 | 6 | 9 | 13 | 25 |
| 50–64 | 2,740 | 5.8 | 34 | 2 | 3 | 4 | 7 | 11 | 16 | 34 |
| 65+ | 8,075 | 6.9 | 40 | 2 | 3 | 5 | 9 | 15 | 19 | 29 |
| **GRAND TOTAL** | 13,448 | 6.3 | 35 | 2 | 3 | 4 | 7 | 13 | 17 | 29 |

## 44.41: SUT GASTRIC ULCER SITE. Formerly included in operation group(s) 606.

| Type of Patients | Observed Patients | Avg. Stay | Vari-ance | 10th | 25th | 50th | 75th | 90th | 95th | 99th |
|---|---|---|---|---|---|---|---|---|---|---|
| **1. SINGLE DX** | | | | | | | | | | |
| 0–19 Years | 1 | 6.0 | 0 | 6 | 6 | 6 | 6 | 6 | 6 | 6 |
| 20–34 | 11 | 5.0 | 2 | 4 | 4 | 4 | 7 | 7 | 7 | 8 |
| 35–49 | 28 | 5.8 | 2 | 4 | 5 | 6 | 6 | 8 | 8 | 9 |
| 50–64 | 17 | 5.4 | 2 | 4 | 5 | 5 | 6 | 7 | 7 | 10 |
| 65+ | 3 | 5.4 | 2 | 4 | 4 | 5 | 7 | 7 | 7 | 7 |
| **2. MULTIPLE DX** | | | | | | | | | | |
| 0–19 Years | 11 | 15.7 | 95 | 5 | 6 | 15 | 18 | 37 | 37 | 37 |
| 20–34 | 65 | 5.7 | 15 | 3 | 3 | 5 | 7 | 8 | 11 | 24 |
| 35–49 | 202 | 9.9 | 65 | 5 | 6 | 7 | 10 | 18 | 29 | 41 |
| 50–64 | 188 | 10.7 | 90 | 5 | 5 | 7 | 11 | 23 | 35 | 50 |
| 65+ | 433 | 12.1 | 94 | 5 | 7 | 10 | 13 | 18 | 27 | 52 |
| **TOTAL SINGLE DX** | 60 | 5.5 | 2 | 4 | 4 | 5 | 6 | 7 | 8 | 9 |
| **TOTAL MULTIPLE DX** | 899 | 10.9 | 85 | 5 | 6 | 8 | 12 | 19 | 28 | 49 |
| **TOTAL** | | | | | | | | | | |
| 0–19 Years | 12 | 14.9 | 94 | 5 | 6 | 15 | 18 | 37 | 37 | 37 |
| 20–34 | 76 | 5.6 | 13 | 3 | 3 | 5 | 7 | 8 | 9 | 22 |
| 35–49 | 230 | 9.4 | 60 | 5 | 5 | 6 | 9 | 18 | 29 | 36 |
| 50–64 | 205 | 10.3 | 85 | 5 | 5 | 6 | 11 | 23 | 31 | 50 |
| 65+ | 436 | 12.1 | 94 | 5 | 7 | 10 | 13 | 18 | 27 | 52 |
| **GRAND TOTAL** | 959 | 10.6 | 82 | 5 | 6 | 8 | 12 | 18 | 27 | 49 |

Length of Stay by Diagnosis and Operation, United States, 2000

# United States, October 1998–September 1999 Data, by Operation

## 44.5: REVISION GASTRIC ANAST. Formerly included in operation group(s) 606.

| Type of Patients | Observed Patients | Avg. Stay | Variance | 10th | 25th | 50th | 75th | 90th | 95th | 99th |
|---|---|---|---|---|---|---|---|---|---|---|
| **1. SINGLE DX** | | | | | | | | | | |
| 0–19 Years | 0 | | | | | | | | | |
| 20–34 | 1 | 9.0 | 0 | 9 | 9 | 9 | 9 | 9 | 9 | 9 |
| 35–49 | 6 | 3.9 | 3 | 2 | 2 | 3 | 6 | 6 | 6 | 6 |
| 50–64 | 6 | 8.0 | 6 | 3 | 2 | 9 | 9 | 9 | 10 | 10 |
| 65+ | 1 | 5.0 | 0 | 5 | 5 | 5 | 5 | 5 | 5 | 5 |
| **2. MULTIPLE DX** | | | | | | | | | | |
| 0–19 Years | 10 | 7.9 | 88 | 1 | 3 | 3 | 11 | 32 | 32 | 32 |
| 20–34 | 45 | 9.1 | 54 | 3 | 3 | 6 | 15 | 20 | 20 | 26 |
| 35–49 | 184 | 8.9 | 140 | 3 | 3 | 5 | 8 | 23 | 29 | 70 |
| 50–64 | 189 | 11.1 | 110 | 2 | 4 | 7 | 14 | 24 | 31 | 50 |
| 65+ | 98 | 15.6 | 144 | 5 | 8 | 12 | 19 | 31 | 40 | 54 |
| **TOTAL SINGLE DX** | 14 | 6.2 | 8 | 2 | 3 | 6 | 9 | 9 | 9 | 10 |
| **TOTAL MULTIPLE DX** | 526 | 10.7 | 126 | 3 | 4 | 7 | 13 | 26 | 31 | 54 |
| **TOTAL** | | | | | | | | | | |
| 0–19 Years | 10 | 7.9 | 88 | 1 | 3 | 3 | 11 | 32 | 32 | 32 |
| 20–34 | 46 | 9.1 | 54 | 3 | 3 | 6 | 15 | 20 | 20 | 26 |
| 35–49 | 190 | 8.8 | 138 | 3 | 3 | 5 | 7 | 23 | 29 | 70 |
| 50–64 | 195 | 11.0 | 107 | 2 | 4 | 7 | 14 | 24 | 31 | 50 |
| 65+ | 99 | 15.4 | 143 | 5 | 7 | 12 | 18 | 31 | 40 | 54 |
| **GRAND TOTAL** | 540 | 10.6 | 124 | 3 | 4 | 7 | 13 | 25 | 31 | 54 |

## 44.61: SUTURE GASTRIC LAC. Formerly included in operation group(s) 606.

| Type of Patients | Observed Patients | Avg. Stay | Variance | 10th | 25th | 50th | 75th | 90th | 95th | 99th |
|---|---|---|---|---|---|---|---|---|---|---|
| **1. SINGLE DX** | | | | | | | | | | |
| 0–19 Years | 5 | 4.9 | 10 | 3 | 3 | 3 | 5 | 13 | 13 | 13 |
| 20–34 | 4 | 4.0 | 1 | 3 | 3 | 3 | 5 | 5 | 5 | 5 |
| 35–49 | 3 | 5.8 | <1 | 5 | 6 | 6 | 6 | 6 | 6 | 6 |
| 50–64 | 0 | | | | | | | | | |
| 65+ | 1 | 10.0 | 0 | 10 | 10 | 10 | 10 | 10 | 10 | 10 |
| **2. MULTIPLE DX** | | | | | | | | | | |
| 0–19 Years | 50 | 9.9 | 133 | 5 | 6 | 7 | 10 | 14 | 16 | 93 |
| 20–34 | 100 | 8.6 | 56 | 3 | 5 | 7 | 10 | 14 | 20 | 57 |
| 35–49 | 54 | 9.4 | 72 | 4 | 5 | 7 | 9 | 28 | 30 | 40 |
| 50–64 | 36 | 10.4 | 90 | 3 | 5 | 8 | 11 | 18 | 30 | 58 |
| 65+ | 49 | 11.6 | 87 | 3 | 5 | 11 | 15 | 22 | 26 | 55 |
| **TOTAL SINGLE DX** | 13 | 5.2 | 5 | 3 | 3 | 5 | 6 | 7 | 10 | 13 |
| **TOTAL MULTIPLE DX** | 289 | 9.7 | 84 | 4 | 5 | 7 | 10 | 17 | 23 | 55 |
| **TOTAL** | | | | | | | | | | |
| 0–19 Years | 55 | 9.5 | 126 | 4 | 6 | 7 | 10 | 14 | 15 | 93 |
| 20–34 | 104 | 8.4 | 55 | 3 | 5 | 7 | 9 | 14 | 18 | 57 |
| 35–49 | 57 | 9.1 | 66 | 4 | 5 | 7 | 9 | 13 | 30 | 40 |
| 50–64 | 36 | 10.4 | 90 | 4 | 5 | 8 | 11 | 18 | 30 | 58 |
| 65+ | 50 | 11.6 | 86 | 3 | 5 | 10 | 14 | 22 | 26 | 55 |
| **GRAND TOTAL** | 302 | 9.5 | 81 | 5 | 5 | 7 | 10 | 16 | 23 | 55 |

## 44.6: OTHER GASTRIC REPAIR. Formerly included in operation group(s) 606.

| Type of Patients | Observed Patients | Avg. Stay | Variance | 10th | 25th | 50th | 75th | 90th | 95th | 99th |
|---|---|---|---|---|---|---|---|---|---|---|
| **1. SINGLE DX** | | | | | | | | | | |
| 0–19 Years | 412 | 2.7 | 3 | 1 | 1 | 2 | 3 | 5 | 6 | 8 |
| 20–34 | 410 | 2.1 | 1 | 1 | 1 | 2 | 2 | 4 | 5 | 6 |
| 35–49 | 642 | 2.3 | 2 | 1 | 1 | 2 | 3 | 4 | 5 | 6 |
| 50–64 | 265 | 1.9 | 2 | 1 | 1 | 2 | 2 | 3 | 3 | 6 |
| 65+ | 72 | 2.3 | 3 | 1 | 1 | 2 | 3 | 4 | 5 | 9 |
| **2. MULTIPLE DX** | | | | | | | | | | |
| 0–19 Years | 2,659 | 10.9 | 173 | 2 | 3 | 6 | 13 | 28 | 41 | 90 |
| 20–34 | 1,568 | 3.7 | 22 | 1 | 2 | 2 | 4 | 7 | 9 | 24 |
| 35–49 | 3,781 | 3.4 | 22 | 1 | 2 | 2 | 4 | 6 | 8 | 24 |
| 50–64 | 2,863 | 3.8 | 36 | 1 | 2 | 2 | 4 | 6 | 10 | 32 |
| 65+ | 1,743 | 6.7 | 78 | 1 | 2 | 4 | 7 | 14 | 21 | 61 |
| **TOTAL SINGLE DX** | 1,801 | 2.3 | 2 | 1 | 1 | 2 | 3 | 4 | 5 | 7 |
| **TOTAL MULTIPLE DX** | 12,614 | 5.4 | 70 | 1 | 2 | 3 | 5 | 11 | 19 | 53 |
| **TOTAL** | | | | | | | | | | |
| 0–19 Years | 3,071 | 9.7 | 156 | 2 | 3 | 5 | 11 | 25 | 37 | 81 |
| 20–34 | 1,978 | 3.4 | 18 | 1 | 2 | 2 | 3 | 7 | 8 | 22 |
| 35–49 | 4,423 | 3.2 | 19 | 1 | 1 | 2 | 4 | 6 | 8 | 22 |
| 50–64 | 3,128 | 3.7 | 33 | 1 | 1 | 2 | 4 | 6 | 9 | 28 |
| 65+ | 1,815 | 6.5 | 76 | 2 | 2 | 4 | 7 | 13 | 20 | 57 |
| **GRAND TOTAL** | 14,415 | 5.0 | 62 | 1 | 2 | 3 | 5 | 10 | 17 | 48 |

## 44.63: CLOSE STOM FISTULA NEC. Formerly included in operation group(s) 606.

| Type of Patients | Observed Patients | Avg. Stay | Variance | 10th | 25th | 50th | 75th | 90th | 95th | 99th |
|---|---|---|---|---|---|---|---|---|---|---|
| **1. SINGLE DX** | | | | | | | | | | |
| 0–19 Years | 33 | 1.8 | 2 | 1 | 1 | 1 | 2 | 5 | 5 | 6 |
| 20–34 | 1 | 4.0 | 0 | 4 | 4 | 4 | 4 | 5 | 4 | 4 |
| 35–49 | 2 | 3.7 | 10 | 1 | 1 | 6 | 6 | 6 | 6 | 6 |
| 50–64 | 0 | | | | | | | | | |
| 65+ | 0 | | | | | | | | | |
| **2. MULTIPLE DX** | | | | | | | | | | |
| 0–19 Years | 91 | 3.8 | 51 | 1 | 1 | 1 | 3 | 9 | 17 | 41 |
| 20–34 | 15 | 9.2 | 108 | 2 | 3 | 7 | 8 | 32 | 33 | 40 |
| 35–49 | 25 | 9.9 | 106 | 4 | 4 | 4 | 16 | 18 | 40 | 53 |
| 50–64 | 32 | 7.2 | 52 | 4 | 4 | 8 | 11 | 12 | 17 | 50 |
| 65+ | 103 | 13.5 | 186 | 3 | 4 | 8 | 16 | 43 | 43 | 45 |
| **TOTAL SINGLE DX** | 36 | 2.0 | 2 | 1 | 1 | 1 | 3 | 5 | 5 | 6 |
| **TOTAL MULTIPLE DX** | 266 | 8.5 | 113 | 1 | 2 | 4 | 10 | 20 | 41 | 47 |
| **TOTAL** | | | | | | | | | | |
| 0–19 Years | 124 | 3.2 | 36 | 1 | 1 | 2 | 2 | 6 | 12 | 30 |
| 20–34 | 16 | 7.9 | 86 | 2 | 3 | 5 | 7 | 12 | 33 | 40 |
| 35–49 | 27 | 9.8 | 105 | 4 | 4 | 4 | 16 | 18 | 30 | 53 |
| 50–64 | 32 | 7.2 | 52 | 2 | 4 | 4 | 11 | 12 | 17 | 50 |
| 65+ | 103 | 13.5 | 186 | 3 | 4 | 8 | 16 | 43 | 43 | 45 |
| **GRAND TOTAL** | 302 | 7.6 | 104 | 1 | 2 | 4 | 8 | 18 | 33 | 45 |

Length of Stay by Diagnosis and Operation, United States, 2000

# United States, October 1998–September 1999 Data, by Operation

## 44.66: CREAT EG SPHINCT COMPET. Formerly included in operation group(s) 606.

| Type of Patients | Observed Patients | Avg. Stay | Vari-ance | Percentiles | | | | | | |
|---|---|---|---|---|---|---|---|---|---|---|
| | | | | 10th | 25th | 50th | 75th | 90th | 95th | 99th |
| **1. SINGLE DX** | | | | | | | | | | |
| 0–19 Years | 357 | 2.9 | 3 | 1 | 2 | 2 | 4 | 5 | 6 | 8 |
| 20–34 | 314 | 1.8 | <1 | 1 | 1 | 1 | 2 | 3 | 3 | 5 |
| 35–49 | 551 | 2.0 | 1 | 1 | 1 | 2 | 2 | 4 | 4 | 5 |
| 50–64 | 251 | 1.9 | 2 | 1 | 1 | 2 | 3 | 3 | 4 | 7 |
| 65+ | 65 | 2.1 | 2 | 1 | 1 | 2 | 3 | 4 | 4 | 5 |
| **2. MULTIPLE DX** | | | | | | | | | | |
| 0–19 Years | 2,341 | 11.5 | 179 | 2 | 4 | 6 | 14 | 29 | 42 | 96 |
| 20–34 | 982 | 3.1 | 19 | 1 | 1 | 2 | 3 | 5 | 7 | 24 |
| 35–49 | 2,890 | 3.0 | 20 | 1 | 1 | 2 | 3 | 5 | 7 | 20 |
| 50–64 | 2,483 | 3.2 | 17 | 1 | 1 | 2 | 4 | 6 | 7 | 15 |
| 65+ | 1,426 | 5.5 | 63 | 2 | 2 | 3 | 6 | 10 | 15 | 61 |
| **TOTAL SINGLE DX** | 1,538 | 2.1 | 2 | 1 | 1 | 2 | 3 | 4 | 4 | 7 |
| **TOTAL MULTIPLE DX** | 10,122 | 5.1 | 69 | 1 | 2 | 3 | 5 | 10 | 19 | 54 |
| **TOTAL** | | | | | | | | | | |
| 0–19 Years | 2,698 | 10.3 | 163 | 2 | 3 | 6 | 12 | 27 | 38 | 90 |
| 20–34 | 1,296 | 2.8 | 15 | 1 | 1 | 2 | 3 | 5 | 6 | 23 |
| 35–49 | 3,441 | 2.9 | 16 | 1 | 1 | 2 | 3 | 5 | 7 | 18 |
| 50–64 | 2,734 | 3.0 | 16 | 1 | 1 | 2 | 3 | 6 | 7 | 15 |
| 65+ | 1,491 | 5.3 | 61 | 1 | 2 | 3 | 6 | 10 | 14 | 61 |
| **GRAND TOTAL** | 11,660 | 4.7 | 60 | 1 | 2 | 2 | 5 | 9 | 16 | 47 |

## 44.9: OTHER STOMACH OPERATIONS. Formerly included in operation group(s) 606.

| Type of Patients | Observed Patients | Avg. Stay | Vari-ance | Percentiles | | | | | | |
|---|---|---|---|---|---|---|---|---|---|---|
| | | | | 10th | 25th | 50th | 75th | 90th | 95th | 99th |
| **1. SINGLE DX** | | | | | | | | | | |
| 0–19 Years | 2 | 4.9 | 16 | 1 | 1 | 8 | 8 | 8 | 8 | 8 |
| 20–34 | 0 | | | | | | | | | |
| 35–49 | 2 | 3.0 | 0 | 3 | 3 | 3 | 3 | 3 | 3 | 3 |
| 50–64 | 2 | 4.7 | <1 | 4 | 4 | 5 | 5 | 5 | 5 | 5 |
| 65+ | 0 | | | | | | | | | |
| **2. MULTIPLE DX** | | | | | | | | | | |
| 0–19 Years | 9 | 16.7 | 156 | 3 | 7 | 12 | 31 | 31 | 39 | 39 |
| 20–34 | 12 | 7.6 | 25 | 2 | 4 | 8 | 8 | 13 | 21 | 21 |
| 35–49 | 30 | 5.2 | 29 | 1 | 2 | 4 | 6 | 9 | 22 | 23 |
| 50–64 | 20 | 7.3 | 23 | 2 | 5 | 7 | 7 | 18 | 18 | 20 |
| 65+ | 39 | 14.4 | 133 | 5 | 7 | 12 | 13 | 28 | 49 | 49 |
| **TOTAL SINGLE DX** | 6 | 4.0 | 4 | 1 | 3 | 3 | 5 | 8 | 8 | 8 |
| **TOTAL MULTIPLE DX** | 110 | 9.8 | 85 | 2 | 4 | 7 | 12 | 21 | 31 | 49 |
| **TOTAL** | | | | | | | | | | |
| 0–19 Years | 11 | 14.8 | 151 | 1 | 7 | 12 | 31 | 31 | 39 | 39 |
| 20–34 | 12 | 7.6 | 25 | 2 | 4 | 8 | 8 | 13 | 21 | 21 |
| 35–49 | 32 | 5.0 | 27 | 2 | 2 | 4 | 6 | 9 | 22 | 23 |
| 50–64 | 22 | 7.2 | 22 | 2 | 5 | 7 | 7 | 18 | 18 | 20 |
| 65+ | 39 | 14.4 | 133 | 5 | 7 | 12 | 13 | 28 | 49 | 49 |
| **GRAND TOTAL** | 116 | 9.5 | 83 | 2 | 4 | 7 | 12 | 20 | 28 | 49 |

## 44.69: GASTRIC REPAIR NEC. Formerly included in operation group(s) 606.

| Type of Patients | Observed Patients | Avg. Stay | Vari-ance | Percentiles | | | | | | |
|---|---|---|---|---|---|---|---|---|---|---|
| | | | | 10th | 25th | 50th | 75th | 90th | 95th | 99th |
| **1. SINGLE DX** | | | | | | | | | | |
| 0–19 Years | 9 | 2.7 | 4 | 1 | 2 | 2 | 2 | 5 | 5 | 11 |
| 20–34 | 90 | 3.1 | 2 | 2 | 2 | 3 | 4 | 5 | 5 | 7 |
| 35–49 | 85 | 3.8 | 2 | 2 | 3 | 4 | 5 | 5 | 5 | 7 |
| 50–64 | 13 | 2.6 | 2 | 1 | 2 | 2 | 3 | 5 | 5 | 7 |
| 65+ | 2 | 4.2 | 5 | 2 | 2 | 6 | 6 | 6 | 6 | 6 |
| **2. MULTIPLE DX** | | | | | | | | | | |
| 0–19 Years | 104 | 9.0 | 109 | 2 | 3 | 5 | 9 | 25 | 33 | 54 |
| 20–34 | 458 | 4.0 | 11 | 2 | 2 | 3 | 4 | 8 | 8 | 12 |
| 35–49 | 755 | 3.9 | 12 | 2 | 3 | 3 | 4 | 6 | 8 | 18 |
| 50–64 | 253 | 8.2 | 187 | 2 | 2 | 4 | 5 | 17 | 53 | 61 |
| 65+ | 85 | 9.1 | 51 | 4 | 5 | 6 | 10 | 18 | 24 | 34 |
| **TOTAL SINGLE DX** | 199 | 3.4 | 2 | 2 | 2 | 3 | 5 | 5 | 5 | 7 |
| **TOTAL MULTIPLE DX** | 1,655 | 5.4 | 53 | 2 | 3 | 3 | 5 | 9 | 16 | 53 |
| **TOTAL** | | | | | | | | | | |
| 0–19 Years | 113 | 8.6 | 105 | 2 | 2 | 5 | 9 | 25 | 33 | 54 |
| 20–34 | 548 | 3.9 | 10 | 2 | 2 | 3 | 4 | 8 | 8 | 12 |
| 35–49 | 840 | 3.9 | 11 | 2 | 3 | 3 | 5 | 6 | 7 | 17 |
| 50–64 | 266 | 8.0 | 181 | 2 | 3 | 4 | 5 | 17 | 53 | 61 |
| 65+ | 87 | 9.0 | 50 | 4 | 5 | 6 | 10 | 18 | 24 | 34 |
| **GRAND TOTAL** | 1,854 | 5.1 | 47 | 2 | 2 | 3 | 5 | 8 | 12 | 53 |

## 45.0: ENTEROTOMY. Formerly included in operation group(s) 610.

| Type of Patients | Observed Patients | Avg. Stay | Vari-ance | Percentiles | | | | | | |
|---|---|---|---|---|---|---|---|---|---|---|
| | | | | 10th | 25th | 50th | 75th | 90th | 95th | 99th |
| **1. SINGLE DX** | | | | | | | | | | |
| 0–19 Years | 4 | 3.6 | <1 | 3 | 3 | 4 | 4 | 4 | 5 | 5 |
| 20–34 | 4 | 4.8 | 2 | 3 | 3 | 6 | 6 | 6 | 6 | 6 |
| 35–49 | 8 | 4.1 | 2 | 2 | 4 | 4 | 5 | 5 | 5 | 7 |
| 50–64 | 6 | 7.4 | 10 | 2 | 4 | 7 | 8 | 14 | 14 | 14 |
| 65+ | 4 | 5.3 | 40 | 2 | 2 | 2 | 5 | 19 | 19 | 19 |
| **2. MULTIPLE DX** | | | | | | | | | | |
| 0–19 Years | 61 | 13.2 | 186 | 3 | 5 | 8 | 14 | 37 | 41 | 57 |
| 20–34 | 46 | 8.5 | 58 | 2 | 4 | 7 | 9 | 19 | 24 | 51 |
| 35–49 | 82 | 9.8 | 42 | 3 | 5 | 7 | 13 | 21 | 23 | 25 |
| 50–64 | 97 | 9.7 | 41 | 3 | 6 | 9 | 12 | 15 | 20 | 39 |
| 65+ | 237 | 11.7 | 76 | 4 | 6 | 10 | 14 | 22 | 28 | 42 |
| **TOTAL SINGLE DX** | 26 | 5.1 | 11 | 2 | 3 | 4 | 6 | 8 | 14 | 19 |
| **TOTAL MULTIPLE DX** | 523 | 11.0 | 77 | 3 | 5 | 9 | 13 | 21 | 26 | 42 |
| **TOTAL** | | | | | | | | | | |
| 0–19 Years | 65 | 12.7 | 181 | 3 | 4 | 8 | 14 | 35 | 41 | 57 |
| 20–34 | 50 | 8.3 | 55 | 2 | 4 | 6 | 9 | 19 | 24 | 51 |
| 35–49 | 90 | 9.4 | 42 | 3 | 5 | 7 | 12 | 21 | 23 | 25 |
| 50–64 | 103 | 9.6 | 39 | 3 | 6 | 8 | 12 | 15 | 20 | 39 |
| 65+ | 241 | 11.6 | 76 | 3 | 6 | 9 | 14 | 22 | 28 | 42 |
| **GRAND TOTAL** | 549 | 10.7 | 76 | 3 | 5 | 8 | 13 | 21 | 26 | 42 |

Length of Stay by Diagnosis and Operation, United States, 2000

# United States, October 1998–September 1999 Data, by Operation

## 45.14: CLSD (ENDO) SM INTEST BX. Formerly included in operation group(s) 607.

| Type of Patients | Observed Patients | Avg. Stay | Variance | 10th | 25th | 50th | 75th | 90th | 95th | 99th |
|---|---|---|---|---|---|---|---|---|---|---|
| **1. SINGLE DX** | | | | | | | | | | |
| 0–19 Years | 5 | 1.5 | <1 | 1 | 1 | 1 | 2 | 2 | 2 | 2 |
| 20–34 | 5 | 2.4 | <1 | 2 | 3 | 3 | 3 | 3 | 4 | 4 |
| 35–49 | 4 | 2.9 | <1 | 2 | 3 | 3 | 3 | 4 | 4 | 4 |
| 50–64 | 4 | 1.9 | <1 | 1 | 2 | 2 | 2 | 2 | 2 | 2 |
| 65+ | 1 | 6.0 | 0 | 6 | 6 | 6 | 6 | 6 | 6 | 6 |
| **2. MULTIPLE DX** | | | | | | | | | | |
| 0–19 Years | 29 | 8.2 | 57 | 1 | 3 | 5 | 18 | 21 | 21 | 21 |
| 20–34 | 57 | 15.8 | 397 | 2 | 3 | 7 | 13 | 57 | 57 | 57 |
| 35–49 | 78 | 6.3 | 44 | 2 | 3 | 5 | 7 | 14 | 20 | 41 |
| 50–64 | 99 | 4.4 | 11 | 2 | 2 | 3 | 4 | 10 | 11 | 14 |
| 65+ | 212 | 6.2 | 23 | 2 | 3 | 5 | 7 | 12 | 16 | 26 |
| **TOTAL SINGLE DX** | 19 | 2.3 | <1 | 1 | 2 | 2 | 3 | 3 | 4 | 6 |
| **TOTAL MULTIPLE DX** | 475 | 7.1 | 81 | 2 | 3 | 4 | 8 | 14 | 21 | 57 |
| **TOTAL** | | | | | | | | | | |
| 0–19 Years | 34 | 7.7 | 56 | 1 | 1 | 5 | 17 | 21 | 21 | 21 |
| 20–34 | 62 | 14.5 | 373 | 2 | 3 | 6 | 13 | 57 | 57 | 57 |
| 35–49 | 82 | 6.1 | 42 | 2 | 3 | 5 | 7 | 14 | 20 | 41 |
| 50–64 | 103 | 4.4 | 11 | 2 | 2 | 3 | 4 | 10 | 11 | 14 |
| 65+ | 213 | 6.2 | 23 | 2 | 3 | 5 | 7 | 12 | 16 | 26 |
| **GRAND TOTAL** | 494 | 7.0 | 79 | 2 | 3 | 4 | 7 | 13 | 20 | 57 |

## 45.16: EGD WITH CLOSED BIOPSY. Formerly included in operation group(s) 607.

| Type of Patients | Observed Patients | Avg. Stay | Variance | 10th | 25th | 50th | 75th | 90th | 95th | 99th |
|---|---|---|---|---|---|---|---|---|---|---|
| **1. SINGLE DX** | | | | | | | | | | |
| 0–19 Years | 762 | 1.7 | 3 | 1 | 1 | 1 | 2 | 4 | 5 | 8 |
| 20–34 | 281 | 2.4 | 3 | 1 | 2 | 2 | 3 | 4 | 5 | 8 |
| 35–49 | 378 | 2.4 | 3 | 1 | 2 | 2 | 3 | 4 | 5 | 8 |
| 50–64 | 205 | 2.7 | 2 | 1 | 2 | 3 | 4 | 4 | 5 | 9 |
| 65+ | 171 | 3.6 | 8 | 1 | 3 | 3 | 4 | 7 | 9 | 13 |
| **2. MULTIPLE DX** | | | | | | | | | | |
| 0–19 Years | 3,805 | 4.9 | 39 | 1 | 2 | 3 | 6 | 11 | 16 | 33 |
| 20–34 | 6,748 | 4.2 | 20 | 1 | 2 | 3 | 5 | 8 | 11 | 21 |
| 35–49 | 18,180 | 4.6 | 22 | 2 | 2 | 4 | 6 | 9 | 12 | 23 |
| 50–64 | 22,615 | 4.9 | 19 | 2 | 2 | 4 | 6 | 9 | 13 | 22 |
| 65+ | 57,914 | 5.9 | 25 | 2 | 3 | 5 | 7 | 11 | 15 | 25 |
| **TOTAL SINGLE DX** | 1,797 | 2.1 | 3 | 1 | 1 | 2 | 3 | 4 | 5 | 9 |
| **TOTAL MULTIPLE DX** | 109,262 | 5.3 | 24 | 2 | 2 | 4 | 7 | 10 | 14 | 25 |
| **TOTAL** | | | | | | | | | | |
| 0–19 Years | 4,567 | 4.1 | 32 | 1 | 1 | 2 | 5 | 9 | 14 | 29 |
| 20–34 | 7,029 | 4.1 | 19 | 1 | 2 | 3 | 5 | 8 | 11 | 21 |
| 35–49 | 18,558 | 4.6 | 22 | 1 | 2 | 4 | 6 | 9 | 12 | 23 |
| 50–64 | 22,820 | 4.9 | 19 | 2 | 2 | 4 | 6 | 9 | 13 | 22 |
| 65+ | 58,085 | 5.9 | 25 | 2 | 3 | 5 | 7 | 11 | 15 | 25 |
| **GRAND TOTAL** | 111,059 | 5.2 | 24 | 1 | 2 | 4 | 6 | 10 | 14 | 24 |

## 45.1: SMALL BOWEL DXTIC PX. Formerly included in operation group(s) 607, 618, 631.

| Type of Patients | Observed Patients | Avg. Stay | Variance | 10th | 25th | 50th | 75th | 90th | 95th | 99th |
|---|---|---|---|---|---|---|---|---|---|---|
| **1. SINGLE DX** | | | | | | | | | | |
| 0–19 Years | 1,002 | 1.8 | 3 | 1 | 1 | 1 | 2 | 2 | 5 | 10 |
| 20–34 | 537 | 2.3 | 3 | 1 | 1 | 2 | 3 | 4 | 5 | 7 |
| 35–49 | 677 | 2.6 | 3 | 1 | 1 | 2 | 3 | 4 | 6 | 8 |
| 50–64 | 392 | 2.6 | 3 | 1 | 1 | 2 | 3 | 4 | 5 | 9 |
| 65+ | 355 | 3.4 | 10 | 2 | 2 | 2 | 4 | 7 | 9 | 15 |
| **2. MULTIPLE DX** | | | | | | | | | | |
| 0–19 Years | 4,799 | 4.8 | 38 | 1 | 1 | 3 | 6 | 11 | 16 | 33 |
| 20–34 | 10,548 | 4.3 | 23 | 1 | 2 | 3 | 5 | 8 | 12 | 23 |
| 35–49 | 28,987 | 4.7 | 22 | 1 | 2 | 3 | 6 | 9 | 12 | 23 |
| 50–64 | 35,240 | 5.0 | 22 | 1 | 2 | 4 | 6 | 10 | 13 | 23 |
| 65+ | 93,252 | 6.0 | 26 | 2 | 3 | 5 | 7 | 12 | 15 | 26 |
| **TOTAL SINGLE DX** | 2,963 | 2.3 | 4 | 1 | 1 | 2 | 3 | 4 | 6 | 11 |
| **TOTAL MULTIPLE DX** | 172,826 | 5.4 | 25 | 2 | 2 | 4 | 7 | 11 | 14 | 25 |
| **TOTAL** | | | | | | | | | | |
| 0–19 Years | 5,801 | 4.1 | 32 | 1 | 1 | 2 | 5 | 9 | 14 | 29 |
| 20–34 | 11,085 | 4.2 | 23 | 1 | 2 | 3 | 5 | 8 | 11 | 21 |
| 35–49 | 29,664 | 4.6 | 22 | 1 | 2 | 3 | 6 | 9 | 12 | 22 |
| 50–64 | 35,632 | 5.0 | 21 | 1 | 2 | 4 | 6 | 10 | 13 | 23 |
| 65+ | 93,607 | 6.0 | 26 | 2 | 3 | 5 | 7 | 12 | 15 | 26 |
| **GRAND TOTAL** | 175,789 | 5.4 | 25 | 2 | 2 | 4 | 7 | 10 | 14 | 25 |

## 45.13: SM BOWEL ENDOSCOPY NEC. Formerly included in operation group(s) 618.

| Type of Patients | Observed Patients | Avg. Stay | Variance | 10th | 25th | 50th | 75th | 90th | 95th | 99th |
|---|---|---|---|---|---|---|---|---|---|---|
| **1. SINGLE DX** | | | | | | | | | | |
| 0–19 Years | 230 | 1.8 | 4 | 1 | 1 | 1 | 2 | 3 | 5 | 11 |
| 20–34 | 248 | 2.3 | 3 | 1 | 1 | 2 | 3 | 4 | 5 | 7 |
| 35–49 | 294 | 2.8 | 3 | 1 | 1 | 3 | 3 | 5 | 6 | 9 |
| 50–64 | 177 | 2.4 | 3 | 1 | 1 | 2 | 3 | 5 | 5 | 9 |
| 65+ | 182 | 3.3 | 11 | 2 | 2 | 2 | 4 | 6 | 9 | 15 |
| **2. MULTIPLE DX** | | | | | | | | | | |
| 0–19 Years | 938 | 4.1 | 27 | 1 | 1 | 3 | 5 | 8 | 13 | 27 |
| 20–34 | 3,702 | 4.3 | 20 | 1 | 2 | 3 | 5 | 8 | 12 | 23 |
| 35–49 | 10,667 | 4.8 | 21 | 1 | 2 | 4 | 6 | 10 | 12 | 22 |
| 50–64 | 12,462 | 5.3 | 25 | 2 | 2 | 4 | 6 | 10 | 14 | 24 |
| 65+ | 35,010 | 6.2 | 28 | 2 | 3 | 5 | 8 | 12 | 16 | 27 |
| **TOTAL SINGLE DX** | 1,131 | 2.6 | 5 | 1 | 1 | 2 | 3 | 4 | 6 | 14 |
| **TOTAL MULTIPLE DX** | 62,779 | 5.6 | 26 | 2 | 3 | 4 | 7 | 11 | 15 | 26 |
| **TOTAL** | | | | | | | | | | |
| 0–19 Years | 1,168 | 3.7 | 23 | 1 | 1 | 2 | 4 | 8 | 11 | 27 |
| 20–34 | 3,950 | 4.2 | 19 | 1 | 2 | 3 | 5 | 8 | 12 | 22 |
| 35–49 | 10,961 | 4.8 | 21 | 1 | 2 | 3 | 6 | 10 | 12 | 22 |
| 50–64 | 12,639 | 5.2 | 25 | 2 | 2 | 4 | 6 | 10 | 14 | 24 |
| 65+ | 35,192 | 6.1 | 28 | 2 | 3 | 5 | 8 | 12 | 16 | 27 |
| **GRAND TOTAL** | 63,910 | 5.6 | 26 | 2 | 3 | 4 | 7 | 11 | 15 | 25 |

Length of Stay by Diagnosis and Operation, United States, 2000

# United States, October 1998–September 1999 Data, by Operation

## 45.2: LG INTESTINE DXTIC PX. Formerly included in operation group(s) 607, 618, 631.

| Type of Patients | Observed Patients | Avg. Stay | Variance | 10th | 25th | 50th | 75th | 90th | 95th | 99th |
|---|---|---|---|---|---|---|---|---|---|---|
| **1. SINGLE DX** | | | | | | | | | | |
| 0–19 Years | 402 | 2.4 | 7 | 1 | 1 | 1 | 3 | 5 | 7 | 13 |
| 20–34 | 562 | 3.0 | 6 | 1 | 1 | 2 | 4 | 6 | 7 | 12 |
| 35–49 | 619 | 3.4 | 6 | 1 | 2 | 3 | 5 | 6 | 8 | 13 |
| 50–64 | 454 | 2.9 | 4 | 1 | 1 | 2 | 3 | 6 | 7 | 9 |
| 65+ | 380 | 3.8 | 5 | 1 | 2 | 4 | 5 | 5 | 7 | 10 |
| **2. MULTIPLE DX** | | | | | | | | | | |
| 0–19 Years | 1,377 | 5.4 | 61 | 1 | 2 | 3 | 6 | 11 | 17 | 48 |
| 20–34 | 4,077 | 4.7 | 19 | 1 | 2 | 3 | 6 | 9 | 12 | 23 |
| 35–49 | 8,874 | 5.1 | 22 | 2 | 2 | 4 | 6 | 10 | 14 | 24 |
| 50–64 | 12,446 | 5.3 | 27 | 2 | 3 | 4 | 6 | 10 | 14 | 25 |
| 65+ | 42,132 | 5.9 | 25 | 2 | 3 | 5 | 7 | 11 | 15 | 25 |
| **TOTAL SINGLE DX** | 2,417 | 3.1 | 6 | 1 | 1 | 2 | 4 | 6 | 7 | 12 |
| **TOTAL MULTIPLE DX** | 68,906 | 5.6 | 26 | 2 | 3 | 4 | 7 | 11 | 14 | 25 |
| **TOTAL** | | | | | | | | | | |
| 0–19 Years | 1,779 | 4.5 | 47 | 1 | 1 | 3 | 5 | 10 | 14 | 33 |
| 20–34 | 4,639 | 4.5 | 17 | 1 | 2 | 3 | 5 | 9 | 12 | 22 |
| 35–49 | 9,493 | 5.0 | 22 | 2 | 2 | 4 | 6 | 10 | 14 | 24 |
| 50–64 | 12,900 | 5.2 | 27 | 2 | 2 | 4 | 6 | 10 | 13 | 25 |
| 65+ | 42,512 | 5.9 | 24 | 2 | 3 | 5 | 7 | 11 | 15 | 25 |
| **GRAND TOTAL** | 71,323 | 5.5 | 25 | 2 | 3 | 4 | 7 | 11 | 14 | 25 |

## 45.22: ENDO LG BOWEL THRU STOMA. Formerly included in operation group(s) 631.

| Type of Patients | Observed Patients | Avg. Stay | Variance | 10th | 25th | 50th | 75th | 90th | 95th | 99th |
|---|---|---|---|---|---|---|---|---|---|---|
| **1. SINGLE DX** | | | | | | | | | | |
| 0–19 Years | 1 | 11.0 | 0 | 11 | 11 | 11 | 11 | 11 | 11 | 11 |
| 20–34 | 0 | | | | | | | | | |
| 35–49 | 0 | | | | | | | | | |
| 50–64 | 1 | 2.0 | 0 | 2 | 2 | 2 | 2 | 2 | 2 | 2 |
| 65+ | 0 | | | | | | | | | |
| **2. MULTIPLE DX** | | | | | | | | | | |
| 0–19 Years | 5 | 9.4 | 151 | 2 | 2 | 2 | 12 | 33 | 33 | 33 |
| 20–34 | 5 | 6.0 | 13 | 3 | 3 | 4 | 11 | 11 | 11 | 11 |
| 35–49 | 29 | 4.2 | 17 | 1 | 1 | 3 | 5 | 9 | 13 | 23 |
| 50–64 | 64 | 4.8 | 20 | 2 | 2 | 3 | 5 | 11 | 15 | 20 |
| 65+ | 226 | 5.5 | 20 | 2 | 3 | 4 | 8 | 11 | 14 | 20 |
| **TOTAL SINGLE DX** | 2 | 10.1 | 8 | 2 | 11 | 11 | 11 | 11 | 11 | 11 |
| **TOTAL MULTIPLE DX** | 329 | 5.3 | 24 | 1 | 2 | 4 | 7 | 11 | 15 | 23 |
| **TOTAL** | | | | | | | | | | |
| 0–19 Years | 6 | 9.8 | 114 | 2 | 2 | 3 | 12 | 33 | 33 | 33 |
| 20–34 | 5 | 6.0 | 13 | 3 | 3 | 4 | 11 | 11 | 11 | 11 |
| 35–49 | 29 | 4.2 | 17 | 2 | 1 | 3 | 5 | 9 | 11 | 23 |
| 50–64 | 65 | 4.8 | 20 | 1 | 2 | 3 | 5 | 11 | 15 | 20 |
| 65+ | 226 | 5.5 | 20 | 2 | 3 | 4 | 8 | 11 | 14 | 20 |
| **GRAND TOTAL** | 331 | 5.4 | 24 | 1 | 2 | 4 | 7 | 11 | 15 | 23 |

## 45.23: COLONOSCOPY. Formerly included in operation group(s) 618.

| Type of Patients | Observed Patients | Avg. Stay | Variance | 10th | 25th | 50th | 75th | 90th | 95th | 99th |
|---|---|---|---|---|---|---|---|---|---|---|
| **1. SINGLE DX** | | | | | | | | | | |
| 0–19 Years | 46 | 1.9 | 3 | 1 | 1 | 2 | 2 | 3 | 5 | 14 |
| 20–34 | 130 | 2.7 | 5 | 1 | 1 | 2 | 4 | 5 | 6 | 13 |
| 35–49 | 207 | 2.7 | 4 | 1 | 2 | 2 | 3 | 6 | 7 | 9 |
| 50–64 | 216 | 2.3 | 2 | 1 | 2 | 2 | 3 | 4 | 5 | 7 |
| 65+ | 220 | 3.6 | 3 | 1 | 2 | 4 | 5 | 5 | 5 | 8 |
| **2. MULTIPLE DX** | | | | | | | | | | |
| 0–19 Years | 219 | 3.6 | 15 | 1 | 2 | 2 | 4 | 8 | 10 | 29 |
| 20–34 | 1,033 | 4.8 | 19 | 1 | 2 | 4 | 6 | 10 | 11 | 25 |
| 35–49 | 3,190 | 4.8 | 18 | 2 | 2 | 4 | 6 | 9 | 12 | 22 |
| 50–64 | 5,501 | 5.2 | 31 | 2 | 2 | 4 | 6 | 10 | 13 | 28 |
| 65+ | 21,415 | 5.5 | 21 | 2 | 3 | 4 | 7 | 10 | 13 | 23 |
| **TOTAL SINGLE DX** | 819 | 2.9 | 4 | 1 | 1 | 2 | 4 | 5 | 5 | 9 |
| **TOTAL MULTIPLE DX** | 31,358 | 5.3 | 22 | 2 | 3 | 4 | 7 | 10 | 13 | 24 |
| **TOTAL** | | | | | | | | | | |
| 0–19 Years | 265 | 3.2 | 13 | 1 | 1 | 2 | 4 | 6 | 10 | 18 |
| 20–34 | 1,163 | 4.4 | 18 | 1 | 2 | 3 | 5 | 9 | 11 | 22 |
| 35–49 | 3,397 | 4.7 | 18 | 1 | 2 | 3 | 6 | 9 | 12 | 20 |
| 50–64 | 5,717 | 5.1 | 30 | 1 | 2 | 4 | 6 | 10 | 13 | 26 |
| 65+ | 21,635 | 5.4 | 20 | 2 | 3 | 4 | 7 | 10 | 13 | 23 |
| **GRAND TOTAL** | 32,177 | 5.2 | 22 | 2 | 2 | 4 | 6 | 10 | 13 | 23 |

## 45.24: FLEXIBLE SIGMOIDOSCOPY. Formerly included in operation group(s) 631.

| Type of Patients | Observed Patients | Avg. Stay | Variance | 10th | 25th | 50th | 75th | 90th | 95th | 99th |
|---|---|---|---|---|---|---|---|---|---|---|
| **1. SINGLE DX** | | | | | | | | | | |
| 0–19 Years | 36 | 1.9 | 3 | 1 | 1 | 1 | 2 | 4 | 6 | 8 |
| 20–34 | 86 | 2.7 | 6 | 1 | 1 | 2 | 3 | 5 | 6 | 18 |
| 35–49 | 96 | 2.6 | 2 | 1 | 2 | 2 | 3 | 5 | 6 | 8 |
| 50–64 | 60 | 3.4 | 5 | 1 | 2 | 3 | 4 | 6 | 7 | 11 |
| 65+ | 66 | 4.9 | 25 | 1 | 2 | 3 | 7 | 10 | 11 | 27 |
| **2. MULTIPLE DX** | | | | | | | | | | |
| 0–19 Years | 146 | 5.2 | 68 | 1 | 1 | 3 | 5 | 13 | 50 | >99 |
| 20–34 | 556 | 4.5 | 21 | 1 | 2 | 3 | 5 | 9 | 13 | 22 |
| 35–49 | 1,186 | 4.7 | 25 | 1 | 2 | 3 | 5 | 9 | 13 | 24 |
| 50–64 | 1,438 | 6.0 | 42 | 1 | 3 | 4 | 7 | 14 | 17 | 27 |
| 65+ | 5,528 | 6.6 | 31 | 2 | 3 | 5 | 8 | 13 | 16 | 29 |
| **TOTAL SINGLE DX** | 344 | 3.0 | 8 | 1 | 1 | 2 | 3 | 6 | 9 | 12 |
| **TOTAL MULTIPLE DX** | 8,854 | 6.1 | 33 | 2 | 3 | 4 | 7 | 12 | 16 | 29 |
| **TOTAL** | | | | | | | | | | |
| 0–19 Years | 182 | 4.4 | 55 | 1 | 1 | 2 | 5 | 11 | 20 | >99 |
| 20–34 | 642 | 4.3 | 19 | 1 | 2 | 3 | 5 | 9 | 13 | 22 |
| 35–49 | 1,282 | 4.6 | 24 | 1 | 2 | 4 | 5 | 9 | 13 | 24 |
| 50–64 | 1,498 | 5.9 | 41 | 1 | 2 | 4 | 7 | 13 | 17 | 27 |
| 65+ | 5,594 | 6.6 | 31 | 2 | 3 | 5 | 8 | 13 | 16 | 29 |
| **GRAND TOTAL** | 9,198 | 5.9 | 32 | 2 | 2 | 4 | 7 | 12 | 16 | 29 |

Length of Stay by Diagnosis and Operation, United States, 2000

# United States, October 1998–September 1999 Data, by Operation

## 45.25: CLSD (ENDO) LG INTEST BX. Formerly included in operation group(s) 607.

| Type of Patients | Observed Patients | Avg. Stay | Vari-ance | Percentiles | | | | | | |
|---|---|---|---|---|---|---|---|---|---|---|
| | | | | 10th | 25th | 50th | 75th | 90th | 95th | 99th |
| **1. SINGLE DX** | | | | | | | | | | |
| 0–19 Years | 312 | 2.5 | 8 | 1 | 1 | 1 | 3 | 6 | 8 | 13 |
| 20–34 | 345 | 3.3 | 6 | 1 | 2 | 3 | 4 | 6 | 9 | 12 |
| 35–49 | 315 | 3.9 | 8 | 1 | 2 | 3 | 5 | 7 | 10 | 15 |
| 50–64 | 176 | 3.4 | 5 | 1 | 2 | 3 | 4 | 7 | 8 | 10 |
| 65+ | 93 | 4.1 | 7 | 1 | 2 | 3 | 6 | 7 | 9 | 10 |
| **2. MULTIPLE DX** | | | | | | | | | | |
| 0–19 Years | 992 | 5.7 | 68 | 1 | 2 | 4 | 7 | 12 | 18 | 36 |
| 20–34 | 2,475 | 4.7 | 18 | 2 | 2 | 3 | 6 | 9 | 12 | 23 |
| 35–49 | 4,451 | 5.4 | 24 | 2 | 3 | 4 | 6 | 11 | 16 | 26 |
| 50–64 | 5,419 | 5.3 | 20 | 2 | 3 | 4 | 6 | 10 | 13 | 23 |
| 65+ | 14,922 | 6.4 | 28 | 2 | 3 | 5 | 8 | 12 | 16 | 26 |
| **TOTAL SINGLE DX** | 1,241 | 3.2 | 7 | 1 | 1 | 2 | 4 | 6 | 9 | 13 |
| **TOTAL MULTIPLE DX** | 28,259 | 5.8 | 27 | 2 | 3 | 4 | 7 | 11 | 15 | 26 |
| **TOTAL** | | | | | | | | | | |
| 0–19 Years | 1,304 | 4.7 | 52 | 1 | 1 | 3 | 5 | 10 | 15 | 31 |
| 20–34 | 2,820 | 4.6 | 17 | 1 | 2 | 3 | 5 | 9 | 12 | 23 |
| 35–49 | 4,766 | 5.3 | 23 | 2 | 3 | 4 | 6 | 10 | 15 | 26 |
| 50–64 | 5,595 | 5.2 | 20 | 2 | 3 | 4 | 6 | 10 | 13 | 22 |
| 65+ | 15,015 | 6.4 | 27 | 2 | 3 | 5 | 8 | 12 | 16 | 26 |
| **GRAND TOTAL** | 29,500 | 5.7 | 26 | 2 | 3 | 4 | 7 | 11 | 15 | 25 |

## 45.30: ENDO EXC/DESTR DUOD LES. Formerly included in operation group(s) 607.

| Type of Patients | Observed Patients | Avg. Stay | Vari-ance | Percentiles | | | | | | |
|---|---|---|---|---|---|---|---|---|---|---|
| | | | | 10th | 25th | 50th | 75th | 90th | 95th | 99th |
| **1. SINGLE DX** | | | | | | | | | | |
| 0–19 Years | 0 | | | | | | | | | |
| 20–34 | 0 | | | | | | | | | |
| 35–49 | 1 | 3.0 | 0 | 3 | 3 | 3 | 3 | 3 | 3 | 3 |
| 50–64 | 2 | 1.5 | <1 | 1 | 1 | 2 | 2 | 2 | 2 | 2 |
| 65+ | 2 | 2.0 | 0 | 2 | 2 | 2 | 2 | 2 | 2 | 2 |
| **2. MULTIPLE DX** | | | | | | | | | | |
| 0–19 Years | 4 | 3.7 | 14 | 1 | 1 | 3 | 3 | 11 | 11 | 11 |
| 20–34 | 11 | 2.8 | 1 | 2 | 2 | 3 | 3 | 4 | 6 | 6 |
| 35–49 | 45 | 3.7 | 8 | 2 | 2 | 3 | 4 | 7 | 8 | 15 |
| 50–64 | 82 | 4.2 | 13 | 2 | 2 | 3 | 5 | 7 | 10 | 23 |
| 65+ | 265 | 5.4 | 18 | 2 | 3 | 5 | 7 | 10 | 13 | 21 |
| **TOTAL SINGLE DX** | 5 | 2.0 | <1 | 2 | 2 | 2 | 2 | 3 | 3 | 3 |
| **TOTAL MULTIPLE DX** | 407 | 4.9 | 16 | 2 | 2 | 4 | 6 | 9 | 13 | 21 |
| **TOTAL** | | | | | | | | | | |
| 0–19 Years | 4 | 3.7 | 14 | 2 | 2 | 3 | 3 | 11 | 11 | 11 |
| 20–34 | 11 | 2.8 | 1 | 2 | 2 | 3 | 3 | 4 | 6 | 6 |
| 35–49 | 46 | 3.7 | 8 | 2 | 2 | 3 | 4 | 7 | 8 | 15 |
| 50–64 | 84 | 4.2 | 13 | 2 | 2 | 3 | 5 | 7 | 10 | 23 |
| 65+ | 267 | 5.4 | 18 | 2 | 3 | 5 | 7 | 9 | 13 | 21 |
| **GRAND TOTAL** | 412 | 4.8 | 16 | 2 | 2 | 4 | 6 | 9 | 13 | 21 |

## 45.3: LOC EXC/DESTR SMB LES. Formerly included in operation group(s) 607.

| Type of Patients | Observed Patients | Avg. Stay | Vari-ance | Percentiles | | | | | | |
|---|---|---|---|---|---|---|---|---|---|---|
| | | | | 10th | 25th | 50th | 75th | 90th | 95th | 99th |
| **1. SINGLE DX** | | | | | | | | | | |
| 0–19 Years | 45 | 3.8 | 10 | 1 | 2 | 3 | 4 | 7 | 14 | 14 |
| 20–34 | 15 | 3.1 | 6 | 1 | 2 | 3 | 4 | 6 | 6 | 6 |
| 35–49 | 11 | 4.6 | 4 | 2 | 3 | 6 | 6 | 6 | 6 | 7 |
| 50–64 | 15 | 4.4 | 5 | 2 | 3 | 4 | 6 | 8 | 9 | 11 |
| 65+ | 5 | 4.2 | 8 | 1 | 2 | 3 | 6 | 9 | 9 | 9 |
| **2. MULTIPLE DX** | | | | | | | | | | |
| 0–19 Years | 181 | 7.4 | 84 | 2 | 4 | 5 | 7 | 13 | 21 | 61 |
| 20–34 | 71 | 5.5 | 10 | 2 | 3 | 6 | 7 | 9 | 10 | 20 |
| 35–49 | 137 | 5.9 | 25 | 2 | 3 | 5 | 8 | 10 | 15 | 26 |
| 50–64 | 211 | 6.6 | 41 | 2 | 3 | 5 | 8 | 12 | 18 | 26 |
| 65+ | 482 | 7.1 | 35 | 3 | 3 | 5 | 8 | 15 | 18 | 27 |
| **TOTAL SINGLE DX** | 91 | 3.9 | 7 | 1 | 2 | 3 | 5 | 7 | 9 | 14 |
| **TOTAL MULTIPLE DX** | 1,082 | 6.8 | 42 | 2 | 3 | 5 | 8 | 13 | 18 | 33 |
| **TOTAL** | | | | | | | | | | |
| 0–19 Years | 226 | 6.6 | 71 | 2 | 3 | 5 | 7 | 12 | 16 | 61 |
| 20–34 | 86 | 5.1 | 10 | 2 | 3 | 5 | 7 | 9 | 10 | 20 |
| 35–49 | 148 | 5.8 | 23 | 2 | 3 | 5 | 8 | 11 | 15 | 25 |
| 50–64 | 226 | 6.5 | 39 | 2 | 3 | 4 | 8 | 11 | 18 | 26 |
| 65+ | 487 | 7.1 | 35 | 3 | 3 | 5 | 8 | 15 | 18 | 27 |
| **GRAND TOTAL** | 1,173 | 6.6 | 40 | 2 | 3 | 5 | 8 | 13 | 17 | 30 |

## 45.33: LOC EXC SM BOWEL LES NEC. Formerly included in operation group(s) 607.

| Type of Patients | Observed Patients | Avg. Stay | Vari-ance | Percentiles | | | | | | |
|---|---|---|---|---|---|---|---|---|---|---|
| | | | | 10th | 25th | 50th | 75th | 90th | 95th | 99th |
| **1. SINGLE DX** | | | | | | | | | | |
| 0–19 Years | 42 | 3.0 | 2 | 1 | 2 | 3 | 4 | 5 | 6 | 7 |
| 20–34 | 13 | 2.9 | 2 | 2 | 2 | 3 | 3 | 6 | 6 | 6 |
| 35–49 | 8 | 4.8 | 4 | 2 | 3 | 6 | 6 | 6 | 7 | 7 |
| 50–64 | 8 | 3.7 | 4 | 3 | 3 | 3 | 4 | 4 | 11 | 11 |
| 65+ | 0 | | | | | | | | | |
| **2. MULTIPLE DX** | | | | | | | | | | |
| 0–19 Years | 159 | 7.1 | 91 | 2 | 4 | 5 | 6 | 12 | 23 | 61 |
| 20–34 | 50 | 5.4 | 7 | 2 | 3 | 6 | 7 | 9 | 9 | 11 |
| 35–49 | 63 | 6.2 | 18 | 3 | 4 | 5 | 8 | 10 | 12 | 19 |
| 50–64 | 58 | 8.6 | 31 | 3 | 4 | 7 | 10 | 16 | 22 | 26 |
| 65+ | 77 | 9.4 | 55 | 3 | 5 | 6 | 14 | 18 | 26 | 29 |
| **TOTAL SINGLE DX** | 71 | 3.3 | 3 | 1 | 2 | 3 | 4 | 6 | 6 | 7 |
| **TOTAL MULTIPLE DX** | 407 | 7.6 | 55 | 2 | 4 | 5 | 9 | 15 | 21 | 44 |
| **TOTAL** | | | | | | | | | | |
| 0–19 Years | 201 | 6.3 | 76 | 2 | 3 | 4 | 6 | 10 | 16 | 61 |
| 20–34 | 63 | 5.0 | 7 | 2 | 3 | 5 | 7 | 9 | 9 | 11 |
| 35–49 | 71 | 6.0 | 16 | 3 | 3 | 6 | 8 | 9 | 11 | 19 |
| 50–64 | 66 | 8.1 | 30 | 3 | 4 | 6 | 10 | 16 | 22 | 22 |
| 65+ | 77 | 9.4 | 55 | 3 | 5 | 6 | 14 | 18 | 26 | 29 |
| **GRAND TOTAL** | 478 | 7.0 | 50 | 2 | 3 | 5 | 8 | 14 | 18 | 33 |

Length of Stay by Diagnosis and Operation, United States, 2000

# United States, October 1998–September 1999 Data, by Operation

## 45.4: LOC DESTR LG BOWEL LES. Formerly included in operation group(s) 607.

| Type of Patients | Observed Patients | Avg. Stay | Variance | Percentiles | | | | | | |
|---|---|---|---|---|---|---|---|---|---|---|
| | | | | 10th | 25th | 50th | 75th | 90th | 95th | 99th |
| **1. SINGLE DX** | | | | | | | | | | |
| 0–19 Years | 25 | 1.5 | 1 | 1 | 1 | 1 | 1 | 4 | 4 | 5 |
| 20–34 | 24 | 3.2 | 4 | 1 | 1 | 3 | 5 | 6 | 7 | 7 |
| 35–49 | 34 | 2.0 | 3 | 1 | 1 | 1 | 3 | 5 | 5 | 8 |
| 50–64 | 63 | 1.5 | 2 | 1 | 1 | 1 | 1 | 3 | 4 | 6 |
| 65+ | 67 | 1.8 | 2 | 1 | 1 | 1 | 2 | 4 | 5 | 7 |
| **2. MULTIPLE DX** | | | | | | | | | | |
| 0–19 Years | 42 | 3.8 | 16 | 1 | 1 | 3 | 5 | 8 | 8 | 24 |
| 20–34 | 227 | 3.7 | 8 | 1 | 2 | 3 | 5 | 7 | 8 | 15 |
| 35–49 | 1,102 | 4.5 | 15 | 1 | 2 | 3 | 6 | 9 | 12 | 19 |
| 50–64 | 3,186 | 4.7 | 15 | 1 | 2 | 4 | 6 | 9 | 11 | 20 |
| 65+ | 11,692 | 5.7 | 24 | 2 | 3 | 4 | 7 | 11 | 14 | 26 |
| **TOTAL SINGLE DX** | 213 | 1.8 | 2 | 1 | 1 | 1 | 2 | 4 | 5 | 7 |
| **TOTAL MULTIPLE DX** | 16,249 | 5.4 | 21 | 2 | 3 | 4 | 7 | 10 | 13 | 24 |
| **TOTAL** | | | | | | | | | | |
| 0–19 Years | 67 | 2.3 | 7 | 1 | 1 | 1 | 3 | 4 | 8 | 15 |
| 20–34 | 251 | 3.6 | 8 | 1 | 2 | 3 | 5 | 7 | 8 | 13 |
| 35–49 | 1,136 | 4.5 | 15 | 1 | 2 | 3 | 6 | 9 | 12 | 19 |
| 50–64 | 3,249 | 4.6 | 15 | 1 | 2 | 3 | 6 | 9 | 11 | 20 |
| 65+ | 11,759 | 5.7 | 24 | 2 | 3 | 4 | 7 | 11 | 14 | 26 |
| **GRAND TOTAL** | 16,462 | 5.3 | 21 | 2 | 2 | 4 | 7 | 10 | 13 | 23 |

## 45.41: LOC EXC LG BOWEL LES. Formerly included in operation group(s) 607.

| Type of Patients | Observed Patients | Avg. Stay | Variance | Percentiles | | | | | | |
|---|---|---|---|---|---|---|---|---|---|---|
| | | | | 10th | 25th | 50th | 75th | 90th | 95th | 99th |
| **1. SINGLE DX** | | | | | | | | | | |
| 0–19 Years | 6 | 3.7 | 1 | 3 | 3 | 4 | 4 | 4 | 5 | 7 |
| 20–34 | 13 | 3.7 | 5 | 1 | 1 | 3 | 6 | 7 | 7 | 7 |
| 35–49 | 9 | 3.7 | 2 | 3 | 3 | 3 | 4 | 5 | 5 | 7 |
| 50–64 | 13 | 2.6 | 3 | 1 | 1 | 3 | 3 | 5 | 5 | 6 |
| 65+ | 15 | 3.2 | 3 | 1 | 1 | 4 | 5 | 5 | 5 | 5 |
| **2. MULTIPLE DX** | | | | | | | | | | |
| 0–19 Years | 4 | 9.9 | 34 | 5 | 8 | 8 | 8 | 24 | 24 | 24 |
| 20–34 | 28 | 3.0 | 4 | 1 | 1 | 2 | 4 | 6 | 7 | 11 |
| 35–49 | 41 | 5.4 | 32 | 2 | 3 | 4 | 6 | 7 | 12 | 29 |
| 50–64 | 97 | 6.0 | 13 | 2 | 4 | 5 | 8 | 10 | 14 | 18 |
| 65+ | 150 | 7.5 | 28 | 3 | 4 | 6 | 9 | 16 | 21 | 26 |
| **TOTAL SINGLE DX** | 56 | 3.3 | 3 | 1 | 2 | 3 | 5 | 5 | 6 | 7 |
| **TOTAL MULTIPLE DX** | 320 | 6.4 | 24 | 2 | 3 | 5 | 8 | 11 | 18 | 26 |
| **TOTAL** | | | | | | | | | | |
| 0–19 Years | 10 | 6.1 | 23 | 3 | 4 | 4 | 8 | 8 | 15 | 24 |
| 20–34 | 41 | 3.2 | 4 | 1 | 3 | 3 | 5 | 6 | 7 | 7 |
| 35–49 | 50 | 5.1 | 28 | 3 | 3 | 5 | 6 | 7 | 9 | 29 |
| 50–64 | 110 | 5.6 | 13 | 2 | 3 | 5 | 7 | 10 | 11 | 18 |
| 65+ | 165 | 7.1 | 27 | 3 | 4 | 6 | 8 | 14 | 21 | 26 |
| **GRAND TOTAL** | 376 | 6.0 | 22 | 2 | 3 | 5 | 7 | 10 | 16 | 26 |

## 45.42: ENDO COLON POLYPECTOMY. Formerly included in operation group(s) 607.

| Type of Patients | Observed Patients | Avg. Stay | Variance | Percentiles | | | | | | |
|---|---|---|---|---|---|---|---|---|---|---|
| | | | | 10th | 25th | 50th | 75th | 90th | 95th | 99th |
| **1. SINGLE DX** | | | | | | | | | | |
| 0–19 Years | 16 | 1.1 | <1 | 1 | 1 | 1 | 1 | 1 | 2 | 3 |
| 20–34 | 5 | 2.8 | 5 | 1 | 1 | 2 | 3 | 7 | 7 | 7 |
| 35–49 | 11 | 1.4 | 2 | 1 | 1 | 1 | 1 | 1 | 2 | 8 |
| 50–64 | 25 | 1.3 | 3 | 1 | 1 | 1 | 1 | 1 | 2 | 14 |
| 65+ | 42 | 1.4 | 1 | 1 | 1 | 1 | 1 | 2 | 3 | 7 |
| **2. MULTIPLE DX** | | | | | | | | | | |
| 0–19 Years | 35 | 2.5 | 2 | 1 | 1 | 2 | 3 | 5 | 5 | 6 |
| 20–34 | 157 | 3.4 | 8 | 1 | 2 | 3 | 5 | 6 | 7 | 15 |
| 35–49 | 919 | 4.4 | 13 | 1 | 2 | 3 | 6 | 8 | 11 | 18 |
| 50–64 | 2,561 | 4.8 | 16 | 2 | 2 | 4 | 6 | 9 | 11 | 20 |
| 65+ | 9,425 | 5.6 | 23 | 2 | 3 | 4 | 7 | 11 | 14 | 25 |
| **TOTAL SINGLE DX** | 99 | 1.3 | 1 | 1 | 1 | 1 | 1 | 2 | 3 | 7 |
| **TOTAL MULTIPLE DX** | 13,097 | 5.4 | 21 | 2 | 3 | 4 | 7 | 10 | 13 | 24 |
| **TOTAL** | | | | | | | | | | |
| 0–19 Years | 51 | 1.5 | 1 | 1 | 1 | 1 | 2 | 3 | 4 | 5 |
| 20–34 | 162 | 3.4 | 8 | 1 | 2 | 3 | 5 | 6 | 7 | 15 |
| 35–49 | 930 | 4.4 | 13 | 1 | 2 | 3 | 6 | 8 | 11 | 18 |
| 50–64 | 2,586 | 4.8 | 16 | 1 | 2 | 4 | 6 | 9 | 11 | 20 |
| 65+ | 9,467 | 5.6 | 23 | 2 | 3 | 4 | 7 | 11 | 14 | 25 |
| **GRAND TOTAL** | 13,196 | 5.3 | 21 | 2 | 2 | 4 | 7 | 10 | 13 | 23 |

## 45.43: ENDO DESTR COLON LES NEC. Formerly included in operation group(s) 607.

| Type of Patients | Observed Patients | Avg. Stay | Variance | Percentiles | | | | | | |
|---|---|---|---|---|---|---|---|---|---|---|
| | | | | 10th | 25th | 50th | 75th | 90th | 95th | 99th |
| **1. SINGLE DX** | | | | | | | | | | |
| 0–19 Years | 2 | 2.6 | <1 | 2 | 2 | 3 | 3 | 3 | 3 | 3 |
| 20–34 | 6 | 2.6 | 2 | 1 | 2 | 2 | 3 | 5 | 5 | 5 |
| 35–49 | 14 | 1.7 | 1 | 1 | 1 | 1 | 2 | 2 | 3 | 5 |
| 50–64 | 25 | 1.3 | <1 | 1 | 1 | 1 | 2 | 2 | 3 | 6 |
| 65+ | 10 | 1.6 | <1 | 1 | 1 | 2 | 2 | 2 | 3 | 3 |
| **2. MULTIPLE DX** | | | | | | | | | | |
| 0–19 Years | 3 | 2.1 | 1 | 1 | 1 | 3 | 3 | 3 | 3 | 3 |
| 20–34 | 40 | 5.0 | 13 | 1 | 2 | 5 | 8 | 8 | 8 | 20 |
| 35–49 | 141 | 4.1 | 16 | 1 | 2 | 3 | 6 | 10 | 14 | 14 |
| 50–64 | 524 | 4.0 | 10 | 1 | 2 | 3 | 6 | 8 | 8 | 14 |
| 65+ | 2,102 | 5.8 | 27 | 2 | 3 | 4 | 7 | 11 | 13 | 28 |
| **TOTAL SINGLE DX** | 57 | 1.6 | 1 | 1 | 1 | 1 | 2 | 3 | 4 | 5 |
| **TOTAL MULTIPLE DX** | 2,810 | 5.4 | 23 | 2 | 2 | 4 | 7 | 11 | 12 | 22 |
| **TOTAL** | | | | | | | | | | |
| 0–19 Years | 5 | 2.4 | <1 | 1 | 2 | 3 | 3 | 3 | 3 | 3 |
| 20–34 | 46 | 4.8 | 12 | 1 | 2 | 4 | 8 | 8 | 8 | 20 |
| 35–49 | 155 | 3.9 | 15 | 1 | 2 | 3 | 6 | 9 | 14 | 14 |
| 50–64 | 549 | 3.8 | 9 | 1 | 2 | 3 | 6 | 8 | 9 | 14 |
| 65+ | 2,112 | 5.8 | 27 | 2 | 3 | 4 | 7 | 11 | 13 | 28 |
| **GRAND TOTAL** | 2,867 | 5.3 | 23 | 1 | 2 | 4 | 7 | 11 | 12 | 22 |

Length of Stay by Diagnosis and Operation, United States, 2000

# United States, October 1998–September 1999 Data, by Operation

## 45.5: INTESTINAL SEG ISOLATION. Formerly included in operation group(s) 610.

| Type of Patients | Observed Patients | Avg. Stay | Variance | 10th | 25th | 50th | 75th | 90th | 95th | 99th |
|---|---|---|---|---|---|---|---|---|---|---|
| **1. SINGLE DX** | | | | | | | | | | |
| 0–19 Years | 0 | | | | | | | | | |
| 20–34 | 0 | | | | | | | | | |
| 35–49 | 3 | 5.0 | <1 | | 5 | 5 | 5 | | 6 | 6 |
| 50–64 | 1 | 6.0 | 0 | | 6 | 6 | 6 | | 6 | 6 |
| 65+ | 0 | | | | | | | | | |
| **2. MULTIPLE DX** | | | | | | | | | | |
| 0–19 Years | 13 | 6.3 | 25 | 3 | 3 | 5 | 9 | 11 | 16 | 30 |
| 20–34 | 6 | 8.9 | 57 | 4 | 5 | 8 | 8 | 10 | 31 | 31 |
| 35–49 | 10 | 10.3 | 45 | 5 | 5 | 9 | 11 | 19 | 19 | 32 |
| 50–64 | 17 | 14.5 | 95 | 6 | 6 | 11 | 29 | 29 | 29 | 29 |
| 65+ | 23 | 9.7 | 22 | 5 | 7 | 9 | 10 | 18 | 22 | 22 |
| **TOTAL SINGLE DX** | 4 | 5.7 | <1 | 5 | 6 | 6 | 6 | 6 | 6 | 6 |
| **TOTAL MULTIPLE DX** | 69 | 10.8 | 56 | 3 | 6 | 9 | 12 | 22 | 29 | 31 |
| **TOTAL** | | | | | | | | | | |
| 0–19 Years | 13 | 6.3 | 25 | 3 | 3 | 5 | 9 | 11 | 16 | 30 |
| 20–34 | 6 | 8.9 | 57 | 4 | 5 | 8 | 8 | 10 | 31 | 31 |
| 35–49 | 13 | 9.3 | 41 | 5 | 5 | 8 | 11 | 19 | 19 | 32 |
| 50–64 | 18 | 12.5 | 85 | 6 | 6 | 7 | 29 | 29 | 29 | 29 |
| 65+ | 23 | 9.7 | 22 | 5 | 7 | 9 | 10 | 18 | 22 | 22 |
| **GRAND TOTAL** | 73 | 10.2 | 52 | 4 | 6 | 8 | 11 | 22 | 29 | 31 |

## 45.61: MULT SEG SM BOWEL RESECT. Formerly included in operation group(s) 608.

| Type of Patients | Observed Patients | Avg. Stay | Variance | 10th | 25th | 50th | 75th | 90th | 95th | 99th |
|---|---|---|---|---|---|---|---|---|---|---|
| **1. SINGLE DX** | | | | | | | | | | |
| 0–19 Years | 2 | 13.5 | 3 | 12 | 12 | 15 | 15 | 15 | 15 | 15 |
| 20–34 | 1 | 6.0 | 0 | 6 | 6 | 6 | 6 | 6 | 6 | 6 |
| 35–49 | 3 | 6.3 | 3 | 4 | 6 | 6 | 8 | 8 | 8 | 8 |
| 50–64 | 2 | 17.8 | 103 | 7 | 8 | 26 | 26 | 26 | 26 | 26 |
| 65+ | 1 | 7.0 | 0 | 7 | 7 | 7 | 7 | 7 | 7 | 7 |
| **2. MULTIPLE DX** | | | | | | | | | | |
| 0–19 Years | 30 | 15.9 | 204 | 5 | 9 | 17 | >99 | >99 | >99 | >99 |
| 20–34 | 64 | 10.2 | 18 | 6 | 7 | 8 | 14 | 17 | 17 | 19 |
| 35–49 | 78 | 16.7 | 178 | 4 | 6 | 11 | 25 | 39 | 39 | 53 |
| 50–64 | 135 | 13.6 | 109 | 6 | 8 | 11 | 14 | 24 | 29 | 69 |
| 65+ | 236 | 16.1 | 131 | 6 | 9 | 12 | 22 | 32 | 34 | 58 |
| **TOTAL SINGLE DX** | 9 | 8.5 | 25 | 6 | 6 | 7 | 8 | 15 | 26 | 26 |
| **TOTAL MULTIPLE DX** | 543 | 14.8 | 126 | 6 | 8 | 11 | 18 | 32 | 39 | >99 |
| **TOTAL** | | | | | | | | | | |
| 0–19 Years | 32 | 15.8 | 193 | 5 | 7 | 17 | >99 | >99 | >99 | >99 |
| 20–34 | 65 | 10.0 | 18 | 6 | 7 | 8 | 14 | 17 | 17 | 19 |
| 35–49 | 81 | 16.3 | 175 | 4 | 6 | 10 | 25 | 39 | 39 | 53 |
| 50–64 | 137 | 13.7 | 109 | 6 | 8 | 11 | 14 | 24 | 29 | 69 |
| 65+ | 237 | 16.0 | 130 | 6 | 9 | 12 | 22 | 32 | 32 | 58 |
| **GRAND TOTAL** | 552 | 14.6 | 124 | 6 | 8 | 11 | 18 | 32 | 39 | >99 |

## 45.6: OTHER SM BOWEL EXCISION. Formerly included in operation group(s) 608.

| Type of Patients | Observed Patients | Avg. Stay | Variance | 10th | 25th | 50th | 75th | 90th | 95th | 99th |
|---|---|---|---|---|---|---|---|---|---|---|
| **1. SINGLE DX** | | | | | | | | | | |
| 0–19 Years | 109 | 6.8 | 23 | 2 | 4 | 6 | 8 | 15 | 18 | 22 |
| 20–34 | 68 | 5.2 | 3 | 3 | 4 | 5 | 6 | 8 | 8 | 10 |
| 35–49 | 94 | 6.3 | 9 | 3 | 4 | 5 | 7 | 12 | 13 | 14 |
| 50–64 | 78 | 6.5 | 12 | 3 | 4 | 6 | 8 | 10 | 12 | 26 |
| 65+ | 48 | 6.5 | 12 | 3 | 5 | 6 | 7 | 12 | 14 | 15 |
| **2. MULTIPLE DX** | | | | | | | | | | |
| 0–19 Years | 912 | 17.7 | 438 | 5 | 6 | 10 | 29 | >99 | >99 | >99 |
| 20–34 | 955 | 9.5 | 69 | 4 | 6 | 7 | 11 | 16 | 21 | 56 |
| 35–49 | 1,889 | 10.6 | 68 | 5 | 6 | 8 | 13 | 20 | 26 | 41 |
| 50–64 | 2,585 | 12.2 | 99 | 6 | 6 | 9 | 14 | 24 | 32 | 55 |
| 65+ | 5,097 | 13.3 | 94 | 6 | 8 | 10 | 16 | 24 | 31 | 61 |
| **TOTAL SINGLE DX** | 397 | 6.4 | 14 | 3 | 4 | 5 | 7 | 11 | 14 | 22 |
| **TOTAL MULTIPLE DX** | 11,438 | 12.5 | 118 | 5 | 7 | 9 | 15 | 25 | 33 | 98 |
| **TOTAL** | | | | | | | | | | |
| 0–19 Years | 1,021 | 16.3 | 398 | 4 | 6 | 9 | 25 | 94 | >99 | >99 |
| 20–34 | 1,023 | 9.3 | 67 | 4 | 5 | 7 | 11 | 16 | 20 | 54 |
| 35–49 | 1,983 | 10.4 | 65 | 4 | 6 | 8 | 13 | 20 | 25 | 41 |
| 50–64 | 2,663 | 12.0 | 97 | 6 | 6 | 9 | 14 | 24 | 32 | 55 |
| 65+ | 5,145 | 13.2 | 94 | 6 | 8 | 10 | 16 | 24 | 30 | 61 |
| **GRAND TOTAL** | 11,835 | 12.3 | 116 | 6 | 6 | 9 | 14 | 24 | 33 | 97 |

## 45.62: PART SM BOWEL RESECT NEC. Formerly included in operation group(s) 608.

| Type of Patients | Observed Patients | Avg. Stay | Variance | 10th | 25th | 50th | 75th | 90th | 95th | 99th |
|---|---|---|---|---|---|---|---|---|---|---|
| **1. SINGLE DX** | | | | | | | | | | |
| 0–19 Years | 107 | 6.7 | 23 | 2 | 4 | 6 | 8 | 14 | 18 | 22 |
| 20–34 | 67 | 5.2 | 3 | 3 | 4 | 5 | 6 | 8 | 8 | 10 |
| 35–49 | 91 | 6.3 | 9 | 3 | 5 | 5 | 7 | 12 | 13 | 14 |
| 50–64 | 75 | 6.3 | 7 | 3 | 4 | 5 | 7 | 10 | 11 | 17 |
| 65+ | 47 | 6.5 | 13 | 3 | 4 | 5 | 8 | 12 | 14 | 15 |
| **2. MULTIPLE DX** | | | | | | | | | | |
| 0–19 Years | 878 | 17.8 | 448 | 5 | 6 | 10 | 28 | 97 | >99 | >99 |
| 20–34 | 885 | 9.5 | 74 | 4 | 6 | 7 | 11 | 16 | 21 | 58 |
| 35–49 | 1,794 | 10.1 | 57 | 5 | 6 | 8 | 12 | 19 | 24 | 41 |
| 50–64 | 2,432 | 12.1 | 97 | 5 | 6 | 8 | 14 | 24 | 32 | 55 |
| 65+ | 4,817 | 13.1 | 92 | 6 | 8 | 10 | 16 | 23 | 29 | 63 |
| **TOTAL SINGLE DX** | 387 | 6.3 | 13 | 3 | 4 | 5 | 7 | 10 | 13 | 21 |
| **TOTAL MULTIPLE DX** | 10,806 | 12.4 | 117 | 5 | 7 | 9 | 14 | 24 | 33 | 97 |
| **TOTAL** | | | | | | | | | | |
| 0–19 Years | 985 | 16.3 | 405 | 4 | 6 | 9 | 24 | 88 | >99 | >99 |
| 20–34 | 952 | 9.2 | 71 | 4 | 5 | 7 | 11 | 15 | 21 | 58 |
| 35–49 | 1,885 | 9.9 | 55 | 4 | 6 | 8 | 12 | 18 | 23 | 39 |
| 50–64 | 2,507 | 11.9 | 95 | 5 | 6 | 9 | 13 | 23 | 32 | 55 |
| 65+ | 4,864 | 13.0 | 92 | 6 | 8 | 10 | 15 | 23 | 29 | 63 |
| **GRAND TOTAL** | 11,193 | 12.2 | 115 | 5 | 6 | 9 | 14 | 23 | 32 | 94 |

# United States, October 1998–September 1999 Data, by Operation

## 45.7: PART LG BOWEL EXCISION. Formerly included in operation group(s) 609.

| Type of Patients | Observed Patients | Avg. Stay | Variance | Percentiles | | | | | | |
|---|---|---|---|---|---|---|---|---|---|---|
| | | | | 10th | 25th | 50th | 75th | 90th | 95th | 99th |
| **1. SINGLE DX** | | | | | | | | | | |
| 0–19 Years | 152 | 5.7 | 6 | 4 | 4 | 5 | 7 | 9 | 11 | 14 |
| 20–34 | 255 | 5.6 | 4 | 4 | 5 | 5 | 6 | 8 | 11 | 13 |
| 35–49 | 743 | 5.6 | 4 | 3 | 4 | 5 | 7 | 8 | 9 | 13 |
| 50–64 | 937 | 5.6 | 4 | 4 | 4 | 5 | 7 | 8 | 9 | 11 |
| 65+ | 649 | 6.1 | 5 | 4 | 5 | 6 | 7 | 8 | 9 | 15 |
| **2. MULTIPLE DX** | | | | | | | | | | |
| 0–19 Years | 734 | 13.7 | 294 | 5 | 6 | 8 | 14 | 33 | 83 | >99 |
| 20–34 | 1,988 | 9.6 | 64 | 4 | 5 | 7 | 10 | 18 | 25 | 41 |
| 35–49 | 6,839 | 8.5 | 39 | 4 | 5 | 7 | 9 | 14 | 19 | 43 |
| 50–64 | 13,794 | 8.7 | 39 | 4 | 5 | 7 | 10 | 14 | 19 | 35 |
| 65+ | 31,709 | 10.6 | 55 | 5 | 6 | 8 | 12 | 18 | 24 | 43 |
| **TOTAL SINGLE DX** | 2,736 | 5.7 | 4 | 4 | 4 | 5 | 7 | 8 | 9 | 12 |
| **TOTAL MULTIPLE DX** | 55,064 | 9.8 | 53 | 5 | 6 | 8 | 11 | 17 | 23 | 42 |
| **TOTAL** | | | | | | | | | | |
| 0–19 Years | 886 | 12.4 | 256 | 4 | 5 | 7 | 12 | 30 | 66 | >99 |
| 20–34 | 2,243 | 9.1 | 58 | 4 | 5 | 7 | 10 | 16 | 23 | 41 |
| 35–49 | 7,582 | 8.2 | 36 | 4 | 5 | 7 | 9 | 14 | 18 | 38 |
| 50–64 | 14,731 | 8.5 | 37 | 4 | 5 | 7 | 9 | 14 | 19 | 34 |
| 65+ | 32,358 | 10.5 | 55 | 5 | 6 | 8 | 12 | 18 | 24 | 42 |
| **GRAND TOTAL** | 57,800 | 9.6 | 52 | 5 | 6 | 8 | 11 | 16 | 22 | 41 |

## 45.71: MULT SEG LG BOWEL RESECT. Formerly included in operation group(s) 609.

| Type of Patients | Observed Patients | Avg. Stay | Variance | Percentiles | | | | | | |
|---|---|---|---|---|---|---|---|---|---|---|
| | | | | 10th | 25th | 50th | 75th | 90th | 95th | 99th |
| **1. SINGLE DX** | | | | | | | | | | |
| 0–19 Years | 1 | 4.0 | 0 | 4 | 4 | 4 | 4 | 4 | 4 | 4 |
| 20–34 | 0 | | | | | | | | | |
| 35–49 | 3 | 8.0 | 3 | 5 | 9 | 9 | 9 | 9 | 9 | 9 |
| 50–64 | 2 | 6.5 | <1 | 4 | 4 | 8 | 8 | 8 | 8 | 8 |
| 65+ | 4 | 6.9 | <1 | 6 | 7 | 7 | 7 | 7 | 7 | 7 |
| **2. MULTIPLE DX** | | | | | | | | | | |
| 0–19 Years | 7 | 12.4 | 61 | 6 | 6 | 9 | 13 | 27 | 27 | 27 |
| 20–34 | 13 | 8.2 | 14 | 6 | 6 | 8 | 8 | 11 | 13 | 32 |
| 35–49 | 34 | 12.0 | 82 | 5 | 7 | 10 | 15 | 16 | 18 | 50 |
| 50–64 | 73 | 10.4 | 68 | 6 | 6 | 8 | 12 | 20 | 20 | 50 |
| 65+ | 185 | 11.3 | 63 | 5 | 7 | 9 | 15 | 19 | 25 | 37 |
| **TOTAL SINGLE DX** | 10 | 7.1 | 3 | 5 | 7 | 7 | 9 | 9 | 9 | 9 |
| **TOTAL MULTIPLE DX** | 312 | 11.0 | 64 | 5 | 6 | 8 | 14 | 19 | 22 | 49 |
| **TOTAL** | | | | | | | | | | |
| 0–19 Years | 8 | 11.9 | 61 | 4 | 6 | 9 | 18 | 27 | 27 | 27 |
| 20–34 | 13 | 8.2 | 14 | 6 | 6 | 8 | 8 | 11 | 13 | 32 |
| 35–49 | 37 | 11.7 | 76 | 5 | 7 | 10 | 15 | 15 | 18 | 50 |
| 50–64 | 75 | 10.3 | 67 | 4 | 6 | 8 | 12 | 20 | 20 | 50 |
| 65+ | 189 | 11.2 | 63 | 5 | 7 | 9 | 15 | 19 | 25 | 37 |
| **GRAND TOTAL** | 322 | 10.9 | 63 | 6 | 6 | 8 | 13 | 18 | 21 | 49 |

## 45.72: CECECTOMY. Formerly included in operation group(s) 609.

| Type of Patients | Observed Patients | Avg. Stay | Variance | Percentiles | | | | | | |
|---|---|---|---|---|---|---|---|---|---|---|
| | | | | 10th | 25th | 50th | 75th | 90th | 95th | 99th |
| **1. SINGLE DX** | | | | | | | | | | |
| 0–19 Years | 41 | 6.2 | 10 | 3 | 5 | 6 | 7 | 11 | 14 | 14 |
| 20–34 | 67 | 5.1 | 6 | 3 | 4 | 5 | 6 | 7 | 8 | 19 |
| 35–49 | 52 | 4.8 | 3 | 3 | 4 | 4 | 6 | 7 | 8 | 11 |
| 50–64 | 39 | 4.7 | 3 | 2 | 5 | 5 | 5 | 7 | 7 | 8 |
| 65+ | 31 | 5.6 | 3 | 4 | 5 | 6 | 6 | 9 | 10 | 11 |
| **2. MULTIPLE DX** | | | | | | | | | | |
| 0–19 Years | 204 | 11.6 | 213 | 4 | 6 | 8 | 10 | 27 | 59 | >99 |
| 20–34 | 407 | 8.8 | 61 | 4 | 4 | 7 | 9 | 15 | 21 | 41 |
| 35–49 | 472 | 7.6 | 29 | 4 | 5 | 7 | 8 | 12 | 15 | 32 |
| 50–64 | 597 | 8.3 | 27 | 4 | 5 | 7 | 11 | 13 | 17 | 27 |
| 65+ | 1,074 | 11.0 | 72 | 4 | 6 | 8 | 13 | 20 | 25 | 55 |
| **TOTAL SINGLE DX** | 230 | 5.3 | 6 | 3 | 4 | 5 | 6 | 8 | 10 | 14 |
| **TOTAL MULTIPLE DX** | 2,754 | 9.5 | 66 | 4 | 5 | 7 | 11 | 17 | 23 | 45 |
| **TOTAL** | | | | | | | | | | |
| 0–19 Years | 245 | 10.7 | 181 | 4 | 5 | 6 | 10 | 21 | 34 | >99 |
| 20–34 | 474 | 8.4 | 56 | 4 | 4 | 6 | 9 | 14 | 21 | 41 |
| 35–49 | 524 | 7.3 | 28 | 4 | 5 | 6 | 8 | 12 | 15 | 31 |
| 50–64 | 636 | 8.1 | 26 | 3 | 5 | 7 | 10 | 13 | 17 | 27 |
| 65+ | 1,105 | 10.8 | 71 | 4 | 6 | 8 | 13 | 20 | 25 | 55 |
| **GRAND TOTAL** | 2,984 | 9.2 | 63 | 4 | 5 | 7 | 10 | 16 | 22 | 43 |

## 45.73: RIGHT HEMICOLECTOMY. Formerly included in operation group(s) 609.

| Type of Patients | Observed Patients | Avg. Stay | Variance | Percentiles | | | | | | |
|---|---|---|---|---|---|---|---|---|---|---|
| | | | | 10th | 25th | 50th | 75th | 90th | 95th | 99th |
| **1. SINGLE DX** | | | | | | | | | | |
| 0–19 Years | 52 | 6.0 | 4 | 4 | 5 | 5 | 7 | 9 | 10 | 12 |
| 20–34 | 62 | 5.4 | 2 | 4 | 5 | 5 | 6 | 7 | 8 | 13 |
| 35–49 | 162 | 5.7 | 2 | 4 | 5 | 5 | 7 | 8 | 8 | 10 |
| 50–64 | 265 | 5.4 | 3 | 4 | 4 | 5 | 6 | 9 | 8 | 9 |
| 65+ | 254 | 5.5 | 3 | 3 | 4 | 5 | 6 | 7 | 8 | 10 |
| **2. MULTIPLE DX** | | | | | | | | | | |
| 0–19 Years | 228 | 14.2 | 299 | 5 | 6 | 8 | 14 | 39 | 76 | >99 |
| 20–34 | 661 | 9.7 | 80 | 4 | 5 | 7 | 10 | 17 | 26 | 58 |
| 35–49 | 1,715 | 9.3 | 66 | 4 | 5 | 7 | 10 | 16 | 24 | 43 |
| 50–64 | 4,357 | 8.6 | 47 | 4 | 5 | 7 | 10 | 14 | 20 | 37 |
| 65+ | 13,021 | 9.9 | 43 | 5 | 6 | 8 | 12 | 17 | 22 | 36 |
| **TOTAL SINGLE DX** | 795 | 5.5 | 3 | 4 | 4 | 5 | 6 | 8 | 9 | 10 |
| **TOTAL MULTIPLE DX** | 19,982 | 9.6 | 50 | 5 | 6 | 8 | 11 | 16 | 22 | 41 |
| **TOTAL** | | | | | | | | | | |
| 0–19 Years | 280 | 12.7 | 257 | 5 | 6 | 7 | 13 | 28 | 65 | >99 |
| 20–34 | 723 | 9.1 | 71 | 5 | 5 | 6 | 9 | 15 | 24 | 58 |
| 35–49 | 1,877 | 8.9 | 60 | 4 | 5 | 7 | 9 | 14 | 22 | 43 |
| 50–64 | 4,622 | 8.5 | 45 | 4 | 5 | 7 | 10 | 14 | 19 | 35 |
| 65+ | 13,275 | 9.8 | 42 | 5 | 6 | 8 | 12 | 17 | 22 | 36 |
| **GRAND TOTAL** | 20,777 | 9.4 | 49 | 4 | 6 | 7 | 11 | 16 | 21 | 40 |

Length of Stay by Diagnosis and Operation

# United States, October 1998–September 1999 Data, by Operation

## 45.74: TRANSVERSE COLON RESECT. Formerly included in operation group(s) 609.

| Type of Patients | Observed Patients | Avg. Stay | Variance | 10th | 25th | 50th | 75th | 90th | 95th | 99th |
|---|---|---|---|---|---|---|---|---|---|---|
| **1. SINGLE DX** | | | | | | | | | | |
| 0–19 Years | 3 | 4.8 | 2 | 4 | 4 | 4 | 6 | 8 | 8 | 8 |
| 20–34 | 6 | 5.0 | 6 | 2 | 2 | 6 | 7 | 8 | 8 | 8 |
| 35–49 | 13 | 7.7 | 14 | 4 | 5 | 6 | 9 | 14 | 14 | 14 |
| 50–64 | 29 | 6.6 | 7 | 4 | 5 | 6 | 8 | 9 | 9 | 18 |
| 65+ | 25 | 6.0 | 3 | 3 | 5 | 6 | 7 | 9 | 9 | 9 |
| **2. MULTIPLE DX** | | | | | | | | | | |
| 0–19 Years | 31 | 17.1 | 575 | 5 | 6 | 6 | 11 | 42 | 87 | 96 |
| 20–34 | 59 | 10.1 | 43 | 6 | 7 | 7 | 10 | 20 | 22 | 48 |
| 35–49 | 177 | 9.3 | 33 | 5 | 6 | 7 | 10 | 16 | 19 | 29 |
| 50–64 | 426 | 9.0 | 48 | 5 | 6 | 7 | 10 | 16 | 21 | 43 |
| 65+ | 1,301 | 10.3 | 44 | 5 | 6 | 8 | 12 | 18 | 27 | 44 |
| **TOTAL SINGLE DX** | 76 | 6.5 | 8 | 4 | 5 | 6 | 8 | 9 | 14 | 18 |
| **TOTAL MULTIPLE DX** | 1,994 | 10.0 | 51 | 5 | 6 | 8 | 12 | 18 | 24 | 44 |
| **TOTAL** | | | | | | | | | | |
| 0–19 Years | 34 | 16.4 | 548 | 4 | 5 | 6 | 10 | 42 | 87 | 87 |
| 20–34 | 65 | 9.7 | 43 | 5 | 7 | 7 | 9 | 20 | 22 | 48 |
| 35–49 | 190 | 9.1 | 31 | 5 | 6 | 7 | 10 | 16 | 18 | 29 |
| 50–64 | 455 | 8.8 | 45 | 5 | 6 | 7 | 9 | 14 | 21 | 43 |
| 65+ | 1,326 | 10.3 | 44 | 5 | 6 | 8 | 12 | 18 | 27 | 43 |
| **GRAND TOTAL** | 2,070 | 9.9 | 50 | 5 | 6 | 8 | 11 | 17 | 23 | 43 |

## 45.76: SIGMOIDECTOMY. Formerly included in operation group(s) 609.

| Type of Patients | Observed Patients | Avg. Stay | Variance | 10th | 25th | 50th | 75th | 90th | 95th | 99th |
|---|---|---|---|---|---|---|---|---|---|---|
| **1. SINGLE DX** | | | | | | | | | | |
| 0–19 Years | 19 | 4.3 | 2 | 3 | 4 | 4 | 4 | 5 | 8 | 9 |
| 20–34 | 78 | 5.9 | 5 | 4 | 5 | 5 | 7 | 10 | 10 | 15 |
| 35–49 | 348 | 5.4 | 4 | 3 | 4 | 5 | 6 | 8 | 8 | 13 |
| 50–64 | 433 | 5.6 | 3 | 4 | 5 | 5 | 7 | 8 | 9 | 12 |
| 65+ | 223 | 6.3 | 4 | 4 | 5 | 6 | 7 | 8 | 9 | 12 |
| **2. MULTIPLE DX** | | | | | | | | | | |
| 0–19 Years | 83 | 12.2 | 80 | 5 | 7 | 9 | 15 | 19 | 32 | >99 |
| 20–34 | 490 | 8.9 | 29 | 5 | 6 | 7 | 11 | 15 | 21 | 29 |
| 35–49 | 2,933 | 8.1 | 25 | 4 | 5 | 7 | 9 | 14 | 17 | 28 |
| 50–64 | 5,267 | 8.5 | 30 | 5 | 6 | 7 | 9 | 14 | 18 | 29 |
| 65+ | 9,436 | 11.1 | 65 | 5 | 7 | 9 | 13 | 19 | 25 | 47 |
| **TOTAL SINGLE DX** | 1,101 | 5.6 | 4 | 4 | 4 | 5 | 7 | 8 | 9 | 12 |
| **TOTAL MULTIPLE DX** | 18,209 | 9.7 | 48 | 5 | 6 | 8 | 11 | 17 | 22 | 41 |
| **TOTAL** | | | | | | | | | | |
| 0–19 Years | 102 | 10.5 | 74 | 4 | 5 | 9 | 13 | 19 | 32 | >99 |
| 20–34 | 568 | 8.5 | 26 | 4 | 5 | 7 | 10 | 14 | 17 | 28 |
| 35–49 | 3,281 | 7.7 | 23 | 4 | 5 | 6 | 9 | 13 | 16 | 27 |
| 50–64 | 5,700 | 8.3 | 28 | 4 | 5 | 7 | 9 | 14 | 17 | 29 |
| 65+ | 9,659 | 10.9 | 64 | 5 | 6 | 9 | 12 | 19 | 25 | 46 |
| **GRAND TOTAL** | 19,310 | 9.4 | 46 | 5 | 6 | 7 | 11 | 16 | 21 | 40 |

## 45.75: LEFT HEMICOLECTOMY. Formerly included in operation group(s) 609.

| Type of Patients | Observed Patients | Avg. Stay | Variance | 10th | 25th | 50th | 75th | 90th | 95th | 99th |
|---|---|---|---|---|---|---|---|---|---|---|
| **1. SINGLE DX** | | | | | | | | | | |
| 0–19 Years | 9 | 6.1 | 2 | 4 | 5 | 7 | 7 | 7 | 7 | 7 |
| 20–34 | 14 | 5.8 | 3 | 4 | 5 | 6 | 6 | 8 | 8 | 13 |
| 35–49 | 98 | 6.1 | 4 | 4 | 5 | 6 | 7 | 8 | 8 | 13 |
| 50–64 | 92 | 6.3 | 5 | 4 | 5 | 6 | 7 | 8 | 8 | 10 |
| 65+ | 64 | 7.4 | 12 | 4 | 6 | 7 | 8 | 10 | 15 | 22 |
| **2. MULTIPLE DX** | | | | | | | | | | |
| 0–19 Years | 49 | 24.6 | 814 | 5 | 6 | 10 | 32 | 86 | 95 | 95 |
| 20–34 | 150 | 11.4 | 74 | 5 | 6 | 8 | 14 | 32 | 32 | 39 |
| 35–49 | 881 | 9.5 | 46 | 5 | 6 | 7 | 11 | 16 | 26 | 35 |
| 50–64 | 1,936 | 9.2 | 39 | 5 | 6 | 7 | 10 | 16 | 21 | 35 |
| 65+ | 4,432 | 11.3 | 59 | 6 | 7 | 9 | 13 | 19 | 24 | 46 |
| **TOTAL SINGLE DX** | 277 | 6.4 | 6 | 4 | 5 | 6 | 7 | 8 | 9 | 21 |
| **TOTAL MULTIPLE DX** | 7,448 | 10.6 | 61 | 5 | 6 | 8 | 12 | 18 | 25 | 46 |
| **TOTAL** | | | | | | | | | | |
| 0–19 Years | 58 | 23.2 | 777 | 5 | 6 | 10 | 32 | 83 | 95 | 95 |
| 20–34 | 164 | 10.9 | 70 | 5 | 6 | 8 | 12 | 32 | 32 | 33 |
| 35–49 | 979 | 9.1 | 42 | 5 | 6 | 7 | 10 | 15 | 24 | 34 |
| 50–64 | 2,028 | 9.0 | 38 | 5 | 6 | 7 | 10 | 16 | 22 | 35 |
| 65+ | 4,496 | 11.2 | 58 | 6 | 7 | 9 | 13 | 19 | 24 | 46 |
| **GRAND TOTAL** | 7,725 | 10.4 | 59 | 5 | 6 | 8 | 12 | 18 | 24 | 44 |

## 45.79: PART LG BOWEL EXC NEC. Formerly included in operation group(s) 609.

| Type of Patients | Observed Patients | Avg. Stay | Variance | 10th | 25th | 50th | 75th | 90th | 95th | 99th |
|---|---|---|---|---|---|---|---|---|---|---|
| **1. SINGLE DX** | | | | | | | | | | |
| 0–19 Years | 27 | 5.2 | 2 | 4 | 5 | 5 | 6 | 6 | 8 | 9 |
| 20–34 | 28 | 5.9 | 2 | 5 | 5 | 5 | 7 | 7 | 8 | 9 |
| 35–49 | 67 | 5.7 | 4 | 4 | 5 | 5 | 7 | 8 | 9 | 11 |
| 50–64 | 77 | 5.6 | 6 | 4 | 5 | 5 | 7 | 9 | 9 | 12 |
| 65+ | 48 | 6.6 | 6 | 4 | 5 | 7 | 8 | 9 | 10 | 19 |
| **2. MULTIPLE DX** | | | | | | | | | | |
| 0–19 Years | 132 | 11.8 | 200 | 4 | 5 | 7 | 12 | 48 | >99 | 95 |
| 20–34 | 208 | 11.0 | 90 | 4 | 6 | 7 | 15 | 19 | 31 | 41 |
| 35–49 | 627 | 8.2 | 32 | 4 | 5 | 7 | 9 | 13 | 18 | 29 |
| 50–64 | 1,138 | 9.1 | 46 | 5 | 6 | 7 | 10 | 15 | 21 | 40 |
| 65+ | 2,260 | 11.4 | 76 | 5 | 6 | 9 | 14 | 21 | 28 | 53 |
| **TOTAL SINGLE DX** | 247 | 5.9 | 4 | 4 | 5 | 5 | 7 | 8 | 9 | 11 |
| **TOTAL MULTIPLE DX** | 4,365 | 10.3 | 68 | 5 | 6 | 8 | 12 | 19 | 27 | 50 |
| **TOTAL** | | | | | | | | | | |
| 0–19 Years | 159 | 10.8 | 177 | 4 | 5 | 7 | 12 | 33 | >99 | >99 |
| 20–34 | 236 | 10.4 | 82 | 4 | 6 | 7 | 12 | 19 | 31 | 41 |
| 35–49 | 694 | 7.9 | 29 | 4 | 5 | 7 | 9 | 12 | 18 | 29 |
| 50–64 | 1,215 | 9.0 | 44 | 4 | 5 | 7 | 10 | 15 | 20 | 40 |
| 65+ | 2,308 | 11.3 | 75 | 5 | 6 | 8 | 13 | 20 | 28 | 53 |
| **GRAND TOTAL** | 4,612 | 10.0 | 65 | 4 | 6 | 8 | 11 | 18 | 26 | 49 |

Length of Stay by Diagnosis and Operation, United States, 2000

United States, October 1998–September 1999 Data, by Operation

## 45.8: TOT INTRA-ABD COLECTOMY. Formerly included in operation group(s) 609.

| Type of Patients | Observed Patients | Avg. Stay | Vari-ance | 10th | 25th | 50th | 75th | 90th | 95th | 99th |
|---|---|---|---|---|---|---|---|---|---|---|
| **1. SINGLE DX** | | | | | | | | | | |
| 0–19 Years | 43 | 7.2 | 8 | 5 | 6 | 7 | 8 | 9 | 10 | 24 |
| 20–34 | 63 | 7.0 | 6 | 5 | 5 | 6 | 8 | 10 | 10 | 19 |
| 35–49 | 54 | 7.5 | 6 | 5 | 6 | 7 | 10 | 10 | 10 | 15 |
| 50–64 | 19 | 6.3 | 2 | 5 | 5 | 6 | 8 | 8 | 8 | 8 |
| 65+ | 8 | 6.2 | 9 | 3 | 5 | 5 | 7 | 14 | 14 | 14 |
| **2. MULTIPLE DX** | | | | | | | | | | |
| 0–19 Years | 145 | 16.0 | 169 | 6 | 8 | 11 | 19 | 40 | 40 | 66 |
| 20–34 | 342 | 10.2 | 61 | 4 | 6 | 7 | 13 | 19 | 23 | 41 |
| 35–49 | 505 | 11.8 | 99 | 5 | 6 | 8 | 13 | 23 | 36 | 46 |
| 50–64 | 532 | 12.6 | 87 | 5 | 7 | 9 | 15 | 25 | 31 | 47 |
| 65+ | 915 | 15.2 | 108 | 7 | 9 | 12 | 18 | 28 | 37 | 58 |
| **TOTAL SINGLE DX** | 187 | 7.1 | 7 | 5 | 5 | 7 | 8 | 10 | 10 | 19 |
| **TOTAL MULTIPLE DX** | 2,439 | 13.3 | 103 | 5 | 7 | 10 | 16 | 26 | 34 | 50 |
| **TOTAL** | | | | | | | | | | |
| 0–19 Years | 188 | 13.7 | 141 | 5 | 7 | 8 | 17 | 26 | 40 | 64 |
| 20–34 | 405 | 9.7 | 54 | 5 | 6 | 7 | 11 | 18 | 21 | 37 |
| 35–49 | 559 | 11.3 | 91 | 5 | 6 | 8 | 12 | 22 | 32 | 46 |
| 50–64 | 551 | 12.5 | 86 | 5 | 6 | 9 | 15 | 25 | 31 | 47 |
| 65+ | 923 | 15.1 | 108 | 7 | 9 | 12 | 18 | 28 | 36 | 58 |
| **GRAND TOTAL** | 2,626 | 12.9 | 98 | 5 | 7 | 10 | 15 | 25 | 32 | 49 |

## 45.9: INTESTINAL ANASTOMOSIS. Formerly included in operation group(s) 611.

| Type of Patients | Observed Patients | Avg. Stay | Vari-ance | 10th | 25th | 50th | 75th | 90th | 95th | 99th |
|---|---|---|---|---|---|---|---|---|---|---|
| **1. SINGLE DX** | | | | | | | | | | |
| 0–19 Years | 24 | 13.6 | 97 | 5 | 5 | 9 | 21 | 30 | 30 | 30 |
| 20–34 | 13 | 5.0 | 1 | 4 | 4 | 4 | 6 | 7 | 7 | 7 |
| 35–49 | 22 | 5.7 | 2 | 4 | 5 | 6 | 6 | 8 | 8 | 8 |
| 50–64 | 29 | 6.8 | 11 | 5 | 5 | 6 | 7 | 8 | 11 | 23 |
| 65+ | 14 | 6.0 | 3 | 4 | 5 | 5 | 8 | 8 | 8 | 10 |
| **2. MULTIPLE DX** | | | | | | | | | | |
| 0–19 Years | 203 | 20.5 | 319 | 6 | 8 | 14 | 26 | 54 | 65 | 73 |
| 20–34 | 148 | 9.2 | 78 | 4 | 4 | 6 | 10 | 15 | 27 | 41 |
| 35–49 | 334 | 10.7 | 66 | 5 | 6 | 9 | 12 | 19 | 24 | 37 |
| 50–64 | 579 | 11.3 | 52 | 6 | 6 | 9 | 14 | 19 | 24 | 40 |
| 65+ | 962 | 12.3 | 58 | 6 | 7 | 10 | 15 | 21 | 26 | 47 |
| **TOTAL SINGLE DX** | 102 | 8.1 | 41 | 4 | 5 | 6 | 7 | 21 | 28 | 30 |
| **TOTAL MULTIPLE DX** | 2,226 | 12.3 | 91 | 5 | 7 | 9 | 14 | 22 | 29 | 57 |
| **TOTAL** | | | | | | | | | | |
| 0–19 Years | 227 | 19.8 | 299 | 5 | 7 | 12 | 26 | 53 | 65 | 73 |
| 20–34 | 161 | 8.8 | 73 | 4 | 4 | 6 | 9 | 15 | 27 | 41 |
| 35–49 | 356 | 10.5 | 64 | 5 | 6 | 8 | 12 | 18 | 24 | 37 |
| 50–64 | 608 | 11.1 | 51 | 6 | 6 | 9 | 14 | 19 | 24 | 40 |
| 65+ | 976 | 12.2 | 58 | 6 | 7 | 10 | 15 | 21 | 26 | 47 |
| **GRAND TOTAL** | 2,328 | 12.2 | 90 | 5 | 7 | 9 | 14 | 21 | 29 | 57 |

## 45.91: SM-TO-SM BOWEL ANAST. Formerly included in operation group(s) 611.

| Type of Patients | Observed Patients | Avg. Stay | Vari-ance | 10th | 25th | 50th | 75th | 90th | 95th | 99th |
|---|---|---|---|---|---|---|---|---|---|---|
| **1. SINGLE DX** | | | | | | | | | | |
| 0–19 Years | 8 | 18.7 | 89 | 6 | 9 | 21 | 30 | 30 | 30 | 30 |
| 20–34 | 2 | 5.5 | <1 | 5 | 5 | 5 | 6 | 5 | 5 | 5 |
| 35–49 | 2 | 4.7 | <1 | 4 | 4 | 5 | 5 | 5 | 5 | 5 |
| 50–64 | 1 | 7.0 | 0 | 7 | 7 | 7 | 7 | 7 | 7 | 7 |
| 65+ | 1 | 5.0 | 0 | 5 | 5 | 5 | 5 | 5 | 5 | 5 |
| **2. MULTIPLE DX** | | | | | | | | | | |
| 0–19 Years | 123 | 27.7 | 372 | 6 | 14 | 21 | 37 | 64 | 66 | 74 |
| 20–34 | 41 | 13.0 | 129 | 5 | 6 | 9 | 15 | 41 | 41 | 41 |
| 35–49 | 91 | 13.1 | 82 | 6 | 7 | 12 | 14 | 21 | 34 | 48 |
| 50–64 | 142 | 14.1 | 72 | 5 | 7 | 13 | 18 | 25 | 33 | 35 |
| 65+ | 216 | 13.4 | 51 | 7 | 8 | 11 | 16 | 23 | 26 | 40 |
| **TOTAL SINGLE DX** | 14 | 13.7 | 91 | 5 | 6 | 7 | 21 | 30 | 30 | 30 |
| **TOTAL MULTIPLE DX** | 613 | 16.1 | 157 | 6 | 8 | 12 | 19 | 31 | 41 | 66 |
| **TOTAL** | | | | | | | | | | |
| 0–19 Years | 131 | 26.7 | 348 | 6 | 14 | 21 | 34 | 57 | 65 | 74 |
| 20–34 | 43 | 12.7 | 125 | 5 | 6 | 8 | 13 | 41 | 41 | 41 |
| 35–49 | 93 | 13.1 | 82 | 6 | 7 | 12 | 14 | 21 | 34 | 48 |
| 50–64 | 143 | 13.8 | 71 | 5 | 7 | 12 | 18 | 25 | 32 | 35 |
| 65+ | 217 | 13.3 | 52 | 7 | 8 | 11 | 16 | 23 | 26 | 40 |
| **GRAND TOTAL** | 627 | 16.1 | 155 | 6 | 8 | 12 | 19 | 31 | 41 | 66 |

## 45.93: SMALL-TO-LARGE BOWEL NEC. Formerly included in operation group(s) 611.

| Type of Patients | Observed Patients | Avg. Stay | Vari-ance | 10th | 25th | 50th | 75th | 90th | 95th | 99th |
|---|---|---|---|---|---|---|---|---|---|---|
| **1. SINGLE DX** | | | | | | | | | | |
| 0–19 Years | 2 | 5.2 | <1 | 5 | 5 | 5 | 5 | 6 | 6 | 6 |
| 20–34 | 2 | 4.0 | 0 | 4 | 4 | 4 | 4 | 4 | 4 | 4 |
| 35–49 | 4 | 5.9 | 4 | 3 | 5 | 7 | 7 | 8 | 8 | 8 |
| 50–64 | 6 | 12.2 | 50 | 6 | 8 | 8 | 23 | 23 | 23 | 23 |
| 65+ | 1 | 10.0 | 0 | 10 | 10 | 10 | 10 | 10 | 10 | 10 |
| **2. MULTIPLE DX** | | | | | | | | | | |
| 0–19 Years | 23 | 9.7 | 23 | 5 | 7 | 10 | 11 | 11 | 19 | 39 |
| 20–34 | 40 | 7.1 | 31 | 4 | 4 | 4 | 8 | 13 | 26 | 27 |
| 35–49 | 92 | 11.2 | 51 | 5 | 7 | 9 | 13 | 18 | 29 | 37 |
| 50–64 | 189 | 12.4 | 50 | 6 | 8 | 11 | 15 | 19 | 24 | 40 |
| 65+ | 310 | 14.2 | 63 | 7 | 8 | 13 | 19 | 21 | 26 | 54 |
| **TOTAL SINGLE DX** | 15 | 8.3 | 32 | 4 | 5 | 7 | 8 | 23 | 23 | 23 |
| **TOTAL MULTIPLE DX** | 654 | 12.6 | 58 | 5 | 7 | 11 | 16 | 20 | 26 | 45 |
| **TOTAL** | | | | | | | | | | |
| 0–19 Years | 25 | 9.6 | 23 | 5 | 7 | 10 | 11 | 11 | 19 | 39 |
| 20–34 | 42 | 7.1 | 31 | 4 | 4 | 4 | 8 | 13 | 26 | 27 |
| 35–49 | 96 | 11.1 | 51 | 5 | 6 | 9 | 13 | 18 | 29 | 37 |
| 50–64 | 195 | 12.4 | 50 | 6 | 8 | 11 | 15 | 19 | 24 | 40 |
| 65+ | 311 | 14.2 | 63 | 7 | 8 | 13 | 19 | 21 | 26 | 54 |
| **GRAND TOTAL** | 669 | 12.6 | 58 | 5 | 7 | 11 | 16 | 20 | 26 | 45 |

Length of Stay by Diagnosis and Operation, United States, 2000

# United States, October 1998–September 1999 Data, by Operation

## 45.94: LG-TO-LG BOWEL ANAST. Formerly included in operation group(s) 611.

| Type of Patients | Observed Patients | Avg. Stay | Variance | 10th | 25th | 50th | 75th | 90th | 95th | 99th |
|---|---|---|---|---|---|---|---|---|---|---|
| **1. SINGLE DX** | | | | | | | | | | |
| 0-19 Years | 2 | 7.2 | 11 | 4 | 4 | 10 | 10 | 10 | 10 | 10 |
| 20-34 | 1 | 5.0 | 0 | 5 | 5 | 5 | 5 | 5 | 5 | 5 |
| 35-49 | 10 | 5.6 | <1 | 4 | 5 | 6 | 6 | 6 | 7 | 7 |
| 50-64 | 18 | 5.6 | 1 | 5 | 5 | 6 | 6 | 6 | 9 | 9 |
| 65+ | 9 | 6.1 | 2 | 4 | 5 | 5 | 8 | 8 | 8 | 8 |
| **2. MULTIPLE DX** | | | | | | | | | | |
| 0-19 Years | 21 | 14.2 | 174 | 5 | 5 | 9 | 18 | 33 | 33 | 58 |
| 20-34 | 23 | 6.7 | 14 | 4 | 5 | 6 | 8 | 9 | 11 | 26 |
| 35-49 | 98 | 7.9 | 20 | 5 | 5 | 7 | 9 | 12 | 16 | 30 |
| 50-64 | 201 | 8.0 | 22 | 5 | 6 | 7 | 9 | 12 | 17 | 41 |
| 65+ | 342 | 9.3 | 29 | 5 | 6 | 8 | 10 | 16 | 21 | 33 |
| **TOTAL SINGLE DX** | 40 | 5.8 | 2 | 4 | 5 | 6 | 6 | 8 | 9 | 10 |
| **TOTAL MULTIPLE DX** | 685 | 8.8 | 30 | 5 | 6 | 7 | 9 | 14 | 19 | 33 |
| **TOTAL** | | | | | | | | | | |
| 0-19 Years | 23 | 13.5 | 162 | 5 | 5 | 9 | 17 | 33 | 33 | 58 |
| 20-34 | 24 | 6.7 | 14 | 5 | 5 | 6 | 8 | 9 | 11 | 26 |
| 35-49 | 108 | 7.7 | 18 | 4 | 5 | 6 | 8 | 12 | 14 | 30 |
| 50-64 | 219 | 7.8 | 21 | 5 | 6 | 7 | 9 | 11 | 16 | 19 |
| 65+ | 351 | 9.3 | 28 | 5 | 6 | 8 | 10 | 15 | 21 | 33 |
| **GRAND TOTAL** | 725 | 8.6 | 29 | 5 | 6 | 7 | 9 | 14 | 18 | 33 |

## 46.01: SM BOWEL EXTERIORIZATION. Formerly included in operation group(s) 610.

| Type of Patients | Observed Patients | Avg. Stay | Variance | 10th | 25th | 50th | 75th | 90th | 95th | 99th |
|---|---|---|---|---|---|---|---|---|---|---|
| **1. SINGLE DX** | | | | | | | | | | |
| 0-19 Years | 2 | 7.2 | 4 | 6 | 6 | 6 | 9 | 9 | 9 | 9 |
| 20-34 | 7 | 4.7 | 14 | 2 | 2 | 2 | 5 | 13 | 13 | 13 |
| 35-49 | 10 | 5.5 | 3 | 4 | 4 | 6 | 7 | 13 | 13 | 13 |
| 50-64 | 2 | 7.0 | 0 | 7 | 7 | 7 | 7 | 7 | 7 | 7 |
| 65+ | 2 | 5.0 | 0 | 5 | 5 | 5 | 5 | 5 | 5 | 5 |
| **2. MULTIPLE DX** | | | | | | | | | | |
| 0-19 Years | 44 | 24.3 | 641 | 5 | 7 | 21 | 43 | >99 | >99 | >99 |
| 20-34 | 44 | 12.0 | 125 | 3 | 4 | 8 | 14 | 37 | 38 | 42 |
| 35-49 | 88 | 12.8 | 109 | 3 | 5 | 11 | 16 | 27 | 33 | 60 |
| 50-64 | 138 | 10.9 | 61 | 5 | 6 | 8 | 12 | 27 | 28 | 32 |
| 65+ | 161 | 12.6 | 63 | 6 | 7 | 10 | 16 | 22 | 26 | 44 |
| **TOTAL SINGLE DX** | 23 | 5.4 | 4 | 4 | 4 | 5 | 6 | 7 | 9 | 13 |
| **TOTAL MULTIPLE DX** | 475 | 13.0 | 135 | 4 | 6 | 9 | 16 | 28 | 37 | >99 |
| **TOTAL** | | | | | | | | | | |
| 0-19 Years | 46 | 23.9 | 633 | 5 | 7 | 21 | 43 | >99 | >99 | >99 |
| 20-34 | 51 | 11.4 | 120 | 3 | 4 | 7 | 14 | 37 | 38 | 42 |
| 35-49 | 98 | 11.8 | 101 | 4 | 4 | 9 | 14 | 24 | 33 | 60 |
| 50-64 | 140 | 10.9 | 60 | 5 | 6 | 8 | 12 | 25 | 28 | 32 |
| 65+ | 163 | 12.4 | 62 | 5 | 7 | 10 | 15 | 22 | 26 | 44 |
| **GRAND TOTAL** | 498 | 12.6 | 131 | 4 | 6 | 9 | 15 | 28 | 35 | >99 |

## 46.0: EXTERIORIZATION OF BOWEL. Formerly included in operation group(s) 610.

| Type of Patients | Observed Patients | Avg. Stay | Variance | 10th | 25th | 50th | 75th | 90th | 95th | 99th |
|---|---|---|---|---|---|---|---|---|---|---|
| **1. SINGLE DX** | | | | | | | | | | |
| 0-19 Years | 20 | 5.0 | 8 | 2 | 2 | 5 | 6 | 9 | 11 | 11 |
| 20-34 | 13 | 6.0 | 5 | 3 | 4 | 7 | 7 | 7 | 7 | 13 |
| 35-49 | 20 | 5.9 | 3 | 4 | 4 | 6 | 7 | 7 | 7 | 13 |
| 50-64 | 10 | 4.9 | 5 | 3 | 3 | 5 | 6 | 6 | 6 | 13 |
| 65+ | 12 | 5.0 | 5 | 3 | 4 | 5 | 5 | 6 | 12 | 12 |
| **2. MULTIPLE DX** | | | | | | | | | | |
| 0-19 Years | 134 | 17.1 | 329 | 4 | 7 | 12 | 23 | 65 | >99 | >99 |
| 20-34 | 99 | 10.4 | 95 | 4 | 4 | 7 | 11 | 21 | 38 | 42 |
| 35-49 | 296 | 11.1 | 91 | 3 | 4 | 8 | 14 | 23 | 31 | 46 |
| 50-64 | 518 | 10.9 | 83 | 3 | 5 | 8 | 13 | 22 | 28 | 43 |
| 65+ | 1,068 | 11.8 | 69 | 4 | 7 | 10 | 14 | 22 | 27 | 44 |
| **TOTAL SINGLE DX** | 75 | 5.3 | 5 | 2 | 4 | 5 | 7 | 7 | 11 | 13 |
| **TOTAL MULTIPLE DX** | 2,115 | 11.7 | 92 | 4 | 6 | 9 | 14 | 23 | 30 | 52 |
| **TOTAL** | | | | | | | | | | |
| 0-19 Years | 154 | 14.4 | 281 | 3 | 6 | 8 | 16 | 52 | >99 | >99 |
| 20-34 | 112 | 10.0 | 88 | 4 | 4 | 7 | 11 | 20 | 37 | 42 |
| 35-49 | 316 | 10.7 | 87 | 4 | 4 | 7 | 14 | 23 | 30 | 46 |
| 50-64 | 528 | 10.8 | 83 | 3 | 5 | 8 | 13 | 22 | 28 | 43 |
| 65+ | 1,080 | 11.7 | 69 | 4 | 7 | 9 | 14 | 22 | 27 | 44 |
| **GRAND TOTAL** | 2,190 | 11.4 | 90 | 3 | 6 | 9 | 14 | 23 | 30 | 52 |

## 46.03: LG BOWEL EXTERIORIZATION. Formerly included in operation group(s) 610.

| Type of Patients | Observed Patients | Avg. Stay | Variance | 10th | 25th | 50th | 75th | 90th | 95th | 99th |
|---|---|---|---|---|---|---|---|---|---|---|
| **1. SINGLE DX** | | | | | | | | | | |
| 0-19 Years | 17 | 5.0 | 8 | 2 | 2 | 5 | 6 | 8 | 11 | 11 |
| 20-34 | 3 | 5.3 | 2 | 4 | 5 | 5 | 7 | 7 | 7 | 7 |
| 35-49 | 9 | 6.3 | 1 | 4 | 6 | 7 | 7 | 7 | 7 | 7 |
| 50-64 | 8 | 4.6 | 5 | 3 | 3 | 4 | 6 | 6 | 6 | 13 |
| 65+ | 8 | 5.2 | 10 | 2 | 3 | 5 | 6 | 12 | 12 | 12 |
| **2. MULTIPLE DX** | | | | | | | | | | |
| 0-19 Years | 88 | 14.3 | 172 | 4 | 7 | 12 | 15 | 27 | 52 | 65 |
| 20-34 | 50 | 9.4 | 76 | 3 | 4 | 7 | 11 | 13 | 21 | 51 |
| 35-49 | 202 | 10.6 | 86 | 3 | 3 | 7 | 14 | 23 | 30 | 46 |
| 50-64 | 367 | 10.7 | 88 | 3 | 5 | 8 | 13 | 21 | 31 | 43 |
| 65+ | 885 | 11.6 | 70 | 4 | 7 | 9 | 14 | 22 | 27 | 43 |
| **TOTAL SINGLE DX** | 45 | 5.2 | 6 | 2 | 3 | 5 | 7 | 8 | 11 | 12 |
| **TOTAL MULTIPLE DX** | 1,592 | 11.3 | 82 | 3 | 6 | 9 | 14 | 22 | 28 | 46 |
| **TOTAL** | | | | | | | | | | |
| 0-19 Years | 105 | 11.6 | 142 | 2 | 5 | 8 | 15 | 19 | 38 | 65 |
| 20-34 | 53 | 9.2 | 75 | 4 | 4 | 7 | 11 | 13 | 21 | 51 |
| 35-49 | 211 | 10.4 | 83 | 3 | 5 | 7 | 14 | 23 | 30 | 46 |
| 50-64 | 375 | 10.5 | 87 | 3 | 5 | 8 | 13 | 21 | 31 | 43 |
| 65+ | 893 | 11.6 | 70 | 4 | 7 | 9 | 14 | 22 | 27 | 43 |
| **GRAND TOTAL** | 1,637 | 11.1 | 80 | 3 | 6 | 9 | 14 | 22 | 28 | 46 |

Length of Stay by Diagnosis and Operation, United States, 2000

# United States, October 1998–September 1999 Data, by Operation

## 46.1: COLOSTOMY. Formerly included in operation group(s) 612.

| Type of Patients | Observed Patients | Avg. Stay | Variance | Percentiles | | | | | | |
|---|---|---|---|---|---|---|---|---|---|---|
| | | | | 10th | 25th | 50th | 75th | 90th | 95th | 99th |
| **1. SINGLE DX** | | | | | | | | | | |
| 0–19 Years | 57 | 5.5 | 8 | 3 | 4 | 5 | 7 | 8 | 10 | 15 |
| 20–34 | 4 | 5.9 | 13 | 2 | 3 | 6 | 6 | 6 | 17 | 17 |
| 35–49 | 14 | 5.4 | 6 | 4 | 4 | 4 | 5 | 8 | 14 | 14 |
| 50–64 | 14 | 4.8 | 5 | 2 | 3 | 4 | 7 | 7 | 7 | 8 |
| 65+ | 14 | 5.5 | 8 | 3 | 4 | 4 | 6 | 11 | 11 | 12 |
| **2. MULTIPLE DX** | | | | | | | | | | |
| 0–19 Years | 247 | 11.7 | 158 | 3 | 5 | 8 | 15 | 21 | 31 | 97 |
| 20–34 | 101 | 13.3 | 56 | 3 | 7 | 13 | 20 | 20 | 20 | 36 |
| 35–49 | 322 | 10.1 | 63 | 4 | 5 | 8 | 13 | 19 | 26 | 47 |
| 50–64 | 519 | 11.5 | 55 | 5 | 7 | 10 | 14 | 19 | 24 | 41 |
| 65+ | 1,230 | 12.4 | 90 | 5 | 7 | 10 | 15 | 23 | 30 | 57 |
| **TOTAL SINGLE DX** | 103 | 5.4 | 7 | 3 | 4 | 4 | 7 | 8 | 11 | 15 |
| **TOTAL MULTIPLE DX** | 2,419 | 11.9 | 85 | 4 | 6 | 9 | 15 | 21 | 29 | 56 |
| **TOTAL** | | | | | | | | | | |
| 0–19 Years | 304 | 10.6 | 136 | 3 | 5 | 7 | 14 | 21 | 30 | 95 |
| 20–34 | 105 | 12.8 | 56 | 3 | 6 | 12 | 20 | 20 | 20 | 36 |
| 35–49 | 336 | 9.9 | 62 | 4 | 5 | 7 | 13 | 19 | 24 | 47 |
| 50–64 | 533 | 11.2 | 54 | 4 | 6 | 9 | 14 | 19 | 23 | 41 |
| 65+ | 1,244 | 12.4 | 90 | 5 | 7 | 10 | 14 | 22 | 30 | 57 |
| **GRAND TOTAL** | 2,522 | 11.6 | 83 | 4 | 6 | 9 | 14 | 21 | 28 | 55 |

## 46.11: TEMPORARY COLOSTOMY. Formerly included in operation group(s) 612.

| Type of Patients | Observed Patients | Avg. Stay | Variance | Percentiles | | | | | | |
|---|---|---|---|---|---|---|---|---|---|---|
| | | | | 10th | 25th | 50th | 75th | 90th | 95th | 99th |
| **1. SINGLE DX** | | | | | | | | | | |
| 0–19 Years | 17 | 6.1 | 13 | 2 | 4 | 5 | 6 | 14 | 15 | 15 |
| 20–34 | 4 | 5.9 | 13 | 2 | 3 | 6 | 6 | 6 | 17 | 17 |
| 35–49 | 5 | 7.1 | 15 | 4 | 5 | 6 | 6 | 14 | 14 | 14 |
| 50–64 | 2 | 3.6 | 2 | 3 | 3 | 3 | 3 | 7 | 7 | 7 |
| 65+ | 4 | 3.9 | 2 | 3 | 3 | 3 | 5 | 7 | 7 | 7 |
| **2. MULTIPLE DX** | | | | | | | | | | |
| 0–19 Years | 105 | 12.0 | 91 | 5 | 6 | 9 | 17 | 21 | 31 | >99 |
| 20–34 | 39 | 8.4 | 39 | 3 | 3 | 8 | 10 | 15 | 16 | 36 |
| 35–49 | 101 | 10.3 | 57 | 3 | 6 | 8 | 13 | 20 | 28 | 37 |
| 50–64 | 149 | 10.8 | 53 | 6 | 6 | 10 | 13 | 21 | 23 | 46 |
| 65+ | 246 | 12.7 | 71 | 5 | 7 | 10 | 16 | 21 | 29 | 43 |
| **TOTAL SINGLE DX** | 32 | 5.7 | 12 | 3 | 3 | 5 | 6 | 14 | 15 | 17 |
| **TOTAL MULTIPLE DX** | 640 | 11.5 | 67 | 4 | 6 | 10 | 14 | 21 | 26 | 48 |
| **TOTAL** | | | | | | | | | | |
| 0–19 Years | 122 | 11.2 | 84 | 4 | 5 | 8 | 15 | 21 | 26 | >99 |
| 20–34 | 43 | 7.9 | 34 | 3 | 3 | 6 | 10 | 15 | 17 | 28 |
| 35–49 | 106 | 10.2 | 56 | 3 | 6 | 7 | 13 | 20 | 28 | 37 |
| 50–64 | 151 | 10.6 | 53 | 3 | 6 | 10 | 13 | 21 | 23 | 46 |
| 65+ | 250 | 12.6 | 71 | 4 | 7 | 10 | 15 | 21 | 29 | 43 |
| **GRAND TOTAL** | 672 | 11.2 | 66 | 4 | 6 | 10 | 14 | 21 | 26 | 47 |

## 46.10: COLOSTOMY NOS. Formerly included in operation group(s) 612.

| Type of Patients | Observed Patients | Avg. Stay | Variance | Percentiles | | | | | | |
|---|---|---|---|---|---|---|---|---|---|---|
| | | | | 10th | 25th | 50th | 75th | 90th | 95th | 99th |
| **1. SINGLE DX** | | | | | | | | | | |
| 0–19 Years | 35 | 5.2 | 5 | 3 | 4 | 4 | 8 | 8 | 9 | 10 |
| 20–34 | 0 | | | | | | | | | |
| 35–49 | 7 | 5.4 | 3 | 4 | 4 | 4 | 7 | 8 | 8 | 8 |
| 50–64 | 7 | 5.0 | 5 | 2 | 2 | 6 | 7 | 7 | 7 | 8 |
| 65+ | 6 | 5.1 | 2 | 3 | 4 | 6 | 6 | 7 | 7 | 7 |
| **2. MULTIPLE DX** | | | | | | | | | | |
| 0–19 Years | 94 | 11.6 | 216 | 3 | 4 | 7 | 12 | 19 | 40 | 79 |
| 20–34 | 43 | 9.8 | 66 | 4 | 5 | 7 | 10 | 19 | 36 | 36 |
| 35–49 | 123 | 11.7 | 86 | 3 | 6 | 8 | 14 | 23 | 29 | 56 |
| 50–64 | 205 | 11.8 | 45 | 5 | 7 | 9 | 18 | 19 | 24 | 33 |
| 65+ | 527 | 12.7 | 95 | 5 | 7 | 10 | 15 | 23 | 33 | 57 |
| **TOTAL SINGLE DX** | 55 | 5.1 | 5 | 2 | 4 | 4 | 7 | 8 | 8 | 10 |
| **TOTAL MULTIPLE DX** | 992 | 12.2 | 95 | 4 | 6 | 9 | 15 | 22 | 29 | 57 |
| **TOTAL** | | | | | | | | | | |
| 0–19 Years | 129 | 9.9 | 169 | 3 | 4 | 6 | 10 | 18 | 26 | 79 |
| 20–34 | 43 | 9.8 | 66 | 4 | 5 | 7 | 10 | 19 | 36 | 36 |
| 35–49 | 130 | 11.3 | 84 | 5 | 6 | 8 | 14 | 23 | 29 | 56 |
| 50–64 | 212 | 11.2 | 45 | 5 | 6 | 9 | 16 | 19 | 23 | 33 |
| 65+ | 533 | 12.6 | 95 | 5 | 7 | 10 | 15 | 23 | 33 | 57 |
| **GRAND TOTAL** | 1,047 | 11.7 | 92 | 4 | 6 | 9 | 14 | 21 | 29 | 57 |

## 46.13: PERMANENT COLOSTOMY. Formerly included in operation group(s) 612.

| Type of Patients | Observed Patients | Avg. Stay | Variance | Percentiles | | | | | | |
|---|---|---|---|---|---|---|---|---|---|---|
| | | | | 10th | 25th | 50th | 75th | 90th | 95th | 99th |
| **1. SINGLE DX** | | | | | | | | | | |
| 0–19 Years | 5 | 6.0 | 2 | 4 | 5 | 6 | 7 | 8 | 8 | 8 |
| 20–34 | 0 | | | | | | | | | |
| 35–49 | 2 | 4.0 | 0 | 4 | 4 | 4 | 4 | 4 | 4 | 4 |
| 50–64 | 5 | 5.5 | 4 | 3 | 4 | 7 | 7 | 8 | 8 | 8 |
| 65+ | 4 | 6.5 | 12 | 4 | 4 | 4 | 11 | 11 | 12 | 12 |
| **2. MULTIPLE DX** | | | | | | | | | | |
| 0–19 Years | 47 | 11.6 | 216 | 2 | 3 | 7 | 14 | 28 | 39 | 76 |
| 20–34 | 19 | 17.9 | 18 | 12 | 20 | 20 | 20 | 20 | 20 | 20 |
| 35–49 | 98 | 8.1 | 38 | 4 | 4 | 5 | 11 | 15 | 17 | 50 |
| 50–64 | 164 | 11.8 | 70 | 4 | 7 | 9 | 14 | 18 | 29 | 47 |
| 65+ | 456 | 12.1 | 95 | 5 | 7 | 9 | 14 | 23 | 29 | 59 |
| **TOTAL SINGLE DX** | 16 | 5.8 | 8 | 4 | 4 | 4 | 7 | 11 | 11 | 12 |
| **TOTAL MULTIPLE DX** | 784 | 12.0 | 87 | 4 | 6 | 9 | 15 | 20 | 28 | 54 |
| **TOTAL** | | | | | | | | | | |
| 0–19 Years | 52 | 11.2 | 204 | 2 | 3 | 7 | 13 | 28 | 39 | 76 |
| 20–34 | 19 | 17.9 | 18 | 12 | 20 | 20 | 20 | 20 | 20 | 20 |
| 35–49 | 100 | 7.9 | 37 | 4 | 5 | 5 | 11 | 15 | 17 | 50 |
| 50–64 | 169 | 11.7 | 70 | 5 | 7 | 9 | 14 | 18 | 29 | 47 |
| 65+ | 460 | 12.0 | 94 | 5 | 7 | 9 | 14 | 22 | 29 | 59 |
| **GRAND TOTAL** | 800 | 11.9 | 86 | 4 | 6 | 9 | 15 | 20 | 28 | 50 |

Length of Stay by Diagnosis and Operation, United States, 2000

# United States, October 1998–September 1999 Data, by Operation

## 46.2: ILEOSTOMY. Formerly included in operation group(s) 612.

| Type of Patients | Observed Patients | Avg. Stay | Variance | Percentiles | | | | | | |
|---|---|---|---|---|---|---|---|---|---|---|
| | | | | 10th | 25th | 50th | 75th | 90th | 95th | 99th |
| **1. SINGLE DX** | | | | | | | | | | |
| 0–19 Years | 6 | 6.0 | 5 | 4 | 4 | 4 | 9 | 9 | 9 | 9 |
| 20–34 | 3 | 6.7 | 2 | 5 | 5 | 7 | 8 | 8 | 8 | 8 |
| 35–49 | 5 | 5.3 | 2 | 4 | 5 | 5 | 5 | 6 | 10 | 10 |
| 50–64 | 4 | 8.6 | 14 | 3 | 6 | 11 | 11 | 12 | 12 | 12 |
| 65+ | 2 | 6.0 | 0 | 6 | 6 | 6 | 6 | 6 | 6 | 6 |
| **2. MULTIPLE DX** | | | | | | | | | | |
| 0–19 Years | 56 | 29.6 | 753 | 5 | 16 | 32 | >99 | >99 | >99 | >99 |
| 20–34 | 51 | 8.7 | 22 | 4 | 6 | 7 | 10 | 15 | 20 | 29 |
| 35–49 | 102 | 12.4 | 125 | 4 | 6 | 8 | 16 | 24 | 35 | 49 |
| 50–64 | 105 | 12.6 | 54 | 6 | 7 | 10 | 18 | 22 | 29 | 35 |
| 65+ | 149 | 12.6 | 79 | 4 | 7 | 10 | 17 | 27 | 30 | 37 |
| **TOTAL SINGLE DX** | 20 | 6.1 | 5 | 4 | 4 | 5 | 7 | 9 | 11 | 12 |
| **TOTAL MULTIPLE DX** | 463 | 14.5 | 209 | 5 | 7 | 10 | 19 | 43 | >99 | >99 |
| **TOTAL** | | | | | | | | | | |
| 0–19 Years | 62 | 27.2 | 727 | 5 | 9 | 25 | >99 | >99 | >99 | >99 |
| 20–34 | 54 | 8.6 | 22 | 4 | 6 | 7 | 10 | 14 | 20 | 29 |
| 35–49 | 107 | 11.7 | 118 | 4 | 6 | 8 | 16 | 24 | 35 | 49 |
| 50–64 | 109 | 12.5 | 54 | 5 | 7 | 10 | 18 | 22 | 29 | 35 |
| 65+ | 151 | 12.5 | 79 | 4 | 7 | 10 | 17 | 27 | 30 | 37 |
| **GRAND TOTAL** | 483 | 14.2 | 203 | 5 | 7 | 10 | 19 | 36 | >99 | >99 |

## 46.32: PERC (ENDO) JEJUNOSTOMY. Formerly included in operation group(s) 612.

| Type of Patients | Observed Patients | Avg. Stay | Variance | Percentiles | | | | | | |
|---|---|---|---|---|---|---|---|---|---|---|
| | | | | 10th | 25th | 50th | 75th | 90th | 95th | 99th |
| **1. SINGLE DX** | | | | | | | | | | |
| 0–19 Years | 0 | | | | | | | | | |
| 20–34 | 0 | | | | | | | | | |
| 35–49 | 0 | | | | | | | | | |
| 50–64 | 3 | 2.9 | 6 | 2 | 2 | 2 | 2 | 9 | 9 | 9 |
| 65+ | 3 | 5.2 | <1 | 3 | 5 | 5 | 6 | 6 | 6 | 6 |
| **2. MULTIPLE DX** | | | | | | | | | | |
| 0–19 Years | 47 | 9.0 | 32 | 1 | 5 | 10 | 14 | 16 | 21 | 23 |
| 20–34 | 33 | 10.9 | 104 | 3 | 4 | 10 | 12 | 17 | 29 | 54 |
| 35–49 | 56 | 12.4 | 97 | 2 | 3 | 9 | 24 | 24 | 24 | >99 |
| 50–64 | 85 | 10.7 | 97 | 2 | 5 | 7 | 15 | 24 | 39 | >99 |
| 65+ | 315 | 11.6 | 85 | 3 | 5 | 9 | 16 | 21 | 28 | 50 |
| **TOTAL SINGLE DX** | 6 | 4.4 | 4 | 2 | 2 | 5 | 6 | 6 | 6 | 9 |
| **TOTAL MULTIPLE DX** | 536 | 11.3 | 85 | 2 | 5 | 9 | 16 | 24 | 28 | 60 |
| **TOTAL** | | | | | | | | | | |
| 0–19 Years | 47 | 9.0 | 32 | 1 | 5 | 10 | 14 | 16 | 21 | 23 |
| 20–34 | 33 | 10.9 | 104 | 3 | 4 | 10 | 12 | 17 | 29 | 54 |
| 35–49 | 56 | 12.4 | 97 | 2 | 3 | 9 | 24 | 24 | 24 | >99 |
| 50–64 | 88 | 10.4 | 96 | 2 | 4 | 7 | 15 | 24 | 39 | >99 |
| 65+ | 318 | 11.5 | 84 | 3 | 5 | 9 | 16 | 21 | 28 | 50 |
| **GRAND TOTAL** | 542 | 11.2 | 85 | 2 | 5 | 9 | 15 | 24 | 27 | 56 |

## 46.3: OTHER ENTEROSTOMY. Formerly included in operation group(s) 612.

| Type of Patients | Observed Patients | Avg. Stay | Variance | Percentiles | | | | | | |
|---|---|---|---|---|---|---|---|---|---|---|
| | | | | 10th | 25th | 50th | 75th | 90th | 95th | 99th |
| **1. SINGLE DX** | | | | | | | | | | |
| 0–19 Years | 3 | 4.5 | <1 | 4 | 4 | 4 | 4 | 6 | 6 | 6 |
| 20–34 | 3 | 3.0 | <1 | 2 | 3 | 3 | 4 | 4 | 4 | 4 |
| 35–49 | 3 | 2.4 | <1 | 2 | 2 | 2 | 2 | 3 | 3 | 3 |
| 50–64 | 3 | 2.9 | 6 | 2 | 2 | 2 | 2 | 9 | 9 | 9 |
| 65+ | 7 | 5.4 | 3 | 3 | 5 | 6 | 6 | 8 | 8 | 8 |
| **2. MULTIPLE DX** | | | | | | | | | | |
| 0–19 Years | 141 | 12.0 | 114 | 2 | 5 | 10 | 15 | 20 | 28 | 59 |
| 20–34 | 91 | 11.7 | 74 | 4 | 5 | 11 | 16 | 19 | 24 | 46 |
| 35–49 | 162 | 11.5 | 111 | 4 | 5 | 9 | 16 | 24 | 31 | 58 |
| 50–64 | 259 | 11.0 | 102 | 2 | 4 | 9 | 16 | 24 | 26 | 90 |
| 65+ | 762 | 11.7 | 89 | 3 | 5 | 9 | 15 | 21 | 30 | 50 |
| **TOTAL SINGLE DX** | 19 | 4.3 | 4 | 2 | 3 | 4 | 6 | 6 | 8 | 9 |
| **TOTAL MULTIPLE DX** | 1,415 | 11.6 | 96 | 2 | 5 | 9 | 16 | 23 | 29 | 54 |
| **TOTAL** | | | | | | | | | | |
| 0–19 Years | 144 | 11.8 | 113 | 2 | 5 | 10 | 15 | 20 | 26 | 59 |
| 20–34 | 94 | 11.5 | 74 | 2 | 4 | 11 | 16 | 18 | 24 | 46 |
| 35–49 | 165 | 11.4 | 111 | 3 | 4 | 9 | 16 | 24 | 31 | 58 |
| 50–64 | 262 | 10.9 | 102 | 2 | 3 | 9 | 16 | 24 | 26 | 90 |
| 65+ | 769 | 11.6 | 89 | 3 | 5 | 9 | 15 | 21 | 30 | 50 |
| **GRAND TOTAL** | 1,434 | 11.5 | 96 | 2 | 5 | 9 | 16 | 23 | 29 | 54 |

## 46.39: ENTEROSTOMY NEC. Formerly included in operation group(s) 612.

| Type of Patients | Observed Patients | Avg. Stay | Variance | Percentiles | | | | | | |
|---|---|---|---|---|---|---|---|---|---|---|
| | | | | 10th | 25th | 50th | 75th | 90th | 95th | 99th |
| **1. SINGLE DX** | | | | | | | | | | |
| 0–19 Years | 3 | 4.5 | <1 | 4 | 4 | 4 | 4 | 6 | 6 | 6 |
| 20–34 | 3 | 3.0 | <1 | 2 | 3 | 3 | 4 | 4 | 4 | 4 |
| 35–49 | 3 | 2.4 | <1 | 2 | 2 | 2 | 3 | 3 | 3 | 3 |
| 50–64 | 0 | | | | | | | | | |
| 65+ | 4 | 5.8 | 6 | 3 | 3 | 6 | 8 | 8 | 8 | 8 |
| **2. MULTIPLE DX** | | | | | | | | | | |
| 0–19 Years | 94 | 13.5 | 148 | 4 | 5 | 11 | 18 | 20 | 44 | 90 |
| 20–34 | 58 | 12.1 | 57 | 4 | 6 | 13 | 16 | 20 | 24 | 36 |
| 35–49 | 106 | 10.9 | 120 | 2 | 3 | 8 | 15 | 18 | 31 | 58 |
| 50–64 | 174 | 11.1 | 104 | 2 | 3 | 9 | 16 | 24 | 25 | 44 |
| 65+ | 446 | 11.7 | 92 | 3 | 5 | 9 | 15 | 21 | 30 | 50 |
| **TOTAL SINGLE DX** | 13 | 4.2 | 4 | 2 | 3 | 4 | 6 | 6 | 8 | 8 |
| **TOTAL MULTIPLE DX** | 878 | 11.7 | 102 | 3 | 5 | 9 | 16 | 22 | 30 | 52 |
| **TOTAL** | | | | | | | | | | |
| 0–19 Years | 97 | 13.2 | 147 | 4 | 5 | 10 | 18 | 20 | 44 | 90 |
| 20–34 | 61 | 11.9 | 57 | 3 | 5 | 12 | 16 | 19 | 24 | 36 |
| 35–49 | 109 | 10.8 | 119 | 2 | 4 | 8 | 14 | 18 | 31 | 58 |
| 50–64 | 174 | 11.1 | 104 | 2 | 3 | 9 | 16 | 24 | 25 | 44 |
| 65+ | 450 | 11.7 | 91 | 3 | 5 | 9 | 15 | 21 | 30 | 50 |
| **GRAND TOTAL** | 891 | 11.6 | 102 | 3 | 5 | 9 | 16 | 22 | 30 | 52 |

Length of Stay by Diagnosis and Operation, United States, 2000

# United States, October 1998–September 1999 Data, by Operation

## 46.42: PERICOLOSTOMY HERNIA REP. Formerly included in operation group(s) 611.

| Type of Patients | Observed Patients | Avg. Stay | Variance | 10th | 25th | 50th | 75th | 90th | 95th | 99th |
|---|---|---|---|---|---|---|---|---|---|---|
| **1. SINGLE DX** | | | | | | | | | | |
| 0–19 Years | 0 | | | | | | | | | |
| 20–34 | 1 | 7.0 | 0 | 7 | 7 | 7 | 7 | 7 | 7 | 7 |
| 35–49 | 5 | 2.2 | <1 | 1 | 1 | 3 | 3 | 3 | 3 | 3 |
| 50–64 | 7 | 4.0 | 5 | 3 | 3 | 3 | 4 | 5 | 10 | 10 |
| 65+ | 12 | 2.8 | 1 | 1 | 2 | 3 | 3 | 5 | 5 | 5 |
| **2. MULTIPLE DX** | | | | | | | | | | |
| 0–19 Years | 1 | 4.0 | 0 | 4 | 4 | 4 | 4 | 4 | 4 | 4 |
| 20–34 | 19 | 5.1 | 7 | 2 | 3 | 4 | 8 | 8 | 9 | 12 |
| 35–49 | 42 | 5.2 | 12 | 1 | 3 | 5 | 7 | 9 | 11 | 16 |
| 50–64 | 117 | 5.5 | 18 | 2 | 3 | 4 | 7 | 10 | 14 | 25 |
| 65+ | 284 | 6.5 | 19 | 2 | 4 | 5 | 8 | 12 | 15 | 23 |
| **TOTAL SINGLE DX** | 25 | 3.2 | 3 | 1 | 2 | 3 | 3 | 5 | 7 | 10 |
| **TOTAL MULTIPLE DX** | 463 | 6.1 | 18 | 2 | 3 | 5 | 8 | 12 | 14 | 22 |
| **TOTAL** | | | | | | | | | | |
| 0–19 Years | 1 | 4.0 | 0 | 4 | 4 | 4 | 4 | 4 | 4 | 4 |
| 20–34 | 20 | 5.3 | 7 | 2 | 3 | 4 | 7 | 8 | 9 | 12 |
| 35–49 | 47 | 5.0 | 11 | 2 | 3 | 4 | 6 | 9 | 11 | 16 |
| 50–64 | 124 | 5.4 | 18 | 2 | 3 | 4 | 7 | 10 | 14 | 25 |
| 65+ | 296 | 6.4 | 19 | 2 | 4 | 5 | 8 | 12 | 15 | 23 |
| **GRAND TOTAL** | 488 | 6.0 | 18 | 2 | 3 | 5 | 8 | 11 | 14 | 22 |

## 46.43: LG BOWEL STOMA REV NEC. Formerly included in operation group(s) 611.

| Type of Patients | Observed Patients | Avg. Stay | Variance | 10th | 25th | 50th | 75th | 90th | 95th | 99th |
|---|---|---|---|---|---|---|---|---|---|---|
| **1. SINGLE DX** | | | | | | | | | | |
| 0–19 Years | 6 | 3.6 | <1 | 3 | 3 | 3 | 5 | 5 | 5 | 5 |
| 20–34 | 3 | 3.4 | 1 | 1 | 4 | 4 | 4 | 4 | 4 | 4 |
| 35–49 | 7 | 2.3 | <1 | 1 | 1 | 1 | 4 | 4 | 4 | 4 |
| 50–64 | 10 | 1.6 | <1 | 1 | 1 | 2 | 2 | 3 | 3 | 3 |
| 65+ | 5 | 3.0 | 5 | 1 | 2 | 2 | 6 | 7 | 7 | 7 |
| **2. MULTIPLE DX** | | | | | | | | | | |
| 0–19 Years | 40 | 6.0 | 22 | 2 | 3 | 5 | 8 | 9 | 14 | 28 |
| 20–34 | 15 | 6.5 | 38 | 1 | 1 | 4 | 10 | 13 | 20 | 28 |
| 35–49 | 56 | 8.6 | 138 | 1 | 5 | 5 | 9 | 18 | 23 | 62 |
| 50–64 | 79 | 4.2 | 47 | 1 | 1 | 2 | 5 | 8 | 12 | 35 |
| 65+ | 210 | 7.0 | 35 | 2 | 3 | 5 | 9 | 15 | 19 | 28 |
| **TOTAL SINGLE DX** | 31 | 2.8 | 2 | 1 | 2 | 3 | 4 | 4 | 5 | 7 |
| **TOTAL MULTIPLE DX** | 400 | 6.4 | 53 | 1 | 2 | 4 | 8 | 14 | 19 | 35 |
| **TOTAL** | | | | | | | | | | |
| 0–19 Years | 46 | 5.6 | 19 | 2 | 3 | 5 | 7 | 9 | 12 | 28 |
| 20–34 | 18 | 5.1 | 24 | 1 | 2 | 4 | 5 | 10 | 14 | 28 |
| 35–49 | 63 | 8.1 | 129 | 1 | 1 | 2 | 8 | 18 | 23 | 62 |
| 50–64 | 89 | 4.1 | 44 | 1 | 1 | 2 | 5 | 8 | 12 | 35 |
| 65+ | 215 | 6.9 | 35 | 2 | 3 | 5 | 9 | 15 | 19 | 28 |
| **GRAND TOTAL** | 431 | 6.2 | 50 | 1 | 2 | 4 | 8 | 14 | 19 | 35 |

## 46.4: INTESTINAL STOMA REV. Formerly included in operation group(s) 611.

| Type of Patients | Observed Patients | Avg. Stay | Variance | 10th | 25th | 50th | 75th | 90th | 95th | 99th |
|---|---|---|---|---|---|---|---|---|---|---|
| **1. SINGLE DX** | | | | | | | | | | |
| 0–19 Years | 12 | 3.7 | 1 | 2 | 3 | 3 | 5 | 5 | 5 | 5 |
| 20–34 | 13 | 3.7 | 2 | 2 | 3 | 4 | 4 | 4 | 7 | 7 |
| 35–49 | 26 | 2.7 | 6 | 1 | 1 | 2 | 3 | 4 | 8 | 15 |
| 50–64 | 30 | 2.7 | 2 | 1 | 2 | 3 | 3 | 4 | 4 | 8 |
| 65+ | 20 | 2.9 | 2 | 1 | 2 | 3 | 3 | 5 | 6 | 7 |
| **2. MULTIPLE DX** | | | | | | | | | | |
| 0–19 Years | 88 | 8.3 | 100 | 2 | 3 | 6 | 11 | 14 | 28 | 37 |
| 20–34 | 86 | 5.9 | 16 | 1 | 4 | 5 | 6 | 11 | 15 | 20 |
| 35–49 | 193 | 7.1 | 59 | 1 | 3 | 5 | 8 | 13 | 19 | 54 |
| 50–64 | 309 | 6.3 | 41 | 1 | 2 | 4 | 7 | 14 | 21 | 24 |
| 65+ | 649 | 6.8 | 35 | 2 | 3 | 5 | 8 | 13 | 18 | 28 |
| **TOTAL SINGLE DX** | 101 | 3.0 | 3 | 1 | 2 | 3 | 4 | 5 | 5 | 10 |
| **TOTAL MULTIPLE DX** | 1,325 | 6.7 | 42 | 2 | 3 | 5 | 8 | 13 | 19 | 29 |
| **TOTAL** | | | | | | | | | | |
| 0–19 Years | 100 | 7.8 | 90 | 2 | 3 | 5 | 9 | 13 | 24 | 37 |
| 20–34 | 99 | 5.6 | 15 | 2 | 3 | 5 | 6 | 11 | 15 | 19 |
| 35–49 | 219 | 6.6 | 55 | 1 | 2 | 5 | 8 | 13 | 17 | 54 |
| 50–64 | 339 | 5.9 | 37 | 1 | 2 | 4 | 7 | 13 | 21 | 24 |
| 65+ | 669 | 6.7 | 34 | 2 | 3 | 5 | 8 | 13 | 18 | 27 |
| **GRAND TOTAL** | 1,426 | 6.5 | 40 | 2 | 3 | 5 | 8 | 13 | 18 | 28 |

## 46.41: SM BOWEL STOMA REVISION. Formerly included in operation group(s) 611.

| Type of Patients | Observed Patients | Avg. Stay | Variance | 10th | 25th | 50th | 75th | 90th | 95th | 99th |
|---|---|---|---|---|---|---|---|---|---|---|
| **1. SINGLE DX** | | | | | | | | | | |
| 0–19 Years | 4 | 4.3 | 2 | 2 | 5 | 5 | 5 | 5 | 5 | 5 |
| 20–34 | 9 | 3.6 | 1 | 2 | 3 | 4 | 4 | 4 | 7 | 7 |
| 35–49 | 14 | 2.9 | 9 | 1 | 1 | 1 | 4 | 8 | 10 | 15 |
| 50–64 | 12 | 2.8 | 1 | 1 | 3 | 3 | 3 | 4 | 4 | 4 |
| 65+ | 3 | 2.7 | <1 | 2 | 2 | 3 | 3 | 3 | 3 | 3 |
| **2. MULTIPLE DX** | | | | | | | | | | |
| 0–19 Years | 44 | 10.2 | 147 | 2 | 3 | 7 | 11 | 22 | 37 | 91 |
| 20–34 | 44 | 6.5 | 14 | 3 | 4 | 6 | 6 | 12 | 15 | 19 |
| 35–49 | 90 | 6.9 | 33 | 2 | 4 | 6 | 8 | 13 | 17 | 29 |
| 50–64 | 104 | 8.6 | 46 | 2 | 4 | 7 | 10 | 21 | 21 | 24 |
| 65+ | 135 | 7.2 | 73 | 2 | 3 | 4 | 8 | 14 | 20 | 34 |
| **TOTAL SINGLE DX** | 42 | 3.0 | 3 | 1 | 2 | 3 | 3 | 5 | 6 | 10 |
| **TOTAL MULTIPLE DX** | 417 | 7.7 | 58 | 2 | 4 | 6 | 9 | 17 | 21 | 37 |
| **TOTAL** | | | | | | | | | | |
| 0–19 Years | 48 | 9.8 | 139 | 2 | 3 | 6 | 11 | 22 | 37 | 37 |
| 20–34 | 53 | 6.2 | 13 | 3 | 4 | 5 | 6 | 11 | 15 | 19 |
| 35–49 | 104 | 6.3 | 32 | 2 | 3 | 5 | 8 | 12 | 17 | 29 |
| 50–64 | 116 | 7.4 | 42 | 2 | 3 | 5 | 10 | 21 | 21 | 24 |
| 65+ | 138 | 7.1 | 72 | 2 | 3 | 4 | 8 | 14 | 20 | 34 |
| **GRAND TOTAL** | 459 | 7.2 | 54 | 2 | 3 | 5 | 8 | 15 | 21 | 34 |

Length of Stay by Diagnosis and Operation, United States, 2000

## 46.5: INTESTINAL STOMA CLOSURE. Formerly included in operation group(s) 611.

| Type of Patients | Observed Patients | Avg. Stay | Variance | Percentiles | | | | | | |
|---|---|---|---|---|---|---|---|---|---|---|
| | | | | 10th | 25th | 50th | 75th | 90th | 95th | 99th |
| **1. SINGLE DX** | | | | | | | | | | |
| 0–19 Years | 185 | 4.3 | 4 | 2 | 3 | 4 | 5 | 7 | 8 | 11 |
| 20–34 | 199 | 4.7 | 3 | 3 | 3 | 5 | 5 | 7 | 8 | 10 |
| 35–49 | 261 | 4.8 | 3 | 3 | 4 | 4 | 6 | 7 | 8 | 10 |
| 50–64 | 164 | 5.2 | 6 | 2 | 3 | 5 | 7 | 8 | 10 | 12 |
| 65+ | 68 | 5.0 | 4 | 3 | 3 | 5 | 6 | 7 | 8 | 12 |
| **2. MULTIPLE DX** | | | | | | | | | | |
| 0–19 Years | 629 | 8.1 | 78 | 3 | 4 | 6 | 8 | 15 | 22 | 58 |
| 20–34 | 519 | 6.5 | 23 | 3 | 4 | 6 | 8 | 10 | 15 | 28 |
| 35–49 | 1,226 | 6.4 | 16 | 3 | 4 | 6 | 8 | 9 | 11 | 20 |
| 50–64 | 1,614 | 6.7 | 20 | 3 | 4 | 6 | 8 | 10 | 13 | 25 |
| 65+ | 2,037 | 7.6 | 23 | 4 | 5 | 7 | 9 | 12 | 16 | 28 |
| **TOTAL SINGLE DX** | 877 | 4.8 | 4 | 3 | 3 | 5 | 6 | 7 | 8 | 11 |
| **TOTAL MULTIPLE DX** | 6,025 | 7.1 | 27 | 3 | 4 | 6 | 8 | 11 | 15 | 29 |
| **TOTAL** | | | | | | | | | | |
| 0–19 Years | 814 | 7.1 | 61 | 3 | 4 | 5 | 7 | 12 | 18 | 47 |
| 20–34 | 718 | 6.0 | 18 | 3 | 3 | 5 | 7 | 9 | 12 | 28 |
| 35–49 | 1,487 | 6.1 | 14 | 3 | 4 | 6 | 7 | 9 | 11 | 18 |
| 50–64 | 1,778 | 6.5 | 18 | 3 | 4 | 6 | 8 | 10 | 13 | 25 |
| 65+ | 2,105 | 7.5 | 22 | 4 | 5 | 7 | 9 | 12 | 16 | 28 |
| **GRAND TOTAL** | 6,902 | 6.7 | 24 | 3 | 4 | 6 | 8 | 10 | 14 | 28 |

## 46.51: SM BOWEL STOMA CLOSURE. Formerly included in operation group(s) 611.

| Type of Patients | Observed Patients | Avg. Stay | Variance | Percentiles | | | | | | |
|---|---|---|---|---|---|---|---|---|---|---|
| | | | | 10th | 25th | 50th | 75th | 90th | 95th | 99th |
| **1. SINGLE DX** | | | | | | | | | | |
| 0–19 Years | 69 | 4.8 | 5 | 2 | 3 | 4 | 6 | 8 | 11 | 11 |
| 20–34 | 69 | 3.7 | 3 | 2 | 3 | 3 | 4 | 6 | 8 | 8 |
| 35–49 | 58 | 4.7 | 5 | 2 | 3 | 4 | 5 | 7 | 8 | 14 |
| 50–64 | 33 | 3.4 | 3 | 2 | 2 | 3 | 4 | 5 | 8 | 10 |
| 65+ | 7 | 2.9 | 1 | 2 | 2 | 3 | 3 | 3 | 5 | 5 |
| **2. MULTIPLE DX** | | | | | | | | | | |
| 0–19 Years | 296 | 10.5 | 142 | 3 | 4 | 6 | 12 | 21 | 40 | 61 |
| 20–34 | 275 | 5.9 | 17 | 3 | 3 | 5 | 8 | 10 | 16 | 22 |
| 35–49 | 396 | 6.6 | 31 | 3 | 4 | 6 | 8 | 11 | 14 | 29 |
| 50–64 | 428 | 6.4 | 35 | 3 | 4 | 6 | 7 | 11 | 20 | 36 |
| 65+ | 408 | 7.3 | 37 | 3 | 4 | 6 | 8 | 15 | 21 | 30 |
| **TOTAL SINGLE DX** | 236 | 4.2 | 4 | 2 | 3 | 4 | 5 | 7 | 8 | 11 |
| **TOTAL MULTIPLE DX** | 1,803 | 7.3 | 52 | 3 | 4 | 5 | 8 | 14 | 20 | 40 |
| **TOTAL** | | | | | | | | | | |
| 0–19 Years | 365 | 9.2 | 116 | 3 | 4 | 6 | 10 | 17 | 35 | 58 |
| 20–34 | 344 | 5.4 | 15 | 3 | 3 | 4 | 7 | 9 | 14 | 20 |
| 35–49 | 454 | 6.4 | 28 | 3 | 4 | 5 | 8 | 10 | 13 | 29 |
| 50–64 | 461 | 6.2 | 34 | 3 | 3 | 4 | 7 | 11 | 20 | 36 |
| 65+ | 415 | 7.3 | 37 | 3 | 4 | 5 | 8 | 15 | 21 | 30 |
| **GRAND TOTAL** | 2,039 | 6.9 | 47 | 3 | 3 | 5 | 8 | 13 | 17 | 40 |

## 46.52: LG BOWEL STOMA CLOSURE. Formerly included in operation group(s) 611.

| Type of Patients | Observed Patients | Avg. Stay | Variance | Percentiles | | | | | | |
|---|---|---|---|---|---|---|---|---|---|---|
| | | | | 10th | 25th | 50th | 75th | 90th | 95th | 99th |
| **1. SINGLE DX** | | | | | | | | | | |
| 0–19 Years | 116 | 4.1 | 2 | 3 | 3 | 4 | 5 | 6 | 6 | 9 |
| 20–34 | 130 | 5.2 | 3 | 3 | 4 | 5 | 6 | 7 | 8 | 10 |
| 35–49 | 203 | 4.8 | 2 | 3 | 4 | 5 | 6 | 7 | 8 | 9 |
| 50–64 | 131 | 5.6 | 5 | 3 | 4 | 5 | 7 | 8 | 11 | 12 |
| 65+ | 61 | 5.2 | 4 | 3 | 3 | 5 | 6 | 7 | 8 | 12 |
| **2. MULTIPLE DX** | | | | | | | | | | |
| 0–19 Years | 332 | 5.9 | 12 | 3 | 4 | 5 | 7 | 9 | 11 | 26 |
| 20–34 | 244 | 7.3 | 29 | 4 | 5 | 6 | 8 | 9 | 15 | 29 |
| 35–49 | 828 | 6.3 | 10 | 3 | 5 | 6 | 8 | 9 | 10 | 18 |
| 50–64 | 1,186 | 6.7 | 14 | 3 | 5 | 6 | 8 | 10 | 12 | 20 |
| 65+ | 1,629 | 7.7 | 20 | 4 | 5 | 7 | 9 | 11 | 15 | 26 |
| **TOTAL SINGLE DX** | 641 | 4.9 | 3 | 3 | 4 | 5 | 6 | 7 | 8 | 11 |
| **TOTAL MULTIPLE DX** | 4,219 | 7.0 | 16 | 4 | 5 | 6 | 8 | 10 | 13 | 26 |
| **TOTAL** | | | | | | | | | | |
| 0–19 Years | 448 | 5.4 | 10 | 3 | 4 | 5 | 6 | 8 | 10 | 18 |
| 20–34 | 374 | 6.5 | 20 | 4 | 5 | 6 | 7 | 9 | 10 | 28 |
| 35–49 | 1,031 | 6.0 | 9 | 4 | 5 | 6 | 7 | 9 | 10 | 16 |
| 50–64 | 1,317 | 6.6 | 13 | 3 | 5 | 6 | 8 | 10 | 11 | 20 |
| 65+ | 1,690 | 7.6 | 19 | 4 | 5 | 7 | 9 | 11 | 15 | 26 |
| **GRAND TOTAL** | 4,860 | 6.7 | 15 | 3 | 5 | 6 | 8 | 10 | 12 | 24 |

## 46.6: FIXATION OF INTESTINE. Formerly included in operation group(s) 611.

| Type of Patients | Observed Patients | Avg. Stay | Variance | Percentiles | | | | | | |
|---|---|---|---|---|---|---|---|---|---|---|
| | | | | 10th | 25th | 50th | 75th | 90th | 95th | 99th |
| **1. SINGLE DX** | | | | | | | | | | |
| 0–19 Years | 2 | 4.0 | 8 | 2 | 2 | 2 | 7 | 7 | 7 | 7 |
| 20–34 | 1 | 5.0 | 0 | 5 | 5 | 5 | 5 | 5 | 5 | 5 |
| 35–49 | 1 | 5.0 | 0 | 5 | 5 | 5 | 5 | 5 | 5 | 5 |
| 50–64 | 3 | 1.6 | 3 | 1 | 1 | 1 | 1 | 2 | 8 | 8 |
| 65+ | 0 | | | | | | | | | |
| **2. MULTIPLE DX** | | | | | | | | | | |
| 0–19 Years | 7 | 11.2 | 18 | 4 | 10 | 10 | 14 | 19 | 19 | 19 |
| 20–34 | 6 | 6.1 | 31 | 3 | 3 | 4 | 6 | 19 | 19 | 19 |
| 35–49 | 18 | 9.4 | 83 | 2 | 3 | 5 | 24 | 24 | 24 | 32 |
| 50–64 | 18 | 7.6 | 29 | 2 | 2 | 9 | 12 | 13 | 17 | 32 |
| 65+ | 25 | 12.5 | 94 | 4 | 9 | 9 | 14 | 23 | 43 | 43 |
| **TOTAL SINGLE DX** | 7 | 3.6 | 5 | 1 | 1 | 5 | 5 | 5 | 7 | 8 |
| **TOTAL MULTIPLE DX** | 74 | 9.7 | 66 | 2 | 4 | 9 | 13 | 23 | 24 | 43 |
| **TOTAL** | | | | | | | | | | |
| 0–19 Years | 9 | 9.5 | 25 | 2 | 7 | 10 | 14 | 14 | 19 | 19 |
| 20–34 | 7 | 5.4 | 10 | 2 | 5 | 5 | 5 | 5 | 6 | 19 |
| 35–49 | 19 | 9.0 | 77 | 1 | 3 | 5 | 16 | 24 | 24 | 24 |
| 50–64 | 21 | 6.5 | 30 | 1 | 2 | 5 | 9 | 13 | 17 | 17 |
| 65+ | 25 | 12.5 | 94 | 4 | 9 | 9 | 14 | 23 | 43 | 43 |
| **GRAND TOTAL** | 81 | 8.6 | 61 | 2 | 3 | 7 | 11 | 19 | 24 | 43 |

Length of Stay by Diagnosis and Operation, United States, 2000

## United States, October 1998–September 1999 Data, by Operation

### 46.74: CLOSURE SMB FISTULA NEC. Formerly included in operation group(s) 611.

| Type of Patients | Observed Patients | Avg. Stay | Variance | 10th | 25th | 50th | 75th | 90th | 95th | 99th |
|---|---|---|---|---|---|---|---|---|---|---|
| **1. SINGLE DX** | | | | | | | | | | |
| 0–19 Years | 2 | 6.6 | <1 | 6 | 6 | 7 | 7 | 7 | 7 | 7 |
| 20–34 | 2 | 4.6 | 7 | 3 | 3 | 3 | 7 | 7 | 7 | 7 |
| 35–49 | 4 | 7.7 | 3 | 7 | 7 | 7 | 10 | 10 | 10 | 10 |
| 50–64 | 1 | 2.0 | 0 | 2 | 2 | 2 | 2 | 2 | 2 | 2 |
| 65+ | 1 | 8.0 | 0 | 8 | 8 | 8 | 8 | 8 | 8 | 8 |
| **2. MULTIPLE DX** | | | | | | | | | | |
| 0–19 Years | 30 | 29.7 | 927 | 4 | 8 | 17 | 79 | 79 | >99 | >99 |
| 20–34 | 29 | 8.3 | 69 | 2 | 2 | 5 | 12 | 26 | 28 | 31 |
| 35–49 | 74 | 19.0 | 236 | 6 | 10 | 14 | 23 | 47 | 55 | >99 |
| 50–64 | 122 | 14.7 | 138 | 5 | 7 | 11 | 20 | 26 | 40 | 68 |
| 65+ | 117 | 14.9 | 177 | 3 | 6 | 10 | 23 | 35 | 42 | 61 |
| **TOTAL SINGLE DX** | 10 | 6.9 | 5 | 3 | 7 | 7 | 8 | 10 | 10 | 10 |
| **TOTAL MULTIPLE DX** | 372 | 16.5 | 267 | 3 | 7 | 11 | 21 | 42 | 68 | >99 |
| **TOTAL** | | | | | | | | | | |
| 0–19 Years | 32 | 28.9 | 912 | 4 | 8 | 17 | 79 | 79 | >99 | >99 |
| 20–34 | 31 | 8.2 | 68 | 2 | 2 | 5 | 12 | 22 | 28 | 31 |
| 35–49 | 78 | 18.0 | 226 | 5 | 7 | 13 | 23 | 47 | 55 | >99 |
| 50–64 | 123 | 14.7 | 138 | 5 | 7 | 11 | 20 | 26 | 40 | 68 |
| 65+ | 118 | 14.8 | 176 | 3 | 6 | 9 | 23 | 35 | 42 | 61 |
| **GRAND TOTAL** | 382 | 16.3 | 263 | 3 | 7 | 11 | 20 | 41 | 67 | >99 |

### 46.75: SUTURE LG BOWEL LAC. Formerly included in operation group(s) 611.

| Type of Patients | Observed Patients | Avg. Stay | Variance | 10th | 25th | 50th | 75th | 90th | 95th | 99th |
|---|---|---|---|---|---|---|---|---|---|---|
| **1. SINGLE DX** | | | | | | | | | | |
| 0–19 Years | 7 | 5.3 | 3 | 3 | 4 | 5 | 6 | 8 | 8 | 8 |
| 20–34 | 17 | 2.6 | 5 | 1 | 1 | 1 | 4 | 5 | 8 | 9 |
| 35–49 | 10 | 4.1 | 2 | 3 | 4 | 5 | 5 | 6 | 6 | 6 |
| 50–64 | 5 | 4.4 | 4 | 3 | 3 | 3 | 5 | 8 | 8 | 8 |
| 65+ | 2 | 7.1 | 3 | 6 | 6 | 6 | 9 | 9 | 9 | 9 |
| **2. MULTIPLE DX** | | | | | | | | | | |
| 0–19 Years | 93 | 8.7 | 46 | 3 | 5 | 6 | 9 | 14 | 25 | 34 |
| 20–34 | 180 | 9.8 | 65 | 4 | 5 | 6 | 11 | 23 | 28 | 28 |
| 35–49 | 152 | 8.5 | 38 | 3 | 5 | 7 | 9 | 20 | 22 | 24 |
| 50–64 | 122 | 10.7 | 47 | 4 | 6 | 8 | 14 | 23 | 23 | 34 |
| 65+ | 253 | 9.2 | 49 | 4 | 6 | 7 | 10 | 14 | 19 | 47 |
| **TOTAL SINGLE DX** | 41 | 3.3 | 5 | 1 | 1 | 3 | 4 | 7 | 8 | 9 |
| **TOTAL MULTIPLE DX** | 800 | 9.4 | 50 | 4 | 5 | 7 | 11 | 20 | 23 | 35 |
| **TOTAL** | | | | | | | | | | |
| 0–19 Years | 100 | 8.5 | 45 | 3 | 5 | 6 | 9 | 14 | 25 | 34 |
| 20–34 | 197 | 8.8 | 63 | 3 | 4 | 6 | 9 | 23 | 28 | 28 |
| 35–49 | 162 | 8.3 | 37 | 4 | 6 | 7 | 9 | 20 | 22 | 24 |
| 50–64 | 127 | 10.4 | 46 | 4 | 6 | 8 | 14 | 23 | 23 | 34 |
| 65+ | 255 | 9.2 | 49 | 4 | 6 | 7 | 10 | 14 | 19 | 47 |
| **GRAND TOTAL** | 841 | 9.0 | 50 | 3 | 5 | 7 | 10 | 20 | 23 | 34 |

### 46.7: OTHER INTESTINAL REPAIR. Formerly included in operation group(s) 611.

| Type of Patients | Observed Patients | Avg. Stay | Variance | 10th | 25th | 50th | 75th | 90th | 95th | 99th |
|---|---|---|---|---|---|---|---|---|---|---|
| **1. SINGLE DX** | | | | | | | | | | |
| 0–19 Years | 44 | 5.9 | 5 | 4 | 4 | 5 | 8 | 10 | 10 | 10 |
| 20–34 | 49 | 3.3 | 5 | 1 | 1 | 3 | 4 | 7 | 7 | 9 |
| 35–49 | 40 | 6.0 | 4 | 4 | 5 | 6 | 6 | 10 | 11 | 11 |
| 50–64 | 16 | 4.0 | 2 | 3 | 3 | 4 | 4 | 5 | 8 | 8 |
| 65+ | 7 | 7.6 | 8 | 3 | 6 | 8 | 9 | 12 | 12 | 12 |
| **2. MULTIPLE DX** | | | | | | | | | | |
| 0–19 Years | 392 | 12.8 | 243 | 4 | 5 | 7 | 15 | 34 | 79 | >99 |
| 20–34 | 544 | 8.8 | 73 | 3 | 4 | 6 | 9 | 21 | 25 | 49 |
| 35–49 | 686 | 10.3 | 85 | 4 | 5 | 7 | 12 | 22 | 29 | 48 |
| 50–64 | 643 | 11.6 | 86 | 4 | 6 | 8 | 15 | 23 | 28 | 53 |
| 65+ | 1,012 | 12.1 | 101 | 4 | 6 | 9 | 15 | 21 | 33 | 56 |
| **TOTAL SINGLE DX** | 156 | 4.8 | 6 | 1 | 3 | 4 | 6 | 8 | 10 | 11 |
| **TOTAL MULTIPLE DX** | 3,277 | 11.1 | 107 | 4 | 5 | 8 | 14 | 23 | 31 | 72 |
| **TOTAL** | | | | | | | | | | |
| 0–19 Years | 436 | 12.2 | 224 | 4 | 5 | 7 | 13 | 34 | 79 | >99 |
| 20–34 | 593 | 8.3 | 69 | 2 | 4 | 6 | 9 | 20 | 23 | 43 |
| 35–49 | 726 | 10.0 | 81 | 4 | 5 | 7 | 11 | 21 | 28 | 48 |
| 50–64 | 659 | 11.3 | 85 | 4 | 6 | 8 | 15 | 22 | 27 | 53 |
| 65+ | 1,019 | 12.0 | 100 | 4 | 6 | 9 | 15 | 21 | 33 | 56 |
| **GRAND TOTAL** | 3,433 | 10.8 | 103 | 4 | 5 | 7 | 13 | 22 | 30 | 70 |

### 46.73: SMALL BOWEL SUTURE NEC. Formerly included in operation group(s) 611.

| Type of Patients | Observed Patients | Avg. Stay | Variance | 10th | 25th | 50th | 75th | 90th | 95th | 99th |
|---|---|---|---|---|---|---|---|---|---|---|
| **1. SINGLE DX** | | | | | | | | | | |
| 0–19 Years | 25 | 5.2 | 5 | 3 | 4 | 4 | 7 | 10 | 10 | 10 |
| 20–34 | 25 | 4.2 | 3 | 2 | 3 | 4 | 5 | 6 | 7 | 8 |
| 35–49 | 18 | 5.7 | 1 | 4 | 6 | 6 | 6 | 6 | 6 | 10 |
| 50–64 | 3 | 3.7 | <1 | 2 | 4 | 4 | 4 | 4 | 4 | 4 |
| 65+ | 1 | 8.0 | 0 | 8 | 8 | 8 | 8 | 8 | 8 | 8 |
| **2. MULTIPLE DX** | | | | | | | | | | |
| 0–19 Years | 165 | 8.5 | 92 | 4 | 5 | 6 | 9 | 17 | 21 | >99 |
| 20–34 | 248 | 6.6 | 44 | 2 | 4 | 6 | 7 | 9 | 14 | 31 |
| 35–49 | 315 | 8.9 | 55 | 4 | 5 | 6 | 10 | 18 | 27 | 38 |
| 50–64 | 252 | 10.5 | 94 | 4 | 6 | 7 | 12 | 22 | 33 | 62 |
| 65+ | 383 | 11.4 | 73 | 4 | 6 | 9 | 14 | 20 | 29 | 41 |
| **TOTAL SINGLE DX** | 72 | 5.1 | 3 | 3 | 4 | 5 | 6 | 7 | 8 | 10 |
| **TOTAL MULTIPLE DX** | 1,363 | 9.4 | 72 | 3 | 5 | 7 | 11 | 18 | 26 | 43 |
| **TOTAL** | | | | | | | | | | |
| 0–19 Years | 190 | 8.0 | 80 | 4 | 5 | 6 | 9 | 16 | 18 | 84 |
| 20–34 | 273 | 6.4 | 41 | 2 | 4 | 6 | 7 | 9 | 11 | 31 |
| 35–49 | 333 | 8.6 | 52 | 4 | 5 | 6 | 9 | 18 | 26 | 38 |
| 50–64 | 255 | 10.5 | 93 | 3 | 5 | 7 | 12 | 22 | 33 | 62 |
| 65+ | 384 | 11.4 | 73 | 4 | 6 | 9 | 14 | 20 | 29 | 41 |
| **GRAND TOTAL** | 1,435 | 9.2 | 69 | 3 | 5 | 7 | 10 | 18 | 25 | 42 |

Length of Stay by Diagnosis and Operation, United States, 2000

# United States, October 1998–September 1999 Data, by Operation

## 46.79: REPAIR OF INTESTINE NEC. Formerly included in operation group(s) 611.

| Type of Patients | Observed Patients | Avg. Stay | Variance | Percentiles | | | | | | |
|---|---|---|---|---|---|---|---|---|---|---|
| | | | | 10th | 25th | 50th | 75th | 90th | 95th | 99th |
| **1. SINGLE DX** | | | | | | | | | | |
| 0–19 Years | 7 | 7.0 | 3 | 4 | 6 | 8 | 8 | 8 | 8 | 8 |
| 20–34 | 2 | 5.3 | 1 | 4 | 4 | 6 | 6 | 6 | 6 | 6 |
| 35–49 | 2 | 6.3 | <1 | 6 | 6 | 6 | 6 | 7 | 7 | 7 |
| 50–64 | 7 | 3.9 | <1 | 2 | 4 | 4 | 4 | 4 | 5 | 7 |
| 65+ | 2 | 4.7 | 3 | 3 | 3 | 6 | 6 | 6 | 6 | 6 |
| **2. MULTIPLE DX** | | | | | | | | | | |
| 0–19 Years | 63 | 12.5 | 147 | 4 | 4 | 9 | 23 | 70 | >99 | >99 |
| 20–34 | 48 | 11.1 | 92 | 4 | 5 | 7 | 21 | 21 | 21 | 68 |
| 35–49 | 93 | 11.2 | 97 | 4 | 6 | 8 | 15 | 21 | 26 | 60 |
| 50–64 | 97 | 11.6 | 62 | 4 | 6 | 8 | 16 | 22 | 22 | 41 |
| 65+ | 177 | 13.3 | 98 | 4 | 7 | 11 | 16 | 21 | 32 | 58 |
| **TOTAL SINGLE DX** | 20 | 5.0 | 4 | 4 | 4 | 4 | 6 | 8 | 8 | 8 |
| **TOTAL MULTIPLE DX** | 478 | 12.2 | 98 | 4 | 6 | 9 | 16 | 22 | 32 | >99 |
| **TOTAL** | | | | | | | | | | |
| 0–19 Years | 70 | 11.9 | 134 | 4 | 4 | 8 | 22 | 48 | >99 | >99 |
| 20–34 | 50 | 11.0 | 91 | 4 | 5 | 7 | 21 | 21 | 21 | 68 |
| 35–49 | 95 | 11.1 | 96 | 4 | 6 | 8 | 15 | 21 | 26 | 60 |
| 50–64 | 104 | 10.5 | 61 | 4 | 6 | 7 | 14 | 22 | 22 | 41 |
| 65+ | 179 | 13.3 | 98 | 4 | 7 | 11 | 16 | 21 | 32 | 58 |
| **GRAND TOTAL** | 498 | 11.8 | 95 | 4 | 6 | 9 | 16 | 22 | 30 | >99 |

## 46.81: INTRA-ABD SM BOWEL MANIP. Formerly included in operation group(s) 611.

| Type of Patients | Observed Patients | Avg. Stay | Variance | Percentiles | | | | | | |
|---|---|---|---|---|---|---|---|---|---|---|
| | | | | 10th | 25th | 50th | 75th | 90th | 95th | 99th |
| **1. SINGLE DX** | | | | | | | | | | |
| 0–19 Years | 57 | 3.2 | 2 | 2 | 2 | 3 | 5 | 5 | 6 | 7 |
| 20–34 | 6 | 5.3 | 3 | 3 | 4 | 6 | 6 | 8 | 8 | 8 |
| 35–49 | 4 | 7.8 | <1 | 7 | 8 | 8 | 8 | 8 | 8 | 8 |
| 50–64 | 6 | 5.6 | 6 | 2 | 6 | 6 | 7 | 8 | 8 | 8 |
| 65+ | 1 | 6.0 | 0 | 6 | 6 | 6 | 6 | 6 | 6 | 6 |
| **2. MULTIPLE DX** | | | | | | | | | | |
| 0–19 Years | 153 | 14.5 | 513 | 3 | 4 | 6 | 11 | 79 | 79 | 91 |
| 20–34 | 31 | 8.9 | 168 | 3 | 3 | 6 | 8 | 16 | 36 | 80 |
| 35–49 | 92 | 8.4 | 24 | 4 | 5 | 7 | 11 | 16 | 18 | 20 |
| 50–64 | 103 | 11.7 | 77 | 4 | 6 | 9 | 15 | 19 | 23 | 47 |
| 65+ | 203 | 11.7 | 53 | 5 | 7 | 10 | 14 | 19 | 28 | 38 |
| **TOTAL SINGLE DX** | 74 | 4.0 | 5 | 2 | 2 | 3 | 5 | 8 | 8 | 8 |
| **TOTAL MULTIPLE DX** | 582 | 11.6 | 167 | 3 | 5 | 8 | 14 | 19 | 30 | 79 |
| **TOTAL** | | | | | | | | | | |
| 0–19 Years | 210 | 10.5 | 359 | 2 | 3 | 5 | 8 | 16 | 79 | 79 |
| 20–34 | 37 | 8.3 | 145 | 3 | 3 | 6 | 8 | 14 | 30 | 80 |
| 35–49 | 96 | 8.3 | 22 | 4 | 5 | 7 | 10 | 16 | 18 | 20 |
| 50–64 | 109 | 11.5 | 76 | 4 | 6 | 9 | 15 | 19 | 23 | 47 |
| 65+ | 204 | 11.7 | 53 | 5 | 7 | 10 | 14 | 19 | 28 | 38 |
| **GRAND TOTAL** | 656 | 10.6 | 151 | 3 | 5 | 8 | 12 | 18 | 27 | 79 |

## 46.8: BOWEL DILATION & MANIP. Formerly included in operation group(s) 611.

| Type of Patients | Observed Patients | Avg. Stay | Variance | Percentiles | | | | | | |
|---|---|---|---|---|---|---|---|---|---|---|
| | | | | 10th | 25th | 50th | 75th | 90th | 95th | 99th |
| **1. SINGLE DX** | | | | | | | | | | |
| 0–19 Years | 145 | 2.8 | 2 | 2 | 2 | 3 | 3 | 5 | 5 | 7 |
| 20–34 | 12 | 5.0 | 23 | 1 | 1 | 4 | 6 | 8 | 20 | 20 |
| 35–49 | 12 | 6.7 | 8 | 3 | 3 | 8 | 8 | 10 | 10 | 10 |
| 50–64 | 14 | 3.2 | 6 | 1 | 1 | 2 | 4 | 7 | 8 | 8 |
| 65+ | 5 | 2.3 | 5 | 1 | 1 | 1 | 4 | 6 | 6 | 6 |
| **2. MULTIPLE DX** | | | | | | | | | | |
| 0–19 Years | 266 | 9.9 | 298 | 2 | 3 | 5 | 8 | 15 | 79 | 79 |
| 20–34 | 66 | 7.4 | 87 | 2 | 3 | 4 | 8 | 17 | 17 | 36 |
| 35–49 | 199 | 6.8 | 24 | 2 | 3 | 6 | 12 | 13 | 17 | 22 |
| 50–64 | 276 | 9.6 | 59 | 2 | 4 | 8 | 12 | 18 | 21 | 40 |
| 65+ | 961 | 8.2 | 45 | 2 | 4 | 6 | 11 | 16 | 19 | 37 |
| **TOTAL SINGLE DX** | 188 | 3.3 | 5 | 1 | 2 | 3 | 4 | 6 | 8 | 10 |
| **TOTAL MULTIPLE DX** | 1,768 | 8.5 | 84 | 2 | 4 | 6 | 10 | 16 | 20 | 52 |
| **TOTAL** | | | | | | | | | | |
| 0–19 Years | 411 | 6.9 | 182 | 2 | 2 | 3 | 6 | 9 | 16 | 79 |
| 20–34 | 78 | 7.0 | 78 | 2 | 3 | 4 | 8 | 17 | 17 | 36 |
| 35–49 | 211 | 6.8 | 22 | 2 | 3 | 6 | 12 | 13 | 16 | 20 |
| 50–64 | 290 | 9.2 | 58 | 2 | 4 | 8 | 12 | 18 | 21 | 33 |
| 65+ | 966 | 8.1 | 45 | 2 | 4 | 6 | 11 | 16 | 19 | 37 |
| **GRAND TOTAL** | 1,956 | 7.8 | 77 | 2 | 3 | 5 | 9 | 16 | 19 | 42 |

## 46.85: DILATION OF INTESTINE. Formerly included in operation group(s) 611.

| Type of Patients | Observed Patients | Avg. Stay | Variance | Percentiles | | | | | | |
|---|---|---|---|---|---|---|---|---|---|---|
| | | | | 10th | 25th | 50th | 75th | 90th | 95th | 99th |
| **1. SINGLE DX** | | | | | | | | | | |
| 0–19 Years | 9 | 1.9 | 3 | 1 | 1 | 1 | 2 | 3 | 8 | 8 |
| 20–34 | 2 | 1.6 | 2 | 1 | 1 | 1 | 1 | 5 | 5 | 5 |
| 35–49 | 4 | 2.5 | 2 | 1 | 1 | 3 | 4 | 4 | 4 | 4 |
| 50–64 | 2 | 1.9 | <1 | 1 | 1 | 2 | 2 | 2 | 2 | 2 |
| 65+ | 4 | 1.5 | 1 | 1 | 1 | 1 | 1 | 4 | 4 | 4 |
| **2. MULTIPLE DX** | | | | | | | | | | |
| 0–19 Years | 12 | 3.1 | <1 | 2 | 3 | 3 | 3 | 4 | 4 | 6 |
| 20–34 | 30 | 6.8 | 31 | 2 | 3 | 4 | 10 | 17 | 17 | 17 |
| 35–49 | 83 | 4.9 | 20 | 2 | 3 | 4 | 6 | 10 | 13 | 25 |
| 50–64 | 144 | 7.1 | 30 | 2 | 4 | 5 | 8 | 14 | 16 | 30 |
| 65+ | 670 | 6.6 | 28 | 2 | 4 | 5 | 8 | 14 | 17 | 26 |
| **TOTAL SINGLE DX** | 21 | 1.9 | 2 | 1 | 1 | 1 | 2 | 3 | 4 | 8 |
| **TOTAL MULTIPLE DX** | 939 | 6.5 | 28 | 2 | 3 | 5 | 8 | 13 | 17 | 26 |
| **TOTAL** | | | | | | | | | | |
| 0–19 Years | 21 | 2.5 | 2 | 1 | 1 | 3 | 3 | 4 | 6 | 8 |
| 20–34 | 32 | 6.2 | 30 | 1 | 2 | 4 | 8 | 17 | 17 | 17 |
| 35–49 | 87 | 4.8 | 20 | 1 | 2 | 4 | 5 | 10 | 13 | 25 |
| 50–64 | 146 | 6.9 | 30 | 2 | 3 | 5 | 9 | 14 | 16 | 30 |
| 65+ | 674 | 6.6 | 28 | 2 | 4 | 5 | 8 | 14 | 17 | 26 |
| **GRAND TOTAL** | 960 | 6.4 | 28 | 2 | 3 | 5 | 8 | 13 | 17 | 26 |

Length of Stay by Diagnosis and Operation, United States, 2000

# United States, October 1998–September 1999 Data, by Operation

## 46.9: OTHER INTESTINAL OPS. Formerly included in operation group(s) 611.

| Type of Patients | Observed Patients | Avg. Stay | Variance | 10th | 25th | 50th | 75th | 90th | 95th | 99th |
|---|---|---|---|---|---|---|---|---|---|---|
| **1. SINGLE DX** | | | | | | | | | | |
| 0–19 Years | 2 | 3.2 | 1 | 2 | 2 | 4 | 4 | 4 | 4 | 4 |
| 20–34 | 5 | 6.1 | 5 | 3 | 5 | 7 | 7 | 7 | 10 | 10 |
| 35–49 | 2 | 7.4 | 2 | 5 | 8 | 8 | 8 | 8 | 8 | 8 |
| 50–64 | 0 | | | | | | | | | |
| 65+ | 0 | | | | | | | | | |
| **2. MULTIPLE DX** | | | | | | | | | | |
| 0–19 Years | 18 | 24.6 | 186 | 5 | 8 | 30 | 36 | 36 | 36 | 49 |
| 20–34 | 40 | 9.3 | 42 | 3 | 5 | 7 | 12 | 18 | 23 | 30 |
| 35–49 | 76 | 8.4 | 39 | 4 | 5 | 6 | 9 | 18 | 22 | 32 |
| 50–64 | 87 | 17.0 | 103 | 5 | 8 | 19 | 21 | 31 | 33 | 43 |
| 65+ | 78 | 13.3 | 61 | 6 | 8 | 12 | 17 | 22 | 27 | 42 |
| **TOTAL SINGLE DX** | 9 | 5.8 | 5 | 3 | 4 | 7 | 7 | 8 | 10 | 10 |
| **TOTAL MULTIPLE DX** | 299 | 14.1 | 99 | 5 | 6 | 11 | 19 | 31 | 33 | 42 |
| **TOTAL** | | | | | | | | | | |
| 0–19 Years | 20 | 23.4 | 200 | 4 | 8 | 30 | 36 | 36 | 36 | 49 |
| 20–34 | 45 | 8.9 | 39 | 3 | 5 | 7 | 12 | 18 | 23 | 30 |
| 35–49 | 78 | 8.4 | 38 | 4 | 5 | 6 | 8 | 17 | 22 | 32 |
| 50–64 | 87 | 17.0 | 103 | 5 | 8 | 19 | 21 | 31 | 33 | 43 |
| 65+ | 78 | 13.3 | 61 | 6 | 8 | 12 | 17 | 22 | 27 | 42 |
| **GRAND TOTAL** | 308 | 13.9 | 99 | 4 | 6 | 10 | 19 | 31 | 33 | 42 |

## 47.01: LAPSCP APPENDECTOMY. Formerly included in operation group(s) 613.

| Type of Patients | Observed Patients | Avg. Stay | Variance | 10th | 25th | 50th | 75th | 90th | 95th | 99th |
|---|---|---|---|---|---|---|---|---|---|---|
| **1. SINGLE DX** | | | | | | | | | | |
| 0–19 Years | 3,094 | 2.1 | 2 | 1 | 1 | 2 | 2 | 4 | 5 | 8 |
| 20–34 | 3,265 | 1.8 | 2 | 1 | 1 | 1 | 2 | 3 | 4 | 6 |
| 35–49 | 1,655 | 1.9 | 1 | 1 | 2 | 2 | 2 | 3 | 4 | 6 |
| 50–64 | 440 | 2.4 | 3 | 1 | 2 | 2 | 3 | 5 | 7 | 7 |
| 65+ | 65 | 2.2 | 2 | 1 | 2 | 2 | 3 | 5 | 5 | 7 |
| **2. MULTIPLE DX** | | | | | | | | | | |
| 0–19 Years | 1,806 | 3.3 | 9 | 1 | 2 | 2 | 4 | 7 | 9 | 16 |
| 20–34 | 2,450 | 2.5 | 5 | 1 | 1 | 2 | 3 | 5 | 6 | 11 |
| 35–49 | 2,169 | 2.9 | 6 | 1 | 2 | 2 | 4 | 6 | 8 | 13 |
| 50–64 | 1,023 | 3.5 | 10 | 1 | 2 | 3 | 4 | 7 | 10 | 15 |
| 65+ | 587 | 4.4 | 16 | 2 | 2 | 4 | 6 | 9 | 11 | 18 |
| **TOTAL SINGLE DX** | 8,519 | 1.9 | 2 | 1 | 1 | 2 | 2 | 3 | 5 | 7 |
| **TOTAL MULTIPLE DX** | 8,035 | 3.1 | 8 | 1 | 1 | 2 | 4 | 6 | 8 | 13 |
| **TOTAL** | | | | | | | | | | |
| 0–19 Years | 4,900 | 2.5 | 5 | 1 | 1 | 2 | 3 | 5 | 7 | 10 |
| 20–34 | 5,715 | 2.1 | 3 | 1 | 1 | 2 | 2 | 4 | 5 | 9 |
| 35–49 | 3,824 | 2.5 | 4 | 1 | 1 | 2 | 3 | 5 | 6 | 11 |
| 50–64 | 1,463 | 3.2 | 8 | 1 | 2 | 3 | 4 | 7 | 8 | 14 |
| 65+ | 652 | 4.2 | 15 | 2 | 2 | 3 | 6 | 8 | 10 | 17 |
| **GRAND TOTAL** | 16,554 | 2.5 | 5 | 1 | 1 | 2 | 3 | 5 | 7 | 11 |

## 47.0: APPENDECTOMY. Formerly included in operation group(s) 613.

| Type of Patients | Observed Patients | Avg. Stay | Variance | 10th | 25th | 50th | 75th | 90th | 95th | 99th |
|---|---|---|---|---|---|---|---|---|---|---|
| **1. SINGLE DX** | | | | | | | | | | |
| 0–19 Years | 16,533 | 2.4 | 3 | 1 | 1 | 2 | 3 | 4 | 6 | 8 |
| 20–34 | 11,923 | 2.0 | 2 | 1 | 1 | 2 | 2 | 3 | 4 | 6 |
| 35–49 | 6,229 | 2.3 | 2 | 1 | 1 | 2 | 3 | 4 | 5 | 8 |
| 50–64 | 1,815 | 2.7 | 3 | 1 | 2 | 2 | 3 | 5 | 6 | 8 |
| 65+ | 327 | 2.9 | 4 | 1 | 2 | 2 | 4 | 5 | 7 | 9 |
| **2. MULTIPLE DX** | | | | | | | | | | |
| 0–19 Years | 9,615 | 4.3 | 14 | 1 | 2 | 3 | 6 | 8 | 10 | 18 |
| 20–34 | 8,360 | 3.3 | 10 | 1 | 2 | 2 | 4 | 6 | 8 | 14 |
| 35–49 | 7,918 | 4.0 | 13 | 1 | 2 | 3 | 5 | 8 | 10 | 16 |
| 50–64 | 4,769 | 4.7 | 15 | 1 | 2 | 4 | 6 | 9 | 11 | 20 |
| 65+ | 3,259 | 6.1 | 24 | 2 | 3 | 5 | 7 | 11 | 14 | 25 |
| **TOTAL SINGLE DX** | 36,827 | 2.3 | 2 | 1 | 1 | 2 | 3 | 4 | 5 | 8 |
| **TOTAL MULTIPLE DX** | 33,921 | 4.2 | 14 | 1 | 2 | 3 | 5 | 8 | 10 | 18 |
| **TOTAL** | | | | | | | | | | |
| 0–19 Years | 26,148 | 3.0 | 8 | 1 | 1 | 2 | 4 | 6 | 8 | 13 |
| 20–34 | 20,283 | 2.5 | 5 | 1 | 1 | 2 | 3 | 5 | 6 | 11 |
| 35–49 | 14,147 | 3.2 | 8 | 1 | 1 | 2 | 4 | 6 | 8 | 13 |
| 50–64 | 6,584 | 4.1 | 12 | 1 | 2 | 3 | 5 | 8 | 10 | 17 |
| 65+ | 3,586 | 5.8 | 23 | 2 | 3 | 5 | 7 | 11 | 14 | 24 |
| **GRAND TOTAL** | 70,748 | 3.1 | 9 | 1 | 1 | 2 | 4 | 6 | 8 | 14 |

## 47.09: OTHER APPENDECTOMY. Formerly included in operation group(s) 613.

| Type of Patients | Observed Patients | Avg. Stay | Variance | 10th | 25th | 50th | 75th | 90th | 95th | 99th |
|---|---|---|---|---|---|---|---|---|---|---|
| **1. SINGLE DX** | | | | | | | | | | |
| 0–19 Years | 13,439 | 2.4 | 3 | 1 | 2 | 3 | 3 | 5 | 6 | 8 |
| 20–34 | 8,658 | 2.1 | 1 | 1 | 2 | 3 | 3 | 4 | 5 | 6 |
| 35–49 | 4,574 | 2.4 | 2 | 1 | 2 | 3 | 3 | 4 | 5 | 8 |
| 50–64 | 1,375 | 2.8 | 3 | 1 | 3 | 3 | 5 | 6 | 6 | 8 |
| 65+ | 262 | 3.1 | 4 | 1 | 2 | 4 | 4 | 6 | 7 | 9 |
| **2. MULTIPLE DX** | | | | | | | | | | |
| 0–19 Years | 7,809 | 4.5 | 14 | 1 | 2 | 3 | 6 | 9 | 11 | 18 |
| 20–34 | 5,910 | 3.6 | 11 | 1 | 2 | 3 | 4 | 7 | 9 | 15 |
| 35–49 | 5,749 | 4.4 | 15 | 2 | 2 | 4 | 6 | 8 | 10 | 17 |
| 50–64 | 3,746 | 5.1 | 16 | 2 | 3 | 5 | 6 | 9 | 12 | 22 |
| 65+ | 2,672 | 6.4 | 25 | 2 | 3 | 5 | 8 | 11 | 14 | 26 |
| **TOTAL SINGLE DX** | 28,308 | 2.3 | 2 | 1 | 2 | 3 | 3 | 4 | 5 | 8 |
| **TOTAL MULTIPLE DX** | 25,886 | 4.5 | 16 | 1 | 2 | 4 | 6 | 9 | 11 | 19 |
| **TOTAL** | | | | | | | | | | |
| 0–19 Years | 21,248 | 3.1 | 8 | 1 | 2 | 3 | 4 | 6 | 8 | 14 |
| 20–34 | 14,568 | 2.7 | 6 | 1 | 2 | 3 | 3 | 5 | 6 | 12 |
| 35–49 | 10,323 | 3.4 | 10 | 2 | 3 | 4 | 4 | 7 | 8 | 13 |
| 50–64 | 5,121 | 4.4 | 13 | 2 | 3 | 5 | 5 | 8 | 10 | 18 |
| 65+ | 2,934 | 6.1 | 24 | 2 | 3 | 5 | 7 | 11 | 14 | 25 |
| **GRAND TOTAL** | 54,194 | 3.3 | 10 | 1 | 2 | 4 | 4 | 7 | 8 | 14 |

Length of Stay by Diagnosis and Operation, United States, 2000

# United States, October 1998–September 1999 Data, by Operation

## 47.1: INCIDENTAL APPENDECTOMY. Formerly included in operation group(s) 613.

| Type of Patients | Observed Patients | Avg. Stay | Variance | Percentiles | | | | | | |
|---|---|---|---|---|---|---|---|---|---|---|
| | | | | 10th | 25th | 50th | 75th | 90th | 95th | 99th |
| **1. SINGLE DX** | | | | | | | | | | |
| 0–19 Years | 73 | 2.9 | 4 | 1 | 1 | 2 | 4 | 7 | 7 | 8 |
| 20–34 | 66 | 2.1 | 1 | 1 | 1 | 2 | 2 | 3 | 4 | 6 |
| 35–49 | 37 | 2.3 | 2 | 1 | 1 | 2 | 3 | 4 | 7 | 7 |
| 50–64 | 5 | 2.7 | 2 | 1 | 2 | 2 | 4 | 5 | 5 | 5 |
| 65+ | 2 | 7.8 | 6 | 4 | 9 | 9 | 9 | 9 | 9 | 9 |
| **2. MULTIPLE DX** | | | | | | | | | | |
| 0–19 Years | 102 | 6.9 | 158 | 1 | 2 | 3 | 7 | 10 | 30 | 60 |
| 20–34 | 145 | 3.2 | 8 | 1 | 2 | 3 | 3 | 6 | 7 | 17 |
| 35–49 | 94 | 5.1 | 22 | 1 | 2 | 4 | 6 | 9 | 10 | 28 |
| 50–64 | 36 | 5.7 | 9 | 2 | 3 | 5 | 8 | 9 | 10 | 15 |
| 65+ | 23 | 8.8 | 33 | 2 | 4 | 8 | 12 | 17 | 21 | 28 |
| **TOTAL SINGLE DX** | 183 | 2.5 | 3 | 1 | 1 | 2 | 3 | 5 | 7 | 8 |
| **TOTAL MULTIPLE DX** | 400 | 5.0 | 49 | 1 | 2 | 3 | 6 | 9 | 12 | 60 |
| **TOTAL** | | | | | | | | | | |
| 0–19 Years | 175 | 5.1 | 92 | 2 | 2 | 3 | 5 | 8 | 10 | 60 |
| 20–34 | 211 | 2.8 | 6 | 1 | 2 | 2 | 3 | 5 | 7 | 17 |
| 35–49 | 131 | 4.4 | 19 | 1 | 2 | 3 | 5 | 9 | 10 | 28 |
| 50–64 | 41 | 5.4 | 10 | 2 | 3 | 5 | 8 | 9 | 10 | 15 |
| 65+ | 25 | 8.8 | 31 | 2 | 4 | 8 | 12 | 15 | 18 | 28 |
| **GRAND TOTAL** | 583 | 4.2 | 35 | 1 | 2 | 3 | 5 | 8 | 10 | 28 |

## 47.2: DRAIN APPENDICEAL ABSC. Formerly included in operation group(s) 614.

| Type of Patients | Observed Patients | Avg. Stay | Variance | Percentiles | | | | | | |
|---|---|---|---|---|---|---|---|---|---|---|
| | | | | 10th | 25th | 50th | 75th | 90th | 95th | 99th |
| **1. SINGLE DX** | | | | | | | | | | |
| 0–19 Years | 39 | 6.9 | 9 | 3 | 5 | 7 | 9 | 12 | 12 | 16 |
| 20–34 | 13 | 5.4 | 14 | 2 | 2 | 4 | 9 | 12 | 12 | 12 |
| 35–49 | 16 | 4.9 | 4 | 2 | 4 | 4 | 7 | 7 | 8 | 9 |
| 50–64 | 10 | 3.7 | 3 | 2 | 2 | 4 | 5 | 6 | 6 | 6 |
| 65+ | 2 | 4.6 | <1 | 3 | 5 | 5 | 5 | 5 | 5 | 5 |
| **2. MULTIPLE DX** | | | | | | | | | | |
| 0–19 Years | 46 | 7.2 | 11 | 3 | 5 | 7 | 8 | 10 | 12 | 22 |
| 20–34 | 23 | 7.4 | 9 | 5 | 6 | 7 | 9 | 11 | 11 | 16 |
| 35–49 | 45 | 7.4 | 13 | 3 | 4 | 7 | 10 | 11 | 15 | 16 |
| 50–64 | 25 | 6.3 | 14 | 3 | 4 | 6 | 6 | 9 | 18 | 18 |
| 65+ | 28 | 8.7 | 27 | 5 | 6 | 7 | 10 | 16 | 22 | 27 |
| **TOTAL SINGLE DX** | 80 | 6.0 | 9 | 2 | 4 | 5 | 8 | 10 | 12 | 16 |
| **TOTAL MULTIPLE DX** | 167 | 7.3 | 14 | 3 | 5 | 7 | 9 | 11 | 15 | 22 |
| **TOTAL** | | | | | | | | | | |
| 0–19 Years | 85 | 7.1 | 10 | 3 | 5 | 7 | 8 | 10 | 12 | 20 |
| 20–34 | 36 | 6.6 | 12 | 2 | 4 | 6 | 9 | 11 | 12 | 16 |
| 35–49 | 61 | 6.7 | 11 | 2 | 4 | 6 | 10 | 11 | 15 | 16 |
| 50–64 | 35 | 5.7 | 13 | 2 | 3 | 6 | 6 | 9 | 18 | 18 |
| 65+ | 30 | 8.4 | 26 | 3 | 6 | 7 | 10 | 15 | 22 | 27 |
| **GRAND TOTAL** | 247 | 6.8 | 13 | 3 | 5 | 6 | 9 | 11 | 12 | 20 |

## 47.11: LAPSCP INCIDENTAL APPY. Formerly included in operation group(s) 613.

| Type of Patients | Observed Patients | Avg. Stay | Variance | Percentiles | | | | | | |
|---|---|---|---|---|---|---|---|---|---|---|
| | | | | 10th | 25th | 50th | 75th | 90th | 95th | 99th |
| **1. SINGLE DX** | | | | | | | | | | |
| 0–19 Years | 44 | 1.8 | <1 | 1 | 1 | 2 | 2 | 3 | 3 | 5 |
| 20–34 | 38 | 2.3 | 2 | 1 | 1 | 2 | 3 | 4 | 5 | 8 |
| 35–49 | 17 | 2.1 | 3 | 1 | 1 | 1 | 2 | 4 | 7 | 7 |
| 50–64 | 3 | 1.6 | <1 | 1 | 1 | 2 | 2 | 2 | 2 | 2 |
| 65+ | 0 | | | | | | | | | |
| **2. MULTIPLE DX** | | | | | | | | | | |
| 0–19 Years | 60 | 3.7 | 10 | 1 | 1 | 2 | 5 | 10 | 10 | 15 |
| 20–34 | 93 | 2.6 | 4 | 1 | 1 | 2 | 3 | 6 | 7 | 8 |
| 35–49 | 47 | 4.4 | 31 | 1 | 2 | 4 | 5 | 6 | 9 | 28 |
| 50–64 | 12 | 4.4 | 5 | 2 | 3 | 5 | 5 | 7 | 9 | 9 |
| 65+ | 4 | 4.2 | 15 | 2 | 2 | 2 | 3 | 11 | 11 | 11 |
| **TOTAL SINGLE DX** | 102 | 2.0 | 2 | 1 | 1 | 2 | 3 | 3 | 5 | 7 |
| **TOTAL MULTIPLE DX** | 216 | 3.4 | 12 | 1 | 2 | 2 | 4 | 7 | 10 | 28 |
| **TOTAL** | | | | | | | | | | |
| 0–19 Years | 104 | 2.9 | 7 | 1 | 1 | 2 | 3 | 7 | 10 | 10 |
| 20–34 | 131 | 2.5 | 3 | 1 | 1 | 2 | 3 | 5 | 6 | 8 |
| 35–49 | 64 | 3.8 | 25 | 1 | 1 | 3 | 5 | 6 | 7 | 28 |
| 50–64 | 15 | 3.8 | 5 | 2 | 2 | 3 | 5 | 7 | 8 | 9 |
| 65+ | 4 | 4.2 | 15 | 2 | 2 | 2 | 3 | 11 | 11 | 11 |
| **GRAND TOTAL** | 318 | 3.0 | 9 | 1 | 1 | 2 | 3 | 6 | 8 | 12 |

## 47.9: OTHER APPENDICEAL OPS. Formerly included in operation group(s) 614.

| Type of Patients | Observed Patients | Avg. Stay | Variance | Percentiles | | | | | | |
|---|---|---|---|---|---|---|---|---|---|---|
| | | | | 10th | 25th | 50th | 75th | 90th | 95th | 99th |
| **1. SINGLE DX** | | | | | | | | | | |
| 0–19 Years | 9 | 4.6 | <1 | 3 | 5 | 5 | 5 | 5 | 5 | 5 |
| 20–34 | 2 | 7.4 | 3 | 8 | 8 | 8 | 8 | 8 | 8 | 8 |
| 35–49 | 2 | 3.1 | 1 | 2 | 2 | 4 | 4 | 4 | 4 | 4 |
| 50–64 | 0 | | | | | | | | | |
| 65+ | 0 | | | | | | | | | |
| **2. MULTIPLE DX** | | | | | | | | | | |
| 0–19 Years | 59 | 4.0 | 3 | 2 | 3 | 4 | 5 | 5 | 7 | 10 |
| 20–34 | 4 | 5.3 | 5 | 3 | 3 | 5 | 8 | 8 | 8 | 8 |
| 35–49 | 5 | 5.7 | 19 | 2 | 2 | 4 | 10 | 13 | 13 | 13 |
| 50–64 | 1 | 3.0 | 0 | 3 | 3 | 3 | 3 | 3 | 3 | 3 |
| 65+ | 0 | | | | | | | | | |
| **TOTAL SINGLE DX** | 13 | 5.3 | 3 | 3 | 5 | 5 | 8 | 8 | 8 | 8 |
| **TOTAL MULTIPLE DX** | 69 | 4.0 | 4 | 2 | 3 | 4 | 5 | 6 | 10 | 11 |
| **TOTAL** | | | | | | | | | | |
| 0–19 Years | 68 | 4.1 | 3 | 2 | 3 | 4 | 5 | 5 | 7 | 10 |
| 20–34 | 6 | 7.0 | 4 | 8 | 8 | 8 | 8 | 8 | 8 | 8 |
| 35–49 | 7 | 5.4 | 17 | 2 | 2 | 4 | 10 | 10 | 13 | 13 |
| 50–64 | 1 | 3.0 | 0 | 3 | 3 | 3 | 3 | 3 | 3 | 3 |
| 65+ | 0 | | | | | | | | | |
| **GRAND TOTAL** | 82 | 4.3 | 4 | 2 | 3 | 4 | 5 | 8 | 8 | 11 |

Length of Stay by Diagnosis and Operation, United States, 2000

# United States, October 1998–September 1999 Data, by Operation

## 48.2: RECTAL/PERIRECT DXTIC PX. Formerly included in operation group(s) 615, 618, 631.

| Type of Patients | Observed Patients | Avg. Stay | Vari-ance | 10th | 25th | 50th | 75th | 90th | 95th | 99th |
|---|---|---|---|---|---|---|---|---|---|---|
| **1. SINGLE DX** | | | | | | | | | | |
| 0–19 Years | 184 | 2.9 | 12 | 1 | 1 | 1 | 3 | 6 | 11 | 19 |
| 20–34 | 33 | 10.1 | 152 | 1 | 1 | 3 | 29 | 29 | 29 | 29 |
| 35–49 | 42 | 2.4 | 11 | 1 | 1 | 2 | 2 | 3 | 6 | 23 |
| 50–64 | 35 | 2.3 | 3 | 1 | 1 | 2 | 3 | 5 | 6 | 6 |
| 65+ | 26 | 1.4 | 3 | 1 | 1 | 1 | 1 | 1 | 3 | 15 |
| **2. MULTIPLE DX** | | | | | | | | | | |
| 0–19 Years | 486 | 8.1 | 124 | 1 | 2 | 5 | 9 | 18 | 28 | 61 |
| 20–34 | 285 | 4.8 | 31 | 1 | 2 | 3 | 5 | 10 | 16 | 25 |
| 35–49 | 496 | 5.8 | 35 | 1 | 2 | 4 | 8 | 12 | 15 | 28 |
| 50–64 | 593 | 6.2 | 38 | 1 | 3 | 4 | 7 | 14 | 19 | 28 |
| 65+ | 1,873 | 6.0 | 25 | 2 | 3 | 5 | 8 | 12 | 15 | 24 |
| **TOTAL SINGLE DX** | 320 | 3.1 | 25 | 1 | 1 | 1 | 3 | 6 | 14 | 29 |
| **TOTAL MULTIPLE DX** | 3,733 | 6.2 | 43 | 1 | 3 | 4 | 8 | 13 | 17 | 30 |
| **TOTAL** | | | | | | | | | | |
| 0–19 Years | 670 | 6.3 | 92 | 1 | 3 | 3 | 7 | 14 | 22 | 58 |
| 20–34 | 318 | 5.5 | 50 | 1 | 2 | 3 | 5 | 11 | 25 | 29 |
| 35–49 | 538 | 5.6 | 34 | 1 | 2 | 4 | 7 | 12 | 15 | 26 |
| 50–64 | 628 | 6.0 | 37 | 1 | 2 | 4 | 7 | 13 | 19 | 26 |
| 65+ | 1,899 | 5.8 | 24 | 1 | 3 | 5 | 8 | 12 | 15 | 23 |
| **GRAND TOTAL** | 4,053 | 5.9 | 42 | 1 | 2 | 4 | 7 | 12 | 16 | 29 |

## 48.23: RIGID PROCTSIGMOIDOSCOPY. Formerly included in operation group(s) 631.

| Type of Patients | Observed Patients | Avg. Stay | Vari-ance | 10th | 25th | 50th | 75th | 90th | 95th | 99th |
|---|---|---|---|---|---|---|---|---|---|---|
| **1. SINGLE DX** | | | | | | | | | | |
| 0–19 Years | 20 | 5.4 | 32 | 1 | 2 | 2 | 14 | 14 | 14 | 14 |
| 20–34 | 19 | 2.4 | 2 | 1 | 1 | 3 | 3 | 4 | 6 | 6 |
| 35–49 | 24 | 1.7 | 2 | 1 | 1 | 1 | 2 | 3 | 3 | 8 |
| 50–64 | 19 | 2.0 | 2 | 1 | 1 | 2 | 3 | 4 | 4 | 6 |
| 65+ | 12 | 2.6 | 6 | 1 | 1 | 2 | 3 | 3 | 11 | 11 |
| **2. MULTIPLE DX** | | | | | | | | | | |
| 0–19 Years | 49 | 5.0 | 22 | 1 | 1 | 4 | 6 | 9 | 18 | 18 |
| 20–34 | 106 | 4.1 | 19 | 1 | 2 | 2 | 5 | 11 | 12 | 26 |
| 35–49 | 150 | 6.3 | 56 | 1 | 2 | 4 | 9 | 12 | 14 | 28 |
| 50–64 | 179 | 5.8 | 31 | 1 | 2 | 4 | 7 | 12 | 19 | 30 |
| 65+ | 548 | 5.9 | 30 | 2 | 3 | 4 | 7 | 11 | 16 | 29 |
| **TOTAL SINGLE DX** | 94 | 3.0 | 17 | 1 | 1 | 2 | 3 | 6 | 14 | 14 |
| **TOTAL MULTIPLE DX** | 1,032 | 5.7 | 33 | 1 | 2 | 4 | 7 | 12 | 16 | 28 |
| **TOTAL** | | | | | | | | | | |
| 0–19 Years | 69 | 5.2 | 26 | 1 | 1 | 4 | 7 | 14 | 14 | 18 |
| 20–34 | 125 | 3.8 | 17 | 1 | 2 | 2 | 4 | 8 | 11 | 19 |
| 35–49 | 174 | 5.6 | 50 | 1 | 2 | 4 | 8 | 11 | 13 | 28 |
| 50–64 | 198 | 5.4 | 29 | 1 | 2 | 4 | 7 | 12 | 18 | 19 |
| 65+ | 560 | 5.8 | 29 | 2 | 2 | 4 | 7 | 11 | 16 | 29 |
| **GRAND TOTAL** | 1,126 | 5.5 | 32 | 1 | 2 | 4 | 7 | 11 | 16 | 26 |

## 48.0: PROCTOTOMY. Formerly included in operation group(s) 615.

| Type of Patients | Observed Patients | Avg. Stay | Vari-ance | 10th | 25th | 50th | 75th | 90th | 95th | 99th |
|---|---|---|---|---|---|---|---|---|---|---|
| **1. SINGLE DX** | | | | | | | | | | |
| 0–19 Years | 4 | 2.3 | 2 | 1 | 1 | 1 | 4 | 4 | 4 | 4 |
| 20–34 | 12 | 1.6 | 2 | 1 | 1 | 1 | 2 | 4 | 5 | 5 |
| 35–49 | 30 | 1.5 | 2 | 1 | 1 | 1 | 1 | 3 | 4 | 12 |
| 50–64 | 9 | 2.3 | 5 | 1 | 1 | 1 | 3 | 5 | 8 | 8 |
| 65+ | 2 | 1.4 | <1 | 1 | 1 | 1 | 2 | 2 | 2 | 2 |
| **2. MULTIPLE DX** | | | | | | | | | | |
| 0–19 Years | 15 | 5.8 | 58 | 1 | 2 | 3 | 7 | 11 | 33 | 33 |
| 20–34 | 44 | 3.4 | 12 | 1 | 2 | 2 | 3 | 5 | 13 | 20 |
| 35–49 | 85 | 3.0 | 8 | 1 | 2 | 3 | 3 | 3 | 7 | 18 |
| 50–64 | 61 | 10.3 | 244 | 1 | 1 | 3 | 8 | 45 | 45 | 45 |
| 65+ | 47 | 8.2 | 60 | 2 | 3 | 6 | 9 | 16 | 25 | 37 |
| **TOTAL SINGLE DX** | 57 | 1.6 | 3 | 1 | 1 | 1 | 1 | 3 | 4 | 8 |
| **TOTAL MULTIPLE DX** | 252 | 5.3 | 72 | 1 | 2 | 3 | 4 | 11 | 20 | 45 |
| **TOTAL** | | | | | | | | | | |
| 0–19 Years | 19 | 5.2 | 51 | 1 | 2 | 3 | 4 | 11 | 33 | 33 |
| 20–34 | 56 | 3.2 | 12 | 1 | 1 | 2 | 3 | 5 | 13 | 20 |
| 35–49 | 115 | 2.6 | 7 | 1 | 1 | 3 | 3 | 3 | 7 | 18 |
| 50–64 | 70 | 9.4 | 223 | 1 | 1 | 3 | 7 | 45 | 45 | 45 |
| 65+ | 49 | 8.0 | 60 | 2 | 3 | 6 | 9 | 16 | 25 | 37 |
| **GRAND TOTAL** | 309 | 4.6 | 61 | 1 | 1 | 3 | 3 | 9 | 16 | 45 |

## 48.1: PROCTOSTOMY. Formerly included in operation group(s) 618.

| Type of Patients | Observed Patients | Avg. Stay | Vari-ance | 10th | 25th | 50th | 75th | 90th | 95th | 99th |
|---|---|---|---|---|---|---|---|---|---|---|
| **1. SINGLE DX** | | | | | | | | | | |
| 0–19 Years | 0 | | | | | | | | | |
| 20–34 | 0 | | | | | | | | | |
| 35–49 | 0 | | | | | | | | | |
| 50–64 | 0 | | | | | | | | | |
| 65+ | 0 | | | | | | | | | |
| **2. MULTIPLE DX** | | | | | | | | | | |
| 0–19 Years | 0 | | | | | | | | | |
| 20–34 | 0 | | | | | | | | | |
| 35–49 | 0 | | | | | | | | | |
| 50–64 | 0 | | | | | | | | | |
| 65+ | 2 | 10.3 | 2 | 8 | 11 | 11 | 11 | 11 | 11 | 11 |
| **TOTAL SINGLE DX** | 0 | | | | | | | | | |
| **TOTAL MULTIPLE DX** | 2 | 10.3 | 2 | 8 | 11 | 11 | 11 | 11 | 11 | 11 |
| **TOTAL** | | | | | | | | | | |
| 0–19 Years | 0 | | | | | | | | | |
| 20–34 | 0 | | | | | | | | | |
| 35–49 | 0 | | | | | | | | | |
| 50–64 | 0 | | | | | | | | | |
| 65+ | 2 | 10.3 | 2 | 8 | 11 | 11 | 11 | 11 | 11 | 11 |
| **GRAND TOTAL** | 2 | 10.3 | 2 | 8 | 11 | 11 | 11 | 11 | 11 | 11 |

## United States, October 1998–September 1999 Data, by Operation

### 48.24: CLSD (ENDO) RECTAL BX. Formerly included in operation group(s) 615.

| Type of Patients | Observed Patients | Avg. Stay | Variance | Percentiles | | | | | | |
|---|---|---|---|---|---|---|---|---|---|---|
| | | | | 10th | 25th | 50th | 75th | 90th | 95th | 99th |
| **1. SINGLE DX** | | | | | | | | | | |
| 0–19 Years | 133 | 2.6 | 9 | 1 | 1 | 1 | 3 | 5 | 7 | 19 |
| 20–34 | 13 | 14.2 | 185 | 1 | 1 | 4 | 29 | 29 | 29 | 29 |
| 35–49 | 16 | 3.7 | 26 | 1 | 2 | 2 | 3 | 7 | 23 | 23 |
| 50–64 | 16 | 2.7 | 4 | 1 | 1 | 2 | 5 | 6 | 6 | 6 |
| 65+ | 9 | 3.4 | 23 | 1 | 1 | 1 | 2 | 11 | 15 | 15 |
| **2. MULTIPLE DX** | | | | | | | | | | |
| 0–19 Years | 370 | 7.4 | 89 | 1 | 2 | 4 | 8 | 16 | 24 | 57 |
| 20–34 | 175 | 5.2 | 35 | 1 | 2 | 5 | 5 | 10 | 16 | 25 |
| 35–49 | 328 | 5.2 | 22 | 1 | 2 | 4 | 7 | 10 | 13 | 29 |
| 50–64 | 397 | 6.1 | 40 | 2 | 3 | 4 | 7 | 13 | 19 | 28 |
| 65+ | 1,282 | 6.1 | 22 | 2 | 3 | 5 | 8 | 12 | 15 | 23 |
| **TOTAL SINGLE DX** | 187 | 3.8 | 38 | 1 | 1 | 2 | 3 | 6 | 19 | 29 |
| **TOTAL MULTIPLE DX** | 2,552 | 6.1 | 37 | 2 | 3 | 4 | 7 | 12 | 16 | 30 |
| **TOTAL** | | | | | | | | | | |
| 0–19 Years | 503 | 5.8 | 66 | 1 | 2 | 3 | 6 | 12 | 20 | 47 |
| 20–34 | 188 | 6.4 | 65 | 1 | 2 | 6 | 6 | 16 | 29 | 29 |
| 35–49 | 344 | 5.2 | 22 | 1 | 2 | 4 | 7 | 10 | 13 | 23 |
| 50–64 | 413 | 6.0 | 39 | 2 | 3 | 4 | 7 | 13 | 19 | 28 |
| 65+ | 1,291 | 6.1 | 23 | 2 | 3 | 5 | 8 | 12 | 15 | 23 |
| **GRAND TOTAL** | 2,739 | 5.9 | 38 | 1 | 2 | 4 | 7 | 12 | 16 | 29 |

### 48.3: LOC DESTR RECTAL LESION. Formerly included in operation group(s) 615.

| Type of Patients | Observed Patients | Avg. Stay | Variance | Percentiles | | | | | | |
|---|---|---|---|---|---|---|---|---|---|---|
| | | | | 10th | 25th | 50th | 75th | 90th | 95th | 99th |
| **1. SINGLE DX** | | | | | | | | | | |
| 0–19 Years | 12 | 2.0 | 5 | 1 | 1 | 1 | 3 | 8 | 8 | 8 |
| 20–34 | 9 | 2.4 | 3 | 1 | 1 | 2 | 4 | 6 | 6 | 6 |
| 35–49 | 28 | 1.5 | <1 | 1 | 1 | 1 | 2 | 3 | 3 | 4 |
| 50–64 | 56 | 1.4 | <1 | 1 | 1 | 1 | 1 | 3 | 4 | 5 |
| 65+ | 62 | 1.6 | <1 | 1 | 1 | 1 | 2 | 3 | 3 | 5 |
| **2. MULTIPLE DX** | | | | | | | | | | |
| 0–19 Years | 20 | 2.2 | 3 | 1 | 1 | 1 | 4 | 5 | 5 | 6 |
| 20–34 | 48 | 5.3 | 43 | 1 | 2 | 2 | 7 | 11 | 23 | 30 |
| 35–49 | 202 | 3.8 | 18 | 1 | 2 | 3 | 4 | 7 | 9 | 14 |
| 50–64 | 453 | 3.8 | 10 | 1 | 2 | 3 | 5 | 7 | 9 | 15 |
| 65+ | 1,548 | 5.7 | 37 | 1 | 3 | 4 | 6 | 13 | 20 | 25 |
| **TOTAL SINGLE DX** | 167 | 1.6 | 1 | 1 | 1 | 1 | 2 | 3 | 4 | 6 |
| **TOTAL MULTIPLE DX** | 2,271 | 5.2 | 31 | 1 | 2 | 3 | 6 | 11 | 19 | 23 |
| **TOTAL** | | | | | | | | | | |
| 0–19 Years | 32 | 2.1 | 3 | 1 | 1 | 1 | 3 | 5 | 6 | 8 |
| 20–34 | 57 | 5.0 | 40 | 1 | 2 | 2 | 7 | 9 | 23 | 30 |
| 35–49 | 230 | 3.5 | 17 | 1 | 1 | 3 | 4 | 7 | 9 | 14 |
| 50–64 | 509 | 3.5 | 10 | 1 | 2 | 3 | 5 | 7 | 8 | 14 |
| 65+ | 1,610 | 5.6 | 37 | 1 | 2 | 4 | 6 | 13 | 20 | 25 |
| **GRAND TOTAL** | 2,438 | 4.9 | 30 | 1 | 2 | 3 | 6 | 11 | 17 | 23 |

### 48.35: LOC EXC RECTAL LES/TISS. Formerly included in operation group(s) 615.

| Type of Patients | Observed Patients | Avg. Stay | Variance | Percentiles | | | | | | |
|---|---|---|---|---|---|---|---|---|---|---|
| | | | | 10th | 25th | 50th | 75th | 90th | 95th | 99th |
| **1. SINGLE DX** | | | | | | | | | | |
| 0–19 Years | 2 | 6.6 | 10 | 1 | 8 | 8 | 8 | 8 | 8 | 8 |
| 20–34 | 7 | 2.7 | 4 | 1 | 1 | 1 | 3 | 6 | 6 | 6 |
| 35–49 | 25 | 1.7 | <1 | 1 | 1 | 1 | 2 | 3 | 3 | 4 |
| 50–64 | 46 | 1.4 | <1 | 1 | 1 | 1 | 1 | 3 | 4 | 6 |
| 65+ | 50 | 1.6 | <1 | 1 | 1 | 1 | 2 | 3 | 3 | 5 |
| **2. MULTIPLE DX** | | | | | | | | | | |
| 0–19 Years | 7 | 4.4 | <1 | 4 | 4 | 5 | 5 | 5 | 6 | 6 |
| 20–34 | 15 | 2.9 | 7 | 1 | 1 | 2 | 4 | 5 | 11 | 11 |
| 35–49 | 58 | 4.3 | 40 | 2 | 2 | 3 | 5 | 7 | 9 | 43 |
| 50–64 | 147 | 3.1 | 10 | 1 | 2 | 2 | 4 | 7 | 9 | 15 |
| 65+ | 576 | 6.8 | 59 | 1 | 2 | 3 | 8 | 20 | 20 | 26 |
| **TOTAL SINGLE DX** | 130 | 1.7 | 2 | 1 | 1 | 1 | 2 | 3 | 4 | 8 |
| **TOTAL MULTIPLE DX** | 803 | 6.0 | 51 | 1 | 1 | 3 | 7 | 20 | 20 | 26 |
| **TOTAL** | | | | | | | | | | |
| 0–19 Years | 9 | 4.8 | 3 | 4 | 4 | 5 | 5 | 8 | 8 | 8 |
| 20–34 | 22 | 2.9 | 7 | 1 | 1 | 2 | 4 | 6 | 9 | 11 |
| 35–49 | 83 | 3.6 | 31 | 1 | 1 | 2 | 4 | 7 | 7 | 43 |
| 50–64 | 193 | 2.6 | 8 | 1 | 1 | 2 | 3 | 6 | 7 | 13 |
| 65+ | 626 | 6.4 | 57 | 1 | 2 | 3 | 8 | 20 | 20 | 26 |
| **GRAND TOTAL** | 933 | 5.4 | 47 | 1 | 1 | 3 | 6 | 18 | 20 | 26 |

### 48.36: ENDO RECTAL POLYPECTOMY. Formerly included in operation group(s) 615.

| Type of Patients | Observed Patients | Avg. Stay | Variance | Percentiles | | | | | | |
|---|---|---|---|---|---|---|---|---|---|---|
| | | | | 10th | 25th | 50th | 75th | 90th | 95th | 99th |
| **1. SINGLE DX** | | | | | | | | | | |
| 0–19 Years | 9 | 1.1 | <1 | 1 | 1 | 1 | 1 | 2 | 2 | 2 |
| 20–34 | 0 | | | | | | | | | |
| 35–49 | 3 | 1.0 | 0 | 1 | 1 | 1 | 1 | 1 | 1 | 1 |
| 50–64 | 9 | 1.4 | 1 | 1 | 1 | 1 | 2 | 3 | 5 | 5 |
| 65+ | 10 | 1.5 | <1 | 1 | 1 | 1 | 2 | 3 | 3 | 3 |
| **2. MULTIPLE DX** | | | | | | | | | | |
| 0–19 Years | 13 | 1.2 | <1 | 1 | 1 | 1 | 1 | 2 | 2 | 3 |
| 20–34 | 28 | 4.4 | 28 | 2 | 2 | 2 | 7 | 8 | 8 | 30 |
| 35–49 | 134 | 3.6 | 9 | 2 | 2 | 3 | 4 | 7 | 9 | 12 |
| 50–64 | 290 | 4.1 | 10 | 2 | 2 | 2 | 4 | 8 | 9 | 14 |
| 65+ | 866 | 5.1 | 20 | 2 | 3 | 4 | 6 | 10 | 13 | 19 |
| **TOTAL SINGLE DX** | 31 | 1.3 | <1 | 1 | 1 | 1 | 1 | 2 | 3 | 5 |
| **TOTAL MULTIPLE DX** | 1,331 | 4.6 | 17 | 1 | 2 | 4 | 6 | 9 | 11 | 18 |
| **TOTAL** | | | | | | | | | | |
| 0–19 Years | 22 | 1.2 | <1 | 1 | 1 | 1 | 1 | 2 | 2 | 3 |
| 20–34 | 28 | 4.4 | 28 | 2 | 2 | 2 | 7 | 8 | 8 | 30 |
| 35–49 | 137 | 3.4 | 8 | 1 | 2 | 3 | 5 | 8 | 9 | 12 |
| 50–64 | 299 | 4.0 | 10 | 2 | 2 | 3 | 5 | 8 | 9 | 14 |
| 65+ | 876 | 5.0 | 20 | 2 | 2 | 4 | 6 | 10 | 13 | 19 |
| **GRAND TOTAL** | 1,362 | 4.5 | 17 | 1 | 2 | 4 | 6 | 8 | 11 | 17 |

Length of Stay by Diagnosis and Operation, United States, 2000

# United States, October 1998–September 1999 Data, by Operation

## 48.4: PULL-THRU RECT RESECTION. Formerly included in operation group(s) 617.

| Type of Patients | Observed Patients | Avg. Stay | Variance | 10th | 25th | 50th | 75th | 90th | 95th | 99th |
|---|---|---|---|---|---|---|---|---|---|---|
| **1. SINGLE DX** | | | | | | | | | | |
| 0–19 Years | 130 | 5.3 | 4 | 3 | 4 | 5 | 6 | 8 | 9 | 10 |
| 20–34 | 2 | 8.5 | <1 | 8 | 8 | 8 | 9 | 9 | 9 | 9 |
| 35–49 | 6 | 3.0 | 4 | 1 | 2 | 2 | 3 | 7 | 7 | 7 |
| 50–64 | 5 | 4.7 | 3 | 3 | 5 | 5 | 5 | 6 | 6 | 9 |
| 65+ | 2 | 2.5 | 1 | 2 | 2 | 2 | 4 | 4 | 4 | 4 |
| **2. MULTIPLE DX** | | | | | | | | | | |
| 0–19 Years | 202 | 8.4 | 81 | 3 | 5 | 6 | 8 | 13 | 20 | 58 |
| 20–34 | 15 | 7.7 | 11 | 3 | 6 | 7 | 9 | 13 | 13 | 15 |
| 35–49 | 12 | 7.7 | 35 | 5 | 6 | 7 | 7 | 8 | 13 | 36 |
| 50–64 | 25 | 5.6 | 30 | 1 | 1 | 3 | 8 | 15 | 15 | 21 |
| 65+ | 110 | 6.3 | 26 | 2 | 3 | 4 | 9 | 14 | 16 | 24 |
| **TOTAL SINGLE DX** | 145 | 5.2 | 4 | 3 | 4 | 5 | 6 | 8 | 9 | 10 |
| **TOTAL MULTIPLE DX** | 364 | 7.4 | 57 | 2 | 4 | 6 | 8 | 14 | 18 | 54 |
| **TOTAL** | | | | | | | | | | |
| 0–19 Years | 332 | 7.0 | 49 | 3 | 4 | 6 | 7 | 10 | 14 | 54 |
| 20–34 | 17 | 7.8 | 10 | 3 | 6 | 8 | 9 | 13 | 13 | 15 |
| 35–49 | 18 | 6.9 | 33 | 3 | 6 | 7 | 7 | 8 | 13 | 36 |
| 50–64 | 30 | 5.5 | 27 | 1 | 1 | 5 | 7 | 15 | 15 | 21 |
| 65+ | 112 | 6.3 | 26 | 2 | 3 | 4 | 8 | 14 | 16 | 24 |
| **GRAND TOTAL** | 509 | 6.7 | 41 | 2 | 4 | 6 | 8 | 11 | 15 | 41 |

## 48.6: OTHER RECTAL RESECTION. Formerly included in operation group(s) 617.

| Type of Patients | Observed Patients | Avg. Stay | Variance | 10th | 25th | 50th | 75th | 90th | 95th | 99th |
|---|---|---|---|---|---|---|---|---|---|---|
| **1. SINGLE DX** | | | | | | | | | | |
| 0–19 Years | 32 | 6.4 | 2 | 5 | 5 | 7 | 7 | 9 | 9 | 9 |
| 20–34 | 17 | 6.3 | 4 | 4 | 5 | 7 | 8 | 8 | 9 | 9 |
| 35–49 | 92 | 5.5 | 2 | 3 | 5 | 6 | 6 | 8 | 8 | 10 |
| 50–64 | 159 | 5.8 | 5 | 4 | 5 | 6 | 7 | 8 | 9 | 13 |
| 65+ | 101 | 5.9 | 6 | 3 | 5 | 6 | 7 | 8 | 10 | 14 |
| **2. MULTIPLE DX** | | | | | | | | | | |
| 0–19 Years | 74 | 10.5 | 52 | 5 | 5 | 8 | 14 | 20 | 31 | 32 |
| 20–34 | 124 | 7.1 | 20 | 4 | 5 | 6 | 8 | 11 | 13 | 37 |
| 35–49 | 618 | 8.4 | 43 | 4 | 5 | 7 | 9 | 12 | 19 | 40 |
| 50–64 | 1,724 | 8.7 | 36 | 5 | 6 | 7 | 9 | 15 | 22 | 27 |
| 65+ | 3,387 | 9.2 | 34 | 5 | 6 | 8 | 10 | 15 | 19 | 35 |
| **TOTAL SINGLE DX** | 401 | 5.8 | 4 | 4 | 5 | 6 | 7 | 8 | 9 | 13 |
| **TOTAL MULTIPLE DX** | 5,927 | 8.9 | 36 | 5 | 6 | 7 | 10 | 15 | 22 | 35 |
| **TOTAL** | | | | | | | | | | |
| 0–19 Years | 106 | 9.4 | 41 | 5 | 5 | 7 | 12 | 18 | 20 | 32 |
| 20–34 | 141 | 7.0 | 19 | 4 | 5 | 6 | 8 | 11 | 13 | 37 |
| 35–49 | 710 | 8.0 | 39 | 4 | 5 | 7 | 8 | 12 | 16 | 40 |
| 50–64 | 1,883 | 8.5 | 35 | 5 | 6 | 7 | 9 | 14 | 22 | 27 |
| 65+ | 3,488 | 9.1 | 33 | 5 | 6 | 8 | 10 | 15 | 19 | 35 |
| **GRAND TOTAL** | 6,328 | 8.7 | 35 | 5 | 6 | 7 | 9 | 14 | 21 | 35 |

## 48.5: ABD-PERINEAL RECT RESECT. Formerly included in operation group(s) 617.

| Type of Patients | Observed Patients | Avg. Stay | Variance | 10th | 25th | 50th | 75th | 90th | 95th | 99th |
|---|---|---|---|---|---|---|---|---|---|---|
| **1. SINGLE DX** | | | | | | | | | | |
| 0–19 Years | 2 | 6.7 | 6 | 5 | 5 | 5 | 9 | 9 | 9 | 9 |
| 20–34 | 3 | 6.5 | 7 | 5 | 5 | 5 | 10 | 10 | 10 | 10 |
| 35–49 | 28 | 6.9 | 3 | 4 | 6 | 7 | 8 | 8 | 10 | 11 |
| 50–64 | 54 | 6.4 | 2 | 5 | 6 | 6 | 7 | 8 | 8 | 12 |
| 65+ | 31 | 6.9 | 6 | 4 | 6 | 7 | 8 | 9 | 10 | 17 |
| **2. MULTIPLE DX** | | | | | | | | | | |
| 0–19 Years | 7 | 7.3 | 8 | 4 | 4 | 6 | 11 | 11 | 11 | 11 |
| 20–34 | 62 | 10.6 | 132 | 5 | 7 | 7 | 10 | 15 | 42 | 73 |
| 35–49 | 288 | 9.2 | 35 | 5 | 6 | 7 | 10 | 16 | 25 | 28 |
| 50–64 | 729 | 9.5 | 47 | 5 | 6 | 8 | 10 | 14 | 19 | 32 |
| 65+ | 1,480 | 10.7 | 39 | 6 | 7 | 9 | 12 | 17 | 22 | 37 |
| **TOTAL SINGLE DX** | 118 | 6.6 | 4 | 4 | 6 | 7 | 8 | 8 | 10 | 12 |
| **TOTAL MULTIPLE DX** | 2,566 | 10.2 | 45 | 5 | 7 | 8 | 11 | 16 | 22 | 38 |
| **TOTAL** | | | | | | | | | | |
| 0–19 Years | 9 | 7.1 | 7 | 4 | 5 | 6 | 9 | 11 | 11 | 11 |
| 20–34 | 65 | 10.6 | 130 | 5 | 7 | 7 | 10 | 15 | 42 | 73 |
| 35–49 | 316 | 9.1 | 34 | 5 | 6 | 7 | 10 | 14 | 25 | 28 |
| 50–64 | 783 | 9.3 | 45 | 5 | 6 | 8 | 10 | 13 | 18 | 29 |
| 65+ | 1,511 | 10.6 | 39 | 6 | 7 | 9 | 12 | 17 | 22 | 37 |
| **GRAND TOTAL** | 2,684 | 10.1 | 44 | 5 | 7 | 8 | 11 | 16 | 22 | 37 |

## 48.62: ANT RECT RESECT W COLOST. Formerly included in operation group(s) 617.

| Type of Patients | Observed Patients | Avg. Stay | Variance | 10th | 25th | 50th | 75th | 90th | 95th | 99th |
|---|---|---|---|---|---|---|---|---|---|---|
| **1. SINGLE DX** | | | | | | | | | | |
| 0–19 Years | 1 | 5.0 | 0 | 5 | 5 | 5 | 5 | 5 | 5 | 5 |
| 20–34 | 0 | | | | | | | | | |
| 35–49 | 4 | 6.3 | <1 | 6 | 6 | 6 | 7 | 7 | 7 | 7 |
| 50–64 | 5 | 7.7 | 6 | 6 | 6 | 7 | 11 | 11 | 11 | 11 |
| 65+ | 5 | 6.0 | <1 | 6 | 6 | 6 | 6 | 6 | 6 | 8 |
| **2. MULTIPLE DX** | | | | | | | | | | |
| 0–19 Years | 0 | | | | | | | | | |
| 20–34 | 10 | 6.9 | 6 | 5 | 5 | 6 | 7 | 11 | 12 | 12 |
| 35–49 | 57 | 10.1 | 28 | 7 | 7 | 9 | 11 | 12 | 20 | 42 |
| 50–64 | 160 | 8.9 | 47 | 5 | 5 | 7 | 9 | 15 | 21 | 35 |
| 65+ | 351 | 12.3 | 70 | 6 | 7 | 10 | 14 | 24 | 35 | 41 |
| **TOTAL SINGLE DX** | 15 | 6.1 | <1 | 6 | 6 | 6 | 6 | 7 | 8 | 11 |
| **TOTAL MULTIPLE DX** | 578 | 10.9 | 59 | 5 | 6 | 8 | 12 | 19 | 26 | 39 |
| **TOTAL** | | | | | | | | | | |
| 0–19 Years | 1 | 5.0 | 0 | 5 | 5 | 5 | 5 | 5 | 5 | 5 |
| 20–34 | 10 | 6.9 | 6 | 5 | 6 | 6 | 7 | 11 | 12 | 12 |
| 35–49 | 61 | 10.0 | 28 | 6 | 7 | 9 | 11 | 12 | 20 | 39 |
| 50–64 | 165 | 8.9 | 47 | 6 | 7 | 9 | 12 | 14 | 21 | 35 |
| 65+ | 356 | 12.0 | 68 | 6 | 7 | 10 | 14 | 23 | 35 | 39 |
| **GRAND TOTAL** | 593 | 10.7 | 58 | 5 | 6 | 8 | 12 | 18 | 26 | 39 |

Length of Stay by Diagnosis and Operation, United States, 2000

# United States, October 1998–September 1999 Data, by Operation

## 48.63: ANTERIOR RECT RESECT NEC. Formerly included in operation group(s) 617.

| Type of Patients | Observed Patients | Avg. Stay | Variance | Percentiles | | | | | | |
|---|---|---|---|---|---|---|---|---|---|---|
| | | | | 10th | 25th | 50th | 75th | 90th | 95th | 99th |
| **1. SINGLE DX** | | | | | | | | | | |
| 0–19 Years | 2 | 4.6 | 1 | 4 | 4 | 4 | 6 | 6 | 6 | 6 |
| 20–34 | 8 | 6.7 | 3 | 4 | 5 | 7 | 8 | 9 | 9 | 9 |
| 35–49 | 71 | 5.6 | 2 | 4 | 5 | 6 | 6 | 8 | 8 | 10 |
| 50–64 | 116 | 5.9 | 2 | 4 | 5 | 6 | 7 | 7 | 8 | 9 |
| 65+ | 74 | 6.8 | 4 | 5 | 6 | 6 | 8 | 9 | 11 | 14 |
| **2. MULTIPLE DX** | | | | | | | | | | |
| 0–19 Years | 2 | 7.6 | 0 | 7 | 7 | 8 | 8 | 8 | 8 | 8 |
| 20–34 | 57 | 7.0 | 9 | 4 | 5 | 6 | 8 | 11 | 12 | 18 |
| 35–49 | 429 | 7.1 | 13 | 4 | 5 | 6 | 8 | 10 | 13 | 24 |
| 50–64 | 1,267 | 8.9 | 36 | 5 | 6 | 7 | 9 | 18 | 22 | 27 |
| 65+ | 2,398 | 8.8 | 24 | 5 | 6 | 8 | 10 | 14 | 18 | 29 |
| **TOTAL SINGLE DX** | 271 | 6.0 | 3 | 4 | 5 | 6 | 7 | 8 | 9 | 12 |
| **TOTAL MULTIPLE DX** | 4,153 | 8.6 | 27 | 5 | 6 | 7 | 9 | 14 | 20 | 27 |
| **TOTAL** | | | | | | | | | | |
| 0–19 Years | 4 | 5.6 | 3 | 4 | 4 | 6 | 7 | 8 | 8 | 8 |
| 20–34 | 65 | 7.0 | 8 | 4 | 5 | 6 | 8 | 11 | 12 | 18 |
| 35–49 | 500 | 6.8 | 12 | 4 | 5 | 6 | 7 | 10 | 12 | 23 |
| 50–64 | 1,383 | 8.7 | 35 | 5 | 6 | 7 | 9 | 16 | 22 | 24 |
| 65+ | 2,472 | 8.7 | 23 | 5 | 6 | 8 | 10 | 14 | 17 | 27 |
| **GRAND TOTAL** | 4,424 | 8.5 | 26 | 5 | 6 | 7 | 9 | 14 | 19 | 27 |

## 48.69: RECTAL RESECTION NEC. Formerly included in operation group(s) 617.

| Type of Patients | Observed Patients | Avg. Stay | Variance | Percentiles | | | | | | |
|---|---|---|---|---|---|---|---|---|---|---|
| | | | | 10th | 25th | 50th | 75th | 90th | 95th | 99th |
| **1. SINGLE DX** | | | | | | | | | | |
| 0–19 Years | 5 | 5.3 | 4 | 3 | 3 | 6 | 6 | 8 | 8 | 8 |
| 20–34 | 9 | 6.1 | 4 | 4 | 4 | 6 | 8 | 9 | 8 | 8 |
| 35–49 | 15 | 5.6 | | 3 | 5 | 5 | 6 | 9 | 9 | 9 |
| 50–64 | 34 | 5.6 | 15 | 1 | 2 | 5 | 6 | 13 | 13 | 13 |
| 65+ | 21 | 3.1 | 4 | 1 | 1 | 3 | 5 | 5 | 6 | 8 |
| **2. MULTIPLE DX** | | | | | | | | | | |
| 0–19 Years | 19 | 13.5 | 130 | 5 | 7 | 7 | 31 | 32 | 32 | 32 |
| 20–34 | 57 | 7.2 | 33 | 4 | 5 | 5 | 8 | 10 | 14 | 37 |
| 35–49 | 128 | 11.3 | 127 | 3 | 5 | 7 | 10 | 40 | 40 | 40 |
| 50–64 | 294 | 7.6 | 25 | 4 | 5 | 7 | 9 | 11 | 13 | 26 |
| 65+ | 618 | 9.2 | 47 | 3 | 5 | 7 | 11 | 17 | 23 | 35 |
| **TOTAL SINGLE DX** | 84 | 4.8 | 10 | 1 | 2 | 5 | 6 | 8 | 13 | 13 |
| **TOTAL MULTIPLE DX** | 1,116 | 9.0 | 53 | 3 | 5 | 7 | 10 | 15 | 24 | 40 |
| **TOTAL** | | | | | | | | | | |
| 0–19 Years | 24 | 12.5 | 121 | 3 | 6 | 7 | 13 | 32 | 32 | 32 |
| 20–34 | 66 | 7.1 | 30 | 4 | 5 | 5 | 8 | 10 | 14 | 37 |
| 35–49 | 143 | 11.0 | 121 | 3 | 5 | 7 | 10 | 40 | 40 | 40 |
| 50–64 | 328 | 7.5 | 25 | 4 | 5 | 7 | 9 | 11 | 13 | 26 |
| 65+ | 639 | 9.0 | 47 | 3 | 5 | 7 | 11 | 17 | 22 | 35 |
| **GRAND TOTAL** | 1,200 | 8.8 | 51 | 3 | 5 | 7 | 10 | 15 | 22 | 40 |

## 48.7: REPAIR OF RECTUM. Formerly included in operation group(s) 618.

| Type of Patients | Observed Patients | Avg. Stay | Variance | Percentiles | | | | | | |
|---|---|---|---|---|---|---|---|---|---|---|
| | | | | 10th | 25th | 50th | 75th | 90th | 95th | 99th |
| **1. SINGLE DX** | | | | | | | | | | |
| 0–19 Years | 22 | 3.0 | 2 | 2 | 2 | 3 | 4 | 5 | 5 | 5 |
| 20–34 | 15 | 2.7 | 3 | 1 | 2 | 2 | 3 | 6 | 7 | 7 |
| 35–49 | 19 | 3.5 | 5 | 1 | 2 | 3 | 6 | 6 | 7 | 8 |
| 50–64 | 14 | 4.5 | 4 | 2 | 2 | 5 | 6 | 6 | 7 | 9 |
| 65+ | 17 | 7.4 | 3 | 5 | 8 | 8 | 8 | 8 | 8 | 8 |
| **2. MULTIPLE DX** | | | | | | | | | | |
| 0–19 Years | 72 | 4.4 | 10 | 1 | 2 | 4 | 6 | 10 | 10 | 16 |
| 20–34 | 63 | 5.4 | 33 | 2 | 4 | 5 | 5 | 7 | 13 | 45 |
| 35–49 | 132 | 5.3 | 18 | 1 | 2 | 4 | 7 | 10 | 12 | 21 |
| 50–64 | 169 | 5.9 | 16 | 1 | 3 | 5 | 9 | 10 | 11 | 17 |
| 65+ | 434 | 6.0 | 19 | 2 | 3 | 5 | 7 | 10 | 13 | 22 |
| **TOTAL SINGLE DX** | 87 | 5.7 | 7 | 2 | 3 | 7 | 8 | 8 | 8 | 8 |
| **TOTAL MULTIPLE DX** | 870 | 5.8 | 20 | 2 | 3 | 5 | 7 | 10 | 12 | 21 |
| **TOTAL** | | | | | | | | | | |
| 0–19 Years | 94 | 4.1 | 8 | 1 | 2 | 4 | 5 | 8 | 10 | 15 |
| 20–34 | 78 | 5.0 | 29 | 2 | 3 | 5 | 5 | 7 | 10 | 45 |
| 35–49 | 151 | 5.2 | 17 | 2 | 3 | 4 | 7 | 10 | 12 | 20 |
| 50–64 | 183 | 5.8 | 16 | 2 | 3 | 5 | 8 | 10 | 11 | 17 |
| 65+ | 451 | 6.2 | 17 | 2 | 4 | 5 | 8 | 10 | 12 | 22 |
| **GRAND TOTAL** | 957 | 5.8 | 18 | 2 | 3 | 5 | 7 | 10 | 12 | 21 |

## 48.76: PROCTOPEXY NEC. Formerly included in operation group(s) 618.

| Type of Patients | Observed Patients | Avg. Stay | Variance | Percentiles | | | | | | |
|---|---|---|---|---|---|---|---|---|---|---|
| | | | | 10th | 25th | 50th | 75th | 90th | 95th | 99th |
| **1. SINGLE DX** | | | | | | | | | | |
| 0–19 Years | 5 | 3.8 | <1 | 3 | 3 | 4 | 4 | 5 | 5 | 5 |
| 20–34 | 7 | 3.3 | 5 | 1 | 1 | 3 | 4 | 6 | 7 | 7 |
| 35–49 | 5 | 3.9 | 6 | 1 | 3 | 3 | 4 | 8 | 8 | 31 |
| 50–64 | 2 | 5.6 | <1 | 5 | 5 | 6 | 6 | 6 | 6 | 6 |
| 65+ | 9 | 2.5 | <1 | 1 | 1 | 3 | 3 | 3 | 5 | 5 |
| **2. MULTIPLE DX** | | | | | | | | | | |
| 0–19 Years | 8 | 3.2 | 16 | 1 | 1 | 1 | 4 | 13 | 13 | 13 |
| 20–34 | 16 | 4.5 | 2 | 1 | 5 | 5 | 5 | 5 | 5 | 6 |
| 35–49 | 46 | 7.0 | 37 | 2 | 3 | 6 | 10 | 14 | 18 | 31 |
| 50–64 | 69 | 6.7 | 16 | 2 | 3 | 5 | 10 | 11 | 11 | 13 |
| 65+ | 226 | 4.8 | 11 | 2 | 2 | 4 | 6 | 9 | 11 | 17 |
| **TOTAL SINGLE DX** | 28 | 3.4 | 3 | 1 | 3 | 3 | 5 | 6 | 6 | 8 |
| **TOTAL MULTIPLE DX** | 365 | 5.3 | 15 | 2 | 3 | 4 | 7 | 10 | 12 | 18 |
| **TOTAL** | | | | | | | | | | |
| 0–19 Years | 13 | 3.3 | 13 | 1 | 1 | 2 | 4 | 5 | 13 | 13 |
| 20–34 | 23 | 4.4 | 2 | 1 | 4 | 5 | 5 | 6 | 5 | 6 |
| 35–49 | 51 | 6.9 | 36 | 2 | 3 | 5 | 10 | 14 | 18 | 31 |
| 50–64 | 71 | 6.7 | 16 | 2 | 3 | 6 | 10 | 11 | 11 | 13 |
| 65+ | 235 | 4.7 | 11 | 2 | 2 | 4 | 6 | 9 | 11 | 17 |
| **GRAND TOTAL** | 393 | 5.2 | 14 | 2 | 3 | 4 | 7 | 10 | 12 | 18 |

Length of Stay by Diagnosis and Operation, United States, 2000

# United States, October 1998–September 1999 Data, by Operation

## 48.8: PERIRECT TISS INC/EXC. Formerly included in operation group(s) 616.

| Type of Patients | Observed Patients | Avg. Stay | Vari-ance | 10th | 25th | 50th | 75th | 90th | 95th | 99th |
|---|---|---|---|---|---|---|---|---|---|---|
| **1. SINGLE DX** | | | | | | | | | | |
| 0–19 Years | 110 | 1.9 | 1 | 1 | 1 | 2 | 2 | 3 | 4 | 6 |
| 20–34 | 266 | 1.7 | 1 | 1 | 1 | 2 | 2 | 3 | 4 | 6 |
| 35–49 | 325 | 2.0 | 1 | 1 | 1 | 2 | 2 | 3 | 4 | 7 |
| 50–64 | 127 | 2.0 | 2 | 1 | 1 | 2 | 2 | 3 | 4 | 10 |
| 65+ | 16 | 1.6 | <1 | 1 | 1 | 1 | 2 | 2 | 3 | 5 |
| **2. MULTIPLE DX** | | | | | | | | | | |
| 0–19 Years | 171 | 4.7 | 31 | 2 | 2 | 3 | 5 | 9 | 13 | 29 |
| 20–34 | 438 | 3.7 | 16 | 1 | 2 | 3 | 4 | 6 | 10 | 23 |
| 35–49 | 863 | 3.9 | 16 | 1 | 2 | 3 | 5 | 9 | 13 | 19 |
| 50–64 | 696 | 4.0 | 13 | 1 | 2 | 3 | 5 | 7 | 10 | 18 |
| 65+ | 465 | 5.8 | 30 | 2 | 3 | 4 | 7 | 14 | 16 | 23 |
| **TOTAL SINGLE DX** | 844 | 1.9 | 1 | 1 | 1 | 2 | 2 | 3 | 4 | 6 |
| **TOTAL MULTIPLE DX** | 2,633 | 4.3 | 19 | 1 | 2 | 3 | 5 | 9 | 13 | 20 |
| **TOTAL** | | | | | | | | | | |
| 0–19 Years | 281 | 3.5 | 20 | 1 | 1 | 2 | 4 | 6 | 10 | 29 |
| 20–34 | 704 | 2.8 | 10 | 1 | 1 | 2 | 3 | 5 | 7 | 17 |
| 35–49 | 1,188 | 3.4 | 13 | 1 | 2 | 3 | 4 | 7 | 10 | 16 |
| 50–64 | 823 | 3.7 | 12 | 1 | 2 | 3 | 5 | 7 | 10 | 17 |
| 65+ | 481 | 5.7 | 30 | 2 | 3 | 4 | 7 | 14 | 16 | 23 |
| **GRAND TOTAL** | 3,477 | 3.6 | 16 | 1 | 1 | 2 | 4 | 7 | 11 | 18 |

## 48.81: PERIRECTAL INCISION. Formerly included in operation group(s) 616.

| Type of Patients | Observed Patients | Avg. Stay | Vari-ance | 10th | 25th | 50th | 75th | 90th | 95th | 99th |
|---|---|---|---|---|---|---|---|---|---|---|
| **1. SINGLE DX** | | | | | | | | | | |
| 0–19 Years | 105 | 1.9 | 1 | 1 | 1 | 2 | 2 | 3 | 4 | 6 |
| 20–34 | 261 | 1.7 | <1 | 1 | 1 | 1 | 2 | 3 | 4 | 6 |
| 35–49 | 321 | 2.0 | 1 | 1 | 1 | 2 | 2 | 3 | 4 | 7 |
| 50–64 | 123 | 2.0 | 2 | 1 | 1 | 2 | 3 | 3 | 4 | 10 |
| 65+ | 14 | 1.6 | <1 | 1 | 1 | 1 | 2 | 2 | 3 | 5 |
| **2. MULTIPLE DX** | | | | | | | | | | |
| 0–19 Years | 165 | 4.8 | 32 | 1 | 2 | 4 | 5 | 9 | 11 | 29 |
| 20–34 | 419 | 3.7 | 15 | 1 | 2 | 3 | 4 | 6 | 10 | 23 |
| 35–49 | 839 | 3.9 | 16 | 1 | 2 | 3 | 5 | 9 | 13 | 17 |
| 50–64 | 674 | 4.0 | 13 | 1 | 2 | 3 | 5 | 7 | 10 | 18 |
| 65+ | 430 | 5.7 | 30 | 2 | 3 | 4 | 7 | 13 | 16 | 21 |
| **TOTAL SINGLE DX** | 824 | 1.9 | 1 | 1 | 1 | 2 | 2 | 3 | 4 | 6 |
| **TOTAL MULTIPLE DX** | 2,527 | 4.2 | 19 | 1 | 2 | 3 | 5 | 9 | 13 | 20 |
| **TOTAL** | | | | | | | | | | |
| 0–19 Years | 270 | 3.6 | 21 | 1 | 1 | 2 | 4 | 6 | 10 | 29 |
| 20–34 | 680 | 2.8 | 9 | 1 | 1 | 2 | 3 | 5 | 7 | 17 |
| 35–49 | 1,160 | 3.3 | 12 | 1 | 1 | 3 | 4 | 7 | 9 | 16 |
| 50–64 | 797 | 3.7 | 12 | 1 | 2 | 3 | 5 | 7 | 9 | 17 |
| 65+ | 444 | 5.6 | 29 | 1 | 2 | 4 | 6 | 12 | 16 | 21 |
| **GRAND TOTAL** | 3,351 | 3.6 | 15 | 1 | 1 | 2 | 4 | 7 | 10 | 18 |

## 48.9: OTH RECTAL/PERIRECT OP. Formerly included in operation group(s) 618.

| Type of Patients | Observed Patients | Avg. Stay | Vari-ance | 10th | 25th | 50th | 75th | 90th | 95th | 99th |
|---|---|---|---|---|---|---|---|---|---|---|
| **1. SINGLE DX** | | | | | | | | | | |
| 0–19 Years | 13 | 3.5 | 5 | 1 | 2 | 3 | 6 | 7 | 7 | 7 |
| 20–34 | 2 | 1.0 | 0 | 1 | 1 | 1 | 1 | 1 | 1 | 1 |
| 35–49 | 0 | | | | | | | | | |
| 50–64 | 3 | 1.7 | <1 | 1 | 1 | 2 | 2 | 2 | 2 | 2 |
| 65+ | 2 | 1.0 | 0 | 1 | 1 | 1 | 1 | 1 | 1 | 1 |
| **2. MULTIPLE DX** | | | | | | | | | | |
| 0–19 Years | 20 | 8.6 | 44 | 1 | 2 | 8 | 15 | 15 | 24 | 24 |
| 20–34 | 8 | 4.2 | 12 | 1 | 1 | 4 | 6 | 9 | 12 | 12 |
| 35–49 | 19 | 4.8 | 15 | 1 | 2 | 4 | 8 | 10 | 12 | 16 |
| 50–64 | 18 | 3.6 | 2 | 1 | 3 | 4 | 4 | 6 | 7 | 7 |
| 65+ | 8 | 2.7 | <1 | 1 | 2 | 3 | 3 | 3 | 5 | 5 |
| **TOTAL SINGLE DX** | 20 | 2.7 | 4 | 1 | 1 | 2 | 4 | 6 | 7 | 7 |
| **TOTAL MULTIPLE DX** | 73 | 5.3 | 23 | 1 | 2 | 4 | 7 | 15 | 15 | 24 |
| **TOTAL** | | | | | | | | | | |
| 0–19 Years | 33 | 7.2 | 38 | 1 | 2 | 6 | 14 | 15 | 18 | 24 |
| 20–34 | 10 | 3.3 | 11 | 1 | 1 | 2 | 6 | 9 | 12 | 12 |
| 35–49 | 19 | 4.8 | 15 | 1 | 2 | 4 | 8 | 10 | 12 | 16 |
| 50–64 | 21 | 3.5 | 3 | 1 | 3 | 4 | 4 | 6 | 7 | 7 |
| 65+ | 10 | 2.4 | 1 | 1 | 2 | 3 | 3 | 3 | 3 | 5 |
| **GRAND TOTAL** | 93 | 4.9 | 21 | 1 | 2 | 3 | 6 | 12 | 15 | 24 |

## 49.0: PERIANAL TISS INC/EXC. Formerly included in operation group(s) 622.

| Type of Patients | Observed Patients | Avg. Stay | Vari-ance | 10th | 25th | 50th | 75th | 90th | 95th | 99th |
|---|---|---|---|---|---|---|---|---|---|---|
| **1. SINGLE DX** | | | | | | | | | | |
| 0–19 Years | 74 | 1.9 | 1 | 1 | 1 | 2 | 2 | 3 | 5 | 5 |
| 20–34 | 133 | 1.6 | <1 | 1 | 1 | 1 | 2 | 3 | 3 | 4 |
| 35–49 | 135 | 2.2 | 2 | 1 | 2 | 2 | 3 | 4 | 4 | 8 |
| 50–64 | 44 | 2.8 | 3 | 1 | 2 | 2 | 4 | 5 | 8 | 8 |
| 65+ | 14 | 2.4 | 1 | 1 | 2 | 3 | 4 | 4 | 4 | 5 |
| **2. MULTIPLE DX** | | | | | | | | | | |
| 0–19 Years | 107 | 3.6 | 13 | 1 | 2 | 3 | 4 | 6 | 8 | 19 |
| 20–34 | 254 | 3.4 | 14 | 1 | 1 | 2 | 4 | 7 | 12 | 17 |
| 35–49 | 408 | 3.7 | 14 | 1 | 2 | 3 | 5 | 8 | 10 | 21 |
| 50–64 | 333 | 4.2 | 13 | 1 | 2 | 3 | 5 | 8 | 12 | 20 |
| 65+ | 193 | 5.0 | 19 | 1 | 2 | 4 | 6 | 10 | 13 | 21 |
| **TOTAL SINGLE DX** | 400 | 2.0 | 2 | 1 | 1 | 2 | 2 | 4 | 4 | 8 |
| **TOTAL MULTIPLE DX** | 1,295 | 3.9 | 15 | 1 | 2 | 3 | 4 | 7 | 12 | 21 |
| **TOTAL** | | | | | | | | | | |
| 0–19 Years | 181 | 2.7 | 7 | 1 | 1 | 2 | 3 | 5 | 6 | 15 |
| 20–34 | 387 | 2.7 | 10 | 1 | 1 | 2 | 3 | 5 | 7 | 17 |
| 35–49 | 543 | 3.3 | 11 | 1 | 2 | 3 | 4 | 5 | 8 | 21 |
| 50–64 | 377 | 4.0 | 12 | 1 | 2 | 3 | 4 | 8 | 10 | 17 |
| 65+ | 207 | 4.8 | 18 | 1 | 2 | 4 | 6 | 10 | 13 | 21 |
| **GRAND TOTAL** | 1,695 | 3.4 | 12 | 1 | 1 | 2 | 4 | 6 | 9 | 18 |

# United States, October 1998–September 1999 Data, by Operation

## 49.01: INC PERIANAL ABSCESS. Formerly included in operation group(s) 622.

| Type of Patients | Observed Patients | Avg. Stay | Variance | 10th | 25th | 50th | 75th | 90th | 95th | 99th |
|---|---|---|---|---|---|---|---|---|---|---|
| **1. SINGLE DX** | | | | | | | | | | |
| 0–19 Years | 70 | 1.8 | 1 | 1 | 1 | 1 | 2 | 3 | 5 | 5 |
| 20–34 | 126 | 1.5 | <1 | 1 | 1 | 1 | 2 | 3 | 3 | 4 |
| 35–49 | 124 | 2.2 | 1 | 1 | 1 | 2 | 4 | 4 | 4 | 8 |
| 50–64 | 44 | 2.8 | 3 | 1 | 2 | 2 | 4 | 5 | 8 | 8 |
| 65+ | 13 | 2.3 | 1 | 2 | 2 | 2 | 4 | 4 | 4 | 5 |
| **2. MULTIPLE DX** | | | | | | | | | | |
| 0–19 Years | 97 | 3.6 | 14 | 1 | 2 | 3 | 4 | 6 | 10 | 19 |
| 20–34 | 228 | 3.4 | 14 | 1 | 1 | 2 | 4 | 7 | 11 | 17 |
| 35–49 | 372 | 3.8 | 15 | 1 | 2 | 3 | 5 | 6 | 10 | 21 |
| 50–64 | 305 | 4.0 | 11 | 1 | 2 | 3 | 6 | 7 | 10 | 20 |
| 65+ | 171 | 5.0 | 16 | 2 | 2 | 4 | 6 | 10 | 14 | 21 |
| **TOTAL SINGLE DX** | 377 | 2.0 | 2 | 1 | 1 | 1 | 2 | 4 | 4 | 8 |
| **TOTAL MULTIPLE DX** | 1,173 | 3.9 | 14 | 1 | 2 | 3 | 5 | 7 | 11 | 21 |
| **TOTAL** | | | | | | | | | | |
| 0–19 Years | 167 | 2.6 | 8 | 1 | 1 | 2 | 3 | 5 | 6 | 15 |
| 20–34 | 354 | 2.6 | 9 | 1 | 1 | 2 | 3 | 5 | 7 | 17 |
| 35–49 | 496 | 3.4 | 12 | 1 | 2 | 3 | 4 | 5 | 8 | 21 |
| 50–64 | 349 | 3.8 | 10 | 1 | 2 | 3 | 4 | 7 | 9 | 17 |
| 65+ | 184 | 4.8 | 16 | 2 | 2 | 4 | 6 | 9 | 12 | 21 |
| **GRAND TOTAL** | 1,550 | 3.3 | 11 | 1 | 1 | 2 | 4 | 6 | 9 | 19 |

## 49.1: INC/EXC OF ANAL FISTULA. Formerly included in operation group(s) 619.

| Type of Patients | Observed Patients | Avg. Stay | Variance | 10th | 25th | 50th | 75th | 90th | 95th | 99th |
|---|---|---|---|---|---|---|---|---|---|---|
| **1. SINGLE DX** | | | | | | | | | | |
| 0–19 Years | 13 | 1.6 | <1 | 1 | 1 | 1 | 2 | 3 | 3 | 4 |
| 20–34 | 11 | 1.5 | <1 | 1 | 1 | 1 | 2 | 2 | 2 | 6 |
| 35–49 | 31 | 1.6 | 1 | 1 | 1 | 1 | 4 | 3 | 4 | 9 |
| 50–64 | 10 | 1.3 | <1 | 1 | 1 | 1 | 1 | 3 | 4 | 3 |
| 65+ | 9 | 2.2 | 3 | 1 | 2 | 1 | 5 | 5 | 5 | 5 |
| **2. MULTIPLE DX** | | | | | | | | | | |
| 0–19 Years | 30 | 4.9 | 30 | 1 | 2 | 3 | 4 | 20 | 20 | 20 |
| 20–34 | 89 | 2.7 | 13 | 1 | 1 | 2 | 3 | 6 | 7 | 15 |
| 35–49 | 168 | 3.3 | 33 | 1 | 2 | 2 | 3 | 6 | 9 | 23 |
| 50–64 | 100 | 3.0 | 19 | 1 | 2 | 2 | 3 | 6 | 9 | 22 |
| 65+ | 112 | 4.2 | 30 | 1 | 1 | 2 | 5 | 9 | 14 | 33 |
| **TOTAL SINGLE DX** | 74 | 1.6 | 1 | 1 | 1 | 1 | 2 | 3 | 5 | 5 |
| **TOTAL MULTIPLE DX** | 499 | 3.5 | 26 | 1 | 1 | 2 | 3 | 7 | 12 | 23 |
| **TOTAL** | | | | | | | | | | |
| 0–19 Years | 43 | 4.0 | 25 | 1 | 1 | 3 | 4 | 11 | 20 | 20 |
| 20–34 | 100 | 2.4 | 10 | 1 | 1 | 2 | 2 | 4 | 6 | 15 |
| 35–49 | 199 | 2.9 | 26 | 1 | 2 | 2 | 3 | 6 | 8 | 23 |
| 50–64 | 110 | 2.8 | 17 | 1 | 1 | 1 | 3 | 5 | 9 | 22 |
| 65+ | 121 | 3.9 | 26 | 1 | 1 | 2 | 5 | 8 | 14 | 23 |
| **GRAND TOTAL** | 573 | 3.1 | 22 | 1 | 1 | 2 | 3 | 6 | 9 | 23 |

## 49.2: ANAL & PERIANAL DXTIC PX. Formerly included in operation group(s) 620, 622, 631.

| Type of Patients | Observed Patients | Avg. Stay | Variance | 10th | 25th | 50th | 75th | 90th | 95th | 99th |
|---|---|---|---|---|---|---|---|---|---|---|
| **1. SINGLE DX** | | | | | | | | | | |
| 0–19 Years | 5 | 2.3 | 3 | 1 | 2 | 2 | 2 | 2 | 7 | 7 |
| 20–34 | 2 | 1.5 | <1 | 1 | 1 | 1 | 1 | 2 | 3 | 3 |
| 35–49 | 5 | 1.5 | <1 | 1 | 1 | 1 | 2 | 2 | 2 | 2 |
| 50–64 | 4 | 2.2 | <1 | 1 | 2 | 2 | 3 | 3 | 3 | 3 |
| 65+ | 2 | 2.0 | 0 | 2 | 2 | 2 | 2 | 2 | 2 | 2 |
| **2. MULTIPLE DX** | | | | | | | | | | |
| 0–19 Years | 21 | 2.7 | 8 | 1 | 1 | 1 | 3 | 7 | 8 | 16 |
| 20–34 | 23 | 3.6 | 25 | 2 | 2 | 2 | 3 | 7 | 11 | 39 |
| 35–49 | 50 | 5.1 | 36 | 1 | 2 | 3 | 6 | 10 | 17 | 37 |
| 50–64 | 60 | 4.2 | 11 | 1 | 2 | 3 | 6 | 6 | 11 | 18 |
| 65+ | 112 | 4.4 | 17 | 1 | 2 | 3 | 6 | 10 | 16 | 16 |
| **TOTAL SINGLE DX** | 18 | 2.1 | 1 | 1 | 2 | 2 | 2 | 3 | 3 | 7 |
| **TOTAL MULTIPLE DX** | 266 | 4.2 | 18 | 1 | 2 | 3 | 5 | 8 | 15 | 18 |
| **TOTAL** | | | | | | | | | | |
| 0–19 Years | 26 | 2.6 | 7 | 1 | 2 | 2 | 3 | 7 | 7 | 16 |
| 20–34 | 25 | 3.5 | 24 | 2 | 2 | 2 | 3 | 7 | 11 | 39 |
| 35–49 | 55 | 4.9 | 35 | 1 | 2 | 3 | 5 | 10 | 17 | 37 |
| 50–64 | 64 | 4.1 | 10 | 1 | 2 | 3 | 6 | 6 | 10 | 18 |
| 65+ | 114 | 4.3 | 16 | 1 | 2 | 3 | 6 | 10 | 16 | 16 |
| **GRAND TOTAL** | 284 | 4.1 | 18 | 1 | 2 | 3 | 5 | 8 | 14 | 18 |

## 49.3: LOC DESTR ANAL LES NEC. Formerly included in operation group(s) 620.

| Type of Patients | Observed Patients | Avg. Stay | Variance | 10th | 25th | 50th | 75th | 90th | 95th | 99th |
|---|---|---|---|---|---|---|---|---|---|---|
| **1. SINGLE DX** | | | | | | | | | | |
| 0–19 Years | 12 | 1.3 | <1 | 1 | 1 | 1 | 1 | 2 | 4 | 4 |
| 20–34 | 14 | 2.4 | 2 | 1 | 1 | 2 | 3 | 5 | 5 | 5 |
| 35–49 | 11 | 1.4 | <1 | 1 | 1 | 1 | 1 | 3 | 3 | 9 |
| 50–64 | 6 | 2.6 | 9 | 1 | 1 | 1 | 2 | 8 | 9 | 9 |
| 65+ | 10 | 3.0 | 10 | 1 | 1 | 1 | 8 | 8 | 8 | 8 |
| **2. MULTIPLE DX** | | | | | | | | | | |
| 0–19 Years | 16 | 1.4 | <1 | 1 | 1 | 1 | 1 | 3 | 3 | 3 |
| 20–34 | 72 | 4.1 | 10 | 1 | 2 | 3 | 6 | 8 | 10 | 17 |
| 35–49 | 152 | 3.0 | 8 | 1 | 2 | 3 | 4 | 5 | 7 | 14 |
| 50–64 | 108 | 3.7 | 15 | 1 | 1 | 2 | 4 | 8 | 11 | 16 |
| 65+ | 159 | 3.9 | 12 | 1 | 2 | 2 | 6 | 10 | 12 | >99 |
| **TOTAL SINGLE DX** | 53 | 1.8 | 3 | 1 | 1 | 1 | 2 | 4 | 7 | 9 |
| **TOTAL MULTIPLE DX** | 507 | 3.4 | 11 | 1 | 1 | 2 | 4 | 7 | 10 | 28 |
| **TOTAL** | | | | | | | | | | |
| 0–19 Years | 28 | 1.4 | <1 | 1 | 1 | 1 | 1 | 3 | 3 | 4 |
| 20–34 | 86 | 3.9 | 10 | 1 | 2 | 3 | 6 | 6 | 10 | 17 |
| 35–49 | 163 | 2.9 | 8 | 1 | 1 | 3 | 4 | 5 | 7 | 14 |
| 50–64 | 114 | 3.6 | 15 | 1 | 2 | 3 | 4 | 8 | 11 | 16 |
| 65+ | 169 | 3.8 | 12 | 1 | 2 | 2 | 6 | 9 | 12 | >99 |
| **GRAND TOTAL** | 560 | 3.2 | 10 | 1 | 1 | 2 | 3 | 7 | 10 | 27 |

Length of Stay by Diagnosis and Operation, United States, 2000

# United States, October 1998–September 1999 Data, by Operation

## 49.39: OTH LOC DESTR ANAL LES. Formerly included in operation group(s) 620.

| Type of Patients | Observed Patients | Avg. Stay | Variance | 10th | 25th | 50th | 75th | 90th | 95th | 99th |
|---|---|---|---|---|---|---|---|---|---|---|
| **1. SINGLE DX** | | | | | | | | | | |
| 0–19 Years | 10 | 1.3 | <1 | 1 | 1 | 1 | 1 | 2 | 4 | 4 |
| 20–34 | 14 | 2.4 | 2 | 1 | 1 | 2 | 3 | 5 | 5 | 5 |
| 35–49 | 11 | 1.4 | <1 | 1 | 1 | 1 | 1 | 3 | 3 | 3 |
| 50–64 | 5 | 1.7 | <1 | 1 | 1 | 1 | 1 | 7 | 7 | 7 |
| 65+ | 10 | 3.0 | 10 | 1 | 1 | 1 | 8 | 8 | 8 | 8 |
| **2. MULTIPLE DX** | | | | | | | | | | |
| 0–19 Years | 14 | 1.5 | <1 | 1 | 1 | 1 | 2 | 3 | 3 | 3 |
| 20–34 | 69 | 4.2 | 11 | 1 | 2 | 3 | 6 | 9 | 10 | 17 |
| 35–49 | 143 | 3.0 | 11 | 1 | 2 | 3 | 3 | 5 | 7 | 14 |
| 50–64 | 96 | 3.8 | 17 | 1 | 2 | 2 | 4 | 9 | 11 | 28 |
| 65+ | 139 | 3.7 | 12 | 1 | 2 | 2 | 5 | 9 | 13 | >99 |
| **TOTAL SINGLE DX** | 50 | 1.7 | 3 | 1 | 1 | 1 | 2 | 4 | 5 | 8 |
| **TOTAL MULTIPLE DX** | 461 | 3.4 | 11 | 1 | 2 | 3 | 4 | 7 | 10 | 35 |
| **TOTAL** | | | | | | | | | | |
| 0–19 Years | 24 | 1.4 | <1 | 1 | 1 | 1 | 1 | 3 | 3 | 4 |
| 20–34 | 83 | 4.0 | 10 | 1 | 2 | 3 | 6 | 8 | 10 | 17 |
| 35–49 | 154 | 2.9 | 7 | 1 | 2 | 3 | 3 | 5 | 7 | 14 |
| 50–64 | 101 | 3.7 | 16 | 1 | 1 | 2 | 4 | 8 | 11 | 28 |
| 65+ | 149 | 3.7 | 12 | 1 | 2 | 2 | 5 | 9 | 12 | >99 |
| **GRAND TOTAL** | 511 | 3.2 | 10 | 1 | 1 | 2 | 3 | 7 | 9 | 28 |

## 49.46: EXC OF HEMORRHOIDS. Formerly included in operation group(s) 621.

| Type of Patients | Observed Patients | Avg. Stay | Variance | 10th | 25th | 50th | 75th | 90th | 95th | 99th |
|---|---|---|---|---|---|---|---|---|---|---|
| **1. SINGLE DX** | | | | | | | | | | |
| 0–19 Years | 7 | 1.1 | <1 | 1 | 1 | 1 | 1 | 1 | 2 | 2 |
| 20–34 | 78 | 1.6 | <1 | 1 | 1 | 1 | 2 | 3 | 4 | 5 |
| 35–49 | 136 | 1.8 | <1 | 1 | 1 | 2 | 2 | 3 | 4 | 5 |
| 50–64 | 66 | 1.6 | <1 | 1 | 1 | 1 | 2 | 3 | 3 | 5 |
| 65+ | 24 | 1.8 | 1 | 1 | 1 | 2 | 2 | 4 | 4 | 6 |
| **2. MULTIPLE DX** | | | | | | | | | | |
| 0–19 Years | 9 | 2.6 | 3 | 1 | 2 | 2 | 4 | 6 | 6 | 6 |
| 20–34 | 410 | 2.2 | 6 | 1 | 2 | 2 | 3 | 4 | 5 | 9 |
| 35–49 | 1,143 | 2.5 | 6 | 1 | 2 | 2 | 3 | 5 | 6 | 12 |
| 50–64 | 773 | 3.0 | 8 | 1 | 2 | 2 | 4 | 6 | 8 | 14 |
| 65+ | 898 | 3.5 | 16 | 1 | 2 | 2 | 4 | 7 | 12 | 19 |
| **TOTAL SINGLE DX** | 311 | 1.7 | <1 | 1 | 1 | 1 | 2 | 3 | 4 | 5 |
| **TOTAL MULTIPLE DX** | 3,233 | 2.8 | 10 | 1 | 1 | 2 | 3 | 6 | 8 | 15 |
| **TOTAL** | | | | | | | | | | |
| 0–19 Years | 16 | 1.6 | 2 | 1 | 1 | 1 | 2 | 3 | 6 | 6 |
| 20–34 | 488 | 2.1 | 5 | 1 | 1 | 2 | 2 | 4 | 5 | 7 |
| 35–49 | 1,279 | 2.4 | 6 | 1 | 2 | 2 | 3 | 4 | 6 | 11 |
| 50–64 | 839 | 2.9 | 8 | 1 | 2 | 2 | 4 | 6 | 8 | 12 |
| 65+ | 922 | 3.5 | 15 | 1 | 2 | 2 | 4 | 7 | 12 | 19 |
| **GRAND TOTAL** | 3,544 | 2.8 | 9 | 1 | 1 | 2 | 3 | 6 | 7 | 14 |

## 49.4: HEMORRHOID PROCEDURES. Formerly included in operation group(s) 621, 622, 631.

| Type of Patients | Observed Patients | Avg. Stay | Variance | 10th | 25th | 50th | 75th | 90th | 95th | 99th |
|---|---|---|---|---|---|---|---|---|---|---|
| **1. SINGLE DX** | | | | | | | | | | |
| 0–19 Years | 10 | 1.2 | <1 | 1 | 1 | 1 | 1 | 2 | 2 | 2 |
| 20–34 | 86 | 1.6 | <1 | 1 | 1 | 1 | 2 | 3 | 4 | 5 |
| 35–49 | 148 | 1.7 | <1 | 1 | 1 | 2 | 2 | 3 | 3 | 5 |
| 50–64 | 70 | 1.6 | <1 | 1 | 1 | 1 | 2 | 3 | 3 | 5 |
| 65+ | 25 | 1.8 | 1 | 1 | 1 | 1 | 2 | 4 | 4 | 6 |
| **2. MULTIPLE DX** | | | | | | | | | | |
| 0–19 Years | 15 | 2.6 | 2 | 1 | 2 | 2 | 3 | 4 | 6 | 6 |
| 20–34 | 469 | 2.4 | 6 | 1 | 1 | 2 | 3 | 4 | 5 | 10 |
| 35–49 | 1,242 | 2.5 | 7 | 1 | 1 | 2 | 3 | 5 | 7 | 12 |
| 50–64 | 878 | 3.1 | 10 | 1 | 1 | 2 | 4 | 6 | 8 | 16 |
| 65+ | 1,084 | 3.8 | 17 | 1 | 1 | 2 | 5 | 9 | 12 | 19 |
| **TOTAL SINGLE DX** | 339 | 1.7 | <1 | 1 | 1 | 1 | 2 | 3 | 3 | 5 |
| **TOTAL MULTIPLE DX** | 3,688 | 3.0 | 11 | 1 | 1 | 2 | 3 | 6 | 9 | 16 |
| **TOTAL** | | | | | | | | | | |
| 0–19 Years | 25 | 1.8 | 1 | 1 | 1 | 1 | 2 | 3 | 4 | 6 |
| 20–34 | 555 | 2.3 | 5 | 1 | 1 | 2 | 3 | 4 | 5 | 9 |
| 35–49 | 1,390 | 2.5 | 7 | 1 | 1 | 2 | 3 | 5 | 6 | 12 |
| 50–64 | 948 | 3.0 | 10 | 1 | 1 | 2 | 4 | 6 | 8 | 16 |
| 65+ | 1,109 | 3.8 | 17 | 1 | 1 | 2 | 5 | 9 | 12 | 19 |
| **GRAND TOTAL** | 4,027 | 2.9 | 10 | 1 | 1 | 2 | 3 | 6 | 8 | 15 |

## 49.5: ANAL SPHINCTER DIVISION. Formerly included in operation group(s) 622.

| Type of Patients | Observed Patients | Avg. Stay | Variance | 10th | 25th | 50th | 75th | 90th | 95th | 99th |
|---|---|---|---|---|---|---|---|---|---|---|
| **1. SINGLE DX** | | | | | | | | | | |
| 0–19 Years | 0 | | | | | | | | | |
| 20–34 | 8 | 2.2 | <1 | 2 | 2 | 2 | 2 | 3 | 4 | 4 |
| 35–49 | 16 | 1.0 | <1 | 1 | 1 | 1 | 1 | 1 | 1 | 2 |
| 50–64 | 1 | 2.0 | 0 | 2 | 2 | 2 | 2 | 2 | 2 | 2 |
| 65+ | 2 | 1.5 | <1 | 1 | 1 | 2 | 2 | 2 | 2 | 2 |
| **2. MULTIPLE DX** | | | | | | | | | | |
| 0–19 Years | 2 | 9.3 | 6 | 10 | 10 | 10 | 10 | 10 | 10 | 10 |
| 20–34 | 21 | 2.9 | 5 | 1 | 1 | 2 | 4 | 7 | 7 | 12 |
| 35–49 | 57 | 1.6 | 2 | 1 | 1 | 1 | 3 | 3 | 5 | 7 |
| 50–64 | 35 | 2.3 | 3 | 1 | 2 | 2 | 3 | 5 | 7 | 8 |
| 65+ | 71 | 4.6 | 18 | 1 | 2 | 2 | 7 | 10 | 15 | 15 |
| **TOTAL SINGLE DX** | 27 | 1.3 | <1 | 1 | 1 | 1 | 2 | 2 | 2 | 4 |
| **TOTAL MULTIPLE DX** | 186 | 2.6 | 8 | 1 | 1 | 1 | 3 | 7 | 9 | 15 |
| **TOTAL** | | | | | | | | | | |
| 0–19 Years | 2 | 9.3 | 6 | 10 | 10 | 10 | 10 | 10 | 10 | 10 |
| 20–34 | 29 | 2.7 | 4 | 1 | 1 | 2 | 3 | 5 | 7 | 12 |
| 35–49 | 73 | 1.5 | 1 | 1 | 1 | 1 | 3 | 3 | 4 | 7 |
| 50–64 | 36 | 2.3 | 3 | 1 | 2 | 2 | 3 | 5 | 7 | 8 |
| 65+ | 73 | 4.6 | 18 | 1 | 2 | 2 | 7 | 10 | 15 | 15 |
| **GRAND TOTAL** | 213 | 2.4 | 7 | 1 | 1 | 1 | 3 | 6 | 9 | 15 |

Length of Stay by Diagnosis and Operation

# United States, October 1998–September 1999 Data, by Operation

## 49.6: EXCISION OF ANUS. Formerly included in operation group(s) 622.

| Type of Patients | Observed Patients | Avg. Stay | Variance | 10th | 25th | 50th | 75th | 90th | 95th | 99th |
|---|---|---|---|---|---|---|---|---|---|---|
| **1. SINGLE DX** | | | | | | | | | | |
| 0–19 Years | 1 | 4.0 | 0 | 4 | 4 | 4 | 4 | 4 | 4 | 4 |
| 20–34 | 0 | | | | | | | | | |
| 35–49 | 1 | 3.0 | 0 | 3 | 3 | 3 | 3 | 3 | 3 | 3 |
| 50–64 | 0 | | | | | | | | | |
| 65+ | 2 | 1.0 | 0 | 1 | 1 | 1 | 1 | 1 | 1 | 1 |
| **2. MULTIPLE DX** | | | | | | | | | | |
| 0–19 Years | 1 | 3.0 | 0 | 3 | 3 | 3 | 3 | 3 | 3 | 3 |
| 20–34 | 0 | | | | | | | | | |
| 35–49 | 1 | 5.0 | 0 | 5 | 5 | 5 | 5 | 5 | 5 | 5 |
| 50–64 | 2 | 5.4 | 17 | 2 | 2 | 2 | 9 | 9 | 9 | 9 |
| 65+ | 8 | 6.4 | 15 | 2 | 3 | 6 | 8 | 15 | 15 | 15 |
| **TOTAL SINGLE DX** | 4 | 2.2 | 2 | 1 | 1 | 3 | 3 | 4 | 4 | 4 |
| **TOTAL MULTIPLE DX** | 12 | 5.3 | 7 | 3 | 3 | 5 | 6 | 8 | 9 | 15 |
| **TOTAL** | | | | | | | | | | |
| 0–19 Years | 2 | 3.3 | <1 | 3 | 3 | 3 | 4 | 4 | 4 | 4 |
| 20–34 | 0 | | | | | | | | | |
| 35–49 | 2 | 4.7 | <1 | 5 | 5 | 5 | 5 | 5 | 5 | 5 |
| 50–64 | 2 | 5.4 | 17 | 2 | 2 | 2 | 9 | 9 | 15 | 15 |
| 65+ | 10 | 4.9 | 17 | 1 | 1 | 6 | 8 | 8 | 15 | 15 |
| **GRAND TOTAL** | 16 | 4.7 | 8 | 3 | 3 | 5 | 5 | 8 | 9 | 15 |

## 49.7: REPAIR OF ANUS. Formerly included in operation group(s) 622.

| Type of Patients | Observed Patients | Avg. Stay | Variance | 10th | 25th | 50th | 75th | 90th | 95th | 99th |
|---|---|---|---|---|---|---|---|---|---|---|
| **1. SINGLE DX** | | | | | | | | | | |
| 0–19 Years | 90 | 3.9 | 7 | 1 | 1 | 3 | 7 | 8 | 8 | 8 |
| 20–34 | 34 | 2.8 | 2 | 2 | 2 | 2 | 4 | 4 | 5 | 7 |
| 35–49 | 59 | 2.6 | 1 | 1 | 2 | 3 | 3 | 4 | 5 | 5 |
| 50–64 | 27 | 2.3 | 1 | 1 | 2 | 2 | 3 | 4 | 5 | 5 |
| 65+ | 18 | 2.5 | <1 | 2 | 2 | 2 | 3 | 4 | 4 | 5 |
| **2. MULTIPLE DX** | | | | | | | | | | |
| 0–19 Years | 261 | 4.5 | 14 | 1 | 2 | 3 | 6 | 9 | 11 | 18 |
| 20–34 | 106 | 2.9 | 5 | 1 | 2 | 2 | 3 | 5 | 5 | 10 |
| 35–49 | 188 | 3.2 | 3 | 1 | 2 | 3 | 4 | 5 | 6 | 8 |
| 50–64 | 129 | 3.3 | 6 | 1 | 2 | 2 | 4 | 6 | 8 | 16 |
| 65+ | 136 | 3.8 | 12 | 1 | 2 | 2 | 5 | 9 | 10 | 17 |
| **TOTAL SINGLE DX** | 228 | 3.2 | 5 | 1 | 2 | 3 | 4 | 8 | 8 | 8 |
| **TOTAL MULTIPLE DX** | 820 | 3.7 | 9 | 1 | 2 | 3 | 5 | 7 | 9 | 18 |
| **TOTAL** | | | | | | | | | | |
| 0–19 Years | 351 | 4.3 | 12 | 1 | 2 | 3 | 6 | 8 | 9 | 18 |
| 20–34 | 140 | 2.9 | 4 | 1 | 2 | 2 | 4 | 4 | 5 | 9 |
| 35–49 | 247 | 3.1 | 3 | 1 | 2 | 3 | 4 | 5 | 6 | 8 |
| 50–64 | 156 | 3.1 | 5 | 1 | 2 | 2 | 4 | 6 | 8 | 16 |
| 65+ | 154 | 3.7 | 11 | 2 | 2 | 2 | 4 | 9 | 9 | 17 |
| **GRAND TOTAL** | 1,048 | 3.6 | 8 | 1 | 2 | 3 | 5 | 7 | 9 | 17 |

## 49.79: ANAL SPHINCTER REP NEC. Formerly included in operation group(s) 622.

| Type of Patients | Observed Patients | Avg. Stay | Variance | 10th | 25th | 50th | 75th | 90th | 95th | 99th |
|---|---|---|---|---|---|---|---|---|---|---|
| **1. SINGLE DX** | | | | | | | | | | |
| 0–19 Years | 81 | 3.0 | 3 | 1 | 2 | 3 | 4 | 5 | 7 | 8 |
| 20–34 | 27 | 3.1 | 2 | 2 | 2 | 3 | 4 | 4 | 5 | 7 |
| 35–49 | 49 | 2.6 | 1 | 2 | 2 | 2 | 3 | 4 | 5 | 7 |
| 50–64 | 23 | 2.5 | 1 | 1 | 2 | 2 | 3 | 4 | 5 | 5 |
| 65+ | 18 | 2.5 | <1 | 2 | 2 | 2 | 3 | 4 | 4 | 5 |
| **2. MULTIPLE DX** | | | | | | | | | | |
| 0–19 Years | 249 | 4.7 | 14 | 1 | 2 | 4 | 6 | 9 | 12 | 18 |
| 20–34 | 90 | 2.6 | 2 | 1 | 2 | 2 | 3 | 4 | 5 | 7 |
| 35–49 | 160 | 3.0 | 2 | 1 | 3 | 3 | 4 | 5 | 6 | 8 |
| 50–64 | 100 | 3.1 | 4 | 2 | 2 | 2 | 4 | 6 | 8 | 8 |
| 65+ | 118 | 3.5 | 10 | 1 | 1 | 2 | 4 | 9 | 9 | 13 |
| **TOTAL SINGLE DX** | 198 | 2.8 | 2 | 1 | 2 | 2 | 4 | 5 | 5 | 8 |
| **TOTAL MULTIPLE DX** | 717 | 3.7 | 9 | 1 | 2 | 3 | 4 | 7 | 9 | 18 |
| **TOTAL** | | | | | | | | | | |
| 0–19 Years | 330 | 4.3 | 12 | 1 | 2 | 3 | 5 | 9 | 11 | 18 |
| 20–34 | 117 | 2.7 | 2 | 2 | 2 | 2 | 4 | 4 | 5 | 7 |
| 35–49 | 209 | 2.9 | 2 | 1 | 2 | 3 | 3 | 6 | 6 | 8 |
| 50–64 | 123 | 3.0 | 4 | 2 | 2 | 3 | 3 | 6 | 8 | 8 |
| 65+ | 136 | 3.3 | 9 | 1 | 2 | 2 | 4 | 8 | 9 | 11 |
| **GRAND TOTAL** | 915 | 3.5 | 7 | 1 | 2 | 3 | 4 | 6 | 9 | 18 |

## 49.9: OTH OPERATIONS ON ANUS. Formerly included in operation group(s) 622.

| Type of Patients | Observed Patients | Avg. Stay | Variance | 10th | 25th | 50th | 75th | 90th | 95th | 99th |
|---|---|---|---|---|---|---|---|---|---|---|
| **1. SINGLE DX** | | | | | | | | | | |
| 0–19 Years | 5 | 3.0 | 2 | 1 | 2 | 4 | 4 | 4 | 4 | 4 |
| 20–34 | 8 | 1.6 | 2 | 1 | 1 | 1 | 1 | 3 | 6 | 6 |
| 35–49 | 16 | 1.7 | <1 | 1 | 1 | 2 | 2 | 3 | 3 | 3 |
| 50–64 | 3 | 2.1 | 1 | 1 | 1 | 3 | 3 | 3 | 3 | 3 |
| 65+ | 3 | 1.0 | 0 | 1 | 1 | 1 | 1 | 1 | 1 | 1 |
| **2. MULTIPLE DX** | | | | | | | | | | |
| 0–19 Years | 8 | 2.1 | 3 | 1 | 1 | 1 | 3 | 5 | 5 | 5 |
| 20–34 | 13 | 3.0 | 2 | 1 | 2 | 3 | 3 | 5 | 6 | 6 |
| 35–49 | 39 | 2.3 | 6 | 1 | 1 | 1 | 2 | 5 | 6 | 8 |
| 50–64 | 22 | 4.7 | 8 | 1 | 3 | 5 | 5 | 5 | 12 | 16 |
| 65+ | 47 | 4.7 | 22 | 1 | 1 | 4 | 5 | 8 | 10 | 40 |
| **TOTAL SINGLE DX** | 35 | 1.8 | 1 | 1 | 1 | 1 | 2 | 3 | 4 | 6 |
| **TOTAL MULTIPLE DX** | 129 | 3.5 | 12 | 1 | 2 | 3 | 5 | 5 | 8 | 15 |
| **TOTAL** | | | | | | | | | | |
| 0–19 Years | 13 | 2.4 | 2 | 1 | 1 | 2 | 4 | 4 | 5 | 5 |
| 20–34 | 21 | 2.2 | 2 | 1 | 1 | 2 | 3 | 5 | 6 | 6 |
| 35–49 | 55 | 2.2 | 5 | 1 | 1 | 2 | 2 | 5 | 5 | 8 |
| 50–64 | 25 | 4.5 | 8 | 1 | 3 | 5 | 5 | 5 | 12 | 16 |
| 65+ | 50 | 4.6 | 21 | 1 | 1 | 4 | 5 | 8 | 10 | 40 |
| **GRAND TOTAL** | 164 | 3.2 | 11 | 1 | 1 | 2 | 4 | 5 | 7 | 14 |

Length of Stay by Diagnosis and Operation, United States, 2000

# United States, October 1998–September 1999 Data, by Operation

## 50.0: HEPATOTOMY. Formerly included in operation group(s) 623.

| Type of Patients | Observed Patients | Avg. Stay | Vari-ance | Percentiles | | | | | | |
|---|---|---|---|---|---|---|---|---|---|---|
| | | | | 10th | 25th | 50th | 75th | 90th | 95th | 99th |
| **1. SINGLE DX** | | | | | | | | | | |
| 0–19 Years | 1 | 3.0 | 0 | 3 | 3 | 3 | 3 | 3 | 3 | 3 |
| 20–34 | 3 | 4.8 | <1 | 4 | 5 | 5 | 5 | 5 | 5 | 5 |
| 35–49 | 5 | 3.8 | <1 | 2 | 4 | 4 | 4 | 4 | 4 | 6 |
| 50–64 | 0 | | | | | | | | | |
| 65+ | 0 | | | | | | | | | |
| **2. MULTIPLE DX** | | | | | | | | | | |
| 0–19 Years | 8 | 26.8 | 222 | 8 | 12 | 29 | 42 | 46 | 46 | 46 |
| 20–34 | 25 | 8.7 | 58 | 3 | 4 | 6 | 11 | 16 | 23 | 51 |
| 35–49 | 24 | 9.9 | 50 | 3 | 5 | 11 | 11 | 12 | 29 | >99 |
| 50–64 | 44 | 14.5 | 73 | 5 | 8 | 16 | 16 | 23 | 30 | 44 |
| 65+ | 94 | 14.1 | 62 | 7 | 9 | 12 | 17 | 24 | 30 | 42 |
| **TOTAL SINGLE DX** | 9 | 3.8 | <1 | 3 | 4 | 4 | 4 | 4 | 5 | 6 |
| **TOTAL MULTIPLE DX** | 195 | 13.0 | 76 | 4 | 8 | 11 | 16 | 24 | 30 | 46 |
| **TOTAL** | | | | | | | | | | |
| 0–19 Years | 9 | 18.2 | 274 | 3 | 3 | 12 | 32 | 46 | 46 | 46 |
| 20–34 | 28 | 8.5 | 55 | 4 | 4 | 6 | 11 | 16 | 23 | 51 |
| 35–49 | 29 | 8.1 | 43 | 3 | 4 | 8 | 11 | 11 | 17 | 40 |
| 50–64 | 44 | 14.5 | 73 | 5 | 8 | 16 | 16 | 23 | 30 | 44 |
| 65+ | 94 | 14.1 | 62 | 7 | 9 | 12 | 17 | 24 | 30 | 42 |
| **GRAND TOTAL** | 204 | 12.1 | 76 | 4 | 5 | 11 | 16 | 22 | 30 | 44 |

## 50.1: HEPATIC DXTIC PX. Formerly included in operation group(s) 624, 631.

| Type of Patients | Observed Patients | Avg. Stay | Vari-ance | Percentiles | | | | | | |
|---|---|---|---|---|---|---|---|---|---|---|
| | | | | 10th | 25th | 50th | 75th | 90th | 95th | 99th |
| **1. SINGLE DX** | | | | | | | | | | |
| 0–19 Years | 190 | 3.4 | 14 | 1 | 1 | 1 | 5 | 9 | 13 | 17 |
| 20–34 | 53 | 2.7 | 7 | 1 | 1 | 1 | 3 | 7 | 8 | 12 |
| 35–49 | 142 | 1.7 | 3 | 1 | 1 | 1 | 1 | 4 | 6 | 9 |
| 50–64 | 70 | 2.5 | 6 | 1 | 1 | 1 | 3 | 5 | 7 | 12 |
| 65+ | 31 | 6.8 | 37 | 1 | 1 | 4 | 15 | 15 | 15 | 16 |
| **2. MULTIPLE DX** | | | | | | | | | | |
| 0–19 Years | 789 | 7.4 | 101 | 1 | 2 | 4 | 8 | 18 | 25 | 57 |
| 20–34 | 340 | 9.7 | 87 | 2 | 3 | 7 | 13 | 26 | 26 | 49 |
| 35–49 | 1,342 | 6.5 | 40 | 1 | 3 | 5 | 8 | 14 | 19 | 31 |
| 50–64 | 1,810 | 7.2 | 33 | 2 | 3 | 6 | 9 | 13 | 16 | 30 |
| 65+ | 2,848 | 8.2 | 36 | 2 | 4 | 7 | 10 | 15 | 20 | 33 |
| **TOTAL SINGLE DX** | 486 | 3.0 | 12 | 1 | 1 | 1 | 3 | 7 | 12 | 16 |
| **TOTAL MULTIPLE DX** | 7,129 | 7.6 | 48 | 1 | 3 | 6 | 9 | 15 | 20 | 35 |
| **TOTAL** | | | | | | | | | | |
| 0–19 Years | 979 | 6.7 | 89 | 1 | 1 | 4 | 7 | 16 | 23 | 50 |
| 20–34 | 393 | 8.7 | 81 | 1 | 2 | 6 | 10 | 25 | 26 | 49 |
| 35–49 | 1,484 | 5.9 | 38 | 1 | 2 | 4 | 7 | 13 | 18 | 30 |
| 50–64 | 1,880 | 7.0 | 33 | 2 | 3 | 6 | 9 | 13 | 16 | 29 |
| 65+ | 2,879 | 8.1 | 37 | 2 | 4 | 7 | 10 | 15 | 20 | 33 |
| **GRAND TOTAL** | 7,615 | 7.3 | 47 | 1 | 3 | 6 | 9 | 15 | 19 | 34 |

## 50.11: CLSD (PERC) LIVER BIOPSY. Formerly included in operation group(s) 624.

| Type of Patients | Observed Patients | Avg. Stay | Vari-ance | Percentiles | | | | | | |
|---|---|---|---|---|---|---|---|---|---|---|
| | | | | 10th | 25th | 50th | 75th | 90th | 95th | 99th |
| **1. SINGLE DX** | | | | | | | | | | |
| 0–19 Years | 165 | 3.2 | 14 | 1 | 1 | 1 | 4 | 7 | 13 | 17 |
| 20–34 | 51 | 2.6 | 7 | 1 | 1 | 1 | 3 | 7 | 9 | 12 |
| 35–49 | 135 | 1.6 | 3 | 1 | 1 | 1 | 1 | 3 | 5 | 9 |
| 50–64 | 67 | 2.5 | 6 | 1 | 1 | 1 | 3 | 5 | 7 | 14 |
| 65+ | 25 | 6.8 | 40 | 1 | 1 | 3 | 15 | 15 | 15 | 16 |
| **2. MULTIPLE DX** | | | | | | | | | | |
| 0–19 Years | 652 | 6.2 | 66 | 1 | 1 | 4 | 7 | 16 | 21 | 45 |
| 20–34 | 317 | 9.2 | 69 | 1 | 3 | 6 | 11 | 25 | 26 | 30 |
| 35–49 | 1,209 | 6.2 | 38 | 1 | 2 | 4 | 8 | 14 | 18 | 29 |
| 50–64 | 1,637 | 7.0 | 31 | 2 | 3 | 6 | 9 | 13 | 16 | 27 |
| 65+ | 2,614 | 8.0 | 34 | 2 | 4 | 7 | 10 | 15 | 19 | 32 |
| **TOTAL SINGLE DX** | 443 | 2.8 | 12 | 1 | 1 | 1 | 3 | 7 | 13 | 16 |
| **TOTAL MULTIPLE DX** | 6,429 | 7.3 | 41 | 1 | 3 | 6 | 9 | 15 | 19 | 31 |
| **TOTAL** | | | | | | | | | | |
| 0–19 Years | 817 | 5.7 | 58 | 1 | 1 | 3 | 6 | 15 | 20 | 44 |
| 20–34 | 368 | 8.1 | 65 | 1 | 2 | 6 | 10 | 24 | 26 | 30 |
| 35–49 | 1,344 | 5.7 | 36 | 1 | 1 | 4 | 7 | 13 | 17 | 29 |
| 50–64 | 1,704 | 6.8 | 31 | 2 | 3 | 6 | 9 | 13 | 16 | 27 |
| 65+ | 2,639 | 8.0 | 34 | 2 | 4 | 7 | 10 | 15 | 19 | 32 |
| **GRAND TOTAL** | 6,872 | 7.0 | 40 | 1 | 3 | 6 | 9 | 14 | 18 | 31 |

## 50.12: OPEN BIOPSY OF LIVER. Formerly included in operation group(s) 624.

| Type of Patients | Observed Patients | Avg. Stay | Vari-ance | Percentiles | | | | | | |
|---|---|---|---|---|---|---|---|---|---|---|
| | | | | 10th | 25th | 50th | 75th | 90th | 95th | 99th |
| **1. SINGLE DX** | | | | | | | | | | |
| 0–19 Years | 25 | 4.7 | 12 | 1 | 2 | 3 | 9 | 9 | 11 | 11 |
| 20–34 | 2 | 6.7 | 3 | 5 | 5 | 8 | 8 | 8 | 8 | 8 |
| 35–49 | 7 | 4.0 | 8 | 1 | 1 | 5 | 6 | 6 | 9 | 9 |
| 50–64 | 3 | 3.3 | 7 | 1 | 2 | 2 | 7 | 7 | 7 | 7 |
| 65+ | 6 | 6.4 | 9 | 4 | 4 | 7 | 8 | 11 | 11 | 11 |
| **2. MULTIPLE DX** | | | | | | | | | | |
| 0–19 Years | 137 | 13.7 | 241 | 2 | 4 | 7 | 15 | 41 | 49 | 79 |
| 20–34 | 23 | 17.9 | 278 | 3 | 5 | 15 | 21 | 49 | 49 | 49 |
| 35–49 | 132 | 7.9 | 46 | 2 | 3 | 6 | 10 | 17 | 19 | 39 |
| 50–64 | 172 | 8.7 | 51 | 3 | 5 | 9 | 9 | 13 | 18 | 43 |
| 65+ | 234 | 10.0 | 63 | 3 | 5 | 7 | 12 | 20 | 24 | 41 |
| **TOTAL SINGLE DX** | 43 | 4.7 | 11 | 1 | 2 | 5 | 8 | 9 | 10 | 11 |
| **TOTAL MULTIPLE DX** | 698 | 10.4 | 112 | 3 | 5 | 7 | 11 | 21 | 32 | 60 |
| **TOTAL** | | | | | | | | | | |
| 0–19 Years | 162 | 12.5 | 219 | 2 | 4 | 7 | 14 | 32 | 44 | 78 |
| 20–34 | 25 | 17.5 | 271 | 3 | 5 | 10 | 21 | 49 | 49 | 49 |
| 35–49 | 139 | 7.7 | 45 | 2 | 3 | 6 | 10 | 17 | 19 | 39 |
| 50–64 | 175 | 8.6 | 50 | 3 | 5 | 9 | 9 | 13 | 18 | 43 |
| 65+ | 240 | 9.9 | 63 | 3 | 5 | 7 | 12 | 20 | 24 | 41 |
| **GRAND TOTAL** | 741 | 10.1 | 108 | 3 | 4 | 7 | 11 | 20 | 32 | 57 |

Length of Stay by Diagnosis and Operation, United States, 2000

## United States, October 1998–September 1999 Data, by Operation

### 50.2: LOC EXC/DESTR LIVER LES. Formerly included in operation group(s) 624.

| Type of Patients | Observed Patients | Avg. Stay | Variance | Percentiles | | | | | | |
|---|---|---|---|---|---|---|---|---|---|---|
| | | | | 10th | 25th | 50th | 75th | 90th | 95th | 99th |
| **1. SINGLE DX** | | | | | | | | | | |
| 0–19 Years | 16 | 5.6 | 13 | 2 | 4 | 4 | 8 | 11 | 11 | 15 |
| 20–34 | 28 | 4.3 | 2 | 2 | 3 | 4 | 5 | 6 | 7 | 9 |
| 35–49 | 23 | 4.5 | 3 | 2 | 3 | 5 | 6 | 7 | 7 | 8 |
| 50–64 | 13 | 4.1 | 4 | 2 | 2 | 4 | 5 | 6 | 9 | 9 |
| 65+ | 9 | 4.7 | 3 | 2 | 4 | 5 | 5 | 6 | 8 | 8 |
| **2. MULTIPLE DX** | | | | | | | | | | |
| 0–19 Years | 59 | 8.6 | 116 | 4 | 5 | 6 | 8 | 11 | 14 | 74 |
| 20–34 | 104 | 7.4 | 34 | 2 | 4 | 6 | 9 | 15 | 15 | 27 |
| 35–49 | 251 | 5.7 | 25 | 2 | 3 | 5 | 7 | 10 | 12 | 22 |
| 50–64 | 368 | 7.4 | 44 | 3 | 4 | 6 | 8 | 13 | 23 | 29 |
| 65+ | 447 | 8.2 | 50 | 3 | 5 | 6 | 9 | 17 | 26 | >99 |
| **TOTAL SINGLE DX** | 89 | 4.7 | 6 | 2 | 3 | 4 | 6 | 7 | 9 | 11 |
| **TOTAL MULTIPLE DX** | 1,229 | 7.4 | 46 | 3 | 4 | 6 | 8 | 13 | 19 | 57 |
| **TOTAL** | | | | | | | | | | |
| 0–19 Years | 75 | 7.9 | 94 | 3 | 5 | 6 | 8 | 11 | 12 | 74 |
| 20–34 | 132 | 6.7 | 28 | 2 | 4 | 5 | 8 | 15 | 15 | 27 |
| 35–49 | 274 | 5.6 | 23 | 2 | 3 | 5 | 6 | 10 | 12 | 22 |
| 50–64 | 381 | 7.3 | 44 | 3 | 4 | 6 | 8 | 13 | 23 | 29 |
| 65+ | 456 | 8.2 | 49 | 3 | 5 | 6 | 9 | 17 | 26 | >99 |
| **GRAND TOTAL** | 1,318 | 7.2 | 44 | 3 | 4 | 6 | 8 | 13 | 18 | 57 |

### 50.29: DESTR HEPATIC LESION NEC. Formerly included in operation group(s) 624.

| Type of Patients | Observed Patients | Avg. Stay | Variance | Percentiles | | | | | | |
|---|---|---|---|---|---|---|---|---|---|---|
| | | | | 10th | 25th | 50th | 75th | 90th | 95th | 99th |
| **1. SINGLE DX** | | | | | | | | | | |
| 0–19 Years | 8 | 3.9 | 6 | 1 | 2 | 4 | 4 | 8 | 8 | 8 |
| 20–34 | 8 | 3.6 | 2 | 2 | 2 | 4 | 5 | 5 | 5 | 5 |
| 35–49 | 6 | 4.0 | 7 | 1 | 2 | 2 | 7 | 7 | 7 | 7 |
| 50–64 | 4 | 3.5 | 5 | 1 | 2 | 2 | 5 | 6 | 6 | 6 |
| 65+ | 3 | 4.0 | 2 | 2 | 3 | 5 | 5 | 5 | 5 | 5 |
| **2. MULTIPLE DX** | | | | | | | | | | |
| 0–19 Years | 23 | 8.6 | 177 | 5 | 5 | 6 | 7 | 7 | 11 | 74 |
| 20–34 | 38 | 6.5 | 29 | 1 | 2 | 5 | 12 | 15 | 15 | 15 |
| 35–49 | 91 | 4.3 | 10 | 1 | 2 | 3 | 5 | 8 | 10 | 17 |
| 50–64 | 122 | 6.3 | 17 | 1 | 3 | 6 | 9 | 11 | 12 | 22 |
| 65+ | 164 | 6.5 | 30 | 2 | 3 | 5 | 8 | 17 | >99 | >99 |
| **TOTAL SINGLE DX** | 29 | 3.8 | 4 | 2 | 2 | 4 | 5 | 7 | 8 | 8 |
| **TOTAL MULTIPLE DX** | 438 | 6.1 | 33 | 2 | 3 | 5 | 8 | 12 | 17 | >99 |
| **TOTAL** | | | | | | | | | | |
| 0–19 Years | 31 | 7.7 | 145 | 2 | 5 | 6 | 7 | 8 | 11 | 74 |
| 20–34 | 46 | 6.2 | 26 | 1 | 2 | 5 | 10 | 15 | 15 | 15 |
| 35–49 | 97 | 4.3 | 10 | 2 | 2 | 3 | 5 | 7 | 10 | 17 |
| 50–64 | 126 | 6.3 | 17 | 1 | 3 | 6 | 9 | 11 | 12 | 22 |
| 65+ | 167 | 6.5 | 30 | 2 | 3 | 5 | 8 | 17 | >99 | >99 |
| **GRAND TOTAL** | 467 | 6.0 | 32 | 2 | 3 | 5 | 7 | 12 | 16 | >99 |

### 50.22: PARTIAL HEPATECTOMY. Formerly included in operation group(s) 624.

| Type of Patients | Observed Patients | Avg. Stay | Variance | Percentiles | | | | | | |
|---|---|---|---|---|---|---|---|---|---|---|
| | | | | 10th | 25th | 50th | 75th | 90th | 95th | 99th |
| **1. SINGLE DX** | | | | | | | | | | |
| 0–19 Years | 7 | 6.8 | 14 | 4 | 4 | 4 | 11 | 11 | 15 | 15 |
| 20–34 | 20 | 4.5 | 2 | 2 | 4 | 4 | 6 | 6 | 7 | 9 |
| 35–49 | 17 | 4.6 | 3 | 3 | 3 | 5 | 6 | 7 | 7 | 8 |
| 50–64 | 7 | 5.2 | 2 | 4 | 4 | 5 | 6 | 9 | 9 | 9 |
| 65+ | 5 | 5.5 | 3 | 4 | 4 | 6 | 6 | 8 | 8 | 8 |
| **2. MULTIPLE DX** | | | | | | | | | | |
| 0–19 Years | 35 | 8.7 | 76 | 4 | 5 | 8 | 9 | 12 | 14 | 56 |
| 20–34 | 64 | 8.1 | 37 | 4 | 5 | 6 | 8 | 13 | 19 | 32 |
| 35–49 | 154 | 6.9 | 33 | 4 | 4 | 5 | 7 | 10 | 14 | 28 |
| 50–64 | 237 | 7.9 | 54 | 4 | 4 | 6 | 8 | 13 | 25 | 33 |
| 65+ | 269 | 9.4 | 60 | 5 | 5 | 6 | 10 | 17 | 23 | 50 |
| **TOTAL SINGLE DX** | 56 | 5.1 | 6 | 4 | 4 | 4 | 6 | 8 | 11 | 15 |
| **TOTAL MULTIPLE DX** | 759 | 8.3 | 53 | 4 | 5 | 6 | 9 | 14 | 22 | 44 |
| **TOTAL** | | | | | | | | | | |
| 0–19 Years | 42 | 8.3 | 61 | 4 | 5 | 7 | 10 | 11 | 14 | 56 |
| 20–34 | 84 | 7.0 | 30 | 4 | 4 | 6 | 7 | 12 | 18 | 32 |
| 35–49 | 171 | 6.6 | 30 | 3 | 5 | 5 | 7 | 10 | 13 | 27 |
| 50–64 | 244 | 7.9 | 53 | 4 | 4 | 6 | 8 | 13 | 25 | 33 |
| 65+ | 274 | 9.3 | 59 | 5 | 5 | 7 | 10 | 17 | 23 | 50 |
| **GRAND TOTAL** | 815 | 8.0 | 50 | 4 | 5 | 6 | 8 | 13 | 20 | 36 |

### 50.3: HEPATIC LOBECTOMY. Formerly included in operation group(s) 624.

| Type of Patients | Observed Patients | Avg. Stay | Variance | Percentiles | | | | | | |
|---|---|---|---|---|---|---|---|---|---|---|
| | | | | 10th | 25th | 50th | 75th | 90th | 95th | 99th |
| **1. SINGLE DX** | | | | | | | | | | |
| 0–19 Years | 14 | 7.6 | 4 | 4 | 6 | 8 | 9 | 10 | 10 | 11 |
| 20–34 | 11 | 5.6 | 3 | 4 | 4 | 5 | 6 | 8 | 10 | 10 |
| 35–49 | 8 | 6.8 | 7 | 5 | 5 | 8 | 8 | 8 | 11 | 11 |
| 50–64 | 5 | 7.5 | 7 | 4 | 5 | 7 | 10 | 10 | 10 | 10 |
| 65+ | 2 | 5.0 | 3 | 4 | 4 | 4 | 7 | 7 | 7 | 7 |
| **2. MULTIPLE DX** | | | | | | | | | | |
| 0–19 Years | 44 | 10.5 | 54 | 5 | 5 | 8 | 12 | 22 | 24 | 36 |
| 20–34 | 48 | 9.7 | 66 | 6 | 6 | 8 | 10 | 15 | 22 | 52 |
| 35–49 | 121 | 8.4 | 37 | 4 | 4 | 7 | 11 | 12 | 20 | 28 |
| 50–64 | 168 | 9.5 | 52 | 4 | 5 | 7 | 11 | 18 | 21 | 39 |
| 65+ | 220 | 10.6 | 75 | 5 | 6 | 8 | 11 | 21 | 37 | 37 |
| **TOTAL SINGLE DX** | 40 | 7.0 | 5 | 4 | 5 | 6 | 9 | 10 | 10 | 11 |
| **TOTAL MULTIPLE DX** | 601 | 9.7 | 59 | 4 | 6 | 8 | 10 | 17 | 25 | 37 |
| **TOTAL** | | | | | | | | | | |
| 0–19 Years | 58 | 9.3 | 37 | 5 | 6 | 8 | 10 | 14 | 22 | 36 |
| 20–34 | 59 | 8.8 | 54 | 4 | 5 | 7 | 9 | 13 | 15 | 52 |
| 35–49 | 129 | 8.3 | 36 | 4 | 4 | 7 | 10 | 12 | 20 | 27 |
| 50–64 | 173 | 9.4 | 51 | 5 | 5 | 7 | 11 | 18 | 21 | 39 |
| 65+ | 222 | 10.6 | 75 | 5 | 6 | 8 | 11 | 21 | 37 | 37 |
| **GRAND TOTAL** | 641 | 9.5 | 55 | 4 | 6 | 8 | 10 | 16 | 23 | 37 |

Length of Stay by Diagnosis and Operation, United States, 2000

# United States, October 1998–September 1999 Data, by Operation

## 50.4: TOTAL HEPATECTOMY. Formerly included in operation group(s) 624.

| Type of Patients | Observed Patients | Avg. Stay | Variance | Percentiles | | | | | | |
|---|---|---|---|---|---|---|---|---|---|---|
| | | | | 10th | 25th | 50th | 75th | 90th | 95th | 99th |
| **1. SINGLE DX** | | | | | | | | | | |
| 0–19 Years | 0 | | | | | | | | | |
| 20–34 | 1 | 1.0 | 0 | | | | | | | |
| 35–49 | 3 | 2.6 | 2 | 1 | 1 | 3 | 4 | 4 | 4 | 4 |
| 50–64 | 1 | 1.0 | 0 | 1 | 1 | 1 | 1 | 1 | 1 | 1 |
| 65+ | 0 | | | | | | | | | |
| **2. MULTIPLE DX** | | | | | | | | | | |
| 0–19 Years | 8 | 18.0 | 49 | 5 | 16 | 23 | 23 | 23 | 23 | 23 |
| 20–34 | 5 | 5.0 | 120 | 1 | 1 | 1 | 1 | 32 | 32 | 32 |
| 35–49 | 4 | 6.8 | 5 | 4 | 6 | 6 | 6 | 11 | 11 | 11 |
| 50–64 | 8 | 13.0 | 441 | 1 | 1 | 5 | 18 | 18 | 85 | 85 |
| 65+ | 3 | 9.2 | 1 | 8 | 8 | 9 | 9 | 11 | 11 | 11 |
| **TOTAL SINGLE DX** | 5 | 1.7 | 1 | 1 | 1 | 1 | 3 | 4 | 4 | 4 |
| **TOTAL MULTIPLE DX** | 28 | 12.8 | 164 | 1 | 1 | 11 | 23 | 23 | 23 | 85 |
| **TOTAL** | | | | | | | | | | |
| 0–19 Years | 8 | 18.0 | 49 | 5 | 16 | 23 | 23 | 23 | 23 | 23 |
| 20–34 | 6 | 3.8 | 86 | 1 | 1 | 1 | 1 | 1 | 32 | 32 |
| 35–49 | 7 | 5.7 | 8 | 3 | 4 | 6 | 6 | 10 | 11 | 11 |
| 50–64 | 9 | 12.3 | 422 | 1 | 1 | 5 | 18 | 18 | 85 | 85 |
| 65+ | 3 | 9.2 | 1 | 8 | 8 | 9 | 9 | 11 | 11 | 11 |
| **GRAND TOTAL** | 33 | 11.6 | 158 | 1 | 1 | 9 | 18 | 23 | 23 | 85 |

## 50.5: LIVER TRANSPLANT. Formerly included in operation group(s) 624.

| Type of Patients | Observed Patients | Avg. Stay | Variance | Percentiles | | | | | | |
|---|---|---|---|---|---|---|---|---|---|---|
| | | | | 10th | 25th | 50th | 75th | 90th | 95th | 99th |
| **1. SINGLE DX** | | | | | | | | | | |
| 0–19 Years | 1 | 10.0 | 0 | 10 | 10 | 10 | 10 | 10 | 10 | 10 |
| 20–34 | 1 | 7.0 | 0 | 7 | 7 | 7 | 7 | 7 | 7 | 7 |
| 35–49 | 4 | 8.2 | 8 | 6 | 6 | 6 | 10 | 12 | 12 | 12 |
| 50–64 | 1 | 9.0 | 0 | 9 | 9 | 9 | 9 | 9 | 9 | 9 |
| 65+ | 1 | 9.0 | 0 | 9 | 9 | 9 | 9 | 9 | 9 | 9 |
| **2. MULTIPLE DX** | | | | | | | | | | |
| 0–19 Years | 192 | 26.5 | 337 | 10 | 14 | 22 | 35 | 61 | 92 | >99 |
| 20–34 | 52 | 20.3 | 312 | 7 | 12 | 14 | 21 | 43 | 64 | 83 |
| 35–49 | 373 | 17.7 | 195 | 6 | 9 | 13 | 21 | 38 | 54 | >99 |
| 50–64 | 354 | 18.9 | 228 | 7 | 10 | 14 | 23 | 38 | 55 | 98 |
| 65+ | 76 | 18.2 | 181 | 8 | 10 | 13 | 20 | 42 | 51 | 74 |
| **TOTAL SINGLE DX** | 8 | 8.7 | 3 | 6 | 7 | 9 | 10 | 10 | 12 | 12 |
| **TOTAL MULTIPLE DX** | 1,047 | 20.9 | 268 | 8 | 10 | 15 | 26 | 47 | 68 | >99 |
| **TOTAL** | | | | | | | | | | |
| 0–19 Years | 193 | 26.4 | 336 | 10 | 14 | 22 | 34 | 61 | 92 | >99 |
| 20–34 | 53 | 20.0 | 309 | 7 | 12 | 13 | 21 | 43 | 64 | 83 |
| 35–49 | 377 | 17.6 | 194 | 6 | 9 | 13 | 21 | 38 | 54 | >99 |
| 50–64 | 355 | 18.8 | 228 | 7 | 10 | 14 | 23 | 38 | 55 | 98 |
| 65+ | 77 | 18.1 | 180 | 8 | 10 | 13 | 20 | 39 | 51 | 74 |
| **GRAND TOTAL** | 1,055 | 20.8 | 267 | 7 | 10 | 15 | 26 | 46 | 67 | >99 |

## 50.59: LIVER TRANSPLANT NEC. Formerly included in operation group(s) 624.

| Type of Patients | Observed Patients | Avg. Stay | Variance | Percentiles | | | | | | |
|---|---|---|---|---|---|---|---|---|---|---|
| | | | | 10th | 25th | 50th | 75th | 90th | 95th | 99th |
| **1. SINGLE DX** | | | | | | | | | | |
| 0–19 Years | 1 | 10.0 | 0 | 10 | 10 | 10 | 10 | 10 | 10 | 10 |
| 20–34 | 1 | 7.0 | 0 | 7 | 7 | 7 | 7 | 7 | 7 | 7 |
| 35–49 | 4 | 8.2 | 8 | 6 | 6 | 6 | 10 | 12 | 12 | 12 |
| 50–64 | 1 | 9.0 | 0 | 9 | 9 | 9 | 9 | 9 | 9 | 9 |
| 65+ | 1 | 9.0 | 0 | 9 | 9 | 9 | 9 | 9 | 9 | 9 |
| **2. MULTIPLE DX** | | | | | | | | | | |
| 0–19 Years | 187 | 26.5 | 338 | 10 | 14 | 22 | 35 | 61 | 92 | >99 |
| 20–34 | 51 | 20.6 | 314 | 7 | 12 | 15 | 21 | 43 | 70 | 83 |
| 35–49 | 369 | 17.7 | 195 | 6 | 9 | 13 | 21 | 39 | 54 | >99 |
| 50–64 | 348 | 19.0 | 231 | 7 | 10 | 14 | 23 | 39 | 55 | 98 |
| 65+ | 75 | 18.0 | 181 | 8 | 10 | 13 | 20 | 42 | 51 | 74 |
| **TOTAL SINGLE DX** | 8 | 8.7 | 3 | 6 | 7 | 9 | 10 | 10 | 12 | 12 |
| **TOTAL MULTIPLE DX** | 1,030 | 21.0 | 269 | 8 | 11 | 16 | 26 | 47 | 68 | >99 |
| **TOTAL** | | | | | | | | | | |
| 0–19 Years | 188 | 26.4 | 338 | 10 | 14 | 22 | 34 | 61 | 92 | >99 |
| 20–34 | 52 | 20.2 | 311 | 7 | 12 | 14 | 21 | 43 | 64 | 83 |
| 35–49 | 373 | 17.6 | 195 | 6 | 9 | 13 | 21 | 38 | 54 | >99 |
| 50–64 | 349 | 19.0 | 230 | 7 | 10 | 14 | 23 | 39 | 55 | 98 |
| 65+ | 76 | 17.9 | 180 | 8 | 10 | 13 | 20 | 42 | 51 | 74 |
| **GRAND TOTAL** | 1,038 | 20.9 | 268 | 8 | 10 | 15 | 26 | 47 | 68 | >99 |

## 50.6: REPAIR OF LIVER. Formerly included in operation group(s) 624.

| Type of Patients | Observed Patients | Avg. Stay | Variance | Percentiles | | | | | | |
|---|---|---|---|---|---|---|---|---|---|---|
| | | | | 10th | 25th | 50th | 75th | 90th | 95th | 99th |
| **1. SINGLE DX** | | | | | | | | | | |
| 0–19 Years | 11 | 3.3 | 1 | 2 | 3 | 3 | 4 | 5 | 5 | 7 |
| 20–34 | 8 | 3.5 | 1 | 3 | 3 | 3 | 5 | 5 | 5 | 5 |
| 35–49 | 4 | 2.8 | 2 | 1 | 2 | 4 | 4 | 4 | 4 | 4 |
| 50–64 | 0 | | | | | | | | | |
| 65+ | 0 | | | | | | | | | |
| **2. MULTIPLE DX** | | | | | | | | | | |
| 0–19 Years | 106 | 10.8 | 81 | 4 | 6 | 8 | 12 | 19 | 21 | 47 |
| 20–34 | 216 | 7.9 | 46 | 3 | 4 | 5 | 9 | 17 | 24 | 34 |
| 35–49 | 176 | 8.7 | 66 | 3 | 4 | 6 | 10 | 18 | 23 | 47 |
| 50–64 | 69 | 11.4 | 143 | 3 | 4 | 8 | 14 | 27 | 33 | 81 |
| 65+ | 52 | 8.4 | 30 | 3 | 5 | 6 | 10 | 16 | 18 | 28 |
| **TOTAL SINGLE DX** | 23 | 3.3 | 1 | 2 | 3 | 3 | 4 | 5 | 5 | 7 |
| **TOTAL MULTIPLE DX** | 619 | 8.9 | 66 | 3 | 4 | 6 | 10 | 19 | 24 | 41 |
| **TOTAL** | | | | | | | | | | |
| 0–19 Years | 117 | 9.7 | 76 | 3 | 4 | 7 | 12 | 19 | 21 | 47 |
| 20–34 | 224 | 7.8 | 46 | 3 | 4 | 5 | 9 | 17 | 24 | 34 |
| 35–49 | 180 | 8.6 | 66 | 3 | 4 | 6 | 10 | 17 | 23 | 47 |
| 50–64 | 69 | 11.4 | 143 | 3 | 4 | 8 | 14 | 27 | 33 | 81 |
| 65+ | 52 | 8.4 | 30 | 3 | 5 | 6 | 10 | 16 | 18 | 28 |
| **GRAND TOTAL** | 642 | 8.7 | 64 | 3 | 4 | 6 | 10 | 18 | 24 | 40 |

Length of Stay by Diagnosis and Operation, United States, 2000

# United States, October 1998–September 1999 Data, by Operation

## 50.61: CLOSURE OF LIVER LAC. Formerly included in operation group(s) 624.

| Type of Patients | Observed Patients | Avg. Stay | Vari-ance | 10th | 25th | 50th | 75th | 90th | 95th | 99th |
|---|---|---|---|---|---|---|---|---|---|---|
| **1. SINGLE DX** | | | | | | | | | | |
| 0–19 Years | 8 | 3.4 | <1 | 3 | 3 | 3 | 4 | 4 | 4 | 7 |
| 20–34 | 8 | 3.5 | 1 | 3 | 3 | 3 | 5 | 5 | 5 | 5 |
| 35–49 | 4 | 2.8 | 2 | 1 | 2 | 4 | 4 | 4 | 4 | 4 |
| 50–64 | 0 | | | | | | | | | |
| 65+ | 0 | | | | | | | | | |
| **2. MULTIPLE DX** | | | | | | | | | | |
| 0–19 Years | 94 | 10.5 | 87 | 4 | 6 | 8 | 12 | 19 | 28 | 47 |
| 20–34 | 198 | 7.7 | 47 | 3 | 4 | 5 | 9 | 17 | 24 | 34 |
| 35–49 | 161 | 9.0 | 68 | 4 | 4 | 6 | 10 | 17 | 24 | 47 |
| 50–64 | 52 | 13.0 | 182 | 2 | 5 | 8 | 20 | 29 | 36 | 81 |
| 65+ | 35 | 8.0 | 22 | 3 | 5 | 6 | 10 | 16 | 16 | 25 |
| **TOTAL SINGLE DX** | 20 | 3.4 | <1 | 3 | 3 | 3 | 4 | 4 | 5 | 7 |
| **TOTAL MULTIPLE DX** | 540 | 8.9 | 69 | 3 | 4 | 6 | 10 | 18 | 25 | 42 |
| **TOTAL** | | | | | | | | | | |
| 0–19 Years | 102 | 9.6 | 81 | 3 | 4 | 7 | 12 | 19 | 21 | 47 |
| 20–34 | 206 | 7.6 | 46 | 3 | 4 | 5 | 9 | 17 | 24 | 34 |
| 35–49 | 165 | 8.9 | 67 | 3 | 4 | 6 | 10 | 17 | 21 | 47 |
| 50–64 | 52 | 13.0 | 182 | 2 | 4 | 8 | 20 | 29 | 36 | 81 |
| 65+ | 35 | 8.0 | 22 | 3 | 5 | 6 | 10 | 16 | 16 | 25 |
| **GRAND TOTAL** | 560 | 8.7 | 68 | 3 | 4 | 6 | 10 | 18 | 24 | 42 |

## 50.91: PERC LIVER ASPIRATION. Formerly included in operation group(s) 623.

| Type of Patients | Observed Patients | Avg. Stay | Vari-ance | 10th | 25th | 50th | 75th | 90th | 95th | 99th |
|---|---|---|---|---|---|---|---|---|---|---|
| **1. SINGLE DX** | | | | | | | | | | |
| 0–19 Years | 3 | 8.5 | 3 | 5 | 9 | 9 | 9 | 11 | 11 | 11 |
| 20–34 | 8 | 6.3 | 11 | 2 | 4 | 7 | 8 | 11 | 11 | 11 |
| 35–49 | 14 | 2.8 | 5 | 1 | 1 | 2 | 5 | 5 | 7 | 10 |
| 50–64 | 6 | 5.5 | 14 | 2 | 2 | 7 | 7 | 11 | 12 | 12 |
| 65+ | 7 | 3.0 | 3 | 2 | 2 | 2 | 5 | 6 | 6 | 6 |
| **2. MULTIPLE DX** | | | | | | | | | | |
| 0–19 Years | 33 | 15.9 | 196 | 2 | 4 | 10 | 29 | 39 | 39 | 39 |
| 20–34 | 52 | 9.2 | 52 | 3 | 4 | 6 | 13 | 15 | 29 | 29 |
| 35–49 | 88 | 11.7 | 44 | 4 | 7 | 9 | 18 | 19 | 19 | 36 |
| 50–64 | 154 | 10.6 | 75 | 4 | 6 | 9 | 11 | 22 | 27 | 52 |
| 65+ | 264 | 11.2 | 44 | 4 | 7 | 10 | 15 | 21 | 24 | 33 |
| **TOTAL SINGLE DX** | 38 | 4.8 | 11 | 1 | 2 | 4 | 7 | 9 | 11 | 12 |
| **TOTAL MULTIPLE DX** | 591 | 11.3 | 64 | 3 | 6 | 9 | 15 | 21 | 27 | 39 |
| **TOTAL** | | | | | | | | | | |
| 0–19 Years | 36 | 15.0 | 177 | 2 | 5 | 9 | 27 | 39 | 39 | 39 |
| 20–34 | 60 | 8.9 | 48 | 3 | 4 | 6 | 12 | 15 | 29 | 29 |
| 35–49 | 102 | 10.8 | 48 | 3 | 7 | 9 | 17 | 19 | 19 | 36 |
| 50–64 | 160 | 10.4 | 73 | 3 | 6 | 9 | 11 | 20 | 27 | 52 |
| 65+ | 271 | 11.0 | 45 | 3 | 7 | 10 | 15 | 21 | 24 | 32 |
| **GRAND TOTAL** | 629 | 10.9 | 63 | 3 | 6 | 9 | 14 | 20 | 27 | 39 |

## 50.9: OTHER LIVER OPERATIONS. Formerly included in operation group(s) 623, 624.

| Type of Patients | Observed Patients | Avg. Stay | Vari-ance | 10th | 25th | 50th | 75th | 90th | 95th | 99th |
|---|---|---|---|---|---|---|---|---|---|---|
| **1. SINGLE DX** | | | | | | | | | | |
| 0–19 Years | 3 | 8.5 | 3 | 5 | 9 | 9 | 9 | 11 | 11 | 11 |
| 20–34 | 8 | 6.3 | 11 | 2 | 4 | 7 | 8 | 11 | 11 | 11 |
| 35–49 | 14 | 2.8 | 5 | 1 | 1 | 2 | 5 | 5 | 7 | 10 |
| 50–64 | 6 | 5.5 | 14 | 2 | 2 | 7 | 7 | 11 | 12 | 12 |
| 65+ | 8 | 2.9 | 3 | 2 | 2 | 3 | 3 | 6 | 6 | 6 |
| **2. MULTIPLE DX** | | | | | | | | | | |
| 0–19 Years | 33 | 15.9 | 196 | 2 | 4 | 10 | 29 | 39 | 39 | 39 |
| 20–34 | 53 | 9.2 | 52 | 3 | 4 | 6 | 13 | 15 | 29 | 29 |
| 35–49 | 116 | 11.1 | 48 | 2 | 7 | 9 | 17 | 19 | 19 | 36 |
| 50–64 | 203 | 10.6 | 69 | 2 | 4 | 7 | 10 | 17 | 27 | 52 |
| 65+ | 329 | 9.6 | 49 | 2 | 4 | 8 | 14 | 20 | 24 | 32 |
| **TOTAL SINGLE DX** | 39 | 4.8 | 11 | 1 | 2 | 4 | 7 | 9 | 11 | 12 |
| **TOTAL MULTIPLE DX** | 734 | 10.0 | 64 | 2 | 4 | 8 | 13 | 19 | 27 | 39 |
| **TOTAL** | | | | | | | | | | |
| 0–19 Years | 36 | 15.0 | 177 | 2 | 5 | 9 | 27 | 39 | 39 | 39 |
| 20–34 | 61 | 8.9 | 48 | 2 | 4 | 6 | 12 | 15 | 29 | 29 |
| 35–49 | 130 | 10.4 | 50 | 3 | 5 | 8 | 17 | 19 | 19 | 36 |
| 50–64 | 209 | 8.9 | 68 | 2 | 4 | 7 | 10 | 16 | 27 | 52 |
| 65+ | 337 | 9.5 | 49 | 2 | 4 | 8 | 14 | 20 | 24 | 32 |
| **GRAND TOTAL** | 773 | 9.8 | 63 | 2 | 4 | 8 | 13 | 19 | 25 | 39 |

## 51.0: GB INC & CHOLECYSTOSTOMY. Formerly included in operation group(s) 629.

| Type of Patients | Observed Patients | Avg. Stay | Vari-ance | 10th | 25th | 50th | 75th | 90th | 95th | 99th |
|---|---|---|---|---|---|---|---|---|---|---|
| **1. SINGLE DX** | | | | | | | | | | |
| 0–19 Years | 0 | | | | | | | | | |
| 20–34 | 0 | | | | | | | | | |
| 35–49 | 3 | 3.9 | <1 | 3 | 3 | 4 | 5 | 5 | 5 | 5 |
| 50–64 | 3 | 3.7 | 12 | 2 | 2 | 4 | 2 | 10 | 10 | 10 |
| 65+ | 2 | 3.1 | 1 | 2 | 2 | 4 | 4 | 4 | 4 | 4 |
| **2. MULTIPLE DX** | | | | | | | | | | |
| 0–19 Years | 4 | 10.4 | 21 | 6 | 6 | 10 | 12 | 19 | 19 | 19 |
| 20–34 | 27 | 10.1 | 78 | 3 | 3 | 6 | 14 | 22 | 27 | 46 |
| 35–49 | 40 | 12.1 | 132 | 4 | 4 | 6 | 16 | 32 | 32 | 51 |
| 50–64 | 95 | 10.6 | 94 | 3 | 5 | 7 | 13 | 25 | 37 | 37 |
| 65+ | 354 | 10.5 | 47 | 4 | 6 | 8 | 13 | 18 | 24 | 36 |
| **TOTAL SINGLE DX** | 8 | 3.7 | 7 | 2 | 2 | 2 | 4 | 4 | 10 | 10 |
| **TOTAL MULTIPLE DX** | 520 | 10.6 | 64 | 4 | 6 | 8 | 13 | 20 | 32 | 37 |
| **TOTAL** | | | | | | | | | | |
| 0–19 Years | 4 | 10.4 | 21 | 6 | 6 | 10 | 12 | 19 | 19 | 19 |
| 20–34 | 27 | 10.1 | 78 | 3 | 3 | 6 | 14 | 22 | 27 | 46 |
| 35–49 | 43 | 11.9 | 130 | 3 | 4 | 6 | 16 | 32 | 32 | 51 |
| 50–64 | 98 | 10.3 | 93 | 3 | 4 | 7 | 12 | 25 | 37 | 37 |
| 65+ | 356 | 10.4 | 47 | 4 | 6 | 8 | 13 | 18 | 24 | 36 |
| **GRAND TOTAL** | 528 | 10.6 | 64 | 3 | 6 | 8 | 13 | 20 | 32 | 37 |

Length of Stay by Diagnosis and Operation, United States, 2000

# United States, October 1998–September 1999 Data, by Operation

## 51.1: BILIARY TRACT DXTIC PX. Formerly included in operation group(s) 628, 629, 631.

| Type of Patients | Observed Patients | Avg. Stay | Variance | 10th | 25th | 50th | 75th | 90th | 95th | 99th |
|---|---|---|---|---|---|---|---|---|---|---|
| **1. SINGLE DX** | | | | | | | | | | |
| 0–19 Years | 42 | 3.3 | 9 | 1 | 1 | 2 | 4 | 8 | 11 | 15 |
| 20–34 | 182 | 2.6 | 4 | 1 | 1 | 2 | 3 | 5 | 6 | 11 |
| 35–49 | 187 | 3.2 | 6 | 1 | 2 | 3 | 4 | 7 | 9 | 12 |
| 50–64 | 130 | 3.9 | 4 | 2 | 2 | 4 | 5 | 6 | 8 | 11 |
| 65+ | 84 | 2.7 | 5 | 1 | 1 | 2 | 3 | 5 | 8 | 12 |
| **2. MULTIPLE DX** | | | | | | | | | | |
| 0–19 Years | 115 | 5.7 | 66 | 1 | 2 | 3 | 6 | 12 | 16 | 48 |
| 20–34 | 730 | 4.8 | 16 | 2 | 2 | 3 | 6 | 9 | 12 | 21 |
| 35–49 | 1,639 | 5.5 | 20 | 2 | 3 | 4 | 7 | 10 | 13 | 25 |
| 50–64 | 2,006 | 5.5 | 21 | 2 | 3 | 4 | 7 | 10 | 14 | 27 |
| 65+ | 3,900 | 6.4 | 23 | 2 | 3 | 5 | 8 | 12 | 15 | 25 |
| **TOTAL SINGLE DX** | 625 | 3.2 | 5 | 1 | 2 | 3 | 4 | 6 | 7 | 11 |
| **TOTAL MULTIPLE DX** | 8,390 | 5.9 | 22 | 2 | 3 | 5 | 7 | 11 | 14 | 25 |
| **TOTAL** | | | | | | | | | | |
| 0–19 Years | 157 | 5.2 | 55 | 1 | 2 | 3 | 6 | 12 | 16 | 48 |
| 20–34 | 912 | 4.3 | 14 | 1 | 2 | 3 | 5 | 8 | 10 | 20 |
| 35–49 | 1,826 | 5.3 | 19 | 2 | 3 | 4 | 7 | 10 | 13 | 24 |
| 50–64 | 2,136 | 5.4 | 20 | 2 | 3 | 4 | 7 | 10 | 14 | 26 |
| 65+ | 3,984 | 6.4 | 23 | 2 | 3 | 5 | 8 | 12 | 15 | 25 |
| **GRAND TOTAL** | 9,015 | 5.7 | 22 | 2 | 3 | 4 | 7 | 11 | 14 | 25 |

## 51.14: CLSD BD/SPHINCT ODDI BX. Formerly included in operation group(s) 628.

| Type of Patients | Observed Patients | Avg. Stay | Variance | 10th | 25th | 50th | 75th | 90th | 95th | 99th |
|---|---|---|---|---|---|---|---|---|---|---|
| **1. SINGLE DX** | | | | | | | | | | |
| 0–19 Years | 0 | | | | | | | | | |
| 20–34 | 1 | 5.0 | 0 | 5 | 5 | 5 | 5 | 5 | 5 | 5 |
| 35–49 | 1 | 1.0 | 0 | 1 | 1 | 1 | 1 | 1 | 1 | 1 |
| 50–64 | 5 | 3.7 | 2 | 2 | 2 | 5 | 5 | 5 | 5 | 5 |
| 65+ | 4 | 4.0 | 8 | 1 | 2 | 4 | 4 | 9 | 9 | 9 |
| **2. MULTIPLE DX** | | | | | | | | | | |
| 0–19 Years | 0 | | | | | | | | | |
| 20–34 | 7 | 6.8 | 107 | 1 | 1 | 5 | 6 | 32 | 32 | 32 |
| 35–49 | 30 | 5.8 | 38 | 1 | 1 | 4 | 7 | 18 | 19 | 21 |
| 50–64 | 79 | 5.5 | 15 | 2 | 2 | 3 | 10 | 10 | 10 | 19 |
| 65+ | 253 | 5.4 | 13 | 2 | 3 | 4 | 7 | 10 | 13 | 16 |
| **TOTAL SINGLE DX** | 11 | 3.6 | 5 | 1 | 2 | 4 | 5 | 5 | 9 | 9 |
| **TOTAL MULTIPLE DX** | 369 | 5.5 | 16 | 2 | 3 | 4 | 8 | 10 | 13 | 19 |
| **TOTAL** | | | | | | | | | | |
| 0–19 Years | 0 | | | | | | | | | |
| 20–34 | 8 | 6.6 | 97 | 1 | 1 | 5 | 6 | 32 | 32 | 32 |
| 35–49 | 31 | 5.7 | 38 | 1 | 1 | 4 | 7 | 18 | 19 | 21 |
| 50–64 | 84 | 5.4 | 15 | 2 | 2 | 3 | 10 | 10 | 10 | 19 |
| 65+ | 257 | 5.4 | 13 | 2 | 3 | 4 | 7 | 10 | 13 | 16 |
| **GRAND TOTAL** | 380 | 5.4 | 16 | 2 | 3 | 4 | 8 | 10 | 13 | 19 |

## 51.10: ERCP. Formerly included in operation group(s) 628.

| Type of Patients | Observed Patients | Avg. Stay | Variance | 10th | 25th | 50th | 75th | 90th | 95th | 99th |
|---|---|---|---|---|---|---|---|---|---|---|
| **1. SINGLE DX** | | | | | | | | | | |
| 0–19 Years | 39 | 3.3 | 9 | 1 | 1 | 2 | 4 | 8 | 11 | 15 |
| 20–34 | 175 | 2.6 | 4 | 1 | 1 | 2 | 3 | 5 | 6 | 11 |
| 35–49 | 179 | 3.2 | 6 | 1 | 2 | 3 | 4 | 7 | 8 | 11 |
| 50–64 | 122 | 4.0 | 4 | 1 | 2 | 4 | 5 | 6 | 8 | 11 |
| 65+ | 75 | 2.6 | 5 | 1 | 1 | 2 | 3 | 5 | 8 | 12 |
| **2. MULTIPLE DX** | | | | | | | | | | |
| 0–19 Years | 114 | 5.7 | 66 | 1 | 2 | 3 | 6 | 12 | 16 | 48 |
| 20–34 | 696 | 4.8 | 16 | 2 | 2 | 4 | 6 | 9 | 12 | 21 |
| 35–49 | 1,556 | 5.5 | 20 | 2 | 3 | 4 | 7 | 10 | 13 | 25 |
| 50–64 | 1,868 | 5.5 | 21 | 2 | 3 | 4 | 7 | 10 | 14 | 27 |
| 65+ | 3,515 | 6.5 | 24 | 2 | 3 | 5 | 8 | 12 | 15 | 27 |
| **TOTAL SINGLE DX** | 590 | 3.2 | 5 | 1 | 2 | 2 | 4 | 6 | 7 | 11 |
| **TOTAL MULTIPLE DX** | 7,749 | 5.9 | 23 | 2 | 3 | 5 | 7 | 11 | 14 | 25 |
| **TOTAL** | | | | | | | | | | |
| 0–19 Years | 153 | 5.2 | 55 | 1 | 2 | 3 | 6 | 12 | 16 | 48 |
| 20–34 | 871 | 4.3 | 14 | 1 | 2 | 3 | 5 | 8 | 10 | 20 |
| 35–49 | 1,735 | 5.3 | 19 | 2 | 3 | 4 | 7 | 10 | 13 | 24 |
| 50–64 | 1,990 | 5.4 | 20 | 2 | 3 | 4 | 6 | 10 | 14 | 27 |
| 65+ | 3,590 | 6.4 | 23 | 2 | 3 | 5 | 8 | 12 | 15 | 26 |
| **GRAND TOTAL** | 8,339 | 5.7 | 22 | 2 | 3 | 4 | 7 | 11 | 14 | 25 |

## 51.2: CHOLECYSTECTOMY. Formerly included in operation group(s) 625, 626.

| Type of Patients | Observed Patients | Avg. Stay | Variance | 10th | 25th | 50th | 75th | 90th | 95th | 99th |
|---|---|---|---|---|---|---|---|---|---|---|
| **1. SINGLE DX** | | | | | | | | | | |
| 0–19 Years | 999 | 2.1 | 2 | 1 | 1 | 2 | 2 | 4 | 4 | 9 |
| 20–34 | 6,595 | 2.1 | 2 | 1 | 1 | 2 | 3 | 4 | 4 | 7 |
| 35–49 | 5,714 | 1.9 | 2 | 1 | 1 | 2 | 2 | 3 | 5 | 6 |
| 50–64 | 3,082 | 2.0 | 2 | 1 | 1 | 2 | 3 | 4 | 6 | 7 |
| 65+ | 1,630 | 2.1 | 3 | 1 | 1 | 2 | 3 | 4 | 6 | 9 |
| **2. MULTIPLE DX** | | | | | | | | | | |
| 0–19 Years | 1,745 | 3.8 | 13 | 1 | 2 | 3 | 5 | 7 | 9 | 16 |
| 20–34 | 13,176 | 3.5 | 10 | 1 | 2 | 3 | 4 | 6 | 8 | 16 |
| 35–49 | 19,408 | 3.7 | 13 | 1 | 2 | 3 | 5 | 7 | 10 | 18 |
| 50–64 | 22,056 | 4.2 | 15 | 1 | 3 | 3 | 5 | 8 | 10 | 18 |
| 65+ | 34,470 | 6.1 | 31 | 1 | 3 | 5 | 8 | 12 | 16 | 28 |
| **TOTAL SINGLE DX** | 18,020 | 2.0 | 2 | 1 | 1 | 2 | 3 | 4 | 5 | 7 |
| **TOTAL MULTIPLE DX** | 90,855 | 4.6 | 21 | 1 | 2 | 3 | 6 | 9 | 12 | 22 |
| **TOTAL** | | | | | | | | | | |
| 0–19 Years | 2,744 | 3.1 | 10 | 1 | 1 | 3 | 4 | 6 | 8 | 14 |
| 20–34 | 19,771 | 3.0 | 8 | 1 | 1 | 3 | 4 | 6 | 7 | 13 |
| 35–49 | 25,122 | 3.2 | 10 | 1 | 2 | 3 | 4 | 6 | 8 | 16 |
| 50–64 | 25,138 | 3.9 | 14 | 1 | 2 | 3 | 5 | 8 | 10 | 18 |
| 65+ | 36,100 | 5.9 | 31 | 1 | 2 | 5 | 8 | 12 | 16 | 28 |
| **GRAND TOTAL** | 108,875 | 4.1 | 18 | 1 | 2 | 3 | 5 | 8 | 11 | 20 |

Length of Stay by Diagnosis and Operation, United States, 2000

## United States, October 1998–September 1999 Data, by Operation

### 51.22: CHOLECYSTECTOMY NOS. Formerly included in operation group(s) 625.

| Type of Patients | Observed Patients | Avg. Stay | Vari-ance | Percentiles | | | | | | |
|---|---|---|---|---|---|---|---|---|---|---|
| | | | | 10th | 25th | 50th | 75th | 90th | 95th | 99th |
| **1. SINGLE DX** | | | | | | | | | | |
| 0–19 Years | 43 | 3.7 | 4 | 2 | 2 | 3 | 5 | 7 | 8 | 10 |
| 20–34 | 297 | 3.8 | 4 | 2 | 3 | 3 | 5 | 7 | 8 | 11 |
| 35–49 | 343 | 3.7 | 4 | 1 | 2 | 3 | 5 | 6 | 7 | 12 |
| 50–64 | 217 | 3.7 | 5 | 2 | 3 | 3 | 5 | 6 | 7 | 11 |
| 65+ | 149 | 4.5 | 6 | 2 | 3 | 4 | 6 | 8 | 9 | 10 |
| **2. MULTIPLE DX** | | | | | | | | | | |
| 0–19 Years | 239 | 5.9 | 28 | 2 | 3 | 5 | 7 | 9 | 12 | 22 |
| 20–34 | 1,813 | 5.4 | 21 | 2 | 3 | 4 | 6 | 9 | 12 | 27 |
| 35–49 | 3,742 | 5.8 | 24 | 2 | 3 | 5 | 7 | 10 | 13 | 24 |
| 50–64 | 5,183 | 6.2 | 24 | 2 | 3 | 5 | 8 | 11 | 14 | 26 |
| 65+ | 9,300 | 8.6 | 42 | 3 | 5 | 7 | 10 | 16 | 20 | 33 |
| **TOTAL SINGLE DX** | 1,049 | 3.8 | 5 | 2 | 2 | 3 | 5 | 7 | 8 | 11 |
| **TOTAL MULTIPLE DX** | 20,277 | 7.2 | 34 | 3 | 4 | 6 | 9 | 13 | 17 | 30 |
| **TOTAL** | | | | | | | | | | |
| 0–19 Years | 282 | 5.6 | 25 | 2 | 3 | 5 | 7 | 8 | 11 | 22 |
| 20–34 | 2,110 | 5.2 | 19 | 2 | 3 | 4 | 6 | 9 | 12 | 25 |
| 35–49 | 4,085 | 5.6 | 23 | 2 | 3 | 5 | 7 | 10 | 13 | 23 |
| 50–64 | 5,400 | 6.1 | 24 | 2 | 3 | 5 | 8 | 11 | 13 | 26 |
| 65+ | 9,449 | 8.6 | 42 | 3 | 5 | 7 | 10 | 15 | 20 | 33 |
| **GRAND TOTAL** | 21,326 | 7.0 | 33 | 2 | 4 | 6 | 8 | 13 | 17 | 29 |

### 51.3: BILIARY TRACT ANAST. Formerly included in operation group(s) 629.

| Type of Patients | Observed Patients | Avg. Stay | Vari-ance | Percentiles | | | | | | |
|---|---|---|---|---|---|---|---|---|---|---|
| | | | | 10th | 25th | 50th | 75th | 90th | 95th | 99th |
| **1. SINGLE DX** | | | | | | | | | | |
| 0–19 Years | 34 | 7.2 | 6 | 5 | 5 | 6 | 9 | 11 | 12 | 12 |
| 20–34 | 7 | 8.6 | 69 | 2 | 5 | 6 | 8 | 29 | 29 | 29 |
| 35–49 | 14 | 5.3 | 4 | 3 | 3 | 6 | 7 | 7 | 8 | 9 |
| 50–64 | 9 | 7.3 | 2 | 5 | 7 | 8 | 8 | 8 | 8 | 10 |
| 65+ | 9 | 10.8 | 21 | 6 | 10 | 10 | 17 | 17 | 17 | 17 |
| **2. MULTIPLE DX** | | | | | | | | | | |
| 0–19 Years | 94 | 18.9 | 310 | 5 | 8 | 11 | 17 | 53 | 53 | 53 |
| 20–34 | 73 | 8.6 | 38 | 3 | 5 | 7 | 10 | 15 | 17 | 39 |
| 35–49 | 188 | 11.1 | 54 | 5 | 7 | 8 | 14 | 20 | 27 | 36 |
| 50–64 | 434 | 10.7 | 36 | 6 | 7 | 9 | 12 | 18 | 24 | 31 |
| 65+ | 881 | 12.9 | 64 | 6 | 7 | 11 | 16 | 22 | 26 | 43 |
| **TOTAL SINGLE DX** | 73 | 7.4 | 13 | 3 | 5 | 7 | 8 | 11 | 17 | 17 |
| **TOTAL MULTIPLE DX** | 1,670 | 12.4 | 78 | 5 | 7 | 10 | 15 | 22 | 28 | 53 |
| **TOTAL** | | | | | | | | | | |
| 0–19 Years | 128 | 17.0 | 280 | 5 | 7 | 10 | 14 | 53 | 53 | 53 |
| 20–34 | 80 | 8.6 | 39 | 3 | 5 | 7 | 10 | 15 | 19 | 39 |
| 35–49 | 202 | 10.6 | 53 | 4 | 6 | 8 | 13 | 19 | 27 | 36 |
| 50–64 | 443 | 10.6 | 35 | 6 | 7 | 9 | 12 | 18 | 24 | 31 |
| 65+ | 890 | 12.9 | 63 | 6 | 7 | 11 | 16 | 22 | 26 | 43 |
| **GRAND TOTAL** | 1,743 | 12.3 | 76 | 5 | 7 | 10 | 15 | 22 | 27 | 53 |

### 51.23: LAPSCP CHOLECYSTECTOMY. Formerly included in operation group(s) 626.

| Type of Patients | Observed Patients | Avg. Stay | Vari-ance | Percentiles | | | | | | |
|---|---|---|---|---|---|---|---|---|---|---|
| | | | | 10th | 25th | 50th | 75th | 90th | 95th | 99th |
| **1. SINGLE DX** | | | | | | | | | | |
| 0–19 Years | 955 | 2.0 | 2 | 1 | 1 | 2 | 2 | 4 | 4 | 8 |
| 20–34 | 6,291 | 2.0 | 1 | 1 | 1 | 2 | 2 | 3 | 4 | 6 |
| 35–49 | 5,368 | 1.8 | 1 | 1 | 1 | 2 | 2 | 3 | 4 | 6 |
| 50–64 | 2,861 | 1.9 | 2 | 1 | 1 | 2 | 2 | 4 | 4 | 6 |
| 65+ | 1,478 | 1.9 | 2 | 1 | 1 | 2 | 2 | 4 | 5 | 7 |
| **2. MULTIPLE DX** | | | | | | | | | | |
| 0–19 Years | 1,503 | 3.5 | 10 | 1 | 2 | 3 | 4 | 6 | 8 | 14 |
| 20–34 | 11,350 | 3.2 | 8 | 1 | 2 | 2 | 4 | 6 | 8 | 14 |
| 35–49 | 15,641 | 3.2 | 9 | 1 | 2 | 3 | 4 | 6 | 8 | 14 |
| 50–64 | 16,839 | 3.6 | 11 | 1 | 2 | 3 | 5 | 7 | 9 | 16 |
| 65+ | 25,110 | 5.1 | 23 | 1 | 2 | 4 | 7 | 10 | 13 | 23 |
| **TOTAL SINGLE DX** | 16,953 | 1.9 | 2 | 1 | 1 | 2 | 2 | 3 | 4 | 6 |
| **TOTAL MULTIPLE DX** | 70,443 | 3.9 | 14 | 1 | 2 | 3 | 5 | 8 | 10 | 18 |
| **TOTAL** | | | | | | | | | | |
| 0–19 Years | 2,458 | 2.9 | 7 | 1 | 1 | 2 | 4 | 5 | 7 | 12 |
| 20–34 | 17,641 | 2.8 | 6 | 1 | 1 | 2 | 3 | 5 | 7 | 11 |
| 35–49 | 21,009 | 2.8 | 7 | 1 | 1 | 2 | 4 | 5 | 7 | 13 |
| 50–64 | 19,700 | 3.3 | 10 | 1 | 2 | 3 | 4 | 7 | 9 | 15 |
| 65+ | 26,588 | 4.9 | 22 | 1 | 2 | 4 | 6 | 10 | 13 | 23 |
| **GRAND TOTAL** | 87,396 | 3.5 | 12 | 1 | 2 | 2 | 4 | 7 | 9 | 17 |

### 51.32: GB-TO-INTESTINE ANAST. Formerly included in operation group(s) 629.

| Type of Patients | Observed Patients | Avg. Stay | Vari-ance | Percentiles | | | | | | |
|---|---|---|---|---|---|---|---|---|---|---|
| | | | | 10th | 25th | 50th | 75th | 90th | 95th | 99th |
| **1. SINGLE DX** | | | | | | | | | | |
| 0–19 Years | 5 | 8.3 | 11 | 5 | 6 | 6 | 12 | 12 | 12 | 12 |
| 20–34 | 2 | 5.5 | <1 | 5 | 5 | 5 | 6 | 6 | 6 | 6 |
| 35–49 | 0 | | | | | | | | | |
| 50–64 | 3 | 7.5 | 1 | 7 | 7 | 7 | 7 | 10 | 10 | 10 |
| 65+ | 3 | 7.7 | <1 | 6 | 8 | 8 | 8 | 8 | 8 | 8 |
| **2. MULTIPLE DX** | | | | | | | | | | |
| 0–19 Years | 10 | 8.9 | 7 | 6 | 7 | 8 | 12 | 12 | 12 | 12 |
| 20–34 | 6 | 8.6 | 3 | 7 | 8 | 8 | 10 | 11 | 11 | 11 |
| 35–49 | 39 | 15.1 | 139 | 4 | 6 | 10 | 24 | 36 | 44 | 44 |
| 50–64 | 111 | 10.8 | 40 | 5 | 6 | 9 | 14 | 21 | 26 | 30 |
| 65+ | 207 | 14.5 | 108 | 6 | 8 | 12 | 19 | 24 | 30 | 49 |
| **TOTAL SINGLE DX** | 13 | 7.6 | 4 | 5 | 6 | 7 | 8 | 12 | 12 | 12 |
| **TOTAL MULTIPLE DX** | 373 | 13.2 | 89 | 5 | 7 | 11 | 17 | 23 | 29 | 44 |
| **TOTAL** | | | | | | | | | | |
| 0–19 Years | 15 | 8.8 | 7 | 5 | 7 | 8 | 12 | 12 | 12 | 12 |
| 20–34 | 8 | 8.1 | 4 | 5 | 7 | 8 | 10 | 10 | 11 | 11 |
| 35–49 | 39 | 15.1 | 139 | 4 | 6 | 10 | 24 | 36 | 44 | 44 |
| 50–64 | 114 | 10.7 | 40 | 5 | 6 | 10 | 13 | 20 | 26 | 30 |
| 65+ | 210 | 14.4 | 107 | 6 | 8 | 12 | 18 | 24 | 30 | 49 |
| **GRAND TOTAL** | 386 | 13.0 | 87 | 5 | 7 | 10 | 17 | 23 | 29 | 44 |

Length of Stay by Diagnosis and Operation, United States, 2000

# United States, October 1998–September 1999 Data, by Operation

## 51.36: CHOLEDOCHOENTEROSTOMY. Formerly included in operation group(s) 629.

| Type of Patients | Observed Patients | Avg. Stay | Variance | 10th | 25th | 50th | 75th | 90th | 95th | 99th |
|---|---|---|---|---|---|---|---|---|---|---|
| **1. SINGLE DX** | | | | | | | | | | |
| 0–19 Years | 0 | | | | | | | | | |
| 20–34 | 0 | | | | | | | | | |
| 35–49 | 10 | 5.0 | 3 | 3 | 3 | 6 | 7 | 7 | 7 | 8 |
| 50–64 | 4 | 5.4 | 2 | 4 | 4 | 5 | 6 | 7 | 7 | 7 |
| 65+ | 6 | 12.1 | 24 | 6 | 6 | 10 | 17 | 17 | 17 | 17 |
| **2. MULTIPLE DX** | | | | | | | | | | |
| 0–19 Years | 17 | 28.6 | 503 | 4 | 8 | 11 | 53 | 53 | 53 | 53 |
| 20–34 | 38 | 8.9 | 45 | 4 | 5 | 6 | 11 | 15 | 15 | 39 |
| 35–49 | 112 | 10.1 | 33 | 5 | 6 | 8 | 13 | 18 | 21 | 29 |
| 50–64 | 237 | 10.1 | 22 | 6 | 7 | 9 | 12 | 17 | 19 | 25 |
| 65+ | 580 | 12.4 | 51 | 6 | 7 | 11 | 15 | 21 | 24 | 43 |
| **TOTAL SINGLE DX** | 20 | 7.2 | 20 | 3 | 4 | 6 | 7 | 17 | 17 | 17 |
| **TOTAL MULTIPLE DX** | 984 | 12.3 | 80 | 5 | 7 | 10 | 15 | 20 | 26 | 53 |
| **TOTAL** | | | | | | | | | | |
| 0–19 Years | 17 | 28.6 | 503 | 4 | 8 | 11 | 53 | 53 | 53 | 53 |
| 20–34 | 38 | 8.9 | 45 | 4 | 5 | 6 | 11 | 15 | 15 | 39 |
| 35–49 | 122 | 9.6 | 33 | 4 | 6 | 8 | 12 | 18 | 20 | 29 |
| 50–64 | 241 | 10.1 | 22 | 6 | 7 | 9 | 12 | 17 | 19 | 25 |
| 65+ | 586 | 12.4 | 50 | 6 | 7 | 11 | 15 | 21 | 24 | 43 |
| **GRAND TOTAL** | 1,004 | 12.2 | 79 | 5 | 7 | 10 | 15 | 20 | 26 | 53 |

## 51.4: INC BILE DUCT OBSTR. Formerly included in operation group(s) 629.

| Type of Patients | Observed Patients | Avg. Stay | Variance | 10th | 25th | 50th | 75th | 90th | 95th | 99th |
|---|---|---|---|---|---|---|---|---|---|---|
| **1. SINGLE DX** | | | | | | | | | | |
| 0–19 Years | 2 | 3.8 | 2 | 3 | 3 | 3 | 6 | 6 | 6 | 6 |
| 20–34 | 12 | 5.7 | 11 | 2 | 4 | 4 | 7 | 12 | 12 | 14 |
| 35–49 | 6 | 5.4 | 4 | 3 | 5 | 5 | 6 | 9 | 9 | 9 |
| 50–64 | 2 | 5.8 | 19 | 2 | 2 | 2 | 10 | 10 | 10 | 10 |
| 65+ | 7 | 3.9 | 2 | 2 | 3 | 4 | 5 | 6 | 6 | 6 |
| **2. MULTIPLE DX** | | | | | | | | | | |
| 0–19 Years | 12 | 17.6 | 238 | 2 | 8 | 17 | 17 | 47 | 47 | 47 |
| 20–34 | 35 | 7.8 | 20 | 4 | 4 | 6 | 12 | 14 | 14 | 23 |
| 35–49 | 72 | 7.5 | 51 | 3 | 5 | 6 | 7 | 12 | 18 | 42 |
| 50–64 | 92 | 9.0 | 37 | 4 | 5 | 7 | 10 | 17 | 23 | 30 |
| 65+ | 251 | 10.5 | 53 | 4 | 6 | 9 | 12 | 20 | 25 | 38 |
| **TOTAL SINGLE DX** | 29 | 5.1 | 7 | 2 | 3 | 4 | 6 | 9 | 10 | 14 |
| **TOTAL MULTIPLE DX** | 462 | 9.4 | 56 | 4 | 5 | 7 | 12 | 18 | 25 | 42 |
| **TOTAL** | | | | | | | | | | |
| 0–19 Years | 14 | 16.3 | 232 | 2 | 6 | 8 | 17 | 47 | 47 | 47 |
| 20–34 | 47 | 7.2 | 18 | 4 | 4 | 6 | 9 | 14 | 14 | 23 |
| 35–49 | 78 | 7.5 | 50 | 3 | 5 | 6 | 7 | 12 | 18 | 42 |
| 50–64 | 94 | 8.9 | 37 | 4 | 5 | 7 | 10 | 17 | 23 | 30 |
| 65+ | 258 | 10.3 | 52 | 4 | 6 | 9 | 12 | 20 | 25 | 38 |
| **GRAND TOTAL** | 491 | 9.2 | 55 | 3 | 5 | 7 | 11 | 17 | 25 | 42 |

## 51.5: OTHER BILE DUCT INCISION. Formerly included in operation group(s) 629.

| Type of Patients | Observed Patients | Avg. Stay | Variance | 10th | 25th | 50th | 75th | 90th | 95th | 99th |
|---|---|---|---|---|---|---|---|---|---|---|
| **1. SINGLE DX** | | | | | | | | | | |
| 0–19 Years | 2 | 7.6 | 33 | 1 | 1 | 11 | 11 | 11 | 11 | 11 |
| 20–34 | 8 | 7.5 | 101 | 2 | 2 | 4 | 7 | 30 | 30 | 30 |
| 35–49 | 1 | 2.0 | | 2 | 2 | 2 | 2 | 2 | 2 | 2 |
| 50–64 | 4 | 6.1 | 13 | 1 | 5 | 5 | 11 | 11 | 11 | 11 |
| 65+ | 2 | 4.9 | 6 | 3 | 3 | 3 | 7 | 7 | 7 | 7 |
| **2. MULTIPLE DX** | | | | | | | | | | |
| 0–19 Years | 7 | 7.8 | 162 | 1 | 3 | 4 | 13 | 13 | 13 | 71 |
| 20–34 | 26 | 5.1 | 11 | 1 | 3 | 5 | 6 | 8 | 11 | 20 |
| 35–49 | 26 | 7.1 | 26 | 3 | 4 | 7 | 8 | 12 | 14 | 31 |
| 50–64 | 46 | 9.0 | 73 | 2 | 4 | 6 | 10 | 22 | 30 | 37 |
| 65+ | 87 | 13.6 | 116 | 3 | 6 | 9 | 23 | 30 | 37 | >99 |
| **TOTAL SINGLE DX** | 17 | 6.7 | 60 | 1 | 2 | 4 | 7 | 11 | 30 | 30 |
| **TOTAL MULTIPLE DX** | 192 | 10.1 | 88 | 2 | 4 | 7 | 12 | 30 | 30 | 71 |
| **TOTAL** | | | | | | | | | | |
| 0–19 Years | 9 | 7.7 | 130 | 1 | 3 | 4 | 11 | 13 | 13 | 71 |
| 20–34 | 34 | 5.5 | 26 | 1 | 3 | 4 | 6 | 8 | 17 | 30 |
| 35–49 | 27 | 7.0 | 26 | 2 | 4 | 7 | 8 | 12 | 14 | 31 |
| 50–64 | 50 | 8.9 | 70 | 2 | 4 | 6 | 10 | 22 | 30 | 37 |
| 65+ | 89 | 13.5 | 115 | 3 | 6 | 9 | 22 | 30 | 37 | >99 |
| **GRAND TOTAL** | 209 | 9.9 | 87 | 2 | 4 | 7 | 12 | 30 | 30 | 42 |

## 51.6: LOC EXC BD & S OF O LES. Formerly included in operation group(s) 628, 629.

| Type of Patients | Observed Patients | Avg. Stay | Variance | 10th | 25th | 50th | 75th | 90th | 95th | 99th |
|---|---|---|---|---|---|---|---|---|---|---|
| **1. SINGLE DX** | | | | | | | | | | |
| 0–19 Years | 14 | 7.5 | 23 | 6 | 6 | 6 | 6 | 8 | 23 | 23 |
| 20–34 | 2 | 5.4 | <1 | 5 | 5 | 5 | 6 | 6 | 6 | 6 |
| 35–49 | 2 | 4.6 | <1 | 4 | 4 | 5 | 5 | 5 | 5 | 5 |
| 50–64 | 0 | | | | | | | | | |
| 65+ | 1 | 9.0 | 0 | 9 | 9 | 9 | 9 | 9 | 9 | 9 |
| **2. MULTIPLE DX** | | | | | | | | | | |
| 0–19 Years | 23 | 9.9 | 38 | 5 | 5 | 8 | 14 | 15 | 17 | 35 |
| 20–34 | 15 | 6.6 | 13 | 3 | 3 | 5 | 10 | 12 | 12 | 14 |
| 35–49 | 26 | 6.5 | 34 | 1 | 1 | 6 | 7 | 12 | 24 | 24 |
| 50–64 | 36 | 10.2 | 116 | 4 | 5 | 6 | 11 | 22 | 49 | 49 |
| 65+ | 67 | 9.7 | 52 | 3 | 6 | 8 | 12 | 19 | 22 | 34 |
| **TOTAL SINGLE DX** | 19 | 7.5 | 19 | 5 | 6 | 6 | 8 | 9 | 23 | 23 |
| **TOTAL MULTIPLE DX** | 167 | 9.2 | 58 | 3 | 5 | 7 | 11 | 18 | 23 | 49 |
| **TOTAL** | | | | | | | | | | |
| 0–19 Years | 37 | 8.8 | 32 | 5 | 6 | 6 | 9 | 14 | 23 | 35 |
| 20–34 | 17 | 6.4 | 11 | 3 | 4 | 5 | 8 | 12 | 12 | 14 |
| 35–49 | 28 | 6.4 | 33 | 1 | 1 | 6 | 7 | 12 | 24 | 24 |
| 50–64 | 36 | 10.2 | 116 | 4 | 5 | 6 | 11 | 22 | 49 | 49 |
| 65+ | 68 | 9.6 | 49 | 3 | 6 | 8 | 12 | 19 | 22 | 34 |
| **GRAND TOTAL** | 186 | 8.9 | 52 | 3 | 5 | 7 | 10 | 17 | 23 | 49 |

# United States, October 1998–September 1999 Data, by Operation

## 51.7: REPAIR OF BILE DUCTS. Formerly included in operation group(s) 629.

| Type of Patients | Observed Patients | Avg. Stay | Variance | Percentiles | | | | | | |
|---|---|---|---|---|---|---|---|---|---|---|
| | | | | 10th | 25th | 50th | 75th | 90th | 95th | 99th |
| **1. SINGLE DX** | | | | | | | | | | |
| 0–19 Years | 4 | 2.9 | 2 | 2 | 2 | 2 | 4 | 6 | 6 | 6 |
| 20–34 | 2 | 3.9 | 1 | 3 | 3 | 3 | 5 | 5 | 5 | 5 |
| 35–49 | 3 | 2.6 | <1 | 2 | 2 | 2 | 3 | 4 | 4 | 4 |
| 50–64 | 1 | 4.0 | 0 | 4 | 4 | 4 | 4 | 4 | 4 | 4 |
| 65+ | 0 | | | | | | | | | |
| **2. MULTIPLE DX** | | | | | | | | | | |
| 0–19 Years | 13 | 10.3 | 50 | 3 | 4 | 9 | 15 | 18 | 26 | 26 |
| 20–34 | 48 | 6.0 | 18 | 3 | 3 | 5 | 7 | 11 | 16 | 18 |
| 35–49 | 56 | 7.4 | 44 | 4 | 4 | 5 | 7 | 11 | 24 | 42 |
| 50–64 | 55 | 9.8 | 97 | 3 | 4 | 7 | 10 | 18 | 30 | 49 |
| 65+ | 56 | 11.5 | 71 | 4 | 7 | 10 | 14 | 18 | 22 | 54 |
| **TOTAL SINGLE DX** | 10 | 3.1 | 2 | 2 | 2 | 3 | 4 | 5 | 6 | 6 |
| **TOTAL MULTIPLE DX** | 228 | 8.6 | 60 | 3 | 4 | 7 | 10 | 16 | 24 | 49 |
| **TOTAL** | | | | | | | | | | |
| 0–19 Years | 17 | 8.3 | 48 | 2 | 3 | 6 | 12 | 18 | 26 | 26 |
| 20–34 | 50 | 6.0 | 17 | 3 | 3 | 5 | 7 | 11 | 16 | 18 |
| 35–49 | 59 | 7.3 | 43 | 3 | 4 | 5 | 7 | 11 | 24 | 42 |
| 50–64 | 56 | 9.7 | 96 | 3 | 4 | 7 | 9 | 16 | 30 | 49 |
| 65+ | 56 | 11.5 | 71 | 4 | 7 | 10 | 14 | 18 | 22 | 54 |
| **GRAND TOTAL** | 238 | 8.4 | 59 | 3 | 4 | 6 | 10 | 16 | 23 | 49 |

## 51.8: SPHINCTER OF ODDI OP NEC. Formerly included in operation group(s) 628, 629.

| Type of Patients | Observed Patients | Avg. Stay | Variance | Percentiles | | | | | | |
|---|---|---|---|---|---|---|---|---|---|---|
| | | | | 10th | 25th | 50th | 75th | 90th | 95th | 99th |
| **1. SINGLE DX** | | | | | | | | | | |
| 0–19 Years | 31 | 2.4 | 2 | 1 | 2 | 2 | 3 | 5 | 5 | 7 |
| 20–34 | 285 | 2.6 | 2 | 1 | 2 | 2 | 3 | 4 | 6 | 8 |
| 35–49 | 267 | 2.3 | 2 | 1 | 2 | 2 | 3 | 4 | 5 | 8 |
| 50–64 | 176 | 2.0 | 2 | 1 | 1 | 1 | 3 | 4 | 5 | 7 |
| 65+ | 146 | 2.4 | 3 | 1 | 1 | 2 | 3 | 4 | 5 | 9 |
| **2. MULTIPLE DX** | | | | | | | | | | |
| 0–19 Years | 130 | 4.9 | 24 | 1 | 2 | 4 | 6 | 11 | 16 | 28 |
| 20–34 | 992 | 4.2 | 13 | 1 | 2 | 3 | 5 | 8 | 10 | 17 |
| 35–49 | 1,493 | 4.6 | 18 | 1 | 2 | 4 | 6 | 9 | 11 | 19 |
| 50–64 | 1,936 | 4.7 | 18 | 1 | 2 | 4 | 6 | 9 | 13 | 22 |
| 65+ | 5,145 | 5.9 | 30 | 1 | 3 | 5 | 7 | 11 | 15 | 26 |
| **TOTAL SINGLE DX** | 905 | 2.4 | 2 | 1 | 1 | 2 | 3 | 4 | 5 | 8 |
| **TOTAL MULTIPLE DX** | 9,696 | 5.2 | 24 | 1 | 2 | 4 | 7 | 10 | 14 | 23 |
| **TOTAL** | | | | | | | | | | |
| 0–19 Years | 161 | 4.4 | 20 | 1 | 2 | 3 | 5 | 10 | 16 | 21 |
| 20–34 | 1,277 | 3.8 | 11 | 1 | 2 | 3 | 5 | 7 | 10 | 16 |
| 35–49 | 1,760 | 4.3 | 17 | 1 | 2 | 3 | 5 | 9 | 11 | 17 |
| 50–64 | 2,112 | 4.4 | 17 | 1 | 2 | 4 | 5 | 9 | 13 | 21 |
| 65+ | 5,291 | 5.7 | 29 | 1 | 2 | 4 | 7 | 11 | 15 | 25 |
| **GRAND TOTAL** | 10,601 | 5.0 | 23 | 1 | 2 | 4 | 6 | 10 | 13 | 22 |

## 51.84: ENDO AMPULLA & BD DILAT. Formerly included in operation group(s) 628.

| Type of Patients | Observed Patients | Avg. Stay | Variance | Percentiles | | | | | | |
|---|---|---|---|---|---|---|---|---|---|---|
| | | | | 10th | 25th | 50th | 75th | 90th | 95th | 99th |
| **1. SINGLE DX** | | | | | | | | | | |
| 0–19 Years | 0 | | | | | | | | | |
| 20–34 | 4 | 2.4 | <1 | 2 | 2 | 2 | 3 | 4 | 4 | 4 |
| 35–49 | 8 | 2.0 | 2 | 1 | 1 | 1 | 3 | 4 | 4 | 4 |
| 50–64 | 6 | 1.1 | <1 | 1 | 1 | 1 | 1 | 1 | 3 | 3 |
| 65+ | 2 | 2.6 | <1 | 2 | 2 | 3 | 3 | 3 | 3 | 3 |
| **2. MULTIPLE DX** | | | | | | | | | | |
| 0–19 Years | 4 | 4.2 | 1 | 2 | 2 | 4 | 5 | 5 | 5 | 5 |
| 20–34 | 18 | 2.9 | 5 | 2 | 2 | 2 | 2 | 7 | 8 | 10 |
| 35–49 | 69 | 4.1 | 11 | 1 | 2 | 3 | 5 | 8 | 12 | 15 |
| 50–64 | 89 | 4.8 | 18 | 2 | 3 | 4 | 6 | 10 | 11 | 15 |
| 65+ | 175 | 5.7 | 17 | 2 | 3 | 5 | 7 | 9 | 13 | 24 |
| **TOTAL SINGLE DX** | 20 | 1.8 | 1 | 1 | 1 | 2 | 2 | 3 | 4 | 4 |
| **TOTAL MULTIPLE DX** | 355 | 5.0 | 16 | 2 | 2 | 4 | 6 | 9 | 12 | 22 |
| **TOTAL** | | | | | | | | | | |
| 0–19 Years | 4 | 4.2 | 1 | 2 | 2 | 4 | 5 | 5 | 5 | 5 |
| 20–34 | 22 | 2.8 | 4 | 2 | 2 | 2 | 2 | 6 | 7 | 10 |
| 35–49 | 77 | 3.9 | 11 | 1 | 2 | 3 | 5 | 7 | 12 | 15 |
| 50–64 | 95 | 4.4 | 17 | 2 | 2 | 4 | 5 | 10 | 11 | 15 |
| 65+ | 177 | 5.6 | 17 | 2 | 3 | 5 | 7 | 9 | 13 | 24 |
| **GRAND TOTAL** | 375 | 4.8 | 15 | 1 | 2 | 4 | 6 | 9 | 12 | 22 |

## 51.85: ENDO SPHINCTOT/PAPILLOT. Formerly included in operation group(s) 628.

| Type of Patients | Observed Patients | Avg. Stay | Variance | Percentiles | | | | | | |
|---|---|---|---|---|---|---|---|---|---|---|
| | | | | 10th | 25th | 50th | 75th | 90th | 95th | 99th |
| **1. SINGLE DX** | | | | | | | | | | |
| 0–19 Years | 17 | 2.6 | 2 | 2 | 2 | 2 | 3 | 5 | 7 | 7 |
| 20–34 | 140 | 2.7 | 2 | 1 | 1 | 2 | 4 | 4 | 5 | 7 |
| 35–49 | 143 | 2.4 | 3 | 1 | 2 | 2 | 3 | 5 | 5 | 9 |
| 50–64 | 101 | 2.4 | 2 | 1 | 1 | 2 | 3 | 4 | 5 | 6 |
| 65+ | 65 | 2.1 | 3 | 1 | 1 | 1 | 3 | 4 | 5 | 9 |
| **2. MULTIPLE DX** | | | | | | | | | | |
| 0–19 Years | 67 | 3.6 | 17 | 1 | 2 | 2 | 5 | 7 | 10 | 21 |
| 20–34 | 571 | 4.1 | 14 | 1 | 3 | 3 | 5 | 7 | 9 | 20 |
| 35–49 | 882 | 4.2 | 13 | 1 | 3 | 3 | 6 | 8 | 12 | 15 |
| 50–64 | 1,064 | 4.4 | 16 | 1 | 3 | 3 | 6 | 9 | 12 | 21 |
| 65+ | 2,616 | 5.6 | 21 | 1 | 3 | 5 | 7 | 11 | 14 | 21 |
| **TOTAL SINGLE DX** | 466 | 2.5 | 3 | 1 | 1 | 2 | 3 | 4 | 5 | 8 |
| **TOTAL MULTIPLE DX** | 5,200 | 4.9 | 18 | 1 | 2 | 4 | 6 | 9 | 13 | 21 |
| **TOTAL** | | | | | | | | | | |
| 0–19 Years | 84 | 3.4 | 14 | 1 | 2 | 2 | 4 | 6 | 8 | 21 |
| 20–34 | 711 | 3.8 | 12 | 1 | 3 | 3 | 5 | 7 | 9 | 16 |
| 35–49 | 1,025 | 4.0 | 12 | 1 | 3 | 3 | 6 | 8 | 10 | 15 |
| 50–64 | 1,165 | 4.3 | 16 | 1 | 2 | 3 | 5 | 8 | 11 | 21 |
| 65+ | 2,681 | 5.5 | 21 | 1 | 3 | 5 | 7 | 11 | 14 | 21 |
| **GRAND TOTAL** | 5,666 | 4.7 | 17 | 1 | 2 | 4 | 6 | 9 | 13 | 20 |

Length of Stay by Diagnosis and Operation, United States, 2000

# United States, October 1998–September 1999 Data, by Operation

## 51.87: ENDO INSERT BD STENT. Formerly included in operation group(s) 628.

| Type of Patients | Observed Patients | Avg. Stay | Vari-ance | 10th | 25th | 50th | 75th | 90th | 95th | 99th |
|---|---|---|---|---|---|---|---|---|---|---|
| **1. SINGLE DX** | | | | | | | | | | |
| 0–19 Years | 4 | 1.8 | 1 | 1 | | 1 | 2 | 4 | 4 | 4 |
| 20–34 | 28 | 3.0 | 4 | 1 | 2 | 3 | 3 | 6 | 9 | 9 |
| 35–49 | 32 | 2.2 | 2 | 1 | 2 | 2 | 3 | 3 | 4 | 8 |
| 50–64 | 21 | 2.5 | 2 | 1 | 1 | 2 | 3 | 5 | 5 | 6 |
| 65+ | 26 | 2.5 | 2 | 2 | 2 | 2 | 2 | 4 | 5 | 9 |
| **2. MULTIPLE DX** | | | | | | | | | | |
| 0–19 Years | 24 | 6.3 | 31 | 2 | 3 | 6 | 7 | 14 | 14 | 29 |
| 20–34 | 132 | 6.0 | 17 | 2 | 3 | 5 | 9 | 11 | 11 | 28 |
| 35–49 | 265 | 6.1 | 34 | 2 | 3 | 5 | 8 | 11 | 15 | 28 |
| 50–64 | 407 | 5.6 | 24 | 1 | 3 | 4 | 7 | 13 | 14 | 26 |
| 65+ | 1,146 | 5.9 | 27 | 1 | 2 | 5 | 8 | 12 | 15 | 23 |
| **TOTAL SINGLE DX** | 111 | 2.6 | 3 | 1 | 2 | 2 | 3 | 4 | 6 | 9 |
| **TOTAL MULTIPLE DX** | 1,974 | 5.9 | 27 | 1 | 3 | 5 | 7 | 12 | 15 | 24 |
| **TOTAL** | | | | | | | | | | |
| 0–19 Years | 28 | 5.6 | 29 | 2 | 2 | 4 | 7 | 12 | 14 | 29 |
| 20–34 | 160 | 5.3 | 16 | 2 | 3 | 4 | 7 | 10 | 11 | 17 |
| 35–49 | 297 | 5.5 | 31 | 1 | 2 | 4 | 7 | 10 | 13 | 23 |
| 50–64 | 428 | 5.5 | 23 | 1 | 2 | 4 | 7 | 13 | 14 | 26 |
| 65+ | 1,172 | 5.7 | 26 | 2 | 2 | 4 | 8 | 12 | 15 | 23 |
| **GRAND TOTAL** | 2,085 | 5.6 | 26 | 1 | 2 | 4 | 7 | 11 | 14 | 23 |

## 51.9: OTHER BILIARY TRACT OPS. Formerly included in operation group(s) 627, 629.

| Type of Patients | Observed Patients | Avg. Stay | Vari-ance | 10th | 25th | 50th | 75th | 90th | 95th | 99th |
|---|---|---|---|---|---|---|---|---|---|---|
| **1. SINGLE DX** | | | | | | | | | | |
| 0–19 Years | 1 | 1.0 | 0 | 1 | 1 | 1 | 1 | 1 | 1 | 1 |
| 20–34 | 7 | 2.1 | 4 | 1 | 1 | 1 | 2 | 7 | 7 | 7 |
| 35–49 | 6 | 3.5 | 8 | 1 | 1 | 4 | 6 | 8 | 8 | 8 |
| 50–64 | 7 | 2.9 | 2 | 1 | 2 | 3 | 4 | 4 | 4 | 4 |
| 65+ | 16 | 1.4 | 1 | 1 | 1 | 1 | 1 | 3 | 5 | 6 |
| **2. MULTIPLE DX** | | | | | | | | | | |
| 0–19 Years | 31 | 7.3 | 58 | 1 | 1 | 6 | 10 | 14 | 16 | 38 |
| 20–34 | 40 | 6.3 | 16 | 2 | 3 | 5 | 11 | 11 | 11 | 16 |
| 35–49 | 144 | 6.8 | 64 | 2 | 3 | 4 | 7 | 13 | 23 | 32 |
| 50–64 | 275 | 8.0 | 43 | 2 | 4 | 6 | 8 | 17 | 22 | 26 |
| 65+ | 550 | 8.2 | 40 | 2 | 4 | 7 | 11 | 15 | 21 | 30 |
| **TOTAL SINGLE DX** | 37 | 2.0 | 3 | 1 | 1 | 1 | 2 | 5 | 6 | 8 |
| **TOTAL MULTIPLE DX** | 1,040 | 7.9 | 44 | 2 | 3 | 6 | 10 | 16 | 21 | 32 |
| **TOTAL** | | | | | | | | | | |
| 0–19 Years | 32 | 7.2 | 57 | 1 | 1 | 6 | 10 | 14 | 16 | 38 |
| 20–34 | 47 | 5.4 | 16 | 1 | 2 | 4 | 9 | 11 | 11 | 16 |
| 35–49 | 150 | 6.7 | 63 | 1 | 3 | 4 | 7 | 12 | 23 | 32 |
| 50–64 | 282 | 8.0 | 43 | 2 | 4 | 6 | 8 | 17 | 22 | 26 |
| 65+ | 566 | 7.9 | 40 | 1 | 3 | 7 | 11 | 15 | 21 | 30 |
| **GRAND TOTAL** | 1,077 | 7.7 | 44 | 1 | 3 | 6 | 10 | 16 | 21 | 32 |

## 51.88: ENDO RMVL BILIARY STONE. Formerly included in operation group(s) 628.

| Type of Patients | Observed Patients | Avg. Stay | Vari-ance | 10th | 25th | 50th | 75th | 90th | 95th | 99th |
|---|---|---|---|---|---|---|---|---|---|---|
| **1. SINGLE DX** | | | | | | | | | | |
| 0–19 Years | 9 | 2.5 | 2 | 1 | 1 | 2 | 3 | 5 | 5 | 5 |
| 20–34 | 101 | 2.1 | 1 | 1 | 1 | 2 | 2 | 3 | 4 | 8 |
| 35–49 | 75 | 2.0 | 1 | 1 | 1 | 2 | 2 | 3 | 4 | 6 |
| 50–64 | 40 | 1.5 | 1 | 1 | 1 | 1 | 1 | 3 | 5 | 7 |
| 65+ | 52 | 2.6 | 3 | 1 | 1 | 2 | 3 | 5 | 5 | 10 |
| **2. MULTIPLE DX** | | | | | | | | | | |
| 0–19 Years | 26 | 4.7 | 13 | 2 | 2 | 4 | 6 | 8 | 16 | 16 |
| 20–34 | 237 | 3.4 | 8 | 1 | 2 | 3 | 4 | 6 | 8 | 12 |
| 35–49 | 228 | 3.7 | 12 | 2 | 2 | 3 | 4 | 8 | 9 | 15 |
| 50–64 | 312 | 4.1 | 14 | 1 | 2 | 3 | 5 | 8 | 10 | 20 |
| 65+ | 1,077 | 5.6 | 27 | 2 | 3 | 4 | 7 | 10 | 14 | 24 |
| **TOTAL SINGLE DX** | 277 | 2.0 | 2 | 1 | 1 | 2 | 2 | 4 | 5 | 7 |
| **TOTAL MULTIPLE DX** | 1,880 | 4.8 | 21 | 1 | 2 | 4 | 6 | 9 | 12 | 20 |
| **TOTAL** | | | | | | | | | | |
| 0–19 Years | 35 | 4.2 | 11 | 1 | 2 | 3 | 5 | 8 | 11 | 16 |
| 20–34 | 338 | 3.0 | 6 | 1 | 2 | 2 | 4 | 5 | 7 | 9 |
| 35–49 | 303 | 3.3 | 10 | 1 | 2 | 2 | 4 | 6 | 8 | 13 |
| 50–64 | 352 | 3.6 | 13 | 1 | 1 | 3 | 5 | 8 | 9 | 20 |
| 65+ | 1,129 | 5.5 | 27 | 2 | 3 | 4 | 7 | 10 | 14 | 21 |
| **GRAND TOTAL** | 2,157 | 4.4 | 19 | 1 | 2 | 3 | 5 | 8 | 11 | 20 |

## 51.98: PERC OP ON BIL TRACT NEC. Formerly included in operation group(s) 627.

| Type of Patients | Observed Patients | Avg. Stay | Vari-ance | 10th | 25th | 50th | 75th | 90th | 95th | 99th |
|---|---|---|---|---|---|---|---|---|---|---|
| **1. SINGLE DX** | | | | | | | | | | |
| 0–19 Years | 1 | 1.0 | 0 | 1 | 1 | 1 | 1 | 1 | 1 | 1 |
| 20–34 | 5 | 3.9 | 6 | 1 | 2 | 3 | 7 | 7 | 7 | 7 |
| 35–49 | 3 | 3.9 | 15 | 1 | 2 | 1 | 8 | 8 | 8 | 8 |
| 50–64 | 5 | 2.9 | 2 | 1 | 2 | 3 | 4 | 4 | 4 | 4 |
| 65+ | 9 | 2.4 | 4 | 1 | 1 | 1 | 3 | 6 | 6 | 6 |
| **2. MULTIPLE DX** | | | | | | | | | | |
| 0–19 Years | 21 | 5.3 | 72 | 1 | 1 | 1 | 7 | 12 | 32 | 38 |
| 20–34 | 21 | 5.7 | 19 | 2 | 2 | 4 | 7 | 16 | 16 | 16 |
| 35–49 | 102 | 6.7 | 83 | 1 | 3 | 3 | 8 | 12 | 23 | 58 |
| 50–64 | 209 | 7.8 | 41 | 2 | 3 | 6 | 8 | 17 | 21 | 24 |
| 65+ | 395 | 8.2 | 43 | 2 | 3 | 7 | 11 | 15 | 21 | 30 |
| **TOTAL SINGLE DX** | 23 | 3.0 | 5 | 1 | 1 | 2 | 4 | 7 | 7 | 8 |
| **TOTAL MULTIPLE DX** | 748 | 7.8 | 47 | 1 | 3 | 6 | 10 | 16 | 21 | 32 |
| **TOTAL** | | | | | | | | | | |
| 0–19 Years | 22 | 5.2 | 70 | 1 | 1 | 1 | 7 | 12 | 32 | 38 |
| 20–34 | 26 | 5.3 | 17 | 1 | 3 | 4 | 7 | 10 | 16 | 16 |
| 35–49 | 105 | 6.6 | 82 | 1 | 3 | 3 | 8 | 12 | 23 | 58 |
| 50–64 | 214 | 7.7 | 40 | 2 | 3 | 6 | 8 | 17 | 21 | 24 |
| 65+ | 404 | 8.1 | 43 | 2 | 3 | 7 | 11 | 15 | 21 | 30 |
| **GRAND TOTAL** | 771 | 7.7 | 47 | 1 | 3 | 6 | 10 | 16 | 21 | 32 |

Length of Stay by Diagnosis and Operation, United States, 2000

# United States, October 1998–September 1999 Data, by Operation

## 52.0: PANCREATOTOMY. Formerly included in operation group(s) 630.

| Type of Patients | Observed Patients | Avg. Stay | Variance | 10th | 25th | 50th | 75th | 90th | 95th | 99th |
|---|---|---|---|---|---|---|---|---|---|---|
| **1. SINGLE DX** | | | | | | | | | | |
| 0–19 Years | 0 | | | | | | | | | |
| 20–34 | 7 | 4.2 | 5 | 1 | 2 | 6 | 6 | 7 | 7 | 7 |
| 35–49 | 7 | 6.1 | 17 | 1 | 2 | 5 | 10 | 11 | 11 | 11 |
| 50–64 | 6 | 3.2 | 4 | 2 | 2 | 2 | 4 | 6 | 8 | 8 |
| 65+ | 1 | 11.0 | 0 | 11 | 11 | 11 | 11 | 11 | 11 | 11 |
| **2. MULTIPLE DX** | | | | | | | | | | |
| 0–19 Years | 11 | 19.4 | 202 | 6 | 9 | 10 | 33 | 33 | 56 | 56 |
| 20–34 | 57 | 15.6 | 95 | 5 | 9 | 14 | 19 | 26 | 38 | 41 |
| 35–49 | 183 | 16.0 | 167 | 5 | 8 | 11 | 20 | 36 | 43 | 74 |
| 50–64 | 156 | 17.0 | 154 | 5 | 8 | 13 | 25 | 30 | 39 | 57 |
| 65+ | 100 | 12.9 | 90 | 4 | 6 | 11 | 19 | 24 | 32 | >99 |
| **TOTAL SINGLE DX** | 21 | 4.5 | 10 | 2 | 2 | 3 | 6 | 10 | 11 | 11 |
| **TOTAL MULTIPLE DX** | 507 | 15.9 | 144 | 5 | 8 | 13 | 21 | 32 | 39 | 65 |
| **TOTAL** | | | | | | | | | | |
| 0–19 Years | 11 | 19.4 | 202 | 6 | 9 | 10 | 33 | 33 | 56 | 56 |
| 20–34 | 64 | 15.0 | 96 | 5 | 9 | 14 | 19 | 26 | 38 | 41 |
| 35–49 | 190 | 15.8 | 166 | 5 | 7 | 11 | 20 | 36 | 43 | 74 |
| 50–64 | 162 | 16.5 | 155 | 4 | 8 | 13 | 25 | 28 | 37 | 57 |
| 65+ | 101 | 12.8 | 89 | 4 | 6 | 11 | 19 | 24 | 32 | >99 |
| **GRAND TOTAL** | 528 | 15.5 | 144 | 4 | 7 | 12 | 21 | 32 | 39 | 65 |

## 52.01: DRAIN PANC CYST BY CATH. Formerly included in operation group(s) 630.

| Type of Patients | Observed Patients | Avg. Stay | Variance | 10th | 25th | 50th | 75th | 90th | 95th | 99th |
|---|---|---|---|---|---|---|---|---|---|---|
| **1. SINGLE DX** | | | | | | | | | | |
| 0–19 Years | 0 | | | | | | | | | |
| 20–34 | 5 | 3.1 | 5 | 1 | 2 | 3 | 3 | 7 | 7 | 7 |
| 35–49 | 4 | 5.9 | 14 | 1 | 1 | 5 | 10 | 10 | 10 | 10 |
| 50–64 | 6 | 3.2 | 4 | 2 | 2 | 2 | 4 | 6 | 8 | 8 |
| 65+ | 1 | 11.0 | 0 | 11 | 11 | 11 | 11 | 11 | 11 | 11 |
| **2. MULTIPLE DX** | | | | | | | | | | |
| 0–19 Years | 5 | 18.9 | 355 | 6 | 9 | 15 | 15 | 56 | 56 | 56 |
| 20–34 | 42 | 15.6 | 105 | 5 | 9 | 14 | 19 | 27 | 38 | 65 |
| 35–49 | 131 | 13.2 | 119 | 4 | 7 | 9 | 16 | 25 | 36 | 65 |
| 50–64 | 114 | 16.4 | 157 | 4 | 8 | 13 | 23 | 33 | 39 | 55 |
| 65+ | 70 | 12.6 | 76 | 4 | 6 | 11 | 19 | 24 | 32 | >99 |
| **TOTAL SINGLE DX** | 16 | 4.0 | 9 | 2 | 2 | 2 | 6 | 10 | 10 | 11 |
| **TOTAL MULTIPLE DX** | 362 | 14.5 | 126 | 4 | 7 | 12 | 19 | 29 | 38 | 62 |
| **TOTAL** | | | | | | | | | | |
| 0–19 Years | 5 | 18.9 | 355 | 6 | 9 | 15 | 15 | 56 | 56 | 56 |
| 20–34 | 47 | 15.1 | 107 | 5 | 9 | 14 | 17 | 27 | 38 | 41 |
| 35–49 | 135 | 13.1 | 118 | 4 | 6 | 9 | 16 | 25 | 36 | 65 |
| 50–64 | 120 | 15.6 | 157 | 3 | 7 | 13 | 21 | 33 | 39 | 55 |
| 65+ | 71 | 12.6 | 75 | 4 | 6 | 11 | 19 | 24 | 32 | >99 |
| **GRAND TOTAL** | 378 | 14.2 | 125 | 4 | 7 | 11 | 19 | 27 | 37 | 62 |

## 52.1: PANCREATIC DXTIC PX. Formerly included in operation group(s) 628, 630, 631.

| Type of Patients | Observed Patients | Avg. Stay | Variance | 10th | 25th | 50th | 75th | 90th | 95th | 99th |
|---|---|---|---|---|---|---|---|---|---|---|
| **1. SINGLE DX** | | | | | | | | | | |
| 0–19 Years | 1 | 1.0 | 0 | 1 | 1 | 1 | 1 | 1 | 1 | 1 |
| 20–34 | 0 | | | | | | | | | |
| 35–49 | 11 | 3.1 | 2 | 2 | 3 | 3 | 3 | 5 | 6 | 8 |
| 50–64 | 11 | 6.3 | 23 | 2 | 2 | 4 | 12 | 12 | 15 | 15 |
| 65+ | 14 | 3.1 | 7 | 1 | 1 | 2 | 4 | 8 | 9 | 9 |
| **2. MULTIPLE DX** | | | | | | | | | | |
| 0–19 Years | 5 | 6.8 | 56 | 1 | 1 | 1 | 8 | 19 | 19 | 19 |
| 20–34 | 54 | 6.0 | 26 | 2 | 3 | 4 | 7 | 14 | 19 | 23 |
| 35–49 | 158 | 10.1 | 63 | 2 | 4 | 8 | 19 | 20 | 22 | 35 |
| 50–64 | 264 | 7.4 | 57 | 2 | 3 | 5 | 9 | 15 | 18 | 56 |
| 65+ | 616 | 8.3 | 45 | 2 | 4 | 6 | 10 | 18 | 22 | 32 |
| **TOTAL SINGLE DX** | 37 | 4.1 | 12 | 1 | 2 | 3 | 4 | 11 | 12 | 15 |
| **TOTAL MULTIPLE DX** | 1,097 | 8.3 | 51 | 2 | 4 | 6 | 10 | 19 | 21 | 34 |
| **TOTAL** | | | | | | | | | | |
| 0–19 Years | 6 | 6.3 | 54 | 1 | 1 | 1 | 8 | 19 | 19 | 19 |
| 20–34 | 54 | 6.0 | 26 | 2 | 3 | 4 | 7 | 14 | 19 | 23 |
| 35–49 | 169 | 9.6 | 62 | 2 | 4 | 7 | 16 | 19 | 22 | 35 |
| 50–64 | 275 | 7.4 | 55 | 2 | 3 | 5 | 9 | 15 | 18 | 56 |
| 65+ | 630 | 8.2 | 45 | 2 | 4 | 6 | 10 | 18 | 22 | 32 |
| **GRAND TOTAL** | 1,134 | 8.2 | 50 | 2 | 4 | 6 | 10 | 18 | 21 | 33 |

## 52.11: PANC ASP (NEEDLE) BX. Formerly included in operation group(s) 630.

| Type of Patients | Observed Patients | Avg. Stay | Variance | 10th | 25th | 50th | 75th | 90th | 95th | 99th |
|---|---|---|---|---|---|---|---|---|---|---|
| **1. SINGLE DX** | | | | | | | | | | |
| 0–19 Years | 1 | 1.0 | 0 | 1 | 1 | 1 | 1 | 1 | 1 | 1 |
| 20–34 | 0 | | | | | | | | | |
| 35–49 | 6 | 2.9 | 6 | 1 | 2 | 3 | 3 | 6 | 8 | 8 |
| 50–64 | 7 | 5.8 | 23 | 2 | 3 | 4 | 10 | 15 | 15 | 15 |
| 65+ | 9 | 2.7 | 6 | 1 | 1 | 2 | 4 | 8 | 9 | 9 |
| **2. MULTIPLE DX** | | | | | | | | | | |
| 0–19 Years | 2 | 6.6 | 11 | 8 | 8 | 8 | 8 | 8 | 8 | 8 |
| 20–34 | 39 | 5.4 | 25 | 2 | 3 | 4 | 5 | 12 | 21 | 24 |
| 35–49 | 112 | 8.2 | 60 | 2 | 3 | 6 | 10 | 20 | 26 | 35 |
| 50–64 | 174 | 6.6 | 20 | 2 | 3 | 6 | 8 | 15 | 16 | 21 |
| 65+ | 420 | 7.1 | 30 | 2 | 4 | 6 | 9 | 13 | 18 | 29 |
| **TOTAL SINGLE DX** | 23 | 3.6 | 12 | 1 | 1 | 3 | 4 | 8 | 11 | 15 |
| **TOTAL MULTIPLE DX** | 747 | 7.1 | 32 | 2 | 3 | 6 | 9 | 14 | 18 | 29 |
| **TOTAL** | | | | | | | | | | |
| 0–19 Years | 3 | 5.3 | 15 | 1 | 1 | 1 | 8 | 8 | 8 | 8 |
| 20–34 | 39 | 5.4 | 25 | 2 | 3 | 5 | 5 | 12 | 21 | 24 |
| 35–49 | 118 | 8.0 | 59 | 1 | 3 | 6 | 10 | 20 | 26 | 35 |
| 50–64 | 181 | 6.6 | 20 | 2 | 3 | 6 | 8 | 15 | 16 | 21 |
| 65+ | 429 | 7.0 | 30 | 2 | 4 | 6 | 9 | 13 | 18 | 29 |
| **GRAND TOTAL** | 770 | 6.9 | 32 | 2 | 3 | 5 | 9 | 14 | 18 | 29 |

Length of Stay by Diagnosis and Operation, United States, 2000

# United States, October 1998–September 1999 Data, by Operation

## 52.2: PANC/PANC DUCT LES DESTR. Formerly included in operation group(s) 628, 630.

| Type of Patients | Observed Patients | Avg. Stay | Vari-ance | Percentiles | | | | | | |
|---|---|---|---|---|---|---|---|---|---|---|
| | | | | 10th | 25th | 50th | 75th | 90th | 95th | 99th |
| **1. SINGLE DX** | | | | | | | | | | |
| 0–19 Years | 2 | 9.6 | 2 | 10 | 10 | 10 | 10 | 10 | 10 | 10 |
| 20–34 | 7 | 5.1 | 5 | 3 | 3 | 5 | 8 | 8 | 8 | 8 |
| 35–49 | 3 | 6.7 | 1 | 6 | 6 | 6 | 7 | 9 | 9 | 9 |
| 50–64 | 3 | 8.6 | 1 | 8 | 9 | 9 | 9 | 9 | 9 | 9 |
| 65+ | 1 | 6.0 | 0 | 6 | 6 | 6 | 6 | 6 | 6 | 6 |
| **2. MULTIPLE DX** | | | | | | | | | | |
| 0–19 Years | 8 | 9.0 | 32 | 4 | 6 | 6 | 12 | 17 | 23 | 23 |
| 20–34 | 36 | 19.8 | 268 | 5 | 8 | 14 | 32 | 47 | 55 | 61 |
| 35–49 | 72 | 24.1 | 448 | 5 | 8 | 17 | 30 | 61 | 72 | >99 |
| 50–64 | 87 | 18.6 | 217 | 5 | 6 | 14 | 28 | 44 | 51 | 69 |
| 65+ | 61 | 23.0 | 480 | 7 | 8 | 12 | 35 | 65 | 80 | >99 |
| **TOTAL SINGLE DX** | 16 | 7.5 | 6 | 3 | 5 | 9 | 9 | 10 | 10 | 10 |
| **TOTAL MULTIPLE DX** | 264 | 21.1 | 351 | 5 | 8 | 14 | 29 | 54 | 68 | >99 |
| **TOTAL** | | | | | | | | | | |
| 0–19 Years | 10 | 9.3 | 19 | 6 | 6 | 10 | 10 | 17 | 17 | 23 |
| 20–34 | 43 | 17.7 | 257 | 3 | 5 | 11 | 26 | 38 | 55 | 61 |
| 35–49 | 75 | 23.6 | 444 | 5 | 8 | 16 | 29 | 60 | 72 | >99 |
| 50–64 | 90 | 17.9 | 209 | 5 | 8 | 13 | 24 | 42 | 48 | 64 |
| 65+ | 62 | 22.8 | 478 | 7 | 8 | 12 | 35 | 65 | 80 | >99 |
| **GRAND TOTAL** | 280 | 20.1 | 338 | 5 | 8 | 12 | 28 | 52 | 63 | >99 |

## 52.3: PANCREATIC CYST MARSUP. Formerly included in operation group(s) 630.

| Type of Patients | Observed Patients | Avg. Stay | Vari-ance | Percentiles | | | | | | |
|---|---|---|---|---|---|---|---|---|---|---|
| | | | | 10th | 25th | 50th | 75th | 90th | 95th | 99th |
| **1. SINGLE DX** | | | | | | | | | | |
| 0–19 Years | 0 | | | | | | | | | |
| 20–34 | 0 | | | | | | | | | |
| 35–49 | 0 | | | | | | | | | |
| 50–64 | 0 | | | | | | | | | |
| 65+ | 1 | 2.0 | 0 | 2 | 2 | 2 | 2 | 2 | 2 | 2 |
| **2. MULTIPLE DX** | | | | | | | | | | |
| 0–19 Years | 1 | 6.0 | 0 | 6 | 6 | 6 | 6 | 6 | 6 | 6 |
| 20–34 | 11 | 18.3 | 420 | 2 | 2 | 12 | 19 | 54 | 66 | 66 |
| 35–49 | 12 | 16.3 | 162 | 6 | 7 | 14 | 16 | 35 | 49 | 49 |
| 50–64 | 8 | 17.8 | 189 | 4 | 9 | 9 | 36 | 42 | 42 | >99 |
| 65+ | 9 | 13.0 | 280 | 7 | 8 | 10 | 10 | 11 | 82 | 82 |
| **TOTAL SINGLE DX** | 1 | 2.0 | 0 | 2 | 2 | 2 | 2 | 2 | 2 | 2 |
| **TOTAL MULTIPLE DX** | 41 | 15.9 | 273 | 4 | 7 | 10 | 15 | 42 | 54 | 82 |
| **TOTAL** | | | | | | | | | | |
| 0–19 Years | 1 | 6.0 | 0 | 6 | 6 | 6 | 6 | 6 | 6 | 6 |
| 20–34 | 11 | 18.3 | 420 | 2 | 2 | 12 | 19 | 54 | 66 | 66 |
| 35–49 | 12 | 16.3 | 162 | 6 | 7 | 14 | 16 | 35 | 49 | 49 |
| 50–64 | 8 | 17.8 | 189 | 4 | 9 | 9 | 36 | 42 | 42 | >99 |
| 65+ | 10 | 12.6 | 275 | 7 | 8 | 10 | 10 | 11 | 82 | 82 |
| **GRAND TOTAL** | 42 | 15.7 | 272 | 4 | 7 | 10 | 15 | 42 | 54 | 82 |

## 52.4: INT DRAIN PANC CYST. Formerly included in operation group(s) 630.

| Type of Patients | Observed Patients | Avg. Stay | Vari-ance | Percentiles | | | | | | |
|---|---|---|---|---|---|---|---|---|---|---|
| | | | | 10th | 25th | 50th | 75th | 90th | 95th | 99th |
| **1. SINGLE DX** | | | | | | | | | | |
| 0–19 Years | 0 | | | | | | | | | |
| 20–34 | 1 | 5.0 | 0 | 5 | 5 | 5 | 5 | 5 | 5 | 5 |
| 35–49 | 3 | 10.2 | <1 | 9 | 9 | 11 | 11 | 11 | 11 | 11 |
| 50–64 | 2 | 5.6 | <1 | 5 | 5 | 6 | 6 | 6 | 6 | 6 |
| 65+ | 0 | | | | | | | | | |
| **2. MULTIPLE DX** | | | | | | | | | | |
| 0–19 Years | 3 | 5.8 | 2 | 4 | 6 | 6 | 7 | 7 | 7 | 7 |
| 20–34 | 20 | 18.1 | 289 | 5 | 7 | 10 | 31 | 43 | 60 | 60 |
| 35–49 | 72 | 14.0 | 156 | 6 | 7 | 9 | 15 | 39 | 39 | 63 |
| 50–64 | 49 | 41.0 | 678 | 7 | 12 | 64 | 64 | 64 | 64 | 64 |
| 65+ | 34 | 20.6 | 351 | 6 | 10 | 12 | 22 | 44 | 60 | 86 |
| **TOTAL SINGLE DX** | 6 | 7.6 | 7 | 5 | 5 | 6 | 10 | 11 | 11 | 11 |
| **TOTAL MULTIPLE DX** | 178 | 27.2 | 583 | 6 | 8 | 14 | 63 | 64 | 64 | 64 |
| **TOTAL** | | | | | | | | | | |
| 0–19 Years | 3 | 5.8 | 2 | 4 | 6 | 6 | 7 | 7 | 7 | 7 |
| 20–34 | 21 | 17.4 | 282 | 5 | 7 | 8 | 31 | 43 | 60 | 60 |
| 35–49 | 75 | 13.9 | 153 | 6 | 7 | 9 | 15 | 39 | 39 | 63 |
| 50–64 | 51 | 40.6 | 685 | 7 | 11 | 64 | 64 | 64 | 64 | 64 |
| 65+ | 34 | 20.6 | 351 | 6 | 10 | 12 | 22 | 44 | 60 | 86 |
| **GRAND TOTAL** | 184 | 26.9 | 580 | 6 | 8 | 14 | 60 | 64 | 64 | 64 |

## 52.5: PARTIAL PANCREATECTOMY. Formerly included in operation group(s) 630.

| Type of Patients | Observed Patients | Avg. Stay | Vari-ance | Percentiles | | | | | | |
|---|---|---|---|---|---|---|---|---|---|---|
| | | | | 10th | 25th | 50th | 75th | 90th | 95th | 99th |
| **1. SINGLE DX** | | | | | | | | | | |
| 0–19 Years | 6 | 8.3 | 4 | 7 | 7 | 7 | 10 | 10 | 10 | 16 |
| 20–34 | 5 | 6.8 | 1 | 7 | 7 | 7 | 7 | 7 | 7 | 9 |
| 35–49 | 15 | 7.8 | 22 | 5 | 5 | 6 | 8 | 21 | 21 | 21 |
| 50–64 | 9 | 6.9 | 26 | 3 | 5 | 5 | 8 | 8 | 23 | 23 |
| 65+ | 4 | 8.2 | 4 | 6 | 7 | 9 | 9 | 11 | 11 | 11 |
| **2. MULTIPLE DX** | | | | | | | | | | |
| 0–19 Years | 46 | 23.5 | 356 | 9 | 11 | 17 | 26 | 52 | 70 | 70 |
| 20–34 | 73 | 10.9 | 92 | 6 | 7 | 10 | 11 | 16 | 23 | 67 |
| 35–49 | 171 | 11.3 | 136 | 5 | 6 | 8 | 11 | 21 | 28 | 70 |
| 50–64 | 191 | 12.0 | 72 | 6 | 7 | 10 | 12 | 20 | 25 | 50 |
| 65+ | 206 | 11.9 | 76 | 6 | 7 | 9 | 15 | 19 | 26 | 44 |
| **TOTAL SINGLE DX** | 39 | 7.6 | 12 | 5 | 6 | 7 | 8 | 10 | 16 | 23 |
| **TOTAL MULTIPLE DX** | 687 | 12.7 | 126 | 6 | 7 | 10 | 13 | 22 | 31 | 70 |
| **TOTAL** | | | | | | | | | | |
| 0–19 Years | 52 | 21.4 | 335 | 7 | 10 | 13 | 26 | 47 | 70 | 70 |
| 20–34 | 78 | 10.5 | 84 | 6 | 7 | 9 | 10 | 15 | 22 | 67 |
| 35–49 | 186 | 11.1 | 129 | 5 | 6 | 7 | 11 | 21 | 28 | 70 |
| 50–64 | 200 | 11.9 | 71 | 6 | 7 | 10 | 12 | 18 | 25 | 50 |
| 65+ | 210 | 11.9 | 75 | 6 | 7 | 9 | 14 | 19 | 26 | 44 |
| **GRAND TOTAL** | 726 | 12.4 | 122 | 6 | 7 | 9 | 12 | 22 | 29 | 70 |

Length of Stay by Diagnosis and Operation, United States, 2000

# United States, October 1998–September 1999 Data, by Operation

## 52.52: DISTAL PANCREATECTOMY. Formerly included in operation group(s) 630.

| Type of Patients | Observed Patients | Avg. Stay | Variance | 10th | 25th | 50th | 75th | 90th | 95th | 99th |
|---|---|---|---|---|---|---|---|---|---|---|
| **1. SINGLE DX** | | | | | | | | | | |
| 0–19 Years | 6 | 8.3 | 4 | 7 | 7 | 7 | 10 | 10 | 10 | 16 |
| 20–34 | 4 | 6.7 | 2 | 7 | 7 | 7 | 7 | 7 | 9 | 9 |
| 35–49 | 9 | 6.5 | 2 | 5 | 6 | 6 | 7 | 8 | 8 | 9 |
| 50–64 | 7 | 7.0 | 32 | 3 | 5 | 5 | 8 | 8 | 23 | 23 |
| 65+ | 1 | 9.0 | 0 | 9 | 9 | 9 | 9 | 9 | 9 | 9 |
| **2. MULTIPLE DX** | | | | | | | | | | |
| 0–19 Years | 28 | 15.1 | 81 | 9 | 10 | 11 | 17 | 26 | 41 | 47 |
| 20–34 | 61 | 11.0 | 66 | 5 | 7 | 8 | 12 | 22 | 28 | 32 |
| 35–49 | 129 | 9.5 | 50 | 5 | 6 | 8 | 10 | 15 | 21 | 38 |
| 50–64 | 131 | 12.1 | 69 | 7 | 8 | 11 | 12 | 20 | 25 | 41 |
| 65+ | 147 | 11.4 | 79 | 6 | 7 | 9 | 13 | 18 | 24 | 59 |
| **TOTAL SINGLE DX** | 27 | 7.3 | 7 | 5 | 6 | 7 | 8 | 10 | 10 | 23 |
| **TOTAL MULTIPLE DX** | 496 | 11.2 | 68 | 6 | 7 | 9 | 12 | 20 | 25 | 43 |
| **TOTAL** | | | | | | | | | | |
| 0–19 Years | 34 | 13.5 | 71 | 7 | 9 | 11 | 13 | 26 | 36 | 47 |
| 20–34 | 65 | 10.4 | 59 | 6 | 7 | 7 | 10 | 22 | 24 | 32 |
| 35–49 | 138 | 9.3 | 48 | 6 | 6 | 8 | 10 | 15 | 21 | 38 |
| 50–64 | 138 | 11.9 | 68 | 6 | 7 | 10 | 12 | 20 | 25 | 41 |
| 65+ | 148 | 11.4 | 79 | 6 | 7 | 9 | 13 | 18 | 24 | 59 |
| **GRAND TOTAL** | 523 | 11.0 | 66 | 6 | 7 | 9 | 12 | 19 | 25 | 43 |

## 52.6: TOTAL PANCREATECTOMY. Formerly included in operation group(s) 630.

| Type of Patients | Observed Patients | Avg. Stay | Variance | 10th | 25th | 50th | 75th | 90th | 95th | 99th |
|---|---|---|---|---|---|---|---|---|---|---|
| **1. SINGLE DX** | | | | | | | | | | |
| 0–19 Years | 1 | 36.0 | 0 | 36 | 36 | 36 | 36 | 36 | 36 | 36 |
| 20–34 | 0 | | | | | | | | | |
| 35–49 | 2 | 5.3 | 1 | 4 | 4 | 6 | 6 | 6 | 6 | 6 |
| 50–64 | 2 | 13.4 | <1 | 13 | 13 | 13 | 14 | 14 | 14 | 14 |
| 65+ | 0 | | | | | | | | | |
| **2. MULTIPLE DX** | | | | | | | | | | |
| 0–19 Years | 3 | 13.3 | 379 | 1 | 1 | 1 | 24 | 47 | 47 | 47 |
| 20–34 | 5 | 11.3 | 27 | 5 | 6 | 9 | 17 | 17 | 17 | 17 |
| 35–49 | 29 | 16.1 | 110 | 11 | 13 | 12 | 20 | 33 | 35 | 49 |
| 50–64 | 22 | 17.7 | 56 | 11 | 13 | 19 | 20 | 22 | 23 | 52 |
| 65+ | 32 | 20.2 | 162 | 9 | 11 | 18 | 22 | 43 | 50 | 66 |
| **TOTAL SINGLE DX** | 5 | 26.6 | 182 | 6 | 13 | 36 | 36 | 36 | 36 | 36 |
| **TOTAL MULTIPLE DX** | 91 | 17.6 | 116 | 7 | 11 | 17 | 22 | 29 | 43 | 61 |
| **TOTAL** | | | | | | | | | | |
| 0–19 Years | 4 | 26.7 | 274 | 1 | 1 | 36 | 36 | 36 | 47 | 47 |
| 20–34 | 5 | 11.3 | 27 | 5 | 6 | 9 | 17 | 17 | 17 | 17 |
| 35–49 | 31 | 15.5 | 110 | 6 | 7 | 12 | 19 | 32 | 35 | 49 |
| 50–64 | 24 | 17.6 | 55 | 11 | 13 | 19 | 20 | 22 | 23 | 52 |
| 65+ | 32 | 20.2 | 162 | 9 | 11 | 18 | 22 | 43 | 50 | 66 |
| **GRAND TOTAL** | 96 | 18.3 | 125 | 7 | 11 | 17 | 22 | 36 | 43 | 52 |

## 52.7: RAD PANC/DUODENECTOMY. Formerly included in operation group(s) 630.

| Type of Patients | Observed Patients | Avg. Stay | Variance | 10th | 25th | 50th | 75th | 90th | 95th | 99th |
|---|---|---|---|---|---|---|---|---|---|---|
| **1. SINGLE DX** | | | | | | | | | | |
| 0–19 Years | 2 | 11.9 | 5 | 11 | 11 | 11 | 11 | 16 | 16 | 16 |
| 20–34 | 2 | 9.7 | 7 | 8 | 8 | 8 | 12 | 12 | 12 | 12 |
| 35–49 | 6 | 20.0 | 550 | 7 | 8 | 11 | 17 | 73 | 73 | 73 |
| 50–64 | 4 | 9.1 | 16 | 6 | 8 | 8 | 8 | 19 | 19 | 19 |
| 65+ | 2 | 10.2 | 2 | 9 | 9 | 11 | 11 | 11 | 11 | 11 |
| **2. MULTIPLE DX** | | | | | | | | | | |
| 0–19 Years | 3 | 24.1 | 157 | 9 | 9 | 35 | 35 | 35 | 35 | 35 |
| 20–34 | 25 | 18.5 | 182 | 9 | 14 | 15 | 22 | 24 | 44 | 94 |
| 35–49 | 159 | 18.8 | 100 | 8 | 10 | 17 | 25 | 31 | 34 | 40 |
| 50–64 | 426 | 17.1 | 137 | 8 | 10 | 13 | 20 | 30 | 39 | 70 |
| 65+ | 605 | 17.5 | 116 | 8 | 10 | 14 | 21 | 31 | 38 | 56 |
| **TOTAL SINGLE DX** | 16 | 13.2 | 201 | 8 | 8 | 8 | 11 | 17 | 19 | 73 |
| **TOTAL MULTIPLE DX** | 1,218 | 17.7 | 122 | 8 | 10 | 14 | 22 | 31 | 37 | 58 |
| **TOTAL** | | | | | | | | | | |
| 0–19 Years | 5 | 22.7 | 155 | 9 | 11 | 16 | 35 | 35 | 35 | 35 |
| 20–34 | 27 | 18.3 | 179 | 8 | 11 | 15 | 22 | 24 | 44 | 94 |
| 35–49 | 165 | 18.8 | 108 | 8 | 10 | 16 | 25 | 31 | 34 | 53 |
| 50–64 | 430 | 17.0 | 137 | 8 | 10 | 13 | 20 | 30 | 39 | 70 |
| 65+ | 607 | 17.5 | 116 | 8 | 10 | 14 | 21 | 31 | 38 | 56 |
| **GRAND TOTAL** | 1,234 | 17.6 | 123 | 8 | 10 | 14 | 22 | 31 | 37 | 59 |

## 52.8: TRANSPLANT OF PANCREAS. Formerly included in operation group(s) 630.

| Type of Patients | Observed Patients | Avg. Stay | Variance | 10th | 25th | 50th | 75th | 90th | 95th | 99th |
|---|---|---|---|---|---|---|---|---|---|---|
| **1. SINGLE DX** | | | | | | | | | | |
| 0–19 Years | 0 | | | | | | | | | |
| 20–34 | 0 | | | | | | | | | |
| 35–49 | 1 | 8.0 | 0 | 8 | 8 | 8 | 8 | 8 | 8 | 8 |
| 50–64 | 0 | | | | | | | | | |
| 65+ | 0 | | | | | | | | | |
| **2. MULTIPLE DX** | | | | | | | | | | |
| 0–19 Years | 0 | | | | | | | | | |
| 20–34 | 15 | 10.6 | 20 | 4 | 7 | 10 | 14 | 18 | 19 | 19 |
| 35–49 | 63 | 12.5 | 116 | 7 | 8 | 9 | 12 | 20 | 33 | 51 |
| 50–64 | 6 | 10.4 | 57 | 6 | 6 | 8 | 9 | 28 | 28 | 28 |
| 65+ | 0 | | | | | | | | | |
| **TOTAL SINGLE DX** | 1 | 8.0 | 0 | 8 | 8 | 8 | 8 | 8 | 8 | 8 |
| **TOTAL MULTIPLE DX** | 84 | 12.1 | 98 | 6 | 8 | 9 | 12 | 20 | 28 | 96 |
| **TOTAL** | | | | | | | | | | |
| 0–19 Years | 0 | | | | | | | | | |
| 20–34 | 15 | 10.6 | 20 | 4 | 7 | 10 | 14 | 18 | 19 | 19 |
| 35–49 | 64 | 12.5 | 115 | 7 | 8 | 9 | 12 | 20 | 33 | 51 |
| 50–64 | 6 | 10.4 | 57 | 6 | 6 | 8 | 9 | 28 | 28 | 28 |
| 65+ | 0 | | | | | | | | | |
| **GRAND TOTAL** | 85 | 12.1 | 98 | 6 | 8 | 9 | 12 | 20 | 28 | 96 |

Length of Stay by Diagnosis and Operation, United States, 2000

# United States, October 1998–September 1999 Data, by Operation

## 52.9: OTHER OPS ON PANCREAS. Formerly included in operation group(s) 628, 630.

| Type of Patients | Observed Patients | Avg. Stay | Variance | 10th | 25th | 50th | 75th | 90th | 95th | 99th |
|---|---|---|---|---|---|---|---|---|---|---|
| **1. SINGLE DX** | | | | | | | | | | |
| 0–19 Years | 7 | 5.7 | 4 | 2 | 5 | 6 | 6 | 8 | 8 | 8 |
| 20–34 | 14 | 5.2 | 9 | 1 | 3 | 6 | 9 | 9 | 9 | 9 |
| 35–49 | 22 | 4.4 | 7 | 2 | 3 | 4 | 5 | 7 | 12 | 12 |
| 50–64 | 6 | 4.7 | 7 | 1 | 2 | 7 | 7 | 7 | 7 | 7 |
| 65+ | 6 | 2.8 | 3 | 2 | 2 | 2 | 3 | 7 | 7 | 7 |
| **2. MULTIPLE DX** | | | | | | | | | | |
| 0–19 Years | 40 | 10.1 | 147 | 2 | 4 | 5 | 11 | 22 | 32 | 68 |
| 20–34 | 119 | 9.3 | 104 | 2 | 3 | 6 | 11 | 28 | 28 | 36 |
| 35–49 | 311 | 8.6 | 67 | 2 | 4 | 7 | 10 | 18 | 24 | 52 |
| 50–64 | 272 | 7.8 | 55 | 2 | 4 | 6 | 9 | 14 | 20 | 52 |
| 65+ | 348 | 7.1 | 58 | 2 | 3 | 5 | 8 | 14 | 19 | 44 |
| **TOTAL SINGLE DX** | 55 | 4.5 | 7 | 2 | 2 | 4 | 6 | 9 | 9 | 12 |
| **TOTAL MULTIPLE DX** | 1,090 | 8.1 | 69 | 2 | 4 | 6 | 9 | 16 | 24 | 47 |
| **TOTAL** | | | | | | | | | | |
| 0–19 Years | 47 | 9.6 | 133 | 2 | 4 | 5 | 10 | 22 | 32 | 68 |
| 20–34 | 133 | 8.9 | 96 | 2 | 3 | 5 | 10 | 27 | 28 | 36 |
| 35–49 | 333 | 8.3 | 64 | 2 | 4 | 7 | 9 | 15 | 23 | 47 |
| 50–64 | 278 | 7.7 | 54 | 2 | 4 | 6 | 9 | 14 | 20 | 52 |
| 65+ | 354 | 7.1 | 58 | 2 | 3 | 5 | 8 | 14 | 18 | 44 |
| **GRAND TOTAL** | 1,145 | 7.9 | 66 | 2 | 3 | 6 | 9 | 15 | 23 | 47 |

## 52.93: ENDO INSERT PANC STENT. Formerly included in operation group(s) 628.

| Type of Patients | Observed Patients | Avg. Stay | Variance | 10th | 25th | 50th | 75th | 90th | 95th | 99th |
|---|---|---|---|---|---|---|---|---|---|---|
| **1. SINGLE DX** | | | | | | | | | | |
| 0–19 Years | 5 | 4.4 | 4 | 2 | 2 | 5 | 6 | 6 | 6 | 6 |
| 20–34 | 8 | 2.8 | 1 | 1 | 2 | 3 | 4 | 4 | 4 | 4 |
| 35–49 | 12 | 4.0 | 6 | 2 | 3 | 3 | 5 | 5 | 12 | 12 |
| 50–64 | 4 | 4.8 | 7 | 1 | 2 | 7 | 7 | 7 | 7 | 7 |
| 65+ | 5 | 2.8 | 4 | 2 | 2 | 2 | 3 | 7 | 7 | 7 |
| **2. MULTIPLE DX** | | | | | | | | | | |
| 0–19 Years | 20 | 5.0 | 16 | 1 | 3 | 5 | 5 | 7 | 10 | 22 |
| 20–34 | 62 | 8.2 | 100 | 2 | 3 | 3 | 9 | 28 | 28 | 28 |
| 35–49 | 133 | 6.4 | 30 | 2 | 3 | 5 | 8 | 11 | 15 | 35 |
| 50–64 | 132 | 5.8 | 49 | 2 | 2 | 4 | 7 | 12 | 16 | 52 |
| 65+ | 247 | 5.9 | 37 | 1 | 3 | 5 | 7 | 10 | 15 | 24 |
| **TOTAL SINGLE DX** | 34 | 3.7 | 5 | 1 | 2 | 3 | 5 | 7 | 7 | 12 |
| **TOTAL MULTIPLE DX** | 594 | 6.3 | 44 | 2 | 3 | 5 | 7 | 11 | 17 | 31 |
| **TOTAL** | | | | | | | | | | |
| 0–19 Years | 25 | 4.9 | 15 | 1 | 3 | 5 | 5 | 7 | 10 | 22 |
| 20–34 | 70 | 7.7 | 94 | 2 | 3 | 3 | 8 | 27 | 28 | 28 |
| 35–49 | 145 | 6.1 | 28 | 2 | 2 | 5 | 7 | 11 | 15 | 35 |
| 50–64 | 136 | 5.8 | 48 | 1 | 2 | 4 | 7 | 12 | 16 | 52 |
| 65+ | 252 | 5.9 | 37 | 1 | 2 | 5 | 7 | 10 | 15 | 24 |
| **GRAND TOTAL** | 628 | 6.1 | 42 | 2 | 3 | 4 | 7 | 11 | 16 | 28 |

## 52.96: PANCREATIC ANASTOMOSIS. Formerly included in operation group(s) 630.

| Type of Patients | Observed Patients | Avg. Stay | Variance | 10th | 25th | 50th | 75th | 90th | 95th | 99th |
|---|---|---|---|---|---|---|---|---|---|---|
| **1. SINGLE DX** | | | | | | | | | | |
| 0–19 Years | 2 | 6.9 | 1 | 6 | 6 | 6 | 8 | 8 | 8 | 8 |
| 20–34 | 3 | 8.5 | 1 | 7 | 9 | 9 | 9 | 9 | 9 | 9 |
| 35–49 | 9 | 6.3 | 9 | 3 | 4 | 6 | 8 | 12 | 12 | 12 |
| 50–64 | 0 | | | | | | | | | |
| 65+ | 0 | | | | | | | | | |
| **2. MULTIPLE DX** | | | | | | | | | | |
| 0–19 Years | 8 | 20.6 | 99 | 5 | 13 | 25 | 25 | 32 | 33 | 33 |
| 20–34 | 38 | 13.8 | 112 | 5 | 8 | 9 | 15 | 36 | 36 | 58 |
| 35–49 | 133 | 11.2 | 84 | 5 | 6 | 8 | 13 | 22 | 27 | 52 |
| 50–64 | 99 | 11.0 | 66 | 6 | 7 | 8 | 12 | 19 | 23 | 55 |
| 65+ | 54 | 13.5 | 102 | 5 | 7 | 11 | 16 | 34 | 36 | 44 |
| **TOTAL SINGLE DX** | 14 | 7.2 | 6 | 4 | 6 | 7 | 9 | 9 | 12 | 12 |
| **TOTAL MULTIPLE DX** | 332 | 11.9 | 87 | 5 | 7 | 8 | 14 | 23 | 31 | 52 |
| **TOTAL** | | | | | | | | | | |
| 0–19 Years | 10 | 16.1 | 108 | 6 | 6 | 13 | 25 | 32 | 33 | 33 |
| 20–34 | 41 | 13.2 | 102 | 5 | 8 | 9 | 15 | 31 | 36 | 58 |
| 35–49 | 142 | 11.0 | 82 | 5 | 7 | 8 | 12 | 22 | 27 | 52 |
| 50–64 | 99 | 11.0 | 66 | 6 | 7 | 8 | 12 | 19 | 23 | 55 |
| 65+ | 54 | 13.5 | 102 | 5 | 7 | 11 | 16 | 34 | 36 | 44 |
| **GRAND TOTAL** | 346 | 11.7 | 85 | 5 | 7 | 8 | 14 | 23 | 31 | 52 |

## 53.0: UNILAT IH REPAIR. Formerly included in operation group(s) 632.

| Type of Patients | Observed Patients | Avg. Stay | Variance | 10th | 25th | 50th | 75th | 90th | 95th | 99th |
|---|---|---|---|---|---|---|---|---|---|---|
| **1. SINGLE DX** | | | | | | | | | | |
| 0–19 Years | 478 | 1.2 | <1 | 1 | 1 | 1 | 1 | 2 | 2 | 4 |
| 20–34 | 258 | 1.5 | <1 | 1 | 1 | 1 | 2 | 2 | 3 | 5 |
| 35–49 | 307 | 1.7 | 2 | 1 | 1 | 1 | 2 | 3 | 4 | 8 |
| 50–64 | 278 | 1.5 | <1 | 1 | 1 | 1 | 2 | 3 | 4 | 5 |
| 65+ | 389 | 1.6 | 2 | 1 | 1 | 1 | 2 | 3 | 4 | 7 |
| **2. MULTIPLE DX** | | | | | | | | | | |
| 0–19 Years | 572 | 5.4 | 203 | 1 | 1 | 1 | 3 | 3 | 57 | >99 |
| 20–34 | 287 | 2.1 | 4 | 1 | 1 | 1 | 2 | 4 | 6 | 9 |
| 35–49 | 633 | 2.6 | 6 | 1 | 1 | 2 | 3 | 5 | 7 | 13 |
| 50–64 | 1,072 | 3.3 | 14 | 1 | 1 | 2 | 4 | 7 | 10 | 18 |
| 65+ | 4,567 | 4.1 | 25 | 1 | 1 | 2 | 5 | 9 | 13 | 27 |
| **TOTAL SINGLE DX** | 1,710 | 1.5 | <1 | 1 | 1 | 1 | 2 | 2 | 3 | 3 |
| **TOTAL MULTIPLE DX** | 7,131 | 3.9 | 37 | 1 | 1 | 2 | 4 | 8 | 13 | 31 |
| **TOTAL** | | | | | | | | | | |
| 0–19 Years | 1,050 | 3.3 | 105 | 1 | 1 | 1 | 2 | 4 | 8 | 82 |
| 20–34 | 545 | 1.8 | 2 | 1 | 1 | 1 | 2 | 3 | 5 | 7 |
| 35–49 | 940 | 2.3 | 4 | 1 | 1 | 2 | 3 | 4 | 7 | 10 |
| 50–64 | 1,350 | 2.9 | 12 | 1 | 1 | 2 | 3 | 6 | 9 | 15 |
| 65+ | 4,956 | 3.9 | 24 | 1 | 1 | 2 | 5 | 9 | 13 | 27 |
| **GRAND TOTAL** | 8,841 | 3.4 | 31 | 1 | 1 | 2 | 4 | 7 | 11 | 27 |

Length of Stay by Diagnosis and Operation, United States, 2000

# United States, October 1998–September 1999 Data, by Operation

## 53.00: UNILAT IH REPAIR NOS. Formerly included in operation group(s) 632.

| Type of Patients | Observed Patients | Avg. Stay | Vari-ance | 10th | 25th | 50th | 75th | 90th | 95th | 99th |
|---|---|---|---|---|---|---|---|---|---|---|
| **1. SINGLE DX** | | | | | | | | | | |
| 0–19 Years | 133 | 1.3 | <1 | 1 | 1 | 1 | 1 | 2 | 3 | 4 |
| 20–34 | 41 | 1.3 | <1 | 1 | 1 | 1 | 2 | 2 | 2 | 3 |
| 35–49 | 38 | 1.8 | 1 | 1 | 1 | 1 | 3 | 3 | 4 | 5 |
| 50–64 | 29 | 1.5 | <1 | 1 | 1 | 1 | 2 | 3 | 3 | 3 |
| 65+ | 50 | 1.7 | <1 | 1 | 1 | 1 | 2 | 3 | 4 | 5 |
| **2. MULTIPLE DX** | | | | | | | | | | |
| 0–19 Years | 184 | 6.9 | 294 | 1 | 1 | 2 | 4 | 26 | 82 | >99 |
| 20–34 | 50 | 2.5 | 6 | 1 | 1 | 2 | 3 | 6 | 6 | 16 |
| 35–49 | 68 | 2.4 | 6 | 1 | 1 | 1 | 5 | 5 | 7 | 15 |
| 50–64 | 108 | 4.1 | 19 | 1 | 1 | 2 | 5 | 9 | 15 | 21 |
| 65+ | 384 | 5.4 | 40 | 1 | 2 | 4 | 6 | 12 | 13 | 39 |
| **TOTAL SINGLE DX** | 291 | 1.5 | <1 | 1 | 1 | 1 | 2 | 3 | 3 | 4 |
| **TOTAL MULTIPLE DX** | 794 | 5.1 | 90 | 1 | 1 | 3 | 5 | 10 | 16 | 84 |
| **TOTAL** | | | | | | | | | | |
| 0–19 Years | 317 | 4.7 | 186 | 1 | 1 | 1 | 3 | 6 | 59 | >99 |
| 20–34 | 91 | 2.0 | 4 | 1 | 1 | 1 | 2 | 5 | 6 | 14 |
| 35–49 | 106 | 2.2 | 5 | 1 | 1 | 1 | 3 | 6 | 6 | 8 |
| 50–64 | 137 | 3.6 | 16 | 1 | 1 | 2 | 4 | 8 | 10 | 21 |
| 65+ | 434 | 5.0 | 38 | 1 | 2 | 3 | 6 | 11 | 13 | 39 |
| **GRAND TOTAL** | 1,085 | 4.2 | 71 | 1 | 1 | 2 | 4 | 8 | 13 | 73 |

## 53.01: UNILAT REP DIRECT IH. Formerly included in operation group(s) 632.

| Type of Patients | Observed Patients | Avg. Stay | Vari-ance | 10th | 25th | 50th | 75th | 90th | 95th | 99th |
|---|---|---|---|---|---|---|---|---|---|---|
| **1. SINGLE DX** | | | | | | | | | | |
| 0–19 Years | 27 | 1.5 | <1 | 1 | 1 | 1 | 2 | 2 | 3 | 3 |
| 20–34 | 20 | 2.2 | 2 | 1 | 1 | 2 | 3 | 4 | 4 | 6 |
| 35–49 | 23 | 1.6 | <1 | 1 | 1 | 1 | 2 | 2 | 3 | 4 |
| 50–64 | 14 | 1.3 | <1 | 1 | 1 | 1 | 1 | 2 | 3 | 4 |
| 65+ | 37 | 2.0 | 2 | 1 | 1 | 1 | 3 | 3 | 4 | 5 |
| **2. MULTIPLE DX** | | | | | | | | | | |
| 0–19 Years | 62 | 15.9 | 627 | 1 | 1 | 3 | 8 | 57 | 72 | 72 |
| 20–34 | 20 | 2.4 | 2 | 1 | 1 | 2 | 3 | 4 | 5 | 7 |
| 35–49 | 64 | 3.3 | 14 | 1 | 1 | 2 | 3 | 6 | 8 | 26 |
| 50–64 | 95 | 2.9 | 6 | 1 | 1 | 2 | 3 | 6 | 8 | 12 |
| 65+ | 377 | 4.2 | 21 | 1 | 1 | 3 | 5 | 9 | 12 | 22 |
| **TOTAL SINGLE DX** | 121 | 1.7 | 1 | 1 | 1 | 1 | 2 | 3 | 5 | 5 |
| **TOTAL MULTIPLE DX** | 618 | 5.2 | 102 | 1 | 1 | 2 | 5 | 9 | 14 | 71 |
| **TOTAL** | | | | | | | | | | |
| 0–19 Years | 89 | 10.9 | 454 | 1 | 1 | 2 | 4 | 57 | 72 | 72 |
| 20–34 | 40 | 2.3 | 2 | 1 | 1 | 2 | 3 | 4 | 5 | 7 |
| 35–49 | 87 | 2.8 | 11 | 1 | 1 | 2 | 3 | 4 | 8 | 20 |
| 50–64 | 109 | 2.8 | 6 | 1 | 1 | 2 | 3 | 6 | 8 | 12 |
| 65+ | 414 | 3.9 | 19 | 1 | 1 | 3 | 5 | 9 | 12 | 22 |
| **GRAND TOTAL** | 739 | 4.6 | 86 | 1 | 1 | 2 | 4 | 8 | 12 | 57 |

## 53.02: UNILAT REP INDIRECT IH. Formerly included in operation group(s) 632.

| Type of Patients | Observed Patients | Avg. Stay | Vari-ance | 10th | 25th | 50th | 75th | 90th | 95th | 99th |
|---|---|---|---|---|---|---|---|---|---|---|
| **1. SINGLE DX** | | | | | | | | | | |
| 0–19 Years | 288 | 1.1 | <1 | 1 | 1 | 1 | 1 | 1 | 2 | 4 |
| 20–34 | 29 | 1.7 | <1 | 1 | 1 | 2 | 2 | 2 | 3 | 6 |
| 35–49 | 36 | 1.6 | <1 | 1 | 1 | 1 | 2 | 3 | 3 | 5 |
| 50–64 | 25 | 1.5 | <1 | 1 | 1 | 1 | 2 | 3 | 3 | 5 |
| 65+ | 45 | 1.5 | 1 | 1 | 1 | 1 | 2 | 3 | 4 | 6 |
| **2. MULTIPLE DX** | | | | | | | | | | |
| 0–19 Years | 302 | 3.2 | 77 | 1 | 1 | 2 | 4 | 5 | 13 | >99 |
| 20–34 | 42 | 2.5 | 3 | 1 | 1 | 2 | 3 | 5 | 6 | 7 |
| 35–49 | 77 | 2.9 | 8 | 1 | 1 | 2 | 4 | 6 | 7 | 15 |
| 50–64 | 112 | 3.4 | 13 | 1 | 1 | 3 | 5 | 7 | 15 | 17 |
| 65+ | 490 | 3.9 | 13 | 1 | 3 | 4 | 5 | 7 | 9 | 21 |
| **TOTAL SINGLE DX** | 423 | 1.2 | <1 | 1 | 1 | 1 | 1 | 2 | 2 | 4 |
| **TOTAL MULTIPLE DX** | 1,023 | 3.5 | 36 | 1 | 2 | 2 | 4 | 7 | 10 | 41 |
| **TOTAL** | | | | | | | | | | |
| 0–19 Years | 590 | 2.0 | 35 | 1 | 1 | 1 | 2 | 2 | 4 | 56 |
| 20–34 | 71 | 2.1 | 2 | 1 | 1 | 2 | 3 | 3 | 5 | 7 |
| 35–49 | 113 | 2.4 | 5 | 1 | 1 | 2 | 3 | 6 | 6 | 15 |
| 50–64 | 137 | 2.8 | 10 | 1 | 1 | 2 | 3 | 6 | 8 | 15 |
| 65+ | 535 | 3.7 | 13 | 1 | 3 | 3 | 5 | 7 | 9 | 21 |
| **GRAND TOTAL** | 1,446 | 2.6 | 23 | 1 | 1 | 1 | 2 | 6 | 7 | 24 |

## 53.03: UNILAT REP DIR IH/GRAFT. Formerly included in operation group(s) 632.

| Type of Patients | Observed Patients | Avg. Stay | Vari-ance | 10th | 25th | 50th | 75th | 90th | 95th | 99th |
|---|---|---|---|---|---|---|---|---|---|---|
| **1. SINGLE DX** | | | | | | | | | | |
| 0–19 Years | 3 | 1.7 | <1 | 1 | 1 | 2 | 2 | 2 | 2 | 2 |
| 20–34 | 43 | 1.5 | <1 | 1 | 1 | 1 | 2 | 3 | 3 | 6 |
| 35–49 | 70 | 1.8 | 4 | 1 | 1 | 1 | 1 | 4 | 8 | 8 |
| 50–64 | 44 | 1.3 | <1 | 1 | 1 | 1 | 1 | 2 | 8 | 8 |
| 65+ | 82 | 1.8 | 3 | 1 | 1 | 2 | 2 | 3 | 5 | 9 |
| **2. MULTIPLE DX** | | | | | | | | | | |
| 0–19 Years | 7 | 1.8 | <1 | 1 | 1 | 2 | 2 | 3 | 3 | 3 |
| 20–34 | 54 | 1.9 | 2 | 1 | 1 | 2 | 2 | 3 | 5 | 7 |
| 35–49 | 138 | 2.2 | 3 | 1 | 1 | 2 | 4 | 5 | 6 | 10 |
| 50–64 | 262 | 3.3 | 21 | 1 | 1 | 2 | 5 | 6 | 13 | 18 |
| 65+ | 1,052 | 3.9 | 23 | 1 | 1 | 3 | 5 | 8 | 12 | 17 |
| **TOTAL SINGLE DX** | 242 | 1.7 | 2 | 1 | 1 | 2 | 2 | 3 | 5 | 8 |
| **TOTAL MULTIPLE DX** | 1,513 | 3.6 | 21 | 1 | 1 | 2 | 4 | 7 | 11 | 18 |
| **TOTAL** | | | | | | | | | | |
| 0–19 Years | 10 | 1.7 | <1 | 1 | 1 | 2 | 2 | 2 | 3 | 3 |
| 20–34 | 97 | 1.7 | 1 | 1 | 1 | 2 | 2 | 3 | 5 | 7 |
| 35–49 | 208 | 2.0 | 3 | 1 | 1 | 2 | 3 | 4 | 7 | 8 |
| 50–64 | 306 | 3.0 | 19 | 1 | 1 | 2 | 3 | 6 | 13 | 18 |
| 65+ | 1,134 | 3.7 | 22 | 1 | 1 | 2 | 5 | 8 | 11 | 17 |
| **GRAND TOTAL** | 1,755 | 3.3 | 18 | 1 | 1 | 2 | 4 | 7 | 10 | 17 |

Length of Stay by Diagnosis and Operation, United States, 2000

# United States, October 1998–September 1999 Data, by Operation

## 53.04: UNILAT INDIRECT IH/GRAFT. Formerly included in operation group(s) 632.

| Type of Patients | Observed Patients | Avg. Stay | Vari-ance | Percentiles | | | | | | |
|---|---|---|---|---|---|---|---|---|---|---|
| | | | | 10th | 25th | 50th | 75th | 90th | 95th | 99th |
| **1. SINGLE DX** | | | | | | | | | | |
| 0–19 Years | 11 | 1.3 | <1 | 1 | 1 | 1 | 2 | 2 | 2 | 2 |
| 20–34 | 68 | 1.6 | <1 | 1 | 1 | 1 | 1 | 2 | 3 | 4 |
| 35–49 | 60 | 1.8 | <1 | 1 | 1 | 2 | 2 | 3 | 4 | 4 |
| 50–64 | 80 | 1.4 | <1 | 1 | 1 | 1 | 2 | 2 | 3 | 5 |
| 65+ | 96 | 1.4 | <1 | 1 | 1 | 1 | 1 | 2 | 4 | 6 |
| **2. MULTIPLE DX** | | | | | | | | | | |
| 0–19 Years | 8 | 2.0 | <1 | 2 | 2 | 2 | 2 | 2 | 3 | 3 |
| 20–34 | 74 | 1.5 | 1 | 1 | 1 | 1 | 2 | 3 | 4 | 6 |
| 35–49 | 146 | 2.8 | 5 | 1 | 1 | 2 | 4 | 7 | 7 | 8 |
| 50–64 | 218 | 3.0 | 11 | 1 | 1 | 1 | 3 | 7 | 13 | 14 |
| 65+ | 1,158 | 3.7 | 20 | 1 | 1 | 2 | 4 | 9 | 13 | 18 |
| **TOTAL SINGLE DX** | 315 | 1.5 | <1 | 1 | 1 | 1 | 2 | 2 | 4 | 5 |
| **TOTAL MULTIPLE DX** | 1,604 | 3.3 | 16 | 1 | 1 | 2 | 4 | 8 | 11 | 18 |
| **TOTAL** | | | | | | | | | | |
| 0–19 Years | 19 | 1.8 | <1 | 1 | 1 | 2 | 2 | 2 | 2 | 3 |
| 20–34 | 142 | 1.6 | 1 | 1 | 1 | 1 | 2 | 3 | 3 | 5 |
| 35–49 | 206 | 2.5 | 4 | 1 | 1 | 2 | 3 | 4 | 7 | 8 |
| 50–64 | 298 | 2.5 | 8 | 1 | 1 | 2 | 3 | 6 | 8 | 13 |
| 65+ | 1,254 | 3.5 | 19 | 1 | 1 | 2 | 4 | 9 | 13 | 18 |
| **GRAND TOTAL** | 1,919 | 3.0 | 14 | 1 | 1 | 2 | 3 | 7 | 11 | 18 |

## 53.05: UNILAT REP IH/GRAFT NOS. Formerly included in operation group(s) 632.

| Type of Patients | Observed Patients | Avg. Stay | Vari-ance | Percentiles | | | | | | |
|---|---|---|---|---|---|---|---|---|---|---|
| | | | | 10th | 25th | 50th | 75th | 90th | 95th | 99th |
| **1. SINGLE DX** | | | | | | | | | | |
| 0–19 Years | 16 | 1.1 | <1 | 1 | 1 | 1 | 1 | 2 | 2 | 3 |
| 20–34 | 57 | 1.4 | <1 | 1 | 1 | 1 | 2 | 2 | 3 | 4 |
| 35–49 | 80 | 1.6 | <1 | 1 | 1 | 1 | 2 | 3 | 4 | 4 |
| 50–64 | 86 | 1.6 | <1 | 1 | 1 | 1 | 2 | 2 | 3 | 4 |
| 65+ | 79 | 1.5 | 1 | 1 | 1 | 1 | 2 | 2 | 4 | 6 |
| **2. MULTIPLE DX** | | | | | | | | | | |
| 0–19 Years | 9 | 1.4 | <1 | 1 | 1 | 1 | 2 | 2 | 3 | 3 |
| 20–34 | 47 | 2.6 | 10 | 1 | 1 | 2 | 3 | 5 | 6 | 24 |
| 35–49 | 140 | 2.5 | 4 | 1 | 1 | 2 | 3 | 6 | 9 | 11 |
| 50–64 | 277 | 3.2 | 12 | 1 | 1 | 2 | 4 | 7 | 9 | 15 |
| 65+ | 1,106 | 4.5 | 34 | 1 | 1 | 3 | 5 | 10 | 15 | 31 |
| **TOTAL SINGLE DX** | 318 | 1.5 | <1 | 1 | 1 | 1 | 2 | 2 | 3 | 4 |
| **TOTAL MULTIPLE DX** | 1,579 | 4.0 | 27 | 1 | 1 | 2 | 4 | 9 | 13 | 31 |
| **TOTAL** | | | | | | | | | | |
| 0–19 Years | 25 | 1.2 | <1 | 1 | 1 | 1 | 1 | 2 | 2 | 3 |
| 20–34 | 104 | 1.9 | 5 | 1 | 1 | 1 | 2 | 3 | 4 | 11 |
| 35–49 | 220 | 2.2 | 3 | 1 | 1 | 2 | 4 | 6 | 6 | 11 |
| 50–64 | 363 | 2.9 | 10 | 1 | 1 | 2 | 4 | 6 | 9 | 15 |
| 65+ | 1,185 | 4.3 | 32 | 1 | 1 | 2 | 4 | 10 | 14 | 31 |
| **GRAND TOTAL** | 1,897 | 3.7 | 24 | 1 | 1 | 2 | 4 | 8 | 12 | 31 |

## 53.1: BILAT IH REPAIR. Formerly included in operation group(s) 633.

| Type of Patients | Observed Patients | Avg. Stay | Vari-ance | Percentiles | | | | | | |
|---|---|---|---|---|---|---|---|---|---|---|
| | | | | 10th | 25th | 50th | 75th | 90th | 95th | 99th |
| **1. SINGLE DX** | | | | | | | | | | |
| 0–19 Years | 380 | 1.2 | <1 | 1 | 1 | 1 | 1 | 2 | 2 | 4 |
| 20–34 | 20 | 1.0 | <1 | 1 | 1 | 1 | 1 | 1 | 1 | 2 |
| 35–49 | 66 | 1.9 | 2 | 1 | 1 | 1 | 3 | 4 | 4 | 4 |
| 50–64 | 75 | 1.4 | <1 | 1 | 1 | 1 | 2 | 2 | 3 | 7 |
| 65+ | 76 | 1.4 | <1 | 1 | 1 | 1 | 1 | 3 | 3 | 4 |
| **2. MULTIPLE DX** | | | | | | | | | | |
| 0–19 Years | 834 | 15.7 | 804 | 1 | 2 | 2 | 18 | 88 | >99 | >99 |
| 20–34 | 43 | 2.1 | 2 | 1 | 1 | 2 | 2 | 4 | 4 | 7 |
| 35–49 | 127 | 1.8 | 2 | 1 | 1 | 1 | 2 | 3 | 5 | 6 |
| 50–64 | 223 | 2.6 | 10 | 1 | 2 | 2 | 2 | 6 | 6 | 14 |
| 65+ | 787 | 3.0 | 12 | 1 | 1 | 2 | 4 | 7 | 10 | 16 |
| **TOTAL SINGLE DX** | 617 | 1.4 | <1 | 1 | 1 | 1 | 1 | 2 | 4 | 4 |
| **TOTAL MULTIPLE DX** | 2,014 | 8.0 | 373 | 1 | 2 | 2 | 4 | 36 | 80 | >99 |
| **TOTAL** | | | | | | | | | | |
| 0–19 Years | 1,214 | 9.9 | 532 | 1 | 1 | 1 | 3 | 67 | 92 | >99 |
| 20–34 | 63 | 1.7 | 2 | 1 | 1 | 1 | 2 | 3 | 4 | 7 |
| 35–49 | 193 | 1.8 | 2 | 1 | 1 | 1 | 2 | 5 | 5 | 6 |
| 50–64 | 298 | 2.4 | 9 | 1 | 1 | 2 | 2 | 5 | 6 | 11 |
| 65+ | 863 | 2.9 | 11 | 1 | 2 | 2 | 3 | 7 | 10 | 15 |
| **GRAND TOTAL** | 2,631 | 6.1 | 273 | 1 | 1 | 1 | 3 | 9 | 67 | >99 |

## 53.10: BILAT IH REPAIR NOS. Formerly included in operation group(s) 633.

| Type of Patients | Observed Patients | Avg. Stay | Vari-ance | Percentiles | | | | | | |
|---|---|---|---|---|---|---|---|---|---|---|
| | | | | 10th | 25th | 50th | 75th | 90th | 95th | 99th |
| **1. SINGLE DX** | | | | | | | | | | |
| 0–19 Years | 121 | 1.2 | <1 | 1 | 1 | 1 | 1 | 2 | 2 | 6 |
| 20–34 | 0 | | | | | | | | | |
| 35–49 | 3 | 1.0 | 0 | 1 | 1 | 1 | 2 | 3 | 3 | 3 |
| 50–64 | 5 | 1.7 | <1 | 1 | 1 | 1 | 2 | 3 | 3 | 3 |
| 65+ | 4 | 2.0 | <1 | 1 | 2 | 2 | 3 | 3 | 3 | 3 |
| **2. MULTIPLE DX** | | | | | | | | | | |
| 0–19 Years | 333 | 27.1 | >999 | 1 | 1 | 5 | 68 | >99 | >99 | >99 |
| 20–34 | 3 | 2.3 | 2 | 1 | 2 | 2 | 4 | 4 | 4 | 4 |
| 35–49 | 4 | 3.3 | 5 | 1 | 2 | 2 | 5 | 6 | 6 | 6 |
| 50–64 | 13 | 4.5 | 9 | 1 | 2 | 5 | 6 | 8 | 11 | 11 |
| 65+ | 36 | 2.3 | 5 | 1 | 1 | 1 | 2 | 5 | 7 | 10 |
| **TOTAL SINGLE DX** | 133 | 1.2 | <1 | 1 | 1 | 1 | 1 | 2 | 2 | 6 |
| **TOTAL MULTIPLE DX** | 389 | 21.3 | >999 | 1 | 1 | 3 | 63 | 98 | >99 | >99 |
| **TOTAL** | | | | | | | | | | |
| 0–19 Years | 454 | 19.1 | 957 | 1 | 1 | 2 | 57 | 98 | >99 | >99 |
| 20–34 | 3 | 2.3 | 2 | 1 | 2 | 2 | 4 | 4 | 4 | 4 |
| 35–49 | 7 | 1.8 | 3 | 1 | 1 | 1 | 2 | 5 | 6 | 6 |
| 50–64 | 18 | 3.6 | 8 | 1 | 1 | 1 | 2 | 6 | 11 | 11 |
| 65+ | 40 | 2.3 | 5 | 1 | 1 | 1 | 3 | 5 | 7 | 10 |
| **GRAND TOTAL** | 522 | 15.9 | 817 | 1 | 1 | 2 | 36 | 91 | >99 | >99 |

Length of Stay by Diagnosis and Operation, United States, 2000

# United States, October 1998–September 1999 Data, by Operation

## 53.12: BILAT INDIRECT IH REPAIR. Formerly included in operation group(s) 633.

| Type of Patients | Observed Patients | Avg. Stay | Variance | Percentiles | | | | | | |
|---|---|---|---|---|---|---|---|---|---|---|
| | | | | 10th | 25th | 50th | 75th | 90th | 95th | 99th |
| **1. SINGLE DX** | | | | | | | | | | |
| 0–19 Years | 222 | 1.2 | <1 | 1 | 1 | 1 | 1 | 2 | 2 | 3 |
| 20–34 | 2 | 1.0 | 0 | 1 | 1 | 1 | 1 | 1 | 1 | 1 |
| 35–49 | 0 | | | | | | | | | |
| 50–64 | 1 | 3.0 | 0 | 3 | 3 | 3 | 3 | 3 | 3 | 3 |
| 65+ | 4 | 2.4 | 2 | 1 | 1 | 3 | 3 | 4 | 4 | 4 |
| **2. MULTIPLE DX** | | | | | | | | | | |
| 0–19 Years | 430 | 9.9 | 524 | 1 | 1 | 1 | 3 | 65 | 82 | >99 |
| 20–34 | 1 | 2.0 | 0 | 2 | 2 | 2 | 2 | 2 | 2 | 2 |
| 35–49 | 4 | 4.9 | 6 | 1 | 2 | 6 | 6 | 6 | 9 | 9 |
| 50–64 | 4 | 3.3 | 12 | 1 | 1 | 2 | 4 | 10 | 10 | 10 |
| 65+ | 31 | 2.3 | 3 | 1 | 1 | 1 | 4 | 4 | 5 | 9 |
| **TOTAL SINGLE DX** | 229 | 1.2 | <1 | 1 | 1 | 1 | 1 | 2 | 2 | 3 |
| **TOTAL MULTIPLE DX** | 470 | 9.5 | 499 | 1 | 1 | 1 | 3 | 64 | 82 | >99 |
| **TOTAL** | | | | | | | | | | |
| 0–19 Years | 652 | 6.1 | 316 | 1 | 1 | 1 | 2 | 7 | 75 | >99 |
| 20–34 | 3 | 1.2 | <1 | 1 | 1 | 1 | 1 | 2 | 2 | 2 |
| 35–49 | 4 | 4.9 | 6 | 1 | 2 | 6 | 6 | 6 | 9 | 9 |
| 50–64 | 5 | 3.3 | 10 | 1 | 1 | 2 | 4 | 10 | 10 | 10 |
| 65+ | 35 | 2.3 | 3 | 1 | 1 | 1 | 4 | 4 | 5 | 9 |
| **GRAND TOTAL** | 699 | 6.0 | 306 | 1 | 1 | 1 | 2 | 7 | 72 | >99 |

## 53.17: BILAT IH REP-GRAFT NOS. Formerly included in operation group(s) 633.

| Type of Patients | Observed Patients | Avg. Stay | Variance | Percentiles | | | | | | |
|---|---|---|---|---|---|---|---|---|---|---|
| | | | | 10th | 25th | 50th | 75th | 90th | 95th | 99th |
| **1. SINGLE DX** | | | | | | | | | | |
| 0–19 Years | 1 | 1.0 | 0 | 1 | 1 | 1 | 1 | 1 | 1 | 1 |
| 20–34 | 8 | 1.1 | <1 | 1 | 1 | 1 | 1 | 1 | 2 | 2 |
| 35–49 | 13 | 1.7 | <1 | 1 | 1 | 2 | 2 | 3 | 3 | 3 |
| 50–64 | 21 | 1.5 | <1 | 1 | 1 | 1 | 2 | 2 | 2 | 6 |
| 65+ | 18 | 1.2 | <1 | 1 | 1 | 1 | 1 | 1 | 3 | 3 |
| **2. MULTIPLE DX** | | | | | | | | | | |
| 0–19 Years | 2 | 7.2 | 39 | 3 | 3 | >99 | >99 | >99 | >99 | >99 |
| 20–34 | 6 | 1.4 | <1 | 1 | 1 | 1 | 1 | 2 | 2 | 2 |
| 35–49 | 19 | 1.2 | <1 | 1 | 1 | 1 | 1 | 1 | 2 | 2 |
| 50–64 | 54 | 2.2 | 2 | 1 | 1 | 2 | 2 | 4 | 5 | 8 |
| 65+ | 172 | 3.7 | 10 | 1 | 1 | 3 | 3 | 8 | 10 | 14 |
| **TOTAL SINGLE DX** | 61 | 1.3 | <1 | 1 | 1 | 1 | 1 | 2 | 3 | 4 |
| **TOTAL MULTIPLE DX** | 253 | 2.7 | 7 | 1 | 1 | 2 | 3 | 6 | 8 | 13 |
| **TOTAL** | | | | | | | | | | |
| 0–19 Years | 3 | 5.5 | 35 | 1 | 1 | 13 | >99 | >99 | >99 | >99 |
| 20–34 | 14 | 1.2 | <1 | 1 | 1 | 1 | 1 | 2 | 2 | 2 |
| 35–49 | 32 | 1.2 | <1 | 1 | 1 | 1 | 1 | 1 | 2 | 2 |
| 50–64 | 75 | 2.1 | 2 | 1 | 1 | 2 | 2 | 4 | 5 | 8 |
| 65+ | 190 | 3.4 | 9 | 1 | 1 | 3 | 3 | 8 | 10 | 12 |
| **GRAND TOTAL** | 314 | 2.6 | 6 | 1 | 1 | 2 | 3 | 6 | 8 | 12 |

## 53.14: BILAT DIRECT IH REP-GRFT. Formerly included in operation group(s) 633.

| Type of Patients | Observed Patients | Avg. Stay | Variance | Percentiles | | | | | | |
|---|---|---|---|---|---|---|---|---|---|---|
| | | | | 10th | 25th | 50th | 75th | 90th | 95th | 99th |
| **1. SINGLE DX** | | | | | | | | | | |
| 0–19 Years | 0 | | | | | | | | | |
| 20–34 | 5 | 1.2 | <1 | 1 | 1 | 1 | 1 | 2 | 2 | 2 |
| 35–49 | 27 | 2.4 | 2 | 1 | 1 | 1 | 4 | 4 | 4 | 4 |
| 50–64 | 29 | 1.6 | 2 | 1 | 1 | 1 | 2 | 2 | 3 | 7 |
| 65+ | 29 | 1.2 | <1 | 1 | 1 | 1 | 1 | 2 | 2 | 4 |
| **2. MULTIPLE DX** | | | | | | | | | | |
| 0–19 Years | 0 | | | | | | | | | |
| 20–34 | 12 | 2.1 | 1 | 1 | 1 | 2 | 2 | 3 | 7 | 7 |
| 35–49 | 54 | 2.0 | 1 | 1 | 1 | 2 | 2 | 3 | 7 | 8 |
| 50–64 | 71 | 3.2 | 32 | 1 | 1 | 2 | 3 | 6 | 10 | 36 |
| 65+ | 212 | 3.5 | 20 | 1 | 1 | 2 | 4 | 10 | 11 | 15 |
| **TOTAL SINGLE DX** | 90 | 2.1 | 2 | 1 | 1 | 1 | 4 | 4 | 4 | 5 |
| **TOTAL MULTIPLE DX** | 349 | 3.1 | 19 | 1 | 1 | 2 | 3 | 8 | 10 | 15 |
| **TOTAL** | | | | | | | | | | |
| 0–19 Years | 0 | | | | | | | | | |
| 20–34 | 17 | 1.9 | 2 | 1 | 1 | 2 | 2 | 3 | 3 | 7 |
| 35–49 | 81 | 2.3 | 2 | 1 | 1 | 2 | 3 | 4 | 4 | 5 |
| 50–64 | 100 | 2.8 | 25 | 1 | 1 | 1 | 2 | 5 | 7 | 36 |
| 65+ | 241 | 3.3 | 19 | 1 | 1 | 1 | 4 | 10 | 11 | 15 |
| **GRAND TOTAL** | 439 | 2.8 | 14 | 1 | 1 | 2 | 3 | 6 | 10 | 14 |

## 53.2: UNILAT FH REPAIR. Formerly included in operation group(s) 634.

| Type of Patients | Observed Patients | Avg. Stay | Variance | Percentiles | | | | | | |
|---|---|---|---|---|---|---|---|---|---|---|
| | | | | 10th | 25th | 50th | 75th | 90th | 95th | 99th |
| **1. SINGLE DX** | | | | | | | | | | |
| 0–19 Years | 6 | 1.4 | <1 | 1 | 1 | 1 | 2 | 2 | 3 | 3 |
| 20–34 | 17 | 1.4 | <1 | 1 | 1 | 1 | 1 | 3 | 3 | 3 |
| 35–49 | 43 | 1.8 | <1 | 1 | 2 | 2 | 2 | 2 | 7 | 7 |
| 50–64 | 28 | 2.0 | <1 | 2 | 2 | 2 | 3 | 4 | 4 | 4 |
| 65+ | 58 | 2.1 | 3 | 1 | 1 | 1 | 3 | 4 | 5 | 8 |
| **2. MULTIPLE DX** | | | | | | | | | | |
| 0–19 Years | 3 | 1.3 | <1 | 1 | 1 | 1 | 2 | 2 | 2 | 2 |
| 20–34 | 13 | 4.1 | 13 | 1 | 3 | 3 | 7 | 11 | 11 | 11 |
| 35–49 | 49 | 3.0 | 7 | 1 | 2 | 2 | 6 | 8 | 9 | 11 |
| 50–64 | 108 | 4.8 | 24 | 2 | 2 | 4 | 7 | 15 | 15 | 15 |
| 65+ | 678 | 5.4 | 28 | 1 | 2 | 4 | 7 | 11 | 15 | 27 |
| **TOTAL SINGLE DX** | 152 | 1.9 | 1 | 1 | 1 | 1 | 2 | 4 | 4 | 7 |
| **TOTAL MULTIPLE DX** | 851 | 5.1 | 26 | 1 | 2 | 4 | 7 | 11 | 15 | 25 |
| **TOTAL** | | | | | | | | | | |
| 0–19 Years | 9 | 1.4 | <1 | 1 | 1 | 1 | 2 | 2 | 3 | 3 |
| 20–34 | 30 | 2.1 | 5 | 1 | 1 | 1 | 3 | 4 | 4 | 11 |
| 35–49 | 92 | 2.4 | 4 | 1 | 1 | 1 | 3 | 4 | 8 | 10 |
| 50–64 | 136 | 4.0 | 19 | 2 | 2 | 2 | 4 | 15 | 15 | 15 |
| 65+ | 736 | 5.1 | 26 | 1 | 2 | 4 | 7 | 10 | 14 | 27 |
| **GRAND TOTAL** | 1,003 | 4.5 | 23 | 1 | 2 | 3 | 6 | 10 | 15 | 21 |

Length of Stay by Diagnosis and Operation, United States, 2000

## 53.21: UNILAT FH REP W GRAFT. Formerly included in operation group(s) 634.

| Type of Patients | Observed Patients | Avg. Stay | Variance | Percentiles | | | | | | |
|---|---|---|---|---|---|---|---|---|---|---|
| | | | | 10th | 25th | 50th | 75th | 90th | 95th | 99th |
| **1. SINGLE DX** | | | | | | | | | | |
| 0–19 Years | 0 | | | | | | | | | |
| 20–34 | 7 | 1.4 | <1 | 1 | 1 | 1 | 2 | 3 | 3 | 3 |
| 35–49 | 26 | 1.8 | <1 | 1 | 1 | 1 | 2 | 3 | 3 | 7 |
| 50–64 | 13 | 2.1 | <1 | 1 | 2 | 2 | 2 | 4 | 4 | 4 |
| 65+ | 35 | 2.0 | 2 | 1 | 1 | 1 | 4 | 4 | 4 | 7 |
| **2. MULTIPLE DX** | | | | | | | | | | |
| 0–19 Years | 2 | 1.5 | <1 | 1 | 1 | 1 | 2 | 2 | 2 | 2 |
| 20–34 | 5 | 4.7 | 19 | 1 | 1 | 4 | 11 | 11 | 11 | 11 |
| 35–49 | 27 | 3.1 | 7 | 1 | 1 | 2 | 4 | 8 | 8 | 14 |
| 50–64 | 61 | 2.5 | 4 | 1 | 1 | 2 | 2 | 5 | 6 | 9 |
| 65+ | 319 | 4.4 | 17 | 1 | 2 | 3 | 6 | 9 | 11 | 20 |
| **TOTAL SINGLE DX** | 81 | 1.9 | 1 | 1 | 1 | 2 | 2 | 4 | 4 | 5 |
| **TOTAL MULTIPLE DX** | 414 | 3.9 | 14 | 1 | 2 | 2 | 5 | 8 | 11 | 16 |
| **TOTAL** | | | | | | | | | | |
| 0–19 Years | 2 | 1.5 | <1 | 1 | 1 | 1 | 2 | 2 | 2 | 2 |
| 20–34 | 12 | 1.9 | 5 | 1 | 1 | 1 | 2 | 3 | 4 | 11 |
| 35–49 | 53 | 2.5 | 5 | 1 | 1 | 2 | 3 | 5 | 8 | 9 |
| 50–64 | 74 | 2.3 | 3 | 1 | 1 | 2 | 2 | 4 | 6 | 9 |
| 65+ | 354 | 4.1 | 16 | 1 | 2 | 3 | 6 | 8 | 11 | 18 |
| **GRAND TOTAL** | 495 | 3.4 | 12 | 1 | 1 | 2 | 4 | 7 | 9 | 16 |

## 53.29: UNILAT FH REP NEC. Formerly included in operation group(s) 634.

| Type of Patients | Observed Patients | Avg. Stay | Variance | Percentiles | | | | | | |
|---|---|---|---|---|---|---|---|---|---|---|
| | | | | 10th | 25th | 50th | 75th | 90th | 95th | 99th |
| **1. SINGLE DX** | | | | | | | | | | |
| 0–19 Years | 6 | 1.4 | <1 | 1 | 1 | 1 | 2 | 2 | 3 | 3 |
| 20–34 | 10 | 1.3 | <1 | 1 | 1 | 1 | 2 | 2 | 3 | 3 |
| 35–49 | 17 | 1.8 | <1 | 1 | 1 | 2 | 2 | 2 | 3 | 3 |
| 50–64 | 15 | 1.5 | <1 | 1 | 1 | 1 | 2 | 2 | 3 | 3 |
| 65+ | 23 | 2.2 | 4 | 1 | 1 | 1 | 2 | 6 | 8 | 8 |
| **2. MULTIPLE DX** | | | | | | | | | | |
| 0–19 Years | 1 | 1.0 | 0 | 1 | 1 | 1 | 1 | 1 | 1 | 1 |
| 20–34 | 8 | 3.6 | 8 | 1 | 3 | 3 | 5 | 9 | 9 | 9 |
| 35–49 | 22 | 2.8 | 6 | 1 | 2 | 2 | 3 | 4 | 8 | 11 |
| 50–64 | 47 | 8.0 | 33 | 2 | 2 | 6 | 15 | 15 | 15 | 15 |
| 65+ | 359 | 6.4 | 37 | 1 | 3 | 5 | 8 | 12 | 16 | 31 |
| **TOTAL SINGLE DX** | 71 | 1.8 | 2 | 1 | 1 | 2 | 2 | 3 | 3 | 8 |
| **TOTAL MULTIPLE DX** | 437 | 6.5 | 36 | 1 | 3 | 5 | 8 | 15 | 15 | 27 |
| **TOTAL** | | | | | | | | | | |
| 0–19 Years | 7 | 1.3 | <1 | 1 | 1 | 1 | 1 | 2 | 3 | 3 |
| 20–34 | 18 | 2.5 | 6 | 1 | 1 | 1 | 3 | 7 | 9 | 9 |
| 35–49 | 39 | 2.2 | 3 | 1 | 1 | 2 | 2 | 3 | 4 | 10 |
| 50–64 | 62 | 7.1 | 33 | 1 | 3 | 5 | 15 | 15 | 15 | 15 |
| 65+ | 382 | 6.2 | 36 | 1 | 3 | 5 | 8 | 12 | 15 | 30 |
| **GRAND TOTAL** | 508 | 5.9 | 34 | 1 | 2 | 4 | 8 | 15 | 15 | 27 |

## 53.3: BILAT FH REPAIR. Formerly included in operation group(s) 634.

| Type of Patients | Observed Patients | Avg. Stay | Variance | Percentiles | | | | | | |
|---|---|---|---|---|---|---|---|---|---|---|
| | | | | 10th | 25th | 50th | 75th | 90th | 95th | 99th |
| **1. SINGLE DX** | | | | | | | | | | |
| 0–19 Years | 1 | 1.0 | 0 | 1 | 1 | 1 | 1 | 1 | 1 | 1 |
| 20–34 | 0 | | | | | | | | | |
| 35–49 | 1 | 2.0 | 0 | 2 | 2 | 2 | 2 | 2 | 2 | 2 |
| 50–64 | 1 | 2.0 | 0 | 2 | 2 | 2 | 2 | 2 | 2 | 2 |
| 65+ | 1 | 7.0 | 0 | 7 | 7 | 7 | 7 | 7 | 7 | 7 |
| **2. MULTIPLE DX** | | | | | | | | | | |
| 0–19 Years | 0 | | | | | | | | | |
| 20–34 | 0 | | | | | | | | | |
| 35–49 | 2 | 1.0 | 0 | 1 | 1 | 1 | 1 | 1 | 1 | 1 |
| 50–64 | 1 | 2.0 | 0 | 2 | 2 | 2 | 2 | 2 | 2 | 2 |
| 65+ | 13 | 4.3 | 18 | 1 | 1 | 5 | 5 | 7 | 9 | 20 |
| **TOTAL SINGLE DX** | 4 | 3.5 | 6 | 2 | 2 | 2 | 7 | 7 | 7 | 7 |
| **TOTAL MULTIPLE DX** | 16 | 2.7 | 12 | 1 | 1 | 1 | 5 | 6 | 7 | 20 |
| **TOTAL** | | | | | | | | | | |
| 0–19 Years | 1 | 1.0 | 0 | 1 | 1 | 1 | 1 | 1 | 1 | 1 |
| 20–34 | 0 | | | | | | | | | |
| 35–49 | 3 | 1.1 | <1 | 1 | 1 | 1 | 2 | 2 | 2 | 2 |
| 50–64 | 2 | 2.0 | 0 | 2 | 2 | 2 | 2 | 2 | 2 | 2 |
| 65+ | 14 | 4.5 | 17 | 1 | 1 | 5 | 6 | 7 | 9 | 20 |
| **GRAND TOTAL** | 20 | 2.8 | 11 | 1 | 1 | 1 | 5 | 6 | 7 | 20 |

## 53.4: UMBILICAL HERNIA REPAIR. Formerly included in operation group(s) 635.

| Type of Patients | Observed Patients | Avg. Stay | Variance | Percentiles | | | | | | |
|---|---|---|---|---|---|---|---|---|---|---|
| | | | | 10th | 25th | 50th | 75th | 90th | 95th | 99th |
| **1. SINGLE DX** | | | | | | | | | | |
| 0–19 Years | 110 | 1.3 | 2 | 1 | 1 | 1 | 1 | 2 | 4 | 6 |
| 20–34 | 116 | 1.5 | <1 | 1 | 1 | 1 | 2 | 3 | 3 | 4 |
| 35–49 | 219 | 1.5 | <1 | 1 | 1 | 1 | 2 | 2 | 3 | 5 |
| 50–64 | 118 | 1.8 | 3 | 1 | 1 | 1 | 2 | 3 | 4 | 5 |
| 65+ | 78 | 1.9 | 2 | 1 | 1 | 2 | 2 | 4 | 4 | 7 |
| **2. MULTIPLE DX** | | | | | | | | | | |
| 0–19 Years | 192 | 8.6 | 166 | 1 | 1 | 3 | 14 | 26 | 72 | >99 |
| 20–34 | 213 | 2.4 | 4 | 1 | 1 | 2 | 3 | 5 | 6 | 9 |
| 35–49 | 772 | 3.5 | 9 | 1 | 2 | 3 | 5 | 6 | 9 | 14 |
| 50–64 | 823 | 3.8 | 15 | 1 | 2 | 3 | 5 | 7 | 10 | 21 |
| 65+ | 1,153 | 4.9 | 26 | 1 | 2 | 3 | 6 | 10 | 14 | 29 |
| **TOTAL SINGLE DX** | 641 | 1.5 | 1 | 1 | 1 | 1 | 2 | 3 | 4 | 5 |
| **TOTAL MULTIPLE DX** | 3,153 | 4.3 | 28 | 1 | 2 | 3 | 5 | 9 | 13 | 29 |
| **TOTAL** | | | | | | | | | | |
| 0–19 Years | 302 | 5.4 | 106 | 1 | 1 | 1 | 5 | 17 | 26 | >99 |
| 20–34 | 329 | 2.0 | 3 | 1 | 1 | 2 | 2 | 4 | 6 | 7 |
| 35–49 | 991 | 3.1 | 8 | 1 | 1 | 2 | 4 | 6 | 8 | 12 |
| 50–64 | 941 | 3.6 | 15 | 1 | 1 | 3 | 6 | 7 | 10 | 20 |
| 65+ | 1,231 | 4.7 | 25 | 1 | 2 | 3 | 6 | 10 | 13 | 29 |
| **GRAND TOTAL** | 3,794 | 3.8 | 24 | 1 | 1 | 2 | 5 | 8 | 12 | 27 |

Length of Stay by Diagnosis and Operation, United States, 2000

# United States, October 1998–September 1999 Data, by Operation

## 53.41: UMB HERNIA REPAIR-GRAFT. Formerly included in operation group(s) 635.

| Type of Patients | Observed Patients | Avg. Stay | Vari-ance | Percentiles | | | | | | |
|---|---|---|---|---|---|---|---|---|---|---|
| | | | | 10th | 25th | 50th | 75th | 90th | 95th | 99th |
| 1. SINGLE DX | | | | | | | | | | |
| 0–19 Years | 0 | | | | | | | | | |
| 20–34 | 20 | 1.3 | <1 | 1 | 1 | 1 | 1 | 3 | 3 | 3 |
| 35–49 | 57 | 1.2 | <1 | 1 | 1 | 1 | 1 | 2 | 3 | 4 |
| 50–64 | 52 | 1.9 | 1 | 1 | 1 | 2 | 2 | 3 | 3 | 5 |
| 65+ | 27 | 1.8 | 1 | 1 | 1 | 2 | 2 | 3 | 3 | 8 |
| 2. MULTIPLE DX | | | | | | | | | | |
| 0–19 Years | 12 | 34.8 | 452 | 18 | 26 | 51 | >99 | >99 | >99 | >99 |
| 20–34 | 44 | 2.0 | 1 | 1 | 1 | 2 | 3 | 3 | 4 | 7 |
| 35–49 | 200 | 3.1 | 6 | 1 | 1 | 2 | 4 | 7 | 10 | 11 |
| 50–64 | 244 | 3.0 | 11 | 1 | 2 | 2 | 3 | 7 | 9 | 19 |
| 65+ | 329 | 3.8 | 13 | 1 | 2 | 2 | 5 | 7 | 10 | 22 |
| TOTAL SINGLE DX | 156 | 1.5 | <1 | 1 | 1 | 1 | 2 | 3 | 4 | 4 |
| TOTAL MULTIPLE DX | 829 | 3.6 | 23 | 1 | 1 | 2 | 4 | 7 | 10 | 31 |
| TOTAL | | | | | | | | | | |
| 0–19 Years | 12 | 34.8 | 452 | 18 | 26 | 51 | >99 | >99 | >99 | >99 |
| 20–34 | 64 | 1.9 | 1 | 1 | 1 | 1 | 3 | 3 | 4 | 7 |
| 35–49 | 257 | 2.6 | 5 | 1 | 1 | 2 | 3 | 5 | 8 | 11 |
| 50–64 | 296 | 2.9 | 10 | 1 | 2 | 2 | 3 | 7 | 9 | 17 |
| 65+ | 356 | 3.7 | 13 | 1 | 2 | 2 | 5 | 7 | 10 | 19 |
| GRAND TOTAL | 985 | 3.2 | 20 | 1 | 1 | 2 | 4 | 7 | 10 | 26 |

## 53.49: UMB HERNIA REPAIR NEC. Formerly included in operation group(s) 635.

| Type of Patients | Observed Patients | Avg. Stay | Vari-ance | Percentiles | | | | | | |
|---|---|---|---|---|---|---|---|---|---|---|
| | | | | 10th | 25th | 50th | 75th | 90th | 95th | 99th |
| 1. SINGLE DX | | | | | | | | | | |
| 0–19 Years | 110 | 1.3 | 2 | 1 | 1 | 1 | 1 | 2 | 4 | 6 |
| 20–34 | 96 | 1.5 | <1 | 1 | 1 | 1 | 2 | 3 | 3 | 4 |
| 35–49 | 162 | 1.6 | <1 | 1 | 1 | 1 | 2 | 2 | 3 | 5 |
| 50–64 | 66 | 1.7 | 4 | 1 | 1 | 1 | 2 | 3 | 4 | 5 |
| 65+ | 51 | 2.0 | 2 | 1 | 1 | 1 | 2 | 4 | 4 | 7 |
| 2. MULTIPLE DX | | | | | | | | | | |
| 0–19 Years | 180 | 7.5 | 123 | 1 | 1 | 3 | 12 | 17 | 25 | >99 |
| 20–34 | 169 | 2.6 | 5 | 1 | 2 | 2 | 3 | 6 | 6 | 11 |
| 35–49 | 572 | 3.7 | 10 | 1 | 2 | 3 | 5 | 6 | 7 | 14 |
| 50–64 | 579 | 4.3 | 18 | 1 | 2 | 3 | 6 | 7 | 11 | 22 |
| 65+ | 824 | 5.4 | 32 | 1 | 2 | 4 | 7 | 11 | 15 | 29 |
| TOTAL SINGLE DX | 485 | 1.6 | 1 | 1 | 1 | 1 | 2 | 3 | 4 | 5 |
| TOTAL MULTIPLE DX | 2,324 | 4.6 | 30 | 1 | 2 | 3 | 6 | 9 | 14 | 29 |
| TOTAL | | | | | | | | | | |
| 0–19 Years | 290 | 4.7 | 77 | 1 | 1 | 1 | 4 | 15 | 20 | 74 |
| 20–34 | 265 | 2.1 | 3 | 1 | 1 | 1 | 2 | 4 | 6 | 7 |
| 35–49 | 734 | 3.3 | 9 | 1 | 1 | 2 | 4 | 6 | 8 | 14 |
| 50–64 | 645 | 4.0 | 17 | 1 | 2 | 3 | 5 | 7 | 10 | 22 |
| 65+ | 875 | 5.2 | 30 | 1 | 2 | 4 | 7 | 11 | 14 | 29 |
| GRAND TOTAL | 2,809 | 4.0 | 26 | 1 | 1 | 2 | 5 | 8 | 13 | 27 |

## 53.5: REP OTH ABD WALL HERNIA. Formerly included in operation group(s) 636.

| Type of Patients | Observed Patients | Avg. Stay | Vari-ance | Percentiles | | | | | | |
|---|---|---|---|---|---|---|---|---|---|---|
| | | | | 10th | 25th | 50th | 75th | 90th | 95th | 99th |
| 1. SINGLE DX | | | | | | | | | | |
| 0–19 Years | 44 | 1.8 | 3 | 1 | 1 | 1 | 2 | 3 | 4 | 11 |
| 20–34 | 135 | 1.7 | 1 | 1 | 1 | 1 | 2 | 3 | 3 | 6 |
| 35–49 | 257 | 2.3 | 2 | 1 | 1 | 1 | 3 | 4 | 5 | 7 |
| 50–64 | 189 | 2.3 | 2 | 1 | 1 | 2 | 3 | 4 | 5 | 7 |
| 65+ | 151 | 2.2 | 2 | 1 | 1 | 2 | 3 | 4 | 5 | 7 |
| 2. MULTIPLE DX | | | | | | | | | | |
| 0–19 Years | 95 | 2.8 | 21 | 1 | 1 | 1 | 3 | 6 | 8 | 40 |
| 20–34 | 314 | 2.8 | 6 | 1 | 2 | 2 | 3 | 5 | 7 | 12 |
| 35–49 | 1,104 | 3.6 | 17 | 1 | 2 | 2 | 4 | 7 | 9 | 18 |
| 50–64 | 1,268 | 4.0 | 13 | 1 | 3 | 3 | 5 | 8 | 10 | 17 |
| 65+ | 1,853 | 5.1 | 30 | 1 | 4 | 4 | 7 | 10 | 14 | 26 |
| TOTAL SINGLE DX | 776 | 2.1 | 2 | 1 | 1 | 2 | 3 | 4 | 5 | 7 |
| TOTAL MULTIPLE DX | 4,634 | 4.2 | 20 | 1 | 3 | 3 | 5 | 8 | 11 | 21 |
| TOTAL | | | | | | | | | | |
| 0–19 Years | 139 | 2.4 | 13 | 1 | 1 | 1 | 3 | 5 | 7 | 19 |
| 20–34 | 449 | 2.5 | 4 | 1 | 2 | 2 | 3 | 4 | 6 | 12 |
| 35–49 | 1,361 | 3.4 | 14 | 1 | 2 | 2 | 4 | 7 | 8 | 18 |
| 50–64 | 1,457 | 3.8 | 11 | 1 | 2 | 3 | 4 | 8 | 9 | 17 |
| 65+ | 2,004 | 4.9 | 29 | 1 | 3 | 4 | 7 | 10 | 14 | 26 |
| GRAND TOTAL | 5,410 | 3.9 | 18 | 1 | 2 | 3 | 5 | 8 | 11 | 19 |

## 53.51: INCISIONAL HERNIA REPAIR. Formerly included in operation group(s) 636.

| Type of Patients | Observed Patients | Avg. Stay | Vari-ance | Percentiles | | | | | | |
|---|---|---|---|---|---|---|---|---|---|---|
| | | | | 10th | 25th | 50th | 75th | 90th | 95th | 99th |
| 1. SINGLE DX | | | | | | | | | | |
| 0–19 Years | 17 | 1.8 | 4 | 1 | 1 | 1 | 2 | 3 | 7 | 11 |
| 20–34 | 60 | 2.1 | <1 | 1 | 2 | 2 | 3 | 3 | 4 | 5 |
| 35–49 | 137 | 2.2 | 1 | 1 | 2 | 2 | 3 | 4 | 5 | 6 |
| 50–64 | 110 | 2.2 | 1 | 1 | 2 | 2 | 3 | 4 | 5 | 7 |
| 65+ | 101 | 2.3 | 2 | 1 | 1 | 2 | 3 | 4 | 5 | 7 |
| 2. MULTIPLE DX | | | | | | | | | | |
| 0–19 Years | 51 | 2.2 | 5 | 1 | 1 | 1 | 2 | 5 | 6 | 9 |
| 20–34 | 193 | 2.8 | 6 | 1 | 2 | 2 | 3 | 5 | 8 | 12 |
| 35–49 | 710 | 3.6 | 10 | 1 | 2 | 3 | 5 | 7 | 10 | 14 |
| 50–64 | 828 | 3.9 | 14 | 1 | 2 | 3 | 5 | 7 | 10 | 18 |
| 65+ | 1,209 | 5.0 | 29 | 1 | 3 | 4 | 7 | 10 | 14 | 26 |
| TOTAL SINGLE DX | 425 | 2.2 | 2 | 1 | 1 | 2 | 3 | 4 | 5 | 7 |
| TOTAL MULTIPLE DX | 2,991 | 4.2 | 19 | 1 | 2 | 3 | 5 | 8 | 11 | 21 |
| TOTAL | | | | | | | | | | |
| 0–19 Years | 68 | 2.0 | 4 | 1 | 1 | 1 | 2 | 4 | 6 | 11 |
| 20–34 | 253 | 2.6 | 5 | 1 | 2 | 2 | 3 | 5 | 8 | 12 |
| 35–49 | 847 | 3.3 | 9 | 1 | 2 | 2 | 4 | 6 | 8 | 13 |
| 50–64 | 938 | 3.6 | 12 | 1 | 2 | 3 | 4 | 7 | 9 | 17 |
| 65+ | 1,310 | 4.8 | 27 | 1 | 2 | 3 | 6 | 10 | 13 | 26 |
| GRAND TOTAL | 3,416 | 3.9 | 17 | 1 | 2 | 3 | 5 | 8 | 11 | 19 |

Length of Stay by Diagnosis and Operation, United States, 2000

# United States, October 1998–September 1999 Data, by Operation

## 53.59: ABD WALL HERNIA REP NEC. Formerly included in operation group(s) 636.

| Type of Patients | Observed Patients | Avg. Stay | Variance | 10th | 25th | 50th | 75th | 90th | 95th | 99th |
|---|---|---|---|---|---|---|---|---|---|---|
| **1. SINGLE DX** | | | | | | | | | | |
| 0–19 Years | 27 | 1.9 | 1 | 1 | 1 | 1 | 3 | 3 | 4 | 5 |
| 20–34 | 75 | 1.5 | 1 | 1 | 1 | 1 | 2 | 2 | 4 | 8 |
| 35–49 | 120 | 2.3 | 3 | 1 | 1 | 2 | 3 | 5 | 6 | 8 |
| 50–64 | 79 | 2.6 | 4 | 1 | 1 | 2 | 3 | 6 | 7 | 8 |
| 65+ | 50 | 2.1 | 2 | 1 | 1 | 1 | 3 | 5 | 5 | 8 |
| **2. MULTIPLE DX** | | | | | | | | | | |
| 0–19 Years | 44 | 3.8 | 45 | 1 | 1 | 2 | 3 | 8 | 10 | 40 |
| 20–34 | 121 | 2.7 | 5 | 1 | 2 | 2 | 3 | 5 | 6 | 11 |
| 35–49 | 394 | 3.7 | 26 | 1 | 1 | 2 | 4 | 7 | 9 | 19 |
| 50–64 | 440 | 4.1 | 11 | 1 | 2 | 4 | 5 | 9 | 10 | 19 |
| 65+ | 644 | 5.3 | 33 | 1 | 2 | 4 | 7 | 10 | 15 | 29 |
| **TOTAL SINGLE DX** | 351 | 2.0 | 2 | 1 | 1 | 1 | 3 | 4 | 6 | 8 |
| **TOTAL MULTIPLE DX** | 1,643 | 4.3 | 23 | 1 | 2 | 3 | 5 | 9 | 12 | 21 |
| **TOTAL** | | | | | | | | | | |
| 0–19 Years | 71 | 3.0 | 27 | 1 | 1 | 3 | 3 | 5 | 8 | 40 |
| 20–34 | 196 | 2.2 | 4 | 1 | 1 | 2 | 2 | 4 | 6 | 9 |
| 35–49 | 514 | 3.5 | 23 | 1 | 1 | 2 | 4 | 7 | 9 | 19 |
| 50–64 | 519 | 4.0 | 10 | 1 | 2 | 3 | 5 | 8 | 10 | 15 |
| 65+ | 694 | 5.1 | 31 | 1 | 2 | 3 | 6 | 10 | 14 | 29 |
| **GRAND TOTAL** | 1,994 | 3.9 | 20 | 1 | 1 | 3 | 5 | 8 | 10 | 19 |

## 53.61: INC HERNIA REPAIR-GRAFT. Formerly included in operation group(s) 636.

| Type of Patients | Observed Patients | Avg. Stay | Variance | 10th | 25th | 50th | 75th | 90th | 95th | 99th |
|---|---|---|---|---|---|---|---|---|---|---|
| **1. SINGLE DX** | | | | | | | | | | |
| 0–19 Years | 3 | 1.1 | <1 | 1 | 1 | 1 | 1 | 1 | 1 | 5 |
| 20–34 | 147 | 2.5 | 1 | 1 | 2 | 2 | 3 | 4 | 5 | 7 |
| 35–49 | 540 | 2.5 | 2 | 1 | 2 | 2 | 3 | 4 | 5 | 7 |
| 50–64 | 452 | 2.4 | 2 | 1 | 1 | 2 | 3 | 4 | 5 | 7 |
| 65+ | 369 | 2.5 | 3 | 1 | 1 | 2 | 3 | 5 | 6 | 8 |
| **2. MULTIPLE DX** | | | | | | | | | | |
| 0–19 Years | 12 | 5.3 | 26 | 1 | 3 | 3 | 13 | 13 | 13 | 13 |
| 20–34 | 315 | 3.2 | 5 | 2 | 2 | 3 | 4 | 5 | 7 | 12 |
| 35–49 | 1,932 | 3.6 | 6 | 1 | 2 | 3 | 5 | 7 | 8 | 12 |
| 50–64 | 2,927 | 4.0 | 12 | 1 | 2 | 3 | 5 | 7 | 9 | 17 |
| 65+ | 3,899 | 4.1 | 15 | 1 | 2 | 3 | 5 | 8 | 10 | 18 |
| **TOTAL SINGLE DX** | 1,511 | 2.5 | 2 | 1 | 1 | 2 | 3 | 4 | 5 | 7 |
| **TOTAL MULTIPLE DX** | 9,085 | 3.9 | 12 | 1 | 2 | 3 | 5 | 7 | 9 | 17 |
| **TOTAL** | | | | | | | | | | |
| 0–19 Years | 15 | 2.8 | 15 | 1 | 1 | 1 | 2 | 13 | 13 | 13 |
| 20–34 | 462 | 3.0 | 4 | 1 | 2 | 3 | 4 | 5 | 6 | 10 |
| 35–49 | 2,472 | 3.4 | 6 | 1 | 2 | 3 | 4 | 7 | 8 | 11 |
| 50–64 | 3,379 | 3.8 | 11 | 1 | 2 | 3 | 5 | 7 | 9 | 17 |
| 65+ | 4,268 | 4.0 | 14 | 1 | 2 | 3 | 5 | 8 | 10 | 17 |
| **GRAND TOTAL** | 10,596 | 3.7 | 11 | 1 | 2 | 3 | 5 | 7 | 9 | 16 |

## 53.6: REP OTH ABD HERNIA-GRAFT. Formerly included in operation group(s) 636.

| Type of Patients | Observed Patients | Avg. Stay | Variance | 10th | 25th | 50th | 75th | 90th | 95th | 99th |
|---|---|---|---|---|---|---|---|---|---|---|
| **1. SINGLE DX** | | | | | | | | | | |
| 0–19 Years | 3 | 1.1 | <1 | 1 | 1 | 1 | 3 | 3 | 4 | 5 |
| 20–34 | 201 | 2.3 | 1 | 1 | 1 | 2 | 3 | 4 | 5 | 6 |
| 35–49 | 721 | 2.5 | 2 | 1 | 2 | 2 | 3 | 4 | 5 | 7 |
| 50–64 | 613 | 2.4 | 2 | 1 | 1 | 2 | 3 | 4 | 5 | 8 |
| 65+ | 464 | 2.5 | 3 | 1 | 1 | 2 | 3 | 5 | 6 | 8 |
| **2. MULTIPLE DX** | | | | | | | | | | |
| 0–19 Years | 25 | 6.2 | 70 | 1 | 1 | 3 | 7 | 13 | 13 | 44 |
| 20–34 | 447 | 3.2 | 8 | 1 | 2 | 2 | 4 | 5 | 7 | 13 |
| 35–49 | 2,523 | 3.6 | 8 | 1 | 2 | 3 | 5 | 7 | 9 | 13 |
| 50–64 | 3,744 | 4.0 | 13 | 1 | 2 | 3 | 5 | 7 | 9 | 19 |
| 65+ | 4,976 | 4.3 | 17 | 1 | 2 | 3 | 5 | 8 | 11 | 21 |
| **TOTAL SINGLE DX** | 2,002 | 2.5 | 2 | 1 | 1 | 2 | 3 | 4 | 5 | 7 |
| **TOTAL MULTIPLE DX** | 11,715 | 4.0 | 13 | 1 | 2 | 3 | 5 | 8 | 10 | 18 |
| **TOTAL** | | | | | | | | | | |
| 0–19 Years | 28 | 3.7 | 42 | 1 | 1 | 1 | 3 | 13 | 13 | 40 |
| 20–34 | 648 | 2.9 | 6 | 1 | 2 | 2 | 3 | 5 | 6 | 10 |
| 35–49 | 3,244 | 3.3 | 6 | 1 | 2 | 3 | 4 | 7 | 8 | 12 |
| 50–64 | 4,357 | 3.8 | 12 | 1 | 2 | 3 | 5 | 7 | 9 | 17 |
| 65+ | 5,440 | 4.2 | 16 | 1 | 2 | 3 | 5 | 8 | 10 | 19 |
| **GRAND TOTAL** | 13,717 | 3.8 | 12 | 1 | 2 | 3 | 5 | 7 | 9 | 17 |

## 53.69: ABD HERNIA REP-GRFT NEC. Formerly included in operation group(s) 636.

| Type of Patients | Observed Patients | Avg. Stay | Variance | 10th | 25th | 50th | 75th | 90th | 95th | 99th |
|---|---|---|---|---|---|---|---|---|---|---|
| **1. SINGLE DX** | | | | | | | | | | |
| 0–19 Years | 0 | | | | | | | | | |
| 20–34 | 54 | 1.8 | <1 | 1 | 1 | 2 | 2 | 3 | 4 | 4 |
| 35–49 | 181 | 2.4 | 2 | 1 | 1 | 2 | 3 | 4 | 5 | 8 |
| 50–64 | 161 | 2.5 | 4 | 1 | 1 | 2 | 3 | 5 | 6 | 9 |
| 65+ | 95 | 2.7 | 6 | 1 | 1 | 2 | 3 | 5 | 6 | 9 |
| **2. MULTIPLE DX** | | | | | | | | | | |
| 0–19 Years | 13 | 7.9 | 157 | 1 | 1 | 5 | 7 | 40 | 40 | 44 |
| 20–34 | 132 | 3.0 | 15 | 1 | 2 | 2 | 3 | 5 | 6 | 32 |
| 35–49 | 591 | 3.6 | 11 | 1 | 1 | 2 | 5 | 8 | 10 | 14 |
| 50–64 | 817 | 3.8 | 16 | 1 | 2 | 3 | 5 | 9 | 10 | 21 |
| 65+ | 1,077 | 4.9 | 23 | 1 | 2 | 4 | 6 | 9 | 13 | 31 |
| **TOTAL SINGLE DX** | 491 | 2.4 | 3 | 1 | 1 | 2 | 3 | 4 | 5 | 9 |
| **TOTAL MULTIPLE DX** | 2,630 | 4.2 | 18 | 1 | 2 | 3 | 5 | 9 | 11 | 24 |
| **TOTAL** | | | | | | | | | | |
| 0–19 Years | 13 | 7.9 | 157 | 1 | 1 | 5 | 7 | 40 | 40 | 44 |
| 20–34 | 186 | 2.7 | 12 | 1 | 1 | 2 | 3 | 4 | 6 | 9 |
| 35–49 | 772 | 3.3 | 9 | 1 | 1 | 3 | 4 | 7 | 8 | 13 |
| 50–64 | 978 | 3.6 | 14 | 1 | 2 | 3 | 5 | 7 | 10 | 20 |
| 65+ | 1,172 | 4.8 | 22 | 1 | 2 | 4 | 6 | 9 | 13 | 31 |
| **GRAND TOTAL** | 3,121 | 3.9 | 16 | 1 | 2 | 3 | 5 | 8 | 10 | 23 |

Length of Stay by Diagnosis and Operation, United States, 2000

# United States, October 1998–September 1999 Data, by Operation

## 53.7: ABD REP-DIAPH HERNIA. Formerly included in operation group(s) 637.

| Type of Patients | Observed Patients | Avg. Stay | Variance | 10th | 25th | 50th | 75th | 90th | 95th | 99th |
|---|---|---|---|---|---|---|---|---|---|---|
| **1. SINGLE DX** | | | | | | | | | | |
| 0–19 Years | 46 | 6.2 | 26 | 2 | 3 | 5 | 7 | 15 | 15 | 31 |
| 20–34 | 6 | 1.9 | 5 | 1 | 1 | 1 | 1 | 7 | 7 | 9 |
| 35–49 | 16 | 3.6 | 7 | 1 | 1 | 3 | 5 | 9 | 9 | 11 |
| 50–64 | 18 | 4.5 | 4 | 2 | 2 | 6 | 6 | 8 | 8 | 8 |
| 65+ | 21 | 3.7 | 2 | 2 | 3 | 4 | 4 | 6 | 7 | 7 |
| **2. MULTIPLE DX** | | | | | | | | | | |
| 0–19 Years | 222 | 16.5 | 236 | 3 | 5 | 9 | 24 | 40 | 66 | >99 |
| 20–34 | 55 | 5.5 | 16 | 2 | 4 | 5 | 6 | 10 | 11 | 12 |
| 35–49 | 182 | 6.7 | 43 | 2 | 3 | 5 | 7 | 14 | 19 | 42 |
| 50–64 | 291 | 8.2 | 101 | 2 | 3 | 6 | 10 | 13 | 24 | 71 |
| 65+ | 605 | 8.9 | 75 | 2 | 4 | 7 | 11 | 18 | 23 | 42 |
| **TOTAL SINGLE DX** | 107 | 4.9 | 17 | 1 | 2 | 4 | 6 | 8 | 15 | 15 |
| **TOTAL MULTIPLE DX** | 1,355 | 9.3 | 105 | 2 | 4 | 6 | 10 | 21 | 32 | 71 |
| **TOTAL** | | | | | | | | | | |
| 0–19 Years | 268 | 14.0 | 205 | 3 | 4 | 8 | 22 | 38 | 60 | >99 |
| 20–34 | 61 | 4.9 | 16 | 1 | 3 | 5 | 6 | 9 | 11 | 12 |
| 35–49 | 198 | 6.4 | 41 | 2 | 3 | 5 | 7 | 13 | 17 | 42 |
| 50–64 | 309 | 8.0 | 96 | 2 | 3 | 6 | 10 | 12 | 22 | 71 |
| 65+ | 626 | 8.8 | 74 | 2 | 4 | 7 | 11 | 17 | 23 | 42 |
| **GRAND TOTAL** | 1,462 | 9.0 | 99 | 2 | 4 | 6 | 10 | 20 | 30 | 66 |

## 53.80: REP DH, THOR APPR NOS. Formerly included in operation group(s) 637.

| Type of Patients | Observed Patients | Avg. Stay | Variance | 10th | 25th | 50th | 75th | 90th | 95th | 99th |
|---|---|---|---|---|---|---|---|---|---|---|
| **1. SINGLE DX** | | | | | | | | | | |
| 0–19 Years | 17 | 7.2 | 41 | 2 | 2 | 4 | 17 | 17 | 17 | 17 |
| 20–34 | 3 | 4.4 | 9 | 1 | 1 | 5 | 5 | 10 | 10 | 10 |
| 35–49 | 9 | 2.2 | 2 | 1 | 1 | 1 | 4 | 4 | 5 | 5 |
| 50–64 | 5 | 4.1 | 5 | 1 | 2 | 5 | 5 | 5 | 8 | 8 |
| 65+ | 4 | 5.2 | <1 | 5 | 5 | 5 | 5 | 6 | 6 | 6 |
| **2. MULTIPLE DX** | | | | | | | | | | |
| 0–19 Years | 62 | 13.0 | 251 | 3 | 4 | 8 | 13 | 44 | 80 | >99 |
| 20–34 | 25 | 4.4 | 22 | 2 | 2 | 2 | 5 | 10 | 15 | 27 |
| 35–49 | 48 | 12.4 | 35 | 2 | 8 | 13 | 17 | 17 | 17 | 20 |
| 50–64 | 77 | 6.0 | 27 | 2 | 3 | 5 | 12 | 17 | 14 | 28 |
| 65+ | 90 | 8.1 | 26 | 3 | 5 | 7 | 12 | 14 | 21 | 30 |
| **TOTAL SINGLE DX** | 38 | 5.6 | 30 | 1 | 2 | 4 | 5 | 17 | 17 | 17 |
| **TOTAL MULTIPLE DX** | 302 | 9.6 | 73 | 2 | 4 | 7 | 13 | 17 | 21 | 80 |
| **TOTAL** | | | | | | | | | | |
| 0–19 Years | 79 | 11.2 | 193 | 2 | 4 | 6 | 17 | 27 | 60 | >99 |
| 20–34 | 28 | 4.4 | 20 | 2 | 2 | 2 | 5 | 10 | 15 | 27 |
| 35–49 | 57 | 11.5 | 40 | 2 | 6 | 13 | 17 | 17 | 17 | 20 |
| 50–64 | 82 | 5.9 | 26 | 2 | 3 | 5 | 7 | 9 | 14 | 28 |
| 65+ | 94 | 8.1 | 25 | 3 | 5 | 7 | 12 | 14 | 21 | 30 |
| **GRAND TOTAL** | 340 | 9.2 | 70 | 2 | 4 | 7 | 13 | 17 | 21 | 80 |

## 53.8: REPAIR DH, THOR APPR. Formerly included in operation group(s) 637.

| Type of Patients | Observed Patients | Avg. Stay | Variance | 10th | 25th | 50th | 75th | 90th | 95th | 99th |
|---|---|---|---|---|---|---|---|---|---|---|
| **1. SINGLE DX** | | | | | | | | | | |
| 0–19 Years | 26 | 5.9 | 33 | 2 | 2 | 3 | 5 | 17 | 17 | 17 |
| 20–34 | 3 | 4.4 | 9 | 1 | 1 | 5 | 5 | 10 | 10 | 10 |
| 35–49 | 9 | 2.2 | 2 | 1 | 1 | 1 | 4 | 4 | 8 | 8 |
| 50–64 | 5 | 4.1 | 5 | 1 | 2 | 5 | 5 | 8 | 8 | 8 |
| 65+ | 4 | 5.2 | <1 | 5 | 5 | 5 | 5 | 6 | 6 | 6 |
| **2. MULTIPLE DX** | | | | | | | | | | |
| 0–19 Years | 101 | 16.0 | 285 | 3 | 5 | 8 | 26 | 53 | 53 | >99 |
| 20–34 | 27 | 4.4 | 21 | 2 | 2 | 2 | 5 | 10 | 15 | 27 |
| 35–49 | 55 | 12.2 | 36 | 4 | 7 | 13 | 17 | 17 | 17 | 20 |
| 50–64 | 88 | 6.4 | 28 | 2 | 3 | 6 | 8 | 12 | 15 | 28 |
| 65+ | 102 | 8.4 | 26 | 3 | 5 | 7 | 12 | 15 | 21 | 30 |
| **TOTAL SINGLE DX** | 47 | 5.0 | 25 | 2 | 2 | 3 | 5 | 17 | 17 | 17 |
| **TOTAL MULTIPLE DX** | 373 | 10.8 | 112 | 2 | 5 | 7 | 14 | 20 | 28 | 80 |
| **TOTAL** | | | | | | | | | | |
| 0–19 Years | 127 | 13.6 | 244 | 2 | 4 | 7 | 17 | 38 | 53 | >99 |
| 20–34 | 30 | 4.4 | 20 | 2 | 2 | 5 | 5 | 10 | 15 | 27 |
| 35–49 | 64 | 11.4 | 40 | 2 | 6 | 13 | 17 | 17 | 17 | 20 |
| 50–64 | 93 | 6.3 | 27 | 2 | 3 | 5 | 7 | 12 | 15 | 28 |
| 65+ | 106 | 8.3 | 25 | 3 | 5 | 7 | 12 | 15 | 21 | 30 |
| **GRAND TOTAL** | 420 | 10.2 | 106 | 2 | 4 | 7 | 13 | 17 | 27 | 73 |

## 53.9: OTHER HERNIA REPAIR. Formerly included in operation group(s) 637.

| Type of Patients | Observed Patients | Avg. Stay | Variance | 10th | 25th | 50th | 75th | 90th | 95th | 99th |
|---|---|---|---|---|---|---|---|---|---|---|
| **1. SINGLE DX** | | | | | | | | | | |
| 0–19 Years | 2 | 2.1 | 2 | 1 | 1 | 1 | 4 | 4 | 4 | 4 |
| 20–34 | 8 | 3.5 | 4 | 2 | 2 | 2 | 6 | 6 | 7 | 7 |
| 35–49 | 11 | 2.6 | 2 | 2 | 2 | 2 | 3 | 3 | 9 | 9 |
| 50–64 | 8 | 2.0 | 2 | 1 | 1 | 2 | 7 | 7 | 7 | 7 |
| 65+ | 4 | 5.1 | 6 | 2 | 5 | 7 | 7 | 7 | 7 | 7 |
| **2. MULTIPLE DX** | | | | | | | | | | |
| 0–19 Years | 18 | 19.3 | 594 | 4 | 6 | 7 | 22 | 77 | 77 | 77 |
| 20–34 | 24 | 3.6 | 18 | 1 | 1 | 5 | 6 | 8 | 11 | 21 |
| 35–49 | 54 | 5.7 | 13 | 2 | 2 | 6 | 8 | 10 | 12 | 17 |
| 50–64 | 60 | 6.1 | 14 | 1 | 3 | 6 | 8 | 11 | 15 | 15 |
| 65+ | 153 | 9.3 | 58 | 3 | 5 | 7 | 10 | 18 | 22 | 40 |
| **TOTAL SINGLE DX** | 33 | 3.4 | 6 | 1 | 2 | 2 | 6 | 7 | 7 | 9 |
| **TOTAL MULTIPLE DX** | 309 | 8.1 | 72 | 2 | 4 | 7 | 9 | 15 | 22 | 40 |
| **TOTAL** | | | | | | | | | | |
| 0–19 Years | 20 | 17.1 | 550 | 1 | 4 | 7 | 22 | 77 | 77 | 77 |
| 20–34 | 32 | 3.6 | 15 | 1 | 2 | 5 | 6 | 8 | 11 | 21 |
| 35–49 | 65 | 5.4 | 13 | 1 | 2 | 5 | 7 | 10 | 12 | 16 |
| 50–64 | 68 | 5.5 | 14 | 1 | 3 | 5 | 7 | 10 | 15 | 15 |
| 65+ | 157 | 9.0 | 55 | 2 | 5 | 7 | 10 | 18 | 22 | 40 |
| **GRAND TOTAL** | 342 | 7.5 | 67 | 1 | 3 | 6 | 9 | 15 | 21 | 40 |

Length of Stay by Diagnosis and Operation, United States, 2000

# United States, October 1998–September 1999 Data, by Operation

## 54.0: ABDOMINAL WALL INCISION. Formerly included in operation group(s) 638.

| Type of Patients | Observed Patients | Avg. Stay | Vari-ance | Percentiles | | | | | | |
|---|---|---|---|---|---|---|---|---|---|---|
| | | | | 10th | 25th | 50th | 75th | 90th | 95th | 99th |
| **1. SINGLE DX** | | | | | | | | | | |
| 0–19 Years | 65 | 3.0 | 9 | 1 | 1 | 2 | 4 | 5 | 12 | 14 |
| 20–34 | 58 | 2.9 | 2 | 1 | 2 | 3 | 4 | 5 | 6 | 6 |
| 35–49 | 64 | 2.7 | 4 | 1 | 2 | 2 | 3 | 5 | 6 | 12 |
| 50–64 | 36 | 3.4 | 4 | 1 | 2 | 3 | 4 | 7 | 7 | 8 |
| 65+ | 37 | 2.9 | 11 | 1 | 1 | 2 | 4 | 5 | 7 | 19 |
| **2. MULTIPLE DX** | | | | | | | | | | |
| 0–19 Years | 142 | 5.9 | 82 | 1 | 2 | 4 | 6 | 12 | 14 | 52 |
| 20–34 | 281 | 5.6 | 39 | 1 | 2 | 4 | 7 | 10 | 14 | 32 |
| 35–49 | 588 | 6.3 | 40 | 2 | 3 | 4 | 8 | 13 | 16 | 39 |
| 50–64 | 550 | 6.2 | 41 | 1 | 2 | 4 | 8 | 14 | 18 | 29 |
| 65+ | 713 | 9.0 | 83 | 2 | 4 | 6 | 11 | 20 | 25 | 47 |
| **TOTAL SINGLE DX** | 260 | 2.9 | 6 | 1 | 1 | 2 | 4 | 5 | 7 | 14 |
| **TOTAL MULTIPLE DX** | 2,274 | 6.9 | 57 | 1 | 3 | 5 | 8 | 15 | 21 | 38 |
| **TOTAL** | | | | | | | | | | |
| 0–19 Years | 207 | 5.0 | 62 | 1 | 2 | 3 | 6 | 12 | 14 | 41 |
| 20–34 | 339 | 5.0 | 33 | 1 | 2 | 4 | 6 | 9 | 11 | 27 |
| 35–49 | 652 | 6.0 | 38 | 1 | 3 | 4 | 7 | 12 | 16 | 33 |
| 50–64 | 586 | 6.0 | 39 | 1 | 2 | 4 | 8 | 14 | 16 | 29 |
| 65+ | 750 | 8.8 | 81 | 2 | 3 | 6 | 11 | 19 | 25 | 47 |
| **GRAND TOTAL** | 2,534 | 6.5 | 53 | 1 | 2 | 4 | 8 | 14 | 19 | 36 |

## 54.1: LAPAROTOMY. Formerly included in operation group(s) 639.

| Type of Patients | Observed Patients | Avg. Stay | Vari-ance | Percentiles | | | | | | |
|---|---|---|---|---|---|---|---|---|---|---|
| | | | | 10th | 25th | 50th | 75th | 90th | 95th | 99th |
| **1. SINGLE DX** | | | | | | | | | | |
| 0–19 Years | 171 | 4.1 | 11 | 1 | 2 | 3 | 5 | 8 | 11 | 16 |
| 20–34 | 255 | 3.0 | 5 | 1 | 2 | 2 | 4 | 5 | 5 | 20 |
| 35–49 | 197 | 3.8 | 7 | 1 | 2 | 3 | 6 | 6 | 8 | 15 |
| 50–64 | 75 | 3.9 | 7 | 1 | 1 | 4 | 5 | 6 | 8 | 10 |
| 65+ | 50 | 4.3 | 7 | 2 | 2 | 4 | 5 | 8 | 9 | 15 |
| **2. MULTIPLE DX** | | | | | | | | | | |
| 0–19 Years | 689 | 10.2 | 225 | 2 | 3 | 5 | 10 | 23 | 39 | 89 |
| 20–34 | 1,317 | 6.0 | 41 | 2 | 3 | 4 | 7 | 12 | 17 | 37 |
| 35–49 | 1,615 | 7.9 | 59 | 3 | 4 | 6 | 9 | 16 | 22 | 38 |
| 50–64 | 1,383 | 10.7 | 109 | 3 | 4 | 8 | 13 | 22 | 33 | 54 |
| 65+ | 1,811 | 11.8 | 112 | 3 | 5 | 8 | 15 | 23 | 31 | 58 |
| **TOTAL SINGLE DX** | 748 | 3.6 | 8 | 1 | 2 | 3 | 5 | 6 | 8 | 16 |
| **TOTAL MULTIPLE DX** | 6,815 | 9.4 | 103 | 2 | 4 | 6 | 11 | 20 | 27 | 57 |
| **TOTAL** | | | | | | | | | | |
| 0–19 Years | 860 | 9.1 | 192 | 2 | 3 | 5 | 8 | 19 | 34 | 80 |
| 20–34 | 1,572 | 5.5 | 36 | 2 | 3 | 4 | 6 | 10 | 15 | 35 |
| 35–49 | 1,812 | 7.4 | 55 | 2 | 3 | 5 | 9 | 15 | 21 | 37 |
| 50–64 | 1,458 | 10.3 | 106 | 3 | 4 | 7 | 12 | 21 | 30 | 53 |
| 65+ | 1,861 | 11.5 | 111 | 3 | 5 | 8 | 14 | 23 | 30 | 58 |
| **GRAND TOTAL** | 7,563 | 8.7 | 96 | 2 | 3 | 6 | 10 | 18 | 26 | 57 |

## 54.11: EXPLORATORY LAPAROTOMY. Formerly included in operation group(s) 639.

| Type of Patients | Observed Patients | Avg. Stay | Vari-ance | Percentiles | | | | | | |
|---|---|---|---|---|---|---|---|---|---|---|
| | | | | 10th | 25th | 50th | 75th | 90th | 95th | 99th |
| **1. SINGLE DX** | | | | | | | | | | |
| 0–19 Years | 126 | 3.4 | 10 | 1 | 2 | 3 | 4 | 6 | 11 | 16 |
| 20–34 | 187 | 3.0 | 7 | 1 | 2 | 3 | 3 | 5 | 8 | 20 |
| 35–49 | 130 | 3.3 | 8 | 1 | 1 | 3 | 4 | 7 | 8 | 14 |
| 50–64 | 53 | 4.1 | 7 | 1 | 2 | 4 | 5 | 7 | 8 | 19 |
| 65+ | 38 | 4.7 | 8 | 2 | 2 | 4 | 5 | 8 | 9 | 15 |
| **2. MULTIPLE DX** | | | | | | | | | | |
| 0–19 Years | 448 | 10.5 | 272 | 2 | 3 | 5 | 9 | 29 | 52 | 91 |
| 20–34 | 901 | 5.6 | 27 | 2 | 3 | 4 | 7 | 11 | 14 | 30 |
| 35–49 | 978 | 7.3 | 54 | 2 | 3 | 5 | 9 | 15 | 20 | 34 |
| 50–64 | 877 | 9.4 | 74 | 3 | 4 | 7 | 11 | 18 | 25 | 45 |
| 65+ | 1,295 | 11.4 | 101 | 4 | 5 | 8 | 14 | 22 | 29 | 61 |
| **TOTAL SINGLE DX** | 534 | 3.4 | 8 | 1 | 2 | 3 | 4 | 6 | 8 | 16 |
| **TOTAL MULTIPLE DX** | 4,499 | 8.8 | 94 | 2 | 3 | 6 | 10 | 18 | 25 | 56 |
| **TOTAL** | | | | | | | | | | |
| 0–19 Years | 574 | 9.0 | 224 | 2 | 3 | 4 | 7 | 23 | 39 | 89 |
| 20–34 | 1,088 | 5.1 | 25 | 2 | 3 | 4 | 6 | 10 | 13 | 28 |
| 35–49 | 1,108 | 6.9 | 50 | 2 | 3 | 5 | 8 | 14 | 20 | 33 |
| 50–64 | 930 | 9.0 | 72 | 3 | 4 | 7 | 11 | 18 | 23 | 44 |
| 65+ | 1,333 | 11.2 | 99 | 3 | 5 | 8 | 14 | 22 | 29 | 61 |
| **GRAND TOTAL** | 5,033 | 8.2 | 87 | 2 | 3 | 5 | 9 | 17 | 23 | 52 |

## 54.12: REOPEN RECENT LAP SITE. Formerly included in operation group(s) 639.

| Type of Patients | Observed Patients | Avg. Stay | Vari-ance | Percentiles | | | | | | |
|---|---|---|---|---|---|---|---|---|---|---|
| | | | | 10th | 25th | 50th | 75th | 90th | 95th | 99th |
| **1. SINGLE DX** | | | | | | | | | | |
| 0–19 Years | 10 | 5.5 | 7 | 2 | 4 | 5 | 7 | 10 | 11 | 10 |
| 20–34 | 13 | 3.1 | 2 | 2 | 2 | 3 | 5 | 5 | 5 | 5 |
| 35–49 | 31 | 4.4 | 4 | 1 | 3 | 6 | 6 | 6 | 8 | 7 |
| 50–64 | 5 | 1.5 | 2 | 1 | 1 | 1 | 1 | 5 | 8 | 10 |
| 65+ | 5 | 3.8 | 1 | 2 | 4 | 4 | 4 | 5 | 9 | 6 |
| **2. MULTIPLE DX** | | | | | | | | | | |
| 0–19 Years | 55 | 8.8 | 61 | 3 | 5 | 6 | 9 | 18 | 22 | 47 |
| 20–34 | 83 | 6.7 | 55 | 2 | 4 | 6 | 7 | 10 | 16 | 66 |
| 35–49 | 163 | 7.2 | 46 | 2 | 5 | 5 | 9 | 14 | 18 | 33 |
| 50–64 | 111 | 11.2 | 114 | 2 | 5 | 8 | 15 | 16 | 38 | 51 |
| 65+ | 105 | 9.9 | 71 | 2 | 4 | 8 | 13 | 20 | 28 | 58 |
| **TOTAL SINGLE DX** | 64 | 4.0 | 5 | 1 | 2 | 4 | 6 | 6 | 6 | 10 |
| **TOTAL MULTIPLE DX** | 517 | 8.7 | 71 | 2 | 4 | 6 | 11 | 16 | 24 | 47 |
| **TOTAL** | | | | | | | | | | |
| 0–19 Years | 65 | 8.3 | 54 | 3 | 5 | 6 | 9 | 18 | 22 | 47 |
| 20–34 | 96 | 6.0 | 46 | 1 | 3 | 5 | 6 | 10 | 12 | 24 |
| 35–49 | 194 | 6.5 | 37 | 1 | 3 | 6 | 8 | 12 | 16 | 31 |
| 50–64 | 116 | 10.6 | 112 | 1 | 4 | 8 | 15 | 16 | 38 | 51 |
| 65+ | 110 | 9.6 | 69 | 2 | 4 | 7 | 13 | 20 | 28 | 58 |
| **GRAND TOTAL** | 581 | 7.9 | 63 | 2 | 4 | 6 | 9 | 15 | 22 | 38 |

Length of Stay by Diagnosis and Operation, United States, 2000

## United States, October 1998–September 1999 Data, by Operation

### 54.19: LAPAROTOMY NEC. Formerly included in operation group(s) 639.

| Type of Patients | Observed Patients | Avg. Stay | Variance | 10th | 25th | 50th | 75th | 90th | 95th | 99th |
|---|---|---|---|---|---|---|---|---|---|---|
| **1. SINGLE DX** | | | | | | | | | | |
| 0–19 Years | 35 | 6.0 | 10 | 3 | 4 | 6 | 7 | 8 | 12 | 20 |
| 20–34 | 55 | 2.9 | 3 | 1 | 2 | 2 | 4 | 5 | 6 | 10 |
| 35–49 | 36 | 4.5 | 11 | 2 | 2 | 4 | 5 | 7 | 8 | 19 |
| 50–64 | 17 | 4.2 | 6 | 2 | 2 | 4 | 6 | 8 | 8 | 9 |
| 65+ | 7 | 3.5 | 3 | 1 | 1 | 4 | 4 | 6 | 6 | 6 |
| **2. MULTIPLE DX** | | | | | | | | | | |
| 0–19 Years | 186 | 10.0 | 182 | 3 | 4 | 6 | 10 | 19 | 30 | 87 |
| 20–34 | 333 | 7.1 | 73 | 1 | 2 | 4 | 8 | 15 | 21 | 51 |
| 35–49 | 474 | 9.2 | 73 | 2 | 4 | 7 | 11 | 19 | 26 | 44 |
| 50–64 | 395 | 13.1 | 165 | 3 | 5 | 9 | 17 | 26 | 43 | 68 |
| 65+ | 411 | 13.4 | 152 | 3 | 5 | 9 | 17 | 27 | 38 | 58 |
| **TOTAL SINGLE DX** | 150 | 4.1 | 8 | 1 | 2 | 4 | 5 | 7 | 8 | 19 |
| **TOTAL MULTIPLE DX** | 1,799 | 10.8 | 132 | 2 | 4 | 8 | 13 | 22 | 33 | 65 |
| **TOTAL** | | | | | | | | | | |
| 0–19 Years | 221 | 9.5 | 163 | 3 | 4 | 6 | 10 | 19 | 25 | 80 |
| 20–34 | 388 | 6.4 | 65 | 2 | 2 | 4 | 7 | 13 | 20 | 51 |
| 35–49 | 510 | 8.9 | 70 | 2 | 4 | 7 | 10 | 18 | 24 | 44 |
| 50–64 | 412 | 12.8 | 162 | 3 | 5 | 9 | 17 | 25 | 43 | 68 |
| 65+ | 418 | 13.1 | 151 | 2 | 5 | 9 | 17 | 27 | 38 | 57 |
| **GRAND TOTAL** | 1,949 | 10.3 | 126 | 2 | 4 | 7 | 12 | 22 | 31 | 59 |

### 54.21: LAPAROSCOPY. Formerly included in operation group(s) 640.

| Type of Patients | Observed Patients | Avg. Stay | Variance | 10th | 25th | 50th | 75th | 90th | 95th | 99th |
|---|---|---|---|---|---|---|---|---|---|---|
| **1. SINGLE DX** | | | | | | | | | | |
| 0–19 Years | 196 | 1.9 | 2 | 1 | 1 | 2 | 2 | 4 | 5 | 6 |
| 20–34 | 432 | 2.2 | 2 | 1 | 1 | 2 | 3 | 4 | 6 | 7 |
| 35–49 | 194 | 2.9 | 7 | 1 | 1 | 2 | 3 | 4 | 5 | 9 |
| 50–64 | 53 | 2.5 | 1 | 1 | 2 | 3 | 3 | 4 | 5 | 6 |
| 65+ | 14 | 2.6 | 2 | 1 | 1 | 3 | 4 | 5 | 5 | 5 |
| **2. MULTIPLE DX** | | | | | | | | | | |
| 0–19 Years | 420 | 4.0 | 25 | 1 | 1 | 3 | 5 | 7 | 10 | 20 |
| 20–34 | 1,327 | 3.8 | 34 | 1 | 1 | 2 | 4 | 7 | 9 | 24 |
| 35–49 | 890 | 3.8 | 16 | 1 | 2 | 3 | 5 | 8 | 10 | 22 |
| 50–64 | 418 | 5.6 | 29 | 1 | 2 | 3 | 8 | 13 | 16 | 26 |
| 65+ | 412 | 7.3 | 47 | 1 | 2 | 5 | 9 | 16 | 21 | 32 |
| **TOTAL SINGLE DX** | 889 | 2.3 | 3 | 1 | 1 | 2 | 3 | 4 | 7 | 9 |
| **TOTAL MULTIPLE DX** | 3,467 | 4.3 | 30 | 1 | 2 | 3 | 5 | 9 | 14 | 24 |
| **TOTAL** | | | | | | | | | | |
| 0–19 Years | 616 | 3.3 | 19 | 1 | 1 | 2 | 4 | 6 | 9 | 20 |
| 20–34 | 1,759 | 3.4 | 26 | 1 | 1 | 3 | 4 | 8 | 8 | 24 |
| 35–49 | 1,084 | 3.6 | 15 | 1 | 2 | 3 | 7 | 8 | 10 | 21 |
| 50–64 | 471 | 5.3 | 27 | 1 | 2 | 5 | 9 | 12 | 16 | 24 |
| 65+ | 426 | 7.2 | 47 | 1 | 2 | 5 | 9 | 16 | 21 | 32 |
| **GRAND TOTAL** | 4,356 | 3.9 | 25 | 1 | 1 | 2 | 4 | 8 | 11 | 24 |

### 54.2: ABD REGION DXTIC PX. Formerly included in operation group(s) 631, 638, 640.

| Type of Patients | Observed Patients | Avg. Stay | Variance | 10th | 25th | 50th | 75th | 90th | 95th | 99th |
|---|---|---|---|---|---|---|---|---|---|---|
| **1. SINGLE DX** | | | | | | | | | | |
| 0–19 Years | 222 | 2.2 | 3 | 1 | 1 | 2 | 3 | 4 | 6 | 9 |
| 20–34 | 455 | 2.2 | 2 | 1 | 1 | 2 | 3 | 4 | 5 | 7 |
| 35–49 | 216 | 2.9 | 6 | 1 | 1 | 2 | 3 | 4 | 5 | 9 |
| 50–64 | 74 | 2.7 | 2 | 1 | 1 | 3 | 3 | 4 | 5 | 6 |
| 65+ | 32 | 2.7 | 7 | 1 | 1 | 2 | 3 | 5 | 10 | 14 |
| **2. MULTIPLE DX** | | | | | | | | | | |
| 0–19 Years | 518 | 4.6 | 45 | 1 | 1 | 3 | 6 | 9 | 12 | 31 |
| 20–34 | 1,520 | 4.1 | 36 | 1 | 1 | 2 | 4 | 8 | 17 | 24 |
| 35–49 | 1,230 | 4.6 | 28 | 1 | 2 | 3 | 6 | 10 | 15 | 24 |
| 50–64 | 978 | 7.4 | 38 | 1 | 3 | 6 | 11 | 16 | 20 | 26 |
| 65+ | 1,422 | 8.4 | 54 | 2 | 4 | 6 | 11 | 16 | 22 | 38 |
| **TOTAL SINGLE DX** | 999 | 2.4 | 3 | 1 | 1 | 2 | 3 | 5 | 7 | 9 |
| **TOTAL MULTIPLE DX** | 5,668 | 5.7 | 43 | 1 | 2 | 3 | 7 | 13 | 18 | 30 |
| **TOTAL** | | | | | | | | | | |
| 0–19 Years | 740 | 3.9 | 34 | 1 | 1 | 2 | 5 | 7 | 10 | 26 |
| 20–34 | 1,975 | 3.6 | 28 | 1 | 2 | 3 | 4 | 7 | 11 | 24 |
| 35–49 | 1,446 | 4.3 | 25 | 1 | 2 | 3 | 5 | 9 | 14 | 23 |
| 50–64 | 1,052 | 7.1 | 37 | 1 | 3 | 5 | 10 | 16 | 20 | 31 |
| 65+ | 1,454 | 8.3 | 54 | 2 | 4 | 6 | 11 | 16 | 22 | 38 |
| **GRAND TOTAL** | 6,667 | 5.2 | 38 | 1 | 2 | 3 | 6 | 12 | 17 | 28 |

### 54.23: PERITONEAL BIOPSY. Formerly included in operation group(s) 638.

| Type of Patients | Observed Patients | Avg. Stay | Variance | 10th | 25th | 50th | 75th | 90th | 95th | 99th |
|---|---|---|---|---|---|---|---|---|---|---|
| **1. SINGLE DX** | | | | | | | | | | |
| 0–19 Years | 7 | 3.8 | 5 | 1 | 1 | 4 | 4 | 7 | 7 | 9 |
| 20–34 | 5 | 3.8 | 4 | 1 | 3 | 5 | 5 | 5 | 5 | 5 |
| 35–49 | 4 | 3.1 | <1 | 3 | 3 | 3 | 4 | 5 | 5 | 5 |
| 50–64 | 14 | 3.2 | 2 | 2 | 2 | 3 | 4 | 5 | 5 | 6 |
| 65+ | 6 | 2.4 | 2 | 2 | 2 | 2 | 2 | 3 | 6 | 6 |
| **2. MULTIPLE DX** | | | | | | | | | | |
| 0–19 Years | 40 | 11.8 | 90 | 3 | 4 | 9 | 18 | 26 | 27 | 52 |
| 20–34 | 53 | 5.6 | 28 | 1 | 2 | 4 | 7 | 14 | 18 | 19 |
| 35–49 | 109 | 6.9 | 45 | 2 | 3 | 7 | 13 | 14 | 15 | 33 |
| 50–64 | 272 | 9.3 | 45 | 3 | 4 | 7 | 13 | 18 | 23 | 31 |
| 65+ | 360 | 10.1 | 79 | 4 | 4 | 7 | 13 | 21 | 32 | 41 |
| **TOTAL SINGLE DX** | 36 | 3.2 | 2 | 1 | 2 | 3 | 4 | 5 | 5 | 7 |
| **TOTAL MULTIPLE DX** | 834 | 9.3 | 62 | 2 | 4 | 7 | 12 | 19 | 24 | 38 |
| **TOTAL** | | | | | | | | | | |
| 0–19 Years | 47 | 10.4 | 84 | 2 | 4 | 8 | 12 | 26 | 26 | 52 |
| 20–34 | 58 | 5.5 | 26 | 1 | 2 | 4 | 8 | 14 | 18 | 19 |
| 35–49 | 113 | 6.3 | 40 | 2 | 3 | 7 | 13 | 18 | 23 | 33 |
| 50–64 | 286 | 9.0 | 45 | 3 | 4 | 7 | 13 | 18 | 30 | 31 |
| 65+ | 366 | 10.0 | 79 | 4 | 4 | 7 | 12 | 21 | 32 | 41 |
| **GRAND TOTAL** | 870 | 9.0 | 61 | 2 | 4 | 7 | 12 | 18 | 23 | 38 |

Length of Stay by Diagnosis and Operation, United States, 2000

# United States, October 1998–September 1999 Data, by Operation

## 54.24: CLSD BX INTRA-ABD MASS. Formerly included in operation group(s) 638.

| Type of Patients | Observed Patients | Avg. Stay | Vari-ance | Percentiles | | | | | | |
|---|---|---|---|---|---|---|---|---|---|---|
| | | | | 10th | 25th | 50th | 75th | 90th | 95th | 99th |
| **1. SINGLE DX** | | | | | | | | | | |
| 0–19 Years | 11 | 5.0 | 11 | 1 | 2 | 5 | 8 | 11 | 11 | 11 |
| 20–34 | 7 | 3.5 | 4 | 1 | 3 | 3 | 4 | 5 | 10 | 10 |
| 35–49 | 12 | 2.9 | 2 | 1 | 2 | 3 | 4 | 4 | 5 | 5 |
| 50–64 | 6 | 2.4 | 3 | 1 | 1 | 2 | 3 | 4 | 6 | 6 |
| 65+ | 11 | 3.7 | 21 | 1 | 1 | 1 | 2 | 10 | 14 | 14 |
| **2. MULTIPLE DX** | | | | | | | | | | |
| 0–19 Years | 18 | 7.3 | 53 | 2 | 2 | 6 | 7 | 14 | 25 | 34 |
| 20–34 | 45 | 4.7 | 28 | 1 | 1 | 6 | 7 | 10 | 13 | 38 |
| 35–49 | 118 | 8.9 | 50 | 2 | 4 | 6 | 12 | 18 | 18 | 36 |
| 50–64 | 203 | 8.5 | 33 | 2 | 4 | 8 | 13 | 16 | 22 | 22 |
| 65+ | 520 | 7.9 | 33 | 2 | 4 | 7 | 10 | 14 | 18 | 29 |
| **TOTAL SINGLE DX** | 47 | 4.1 | 10 | 1 | 1 | 3 | 5 | 8 | 11 | 14 |
| **TOTAL MULTIPLE DX** | 904 | 8.1 | 36 | 2 | 4 | 7 | 11 | 16 | 19 | 28 |
| **TOTAL** | | | | | | | | | | |
| 0–19 Years | 29 | 6.0 | 30 | 1 | 2 | 5 | 8 | 11 | 14 | 34 |
| 20–34 | 52 | 4.4 | 24 | 1 | 1 | 3 | 5 | 9 | 12 | 22 |
| 35–49 | 130 | 8.7 | 49 | 2 | 4 | 6 | 11 | 18 | 18 | 36 |
| 50–64 | 209 | 8.4 | 33 | 2 | 4 | 7 | 13 | 16 | 22 | 22 |
| 65+ | 531 | 7.8 | 33 | 2 | 4 | 7 | 10 | 14 | 18 | 29 |
| **GRAND TOTAL** | 951 | 7.9 | 36 | 2 | 4 | 6 | 10 | 16 | 19 | 28 |

## 54.3: EXC/DESTR ABD WALL LES. Formerly included in operation group(s) 638.

| Type of Patients | Observed Patients | Avg. Stay | Vari-ance | Percentiles | | | | | | |
|---|---|---|---|---|---|---|---|---|---|---|
| | | | | 10th | 25th | 50th | 75th | 90th | 95th | 99th |
| **1. SINGLE DX** | | | | | | | | | | |
| 0–19 Years | 35 | 3.1 | 4 | 1 | 1 | 3 | 4 | 6 | 6 | 8 |
| 20–34 | 49 | 2.0 | 1 | 1 | 1 | 2 | 3 | 3 | 4 | 7 |
| 35–49 | 44 | 2.3 | 3 | 1 | 1 | 2 | 3 | 4 | 6 | 8 |
| 50–64 | 22 | 3.0 | 5 | 1 | 2 | 2 | 4 | 4 | 6 | 14 |
| 65+ | 12 | 1.5 | <1 | 1 | 1 | 1 | 2 | 2 | 3 | 3 |
| **2. MULTIPLE DX** | | | | | | | | | | |
| 0–19 Years | 68 | 6.2 | 66 | 1 | 2 | 4 | 7 | 14 | 18 | 60 |
| 20–34 | 179 | 3.9 | 10 | 1 | 2 | 3 | 5 | 8 | 11 | 15 |
| 35–49 | 286 | 6.1 | 32 | 2 | 3 | 4 | 7 | 12 | 16 | 32 |
| 50–64 | 355 | 7.1 | 57 | 2 | 3 | 5 | 8 | 18 | 22 | 37 |
| 65+ | 402 | 7.0 | 43 | 2 | 3 | 5 | 9 | 14 | 22 | 30 |
| **TOTAL SINGLE DX** | 162 | 2.4 | 3 | 1 | 1 | 2 | 3 | 5 | 6 | 8 |
| **TOTAL MULTIPLE DX** | 1,290 | 6.4 | 42 | 1 | 3 | 4 | 8 | 13 | 18 | 32 |
| **TOTAL** | | | | | | | | | | |
| 0–19 Years | 103 | 4.8 | 40 | 1 | 2 | 3 | 6 | 8 | 14 | 30 |
| 20–34 | 228 | 3.6 | 9 | 1 | 1 | 3 | 4 | 7 | 10 | 15 |
| 35–49 | 330 | 5.6 | 30 | 1 | 3 | 4 | 7 | 12 | 16 | 32 |
| 50–64 | 377 | 6.9 | 55 | 2 | 3 | 4 | 8 | 17 | 21 | 37 |
| 65+ | 414 | 6.5 | 42 | 1 | 3 | 4 | 8 | 14 | 20 | 30 |
| **GRAND TOTAL** | 1,452 | 5.8 | 39 | 1 | 2 | 4 | 7 | 12 | 18 | 31 |

## 54.4: EXC/DESTR PERITON TISS. Formerly included in operation group(s) 638.

| Type of Patients | Observed Patients | Avg. Stay | Vari-ance | Percentiles | | | | | | |
|---|---|---|---|---|---|---|---|---|---|---|
| | | | | 10th | 25th | 50th | 75th | 90th | 95th | 99th |
| **1. SINGLE DX** | | | | | | | | | | |
| 0–19 Years | 80 | 4.1 | 3 | 2 | 3 | 4 | 5 | 6 | 7 | 9 |
| 20–34 | 67 | 2.8 | 2 | 1 | 2 | 3 | 3 | 4 | 5 | 6 |
| 35–49 | 82 | 3.6 | 5 | 2 | 2 | 3 | 4 | 7 | 10 | 10 |
| 50–64 | 56 | 3.7 | 4 | 1 | 3 | 3 | 4 | 6 | 8 | 12 |
| 65+ | 16 | 3.9 | 1 | 3 | 3 | 4 | 5 | 5 | 6 | 6 |
| **2. MULTIPLE DX** | | | | | | | | | | |
| 0–19 Years | 202 | 10.2 | 214 | 2 | 3 | 6 | 10 | 20 | 51 | 92 |
| 20–34 | 278 | 3.9 | 13 | 1 | 2 | 3 | 5 | 7 | 8 | 18 |
| 35–49 | 517 | 5.4 | 36 | 2 | 2 | 4 | 6 | 10 | 13 | 34 |
| 50–64 | 609 | 6.7 | 28 | 1 | 4 | 6 | 8 | 12 | 15 | 27 |
| 65+ | 678 | 9.8 | 68 | 3 | 5 | 7 | 11 | 21 | 26 | 37 |
| **TOTAL SINGLE DX** | 301 | 3.6 | 3 | 2 | 2 | 3 | 4 | 6 | 7 | 10 |
| **TOTAL MULTIPLE DX** | 2,284 | 7.2 | 59 | 2 | 3 | 5 | 8 | 13 | 19 | 39 |
| **TOTAL** | | | | | | | | | | |
| 0–19 Years | 282 | 8.2 | 154 | 2 | 3 | 5 | 8 | 15 | 25 | 67 |
| 20–34 | 345 | 3.6 | 10 | 1 | 2 | 3 | 5 | 7 | 8 | 18 |
| 35–49 | 599 | 5.2 | 32 | 2 | 2 | 4 | 6 | 10 | 12 | 34 |
| 50–64 | 665 | 6.5 | 27 | 3 | 3 | 6 | 8 | 11 | 14 | 24 |
| 65+ | 694 | 9.6 | 67 | 3 | 5 | 7 | 11 | 20 | 26 | 37 |
| **GRAND TOTAL** | 2,585 | 6.7 | 54 | 2 | 3 | 5 | 8 | 12 | 18 | 37 |

## 54.5: PERITONEAL ADHESIOLYSIS. Formerly included in operation group(s) 642.

| Type of Patients | Observed Patients | Avg. Stay | Vari-ance | Percentiles | | | | | | |
|---|---|---|---|---|---|---|---|---|---|---|
| | | | | 10th | 25th | 50th | 75th | 90th | 95th | 99th |
| **1. SINGLE DX** | | | | | | | | | | |
| 0–19 Years | 173 | 5.8 | 46 | 1 | 4 | 5 | 6 | 9 | 12 | 18 |
| 20–34 | 275 | 4.4 | 15 | 1 | 2 | 3 | 5 | 9 | 10 | 24 |
| 35–49 | 503 | 3.9 | 10 | 2 | 2 | 3 | 5 | 8 | 10 | 17 |
| 50–64 | 211 | 5.8 | 14 | 2 | 3 | 5 | 7 | 11 | 13 | 18 |
| 65+ | 121 | 6.5 | 11 | 3 | 4 | 6 | 8 | 12 | 13 | 16 |
| **2. MULTIPLE DX** | | | | | | | | | | |
| 0–19 Years | 926 | 10.3 | 122 | 2 | 5 | 7 | 12 | 22 | 31 | 59 |
| 20–34 | 2,457 | 5.4 | 37 | 1 | 2 | 3 | 7 | 11 | 16 | 34 |
| 35–49 | 4,945 | 6.4 | 33 | 3 | 5 | 5 | 8 | 12 | 17 | 29 |
| 50–64 | 4,157 | 8.6 | 45 | 3 | 4 | 7 | 10 | 16 | 21 | 34 |
| 65+ | 6,641 | 11.1 | 58 | 4 | 7 | 9 | 13 | 20 | 25 | 41 |
| **TOTAL SINGLE DX** | 1,283 | 4.8 | 18 | 1 | 2 | 4 | 6 | 9 | 11 | 18 |
| **TOTAL MULTIPLE DX** | 19,126 | 8.5 | 54 | 2 | 4 | 7 | 11 | 16 | 22 | 38 |
| **TOTAL** | | | | | | | | | | |
| 0–19 Years | 1,099 | 9.6 | 112 | 2 | 4 | 6 | 11 | 20 | 31 | 59 |
| 20–34 | 2,732 | 5.3 | 35 | 1 | 2 | 3 | 7 | 10 | 16 | 34 |
| 35–49 | 5,448 | 6.1 | 31 | 2 | 3 | 5 | 8 | 12 | 16 | 28 |
| 50–64 | 4,368 | 8.4 | 44 | 2 | 4 | 7 | 10 | 15 | 21 | 33 |
| 65+ | 6,762 | 11.0 | 57 | 4 | 6 | 9 | 13 | 20 | 25 | 41 |
| **GRAND TOTAL** | 20,409 | 8.2 | 52 | 2 | 4 | 7 | 10 | 16 | 21 | 37 |

Length of Stay by Diagnosis and Operation, United States, 2000

## United States, October 1998–September 1999 Data, by Operation

### 54.51: LAPSCP PERITON ADHESIO. Formerly included in operation group(s) 642.

| Type of Patients | Observed Patients | Avg. Stay | Vari-ance | Percentiles | | | | | | |
|---|---|---|---|---|---|---|---|---|---|---|
| | | | | 10th | 25th | 50th | 75th | 90th | 95th | 99th |
| **1. SINGLE DX** | | | | | | | | | | |
| 0–19 Years | 45 | 6.5 | 95 | 1 | 4 | 5 | 6 | 11 | 13 | 97 |
| 20–34 | 96 | 2.9 | 3 | 1 | 2 | 3 | 4 | 5 | 6 | 10 |
| 35–49 | 136 | 2.7 | 4 | 1 | 1 | 2 | 4 | 4 | 6 | 11 |
| 50–64 | 43 | 4.2 | 8 | 1 | 2 | 3 | 6 | 7 | 10 | 14 |
| 65+ | 20 | 4.9 | 9 | 1 | 2 | 5 | 6 | 10 | 10 | 11 |
| **2. MULTIPLE DX** | | | | | | | | | | |
| 0–19 Years | 165 | 9.8 | 199 | 1 | 1 | 4 | 9 | 26 | 53 | 59 |
| 20–34 | 790 | 3.0 | 8 | 1 | 1 | 2 | 3 | 6 | 6 | 15 |
| 35–49 | 993 | 4.1 | 17 | 1 | 2 | 3 | 5 | 9 | 12 | 18 |
| 50–64 | 484 | 5.2 | 27 | 1 | 2 | 4 | 7 | 11 | 13 | 29 |
| 65+ | 540 | 7.4 | 35 | 1 | 3 | 6 | 10 | 15 | 19 | 25 |
| **TOTAL SINGLE DX** | 340 | 3.8 | 25 | 1 | 2 | 3 | 5 | 7 | 9 | 13 |
| **TOTAL MULTIPLE DX** | 2,972 | 4.9 | 34 | 1 | 2 | 3 | 6 | 10 | 14 | 29 |
| **TOTAL** | | | | | | | | | | |
| 0–19 Years | 210 | 8.9 | 170 | 1 | 2 | 5 | 9 | 19 | 50 | 59 |
| 20–34 | 886 | 3.0 | 8 | 1 | 2 | 3 | 3 | 6 | 8 | 14 |
| 35–49 | 1,129 | 3.9 | 15 | 1 | 2 | 3 | 5 | 8 | 11 | 18 |
| 50–64 | 527 | 5.1 | 26 | 1 | 2 | 4 | 7 | 11 | 13 | 29 |
| 65+ | 560 | 7.3 | 34 | 1 | 3 | 6 | 10 | 15 | 19 | 25 |
| **GRAND TOTAL** | 3,312 | 4.7 | 33 | 1 | 2 | 3 | 6 | 10 | 13 | 28 |

### 54.6: ABD WALL/PERITON SUTURE. Formerly included in operation group(s) 642.

| Type of Patients | Observed Patients | Avg. Stay | Vari-ance | Percentiles | | | | | | |
|---|---|---|---|---|---|---|---|---|---|---|
| | | | | 10th | 25th | 50th | 75th | 90th | 95th | 99th |
| **1. SINGLE DX** | | | | | | | | | | |
| 0–19 Years | 13 | 2.0 | <1 | 1 | 1 | 2 | 2 | 3 | 3 | 5 |
| 20–34 | 43 | 2.6 | 7 | 1 | 2 | 3 | 3 | 4 | 4 | 8 |
| 35–49 | 40 | 3.3 | 7 | 1 | 2 | 2 | 4 | 7 | 8 | 13 |
| 50–64 | 19 | 2.5 | 3 | 1 | 2 | 2 | 4 | 6 | 6 | 6 |
| 65+ | 19 | 3.0 | 8 | 1 | 1 | 2 | 4 | 6 | 7 | 14 |
| **2. MULTIPLE DX** | | | | | | | | | | |
| 0–19 Years | 75 | 6.4 | 113 | 1 | 2 | 3 | 4 | 13 | 31 | 58 |
| 20–34 | 136 | 4.9 | 21 | 1 | 2 | 3 | 6 | 15 | 15 | 17 |
| 35–49 | 199 | 5.8 | 28 | 1 | 3 | 4 | 7 | 12 | 16 | 24 |
| 50–64 | 169 | 7.0 | 45 | 2 | 3 | 5 | 8 | 14 | 20 | 35 |
| 65+ | 266 | 7.8 | 41 | 2 | 4 | 7 | 9 | 17 | 20 | 38 |
| **TOTAL SINGLE DX** | 134 | 2.8 | 4 | 1 | 2 | 3 | 3 | 5 | 7 | 13 |
| **TOTAL MULTIPLE DX** | 845 | 6.6 | 42 | 1 | 3 | 5 | 8 | 14 | 19 | 34 |
| **TOTAL** | | | | | | | | | | |
| 0–19 Years | 88 | 5.8 | 99 | 1 | 2 | 3 | 4 | 12 | 27 | 58 |
| 20–34 | 179 | 4.2 | 16 | 1 | 2 | 3 | 4 | 10 | 15 | 15 |
| 35–49 | 239 | 5.5 | 26 | 1 | 2 | 4 | 7 | 12 | 14 | 22 |
| 50–64 | 188 | 6.6 | 43 | 1 | 3 | 5 | 8 | 13 | 19 | 34 |
| 65+ | 285 | 7.5 | 40 | 2 | 4 | 6 | 8 | 16 | 20 | 32 |
| **GRAND TOTAL** | 979 | 6.1 | 39 | 1 | 2 | 4 | 8 | 13 | 17 | 32 |

### 54.59: PERITON ADHESIOLYSIS NEC. Formerly included in operation group(s) 642.

| Type of Patients | Observed Patients | Avg. Stay | Vari-ance | Percentiles | | | | | | |
|---|---|---|---|---|---|---|---|---|---|---|
| | | | | 10th | 25th | 50th | 75th | 90th | 95th | 99th |
| **1. SINGLE DX** | | | | | | | | | | |
| 0–19 Years | 128 | 5.3 | 8 | 2 | 4 | 5 | 6 | 8 | 10 | 18 |
| 20–34 | 179 | 5.3 | 21 | 2 | 2 | 4 | 7 | 10 | 11 | 24 |
| 35–49 | 367 | 4.4 | 12 | 1 | 2 | 4 | 6 | 8 | 11 | 17 |
| 50–64 | 168 | 6.1 | 15 | 2 | 3 | 5 | 8 | 11 | 14 | 18 |
| 65+ | 101 | 6.7 | 11 | 3 | 5 | 6 | 8 | 12 | 13 | 16 |
| **2. MULTIPLE DX** | | | | | | | | | | |
| 0–19 Years | 761 | 10.4 | 101 | 3 | 5 | 7 | 12 | 21 | 31 | 61 |
| 20–34 | 1,667 | 6.7 | 47 | 2 | 3 | 5 | 8 | 13 | 20 | 34 |
| 35–49 | 3,952 | 7.0 | 35 | 2 | 3 | 5 | 9 | 13 | 17 | 32 |
| 50–64 | 3,673 | 9.0 | 46 | 3 | 5 | 7 | 11 | 16 | 22 | 37 |
| 65+ | 6,101 | 11.4 | 58 | 5 | 7 | 10 | 14 | 20 | 25 | 42 |
| **TOTAL SINGLE DX** | 943 | 5.2 | 14 | 1 | 2 | 5 | 7 | 9 | 12 | 18 |
| **TOTAL MULTIPLE DX** | 16,154 | 9.2 | 54 | 3 | 5 | 8 | 11 | 17 | 23 | 39 |
| **TOTAL** | | | | | | | | | | |
| 0–19 Years | 889 | 9.8 | 92 | 3 | 5 | 7 | 11 | 20 | 29 | 59 |
| 20–34 | 1,846 | 6.6 | 45 | 2 | 3 | 4 | 8 | 13 | 19 | 34 |
| 35–49 | 4,319 | 6.7 | 34 | 2 | 3 | 5 | 9 | 13 | 17 | 30 |
| 50–64 | 3,841 | 8.9 | 44 | 3 | 5 | 7 | 11 | 16 | 22 | 35 |
| 65+ | 6,202 | 11.3 | 58 | 5 | 7 | 10 | 14 | 20 | 25 | 42 |
| **GRAND TOTAL** | 17,097 | 9.0 | 53 | 2 | 4 | 7 | 11 | 17 | 23 | 38 |

### 54.61: RECLOSE POSTOP DISRUPT. Formerly included in operation group(s) 642.

| Type of Patients | Observed Patients | Avg. Stay | Vari-ance | Percentiles | | | | | | |
|---|---|---|---|---|---|---|---|---|---|---|
| | | | | 10th | 25th | 50th | 75th | 90th | 95th | 99th |
| **1. SINGLE DX** | | | | | | | | | | |
| 0–19 Years | 8 | 2.3 | <1 | 2 | 2 | 2 | 3 | 3 | 3 | 3 |
| 20–34 | 20 | 2.7 | 2 | 2 | 2 | 2 | 3 | 4 | 6 | 8 |
| 35–49 | 19 | 4.2 | 10 | 1 | 2 | 3 | 5 | 7 | 13 | 13 |
| 50–64 | 15 | 2.3 | 2 | 1 | 2 | 2 | 4 | 4 | 6 | 6 |
| 65+ | 16 | 2.4 | 2 | 1 | 2 | 3 | 3 | 4 | 5 | 6 |
| **2. MULTIPLE DX** | | | | | | | | | | |
| 0–19 Years | 23 | 4.4 | 35 | 1 | 2 | 3 | 4 | 6 | 11 | 36 |
| 20–34 | 41 | 6.7 | 28 | 2 | 2 | 4 | 15 | 15 | 15 | 15 |
| 35–49 | 105 | 7.0 | 25 | 2 | 3 | 7 | 10 | 12 | 16 | 22 |
| 50–64 | 127 | 7.2 | 49 | 2 | 4 | 7 | 9 | 14 | 20 | 35 |
| 65+ | 223 | 8.1 | 33 | 2 | 4 | 7 | 9 | 17 | 20 | 30 |
| **TOTAL SINGLE DX** | 78 | 2.8 | 4 | 1 | 2 | 2 | 3 | 5 | 7 | 13 |
| **TOTAL MULTIPLE DX** | 519 | 7.4 | 36 | 2 | 4 | 6 | 9 | 15 | 19 | 30 |
| **TOTAL** | | | | | | | | | | |
| 0–19 Years | 31 | 3.9 | 27 | 2 | 2 | 2 | 4 | 6 | 10 | 36 |
| 20–34 | 61 | 5.0 | 21 | 2 | 3 | 3 | 6 | 15 | 15 | 15 |
| 35–49 | 124 | 6.7 | 24 | 2 | 3 | 6 | 8 | 12 | 16 | 22 |
| 50–64 | 142 | 6.7 | 46 | 2 | 3 | 4 | 9 | 13 | 20 | 35 |
| 65+ | 239 | 7.7 | 33 | 2 | 3 | 7 | 9 | 17 | 20 | 27 |
| **GRAND TOTAL** | 597 | 6.8 | 34 | 2 | 3 | 5 | 8 | 14 | 18 | 27 |

Length of Stay by Diagnosis and Operation, United States, 2000

## 54.7: OTH ABD WALL PERITON REP. Formerly included in operation group(s) 642.

| Type of Patients | Observed Patients | Avg. Stay | Vari-ance | 10th | 25th | 50th | 75th | 90th | 95th | 99th |
|---|---|---|---|---|---|---|---|---|---|---|
| **1. SINGLE DX** | | | | | | | | | | |
| 0–19 Years | 14 | 18.6 | 59 | 10 | 16 | 16 | 26 | 29 | 29 | 29 |
| 20–34 | 10 | 4.4 | 5 | 2 | 2 | 5 | 5 | 6 | 8 | 8 |
| 35–49 | 7 | 3.4 | 3 | 1 | 2 | 3 | 5 | 6 | 6 | 6 |
| 50–64 | 6 | 2.4 | 3 | 1 | 1 | 2 | 3 | 6 | 6 | 6 |
| 65+ | 3 | 3.2 | 2 | 2 | 2 | 3 | 5 | 5 | 5 | 5 |
| **2. MULTIPLE DX** | | | | | | | | | | |
| 0–19 Years | 305 | 34.1 | 533 | 19 | 19 | 33 | 55 | 94 | >99 | >99 |
| 20–34 | 57 | 5.3 | 5 | 3 | 3 | 5 | 6 | 8 | 9 | 9 |
| 35–49 | 77 | 8.8 | 101 | 2 | 4 | 6 | 8 | 26 | 34 | 49 |
| 50–64 | 53 | 8.6 | 40 | 2 | 4 | 7 | 12 | 19 | 24 | 24 |
| 65+ | 42 | 7.1 | 24 | 3 | 4 | 6 | 8 | 14 | 16 | >99 |
| **TOTAL SINGLE DX** | 40 | 12.2 | 91 | 2 | 4 | 10 | 17 | 29 | 29 | 29 |
| **TOTAL MULTIPLE DX** | 534 | 20.7 | 471 | 3 | 5 | 12 | 34 | 71 | 97 | >99 |
| **TOTAL** | | | | | | | | | | |
| 0–19 Years | 319 | 32.7 | 508 | 6 | 18 | 29 | 54 | 93 | >99 | >99 |
| 20–34 | 67 | 5.2 | 5 | 3 | 3 | 5 | 6 | 8 | 9 | 12 |
| 35–49 | 84 | 8.4 | 96 | 2 | 3 | 6 | 8 | 24 | 28 | 49 |
| 50–64 | 59 | 8.1 | 39 | 2 | 3 | 6 | 11 | 15 | 24 | 24 |
| 65+ | 45 | 7.0 | 24 | 3 | 4 | 6 | 8 | 14 | 16 | >99 |
| **GRAND TOTAL** | 574 | 20.0 | 445 | 3 | 5 | 12 | 33 | 70 | 94 | >99 |

## 54.91: PERC ABD DRAINAGE. Formerly included in operation group(s) 638.

| Type of Patients | Observed Patients | Avg. Stay | Vari-ance | 10th | 25th | 50th | 75th | 90th | 95th | 99th |
|---|---|---|---|---|---|---|---|---|---|---|
| **1. SINGLE DX** | | | | | | | | | | |
| 0–19 Years | 56 | 5.8 | 10 | 2 | 4 | 5 | 8 | 11 | 13 | 13 |
| 20–34 | 85 | 4.4 | 11 | 1 | 2 | 3 | 6 | 9 | 9 | 19 |
| 35–49 | 95 | 3.9 | 5 | 2 | 2 | 3 | 6 | 7 | 8 | 12 |
| 50–64 | 60 | 6.0 | 18 | 2 | 2 | 4 | 11 | 12 | 14 | 18 |
| 65+ | 30 | 5.2 | 37 | 1 | 2 | 4 | 7 | 8 | 9 | 32 |
| **2. MULTIPLE DX** | | | | | | | | | | |
| 0–19 Years | 409 | 7.5 | 65 | 2 | 4 | 6 | 9 | 13 | 17 | 50 |
| 20–34 | 966 | 6.5 | 36 | 2 | 3 | 5 | 8 | 12 | 16 | 25 |
| 35–49 | 4,693 | 6.2 | 29 | 2 | 3 | 5 | 8 | 12 | 16 | 28 |
| 50–64 | 5,292 | 6.3 | 28 | 2 | 3 | 5 | 8 | 12 | 16 | 26 |
| 65+ | 5,931 | 7.3 | 38 | 2 | 3 | 6 | 9 | 14 | 19 | 30 |
| **TOTAL SINGLE DX** | 326 | 4.8 | 13 | 1 | 2 | 4 | 6 | 9 | 11 | 14 |
| **TOTAL MULTIPLE DX** | 17,291 | 6.7 | 33 | 2 | 3 | 5 | 8 | 13 | 17 | 28 |
| **TOTAL** | | | | | | | | | | |
| 0–19 Years | 465 | 7.4 | 60 | 2 | 4 | 6 | 9 | 12 | 16 | 50 |
| 20–34 | 1,051 | 6.2 | 33 | 1 | 3 | 5 | 8 | 12 | 16 | 25 |
| 35–49 | 4,788 | 6.1 | 29 | 2 | 3 | 5 | 8 | 12 | 16 | 28 |
| 50–64 | 5,352 | 6.3 | 28 | 2 | 3 | 5 | 8 | 12 | 16 | 26 |
| 65+ | 5,961 | 7.3 | 38 | 2 | 3 | 6 | 9 | 14 | 19 | 30 |
| **GRAND TOTAL** | 17,617 | 6.6 | 33 | 2 | 3 | 5 | 8 | 13 | 17 | 28 |

## 54.9: OTHER ABD REGION OPS. Formerly included in operation group(s) 638, 641, 642.

| Type of Patients | Observed Patients | Avg. Stay | Vari-ance | 10th | 25th | 50th | 75th | 90th | 95th | 99th |
|---|---|---|---|---|---|---|---|---|---|---|
| **1. SINGLE DX** | | | | | | | | | | |
| 0–19 Years | 254 | 4.7 | 9 | 1 | 3 | 4 | 6 | 9 | 9 | 13 |
| 20–34 | 126 | 3.8 | 9 | 1 | 2 | 3 | 4 | 9 | 9 | 14 |
| 35–49 | 133 | 3.5 | 4 | 1 | 2 | 3 | 4 | 7 | 8 | 10 |
| 50–64 | 78 | 5.5 | 18 | 1 | 2 | 3 | 8 | 11 | 14 | 18 |
| 65+ | 50 | 5.1 | 35 | 1 | 2 | 3 | 7 | 9 | 23 | 32 |
| **2. MULTIPLE DX** | | | | | | | | | | |
| 0–19 Years | 1,828 | 7.6 | 107 | 2 | 2 | 5 | 9 | 17 | 26 | 76 |
| 20–34 | 2,090 | 5.9 | 34 | 1 | 3 | 4 | 7 | 11 | 15 | 28 |
| 35–49 | 6,909 | 6.0 | 30 | 2 | 3 | 5 | 8 | 12 | 16 | 28 |
| 50–64 | 7,967 | 6.5 | 47 | 2 | 3 | 5 | 8 | 13 | 17 | 29 |
| 65+ | 8,458 | 7.4 | 42 | 2 | 3 | 6 | 9 | 14 | 20 | 34 |
| **TOTAL SINGLE DX** | 641 | 4.4 | 11 | 1 | 2 | 4 | 5 | 9 | 10 | 14 |
| **TOTAL MULTIPLE DX** | 27,252 | 6.7 | 45 | 2 | 3 | 5 | 8 | 13 | 18 | 33 |
| **TOTAL** | | | | | | | | | | |
| 0–19 Years | 2,082 | 7.2 | 94 | 1 | 2 | 4 | 5 | 15 | 23 | 67 |
| 20–34 | 2,216 | 5.7 | 32 | 1 | 2 | 4 | 7 | 11 | 15 | 27 |
| 35–49 | 7,042 | 6.0 | 30 | 2 | 3 | 4 | 7 | 12 | 16 | 28 |
| 50–64 | 8,045 | 6.5 | 47 | 2 | 3 | 5 | 8 | 13 | 17 | 29 |
| 65+ | 8,508 | 7.4 | 42 | 2 | 3 | 6 | 9 | 14 | 20 | 34 |
| **GRAND TOTAL** | 27,893 | 6.6 | 44 | 2 | 3 | 5 | 8 | 13 | 18 | 32 |

## 54.92: RMVL FB PERITON CAVITY. Formerly included in operation group(s) 642.

| Type of Patients | Observed Patients | Avg. Stay | Vari-ance | 10th | 25th | 50th | 75th | 90th | 95th | 99th |
|---|---|---|---|---|---|---|---|---|---|---|
| **1. SINGLE DX** | | | | | | | | | | |
| 0–19 Years | 6 | 1.7 | <1 | 1 | 1 | 1 | 2 | 4 | 4 | 4 |
| 20–34 | 7 | 1.9 | <1 | 1 | 1 | 2 | 2 | 3 | 3 | 3 |
| 35–49 | 6 | 2.5 | <1 | 2 | 2 | 2 | 3 | 3 | 3 | 4 |
| 50–64 | 1 | 1.0 | 0 | 1 | 1 | 1 | 1 | 1 | 1 | 1 |
| 65+ | 1 | 1.0 | 0 | 1 | 1 | 1 | 1 | 1 | 1 | 1 |
| **2. MULTIPLE DX** | | | | | | | | | | |
| 0–19 Years | 28 | 7.2 | 61 | 2 | 3 | 4 | 10 | 22 | 29 | 33 |
| 20–34 | 53 | 5.8 | 41 | 2 | 3 | 4 | 7 | 9 | 12 | 55 |
| 35–49 | 116 | 6.2 | 37 | 2 | 3 | 4 | 7 | 12 | 20 | 24 |
| 50–64 | 88 | 23.3 | 996 | 3 | 4 | 7 | 20 | 85 | 85 | 85 |
| 65+ | 73 | 8.4 | 98 | 3 | 4 | 4 | 8 | 17 | 26 | 65 |
| **TOTAL SINGLE DX** | 21 | 2.1 | <1 | 1 | 1 | 2 | 3 | 3 | 3 | 4 |
| **TOTAL MULTIPLE DX** | 358 | 11.0 | 346 | 2 | 3 | 5 | 9 | 20 | 85 | 85 |
| **TOTAL** | | | | | | | | | | |
| 0–19 Years | 34 | 6.2 | 54 | 1 | 2 | 4 | 8 | 10 | 29 | 33 |
| 20–34 | 60 | 5.1 | 36 | 1 | 2 | 4 | 5 | 9 | 12 | 29 |
| 35–49 | 122 | 5.6 | 33 | 2 | 3 | 4 | 6 | 10 | 19 | 24 |
| 50–64 | 89 | 22.8 | 985 | 1 | 4 | 7 | 20 | 85 | 85 | 85 |
| 65+ | 74 | 8.3 | 97 | 3 | 4 | 4 | 8 | 17 | 26 | 65 |
| **GRAND TOTAL** | 379 | 10.0 | 315 | 2 | 3 | 4 | 8 | 20 | 55 | 85 |

# United States, October 1998–September 1999 Data, by Operation

## 54.93: CREATE CUTANEOPERIT FIST. Formerly included in operation group(s) 642.

| Type of Patients | Observed Patients | Variance | Avg. Stay | 10th | 25th | 50th | 75th | 90th | 95th | 99th |
|---|---|---|---|---|---|---|---|---|---|---|
| **1. SINGLE DX** | | | | | | | | | | |
| 0–19 Years | 16 | 19 | 3.5 | 1 | 1 | 1 | 7 | 11 | 16 | 16 |
| 20–34 | 13 | <1 | 2.0 | 1 | 1 | 1 | 3 | 4 | 6 | 6 |
| 35–49 | 20 | 1 | 2.2 | 1 | 1 | 2 | 3 | 4 | 4 | 5 |
| 50–64 | 6 | 2 | 1.4 | 1 | 1 | 1 | 1 | 5 | 5 | 5 |
| 65+ | 9 | 74 | 6.4 | 1 | 1 | 2 | 7 | 23 | 23 | 23 |
| **2. MULTIPLE DX** | | | | | | | | | | |
| 0–19 Years | 230 | 303 | 14.9 | 2 | 4 | 10 | 21 | 33 | 75 | 94 |
| 20–34 | 210 | 52 | 6.7 | 1 | 2 | 4 | 9 | 13 | 19 | 36 |
| 35–49 | 409 | 43 | 6.8 | 1 | 2 | 5 | 9 | 15 | 20 | 32 |
| 50–64 | 605 | 65 | 8.2 | 1 | 3 | 6 | 11 | 18 | 24 | 39 |
| 65+ | 606 | 80 | 9.5 | 2 | 4 | 7 | 11 | 22 | 30 | 41 |
| **TOTAL SINGLE DX** | 64 | 17 | 3.0 | 1 | 1 | 1 | 3 | 7 | 11 | 23 |
| **TOTAL MULTIPLE DX** | 2,060 | 99 | 9.0 | 1 | 3 | 6 | 11 | 20 | 28 | 52 |
| **TOTAL** | | | | | | | | | | |
| 0–19 Years | 246 | 293 | 14.2 | 1 | 3 | 9 | 18 | 33 | 67 | 94 |
| 20–34 | 223 | 51 | 6.5 | 1 | 2 | 4 | 9 | 13 | 19 | 36 |
| 35–49 | 429 | 42 | 6.7 | 1 | 2 | 5 | 9 | 15 | 20 | 32 |
| 50–64 | 611 | 65 | 8.2 | 1 | 3 | 6 | 11 | 18 | 24 | 39 |
| 65+ | 615 | 80 | 9.4 | 2 | 4 | 7 | 11 | 22 | 30 | 41 |
| **GRAND TOTAL** | 2,124 | 98 | 8.9 | 1 | 3 | 6 | 11 | 20 | 28 | 52 |

## 54.94: CREAT PERITONEOVAS SHUNT. Formerly included in operation group(s) 642.

| Type of Patients | Observed Patients | Variance | Avg. Stay | 10th | 25th | 50th | 75th | 90th | 95th | 99th |
|---|---|---|---|---|---|---|---|---|---|---|
| **1. SINGLE DX** | | | | | | | | | | |
| 0–19 Years | 3 | <1 | 3.3 | 2 | 3 | 4 | 4 | 4 | 4 | 4 |
| 20–34 | 2 | <1 | 4.7 | 3 | 5 | 5 | 5 | 5 | 5 | 5 |
| 35–49 | 1 | 0 | 2.0 | 2 | 2 | 2 | 2 | 2 | 2 | 2 |
| 50–64 | 1 | 0 | 2.0 | 2 | 2 | 2 | 2 | 2 | 2 | 2 |
| 65+ | 0 | | | | | | | | | |
| **2. MULTIPLE DX** | | | | | | | | | | |
| 0–19 Years | 18 | 44 | 10.8 | 2 | 9 | 13 | 22 | >99 | >99 | >99 |
| 20–34 | 17 | 11 | 7.9 | 3 | 8 | 9 | 9 | 10 | 10 | 20 |
| 35–49 | 63 | 34 | 8.4 | 2 | 5 | 7 | 12 | 15 | 22 | 30 |
| 50–64 | 132 | 63 | 8.7 | 2 | 4 | 6 | 11 | 21 | 25 | 32 |
| 65+ | 148 | 56 | 9.6 | 2 | 3 | 8 | 14 | 20 | 22 | 33 |
| **TOTAL SINGLE DX** | 7 | 2 | 3.4 | 2 | 2 | 3 | 5 | 5 | 5 | 5 |
| **TOTAL MULTIPLE DX** | 378 | 48 | 9.0 | 2 | 4 | 8 | 12 | 20 | 24 | 58 |
| **TOTAL** | | | | | | | | | | |
| 0–19 Years | 21 | 44 | 9.9 | 2 | 5 | 11 | 17 | >99 | >99 | >99 |
| 20–34 | 19 | 11 | 7.7 | 3 | 5 | 9 | 9 | 10 | 10 | 20 |
| 35–49 | 64 | 34 | 8.3 | 2 | 5 | 7 | 12 | 15 | 15 | 30 |
| 50–64 | 133 | 63 | 8.7 | 2 | 4 | 6 | 11 | 21 | 25 | 32 |
| 65+ | 148 | 56 | 9.6 | 2 | 3 | 8 | 14 | 20 | 22 | 33 |
| **GRAND TOTAL** | 385 | 48 | 8.9 | 2 | 4 | 8 | 12 | 20 | 24 | 58 |

## 54.95: PERITONEAL INCISION. Formerly included in operation group(s) 642.

| Type of Patients | Observed Patients | Variance | Avg. Stay | 10th | 25th | 50th | 75th | 90th | 95th | 99th |
|---|---|---|---|---|---|---|---|---|---|---|
| **1. SINGLE DX** | | | | | | | | | | |
| 0–19 Years | 166 | 6 | 4.6 | 1 | 3 | 4 | 5 | 8 | 9 | 10 |
| 20–34 | 12 | <1 | 2.4 | 2 | 2 | 2 | 3 | 4 | 4 | 5 |
| 35–49 | 6 | 2 | 3.3 | 1 | 3 | 3 | 3 | 6 | 6 | 6 |
| 50–64 | 5 | 2 | 4.3 | 2 | 4 | 4 | 5 | 5 | 7 | 7 |
| 65+ | 5 | <1 | 1.9 | 1 | 1 | 2 | 3 | 3 | 3 | 3 |
| **2. MULTIPLE DX** | | | | | | | | | | |
| 0–19 Years | 729 | 85 | 6.5 | 1 | 2 | 3 | 7 | 16 | 23 | 61 |
| 20–34 | 201 | 44 | 6.6 | 1 | 2 | 5 | 9 | 11 | 20 | 36 |
| 35–49 | 313 | 74 | 7.6 | 2 | 3 | 5 | 9 | 16 | 21 | 47 |
| 50–64 | 321 | 65 | 7.9 | 2 | 3 | 5 | 10 | 18 | 24 | 36 |
| 65+ | 308 | 80 | 9.0 | 2 | 3 | 7 | 12 | 20 | 25 | 38 |
| **TOTAL SINGLE DX** | 194 | 5 | 4.3 | 1 | 3 | 4 | 5 | 8 | 9 | 10 |
| **TOTAL MULTIPLE DX** | 1,872 | 75 | 7.3 | 1 | 2 | 5 | 9 | 17 | 22 | 44 |
| **TOTAL** | | | | | | | | | | |
| 0–19 Years | 895 | 67 | 6.1 | 1 | 2 | 4 | 7 | 13 | 21 | 44 |
| 20–34 | 213 | 41 | 6.2 | 1 | 2 | 5 | 8 | 11 | 19 | 35 |
| 35–49 | 319 | 72 | 7.5 | 2 | 3 | 5 | 9 | 15 | 21 | 47 |
| 50–64 | 326 | 64 | 7.9 | 2 | 3 | 5 | 10 | 17 | 24 | 36 |
| 65+ | 313 | 80 | 9.0 | 2 | 3 | 7 | 12 | 20 | 25 | 38 |
| **GRAND TOTAL** | 2,066 | 67 | 6.9 | 1 | 2 | 5 | 8 | 15 | 22 | 42 |

## 54.98: PERITONEAL DIALYSIS. Formerly included in operation group(s) 641.

| Type of Patients | Observed Patients | Variance | Avg. Stay | 10th | 25th | 50th | 75th | 90th | 95th | 99th |
|---|---|---|---|---|---|---|---|---|---|---|
| **1. SINGLE DX** | | | | | | | | | | |
| 0–19 Years | 4 | 2 | 1.7 | 1 | 1 | 1 | 1 | 5 | 5 | 5 |
| 20–34 | 3 | 19 | 6.7 | 1 | 3 | 10 | 10 | 10 | 10 | 10 |
| 35–49 | 4 | <1 | 3.2 | 3 | 3 | 3 | 3 | 4 | 4 | 4 |
| 50–64 | 3 | 1 | 5.1 | 1 | 1 | 9 | 9 | 10 | 10 | 10 |
| 65+ | 2 | 10 | 7.2 | 2 | 2 | 9 | 9 | 9 | 9 | 9 |
| **2. MULTIPLE DX** | | | | | | | | | | |
| 0–19 Years | 392 | 57 | 5.3 | 1 | 2 | 3 | 6 | 12 | 16 | 43 |
| 20–34 | 613 | 18 | 4.3 | 2 | 3 | 3 | 5 | 7 | 11 | 22 |
| 35–49 | 1,259 | 18 | 4.7 | 2 | 3 | 4 | 6 | 9 | 12 | 19 |
| 50–64 | 1,459 | 20 | 5.1 | 2 | 3 | 4 | 6 | 10 | 14 | 21 |
| 65+ | 1,351 | 24 | 5.9 | 2 | 3 | 5 | 7 | 11 | 15 | 27 |
| **TOTAL SINGLE DX** | 16 | 13 | 4.7 | 1 | 1 | 3 | 9 | 10 | 10 | 10 |
| **TOTAL MULTIPLE DX** | 5,074 | 23 | 5.1 | 2 | 2 | 4 | 6 | 10 | 13 | 23 |
| **TOTAL** | | | | | | | | | | |
| 0–19 Years | 396 | 56 | 5.3 | 1 | 2 | 3 | 6 | 12 | 16 | 43 |
| 20–34 | 616 | 18 | 4.3 | 2 | 3 | 3 | 5 | 7 | 11 | 22 |
| 35–49 | 1,263 | 18 | 4.7 | 1 | 2 | 4 | 6 | 9 | 12 | 19 |
| 50–64 | 1,462 | 20 | 5.1 | 2 | 2 | 4 | 6 | 10 | 14 | 21 |
| 65+ | 1,353 | 24 | 5.9 | 2 | 3 | 5 | 7 | 11 | 15 | 26 |
| **GRAND TOTAL** | 5,090 | 23 | 5.1 | 2 | 2 | 4 | 6 | 10 | 13 | 23 |

# United States, October 1998–September 1999 Data, by Operation

## 55.0: NEPHROTOMY & NEPHROSTOMY. Formerly included in operation group(s) 644, 646.

| Type of Patients | Observed Patients | Avg. Stay | Vari- ance | Percentiles | | | | | | |
|---|---|---|---|---|---|---|---|---|---|---|
| | | | | 10th | 25th | 50th | 75th | 90th | 95th | 99th |
| **1. SINGLE DX** | | | | | | | | | | |
| 0–19 Years | 50 | 3.6 | 8 | 1 | 1 | 2 | 8 | 8 | 8 | 8 |
| 20–34 | 189 | 2.9 | 2 | 1 | 2 | 3 | 4 | 5 | 6 | 6 |
| 35–49 | 319 | 3.1 | 5 | 1 | 2 | 2 | 4 | 7 | 9 | 9 |
| 50–64 | 223 | 2.4 | 2 | 1 | 2 | 2 | 3 | 4 | 5 | 7 |
| 65+ | 74 | 3.1 | 3 | 1 | 2 | 3 | 4 | 6 | 8 | 8 |
| **2. MULTIPLE DX** | | | | | | | | | | |
| 0–19 Years | 249 | 7.1 | 89 | 2 | 2 | 4 | 7 | 16 | 24 | 52 |
| 20–34 | 647 | 5.4 | 29 | 1 | 2 | 4 | 6 | 11 | 16 | 30 |
| 35–49 | 1,371 | 5.3 | 32 | 1 | 2 | 4 | 7 | 11 | 14 | 32 |
| 50–64 | 1,538 | 7.2 | 54 | 2 | 3 | 5 | 10 | 16 | 24 | 31 |
| 65+ | 2,327 | 8.1 | 49 | 2 | 3 | 6 | 10 | 16 | 22 | 32 |
| **TOTAL SINGLE DX** | 855 | 2.9 | 4 | 1 | 2 | 2 | 4 | 5 | 8 | 9 |
| **TOTAL MULTIPLE DX** | 6,132 | 7.0 | 48 | 2 | 2 | 5 | 9 | 15 | 21 | 32 |
| **TOTAL** | | | | | | | | | | |
| 0–19 Years | 299 | 6.4 | 75 | 1 | 2 | 4 | 8 | 11 | 24 | 47 |
| 20–34 | 836 | 4.8 | 23 | 1 | 2 | 3 | 5 | 10 | 15 | 23 |
| 35–49 | 1,690 | 4.9 | 27 | 1 | 2 | 3 | 6 | 10 | 13 | 27 |
| 50–64 | 1,761 | 6.8 | 51 | 1 | 2 | 4 | 9 | 16 | 24 | 30 |
| 65+ | 2,401 | 7.9 | 49 | 2 | 3 | 6 | 10 | 16 | 22 | 32 |
| **GRAND TOTAL** | 6,987 | 6.5 | 44 | 1 | 2 | 4 | 8 | 14 | 19 | 31 |

## 55.01: NEPHROTOMY. Formerly included in operation group(s) 646.

| Type of Patients | Observed Patients | Avg. Stay | Vari- ance | Percentiles | | | | | | |
|---|---|---|---|---|---|---|---|---|---|---|
| | | | | 10th | 25th | 50th | 75th | 90th | 95th | 99th |
| **1. SINGLE DX** | | | | | | | | | | |
| 0–19 Years | 6 | 3.0 | 1 | 1 | 3 | 3 | 4 | 4 | 4 | 4 |
| 20–34 | 34 | 3.2 | 2 | 2 | 2 | 3 | 4 | 5 | 6 | 8 |
| 35–49 | 49 | 2.3 | 1 | 1 | 1 | 2 | 3 | 4 | 4 | 5 |
| 50–64 | 39 | 2.7 | 2 | 1 | 1 | 2 | 3 | 4 | 6 | 6 |
| 65+ | 11 | 2.9 | 4 | 1 | 1 | 2 | 5 | 5 | 7 | 7 |
| **2. MULTIPLE DX** | | | | | | | | | | |
| 0–19 Years | 24 | 6.1 | 11 | 3 | 4 | 5 | 9 | 9 | 10 | 19 |
| 20–34 | 78 | 6.2 | 17 | 2 | 3 | 5 | 8 | 11 | 13 | 23 |
| 35–49 | 169 | 4.8 | 20 | 1 | 2 | 4 | 5 | 9 | 13 | 16 |
| 50–64 | 154 | 5.1 | 34 | 1 | 2 | 3 | 7 | 10 | 13 | 25 |
| 65+ | 121 | 5.3 | 11 | 2 | 3 | 5 | 7 | 9 | 12 | 16 |
| **TOTAL SINGLE DX** | 139 | 2.7 | 2 | 1 | 2 | 2 | 3 | 4 | 5 | 6 |
| **TOTAL MULTIPLE DX** | 546 | 5.3 | 22 | 2 | 3 | 4 | 7 | 10 | 13 | 21 |
| **TOTAL** | | | | | | | | | | |
| 0–19 Years | 30 | 5.8 | 11 | 3 | 4 | 5 | 8 | 9 | 10 | 19 |
| 20–34 | 112 | 5.4 | 15 | 2 | 3 | 5 | 6 | 11 | 13 | 23 |
| 35–49 | 218 | 4.2 | 16 | 2 | 3 | 4 | 5 | 8 | 13 | 16 |
| 50–64 | 193 | 4.7 | 29 | 1 | 2 | 3 | 5 | 10 | 11 | 25 |
| 65+ | 132 | 5.1 | 11 | 2 | 3 | 5 | 7 | 9 | 12 | 16 |
| **GRAND TOTAL** | 685 | 4.8 | 19 | 1 | 2 | 4 | 6 | 9 | 12 | 20 |

## 55.02: NEPHROSTOMY. Formerly included in operation group(s) 646.

| Type of Patients | Observed Patients | Avg. Stay | Vari- ance | Percentiles | | | | | | |
|---|---|---|---|---|---|---|---|---|---|---|
| | | | | 10th | 25th | 50th | 75th | 90th | 95th | 99th |
| **1. SINGLE DX** | | | | | | | | | | |
| 0–19 Years | 3 | 2.3 | <1 | 2 | 2 | 2 | 2 | 5 | 5 | 5 |
| 20–34 | 2 | 4.3 | 2 | 2 | 5 | 5 | 5 | 5 | 5 | 5 |
| 35–49 | 13 | 3.1 | 3 | 2 | 2 | 2 | 3 | 7 | 7 | 7 |
| 50–64 | 9 | 3.0 | 3 | 1 | 1 | 2 | 5 | 5 | 6 | 6 |
| 65+ | 1 | 2.0 | 0 | 2 | 2 | 2 | 2 | 2 | 2 | 2 |
| **2. MULTIPLE DX** | | | | | | | | | | |
| 0–19 Years | 26 | 10.1 | 124 | 1 | 3 | 7 | 11 | 24 | 30 | 52 |
| 20–34 | 39 | 6.6 | 60 | 1 | 2 | 5 | 8 | 11 | 23 | 59 |
| 35–49 | 90 | 7.2 | 52 | 1 | 3 | 4 | 12 | 15 | 22 | 34 |
| 50–64 | 106 | 7.6 | 30 | 3 | 3 | 6 | 11 | 15 | 15 | 26 |
| 65+ | 209 | 10.1 | 51 | 3 | 5 | 9 | 13 | 20 | 24 | 35 |
| **TOTAL SINGLE DX** | 28 | 3.0 | 3 | 2 | 2 | 2 | 4 | 6 | 7 | 7 |
| **TOTAL MULTIPLE DX** | 470 | 8.6 | 54 | 2 | 3 | 6 | 12 | 16 | 23 | 34 |
| **TOTAL** | | | | | | | | | | |
| 0–19 Years | 29 | 8.9 | 112 | 1 | 2 | 5 | 10 | 24 | 24 | 52 |
| 20–34 | 41 | 6.4 | 56 | 1 | 2 | 5 | 7 | 11 | 23 | 59 |
| 35–49 | 103 | 6.4 | 45 | 2 | 3 | 3 | 9 | 14 | 20 | 34 |
| 50–64 | 115 | 7.3 | 30 | 2 | 3 | 6 | 11 | 15 | 15 | 26 |
| 65+ | 210 | 9.9 | 52 | 2 | 5 | 9 | 13 | 20 | 24 | 35 |
| **GRAND TOTAL** | 498 | 8.1 | 52 | 2 | 3 | 6 | 12 | 16 | 22 | 34 |

## 55.03: PERC NEPHROSTOMY-NO FRAG. Formerly included in operation group(s) 644.

| Type of Patients | Observed Patients | Avg. Stay | Vari- ance | Percentiles | | | | | | |
|---|---|---|---|---|---|---|---|---|---|---|
| | | | | 10th | 25th | 50th | 75th | 90th | 95th | 99th |
| **1. SINGLE DX** | | | | | | | | | | |
| 0–19 Years | 32 | 4.5 | 10 | 1 | 1 | 3 | 8 | 8 | 8 | 8 |
| 20–34 | 89 | 2.8 | 2 | 1 | 2 | 3 | 3 | 5 | 6 | 7 |
| 35–49 | 142 | 2.6 | 2 | 1 | 2 | 3 | 3 | 4 | 5 | 8 |
| 50–64 | 88 | 2.1 | 1 | 1 | 1 | 2 | 3 | 4 | 5 | 5 |
| 65+ | 35 | 3.1 | 5 | 1 | 2 | 2 | 3 | 8 | 8 | 12 |
| **2. MULTIPLE DX** | | | | | | | | | | |
| 0–19 Years | 172 | 6.0 | 76 | 1 | 2 | 4 | 6 | 10 | 19 | 53 |
| 20–34 | 396 | 5.5 | 32 | 1 | 2 | 4 | 7 | 11 | 16 | 31 |
| 35–49 | 803 | 5.5 | 34 | 1 | 3 | 4 | 7 | 11 | 14 | 32 |
| 50–64 | 977 | 8.2 | 65 | 1 | 3 | 6 | 11 | 19 | 24 | 31 |
| 65+ | 1,739 | 8.2 | 50 | 2 | 3 | 6 | 11 | 17 | 22 | 32 |
| **TOTAL SINGLE DX** | 386 | 2.8 | 4 | 1 | 2 | 3 | 3 | 5 | 8 | 8 |
| **TOTAL MULTIPLE DX** | 4,087 | 7.4 | 52 | 2 | 3 | 5 | 9 | 16 | 22 | 32 |
| **TOTAL** | | | | | | | | | | |
| 0–19 Years | 204 | 5.7 | 63 | 1 | 2 | 4 | 7 | 9 | 17 | 36 |
| 20–34 | 485 | 5.0 | 27 | 1 | 2 | 3 | 6 | 10 | 16 | 31 |
| 35–49 | 945 | 5.1 | 31 | 1 | 2 | 3 | 6 | 10 | 14 | 32 |
| 50–64 | 1,065 | 7.8 | 63 | 1 | 2 | 5 | 10 | 18 | 24 | 31 |
| 65+ | 1,774 | 8.2 | 50 | 2 | 3 | 6 | 10 | 16 | 22 | 32 |
| **GRAND TOTAL** | 4,473 | 7.0 | 50 | 1 | 2 | 5 | 9 | 15 | 21 | 32 |

Length of Stay by Diagnosis and Operation, United States, 2000

# United States, October 1998–September 1999 Data, by Operation

## 55.04: PERC NEPHROSTOMY W FRAG. Formerly included in operation group(s) 644.

| Type of Patients | Observed Patients | Avg. Stay | Variance | 10th | 25th | 50th | 75th | 90th | 95th | 99th |
|---|---|---|---|---|---|---|---|---|---|---|
| **1. SINGLE DX** | | | | | | | | | | |
| 0–19 Years | 9 | 1.5 | <1 | 1 | 1 | 1 | 2 | 2 | 4 | 5 |
| 20–34 | 64 | 2.7 | 2 | 1 | 1 | 3 | 4 | 5 | 5 | 6 |
| 35–49 | 115 | 3.8 | 8 | 2 | 2 | 3 | 4 | 9 | 9 | 9 |
| 50–64 | 87 | 2.6 | 3 | 1 | 2 | 2 | 3 | 4 | 5 | 10 |
| 65+ | 27 | 3.2 | 2 | 2 | 3 | 3 | 4 | 5 | 6 | 6 |
| **2. MULTIPLE DX** | | | | | | | | | | |
| 0–19 Years | 27 | 12.3 | 213 | 2 | 3 | 5 | 12 | 37 | 37 | 47 |
| 20–34 | 134 | 3.9 | 12 | 2 | 2 | 3 | 5 | 6 | 8 | 18 |
| 35–49 | 309 | 4.4 | 19 | 1 | 2 | 3 | 5 | 8 | 13 | 22 |
| 50–64 | 301 | 4.6 | 23 | 2 | 2 | 3 | 6 | 16 | 16 | 17 |
| 65+ | 258 | 5.8 | 43 | 2 | 2 | 4 | 6 | 10 | 25 | 28 |
| **TOTAL SINGLE DX** | 302 | 3.2 | 5 | 1 | 2 | 3 | 4 | 6 | 9 | 9 |
| **TOTAL MULTIPLE DX** | 1,029 | 4.9 | 32 | 1 | 2 | 3 | 5 | 10 | 16 | 27 |
| **TOTAL** | | | | | | | | | | |
| 0–19 Years | 36 | 8.2 | 160 | 1 | 3 | 3 | 6 | 37 | 37 | 47 |
| 20–34 | 198 | 3.5 | 9 | 1 | 2 | 3 | 4 | 5 | 7 | 18 |
| 35–49 | 424 | 4.2 | 16 | 1 | 2 | 3 | 5 | 9 | 10 | 21 |
| 50–64 | 388 | 4.3 | 20 | 1 | 2 | 3 | 4 | 16 | 16 | 16 |
| 65+ | 285 | 5.5 | 39 | 2 | 2 | 4 | 6 | 10 | 25 | 25 |
| **GRAND TOTAL** | 1,331 | 4.5 | 26 | 1 | 2 | 3 | 5 | 9 | 16 | 25 |

## 55.11: PYELOTOMY. Formerly included in operation group(s) 646.

| Type of Patients | Observed Patients | Avg. Stay | Variance | 10th | 25th | 50th | 75th | 90th | 95th | 99th |
|---|---|---|---|---|---|---|---|---|---|---|
| **1. SINGLE DX** | | | | | | | | | | |
| 0–19 Years | 15 | 1.5 | <1 | 1 | 1 | 1 | 2 | 2 | 4 | 4 |
| 20–34 | 22 | 2.9 | 2 | 1 | 2 | 3 | 3 | 5 | 5 | 9 |
| 35–49 | 37 | 3.0 | 2 | 1 | 2 | 3 | 4 | 5 | 6 | 7 |
| 50–64 | 20 | 4.3 | 5 | 1 | 3 | 4 | 7 | 7 | 7 | 7 |
| 65+ | 5 | 5.4 | 3 | 4 | 4 | 5 | 8 | 8 | 8 | 8 |
| **2. MULTIPLE DX** | | | | | | | | | | |
| 0–19 Years | 25 | 5.9 | 26 | 2 | 3 | 4 | 7 | 16 | 16 | 21 |
| 20–34 | 60 | 4.0 | 6 | 1 | 2 | 4 | 6 | 7 | 7 | 13 |
| 35–49 | 97 | 4.2 | 6 | 1 | 3 | 4 | 5 | 7 | 8 | 14 |
| 50–64 | 90 | 5.5 | 10 | 3 | 4 | 6 | 6 | 9 | 10 | 17 |
| 65+ | 117 | 6.4 | 28 | 1 | 3 | 5 | 8 | 13 | 17 | 30 |
| **TOTAL SINGLE DX** | 99 | 3.0 | 3 | 1 | 2 | 3 | 4 | 6 | 7 | 8 |
| **TOTAL MULTIPLE DX** | 389 | 5.1 | 14 | 1 | 3 | 4 | 6 | 9 | 12 | 21 |
| **TOTAL** | | | | | | | | | | |
| 0–19 Years | 40 | 4.2 | 21 | 1 | 1 | 3 | 5 | 7 | 16 | 21 |
| 20–34 | 82 | 3.7 | 5 | 1 | 2 | 3 | 5 | 6 | 7 | 13 |
| 35–49 | 134 | 3.9 | 5 | 1 | 2 | 4 | 5 | 6 | 7 | 14 |
| 50–64 | 110 | 5.3 | 10 | 2 | 4 | 5 | 6 | 7 | 10 | 14 |
| 65+ | 122 | 6.4 | 28 | 1 | 3 | 5 | 8 | 13 | 17 | 30 |
| **GRAND TOTAL** | 488 | 4.7 | 13 | 1 | 2 | 4 | 6 | 8 | 10 | 18 |

## 55.1: PYELOTOMY & PYELOSTOMY. Formerly included in operation group(s) 646.

| Type of Patients | Observed Patients | Avg. Stay | Variance | 10th | 25th | 50th | 75th | 90th | 95th | 99th |
|---|---|---|---|---|---|---|---|---|---|---|
| **1. SINGLE DX** | | | | | | | | | | |
| 0–19 Years | 16 | 1.5 | <1 | 1 | 1 | 1 | 2 | 2 | 4 | 4 |
| 20–34 | 23 | 2.9 | 2 | 1 | 2 | 3 | 4 | 5 | 5 | 9 |
| 35–49 | 37 | 3.0 | 2 | 1 | 2 | 3 | 4 | 5 | 6 | 7 |
| 50–64 | 20 | 4.3 | 5 | 1 | 3 | 4 | 7 | 7 | 7 | 7 |
| 65+ | 6 | 4.9 | 4 | 2 | 4 | 5 | 5 | 8 | 8 | 8 |
| **2. MULTIPLE DX** | | | | | | | | | | |
| 0–19 Years | 39 | 5.6 | 58 | 1 | 2 | 3 | 5 | 16 | 16 | 22 |
| 20–34 | 68 | 4.1 | 7 | 1 | 2 | 4 | 6 | 7 | 7 | 13 |
| 35–49 | 108 | 4.2 | 9 | 1 | 2 | 3 | 5 | 7 | 7 | 17 |
| 50–64 | 104 | 5.4 | 10 | 2 | 4 | 6 | 6 | 8 | 10 | 14 |
| 65+ | 149 | 6.7 | 33 | 1 | 3 | 5 | 8 | 13 | 19 | 27 |
| **TOTAL SINGLE DX** | 102 | 3.0 | 3 | 1 | 2 | 3 | 4 | 6 | 7 | 8 |
| **TOTAL MULTIPLE DX** | 468 | 5.2 | 20 | 1 | 3 | 4 | 6 | 9 | 13 | 22 |
| **TOTAL** | | | | | | | | | | |
| 0–19 Years | 55 | 4.4 | 44 | 1 | 1 | 2 | 5 | 9 | 16 | 22 |
| 20–34 | 91 | 3.8 | 6 | 1 | 2 | 3 | 5 | 6 | 7 | 13 |
| 35–49 | 145 | 4.0 | 8 | 1 | 2 | 4 | 5 | 7 | 8 | 17 |
| 50–64 | 124 | 5.2 | 10 | 2 | 3 | 5 | 6 | 7 | 10 | 14 |
| 65+ | 155 | 6.7 | 32 | 1 | 3 | 5 | 8 | 13 | 18 | 27 |
| **GRAND TOTAL** | 570 | 4.8 | 18 | 1 | 2 | 4 | 6 | 8 | 12 | 22 |

## 55.2: RENAL DIAGNOSTIC PX. Formerly included in operation group(s) 646, 651, 664.

| Type of Patients | Observed Patients | Avg. Stay | Variance | 10th | 25th | 50th | 75th | 90th | 95th | 99th |
|---|---|---|---|---|---|---|---|---|---|---|
| **1. SINGLE DX** | | | | | | | | | | |
| 0–19 Years | 260 | 2.2 | 4 | 1 | 1 | 1 | 3 | 4 | 7 | 13 |
| 20–34 | 92 | 2.8 | 10 | 1 | 1 | 1 | 4 | 8 | 11 | 14 |
| 35–49 | 73 | 1.5 | 3 | 1 | 1 | 1 | 1 | 2 | 4 | 10 |
| 50–64 | 43 | 1.5 | 2 | 1 | 1 | 1 | 1 | 2 | 4 | 8 |
| 65+ | 20 | 10.6 | 51 | 16 | 16 | 16 | 16 | 16 | 16 | 16 |
| **2. MULTIPLE DX** | | | | | | | | | | |
| 0–19 Years | 879 | 5.6 | 39 | 1 | 1 | 4 | 7 | 13 | 17 | 30 |
| 20–34 | 908 | 5.3 | 30 | 1 | 2 | 4 | 8 | 12 | 14 | 23 |
| 35–49 | 1,264 | 5.3 | 31 | 1 | 2 | 3 | 7 | 12 | 16 | 29 |
| 50–64 | 1,048 | 5.9 | 33 | 1 | 2 | 6 | 9 | 12 | 16 | 30 |
| 65+ | 983 | 6.9 | 45 | 2 | 2 | 6 | 9 | 14 | 18 | 31 |
| **TOTAL SINGLE DX** | 488 | 3.2 | 19 | 1 | 1 | 1 | 3 | 10 | 16 | 16 |
| **TOTAL MULTIPLE DX** | 5,082 | 5.8 | 36 | 1 | 2 | 4 | 8 | 13 | 16 | 30 |
| **TOTAL** | | | | | | | | | | |
| 0–19 Years | 1,139 | 4.8 | 33 | 1 | 1 | 3 | 6 | 11 | 15 | 25 |
| 20–34 | 1,000 | 5.1 | 29 | 1 | 1 | 4 | 7 | 11 | 14 | 21 |
| 35–49 | 1,337 | 4.9 | 30 | 1 | 1 | 4 | 8 | 11 | 15 | 28 |
| 50–64 | 1,091 | 5.6 | 32 | 1 | 2 | 6 | 8 | 12 | 16 | 29 |
| 65+ | 1,003 | 7.2 | 46 | 1 | 2 | 6 | 10 | 16 | 18 | 31 |
| **GRAND TOTAL** | 5,570 | 5.5 | 35 | 1 | 1 | 4 | 7 | 12 | 16 | 28 |

Length of Stay by Diagnosis and Operation, United States, 2000

## United States, October 1998–September 1999 Data, by Operation

### 55.23: CLSD (PERC) RENAL BIOPSY. Formerly included in operation group(s) 646.

| Type of Patients | Observed Patients | Avg. Stay | Vari-ance | 10th | 25th | 50th | 75th | 90th | 95th | 99th |
|---|---|---|---|---|---|---|---|---|---|---|
| **1. SINGLE DX** | | | | | | | | | | |
| 0–19 Years | 246 | 2.2 | <1 | 1 | 1 | 1 | 3 | 4 | 7 | 13 |
| 20–34 | 89 | 2.6 | <1 | 1 | 1 | 1 | 3 | 5 | 11 | 11 |
| 35–49 | 66 | 1.5 | <1 | 1 | 1 | 1 | 1 | 2 | 6 | 10 |
| 50–64 | 39 | 1.4 | <1 | 1 | 1 | 1 | 1 | 2 | 4 | 8 |
| 65+ | 18 | 10.7 | 50 | 1 | 1 | 16 | 16 | 16 | 16 | 16 |
| **2. MULTIPLE DX** | | | | | | | | | | |
| 0–19 Years | 811 | 5.1 | 25 | 1 | 1 | 4 | 7 | 11 | 15 | 25 |
| 20–34 | 871 | 5.1 | 27 | 1 | 2 | 4 | 7 | 10 | 14 | 20 |
| 35–49 | 1,207 | 5.3 | 30 | 1 | 1 | 4 | 7 | 11 | 15 | 27 |
| 50–64 | 976 | 5.8 | 32 | 1 | 1 | 4 | 8 | 12 | 16 | 29 |
| 65+ | 929 | 6.8 | 45 | 1 | 2 | 6 | 9 | 14 | 18 | 31 |
| **TOTAL SINGLE DX** | 458 | 3.2 | 19 | 1 | 1 | 1 | 3 | 11 | 16 | 16 |
| **TOTAL MULTIPLE DX** | 4,794 | 5.6 | 32 | 1 | 2 | 4 | 3 | 12 | 16 | 28 |
| **TOTAL** | | | | | | | | | | |
| 0–19 Years | 1,057 | 4.4 | 22 | 3 | 3 | 3 | 6 | 10 | 14 | 24 |
| 20–34 | 960 | 4.8 | 25 | 1 | 3 | 4 | 7 | 10 | 13 | 20 |
| 35–49 | 1,273 | 4.9 | 29 | 1 | 3 | 3 | 7 | 11 | 14 | 26 |
| 50–64 | 1,015 | 5.5 | 31 | 1 | 3 | 4 | 8 | 12 | 15 | 28 |
| 65+ | 947 | 7.2 | 47 | 2 | 2 | 6 | 10 | 16 | 18 | 31 |
| **GRAND TOTAL** | 5,252 | 5.3 | 31 | 1 | 3 | 4 | 7 | 12 | 16 | 26 |

### 55.39: LOC DESTR RENAL LES NEC. Formerly included in operation group(s) 646.

| Type of Patients | Observed Patients | Avg. Stay | Vari-ance | 10th | 25th | 50th | 75th | 90th | 95th | 99th |
|---|---|---|---|---|---|---|---|---|---|---|
| **1. SINGLE DX** | | | | | | | | | | |
| 0–19 Years | 5 | 3.3 | <1 | 3 | 3 | 3 | 3 | 4 | 6 | 6 |
| 20–34 | 10 | 3.7 | <1 | 2 | 3 | 3 | 4 | 5 | 5 | 5 |
| 35–49 | 12 | 4.0 | <1 | 3 | 3 | 4 | 5 | 5 | 5 | 5 |
| 50–64 | 10 | 1.9 | <1 | 1 | 1 | 2 | 3 | 3 | 3 | 4 |
| 65+ | 8 | 3.5 | 2 | 2 | 2 | 4 | 5 | 5 | 5 | 5 |
| **2. MULTIPLE DX** | | | | | | | | | | |
| 0–19 Years | 24 | 7.2 | 46 | 2 | 4 | 5 | 7 | 19 | 19 | 41 |
| 20–34 | 20 | 5.4 | 15 | 1 | 3 | 4 | 8 | 12 | 12 | 12 |
| 35–49 | 46 | 4.9 | 8 | 2 | 2 | 5 | 9 | 9 | 9 | 10 |
| 50–64 | 68 | 4.3 | 9 | 1 | 3 | 4 | 5 | 7 | 8 | 20 |
| 65+ | 123 | 4.8 | 12 | 2 | 3 | 4 | 6 | 8 | 12 | 19 |
| **TOTAL SINGLE DX** | 45 | 3.3 | 1 | 2 | 3 | 3 | 4 | 5 | 5 | 6 |
| **TOTAL MULTIPLE DX** | 281 | 5.0 | 14 | 2 | 3 | 4 | 6 | 9 | 12 | 19 |
| **TOTAL** | | | | | | | | | | |
| 0–19 Years | 29 | 6.4 | 39 | 2 | 3 | 5 | 5 | 19 | 19 | 41 |
| 20–34 | 30 | 4.9 | 12 | 1 | 3 | 4 | 5 | 12 | 12 | 12 |
| 35–49 | 58 | 4.8 | 7 | 2 | 3 | 5 | 7 | 9 | 9 | 10 |
| 50–64 | 78 | 4.1 | 9 | 1 | 2 | 4 | 5 | 7 | 7 | 20 |
| 65+ | 131 | 4.7 | 12 | 2 | 3 | 4 | 6 | 8 | 12 | 19 |
| **GRAND TOTAL** | 326 | 4.8 | 13 | 2 | 3 | 4 | 5 | 9 | 11 | 19 |

### 55.3: LOC EXC/DESTR RENAL LES. Formerly included in operation group(s) 646.

| Type of Patients | Observed Patients | Avg. Stay | Vari-ance | 10th | 25th | 50th | 75th | 90th | 95th | 99th |
|---|---|---|---|---|---|---|---|---|---|---|
| **1. SINGLE DX** | | | | | | | | | | |
| 0–19 Years | 5 | 3.3 | <1 | 3 | 3 | 3 | 3 | 4 | 6 | 6 |
| 20–34 | 12 | 3.5 | <1 | 2 | 3 | 3 | 4 | 5 | 5 | 5 |
| 35–49 | 15 | 3.8 | <1 | 3 | 3 | 4 | 4 | 5 | 5 | 5 |
| 50–64 | 10 | 1.9 | <1 | 1 | 1 | 2 | 3 | 3 | 4 | 4 |
| 65+ | 11 | 3.4 | 2 | 1 | 2 | 4 | 5 | 5 | 5 | 5 |
| **2. MULTIPLE DX** | | | | | | | | | | |
| 0–19 Years | 25 | 7.1 | 46 | 2 | 4 | 5 | 7 | 19 | 19 | 41 |
| 20–34 | 22 | 5.4 | 14 | 1 | 3 | 5 | 8 | 12 | 12 | 12 |
| 35–49 | 52 | 4.8 | 8 | 2 | 2 | 5 | 8 | 9 | 9 | 10 |
| 50–64 | 82 | 4.5 | 13 | 1 | 3 | 4 | 5 | 7 | 11 | 20 |
| 65+ | 133 | 4.6 | 12 | 1 | 3 | 4 | 6 | 8 | 12 | 20 |
| **TOTAL SINGLE DX** | 53 | 3.3 | 1 | 1 | 3 | 3 | 4 | 5 | 5 | 6 |
| **TOTAL MULTIPLE DX** | 314 | 4.9 | 15 | 1 | 3 | 4 | 6 | 9 | 12 | 20 |
| **TOTAL** | | | | | | | | | | |
| 0–19 Years | 30 | 6.4 | 39 | 2 | 3 | 5 | 5 | 19 | 19 | 41 |
| 20–34 | 34 | 4.8 | 11 | 1 | 3 | 4 | 5 | 12 | 12 | 12 |
| 35–49 | 67 | 4.7 | 7 | 2 | 3 | 4 | 7 | 9 | 9 | 10 |
| 50–64 | 92 | 4.3 | 13 | 1 | 3 | 4 | 5 | 7 | 11 | 20 |
| 65+ | 144 | 4.5 | 11 | 1 | 2 | 4 | 6 | 8 | 12 | 20 |
| **GRAND TOTAL** | 367 | 4.7 | 14 | 1 | 3 | 4 | 5 | 9 | 11 | 19 |

### 55.4: PARTIAL NEPHRECTOMY. Formerly included in operation group(s) 646.

| Type of Patients | Observed Patients | Avg. Stay | Vari-ance | 10th | 25th | 50th | 75th | 90th | 95th | 99th |
|---|---|---|---|---|---|---|---|---|---|---|
| **1. SINGLE DX** | | | | | | | | | | |
| 0–19 Years | 29 | 4.2 | 11 | 1 | 2 | 4 | 5 | 10 | 10 | 10 |
| 20–34 | 9 | 2.9 | 3 | 1 | 1 | 3 | 4 | 6 | 6 | 6 |
| 35–49 | 27 | 4.1 | <1 | 3 | 3 | 4 | 5 | 5 | 8 | 8 |
| 50–64 | 23 | 5.1 | 2 | 3 | 4 | 5 | 5 | 8 | 8 | 8 |
| 65+ | 16 | 4.7 | 1 | 3 | 4 | 5 | 5 | 6 | 6 | 6 |
| **2. MULTIPLE DX** | | | | | | | | | | |
| 0–19 Years | 178 | 3.9 | 11 | 2 | 2 | 3 | 4 | 7 | 13 | 18 |
| 20–34 | 52 | 5.3 | 25 | 3 | 4 | 5 | 5 | 6 | 7 | 26 |
| 35–49 | 157 | 5.0 | 6 | 3 | 4 | 4 | 5 | 7 | 8 | 14 |
| 50–64 | 267 | 5.6 | 11 | 3 | 4 | 5 | 6 | 8 | 10 | 24 |
| 65+ | 293 | 6.5 | 41 | 3 | 4 | 5 | 7 | 10 | 14 | 30 |
| **TOTAL SINGLE DX** | 104 | 4.5 | 4 | 2 | 3 | 4 | 5 | 8 | 10 | 10 |
| **TOTAL MULTIPLE DX** | 947 | 5.5 | 22 | 3 | 4 | 5 | 6 | 8 | 11 | 28 |
| **TOTAL** | | | | | | | | | | |
| 0–19 Years | 207 | 4.0 | 11 | 1 | 2 | 3 | 4 | 9 | 11 | 18 |
| 20–34 | 61 | 5.1 | 24 | 1 | 3 | 5 | 5 | 6 | 7 | 26 |
| 35–49 | 184 | 4.9 | 6 | 3 | 4 | 4 | 5 | 6 | 8 | 14 |
| 50–64 | 290 | 5.6 | 9 | 3 | 4 | 5 | 6 | 8 | 10 | 24 |
| 65+ | 309 | 6.4 | 38 | 3 | 4 | 5 | 7 | 9 | 14 | 30 |
| **GRAND TOTAL** | 1,051 | 5.4 | 20 | 3 | 4 | 4 | 6 | 8 | 11 | 28 |

Length of Stay by Diagnosis and Operation, United States, 2000

# United States, October 1998–September 1999 Data, by Operation

## 55.5: COMPLETE NEPHRECTOMY. Formerly included in operation group(s) 643.

| Type of Patients | Observed Patients | Avg. Stay | Variance | 10th | 25th | 50th | 75th | 90th | 95th | 99th |
|---|---|---|---|---|---|---|---|---|---|---|
| **1. SINGLE DX** | | | | | | | | | | |
| 0–19 Years | 175 | 3.9 | 6 | 1 | 2 | 4 | 5 | 7 | 8 | 10 |
| 20–34 | 327 | 3.9 | 2 | 2 | 3 | 4 | 5 | 6 | 6 | 7 |
| 35–49 | 578 | 4.1 | 2 | 3 | 3 | 4 | 5 | 6 | 6 | 7 |
| 50–64 | 402 | 4.1 | 2 | 3 | 3 | 4 | 5 | 6 | 6 | 8 |
| 65+ | 195 | 4.6 | 2 | 3 | 4 | 5 | 5 | 6 | 7 | 8 |
| **2. MULTIPLE DX** | | | | | | | | | | |
| 0–19 Years | 712 | 5.5 | 34 | 1 | 4 | 4 | 7 | 11 | 15 | 37 |
| 20–34 | 685 | 6.1 | 35 | 2 | 3 | 4 | 6 | 10 | 19 | 32 |
| 35–49 | 1,850 | 6.0 | 30 | 3 | 3 | 5 | 6 | 10 | 15 | 32 |
| 50–64 | 2,931 | 6.2 | 22 | 3 | 4 | 5 | 7 | 9 | 13 | 26 |
| 65+ | 4,135 | 7.8 | 41 | 4 | 4 | 6 | 8 | 14 | 19 | 40 |
| **TOTAL SINGLE DX** | 1,677 | 4.1 | 2 | 2 | 3 | 4 | 5 | 6 | 6 | 8 |
| **TOTAL MULTIPLE DX** | 10,313 | 6.7 | 33 | 3 | 4 | 5 | 7 | 11 | 16 | 33 |
| **TOTAL** | | | | | | | | | | |
| 0–19 Years | 887 | 5.1 | 29 | 2 | 3 | 4 | 7 | 10 | 13 | 27 |
| 20–34 | 1,012 | 5.4 | 26 | 3 | 3 | 4 | 5 | 8 | 12 | 28 |
| 35–49 | 2,428 | 5.5 | 24 | 3 | 3 | 5 | 6 | 9 | 13 | 27 |
| 50–64 | 3,333 | 5.9 | 20 | 3 | 4 | 5 | 7 | 9 | 12 | 26 |
| 65+ | 4,330 | 7.6 | 40 | 4 | 4 | 6 | 8 | 13 | 19 | 40 |
| **GRAND TOTAL** | 11,990 | 6.3 | 29 | 3 | 4 | 5 | 7 | 10 | 15 | 30 |

## 55.51: NEPHROURETERECTOMY. Formerly included in operation group(s) 643.

| Type of Patients | Observed Patients | Avg. Stay | Variance | 10th | 25th | 50th | 75th | 90th | 95th | 99th |
|---|---|---|---|---|---|---|---|---|---|---|
| **1. SINGLE DX** | | | | | | | | | | |
| 0–19 Years | 173 | 3.9 | 6 | 1 | 2 | 4 | 5 | 7 | 8 | 10 |
| 20–34 | 325 | 3.9 | 2 | 2 | 3 | 4 | 5 | 6 | 6 | 7 |
| 35–49 | 577 | 4.1 | 2 | 3 | 3 | 4 | 5 | 6 | 6 | 7 |
| 50–64 | 399 | 4.1 | 2 | 3 | 3 | 4 | 5 | 6 | 6 | 8 |
| 65+ | 193 | 4.6 | 2 | 3 | 4 | 5 | 5 | 6 | 7 | 8 |
| **2. MULTIPLE DX** | | | | | | | | | | |
| 0–19 Years | 627 | 5.1 | 32 | 1 | 2 | 4 | 7 | 10 | 12 | 30 |
| 20–34 | 535 | 5.7 | 28 | 3 | 3 | 4 | 6 | 8 | 16 | 28 |
| 35–49 | 1,614 | 5.7 | 23 | 3 | 3 | 5 | 6 | 9 | 14 | 27 |
| 50–64 | 2,747 | 6.1 | 20 | 3 | 4 | 5 | 7 | 9 | 12 | 26 |
| 65+ | 4,077 | 7.7 | 40 | 4 | 4 | 6 | 8 | 14 | 19 | 40 |
| **TOTAL SINGLE DX** | 1,667 | 4.1 | 2 | 2 | 3 | 4 | 5 | 6 | 6 | 8 |
| **TOTAL MULTIPLE DX** | 9,600 | 6.6 | 31 | 3 | 4 | 5 | 7 | 11 | 16 | 31 |
| **TOTAL** | | | | | | | | | | |
| 0–19 Years | 800 | 4.8 | 26 | 1 | 3 | 4 | 6 | 9 | 11 | 22 |
| 20–34 | 860 | 5.1 | 20 | 3 | 3 | 4 | 5 | 8 | 11 | 26 |
| 35–49 | 2,191 | 5.3 | 17 | 3 | 4 | 5 | 7 | 10 | 12 | 27 |
| 50–64 | 3,146 | 5.8 | 18 | 4 | 4 | 5 | 6 | 9 | 12 | 26 |
| 65+ | 4,270 | 7.6 | 39 | 4 | 4 | 6 | 8 | 13 | 19 | 40 |
| **GRAND TOTAL** | 11,267 | 6.2 | 27 | 3 | 4 | 5 | 7 | 10 | 15 | 29 |

## 55.53: REJECTED KID NEPHRECTOMY. Formerly included in operation group(s) 643.

| Type of Patients | Observed Patients | Avg. Stay | Variance | 10th | 25th | 50th | 75th | 90th | 95th | 99th |
|---|---|---|---|---|---|---|---|---|---|---|
| **1. SINGLE DX** | | | | | | | | | | |
| 0–19 Years | 0 | | | | | | | | | |
| 20–34 | 0 | | | | | | | | | |
| 35–49 | 0 | | | | | | | | | |
| 50–64 | 2 | 2.9 | 2 | 2 | 2 | 3 | 4 | 4 | 4 | 4 |
| 65+ | 1 | 3.0 | 0 | 3 | 3 | 3 | 3 | 3 | 3 | 3 |
| **2. MULTIPLE DX** | | | | | | | | | | |
| 0–19 Years | 42 | 7.3 | 35 | 2 | 3 | 5 | 8 | 14 | 22 | 27 |
| 20–34 | 118 | 7.0 | 39 | 2 | 3 | 4 | 9 | 13 | 21 | 33 |
| 35–49 | 160 | 8.2 | 69 | 2 | 3 | 6 | 9 | 15 | 31 | 42 |
| 50–64 | 104 | 8.7 | 71 | 2 | 3 | 6 | 12 | 20 | 29 | 39 |
| 65+ | 23 | 6.9 | 24 | 2 | 3 | 6 | 9 | 14 | 20 | 20 |
| **TOTAL SINGLE DX** | 3 | 3.0 | <1 | 2 | 3 | 3 | 3 | 4 | 4 | 4 |
| **TOTAL MULTIPLE DX** | 447 | 7.9 | 56 | 2 | 3 | 5 | 9 | 17 | 23 | 39 |
| **TOTAL** | | | | | | | | | | |
| 0–19 Years | 42 | 7.3 | 35 | 2 | 3 | 5 | 8 | 14 | 22 | 27 |
| 20–34 | 118 | 7.0 | 39 | 2 | 3 | 4 | 9 | 13 | 21 | 33 |
| 35–49 | 160 | 8.2 | 69 | 2 | 3 | 6 | 9 | 15 | 31 | 42 |
| 50–64 | 106 | 8.6 | 71 | 2 | 3 | 6 | 12 | 20 | 29 | 39 |
| 65+ | 24 | 6.7 | 24 | 2 | 3 | 6 | 9 | 14 | 20 | 20 |
| **GRAND TOTAL** | 450 | 7.8 | 56 | 2 | 3 | 5 | 9 | 17 | 23 | 39 |

## 55.6: KIDNEY TRANSPLANT. Formerly included in operation group(s) 645.

| Type of Patients | Observed Patients | Avg. Stay | Variance | 10th | 25th | 50th | 75th | 90th | 95th | 99th |
|---|---|---|---|---|---|---|---|---|---|---|
| **1. SINGLE DX** | | | | | | | | | | |
| 0–19 Years | 20 | 7.5 | 7 | 4 | 6 | 7 | 10 | 10 | 13 | 13 |
| 20–34 | 51 | 5.2 | 2 | 3 | 4 | 5 | 6 | 7 | 8 | 9 |
| 35–49 | 59 | 5.8 | 5 | 4 | 4 | 5 | 7 | 8 | 10 | 15 |
| 50–64 | 38 | 7.3 | 16 | 4 | 4 | 6 | 8 | 14 | 17 | 17 |
| 65+ | 8 | 8.0 | 24 | 3 | 4 | 7 | 9 | 17 | 17 | 17 |
| **2. MULTIPLE DX** | | | | | | | | | | |
| 0–19 Years | 338 | 12.2 | 86 | 5 | 7 | 9 | 15 | 21 | 31 | 45 |
| 20–34 | 779 | 8.9 | 55 | 4 | 5 | 7 | 10 | 16 | 22 | 36 |
| 35–49 | 1,342 | 8.8 | 43 | 4 | 5 | 7 | 10 | 15 | 21 | 37 |
| 50–64 | 1,143 | 8.2 | 24 | 4 | 5 | 7 | 9 | 14 | 18 | 26 |
| 65+ | 239 | 10.3 | 74 | 5 | 6 | 7 | 12 | 17 | 23 | 50 |
| **TOTAL SINGLE DX** | 176 | 6.4 | 8 | 4 | 4 | 6 | 8 | 10 | 13 | 17 |
| **TOTAL MULTIPLE DX** | 3,841 | 9.1 | 49 | 4 | 5 | 7 | 10 | 16 | 21 | 39 |
| **TOTAL** | | | | | | | | | | |
| 0–19 Years | 358 | 11.6 | 78 | 5 | 6 | 9 | 14 | 20 | 27 | 45 |
| 20–34 | 830 | 8.7 | 52 | 5 | 6 | 7 | 9 | 15 | 21 | 34 |
| 35–49 | 1,401 | 8.7 | 42 | 4 | 5 | 7 | 10 | 15 | 19 | 37 |
| 50–64 | 1,181 | 8.2 | 24 | 4 | 5 | 7 | 9 | 14 | 18 | 26 |
| 65+ | 247 | 10.2 | 73 | 5 | 6 | 7 | 12 | 17 | 23 | 50 |
| **GRAND TOTAL** | 4,017 | 9.0 | 47 | 4 | 5 | 7 | 10 | 15 | 21 | 39 |

Length of Stay by Diagnosis and Operation, United States, 2000

# United States, October 1998–September 1999 Data, by Operation

## 55.69: KIDNEY TRANSPLANT NEC. Formerly included in operation group(s) 645.

| Type of Patients | Observed Patients | Avg. Stay | Vari-ance | 10th | 25th | 50th | 75th | 90th | 95th | 99th |
|---|---|---|---|---|---|---|---|---|---|---|
| **1. SINGLE DX** | | | | | | | | | | |
| 0–19 Years | 20 | 7.5 | 7 | 4 | 6 | 7 | 10 | 10 | 13 | 13 |
| 20–34 | 51 | 5.2 | 2 | 3 | 4 | 5 | 6 | 7 | 8 | 9 |
| 35–49 | 59 | 5.8 | 5 | 4 | 4 | 5 | 7 | 8 | 10 | 15 |
| 50–64 | 38 | 7.3 | 16 | 4 | 4 | 6 | 8 | 14 | 17 | 17 |
| 65+ | 8 | 8.0 | 24 | 3 | 4 | 7 | 9 | 17 | 17 | 17 |
| **2. MULTIPLE DX** | | | | | | | | | | |
| 0–19 Years | 338 | 12.2 | 86 | 5 | 7 | 9 | 15 | 21 | 31 | 45 |
| 20–34 | 779 | 8.9 | 55 | 4 | 5 | 7 | 10 | 16 | 22 | 36 |
| 35–49 | 1,339 | 8.8 | 43 | 4 | 5 | 7 | 10 | 15 | 21 | 37 |
| 50–64 | 1,142 | 8.2 | 24 | 4 | 5 | 7 | 9 | 14 | 18 | 26 |
| 65+ | 238 | 10.2 | 74 | 5 | 6 | 7 | 12 | 18 | 23 | 50 |
| **TOTAL SINGLE DX** | 176 | 6.4 | 8 | 4 | 4 | 6 | 8 | 10 | 13 | 17 |
| **TOTAL MULTIPLE DX** | 3,836 | 9.1 | 49 | 4 | 5 | 7 | 10 | 16 | 21 | 39 |
| **TOTAL** | | | | | | | | | | |
| 0–19 Years | 358 | 11.6 | 78 | 5 | 6 | 9 | 14 | 20 | 27 | 45 |
| 20–34 | 830 | 8.7 | 52 | 4 | 5 | 6 | 9 | 15 | 21 | 34 |
| 35–49 | 1,398 | 8.7 | 42 | 4 | 5 | 7 | 10 | 15 | 20 | 37 |
| 50–64 | 1,180 | 8.2 | 24 | 4 | 5 | 7 | 9 | 14 | 18 | 26 |
| 65+ | 246 | 10.2 | 73 | 5 | 6 | 7 | 12 | 17 | 23 | 50 |
| **GRAND TOTAL** | 4,012 | 9.0 | 47 | 4 | 5 | 7 | 10 | 15 | 21 | 39 |

## 55.8: OTHER KIDNEY REPAIR. Formerly included in operation group(s) 646.

| Type of Patients | Observed Patients | Avg. Stay | Vari-ance | 10th | 25th | 50th | 75th | 90th | 95th | 99th |
|---|---|---|---|---|---|---|---|---|---|---|
| **1. SINGLE DX** | | | | | | | | | | |
| 0–19 Years | 438 | 2.6 | 1 | 1 | 2 | 2 | 3 | 4 | 5 | 6 |
| 20–34 | 72 | 3.2 | <1 | 2 | 3 | 3 | 3 | 4 | 5 | 6 |
| 35–49 | 51 | 3.2 | 1 | 2 | 3 | 3 | 4 | 4 | 5 | 6 |
| 50–64 | 18 | 4.2 | 2 | 3 | 3 | 4 | 4 | 7 | 5 | 7 |
| 65+ | 7 | 4.2 | 1 | 3 | 3 | 5 | 5 | 5 | 5 | 5 |
| **2. MULTIPLE DX** | | | | | | | | | | |
| 0–19 Years | 733 | 3.5 | 6 | 2 | 3 | 3 | 4 | 6 | 7 | 17 |
| 20–34 | 179 | 4.7 | 11 | 2 | 3 | 4 | 5 | 8 | 10 | 13 |
| 35–49 | 169 | 4.4 | 8 | 2 | 3 | 4 | 5 | 7 | 8 | 15 |
| 50–64 | 123 | 4.6 | 7 | 2 | 3 | 4 | 5 | 7 | 8 | 19 |
| 65+ | 98 | 5.1 | 5 | 3 | 4 | 4 | 6 | 8 | 9 | 12 |
| **TOTAL SINGLE DX** | 586 | 2.8 | 1 | 2 | 2 | 3 | 3 | 4 | 5 | 7 |
| **TOTAL MULTIPLE DX** | 1,302 | 4.0 | 8 | 2 | 3 | 3 | 5 | 7 | 8 | 15 |
| **TOTAL** | | | | | | | | | | |
| 0–19 Years | 1,171 | 3.1 | 4 | 2 | 3 | 3 | 3 | 5 | 6 | 13 |
| 20–34 | 251 | 4.3 | 8 | 3 | 3 | 4 | 5 | 7 | 9 | 11 |
| 35–49 | 220 | 4.1 | 7 | 3 | 3 | 4 | 5 | 6 | 8 | 15 |
| 50–64 | 141 | 4.6 | 7 | 3 | 3 | 4 | 5 | 7 | 8 | 16 |
| 65+ | 105 | 5.0 | 5 | 3 | 4 | 4 | 6 | 8 | 9 | 12 |
| **GRAND TOTAL** | 1,888 | 3.6 | 6 | 2 | 2 | 3 | 4 | 6 | 7 | 14 |

## 55.7: NEPHROPEXY. Formerly included in operation group(s) 646.

| Type of Patients | Observed Patients | Avg. Stay | Vari-ance | 10th | 25th | 50th | 75th | 90th | 95th | 99th |
|---|---|---|---|---|---|---|---|---|---|---|
| **1. SINGLE DX** | | | | | | | | | | |
| 0–19 Years | 1 | 2.0 | 0 | 2 | 2 | 2 | 2 | 2 | 2 | 2 |
| 20–34 | 0 | | | | | | | | | |
| 35–49 | 1 | 2.0 | 0 | 2 | 2 | 2 | 2 | 2 | 2 | 2 |
| 50–64 | 0 | | | | | | | | | |
| 65+ | 0 | | | | | | | | | |
| **2. MULTIPLE DX** | | | | | | | | | | |
| 0–19 Years | 1 | 7.0 | 0 | 7 | 7 | 7 | 7 | 7 | 7 | 7 |
| 20–34 | 3 | 3.0 | 0 | 3 | 3 | 3 | 3 | 3 | 3 | 3 |
| 35–49 | 9 | 3.4 | <1 | 2 | 3 | 4 | 8 | 8 | 8 | 8 |
| 50–64 | 7 | 4.3 | 7 | 2 | 4 | 4 | 8 | 8 | 8 | 8 |
| 65+ | 1 | 4.0 | 0 | 4 | 4 | 4 | 4 | 4 | 4 | 4 |
| **TOTAL SINGLE DX** | 2 | 2.0 | 0 | 2 | 2 | 2 | 2 | 2 | 2 | 2 |
| **TOTAL MULTIPLE DX** | 21 | 3.7 | 3 | 2 | 3 | 3 | 4 | 7 | 8 | 8 |
| **TOTAL** | | | | | | | | | | |
| 0–19 Years | 2 | 2.5 | 2 | 2 | 2 | 2 | 2 | 2 | 7 | 7 |
| 20–34 | 3 | 3.0 | 0 | 3 | 3 | 3 | 3 | 3 | 3 | 3 |
| 35–49 | 10 | 3.1 | <1 | 2 | 2 | 3 | 4 | 4 | 4 | 4 |
| 50–64 | 7 | 4.3 | 7 | 2 | 4 | 4 | 8 | 8 | 8 | 8 |
| 65+ | 1 | 4.0 | 0 | 4 | 4 | 4 | 4 | 4 | 4 | 4 |
| **GRAND TOTAL** | 23 | 3.3 | 3 | 2 | 2 | 3 | 4 | 4 | 8 | 8 |

## 55.87: CORRECTION OF UPJ. Formerly included in operation group(s) 646.

| Type of Patients | Observed Patients | Avg. Stay | Vari-ance | 10th | 25th | 50th | 75th | 90th | 95th | 99th |
|---|---|---|---|---|---|---|---|---|---|---|
| **1. SINGLE DX** | | | | | | | | | | |
| 0–19 Years | 436 | 2.6 | 1 | 1 | 2 | 2 | 3 | 4 | 5 | 6 |
| 20–34 | 70 | 3.2 | <1 | 2 | 3 | 3 | 3 | 4 | 5 | 6 |
| 35–49 | 51 | 3.2 | 1 | 2 | 3 | 3 | 4 | 4 | 5 | 6 |
| 50–64 | 17 | 4.2 | 2 | 3 | 3 | 4 | 4 | 7 | 7 | 7 |
| 65+ | 7 | 4.2 | 1 | 3 | 3 | 5 | 5 | 5 | 5 | 5 |
| **2. MULTIPLE DX** | | | | | | | | | | |
| 0–19 Years | 697 | 3.4 | 6 | 2 | 3 | 3 | 4 | 6 | 7 | 17 |
| 20–34 | 156 | 4.2 | 4 | 2 | 3 | 4 | 5 | 7 | 10 | 11 |
| 35–49 | 154 | 4.0 | 4 | 2 | 3 | 4 | 5 | 6 | 7 | 11 |
| 50–64 | 107 | 4.2 | 5 | 2 | 3 | 4 | 4 | 6 | 7 | 19 |
| 65+ | 91 | 5.0 | 5 | 3 | 4 | 4 | 6 | 8 | 9 | 11 |
| **TOTAL SINGLE DX** | 581 | 2.8 | 1 | 2 | 2 | 3 | 3 | 4 | 5 | 7 |
| **TOTAL MULTIPLE DX** | 1,205 | 3.8 | 6 | 2 | 2 | 3 | 4 | 6 | 8 | 14 |
| **TOTAL** | | | | | | | | | | |
| 0–19 Years | 1,133 | 3.1 | 4 | 2 | 3 | 3 | 3 | 5 | 6 | 12 |
| 20–34 | 226 | 3.9 | 4 | 2 | 3 | 3 | 4 | 6 | 8 | 11 |
| 35–49 | 205 | 3.8 | 3 | 2 | 3 | 3 | 4 | 6 | 7 | 11 |
| 50–64 | 124 | 4.2 | 5 | 2 | 3 | 4 | 4 | 6 | 7 | 19 |
| 65+ | 98 | 5.0 | 5 | 3 | 4 | 4 | 6 | 8 | 9 | 11 |
| **GRAND TOTAL** | 1,786 | 3.4 | 4 | 2 | 2 | 3 | 4 | 5 | 7 | 11 |

Length of Stay by Diagnosis and Operation, United States, 2000

# United States, October 1998–September 1999 Data, by Operation

## 55.9: OTHER RENAL OPERATIONS. Formerly included in operation group(s) 646.

| Type of Patients | Observed Patients | Avg. Stay | Variance | 10th | 25th | 50th | 75th | 90th | 95th | 99th |
|---|---|---|---|---|---|---|---|---|---|---|
| **1. SINGLE DX** | | | | | | | | | | |
| 0–19 Years | 7 | 4.4 | 8 | 2 | | 3 | 8 | 8 | 8 | 8 |
| 20–34 | 5 | 3.0 | 4 | 1 | 1 | 3 | 5 | 6 | 6 | 6 |
| 35–49 | 10 | 3.4 | 8 | 1 | 1 | 2 | 5 | 6 | 10 | 10 |
| 50–64 | 3 | 1.4 | <1 | 1 | 1 | 1 | 2 | 2 | 2 | 2 |
| 65+ | 9 | 2.2 | 1 | 1 | 2 | 2 | 2 | 4 | 4 | 4 |
| **2. MULTIPLE DX** | | | | | | | | | | |
| 0–19 Years | 29 | 8.7 | 49 | 1 | 3 | 5 | 13 | 19 | 22 | 22 |
| 20–34 | 70 | 5.4 | 20 | 2 | 3 | 4 | 6 | 10 | 17 | 23 |
| 35–49 | 131 | 7.1 | 38 | 2 | 2 | 5 | 10 | 15 | 21 | 31 |
| 50–64 | 173 | 6.1 | 19 | 2 | 3 | 6 | 7 | 10 | 14 | 27 |
| 65+ | 387 | 6.2 | 27 | 2 | 2 | 5 | 8 | 13 | 16 | 26 |
| **TOTAL SINGLE DX** | 34 | 3.0 | 5 | 1 | 1 | 2 | 4 | 8 | 8 | 10 |
| **TOTAL MULTIPLE DX** | 790 | 6.3 | 27 | 2 | 2 | 5 | 8 | 13 | 17 | 26 |
| **TOTAL** | | | | | | | | | | |
| 0–19 Years | 36 | 7.8 | 44 | 1 | 3 | 5 | 13 | 19 | 19 | 22 |
| 20–34 | 75 | 5.3 | 19 | 1 | 3 | 4 | 6 | 9 | 17 | 23 |
| 35–49 | 141 | 6.8 | 37 | 1 | 2 | 5 | 10 | 14 | 21 | 31 |
| 50–64 | 176 | 6.0 | 19 | 2 | 3 | 6 | 7 | 10 | 14 | 27 |
| 65+ | 396 | 6.1 | 27 | 2 | 2 | 5 | 8 | 13 | 16 | 26 |
| **GRAND TOTAL** | 824 | 6.2 | 27 | 2 | 2 | 5 | 8 | 13 | 16 | 26 |

## 56.0: TU RMVL URETERAL OBSTR. Formerly included in operation group(s) 649.

| Type of Patients | Observed Patients | Avg. Stay | Variance | 10th | 25th | 50th | 75th | 90th | 95th | 99th |
|---|---|---|---|---|---|---|---|---|---|---|
| **1. SINGLE DX** | | | | | | | | | | |
| 0–19 Years | 166 | 1.7 | <1 | 1 | 1 | 2 | 2 | 3 | 3 | 4 |
| 20–34 | 1,080 | 1.7 | <1 | 1 | 1 | 2 | 2 | 3 | 4 | 5 |
| 35–49 | 1,279 | 1.6 | <1 | 1 | 1 | 1 | 2 | 3 | 3 | 5 |
| 50–64 | 659 | 1.5 | <1 | 1 | 1 | 1 | 2 | 3 | 3 | 4 |
| 65+ | 146 | 1.6 | <1 | 1 | 1 | 1 | 2 | 3 | 3 | 5 |
| **2. MULTIPLE DX** | | | | | | | | | | |
| 0–19 Years | 227 | 2.3 | 3 | 1 | 1 | 2 | 3 | 4 | 5 | 9 |
| 20–34 | 1,464 | 2.6 | 10 | 1 | 1 | 2 | 3 | 4 | 6 | 15 |
| 35–49 | 2,423 | 2.6 | 12 | 1 | 1 | 2 | 3 | 5 | 6 | 13 |
| 50–64 | 2,289 | 2.8 | 7 | 1 | 1 | 2 | 3 | 6 | 8 | 14 |
| 65+ | 1,825 | 3.9 | 15 | 1 | 2 | 3 | 4 | 8 | 11 | 20 |
| **TOTAL SINGLE DX** | 3,330 | 1.6 | <1 | 1 | 1 | 1 | 2 | 3 | 3 | 5 |
| **TOTAL MULTIPLE DX** | 8,228 | 2.9 | 11 | 1 | 1 | 2 | 3 | 5 | 8 | 15 |
| **TOTAL** | | | | | | | | | | |
| 0–19 Years | 393 | 2.0 | 2 | 1 | 1 | 2 | 2 | 3 | 4 | 7 |
| 20–34 | 2,544 | 2.3 | 7 | 1 | 1 | 2 | 3 | 4 | 5 | 15 |
| 35–49 | 3,702 | 2.3 | 8 | 1 | 1 | 2 | 3 | 5 | 5 | 13 |
| 50–64 | 2,948 | 2.5 | 6 | 1 | 1 | 2 | 3 | 5 | 7 | 13 |
| 65+ | 1,971 | 3.7 | 14 | 1 | 2 | 3 | 4 | 8 | 11 | 20 |
| **GRAND TOTAL** | 11,558 | 2.5 | 8 | 1 | 1 | 2 | 3 | 4 | 7 | 14 |

## 55.93: REPL NEPHROSTOMY TUBE. Formerly included in operation group(s) 646.

| Type of Patients | Observed Patients | Avg. Stay | Variance | 10th | 25th | 50th | 75th | 90th | 95th | 99th |
|---|---|---|---|---|---|---|---|---|---|---|
| **1. SINGLE DX** | | | | | | | | | | |
| 0–19 Years | 3 | 1.9 | <1 | 1 | 2 | 2 | 2 | 2 | 2 | 2 |
| 20–34 | 2 | 3.0 | 8 | 1 | 1 | 1 | 6 | 6 | 6 | 6 |
| 35–49 | 2 | 5.2 | 26 | 1 | 2 | 1 | 10 | 10 | 10 | 10 |
| 50–64 | 0 | | | | | | | | | |
| 65+ | 6 | 2.6 | 2 | 1 | 1 | 2 | 4 | 4 | 4 | 4 |
| **2. MULTIPLE DX** | | | | | | | | | | |
| 0–19 Years | 15 | 5.6 | 41 | 1 | 1 | 3 | 5 | 22 | 22 | 22 |
| 20–34 | 41 | 4.9 | 15 | 1 | 2 | 4 | 5 | 9 | 17 | 18 |
| 35–49 | 78 | 6.4 | 41 | 1 | 2 | 5 | 8 | 15 | 21 | 24 |
| 50–64 | 116 | 5.7 | 14 | 2 | 3 | 6 | 7 | 8 | 10 | 24 |
| 65+ | 280 | 5.8 | 26 | 2 | 2 | 4 | 8 | 13 | 14 | 26 |
| **TOTAL SINGLE DX** | 13 | 2.8 | 5 | 1 | 1 | 2 | 4 | 6 | 10 | 10 |
| **TOTAL MULTIPLE DX** | 530 | 5.8 | 24 | 2 | 2 | 5 | 7 | 12 | 15 | 26 |
| **TOTAL** | | | | | | | | | | |
| 0–19 Years | 18 | 4.9 | 35 | 1 | 1 | 3 | 4 | 10 | 22 | 22 |
| 20–34 | 43 | 4.9 | 15 | 2 | 2 | 4 | 5 | 9 | 17 | 18 |
| 35–49 | 80 | 6.4 | 40 | 1 | 2 | 3 | 7 | 15 | 21 | 24 |
| 50–64 | 116 | 5.7 | 14 | 2 | 3 | 6 | 7 | 8 | 10 | 24 |
| 65+ | 286 | 5.8 | 26 | 2 | 2 | 4 | 8 | 13 | 14 | 26 |
| **GRAND TOTAL** | 543 | 5.7 | 24 | 2 | 2 | 4 | 7 | 12 | 15 | 26 |

## 56.1: URETERAL MEATOTOMY. Formerly included in operation group(s) 650.

| Type of Patients | Observed Patients | Avg. Stay | Variance | 10th | 25th | 50th | 75th | 90th | 95th | 99th |
|---|---|---|---|---|---|---|---|---|---|---|
| **1. SINGLE DX** | | | | | | | | | | |
| 0–19 Years | 1 | 1.0 | 0 | 1 | 1 | 1 | 1 | 1 | 1 | 1 |
| 20–34 | 7 | 1.9 | <1 | 1 | 2 | 2 | 2 | 3 | 3 | 3 |
| 35–49 | 8 | 2.3 | <1 | 2 | 2 | 2 | 2 | 4 | 4 | 4 |
| 50–64 | 3 | 1.8 | <1 | 1 | 1 | 2 | 2 | 2 | 2 | 2 |
| 65+ | 1 | 2.0 | 0 | 2 | 2 | 2 | 2 | 2 | 2 | 2 |
| **2. MULTIPLE DX** | | | | | | | | | | |
| 0–19 Years | 8 | 2.1 | 3 | 1 | 1 | 2 | 2 | 4 | 7 | 7 |
| 20–34 | 11 | 3.1 | 3 | 1 | 2 | 3 | 4 | 4 | 7 | 9 |
| 35–49 | 26 | 2.3 | 2 | 1 | 1 | 2 | 3 | 4 | 4 | 5 |
| 50–64 | 29 | 4.1 | 20 | 1 | 2 | 3 | 3 | 13 | 17 | 17 |
| 65+ | 29 | 4.5 | 12 | 2 | 2 | 4 | 4 | 6 | 17 | 18 |
| **TOTAL SINGLE DX** | 20 | 2.0 | <1 | 1 | 2 | 2 | 2 | 2 | 4 | 4 |
| **TOTAL MULTIPLE DX** | 103 | 3.7 | 12 | 1 | 2 | 3 | 4 | 5 | 13 | 17 |
| **TOTAL** | | | | | | | | | | |
| 0–19 Years | 9 | 1.9 | 2 | 1 | 1 | 1 | 2 | 4 | 4 | 7 |
| 20–34 | 18 | 2.6 | 2 | 2 | 2 | 2 | 3 | 4 | 4 | 9 |
| 35–49 | 34 | 2.3 | 1 | 1 | 1 | 2 | 3 | 4 | 4 | 5 |
| 50–64 | 32 | 3.9 | 19 | 1 | 2 | 3 | 4 | 6 | 17 | 17 |
| 65+ | 30 | 4.5 | 12 | 2 | 2 | 4 | 4 | 6 | 17 | 18 |
| **GRAND TOTAL** | 123 | 3.4 | 10 | 1 | 2 | 3 | 4 | 4 | 8 | 17 |

Length of Stay by Diagnosis and Operation, United States, 2000

# United States, October 1998–September 1999 Data, by Operation

## 56.2: URETEROTOMY. Formerly included in operation group(s) 647.

| Type of Patients | Observed Patients | Avg. Stay | Variance | 10th | 25th | 50th | 75th | 90th | 95th | 99th |
|---|---|---|---|---|---|---|---|---|---|---|
| **1. SINGLE DX** | | | | | | | | | | |
| 0–19 Years | 13 | 1.4 | <1 | 1 | 1 | 1 | 1 | 3 | 4 | 4 |
| 20–34 | 24 | 2.6 | 2 | 1 | 2 | 2 | 3 | 4 | 6 | 6 |
| 35–49 | 34 | 2.7 | 4 | 1 | 2 | 2 | 3 | 5 | 8 | 9 |
| 50–64 | 22 | 3.6 | 2 | 2 | 3 | 3 | 5 | 5 | 6 | 8 |
| 65+ | 10 | 2.8 | 2 | 2 | 3 | 2 | 4 | 5 | 5 | 5 |
| **2. MULTIPLE DX** | | | | | | | | | | |
| 0–19 Years | 51 | 4.1 | 35 | 1 | 1 | 3 | 5 | 8 | 9 | 41 |
| 20–34 | 53 | 3.1 | 3 | 1 | 1 | 2 | 4 | 6 | 9 | 16 |
| 35–49 | 115 | 4.6 | 27 | 1 | 2 | 3 | 5 | 8 | 15 | 34 |
| 50–64 | 142 | 4.7 | 24 | 2 | 2 | 4 | 5 | 8 | 10 | 40 |
| 65+ | 160 | 5.0 | 20 | 2 | 2 | 4 | 6 | 10 | 13 | 22 |
| **TOTAL SINGLE DX** | 103 | 2.7 | 3 | 1 | 1 | 2 | 3 | 5 | 6 | 8 |
| **TOTAL MULTIPLE DX** | 521 | 4.5 | 24 | 1 | 2 | 3 | 5 | 8 | 10 | 34 |
| **TOTAL** | | | | | | | | | | |
| 0–19 Years | 64 | 3.6 | 30 | 1 | 1 | 2 | 5 | 8 | 9 | 41 |
| 20–34 | 77 | 3.0 | 5 | 1 | 2 | 2 | 4 | 6 | 8 | 16 |
| 35–49 | 149 | 4.1 | 22 | 1 | 2 | 3 | 5 | 7 | 10 | 34 |
| 50–64 | 164 | 4.5 | 21 | 2 | 2 | 4 | 5 | 8 | 10 | 40 |
| 65+ | 170 | 4.9 | 19 | 2 | 2 | 4 | 6 | 10 | 13 | 22 |
| **GRAND TOTAL** | 624 | 4.2 | 21 | 1 | 2 | 3 | 5 | 8 | 10 | 33 |

## 56.3: URETERAL DIAGNOSTIC PX. Formerly included in operation group(s) 650, 651, 664.

| Type of Patients | Observed Patients | Avg. Stay | Variance | 10th | 25th | 50th | 75th | 90th | 95th | 99th |
|---|---|---|---|---|---|---|---|---|---|---|
| **1. SINGLE DX** | | | | | | | | | | |
| 0–19 Years | 6 | 1.8 | <1 | 1 | 1 | 1 | 3 | 3 | 3 | 3 |
| 20–34 | 68 | 1.6 | <1 | 1 | 1 | 1 | 3 | 3 | 4 | 5 |
| 35–49 | 83 | 1.5 | <1 | 1 | 1 | 1 | 2 | 3 | 3 | 6 |
| 50–64 | 38 | 2.0 | <1 | 1 | 1 | 2 | 3 | 3 | 4 | 4 |
| 65+ | 11 | 3.8 | <1 | 4 | 4 | 4 | 4 | 4 | 4 | 4 |
| **2. MULTIPLE DX** | | | | | | | | | | |
| 0–19 Years | 16 | 3.8 | 9 | 1 | 2 | 3 | 7 | 9 | 9 | 9 |
| 20–34 | 121 | 2.7 | 3 | 1 | 1 | 3 | 3 | 4 | 7 | 7 |
| 35–49 | 228 | 3.1 | 11 | 1 | 2 | 2 | 4 | 7 | 9 | 12 |
| 50–64 | 204 | 3.8 | 11 | 1 | 2 | 3 | 4 | 10 | 10 | 12 |
| 65+ | 275 | 4.7 | 16 | 1 | 2 | 3 | 6 | 11 | 13 | 19 |
| **TOTAL SINGLE DX** | 206 | 2.1 | 2 | 1 | 1 | 1 | 3 | 4 | 4 | 5 |
| **TOTAL MULTIPLE DX** | 844 | 3.7 | 12 | 1 | 2 | 2 | 5 | 9 | 11 | 14 |
| **TOTAL** | | | | | | | | | | |
| 0–19 Years | 22 | 3.1 | 7 | 1 | 1 | 2 | 3 | 9 | 9 | 9 |
| 20–34 | 189 | 2.4 | 3 | 1 | 1 | 2 | 3 | 4 | 6 | 7 |
| 35–49 | 311 | 2.5 | 8 | 1 | 1 | 2 | 3 | 6 | 7 | 12 |
| 50–64 | 242 | 3.6 | 10 | 1 | 2 | 4 | 4 | 10 | 10 | 12 |
| 65+ | 286 | 4.5 | 13 | 2 | 2 | 4 | 5 | 9 | 12 | 19 |
| **GRAND TOTAL** | 1,050 | 3.2 | 10 | 1 | 1 | 2 | 4 | 7 | 10 | 14 |

## 56.31: URETEROSCOPY. Formerly included in operation group(s) 651.

| Type of Patients | Observed Patients | Avg. Stay | Variance | 10th | 25th | 50th | 75th | 90th | 95th | 99th |
|---|---|---|---|---|---|---|---|---|---|---|
| **1. SINGLE DX** | | | | | | | | | | |
| 0–19 Years | 6 | 1.8 | <1 | 1 | 1 | 1 | 3 | 3 | 3 | 3 |
| 20–34 | 67 | 1.6 | <1 | 1 | 1 | 1 | 3 | 3 | 4 | 5 |
| 35–49 | 81 | 1.5 | <1 | 1 | 1 | 1 | 2 | 3 | 3 | 6 |
| 50–64 | 34 | 1.9 | 1 | 1 | 1 | 2 | 3 | 3 | 4 | 4 |
| 65+ | 9 | 3.8 | <1 | 4 | 4 | 4 | 4 | 4 | 4 | 4 |
| **2. MULTIPLE DX** | | | | | | | | | | |
| 0–19 Years | 14 | 3.6 | 10 | 1 | 1 | 2 | 5 | 8 | 9 | 9 |
| 20–34 | 119 | 2.7 | 3 | 1 | 1 | 2 | 3 | 4 | 7 | 7 |
| 35–49 | 211 | 2.7 | 8 | 1 | 2 | 2 | 3 | 6 | 7 | 9 |
| 50–64 | 163 | 3.6 | 10 | 2 | 2 | 4 | 4 | 10 | 10 | 12 |
| 65+ | 190 | 4.1 | 13 | 1 | 1 | 3 | 6 | 9 | 11 | 14 |
| **TOTAL SINGLE DX** | 197 | 2.1 | 2 | 1 | 1 | 1 | 3 | 4 | 4 | 5 |
| **TOTAL MULTIPLE DX** | 697 | 3.3 | 9 | 1 | 2 | 2 | 4 | 7 | 10 | 13 |
| **TOTAL** | | | | | | | | | | |
| 0–19 Years | 20 | 2.9 | 7 | 1 | 1 | 2 | 3 | 9 | 9 | 9 |
| 20–34 | 186 | 2.3 | 3 | 1 | 1 | 2 | 3 | 4 | 6 | 7 |
| 35–49 | 292 | 2.2 | 6 | 1 | 1 | 2 | 3 | 5 | 7 | 8 |
| 50–64 | 197 | 3.4 | 9 | 1 | 2 | 4 | 4 | 10 | 10 | 12 |
| 65+ | 199 | 4.0 | 9 | 1 | 2 | 4 | 6 | 8 | 10 | 14 |
| **GRAND TOTAL** | 894 | 2.9 | 7 | 1 | 1 | 2 | 4 | 6 | 8 | 12 |

## 56.4: URETERECTOMY. Formerly included in operation group(s) 650.

| Type of Patients | Observed Patients | Avg. Stay | Variance | 10th | 25th | 50th | 75th | 90th | 95th | 99th |
|---|---|---|---|---|---|---|---|---|---|---|
| **1. SINGLE DX** | | | | | | | | | | |
| 0–19 Years | 13 | 2.0 | 2 | 1 | 1 | 1 | 3 | 4 | 7 | 7 |
| 20–34 | 3 | 5.3 | 2 | 2 | 6 | 6 | 6 | 6 | 6 | 6 |
| 35–49 | 12 | 2.5 | 2 | 2 | 1 | 2 | 4 | 5 | 5 | 5 |
| 50–64 | 4 | 5.3 | 11 | 4 | 4 | 4 | 9 | 9 | 9 | 9 |
| 65+ | 14 | 4.4 | 5 | 1 | 3 | 4 | 5 | 8 | 8 | 8 |
| **2. MULTIPLE DX** | | | | | | | | | | |
| 0–19 Years | 162 | 3.8 | 6 | 2 | 2 | 3 | 4 | 6 | 7 | 15 |
| 20–34 | 41 | 5.7 | 6 | 3 | 4 | 6 | 6 | 10 | 10 | 12 |
| 35–49 | 59 | 4.9 | 4 | 3 | 4 | 4 | 6 | 7 | 9 | 11 |
| 50–64 | 103 | 4.6 | 12 | 2 | 3 | 4 | 5 | 7 | 9 | 25 |
| 65+ | 237 | 6.1 | 28 | 2 | 3 | 5 | 7 | 10 | 12 | 31 |
| **TOTAL SINGLE DX** | 46 | 3.4 | 6 | 1 | 1 | 2 | 5 | 8 | 9 | 9 |
| **TOTAL MULTIPLE DX** | 602 | 5.0 | 15 | 2 | 3 | 4 | 6 | 8 | 10 | 19 |
| **TOTAL** | | | | | | | | | | |
| 0–19 Years | 175 | 3.6 | 6 | 2 | 2 | 3 | 4 | 5 | 7 | 15 |
| 20–34 | 44 | 5.7 | 5 | 3 | 4 | 6 | 6 | 6 | 10 | 12 |
| 35–49 | 71 | 4.6 | 12 | 2 | 3 | 4 | 5 | 7 | 9 | 11 |
| 50–64 | 107 | 4.7 | 12 | 2 | 3 | 4 | 6 | 8 | 9 | 25 |
| 65+ | 251 | 6.0 | 27 | 2 | 3 | 5 | 7 | 10 | 12 | 31 |
| **GRAND TOTAL** | 648 | 4.8 | 15 | 2 | 3 | 4 | 6 | 8 | 10 | 16 |

Length of Stay by Diagnosis and Operation, United States, 2000

# United States, October 1998–September 1999 Data, by Operation

## 56.41: PARTIAL URETERECTOMY. Formerly included in operation group(s) 650.

| Type of Patients | Observed Patients | Avg. Stay | Variance | Percentiles | | | | | | |
|---|---|---|---|---|---|---|---|---|---|---|
| | | | | 10th | 25th | 50th | 75th | 90th | 95th | 99th |
| **1. SINGLE DX** | | | | | | | | | | |
| 0–19 Years | 12 | 2.0 | 2 | 1 | 1 | 1 | 3 | 4 | 7 | 7 |
| 20–34 | 3 | 5.3 | 2 | 2 | 6 | 6 | 6 | 6 | 6 | 6 |
| 35–49 | 10 | 2.2 | 2 | 1 | 1 | 2 | 3 | 5 | 5 | 5 |
| 50–64 | 4 | 5.3 | 11 | 1 | 2 | 4 | 9 | 9 | 9 | 9 |
| 65+ | 11 | 4.4 | 6 | 1 | 3 | 4 | 5 | 8 | 8 | 8 |
| **2. MULTIPLE DX** | | | | | | | | | | |
| 0–19 Years | 145 | 3.6 | 5 | 2 | 2 | 3 | 4 | 6 | 7 | 15 |
| 20–34 | 37 | 5.8 | 6 | 3 | 4 | 6 | 6 | 10 | 10 | 12 |
| 35–49 | 53 | 5.0 | 4 | 3 | 4 | 4 | 6 | 7 | 9 | 11 |
| 50–64 | 92 | 4.6 | 13 | 2 | 3 | 4 | 6 | 7 | 11 | 25 |
| 65+ | 190 | 6.0 | 30 | 2 | 3 | 5 | 8 | 10 | 12 | 46 |
| **TOTAL SINGLE DX** | 40 | 3.4 | 7 | 1 | 1 | 2 | 5 | 8 | 9 | 9 |
| **TOTAL MULTIPLE DX** | 517 | 4.9 | 15 | 2 | 3 | 4 | 6 | 8 | 10 | 15 |
| **TOTAL** | | | | | | | | | | |
| 0–19 Years | 157 | 3.4 | 5 | 2 | 2 | 3 | 4 | 6 | 7 | 15 |
| 20–34 | 40 | 5.8 | 5 | 3 | 4 | 6 | 6 | 10 | 10 | 12 |
| 35–49 | 63 | 4.6 | 4 | 3 | 3 | 4 | 6 | 7 | 9 | 11 |
| 50–64 | 96 | 4.7 | 13 | 2 | 3 | 4 | 6 | 8 | 9 | 25 |
| 65+ | 201 | 5.9 | 29 | 2 | 3 | 5 | 8 | 10 | 12 | 20 |
| **GRAND TOTAL** | 557 | 4.7 | 14 | 3 | 3 | 4 | 6 | 8 | 10 | 15 |

## 56.51: FORM CUTAN ILEOURETEROST. Formerly included in operation group(s) 648.

| Type of Patients | Observed Patients | Avg. Stay | Variance | Percentiles | | | | | | |
|---|---|---|---|---|---|---|---|---|---|---|
| | | | | 10th | 25th | 50th | 75th | 90th | 95th | 99th |
| **1. SINGLE DX** | | | | | | | | | | |
| 0–19 Years | 2 | 4.9 | <1 | 5 | 5 | 5 | 5 | 5 | 5 | 5 |
| 20–34 | 1 | 8.0 | 0 | 8 | 8 | 8 | 8 | 8 | 8 | 8 |
| 35–49 | 1 | 14.0 | 0 | 14 | 14 | 13 | 14 | 14 | 14 | 14 |
| 50–64 | 3 | 14.4 | 12 | 10 | 13 | 13 | 18 | 18 | 18 | 18 |
| 65+ | 2 | 7.4 | 3 | 6 | 6 | 6 | 9 | 9 | 9 | 9 |
| **2. MULTIPLE DX** | | | | | | | | | | |
| 0–19 Years | 23 | 4.1 | 13 | 1 | 1 | 3 | 6 | 7 | 12 | 15 |
| 20–34 | 29 | 13.2 | 54 | 7 | 9 | 13 | 13 | 17 | 34 | 43 |
| 35–49 | 76 | 11.1 | 61 | 6 | 7 | 12 | 12 | 15 | 26 | 46 |
| 50–64 | 114 | 12.9 | 62 | 6 | 8 | 12 | 15 | 21 | 23 | 56 |
| 65+ | 238 | 14.0 | 105 | 7 | 9 | 10 | 15 | 27 | 37 | 50 |
| **TOTAL SINGLE DX** | 9 | 9.0 | 23 | 5 | 5 | 6 | 13 | 18 | 18 | 18 |
| **TOTAL MULTIPLE DX** | 480 | 12.6 | 84 | 6 | 8 | 10 | 14 | 21 | 33 | 50 |
| **TOTAL** | | | | | | | | | | |
| 0–19 Years | 25 | 4.2 | 11 | 1 | 1 | 3 | 4 | 6 | 12 | 15 |
| 20–34 | 30 | 13.1 | 54 | 7 | 9 | 9 | 13 | 17 | 34 | 43 |
| 35–49 | 77 | 11.2 | 60 | 6 | 7 | 12 | 12 | 15 | 26 | 46 |
| 50–64 | 117 | 12.9 | 61 | 6 | 8 | 12 | 15 | 21 | 23 | 56 |
| 65+ | 240 | 13.9 | 105 | 7 | 9 | 10 | 15 | 27 | 37 | 50 |
| **GRAND TOTAL** | 489 | 12.5 | 83 | 6 | 8 | 10 | 14 | 21 | 33 | 46 |

## 56.5: CUTAN URETERO-ILEOSTOMY. Formerly included in operation group(s) 648.

| Type of Patients | Observed Patients | Avg. Stay | Variance | Percentiles | | | | | | |
|---|---|---|---|---|---|---|---|---|---|---|
| | | | | 10th | 25th | 50th | 75th | 90th | 95th | 99th |
| **1. SINGLE DX** | | | | | | | | | | |
| 0–19 Years | 4 | 5.3 | 1 | 4 | 5 | 5 | 7 | 7 | 7 | 7 |
| 20–34 | 1 | 8.0 | 0 | 8 | 8 | 8 | 8 | 8 | 8 | 8 |
| 35–49 | 1 | 14.0 | 0 | 14 | 14 | 14 | 14 | 14 | 14 | 14 |
| 50–64 | 3 | 14.4 | 12 | 10 | 13 | 13 | 18 | 18 | 18 | 18 |
| 65+ | 4 | 5.4 | 9 | 1 | 5 | 6 | 5 | 9 | 9 | 9 |
| **2. MULTIPLE DX** | | | | | | | | | | |
| 0–19 Years | 33 | 4.9 | 34 | 1 | 1 | 3 | 4 | 6 | 7 | 15 |
| 20–34 | 47 | 10.7 | 54 | 4 | 6 | 10 | 13 | 17 | 25 | 40 |
| 35–49 | 101 | 10.8 | 55 | 5 | 7 | 11 | 12 | 19 | 24 | 46 |
| 50–64 | 146 | 12.0 | 59 | 6 | 8 | 11 | 15 | 19 | 23 | 56 |
| 65+ | 281 | 13.3 | 118 | 5 | 8 | 10 | 15 | 27 | 40 | 50 |
| **TOTAL SINGLE DX** | 13 | 8.0 | 21 | 4 | 5 | 6 | 10 | 14 | 18 | 18 |
| **TOTAL MULTIPLE DX** | 608 | 11.9 | 87 | 4 | 7 | 10 | 14 | 21 | 32 | 50 |
| **TOTAL** | | | | | | | | | | |
| 0–19 Years | 37 | 5.0 | 29 | 1 | 1 | 4 | 7 | 7 | 12 | 32 |
| 20–34 | 48 | 10.7 | 54 | 4 | 6 | 10 | 13 | 17 | 25 | 40 |
| 35–49 | 102 | 10.8 | 54 | 5 | 7 | 9 | 12 | 19 | 21 | 46 |
| 50–64 | 149 | 12.1 | 58 | 6 | 8 | 11 | 15 | 19 | 23 | 56 |
| 65+ | 285 | 13.2 | 117 | 5 | 8 | 10 | 15 | 25 | 40 | 50 |
| **GRAND TOTAL** | 621 | 11.8 | 86 | 4 | 7 | 10 | 14 | 21 | 32 | 50 |

## 56.6: EXT URIN DIVERSION NEC. Formerly included in operation group(s) 648.

| Type of Patients | Observed Patients | Avg. Stay | Variance | Percentiles | | | | | | |
|---|---|---|---|---|---|---|---|---|---|---|
| | | | | 10th | 25th | 50th | 75th | 90th | 95th | 99th |
| **1. SINGLE DX** | | | | | | | | | | |
| 0–19 Years | 3 | 2.0 | 2 | 1 | 1 | 1 | 3 | 4 | 4 | 4 |
| 20–34 | 0 | | | | | | | | | |
| 35–49 | 1 | 8.0 | 0 | 8 | 8 | 8 | 8 | 8 | 8 | 8 |
| 50–64 | 2 | 3.0 | 0 | 3 | 3 | 3 | 3 | 3 | 3 | 3 |
| 65+ | 0 | | | | | | | | | |
| **2. MULTIPLE DX** | | | | | | | | | | |
| 0–19 Years | 39 | 5.6 | 33 | 1 | 1 | 3 | 8 | 16 | 18 | 23 |
| 20–34 | 8 | 5.5 | 2 | 4 | 4 | 6 | 7 | 7 | 8 | 8 |
| 35–49 | 7 | 8.1 | 30 | 2 | 4 | 7 | 13 | 16 | 16 | 16 |
| 50–64 | 12 | 9.4 | 78 | 3 | 5 | 8 | 13 | 16 | 16 | 49 |
| 65+ | 14 | 5.5 | 28 | 3 | 3 | 3 | 7 | 13 | 15 | 31 |
| **TOTAL SINGLE DX** | 6 | 3.0 | 2 | 1 | 3 | 3 | 3 | 3 | 4 | 8 |
| **TOTAL MULTIPLE DX** | 80 | 6.3 | 37 | 1 | 2 | 4 | 8 | 15 | 17 | 23 |
| **TOTAL** | | | | | | | | | | |
| 0–19 Years | 42 | 5.5 | 33 | 1 | 3 | 4 | 7 | 15 | 18 | 23 |
| 20–34 | 8 | 5.5 | 2 | 4 | 4 | 6 | 7 | 7 | 8 | 8 |
| 35–49 | 8 | 8.1 | 28 | 1 | 4 | 7 | 13 | 16 | 16 | 16 |
| 50–64 | 14 | 6.8 | 56 | 2 | 3 | 3 | 8 | 13 | 16 | 49 |
| 65+ | 14 | 5.5 | 28 | 3 | 3 | 3 | 7 | 13 | 15 | 31 |
| **GRAND TOTAL** | 86 | 5.9 | 35 | 1 | 2 | 3 | 8 | 13 | 17 | 23 |

Length of Stay by Diagnosis and Operation, United States, 2000

## United States, October 1998–September 1999 Data, by Operation

### 56.8: REPAIR OF URETER. Formerly included in operation group(s) 650.

| Type of Patients | Observed Patients | Avg. Stay | Vari-ance | Percentiles | | | | | | |
|---|---|---|---|---|---|---|---|---|---|---|
| | | | | 10th | 25th | 50th | 75th | 90th | 95th | 99th |
| **1. SINGLE DX** | | | | | | | | | | |
| 0–19 Years | 10 | 2.7 | 1 | 1 | 2 | 3 | 3 | 3 | 3 | 7 |
| 20–34 | 3 | 4.3 | 2 | 3 | 3 | 5 | 5 | 6 | 6 | 6 |
| 35–49 | 9 | 3.8 | 4 | 1 | 2 | 4 | 5 | 7 | 7 | 7 |
| 50–64 | 0 | | | | | | | | | |
| 65+ | 0 | | | | | | | | | |
| **2. MULTIPLE DX** | | | | | | | | | | |
| 0–19 Years | 41 | 4.3 | 7 | 2 | 2 | 4 | 6 | 8 | 9 | 12 |
| 20–34 | 16 | 5.5 | 18 | 1 | 2 | 4 | 8 | 13 | 15 | 15 |
| 35–49 | 21 | 5.6 | 29 | 2 | 2 | 3 | 8 | 10 | 23 | 23 |
| 50–64 | 13 | 8.3 | 124 | 4 | 6 | 4 | 6 | 33 | 33 | 33 |
| 65+ | 18 | 8.4 | 20 | 4 | 6 | 6 | 11 | 13 | 21 | 22 |
| **TOTAL SINGLE DX** | 22 | 3.2 | 2 | 1 | 2 | 3 | 4 | 5 | 7 | 7 |
| **TOTAL MULTIPLE DX** | 109 | 5.7 | 31 | 2 | 2 | 4 | 7 | 11 | 15 | 33 |
| **TOTAL** | | | | | | | | | | |
| 0–19 Years | 51 | 4.0 | 6 | 2 | 2 | 3 | 6 | 7 | 8 | 12 |
| 20–34 | 19 | 5.4 | 16 | 1 | 2 | 4 | 8 | 13 | 15 | 15 |
| 35–49 | 30 | 5.2 | 23 | 1 | 2 | 4 | 7 | 9 | 10 | 23 |
| 50–64 | 13 | 8.3 | 124 | 1 | 6 | 4 | 6 | 33 | 33 | 33 |
| 65+ | 18 | 8.4 | 20 | 4 | 6 | 6 | 11 | 13 | 21 | 22 |
| **GRAND TOTAL** | 131 | 5.3 | 27 | 2 | 2 | 4 | 6 | 10 | 13 | 33 |

### 56.9: OTHER URETERAL OPERATION. Formerly included in operation group(s) 650.

| Type of Patients | Observed Patients | Avg. Stay | Vari-ance | Percentiles | | | | | | |
|---|---|---|---|---|---|---|---|---|---|---|
| | | | | 10th | 25th | 50th | 75th | 90th | 95th | 99th |
| **1. SINGLE DX** | | | | | | | | | | |
| 0–19 Years | 0 | | | | | | | | | |
| 20–34 | 1 | 1.0 | 0 | 1 | 1 | 1 | 1 | 1 | 1 | 1 |
| 35–49 | 0 | | | | | | | | | |
| 50–64 | 1 | 2.0 | 0 | 2 | 2 | | 2 | 2 | 2 | 2 |
| 65+ | 1 | 1.0 | 0 | 1 | 1 | 1 | 1 | 1 | 1 | 1 |
| **2. MULTIPLE DX** | | | | | | | | | | |
| 0–19 Years | 7 | 8.9 | 39 | 2 | 3 | 9 | 9 | 20 | 20 | 20 |
| 20–34 | 2 | 2.6 | <1 | 2 | 2 | 2 | 4 | 4 | 4 | 4 |
| 35–49 | 4 | 2.1 | <1 | 1 | 1 | 2 | 2 | 3 | 3 | 3 |
| 50–64 | 10 | 3.9 | 13 | 1 | 2 | 2 | 6 | 10 | 10 | 10 |
| 65+ | 17 | 7.9 | 33 | 1 | 2 | 6 | 15 | 15 | 15 | 15 |
| **TOTAL SINGLE DX** | 3 | 1.4 | <1 | 1 | 1 | 1 | 2 | 2 | 2 | 2 |
| **TOTAL MULTIPLE DX** | 40 | 6.0 | 29 | 1 | 2 | 3 | 9 | 15 | 15 | 20 |
| **TOTAL** | | | | | | | | | | |
| 0–19 Years | 7 | 8.9 | 39 | 2 | 3 | 9 | 9 | 20 | 20 | 20 |
| 20–34 | 3 | 2.4 | 1 | 1 | 2 | 2 | 4 | 4 | 4 | 4 |
| 35–49 | 5 | 2.1 | <1 | 1 | 1 | 2 | 2 | 3 | 3 | 3 |
| 50–64 | 10 | 3.9 | 13 | 1 | 2 | 2 | 6 | 10 | 10 | 10 |
| 65+ | 18 | 7.8 | 33 | 1 | 2 | 6 | 15 | 15 | 15 | 15 |
| **GRAND TOTAL** | 43 | 5.9 | 29 | 1 | 2 | 3 | 9 | 15 | 15 | 20 |

### 56.7: OTHER URETERAL ANAST. Formerly included in operation group(s) 648.

| Type of Patients | Observed Patients | Avg. Stay | Vari-ance | Percentiles | | | | | | |
|---|---|---|---|---|---|---|---|---|---|---|
| | | | | 10th | 25th | 50th | 75th | 90th | 95th | 99th |
| **1. SINGLE DX** | | | | | | | | | | |
| 0–19 Years | 1,284 | 2.7 | 2 | 1 | 2 | 2 | 3 | 4 | 5 | 7 |
| 20–34 | 24 | 4.1 | 3 | 2 | 3 | 4 | 5 | 6 | 7 | 7 |
| 35–49 | 12 | 4.2 | 4 | 2 | 3 | 4 | 4 | 8 | 8 | 8 |
| 50–64 | 11 | 4.7 | 3 | 3 | 4 | 4 | 5 | 8 | 8 | 8 |
| 65+ | 3 | 7.0 | 35 | 3 | 4 | 4 | 16 | 16 | 16 | 16 |
| **2. MULTIPLE DX** | | | | | | | | | | |
| 0–19 Years | 1,661 | 3.8 | 8 | 2 | 2 | 3 | 4 | 7 | 8 | 15 |
| 20–34 | 121 | 5.5 | 14 | 2 | 3 | 4 | 8 | 9 | 10 | 26 |
| 35–49 | 185 | 5.7 | 14 | 3 | 3 | 5 | 7 | 10 | 11 | 18 |
| 50–64 | 117 | 7.3 | 20 | 3 | 5 | 6 | 9 | 14 | 16 | 21 |
| 65+ | 119 | 7.7 | 32 | 3 | 4 | 6 | 9 | 14 | 17 | 27 |
| **TOTAL SINGLE DX** | 1,334 | 2.7 | 2 | 1 | 2 | 2 | 3 | 4 | 5 | 8 |
| **TOTAL MULTIPLE DX** | 2,203 | 4.4 | 12 | 2 | 2 | 3 | 5 | 8 | 10 | 17 |
| **TOTAL** | | | | | | | | | | |
| 0–19 Years | 2,945 | 3.3 | 5 | 1 | 2 | 3 | 4 | 6 | 7 | 12 |
| 20–34 | 145 | 5.3 | 12 | 2 | 3 | 4 | 7 | 9 | 10 | 17 |
| 35–49 | 197 | 5.6 | 13 | 3 | 3 | 4 | 7 | 10 | 11 | 17 |
| 50–64 | 128 | 7.1 | 19 | 3 | 4 | 6 | 8 | 13 | 16 | 21 |
| 65+ | 122 | 7.7 | 32 | 3 | 4 | 6 | 9 | 14 | 17 | 27 |
| **GRAND TOTAL** | 3,537 | 3.7 | 9 | 2 | 2 | 3 | 4 | 7 | 9 | 16 |

### 56.74: URETERONEOCYSTOSTOMY. Formerly included in operation group(s) 648.

| Type of Patients | Observed Patients | Avg. Stay | Vari-ance | Percentiles | | | | | | |
|---|---|---|---|---|---|---|---|---|---|---|
| | | | | 10th | 25th | 50th | 75th | 90th | 95th | 99th |
| **1. SINGLE DX** | | | | | | | | | | |
| 0–19 Years | 1,280 | 2.7 | 2 | 1 | 2 | 2 | 3 | 4 | 5 | 7 |
| 20–34 | 21 | 4.3 | 3 | 2 | 3 | 5 | 6 | 7 | 7 | 7 |
| 35–49 | 10 | 3.7 | 3 | 2 | 3 | 4 | 4 | 5 | 7 | 8 |
| 50–64 | 10 | 4.6 | 3 | 2 | 4 | 4 | 5 | 8 | 8 | 8 |
| 65+ | 3 | 7.0 | 35 | 3 | 4 | 4 | 16 | 16 | 16 | 16 |
| **2. MULTIPLE DX** | | | | | | | | | | |
| 0–19 Years | 1,614 | 3.7 | 7 | 2 | 2 | 3 | 4 | 7 | 8 | 13 |
| 20–34 | 104 | 5.4 | 11 | 2 | 3 | 4 | 7 | 9 | 10 | 16 |
| 35–49 | 152 | 5.2 | 9 | 3 | 4 | 4 | 6 | 9 | 11 | 12 |
| 50–64 | 96 | 6.9 | 17 | 3 | 4 | 6 | 8 | 13 | 16 | 20 |
| 65+ | 84 | 6.1 | 25 | 3 | 4 | 5 | 7 | 10 | 16 | 17 |
| **TOTAL SINGLE DX** | 1,324 | 2.7 | 2 | 1 | 2 | 2 | 3 | 4 | 5 | 7 |
| **TOTAL MULTIPLE DX** | 2,050 | 4.1 | 9 | 2 | 2 | 3 | 5 | 7 | 9 | 16 |
| **TOTAL** | | | | | | | | | | |
| 0–19 Years | 2,894 | 3.2 | 5 | 1 | 2 | 3 | 4 | 5 | 7 | 11 |
| 20–34 | 125 | 5.2 | 10 | 2 | 3 | 4 | 7 | 8 | 9 | 16 |
| 35–49 | 162 | 5.0 | 9 | 3 | 3 | 4 | 6 | 9 | 11 | 12 |
| 50–64 | 106 | 6.7 | 16 | 3 | 4 | 5 | 8 | 13 | 16 | 16 |
| 65+ | 87 | 6.1 | 25 | 3 | 4 | 5 | 7 | 10 | 16 | 17 |
| **GRAND TOTAL** | 3,374 | 3.5 | 7 | 2 | 2 | 3 | 4 | 6 | 8 | 13 |

Length of Stay by Diagnosis and Operation, United States, 2000

# United States, October 1998–September 1999 Data, by Operation

## 57.0: TU BLADDER CLEARANCE. Formerly included in operation group(s) 653.

| Type of Patients | Observed Patients | Avg. Stay | Variance | 10th | 25th | 50th | 75th | 90th | 95th | 99th |
|---|---|---|---|---|---|---|---|---|---|---|
| **1. SINGLE DX** | | | | | | | | | | |
| 0–19 Years | 10 | 1.3 | <1 | 1 | 1 | 1 | 2 | 2 | 2 | 2 |
| 20–34 | 10 | 1.6 | 1 | 1 | 1 | 1 | 1 | 4 | 4 | 4 |
| 35–49 | 11 | 2.4 | 3 | 1 | 1 | 2 | 5 | 5 | 5 | 6 |
| 50–64 | 12 | 2.2 | <1 | 1 | 2 | 2 | 3 | 3 | 3 | 3 |
| 65+ | 22 | 1.5 | <1 | 1 | 1 | 1 | 2 | 3 | 3 | 4 |
| **2. MULTIPLE DX** | | | | | | | | | | |
| 0–19 Years | 30 | 3.3 | 21 | 1 | 1 | 1 | 4 | 7 | 12 | 20 |
| 20–34 | 69 | 3.6 | 14 | 1 | 2 | 2 | 4 | 7 | 13 | 18 |
| 35–49 | 131 | 3.9 | 17 | 1 | 2 | 4 | 4 | 7 | 9 | 30 |
| 50–64 | 243 | 4.7 | 26 | 1 | 2 | 3 | 6 | 10 | 13 | 34 |
| 65+ | 1,070 | 4.9 | 25 | 1 | 2 | 3 | 6 | 12 | 16 | 23 |
| **TOTAL SINGLE DX** | 65 | 1.8 | 1 | 1 | 1 | 1 | 2 | 3 | 4 | 5 |
| **TOTAL MULTIPLE DX** | 1,543 | 4.6 | 24 | 1 | 2 | 3 | 6 | 10 | 15 | 23 |
| **TOTAL** | | | | | | | | | | |
| 0–19 Years | 40 | 2.9 | 18 | 1 | 1 | 1 | 3 | 7 | 12 | 20 |
| 20–34 | 79 | 3.3 | 13 | 1 | 1 | 2 | 4 | 7 | 12 | 18 |
| 35–49 | 142 | 3.8 | 16 | 1 | 2 | 4 | 4 | 7 | 9 | 23 |
| 50–64 | 255 | 4.6 | 25 | 1 | 2 | 3 | 6 | 10 | 13 | 29 |
| 65+ | 1,092 | 4.8 | 25 | 1 | 2 | 3 | 6 | 11 | 16 | 23 |
| **GRAND TOTAL** | 1,608 | 4.5 | 24 | 1 | 2 | 3 | 6 | 10 | 14 | 23 |

## 57.1: CYSTOTOMY & CYSTOSTOMY. Formerly included in operation group(s) 654.

| Type of Patients | Observed Patients | Avg. Stay | Variance | 10th | 25th | 50th | 75th | 90th | 95th | 99th |
|---|---|---|---|---|---|---|---|---|---|---|
| **1. SINGLE DX** | | | | | | | | | | |
| 0–19 Years | 35 | 3.1 | 6 | 1 | 2 | 3 | 3 | 5 | 11 | 11 |
| 20–34 | 17 | 2.4 | 2 | 1 | 1 | 2 | 4 | 4 | 4 | 4 |
| 35–49 | 63 | 1.9 | <1 | 1 | 1 | 2 | 2 | 4 | 4 | 5 |
| 50–64 | 63 | 1.9 | <1 | 1 | 1 | 2 | 2 | 3 | 3 | 4 |
| 65+ | 38 | 2.5 | 3 | 1 | 2 | 2 | 3 | 3 | 5 | 12 |
| **2. MULTIPLE DX** | | | | | | | | | | |
| 0–19 Years | 205 | 8.5 | 136 | 1 | 2 | 5 | 9 | 23 | 35 | 57 |
| 20–34 | 134 | 5.4 | 29 | 1 | 2 | 3 | 8 | 11 | 14 | 23 |
| 35–49 | 370 | 4.5 | 26 | 1 | 2 | 3 | 5 | 9 | 14 | 22 |
| 50–64 | 579 | 4.4 | 38 | 1 | 2 | 3 | 4 | 9 | 15 | 26 |
| 65+ | 1,437 | 7.1 | 42 | 1 | 3 | 5 | 11 | 14 | 20 | 32 |
| **TOTAL SINGLE DX** | 216 | 2.1 | 2 | 1 | 1 | 2 | 3 | 3 | 4 | 5 |
| **TOTAL MULTIPLE DX** | 2,725 | 6.2 | 47 | 1 | 2 | 4 | 8 | 13 | 18 | 32 |
| **TOTAL** | | | | | | | | | | |
| 0–19 Years | 240 | 8.0 | 127 | 1 | 2 | 4 | 8 | 20 | 35 | 57 |
| 20–34 | 151 | 5.1 | 27 | 1 | 2 | 3 | 7 | 10 | 14 | 23 |
| 35–49 | 433 | 4.2 | 23 | 1 | 2 | 3 | 5 | 9 | 13 | 22 |
| 50–64 | 642 | 4.2 | 35 | 1 | 2 | 2 | 4 | 9 | 14 | 26 |
| 65+ | 1,475 | 7.0 | 42 | 1 | 2 | 5 | 10 | 13 | 20 | 32 |
| **GRAND TOTAL** | 2,941 | 5.9 | 45 | 1 | 2 | 3 | 8 | 12 | 18 | 32 |

## 57.17: PERCUTANEOUS CYSTOSTOMY. Formerly included in operation group(s) 654.

| Type of Patients | Observed Patients | Avg. Stay | Variance | 10th | 25th | 50th | 75th | 90th | 95th | 99th |
|---|---|---|---|---|---|---|---|---|---|---|
| **1. SINGLE DX** | | | | | | | | | | |
| 0–19 Years | 3 | 8.5 | 17 | 3 | 3 | 11 | 11 | 11 | 11 | 11 |
| 20–34 | 5 | 2.6 | 1 | 1 | 2 | 2 | 4 | 2 | 2 | 4 |
| 35–49 | 5 | 1.7 | <1 | 1 | 1 | 2 | 2 | 2 | 2 | 2 |
| 50–64 | 0 | | | | | | | | | |
| 65+ | 3 | 1.7 | <1 | 1 | 1 | 2 | 2 | 2 | 2 | 2 |
| **2. MULTIPLE DX** | | | | | | | | | | |
| 0–19 Years | 41 | 8.9 | 118 | 2 | 2 | 5 | 9 | 35 | 35 | 35 |
| 20–34 | 26 | 5.5 | 21 | 1 | 3 | 4 | 9 | 10 | 12 | 22 |
| 35–49 | 50 | 5.9 | 31 | 1 | 4 | 4 | 7 | 12 | 20 | 35 |
| 50–64 | 72 | 6.6 | 23 | 3 | 3 | 6 | 8 | 14 | 16 | 23 |
| 65+ | 364 | 8.2 | 36 | 1 | 4 | 8 | 12 | 13 | 17 | 30 |
| **TOTAL SINGLE DX** | 16 | 2.7 | 6 | 1 | 2 | 2 | 3 | 4 | 11 | 11 |
| **TOTAL MULTIPLE DX** | 553 | 7.7 | 41 | 1 | 3 | 6 | 11 | 13 | 18 | 35 |
| **TOTAL** | | | | | | | | | | |
| 0–19 Years | 44 | 8.9 | 115 | 2 | 2 | 5 | 9 | 35 | 35 | 35 |
| 20–34 | 31 | 5.0 | 19 | 1 | 3 | 3 | 5 | 10 | 12 | 22 |
| 35–49 | 55 | 5.5 | 30 | 1 | 3 | 6 | 6 | 12 | 13 | 35 |
| 50–64 | 72 | 6.6 | 23 | 3 | 3 | 6 | 8 | 14 | 16 | 23 |
| 65+ | 367 | 8.2 | 36 | 2 | 3 | 8 | 12 | 13 | 17 | 30 |
| **GRAND TOTAL** | 569 | 7.6 | 40 | 1 | 3 | 6 | 11 | 13 | 18 | 35 |

## 57.18: S/P CYSTOSTOMY NEC. Formerly included in operation group(s) 654.

| Type of Patients | Observed Patients | Avg. Stay | Variance | 10th | 25th | 50th | 75th | 90th | 95th | 99th |
|---|---|---|---|---|---|---|---|---|---|---|
| **1. SINGLE DX** | | | | | | | | | | |
| 0–19 Years | 5 | 2.4 | 2 | 1 | 1 | 3 | 4 | 4 | 4 | 4 |
| 20–34 | 11 | 1.8 | 1 | 1 | 1 | 1 | 3 | 3 | 4 | 4 |
| 35–49 | 53 | 2.1 | 1 | 1 | 1 | 2 | 3 | 3 | 4 | 5 |
| 50–64 | 55 | 1.9 | <1 | 1 | 1 | 2 | 2 | 3 | 3 | 4 |
| 65+ | 24 | 2.4 | 4 | 1 | 2 | 2 | 3 | 3 | 5 | 12 |
| **2. MULTIPLE DX** | | | | | | | | | | |
| 0–19 Years | 35 | 7.9 | 131 | 1 | 1 | 3 | 8 | 20 | 23 | 63 |
| 20–34 | 72 | 6.3 | 43 | 2 | 2 | 4 | 9 | 11 | 19 | 23 |
| 35–49 | 283 | 4.2 | 28 | 1 | 2 | 2 | 5 | 8 | 15 | 22 |
| 50–64 | 422 | 3.9 | 41 | 1 | 2 | 4 | 5 | 8 | 14 | 32 |
| 65+ | 849 | 6.1 | 39 | 1 | 2 | 4 | 8 | 14 | 19 | 30 |
| **TOTAL SINGLE DX** | 148 | 2.1 | 1 | 1 | 1 | 2 | 2 | 3 | 4 | 5 |
| **TOTAL MULTIPLE DX** | 1,661 | 5.2 | 42 | 1 | 2 | 3 | 6 | 12 | 17 | 30 |
| **TOTAL** | | | | | | | | | | |
| 0–19 Years | 40 | 7.5 | 125 | 1 | 1 | 3 | 8 | 20 | 23 | 63 |
| 20–34 | 83 | 5.8 | 41 | 1 | 2 | 4 | 9 | 11 | 19 | 23 |
| 35–49 | 336 | 3.9 | 25 | 1 | 2 | 2 | 4 | 8 | 13 | 22 |
| 50–64 | 477 | 3.6 | 37 | 1 | 2 | 2 | 3 | 7 | 13 | 26 |
| 65+ | 873 | 6.0 | 39 | 1 | 2 | 4 | 8 | 13 | 19 | 30 |
| **GRAND TOTAL** | 1,809 | 5.0 | 39 | 1 | 2 | 3 | 6 | 11 | 16 | 28 |

Length of Stay by Diagnosis and Operation, United States, 2000

# United States, October 1998–September 1999 Data, by Operation

## 57.3: BLADDER DIAGNOSTIC PX. Formerly included in operation group(s) 651, 652, 654, 664.

| Type of Patients | Observed Patients | Avg. Stay | Variance | Percentiles | | | | | | |
|---|---|---|---|---|---|---|---|---|---|---|
| | | | | 10th | 25th | 50th | 75th | 90th | 95th | 99th |
| **1. SINGLE DX** | | | | | | | | | | |
| 0–19 Years | 60 | 1.9 | 2 | 1 | 1 | 1 | 2 | 4 | 5 | 5 |
| 20–34 | 173 | 1.8 | 1 | 1 | 1 | 1 | 2 | 3 | 5 | 5 |
| 35–49 | 236 | 2.1 | 2 | 1 | 1 | 2 | 3 | 4 | 4 | 6 |
| 50–64 | 122 | 1.6 | 1 | 1 | 1 | 1 | 2 | 3 | 4 | 5 |
| 65+ | 97 | 2.0 | 2 | 1 | 1 | 1 | 2 | 4 | 5 | 10 |
| **2. MULTIPLE DX** | | | | | | | | | | |
| 0–19 Years | 256 | 4.5 | 26 | 1 | 1 | 3 | 6 | 10 | 12 | 25 |
| 20–34 | 769 | 3.7 | 15 | 1 | 2 | 3 | 4 | 7 | 9 | 16 |
| 35–49 | 1,465 | 5.2 | 42 | 1 | 2 | 3 | 6 | 11 | 17 | 36 |
| 50–64 | 1,934 | 5.5 | 25 | 1 | 2 | 4 | 7 | 12 | 15 | 25 |
| 65+ | 6,528 | 7.3 | 38 | 2 | 3 | 6 | 9 | 14 | 18 | 32 |
| **TOTAL SINGLE DX** | 688 | 1.9 | 2 | 1 | 1 | 1 | 2 | 4 | 4 | 6 |
| **TOTAL MULTIPLE DX** | 10,952 | 6.3 | 35 | 1 | 2 | 5 | 8 | 13 | 17 | 30 |
| **TOTAL** | | | | | | | | | | |
| 0–19 Years | 316 | 4.0 | 22 | 1 | 1 | 3 | 5 | 9 | 12 | 25 |
| 20–34 | 942 | 3.3 | 13 | 1 | 1 | 2 | 4 | 6 | 9 | 14 |
| 35–49 | 1,701 | 4.7 | 37 | 1 | 2 | 3 | 5 | 10 | 14 | 32 |
| 50–64 | 2,056 | 5.1 | 24 | 1 | 2 | 4 | 7 | 12 | 14 | 24 |
| 65+ | 6,625 | 7.2 | 37 | 2 | 3 | 6 | 9 | 14 | 18 | 32 |
| **GRAND TOTAL** | 11,640 | 5.9 | 34 | 1 | 2 | 4 | 8 | 13 | 16 | 29 |

## 57.32: CYSTOSCOPY NEC. Formerly included in operation group(s) 651.

| Type of Patients | Observed Patients | Avg. Stay | Variance | Percentiles | | | | | | |
|---|---|---|---|---|---|---|---|---|---|---|
| | | | | 10th | 25th | 50th | 75th | 90th | 95th | 99th |
| **1. SINGLE DX** | | | | | | | | | | |
| 0–19 Years | 59 | 1.9 | 2 | 1 | 1 | 1 | 2 | 4 | 5 | 5 |
| 20–34 | 168 | 1.8 | 1 | 1 | 1 | 1 | 2 | 3 | 4 | 5 |
| 35–49 | 231 | 2.1 | 2 | 1 | 1 | 2 | 3 | 4 | 4 | 6 |
| 50–64 | 110 | 1.7 | 2 | 1 | 1 | 1 | 2 | 3 | 4 | 5 |
| 65+ | 71 | 2.3 | 3 | 1 | 1 | 2 | 3 | 4 | 5 | 10 |
| **2. MULTIPLE DX** | | | | | | | | | | |
| 0–19 Years | 225 | 4.4 | 24 | 1 | 1 | 3 | 6 | 10 | 12 | 25 |
| 20–34 | 702 | 3.6 | 14 | 1 | 2 | 3 | 4 | 7 | 9 | 14 |
| 35–49 | 1,251 | 5.3 | 44 | 1 | 2 | 3 | 6 | 11 | 17 | 36 |
| 50–64 | 1,593 | 5.4 | 24 | 1 | 2 | 4 | 7 | 12 | 15 | 25 |
| 65+ | 5,190 | 7.5 | 37 | 2 | 3 | 6 | 10 | 15 | 18 | 31 |
| **TOTAL SINGLE DX** | 639 | 1.9 | 2 | 1 | 1 | 1 | 2 | 4 | 4 | 6 |
| **TOTAL MULTIPLE DX** | 8,961 | 6.2 | 35 | 1 | 2 | 5 | 8 | 13 | 16 | 30 |
| **TOTAL** | | | | | | | | | | |
| 0–19 Years | 284 | 3.8 | 20 | 1 | 1 | 2 | 4 | 9 | 12 | 25 |
| 20–34 | 870 | 3.2 | 12 | 1 | 1 | 2 | 4 | 6 | 9 | 14 |
| 35–49 | 1,482 | 4.6 | 37 | 1 | 2 | 3 | 5 | 10 | 15 | 32 |
| 50–64 | 1,703 | 5.0 | 23 | 1 | 2 | 4 | 7 | 12 | 14 | 23 |
| 65+ | 5,261 | 7.4 | 37 | 2 | 3 | 6 | 10 | 15 | 18 | 31 |
| **GRAND TOTAL** | 9,600 | 5.9 | 33 | 1 | 2 | 4 | 8 | 13 | 16 | 29 |

## 57.19: CYSTOTOMY NEC. Formerly included in operation group(s) 654.

| Type of Patients | Observed Patients | Avg. Stay | Variance | Percentiles | | | | | | |
|---|---|---|---|---|---|---|---|---|---|---|
| | | | | 10th | 25th | 50th | 75th | 90th | 95th | 99th |
| **1. SINGLE DX** | | | | | | | | | | |
| 0–19 Years | 11 | 2.0 | <1 | 1 | 1 | 2 | 3 | 3 | 4 | 4 |
| 20–34 | 1 | 4.0 | 0 | 4 | 4 | 4 | 4 | 4 | 4 | 4 |
| 35–49 | 5 | 1.2 | <1 | 1 | 1 | 1 | 1 | 2 | 2 | 2 |
| 50–64 | 8 | 1.5 | <1 | 1 | 1 | 1 | 2 | 3 | 3 | 3 |
| 65+ | 11 | 3.2 | <1 | 2 | 3 | 3 | 3 | 5 | 5 | 5 |
| **2. MULTIPLE DX** | | | | | | | | | | |
| 0–19 Years | 50 | 6.5 | 68 | 1 | 2 | 3 | 5 | 24 | 27 | 35 |
| 20–34 | 35 | 4.1 | 13 | 1 | 2 | 3 | 5 | 9 | 14 | 17 |
| 35–49 | 35 | 4.5 | 8 | 2 | 3 | 3 | 6 | 9 | 9 | 17 |
| 50–64 | 84 | 4.9 | 30 | 2 | 3 | 3 | 4 | 9 | 18 | 26 |
| 65+ | 219 | 8.2 | 60 | 2 | 3 | 5 | 11 | 23 | 26 | 32 |
| **TOTAL SINGLE DX** | 36 | 1.9 | 1 | 1 | 1 | 1 | 3 | 3 | 4 | 5 |
| **TOTAL MULTIPLE DX** | 423 | 6.5 | 46 | 1 | 2 | 4 | 7 | 14 | 26 | 32 |
| **TOTAL** | | | | | | | | | | |
| 0–19 Years | 61 | 6.0 | 62 | 1 | 2 | 3 | 5 | 15 | 27 | 35 |
| 20–34 | 36 | 4.1 | 12 | 1 | 1 | 3 | 5 | 9 | 14 | 17 |
| 35–49 | 40 | 4.0 | 8 | 1 | 2 | 3 | 4 | 9 | 9 | 17 |
| 50–64 | 92 | 4.6 | 28 | 1 | 2 | 3 | 4 | 9 | 15 | 26 |
| 65+ | 230 | 8.0 | 59 | 2 | 3 | 5 | 11 | 23 | 26 | 32 |
| **GRAND TOTAL** | 459 | 6.2 | 45 | 1 | 2 | 4 | 7 | 13 | 24 | 32 |

## 57.2: VESICOSTOMY. Formerly included in operation group(s) 654.

| Type of Patients | Observed Patients | Avg. Stay | Variance | Percentiles | | | | | | |
|---|---|---|---|---|---|---|---|---|---|---|
| | | | | 10th | 25th | 50th | 75th | 90th | 95th | 99th |
| **1. SINGLE DX** | | | | | | | | | | |
| 0–19 Years | 7 | 1.9 | 3 | 1 | 1 | 1 | 2 | 3 | 3 | 8 |
| 20–34 | 1 | 8.0 | 0 | 8 | 8 | 8 | 8 | 8 | 8 | 8 |
| 35–49 | 1 | 3.0 | 0 | 3 | 3 | 3 | 3 | 3 | 3 | 3 |
| 50–64 | 1 | 1.0 | 0 | 1 | 1 | 1 | 1 | 1 | 1 | 1 |
| 65+ | 0 | | | | | | | | | |
| **2. MULTIPLE DX** | | | | | | | | | | |
| 0–19 Years | 187 | 7.5 | 105 | 1 | 1 | 4 | 8 | 15 | 32 | 45 |
| 20–34 | 23 | 8.3 | 30 | 4 | 4 | 5 | 10 | 19 | 20 | 20 |
| 35–49 | 12 | 6.9 | 16 | 3 | 4 | 6 | 8 | 14 | 16 | 16 |
| 50–64 | 13 | 3.7 | 11 | 1 | 1 | 3 | 5 | 9 | 11 | 16 |
| 65+ | 10 | 6.8 | 12 | 5 | 5 | 6 | 7 | 9 | 19 | 19 |
| **TOTAL SINGLE DX** | 10 | 2.2 | 5 | 1 | 1 | 1 | 2 | 3 | 8 | 8 |
| **TOTAL MULTIPLE DX** | 245 | 7.2 | 86 | 1 | 1 | 5 | 8 | 15 | 32 | 45 |
| **TOTAL** | | | | | | | | | | |
| 0–19 Years | 194 | 7.3 | 102 | 1 | 1 | 4 | 8 | 15 | 32 | 45 |
| 20–34 | 24 | 8.3 | 30 | 4 | 4 | 5 | 10 | 19 | 20 | 20 |
| 35–49 | 13 | 6.6 | 16 | 3 | 3 | 6 | 8 | 14 | 16 | 16 |
| 50–64 | 14 | 3.6 | 11 | 1 | 1 | 3 | 5 | 9 | 11 | 16 |
| 65+ | 10 | 6.8 | 12 | 5 | 5 | 6 | 7 | 9 | 19 | 19 |
| **GRAND TOTAL** | 255 | 7.0 | 83 | 1 | 1 | 4 | 8 | 15 | 31 | 45 |

Length of Stay by Diagnosis and Operation, United States, 2000

# United States, October 1998–September 1999 Data, by Operation

## 57.33: CLSD (TU) BLADDER BIOPSY. Formerly included in operation group(s) 652.

| Type of Patients | Observed Patients | Avg. Stay | Variance | Percentiles 10th | 25th | 50th | 75th | 90th | 95th | 99th |
|---|---|---|---|---|---|---|---|---|---|---|
| **1. SINGLE DX** | | | | | | | | | | |
| 0–19 Years | 1 | 3.0 | 0 | 3 | 3 | 3 | 3 | 3 | 3 | 3 |
| 20–34 | 5 | 2.7 | 3 | 1 | 1 | 2 | 4 | 5 | 5 | 5 |
| 35–49 | 5 | 1.4 | <1 | 1 | 1 | 1 | 2 | 2 | 2 | 2 |
| 50–64 | 11 | 1.0 | <1 | 1 | 1 | 1 | 1 | 2 | 2 | 2 |
| 65+ | 26 | 1.3 | <1 | 1 | 1 | 1 | 1 | 2 | 3 | 3 |
| **2. MULTIPLE DX** | | | | | | | | | | |
| 0–19 Years | 23 | 6.0 | 67 | 1 | 2 | 3 | 7 | 12 | 18 | 57 |
| 20–34 | 63 | 5.6 | 40 | 1 | 2 | 4 | 6 | 10 | 12 | 42 |
| 35–49 | 199 | 5.2 | 31 | 1 | 2 | 3 | 6 | 11 | 15 | 27 |
| 50–64 | 327 | 5.7 | 29 | 1 | 2 | 4 | 7 | 12 | 16 | 30 |
| 65+ | 1,293 | 6.6 | 39 | 1 | 3 | 5 | 8 | 13 | 19 | 32 |
| **TOTAL SINGLE DX** | 48 | 1.3 | <1 | 1 | 1 | 1 | 1 | 2 | 3 | 5 |
| **TOTAL MULTIPLE DX** | 1,905 | 6.3 | 37 | 1 | 3 | 5 | 8 | 12 | 17 | 32 |
| **TOTAL** | | | | | | | | | | |
| 0–19 Years | 24 | 5.7 | 61 | 1 | 2 | 3 | 7 | 12 | 18 | 57 |
| 20–34 | 68 | 5.4 | 39 | 1 | 2 | 4 | 6 | 10 | 12 | 42 |
| 35–49 | 204 | 5.1 | 31 | 1 | 2 | 3 | 6 | 11 | 14 | 27 |
| 50–64 | 338 | 5.5 | 29 | 1 | 2 | 4 | 7 | 12 | 16 | 30 |
| 65+ | 1,319 | 6.5 | 39 | 1 | 3 | 5 | 8 | 13 | 18 | 32 |
| **GRAND TOTAL** | 1,953 | 6.2 | 37 | 1 | 2 | 5 | 8 | 12 | 17 | 32 |

## 57.49: TU DESTR BLADDER LES NEC. Formerly included in operation group(s) 652.

| Type of Patients | Observed Patients | Avg. Stay | Variance | Percentiles 10th | 25th | 50th | 75th | 90th | 95th | 99th |
|---|---|---|---|---|---|---|---|---|---|---|
| **1. SINGLE DX** | | | | | | | | | | |
| 0–19 Years | 13 | 1.3 | <1 | 1 | 1 | 1 | 1 | 3 | 3 | 3 |
| 20–34 | 7 | 1.5 | <1 | 1 | 1 | 1 | 2 | 3 | 3 | 3 |
| 35–49 | 49 | 1.6 | 1 | 1 | 1 | 1 | 2 | 3 | 4 | 5 |
| 50–64 | 156 | 1.5 | 1 | 1 | 1 | 1 | 2 | 2 | 3 | 7 |
| 65+ | 393 | 1.5 | 1 | 1 | 1 | 1 | 2 | 2 | 4 | 6 |
| **2. MULTIPLE DX** | | | | | | | | | | |
| 0–19 Years | 36 | 3.9 | 18 | 1 | 1 | 3 | 4 | 7 | 7 | 30 |
| 20–34 | 68 | 3.8 | 23 | 1 | 1 | 4 | 4 | 7 | 11 | 15 |
| 35–49 | 377 | 3.6 | 17 | 1 | 1 | 3 | 4 | 8 | 10 | 25 |
| 50–64 | 1,315 | 3.3 | 16 | 1 | 1 | 2 | 4 | 7 | 10 | 18 |
| 65+ | 7,550 | 4.1 | 22 | 1 | 2 | 2 | 5 | 9 | 13 | 21 |
| **TOTAL SINGLE DX** | 618 | 1.5 | 1 | 1 | 1 | 1 | 2 | 2 | 3 | 6 |
| **TOTAL MULTIPLE DX** | 9,346 | 3.9 | 21 | 1 | 2 | 2 | 5 | 9 | 13 | 21 |
| **TOTAL** | | | | | | | | | | |
| 0–19 Years | 49 | 3.2 | 15 | 1 | 1 | 1 | 4 | 7 | 7 | 30 |
| 20–34 | 75 | 3.4 | 21 | 1 | 1 | 2 | 4 | 7 | 11 | 15 |
| 35–49 | 426 | 3.4 | 16 | 1 | 1 | 2 | 4 | 7 | 10 | 25 |
| 50–64 | 1,471 | 3.1 | 15 | 1 | 1 | 2 | 4 | 7 | 9 | 18 |
| 65+ | 7,943 | 3.9 | 21 | 1 | 2 | 2 | 5 | 9 | 13 | 21 |
| **GRAND TOTAL** | 9,964 | 3.8 | 20 | 1 | 1 | 2 | 5 | 8 | 12 | 21 |

## 57.4: TU EXC/DESTR BLADDER LES. Formerly included in operation group(s) 652.

| Type of Patients | Observed Patients | Avg. Stay | Variance | Percentiles 10th | 25th | 50th | 75th | 90th | 95th | 99th |
|---|---|---|---|---|---|---|---|---|---|---|
| **1. SINGLE DX** | | | | | | | | | | |
| 0–19 Years | 13 | 1.3 | <1 | 1 | 1 | 1 | 1 | 3 | 3 | 3 |
| 20–34 | 7 | 1.5 | <1 | 1 | 1 | 1 | 2 | 3 | 3 | 3 |
| 35–49 | 49 | 1.6 | 1 | 1 | 1 | 1 | 2 | 3 | 4 | 5 |
| 50–64 | 156 | 1.5 | 1 | 1 | 1 | 1 | 2 | 2 | 3 | 7 |
| 65+ | 393 | 1.5 | 1 | 1 | 1 | 1 | 2 | 2 | 4 | 6 |
| **2. MULTIPLE DX** | | | | | | | | | | |
| 0–19 Years | 37 | 3.8 | 18 | 1 | 1 | 3 | 4 | 7 | 7 | 30 |
| 20–34 | 68 | 3.8 | 23 | 1 | 1 | 4 | 4 | 7 | 11 | 15 |
| 35–49 | 377 | 3.6 | 17 | 1 | 1 | 3 | 4 | 8 | 10 | 25 |
| 50–64 | 1,316 | 3.3 | 16 | 1 | 1 | 2 | 4 | 7 | 10 | 18 |
| 65+ | 7,550 | 4.1 | 22 | 1 | 2 | 2 | 5 | 9 | 13 | 21 |
| **TOTAL SINGLE DX** | 618 | 1.5 | 1 | 1 | 1 | 1 | 2 | 2 | 3 | 6 |
| **TOTAL MULTIPLE DX** | 9,348 | 3.9 | 21 | 1 | 1 | 2 | 5 | 9 | 13 | 21 |
| **TOTAL** | | | | | | | | | | |
| 0–19 Years | 50 | 3.2 | 15 | 1 | 1 | 1 | 4 | 7 | 7 | 30 |
| 20–34 | 75 | 3.4 | 21 | 1 | 2 | 2 | 4 | 7 | 11 | 15 |
| 35–49 | 426 | 3.4 | 16 | 1 | 2 | 2 | 4 | 7 | 10 | 25 |
| 50–64 | 1,472 | 3.1 | 15 | 1 | 2 | 2 | 4 | 7 | 9 | 18 |
| 65+ | 7,943 | 3.9 | 21 | 1 | 2 | 2 | 5 | 9 | 13 | 21 |
| **GRAND TOTAL** | 9,966 | 3.8 | 20 | 1 | 1 | 2 | 5 | 8 | 12 | 21 |

## 57.5: BLADDER LES DESTR NEC. Formerly included in operation group(s) 654.

| Type of Patients | Observed Patients | Avg. Stay | Variance | Percentiles 10th | 25th | 50th | 75th | 90th | 95th | 99th |
|---|---|---|---|---|---|---|---|---|---|---|
| **1. SINGLE DX** | | | | | | | | | | |
| 0–19 Years | 34 | 2.3 | <1 | 1 | 2 | 2 | 3 | 3 | 4 | 5 |
| 20–34 | 8 | 3.1 | 3 | 1 | 2 | 3 | 4 | 4 | 7 | 7 |
| 35–49 | 9 | 3.3 | 5 | 1 | 2 | 3 | 3 | 4 | 8 | 8 |
| 50–64 | 9 | 1.9 | 2 | 1 | 1 | 1 | 3 | 4 | 4 | 4 |
| 65+ | 3 | 4.8 | 3 | 2 | 4 | 6 | 6 | 6 | 6 | 6 |
| **2. MULTIPLE DX** | | | | | | | | | | |
| 0–19 Years | 52 | 5.3 | 36 | 2 | 3 | 3 | 7 | 7 | 8 | 49 |
| 20–34 | 16 | 3.8 | 5 | 1 | 3 | 3 | 5 | 6 | 7 | 13 |
| 35–49 | 26 | 3.8 | 17 | 2 | 3 | 3 | 5 | 6 | 7 | 24 |
| 50–64 | 77 | 4.3 | 4 | 2 | 3 | 4 | 5 | 6 | 8 | 11 |
| 65+ | 148 | 5.9 | 22 | 2 | 3 | 5 | 7 | 13 | 15 | 21 |
| **TOTAL SINGLE DX** | 63 | 2.6 | 2 | 1 | 2 | 2 | 3 | 4 | 6 | 8 |
| **TOTAL MULTIPLE DX** | 319 | 5.1 | 19 | 2 | 3 | 4 | 6 | 8 | 12 | 22 |
| **TOTAL** | | | | | | | | | | |
| 0–19 Years | 86 | 4.2 | 25 | 2 | 2 | 3 | 5 | 7 | 7 | 34 |
| 20–34 | 24 | 3.5 | 4 | 1 | 2 | 3 | 4 | 6 | 7 | 13 |
| 35–49 | 35 | 3.7 | 14 | 1 | 2 | 3 | 4 | 7 | 8 | 24 |
| 50–64 | 86 | 4.2 | 4 | 2 | 3 | 4 | 5 | 6 | 7 | 11 |
| 65+ | 151 | 5.9 | 21 | 2 | 3 | 5 | 7 | 12 | 15 | 21 |
| **GRAND TOTAL** | 382 | 4.7 | 17 | 2 | 3 | 4 | 6 | 7 | 12 | 21 |

Length of Stay by Diagnosis and Operation, United States, 2000

## United States, October 1998–September 1999 Data, by Operation

### 57.59: OTH BLADDER LESION DESTR. Formerly included in operation group(s) 654.

| Type of Patients | Observed Patients | Avg. Stay | Variance | 10th | 25th | 50th | 75th | 90th | 95th | 99th |
|---|---|---|---|---|---|---|---|---|---|---|
| **1. SINGLE DX** | | | | | | | | | | |
| 0–19 Years | 14 | 2.8 | <1 | 2 | 2 | 3 | 3 | 4 | 4 | 6 |
| 20–34 | 3 | 2.3 | <1 | 2 | 2 | 3 | 3 | 3 | 3 | 3 |
| 35–49 | 4 | 2.4 | <1 | 1 | 2 | 3 | 3 | 3 | 3 | 3 |
| 50–64 | 9 | 1.9 | 2 | 1 | 1 | 2 | 2 | 4 | 4 | 4 |
| 65+ | 3 | 4.8 | 3 | 2 | 4 | 5 | 5 | 6 | 6 | 6 |
| **2. MULTIPLE DX** | | | | | | | | | | |
| 0–19 Years | 29 | 4.0 | 11 | 2 | 3 | 3 | 5 | 7 | 7 | 7 |
| 20–34 | 9 | 4.1 | 5 | 3 | 3 | 3 | 5 | 6 | 7 | 13 |
| 35–49 | 22 | 4.0 | 23 | 1 | 1 | 3 | 5 | 5 | 7 | 24 |
| 50–64 | 74 | 4.3 | 4 | 2 | 2 | 4 | 5 | 6 | 8 | 11 |
| 65+ | 146 | 6.0 | 22 | 2 | 3 | 5 | 7 | 13 | 15 | 21 |
| **TOTAL SINGLE DX** | 33 | 2.7 | 1 | 1 | 2 | 3 | 3 | 4 | 4 | 6 |
| **TOTAL MULTIPLE DX** | 280 | 5.0 | 15 | 2 | 3 | 4 | 6 | 9 | 13 | 19 |
| **TOTAL** | | | | | | | | | | |
| 0–19 Years | 43 | 3.7 | 8 | 2 | 3 | 3 | 4 | 7 | 7 | 7 |
| 20–34 | 12 | 3.7 | 5 | 2 | 3 | 3 | 4 | 6 | 7 | 13 |
| 35–49 | 26 | 3.8 | 20 | 1 | 1 | 3 | 5 | 5 | 7 | 24 |
| 50–64 | 83 | 4.2 | 4 | 2 | 3 | 4 | 5 | 6 | 8 | 11 |
| 65+ | 149 | 5.9 | 22 | 2 | 3 | 5 | 7 | 12 | 15 | 21 |
| **GRAND TOTAL** | 313 | 4.8 | 14 | 2 | 3 | 4 | 6 | 8 | 12 | 19 |

### 57.7: TOTAL CYSTECTOMY. Formerly included in operation group(s) 654.

| Type of Patients | Observed Patients | Avg. Stay | Variance | 10th | 25th | 50th | 75th | 90th | 95th | 99th |
|---|---|---|---|---|---|---|---|---|---|---|
| **1. SINGLE DX** | | | | | | | | | | |
| 0–19 Years | 2 | 3.7 | 6 | 1 | 1 | 5 | 5 | 5 | 5 | 5 |
| 20–34 | 2 | 2.8 | <1 | 2 | 3 | 3 | 3 | 3 | 3 | 3 |
| 35–49 | 9 | 7.3 | 4 | 6 | 7 | 7 | 9 | 10 | 10 | 10 |
| 50–64 | 25 | 7.5 | 3 | 6 | 6 | 7 | 9 | 9 | 10 | 15 |
| 65+ | 39 | 9.2 | 10 | 6 | 7 | 9 | 11 | 14 | 16 | 19 |
| **2. MULTIPLE DX** | | | | | | | | | | |
| 0–19 Years | 1 | 8.0 | 0 | 8 | 8 | 8 | 8 | 8 | 8 | 8 |
| 20–34 | 10 | 10.7 | 17 | 4 | 8 | 10 | 14 | 14 | 20 | 20 |
| 35–49 | 110 | 9.8 | 53 | 4 | 7 | 9 | 11 | 16 | 18 | 42 |
| 50–64 | 509 | 11.8 | 63 | 6 | 8 | 10 | 13 | 18 | 30 | 42 |
| 65+ | 1,203 | 11.7 | 62 | 7 | 8 | 9 | 13 | 19 | 23 | 56 |
| **TOTAL SINGLE DX** | 77 | 8.1 | 9 | 6 | 6 | 7 | 9 | 11 | 14 | 18 |
| **TOTAL MULTIPLE DX** | 1,833 | 11.6 | 61 | 6 | 8 | 9 | 13 | 18 | 25 | 53 |
| **TOTAL** | | | | | | | | | | |
| 0–19 Years | 3 | 5.0 | 9 | 1 | 5 | 5 | 8 | 8 | 8 | 8 |
| 20–34 | 12 | 9.6 | 22 | 3 | 5 | 10 | 14 | 14 | 14 | 20 |
| 35–49 | 119 | 9.7 | 51 | 4 | 7 | 8 | 11 | 16 | 18 | 42 |
| 50–64 | 534 | 11.6 | 61 | 6 | 8 | 9 | 13 | 17 | 29 | 42 |
| 65+ | 1,242 | 11.6 | 60 | 7 | 8 | 9 | 13 | 19 | 23 | 56 |
| **GRAND TOTAL** | 1,910 | 11.5 | 60 | 6 | 8 | 9 | 13 | 18 | 24 | 52 |

### 57.6: PARTIAL CYSTECTOMY. Formerly included in operation group(s) 654.

| Type of Patients | Observed Patients | Avg. Stay | Variance | 10th | 25th | 50th | 75th | 90th | 95th | 99th |
|---|---|---|---|---|---|---|---|---|---|---|
| **1. SINGLE DX** | | | | | | | | | | |
| 0–19 Years | 0 | | | | | | | | | |
| 20–34 | 2 | 5.8 | 8 | 3 | 3 | 8 | 8 | 8 | 8 | 8 |
| 35–49 | 5 | 3.4 | 4 | 1 | 1 | 5 | 5 | 5 | 5 | 5 |
| 50–64 | 8 | 3.5 | 2 | 3 | 3 | 3 | 4 | 4 | 5 | 5 |
| 65+ | 15 | 3.4 | 1 | 2 | 3 | 3 | 4 | 4 | 6 | 6 |
| **2. MULTIPLE DX** | | | | | | | | | | |
| 0–19 Years | 5 | 12.8 | 85 | 4 | 7 | 11 | 15 | 15 | 41 | 41 |
| 20–34 | 13 | 8.5 | 16 | 3 | 6 | 8 | 13 | 13 | 13 | 14 |
| 35–49 | 43 | 7.3 | 31 | 2 | 4 | 5 | 10 | 15 | 17 | 23 |
| 50–64 | 75 | 6.7 | 33 | 2 | 3 | 4 | 8 | 15 | 19 | 28 |
| 65+ | 250 | 6.7 | 30 | 3 | 4 | 5 | 7 | 11 | 17 | 28 |
| **TOTAL SINGLE DX** | 30 | 3.6 | 2 | 2 | 3 | 3 | 4 | 5 | 6 | 10 |
| **TOTAL MULTIPLE DX** | 386 | 6.9 | 31 | 3 | 4 | 5 | 8 | 13 | 19 | 28 |
| **TOTAL** | | | | | | | | | | |
| 0–19 Years | 5 | 12.8 | 85 | 4 | 7 | 11 | 15 | 15 | 41 | 41 |
| 20–34 | 15 | 8.2 | 16 | 3 | 4 | 8 | 13 | 13 | 13 | 14 |
| 35–49 | 48 | 7.0 | 30 | 3 | 3 | 5 | 10 | 15 | 17 | 23 |
| 50–64 | 83 | 6.4 | 30 | 3 | 3 | 4 | 8 | 13 | 19 | 28 |
| 65+ | 265 | 6.5 | 29 | 2 | 4 | 5 | 7 | 11 | 17 | 28 |
| **GRAND TOTAL** | 416 | 6.6 | 30 | 3 | 3 | 5 | 7 | 13 | 17 | 28 |

### 57.71: RADICAL CYSTECTOMY. Formerly included in operation group(s) 654.

| Type of Patients | Observed Patients | Avg. Stay | Variance | 10th | 25th | 50th | 75th | 90th | 95th | 99th |
|---|---|---|---|---|---|---|---|---|---|---|
| **1. SINGLE DX** | | | | | | | | | | |
| 0–19 Years | 1 | 5.0 | 0 | 5 | 5 | 5 | 5 | 5 | 5 | 5 |
| 20–34 | 0 | | | | | | | | | |
| 35–49 | 9 | 7.3 | 4 | 6 | 7 | 7 | 9 | 10 | 10 | 10 |
| 50–64 | 24 | 7.3 | 2 | 6 | 6 | 7 | 8 | 9 | 10 | 13 |
| 65+ | 36 | 9.2 | 10 | 6 | 7 | 9 | 10 | 14 | 16 | 19 |
| **2. MULTIPLE DX** | | | | | | | | | | |
| 0–19 Years | 0 | | | | | | | | | |
| 20–34 | 6 | 9.1 | 21 | 4 | 8 | 8 | 10 | 14 | 20 | 20 |
| 35–49 | 95 | 9.4 | 55 | 4 | 6 | 8 | 11 | 14 | 16 | 42 |
| 50–64 | 474 | 11.8 | 65 | 6 | 8 | 10 | 13 | 18 | 30 | 53 |
| 65+ | 1,125 | 11.8 | 62 | 7 | 8 | 10 | 13 | 19 | 23 | 61 |
| **TOTAL SINGLE DX** | 70 | 8.2 | 7 | 6 | 7 | 8 | 9 | 11 | 14 | 18 |
| **TOTAL MULTIPLE DX** | 1,700 | 11.6 | 62 | 6 | 8 | 9 | 13 | 18 | 25 | 53 |
| **TOTAL** | | | | | | | | | | |
| 0–19 Years | 1 | 5.0 | 0 | 5 | 5 | 5 | 5 | 5 | 5 | 5 |
| 20–34 | 6 | 9.1 | 21 | 4 | 6 | 8 | 10 | 14 | 20 | 20 |
| 35–49 | 104 | 9.3 | 51 | 4 | 6 | 8 | 10 | 13 | 16 | 42 |
| 50–64 | 498 | 11.6 | 63 | 6 | 8 | 9 | 13 | 17 | 30 | 45 |
| 65+ | 1,161 | 11.7 | 60 | 7 | 8 | 9 | 13 | 19 | 23 | 57 |
| **GRAND TOTAL** | 1,770 | 11.5 | 61 | 6 | 8 | 9 | 13 | 18 | 25 | 53 |

Length of Stay by Diagnosis and Operation, United States, 2000

# United States, October 1998–September 1999 Data, by Operation

## 57.8: OTH URIN BLADDER REPAIR. Formerly included in operation group(s) 654.

| Type of Patients | Observed Patients | Avg. Stay | Variance | 10th | 25th | 50th | 75th | 90th | 95th | 99th |
|---|---|---|---|---|---|---|---|---|---|---|
| **1. SINGLE DX** | | | | | | | | | | |
| 0–19 Years | 15 | 7.5 | 20 | 2 | 4 | 6 | 14 | 14 | 14 | 14 |
| 20–34 | 33 | 3.4 | | 1 | 2 | 3 | 4 | 6 | 7 | 11 |
| 35–49 | 77 | 2.6 | 3 | 1 | 1 | 2 | 3 | 4 | 6 | 8 |
| 50–64 | 26 | 1.9 | <1 | 1 | 1 | 2 | 2 | 3 | 3 | 5 |
| 65+ | 31 | 2.0 | 3 | 1 | 1 | 2 | 2 | 3 | 5 | 9 |
| **2. MULTIPLE DX** | | | | | | | | | | |
| 0–19 Years | 336 | 10.5 | 82 | 4 | 6 | 8 | 10 | 22 | 38 | 38 |
| 20–34 | 177 | 8.8 | 66 | 2 | 4 | 6 | 11 | 17 | 25 | 44 |
| 35–49 | 358 | 5.3 | 26 | 1 | 2 | 4 | 7 | 11 | 14 | 25 |
| 50–64 | 324 | 6.6 | 116 | 1 | 2 | 4 | 7 | 10 | 18 | 70 |
| 65+ | 347 | 10.4 | 113 | 2 | 5 | 7 | 12 | 20 | 34 | 53 |
| **TOTAL SINGLE DX** | 182 | 3.0 | 7 | 1 | 2 | 3 | 3 | 6 | 8 | 14 |
| **TOTAL MULTIPLE DX** | 1,542 | 8.3 | 86 | 2 | 3 | 6 | 9 | 17 | 25 | 53 |
| **TOTAL** | | | | | | | | | | |
| 0–19 Years | 351 | 10.4 | 80 | 4 | 6 | 8 | 10 | 20 | 38 | 38 |
| 20–34 | 210 | 8.2 | 62 | 2 | 3 | 6 | 10 | 17 | 22 | 44 |
| 35–49 | 435 | 4.7 | 22 | 2 | 3 | 4 | 6 | 9 | 13 | 25 |
| 50–64 | 350 | 6.2 | 109 | 1 | 2 | 3 | 7 | 10 | 18 | 70 |
| 65+ | 378 | 9.8 | 110 | 2 | 4 | 7 | 11 | 19 | 32 | 53 |
| **GRAND TOTAL** | 1,724 | 7.7 | 81 | 1 | 3 | 5 | 9 | 15 | 24 | 53 |

## 57.84: REP OTH FISTULA BLADDER. Formerly included in operation group(s) 654.

| Type of Patients | Observed Patients | Avg. Stay | Variance | 10th | 25th | 50th | 75th | 90th | 95th | 99th |
|---|---|---|---|---|---|---|---|---|---|---|
| **1. SINGLE DX** | | | | | | | | | | |
| 0–19 Years | 2 | 1.0 | 0 | 1 | 1 | 1 | 1 | 1 | 1 | 1 |
| 20–34 | 22 | 3.0 | 2 | 1 | 2 | 3 | 3 | 6 | 6 | 7 |
| 35–49 | 44 | 2.4 | 2 | 1 | 1 | 3 | 3 | 4 | 5 | 6 |
| 50–64 | 7 | 1.9 | 2 | 1 | 1 | 1 | 2 | 4 | 4 | 5 |
| 65+ | 3 | 1.7 | <1 | 1 | 1 | 2 | 2 | 2 | 2 | 2 |
| **2. MULTIPLE DX** | | | | | | | | | | |
| 0–19 Years | 6 | 2.9 | 3 | 1 | 1 | 3 | 5 | 5 | 5 | 5 |
| 20–34 | 33 | 4.0 | 56 | 1 | 1 | 3 | 4 | 6 | 8 | 56 |
| 35–49 | 127 | 4.1 | 8 | 2 | 3 | 3 | 4 | 7 | 9 | 18 |
| 50–64 | 54 | 5.7 | 38 | 2 | 3 | 3 | 6 | 9 | 16 | 41 |
| 65+ | 28 | 10.3 | 102 | 3 | 3 | 6 | 16 | 32 | 32 | 33 |
| **TOTAL SINGLE DX** | 78 | 2.4 | 2 | 1 | 1 | 2 | 3 | 4 | 5 | 7 |
| **TOTAL MULTIPLE DX** | 248 | 4.9 | 33 | 1 | 3 | 3 | 5 | 9 | 14 | 32 |
| **TOTAL** | | | | | | | | | | |
| 0–19 Years | 8 | 2.7 | 3 | 1 | 1 | 2 | 5 | 5 | 5 | 5 |
| 20–34 | 55 | 3.6 | 38 | 1 | 1 | 3 | 3 | 6 | 7 | 56 |
| 35–49 | 171 | 3.6 | 7 | 1 | 2 | 3 | 4 | 6 | 9 | 14 |
| 50–64 | 61 | 5.1 | 35 | 1 | 2 | 3 | 5 | 8 | 13 | 41 |
| 65+ | 31 | 9.6 | 99 | 2 | 3 | 7 | 12 | 32 | 32 | 33 |
| **GRAND TOTAL** | 326 | 4.3 | 27 | 1 | 2 | 3 | 5 | 7 | 12 | 32 |

## 57.83: ENTEROVESICAL FIST REP. Formerly included in operation group(s) 654.

| Type of Patients | Observed Patients | Avg. Stay | Variance | 10th | 25th | 50th | 75th | 90th | 95th | 99th |
|---|---|---|---|---|---|---|---|---|---|---|
| **1. SINGLE DX** | | | | | | | | | | |
| 0–19 Years | 0 | | | | | | | | | |
| 20–34 | 0 | | | | | | | | | |
| 35–49 | 2 | 8.0 | 0 | 8 | 8 | 8 | 8 | 8 | 8 | 8 |
| 50–64 | 0 | | | | | | | | | |
| 65+ | 1 | 9.0 | 0 | 9 | 9 | 9 | 9 | 9 | 9 | 9 |
| **2. MULTIPLE DX** | | | | | | | | | | |
| 0–19 Years | 14 | 8.8 | 49 | 1 | 2 | 7 | 17 | 17 | 19 | 23 |
| 20–34 | 11 | 13.4 | 135 | 5 | 5 | 7 | 20 | 36 | 36 | 36 |
| 35–49 | 51 | 8.0 | 21 | 4 | 5 | 7 | 8 | 13 | 17 | 17 |
| 50–64 | 88 | 9.3 | 109 | 5 | 5 | 7 | 8 | 11 | 22 | 70 |
| 65+ | 133 | 11.9 | 82 | 5 | 7 | 9 | 15 | 19 | 34 | 58 |
| **TOTAL SINGLE DX** | 3 | 8.2 | <1 | 8 | 8 | 8 | 8 | 9 | 9 | 9 |
| **TOTAL MULTIPLE DX** | 297 | 10.5 | 85 | 5 | 5 | 8 | 10 | 17 | 27 | 58 |
| **TOTAL** | | | | | | | | | | |
| 0–19 Years | 14 | 8.8 | 49 | 1 | 2 | 7 | 17 | 17 | 19 | 23 |
| 20–34 | 11 | 13.4 | 135 | 5 | 5 | 7 | 20 | 36 | 36 | 36 |
| 35–49 | 53 | 8.0 | 20 | 4 | 6 | 7 | 8 | 13 | 17 | 17 |
| 50–64 | 88 | 9.3 | 109 | 5 | 5 | 7 | 8 | 11 | 22 | 61 |
| 65+ | 134 | 11.9 | 82 | 5 | 7 | 9 | 14 | 19 | 34 | 58 |
| **GRAND TOTAL** | 300 | 10.4 | 84 | 5 | 6 | 8 | 10 | 17 | 26 | 58 |

## 57.89: BLADDER REPAIR NEC. Formerly included in operation group(s) 654.

| Type of Patients | Observed Patients | Avg. Stay | Variance | 10th | 25th | 50th | 75th | 90th | 95th | 99th |
|---|---|---|---|---|---|---|---|---|---|---|
| **1. SINGLE DX** | | | | | | | | | | |
| 0–19 Years | 0 | | | | | | | | | |
| 20–34 | 1 | 3.0 | 0 | 3 | 3 | 3 | 3 | 3 | 3 | 3 |
| 35–49 | 24 | 1.9 | 1 | 1 | 1 | 1 | 2 | 3 | 3 | 6 |
| 50–64 | 19 | 1.9 | <1 | 1 | 1 | 2 | 2 | 3 | 3 | 6 |
| 65+ | 25 | 1.7 | <1 | 1 | 1 | 2 | 2 | 2 | 3 | 5 |
| **2. MULTIPLE DX** | | | | | | | | | | |
| 0–19 Years | 32 | 7.4 | 21 | 4 | 4 | 7 | 8 | 12 | 17 | 26 |
| 20–34 | 24 | 7.4 | 36 | 3 | 3 | 6 | 9 | 11 | 23 | 36 |
| 35–49 | 77 | 3.3 | 40 | 1 | 1 | 2 | 3 | 6 | 9 | 25 |
| 50–64 | 121 | 4.8 | 152 | 1 | 2 | 2 | 3 | 6 | 11 | 70 |
| 65+ | 104 | 5.5 | 44 | 2 | 4 | 4 | 6 | 10 | 18 | 47 |
| **TOTAL SINGLE DX** | 69 | 1.8 | <1 | 1 | 1 | 2 | 2 | 3 | 3 | 6 |
| **TOTAL MULTIPLE DX** | 358 | 5.0 | 93 | 1 | 1 | 2 | 5 | 9 | 13 | 70 |
| **TOTAL** | | | | | | | | | | |
| 0–19 Years | 32 | 7.4 | 21 | 4 | 4 | 7 | 8 | 12 | 17 | 26 |
| 20–34 | 25 | 7.4 | 35 | 3 | 3 | 6 | 9 | 11 | 23 | 36 |
| 35–49 | 101 | 2.9 | 30 | 1 | 1 | 2 | 3 | 5 | 8 | 25 |
| 50–64 | 140 | 4.4 | 135 | 1 | 2 | 2 | 5 | 9 | 10 | 70 |
| 65+ | 129 | 4.8 | 38 | 2 | 2 | 4 | 6 | 10 | 17 | 47 |
| **GRAND TOTAL** | 427 | 4.5 | 80 | 1 | 1 | 2 | 4 | 8 | 11 | 70 |

Length of Stay by Diagnosis and Operation, United States, 2000

# United States, October 1998–September 1999 Data, by Operation

## 57.9: OTHER BLADDER OPERATIONS. Formerly included in operation group(s) 664.

| Type of Patients | Observed Patients | Avg. Stay | Variance | 10th | 25th | 50th | 75th | 90th | 95th | 99th |
|---|---|---|---|---|---|---|---|---|---|---|
| **1. SINGLE DX** | | | | | | | | | | |
| 0–19 Years | 13 | 2.2 | <1 | 1 | 1 | 2 | 3 | 3 | 3 | 4 |
| 20–34 | 10 | 3.5 | 15 | 1 | 1 | 3 | 3 | 13 | 13 | 13 |
| 35–49 | 15 | 1.5 | 0 | 1 | 1 | 1 | 1 | 2 | 6 | 6 |
| 50–64 | 25 | 2.1 | 3 | 1 | 1 | 2 | 2 | 3 | 4 | 12 |
| 65+ | 39 | 1.3 | <1 | 1 | 1 | 1 | 1 | 2 | 3 | 6 |
| **2. MULTIPLE DX** | | | | | | | | | | |
| 0–19 Years | 105 | 4.4 | 28 | 1 | 2 | 2 | 6 | 9 | 14 | 32 |
| 20–34 | 131 | 4.6 | 31 | 1 | 1 | 3 | 7 | 11 | 14 | 18 |
| 35–49 | 293 | 4.1 | 15 | 1 | 2 | 3 | 5 | 7 | 11 | 20 |
| 50–64 | 501 | 5.1 | 20 | 1 | 2 | 4 | 6 | 10 | 12 | 21 |
| 65+ | 3,241 | 5.5 | 19 | 2 | 3 | 4 | 7 | 10 | 14 | 20 |
| **TOTAL SINGLE DX** | 102 | 2.0 | 4 | 1 | 1 | 1 | 2 | 3 | 4 | 13 |
| **TOTAL MULTIPLE DX** | 4,271 | 5.3 | 19 | 1 | 2 | 4 | 7 | 10 | 14 | 20 |
| **TOTAL** | | | | | | | | | | |
| 0–19 Years | 118 | 4.0 | 24 | 1 | 2 | 2 | 4 | 7 | 11 | 32 |
| 20–34 | 141 | 4.5 | 30 | 1 | 1 | 3 | 7 | 11 | 14 | 18 |
| 35–49 | 308 | 4.0 | 14 | 1 | 2 | 3 | 5 | 7 | 11 | 20 |
| 50–64 | 526 | 4.9 | 20 | 1 | 2 | 4 | 6 | 9 | 12 | 21 |
| 65+ | 3,280 | 5.5 | 19 | 2 | 3 | 4 | 7 | 10 | 14 | 20 |
| **GRAND TOTAL** | 4,373 | 5.2 | 19 | 1 | 2 | 4 | 7 | 10 | 14 | 20 |

## 57.91: BLADDER SPHINCTEROTOMY. Formerly included in operation group(s) 654.

| Type of Patients | Observed Patients | Avg. Stay | Variance | 10th | 25th | 50th | 75th | 90th | 95th | 99th |
|---|---|---|---|---|---|---|---|---|---|---|
| **1. SINGLE DX** | | | | | | | | | | |
| 0–19 Years | 0 | | | | | | | | | |
| 20–34 | 0 | | | | | | | | | |
| 35–49 | 4 | 1.0 | 0 | 1 | 1 | 1 | 1 | 1 | 1 | 1 |
| 50–64 | 8 | 1.4 | <1 | 1 | 1 | 1 | 1 | 3 | 3 | 3 |
| 65+ | 21 | 1.1 | <1 | 1 | 1 | 1 | 1 | 1 | 2 | 3 |
| **2. MULTIPLE DX** | | | | | | | | | | |
| 0–19 Years | 3 | 3.6 | 4 | 2 | 2 | 3 | 6 | 6 | 6 | 6 |
| 20–34 | 6 | 3.3 | 13 | 1 | 1 | 2 | 2 | 10 | 10 | 10 |
| 35–49 | 51 | 2.8 | 13 | 1 | 1 | 1 | 3 | 6 | 8 | 18 |
| 50–64 | 86 | 2.5 | 11 | 1 | 1 | 1 | 3 | 6 | 8 | 10 |
| 65+ | 415 | 3.9 | 14 | 1 | 1 | 3 | 5 | 8 | 10 | 20 |
| **TOTAL SINGLE DX** | 33 | 1.1 | <1 | 1 | 1 | 1 | 1 | 1 | 3 | 3 |
| **TOTAL MULTIPLE DX** | 561 | 3.6 | 14 | 1 | 1 | 2 | 4 | 8 | 10 | 20 |
| **TOTAL** | | | | | | | | | | |
| 0–19 Years | 3 | 3.6 | 4 | 2 | 2 | 3 | 6 | 6 | 6 | 6 |
| 20–34 | 6 | 3.3 | 13 | 1 | 1 | 2 | 2 | 10 | 10 | 10 |
| 35–49 | 55 | 2.7 | 13 | 1 | 1 | 1 | 3 | 6 | 7 | 18 |
| 50–64 | 94 | 2.4 | 10 | 1 | 1 | 1 | 2 | 5 | 8 | 10 |
| 65+ | 436 | 3.8 | 14 | 1 | 1 | 3 | 5 | 8 | 10 | 20 |
| **GRAND TOTAL** | 594 | 3.5 | 13 | 1 | 1 | 2 | 4 | 7 | 10 | 20 |

## 57.93: CONTROL BLADDER HEMOR. Formerly included in operation group(s) 654.

| Type of Patients | Observed Patients | Avg. Stay | Variance | 10th | 25th | 50th | 75th | 90th | 95th | 99th |
|---|---|---|---|---|---|---|---|---|---|---|
| **1. SINGLE DX** | | | | | | | | | | |
| 0–19 Years | 0 | | | | | | | | | |
| 20–34 | 1 | 1.0 | 0 | 1 | 1 | 1 | 1 | 1 | 1 | 1 |
| 35–49 | 1 | 1.0 | 0 | 1 | 1 | 1 | 1 | 1 | 1 | 1 |
| 50–64 | 4 | 1.3 | <1 | 1 | 1 | 1 | 2 | 2 | 2 | 2 |
| 65+ | 10 | 1.8 | 2 | 1 | 1 | 1 | 2 | 2 | 6 | 6 |
| **2. MULTIPLE DX** | | | | | | | | | | |
| 0–19 Years | 2 | 28.3 | 116 | 1 | 32 | 32 | 32 | 32 | 32 | 32 |
| 20–34 | 5 | 3.6 | 7 | 2 | 2 | 3 | 3 | 9 | 9 | 9 |
| 35–49 | 27 | 3.5 | 5 | 1 | 2 | 3 | 5 | 7 | 8 | 8 |
| 50–64 | 66 | 4.9 | 51 | 1 | 2 | 3 | 5 | 7 | 10 | 42 |
| 65+ | 371 | 4.6 | 16 | 1 | 2 | 3 | 6 | 9 | 12 | 21 |
| **TOTAL SINGLE DX** | 16 | 1.4 | 1 | 1 | 1 | 1 | 1 | 2 | 2 | 6 |
| **TOTAL MULTIPLE DX** | 471 | 4.7 | 24 | 1 | 2 | 3 | 6 | 9 | 13 | 25 |
| **TOTAL** | | | | | | | | | | |
| 0–19 Years | 2 | 28.3 | 116 | 1 | 32 | 32 | 32 | 32 | 32 | 32 |
| 20–34 | 6 | 2.3 | 5 | 1 | 1 | 2 | 3 | 3 | 9 | 9 |
| 35–49 | 28 | 3.2 | 5 | 1 | 2 | 3 | 5 | 7 | 8 | 8 |
| 50–64 | 70 | 4.7 | 49 | 1 | 2 | 3 | 4 | 7 | 10 | 42 |
| 65+ | 381 | 4.6 | 16 | 1 | 2 | 3 | 6 | 9 | 11 | 21 |
| **GRAND TOTAL** | 487 | 4.6 | 24 | 1 | 2 | 3 | 6 | 8 | 12 | 25 |

## 57.94: INSERT INDWELL URIN CATH. Formerly included in operation group(s) 664.

| Type of Patients | Observed Patients | Avg. Stay | Variance | 10th | 25th | 50th | 75th | 90th | 95th | 99th |
|---|---|---|---|---|---|---|---|---|---|---|
| **1. SINGLE DX** | | | | | | | | | | |
| 0–19 Years | 10 | 2.4 | <1 | 1 | 2 | 3 | 3 | 3 | 3 | 4 |
| 20–34 | 7 | 2.5 | 2 | 1 | 2 | 3 | 3 | 3 | 5 | 5 |
| 35–49 | 7 | 1.4 | 2 | 1 | 1 | 1 | 1 | 2 | 6 | 6 |
| 50–64 | 10 | 2.6 | 4 | 1 | 1 | 2 | 3 | 3 | 7 | 12 |
| 65+ | 8 | 1.4 | <1 | 1 | 1 | 2 | 2 | 2 | 3 | 3 |
| **2. MULTIPLE DX** | | | | | | | | | | |
| 0–19 Years | 92 | 3.8 | 13 | 1 | 2 | 2 | 4 | 7 | 10 | 19 |
| 20–34 | 112 | 4.3 | 17 | 1 | 3 | 3 | 7 | 11 | 14 | 14 |
| 35–49 | 187 | 4.3 | 16 | 2 | 3 | 4 | 5 | 8 | 11 | 23 |
| 50–64 | 309 | 5.6 | 18 | 2 | 3 | 5 | 7 | 11 | 13 | 21 |
| 65+ | 2,220 | 5.8 | 19 | 2 | 3 | 5 | 7 | 11 | 14 | 19 |
| **TOTAL SINGLE DX** | 42 | 2.2 | 2 | 1 | 1 | 2 | 3 | 3 | 4 | 7 |
| **TOTAL MULTIPLE DX** | 2,920 | 5.5 | 19 | 2 | 3 | 4 | 7 | 11 | 14 | 19 |
| **TOTAL** | | | | | | | | | | |
| 0–19 Years | 102 | 3.6 | 11 | 1 | 2 | 3 | 4 | 7 | 10 | 19 |
| 20–34 | 119 | 4.2 | 16 | 1 | 3 | 3 | 6 | 11 | 14 | 14 |
| 35–49 | 194 | 4.2 | 16 | 2 | 3 | 4 | 5 | 8 | 11 | 23 |
| 50–64 | 319 | 5.5 | 18 | 2 | 3 | 4 | 7 | 11 | 12 | 21 |
| 65+ | 2,228 | 5.8 | 19 | 2 | 3 | 5 | 7 | 11 | 14 | 19 |
| **GRAND TOTAL** | 2,962 | 5.5 | 19 | 2 | 3 | 4 | 7 | 11 | 14 | 19 |

# United States, October 1998–September 1999 Data, by Operation

## 58.0: URETHROTOMY. Formerly included in operation group(s) 658.

| Type of Patients | Observed Patients | Avg. Stay | Variance | 10th | 25th | 50th | 75th | 90th | 95th | 99th |
|---|---|---|---|---|---|---|---|---|---|---|
| **1. SINGLE DX** | | | | | | | | | | |
| 0–19 Years | 5 | 1.8 | <1 | 1 | 1 | 1 | | 3 | 3 | 3 |
| 20–34 | 3 | 1.9 | <1 | 1 | 1 | 2 | | 3 | 3 | 3 |
| 35–49 | 0 | | | | | | | | | |
| 50–64 | 3 | 3.6 | 24 | 1 | 1 | | 11 | 11 | 11 | 11 |
| 65+ | 1 | 1.0 | 0 | 1 | 1 | | 1 | 1 | 1 | 1 |
| **2. MULTIPLE DX** | | | | | | | | | | |
| 0–19 Years | 14 | 2.7 | 7 | 1 | 1 | 2 | 3 | 8 | 8 | 12 |
| 20–34 | 11 | 3.2 | 6 | 1 | 1 | 2 | 3 | 8 | 8 | 8 |
| 35–49 | 17 | 4.3 | 14 | 2 | 2 | 3 | 5 | 12 | 12 | 13 |
| 50–64 | 9 | 23.5 | 270 | 2 | 4 | 38 | 38 | 38 | 38 | 38 |
| 65+ | 45 | 5.0 | 19 | 1 | 2 | 4 | 7 | 10 | 11 | 23 |
| **TOTAL SINGLE DX** | 12 | 2.0 | 3 | 1 | 1 | 1 | 3 | 3 | 3 | 11 |
| **TOTAL MULTIPLE DX** | 96 | 6.8 | 94 | 1 | 2 | 3 | 8 | 13 | 38 | 38 |
| **TOTAL** | | | | | | | | | | |
| 0–19 Years | 19 | 2.2 | 4 | 1 | 1 | 1 | 3 | 3 | 8 | 12 |
| 20–34 | 14 | 3.0 | 5 | 1 | 1 | 2 | 3 | 8 | 8 | 8 |
| 35–49 | 17 | 4.3 | 14 | 2 | 2 | 3 | 5 | 12 | 12 | 13 |
| 50–64 | 12 | 21.1 | 282 | 1 | 3 | 24 | 38 | 38 | 38 | 38 |
| 65+ | 46 | 4.9 | 18 | 1 | 2 | 4 | 7 | 10 | 11 | 23 |
| **GRAND TOTAL** | 108 | 5.9 | 81 | 1 | 2 | 3 | 6 | 11 | 38 | 38 |

## 58.1: URETHRAL MEATOTOMY. Formerly included in operation group(s) 655.

| Type of Patients | Observed Patients | Avg. Stay | Variance | 10th | 25th | 50th | 75th | 90th | 95th | 99th |
|---|---|---|---|---|---|---|---|---|---|---|
| **1. SINGLE DX** | | | | | | | | | | |
| 0–19 Years | 4 | 1.0 | 0 | 1 | 1 | 1 | 1 | 1 | 1 | 1 |
| 20–34 | 0 | | | | | | | | | |
| 35–49 | 0 | | | | | | | | | |
| 50–64 | 0 | | | | | | | | | |
| **2. MULTIPLE DX** | | | | | | | | | | |
| 0–19 Years | 9 | 3.3 | 20 | 1 | 1 | 1 | 4 | 13 | 13 | 13 |
| 20–34 | 2 | 5.2 | 1 | 4 | 4 | 6 | 6 | 6 | 6 | 6 |
| 35–49 | 5 | 7.9 | 26 | 2 | 2 | 6 | 14 | 14 | 14 | 14 |
| 50–64 | 12 | 5.1 | 17 | 1 | 2 | 5 | 8 | 9 | 15 | 15 |
| 65+ | 14 | 6.9 | 38 | 1 | 2 | 5 | 12 | 16 | 16 | 23 |
| **TOTAL SINGLE DX** | 4 | 1.0 | 0 | 1 | 1 | 1 | 1 | 1 | 1 | 1 |
| **TOTAL MULTIPLE DX** | 42 | 5.6 | 27 | 1 | 1 | 4 | 8 | 14 | 16 | 16 |
| **TOTAL** | | | | | | | | | | |
| 0–19 Years | 13 | 3.0 | 18 | 1 | 1 | 1 | 6 | 13 | 13 | 13 |
| 20–34 | 2 | 5.2 | | 4 | 4 | 6 | 6 | 6 | 6 | 6 |
| 35–49 | 5 | 7.9 | 26 | 2 | 2 | 6 | 14 | 14 | 14 | 14 |
| 50–64 | 12 | 5.1 | 17 | 1 | 2 | 5 | 8 | 9 | 15 | 15 |
| 65+ | 14 | 6.9 | 38 | 1 | 2 | 5 | 12 | 16 | 16 | 23 |
| **GRAND TOTAL** | 46 | 5.4 | 27 | 1 | 1 | 4 | 8 | 14 | 16 | 16 |

## 58.2: URETHRAL DIAGNOSTIC PX. Formerly included in operation group(s) 651, 656, 658, 664.

| Type of Patients | Observed Patients | Avg. Stay | Variance | 10th | 25th | 50th | 75th | 90th | 95th | 99th |
|---|---|---|---|---|---|---|---|---|---|---|
| **1. SINGLE DX** | | | | | | | | | | |
| 0–19 Years | 1 | 4.0 | 0 | 4 | 4 | 4 | 4 | 4 | 4 | 4 |
| 20–34 | 2 | 2.0 | 0 | 2 | 2 | 2 | 2 | 2 | 2 | 2 |
| 35–49 | 5 | 1.0 | 0 | | | 1 | 1 | 1 | 1 | 1 |
| 50–64 | 3 | 3.0 | <1 | 2 | 2 | 3 | 3 | 4 | 4 | 4 |
| 65+ | 0 | | | | | | | | | |
| **2. MULTIPLE DX** | | | | | | | | | | |
| 0–19 Years | 5 | 3.9 | 13 | 1 | 1 | 2 | 9 | 9 | 9 | 9 |
| 20–34 | 7 | 3.5 | 2 | 1 | 3 | 3 | 5 | 5 | 5 | 5 |
| 35–49 | 28 | 3.5 | 12 | 1 | 2 | 3 | 4 | 7 | 7 | 23 |
| 50–64 | 28 | 6.2 | 20 | 1 | 2 | 6 | 9 | 13 | 14 | 16 |
| 65+ | 62 | 5.4 | 20 | 2 | 2 | 5 | 7 | 10 | 16 | 25 |
| **TOTAL SINGLE DX** | 11 | 1.6 | 1 | 1 | 1 | 1 | 2 | 4 | 4 | 4 |
| **TOTAL MULTIPLE DX** | 130 | 4.7 | 17 | 1 | 2 | 4 | 6 | 9 | 13 | 17 |
| **TOTAL** | | | | | | | | | | |
| 0–19 Years | 6 | 3.9 | 11 | 1 | 1 | 3 | 9 | 9 | 9 | 9 |
| 20–34 | 9 | 3.4 | 2 | 1 | 1 | 3 | 5 | 5 | 5 | 5 |
| 35–49 | 33 | 3.1 | 11 | 1 | 1 | 3 | 4 | 7 | 7 | 23 |
| 50–64 | 31 | 6.0 | 19 | 1 | 2 | 5 | 9 | 13 | 14 | 16 |
| 65+ | 62 | 5.4 | 20 | 1 | 2 | 5 | 7 | 10 | 16 | 25 |
| **GRAND TOTAL** | 141 | 4.5 | 16 | 1 | 2 | 3 | 6 | 9 | 13 | 17 |

## 58.3: EXC/DESTR URETHRAL LES. Formerly included in operation group(s) 656.

| Type of Patients | Observed Patients | Avg. Stay | Variance | 10th | 25th | 50th | 75th | 90th | 95th | 99th |
|---|---|---|---|---|---|---|---|---|---|---|
| **1. SINGLE DX** | | | | | | | | | | |
| 0–19 Years | 34 | 1.5 | <1 | 1 | 1 | 1 | 1 | 3 | 4 | 4 |
| 20–34 | 22 | 1.1 | <1 | 1 | 1 | 1 | 1 | 2 | 3 | 3 |
| 35–49 | 35 | 1.4 | <1 | 1 | 1 | 1 | 2 | 3 | 3 | 4 |
| 50–64 | 10 | 1.4 | <1 | 1 | 1 | 1 | 1 | 4 | 4 | 4 |
| 65+ | 8 | 1.4 | 4 | 1 | 1 | 1 | 1 | 1 | 2 | 12 |
| **2. MULTIPLE DX** | | | | | | | | | | |
| 0–19 Years | 87 | 4.2 | 18 | 1 | 1 | 3 | 6 | 10 | 10 | 20 |
| 20–34 | 33 | 1.9 | 2 | 1 | 1 | 1 | 2 | 3 | 4 | 7 |
| 35–49 | 65 | 2.1 | 4 | 1 | 1 | 2 | 3 | 4 | 7 | 13 |
| 50–64 | 53 | 2.4 | 6 | 1 | 1 | 2 | 2 | 4 | 7 | 10 |
| 65+ | 169 | 3.8 | 12 | 1 | 1 | 3 | 5 | 9 | 11 | 16 |
| **TOTAL SINGLE DX** | 109 | 1.4 | <1 | 1 | 1 | 1 | 1 | 2 | 3 | 4 |
| **TOTAL MULTIPLE DX** | 407 | 3.3 | 12 | 1 | 1 | 2 | 4 | 8 | 10 | 17 |
| **TOTAL** | | | | | | | | | | |
| 0–19 Years | 121 | 3.7 | 16 | 1 | 1 | 2 | 6 | 10 | 10 | 19 |
| 20–34 | 55 | 1.5 | <1 | 1 | 1 | 1 | 1 | 3 | 4 | 7 |
| 35–49 | 100 | 1.9 | 3 | 1 | 1 | 1 | 3 | 3 | 4 | 13 |
| 50–64 | 63 | 2.3 | 5 | 1 | 1 | 2 | 2 | 4 | 7 | 10 |
| 65+ | 177 | 3.6 | 12 | 1 | 1 | 2 | 4 | 9 | 11 | 16 |
| **GRAND TOTAL** | 516 | 2.9 | 10 | 1 | 2 | 2 | 3 | 7 | 10 | 16 |

Length of Stay by Diagnosis and Operation, United States, 2000

# United States, October 1998–September 1999 Data, by Operation

## 58.4: REPAIR OF URETHRA. Formerly included in operation group(s) 656.

| Type of Patients | Observed Patients | Avg. Stay | Variance | 10th | 25th | 50th | 75th | 90th | 95th | 99th |
|---|---|---|---|---|---|---|---|---|---|---|
| **1. SINGLE DX** | | | | | | | | | | |
| 0–19 Years | 267 | 1.7 | 2 | 1 | 1 | 1 | 2 | 3 | 5 | 7 |
| 20–34 | 39 | 2.1 | 1 | 1 | 1 | 2 | 2 | 4 | 5 | 6 |
| 35–49 | 51 | 2.2 | 2 | 1 | 1 | 2 | 3 | 4 | 5 | 7 |
| 50–64 | 23 | 2.1 | <1 | 1 | 2 | 2 | 2 | 3 | 4 | 4 |
| 65+ | 8 | 1.6 | <1 | 1 | 1 | 1 | 2 | 3 | 3 | 4 |
| **2. MULTIPLE DX** | | | | | | | | | | |
| 0–19 Years | 397 | 2.4 | 4 | 1 | 1 | 2 | 3 | 4 | 6 | 19 |
| 20–34 | 110 | 3.4 | 18 | 1 | 2 | 3 | 4 | 6 | 8 | 29 |
| 35–49 | 153 | 3.3 | 17 | 1 | 1 | 2 | 4 | 7 | 7 | 33 |
| 50–64 | 120 | 3.5 | 37 | 1 | 1 | 2 | 4 | 7 | 8 | 23 |
| 65+ | 108 | 3.4 | 17 | 1 | 1 | 2 | 4 | 6 | 7 | 27 |
| **TOTAL SINGLE DX** | 388 | 1.8 | 2 | 1 | 1 | 1 | 2 | 3 | 5 | 7 |
| **TOTAL MULTIPLE DX** | 888 | 3.0 | 17 | 1 | 1 | 2 | 3 | 5 | 7 | 19 |
| **TOTAL** | | | | | | | | | | |
| 0–19 Years | 664 | 2.1 | 6 | 1 | 1 | 1 | 2 | 4 | 5 | 15 |
| 20–34 | 149 | 3.1 | 14 | 1 | 2 | 2 | 4 | 5 | 7 | 22 |
| 35–49 | 204 | 3.1 | 14 | 1 | 1 | 2 | 4 | 7 | 7 | 17 |
| 50–64 | 143 | 3.2 | 30 | 1 | 2 | 2 | 3 | 5 | 7 | 23 |
| 65+ | 116 | 3.2 | 15 | 1 | 1 | 2 | 3 | 5 | 7 | 27 |
| **GRAND TOTAL** | 1,276 | 2.6 | 12 | 1 | 1 | 2 | 3 | 5 | 7 | 17 |

## 58.45: HYPOSPAD/EPISPADIAS REP. Formerly included in operation group(s) 656.

| Type of Patients | Observed Patients | Avg. Stay | Variance | 10th | 25th | 50th | 75th | 90th | 95th | 99th |
|---|---|---|---|---|---|---|---|---|---|---|
| **1. SINGLE DX** | | | | | | | | | | |
| 0–19 Years | 209 | 1.7 | 2 | 1 | 1 | 1 | 2 | 3 | 5 | 7 |
| 20–34 | 4 | 1.3 | <1 | 1 | 1 | 1 | 2 | 2 | 2 | 2 |
| 35–49 | 2 | 1.4 | <1 | 1 | 1 | 1 | 1 | 4 | 4 | 4 |
| 50–64 | 0 | | | | | | | | | |
| 65+ | 0 | | | | | | | | | |
| **2. MULTIPLE DX** | | | | | | | | | | |
| 0–19 Years | 292 | 2.0 | 4 | 1 | 1 | 2 | 3 | 4 | 4 | 7 |
| 20–34 | 11 | 2.7 | 2 | 2 | 2 | 3 | 3 | 3 | 4 | 8 |
| 35–49 | 6 | 9.8 | 182 | 1 | 1 | 4 | 4 | 34 | 34 | 34 |
| 50–64 | 5 | 2.9 | 2 | 1 | 1 | 3 | 4 | 5 | 5 | 5 |
| 65+ | 3 | 2.0 | <1 | 1 | 1 | 2 | 3 | 3 | 3 | 3 |
| **TOTAL SINGLE DX** | 215 | 1.7 | 2 | 1 | 1 | 1 | 2 | 3 | 5 | 7 |
| **TOTAL MULTIPLE DX** | 317 | 2.2 | 8 | 1 | 1 | 2 | 3 | 4 | 4 | 8 |
| **TOTAL** | | | | | | | | | | |
| 0–19 Years | 501 | 1.9 | 3 | 1 | 1 | 1 | 2 | 3 | 4 | 7 |
| 20–34 | 15 | 2.6 | 2 | 1 | 2 | 2 | 3 | 3 | 4 | 8 |
| 35–49 | 8 | 6.9 | 134 | 1 | 1 | 4 | 4 | 34 | 34 | 34 |
| 50–64 | 5 | 2.9 | <1 | 1 | 2 | 3 | 3 | 5 | 5 | 5 |
| 65+ | 3 | 2.0 | | 1 | 1 | 2 | 3 | 3 | 3 | 3 |
| **GRAND TOTAL** | 532 | 2.0 | 5 | 1 | 1 | 1 | 2 | 4 | 4 | 8 |

## 58.49: URETHRAL REPAIR NEC. Formerly included in operation group(s) 656.

| Type of Patients | Observed Patients | Avg. Stay | Variance | 10th | 25th | 50th | 75th | 90th | 95th | 99th |
|---|---|---|---|---|---|---|---|---|---|---|
| **1. SINGLE DX** | | | | | | | | | | |
| 0–19 Years | 14 | 1.8 | 1 | 1 | 1 | 1 | 2 | 3 | 5 | 5 |
| 20–34 | 25 | 2.0 | 1 | 1 | 1 | 2 | 2 | 4 | 5 | 5 |
| 35–49 | 34 | 2.0 | 2 | 1 | 2 | 2 | 3 | 3 | 4 | 7 |
| 50–64 | 22 | 2.1 | <1 | 1 | 2 | 2 | 2 | 3 | 4 | 4 |
| 65+ | 7 | 1.6 | <1 | 1 | 1 | 1 | 2 | 3 | 3 | 4 |
| **2. MULTIPLE DX** | | | | | | | | | | |
| 0–19 Years | 36 | 3.4 | 17 | 1 | 1 | 2 | 4 | 6 | 15 | 25 |
| 20–34 | 49 | 3.5 | 27 | 1 | 2 | 3 | 4 | 6 | 6 | 39 |
| 35–49 | 68 | 2.1 | 2 | 1 | 1 | 2 | 2 | 4 | 4 | 7 |
| 50–64 | 62 | 2.1 | 2 | 1 | 1 | 2 | 2 | 4 | 4 | 7 |
| 65+ | 62 | 3.4 | 22 | 1 | 2 | 2 | 3 | 6 | 6 | 27 |
| **TOTAL SINGLE DX** | 102 | 2.0 | 1 | 1 | 1 | 2 | 2 | 3 | 4 | 5 |
| **TOTAL MULTIPLE DX** | 277 | 2.7 | 12 | 1 | 1 | 2 | 3 | 4 | 6 | 16 |
| **TOTAL** | | | | | | | | | | |
| 0–19 Years | 50 | 2.7 | 11 | 1 | 1 | 2 | 3 | 5 | 7 | 16 |
| 20–34 | 74 | 3.0 | 18 | 1 | 2 | 2 | 4 | 4 | 7 | 39 |
| 35–49 | 102 | 2.1 | 2 | 1 | 1 | 2 | 2 | 3 | 4 | 7 |
| 50–64 | 84 | 2.1 | 1 | 1 | 2 | 2 | 2 | 3 | 4 | 7 |
| 65+ | 69 | 3.0 | 18 | 1 | 1 | 2 | 3 | 5 | 6 | 27 |
| **GRAND TOTAL** | 379 | 2.5 | 9 | 1 | 1 | 2 | 3 | 4 | 5 | 13 |

## 58.5: URETHRAL STRICTURE REL. Formerly included in operation group(s) 658.

| Type of Patients | Observed Patients | Avg. Stay | Variance | 10th | 25th | 50th | 75th | 90th | 95th | 99th |
|---|---|---|---|---|---|---|---|---|---|---|
| **1. SINGLE DX** | | | | | | | | | | |
| 0–19 Years | 15 | 1.6 | 2 | 1 | 1 | 1 | 1 | 3 | 6 | 6 |
| 20–34 | 13 | 1.6 | <1 | 1 | 1 | 2 | 2 | 2 | 2 | 3 |
| 35–49 | 14 | 1.9 | 2 | 1 | 1 | 1 | 3 | 4 | 3 | 4 |
| 50–64 | 16 | 1.6 | <1 | 1 | 1 | 1 | 2 | 3 | 3 | 3 |
| 65+ | 20 | 1.3 | <1 | 1 | 1 | 1 | 1 | 2 | 3 | 4 |
| **2. MULTIPLE DX** | | | | | | | | | | |
| 0–19 Years | 26 | 2.2 | 8 | 1 | 1 | 1 | 2 | 5 | 8 | 12 |
| 20–34 | 59 | 4.3 | 21 | 1 | 2 | 3 | 6 | 8 | 12 | 23 |
| 35–49 | 171 | 3.7 | 7 | 1 | 2 | 3 | 5 | 7 | 13 | 14 |
| 50–64 | 252 | 4.5 | 21 | 1 | 2 | 3 | 5 | 10 | 13 | 24 |
| 65+ | 878 | 5.0 | 35 | 1 | 2 | 3 | 7 | 11 | 15 | 30 |
| **TOTAL SINGLE DX** | 78 | 1.6 | <1 | 1 | 1 | 1 | 2 | 3 | 3 | 6 |
| **TOTAL MULTIPLE DX** | 1,386 | 4.6 | 27 | 1 | 2 | 3 | 6 | 10 | 14 | 27 |
| **TOTAL** | | | | | | | | | | |
| 0–19 Years | 41 | 2.0 | 5 | 1 | 1 | 1 | 2 | 5 | 6 | 12 |
| 20–34 | 72 | 3.7 | 18 | 1 | 2 | 3 | 4 | 7 | 12 | 23 |
| 35–49 | 185 | 3.6 | 7 | 1 | 1 | 3 | 6 | 7 | 8 | 14 |
| 50–64 | 268 | 4.3 | 20 | 1 | 2 | 3 | 5 | 9 | 12 | 24 |
| 65+ | 898 | 4.9 | 34 | 1 | 2 | 3 | 6 | 11 | 15 | 29 |
| **GRAND TOTAL** | 1,464 | 4.4 | 26 | 1 | 1 | 3 | 6 | 9 | 13 | 27 |

Length of Stay by Diagnosis and Operation, United States, 2000

# United States, October 1998–September 1999 Data, by Operation

## 58.6: URETHRAL DILATION. Formerly included in operation group(s) 657.

| Type of Patients | Observed Patients | Avg. Stay | Variance | Percentiles | | | | | | |
|---|---|---|---|---|---|---|---|---|---|---|
| | | | | 10th | 25th | 50th | 75th | 90th | 95th | 99th |
| **1. SINGLE DX** | | | | | | | | | | |
| 0–19 Years | 5 | 1.2 | <1 | 1 | 1 | 1 | | 2 | 2 | 2 |
| 20–34 | 8 | 1.6 | 2 | 1 | 1 | 1 | 1 | 2 | 6 | 6 |
| 35–49 | 10 | 1.9 | 3 | 1 | 1 | 1 | 2 | 3 | 7 | 7 |
| 50–64 | 7 | 1.3 | <1 | 1 | 1 | 1 | 1 | 2 | 3 | 3 |
| 65+ | 8 | 1.8 | 1 | 1 | 1 | 1 | 2 | 3 | 4 | 4 |
| **2. MULTIPLE DX** | | | | | | | | | | |
| 0–19 Years | 52 | 2.4 | 8 | 1 | 1 | 1 | 3 | 4 | 5 | 17 |
| 20–34 | 96 | 4.0 | 48 | 1 | 1 | 2 | 5 | 7 | 9 | 20 |
| 35–49 | 171 | 4.6 | 19 | 1 | 1 | 3 | 6 | 9 | 12 | 19 |
| 50–64 | 266 | 4.5 | 22 | 1 | 1 | 3 | 6 | 10 | 13 | 22 |
| 65+ | 1,057 | 6.5 | 25 | 2 | 3 | 5 | 8 | 13 | 16 | 22 |
| **TOTAL SINGLE DX** | 38 | 1.6 | 2 | 1 | 1 | 1 | 2 | 3 | 4 | 7 |
| **TOTAL MULTIPLE DX** | 1,642 | 5.6 | 26 | 1 | 2 | 4 | 7 | 11 | 16 | 22 |
| **TOTAL** | | | | | | | | | | |
| 0–19 Years | 57 | 2.3 | 8 | 1 | 1 | 1 | 3 | 4 | 5 | 17 |
| 20–34 | 104 | 3.8 | 45 | 1 | 1 | 2 | 5 | 7 | 9 | 20 |
| 35–49 | 181 | 4.4 | 18 | 1 | 1 | 3 | 6 | 9 | 12 | 19 |
| 50–64 | 273 | 4.5 | 22 | 1 | 1 | 3 | 6 | 10 | 13 | 22 |
| 65+ | 1,065 | 6.4 | 24 | 2 | 3 | 5 | 8 | 13 | 16 | 22 |
| **GRAND TOTAL** | 1,680 | 5.5 | 26 | 1 | 2 | 4 | 7 | 11 | 15 | 22 |

## 58.9: OTHER URETHRAL OPS. Formerly included in operation group(s) 658.

| Type of Patients | Observed Patients | Avg. Stay | Variance | Percentiles | | | | | | |
|---|---|---|---|---|---|---|---|---|---|---|
| | | | | 10th | 25th | 50th | 75th | 90th | 95th | 99th |
| **1. SINGLE DX** | | | | | | | | | | |
| 0–19 Years | 4 | 2.7 | 3 | 1 | 2 | 2 | 3 | 6 | 6 | 6 |
| 20–34 | 5 | 2.0 | <1 | 1 | 2 | 2 | 2 | 2 | 3 | 3 |
| 35–49 | 6 | 1.7 | <1 | 1 | 1 | 1 | 3 | 3 | 3 | 3 |
| 50–64 | 11 | 1.3 | <1 | 1 | 1 | 1 | 1 | 2 | 2 | 2 |
| 65+ | 17 | 1.4 | 1 | 1 | 1 | 1 | 1 | 3 | 4 | 4 |
| **2. MULTIPLE DX** | | | | | | | | | | |
| 0–19 Years | 21 | 6.7 | 8 | 2 | 5 | 8 | 8 | 9 | 10 | 13 |
| 20–34 | 33 | 2.8 | 4 | 1 | 1 | 2 | 4 | 7 | 7 | 8 |
| 35–49 | 50 | 4.9 | 53 | 1 | 2 | 2 | 5 | 10 | 29 | 29 |
| 50–64 | 148 | 2.2 | 6 | 1 | 1 | 1 | 2 | 4 | 6 | 10 |
| 65+ | 493 | 2.3 | 6 | 1 | 1 | 2 | 2 | 4 | 7 | 17 |
| **TOTAL SINGLE DX** | 43 | 1.5 | <1 | 1 | 1 | 1 | 2 | 3 | 3 | 5 |
| **TOTAL MULTIPLE DX** | 745 | 2.6 | 10 | 1 | 1 | 2 | 3 | 5 | 8 | 17 |
| **TOTAL** | | | | | | | | | | |
| 0–19 Years | 25 | 6.5 | 9 | 2 | 5 | 8 | 8 | 9 | 10 | 13 |
| 20–34 | 38 | 2.7 | 4 | 1 | 2 | 2 | 4 | 5 | 7 | 8 |
| 35–49 | 56 | 4.6 | 48 | 1 | 1 | 2 | 5 | 10 | 29 | 29 |
| 50–64 | 159 | 2.1 | 5 | 1 | 1 | 1 | 2 | 4 | 6 | 10 |
| 65+ | 510 | 2.2 | 6 | 1 | 1 | 2 | 2 | 4 | 7 | 17 |
| **GRAND TOTAL** | 788 | 2.6 | 9 | 1 | 1 | 2 | 3 | 5 | 8 | 17 |

## 58.93: IMPLANTATION OF AUS. Formerly included in operation group(s) 658.

| Type of Patients | Observed Patients | Avg. Stay | Variance | Percentiles | | | | | | |
|---|---|---|---|---|---|---|---|---|---|---|
| | | | | 10th | 25th | 50th | 75th | 90th | 95th | 99th |
| **1. SINGLE DX** | | | | | | | | | | |
| 0–19 Years | 2 | 3.3 | 0 | 1 | 1 | 1 | 6 | 6 | 6 | 6 |
| 20–34 | 2 | 2.3 | <1 | 2 | 2 | 2 | 3 | 3 | 3 | 3 |
| 35–49 | 3 | 2.5 | <1 | 1 | 3 | 3 | 3 | 3 | 3 | 3 |
| 50–64 | 6 | 1.4 | <1 | 1 | 1 | 1 | 2 | 2 | 2 | 2 |
| 65+ | 12 | 1.3 | <1 | 1 | 1 | 1 | 1 | 2 | 4 | 4 |
| **2. MULTIPLE DX** | | | | | | | | | | |
| 0–19 Years | 13 | 4.1 | 8 | 1 | 2 | 3 | 5 | 9 | 9 | 9 |
| 20–34 | 19 | 2.0 | 3 | 1 | 1 | 1 | 2 | 4 | 7 | 8 |
| 35–49 | 17 | 2.7 | 7 | 1 | 1 | 2 | 3 | 10 | 10 | 10 |
| 50–64 | 109 | 1.7 | 2 | 1 | 1 | 1 | 2 | 3 | 3 | 6 |
| 65+ | 372 | 1.9 | 3 | 1 | 1 | 1 | 2 | 3 | 4 | 10 |
| **TOTAL SINGLE DX** | 25 | 1.6 | 1 | 1 | 1 | 1 | 2 | 3 | 3 | 6 |
| **TOTAL MULTIPLE DX** | 530 | 1.9 | 3 | 1 | 1 | 1 | 2 | 3 | 4 | 10 |
| **TOTAL** | | | | | | | | | | |
| 0–19 Years | 15 | 4.1 | 8 | 1 | 2 | 3 | 6 | 9 | 9 | 9 |
| 20–34 | 21 | 2.0 | 3 | 1 | 1 | 1 | 2 | 4 | 7 | 8 |
| 35–49 | 20 | 2.7 | 6 | 1 | 1 | 2 | 3 | 5 | 10 | 10 |
| 50–64 | 115 | 1.7 | 2 | 1 | 1 | 1 | 2 | 3 | 3 | 6 |
| 65+ | 384 | 1.8 | 3 | 1 | 1 | 1 | 2 | 3 | 4 | 9 |
| **GRAND TOTAL** | 555 | 1.9 | 3 | 1 | 1 | 1 | 2 | 3 | 4 | 10 |

## 59.0: RETROPERITON DISSECTION. Formerly included in operation group(s) 663.

| Type of Patients | Observed Patients | Avg. Stay | Variance | Percentiles | | | | | | |
|---|---|---|---|---|---|---|---|---|---|---|
| | | | | 10th | 25th | 50th | 75th | 90th | 95th | 99th |
| **1. SINGLE DX** | | | | | | | | | | |
| 0–19 Years | 2 | 1.0 | 0 | 1 | 1 | 1 | 1 | 1 | 1 | 1 |
| 20–34 | 2 | 2.4 | 3 | 1 | 1 | 1 | 4 | 4 | 4 | 4 |
| 35–49 | 5 | 2.9 | 4 | 2 | 2 | 3 | 4 | 4 | 4 | 4 |
| 50–64 | 3 | 4.5 | 4 | 1 | 4 | 6 | 6 | 6 | 6 | 6 |
| 65+ | 1 | 6.0 | 0 | 6 | 6 | 6 | 6 | 6 | 6 | 6 |
| **2. MULTIPLE DX** | | | | | | | | | | |
| 0–19 Years | 19 | 7.9 | 38 | 2 | 3 | 5 | 11 | 19 | 19 | 22 |
| 20–34 | 42 | 4.8 | 9 | 1 | 3 | 5 | 6 | 9 | 10 | 23 |
| 35–49 | 91 | 6.0 | 22 | 2 | 3 | 5 | 7 | 10 | 18 | 25 |
| 50–64 | 104 | 5.8 | 15 | 2 | 3 | 5 | 10 | 11 | 14 | 23 |
| 65+ | 73 | 8.6 | 72 | 2 | 4 | 8 | 10 | 16 | 18 | 59 |
| **TOTAL SINGLE DX** | 13 | 3.2 | 4 | 1 | 1 | 4 | 4 | 6 | 6 | 6 |
| **TOTAL MULTIPLE DX** | 329 | 6.3 | 29 | 2 | 3 | 5 | 8 | 11 | 16 | 25 |
| **TOTAL** | | | | | | | | | | |
| 0–19 Years | 21 | 7.3 | 38 | 1 | 3 | 5 | 11 | 19 | 19 | 22 |
| 20–34 | 44 | 4.7 | 9 | 1 | 3 | 5 | 6 | 9 | 10 | 23 |
| 35–49 | 96 | 5.9 | 21 | 2 | 3 | 5 | 6 | 9 | 18 | 25 |
| 50–64 | 107 | 5.8 | 14 | 2 | 3 | 5 | 7 | 11 | 14 | 23 |
| 65+ | 74 | 8.5 | 71 | 2 | 4 | 8 | 10 | 16 | 18 | 59 |
| **GRAND TOTAL** | 342 | 6.2 | 29 | 2 | 3 | 5 | 7 | 11 | 15 | 25 |

Length of Stay by Diagnosis and Operation, United States, 2000

# United States, October 1998–September 1999 Data, by Operation

## 59.1: PERIVESICAL INCISION. Formerly included in operation group(s) 663.

| Type of Patients | Observed Patients | Avg. Stay | Variance | 10th | 25th | 50th | 75th | 90th | 95th | 99th |
|---|---|---|---|---|---|---|---|---|---|---|
| **1. SINGLE DX** | | | | | | | | | | |
| 0–19 Years | 0 | | | | | | | | | |
| 20–34 | 0 | | | | | | | | | |
| 35–49 | 0 | | | | | | | | | |
| 50–64 | 0 | | | | | | | | | |
| 65+ | 0 | | | | | | | | | |
| **2. MULTIPLE DX** | | | | | | | | | | |
| 0–19 Years | 0 | | | | | | | | | |
| 20–34 | 3 | 9.5 | 164 | 1 | 1 | 4 | 27 | 27 | 27 | 27 |
| 35–49 | 8 | 4.8 | 15 | 1 | 1 | 3 | 6 | 11 | 11 | 11 |
| 50–64 | 6 | 3.0 | 4 | 1 | 1 | 2 | 6 | 6 | 6 | 6 |
| 65+ | 10 | 10.8 | 28 | 3 | 4 | 13 | 13 | 19 | 19 | 19 |
| **TOTAL SINGLE DX** | 0 | | | | | | | | | |
| **TOTAL MULTIPLE DX** | 27 | 7.4 | 35 | 1 | 2 | 5 | 13 | 13 | 19 | 27 |
| **TOTAL** | | | | | | | | | | |
| 0–19 Years | 0 | | | | | | | | | |
| 20–34 | 3 | 9.5 | 164 | 1 | 1 | 4 | 27 | 27 | 27 | 27 |
| 35–49 | 8 | 4.8 | 15 | 1 | 1 | 3 | 6 | 11 | 11 | 11 |
| 50–64 | 6 | 3.0 | 4 | 1 | 1 | 2 | 6 | 6 | 6 | 6 |
| 65+ | 10 | 10.8 | 28 | 3 | 4 | 13 | 13 | 19 | 19 | 19 |
| **GRAND TOTAL** | 27 | 7.4 | 35 | 1 | 2 | 5 | 13 | 13 | 19 | 27 |

## 59.2: PERIRENAL DXTIC PX. Formerly included in operation group(s) 663, 664.

| Type of Patients | Observed Patients | Avg. Stay | Variance | 10th | 25th | 50th | 75th | 90th | 95th | 99th |
|---|---|---|---|---|---|---|---|---|---|---|
| **1. SINGLE DX** | | | | | | | | | | |
| 0–19 Years | 0 | | | | | | | | | |
| 20–34 | 0 | | | | | | | | | |
| 35–49 | 0 | | | | | | | | | |
| 50–64 | 0 | | | | | | | | | |
| 65+ | 0 | | | | | | | | | |
| **2. MULTIPLE DX** | | | | | | | | | | |
| 0–19 Years | 1 | 12.0 | 0 | 12 | 12 | 12 | 12 | 12 | 12 | 12 |
| 20–34 | 0 | | | | | | | | | |
| 35–49 | 0 | | | | | | | | | |
| 50–64 | 3 | 7.0 | 37 | 4 | 4 | 4 | 4 | 18 | 18 | 18 |
| 65+ | 11 | 5.6 | 5 | 3 | 4 | 5 | 7 | 10 | 10 | 10 |
| **TOTAL SINGLE DX** | 0 | | | | | | | | | |
| **TOTAL MULTIPLE DX** | 15 | 6.2 | 14 | 3 | 4 | 5 | 7 | 12 | 18 | 18 |
| **TOTAL** | | | | | | | | | | |
| 0–19 Years | 1 | 12.0 | 0 | 12 | 12 | 12 | 12 | 12 | 12 | 12 |
| 20–34 | 0 | | | | | | | | | |
| 35–49 | 0 | | | | | | | | | |
| 50–64 | 3 | 7.0 | 37 | 4 | 4 | 4 | 4 | 18 | 18 | 18 |
| 65+ | 11 | 5.6 | 5 | 3 | 4 | 5 | 7 | 10 | 10 | 10 |
| **GRAND TOTAL** | 15 | 6.2 | 14 | 3 | 4 | 5 | 7 | 12 | 18 | 18 |

## 59.3: URETHROVES JUNCT PLICAT. Formerly included in operation group(s) 660.

| Type of Patients | Observed Patients | Avg. Stay | Variance | 10th | 25th | 50th | 75th | 90th | 95th | 99th |
|---|---|---|---|---|---|---|---|---|---|---|
| **1. SINGLE DX** | | | | | | | | | | |
| 0–19 Years | 0 | | | | | | | | | |
| 20–34 | 0 | | | | | | | | | |
| 35–49 | 1 | 2.0 | 0 | 2 | 2 | 2 | 2 | 2 | 2 | 2 |
| 50–64 | 2 | 2.0 | 0 | 1 | 1 | 1 | 3 | 3 | 3 | 3 |
| 65+ | 1 | 2.0 | 0 | 2 | 2 | 2 | 2 | 2 | 2 | 2 |
| **2. MULTIPLE DX** | | | | | | | | | | |
| 0–19 Years | 0 | | | | | | | | | |
| 20–34 | 3 | 5.2 | 26 | 2 | 2 | 2 | 12 | 12 | 12 | 12 |
| 35–49 | 8 | 1.6 | <1 | 1 | 1 | 1 | 2 | 2 | 2 | 2 |
| 50–64 | 8 | 1.3 | <1 | 1 | 1 | 1 | 2 | 2 | 2 | 2 |
| 65+ | 16 | 3.2 | 4 | 1 | 1 | 3 | 6 | 6 | 6 | 6 |
| **TOTAL SINGLE DX** | 4 | 2.0 | <1 | 1 | 2 | 2 | 2 | 3 | 3 | 3 |
| **TOTAL MULTIPLE DX** | 35 | 2.2 | 4 | 1 | 1 | 2 | 2 | 6 | 6 | 12 |
| **TOTAL** | | | | | | | | | | |
| 0–19 Years | 0 | | | | | | | | | |
| 20–34 | 3 | 5.2 | 26 | 2 | 2 | 2 | 12 | 12 | 12 | 12 |
| 35–49 | 9 | 1.7 | <1 | 1 | 1 | 1 | 2 | 2 | 2 | 2 |
| 50–64 | 10 | 1.3 | <1 | 1 | 1 | 1 | 2 | 2 | 2 | 3 |
| 65+ | 17 | 3.2 | 4 | 1 | 1 | 3 | 6 | 6 | 6 | 6 |
| **GRAND TOTAL** | 39 | 2.2 | 3 | 1 | 1 | 2 | 2 | 6 | 6 | 12 |

## 59.4: SUPRAPUBIC SLING OP. Formerly included in operation group(s) 660.

| Type of Patients | Observed Patients | Avg. Stay | Variance | 10th | 25th | 50th | 75th | 90th | 95th | 99th |
|---|---|---|---|---|---|---|---|---|---|---|
| **1. SINGLE DX** | | | | | | | | | | |
| 0–19 Years | 0 | | | | | | | | | |
| 20–34 | 16 | 1.2 | <1 | 1 | 1 | 1 | 1 | 2 | 2 | 3 |
| 35–49 | 139 | 1.5 | <1 | 1 | 1 | 1 | 2 | 2 | 3 | 3 |
| 50–64 | 153 | 1.5 | <1 | 1 | 1 | 1 | 2 | 2 | 3 | 3 |
| 65+ | 100 | 1.8 | <1 | 1 | 1 | 2 | 2 | 3 | 3 | 4 |
| **2. MULTIPLE DX** | | | | | | | | | | |
| 0–19 Years | 10 | 6.7 | 27 | 1 | 2 | 5 | 14 | 14 | 14 | 14 |
| 20–34 | 52 | 2.1 | 2 | 1 | 1 | 2 | 2 | 3 | 4 | 12 |
| 35–49 | 414 | 1.8 | <1 | 1 | 1 | 2 | 2 | 3 | 3 | 5 |
| 50–64 | 701 | 2.0 | 1 | 1 | 1 | 2 | 2 | 3 | 4 | 7 |
| 65+ | 753 | 2.1 | 2 | 1 | 1 | 2 | 3 | 3 | 4 | 8 |
| **TOTAL SINGLE DX** | 408 | 1.5 | <1 | 1 | 1 | 1 | 2 | 2 | 3 | 3 |
| **TOTAL MULTIPLE DX** | 1,930 | 2.0 | 2 | 1 | 1 | 2 | 2 | 3 | 4 | 7 |
| **TOTAL** | | | | | | | | | | |
| 0–19 Years | 10 | 6.7 | 27 | 1 | 2 | 5 | 14 | 14 | 14 | 14 |
| 20–34 | 68 | 1.9 | 2 | 1 | 1 | 2 | 2 | 3 | 3 | 12 |
| 35–49 | 553 | 1.7 | <1 | 1 | 1 | 2 | 2 | 3 | 3 | 4 |
| 50–64 | 854 | 1.9 | 1 | 1 | 1 | 2 | 2 | 3 | 4 | 7 |
| 65+ | 853 | 2.1 | 2 | 1 | 1 | 2 | 3 | 3 | 4 | 7 |
| **GRAND TOTAL** | 2,338 | 1.9 | 2 | 1 | 1 | 2 | 2 | 3 | 4 | 6 |

Length of Stay by Diagnosis and Operation, United States, 2000

# United States, October 1998–September 1999 Data, by Operation

## 59.5: RETROPUBIC URETHRAL SUSP. Formerly included in operation group(s) 659.

| Type of Patients | Observed Patients | Avg. Stay | Variance | 10th | 25th | 50th | 75th | 90th | 95th | 99th |
|---|---|---|---|---|---|---|---|---|---|---|
| **1. SINGLE DX** | | | | | | | | | | |
| 0–19 Years | 1 | 2.0 | 0 | 2 | 2 | 2 | 2 | 2 | 2 | 2 |
| 20–34 | 83 | 2.4 | <1 | 1 | 2 | 2 | 3 | 3 | 3 | 4 |
| 35–49 | 463 | 2.0 | <1 | 1 | 1 | 2 | 2 | 3 | 3 | 5 |
| 50–64 | 398 | 2.3 | <1 | 1 | 1 | 2 | 3 | 3 | 3 | 5 |
| 65+ | 161 | 2.3 | 1 | 1 | 2 | 2 | 3 | 3 | 4 | 5 |
| **2. MULTIPLE DX** | | | | | | | | | | |
| 0–19 Years | 6 | 3.2 | 1 | 2 | 2 | 3 | 3 | 5 | 6 | 6 |
| 20–34 | 181 | 2.5 | 3 | 1 | 2 | 2 | 3 | 4 | 4 | 8 |
| 35–49 | 1,479 | 2.5 | 3 | 1 | 2 | 2 | 3 | 4 | 4 | 9 |
| 50–64 | 1,870 | 2.6 | 2 | 1 | 2 | 2 | 3 | 4 | 5 | 8 |
| 65+ | 1,277 | 3.0 | 6 | 1 | 2 | 3 | 3 | 4 | 6 | 9 |
| **TOTAL SINGLE DX** | 1,106 | 2.2 | <1 | 1 | 2 | 2 | 3 | 3 | 3 | 5 |
| **TOTAL MULTIPLE DX** | 4,813 | 2.6 | 3 | 1 | 2 | 2 | 3 | 4 | 5 | 8 |
| **TOTAL** | | | | | | | | | | |
| 0–19 Years | 7 | 3.1 | 1 | 2 | 2 | 3 | 3 | 5 | 6 | 6 |
| 20–34 | 264 | 2.5 | 2 | 1 | 2 | 2 | 3 | 4 | 4 | 7 |
| 35–49 | 1,942 | 2.4 | 2 | 1 | 2 | 2 | 3 | 4 | 4 | 8 |
| 50–64 | 2,268 | 2.5 | 2 | 1 | 2 | 2 | 3 | 4 | 5 | 8 |
| 65+ | 1,438 | 2.9 | 5 | 1 | 2 | 3 | 3 | 4 | 6 | 8 |
| **GRAND TOTAL** | 5,919 | 2.5 | 2 | 1 | 2 | 2 | 3 | 4 | 4 | 8 |

## 59.6: PARAURETHRAL SUSPENSION. Formerly included in operation group(s) 660.

| Type of Patients | Observed Patients | Avg. Stay | Variance | 10th | 25th | 50th | 75th | 90th | 95th | 99th |
|---|---|---|---|---|---|---|---|---|---|---|
| **1. SINGLE DX** | | | | | | | | | | |
| 0–19 Years | 0 | | | | | | | | | |
| 20–34 | 2 | 3.0 | 0 | 3 | 3 | 3 | 3 | 3 | 3 | 3 |
| 35–49 | 15 | 1.2 | <1 | 1 | 1 | 1 | 1 | 2 | 3 | 3 |
| 50–64 | 12 | 2.0 | <1 | 1 | 1 | 2 | 2 | 3 | 3 | 4 |
| 65+ | 6 | 2.1 | <1 | 1 | 1 | 3 | 3 | 3 | 3 | 3 |
| **2. MULTIPLE DX** | | | | | | | | | | |
| 0–19 Years | 0 | | | | | | | | | |
| 20–34 | 2 | 1.7 | 1 | 1 | 1 | 1 | 3 | 3 | 3 | 3 |
| 35–49 | 57 | 2.0 | 2 | 1 | 1 | 2 | 3 | 3 | 4 | 4 |
| 50–64 | 92 | 1.8 | 1 | 1 | 1 | 2 | 3 | 3 | 4 | 5 |
| 65+ | 104 | 2.2 | 2 | 1 | 2 | 2 | 3 | 3 | 4 | 5 |
| **TOTAL SINGLE DX** | 35 | 1.6 | <1 | 1 | 1 | 1 | 2 | 3 | 3 | 4 |
| **TOTAL MULTIPLE DX** | 255 | 2.0 | 2 | 1 | 1 | 2 | 3 | 3 | 3 | 5 |
| **TOTAL** | | | | | | | | | | |
| 0–19 Years | 0 | | | | | | | | | |
| 20–34 | 4 | 2.2 | 1 | 1 | 1 | 3 | 3 | 3 | 3 | 3 |
| 35–49 | 72 | 1.8 | 1 | 1 | 1 | 1 | 2 | 3 | 3 | 9 |
| 50–64 | 104 | 1.8 | 1 | 1 | 1 | 2 | 3 | 3 | 3 | 5 |
| 65+ | 110 | 2.2 | 2 | 1 | 2 | 2 | 3 | 3 | 3 | 5 |
| **GRAND TOTAL** | 290 | 1.9 | 1 | 1 | 2 | 2 | 3 | 3 | 3 | 5 |

## 59.7: OTH URINARY INCONT REP. Formerly included in operation group(s) 660.

| Type of Patients | Observed Patients | Avg. Stay | Variance | 10th | 25th | 50th | 75th | 90th | 95th | 99th |
|---|---|---|---|---|---|---|---|---|---|---|
| **1. SINGLE DX** | | | | | | | | | | |
| 0–19 Years | 1 | 3.0 | 0 | 3 | 3 | 3 | 3 | 3 | 3 | 3 |
| 20–34 | 68 | 1.6 | <1 | 1 | 1 | 1 | 2 | 2 | 3 | 3 |
| 35–49 | 431 | 1.5 | <1 | 1 | 1 | 1 | 2 | 3 | 3 | 4 |
| 50–64 | 451 | 1.5 | <1 | 1 | 1 | 1 | 2 | 3 | 3 | 3 |
| 65+ | 260 | 1.7 | <1 | 1 | 1 | 2 | 2 | 3 | 3 | 4 |
| **2. MULTIPLE DX** | | | | | | | | | | |
| 0–19 Years | 8 | 4.6 | 10 | 1 | 2 | 3 | 8 | 8 | 10 | 10 |
| 20–34 | 101 | 2.0 | <1 | 1 | 1 | 1 | 2 | 3 | 4 | 5 |
| 35–49 | 1,092 | 2.0 | 1 | 1 | 1 | 1 | 2 | 3 | 4 | 5 |
| 50–64 | 1,713 | 2.0 | 1 | 1 | 1 | 2 | 2 | 3 | 4 | 6 |
| 65+ | 1,698 | 2.3 | 3 | 1 | 1 | 2 | 3 | 4 | 5 | 14 |
| **TOTAL SINGLE DX** | 1,211 | 1.6 | <1 | 1 | 1 | 1 | 2 | 3 | 3 | 4 |
| **TOTAL MULTIPLE DX** | 4,612 | 2.1 | 3 | 1 | 1 | 2 | 3 | 3 | 4 | 7 |
| **TOTAL** | | | | | | | | | | |
| 0–19 Years | 9 | 4.4 | 9 | 1 | 2 | 3 | 8 | 8 | 10 | 10 |
| 20–34 | 169 | 1.8 | <1 | 1 | 1 | 1 | 2 | 3 | 3 | 4 |
| 35–49 | 1,523 | 1.8 | 1 | 1 | 1 | 1 | 2 | 3 | 3 | 5 |
| 50–64 | 2,164 | 1.9 | 2 | 1 | 1 | 2 | 2 | 3 | 3 | 6 |
| 65+ | 1,958 | 2.2 | 3 | 1 | 1 | 2 | 3 | 4 | 5 | 10 |
| **GRAND TOTAL** | 5,823 | 1.9 | 2 | 1 | 1 | 2 | 2 | 3 | 4 | 6 |

## 59.71: LEVATOR MUSC SUSPENSION. Formerly included in operation group(s) 660.

| Type of Patients | Observed Patients | Avg. Stay | Variance | 10th | 25th | 50th | 75th | 90th | 95th | 99th |
|---|---|---|---|---|---|---|---|---|---|---|
| **1. SINGLE DX** | | | | | | | | | | |
| 0–19 Years | 0 | | | | | | | | | |
| 20–34 | 8 | 1.2 | <1 | 1 | 1 | 1 | 1 | 2 | 2 | 2 |
| 35–49 | 50 | 1.5 | <1 | 1 | 1 | 1 | 2 | 3 | 3 | 5 |
| 50–64 | 60 | 1.4 | <1 | 1 | 1 | 1 | 2 | 2 | 3 | 3 |
| 65+ | 26 | 1.6 | <1 | 1 | 1 | 2 | 2 | 3 | 3 | 3 |
| **2. MULTIPLE DX** | | | | | | | | | | |
| 0–19 Years | 2 | 7.2 | 3 | 4 | 8 | 8 | 8 | 8 | 8 | 8 |
| 20–34 | 8 | 1.8 | 1 | 1 | 1 | 1 | 3 | 4 | 4 | 4 |
| 35–49 | 122 | 1.8 | <1 | 1 | 1 | 1 | 2 | 3 | 3 | 4 |
| 50–64 | 218 | 1.8 | <1 | 1 | 1 | 2 | 2 | 3 | 3 | 4 |
| 65+ | 215 | 2.4 | 6 | 1 | 1 | 2 | 3 | 3 | 7 | 14 |
| **TOTAL SINGLE DX** | 144 | 1.4 | <1 | 1 | 1 | 1 | 2 | 2 | 3 | 3 |
| **TOTAL MULTIPLE DX** | 565 | 2.0 | 3 | 1 | 1 | 2 | 2 | 3 | 3 | 9 |
| **TOTAL** | | | | | | | | | | |
| 0–19 Years | 2 | 7.2 | 3 | 4 | 8 | 8 | 8 | 8 | 8 | 8 |
| 20–34 | 16 | 1.4 | <1 | 1 | 1 | 1 | 1 | 2 | 3 | 4 |
| 35–49 | 172 | 1.7 | <1 | 1 | 1 | 1 | 2 | 3 | 3 | 5 |
| 50–64 | 278 | 1.7 | <1 | 1 | 1 | 2 | 2 | 3 | 3 | 4 |
| 65+ | 241 | 2.3 | 6 | 1 | 1 | 2 | 3 | 3 | 6 | 14 |
| **GRAND TOTAL** | 709 | 1.9 | 2 | 1 | 1 | 2 | 2 | 3 | 3 | 8 |

Length of Stay by Diagnosis and Operation, United States, 2000

# United States, October 1998–September 1999 Data, by Operation

## 59.79: URIN INCONT REPAIR NEC. Formerly included in operation group(s) 660.

| Type of Patients | Observed Patients | Avg. Stay | Variance | 10th | 25th | 50th | 75th | 90th | 95th | 99th |
|---|---|---|---|---|---|---|---|---|---|---|
| **1. SINGLE DX** | | | | | | | | | | |
| 0–19 Years | 1 | 3.0 | 0 | 3 | 3 | 3 | 3 | 3 | 3 | 3 |
| 20–34 | 59 | 1.6 | <1 | 1 | 1 | 1 | 2 | 3 | 3 | 3 |
| 35–49 | 380 | 1.5 | <1 | 1 | 1 | 1 | 2 | 3 | 3 | 4 |
| 50–64 | 391 | 1.5 | <1 | 1 | 1 | 1 | 2 | 3 | 3 | 4 |
| 65+ | 228 | 1.8 | <1 | 1 | 1 | 2 | 2 | 3 | 3 | 5 |
| **2. MULTIPLE DX** | | | | | | | | | | |
| 0–19 Years | 6 | 3.4 | 9 | 1 | 1 | 3 | 3 | 7 | 10 | 10 |
| 20–34 | 91 | 1.9 | <1 | 1 | 1 | 1 | 2 | 3 | 3 | 4 |
| 35–49 | 968 | 2.0 | 1 | 1 | 1 | 2 | 2 | 3 | 4 | 6 |
| 50–64 | 1,490 | 2.0 | 3 | 1 | 1 | 2 | 2 | 3 | 4 | 6 |
| 65+ | 1,451 | 2.2 | 3 | 1 | 1 | 2 | 3 | 4 | 5 | 8 |
| **TOTAL SINGLE DX** | 1,059 | 1.6 | <1 | 1 | 1 | 1 | 2 | 3 | 3 | 4 |
| **TOTAL MULTIPLE DX** | 4,006 | 2.1 | 3 | 1 | 1 | 2 | 2 | 3 | 4 | 7 |
| **TOTAL** | | | | | | | | | | |
| 0–19 Years | 7 | 3.3 | 7 | 1 | 1 | 3 | 3 | 7 | 10 | 10 |
| 20–34 | 150 | 1.8 | <1 | 1 | 1 | 2 | 2 | 3 | 3 | 4 |
| 35–49 | 1,348 | 1.8 | 1 | 1 | 1 | 2 | 2 | 3 | 4 | 5 |
| 50–64 | 1,881 | 1.9 | 3 | 1 | 1 | 2 | 2 | 3 | 4 | 6 |
| 65+ | 1,679 | 2.2 | 3 | 1 | 1 | 2 | 3 | 4 | 4 | 8 |
| **GRAND TOTAL** | 5,065 | 1.9 | 2 | 1 | 1 | 2 | 2 | 3 | 4 | 6 |

## 59.9: OTHER URINARY SYSTEM OPS. Formerly included in operation group(s) 662, 663.

| Type of Patients | Observed Patients | Avg. Stay | Variance | 10th | 25th | 50th | 75th | 90th | 95th | 99th |
|---|---|---|---|---|---|---|---|---|---|---|
| **1. SINGLE DX** | | | | | | | | | | |
| 0–19 Years | 1 | 1.0 | 0 | 1 | 1 | 1 | 1 | 1 | 1 | 1 |
| 20–34 | 10 | 1.3 | <1 | 1 | 1 | 1 | 1 | 2 | 3 | 3 |
| 35–49 | 9 | 2.5 | <1 | 2 | 2 | 2 | 4 | 4 | 4 | 4 |
| 50–64 | 10 | 2.0 | <1 | 1 | 1 | 2 | 3 | 3 | 3 | 4 |
| 65+ | 4 | 3.2 | 5 | 1 | 1 | 4 | 5 | 7 | 7 | 7 |
| **2. MULTIPLE DX** | | | | | | | | | | |
| 0–19 Years | 16 | 13.8 | 192 | 1 | 2 | 4 | 31 | 31 | 31 | 31 |
| 20–34 | 34 | 4.4 | 10 | 1 | 2 | 4 | 8 | 8 | 8 | 18 |
| 35–49 | 54 | 5.4 | 68 | 1 | 2 | 3 | 6 | 8 | 10 | 57 |
| 50–64 | 78 | 4.8 | 5 | 2 | 3 | 5 | 6 | 8 | 8 | 12 |
| 65+ | 179 | 6.0 | 32 | 1 | 2 | 4 | 8 | 12 | 24 | 24 |
| **TOTAL SINGLE DX** | 34 | 2.1 | 2 | 1 | 1 | 2 | 2 | 4 | 4 | 7 |
| **TOTAL MULTIPLE DX** | 361 | 5.8 | 41 | 1 | 2 | 4 | 7 | 10 | 18 | 31 |
| **TOTAL** | | | | | | | | | | |
| 0–19 Years | 17 | 13.7 | 191 | 1 | 2 | 4 | 31 | 31 | 31 | 31 |
| 20–34 | 44 | 3.7 | 10 | 1 | 1 | 2 | 6 | 8 | 8 | 10 |
| 35–49 | 63 | 5.0 | 60 | 1 | 2 | 3 | 6 | 7 | 10 | 53 |
| 50–64 | 88 | 4.5 | 5 | 1 | 2 | 5 | 6 | 7 | 8 | 12 |
| 65+ | 183 | 5.9 | 31 | 1 | 2 | 4 | 7 | 12 | 24 | 24 |
| **GRAND TOTAL** | 395 | 5.6 | 39 | 1 | 2 | 4 | 7 | 10 | 18 | 31 |

## 59.8: URETERAL CATHETERIZATION. Formerly included in operation group(s) 661.

| Type of Patients | Observed Patients | Avg. Stay | Variance | 10th | 25th | 50th | 75th | 90th | 95th | 99th |
|---|---|---|---|---|---|---|---|---|---|---|
| **1. SINGLE DX** | | | | | | | | | | |
| 0–19 Years | 72 | 1.7 | 1 | 1 | 1 | 1 | 2 | 3 | 4 | 7 |
| 20–34 | 411 | 1.7 | <1 | 1 | 1 | 1 | 2 | 3 | 3 | 6 |
| 35–49 | 564 | 1.6 | <1 | 1 | 1 | 1 | 2 | 3 | 3 | 5 |
| 50–64 | 274 | 1.8 | 2 | 1 | 1 | 1 | 2 | 3 | 5 | 7 |
| 65+ | 94 | 2.1 | 4 | 1 | 1 | 1 | 3 | 3 | 4 | 8 |
| **2. MULTIPLE DX** | | | | | | | | | | |
| 0–19 Years | 282 | 3.6 | 11 | 1 | 2 | 3 | 4 | 7 | 9 | 18 |
| 20–34 | 1,387 | 2.9 | 7 | 1 | 1 | 2 | 4 | 5 | 7 | 14 |
| 35–49 | 1,991 | 2.9 | 7 | 1 | 1 | 2 | 4 | 6 | 7 | 12 |
| 50–64 | 1,972 | 3.8 | 16 | 1 | 1 | 2 | 5 | 8 | 11 | 22 |
| 65+ | 2,599 | 5.4 | 25 | 2 | 2 | 4 | 7 | 11 | 14 | 22 |
| **TOTAL SINGLE DX** | 1,415 | 1.7 | 1 | 1 | 1 | 1 | 2 | 3 | 4 | 6 |
| **TOTAL MULTIPLE DX** | 8,231 | 3.9 | 16 | 1 | 1 | 3 | 5 | 8 | 11 | 20 |
| **TOTAL** | | | | | | | | | | |
| 0–19 Years | 354 | 3.2 | 10 | 1 | 1 | 2 | 4 | 6 | 8 | 18 |
| 20–34 | 1,798 | 2.6 | 6 | 1 | 1 | 2 | 3 | 5 | 6 | 13 |
| 35–49 | 2,555 | 2.6 | 6 | 1 | 1 | 2 | 3 | 5 | 7 | 11 |
| 50–64 | 2,246 | 3.6 | 15 | 1 | 1 | 2 | 4 | 8 | 11 | 22 |
| 65+ | 2,693 | 5.3 | 25 | 2 | 2 | 4 | 7 | 11 | 14 | 22 |
| **GRAND TOTAL** | 9,646 | 3.6 | 14 | 1 | 1 | 2 | 4 | 7 | 10 | 19 |

## 60.0: INCISION OF PROSTATE. Formerly included in operation group(s) 667.

| Type of Patients | Observed Patients | Avg. Stay | Variance | 10th | 25th | 50th | 75th | 90th | 95th | 99th |
|---|---|---|---|---|---|---|---|---|---|---|
| **1. SINGLE DX** | | | | | | | | | | |
| 0–19 Years | 0 | | | | | | | | | |
| 20–34 | 0 | | | | | | | | | |
| 35–49 | 5 | 1.1 | <1 | 1 | 1 | 1 | 1 | 1 | 2 | 2 |
| 50–64 | 18 | 1.7 | <1 | 1 | 1 | 1 | 3 | 3 | 3 | 3 |
| 65+ | 20 | 1.3 | <1 | 1 | 1 | 1 | 1 | 2 | 3 | 3 |
| **2. MULTIPLE DX** | | | | | | | | | | |
| 0–19 Years | 1 | 2.0 | 0 | 2 | 2 | 2 | 2 | 2 | 2 | 2 |
| 20–34 | 3 | 2.1 | 2 | 1 | 1 | 1 | 4 | 4 | 4 | 4 |
| 35–49 | 28 | 1.9 | 3 | 1 | 1 | 1 | 2 | 4 | 6 | 10 |
| 50–64 | 72 | 3.6 | 24 | 1 | 1 | 2 | 3 | 8 | 14 | 26 |
| 65+ | 179 | 3.5 | 17 | 1 | 1 | 2 | 4 | 9 | 13 | 19 |
| **TOTAL SINGLE DX** | 43 | 1.5 | <1 | 1 | 1 | 1 | 2 | 3 | 3 | 3 |
| **TOTAL MULTIPLE DX** | 283 | 3.4 | 17 | 1 | 1 | 2 | 3 | 7 | 13 | 20 |
| **TOTAL** | | | | | | | | | | |
| 0–19 Years | 1 | 2.0 | 0 | 2 | 2 | 2 | 2 | 2 | 2 | 2 |
| 20–34 | 3 | 2.1 | 2 | 1 | 1 | 1 | 4 | 4 | 4 | 4 |
| 35–49 | 33 | 1.8 | 2 | 1 | 1 | 1 | 2 | 4 | 6 | 6 |
| 50–64 | 90 | 3.2 | 20 | 1 | 1 | 2 | 3 | 7 | 13 | 26 |
| 65+ | 199 | 3.4 | 16 | 1 | 1 | 2 | 3 | 8 | 13 | 19 |
| **GRAND TOTAL** | 326 | 3.2 | 16 | 1 | 1 | 2 | 3 | 7 | 12 | 20 |

Length of Stay by Diagnosis and Operation, United States, 2000

# United States, October 1998–September 1999 Data, by Operation

## 60.1: PROS/SEM VESICL DXTIC PX. Formerly included in operation group(s) 667, 677.

| Type of Patients | Observed Patients | Avg. Stay | Variance | 10th | 25th | 50th | 75th | 90th | 95th | 99th |
|---|---|---|---|---|---|---|---|---|---|---|
| **1. SINGLE DX** | | | | | | | | | | |
| 0–19 Years | 0 | | | | | | | | | |
| 20–34 | 0 | | | | | | | | | |
| 35–49 | 2 | 1.0 | 0 | 1 | 1 | 1 | 1 | 1 | 1 | 1 |
| 50–64 | 9 | 1.9 | 1 | 1 | 1 | 2 | 3 | 4 | 4 | 4 |
| 65+ | 7 | 4.3 | 6 | 1 | 1 | 6 | 6 | 6 | 7 | 7 |
| **2. MULTIPLE DX** | | | | | | | | | | |
| 0–19 Years | 5 | 8.8 | 34 | 2 | 8 | 8 | 9 | 9 | 25 | 25 |
| 20–34 | 1 | 3.0 | 0 | 3 | 3 | 3 | 3 | 3 | 3 | 3 |
| 35–49 | 16 | 4.6 | 8 | 1 | 3 | 4 | 4 | 8 | 12 | 12 |
| 50–64 | 138 | 6.0 | 35 | 1 | 2 | 4 | 8 | 13 | 17 | 24 |
| 65+ | 746 | 8.1 | 39 | 2 | 4 | 7 | 10 | 15 | 20 | 32 |
| **TOTAL SINGLE DX** | 18 | 3.0 | 5 | 1 | 1 | 2 | 6 | 6 | 6 | 7 |
| **TOTAL MULTIPLE DX** | 906 | 7.7 | 39 | 2 | 3 | 6 | 10 | 15 | 19 | 31 |
| **TOTAL** | | | | | | | | | | |
| 0–19 Years | 5 | 8.8 | 34 | 2 | 8 | 8 | 9 | 9 | 25 | 25 |
| 20–34 | 1 | 3.0 | 0 | 3 | 3 | 3 | 3 | 3 | 3 | 3 |
| 35–49 | 18 | 3.7 | 9 | 1 | 1 | 4 | 4 | 8 | 12 | 12 |
| 50–64 | 147 | 5.8 | 34 | 1 | 2 | 4 | 7 | 13 | 17 | 24 |
| 65+ | 753 | 8.0 | 39 | 2 | 4 | 7 | 10 | 15 | 20 | 32 |
| **GRAND TOTAL** | 924 | 7.6 | 39 | 2 | 3 | 6 | 10 | 15 | 19 | 29 |

## 60.2: TU PROSTATECTOMY. Formerly included in operation group(s) 667.

| Type of Patients | Observed Patients | Avg. Stay | Variance | 10th | 25th | 50th | 75th | 90th | 95th | 99th |
|---|---|---|---|---|---|---|---|---|---|---|
| **1. SINGLE DX** | | | | | | | | | | |
| 0–19 Years | 0 | | | | | | | | | |
| 20–34 | 1 | 2.0 | 0 | 2 | 2 | 2 | 2 | 2 | 2 | 2 |
| 35–49 | 35 | 1.5 | <1 | 1 | 1 | 1 | 2 | 2 | 3 | 3 |
| 50–64 | 476 | 1.9 | <1 | 1 | 1 | 2 | 2 | 3 | 4 | 4 |
| 65+ | 989 | 1.9 | <1 | 1 | 1 | 2 | 2 | 3 | 4 | 5 |
| **2. MULTIPLE DX** | | | | | | | | | | |
| 0–19 Years | 2 | 5.2 | 1 | 4 | 4 | 6 | 6 | 6 | 6 | 6 |
| 20–34 | 12 | 3.5 | 14 | 1 | 3 | 3 | 3 | 3 | 7 | 21 |
| 35–49 | 302 | 2.6 | 8 | 1 | 1 | 2 | 2 | 4 | 7 | 16 |
| 50–64 | 5,696 | 2.7 | 9 | 1 | 2 | 2 | 3 | 5 | 7 | 16 |
| 65+ | 26,733 | 3.6 | 16 | 2 | 2 | 2 | 4 | 7 | 11 | 22 |
| **TOTAL SINGLE DX** | 1,501 | 1.9 | <1 | 1 | 1 | 2 | 2 | 3 | 4 | 5 |
| **TOTAL MULTIPLE DX** | 32,745 | 3.4 | 15 | 1 | 2 | 2 | 3 | 7 | 10 | 21 |
| **TOTAL** | | | | | | | | | | |
| 0–19 Years | 2 | 5.2 | 1 | 4 | 4 | 6 | 6 | 6 | 6 | 6 |
| 20–34 | 13 | 3.5 | 13 | 1 | 3 | 3 | 3 | 3 | 7 | 21 |
| 35–49 | 337 | 2.5 | 7 | 1 | 1 | 2 | 2 | 4 | 7 | 16 |
| 50–64 | 6,172 | 2.7 | 8 | 1 | 2 | 2 | 3 | 4 | 7 | 15 |
| 65+ | 27,722 | 3.5 | 16 | 2 | 2 | 2 | 4 | 7 | 11 | 22 |
| **GRAND TOTAL** | 34,246 | 3.3 | 14 | 1 | 2 | 2 | 3 | 7 | 10 | 20 |

## 60.11: CLSD (PERC) PROSTATIC BX. Formerly included in operation group(s) 667.

| Type of Patients | Observed Patients | Avg. Stay | Variance | 10th | 25th | 50th | 75th | 90th | 95th | 99th |
|---|---|---|---|---|---|---|---|---|---|---|
| **1. SINGLE DX** | | | | | | | | | | |
| 0–19 Years | 0 | | | | | | | | | |
| 20–34 | 0 | | | | | | | | | |
| 35–49 | 2 | 1.0 | 0 | 1 | 1 | 1 | 1 | 1 | 1 | 1 |
| 50–64 | 9 | 1.9 | 1 | 1 | 1 | 2 | 3 | 4 | 4 | 4 |
| 65+ | 7 | 4.3 | 6 | 1 | 1 | 6 | 6 | 6 | 7 | 7 |
| **2. MULTIPLE DX** | | | | | | | | | | |
| 0–19 Years | 5 | 8.8 | 34 | 2 | 8 | 8 | 9 | 9 | 25 | 25 |
| 20–34 | 1 | 3.0 | 0 | 3 | 3 | 3 | 3 | 3 | 3 | 3 |
| 35–49 | 15 | 4.7 | 9 | 1 | 3 | 3 | 4 | 10 | 12 | 12 |
| 50–64 | 136 | 6.0 | 35 | 1 | 2 | 4 | 8 | 13 | 17 | 24 |
| 65+ | 736 | 8.1 | 39 | 2 | 4 | 7 | 10 | 15 | 20 | 32 |
| **TOTAL SINGLE DX** | 18 | 3.0 | 5 | 1 | 1 | 2 | 6 | 6 | 6 | 7 |
| **TOTAL MULTIPLE DX** | 893 | 7.7 | 39 | 2 | 3 | 7 | 10 | 15 | 19 | 31 |
| **TOTAL** | | | | | | | | | | |
| 0–19 Years | 5 | 8.8 | 34 | 2 | 8 | 8 | 9 | 9 | 25 | 25 |
| 20–34 | 1 | 3.0 | 0 | 3 | 3 | 3 | 3 | 3 | 3 | 3 |
| 35–49 | 17 | 3.8 | 9 | 1 | 1 | 4 | 4 | 8 | 12 | 12 |
| 50–64 | 145 | 5.8 | 34 | 2 | 2 | 4 | 7 | 13 | 17 | 24 |
| 65+ | 743 | 8.1 | 39 | 2 | 4 | 7 | 10 | 15 | 20 | 32 |
| **GRAND TOTAL** | 911 | 7.6 | 39 | 2 | 3 | 6 | 10 | 15 | 19 | 31 |

## 60.21: TULIP PROCEDURE. Formerly included in operation group(s) 667.

| Type of Patients | Observed Patients | Avg. Stay | Variance | 10th | 25th | 50th | 75th | 90th | 95th | 99th |
|---|---|---|---|---|---|---|---|---|---|---|
| **1. SINGLE DX** | | | | | | | | | | |
| 0–19 Years | 0 | | | | | | | | | |
| 20–34 | 0 | | | | | | | | | |
| 35–49 | 3 | 1.0 | 0 | 1 | 1 | 1 | 1 | 1 | 1 | 1 |
| 50–64 | 23 | 1.1 | <1 | 1 | 1 | 1 | 2 | 2 | 2 | 2 |
| 65+ | 27 | 1.3 | <1 | 1 | 1 | 1 | 2 | 2 | 3 | 3 |
| **2. MULTIPLE DX** | | | | | | | | | | |
| 0–19 Years | 0 | | | | | | | | | |
| 20–34 | 1 | 1.0 | 0 | 1 | 1 | 1 | 1 | 1 | 1 | 1 |
| 35–49 | 10 | 6.0 | 48 | 1 | 2 | 2 | 12 | 12 | 25 | 25 |
| 50–64 | 113 | 2.6 | 7 | 1 | 1 | 2 | 3 | 4 | 6 | 11 |
| 65+ | 707 | 4.5 | 35 | 1 | 1 | 2 | 4 | 15 | 17 | 28 |
| **TOTAL SINGLE DX** | 53 | 1.2 | <1 | 1 | 1 | 1 | 1 | 2 | 2 | 3 |
| **TOTAL MULTIPLE DX** | 831 | 4.2 | 31 | 1 | 1 | 1 | 4 | 12 | 17 | 28 |
| **TOTAL** | | | | | | | | | | |
| 0–19 Years | 0 | | | | | | | | | |
| 20–34 | 1 | 1.0 | 0 | 1 | 1 | 1 | 1 | 1 | 1 | 1 |
| 35–49 | 13 | 4.6 | 40 | 1 | 1 | 1 | 4 | 12 | 25 | 25 |
| 50–64 | 136 | 2.2 | 6 | 1 | 1 | 2 | 3 | 3 | 5 | 10 |
| 65+ | 734 | 4.4 | 34 | 1 | 1 | 2 | 4 | 15 | 17 | 28 |
| **GRAND TOTAL** | 884 | 4.0 | 30 | 1 | 1 | 2 | 3 | 11 | 17 | 28 |

Length of Stay by Diagnosis and Operation, United States, 2000

# United States, October 1998–September 1999 Data, by Operation

## 60.29: TU PROSTATECTOMY NEC. Formerly included in operation group(s) 667.

| Type of Patients | Observed Patients | Avg. Stay | Variance | Percentiles | | | | | | |
|---|---|---|---|---|---|---|---|---|---|---|
| | | | | 10th | 25th | 50th | 75th | 90th | 95th | 99th |
| **1. SINGLE DX** | | | | | | | | | | |
| 0–19 Years | 0 | | | | | | | | | |
| 20–34 | 1 | 2.0 | 0 | 2 | 2 | 2 | 2 | 2 | 2 | 2 |
| 35–49 | 32 | 1.5 | <1 | 1 | 1 | 1 | 2 | 2 | 3 | 3 |
| 50–64 | 453 | 1.9 | <1 | 1 | 1 | 2 | 2 | 3 | 3 | 4 |
| 65+ | 962 | 2.0 | <1 | 1 | 1 | 2 | 2 | 3 | 4 | 5 |
| **2. MULTIPLE DX** | | | | | | | | | | |
| 0–19 Years | 2 | 5.2 | 1 | 4 | 4 | 6 | 6 | 6 | 6 | 6 |
| 20–34 | 11 | 3.6 | 14 | 1 | 3 | 3 | 3 | 3 | 7 | 21 |
| 35–49 | 292 | 2.5 | 6 | 1 | 1 | 2 | 2 | 4 | 7 | 16 |
| 50–64 | 5,583 | 2.7 | 9 | 1 | 1 | 2 | 3 | 5 | 7 | 16 |
| 65+ | 26,026 | 3.5 | 16 | 1 | 2 | 2 | 4 | 7 | 10 | 22 |
| **TOTAL SINGLE DX** | 1,448 | 1.9 | <1 | 1 | 1 | 2 | 2 | 3 | 4 | 5 |
| **TOTAL MULTIPLE DX** | 31,914 | 3.4 | 15 | 2 | 2 | 2 | 3 | 7 | 10 | 21 |
| **TOTAL** | | | | | | | | | | |
| 0–19 Years | 2 | 5.2 | 1 | 4 | 4 | 6 | 6 | 6 | 6 | 6 |
| 20–34 | 12 | 3.5 | 14 | 1 | 3 | 3 | 3 | 3 | 7 | 21 |
| 35–49 | 324 | 2.4 | 6 | 1 | 1 | 2 | 2 | 3 | 7 | 16 |
| 50–64 | 6,036 | 2.7 | 9 | 1 | 2 | 2 | 3 | 4 | 7 | 15 |
| 65+ | 26,988 | 3.5 | 15 | 1 | 2 | 2 | 4 | 7 | 10 | 21 |
| **GRAND TOTAL** | 33,362 | 3.3 | 14 | 2 | 2 | 2 | 3 | 6 | 10 | 20 |

## 60.4: RETROPUBIC PROSTATECTOMY. Formerly included in operation group(s) 666.

| Type of Patients | Observed Patients | Avg. Stay | Variance | Percentiles | | | | | | |
|---|---|---|---|---|---|---|---|---|---|---|
| | | | | 10th | 25th | 50th | 75th | 90th | 95th | 99th |
| **1. SINGLE DX** | | | | | | | | | | |
| 0–19 Years | 2 | 2.3 | 1 | 1 | 1 | 3 | 3 | 3 | 3 | 3 |
| 20–34 | 0 | | | | | | | | | |
| 35–49 | 14 | 4.1 | 2 | 3 | 3 | 4 | 5 | 5 | 7 | 7 |
| 50–64 | 74 | 3.3 | 1 | 2 | 3 | 3 | 4 | 6 | 5 | 8 |
| 65+ | 26 | 3.6 | 2 | 2 | 3 | 4 | 5 | 6 | 6 | 6 |
| **2. MULTIPLE DX** | | | | | | | | | | |
| 0–19 Years | 2 | 3.5 | <1 | 3 | 3 | 3 | 4 | 4 | 4 | 4 |
| 20–34 | 0 | | | | | | | | | |
| 35–49 | 11 | 3.8 | <1 | 3 | 3 | 4 | 4 | 6 | 5 | 5 |
| 50–64 | 291 | 3.9 | 6 | 2 | 3 | 3 | 4 | 6 | 8 | 18 |
| 65+ | 542 | 5.0 | 14 | 2 | 3 | 4 | 6 | 8 | 12 | 19 |
| **TOTAL SINGLE DX** | 116 | 3.5 | 2 | 2 | 3 | 3 | 4 | 5 | 6 | 8 |
| **TOTAL MULTIPLE DX** | 846 | 4.6 | 11 | 2 | 3 | 4 | 5 | 7 | 10 | 18 |
| **TOTAL** | | | | | | | | | | |
| 0–19 Years | 4 | 3.1 | <1 | 1 | 3 | 3 | 4 | 4 | 4 | 4 |
| 20–34 | 0 | | | | | | | | | |
| 35–49 | 25 | 3.9 | 1 | 3 | 3 | 4 | 5 | 5 | 5 | 7 |
| 50–64 | 365 | 3.8 | 5 | 2 | 3 | 3 | 4 | 5 | 7 | 14 |
| 65+ | 568 | 4.9 | 13 | 2 | 3 | 4 | 6 | 8 | 11 | 19 |
| **GRAND TOTAL** | 962 | 4.5 | 10 | 2 | 3 | 4 | 5 | 7 | 10 | 18 |

## 60.3: SUPRAPUBIC PROSTATECTOMY. Formerly included in operation group(s) 666.

| Type of Patients | Observed Patients | Avg. Stay | Variance | Percentiles | | | | | | |
|---|---|---|---|---|---|---|---|---|---|---|
| | | | | 10th | 25th | 50th | 75th | 90th | 95th | 99th |
| **1. SINGLE DX** | | | | | | | | | | |
| 0–19 Years | 0 | | | | | | | | | |
| 20–34 | 0 | | | | | | | | | |
| 35–49 | 0 | | | | | | | | | |
| 50–64 | 12 | 4.0 | 3 | 3 | 3 | 3 | 4 | 5 | 10 | 10 |
| 65+ | 12 | 4.9 | 3 | 4 | 4 | 4 | 6 | 8 | 8 | 8 |
| **2. MULTIPLE DX** | | | | | | | | | | |
| 0–19 Years | 0 | | | | | | | | | |
| 20–34 | 0 | | | | | | | | | |
| 35–49 | 1 | 11.0 | 0 | 11 | 11 | 11 | 11 | 11 | 11 | 11 |
| 50–64 | 168 | 5.4 | 3 | 3 | 4 | 5 | 7 | 7 | 8 | 10 |
| 65+ | 664 | 6.9 | 18 | 3 | 4 | 6 | 8 | 12 | 16 | 19 |
| **TOTAL SINGLE DX** | 24 | 4.4 | 3 | 3 | 3 | 4 | 5 | 7 | 8 | 10 |
| **TOTAL MULTIPLE DX** | 833 | 6.5 | 14 | 3 | 4 | 6 | 7 | 11 | 14 | 19 |
| **TOTAL** | | | | | | | | | | |
| 0–19 Years | 0 | | | | | | | | | |
| 20–34 | 0 | | | | | | | | | |
| 35–49 | 1 | 11.0 | 0 | 11 | 11 | 11 | 11 | 11 | 11 | 11 |
| 50–64 | 180 | 5.3 | 3 | 3 | 4 | 5 | 6 | 7 | 8 | 10 |
| 65+ | 676 | 6.9 | 18 | 3 | 4 | 6 | 8 | 12 | 16 | 19 |
| **GRAND TOTAL** | 857 | 6.5 | 14 | 3 | 4 | 6 | 7 | 10 | 14 | 19 |

## 60.5: RADICAL PROSTATECTOMY. Formerly included in operation group(s) 666.

| Type of Patients | Observed Patients | Avg. Stay | Variance | Percentiles | | | | | | |
|---|---|---|---|---|---|---|---|---|---|---|
| | | | | 10th | 25th | 50th | 75th | 90th | 95th | 99th |
| **1. SINGLE DX** | | | | | | | | | | |
| 0–19 Years | 0 | | | | | | | | | |
| 20–34 | 0 | | | | | | | | | |
| 35–49 | 268 | 3.0 | <1 | 2 | 2 | 3 | 4 | 4 | 4 | 7 |
| 50–64 | 2,383 | 3.1 | 1 | 2 | 2 | 3 | 4 | 4 | 5 | 6 |
| 65+ | 1,144 | 3.2 | 1 | 2 | 2 | 3 | 4 | 5 | 5 | 7 |
| **2. MULTIPLE DX** | | | | | | | | | | |
| 0–19 Years | 1 | 2.0 | 0 | 2 | 2 | 2 | 2 | 2 | 2 | 2 |
| 20–34 | 1 | 8.0 | 0 | 8 | 8 | 8 | 8 | 8 | 8 | 8 |
| 35–49 | 527 | 3.6 | 2 | 2 | 3 | 3 | 4 | 5 | 7 | 9 |
| 50–64 | 7,062 | 3.7 | 3 | 2 | 3 | 3 | 4 | 5 | 7 | 9 |
| 65+ | 5,656 | 3.9 | 4 | 2 | 3 | 3 | 4 | 6 | 7 | 11 |
| **TOTAL SINGLE DX** | 3,795 | 3.1 | 1 | 2 | 2 | 3 | 4 | 4 | 5 | 6 |
| **TOTAL MULTIPLE DX** | 13,247 | 3.8 | 4 | 2 | 3 | 3 | 4 | 6 | 7 | 10 |
| **TOTAL** | | | | | | | | | | |
| 0–19 Years | 1 | 2.0 | 0 | 2 | 2 | 2 | 2 | 2 | 2 | 2 |
| 20–34 | 1 | 8.0 | 0 | 8 | 8 | 8 | 8 | 9 | 8 | 8 |
| 35–49 | 795 | 3.4 | 2 | 2 | 3 | 3 | 4 | 5 | 6 | 8 |
| 50–64 | 9,445 | 3.5 | 3 | 2 | 3 | 3 | 4 | 5 | 6 | 9 |
| 65+ | 6,800 | 3.8 | 4 | 2 | 3 | 3 | 4 | 6 | 7 | 11 |
| **GRAND TOTAL** | 17,042 | 3.6 | 3 | 2 | 3 | 3 | 4 | 5 | 6 | 10 |

Length of Stay by Diagnosis and Operation, United States, 2000

# United States, October 1998–September 1999 Data, by Operation

## 60.6: OTHER PROSTATECTOMY. Formerly included in operation group(s) 666.

| Type of Patients | Observed Patients | Avg. Stay | Variance | Percentiles | | | | | | |
|---|---|---|---|---|---|---|---|---|---|---|
| | | | | 10th | 25th | 50th | 75th | 90th | 95th | 99th |
| **1. SINGLE DX** | | | | | | | | | | |
| 0–19 Years | 0 | | | | | | | | | |
| 20–34 | 0 | | | | | | | | | |
| 35–49 | 1 | 2.0 | 0 | 2 | 2 | 2 | 2 | 2 | 2 | 2 |
| 50–64 | 12 | 2.1 | 1 | 2 | 2 | 2 | 2 | 3 | 5 | 6 |
| 65+ | 10 | 1.9 | <1 | 1 | 1 | 2 | 3 | 3 | 4 | 4 |
| **2. MULTIPLE DX** | | | | | | | | | | |
| 0–19 Years | 1 | 5.0 | 0 | 5 | 5 | 5 | 5 | 5 | 5 | 5 |
| 20–34 | 1 | 7.0 | 0 | 7 | 7 | 7 | 7 | 7 | 7 | 7 |
| 35–49 | 5 | 2.8 | 3 | 2 | 2 | 2 | 2 | 6 | 6 | 6 |
| 50–64 | 49 | 4.1 | 13 | 1 | 1 | 4 | 4 | 8 | 14 | 19 |
| 65+ | 172 | 4.7 | 20 | 1 | 2 | 3 | 5 | 11 | 14 | 20 |
| **TOTAL SINGLE DX** | 23 | 2.0 | <1 | 1 | 1 | 2 | 2 | 3 | 4 | 6 |
| **TOTAL MULTIPLE DX** | 228 | 4.5 | 17 | 1 | 2 | 3 | 5 | 10 | 14 | 20 |
| **TOTAL** | | | | | | | | | | |
| 0–19 Years | 1 | 5.0 | 0 | 5 | 5 | 5 | 5 | 5 | 5 | 5 |
| 20–34 | 1 | 7.0 | 0 | 7 | 7 | 7 | 7 | 7 | 7 | 7 |
| 35–49 | 6 | 2.7 | 3 | 2 | 2 | 2 | 2 | 6 | 6 | 6 |
| 50–64 | 61 | 3.5 | 10 | 1 | 1 | 3 | 4 | 6 | 14 | 14 |
| 65+ | 182 | 4.5 | 19 | 1 | 2 | 3 | 5 | 10 | 14 | 20 |
| **GRAND TOTAL** | 251 | 4.1 | 16 | 1 | 2 | 3 | 5 | 8 | 14 | 19 |

## 60.7: SEMINAL VESICLE OPS. Formerly included in operation group(s) 667.

| Type of Patients | Observed Patients | Avg. Stay | Variance | Percentiles | | | | | | |
|---|---|---|---|---|---|---|---|---|---|---|
| | | | | 10th | 25th | 50th | 75th | 90th | 95th | 99th |
| **1. SINGLE DX** | | | | | | | | | | |
| 0–19 Years | 2 | 4.9 | 9 | 2 | 2 | 2 | 8 | 8 | 8 | 8 |
| 20–34 | 1 | 7.0 | 0 | 7 | 7 | 7 | 7 | 7 | 7 | 7 |
| 35–49 | 0 | | | | | | | | | |
| 50–64 | 1 | 1.0 | 0 | 1 | 1 | 1 | 1 | 1 | 1 | 1 |
| 65+ | 0 | | | | | | | | | |
| **2. MULTIPLE DX** | | | | | | | | | | |
| 0–19 Years | 0 | | | | | | | | | |
| 20–34 | 2 | 2.1 | <1 | 2 | 2 | 2 | 2 | 3 | 3 | 3 |
| 35–49 | 3 | 2.3 | <1 | 2 | 2 | 2 | 3 | 3 | 3 | 3 |
| 50–64 | 1 | 6.0 | 0 | 6 | 6 | 6 | 6 | 6 | 6 | 6 |
| 65+ | 0 | | | | | | | | | |
| **TOTAL SINGLE DX** | 4 | 4.8 | 9 | 2 | 2 | 2 | 8 | 8 | 8 | 8 |
| **TOTAL MULTIPLE DX** | 6 | 2.4 | 1 | 2 | 2 | 2 | 2 | 3 | 6 | 6 |
| **TOTAL** | | | | | | | | | | |
| 0–19 Years | 2 | 4.9 | 9 | 2 | 2 | 2 | 8 | 8 | 8 | 8 |
| 20–34 | 3 | 2.4 | 2 | 2 | 2 | 2 | 3 | 3 | 7 | 7 |
| 35–49 | 3 | 2.3 | <1 | 2 | 2 | 2 | 3 | 3 | 3 | 3 |
| 50–64 | 2 | 3.5 | 9 | 1 | 1 | 4 | 6 | 6 | 6 | 6 |
| 65+ | 0 | | | | | | | | | |
| **GRAND TOTAL** | 10 | 3.7 | 7 | 2 | 2 | 2 | 7 | 8 | 8 | 8 |

## 60.8: PERIPROSTATIC INC OR EXC. Formerly included in operation group(s) 667.

| Type of Patients | Observed Patients | Avg. Stay | Variance | Percentiles | | | | | | |
|---|---|---|---|---|---|---|---|---|---|---|
| | | | | 10th | 25th | 50th | 75th | 90th | 95th | 99th |
| **1. SINGLE DX** | | | | | | | | | | |
| 0–19 Years | 0 | | | | | | | | | |
| 20–34 | 0 | | | | | | | | | |
| 35–49 | 1 | 2.0 | 0 | 2 | 2 | 2 | 2 | 2 | 2 | 2 |
| 50–64 | 0 | | | | | | | | | |
| 65+ | 0 | | | | | | | | | |
| **2. MULTIPLE DX** | | | | | | | | | | |
| 0–19 Years | 0 | | | | | | | | | |
| 20–34 | 0 | | | | | | | | | |
| 35–49 | 0 | | | | | | | | | |
| 50–64 | 0 | | | | | | | | | |
| 65+ | 4 | 5.1 | 16 | 1 | 4 | 4 | 5 | 12 | 12 | 12 |
| **TOTAL SINGLE DX** | 1 | 2.0 | 0 | 2 | 2 | 2 | 2 | 2 | 2 | 2 |
| **TOTAL MULTIPLE DX** | 4 | 5.1 | 16 | 1 | 4 | 4 | 5 | 12 | 12 | 12 |
| **TOTAL** | | | | | | | | | | |
| 0–19 Years | 0 | | | | | | | | | |
| 20–34 | 0 | | | | | | | | | |
| 35–49 | 1 | 2.0 | 0 | 2 | 2 | 2 | 2 | 2 | 2 | 2 |
| 50–64 | 0 | | | | | | | | | |
| 65+ | 4 | 5.1 | 16 | 1 | 4 | 4 | 5 | 12 | 12 | 12 |
| **GRAND TOTAL** | 5 | 4.7 | 15 | 1 | 2 | 4 | 5 | 12 | 12 | 12 |

## 60.9: OTHER PROSTATIC OPS. Formerly included in operation group(s) 667.

| Type of Patients | Observed Patients | Avg. Stay | Variance | Percentiles | | | | | | |
|---|---|---|---|---|---|---|---|---|---|---|
| | | | | 10th | 25th | 50th | 75th | 90th | 95th | 99th |
| **1. SINGLE DX** | | | | | | | | | | |
| 0–19 Years | 0 | | | | | | | | | |
| 20–34 | 0 | | | | | | | | | |
| 35–49 | 2 | 3.3 | 2 | 1 | 1 | 4 | 4 | 4 | 4 | 4 |
| 50–64 | 3 | 1.4 | <1 | 1 | 1 | 1 | 2 | 2 | 2 | 2 |
| 65+ | 7 | 1.4 | 1 | 1 | 1 | 1 | 1 | 3 | 3 | 5 |
| **2. MULTIPLE DX** | | | | | | | | | | |
| 0–19 Years | 1 | 1.0 | 0 | 1 | 1 | 1 | 1 | 1 | 1 | 1 |
| 20–34 | 2 | 3.6 | <1 | 3 | 3 | 4 | 4 | 4 | 4 | 4 |
| 35–49 | 12 | 3.9 | 21 | 1 | 1 | 3 | 5 | 5 | 20 | 20 |
| 50–64 | 47 | 4.6 | 7 | 1 | 2 | 4 | 7 | 7 | 7 | 15 |
| 65+ | 320 | 4.3 | 14 | 1 | 2 | 3 | 5 | 9 | 12 | 19 |
| **TOTAL SINGLE DX** | 12 | 1.7 | 2 | 1 | 1 | 1 | 2 | 4 | 4 | 5 |
| **TOTAL MULTIPLE DX** | 382 | 4.3 | 13 | 1 | 2 | 3 | 5 | 8 | 11 | 19 |
| **TOTAL** | | | | | | | | | | |
| 0–19 Years | 1 | 1.0 | 0 | 1 | 1 | 1 | 1 | 1 | 1 | 1 |
| 20–34 | 2 | 3.6 | <1 | 3 | 3 | 4 | 4 | 4 | 4 | 4 |
| 35–49 | 14 | 3.8 | 19 | 1 | 1 | 3 | 5 | 5 | 20 | 20 |
| 50–64 | 50 | 4.4 | 8 | 1 | 2 | 4 | 7 | 7 | 7 | 15 |
| 65+ | 327 | 4.2 | 14 | 1 | 2 | 3 | 5 | 9 | 12 | 19 |
| **GRAND TOTAL** | 394 | 4.2 | 13 | 1 | 2 | 3 | 5 | 8 | 11 | 19 |

Length of Stay by Diagnosis and Operation, United States, 2000

# United States, October 1998–September 1999 Data, by Operation

## 60.94: CNTRL POSTOP PROS HEMOR. Formerly included in operation group(s) 667.

| Type of Patients | Observed Patients | Avg. Stay | Vari-ance | 10th | 25th | 50th | 75th | 90th | 95th | 99th |
|---|---|---|---|---|---|---|---|---|---|---|
| **1. SINGLE DX** | | | | | | | | | | |
| 0–19 Years | 0 | | | | | | | | | |
| 20–34 | 0 | | | | | | | | | |
| 35–49 | 2 | 3.3 | 2 | 1 | 4 | 4 | 4 | 4 | 4 | 4 |
| 50–64 | 3 | 1.4 | <1 | 1 | 1 | 1 | 2 | 2 | 2 | 2 |
| 65+ | 6 | 1.8 | 2 | 1 | 1 | 1 | 3 | 3 | 5 | 5 |
| **2. MULTIPLE DX** | | | | | | | | | | |
| 0–19 Years | 0 | | | | | | | | | |
| 20–34 | 1 | 3.0 | 0 | 3 | 3 | 3 | 3 | 3 | 3 | 3 |
| 35–49 | 9 | 3.8 | 29 | 1 | 1 | 2 | 4 | 5 | 20 | 20 |
| 50–64 | 42 | 4.5 | 7 | 1 | 3 | 4 | 7 | 7 | 7 | 15 |
| 65+ | 279 | 4.3 | 13 | 1 | 2 | 3 | 5 | 9 | 11 | 17 |
| **TOTAL SINGLE DX** | 11 | 2.1 | 2 | 1 | 1 | 1 | 3 | 4 | 5 | 5 |
| **TOTAL MULTIPLE DX** | 331 | 4.3 | 12 | 1 | 2 | 3 | 5 | 8 | 11 | 17 |
| **TOTAL** | | | | | | | | | | |
| 0–19 Years | 0 | | | | | | | | | |
| 20–34 | 1 | 3.0 | 0 | 3 | 3 | 3 | 3 | 3 | 3 | 3 |
| 35–49 | 11 | 3.8 | 24 | 1 | 1 | 2 | 4 | 5 | 20 | 20 |
| 50–64 | 45 | 4.4 | 7 | 1 | 2 | 4 | 7 | 7 | 7 | 15 |
| 65+ | 285 | 4.2 | 13 | 1 | 2 | 3 | 5 | 9 | 11 | 17 |
| **GRAND TOTAL** | 342 | 4.2 | 12 | 1 | 2 | 3 | 5 | 8 | 11 | 17 |

## 61.0: SCROTUM & TUNICA VAG I&D. Formerly included in operation group(s) 668.

| Type of Patients | Observed Patients | Avg. Stay | Vari-ance | 10th | 25th | 50th | 75th | 90th | 95th | 99th |
|---|---|---|---|---|---|---|---|---|---|---|
| **1. SINGLE DX** | | | | | | | | | | |
| 0–19 Years | 37 | 1.6 | 2 | 1 | 1 | 1 | 2 | 2 | 5 | 8 |
| 20–34 | 35 | 1.5 | <1 | 1 | 1 | 1 | 2 | 2 | 3 | 4 |
| 35–49 | 54 | 2.3 | 2 | 1 | 1 | 2 | 2 | 4 | 6 | 7 |
| 50–64 | 19 | 2.4 | 6 | 1 | 1 | 2 | 3 | 3 | 9 | 13 |
| 65+ | 13 | 3.8 | 4 | 2 | 2 | 4 | 5 | 7 | 7 | 7 |
| **2. MULTIPLE DX** | | | | | | | | | | |
| 0–19 Years | 50 | 3.4 | 6 | 1 | 1 | 3 | 5 | 8 | 8 | 10 |
| 20–34 | 107 | 3.7 | 8 | 1 | 2 | 3 | 5 | 8 | 11 | 15 |
| 35–49 | 248 | 4.4 | 20 | 1 | 2 | 5 | 6 | 9 | 11 | 17 |
| 50–64 | 183 | 5.7 | 22 | 2 | 2 | 5 | 8 | 11 | 14 | 24 |
| 65+ | 132 | 8.7 | 69 | 2 | 3 | 6 | 10 | 21 | 32 | 32 |
| **TOTAL SINGLE DX** | 158 | 2.1 | 2 | 1 | 1 | 2 | 2 | 4 | 5 | 8 |
| **TOTAL MULTIPLE DX** | 720 | 5.3 | 28 | 1 | 2 | 4 | 6 | 10 | 13 | 32 |
| **TOTAL** | | | | | | | | | | |
| 0–19 Years | 87 | 2.5 | 5 | 1 | 1 | 2 | 3 | 5 | 8 | 10 |
| 20–34 | 142 | 3.2 | 8 | 1 | 1 | 2 | 4 | 7 | 9 | 11 |
| 35–49 | 302 | 4.0 | 17 | 1 | 2 | 3 | 5 | 9 | 10 | 17 |
| 50–64 | 202 | 5.5 | 22 | 2 | 2 | 5 | 7 | 10 | 14 | 22 |
| 65+ | 145 | 8.3 | 65 | 2 | 3 | 6 | 10 | 20 | 32 | 32 |
| **GRAND TOTAL** | 878 | 4.7 | 25 | 1 | 2 | 3 | 6 | 10 | 12 | 32 |

## 61.1: SCROTUM/TUNICA DXTIC PX. Formerly included in operation group(s) 668, 677.

| Type of Patients | Observed Patients | Avg. Stay | Vari-ance | 10th | 25th | 50th | 75th | 90th | 95th | 99th |
|---|---|---|---|---|---|---|---|---|---|---|
| **1. SINGLE DX** | | | | | | | | | | |
| 0–19 Years | 0 | | | | | | | | | |
| 20–34 | 0 | | | | | | | | | |
| 35–49 | 0 | | | | | | | | | |
| 50–64 | 0 | | | | | | | | | |
| 65+ | 0 | | | | | | | | | |
| **2. MULTIPLE DX** | | | | | | | | | | |
| 0–19 Years | 2 | 7.4 | 3 | 8 | 8 | 8 | 8 | 8 | 8 | 8 |
| 20–34 | 2 | 1.5 | 1 | 1 | 1 | 1 | 3 | 3 | 3 | 3 |
| 35–49 | 2 | 4.2 | 5 | 3 | 3 | 3 | 7 | 7 | 7 | 7 |
| 50–64 | 2 | 5.4 | 26 | 1 | 1 | 1 | 10 | 10 | 10 | 10 |
| 65+ | 1 | 16.0 | 0 | 16 | 16 | 16 | 16 | 16 | 16 | 16 |
| **TOTAL SINGLE DX** | 0 | | | | | | | | | |
| **TOTAL MULTIPLE DX** | 9 | 6.3 | 17 | 1 | 3 | 8 | 8 | 10 | 16 | 16 |
| **TOTAL** | | | | | | | | | | |
| 0–19 Years | 2 | 7.4 | 3 | 8 | 8 | 8 | 8 | 8 | 8 | 8 |
| 20–34 | 2 | 1.5 | 1 | 1 | 1 | 1 | 3 | 3 | 3 | 3 |
| 35–49 | 2 | 4.2 | 5 | 3 | 3 | 3 | 7 | 7 | 7 | 7 |
| 50–64 | 2 | 5.4 | 26 | 1 | 1 | 1 | 10 | 10 | 10 | 10 |
| 65+ | 1 | 16.0 | 0 | 16 | 16 | 16 | 16 | 16 | 16 | 16 |
| **GRAND TOTAL** | 9 | 6.3 | 17 | 1 | 3 | 8 | 8 | 10 | 16 | 16 |

## 61.2: EXCISION OF HYDROCELE. Formerly included in operation group(s) 668.

| Type of Patients | Observed Patients | Avg. Stay | Vari-ance | 10th | 25th | 50th | 75th | 90th | 95th | 99th |
|---|---|---|---|---|---|---|---|---|---|---|
| **1. SINGLE DX** | | | | | | | | | | |
| 0–19 Years | 14 | 1.0 | 0 | 1 | 1 | 1 | 1 | 1 | 1 | 1 |
| 20–34 | 4 | 2.1 | 2 | 1 | 1 | 1 | 4 | 4 | 4 | 4 |
| 35–49 | 5 | 1.5 | <1 | 1 | 1 | 1 | 2 | 2 | 2 | 2 |
| 50–64 | 1 | 1.0 | 0 | 1 | 1 | 1 | 1 | 1 | 1 | 1 |
| 65+ | 5 | 3.0 | 5 | 2 | 2 | 2 | 6 | 6 | 6 | 6 |
| **2. MULTIPLE DX** | | | | | | | | | | |
| 0–19 Years | 24 | 1.2 | <1 | 1 | 1 | 1 | 1 | 1 | 3 | 6 |
| 20–34 | 7 | 2.4 | 3 | 1 | 1 | 2 | 3 | 5 | 5 | 5 |
| 35–49 | 15 | 5.8 | 24 | 1 | 1 | 3 | 9 | 14 | 14 | 14 |
| 50–64 | 26 | 2.8 | 12 | 1 | 2 | 2 | 3 | 4 | 14 | 17 |
| 65+ | 68 | 3.0 | 6 | 1 | 2 | 2 | 3 | 6 | 8 | 13 |
| **TOTAL SINGLE DX** | 29 | 1.5 | 1 | 1 | 1 | 1 | 1 | 2 | 4 | 6 |
| **TOTAL MULTIPLE DX** | 140 | 2.8 | 9 | 1 | 1 | 2 | 3 | 6 | 9 | 14 |
| **TOTAL** | | | | | | | | | | |
| 0–19 Years | 38 | 1.2 | <1 | 1 | 1 | 1 | 1 | 1 | 3 | 6 |
| 20–34 | 11 | 2.3 | 2 | 1 | 1 | 2 | 3 | 5 | 5 | 5 |
| 35–49 | 20 | 5.0 | 22 | 1 | 1 | 2 | 8 | 14 | 14 | 14 |
| 50–64 | 27 | 2.8 | 12 | 1 | 2 | 2 | 3 | 4 | 14 | 17 |
| 65+ | 73 | 3.0 | 6 | 1 | 2 | 2 | 3 | 6 | 8 | 13 |
| **GRAND TOTAL** | 169 | 2.6 | 8 | 1 | 1 | 2 | 3 | 5 | 9 | 14 |

Length of Stay by Diagnosis and Operation, United States, 2000

# United States, October 1998–September 1999 Data, by Operation

## 61.3: SCROTAL LES EXC/DESTR. Formerly included in operation group(s) 668.

| Type of Patients | Observed Patients | Avg. Stay | Variance | Percentiles | | | | | | |
|---|---|---|---|---|---|---|---|---|---|---|
| | | | | 10th | 25th | 50th | 75th | 90th | 95th | 99th |
| 1. SINGLE DX | | | | | | | | | | |
| 0–19 Years | 5 | 1.1 | <1 | 1 | 1 | 1 | 1 | 1 | 2 | 2 |
| 20–34 | 6 | 1.6 | <1 | 1 | 1 | 1 | 2 | 3 | 3 | 3 |
| 35–49 | 5 | 4.7 | 22 | 2 | 2 | 4 | 4 | 13 | 13 | 13 |
| 50–64 | 6 | 4.3 | 15 | 1 | 1 | 2 | 8 | 11 | 11 | 11 |
| 65+ | 2 | 1.5 | 3 | 1 | 1 | 1 | 1 | 1 | 8 | 8 |
| 2. MULTIPLE DX | | | | | | | | | | |
| 0–19 Years | 5 | 5.4 | 2 | 4 | 4 | 6 | 6 | 6 | 7 | 7 |
| 20–34 | 18 | 21.4 | 599 | 1 | 4 | 9 | 60 | 60 | 60 | 60 |
| 35–49 | 46 | 6.5 | 35 | 1 | 2 | 6 | 7 | 10 | 15 | 35 |
| 50–64 | 56 | 7.2 | 21 | 2 | 4 | 7 | 9 | 13 | 17 | 22 |
| 65+ | 30 | 7.5 | 54 | 2 | 3 | 5 | 7 | 18 | 30 | 30 |
| TOTAL SINGLE DX | 24 | 2.1 | 6 | 1 | 1 | 1 | 2 | 4 | 8 | 13 |
| TOTAL MULTIPLE DX | 155 | 8.9 | 137 | 2 | 3 | 6 | 9 | 16 | 30 | 60 |
| TOTAL | | | | | | | | | | |
| 0–19 Years | 10 | 4.0 | 5 | 1 | 1 | 4 | 6 | 6 | 7 | 7 |
| 20–34 | 24 | 12.2 | 419 | 1 | 1 | 3 | 9 | 60 | 60 | 60 |
| 35–49 | 51 | 6.3 | 34 | 1 | 2 | 6 | 7 | 10 | 14 | 35 |
| 50–64 | 62 | 6.9 | 21 | 2 | 4 | 6 | 9 | 12 | 16 | 22 |
| 65+ | 32 | 6.2 | 49 | 1 | 2 | 4 | 7 | 18 | 23 | 30 |
| GRAND TOTAL | 179 | 7.5 | 118 | 1 | 2 | 5 | 8 | 13 | 23 | 60 |

## 61.9: OTH SCROT/TUNICA VAG OPS. Formerly included in operation group(s) 668.

| Type of Patients | Observed Patients | Avg. Stay | Variance | Percentiles | | | | | | |
|---|---|---|---|---|---|---|---|---|---|---|
| | | | | 10th | 25th | 50th | 75th | 90th | 95th | 99th |
| 1. SINGLE DX | | | | | | | | | | |
| 0–19 Years | 0 | | | | | | | | | |
| 20–34 | 4 | 1.8 | 2 | 1 | 1 | 1 | 2 | 4 | 4 | 4 |
| 35–49 | 0 | | | | | | | | | |
| 50–64 | 1 | 1.0 | 0 | 1 | 1 | 1 | 1 | 1 | 1 | 1 |
| 65+ | 0 | | | | | | | | | |
| 2. MULTIPLE DX | | | | | | | | | | |
| 0–19 Years | 1 | 2.0 | 0 | 2 | 2 | 2 | 2 | 2 | 2 | 2 |
| 20–34 | 3 | 2.0 | 0 | 2 | 2 | 2 | 2 | 2 | 8 | 8 |
| 35–49 | 2 | 3.7 | 17 | 1 | 1 | 1 | 5 | 8 | 8 | 8 |
| 50–64 | 7 | 4.3 | 4 | 3 | 3 | 3 | 5 | 8 | 8 | 8 |
| 65+ | 9 | 6.5 | 5 | 3 | 4 | 8 | 8 | 8 | 10 | 10 |
| TOTAL SINGLE DX | 5 | 1.6 | 1 | 1 | 1 | 1 | 2 | 4 | 4 | 4 |
| TOTAL MULTIPLE DX | 22 | 4.8 | 6 | 2 | 3 | 4 | 8 | 8 | 8 | 10 |
| TOTAL | | | | | | | | | | |
| 0–19 Years | 1 | 2.0 | 0 | 2 | 2 | 2 | 2 | 2 | 2 | 2 |
| 20–34 | 7 | 1.9 | <1 | 1 | 1 | 1 | 2 | 4 | 4 | 4 |
| 35–49 | 2 | 3.7 | 17 | 1 | 1 | 3 | 5 | 8 | 8 | 8 |
| 50–64 | 8 | 4.0 | 5 | 3 | 3 | 3 | 5 | 8 | 8 | 8 |
| 65+ | 9 | 6.5 | 5 | 3 | 4 | 8 | 8 | 8 | 10 | 10 |
| GRAND TOTAL | 27 | 4.4 | 7 | 1 | 2 | 3 | 8 | 8 | 8 | 10 |

## 61.4: SCROTUM & TUNICA VAG REP. Formerly included in operation group(s) 668.

| Type of Patients | Observed Patients | Avg. Stay | Variance | Percentiles | | | | | | |
|---|---|---|---|---|---|---|---|---|---|---|
| | | | | 10th | 25th | 50th | 75th | 90th | 95th | 99th |
| 1. SINGLE DX | | | | | | | | | | |
| 0–19 Years | 12 | 1.3 | <1 | 1 | 1 | 1 | 1 | 1 | 3 | 3 |
| 20–34 | 2 | 4.2 | 2 | 3 | 3 | 3 | 6 | 6 | 6 | 6 |
| 35–49 | 5 | 2.2 | 1 | 2 | 2 | 2 | 2 | 2 | 7 | 7 |
| 50–64 | 1 | 1.0 | 0 | 1 | 1 | 1 | 1 | 1 | 1 | 1 |
| 65+ | 0 | | | | | | | | | |
| 2. MULTIPLE DX | | | | | | | | | | |
| 0–19 Years | 12 | 2.7 | 3 | 1 | 1 | 2 | 5 | 5 | 5 | 6 |
| 20–34 | 19 | 3.5 | 39 | 1 | 1 | 2 | 2 | 5 | 19 | 40 |
| 35–49 | 27 | 12.1 | 164 | 1 | 2 | 5 | 17 | 40 | 40 | 40 |
| 50–64 | 24 | 6.7 | 68 | 2 | 2 | 5 | 8 | 28 | 28 | 29 |
| 65+ | 17 | 8.2 | 37 | 3 | 6 | 7 | 7 | 14 | 17 | 35 |
| TOTAL SINGLE DX | 20 | 2.1 | 1 | 1 | 1 | 2 | 2 | 3 | 6 | 7 |
| TOTAL MULTIPLE DX | 99 | 6.7 | 74 | 1 | 2 | 3 | 7 | 17 | 28 | 40 |
| TOTAL | | | | | | | | | | |
| 0–19 Years | 24 | 2.1 | 2 | 1 | 1 | 1 | 3 | 5 | 5 | 6 |
| 20–34 | 21 | 3.5 | 36 | 1 | 1 | 2 | 2 | 24 | 19 | 30 |
| 35–49 | 32 | 6.6 | 98 | 2 | 2 | 3 | 5 | 24 | 28 | 40 |
| 50–64 | 25 | 6.6 | 68 | 2 | 2 | 3 | 8 | 28 | 28 | 29 |
| 65+ | 17 | 8.2 | 37 | 3 | 6 | 7 | 7 | 14 | 17 | 35 |
| GRAND TOTAL | 119 | 5.5 | 60 | 1 | 2 | 2 | 7 | 14 | 28 | 40 |

## 62.0: INCISION OF TESTIS. Formerly included in operation group(s) 671.

| Type of Patients | Observed Patients | Avg. Stay | Variance | Percentiles | | | | | | |
|---|---|---|---|---|---|---|---|---|---|---|
| | | | | 10th | 25th | 50th | 75th | 90th | 95th | 99th |
| 1. SINGLE DX | | | | | | | | | | |
| 0–19 Years | 13 | 1.2 | <1 | 1 | 1 | 1 | 1 | 2 | 2 | 2 |
| 20–34 | 6 | 1.2 | <1 | 1 | 1 | 1 | 1 | 1 | 1 | 1 |
| 35–49 | 1 | 1.0 | 0 | 1 | 1 | 1 | 1 | 1 | 1 | 1 |
| 50–64 | 0 | | | | | | | | | |
| 65+ | 0 | | | | | | | | | |
| 2. MULTIPLE DX | | | | | | | | | | |
| 0–19 Years | 10 | 2.8 | 3 | 1 | 1 | 2 | 2 | 5 | 5 | 5 |
| 20–34 | 6 | 9.3 | 29 | 3 | 3 | 13 | 13 | 13 | 13 | 13 |
| 35–49 | 2 | 4.4 | 2 | 2 | 4 | 5 | 5 | 5 | 5 | 7 |
| 50–64 | 3 | 4.4 | 8 | 1 | 6 | 6 | 7 | 7 | 7 | 7 |
| 65+ | 5 | 8.5 | 48 | 1 | 6 | 6 | 11 | 22 | 22 | 22 |
| TOTAL SINGLE DX | 20 | 1.2 | <1 | 1 | 1 | 1 | 1 | 2 | 2 | 2 |
| TOTAL MULTIPLE DX | 26 | 4.4 | 14 | 1 | 2 | 5 | 5 | 7 | 13 | 22 |
| TOTAL | | | | | | | | | | |
| 0–19 Years | 23 | 1.7 | 2 | 1 | 1 | 1 | 2 | 5 | 5 | 5 |
| 20–34 | 8 | 2.4 | 11 | 1 | 2 | 5 | 5 | 3 | 13 | 13 |
| 35–49 | 3 | 3.9 | 3 | 2 | 2 | 2 | 5 | 5 | 5 | 7 |
| 50–64 | 3 | 4.4 | 8 | 1 | 6 | 6 | 7 | 7 | 7 | 7 |
| 65+ | 5 | 8.5 | 48 | 1 | 6 | 6 | 11 | 22 | 22 | 22 |
| GRAND TOTAL | 46 | 2.6 | 9 | 1 | 1 | 1 | 4 | 5 | 7 | 13 |

Length of Stay by Diagnosis and Operation, United States, 2000

# United States, October 1998–September 1999 Data, by Operation

## 62.1: TESTES DXTIC PX. Formerly included in operation group(s) 671, 677.

| Type of Patients | Observed Patients | Avg. Stay | Variance | Percentiles | | | | | | |
|---|---|---|---|---|---|---|---|---|---|---|
| | | | | 10th | 25th | 50th | 75th | 90th | 95th | 99th |
| **1. SINGLE DX** | | | | | | | | | | |
| 0–19 Years | 5 | 5.0 | 19 | 1 | 2 | 2 | 11 | 11 | 11 | 11 |
| 20–34 | 1 | 1.0 | 0 | 1 | 1 | 1 | 1 | 1 | 1 | 1 |
| 35–49 | 2 | 1.3 | <1 | 1 | 1 | 1 | 2 | 2 | 2 | 2 |
| 50–64 | 0 | | | | | | | | | |
| 65+ | 0 | | | | | | | | | |
| **2. MULTIPLE DX** | | | | | | | | | | |
| 0–19 Years | 16 | 6.2 | 92 | 1 | 1 | 4 | 7 | 7 | 25 | 53 |
| 20–34 | 3 | 1.7 | 2 | 1 | 1 | 1 | 1 | 4 | 4 | 4 |
| 35–49 | 4 | 5.8 | 8 | 2 | 2 | 8 | 8 | 8 | 8 | 8 |
| 50–64 | 1 | 16.0 | 0 | 16 | 16 | 16 | 16 | 16 | 16 | 16 |
| 65+ | 3 | 1.7 | <1 | 1 | 1 | 2 | 2 | 2 | 2 | 2 |
| **TOTAL SINGLE DX** | 8 | 3.5 | 15 | 1 | 1 | 2 | 3 | 11 | 11 | 11 |
| **TOTAL MULTIPLE DX** | 27 | 6.3 | 69 | 1 | 2 | 4 | 7 | 16 | 16 | 53 |
| **TOTAL** | | | | | | | | | | |
| 0–19 Years | 21 | 6.0 | 79 | 1 | 1 | 4 | 7 | 11 | 17 | 53 |
| 20–34 | 4 | 1.5 | 2 | 1 | 1 | 1 | 1 | 4 | 4 | 4 |
| 35–49 | 6 | 4.5 | 10 | 2 | 2 | 2 | 8 | 8 | 8 | 8 |
| 50–64 | 1 | 16.0 | 0 | 16 | 16 | 16 | 16 | 16 | 16 | 16 |
| 65+ | 3 | 1.7 | <1 | 1 | 1 | 2 | 2 | 2 | 2 | 2 |
| **GRAND TOTAL** | 35 | 5.8 | 60 | 1 | 1 | 4 | 7 | 16 | 16 | 53 |

## 62.2: TESTICULAR LES DESTR/EXC. Formerly included in operation group(s) 671.

| Type of Patients | Observed Patients | Avg. Stay | Variance | Percentiles | | | | | | |
|---|---|---|---|---|---|---|---|---|---|---|
| | | | | 10th | 25th | 50th | 75th | 90th | 95th | 99th |
| **1. SINGLE DX** | | | | | | | | | | |
| 0–19 Years | 40 | 1.2 | <1 | 1 | 1 | 1 | 1 | 1 | 3 | 5 |
| 20–34 | 3 | 1.0 | 0 | 1 | 1 | 1 | 1 | 1 | 1 | 1 |
| 35–49 | 0 | | | | | | | | | |
| 50–64 | 0 | | | | | | | | | |
| 65+ | 2 | 1.9 | <1 | 1 | 2 | 2 | 2 | 2 | 2 | 2 |
| **2. MULTIPLE DX** | | | | | | | | | | |
| 0–19 Years | 21 | 1.1 | <1 | 1 | 1 | 1 | 1 | 1 | 3 | 3 |
| 20–34 | 2 | 3.7 | 12 | 1 | 1 | 6 | 6 | 6 | 6 | 6 |
| 35–49 | 2 | 10.6 | 43 | 2 | 2 | 15 | 15 | 15 | 15 | 15 |
| 50–64 | 0 | | | | | | | | | |
| 65+ | 5 | 6.1 | 16 | 1 | 2 | 8 | 11 | 11 | 11 | 11 |
| **TOTAL SINGLE DX** | 45 | 1.2 | <1 | 1 | 1 | 1 | 1 | 2 | 2 | 5 |
| **TOTAL MULTIPLE DX** | 30 | 2.8 | 16 | 1 | 1 | 1 | 2 | 11 | 15 | 15 |
| **TOTAL** | | | | | | | | | | |
| 0–19 Years | 61 | 1.2 | <1 | 1 | 1 | 1 | 1 | 1 | 3 | 5 |
| 20–34 | 5 | 1.8 | 4 | 1 | 1 | 1 | 1 | 6 | 6 | 6 |
| 35–49 | 2 | 10.6 | 43 | 2 | 2 | 15 | 15 | 15 | 15 | 15 |
| 50–64 | 0 | | | | | | | | | |
| 65+ | 7 | 3.7 | 11 | 1 | 2 | 2 | 4 | 11 | 11 | 11 |
| **GRAND TOTAL** | 75 | 1.8 | 7 | 1 | 1 | 1 | 1 | 3 | 6 | 15 |

## 62.3: UNILATERAL ORCHIECTOMY. Formerly included in operation group(s) 669.

| Type of Patients | Observed Patients | Avg. Stay | Variance | Percentiles | | | | | | |
|---|---|---|---|---|---|---|---|---|---|---|
| | | | | 10th | 25th | 50th | 75th | 90th | 95th | 99th |
| **1. SINGLE DX** | | | | | | | | | | |
| 0–19 Years | 162 | 1.3 | <1 | 1 | 1 | 1 | 1 | 2 | 2 | 4 |
| 20–34 | 120 | 1.7 | 2 | 1 | 1 | 1 | 2 | 3 | 4 | 8 |
| 35–49 | 40 | 2.3 | 3 | 1 | 1 | 2 | 3 | 4 | 5 | 9 |
| 50–64 | 18 | 1.8 | 3 | 1 | 1 | 1 | 1 | 4 | 6 | 8 |
| 65+ | 11 | 2.0 | 2 | 1 | 1 | 1 | 3 | 5 | 5 | 5 |
| **2. MULTIPLE DX** | | | | | | | | | | |
| 0–19 Years | 194 | 2.0 | 3 | 1 | 1 | 2 | 2 | 4 | 5 | 8 |
| 20–34 | 150 | 5.6 | 29 | 1 | 1 | 3 | 8 | 15 | 15 | 19 |
| 35–49 | 172 | 5.0 | 21 | 1 | 2 | 3 | 8 | 9 | 11 | 28 |
| 50–64 | 108 | 5.2 | 34 | 1 | 1 | 2 | 7 | 14 | 17 | 34 |
| 65+ | 243 | 5.7 | 22 | 1 | 2 | 5 | 8 | 12 | 12 | 22 |
| **TOTAL SINGLE DX** | 351 | 1.5 | 1 | 1 | 1 | 1 | 2 | 2 | 4 | 7 |
| **TOTAL MULTIPLE DX** | 867 | 4.5 | 22 | 1 | 1 | 3 | 7 | 10 | 15 | 19 |
| **TOTAL** | | | | | | | | | | |
| 0–19 Years | 356 | 1.6 | 2 | 1 | 1 | 1 | 2 | 3 | 4 | 7 |
| 20–34 | 270 | 3.9 | 20 | 1 | 1 | 2 | 4 | 11 | 15 | 19 |
| 35–49 | 212 | 4.6 | 20 | 1 | 1 | 3 | 7 | 9 | 11 | 24 |
| 50–64 | 126 | 4.6 | 30 | 1 | 2 | 5 | 5 | 13 | 17 | 23 |
| 65+ | 254 | 5.6 | 22 | 1 | 2 | 5 | 8 | 12 | 12 | 22 |
| **GRAND TOTAL** | 1,218 | 3.6 | 17 | 1 | 1 | 2 | 4 | 9 | 12 | 18 |

## 62.4: BILATERAL ORCHIECTOMY. Formerly included in operation group(s) 669.

| Type of Patients | Observed Patients | Avg. Stay | Variance | Percentiles | | | | | | |
|---|---|---|---|---|---|---|---|---|---|---|
| | | | | 10th | 25th | 50th | 75th | 90th | 95th | 99th |
| **1. SINGLE DX** | | | | | | | | | | |
| 0–19 Years | 3 | 1.0 | 0 | 1 | 1 | 1 | 1 | 1 | 1 | 1 |
| 20–34 | 3 | 2.4 | <1 | 1 | 2 | 3 | 3 | 3 | 3 | 3 |
| 35–49 | 3 | 1.3 | <1 | 1 | 1 | 1 | 2 | 2 | 2 | 2 |
| 50–64 | 2 | 1.2 | <1 | 1 | 1 | 1 | 1 | 2 | 2 | 2 |
| 65+ | 21 | 1.5 | <1 | 1 | 1 | 1 | 2 | 3 | 3 | 3 |
| **2. MULTIPLE DX** | | | | | | | | | | |
| 0–19 Years | 3 | 4.0 | 16 | 1 | 1 | 2 | 2 | 8 | 8 | 8 |
| 20–34 | 11 | 2.5 | 10 | 1 | 1 | 1 | 2 | 7 | 7 | 16 |
| 35–49 | 5 | 5.2 | 3 | 2 | 2 | 3 | 4 | 4 | 8 | 8 |
| 50–64 | 69 | 11.2 | 74 | 2 | 5 | 10 | 14 | 19 | 36 | 36 |
| 65+ | 564 | 7.0 | 82 | 1 | 2 | 5 | 9 | 14 | 19 | 47 |
| **TOTAL SINGLE DX** | 32 | 1.4 | <1 | 1 | 1 | 1 | 2 | 3 | 3 | 3 |
| **TOTAL MULTIPLE DX** | 652 | 7.4 | 81 | 1 | 2 | 5 | 9 | 14 | 21 | 40 |
| **TOTAL** | | | | | | | | | | |
| 0–19 Years | 6 | 1.6 | 4 | 1 | 1 | 1 | 1 | 2 | 8 | 8 |
| 20–34 | 14 | 2.5 | 9 | 1 | 1 | 3 | 3 | 7 | 7 | 16 |
| 35–49 | 8 | 2.9 | 3 | 1 | 3 | 3 | 4 | 4 | 8 | 8 |
| 50–64 | 71 | 11.0 | 74 | 1 | 5 | 10 | 14 | 19 | 36 | 36 |
| 65+ | 585 | 6.9 | 81 | 1 | 2 | 4 | 8 | 14 | 19 | 41 |
| **GRAND TOTAL** | 684 | 7.2 | 79 | 1 | 2 | 5 | 9 | 14 | 19 | 40 |

Length of Stay by Diagnosis and Operation, United States, 2000

# United States, October 1998–September 1999 Data, by Operation

## 62.41: RMVL BOTH TESTES. Formerly included in operation group(s) 669.

| Type of Patients | Observed Patients | Avg. Stay | Variance | 10th | 25th | 50th | 75th | 90th | 95th | 99th |
|---|---|---|---|---|---|---|---|---|---|---|
| **1. SINGLE DX** | | | | | | | | | | |
| 0–19 Years | 3 | 1.0 | 0 | 1 | | 1 | 1 | 1 | 1 | 1 |
| 20–34 | 3 | 2.4 | <1 | 1 | 2 | 3 | 3 | 3 | 3 | 3 |
| 35–49 | 3 | 1.3 | <1 | 1 | 2 | 1 | 2 | 2 | 2 | 2 |
| 50–64 | 2 | 1.2 | <1 | 1 | 1 | 1 | 1 | 2 | 2 | 2 |
| 65+ | 21 | 1.5 | <1 | 1 | 1 | 1 | 2 | 3 | 3 | 3 |
| **2. MULTIPLE DX** | | | | | | | | | | |
| 0–19 Years | 0 | | | | | | | | | |
| 20–34 | 5 | 3.6 | 6 | 1 | 2 | 2 | 7 | 7 | 7 | 7 |
| 35–49 | 4 | 3.8 | 3 | 2 | 3 | 3 | 4 | 8 | 8 | 8 |
| 50–64 | 67 | 10.9 | 89 | 1 | 5 | 7 | 15 | 23 | 36 | 36 |
| 65+ | 557 | 7.1 | 83 | 1 | 2 | 5 | 9 | 14 | 19 | 47 |
| **TOTAL SINGLE DX** | 32 | 1.4 | <1 | 1 | 1 | 1 | 2 | 3 | 3 | 3 |
| **TOTAL MULTIPLE DX** | 633 | 7.5 | 84 | 1 | 2 | 5 | 9 | 15 | 21 | 41 |
| **TOTAL** | | | | | | | | | | |
| 0–19 | 3 | 1.0 | 0 | 1 | 1 | 1 | 1 | 1 | 1 | 1 |
| 20–34 | 8 | 3.2 | 4 | 1 | 2 | 3 | 3 | 7 | 7 | 7 |
| 35–49 | 7 | 3.0 | 4 | 1 | 2 | 3 | 4 | 8 | 8 | 8 |
| 50–64 | 69 | 10.7 | 89 | 1 | 5 | 7 | 14 | 23 | 36 | 36 |
| 65+ | 578 | 7.0 | 82 | 1 | 2 | 5 | 9 | 14 | 19 | 41 |
| **GRAND TOTAL** | 665 | 7.3 | 82 | 1 | 2 | 5 | 9 | 15 | 21 | 40 |

## 62.5: ORCHIOPEXY. Formerly included in operation group(s) 670.

| Type of Patients | Observed Patients | Avg. Stay | Variance | 10th | 25th | 50th | 75th | 90th | 95th | 99th |
|---|---|---|---|---|---|---|---|---|---|---|
| **1. SINGLE DX** | | | | | | | | | | |
| 0–19 Years | 371 | 1.1 | <1 | 1 | 1 | 1 | 1 | 1 | 2 | 3 |
| 20–34 | 69 | 1.0 | <1 | 1 | 1 | 1 | 1 | 1 | 1 | 2 |
| 35–49 | 7 | 1.0 | 0 | 1 | 1 | 1 | 1 | 1 | 1 | 1 |
| 50–64 | 2 | 2.8 | <1 | 3 | 3 | 3 | 3 | 3 | 3 | 3 |
| 65+ | 0 | | | | | | | | | |
| **2. MULTIPLE DX** | | | | | | | | | | |
| 0–19 Years | 261 | 1.7 | 3 | 1 | 1 | 1 | 2 | 4 | 4 | 8 |
| 20–34 | 39 | 1.7 | 3 | 1 | 1 | 1 | 2 | 4 | 4 | 6 |
| 35–49 | 12 | 1.7 | <1 | 1 | 1 | 1 | 3 | 3 | 3 | 3 |
| 50–64 | 4 | 3.6 | 6 | 1 | 5 | 4 | 7 | 7 | >99 | >99 |
| 65+ | 2 | 1.0 | 0 | 1 | 1 | 1 | 1 | 1 | 1 | 1 |
| **TOTAL SINGLE DX** | 449 | 1.1 | <1 | 1 | 1 | 1 | 1 | 1 | 2 | 3 |
| **TOTAL MULTIPLE DX** | 318 | 1.7 | 3 | 1 | 1 | 1 | 2 | 4 | 4 | 8 |
| **TOTAL** | | | | | | | | | | |
| 0–19 | 632 | 1.3 | 1 | 1 | 1 | 1 | 1 | 2 | 4 | 7 |
| 20–34 | 108 | 1.3 | 1 | 1 | 1 | 1 | 1 | 2 | 3 | 5 |
| 35–49 | 19 | 1.2 | <1 | 1 | 1 | 1 | 1 | 3 | 3 | 3 |
| 50–64 | 6 | 3.2 | 3 | 1 | 3 | 3 | 4 | 7 | 7 | >99 |
| 65+ | 2 | 1.0 | 0 | 1 | 1 | 1 | 1 | 1 | 1 | 1 |
| **GRAND TOTAL** | 767 | 1.3 | 1 | 1 | 1 | 1 | 1 | 2 | 4 | 7 |

## 62.6: REPAIR OF TESTES. Formerly included in operation group(s) 671.

| Type of Patients | Observed Patients | Avg. Stay | Variance | 10th | 25th | 50th | 75th | 90th | 95th | 99th |
|---|---|---|---|---|---|---|---|---|---|---|
| **1. SINGLE DX** | | | | | | | | | | |
| 0–19 Years | 7 | 1.8 | 2 | 1 | 1 | 1 | 4 | 4 | 4 | 4 |
| 20–34 | 9 | 1.2 | <1 | 1 | 1 | 1 | 1 | 1 | 1 | 1 |
| 35–49 | 1 | 1.0 | 0 | 1 | 1 | 1 | 1 | 1 | 1 | 1 |
| 50–64 | 0 | | | | | | | | | |
| 65+ | 0 | | | | | | | | | |
| **2. MULTIPLE DX** | | | | | | | | | | |
| 0–19 Years | 8 | 1.7 | 1 | 1 | 1 | 1 | 3 | 3 | 4 | 4 |
| 20–34 | 6 | 1.7 | <1 | 1 | 1 | 2 | 2 | 3 | 3 | 3 |
| 35–49 | 3 | 1.8 | <1 | 1 | 2 | 2 | 2 | 2 | 2 | 2 |
| 50–64 | 1 | 1.0 | 0 | 1 | 1 | 1 | 1 | 1 | 1 | 1 |
| 65+ | 0 | | | | | | | | | |
| **TOTAL SINGLE DX** | 17 | 1.4 | 1 | 1 | 1 | 1 | 1 | 4 | 4 | 4 |
| **TOTAL MULTIPLE DX** | 18 | 1.6 | <1 | 1 | 1 | 1 | 2 | 3 | 3 | 4 |
| **TOTAL** | | | | | | | | | | |
| 0–19 | 15 | 1.8 | 1 | 1 | 1 | 1 | 3 | 4 | 4 | 4 |
| 20–34 | 15 | 1.3 | <1 | 1 | 1 | 1 | 1 | 2 | 3 | 4 |
| 35–49 | 4 | 1.7 | <1 | 1 | 2 | 2 | 2 | 2 | 2 | 2 |
| 50–64 | 1 | 1.0 | 0 | 1 | 1 | 1 | 1 | 1 | 1 | 1 |
| 65+ | 0 | | | | | | | | | |
| **GRAND TOTAL** | 35 | 1.5 | <1 | 1 | 1 | 1 | 2 | 3 | 4 | 4 |

## 62.7: INSERT TESTICULAR PROSTH. Formerly included in operation group(s) 671.

| Type of Patients | Observed Patients | Avg. Stay | Variance | 10th | 25th | 50th | 75th | 90th | 95th | 99th |
|---|---|---|---|---|---|---|---|---|---|---|
| **1. SINGLE DX** | | | | | | | | | | |
| 0–19 Years | 4 | 1.0 | 0 | 1 | 1 | 1 | 1 | 1 | 1 | 1 |
| 20–34 | 0 | | | | | | | | | |
| 35–49 | 2 | 2.5 | 4 | 1 | 1 | 1 | 5 | 5 | 5 | 5 |
| 50–64 | 0 | | | | | | | | | |
| 65+ | 0 | | | | | | | | | |
| **2. MULTIPLE DX** | | | | | | | | | | |
| 0–19 Years | 2 | 1.0 | 0 | 1 | 1 | 1 | 1 | 1 | 1 | 1 |
| 20–34 | 0 | | | | | | | | | |
| 35–49 | 1 | 1.0 | 0 | 1 | 1 | 1 | 1 | 1 | 1 | 1 |
| 50–64 | 0 | | | | | | | | | |
| 65+ | 0 | | | | | | | | | |
| **TOTAL SINGLE DX** | 6 | 1.7 | 2 | 1 | 1 | 1 | 1 | 5 | 5 | 5 |
| **TOTAL MULTIPLE DX** | 3 | 1.0 | 0 | 1 | 1 | 1 | 1 | 1 | 1 | 1 |
| **TOTAL** | | | | | | | | | | |
| 0–19 | 6 | 1.0 | 0 | 1 | 1 | 1 | 1 | 1 | 1 | 1 |
| 20–34 | 0 | | | | | | | | | |
| 35–49 | 3 | 1.9 | 3 | 1 | 1 | 1 | 5 | 5 | 5 | 5 |
| 50–64 | 0 | | | | | | | | | |
| 65+ | 0 | | | | | | | | | |
| **GRAND TOTAL** | 9 | 1.2 | <1 | 1 | 1 | 1 | 1 | 5 | 5 | 5 |

Length of Stay by Diagnosis and Operation, United States, 2000

## United States, October 1998–September 1999 Data, by Operation

### 62.9: OTHER TESTICULAR OPS. Formerly included in operation group(s) 671.

| Type of Patients | Observed Patients | Avg. Stay | Vari- ance | 10th | 25th | 50th | 75th | 90th | 95th | 99th |
|---|---|---|---|---|---|---|---|---|---|---|
| **1. SINGLE DX** | | | | | | | | | | |
| 0–19 Years | 1 | 1.0 | 0 | 1 | 1 | 1 | 1 | 1 | 1 | 1 |
| 20–34 | 0 | | | | | | | | | |
| 35–49 | 0 | | | | | | | | | |
| 50–64 | 1 | 1.0 | 0 | 1 | 1 | 1 | 1 | 1 | 1 | 1 |
| 65+ | 0 | | | | | | | | | |
| **2. MULTIPLE DX** | | | | | | | | | | |
| 0–19 Years | 2 | 2.1 | <1 | 2 | 2 | 2 | 2 | 3 | 3 | 3 |
| 20–34 | 0 | | | | | | | | | |
| 35–49 | 2 | 10.1 | 1 | 9 | 9 | 11 | 11 | 11 | 11 | 11 |
| 50–64 | 2 | 6.4 | 4 | 5 | 5 | 5 | 9 | 9 | 9 | 9 |
| 65+ | 2 | 3.5 | 5 | 1 | 1 | 5 | 5 | 5 | 5 | 5 |
| **TOTAL SINGLE DX** | 2 | 1.0 | 0 | 1 | 1 | 1 | 1 | 1 | 1 | 1 |
| **TOTAL MULTIPLE DX** | 8 | 3.8 | 9 | 2 | 2 | 2 | 5 | 9 | 11 | 11 |
| **TOTAL** | | | | | | | | | | |
| 0–19 Years | 3 | 2.0 | <1 | 2 | 2 | 2 | 2 | 3 | 3 | 3 |
| 20–34 | 0 | | | | | | | | | |
| 35–49 | 2 | 10.1 | 1 | 9 | 9 | 11 | 11 | 11 | 11 | 11 |
| 50–64 | 3 | 5.5 | 8 | 1 | 5 | 5 | 9 | 9 | 9 | 9 |
| 65+ | 2 | 3.5 | 5 | 1 | 1 | 5 | 5 | 5 | 5 | 5 |
| **GRAND TOTAL** | 10 | 3.6 | 9 | 1 | 2 | 2 | 5 | 9 | 11 | 11 |

### 63.0: SPERMATIC CORD DXTIC PX. Formerly included in operation group(s) 673, 677.

| Type of Patients | Observed Patients | Avg. Stay | Vari- ance | 10th | 25th | 50th | 75th | 90th | 95th | 99th |
|---|---|---|---|---|---|---|---|---|---|---|
| **1. SINGLE DX** | | | | | | | | | | |
| 0–19 Years | 0 | | | | | | | | | |
| 20–34 | 0 | | | | | | | | | |
| 35–49 | 0 | | | | | | | | | |
| 50–64 | 0 | | | | | | | | | |
| 65+ | 0 | | | | | | | | | |
| **2. MULTIPLE DX** | | | | | | | | | | |
| 0–19 Years | 1 | 1.0 | 0 | 1 | 1 | 1 | 1 | 1 | 1 | 1 |
| 20–34 | 0 | | | | | | | | | |
| 35–49 | 0 | | | | | | | | | |
| 50–64 | 1 | 3.0 | 0 | 3 | 3 | 3 | 3 | 3 | 3 | 3 |
| 65+ | 1 | 11.0 | 0 | 11 | 11 | 11 | 11 | 11 | 11 | 11 |
| **TOTAL SINGLE DX** | 0 | | | | | | | | | |
| **TOTAL MULTIPLE DX** | 3 | 4.0 | 19 | 1 | 1 | 3 | 11 | 11 | 11 | 11 |
| **TOTAL** | | | | | | | | | | |
| 0–19 Years | 1 | 1.0 | 0 | 1 | 1 | 1 | 1 | 1 | 1 | 1 |
| 20–34 | 0 | | | | | | | | | |
| 35–49 | 0 | | | | | | | | | |
| 50–64 | 1 | 3.0 | 0 | 3 | 3 | 3 | 3 | 3 | 3 | 3 |
| 65+ | 1 | 11.0 | 0 | 11 | 11 | 11 | 11 | 11 | 11 | 11 |
| **GRAND TOTAL** | 3 | 4.0 | 19 | 1 | 1 | 3 | 11 | 11 | 11 | 11 |

### 63.1: EXC SPERMATIC VARICOCELE. Formerly included in operation group(s) 673.

| Type of Patients | Observed Patients | Avg. Stay | Vari- ance | 10th | 25th | 50th | 75th | 90th | 95th | 99th |
|---|---|---|---|---|---|---|---|---|---|---|
| **1. SINGLE DX** | | | | | | | | | | |
| 0–19 Years | 42 | 1.1 | <1 | 1 | 1 | 1 | 1 | 1 | 2 | 3 |
| 20–34 | 6 | 1.6 | <1 | 1 | 1 | 1 | 2 | 2 | 3 | 3 |
| 35–49 | 7 | 2.6 | 11 | 1 | 1 | 1 | 2 | 10 | 10 | 10 |
| 50–64 | 13 | 1.8 | 1 | 1 | 1 | 1 | 3 | 4 | 4 | 4 |
| 65+ | 2 | 1.7 | 1 | 1 | 1 | 1 | 3 | 3 | 3 | 3 |
| **2. MULTIPLE DX** | | | | | | | | | | |
| 0–19 Years | 44 | 2.1 | 25 | 1 | 1 | 1 | 2 | 2 | 3 | 9 |
| 20–34 | 23 | 2.6 | 24 | 1 | 1 | 1 | 2 | 3 | 3 | 24 |
| 35–49 | 29 | 3.0 | 9 | 1 | 2 | 2 | 4 | 6 | 11 | 17 |
| 50–64 | 36 | 3.4 | 12 | 1 | 2 | 2 | 4 | 10 | 11 | 20 |
| 65+ | 73 | 3.7 | 11 | 1 | 2 | 2 | 6 | 8 | 9 | 14 |
| **TOTAL SINGLE DX** | 70 | 1.3 | <1 | 1 | 1 | 1 | 1 | 2 | 3 | 4 |
| **TOTAL MULTIPLE DX** | 205 | 3.1 | 16 | 1 | 1 | 2 | 3 | 8 | 9 | 20 |
| **TOTAL** | | | | | | | | | | |
| 0–19 Years | 86 | 1.4 | 8 | 1 | 1 | 1 | 1 | 2 | 2 | 5 |
| 20–34 | 29 | 2.4 | 19 | 1 | 1 | 1 | 2 | 3 | 3 | 24 |
| 35–49 | 36 | 2.9 | 9 | 1 | 2 | 2 | 3 | 7 | 10 | 17 |
| 50–64 | 49 | 2.8 | 9 | 1 | 2 | 2 | 3 | 6 | 10 | 12 |
| 65+ | 75 | 3.7 | 11 | 1 | 2 | 2 | 6 | 8 | 9 | 14 |
| **GRAND TOTAL** | 275 | 2.4 | 11 | 1 | 1 | 1 | 2 | 5 | 8 | 14 |

### 63.2: EXC EPIDIDYMIS CYST. Formerly included in operation group(s) 673.

| Type of Patients | Observed Patients | Avg. Stay | Vari- ance | 10th | 25th | 50th | 75th | 90th | 95th | 99th |
|---|---|---|---|---|---|---|---|---|---|---|
| **1. SINGLE DX** | | | | | | | | | | |
| 0–19 Years | 1 | 1.0 | 0 | 1 | 1 | 1 | 1 | 1 | 1 | 1 |
| 20–34 | 3 | 1.9 | <1 | 1 | 1 | 2 | 3 | 3 | 3 | 3 |
| 35–49 | 3 | 2.3 | 2 | 1 | 1 | 2 | 4 | 4 | 4 | 4 |
| 50–64 | 0 | | | | | | | | | |
| 65+ | 1 | 1.0 | 0 | 1 | 1 | 1 | 1 | 1 | 1 | 1 |
| **2. MULTIPLE DX** | | | | | | | | | | |
| 0–19 Years | 3 | 4.3 | 9 | 1 | 1 | 7 | 7 | 7 | 7 | 7 |
| 20–34 | 2 | 1.0 | 0 | 1 | 1 | 1 | 1 | 1 | 1 | 1 |
| 35–49 | 6 | 1.0 | 0 | 1 | 1 | 1 | 1 | 1 | 1 | 1 |
| 50–64 | 12 | 2.1 | 4 | 1 | 1 | 1 | 2 | 7 | 7 | 7 |
| 65+ | 25 | 2.3 | 5 | 1 | 2 | 2 | 2 | 4 | 5 | 13 |
| **TOTAL SINGLE DX** | 8 | 1.9 | 1 | 1 | 1 | 2 | 3 | 3 | 4 | 4 |
| **TOTAL MULTIPLE DX** | 48 | 2.4 | 6 | 1 | 1 | 1 | 3 | 7 | 7 | 13 |
| **TOTAL** | | | | | | | | | | |
| 0–19 Years | 4 | 4.2 | 9 | 1 | 1 | 7 | 7 | 7 | 7 | 7 |
| 20–34 | 5 | 1.6 | <1 | 1 | 1 | 1 | 2 | 3 | 3 | 3 |
| 35–49 | 9 | 1.3 | <1 | 1 | 1 | 1 | 1 | 2 | 4 | 4 |
| 50–64 | 12 | 2.1 | 4 | 1 | 1 | 1 | 2 | 7 | 7 | 7 |
| 65+ | 26 | 2.3 | 5 | 1 | 2 | 2 | 2 | 4 | 5 | 13 |
| **GRAND TOTAL** | 56 | 2.4 | 5 | 1 | 1 | 1 | 3 | 7 | 7 | 13 |

Length of Stay by Diagnosis and Operation, United States, 2000

# United States, October 1998–September 1999 Data, by Operation

## 63.3: EXC SPERM CORD LES NEC. Formerly included in operation group(s) 673.

| Type of Patients | Observed Patients | Avg. Stay | Variance | Percentiles | | | | | | |
|---|---|---|---|---|---|---|---|---|---|---|
| | | | | 10th | 25th | 50th | 75th | 90th | 95th | 99th |
| **1. SINGLE DX** | | | | | | | | | | |
| 0–19 Years | 7 | 1.1 | <1 | 1 | 1 | 1 | 1 | 1 | 2 | 2 |
| 20–34 | 4 | 1.4 | 2 | 1 | 1 | 1 | 1 | 2 | 6 | 6 |
| 35–49 | 5 | 2.5 | 3 | 1 | 1 | 2 | 4 | 5 | 5 | 5 |
| 50–64 | 2 | 1.0 | 0 | 1 | 1 | 1 | 1 | 1 | 1 | 1 |
| 65+ | 2 | 1.0 | 0 | 1 | 1 | 1 | 1 | 1 | 1 | 1 |
| **2. MULTIPLE DX** | | | | | | | | | | |
| 0–19 Years | 6 | 3.5 | 7 | 1 | 1 | 1 | 5 | 8 | 8 | 8 |
| 20–34 | 3 | 2.8 | 6 | 1 | 1 | 1 | 5 | 6 | 6 | 6 |
| 35–49 | 4 | 1.3 | <1 | 1 | 1 | 2 | 2 | 2 | 2 | 2 |
| 50–64 | 10 | 4.4 | 6 | 1 | 3 | 3 | 6 | 6 | 6 | 10 |
| 65+ | 16 | 2.5 | 6 | 1 | 1 | 2 | 3 | 4 | 6 | 14 |
| **TOTAL SINGLE DX** | 20 | 1.5 | 2 | 1 | 1 | 1 | 1 | 4 | 5 | 6 |
| **TOTAL MULTIPLE DX** | 39 | 3.1 | 6 | 1 | 1 | 2 | 5 | 6 | 8 | 14 |
| **TOTAL** | | | | | | | | | | |
| 0–19 Years | 13 | 2.4 | 5 | 1 | 1 | 1 | 5 | 6 | 8 | 8 |
| 20–34 | 7 | 1.7 | 3 | 1 | 1 | 1 | 4 | 6 | 6 | 6 |
| 35–49 | 9 | 2.1 | 2 | 1 | 1 | 1 | 4 | 6 | 6 | 5 |
| 50–64 | 12 | 4.0 | 6 | 1 | 2 | 3 | 6 | 6 | 10 | 10 |
| 65+ | 18 | 2.4 | 6 | 1 | 1 | 2 | 3 | 4 | 5 | 14 |
| **GRAND TOTAL** | 59 | 2.5 | 5 | 1 | 1 | 1 | 4 | 6 | 6 | 10 |

## 63.4: EPIDIDYMECTOMY. Formerly included in operation group(s) 673.

| Type of Patients | Observed Patients | Avg. Stay | Variance | Percentiles | | | | | | |
|---|---|---|---|---|---|---|---|---|---|---|
| | | | | 10th | 25th | 50th | 75th | 90th | 95th | 99th |
| **1. SINGLE DX** | | | | | | | | | | |
| 0–19 Years | 1 | 1.0 | 0 | 1 | 1 | 1 | 1 | 1 | 1 | 1 |
| 20–34 | 3 | 1.0 | 0 | 1 | 1 | 1 | 1 | 1 | 1 | 1 |
| 35–49 | 2 | 1.0 | 0 | 1 | 1 | 1 | 1 | 1 | 1 | 1 |
| 50–64 | 2 | 2.5 | <1 | 1 | 3 | 3 | 3 | 3 | 3 | 3 |
| 65+ | 1 | 3.0 | 0 | 3 | 3 | 3 | 3 | 3 | 3 | 3 |
| **2. MULTIPLE DX** | | | | | | | | | | |
| 0–19 Years | 1 | 1.0 | 0 | 1 | 1 | 1 | 1 | 1 | 1 | 1 |
| 20–34 | 5 | 6.4 | 23 | 2 | 2 | 4 | 12 | 12 | 12 | 12 |
| 35–49 | 8 | 3.6 | 8 | 1 | 1 | 2 | 5 | 9 | 9 | 9 |
| 50–64 | 7 | 3.1 | 8 | 1 | 1 | 2 | 5 | 9 | 9 | 9 |
| 65+ | 13 | 3.9 | 14 | 1 | 1 | 2 | 6 | 10 | 13 | 13 |
| **TOTAL SINGLE DX** | 9 | 1.7 | <1 | 1 | 1 | 1 | 3 | 3 | 3 | 3 |
| **TOTAL MULTIPLE DX** | 34 | 3.6 | 12 | 1 | 1 | 2 | 5 | 9 | 12 | 13 |
| **TOTAL** | | | | | | | | | | |
| 0–19 Years | 2 | 1.0 | 0 | 1 | 1 | 1 | 1 | 1 | 1 | 1 |
| 20–34 | 8 | 5.0 | 22 | 1 | 2 | 2 | 11 | 12 | 12 | 12 |
| 35–49 | 10 | 3.1 | 8 | 1 | 1 | 2 | 4 | 9 | 9 | 9 |
| 50–64 | 9 | 2.9 | 7 | 1 | 1 | 2 | 3 | 9 | 9 | 9 |
| 65+ | 14 | 3.8 | 13 | 1 | 1 | 2 | 6 | 10 | 13 | 13 |
| **GRAND TOTAL** | 43 | 3.3 | 11 | 1 | 1 | 2 | 4 | 9 | 11 | 13 |

## 63.5: SPERM CORD/EPID REPAIR. Formerly included in operation group(s) 673.

| Type of Patients | Observed Patients | Avg. Stay | Variance | Percentiles | | | | | | |
|---|---|---|---|---|---|---|---|---|---|---|
| | | | | 10th | 25th | 50th | 75th | 90th | 95th | 99th |
| **1. SINGLE DX** | | | | | | | | | | |
| 0–19 Years | 13 | 1.0 | 0 | 1 | 1 | 1 | 1 | 1 | 1 | 1 |
| 20–34 | 1 | 1.0 | 0 | 1 | 1 | 1 | 1 | 1 | 1 | 1 |
| 35–49 | 0 | | | | | | | | | |
| 50–64 | 0 | | | | | | | | | |
| 65+ | 0 | | | | | | | | | |
| **2. MULTIPLE DX** | | | | | | | | | | |
| 0–19 Years | 5 | 1.0 | 0 | 1 | 1 | 1 | 1 | 1 | 1 | 1 |
| 20–34 | 1 | 1.0 | 0 | 1 | 1 | 1 | 1 | 1 | 1 | 1 |
| 35–49 | 0 | | | | | | | | | |
| 50–64 | 1 | 3.0 | 0 | 3 | 3 | 3 | 3 | 3 | 3 | 3 |
| 65+ | 1 | 2.0 | 0 | 2 | 2 | 2 | 2 | 2 | 2 | 2 |
| **TOTAL SINGLE DX** | 14 | 1.0 | 0 | 1 | 1 | 1 | 1 | 1 | 1 | 1 |
| **TOTAL MULTIPLE DX** | 8 | 1.4 | <1 | 1 | 1 | 1 | 2 | 2 | 2 | 3 |
| **TOTAL** | | | | | | | | | | |
| 0–19 Years | 18 | 1.0 | 0 | 1 | 1 | 1 | 1 | 1 | 1 | 1 |
| 20–34 | 2 | 1.0 | 0 | 1 | 1 | 1 | 1 | 1 | 1 | 1 |
| 35–49 | 0 | | | | | | | | | |
| 50–64 | 1 | 3.0 | 0 | 3 | 3 | 3 | 3 | 3 | 3 | 3 |
| 65+ | 1 | 2.0 | 0 | 2 | 2 | 2 | 2 | 2 | 2 | 2 |
| **GRAND TOTAL** | 22 | 1.2 | <1 | 1 | 1 | 1 | 1 | 2 | 2 | 3 |

## 63.6: VASOTOMY. Formerly included in operation group(s) 672.

| Type of Patients | Observed Patients | Avg. Stay | Variance | Percentiles | | | | | | |
|---|---|---|---|---|---|---|---|---|---|---|
| | | | | 10th | 25th | 50th | 75th | 90th | 95th | 99th |
| **1. SINGLE DX** | | | | | | | | | | |
| 0–19 Years | 0 | | | | | | | | | |
| 20–34 | 1 | 1.0 | 0 | 1 | 1 | 1 | 1 | 1 | 1 | 1 |
| 35–49 | 0 | | | | | | | | | |
| 50–64 | 0 | | | | | | | | | |
| 65+ | 0 | | | | | | | | | |
| **2. MULTIPLE DX** | | | | | | | | | | |
| 0–19 Years | 0 | | | | | | | | | |
| 20–34 | 0 | | | | | | | | | |
| 35–49 | 1 | 1.0 | 0 | 1 | 1 | 1 | 1 | 1 | 1 | 1 |
| 50–64 | 0 | | | | | | | | | |
| 65+ | 0 | | | | | | | | | |
| **TOTAL SINGLE DX** | 1 | 1.0 | 0 | 1 | 1 | 1 | 1 | 1 | 1 | 1 |
| **TOTAL MULTIPLE DX** | 1 | 1.0 | 0 | 1 | 1 | 1 | 1 | 1 | 1 | 1 |
| **TOTAL** | | | | | | | | | | |
| 0–19 Years | 0 | | | | | | | | | |
| 20–34 | 1 | 1.0 | 0 | 1 | 1 | 1 | 1 | 1 | 1 | 1 |
| 35–49 | 1 | 1.0 | 0 | 1 | 1 | 1 | 1 | 1 | 1 | 1 |
| 50–64 | 0 | | | | | | | | | |
| 65+ | 0 | | | | | | | | | |
| **GRAND TOTAL** | 2 | 1.0 | 0 | 1 | 1 | 1 | 1 | 1 | 1 | 1 |

Length of Stay by Diagnosis and Operation, United States, 2000

## United States, October 1998–September 1999 Data, by Operation

### 63.7: VASECTOMY & VAS DEF LIG. Formerly included in operation group(s) 672.

| Type of Patients | Observed Patients | Avg. Stay | Variance | Percentiles 10th | 25th | 50th | 75th | 90th | 95th | 99th |
|---|---|---|---|---|---|---|---|---|---|---|
| **1. SINGLE DX** | | | | | | | | | | |
| 0–19 Years | 0 | | | | | | | | | |
| 20–34 | 0 | | | | | | | | | |
| 35–49 | 1 | 1.0 | 0 | 1 | 1 | | 1 | 1 | 1 | 1 |
| 50–64 | 0 | | | | | | | | | |
| 65+ | 0 | | | | | | | | | |
| **2. MULTIPLE DX** | | | | | | | | | | |
| 0–19 Years | 0 | | | | | | | | | |
| 20–34 | 0 | | | | | | | | | |
| 35–49 | 0 | | | | | | | | | |
| 50–64 | 0 | | | | | | | | | |
| 65+ | 0 | | | | | | | | | |
| **TOTAL SINGLE DX** | 1 | 1.0 | 0 | 1 | 1 | | 1 | 1 | 1 | 1 |
| **TOTAL MULTIPLE DX** | 0 | | | | | | | | | |
| **TOTAL** | | | | | | | | | | |
| 0–19 Years | 0 | | | | | | | | | |
| 20–34 | 0 | | | | | | | | | |
| 35–49 | 1 | 1.0 | 0 | 1 | 1 | | 1 | 1 | 1 | 1 |
| 50–64 | 0 | | | | | | | | | |
| 65+ | 0 | | | | | | | | | |
| **GRAND TOTAL** | 1 | 1.0 | 0 | 1 | 1 | | 1 | 1 | 1 | 1 |

### 63.8: VAS DEF & EPID REPAIR. Formerly included in operation group(s) 673.

| Type of Patients | Observed Patients | Avg. Stay | Variance | Percentiles 10th | 25th | 50th | 75th | 90th | 95th | 99th |
|---|---|---|---|---|---|---|---|---|---|---|
| **1. SINGLE DX** | | | | | | | | | | |
| 0–19 Years | 0 | | | | | | | | | |
| 20–34 | 0 | | | | | | | | | |
| 35–49 | 3 | 1.0 | 0 | 1 | 1 | | 1 | 1 | 1 | 1 |
| 50–64 | 0 | | | | | | | | | |
| 65+ | 0 | | | | | | | | | |
| **2. MULTIPLE DX** | | | | | | | | | | |
| 0–19 Years | 0 | | | | | | | | | |
| 20–34 | 1 | 1.0 | 0 | 1 | 1 | | 1 | 1 | | |
| 35–49 | 4 | 1.8 | 2 | 1 | 1 | | 1 | 5 | 5 | 5 |
| 50–64 | 0 | | | | | | | | | |
| 65+ | 0 | | | | | | | | | |
| **TOTAL SINGLE DX** | 3 | 1.0 | 0 | 1 | 1 | | 1 | 1 | 1 | 1 |
| **TOTAL MULTIPLE DX** | 5 | 1.7 | 2 | 1 | 1 | | 1 | 5 | 5 | 5 |
| **TOTAL** | | | | | | | | | | |
| 0–19 Years | 0 | | | | | | | | | |
| 20–34 | 1 | 1.0 | 0 | 1 | 1 | | 1 | 1 | | |
| 35–49 | 7 | 1.6 | 2 | 1 | 1 | | 1 | 5 | 5 | 5 |
| 50–64 | 0 | | | | | | | | | |
| 65+ | 0 | | | | | | | | | |
| **GRAND TOTAL** | 8 | 1.6 | 2 | 1 | 1 | | 1 | 5 | 5 | 5 |

### 63.9: OTH SPERM CORD/EPID OPS. Formerly included in operation group(s) 673.

| Type of Patients | Observed Patients | Avg. Stay | Variance | Percentiles 10th | 25th | 50th | 75th | 90th | 95th | 99th |
|---|---|---|---|---|---|---|---|---|---|---|
| **1. SINGLE DX** | | | | | | | | | | |
| 0–19 Years | 2 | 2.4 | 1 | 1 | 1 | 3 | 3 | 3 | 3 | 3 |
| 20–34 | 2 | 3.8 | 8 | 1 | 1 | 6 | 6 | 6 | 6 | 6 |
| 35–49 | 1 | 1.0 | 0 | 1 | 1 | 1 | 1 | 1 | 1 | 1 |
| 50–64 | 0 | | | | | | | | | |
| 65+ | 1 | 2.0 | 0 | 2 | 2 | 2 | 2 | 2 | 2 | 2 |
| **2. MULTIPLE DX** | | | | | | | | | | |
| 0–19 Years | 4 | 1.3 | 2 | 1 | 1 | 1 | 1 | 1 | 6 | 7 |
| 20–34 | 3 | 9.6 | 54 | 1 | 1 | 10 | 16 | 16 | 16 | 16 |
| 35–49 | 10 | 4.7 | 5 | 2 | 3 | 4 | 7 | 7 | 7 | 7 |
| 50–64 | 4 | 2.8 | 1 | 1 | 3 | 3 | 3 | 5 | 5 | 5 |
| 65+ | 5 | 11.5 | 13 | 3 | 12 | 12 | 12 | 16 | 16 | 16 |
| **TOTAL SINGLE DX** | 6 | 2.6 | 4 | 1 | 1 | 2 | 3 | 6 | 6 | 6 |
| **TOTAL MULTIPLE DX** | 26 | 4.5 | 18 | 1 | 1 | 3 | 7 | 12 | 16 | 16 |
| **TOTAL** | | | | | | | | | | |
| 0–19 Years | 6 | 1.4 | 2 | 1 | 1 | 1 | 1 | 3 | 6 | 7 |
| 20–34 | 5 | 7.4 | 42 | 1 | 2 | 6 | 16 | 16 | 16 | 16 |
| 35–49 | 11 | 4.5 | 5 | 1 | 3 | 4 | 7 | 7 | 7 | 7 |
| 50–64 | 4 | 2.8 | 1 | 1 | 3 | 3 | 3 | 5 | 5 | 5 |
| 65+ | 6 | 10.5 | 21 | 2 | 10 | 12 | 12 | 16 | 16 | 16 |
| **GRAND TOTAL** | 32 | 4.3 | 17 | 1 | 1 | 3 | 7 | 12 | 12 | 16 |

### 64.0: CIRCUMCISION. Formerly included in operation group(s) 677.

| Type of Patients | Observed Patients | Avg. Stay | Variance | Percentiles 10th | 25th | 50th | 75th | 90th | 95th | 99th |
|---|---|---|---|---|---|---|---|---|---|---|
| **1. SINGLE DX** | | | | | | | | | | |
| 0–19 Years | 165,903 | 1.9 | <1 | 1 | 1 | 2 | 2 | 3 | 3 | 4 |
| 20–34 | 5 | 2.2 | 3 | 1 | 1 | 1 | 5 | 5 | 5 | 5 |
| 35–49 | 2 | 1.3 | <1 | 1 | 1 | 1 | 2 | 3 | 3 | 3 |
| 50–64 | 6 | 2.0 | <1 | 1 | 1 | 2 | 3 | 3 | 3 | 3 |
| 65+ | 2 | 8.2 | 8 | 4 | 4 | 10 | 10 | 10 | 10 | 10 |
| **2. MULTIPLE DX** | | | | | | | | | | |
| 0–19 Years | 184,010 | 2.8 | 13 | 1 | 2 | 2 | 3 | 4 | 6 | 16 |
| 20–34 | 22 | 3.9 | 56 | 1 | 1 | 2 | 3 | 6 | 10 | 45 |
| 35–49 | 41 | 2.7 | 11 | 1 | 2 | 2 | 4 | 6 | 8 | 23 |
| 50–64 | 75 | 6.4 | 74 | 2 | 2 | 4 | 7 | 11 | 17 | 68 |
| 65+ | 237 | 6.0 | 22 | 1 | 2 | 5 | 11 | 11 | 11 | 19 |
| **TOTAL SINGLE DX** | 165,918 | 1.9 | <1 | 1 | 1 | 2 | 2 | 3 | 3 | 4 |
| **TOTAL MULTIPLE DX** | 184,385 | 2.8 | 13 | 1 | 2 | 2 | 3 | 4 | 6 | 16 |
| **TOTAL** | | | | | | | | | | |
| 0–19 Years | 349,913 | 2.4 | 7 | 1 | 2 | 2 | 2 | 3 | 4 | 11 |
| 20–34 | 27 | 3.6 | 47 | 1 | 1 | 2 | 3 | 6 | 10 | 45 |
| 35–49 | 43 | 2.6 | 10 | 1 | 1 | 2 | 4 | 6 | 7 | 23 |
| 50–64 | 81 | 6.0 | 70 | 1 | 2 | 4 | 7 | 10 | 17 | 68 |
| 65+ | 239 | 6.1 | 22 | 1 | 2 | 5 | 11 | 11 | 11 | 19 |
| **GRAND TOTAL** | 350,303 | 2.4 | 7 | 1 | 2 | 2 | 2 | 3 | 4 | 11 |

Length of Stay by Diagnosis and Operation, United States, 2000

# United States, October 1998–September 1999 Data, by Operation

## 64.1: PENILE DIAGNOSTIC PX. Formerly included in operation group(s) 676, 677.

| Type of Patients | Observed Patients | Avg. Stay | Variance | Percentiles | | | | | | |
|---|---|---|---|---|---|---|---|---|---|---|
| | | | | 10th | 25th | 50th | 75th | 90th | 95th | 99th |
| **1. SINGLE DX** | | | | | | | | | | |
| 0–19 Years | 0 | | | | | | | | | |
| 20–34 | 0 | | | | | | | | | |
| 35–49 | 0 | | | | | | | | | |
| 50–64 | 1 | 1.0 | 0 | 1 | 1 | 1 | 1 | 1 | 1 | 1 |
| 65+ | 1 | 1.0 | 0 | 1 | 1 | 1 | 1 | 1 | 1 | 1 |
| **2. MULTIPLE DX** | | | | | | | | | | |
| 0–19 Years | 3 | 1.0 | 0 | 1 | 1 | 1 | 1 | 1 | 1 | 1 |
| 20–34 | 3 | 6.1 | 7 | 3 | 3 | 8 | 8 | 8 | 8 | 8 |
| 35–49 | 11 | 6.4 | 10 | 2 | 3 | 7 | 8 | 11 | 11 | 11 |
| 50–64 | 12 | 3.5 | 2 | 1 | 2 | 4 | 4 | 4 | 7 | 7 |
| 65+ | 27 | 4.7 | 47 | 1 | 2 | 3 | 4 | 8 | 28 | 31 |
| **TOTAL SINGLE DX** | 2 | 1.0 | 0 | 1 | 1 | 1 | 1 | 1 | 1 | 1 |
| **TOTAL MULTIPLE DX** | 56 | 4.4 | 27 | 1 | 2 | 3 | 4 | 8 | 11 | 31 |
| **TOTAL** | | | | | | | | | | |
| 0–19 Years | 3 | 1.0 | 0 | 1 | 1 | 1 | 1 | 1 | 1 | 1 |
| 20–34 | 3 | 6.1 | 7 | 3 | 3 | 8 | 8 | 8 | 8 | 8 |
| 35–49 | 11 | 6.4 | 10 | 2 | 3 | 7 | 8 | 11 | 11 | 11 |
| 50–64 | 13 | 3.3 | 3 | 1 | 2 | 4 | 4 | 4 | 7 | 7 |
| 65+ | 28 | 4.7 | 47 | 1 | 2 | 3 | 4 | 8 | 28 | 31 |
| **GRAND TOTAL** | 58 | 4.3 | 26 | 1 | 1 | 3 | 4 | 8 | 11 | 31 |

## 64.2: LOC EXC/DESTR PENILE LES. Formerly included in operation group(s) 676.

| Type of Patients | Observed Patients | Avg. Stay | Variance | Percentiles | | | | | | |
|---|---|---|---|---|---|---|---|---|---|---|
| | | | | 10th | 25th | 50th | 75th | 90th | 95th | 99th |
| **1. SINGLE DX** | | | | | | | | | | |
| 0–19 Years | 10 | 2.5 | 3 | 1 | 1 | 3 | 3 | 5 | 7 | 7 |
| 20–34 | 2 | 3.8 | 3 | 2 | 2 | 5 | 5 | 5 | 5 | 5 |
| 35–49 | 6 | 4.9 | 50 | 2 | 2 | 2 | 4 | 24 | 24 | 24 |
| 50–64 | 8 | 1.9 | 0 | 1 | 1 | 2 | 2 | 2 | 5 | 5 |
| 65+ | 2 | 1.0 | | 1 | 1 | 1 | 1 | 1 | 1 | 1 |
| **2. MULTIPLE DX** | | | | | | | | | | |
| 0–19 Years | 13 | 4.2 | 28 | 1 | 1 | 1 | 6 | 15 | 15 | 15 |
| 20–34 | 20 | 8.9 | 191 | 2 | 2 | 3 | 9 | 23 | 59 | 59 |
| 35–49 | 29 | 6.4 | 53 | 1 | 3 | 3 | 8 | 20 | 21 | 35 |
| 50–64 | 63 | 6.4 | 66 | 1 | 3 | 3 | 8 | 19 | 20 | 41 |
| 65+ | 55 | 9.1 | 90 | 2 | 6 | 6 | 12 | 19 | 30 | 45 |
| **TOTAL SINGLE DX** | 28 | 2.9 | 14 | 1 | 1 | 2 | 3 | 5 | 5 | 5 |
| **TOTAL MULTIPLE DX** | 180 | 7.4 | 88 | 1 | 2 | 3 | 9 | 19 | 23 | 45 |
| **TOTAL** | | | | | | | | | | |
| 0–19 Years | 23 | 3.5 | 19 | 1 | 1 | 3 | 3 | 13 | 15 | 15 |
| 20–34 | 22 | 8.6 | 180 | 2 | 3 | 3 | 7 | 23 | 59 | 59 |
| 35–49 | 35 | 6.1 | 52 | 2 | 3 | 3 | 7 | 20 | 21 | 35 |
| 50–64 | 71 | 6.1 | 63 | 1 | 3 | 4 | 7 | 19 | 20 | 41 |
| 65+ | 57 | 8.8 | 89 | 2 | 5 | 5 | 11 | 19 | 30 | 45 |
| **GRAND TOTAL** | 208 | 6.9 | 82 | 1 | 2 | 3 | 8 | 19 | 23 | 45 |

## 64.3: AMPUTATION OF PENIS. Formerly included in operation group(s) 676.

| Type of Patients | Observed Patients | Avg. Stay | Variance | Percentiles | | | | | | |
|---|---|---|---|---|---|---|---|---|---|---|
| | | | | 10th | 25th | 50th | 75th | 90th | 95th | 99th |
| **1. SINGLE DX** | | | | | | | | | | |
| 0–19 Years | 1 | 4.0 | 0 | 4 | 4 | 4 | 4 | 4 | 4 | 4 |
| 20–34 | 3 | 2.1 | <1 | 1 | 2 | 2 | 3 | 3 | 3 | 3 |
| 35–49 | 5 | 2.4 | <1 | 2 | 2 | 2 | 3 | 3 | 3 | 3 |
| 50–64 | 8 | 3.2 | 12 | 1 | 1 | 1 | 3 | 9 | 9 | 9 |
| 65+ | 7 | 1.3 | <1 | 1 | 1 | 1 | 2 | 2 | 2 | 2 |
| **2. MULTIPLE DX** | | | | | | | | | | |
| 0–19 Years | 1 | 3.0 | 0 | 3 | 3 | 3 | 3 | 3 | 3 | 3 |
| 20–34 | 5 | 2.2 | 5 | 1 | 1 | 1 | 5 | 8 | 8 | 8 |
| 35–49 | 16 | 6.1 | 22 | 2 | 5 | 5 | 11 | 12 | 19 | 19 |
| 50–64 | 48 | 8.0 | 62 | 1 | 2 | 5 | 7 | 24 | 27 | 28 |
| 65+ | 92 | 5.4 | 51 | 1 | 2 | 3 | 7 | 13 | 16 | 45 |
| **TOTAL SINGLE DX** | 24 | 2.5 | 6 | 1 | 1 | 1 | 2 | 9 | 9 | 9 |
| **TOTAL MULTIPLE DX** | 162 | 6.1 | 50 | 1 | 2 | 4 | 7 | 15 | 23 | 28 |
| **TOTAL** | | | | | | | | | | |
| 0–19 Years | 2 | 3.2 | <1 | 3 | 3 | 3 | 3 | 4 | 4 | 4 |
| 20–34 | 8 | 2.2 | 4 | 1 | 3 | 5 | 5 | 4 | 4 | 8 |
| 35–49 | 21 | 5.6 | 21 | 2 | 3 | 5 | 5 | 12 | 19 | 19 |
| 50–64 | 56 | 7.3 | 58 | 1 | 2 | 5 | 9 | 20 | 25 | 28 |
| 65+ | 99 | 5.2 | 49 | 1 | 2 | 3 | 7 | 12 | 15 | 45 |
| **GRAND TOTAL** | 186 | 5.7 | 46 | 1 | 2 | 3 | 7 | 15 | 20 | 28 |

## 64.4: PENILE REP/PLASTIC OPS. Formerly included in operation group(s) 676.

| Type of Patients | Observed Patients | Avg. Stay | Variance | Percentiles | | | | | | |
|---|---|---|---|---|---|---|---|---|---|---|
| | | | | 10th | 25th | 50th | 75th | 90th | 95th | 99th |
| **1. SINGLE DX** | | | | | | | | | | |
| 0–19 Years | 42 | 1.6 | 5 | 1 | 1 | 1 | 1 | 2 | 3 | 17 |
| 20–34 | 28 | 1.9 | 3 | 1 | 1 | 1 | 3 | 3 | 4 | 9 |
| 35–49 | 20 | 1.5 | <1 | 1 | 2 | 2 | 2 | 2 | 2 | 3 |
| 50–64 | 12 | 1.3 | <1 | 1 | 1 | 1 | 1 | 3 | 3 | 3 |
| 65+ | 5 | 1.7 | 2 | 1 | 1 | 1 | 2 | 5 | 5 | 5 |
| **2. MULTIPLE DX** | | | | | | | | | | |
| 0–19 Years | 66 | 2.8 | 18 | 1 | 1 | 1 | 2 | 6 | 11 | 23 |
| 20–34 | 40 | 2.8 | 8 | 1 | 1 | 3 | 4 | 4 | 7 | 17 |
| 35–49 | 42 | 5.3 | 45 | 2 | 2 | 3 | 6 | 9 | 19 | 31 |
| 50–64 | 38 | 4.5 | 57 | 1 | 1 | 2 | 4 | 7 | 30 | 30 |
| 65+ | 17 | 2.3 | 2 | 1 | 2 | 2 | 3 | 5 | 5 | 6 |
| **TOTAL SINGLE DX** | 107 | 1.7 | 3 | 1 | 1 | 1 | 2 | 3 | 3 | 9 |
| **TOTAL MULTIPLE DX** | 203 | 3.5 | 25 | 1 | 1 | 2 | 3 | 7 | 13 | 30 |
| **TOTAL** | | | | | | | | | | |
| 0–19 Years | 108 | 2.3 | 13 | 1 | 1 | 1 | 2 | 4 | 8 | 23 |
| 20–34 | 68 | 2.5 | 7 | 1 | 1 | 2 | 3 | 4 | 5 | 17 |
| 35–49 | 62 | 4.1 | 34 | 1 | 1 | 2 | 3 | 8 | 13 | 31 |
| 50–64 | 50 | 3.9 | 47 | 1 | 1 | 2 | 3 | 7 | 27 | 30 |
| 65+ | 22 | 2.2 | 2 | 1 | 1 | 2 | 3 | 5 | 5 | 6 |
| **GRAND TOTAL** | 310 | 2.9 | 18 | 1 | 1 | 2 | 3 | 5 | 9 | 30 |

Length of Stay by Diagnosis and Operation, United States, 2000

## United States, October 1998–September 1999 Data, by Operation

### 64.96: RMVL INT PENILE PROSTH. Formerly included in operation group(s) 676.

| Type of Patients | Observed Patients | Avg. Stay | Vari-ance | Percentiles | | | | | | |
|---|---|---|---|---|---|---|---|---|---|---|
| | | | | 10th | 25th | 50th | 75th | 90th | 95th | 99th |
| **1. SINGLE DX** | | | | | | | | | | |
| 0-19 Years | 0 | | | | | | | | | |
| 20-34 | 0 | | | | | | | | | |
| 35-49 | 5 | 3.8 | 3 | 1 | 2 | 5 | 5 | 5 | 5 | 5 |
| 50-64 | 13 | 1.9 | 3 | 1 | 1 | 1 | 2 | 4 | 4 | 10 |
| 65+ | 15 | 2.4 | 2 | 1 | 2 | 2 | 2 | 4 | 4 | 7 |
| **2. MULTIPLE DX** | | | | | | | | | | |
| 0-19 Years | 0 | | | | | | | | | |
| 20-34 | 3 | 5.6 | 8 | 3 | 4 | 4 | 9 | 9 | 9 | 9 |
| 35-49 | 49 | 5.0 | 19 | 2 | 2 | 3 | 7 | 13 | 13 | 23 |
| 50-64 | 116 | 4.1 | 10 | 1 | 2 | 3 | 5 | 9 | 10 | 15 |
| 65+ | 123 | 4.9 | 28 | 1 | 2 | 3 | 6 | 13 | 17 | 21 |
| **TOTAL SINGLE DX** | 33 | 2.5 | 2 | 1 | 1 | 2 | 4 | 5 | 5 | 7 |
| **TOTAL MULTIPLE DX** | 291 | 4.5 | 18 | 1 | 2 | 3 | 5 | 9 | 13 | 21 |
| **TOTAL** | | | | | | | | | | |
| 0-19 Years | 0 | | | | | | | | | |
| 20-34 | 3 | 5.6 | 8 | 3 | 4 | 4 | 9 | 9 | 9 | 9 |
| 35-49 | 54 | 4.9 | 17 | 2 | 2 | 3 | 5 | 13 | 13 | 23 |
| 50-64 | 129 | 3.9 | 10 | 1 | 1 | 3 | 5 | 9 | 10 | 15 |
| 65+ | 138 | 4.3 | 23 | 1 | 2 | 3 | 6 | 10 | 16 | 21 |
| **GRAND TOTAL** | 324 | 4.2 | 16 | 1 | 2 | 3 | 5 | 9 | 13 | 21 |

### 64.97: INSERT OR REPL IPP. Formerly included in operation group(s) 675.

| Type of Patients | Observed Patients | Avg. Stay | Vari-ance | Percentiles | | | | | | |
|---|---|---|---|---|---|---|---|---|---|---|
| | | | | 10th | 25th | 50th | 75th | 90th | 95th | 99th |
| **1. SINGLE DX** | | | | | | | | | | |
| 0-19 Years | 0 | | | | | | | | | |
| 20-34 | 3 | 1.4 | <1 | 1 | 1 | 1 | 2 | 2 | 2 | 2 |
| 35-49 | 18 | 1.5 | <1 | 1 | 1 | 1 | 2 | 2 | 2 | 2 |
| 50-64 | 66 | 1.7 | <1 | 1 | 1 | 1 | 2 | 3 | 3 | 5 |
| 65+ | 71 | 1.3 | <1 | 1 | 1 | 1 | 1 | 2 | 5 | 5 |
| **2. MULTIPLE DX** | | | | | | | | | | |
| 0-19 Years | 1 | 5.0 | 0 | 5 | 5 | 5 | 5 | 5 | 5 | 5 |
| 20-34 | 10 | 2.2 | 4 | 1 | 1 | 1 | 2 | 5 | 7 | 7 |
| 35-49 | 157 | 2.1 | 3 | 1 | 1 | 2 | 3 | 4 | 4 | 7 |
| 50-64 | 508 | 1.7 | 4 | 1 | 1 | 1 | 2 | 3 | 4 | 6 |
| 65+ | 507 | 1.7 | 2 | 1 | 1 | 1 | 2 | 3 | 4 | 7 |
| **TOTAL SINGLE DX** | 158 | 1.5 | <1 | 1 | 1 | 1 | 2 | 3 | 3 | 5 |
| **TOTAL MULTIPLE DX** | 1,183 | 1.8 | 3 | 1 | 1 | 1 | 2 | 3 | 4 | 7 |
| **TOTAL** | | | | | | | | | | |
| 0-19 Years | 1 | 5.0 | 0 | 5 | 5 | 5 | 5 | 5 | 5 | 5 |
| 20-34 | 13 | 2.0 | 3 | 1 | 1 | 1 | 2 | 5 | 7 | 7 |
| 35-49 | 175 | 2.1 | 2 | 1 | 1 | 2 | 3 | 4 | 4 | 6 |
| 50-64 | 574 | 1.7 | 3 | 1 | 1 | 1 | 2 | 3 | 4 | 6 |
| 65+ | 578 | 1.6 | 2 | 1 | 1 | 1 | 2 | 3 | 4 | 7 |
| **GRAND TOTAL** | 1,341 | 1.8 | 3 | 1 | 1 | 1 | 2 | 3 | 4 | 7 |

### 64.5: SEX TRANSFORMATION NEC. Formerly included in operation group(s) 676.

| Type of Patients | Observed Patients | Avg. Stay | Vari-ance | Percentiles | | | | | | |
|---|---|---|---|---|---|---|---|---|---|---|
| | | | | 10th | 25th | 50th | 75th | 90th | 95th | 99th |
| **1. SINGLE DX** | | | | | | | | | | |
| 0-19 Years | 0 | | | | | | | | | |
| 20-34 | 0 | | | | | | | | | |
| 35-49 | 0 | | | | | | | | | |
| 50-64 | 0 | | | | | | | | | |
| 65+ | 0 | | | | | | | | | |
| **2. MULTIPLE DX** | | | | | | | | | | |
| 0-19 Years | 0 | | | | | | | | | |
| 20-34 | 1 | 6.0 | 0 | 6 | 6 | 6 | 6 | 6 | 6 | 6 |
| 35-49 | 0 | | | | | | | | | |
| 50-64 | 0 | | | | | | | | | |
| 65+ | 0 | | | | | | | | | |
| **TOTAL SINGLE DX** | 0 | | | | | | | | | |
| **TOTAL MULTIPLE DX** | 1 | 6.0 | 0 | 6 | 6 | 6 | 6 | 6 | 6 | 6 |
| **TOTAL** | | | | | | | | | | |
| 0-19 Years | 0 | | | | | | | | | |
| 20-34 | 1 | 6.0 | 0 | 6 | 6 | 6 | 6 | 6 | 6 | 6 |
| 35-49 | 0 | | | | | | | | | |
| 50-64 | 0 | | | | | | | | | |
| 65+ | 0 | | | | | | | | | |
| **GRAND TOTAL** | 1 | 6.0 | 0 | 6 | 6 | 6 | 6 | 6 | 6 | 6 |

### 64.9: OTHER MALE GENITAL OPS. Formerly included in operation group(s) 675, 676, 677.

| Type of Patients | Observed Patients | Avg. Stay | Vari-ance | Percentiles | | | | | | |
|---|---|---|---|---|---|---|---|---|---|---|
| | | | | 10th | 25th | 50th | 75th | 90th | 95th | 99th |
| **1. SINGLE DX** | | | | | | | | | | |
| 0-19 Years | 24 | 1.4 | 1 | 1 | 1 | 1 | 1 | 3 | 3 | 6 |
| 20-34 | 30 | 1.4 | <1 | 1 | 1 | 1 | 2 | 2 | 3 | 5 |
| 35-49 | 58 | 2.3 | 3 | 1 | 1 | 2 | 3 | 5 | 6 | 6 |
| 50-64 | 102 | 1.7 | 1 | 1 | 1 | 1 | 2 | 3 | 4 | 5 |
| 65+ | 96 | 1.6 | 1 | 1 | 1 | 1 | 2 | 3 | 4 | 6 |
| **2. MULTIPLE DX** | | | | | | | | | | |
| 0-19 Years | 144 | 3.2 | 10 | 1 | 1 | 2 | 4 | 8 | 10 | 14 |
| 20-34 | 109 | 3.4 | 16 | 1 | 1 | 2 | 4 | 9 | 9 | 21 |
| 35-49 | 324 | 3.0 | 9 | 1 | 1 | 2 | 4 | 6 | 9 | 16 |
| 50-64 | 770 | 2.4 | 7 | 1 | 1 | 1 | 3 | 5 | 6 | 14 |
| 65+ | 772 | 2.8 | 16 | 1 | 1 | 1 | 3 | 6 | 8 | 21 |
| **TOTAL SINGLE DX** | 310 | 1.7 | 1 | 1 | 1 | 1 | 2 | 3 | 5 | 6 |
| **TOTAL MULTIPLE DX** | 2,119 | 2.7 | 11 | 1 | 1 | 2 | 3 | 6 | 9 | 16 |
| **TOTAL** | | | | | | | | | | |
| 0-19 Years | 168 | 2.9 | 9 | 1 | 1 | 2 | 3 | 7 | 10 | 12 |
| 20-34 | 139 | 2.9 | 13 | 1 | 1 | 1 | 3 | 8 | 9 | 19 |
| 35-49 | 382 | 2.9 | 8 | 1 | 1 | 2 | 4 | 6 | 7 | 16 |
| 50-64 | 872 | 2.3 | 7 | 1 | 1 | 1 | 3 | 5 | 6 | 13 |
| 65+ | 868 | 2.6 | 14 | 1 | 1 | 1 | 2 | 6 | 8 | 17 |
| **GRAND TOTAL** | 2,429 | 2.6 | 10 | 1 | 1 | 1 | 3 | 5 | 8 | 16 |

Length of Stay by Diagnosis and Operation, United States, 2000

# United States, October 1998–September 1999 Data, by Operation

## 65.0: OOPHOROTOMY. Formerly included in operation group(s) 681.

| Type of Patients | Observed Patients | Avg. Stay | Variance | 10th | 25th | 50th | 75th | 90th | 95th | 99th |
|---|---|---|---|---|---|---|---|---|---|---|
| **1. SINGLE DX** | | | | | | | | | | |
| 0–19 Years | 28 | 1.7 | <1 | 1 | 1 | 2 | 2 | 3 | 3 | 4 |
| 20–34 | 31 | 2.3 | 2 | 1 | 1 | 2 | 3 | 4 | 5 | 8 |
| 35–49 | 12 | 2.4 | 4 | 1 | 1 | 2 | 2 | 7 | 7 | 7 |
| 50–64 | 0 | | | | | | | | | |
| 65+ | 0 | | | | | | | | | |
| **2. MULTIPLE DX** | | | | | | | | | | |
| 0–19 Years | 47 | 2.3 | 3 | 1 | 1 | 2 | 3 | 4 | 6 | 8 |
| 20–34 | 174 | 2.8 | 3 | 1 | 2 | 2 | 3 | 5 | 7 | 9 |
| 35–49 | 88 | 3.1 | 7 | 1 | 2 | 2 | 3 | 6 | 9 | 14 |
| 50–64 | 6 | 3.5 | 6 | 1 | 2 | 3 | 3 | 8 | 8 | 14 |
| 65+ | 3 | 9.5 | 37 | 3 | 3 | 13 | 16 | 16 | 16 | 16 |
| **TOTAL SINGLE DX** | 71 | 2.0 | 2 | 1 | 1 | 2 | 2 | 3 | 5 | 8 |
| **TOTAL MULTIPLE DX** | 318 | 2.9 | 5 | 1 | 2 | 2 | 3 | 6 | 8 | 13 |
| **TOTAL** | | | | | | | | | | |
| 0–19 Years | 75 | 2.1 | 2 | 1 | 1 | 2 | 3 | 3 | 4 | 8 |
| 20–34 | 205 | 2.7 | 3 | 1 | 2 | 2 | 3 | 4 | 7 | 9 |
| 35–49 | 100 | 3.0 | 7 | 1 | 2 | 2 | 3 | 6 | 8 | 14 |
| 50–64 | 6 | 3.5 | 6 | 1 | 2 | 3 | 3 | 8 | 8 | 14 |
| 65+ | 3 | 9.5 | 37 | 3 | 3 | 13 | 16 | 16 | 16 | 16 |
| **GRAND TOTAL** | 389 | 2.7 | 5 | 1 | 1 | 2 | 3 | 5 | 7 | 11 |

## 65.2: LOC EXC/DESTR OVARY LES. Formerly included in operation group(s) 678.

| Type of Patients | Observed Patients | Avg. Stay | Variance | 10th | 25th | 50th | 75th | 90th | 95th | 99th |
|---|---|---|---|---|---|---|---|---|---|---|
| **1. SINGLE DX** | | | | | | | | | | |
| 0–19 Years | 321 | 2.2 | 1 | 1 | 2 | 2 | 2 | 3 | 4 | 6 |
| 20–34 | 895 | 2.1 | <1 | 1 | 1 | 2 | 2 | 3 | 4 | 5 |
| 35–49 | 267 | 2.1 | 1 | 1 | 1 | 2 | 2 | 4 | 5 | 10 |
| 50–64 | 27 | 2.4 | <1 | 2 | 2 | 2 | 3 | 4 | 4 | 5 |
| 65+ | 8 | 4.3 | 6 | 2 | 2 | 5 | 5 | 5 | 12 | 12 |
| **2. MULTIPLE DX** | | | | | | | | | | |
| 0–19 Years | 628 | 2.4 | 2 | 1 | 1 | 2 | 3 | 4 | 5 | 9 |
| 20–34 | 3,145 | 2.6 | 2 | 1 | 2 | 2 | 3 | 4 | 5 | 8 |
| 35–49 | 1,576 | 2.7 | 3 | 1 | 2 | 2 | 3 | 4 | 6 | 10 |
| 50–64 | 186 | 3.6 | 5 | 1 | 2 | 3 | 5 | 7 | 7 | 12 |
| 65+ | 172 | 6.5 | 25 | 2 | 3 | 5 | 9 | 15 | 16 | 25 |
| **TOTAL SINGLE DX** | 1,518 | 2.1 | 1 | 1 | 1 | 2 | 3 | 3 | 4 | 5 |
| **TOTAL MULTIPLE DX** | 5,707 | 2.8 | 4 | 1 | 2 | 2 | 3 | 4 | 6 | 10 |
| **TOTAL** | | | | | | | | | | |
| 0–19 Years | 949 | 2.3 | 2 | 1 | 2 | 2 | 3 | 3 | 5 | 8 |
| 20–34 | 4,040 | 2.5 | 2 | 1 | 2 | 2 | 3 | 4 | 5 | 9 |
| 35–49 | 1,843 | 2.7 | 3 | 1 | 2 | 2 | 3 | 4 | 5 | 9 |
| 50–64 | 213 | 3.4 | 5 | 1 | 2 | 3 | 4 | 6 | 7 | 12 |
| 65+ | 180 | 6.4 | 24 | 2 | 3 | 5 | 9 | 14 | 15 | 25 |
| **GRAND TOTAL** | 7,225 | 2.6 | 3 | 1 | 2 | 2 | 3 | 4 | 5 | 10 |

## 65.1: DXTIC PX ON OVARIES. Formerly included in operation group(s) 678, 681, 704.

| Type of Patients | Observed Patients | Avg. Stay | Variance | 10th | 25th | 50th | 75th | 90th | 95th | 99th |
|---|---|---|---|---|---|---|---|---|---|---|
| **1. SINGLE DX** | | | | | | | | | | |
| 0–19 Years | 8 | 2.2 | <1 | 1 | 1 | 2 | 2 | 3 | 4 | 4 |
| 20–34 | 12 | 1.3 | <1 | 1 | 1 | 1 | 1 | 3 | 5 | 5 |
| 35–49 | 8 | 2.1 | <1 | 1 | 1 | 2 | 2 | 3 | 4 | 4 |
| 50–64 | 1 | 2.0 | 0 | 2 | 2 | 2 | 2 | 2 | 2 | 2 |
| 65+ | 1 | 3.0 | | 3 | 3 | 3 | 3 | 3 | 3 | 3 |
| **2. MULTIPLE DX** | | | | | | | | | | |
| 0–19 Years | 21 | 1.6 | <1 | 1 | 1 | 2 | 2 | 3 | 3 | 3 |
| 20–34 | 76 | 2.4 | 2 | 1 | 1 | 2 | 3 | 3 | 6 | 6 |
| 35–49 | 70 | 3.9 | 14 | 1 | 2 | 3 | 5 | 5 | 7 | 34 |
| 50–64 | 21 | 4.3 | 13 | 2 | 2 | 4 | 6 | 8 | 14 | 16 |
| 65+ | 29 | 6.9 | 24 | 3 | 3 | 6 | 9 | 11 | 14 | 28 |
| **TOTAL SINGLE DX** | 30 | 1.8 | <1 | 1 | 1 | 2 | 2 | 3 | 3 | 4 |
| **TOTAL MULTIPLE DX** | 217 | 3.3 | 11 | 1 | 2 | 2 | 4 | 6 | 9 | 14 |
| **TOTAL** | | | | | | | | | | |
| 0–19 Years | 29 | 1.7 | <1 | 1 | 1 | 2 | 2 | 3 | 3 | 3 |
| 20–34 | 88 | 2.3 | 2 | 1 | 1 | 2 | 3 | 4 | 4 | 6 |
| 35–49 | 78 | 3.7 | 13 | 1 | 2 | 3 | 5 | 5 | 6 | 15 |
| 50–64 | 22 | 4.1 | 13 | 2 | 2 | 4 | 6 | 8 | 14 | 16 |
| 65+ | 30 | 6.8 | 24 | 3 | 3 | 6 | 9 | 10 | 14 | 28 |
| **GRAND TOTAL** | 247 | 3.2 | 10 | 1 | 1 | 2 | 4 | 5 | 9 | 14 |

## 65.25: LAPSCP OV LES EXC NEC. Formerly included in operation group(s) 678.

| Type of Patients | Observed Patients | Avg. Stay | Variance | 10th | 25th | 50th | 75th | 90th | 95th | 99th |
|---|---|---|---|---|---|---|---|---|---|---|
| **1. SINGLE DX** | | | | | | | | | | |
| 0–19 Years | 90 | 2.0 | 1 | 1 | 1 | 2 | 2 | 3 | 4 | 6 |
| 20–34 | 180 | 1.9 | 1 | 1 | 1 | 2 | 2 | 3 | 4 | 5 |
| 35–49 | 57 | 2.5 | 2 | 1 | 1 | 2 | 3 | 5 | 5 | 5 |
| 50–64 | 2 | 1.6 | 1 | 1 | 1 | 2 | 3 | 3 | 3 | 3 |
| 65+ | 0 | | | | | | | | | |
| **2. MULTIPLE DX** | | | | | | | | | | |
| 0–19 Years | 168 | 1.9 | 2 | 1 | 1 | 2 | 2 | 3 | 4 | 8 |
| 20–34 | 706 | 2.3 | 3 | 1 | 1 | 2 | 3 | 4 | 7 | 10 |
| 35–49 | 340 | 2.4 | 4 | 1 | 1 | 2 | 3 | 5 | 6 | 12 |
| 50–64 | 23 | 2.3 | 7 | 1 | 2 | 2 | 5 | 8 | 9 | 12 |
| 65+ | 18 | 4.2 | 23 | 2 | 2 | 5 | 9 | 14 | 16 | 16 |
| **TOTAL SINGLE DX** | 329 | 2.0 | 1 | 1 | 1 | 2 | 2 | 3 | 4 | 6 |
| **TOTAL MULTIPLE DX** | 1,255 | 2.3 | 3 | 1 | 1 | 2 | 3 | 4 | 6 | 9 |
| **TOTAL** | | | | | | | | | | |
| 0–19 Years | 258 | 2.0 | 2 | 1 | 1 | 2 | 2 | 3 | 4 | 7 |
| 20–34 | 886 | 2.2 | 3 | 1 | 1 | 2 | 3 | 4 | 6 | 8 |
| 35–49 | 397 | 2.4 | 3 | 1 | 1 | 2 | 3 | 5 | 6 | 10 |
| 50–64 | 25 | 2.2 | 7 | 1 | 2 | 2 | 5 | 8 | 9 | 12 |
| 65+ | 18 | 4.2 | 23 | 2 | 2 | 5 | 9 | 14 | 16 | 16 |
| **GRAND TOTAL** | 1,584 | 2.2 | 3 | 1 | 1 | 2 | 3 | 4 | 5 | 8 |

Length of Stay by Diagnosis and Operation, United States, 2000

### 65.29: LOC EXC/DESTR OV LES NEC. Formerly included in operation group(s) 678.

| Type of Patients | Observed Patients | Avg. Stay | Variance | Percentiles 10th | 25th | 50th | 75th | 90th | 95th | 99th |
|---|---|---|---|---|---|---|---|---|---|---|
| **1. SINGLE DX** | | | | | | | | | | |
| 0–19 Years | 214 | 2.3 | <1 | 1 | 2 | 2 | 3 | 3 | 4 | 6 |
| 20–34 | 678 | 2.1 | <1 | 1 | 2 | 2 | 3 | 3 | 4 | 5 |
| 35–49 | 197 | 2.0 | 1 | 1 | 1 | 2 | 3 | 3 | 5 | 5 |
| 50–64 | 25 | 2.5 | <1 | 2 | 2 | 2 | 3 | 3 | 4 | 5 |
| 65+ | 8 | 4.3 | 6 | 2 | 2 | 5 | 5 | 5 | 12 | 12 |
| **2. MULTIPLE DX** | | | | | | | | | | |
| 0–19 Years | 426 | 2.7 | 2 | 1 | 2 | 2 | 3 | 4 | 5 | 9 |
| 20–34 | 2,259 | 2.7 | 2 | 2 | 2 | 2 | 3 | 4 | 5 | 8 |
| 35–49 | 1,181 | 2.9 | 3 | 2 | 2 | 2 | 3 | 4 | 6 | 9 |
| 50–64 | 162 | 3.8 | 5 | 2 | 2 | 3 | 5 | 7 | 7 | 12 |
| 65+ | 152 | 6.7 | 25 | 2 | 3 | 5 | 9 | 15 | 16 | 25 |
| **TOTAL SINGLE DX** | **1,122** | **2.2** | **<1** | **1** | **2** | **2** | **3** | **3** | **4** | **5** |
| **TOTAL MULTIPLE DX** | **4,180** | **2.9** | **4** | **2** | **2** | **2** | **3** | **5** | **6** | **12** |
| **TOTAL** | | | | | | | | | | |
| 0–19 Years | 640 | 2.5 | 2 | 1 | 2 | 2 | 3 | 4 | 5 | 9 |
| 20–34 | 2,937 | 2.5 | 2 | 1 | 2 | 2 | 3 | 4 | 5 | 7 |
| 35–49 | 1,378 | 2.7 | 3 | 1 | 2 | 2 | 3 | 4 | 5 | 9 |
| 50–64 | 187 | 3.6 | 4 | 2 | 2 | 3 | 5 | 6 | 7 | 12 |
| 65+ | 160 | 6.6 | 24 | 2 | 3 | 5 | 9 | 14 | 15 | 25 |
| **GRAND TOTAL** | **5,302** | **2.7** | **3** | **1** | **2** | **2** | **3** | **4** | **6** | **10** |

### 65.3: UNILATERAL OOPHORECTOMY. Formerly included in operation group(s) 679.

| Type of Patients | Observed Patients | Avg. Stay | Variance | Percentiles 10th | 25th | 50th | 75th | 90th | 95th | 99th |
|---|---|---|---|---|---|---|---|---|---|---|
| **1. SINGLE DX** | | | | | | | | | | |
| 0–19 Years | 112 | 2.5 | 2 | 1 | 2 | 2 | 3 | 4 | 5 | 7 |
| 20–34 | 264 | 2.1 | <1 | 1 | 2 | 2 | 3 | 3 | 4 | 4 |
| 35–49 | 181 | 2.3 | <1 | 1 | 2 | 2 | 3 | 3 | 4 | 4 |
| 50–64 | 25 | 2.0 | 1 | 1 | 1 | 2 | 3 | 4 | 4 | 4 |
| 65+ | 13 | 3.2 | 5 | 2 | 3 | 3 | 3 | 3 | 4 | 16 |
| **2. MULTIPLE DX** | | | | | | | | | | |
| 0–19 Years | 155 | 2.9 | 3 | 1 | 2 | 3 | 3 | 5 | 7 | 9 |
| 20–34 | 825 | 2.7 | 3 | 1 | 2 | 2 | 3 | 4 | 5 | 8 |
| 35–49 | 903 | 3.0 | 5 | 1 | 2 | 3 | 3 | 5 | 7 | 14 |
| 50–64 | 186 | 3.3 | 11 | 1 | 2 | 2 | 4 | 7 | 8 | 13 |
| 65+ | 197 | 6.0 | 33 | 2 | 2 | 4 | 8 | 14 | 17 | 20 |
| **TOTAL SINGLE DX** | **595** | **2.3** | **1** | **1** | **2** | **2** | **3** | **3** | **4** | **5** |
| **TOTAL MULTIPLE DX** | **2,266** | **3.2** | **7** | **1** | **2** | **3** | **3** | **5** | **8** | **14** |
| **TOTAL** | | | | | | | | | | |
| 0–19 Years | 267 | 2.7 | 3 | 1 | 2 | 3 | 3 | 4 | 5 | 9 |
| 20–34 | 1,089 | 2.6 | 2 | 1 | 2 | 2 | 3 | 4 | 5 | 8 |
| 35–49 | 1,084 | 2.9 | 4 | 1 | 2 | 2 | 3 | 5 | 7 | 11 |
| 50–64 | 211 | 3.1 | 10 | 1 | 2 | 2 | 3 | 6 | 8 | 12 |
| 65+ | 210 | 5.7 | 30 | 2 | 2 | 4 | 7 | 12 | 17 | 19 |
| **GRAND TOTAL** | **2,861** | **3.0** | **6** | **1** | **2** | **2** | **3** | **5** | **7** | **14** |

### 65.31: LAPSCP UNILAT OOPHORECT. Formerly included in operation group(s) 679.

| Type of Patients | Observed Patients | Avg. Stay | Variance | Percentiles 10th | 25th | 50th | 75th | 90th | 95th | 99th |
|---|---|---|---|---|---|---|---|---|---|---|
| **1. SINGLE DX** | | | | | | | | | | |
| 0–19 Years | 15 | 2.3 | 1 | 1 | 1 | 2 | 3 | 3 | 5 | 5 |
| 20–34 | 39 | 1.6 | <1 | 1 | 1 | 1 | 2 | 3 | 3 | 3 |
| 35–49 | 24 | 1.7 | <1 | 1 | 1 | 1 | 2 | 3 | 3 | 4 |
| 50–64 | 3 | 1.7 | <1 | 1 | 1 | 2 | 2 | 2 | 2 | 2 |
| 65+ | 3 | 1.0 | 0 | 1 | 1 | 1 | 1 | 1 | 1 | 1 |
| **2. MULTIPLE DX** | | | | | | | | | | |
| 0–19 Years | 14 | 2.1 | 1 | 1 | 1 | 2 | 3 | 4 | 4 | 5 |
| 20–34 | 118 | 2.1 | 4 | 1 | 1 | 2 | 2 | 4 | 5 | 8 |
| 35–49 | 127 | 2.3 | 3 | 1 | 1 | 2 | 3 | 6 | 6 | 9 |
| 50–64 | 24 | 1.8 | 5 | 1 | 1 | 1 | 2 | 3 | 4 | 18 |
| 65+ | 29 | 2.8 | 5 | 1 | 1 | 2 | 3 | 7 | 8 | 10 |
| **TOTAL SINGLE DX** | **84** | **1.9** | **<1** | **1** | **1** | **2** | **3** | **3** | **3** | **5** |
| **TOTAL MULTIPLE DX** | **312** | **2.2** | **4** | **1** | **1** | **2** | **3** | **4** | **6** | **9** |
| **TOTAL** | | | | | | | | | | |
| 0–19 Years | 29 | 2.2 | 1 | 1 | 1 | 2 | 3 | 3 | 5 | 5 |
| 20–34 | 157 | 2.0 | 3 | 1 | 1 | 2 | 2 | 3 | 4 | 8 |
| 35–49 | 151 | 2.3 | 3 | 1 | 1 | 2 | 3 | 5 | 6 | 9 |
| 50–64 | 27 | 1.8 | 5 | 1 | 1 | 1 | 2 | 3 | 4 | 18 |
| 65+ | 32 | 2.7 | 5 | 1 | 1 | 2 | 3 | 6 | 8 | 10 |
| **GRAND TOTAL** | **396** | **2.2** | **3** | **1** | **1** | **2** | **3** | **4** | **6** | **9** |

### 65.39: UNILAT OOPHORECTOMY NEC. Formerly included in operation group(s) 679.

| Type of Patients | Observed Patients | Avg. Stay | Variance | Percentiles 10th | 25th | 50th | 75th | 90th | 95th | 99th |
|---|---|---|---|---|---|---|---|---|---|---|
| **1. SINGLE DX** | | | | | | | | | | |
| 0–19 Years | 97 | 2.5 | 2 | 1 | 2 | 2 | 3 | 4 | 5 | 7 |
| 20–34 | 225 | 2.2 | <1 | 1 | 2 | 2 | 3 | 3 | 4 | 4 |
| 35–49 | 157 | 2.4 | <1 | 1 | 2 | 2 | 3 | 3 | 4 | 4 |
| 50–64 | 22 | 2.0 | 1 | 1 | 1 | 2 | 3 | 4 | 4 | 4 |
| 65+ | 10 | 3.3 | 5 | 2 | 3 | 3 | 3 | 3 | 4 | 16 |
| **2. MULTIPLE DX** | | | | | | | | | | |
| 0–19 Years | 141 | 3.0 | 3 | 1 | 2 | 3 | 3 | 5 | 7 | 9 |
| 20–34 | 707 | 2.8 | 2 | 2 | 2 | 3 | 3 | 4 | 5 | 8 |
| 35–49 | 776 | 3.2 | 5 | 2 | 2 | 3 | 3 | 5 | 7 | 14 |
| 50–64 | 162 | 3.6 | 11 | 2 | 2 | 3 | 4 | 7 | 8 | 13 |
| 65+ | 168 | 6.4 | 35 | 2 | 3 | 4 | 8 | 14 | 17 | 20 |
| **TOTAL SINGLE DX** | **511** | **2.4** | **1** | **1** | **2** | **2** | **3** | **3** | **4** | **5** |
| **TOTAL MULTIPLE DX** | **1,954** | **3.3** | **8** | **2** | **2** | **3** | **4** | **5** | **8** | **17** |
| **TOTAL** | | | | | | | | | | |
| 0–19 Years | 238 | 2.8 | 3 | 1 | 2 | 3 | 3 | 4 | 6 | 9 |
| 20–34 | 932 | 2.7 | 2 | 2 | 2 | 2 | 3 | 4 | 5 | 8 |
| 35–49 | 933 | 3.0 | 4 | 2 | 2 | 3 | 3 | 5 | 7 | 14 |
| 50–64 | 184 | 3.3 | 10 | 1 | 2 | 2 | 4 | 6 | 8 | 12 |
| 65+ | 178 | 6.0 | 32 | 2 | 3 | 4 | 8 | 14 | 17 | 20 |
| **GRAND TOTAL** | **2,465** | **3.1** | **7** | **2** | **2** | **3** | **3** | **5** | **7** | **14** |

# United States, October 1998–September 1999 Data, by Operation

## 65.49: UNILATERAL S-O NEC. Formerly included in operation group(s) 679.

| Type of Patients | Observed Patients | Avg. Stay | Variance | 10th | 25th | 50th | 75th | 90th | 95th | 99th |
|---|---|---|---|---|---|---|---|---|---|---|
| **1. SINGLE DX** | | | | | | | | | | |
| 0–19 Years | 143 | 2.9 | 2 | 2 | 2 | 3 | 3 | 4 | 5 | 8 |
| 20–34 | 401 | 2.5 | 1 | 1 | 2 | 2 | 3 | 3 | 4 | 7 |
| 35–49 | 410 | 2.5 | 2 | 2 | 2 | 2 | 3 | 4 | 4 | 8 |
| 50–64 | 71 | 2.3 | <1 | 2 | 2 | 2 | 3 | 3 | 4 | 5 |
| 65+ | 23 | 2.6 | <1 | 1 | 2 | 3 | 3 | 3 | 4 | 4 |
| **2. MULTIPLE DX** | | | | | | | | | | |
| 0–19 Years | 350 | 3.7 | 5 | 2 | 2 | 3 | 4 | 6 | 8 | 13 |
| 20–34 | 2,318 | 3.0 | 3 | 2 | 2 | 3 | 3 | 5 | 6 | 9 |
| 35–49 | 3,184 | 3.2 | 5 | 2 | 2 | 3 | 4 | 5 | 7 | 12 |
| 50–64 | 664 | 3.7 | 13 | 2 | 2 | 3 | 4 | 6 | 9 | 19 |
| 65+ | 540 | 6.0 | 26 | 2 | 3 | 4 | 7 | 14 | 17 | 22 |
| **TOTAL SINGLE DX** | 1,048 | 2.6 | 1 | 2 | 2 | 2 | 3 | 4 | 4 | 8 |
| **TOTAL MULTIPLE DX** | 7,056 | 3.4 | 8 | 2 | 2 | 3 | 4 | 6 | 8 | 16 |
| **TOTAL** | | | | | | | | | | |
| 0–19 Years | 493 | 3.5 | 4 | 2 | 2 | 3 | 4 | 5 | 7 | 11 |
| 20–34 | 2,719 | 2.9 | 3 | 2 | 2 | 3 | 3 | 4 | 6 | 9 |
| 35–49 | 3,594 | 3.1 | 5 | 2 | 2 | 3 | 4 | 5 | 7 | 11 |
| 50–64 | 735 | 3.5 | 12 | 2 | 2 | 3 | 4 | 6 | 8 | 19 |
| 65+ | 563 | 5.8 | 25 | 2 | 3 | 4 | 7 | 14 | 17 | 22 |
| **GRAND TOTAL** | 8,104 | 3.3 | 7 | 2 | 2 | 3 | 4 | 5 | 8 | 15 |

## 65.5: BILATERAL OOPHORECTOMY. Formerly included in operation group(s) 680.

| Type of Patients | Observed Patients | Avg. Stay | Variance | 10th | 25th | 50th | 75th | 90th | 95th | 99th |
|---|---|---|---|---|---|---|---|---|---|---|
| **1. SINGLE DX** | | | | | | | | | | |
| 0–19 Years | 7 | 3.3 | 5 | 2 | 2 | 3 | 3 | 8 | 8 | 8 |
| 20–34 | 11 | 2.2 | 2 | 1 | 1 | 2 | 2 | 5 | 5 | 5 |
| 35–49 | 20 | 2.5 | <1 | 1 | 2 | 2 | 3 | 3 | 3 | 5 |
| 50–64 | 14 | 2.5 | <1 | 2 | 2 | 2 | 3 | 3 | 3 | 6 |
| 65+ | 4 | 1.9 | <1 | 1 | 2 | 2 | 3 | 3 | 3 | 3 |
| **2. MULTIPLE DX** | | | | | | | | | | |
| 0–19 Years | 9 | 2.3 | 2 | 1 | 1 | 2 | 3 | 5 | 5 | 7 |
| 20–34 | 72 | 2.7 | 1 | 1 | 2 | 3 | 4 | 4 | 6 | 7 |
| 35–49 | 287 | 3.4 | 6 | 1 | 2 | 3 | 5 | 5 | 10 | 13 |
| 50–64 | 146 | 4.5 | 20 | 2 | 2 | 3 | 5 | 7 | 16 | 23 |
| 65+ | 121 | 4.9 | 13 | 2 | 3 | 4 | 5 | 9 | 11 | 20 |
| **TOTAL SINGLE DX** | 56 | 2.5 | 1 | 1 | 2 | 3 | 3 | 3 | 3 | 8 |
| **TOTAL MULTIPLE DX** | 635 | 3.8 | 10 | 2 | 2 | 3 | 4 | 7 | 10 | 18 |
| **TOTAL** | | | | | | | | | | |
| 0–19 Years | 16 | 2.7 | 3 | 1 | 1 | 2 | 3 | 5 | 8 | 8 |
| 20–34 | 83 | 2.6 | 1 | 1 | 2 | 2 | 4 | 4 | 5 | 7 |
| 35–49 | 307 | 3.3 | 5 | 1 | 2 | 3 | 4 | 5 | 9 | 13 |
| 50–64 | 160 | 4.3 | 18 | 2 | 2 | 3 | 5 | 7 | 14 | 23 |
| 65+ | 125 | 4.8 | 13 | 2 | 3 | 4 | 5 | 9 | 11 | 19 |
| **GRAND TOTAL** | 691 | 3.7 | 9 | 2 | 2 | 3 | 4 | 6 | 9 | 17 |

## 65.4: UNILATERAL S-O. Formerly included in operation group(s) 679.

| Type of Patients | Observed Patients | Avg. Stay | Variance | 10th | 25th | 50th | 75th | 90th | 95th | 99th |
|---|---|---|---|---|---|---|---|---|---|---|
| **1. SINGLE DX** | | | | | | | | | | |
| 0–19 Years | 164 | 2.8 | 2 | 1 | 2 | 2 | 4 | 5 | 5 | 7 |
| 20–34 | 465 | 2.4 | 1 | 1 | 2 | 2 | 3 | 3 | 4 | 7 |
| 35–49 | 483 | 2.4 | <1 | 1 | 2 | 2 | 3 | 4 | 4 | 8 |
| 50–64 | 87 | 2.2 | <1 | 1 | 2 | 2 | 3 | 3 | 3 | 5 |
| 65+ | 28 | 2.5 | <1 | 1 | 2 | 3 | 3 | 3 | 4 | 5 |
| **2. MULTIPLE DX** | | | | | | | | | | |
| 0–19 Years | 398 | 3.5 | 4 | 2 | 2 | 3 | 4 | 6 | 7 | 12 |
| 20–34 | 2,669 | 2.9 | 3 | 1 | 2 | 3 | 3 | 4 | 6 | 10 |
| 35–49 | 3,719 | 3.1 | 5 | 1 | 2 | 3 | 4 | 5 | 7 | 12 |
| 50–64 | 769 | 3.5 | 12 | 2 | 2 | 3 | 4 | 6 | 9 | 19 |
| 65+ | 627 | 5.6 | 25 | 2 | 3 | 4 | 7 | 14 | 16 | 22 |
| **TOTAL SINGLE DX** | 1,227 | 2.5 | 1 | 1 | 1 | 2 | 3 | 4 | 5 | 8 |
| **TOTAL MULTIPLE DX** | 8,182 | 3.3 | 7 | 1 | 2 | 3 | 4 | 6 | 8 | 15 |
| **TOTAL** | | | | | | | | | | |
| 0–19 Years | 562 | 3.3 | 4 | 2 | 2 | 3 | 4 | 5 | 6 | 10 |
| 20–34 | 3,134 | 2.9 | 3 | 1 | 2 | 3 | 3 | 4 | 6 | 9 |
| 35–49 | 4,202 | 3.0 | 5 | 1 | 2 | 3 | 4 | 5 | 7 | 11 |
| 50–64 | 856 | 3.3 | 11 | 2 | 2 | 3 | 4 | 6 | 8 | 17 |
| 65+ | 655 | 5.5 | 25 | 2 | 3 | 4 | 7 | 13 | 16 | 22 |
| **GRAND TOTAL** | 9,409 | 3.2 | 7 | 1 | 2 | 3 | 3 | 5 | 7 | 15 |

## 65.41: LAPSCP UNILATERAL S-O. Formerly included in operation group(s) 679.

| Type of Patients | Observed Patients | Avg. Stay | Variance | 10th | 25th | 50th | 75th | 90th | 95th | 99th |
|---|---|---|---|---|---|---|---|---|---|---|
| **1. SINGLE DX** | | | | | | | | | | |
| 0–19 Years | 21 | 2.8 | 3 | 1 | 1 | 2 | 5 | 5 | 5 | 5 |
| 20–34 | 64 | 2.0 | 1 | 1 | 1 | 2 | 3 | 3 | 4 | 7 |
| 35–49 | 73 | 1.8 | <1 | 1 | 1 | 2 | 2 | 2 | 3 | 4 |
| 50–64 | 16 | 1.7 | <1 | 1 | 1 | 2 | 2 | 2 | 3 | 3 |
| 65+ | 5 | 1.9 | 3 | 1 | 1 | 1 | 4 | 5 | 5 | 5 |
| **2. MULTIPLE DX** | | | | | | | | | | |
| 0–19 Years | 48 | 2.5 | 2 | 1 | 2 | 2 | 3 | 4 | 6 | 7 |
| 20–34 | 351 | 2.5 | 4 | 1 | 1 | 2 | 3 | 4 | 6 | 13 |
| 35–49 | 535 | 2.5 | 5 | 1 | 2 | 2 | 3 | 5 | 7 | 15 |
| 50–64 | 105 | 2.4 | 3 | 1 | 2 | 2 | 3 | 4 | 6 | 8 |
| 65+ | 87 | 2.9 | 14 | 1 | 2 | 2 | 4 | 5 | 8 | 12 |
| **TOTAL SINGLE DX** | 179 | 2.1 | 2 | 1 | 1 | 2 | 2 | 5 | 5 | 5 |
| **TOTAL MULTIPLE DX** | 1,126 | 2.5 | 5 | 1 | 1 | 2 | 3 | 5 | 6 | 13 |
| **TOTAL** | | | | | | | | | | |
| 0–19 Years | 69 | 2.6 | 2 | 1 | 2 | 2 | 4 | 5 | 5 | 7 |
| 20–34 | 415 | 2.4 | 3 | 1 | 1 | 2 | 3 | 4 | 5 | 13 |
| 35–49 | 608 | 2.4 | 4 | 1 | 2 | 2 | 3 | 5 | 6 | 11 |
| 50–64 | 121 | 2.2 | 2 | 1 | 2 | 2 | 2 | 3 | 4 | 8 |
| 65+ | 92 | 2.9 | 14 | 1 | 2 | 2 | 4 | 5 | 8 | 12 |
| **GRAND TOTAL** | 1,305 | 2.4 | 4 | 1 | 1 | 2 | 3 | 5 | 6 | 12 |

Length of Stay by Diagnosis and Operation, United States, 2000

# United States, October 1998–September 1999 Data, by Operation

## 65.51: RMVL BOTH OVARIES NEC. Formerly included in operation group(s) 680.

| Type of Patients | Observed Patients | Avg. Stay | Variance | 10th | 25th | 50th | 75th | 90th | 95th | 99th |
|---|---|---|---|---|---|---|---|---|---|---|
| **1. SINGLE DX** | | | | | | | | | | |
| 0–19 Years | 6 | 3.6 | 5 | 2 | 2 | 3 | 3 | 8 | 8 | 8 |
| 20–34 | 7 | 1.8 | <1 | 1 | 1 | 2 | 2 | 2 | 2 | 4 |
| 35–49 | 12 | 2.8 | <1 | 2 | 3 | 3 | 3 | 3 | 3 | 3 |
| 50–64 | 11 | 2.5 | <1 | 2 | 2 | 2 | 3 | 3 | 3 | 6 |
| 65+ | 2 | 2.7 | <1 | 2 | 2 | 3 | 3 | 3 | 3 | 3 |
| **2. MULTIPLE DX** | | | | | | | | | | |
| 0–19 Years | 4 | 2.3 | 3 | 1 | 1 | 2 | 2 | 5 | 5 | 7 |
| 20–34 | 37 | 2.4 | <1 | 2 | 2 | 2 | 3 | 3 | 4 | 4 |
| 35–49 | 150 | 3.0 | 3 | 1 | 2 | 3 | 4 | 5 | 5 | 12 |
| 50–64 | 107 | 4.8 | 22 | 2 | 2 | 3 | 5 | 9 | 16 | 23 |
| 65+ | 84 | 5.7 | 13 | 3 | 3 | 5 | 7 | 9 | 13 | 18 |
| **TOTAL SINGLE DX** | 38 | 2.7 | 1 | 2 | 2 | 3 | 3 | 3 | 3 | 8 |
| **TOTAL MULTIPLE DX** | 382 | 3.9 | 11 | 2 | 2 | 3 | 4 | 7 | 9 | 20 |
| **TOTAL** | | | | | | | | | | |
| 0–19 Years | 10 | 2.8 | 4 | 1 | 2 | 2 | 3 | 5 | 8 | 8 |
| 20–34 | 44 | 2.3 | <1 | 1 | 2 | 2 | 3 | 3 | 4 | 4 |
| 35–49 | 162 | 3.0 | 3 | 2 | 2 | 3 | 4 | 5 | 5 | 8 |
| 50–64 | 118 | 4.6 | 20 | 2 | 2 | 3 | 5 | 7 | 16 | 23 |
| 65+ | 86 | 5.6 | 13 | 3 | 3 | 4 | 7 | 9 | 13 | 18 |
| **GRAND TOTAL** | 420 | 3.7 | 10 | 2 | 2 | 3 | 4 | 6 | 9 | 18 |

## 65.61: RMVL BOTH OV & FALL NEC. Formerly included in operation group(s) 680.

| Type of Patients | Observed Patients | Avg. Stay | Variance | 10th | 25th | 50th | 75th | 90th | 95th | 99th |
|---|---|---|---|---|---|---|---|---|---|---|
| **1. SINGLE DX** | | | | | | | | | | |
| 0–19 Years | 5 | 2.3 | 1 | 1 | 2 | 2 | 3 | 4 | 4 | 4 |
| 20–34 | 36 | 2.5 | 1 | 1 | 2 | 2 | 3 | 3 | 4 | 6 |
| 35–49 | 150 | 2.5 | <1 | 1 | 2 | 2 | 3 | 4 | 4 | 5 |
| 50–64 | 158 | 2.5 | 2 | 1 | 2 | 2 | 3 | 4 | 6 | 7 |
| 65+ | 55 | 3.0 | 2 | 2 | 3 | 3 | 3 | 4 | 5 | 8 |
| **2. MULTIPLE DX** | | | | | | | | | | |
| 0–19 Years | 8 | 4.8 | 10 | 1 | 2 | 4 | 9 | 9 | 9 | 9 |
| 20–34 | 556 | 3.0 | 6 | 2 | 2 | 3 | 3 | 5 | 6 | 11 |
| 35–49 | 2,994 | 3.3 | 6 | 2 | 2 | 3 | 3 | 5 | 7 | 15 |
| 50–64 | 2,353 | 4.0 | 14 | 2 | 2 | 3 | 4 | 7 | 10 | 18 |
| 65+ | 1,733 | 5.5 | 19 | 2 | 3 | 4 | 7 | 10 | 14 | 24 |
| **TOTAL SINGLE DX** | 404 | 2.6 | 1 | 1 | 2 | 2 | 3 | 4 | 5 | 7 |
| **TOTAL MULTIPLE DX** | 7,644 | 4.0 | 12 | 2 | 2 | 3 | 4 | 7 | 10 | 18 |
| **TOTAL** | | | | | | | | | | |
| 0–19 Years | 13 | 4.0 | 8 | 1 | 2 | 3 | 5 | 9 | 9 | 9 |
| 20–34 | 592 | 2.9 | 4 | 2 | 2 | 3 | 3 | 5 | 6 | 10 |
| 35–49 | 3,144 | 3.3 | 6 | 2 | 2 | 3 | 3 | 5 | 7 | 15 |
| 50–64 | 2,511 | 3.9 | 13 | 2 | 2 | 3 | 4 | 7 | 9 | 18 |
| 65+ | 1,788 | 5.4 | 19 | 2 | 3 | 4 | 7 | 10 | 14 | 24 |
| **GRAND TOTAL** | 8,048 | 3.9 | 11 | 2 | 2 | 3 | 4 | 7 | 10 | 18 |

## 65.6: BILAT SALPINGO-OOPHORECT. Formerly included in operation group(s) 680.

| Type of Patients | Observed Patients | Avg. Stay | Variance | 10th | 25th | 50th | 75th | 90th | 95th | 99th |
|---|---|---|---|---|---|---|---|---|---|---|
| **1. SINGLE DX** | | | | | | | | | | |
| 0–19 Years | 5 | 2.3 | 1 | 1 | 2 | 2 | 3 | 4 | 4 | 4 |
| 20–34 | 58 | 2.3 | <1 | 1 | 2 | 2 | 3 | 3 | 4 | 6 |
| 35–49 | 190 | 2.4 | 1 | 1 | 2 | 2 | 3 | 4 | 5 | 5 |
| 50–64 | 196 | 2.5 | 2 | 1 | 2 | 2 | 3 | 4 | 5 | 7 |
| 65+ | 79 | 2.7 | 2 | 1 | 2 | 3 | 3 | 4 | 5 | 8 |
| **2. MULTIPLE DX** | | | | | | | | | | |
| 0–19 Years | 15 | 4.2 | 12 | 1 | 1 | 3 | 5 | 9 | 9 | 14 |
| 20–34 | 827 | 2.8 | 3 | 1 | 2 | 3 | 3 | 5 | 6 | 9 |
| 35–49 | 3,874 | 3.2 | 5 | 2 | 2 | 3 | 4 | 5 | 7 | 14 |
| 50–64 | 2,776 | 3.8 | 13 | 2 | 2 | 3 | 5 | 6 | 9 | 18 |
| 65+ | 2,023 | 5.2 | 19 | 2 | 3 | 4 | 6 | 10 | 14 | 24 |
| **TOTAL SINGLE DX** | 528 | 2.5 | 1 | 1 | 2 | 2 | 3 | 4 | 5 | 7 |
| **TOTAL MULTIPLE DX** | 9,515 | 3.7 | 11 | 2 | 2 | 3 | 4 | 7 | 9 | 17 |
| **TOTAL** | | | | | | | | | | |
| 0–19 Years | 20 | 3.8 | 11 | 1 | 2 | 3 | 4 | 9 | 9 | 14 |
| 20–34 | 885 | 2.8 | 3 | 1 | 2 | 3 | 3 | 4 | 6 | 9 |
| 35–49 | 4,064 | 3.1 | 5 | 2 | 2 | 3 | 4 | 6 | 7 | 14 |
| 50–64 | 2,972 | 3.7 | 12 | 2 | 2 | 3 | 4 | 6 | 9 | 17 |
| 65+ | 2,102 | 5.1 | 18 | 2 | 3 | 4 | 6 | 10 | 14 | 24 |
| **GRAND TOTAL** | 10,043 | 3.7 | 10 | 2 | 2 | 3 | 4 | 7 | 9 | 17 |

## 65.62: RMVL REM OV & FALL NEC. Formerly included in operation group(s) 680.

| Type of Patients | Observed Patients | Avg. Stay | Variance | 10th | 25th | 50th | 75th | 90th | 95th | 99th |
|---|---|---|---|---|---|---|---|---|---|---|
| **1. SINGLE DX** | | | | | | | | | | |
| 0–19 Years | 0 | | | | | | | | | |
| 20–34 | 10 | 2.7 | <1 | 2 | 2 | 3 | 3 | 4 | 4 | 4 |
| 35–49 | 22 | 2.3 | 1 | 1 | 2 | 2 | 3 | 3 | 5 | 5 |
| 50–64 | 10 | 2.5 | <1 | 2 | 2 | 3 | 3 | 3 | 3 | 3 |
| 65+ | 7 | 2.9 | <1 | 2 | 3 | 3 | 3 | 4 | 4 | 4 |
| **2. MULTIPLE DX** | | | | | | | | | | |
| 0–19 Years | 6 | 5.3 | 18 | 3 | 3 | 3 | 4 | 14 | 14 | 14 |
| 20–34 | 162 | 2.6 | 1 | 1 | 2 | 3 | 3 | 4 | 5 | 7 |
| 35–49 | 478 | 2.9 | 4 | 2 | 2 | 3 | 4 | 5 | 6 | 13 |
| 50–64 | 142 | 3.8 | 9 | 2 | 3 | 3 | 4 | 6 | 10 | 14 |
| 65+ | 106 | 5.1 | 20 | 2 | 3 | 4 | 5 | 9 | 15 | 27 |
| **TOTAL SINGLE DX** | 49 | 2.5 | <1 | 1 | 2 | 2 | 3 | 4 | 4 | 5 |
| **TOTAL MULTIPLE DX** | 894 | 3.3 | 7 | 2 | 2 | 3 | 4 | 5 | 7 | 14 |
| **TOTAL** | | | | | | | | | | |
| 0–19 Years | 6 | 5.3 | 18 | 3 | 3 | 3 | 4 | 14 | 14 | 14 |
| 20–34 | 172 | 2.6 | 1 | 1 | 2 | 2 | 3 | 4 | 5 | 7 |
| 35–49 | 500 | 2.9 | 4 | 2 | 2 | 3 | 4 | 6 | 6 | 13 |
| 50–64 | 152 | 3.7 | 9 | 2 | 3 | 3 | 4 | 6 | 9 | 14 |
| 65+ | 113 | 5.0 | 19 | 2 | 3 | 4 | 5 | 8 | 14 | 27 |
| **GRAND TOTAL** | 943 | 3.2 | 7 | 2 | 2 | 3 | 3 | 5 | 7 | 14 |

Length of Stay by Diagnosis and Operation, United States, 2000

# United States, October 1998–September 1999 Data, by Operation

## 65.63: LAPSCP RMVL BOTH OV/FALL. Formerly included in operation group(s) 680.

| Type of Patients | Observed Patients | Avg. Stay | Variance | Percentiles | | | | | | |
|---|---|---|---|---|---|---|---|---|---|---|
| | | | | 10th | 25th | 50th | 75th | 90th | 95th | 99th |
| **1. SINGLE DX** | | | | | | | | | | |
| 0–19 Years | 0 | | | | | | | | | |
| 20–34 | 7 | 1.8 | <1 | 1 | 1 | 1 | 3 | 3 | 3 | 3 |
| 35–49 | 14 | 1.6 | 1 | 1 | 1 | 1 | 2 | 3 | 3 | 5 |
| 50–64 | 26 | 2.3 | 1 | 1 | 1 | 2 | 3 | 3 | 4 | 4 |
| 65+ | 17 | 1.7 | 2 | 1 | 1 | 1 | 2 | 4 | 5 | 5 |
| **2. MULTIPLE DX** | | | | | | | | | | |
| 0–19 Years | 1 | 1.0 | 0 | 1 | 1 | 1 | 1 | 1 | 1 | 1 |
| 20–34 | 81 | 2.2 | 2 | 1 | 1 | 2 | 3 | 5 | 6 | 7 |
| 35–49 | 343 | 2.3 | 5 | 1 | 1 | 2 | 3 | 4 | 4 | 10 |
| 50–64 | 261 | 1.9 | 2 | 1 | 1 | 2 | 3 | 3 | 4 | 7 |
| 65+ | 173 | 2.4 | 6 | 1 | 1 | 1 | 3 | 4 | 7 | 14 |
| **TOTAL SINGLE DX** | 64 | 1.9 | 1 | 1 | 1 | 1 | 3 | 4 | 4 | 5 |
| **TOTAL MULTIPLE DX** | 859 | 2.2 | 4 | 1 | 1 | 2 | 3 | 4 | 5 | 9 |
| **TOTAL** | | | | | | | | | | |
| 0–19 Years | 1 | 1.0 | 0 | 1 | 1 | 1 | 1 | 1 | 1 | 1 |
| 20–34 | 88 | 2.2 | 2 | 1 | 1 | 2 | 3 | 4 | 5 | 7 |
| 35–49 | 357 | 2.3 | 5 | 1 | 1 | 2 | 3 | 4 | 4 | 10 |
| 50–64 | 287 | 1.9 | 2 | 1 | 1 | 2 | 3 | 3 | 4 | 7 |
| 65+ | 190 | 2.3 | 6 | 1 | 1 | 1 | 3 | 4 | 7 | 14 |
| **GRAND TOTAL** | 923 | 2.2 | 4 | 1 | 1 | 2 | 3 | 4 | 5 | 9 |

## 65.8: TUBO-OVARIAN ADHESIO. Formerly included in operation group(s) 681.

| Type of Patients | Observed Patients | Avg. Stay | Variance | Percentiles | | | | | | |
|---|---|---|---|---|---|---|---|---|---|---|
| | | | | 10th | 25th | 50th | 75th | 90th | 95th | 99th |
| **1. SINGLE DX** | | | | | | | | | | |
| 0–19 Years | 3 | 2.0 | <1 | 1 | 1 | 2 | 3 | 3 | 3 | 3 |
| 20–34 | 21 | 2.0 | <1 | 1 | 2 | 2 | 2 | 2 | 3 | 4 |
| 35–49 | 25 | 2.1 | <1 | 1 | 2 | 2 | 2 | 3 | 5 | 5 |
| 50–64 | 6 | 2.6 | 5 | 1 | 1 | 2 | 5 | 6 | 6 | 6 |
| 65+ | 0 | | | | | | | | | |
| **2. MULTIPLE DX** | | | | | | | | | | |
| 0–19 Years | 34 | 4.7 | 8 | 2 | 2 | 5 | 6 | 11 | 11 | 11 |
| 20–34 | 485 | 2.6 | 3 | 1 | 2 | 2 | 3 | 4 | 6 | 9 |
| 35–49 | 448 | 2.9 | 4 | 1 | 2 | 3 | 3 | 5 | 5 | 10 |
| 50–64 | 71 | 3.2 | 10 | 1 | 2 | 3 | 3 | 6 | 8 | 9 |
| 65+ | 30 | 4.0 | 11 | 2 | 3 | 3 | 5 | 6 | 8 | 27 |
| **TOTAL SINGLE DX** | 55 | 2.1 | <1 | 1 | 2 | 2 | 2 | 3 | 4 | 6 |
| **TOTAL MULTIPLE DX** | 1,068 | 2.9 | 4 | 1 | 2 | 2 | 3 | 5 | 6 | 11 |
| **TOTAL** | | | | | | | | | | |
| 0–19 Years | 37 | 4.6 | 8 | 2 | 2 | 5 | 6 | 11 | 11 | 11 |
| 20–34 | 506 | 2.5 | 3 | 1 | 2 | 2 | 3 | 4 | 6 | 9 |
| 35–49 | 473 | 2.8 | 4 | 1 | 2 | 3 | 3 | 5 | 5 | 10 |
| 50–64 | 77 | 3.2 | 10 | 1 | 2 | 3 | 3 | 6 | 8 | 9 |
| 65+ | 30 | 4.0 | 11 | 2 | 3 | 3 | 5 | 6 | 8 | 27 |
| **GRAND TOTAL** | 1,123 | 2.8 | 4 | 1 | 2 | 2 | 3 | 5 | 6 | 11 |

## 65.7: REPAIR OF OVARY. Formerly included in operation group(s) 681.

| Type of Patients | Observed Patients | Avg. Stay | Variance | Percentiles | | | | | | |
|---|---|---|---|---|---|---|---|---|---|---|
| | | | | 10th | 25th | 50th | 75th | 90th | 95th | 99th |
| **1. SINGLE DX** | | | | | | | | | | |
| 0–19 Years | 11 | 1.4 | <1 | 1 | 1 | 1 | 2 | 2 | 2 | 3 |
| 20–34 | 11 | 2.7 | 1 | 1 | 2 | 2 | 4 | 4 | 4 | 4 |
| 35–49 | 5 | 2.3 | <1 | 2 | 2 | 2 | 3 | 3 | 3 | 3 |
| 50–64 | 0 | | | | | | | | | |
| 65+ | 0 | | | | | | | | | |
| **2. MULTIPLE DX** | | | | | | | | | | |
| 0–19 Years | 27 | 2.9 | <1 | 2 | 3 | 3 | 3 | 4 | 4 | 4 |
| 20–34 | 64 | 3.2 | 3 | 1 | 2 | 3 | 4 | 6 | 6 | 7 |
| 35–49 | 27 | 3.3 | 12 | 2 | 2 | 2 | 5 | 4 | 14 | 18 |
| 50–64 | 2 | 3.5 | 3 | 2 | 2 | 4 | 5 | 5 | 5 | 5 |
| 65+ | 0 | | | | | | | | | |
| **TOTAL SINGLE DX** | 27 | 2.2 | <1 | 1 | 2 | 2 | 3 | 3 | 4 | 4 |
| **TOTAL MULTIPLE DX** | 120 | 3.1 | 4 | 1 | 2 | 3 | 3 | 5 | 6 | 14 |
| **TOTAL** | | | | | | | | | | |
| 0–19 Years | 38 | 2.6 | <1 | 2 | 2 | 3 | 3 | 4 | 4 | 4 |
| 20–34 | 75 | 3.1 | 3 | 1 | 2 | 3 | 4 | 6 | 6 | 7 |
| 35–49 | 32 | 2.9 | 7 | 2 | 2 | 2 | 4 | 4 | 4 | 18 |
| 50–64 | 2 | 3.5 | 3 | 2 | 2 | 4 | 5 | 5 | 5 | 5 |
| 65+ | 0 | | | | | | | | | |
| **GRAND TOTAL** | 147 | 2.9 | 3 | 1 | 2 | 3 | 3 | 4 | 6 | 7 |

## 65.81: LAPSCP ADHESIO OV/FALL. Formerly included in operation group(s) 681.

| Type of Patients | Observed Patients | Avg. Stay | Variance | Percentiles | | | | | | |
|---|---|---|---|---|---|---|---|---|---|---|
| | | | | 10th | 25th | 50th | 75th | 90th | 95th | 99th |
| **1. SINGLE DX** | | | | | | | | | | |
| 0–19 Years | 1 | 2.0 | 0 | 2 | 2 | 2 | 2 | 2 | 2 | 2 |
| 20–34 | 9 | 2.0 | <1 | 2 | 2 | 2 | 2 | 2 | 2 | 6 |
| 35–49 | 5 | 1.6 | <1 | 1 | 1 | 2 | 2 | 2 | 2 | 2 |
| 50–64 | 0 | | | | | | | | | |
| 65+ | 0 | | | | | | | | | |
| **2. MULTIPLE DX** | | | | | | | | | | |
| 0–19 Years | 20 | 3.7 | 3 | 2 | 2 | 4 | 5 | 6 | 6 | 6 |
| 20–34 | 167 | 2.4 | 3 | 1 | 1 | 2 | 3 | 4 | 7 | 9 |
| 35–49 | 143 | 2.4 | 3 | 1 | 1 | 2 | 3 | 5 | 5 | 10 |
| 50–64 | 23 | 2.9 | 5 | 1 | 1 | 2 | 5 | 8 | 8 | 8 |
| 65+ | 7 | 2.8 | 6 | 1 | 1 | 2 | 3 | 8 | 8 | 8 |
| **TOTAL SINGLE DX** | 15 | 2.0 | <1 | 2 | 2 | 2 | 2 | 2 | 2 | 6 |
| **TOTAL MULTIPLE DX** | 360 | 2.5 | 3 | 1 | 1 | 2 | 3 | 5 | 7 | 9 |
| **TOTAL** | | | | | | | | | | |
| 0–19 Years | 21 | 3.7 | 3 | 2 | 2 | 4 | 5 | 6 | 6 | 6 |
| 20–34 | 176 | 2.4 | 3 | 1 | 1 | 2 | 3 | 4 | 7 | 9 |
| 35–49 | 148 | 2.4 | 3 | 1 | 1 | 2 | 3 | 4 | 5 | 10 |
| 50–64 | 23 | 2.9 | 5 | 1 | 1 | 2 | 5 | 8 | 8 | 8 |
| 65+ | 7 | 2.8 | 6 | 1 | 1 | 2 | 3 | 8 | 8 | 8 |
| **GRAND TOTAL** | 375 | 2.5 | 3 | 1 | 1 | 2 | 3 | 5 | 6 | 9 |

243

Length of Stay by Diagnosis and Operation, United States, 2000

**United States, October 1998–September 1999 Data, by Operation**

## 65.89: ADHESIO OV/FALL TUBE NEC. Formerly included in operation group(s) 681.

| Type of Patients | Observed Patients | Avg. Stay | Vari-ance | Percentiles | | | | | | |
|---|---|---|---|---|---|---|---|---|---|---|
| | | | | 10th | 25th | 50th | 75th | 90th | 95th | 99th |
| **1. SINGLE DX** | | | | | | | | | | |
| 0–19 Years | 2 | 2.0 | 1 | 1 | 1 | 1 | 3 | 3 | 3 | 3 |
| 20–34 | 12 | 2.0 | <1 | 1 | 2 | 2 | 2 | 3 | 4 | 4 |
| 35–49 | 20 | 2.2 | <1 | 1 | 2 | 2 | 2 | 3 | 5 | 5 |
| 50–64 | 6 | 2.6 | 5 | 1 | 1 | 2 | 5 | 6 | 6 | 6 |
| 65+ | 0 | | | | | | | | | |
| **2. MULTIPLE DX** | | | | | | | | | | |
| 0–19 Years | 14 | 6.7 | 12 | 2 | 3 | 7 | 11 | 11 | 11 | 11 |
| 20–34 | 318 | 2.6 | 2 | 1 | 2 | 2 | 3 | 4 | 5 | 10 |
| 35–49 | 305 | 3.1 | 4 | 2 | 2 | 3 | 3 | 5 | 5 | 11 |
| 50–64 | 48 | 3.4 | 13 | 1 | 1 | 3 | 3 | 6 | 8 | 9 |
| 65+ | 23 | 4.4 | 12 | 3 | 3 | 4 | 5 | 5 | 8 | 27 |
| **TOTAL SINGLE DX** | 40 | 2.2 | 1 | 1 | 2 | 2 | 2 | 4 | 5 | 6 |
| **TOTAL MULTIPLE DX** | 708 | 3.0 | 5 | 1 | 2 | 3 | 3 | 5 | 6 | 11 |
| **TOTAL** | | | | | | | | | | |
| 0–19 Years | 16 | 6.4 | 13 | 2 | 3 | 6 | 11 | 11 | 11 | 11 |
| 20–34 | 330 | 2.6 | 2 | 1 | 2 | 2 | 3 | 4 | 5 | 10 |
| 35–49 | 325 | 3.0 | 4 | 2 | 2 | 3 | 3 | 5 | 5 | 11 |
| 50–64 | 54 | 3.3 | 12 | 1 | 2 | 3 | 3 | 6 | 8 | 9 |
| 65+ | 23 | 4.4 | 12 | 3 | 3 | 4 | 5 | 5 | 8 | 27 |
| **GRAND TOTAL** | 748 | 3.0 | 6 | 2 | 2 | 3 | 3 | 5 | 6 | 11 |

## 65.91: ASPIRATION OF OVARY. Formerly included in operation group(s) 681.

| Type of Patients | Observed Patients | Avg. Stay | Vari-ance | Percentiles | | | | | | |
|---|---|---|---|---|---|---|---|---|---|---|
| | | | | 10th | 25th | 50th | 75th | 90th | 95th | 99th |
| **1. SINGLE DX** | | | | | | | | | | |
| 0–19 Years | 52 | 2.0 | 2 | 1 | 1 | 1 | 3 | 4 | 5 | 10 |
| 20–34 | 68 | 1.8 | <1 | 1 | 1 | 1 | 2 | 3 | 3 | 6 |
| 35–49 | 19 | 1.7 | <1 | 1 | 1 | 2 | 2 | 3 | 3 | 6 |
| 50–64 | 1 | 6.0 | 0 | 6 | 6 | 6 | 6 | 6 | 6 | 6 |
| 65+ | 0 | | | | | | | | | |
| **2. MULTIPLE DX** | | | | | | | | | | |
| 0–19 Years | 77 | 3.8 | 6 | 1 | 2 | 3 | 7 | 7 | 7 | 8 |
| 20–34 | 309 | 2.6 | 4 | 1 | 1 | 3 | 3 | 6 | 7 | 11 |
| 35–49 | 146 | 3.1 | 5 | 1 | 2 | 2 | 4 | 6 | 8 | 12 |
| 50–64 | 12 | 3.4 | 9 | 1 | 2 | 3 | 5 | 7 | 13 | 13 |
| 65+ | 11 | 8.1 | 56 | 2 | 3 | 3 | 18 | 18 | 24 | 24 |
| **TOTAL SINGLE DX** | 140 | 1.9 | 2 | 1 | 1 | 2 | 2 | 3 | 5 | 6 |
| **TOTAL MULTIPLE DX** | 555 | 3.1 | 6 | 1 | 1 | 2 | 4 | 7 | 7 | 13 |
| **TOTAL** | | | | | | | | | | |
| 0–19 Years | 129 | 3.3 | 6 | 1 | 1 | 3 | 5 | 7 | 7 | 8 |
| 20–34 | 377 | 2.5 | 4 | 1 | 1 | 2 | 3 | 5 | 6 | 11 |
| 35–49 | 165 | 2.9 | 5 | 1 | 2 | 2 | 4 | 6 | 8 | 12 |
| 50–64 | 13 | 3.6 | 9 | 2 | 2 | 3 | 6 | 7 | 13 | 13 |
| 65+ | 11 | 8.1 | 56 | 2 | 3 | 3 | 18 | 18 | 24 | 24 |
| **GRAND TOTAL** | 695 | 2.9 | 6 | 1 | 1 | 2 | 3 | 6 | 7 | 12 |

## 65.9: OTHER OVARIAN OPERATIONS. Formerly included in operation group(s) 681.

| Type of Patients | Observed Patients | Avg. Stay | Vari-ance | Percentiles | | | | | | |
|---|---|---|---|---|---|---|---|---|---|---|
| | | | | 10th | 25th | 50th | 75th | 90th | 95th | 99th |
| **1. SINGLE DX** | | | | | | | | | | |
| 0–19 Years | 58 | 2.0 | 2 | 1 | 1 | 1 | 3 | 3 | 5 | 6 |
| 20–34 | 72 | 1.7 | <1 | 1 | 1 | 2 | 2 | 2 | 3 | 6 |
| 35–49 | 24 | 1.7 | <1 | 1 | 1 | 2 | 2 | 3 | 5 | 5 |
| 50–64 | 1 | 6.0 | 0 | 6 | 6 | 6 | 6 | 6 | 6 | 6 |
| 65+ | 0 | | | | | | | | | |
| **2. MULTIPLE DX** | | | | | | | | | | |
| 0–19 Years | 92 | 3.7 | 7 | 1 | 3 | 3 | 7 | 7 | 7 | 8 |
| 20–34 | 342 | 2.6 | 4 | 1 | 2 | 2 | 3 | 5 | 7 | 11 |
| 35–49 | 151 | 3.1 | 5 | 1 | 2 | 2 | 4 | 6 | 8 | 12 |
| 50–64 | 13 | 3.4 | 8 | 1 | 2 | 3 | 5 | 7 | 13 | 13 |
| 65+ | 11 | 8.1 | 56 | 2 | 3 | 3 | 18 | 18 | 24 | 24 |
| **TOTAL SINGLE DX** | 155 | 1.9 | 1 | 1 | 1 | 2 | 2 | 3 | 4 | 6 |
| **TOTAL MULTIPLE DX** | 609 | 3.0 | 6 | 1 | 1 | 2 | 4 | 7 | 7 | 12 |
| **TOTAL** | | | | | | | | | | |
| 0–19 Years | 150 | 3.1 | 6 | 1 | 1 | 2 | 4 | 7 | 7 | 8 |
| 20–34 | 414 | 2.5 | 4 | 1 | 2 | 2 | 3 | 5 | 6 | 10 |
| 35–49 | 175 | 2.9 | 5 | 1 | 2 | 2 | 3 | 6 | 7 | 12 |
| 50–64 | 14 | 3.6 | 8 | 2 | 2 | 3 | 6 | 7 | 13 | 13 |
| 65+ | 11 | 8.1 | 56 | 2 | 3 | 3 | 18 | 18 | 24 | 24 |
| **GRAND TOTAL** | 764 | 2.8 | 6 | 1 | 1 | 2 | 3 | 6 | 7 | 12 |

## 66.0: SALPINGOSTOMY/SALPINGOT. Formerly included in operation group(s) 684.

| Type of Patients | Observed Patients | Avg. Stay | Vari-ance | Percentiles | | | | | | |
|---|---|---|---|---|---|---|---|---|---|---|
| | | | | 10th | 25th | 50th | 75th | 90th | 95th | 99th |
| **1. SINGLE DX** | | | | | | | | | | |
| 0–19 Years | 60 | 1.9 | <1 | 1 | 2 | 2 | 2 | 2 | 3 | 4 |
| 20–34 | 519 | 1.6 | <1 | 1 | 1 | 1 | 2 | 3 | 3 | 4 |
| 35–49 | 107 | 1.7 | <1 | 1 | 1 | 1 | 2 | 3 | 3 | 4 |
| 50–64 | 0 | | | | | | | | | |
| 65+ | | | | | | | | | | |
| **2. MULTIPLE DX** | | | | | | | | | | |
| 0–19 Years | 92 | 2.8 | 8 | 1 | 2 | 2 | 3 | 4 | 9 | 15 |
| 20–34 | 723 | 1.9 | 1 | 1 | 1 | 2 | 2 | 3 | 4 | 7 |
| 35–49 | 140 | 2.5 | 8 | 1 | 2 | 2 | 3 | 7 | 5 | 12 |
| 50–64 | 3 | 5.0 | 5 | 3 | 7 | 7 | 7 | 7 | 7 | 7 |
| 65+ | 2 | 1.7 | <1 | 1 | 1 | 2 | 2 | 2 | 2 | 2 |
| **TOTAL SINGLE DX** | 686 | 1.6 | <1 | 1 | 1 | 1 | 2 | 3 | 3 | 4 |
| **TOTAL MULTIPLE DX** | 960 | 2.1 | 3 | 1 | 1 | 2 | 3 | 3 | 4 | 9 |
| **TOTAL** | | | | | | | | | | |
| 0–19 Years | 152 | 2.4 | 5 | 1 | 2 | 2 | 3 | 3 | 4 | 15 |
| 20–34 | 1,242 | 1.8 | 1 | 1 | 1 | 1 | 2 | 3 | 4 | 6 |
| 35–49 | 247 | 2.1 | 5 | 1 | 2 | 2 | 3 | 3 | 5 | 10 |
| 50–64 | 3 | 5.0 | 5 | 2 | 2 | 7 | 7 | 7 | 7 | 7 |
| 65+ | 2 | 1.7 | <1 | 1 | 1 | 2 | 2 | 2 | 2 | 2 |
| **GRAND TOTAL** | 1,646 | 1.9 | 2 | 1 | 1 | 2 | 2 | 3 | 4 | 7 |

Length of Stay by Diagnosis and Operation, United States, 2000

# United States, October 1998–September 1999 Data, by Operation

## 66.02: SALPINGOSTOMY. Formerly included in operation group(s) 684.

| Type of Patients | Observed Patients | Avg. Stay | Variance | 10th | 25th | 50th | 75th | 90th | 95th | 99th |
|---|---|---|---|---|---|---|---|---|---|---|
| **1. SINGLE DX** | | | | | | | | | | |
| 0–19 Years | 50 | 1.9 | <1 | 1 | 1 | 2 | 2 | 2 | 3 | 4 |
| 20–34 | 449 | 1.6 | <1 | 1 | 1 | 1 | 2 | 2 | 3 | 4 |
| 35–49 | 83 | 1.6 | <1 | 1 | 1 | 1 | 2 | 3 | 3 | 3 |
| 50–64 | 0 | | | | | | | | | |
| 65+ | 0 | | | | | | | | | |
| **2. MULTIPLE DX** | | | | | | | | | | |
| 0–19 Years | 71 | 2.2 | <1 | 1 | 2 | 2 | 3 | 3 | 3 | 7 |
| 20–34 | 612 | 1.8 | 1 | 1 | 1 | 2 | 2 | 3 | 4 | 5 |
| 35–49 | 120 | 1.9 | 1 | 1 | 1 | 2 | 3 | 3 | 3 | 4 |
| 50–64 | 1 | 2.0 | 0 | 2 | 2 | 2 | 2 | 2 | 2 | 2 |
| 65+ | 0 | | | | | | | | | |
| **TOTAL SINGLE DX** | 582 | 1.6 | <1 | 1 | 1 | 1 | 2 | 3 | 3 | 4 |
| **TOTAL MULTIPLE DX** | 804 | 1.9 | 1 | 1 | 1 | 2 | 2 | 3 | 4 | 5 |
| **TOTAL** | | | | | | | | | | |
| 0–19 Years | 121 | 2.1 | <1 | 1 | 1 | 2 | 2 | 3 | 3 | 4 |
| 20–34 | 1,061 | 1.7 | <1 | 1 | 1 | 1 | 2 | 3 | 3 | 5 |
| 35–49 | 203 | 1.8 | <1 | 1 | 1 | 2 | 2 | 3 | 3 | 4 |
| 50–64 | 1 | 2.0 | 0 | 2 | 2 | 2 | 2 | 2 | 2 | 2 |
| 65+ | 0 | | | | | | | | | |
| **GRAND TOTAL** | 1,386 | 1.7 | <1 | 1 | 1 | 2 | 2 | 3 | 3 | 5 |

## 66.1: FALLOPIAN TUBE DXTIC PX. Formerly included in operation group(s) 684, 704.

| Type of Patients | Observed Patients | Avg. Stay | Variance | 10th | 25th | 50th | 75th | 90th | 95th | 99th |
|---|---|---|---|---|---|---|---|---|---|---|
| **1. SINGLE DX** | | | | | | | | | | |
| 0–19 Years | 0 | | | | | | | | | |
| 20–34 | 1 | 1.0 | 0 | 1 | 1 | 1 | 1 | 1 | 1 | 1 |
| 35–49 | 0 | | | | | | | | | |
| 50–64 | 0 | | | | | | | | | |
| 65+ | 0 | | | | | | | | | |
| **2. MULTIPLE DX** | | | | | | | | | | |
| 0–19 Years | 0 | | | | | | | | | |
| 20–34 | 9 | 2.7 | 4 | 1 | 1 | 2 | 4 | 4 | 7 | 7 |
| 35–49 | 4 | 5.9 | 14 | 1 | 2 | 9 | 9 | 9 | 9 | 9 |
| 50–64 | 1 | 4.0 | 0 | 4 | 4 | 4 | 4 | 4 | 4 | 4 |
| 65+ | 1 | 4.0 | 0 | 4 | 4 | 4 | 4 | 4 | 4 | 4 |
| **TOTAL SINGLE DX** | 1 | 1.0 | 0 | 1 | 1 | 1 | 1 | 1 | 1 | 1 |
| **TOTAL MULTIPLE DX** | 15 | 3.4 | 7 | 1 | 1 | 2 | 4 | 9 | 9 | 9 |
| **TOTAL** | | | | | | | | | | |
| 0–19 Years | 0 | | | | | | | | | |
| 20–34 | 10 | 2.7 | 4 | 1 | 2 | 2 | 4 | 4 | 7 | 7 |
| 35–49 | 4 | 5.9 | 14 | 1 | 2 | 9 | 9 | 9 | 9 | 9 |
| 50–64 | 1 | 4.0 | 0 | 4 | 4 | 4 | 4 | 4 | 4 | 4 |
| 65+ | 1 | 4.0 | 0 | 4 | 4 | 4 | 4 | 4 | 4 | 4 |
| **GRAND TOTAL** | 16 | 3.3 | 7 | 1 | 1 | 2 | 4 | 9 | 9 | 9 |

## 66.2: BILAT ENDO OCCL FALL. Formerly included in operation group(s) 682.

| Type of Patients | Observed Patients | Avg. Stay | Variance | 10th | 25th | 50th | 75th | 90th | 95th | 99th |
|---|---|---|---|---|---|---|---|---|---|---|
| **1. SINGLE DX** | | | | | | | | | | |
| 0–19 Years | 0 | | | | | | | | | |
| 20–34 | 30 | 1.4 | <1 | 1 | 1 | 1 | 2 | 3 | 3 | 3 |
| 35–49 | 15 | 1.2 | <1 | 1 | 1 | 1 | 1 | 2 | 2 | 2 |
| 50–64 | 0 | | | | | | | | | |
| 65+ | 0 | | | | | | | | | |
| **2. MULTIPLE DX** | | | | | | | | | | |
| 0–19 Years | 4 | 1.0 | 0 | 1 | 1 | 1 | 1 | 1 | 1 | 1 |
| 20–34 | 1,256 | 2.0 | <1 | 1 | 2 | 2 | 2 | 3 | 3 | 4 |
| 35–49 | 311 | 2.2 | 2 | 1 | 2 | 2 | 2 | 3 | 4 | 12 |
| 50–64 | 2 | 2.0 | 0 | 2 | 2 | 2 | 2 | 2 | 2 | 2 |
| 65+ | 0 | | | | | | | | | |
| **TOTAL SINGLE DX** | 45 | 1.4 | <1 | 1 | 1 | 1 | 2 | 2 | 3 | 3 |
| **TOTAL MULTIPLE DX** | 1,573 | 2.0 | 1 | 1 | 2 | 2 | 2 | 3 | 3 | 5 |
| **TOTAL** | | | | | | | | | | |
| 0–19 Years | 4 | 1.0 | 0 | 1 | 1 | 1 | 1 | 1 | 1 | 1 |
| 20–34 | 1,286 | 2.0 | <1 | 1 | 1 | 2 | 2 | 3 | 3 | 4 |
| 35–49 | 326 | 2.1 | 2 | 1 | 2 | 2 | 2 | 3 | 4 | 12 |
| 50–64 | 2 | 2.0 | 0 | 2 | 2 | 2 | 2 | 2 | 2 | 2 |
| 65+ | 0 | | | | | | | | | |
| **GRAND TOTAL** | 1,618 | 2.0 | 1 | 1 | 2 | 2 | 2 | 3 | 3 | 5 |

## 66.22: BILAT ENDO LIG/DIV FALL. Formerly included in operation group(s) 682.

| Type of Patients | Observed Patients | Avg. Stay | Variance | 10th | 25th | 50th | 75th | 90th | 95th | 99th |
|---|---|---|---|---|---|---|---|---|---|---|
| **1. SINGLE DX** | | | | | | | | | | |
| 0–19 Years | 0 | | | | | | | | | |
| 20–34 | 4 | 1.7 | <1 | 1 | 1 | 2 | 2 | 2 | 2 | 2 |
| 35–49 | 3 | 1.0 | 0 | 1 | 1 | 1 | 1 | 1 | 1 | 1 |
| 50–64 | 0 | | | | | | | | | |
| 65+ | 0 | | | | | | | | | |
| **2. MULTIPLE DX** | | | | | | | | | | |
| 0–19 Years | 1 | 1.0 | 0 | 1 | 1 | 1 | 1 | 1 | 1 | 1 |
| 20–34 | 550 | 2.1 | <1 | 1 | 2 | 2 | 2 | 3 | 3 | 5 |
| 35–49 | 124 | 2.1 | 1 | 1 | 2 | 2 | 2 | 3 | 3 | 5 |
| 50–64 | 0 | | | | | | | | | |
| 65+ | 0 | | | | | | | | | |
| **TOTAL SINGLE DX** | 7 | 1.5 | <1 | 1 | 1 | 1 | 2 | 2 | 2 | 2 |
| **TOTAL MULTIPLE DX** | 675 | 2.1 | <1 | 1 | 2 | 2 | 2 | 3 | 3 | 5 |
| **TOTAL** | | | | | | | | | | |
| 0–19 Years | 1 | 1.0 | 0 | 1 | 1 | 1 | 1 | 1 | 1 | 1 |
| 20–34 | 554 | 2.1 | <1 | 1 | 2 | 2 | 2 | 3 | 3 | 5 |
| 35–49 | 127 | 2.1 | 1 | 1 | 2 | 2 | 2 | 3 | 3 | 5 |
| 50–64 | 0 | | | | | | | | | |
| 65+ | 0 | | | | | | | | | |
| **GRAND TOTAL** | 682 | 2.1 | <1 | 1 | 2 | 2 | 2 | 3 | 3 | 5 |

245

Length of Stay by Diagnosis and Operation, United States, 2000

# United States, October 1998–September 1999 Data, by Operation

## 66.29: BILAT ENDO OCCL FALL NEC. Formerly included in operation group(s) 682.

| Type of Patients | Observed Patients | Avg. Stay | Vari-ance | Percentiles | | | | | | |
|---|---|---|---|---|---|---|---|---|---|---|
| | | | | 10th | 25th | 50th | 75th | 90th | 95th | 99th |
| **1. SINGLE DX** | | | | | | | | | | |
| 0–19 Years | 0 | | | | | | | | | |
| 20–34 | 25 | 1.4 | <1 | 1 | 1 | 1 | 1 | 3 | 3 | 3 |
| 35–49 | 11 | 1.3 | <1 | 1 | 1 | 1 | 2 | 2 | 2 | 2 |
| 50–64 | 0 | | | | | | | | | |
| 65+ | 0 | | | | | | | | | |
| **2. MULTIPLE DX** | | | | | | | | | | |
| 0–19 Years | 3 | 1.0 | 0 | 1 | 1 | 1 | 1 | 1 | 1 | 1 |
| 20–34 | 689 | 1.9 | <1 | 1 | 2 | 2 | 2 | 3 | 3 | 4 |
| 35–49 | 185 | 2.2 | 3 | 1 | 1 | 2 | 2 | 3 | 5 | 12 |
| 50–64 | 2 | 2.0 | 0 | 2 | 2 | 2 | 2 | 2 | 2 | 2 |
| 65+ | 0 | | | | | | | | | |
| **TOTAL SINGLE DX** | 36 | 1.3 | <1 | 1 | 1 | 1 | 1 | 2 | 3 | 3 |
| **TOTAL MULTIPLE DX** | 879 | 2.0 | 1 | 1 | 1 | 2 | 2 | 3 | 3 | 7 |
| **TOTAL** | | | | | | | | | | |
| 0–19 Years | 3 | 1.0 | 0 | 1 | 1 | 1 | 1 | 1 | 1 | 1 |
| 20–34 | 714 | 1.9 | <1 | 1 | 1 | 2 | 2 | 3 | 3 | 4 |
| 35–49 | 196 | 2.1 | 3 | 1 | 1 | 2 | 2 | 3 | 5 | 12 |
| 50–64 | 2 | 2.0 | 0 | 2 | 2 | 2 | 2 | 2 | 2 | 2 |
| 65+ | 0 | | | | | | | | | |
| **GRAND TOTAL** | 915 | 2.0 | 1 | 1 | 1 | 2 | 2 | 3 | 3 | 6 |

## 66.3: OTH BILAT FALL DESTR/EXC. Formerly included in operation group(s) 683.

| Type of Patients | Observed Patients | Avg. Stay | Vari-ance | Percentiles | | | | | | |
|---|---|---|---|---|---|---|---|---|---|---|
| | | | | 10th | 25th | 50th | 75th | 90th | 95th | 99th |
| **1. SINGLE DX** | | | | | | | | | | |
| 0–19 Years | 0 | | | | | | | | | |
| 20–34 | 145 | 1.9 | <1 | 1 | 2 | 2 | 2 | 3 | 3 | 4 |
| 35–49 | 50 | 1.8 | <1 | 1 | 1 | 2 | 2 | 2 | 3 | 3 |
| 50–64 | 0 | | | | | | | | | |
| 65+ | 0 | | | | | | | | | |
| **2. MULTIPLE DX** | | | | | | | | | | |
| 0–19 Years | 76 | 2.1 | 2 | 1 | 2 | 2 | 2 | 3 | 3 | 12 |
| 20–34 | 21,997 | 2.1 | 2 | 1 | 2 | 2 | 2 | 3 | 3 | 4 |
| 35–49 | 5,034 | 2.2 | 1 | 1 | 2 | 2 | 2 | 3 | 3 | 5 |
| 50–64 | 2 | 2.5 | <1 | 2 | 2 | 2 | 2 | 3 | 3 | 3 |
| 65+ | 0 | | | | | | | | | |
| **TOTAL SINGLE DX** | 195 | 1.9 | <1 | 1 | 2 | 2 | 2 | 3 | 3 | 3 |
| **TOTAL MULTIPLE DX** | 27,109 | 2.1 | 2 | 1 | 2 | 2 | 2 | 3 | 3 | 5 |
| **TOTAL** | | | | | | | | | | |
| 0–19 Years | 76 | 2.1 | 2 | 1 | 2 | 2 | 2 | 3 | 3 | 12 |
| 20–34 | 22,142 | 2.1 | 2 | 1 | 2 | 2 | 2 | 3 | 3 | 4 |
| 35–49 | 5,084 | 2.2 | 1 | 1 | 2 | 2 | 3 | 3 | 3 | 5 |
| 50–64 | 2 | 2.5 | <1 | 2 | 2 | 2 | 2 | 3 | 3 | 3 |
| 65+ | 0 | | | | | | | | | |
| **GRAND TOTAL** | 27,304 | 2.1 | 2 | 1 | 2 | 2 | 2 | 3 | 3 | 5 |

## 66.32: BILAT FALL LIG & DIV NEC. Formerly included in operation group(s) 683.

| Type of Patients | Observed Patients | Avg. Stay | Vari-ance | Percentiles | | | | | | |
|---|---|---|---|---|---|---|---|---|---|---|
| | | | | 10th | 25th | 50th | 75th | 90th | 95th | 99th |
| **1. SINGLE DX** | | | | | | | | | | |
| 0–19 Years | 0 | | | | | | | | | |
| 20–34 | 79 | 2.0 | <1 | 1 | 2 | 2 | 2 | 3 | 3 | 4 |
| 35–49 | 23 | 2.0 | <1 | 2 | 2 | 2 | 2 | 2 | 3 | 3 |
| 50–64 | 0 | | | | | | | | | |
| 65+ | 0 | | | | | | | | | |
| **2. MULTIPLE DX** | | | | | | | | | | |
| 0–19 Years | 28 | 2.2 | 3 | 1 | 2 | 2 | 2 | 2 | 4 | 12 |
| 20–34 | 13,731 | 2.1 | 1 | 1 | 2 | 2 | 2 | 3 | 3 | 4 |
| 35–49 | 3,204 | 2.2 | 1 | 1 | 2 | 2 | 2 | 3 | 3 | 5 |
| 50–64 | 1 | 2.0 | 0 | 2 | 2 | 2 | 2 | 2 | 2 | 2 |
| 65+ | 0 | | | | | | | | | |
| **TOTAL SINGLE DX** | 102 | 2.0 | <1 | 1 | 2 | 2 | 2 | 3 | 3 | 4 |
| **TOTAL MULTIPLE DX** | 16,964 | 2.1 | 1 | 1 | 2 | 2 | 2 | 3 | 3 | 5 |
| **TOTAL** | | | | | | | | | | |
| 0–19 Years | 28 | 2.2 | 3 | 1 | 2 | 2 | 2 | 2 | 4 | 12 |
| 20–34 | 13,810 | 2.1 | 1 | 1 | 2 | 2 | 2 | 3 | 3 | 4 |
| 35–49 | 3,227 | 2.2 | 1 | 1 | 2 | 2 | 2 | 3 | 3 | 5 |
| 50–64 | 1 | 2.0 | 0 | 2 | 2 | 2 | 2 | 2 | 2 | 2 |
| 65+ | 0 | | | | | | | | | |
| **GRAND TOTAL** | 17,066 | 2.1 | 1 | 1 | 2 | 2 | 2 | 3 | 3 | 5 |

## 66.39: BILAT FALL DESTR NEC. Formerly included in operation group(s) 683.

| Type of Patients | Observed Patients | Avg. Stay | Vari-ance | Percentiles | | | | | | |
|---|---|---|---|---|---|---|---|---|---|---|
| | | | | 10th | 25th | 50th | 75th | 90th | 95th | 99th |
| **1. SINGLE DX** | | | | | | | | | | |
| 0–19 Years | 0 | | | | | | | | | |
| 20–34 | 65 | 1.9 | <1 | 1 | 2 | 2 | 2 | 2 | 3 | 3 |
| 35–49 | 27 | 1.7 | <1 | 1 | 1 | 2 | 2 | 3 | 3 | 3 |
| 50–64 | 0 | | | | | | | | | |
| 65+ | 0 | | | | | | | | | |
| **2. MULTIPLE DX** | | | | | | | | | | |
| 0–19 Years | 48 | 2.0 | 1 | 1 | 1 | 2 | 2 | 3 | 3 | 9 |
| 20–34 | 8,237 | 2.1 | 2 | 1 | 2 | 2 | 2 | 3 | 3 | 5 |
| 35–49 | 1,821 | 2.2 | 2 | 1 | 2 | 2 | 2 | 3 | 3 | 4 |
| 50–64 | 1 | 3.0 | 0 | 3 | 3 | 3 | 3 | 3 | 3 | 3 |
| 65+ | 0 | | | | | | | | | |
| **TOTAL SINGLE DX** | 92 | 1.9 | <1 | 1 | 2 | 2 | 2 | 2 | 3 | 3 |
| **TOTAL MULTIPLE DX** | 10,107 | 2.1 | 2 | 1 | 2 | 2 | 2 | 3 | 3 | 5 |
| **TOTAL** | | | | | | | | | | |
| 0–19 Years | 48 | 2.0 | 1 | 1 | 1 | 2 | 2 | 3 | 3 | 9 |
| 20–34 | 8,302 | 2.1 | 2 | 1 | 2 | 2 | 2 | 3 | 3 | 5 |
| 35–49 | 1,848 | 2.2 | 2 | 1 | 2 | 2 | 3 | 3 | 3 | 4 |
| 50–64 | 1 | 3.0 | 0 | 3 | 3 | 3 | 3 | 3 | 3 | 3 |
| 65+ | 0 | | | | | | | | | |
| **GRAND TOTAL** | 10,199 | 2.1 | 2 | 1 | 2 | 2 | 2 | 3 | 3 | 5 |

Length of Stay by Diagnosis and Operation, United States, 2000

# United States, October 1998–September 1999 Data, by Operation

## 66.4: TOT UNILAT SALPINGECTOMY. Formerly included in operation group(s) 684.

| Type of Patients | Observed Patients | Avg. Stay | Variance | Percentiles | | | | | | |
|---|---|---|---|---|---|---|---|---|---|---|
| | | | | 10th | 25th | 50th | 75th | 90th | 95th | 99th |
| **1. SINGLE DX** | | | | | | | | | | |
| 0–19 Years | 18 | 2.0 | 1 | 1 | 1 | 1 | 3 | 3 | 5 | 5 |
| 20–34 | 97 | 2.2 | <1 | 1 | 2 | 2 | 3 | 3 | 3 | 7 |
| 35–49 | 47 | 2.1 | <1 | 1 | 2 | 2 | 3 | 3 | 4 | 4 |
| 50–64 | 3 | 2.0 | <1 | 2 | 2 | 2 | 2 | 3 | 4 | 4 |
| 65+ | 1 | 2.0 | 0 | 2 | 2 | 2 | 2 | 2 | 2 | 2 |
| **2. MULTIPLE DX** | | | | | | | | | | |
| 0–19 Years | 63 | 3.5 | 9 | 2 | 2 | 2 | 3 | 11 | 11 | 11 |
| 20–34 | 331 | 2.9 | 4 | 1 | 2 | 2 | 3 | 5 | 8 | 11 |
| 35–49 | 250 | 3.2 | 5 | 1 | 2 | 3 | 4 | 7 | 7 | 14 |
| 50–64 | 32 | 2.7 | 3 | 2 | 2 | 3 | 5 | 5 | 5 | 12 |
| 65+ | 22 | 12.5 | 58 | 3 | 4 | 13 | 21 | 21 | 21 | 21 |
| **TOTAL SINGLE DX** | 166 | 2.1 | <1 | 1 | 1 | 2 | 3 | 3 | 4 | 5 |
| **TOTAL MULTIPLE DX** | 698 | 3.4 | 10 | 1 | 2 | 2 | 3 | 7 | 11 | 21 |
| **TOTAL** | | | | | | | | | | |
| 0–19 Years | 81 | 3.2 | 8 | 1 | 2 | 2 | 3 | 8 | 11 | 11 |
| 20–34 | 428 | 2.7 | 4 | 1 | 2 | 2 | 3 | 4 | 7 | 11 |
| 35–49 | 297 | 3.0 | 5 | 1 | 2 | 2 | 4 | 5 | 7 | 9 |
| 50–64 | 35 | 2.6 | 3 | 2 | 2 | 2 | 4 | 5 | 5 | 12 |
| 65+ | 23 | 12.3 | 58 | 2 | 4 | 13 | 21 | 21 | 21 | 21 |
| **GRAND TOTAL** | 864 | 3.2 | 9 | 1 | 2 | 2 | 3 | 6 | 9 | 21 |

## 66.6: OTHER SALPINGECTOMY. Formerly included in operation group(s) 683, 684.

| Type of Patients | Observed Patients | Avg. Stay | Variance | Percentiles | | | | | | |
|---|---|---|---|---|---|---|---|---|---|---|
| | | | | 10th | 25th | 50th | 75th | 90th | 95th | 99th |
| **1. SINGLE DX** | | | | | | | | | | |
| 0–19 Years | 148 | 1.9 | <1 | 1 | 1 | 2 | 2 | 3 | 3 | 4 |
| 20–34 | 1,577 | 2.0 | <1 | 1 | 1 | 2 | 2 | 3 | 4 | 5 |
| 35–49 | 471 | 1.8 | <1 | 1 | 1 | 2 | 2 | 3 | 5 | 5 |
| 50–64 | 8 | 1.9 | 2 | 1 | 1 | 1 | 3 | 5 | 5 | 5 |
| 65+ | 2 | 1.8 | 2 | 1 | 1 | 1 | 3 | 3 | 3 | 3 |
| **2. MULTIPLE DX** | | | | | | | | | | |
| 0–19 Years | 297 | 2.5 | 1 | 2 | 2 | 2 | 3 | 4 | 4 | 7 |
| 20–34 | 3,546 | 2.4 | 2 | 2 | 2 | 2 | 3 | 4 | 4 | 7 |
| 35–49 | 1,223 | 2.5 | 2 | 2 | 2 | 2 | 3 | 4 | 5 | 9 |
| 50–64 | 32 | 3.0 | 3 | 2 | 2 | 3 | 4 | 6 | 7 | 7 |
| 65+ | 22 | 3.6 | 9 | 1 | 2 | 3 | 4 | 8 | 10 | 15 |
| **TOTAL SINGLE DX** | 2,206 | 1.9 | <1 | 1 | 1 | 2 | 2 | 3 | 4 | 5 |
| **TOTAL MULTIPLE DX** | 5,120 | 2.5 | 2 | 2 | 2 | 2 | 3 | 4 | 5 | 7 |
| **TOTAL** | | | | | | | | | | |
| 0–19 Years | 445 | 2.3 | 1 | 2 | 2 | 2 | 3 | 3 | 4 | 7 |
| 20–34 | 5,123 | 2.3 | 2 | 1 | 1 | 2 | 3 | 3 | 4 | 6 |
| 35–49 | 1,694 | 2.3 | 2 | 1 | 1 | 2 | 3 | 4 | 7 | 7 |
| 50–64 | 40 | 2.8 | 3 | 2 | 2 | 3 | 3 | 6 | 7 | 7 |
| 65+ | 24 | 3.5 | 9 | 1 | 3 | 3 | 4 | 7 | 10 | 15 |
| **GRAND TOTAL** | 7,326 | 2.3 | 2 | 1 | 1 | 2 | 3 | 4 | 4 | 7 |

## 66.5: TOT BILAT SALPINGECTOMY. Formerly included in operation group(s) 683.

| Type of Patients | Observed Patients | Avg. Stay | Variance | Percentiles | | | | | | |
|---|---|---|---|---|---|---|---|---|---|---|
| | | | | 10th | 25th | 50th | 75th | 90th | 95th | 99th |
| **1. SINGLE DX** | | | | | | | | | | |
| 0–19 Years | 1 | 1.0 | 0 | 1 | 1 | 1 | 1 | 1 | 1 | 1 |
| 20–34 | 20 | 2.7 | 3 | 1 | 2 | 2 | 3 | 6 | 6 | 6 |
| 35–49 | 11 | 2.2 | <1 | 2 | 1 | 2 | 2 | 3 | 3 | 3 |
| 50–64 | | | | | | | | | | |
| 65+ | 0 | 2.0 | 0 | 2 | 2 | 2 | 2 | 2 | 2 | 2 |
| **2. MULTIPLE DX** | | | | | | | | | | |
| 0–19 Years | 2 | 4.1 | 3 | 3 | 3 | 3 | 6 | 6 | 6 | 6 |
| 20–34 | 123 | 2.9 | 5 | 1 | 2 | 2 | 3 | 5 | 6 | 14 |
| 35–49 | 133 | 3.0 | 4 | 2 | 2 | 3 | 3 | 6 | 8 | 11 |
| 50–64 | 20 | 3.2 | 2 | 3 | 3 | 3 | 4 | 4 | 6 | 8 |
| 65+ | 14 | 4.1 | 12 | 1 | 1 | 3 | 6 | 11 | 11 | 11 |
| **TOTAL SINGLE DX** | 33 | 2.4 | 2 | 1 | 2 | 2 | 3 | 6 | 6 | 6 |
| **TOTAL MULTIPLE DX** | 292 | 3.0 | 5 | 1 | 2 | 2 | 3 | 6 | 7 | 12 |
| **TOTAL** | | | | | | | | | | |
| 0–19 Years | 3 | 3.1 | 5 | 1 | 1 | 3 | 3 | 6 | 6 | 6 |
| 20–34 | 143 | 2.9 | 5 | 1 | 2 | 2 | 3 | 6 | 7 | 14 |
| 35–49 | 144 | 2.9 | 3 | 2 | 2 | 3 | 3 | 6 | 6 | 11 |
| 50–64 | 21 | 3.2 | 2 | 3 | 3 | 3 | 4 | 4 | 6 | 8 |
| 65+ | 14 | 4.1 | 12 | 1 | 1 | 3 | 6 | 11 | 11 | 11 |
| **GRAND TOTAL** | 325 | 2.9 | 4 | 1 | 2 | 2 | 3 | 6 | 7 | 12 |

## 66.61: EXC/DESTR FALL LES. Formerly included in operation group(s) 684.

| Type of Patients | Observed Patients | Avg. Stay | Variance | Percentiles | | | | | | |
|---|---|---|---|---|---|---|---|---|---|---|
| | | | | 10th | 25th | 50th | 75th | 90th | 95th | 99th |
| **1. SINGLE DX** | | | | | | | | | | |
| 0–19 Years | 12 | 2.1 | <1 | 2 | 2 | 2 | 2 | 2 | 3 | 4 |
| 20–34 | 28 | 1.8 | <1 | 1 | 1 | 1 | 2 | 3 | 3 | 5 |
| 35–49 | 11 | 2.7 | 2 | 1 | 2 | 2 | 3 | 6 | 6 | 11 |
| 50–64 | 4 | 1.4 | <1 | 1 | 1 | 1 | 1 | 3 | 3 | 3 |
| 65+ | 1 | 3.0 | 0 | 3 | 3 | 3 | 3 | 3 | 3 | 3 |
| **2. MULTIPLE DX** | | | | | | | | | | |
| 0–19 Years | 50 | 2.9 | 3 | 1 | 2 | 2 | 3 | 4 | 7 | 8 |
| 20–34 | 135 | 2.5 | 3 | 1 | 1 | 2 | 3 | 5 | 6 | 8 |
| 35–49 | 67 | 2.6 | 4 | 1 | 2 | 2 | 3 | 4 | 6 | 11 |
| 50–64 | 21 | 3.1 | 3 | 2 | 2 | 2 | 4 | 7 | 7 | 7 |
| 65+ | 15 | 4.2 | 10 | 2 | 3 | 3 | 5 | 8 | 15 | 15 |
| **TOTAL SINGLE DX** | 56 | 1.9 | <1 | 1 | 1 | 2 | 2 | 3 | 3 | 6 |
| **TOTAL MULTIPLE DX** | 288 | 2.7 | 3 | 1 | 2 | 2 | 3 | 5 | 6 | 9 |
| **TOTAL** | | | | | | | | | | |
| 0–19 Years | 62 | 2.7 | 2 | 2 | 2 | 2 | 3 | 4 | 7 | 8 |
| 20–34 | 163 | 2.3 | 2 | 1 | 2 | 2 | 3 | 4 | 5 | 8 |
| 35–49 | 78 | 2.6 | 3 | 1 | 2 | 2 | 3 | 4 | 6 | 11 |
| 50–64 | 25 | 2.7 | 3 | 2 | 2 | 3 | 3 | 6 | 6 | 7 |
| 65+ | 16 | 4.2 | 10 | 2 | 3 | 3 | 5 | 8 | 15 | 15 |
| **GRAND TOTAL** | 344 | 2.6 | 3 | 1 | 2 | 2 | 3 | 4 | 6 | 9 |

Length of Stay by Diagnosis and Operation, United States, 2000

# United States, October 1998–September 1999 Data, by Operation

## 66.62: RMVL FALL & TUBAL PREG. Formerly included in operation group(s) 684.

| Type of Patients | Observed Patients | Avg. Stay | Variance | 10th | 25th | 50th | 75th | 90th | 95th | 99th |
|---|---|---|---|---|---|---|---|---|---|---|
| **1. SINGLE DX** | | | | | | | | | | |
| 0–19 Years | 128 | 1.8 | <1 | 1 | 1 | 2 | 2 | 3 | 3 | 4 |
| 20–34 | 1,449 | 2.0 | <1 | 1 | 1 | 2 | 2 | 3 | 4 | 5 |
| 35–49 | 427 | 1.8 | <1 | 1 | 1 | 2 | 2 | 3 | 3 | 4 |
| 50–64 | 0 | | | | | | | | | |
| 65+ | 0 | | | | | | | | | |
| **2. MULTIPLE DX** | | | | | | | | | | |
| 0–19 Years | 219 | 2.4 | 1 | 1 | 2 | 2 | 3 | 3 | 4 | 6 |
| 20–34 | 3,036 | 2.4 | 2 | 1 | 2 | 2 | 3 | 4 | 4 | 7 |
| 35–49 | 1,021 | 2.5 | 2 | 1 | 2 | 2 | 3 | 4 | 5 | 8 |
| 50–64 | 0 | | | | | | | | | |
| 65+ | 0 | | | | | | | | | |
| **TOTAL SINGLE DX** | 2,004 | 1.9 | <1 | 1 | 1 | 2 | 2 | 3 | 4 | 4 |
| **TOTAL MULTIPLE DX** | 4,276 | 2.4 | 2 | 1 | 2 | 2 | 3 | 4 | 4 | 7 |
| **TOTAL** | | | | | | | | | | |
| 0–19 Years | 347 | 2.2 | 1 | 1 | 2 | 2 | 3 | 3 | 4 | 6 |
| 20–34 | 4,485 | 2.3 | 2 | 1 | 1 | 2 | 3 | 4 | 4 | 6 |
| 35–49 | 1,448 | 2.3 | 2 | 1 | 1 | 2 | 3 | 4 | 4 | 7 |
| 50–64 | 0 | | | | | | | | | |
| 65+ | 0 | | | | | | | | | |
| **GRAND TOTAL** | 6,280 | 2.3 | 2 | 1 | 1 | 2 | 3 | 4 | 4 | 7 |

## 66.69: PARTIAL FALL RMVL NEC. Formerly included in operation group(s) 684.

| Type of Patients | Observed Patients | Avg. Stay | Variance | 10th | 25th | 50th | 75th | 90th | 95th | 99th |
|---|---|---|---|---|---|---|---|---|---|---|
| **1. SINGLE DX** | | | | | | | | | | |
| 0–19 Years | 8 | 1.4 | <1 | 1 | 1 | 1 | 2 | 2 | 2 | 2 |
| 20–34 | 93 | 2.1 | 1 | 1 | 1 | 2 | 3 | 3 | 3 | 8 |
| 35–49 | 30 | 2.2 | 1 | 1 | 1 | 2 | 2 | 3 | 5 | 5 |
| 50–64 | 4 | 2.8 | 3 | 1 | 1 | 2 | 5 | 5 | 5 | 5 |
| 65+ | 1 | 1.0 | 0 | 1 | 1 | 1 | 1 | 1 | 1 | 1 |
| **2. MULTIPLE DX** | | | | | | | | | | |
| 0–19 Years | 28 | 2.5 | 2 | 1 | 2 | 2 | 3 | 3 | 4 | 7 |
| 20–34 | 305 | 2.5 | 2 | 1 | 2 | 2 | 3 | 4 | 5 | 7 |
| 35–49 | 113 | 2.4 | 2 | 1 | 1 | 2 | 3 | 3 | 5 | 7 |
| 50–64 | 11 | 2.8 | 3 | 1 | 2 | 2 | 3 | 6 | 7 | 7 |
| 65+ | 7 | 2.6 | 5 | 1 | 1 | 2 | 3 | 4 | 10 | 10 |
| **TOTAL SINGLE DX** | 136 | 2.1 | 1 | 1 | 1 | 2 | 3 | 3 | 4 | 6 |
| **TOTAL MULTIPLE DX** | 464 | 2.5 | 2 | 1 | 2 | 2 | 3 | 4 | 5 | 7 |
| **TOTAL** | | | | | | | | | | |
| 0–19 Years | 36 | 2.3 | 2 | 1 | 1 | 2 | 3 | 4 | 5 | 7 |
| 20–34 | 398 | 2.4 | 2 | 1 | 2 | 2 | 3 | 4 | 5 | 7 |
| 35–49 | 143 | 2.4 | 2 | 1 | 1 | 2 | 3 | 4 | 5 | 7 |
| 50–64 | 15 | 2.8 | 3 | 1 | 2 | 2 | 4 | 5 | 7 | 7 |
| 65+ | 8 | 2.5 | 5 | 1 | 1 | 2 | 2 | 4 | 10 | 10 |
| **GRAND TOTAL** | 600 | 2.4 | 2 | 1 | 1 | 2 | 3 | 4 | 5 | 7 |

## 66.7: REPAIR OF FALLOPIAN TUBE. Formerly included in operation group(s) 684.

| Type of Patients | Observed Patients | Avg. Stay | Variance | 10th | 25th | 50th | 75th | 90th | 95th | 99th |
|---|---|---|---|---|---|---|---|---|---|---|
| **1. SINGLE DX** | | | | | | | | | | |
| 0–19 Years | 1 | 3.0 | 0 | 3 | 3 | 3 | 3 | 3 | 3 | 3 |
| 20–34 | 172 | 1.6 | <1 | 1 | 1 | 2 | 2 | 2 | 3 | 3 |
| 35–49 | 132 | 1.6 | <1 | 1 | 1 | 1 | 2 | 3 | 3 | 4 |
| 50–64 | 0 | | | | | | | | | |
| 65+ | 0 | | | | | | | | | |
| **2. MULTIPLE DX** | | | | | | | | | | |
| 0–19 Years | 2 | 2.1 | 1 | 1 | 1 | 3 | 3 | 3 | 3 | 3 |
| 20–34 | 292 | 2.1 | <1 | 1 | 2 | 2 | 2 | 3 | 4 | 4 |
| 35–49 | 168 | 2.0 | <1 | 1 | 1 | 2 | 2 | 3 | 4 | 5 |
| 50–64 | 0 | | | | | | | | | |
| 65+ | 0 | | | | | | | | | |
| **TOTAL SINGLE DX** | 305 | 1.7 | <1 | 1 | 1 | 2 | 2 | 3 | 3 | 4 |
| **TOTAL MULTIPLE DX** | 462 | 2.1 | <1 | 1 | 1 | 2 | 2 | 3 | 4 | 4 |
| **TOTAL** | | | | | | | | | | |
| 0–19 Years | 3 | 2.7 | <1 | 1 | 3 | 3 | 3 | 3 | 3 | 3 |
| 20–34 | 464 | 1.9 | <1 | 1 | 1 | 2 | 2 | 3 | 3 | 4 |
| 35–49 | 300 | 1.8 | <1 | 1 | 1 | 2 | 2 | 3 | 3 | 4 |
| 50–64 | 0 | | | | | | | | | |
| 65+ | 0 | | | | | | | | | |
| **GRAND TOTAL** | 767 | 1.9 | <1 | 1 | 1 | 2 | 2 | 3 | 3 | 4 |

## 66.79: FALL TUBE REPAIR NEC. Formerly included in operation group(s) 684.

| Type of Patients | Observed Patients | Avg. Stay | Variance | 10th | 25th | 50th | 75th | 90th | 95th | 99th |
|---|---|---|---|---|---|---|---|---|---|---|
| **1. SINGLE DX** | | | | | | | | | | |
| 0–19 Years | 0 | | | | | | | | | |
| 20–34 | 158 | 1.6 | <1 | 1 | 1 | 2 | 2 | 2 | 3 | 3 |
| 35–49 | 126 | 1.6 | <1 | 1 | 1 | 1 | 2 | 3 | 3 | 4 |
| 50–64 | 0 | | | | | | | | | |
| 65+ | 0 | | | | | | | | | |
| **2. MULTIPLE DX** | | | | | | | | | | |
| 0–19 Years | 1 | 3.0 | 0 | 3 | 3 | 3 | 3 | 3 | 3 | 3 |
| 20–34 | 273 | 2.1 | 1 | 1 | 1 | 2 | 2 | 3 | 4 | 4 |
| 35–49 | 157 | 2.0 | <1 | 1 | 1 | 2 | 2 | 3 | 4 | 5 |
| 50–64 | 0 | | | | | | | | | |
| 65+ | 0 | | | | | | | | | |
| **TOTAL SINGLE DX** | 284 | 1.6 | <1 | 1 | 1 | 2 | 2 | 2 | 3 | 3 |
| **TOTAL MULTIPLE DX** | 431 | 2.1 | <1 | 1 | 1 | 2 | 2 | 3 | 4 | 4 |
| **TOTAL** | | | | | | | | | | |
| 0–19 Years | 1 | 3.0 | 0 | 3 | 3 | 3 | 3 | 3 | 3 | 3 |
| 20–34 | 431 | 1.9 | <1 | 1 | 1 | 2 | 2 | 3 | 3 | 4 |
| 35–49 | 283 | 1.8 | <1 | 1 | 1 | 2 | 2 | 3 | 3 | 4 |
| 50–64 | 0 | | | | | | | | | |
| 65+ | 0 | | | | | | | | | |
| **GRAND TOTAL** | 715 | 1.9 | <1 | 1 | 1 | 2 | 2 | 3 | 3 | 4 |

# United States, October 1998–September 1999 Data, by Operation

## 66.8: FALL TUBE INSUFFLATION. Formerly included in operation group(s) 684.

| Type of Patients | Observed Patients | Avg. Stay | Variance | 10th | 25th | 50th | 75th | 90th | 95th | 99th |
|---|---|---|---|---|---|---|---|---|---|---|
| **1. SINGLE DX** | | | | | | | | | | |
| 0–19 Years | 0 | | | | | | | | | |
| 20–34 | 2 | 1.0 | 0 | 1 | 1 | 1 | 1 | 1 | 1 | 1 |
| 35–49 | 0 | | | | | | | | | |
| 50–64 | 0 | | | | | | | | | |
| 65+ | 0 | | | | | | | | | |
| **2. MULTIPLE DX** | | | | | | | | | | |
| 0–19 Years | 0 | | | | | | | | | |
| 20–34 | 9 | 1.6 | <1 | 1 | 1 | 1 | 2 | 2 | 3 | 3 |
| 35–49 | 2 | 2.0 | 2 | 1 | 1 | 3 | 3 | 3 | 3 | 3 |
| 50–64 | 0 | | | | | | | | | |
| 65+ | 0 | | | | | | | | | |
| **TOTAL SINGLE DX** | 2 | 1.0 | 0 | 1 | 1 | 1 | 1 | 1 | 1 | 1 |
| **TOTAL MULTIPLE DX** | 11 | 1.6 | <1 | 1 | 1 | 1 | 2 | 2 | 3 | 3 |
| **TOTAL** | | | | | | | | | | |
| 0–19 Years | 0 | | | | | | | | | |
| 20–34 | 11 | 1.5 | <1 | 1 | 1 | 1 | 2 | 2 | 2 | 3 |
| 35–49 | 2 | 2.0 | 2 | 1 | 1 | 3 | 3 | 3 | 3 | 3 |
| 50–64 | 0 | | | | | | | | | |
| 65+ | 0 | | | | | | | | | |
| **GRAND TOTAL** | 13 | 1.6 | <1 | 1 | 1 | 1 | 2 | 2 | 3 | 3 |

## 67.0: CERVICAL CANAL DILATION. Formerly included in operation group(s) 697.

| Type of Patients | Observed Patients | Avg. Stay | Variance | 10th | 25th | 50th | 75th | 90th | 95th | 99th |
|---|---|---|---|---|---|---|---|---|---|---|
| **1. SINGLE DX** | | | | | | | | | | |
| 0–19 Years | 0 | | | | | | | | | |
| 20–34 | 4 | 1.4 | <1 | 1 | 1 | 1 | 2 | 2 | 2 | 2 |
| 35–49 | 3 | 2.7 | <1 | 2 | 2 | 3 | 3 | 3 | 3 | 3 |
| 50–64 | 1 | 2.0 | 0 | 2 | 2 | 2 | 3 | 3 | 3 | 3 |
| 65+ | 2 | 1.2 | <1 | 1 | 1 | 1 | 1 | 2 | 2 | 2 |
| **2. MULTIPLE DX** | | | | | | | | | | |
| 0–19 Years | 1 | 4.0 | 0 | 4 | 4 | 4 | 4 | 4 | 4 | 4 |
| 20–34 | 7 | 2.5 | 1 | 1 | 2 | 2 | 4 | 4 | 4 | 4 |
| 35–49 | 15 | 1.4 | <1 | 1 | 1 | 1 | 2 | 2 | 3 | 4 |
| 50–64 | 10 | 2.3 | <1 | 1 | 1 | 2 | 2 | 4 | 4 | 4 |
| 65+ | 4 | 2.0 | 0 | 2 | 2 | 2 | 2 | 2 | 2 | 2 |
| **TOTAL SINGLE DX** | 10 | 1.9 | <1 | 1 | 1 | 2 | 3 | 3 | 3 | 3 |
| **TOTAL MULTIPLE DX** | 37 | 2.3 | 1 | 1 | 1 | 2 | 4 | 4 | 4 | 4 |
| **TOTAL** | | | | | | | | | | |
| 0–19 Years | 1 | 4.0 | 0 | 4 | 4 | 4 | 4 | 4 | 4 | 4 |
| 20–34 | 11 | 2.0 | <1 | 1 | 1 | 2 | 2 | 2 | 2 | 4 |
| 35–49 | 18 | 1.9 | <1 | 1 | 1 | 2 | 2 | 4 | 3 | 4 |
| 50–64 | 11 | 2.3 | 2 | 1 | 1 | 2 | 2 | 4 | 4 | 4 |
| 65+ | 6 | 1.6 | <1 | 2 | 1 | 2 | 2 | 2 | 2 | 2 |
| **GRAND TOTAL** | 47 | 2.2 | 1 | 1 | 1 | 2 | 3 | 4 | 4 | 4 |

## 66.9: OTHER FALLOPIAN TUBE OPS. Formerly included in operation group(s) 684.

| Type of Patients | Observed Patients | Avg. Stay | Variance | 10th | 25th | 50th | 75th | 90th | 95th | 99th |
|---|---|---|---|---|---|---|---|---|---|---|
| **1. SINGLE DX** | | | | | | | | | | |
| 0–19 Years | 2 | 2.0 | 0 | 2 | 2 | 2 | 2 | 2 | 2 | 2 |
| 20–34 | 10 | 1.6 | 1 | 1 | 1 | 1 | 2 | 4 | 4 | 4 |
| 35–49 | 3 | 2.0 | <1 | 1 | 2 | 2 | 3 | 3 | 3 | 3 |
| 50–64 | 0 | | | | | | | | | |
| 65+ | 0 | | | | | | | | | |
| **2. MULTIPLE DX** | | | | | | | | | | |
| 0–19 Years | 2 | 3.0 | 0 | 3 | 3 | 3 | 3 | 3 | 3 | 3 |
| 20–34 | 115 | 2.2 | 1 | 1 | 1 | 2 | 2 | 3 | 4 | 5 |
| 35–49 | 47 | 2.9 | 22 | 1 | 2 | 2 | 2 | 3 | 8 | 43 |
| 50–64 | 0 | | | | | | | | | |
| 65+ | 0 | | | | | | | | | |
| **TOTAL SINGLE DX** | 15 | 1.7 | <1 | 1 | 1 | 2 | 2 | 3 | 4 | 4 |
| **TOTAL MULTIPLE DX** | 164 | 2.4 | 7 | 1 | 2 | 2 | 2 | 3 | 4 | 10 |
| **TOTAL** | | | | | | | | | | |
| 0–19 Years | 4 | 2.6 | <1 | 2 | 2 | 3 | 3 | 3 | 3 | 3 |
| 20–34 | 125 | 2.1 | 1 | 1 | 1 | 2 | 2 | 3 | 4 | 5 |
| 35–49 | 50 | 2.9 | 21 | 1 | 2 | 2 | 3 | 3 | 8 | 43 |
| 50–64 | 0 | | | | | | | | | |
| 65+ | 0 | | | | | | | | | |
| **GRAND TOTAL** | 179 | 2.3 | 6 | 1 | 2 | 2 | 2 | 3 | 4 | 10 |

## 67.1: CERVICAL DIAGNOSTIC PX. Formerly included in operation group(s) 686, 704.

| Type of Patients | Observed Patients | Avg. Stay | Variance | 10th | 25th | 50th | 75th | 90th | 95th | 99th |
|---|---|---|---|---|---|---|---|---|---|---|
| **1. SINGLE DX** | | | | | | | | | | |
| 0–19 Years | 0 | | | | | | | | | |
| 20–34 | 3 | 4.9 | 6 | 2 | 3 | 7 | 7 | 7 | 7 | 7 |
| 35–49 | 10 | 2.6 | 4 | 2 | 2 | 2 | 6 | 6 | 6 | 12 |
| 50–64 | 2 | 4.4 | 4 | 3 | 3 | 3 | 6 | 6 | 6 | 6 |
| 65+ | 2 | 1.5 | <1 | 1 | 1 | 1 | 2 | 2 | 2 | 2 |
| **2. MULTIPLE DX** | | | | | | | | | | |
| 0–19 Years | 4 | 1.3 | <1 | 1 | 1 | 1 | 1 | 3 | 3 | 3 |
| 20–34 | 41 | 4.1 | 8 | 1 | 1 | 3 | 6 | 9 | 9 | 14 |
| 35–49 | 145 | 5.6 | 58 | 1 | 2 | 4 | 7 | 10 | 14 | 43 |
| 50–64 | 103 | 4.4 | 14 | 1 | 2 | 3 | 6 | 9 | 12 | 19 |
| 65+ | 156 | 6.7 | 25 | 2 | 3 | 6 | 9 | 13 | 16 | 25 |
| **TOTAL SINGLE DX** | 17 | 3.1 | 5 | 1 | 2 | 2 | 3 | 7 | 7 | 12 |
| **TOTAL MULTIPLE DX** | 449 | 5.5 | 30 | 1 | 2 | 4 | 8 | 11 | 14 | 25 |
| **TOTAL** | | | | | | | | | | |
| 0–19 Years | 4 | 1.3 | <1 | 1 | 1 | 1 | 1 | 3 | 3 | 3 |
| 20–34 | 44 | 4.2 | 8 | 1 | 2 | 3 | 6 | 9 | 9 | 14 |
| 35–49 | 155 | 5.3 | 54 | 1 | 2 | 3 | 7 | 10 | 14 | 35 |
| 50–64 | 105 | 4.4 | 14 | 1 | 2 | 3 | 6 | 9 | 12 | 19 |
| 65+ | 158 | 6.7 | 25 | 2 | 3 | 6 | 9 | 13 | 16 | 25 |
| **GRAND TOTAL** | 466 | 5.4 | 30 | 1 | 2 | 4 | 7 | 10 | 14 | 25 |

Length of Stay by Diagnosis and Operation, United States, 2000

### 67.12: CERVICAL BIOPSY NEC. Formerly included in operation group(s) 686.

| Type of Patients | Observed Patients | Avg. Stay | Vari-ance | Percentiles | | | | | | |
|---|---|---|---|---|---|---|---|---|---|---|
| | | | | 10th | 25th | 50th | 75th | 90th | 95th | 99th |
| **1. SINGLE DX** | | | | | | | | | | |
| 0–19 Years | 0 | | | | | | | | | |
| 20–34 | 3 | 4.9 | 6 | 2 | 3 | 7 | 7 | 7 | 7 | 7 |
| 35–49 | 9 | 2.7 | 4 | 2 | 3 | 2 | 2 | 6 | 6 | 12 |
| 50–64 | 1 | 3.0 | 0 | 3 | 3 | 3 | 3 | 3 | 3 | 3 |
| 65+ | 2 | 1.5 | <1 | 1 | 1 | 1 | 2 | 2 | 2 | 2 |
| **2. MULTIPLE DX** | | | | | | | | | | |
| 0–19 Years | 2 | 1.0 | 0 | 1 | 1 | 1 | 1 | 1 | 1 | 1 |
| 20–34 | 36 | 4.0 | 7 | 1 | 2 | 3 | 6 | 9 | 9 | 9 |
| 35–49 | 118 | 5.6 | 65 | 1 | 2 | 4 | 7 | 10 | 17 | 43 |
| 50–64 | 81 | 4.7 | 13 | 2 | 2 | 4 | 6 | 9 | 11 | 21 |
| 65+ | 131 | 7.0 | 23 | 1 | 3 | 7 | 10 | 13 | 16 | 25 |
| **TOTAL SINGLE DX** | **15** | **3.2** | **5** | **2** | **2** | **2** | **3** | **7** | **7** | **12** |
| **TOTAL MULTIPLE DX** | **368** | **5.8** | **32** | **1** | **2** | **4** | **8** | **11** | **14** | **25** |
| **TOTAL** | | | | | | | | | | |
| 0–19 Years | 2 | 1.0 | 0 | 1 | 1 | 1 | 1 | 1 | 1 | 1 |
| 20–34 | 39 | 4.1 | 7 | 1 | 2 | 3 | 6 | 9 | 9 | 9 |
| 35–49 | 127 | 5.3 | 59 | 1 | 2 | 3 | 6 | 10 | 14 | 43 |
| 50–64 | 82 | 4.7 | 13 | 2 | 2 | 4 | 6 | 9 | 11 | 21 |
| 65+ | 133 | 6.9 | 23 | 1 | 3 | 7 | 10 | 13 | 16 | 25 |
| **GRAND TOTAL** | **383** | **5.6** | **31** | **1** | **2** | **4** | **8** | **11** | **14** | **25** |

### 67.3: EXC/DESTR CERV LES NEC. Formerly included in operation group(s) 686.

| Type of Patients | Observed Patients | Avg. Stay | Vari-ance | Percentiles | | | | | | |
|---|---|---|---|---|---|---|---|---|---|---|
| | | | | 10th | 25th | 50th | 75th | 90th | 95th | 99th |
| **1. SINGLE DX** | | | | | | | | | | |
| 0–19 Years | 4 | 1.0 | 0 | 1 | 1 | 1 | 1 | 1 | 1 | 1 |
| 20–34 | 17 | 1.3 | <1 | 1 | 1 | 1 | 1 | 2 | 3 | 3 |
| 35–49 | 5 | 1.1 | <1 | 1 | 1 | 1 | 1 | 2 | 2 | 2 |
| 50–64 | 4 | 1.3 | 2 | 1 | 1 | 1 | 1 | 1 | 6 | 6 |
| 65+ | 2 | 3.7 | 4 | 1 | 1 | 5 | 5 | 5 | 5 | 5 |
| **2. MULTIPLE DX** | | | | | | | | | | |
| 0–19 Years | 13 | 2.0 | <1 | 1 | 2 | 2 | 2 | 3 | 3 | 3 |
| 20–34 | 77 | 3.8 | 111 | 1 | 1 | 2 | 3 | 4 | 7 | 82 |
| 35–49 | 104 | 3.1 | 6 | 1 | 1 | 3 | 4 | 6 | 8 | 15 |
| 50–64 | 58 | 3.2 | 5 | 1 | 1 | 3 | 4 | 6 | 6 | 12 |
| 65+ | 66 | 4.9 | 36 | 1 | 2 | 3 | 5 | 10 | 16 | 35 |
| **TOTAL SINGLE DX** | **32** | **1.4** | **<1** | **1** | **1** | **1** | **1** | **2** | **3** | **6** |
| **TOTAL MULTIPLE DX** | **318** | **3.6** | **38** | **1** | **1** | **2** | **4** | **6** | **8** | **22** |
| **TOTAL** | | | | | | | | | | |
| 0–19 Years | 17 | 1.7 | <1 | 1 | 1 | 2 | 2 | 3 | 3 | 3 |
| 20–34 | 94 | 3.5 | 95 | 1 | 1 | 2 | 3 | 4 | 7 | 82 |
| 35–49 | 109 | 2.9 | 5 | 1 | 1 | 3 | 4 | 5 | 7 | 15 |
| 50–64 | 62 | 3.0 | 5 | 1 | 1 | 3 | 4 | 5 | 6 | 11 |
| 65+ | 68 | 4.9 | 36 | 1 | 2 | 3 | 5 | 8 | 16 | 35 |
| **GRAND TOTAL** | **350** | **3.4** | **34** | **1** | **1** | **2** | **4** | **6** | **8** | **22** |

### 67.2: CONIZATION OF CERVIX. Formerly included in operation group(s) 685.

| Type of Patients | Observed Patients | Avg. Stay | Vari-ance | Percentiles | | | | | | |
|---|---|---|---|---|---|---|---|---|---|---|
| | | | | 10th | 25th | 50th | 75th | 90th | 95th | 99th |
| **1. SINGLE DX** | | | | | | | | | | |
| 0–19 Years | 0 | | | | | | | | | |
| 20–34 | 16 | 1.1 | <1 | 1 | 1 | 1 | 1 | 2 | 2 | 3 |
| 35–49 | 14 | 1.2 | <1 | 1 | 1 | 1 | 1 | 2 | 2 | 3 |
| 50–64 | 3 | 1.0 | 0 | 1 | 1 | 1 | 1 | 1 | 1 | 1 |
| 65+ | 2 | 1.0 | 0 | 1 | 1 | 1 | 1 | 1 | 1 | 1 |
| **2. MULTIPLE DX** | | | | | | | | | | |
| 0–19 Years | 3 | 5.3 | 13 | 1 | 1 | 8 | 8 | 8 | 8 | 8 |
| 20–34 | 41 | 2.2 | 3 | 1 | 1 | 1 | 3 | 5 | 5 | 7 |
| 35–49 | 48 | 2.3 | 8 | 1 | 1 | 2 | 3 | 4 | 4 | 18 |
| 50–64 | 18 | 2.6 | 8 | 1 | 1 | 1 | 3 | 4 | 6 | 14 |
| 65+ | 20 | 4.9 | 13 | 1 | 2 | 3 | 10 | 10 | 10 | 12 |
| **TOTAL SINGLE DX** | **35** | **1.2** | **<1** | **1** | **1** | **1** | **1** | **2** | **2** | **3** |
| **TOTAL MULTIPLE DX** | **130** | **2.7** | **9** | **1** | **1** | **2** | **3** | **6** | **8** | **12** |
| **TOTAL** | | | | | | | | | | |
| 0–19 Years | 3 | 5.3 | 13 | 1 | 1 | 8 | 8 | 8 | 8 | 8 |
| 20–34 | 57 | 1.9 | 2 | 1 | 1 | 1 | 2 | 4 | 5 | 7 |
| 35–49 | 62 | 2.2 | 7 | 1 | 1 | 2 | 3 | 3 | 3 | 18 |
| 50–64 | 21 | 2.4 | 7 | 1 | 1 | 1 | 3 | 4 | 6 | 14 |
| 65+ | 22 | 4.7 | 13 | 1 | 2 | 3 | 8 | 10 | 10 | 12 |
| **GRAND TOTAL** | **165** | **2.5** | **8** | **1** | **1** | **1** | **3** | **5** | **8** | **12** |

### 67.4: AMPUTATION OF CERVIX. Formerly included in operation group(s) 686.

| Type of Patients | Observed Patients | Avg. Stay | Vari-ance | Percentiles | | | | | | |
|---|---|---|---|---|---|---|---|---|---|---|
| | | | | 10th | 25th | 50th | 75th | 90th | 95th | 99th |
| **1. SINGLE DX** | | | | | | | | | | |
| 0–19 Years | 0 | | | | | | | | | |
| 20–34 | 0 | | | | | | | | | |
| 35–49 | 3 | 3.6 | 4 | 1 | 3 | 3 | 3 | 7 | 7 | 7 |
| 50–64 | 7 | 1.4 | <1 | 1 | 1 | 1 | 2 | 2 | 3 | 3 |
| 65+ | 1 | 3.0 | 0 | 3 | 3 | 3 | 3 | 3 | 3 | 3 |
| **2. MULTIPLE DX** | | | | | | | | | | |
| 0–19 Years | 1 | 3.0 | 0 | 3 | 3 | 3 | 3 | 3 | 3 | 3 |
| 20–34 | 9 | 4.1 | 2 | 2 | 3 | 5 | 5 | 5 | 5 | 6 |
| 35–49 | 34 | 3.5 | 5 | 2 | 3 | 3 | 5 | 6 | 6 | 8 |
| 50–64 | 27 | 3.4 | 2 | 1 | 2 | 3 | 3 | 4 | 7 | 8 |
| 65+ | 85 | 3.1 | 9 | 1 | 2 | 2 | 3 | 4 | 7 | 16 |
| **TOTAL SINGLE DX** | **11** | **2.3** | **3** | **1** | **1** | **2** | **3** | **3** | **7** | **7** |
| **TOTAL MULTIPLE DX** | **156** | **3.4** | **6** | **1** | **2** | **3** | **4** | **6** | **7** | **16** |
| **TOTAL** | | | | | | | | | | |
| 0–19 Years | 1 | 3.0 | 0 | 3 | 3 | 3 | 3 | 3 | 3 | 3 |
| 20–34 | 9 | 4.1 | 2 | 2 | 2 | 5 | 5 | 5 | 5 | 6 |
| 35–49 | 37 | 3.5 | 5 | 1 | 2 | 3 | 4 | 6 | 6 | 8 |
| 50–64 | 34 | 3.1 | 3 | 1 | 2 | 3 | 3 | 4 | 7 | 8 |
| 65+ | 86 | 3.1 | 9 | 1 | 2 | 2 | 3 | 4 | 7 | 16 |
| **GRAND TOTAL** | **167** | **3.3** | **6** | **1** | **2** | **3** | **4** | **6** | **7** | **16** |

Length of Stay by Diagnosis and Operation, United States, 2000

# United States, October 1998–September 1999 Data, by Operation

## 67.5: INT CERVICAL OS REPAIR. Formerly included in operation group(s) 687.

| Type of Patients | Observed Patients | Avg. Stay | Variance | 10th | 25th | 50th | 75th | 90th | 95th | 99th |
|---|---|---|---|---|---|---|---|---|---|---|
| **1. SINGLE DX** | | | | | | | | | | |
| 0–19 Years | 73 | 2.3 | 3 | 1 | 1 | 2 | 3 | 5 | 5 | 8 |
| 20–34 | 670 | 2.2 | 4 | 1 | 1 | 1 | 3 | 4 | 6 | 8 |
| 35–49 | 118 | 1.9 | 2 | 1 | 1 | 2 | 2 | 4 | 5 | 6 |
| 50–64 | 0 | | | | | | | | | |
| 65+ | 0 | | | | | | | | | |
| **2. MULTIPLE DX** | | | | | | | | | | |
| 0–19 Years | 99 | 4.9 | 32 | 1 | 2 | 3 | 6 | 13 | 21 | 26 |
| 20–34 | 808 | 5.6 | 75 | 1 | 2 | 3 | 6 | 11 | 19 | 48 |
| 35–49 | 226 | 7.9 | 286 | 1 | 2 | 5 | 5 | 13 | 46 | 73 |
| 50–64 | 1 | 5.0 | 0 | 5 | 5 | 5 | 5 | 5 | 5 | 5 |
| 65+ | 0 | | | | | | | | | |
| **TOTAL SINGLE DX** | 861 | 2.1 | 4 | 1 | 1 | 1 | 3 | 4 | 5 | 8 |
| **TOTAL MULTIPLE DX** | 1,134 | 6.1 | 129 | 1 | 1 | 3 | 5 | 11 | 28 | 73 |
| **TOTAL** | | | | | | | | | | |
| 0–19 Years | 172 | 3.7 | 21 | 1 | 1 | 2 | 4 | 8 | 13 | 26 |
| 20–34 | 1,478 | 3.9 | 43 | 1 | 1 | 2 | 4 | 8 | 11 | 43 |
| 35–49 | 344 | 6.2 | 214 | 1 | 1 | 2 | 4 | 8 | 42 | 73 |
| 50–64 | 1 | 5.0 | 0 | 5 | 5 | 5 | 5 | 5 | 5 | 5 |
| 65+ | 0 | | | | | | | | | |
| **GRAND TOTAL** | 1,995 | 4.3 | 77 | 1 | 1 | 2 | 4 | 8 | 13 | 48 |

## 67.6: OTHER REPAIR OF CERVIX. Formerly included in operation group(s) 687.

| Type of Patients | Observed Patients | Avg. Stay | Variance | 10th | 25th | 50th | 75th | 90th | 95th | 99th |
|---|---|---|---|---|---|---|---|---|---|---|
| **1. SINGLE DX** | | | | | | | | | | |
| 0–19 Years | 0 | | | | | | | | | |
| 20–34 | 11 | 4.8 | 4 | 6 | 6 | 6 | 6 | 6 | 6 | 6 |
| 35–49 | 9 | 1.1 | <1 | 1 | 1 | 1 | 1 | 2 | 2 | 2 |
| 50–64 | 2 | 1.4 | <1 | 1 | 1 | 1 | 2 | 2 | 2 | 2 |
| 65+ | 1 | 4.0 | 0 | 4 | 4 | 4 | 4 | 4 | 4 | 4 |
| **2. MULTIPLE DX** | | | | | | | | | | |
| 0–19 Years | 4 | 1.2 | <1 | 1 | 1 | 1 | 1 | 2 | 2 | 2 |
| 20–34 | 23 | 2.5 | 7 | 1 | 1 | 2 | 3 | 5 | 5 | 19 |
| 35–49 | 15 | 1.6 | 1 | 1 | 1 | 1 | 3 | 4 | 5 | 5 |
| 50–64 | 3 | 1.9 | 1 | 1 | 1 | 1 | 3 | 3 | 3 | 3 |
| 65+ | 3 | 6.3 | 8 | 5 | 5 | 5 | 5 | 12 | 12 | 12 |
| **TOTAL SINGLE DX** | 23 | 4.1 | 6 | 1 | 1 | 6 | 6 | 6 | 6 | 6 |
| **TOTAL MULTIPLE DX** | 48 | 2.3 | 6 | 1 | 1 | 1 | 3 | 5 | 5 | 12 |
| **TOTAL** | | | | | | | | | | |
| 0–19 Years | 4 | 1.2 | <1 | 1 | 1 | 1 | 1 | 2 | 2 | 2 |
| 20–34 | 34 | 4.3 | 6 | 1 | 1 | 6 | 6 | 6 | 6 | 6 |
| 35–49 | 24 | 1.4 | 1 | 1 | 1 | 1 | 2 | 3 | 4 | 5 |
| 50–64 | 5 | 1.6 | <1 | 1 | 1 | 1 | 2 | 3 | 3 | 3 |
| 65+ | 4 | 5.9 | 7 | 4 | 5 | 5 | 5 | 12 | 12 | 12 |
| **GRAND TOTAL** | 71 | 3.4 | 6 | 1 | 1 | 2 | 6 | 6 | 6 | 6 |

## 68.0: HYSTEROTOMY. Formerly included in operation group(s) 688.

| Type of Patients | Observed Patients | Avg. Stay | Variance | 10th | 25th | 50th | 75th | 90th | 95th | 99th |
|---|---|---|---|---|---|---|---|---|---|---|
| **1. SINGLE DX** | | | | | | | | | | |
| 0–19 Years | 0 | | | | | | | | | |
| 20–34 | 4 | 3.3 | <1 | 2 | 2 | 4 | 4 | 4 | 4 | 4 |
| 35–49 | 0 | | | | | | | | | |
| 50–64 | 0 | | | | | | | | | |
| 65+ | 0 | | | | | | | | | |
| **2. MULTIPLE DX** | | | | | | | | | | |
| 0–19 Years | 7 | 3.0 | <1 | 2 | 3 | 3 | 3 | 3 | 5 | 5 |
| 20–34 | 25 | 4.3 | 7 | 2 | 2 | 3 | 6 | 7 | 10 | 12 |
| 35–49 | 11 | 3.0 | <1 | 2 | 3 | 3 | 3 | 3 | 6 | 6 |
| 50–64 | | | | | | | | | | |
| 65+ | 1 | 4.0 | 0 | 4 | 4 | 4 | 4 | 4 | 4 | 4 |
| **TOTAL SINGLE DX** | 4 | 3.3 | <1 | 2 | 2 | 4 | 4 | 4 | 4 | 4 |
| **TOTAL MULTIPLE DX** | 44 | 3.4 | 3 | 2 | 2 | 3 | 3 | 6 | 6 | 12 |
| **TOTAL** | | | | | | | | | | |
| 0–19 Years | 7 | 3.0 | <1 | 2 | 2 | 3 | 3 | 3 | 5 | 5 |
| 20–34 | 29 | 4.1 | 6 | 2 | 2 | 3 | 5 | 7 | 10 | 12 |
| 35–49 | 11 | 3.0 | <1 | 2 | 3 | 3 | 3 | 3 | 6 | 6 |
| 50–64 | 0 | | | | | | | | | |
| 65+ | 1 | 4.0 | 0 | 4 | 4 | 4 | 4 | 4 | 4 | 4 |
| **GRAND TOTAL** | 48 | 3.4 | 3 | 2 | 3 | 3 | 3 | 6 | 6 | 12 |

## 68.1: UTER/ADNEXA DXTIC PX. Formerly included in operation group(s) 688, 697, 704.

| Type of Patients | Observed Patients | Avg. Stay | Variance | 10th | 25th | 50th | 75th | 90th | 95th | 99th |
|---|---|---|---|---|---|---|---|---|---|---|
| **1. SINGLE DX** | | | | | | | | | | |
| 0–19 Years | 3 | 2.1 | 2 | 1 | 1 | 1 | 4 | 4 | 4 | 4 |
| 20–34 | 12 | 2.0 | <1 | 1 | 1 | 2 | 3 | 3 | 3 | 3 |
| 35–49 | 11 | 2.0 | 1 | 1 | 1 | 2 | 3 | 3 | 3 | 6 |
| 50–64 | 1 | 1.0 | 0 | 1 | 1 | 1 | 1 | 1 | 1 | 1 |
| 65+ | 4 | 2.4 | 2 | 2 | 1 | 2 | 2 | 5 | 5 | 5 |
| **2. MULTIPLE DX** | | | | | | | | | | |
| 0–19 Years | 12 | 3.6 | 11 | 1 | 1 | 2 | 5 | 11 | 11 | 11 |
| 20–34 | 142 | 3.7 | 23 | 1 | 2 | 3 | 6 | 8 | 10 | 13 |
| 35–49 | 451 | 4.5 | 21 | 1 | 2 | 4 | 6 | 10 | 13 | 25 |
| 50–64 | 221 | 6.6 | 54 | 1 | 2 | 4 | 7 | 20 | 20 | 36 |
| 65+ | 425 | 7.8 | 56 | 2 | 3 | 5 | 10 | 18 | 27 | 32 |
| **TOTAL SINGLE DX** | 31 | 2.0 | 1 | 1 | 1 | 2 | 3 | 3 | 4 | 6 |
| **TOTAL MULTIPLE DX** | 1,251 | 5.9 | 40 | 1 | 2 | 4 | 7 | 13 | 20 | 32 |
| **TOTAL** | | | | | | | | | | |
| 0–19 Years | 15 | 3.3 | 10 | 1 | 2 | 2 | 4 | 11 | 11 | 11 |
| 20–34 | 154 | 3.6 | 22 | 1 | 2 | 3 | 4 | 8 | 10 | 13 |
| 35–49 | 462 | 4.4 | 20 | 1 | 2 | 3 | 6 | 10 | 12 | 23 |
| 50–64 | 222 | 6.5 | 54 | 2 | 4 | 4 | 7 | 20 | 20 | 36 |
| 65+ | 429 | 7.8 | 56 | 2 | 3 | 5 | 10 | 18 | 27 | 32 |
| **GRAND TOTAL** | 1,282 | 5.8 | 40 | 1 | 2 | 4 | 7 | 13 | 19 | 32 |

Length of Stay by Diagnosis and Operation, United States, 2000

# United States, October 1998–September 1999 Data, by Operation

## 68.16: CLSD UTERINE BX. Formerly included in operation group(s) 688.

| Type of Patients | Observed Patients | Avg. Stay | Variance | 10th | 25th | 50th | 75th | 90th | 95th | 99th |
|---|---|---|---|---|---|---|---|---|---|---|
| **1. SINGLE DX** | | | | | | | | | | |
| 0–19 Years | 3 | 2.1 | 2 | 1 | 1 | 1 | 4 | 4 | 4 | 4 |
| 20–34 | 4 | 3.0 | 0 | 3 | 3 | 3 | 3 | 3 | 3 | 3 |
| 35–49 | 6 | 1.6 | <1 | 1 | 1 | 2 | 2 | 2 | 2 | 2 |
| 50–64 | 1 | 1.0 | 0 | 1 | 1 | 1 | 1 | 1 | 1 | 1 |
| 65+ | 4 | 2.4 | 2 | 1 | 1 | 2 | 2 | 5 | 5 | 5 |
| **2. MULTIPLE DX** | | | | | | | | | | |
| 0–19 Years | 8 | 4.1 | 12 | 1 | 2 | 4 | 5 | 11 | 11 | 11 |
| 20–34 | 92 | 4.5 | 33 | 1 | 2 | 5 | 5 | 10 | 12 | 51 |
| 35–49 | 377 | 5.1 | 24 | 1 | 2 | 3 | 7 | 10 | 15 | 25 |
| 50–64 | 196 | 6.9 | 57 | 2 | 3 | 4 | 8 | 20 | 22 | 36 |
| 65+ | 394 | 8.1 | 58 | 2 | 3 | 5 | 11 | 18 | 28 | 32 |
| **TOTAL SINGLE DX** | 18 | 1.9 | 1 | 1 | 1 | 2 | 2 | 3 | 4 | 5 |
| **TOTAL MULTIPLE DX** | 1,067 | 6.5 | 45 | 1 | 2 | 4 | 8 | 14 | 20 | 32 |
| **TOTAL** | | | | | | | | | | |
| 0–19 Years | 11 | 3.7 | 11 | 1 | 1 | 2 | 5 | 11 | 11 | 11 |
| 20–34 | 96 | 4.4 | 32 | 1 | 2 | 3 | 5 | 10 | 12 | 51 |
| 35–49 | 383 | 5.0 | 24 | 1 | 2 | 3 | 7 | 10 | 15 | 25 |
| 50–64 | 197 | 6.9 | 57 | 2 | 2 | 4 | 8 | 20 | 22 | 36 |
| 65+ | 398 | 8.1 | 58 | 2 | 3 | 5 | 11 | 18 | 28 | 32 |
| **GRAND TOTAL** | 1,085 | 6.4 | 45 | 1 | 2 | 4 | 8 | 14 | 20 | 32 |

## 68.29: UTER LES EXC/DESTR NEC. Formerly included in operation group(s) 688.

| Type of Patients | Observed Patients | Avg. Stay | Variance | 10th | 25th | 50th | 75th | 90th | 95th | 99th |
|---|---|---|---|---|---|---|---|---|---|---|
| **1. SINGLE DX** | | | | | | | | | | |
| 0–19 Years | 4 | 2.5 | 2 | 1 | 1 | 3 | 3 | 3 | 5 | 5 |
| 20–34 | 846 | 2.4 | <1 | 2 | 2 | 3 | 3 | 3 | 3 | 4 |
| 35–49 | 893 | 2.4 | <1 | 1 | 2 | 2 | 3 | 3 | 4 | 6 |
| 50–64 | 24 | 2.1 | <1 | 1 | 2 | 2 | 2 | 3 | 4 | 5 |
| 65+ | 3 | 2.2 | 2 | 1 | 1 | 2 | 4 | 4 | 4 | 4 |
| **2. MULTIPLE DX** | | | | | | | | | | |
| 0–19 Years | 28 | 3.2 | 4 | 2 | 2 | 3 | 3 | 4 | 6 | 12 |
| 20–34 | 3,184 | 2.8 | 2 | 2 | 2 | 3 | 3 | 3 | 5 | 8 |
| 35–49 | 4,724 | 2.8 | 2 | 2 | 2 | 3 | 3 | 4 | 5 | 8 |
| 50–64 | 128 | 2.5 | 7 | 1 | 1 | 2 | 3 | 4 | 7 | 12 |
| 65+ | 86 | 5.3 | 18 | 1 | 2 | 4 | 7 | 12 | 13 | 20 |
| **TOTAL SINGLE DX** | 1,770 | 2.4 | <1 | 1 | 2 | 2 | 3 | 3 | 4 | 5 |
| **TOTAL MULTIPLE DX** | 8,150 | 2.8 | 2 | 2 | 2 | 3 | 3 | 4 | 5 | 8 |
| **TOTAL** | | | | | | | | | | |
| 0–19 Years | 32 | 3.1 | 4 | 2 | 2 | 3 | 3 | 4 | 6 | 12 |
| 20–34 | 4,030 | 2.7 | 2 | 2 | 2 | 2 | 3 | 4 | 4 | 7 |
| 35–49 | 5,617 | 2.8 | 2 | 1 | 2 | 3 | 3 | 4 | 5 | 7 |
| 50–64 | 152 | 2.4 | 6 | 1 | 1 | 2 | 3 | 4 | 5 | 12 |
| 65+ | 89 | 5.2 | 18 | 1 | 2 | 4 | 7 | 12 | 13 | 20 |
| **GRAND TOTAL** | 9,920 | 2.7 | 2 | 2 | 2 | 3 | 3 | 4 | 5 | 8 |

## 68.2: UTERINE LES EXC/DESTR. Formerly included in operation group(s) 688.

| Type of Patients | Observed Patients | Avg. Stay | Variance | 10th | 25th | 50th | 75th | 90th | 95th | 99th |
|---|---|---|---|---|---|---|---|---|---|---|
| **1. SINGLE DX** | | | | | | | | | | |
| 0–19 Years | 5 | 2.2 | 2 | 1 | 1 | 3 | 3 | 3 | 5 | 5 |
| 20–34 | 852 | 2.4 | <1 | 2 | 2 | 3 | 3 | 3 | 3 | 5 |
| 35–49 | 902 | 2.4 | <1 | 1 | 2 | 2 | 3 | 3 | 4 | 4 |
| 50–64 | 24 | 2.1 | <1 | 1 | 2 | 2 | 2 | 3 | 4 | 6 |
| 65+ | 3 | 2.2 | 2 | 1 | 1 | 2 | 4 | 4 | 4 | 4 |
| **2. MULTIPLE DX** | | | | | | | | | | |
| 0–19 Years | 42 | 2.8 | 8 | 1 | 1 | 2 | 3 | 5 | 5 | 12 |
| 20–34 | 3,248 | 2.8 | 2 | 2 | 2 | 3 | 3 | 4 | 5 | 8 |
| 35–49 | 4,869 | 2.9 | 2 | 2 | 2 | 3 | 3 | 4 | 5 | 8 |
| 50–64 | 147 | 2.4 | 6 | 1 | 1 | 2 | 3 | 4 | 7 | 12 |
| 65+ | 102 | 5.1 | 18 | 1 | 1 | 4 | 7 | 12 | 13 | 20 |
| **TOTAL SINGLE DX** | 1,786 | 2.3 | <1 | 1 | 2 | 2 | 3 | 3 | 4 | 5 |
| **TOTAL MULTIPLE DX** | 8,408 | 2.8 | 2 | 2 | 2 | 3 | 3 | 4 | 5 | 9 |
| **TOTAL** | | | | | | | | | | |
| 0–19 Years | 47 | 2.7 | 8 | 1 | 1 | 2 | 3 | 5 | 5 | 12 |
| 20–34 | 4,100 | 2.7 | 2 | 2 | 2 | 2 | 3 | 4 | 4 | 7 |
| 35–49 | 5,771 | 2.8 | 2 | 2 | 2 | 3 | 3 | 3 | 5 | 8 |
| 50–64 | 171 | 2.3 | 5 | 1 | 1 | 2 | 3 | 3 | 5 | 12 |
| 65+ | 105 | 5.1 | 18 | 1 | 1 | 4 | 7 | 12 | 13 | 20 |
| **GRAND TOTAL** | 10,194 | 2.7 | 2 | 2 | 2 | 3 | 3 | 4 | 5 | 8 |

## 68.3: SUBTOT ABD HYSTERECTOMY. Formerly included in operation group(s) 689.

| Type of Patients | Observed Patients | Avg. Stay | Variance | 10th | 25th | 50th | 75th | 90th | 95th | 99th |
|---|---|---|---|---|---|---|---|---|---|---|
| **1. SINGLE DX** | | | | | | | | | | |
| 0–19 Years | 1 | 3.0 | 0 | 3 | 3 | 3 | 3 | 3 | 3 | 3 |
| 20–34 | 19 | 2.5 | <1 | 2 | 2 | 3 | 3 | 3 | 3 | 3 |
| 35–49 | 108 | 2.5 | <1 | 1 | 2 | 3 | 3 | 3 | 4 | 5 |
| 50–64 | 20 | 2.1 | 2 | 1 | 1 | 2 | 2 | 3 | 5 | 11 |
| 65+ | 2 | 6.7 | <1 | 6 | 6 | 7 | 7 | 7 | 7 | 7 |
| **2. MULTIPLE DX** | | | | | | | | | | |
| 0–19 Years | 8 | 2.2 | 1 | 2 | 2 | 2 | 2 | 2 | 2 | 8 |
| 20–34 | 352 | 3.4 | 5 | 2 | 2 | 3 | 4 | 5 | 7 | 10 |
| 35–49 | 2,616 | 3.1 | 5 | 2 | 2 | 3 | 4 | 4 | 5 | 10 |
| 50–64 | 568 | 4.3 | 16 | 2 | 2 | 4 | 4 | 9 | 14 | 21 |
| 65+ | 189 | 7.7 | 48 | 2 | 3 | 6 | 9 | 14 | 22 | 40 |
| **TOTAL SINGLE DX** | 150 | 2.5 | 1 | 1 | 2 | 3 | 3 | 3 | 4 | 6 |
| **TOTAL MULTIPLE DX** | 3,733 | 3.5 | 9 | 2 | 2 | 3 | 4 | 5 | 8 | 16 |
| **TOTAL** | | | | | | | | | | |
| 0–19 Years | 9 | 2.2 | 1 | 2 | 2 | 2 | 2 | 2 | 3 | 8 |
| 20–34 | 371 | 3.3 | 5 | 2 | 3 | 3 | 4 | 5 | 7 | 10 |
| 35–49 | 2,724 | 3.1 | 5 | 2 | 2 | 3 | 4 | 4 | 5 | 9 |
| 50–64 | 588 | 4.3 | 16 | 2 | 2 | 4 | 4 | 9 | 14 | 21 |
| 65+ | 191 | 7.7 | 48 | 2 | 3 | 6 | 9 | 14 | 22 | 40 |
| **GRAND TOTAL** | 3,883 | 3.5 | 9 | 2 | 2 | 3 | 4 | 5 | 7 | 16 |

Length of Stay by Diagnosis and Operation, United States, 2000

# United States, October 1998–September 1999 Data, by Operation

## 68.4: TOTAL ABD HYSTERECTOMY. Formerly included in operation group(s) 689.

| Type of Patients | Observed Patients | Avg. Stay | Variance | 10th | 25th | 50th | 75th | 90th | 95th | 99th |
|---|---|---|---|---|---|---|---|---|---|---|
| **1. SINGLE DX** | | | | | | | | | | |
| 0–19 Years | 3 | 2.4 | <1 | 2 | 2 | 2 | 3 | 3 | 3 | 3 |
| 20–34 | 725 | 2.7 | <1 | 2 | 2 | 3 | 3 | 4 | 4 | 5 |
| 35–49 | 2,892 | 2.7 | <1 | 2 | 2 | 3 | 3 | 4 | 4 | 5 |
| 50–64 | 918 | 2.9 | <1 | 2 | 2 | 3 | 3 | 4 | 4 | 6 |
| 65+ | 354 | 3.1 | 1 | 2 | 3 | 3 | 3 | 4 | 5 | 6 |
| **2. MULTIPLE DX** | | | | | | | | | | |
| 0–19 Years | 62 | 4.8 | 61 | 2 | 2 | 2 | 4 | 11 | 13 | 46 |
| 20–34 | 12,984 | 2.9 | 2 | 2 | 2 | 3 | 3 | 4 | 5 | 9 |
| 35–49 | 69,076 | 3.0 | 2 | 2 | 2 | 3 | 4 | 4 | 5 | 9 |
| 50–64 | 20,352 | 3.3 | 4 | 2 | 2 | 3 | 4 | 5 | 6 | 12 |
| 65+ | 8,853 | 4.9 | 14 | 2 | 3 | 4 | 5 | 8 | 12 | 21 |
| **TOTAL SINGLE DX** | 4,892 | 2.8 | <1 | 2 | 2 | 3 | 3 | 4 | 4 | 6 |
| **TOTAL MULTIPLE DX** | 111,327 | 3.2 | 4 | 2 | 2 | 3 | 3 | 4 | 6 | 11 |
| **TOTAL** | | | | | | | | | | |
| 0–19 Years | 65 | 4.8 | 60 | 2 | 2 | 2 | 4 | 11 | 13 | 46 |
| 20–34 | 13,709 | 2.9 | 2 | 2 | 2 | 3 | 3 | 4 | 5 | 9 |
| 35–49 | 71,968 | 3.0 | 2 | 2 | 2 | 3 | 3 | 4 | 5 | 9 |
| 50–64 | 21,270 | 3.3 | 4 | 2 | 2 | 3 | 4 | 5 | 6 | 12 |
| 65+ | 9,207 | 4.8 | 13 | 2 | 3 | 4 | 5 | 8 | 11 | 20 |
| **GRAND TOTAL** | 116,219 | 3.2 | 4 | 2 | 2 | 3 | 3 | 4 | 6 | 11 |

## 68.5: VAGINAL HYSTERECTOMY. Formerly included in operation group(s) 690.

| Type of Patients | Observed Patients | Avg. Stay | Variance | 10th | 25th | 50th | 75th | 90th | 95th | 99th |
|---|---|---|---|---|---|---|---|---|---|---|
| **1. SINGLE DX** | | | | | | | | | | |
| 0–19 Years | 1 | 1.0 | 0 | 1 | 1 | 1 | 1 | 1 | 1 | 1 |
| 20–34 | 905 | 1.7 | <1 | 1 | 1 | 2 | 2 | 2 | 3 | 3 |
| 35–49 | 1,983 | 1.7 | <1 | 1 | 1 | 2 | 2 | 3 | 3 | 3 |
| 50–64 | 767 | 2.0 | <1 | 1 | 1 | 2 | 3 | 3 | 3 | 4 |
| 65+ | 496 | 2.5 | <1 | 1 | 2 | 3 | 3 | 3 | 4 | 5 |
| **2. MULTIPLE DX** | | | | | | | | | | |
| 0–19 Years | 11 | 1.4 | <1 | 1 | 1 | 1 | 2 | 2 | 3 | 3 |
| 20–34 | 8,560 | 1.9 | <1 | 1 | 1 | 2 | 2 | 3 | 3 | 5 |
| 35–49 | 30,978 | 1.9 | <1 | 1 | 1 | 2 | 2 | 3 | 3 | 5 |
| 50–64 | 9,741 | 2.2 | 1 | 1 | 2 | 2 | 3 | 3 | 4 | 5 |
| 65+ | 6,497 | 2.8 | 3 | 2 | 2 | 3 | 3 | 4 | 5 | 7 |
| **TOTAL SINGLE DX** | 4,152 | 1.9 | <1 | 1 | 1 | 2 | 2 | 3 | 3 | 4 |
| **TOTAL MULTIPLE DX** | 55,787 | 2.1 | 1 | 1 | 1 | 2 | 2 | 3 | 4 | 5 |
| **TOTAL** | | | | | | | | | | |
| 0–19 Years | 12 | 1.4 | <1 | 1 | 1 | 1 | 2 | 2 | 3 | 3 |
| 20–34 | 9,465 | 1.9 | <1 | 1 | 1 | 2 | 2 | 3 | 3 | 5 |
| 35–49 | 32,961 | 1.9 | <1 | 1 | 1 | 2 | 2 | 3 | 3 | 5 |
| 50–64 | 10,508 | 2.2 | 1 | 1 | 2 | 2 | 3 | 3 | 4 | 5 |
| 65+ | 6,993 | 2.8 | 2 | 2 | 2 | 3 | 3 | 4 | 5 | 7 |
| **GRAND TOTAL** | 59,939 | 2.1 | 1 | 1 | 1 | 2 | 2 | 3 | 4 | 5 |

## 68.51: LAVH. Formerly included in operation group(s) 690.

| Type of Patients | Observed Patients | Avg. Stay | Variance | 10th | 25th | 50th | 75th | 90th | 95th | 99th |
|---|---|---|---|---|---|---|---|---|---|---|
| **1. SINGLE DX** | | | | | | | | | | |
| 0–19 Years | 0 | | | | | | | | | |
| 20–34 | 164 | 1.6 | <1 | 1 | 1 | 2 | 2 | 2 | 2 | 3 |
| 35–49 | 379 | 1.7 | <1 | 1 | 1 | 2 | 2 | 2 | 3 | 3 |
| 50–64 | 138 | 1.7 | <1 | 1 | 1 | 2 | 2 | 3 | 3 | 3 |
| 65+ | 28 | 2.0 | <1 | 1 | 1 | 2 | 3 | 3 | 3 | 3 |
| **2. MULTIPLE DX** | | | | | | | | | | |
| 0–19 Years | 4 | 1.4 | <1 | 1 | 1 | 1 | 2 | 2 | 2 | 2 |
| 20–34 | 2,939 | 1.8 | <1 | 1 | 2 | 2 | 2 | 3 | 3 | 4 |
| 35–49 | 10,226 | 1.8 | 1 | 1 | 2 | 2 | 2 | 3 | 4 | 5 |
| 50–64 | 2,564 | 2.0 | 1 | 1 | 2 | 2 | 3 | 3 | 4 | 5 |
| 65+ | 706 | 2.5 | 3 | 1 | 2 | 2 | 3 | 4 | 4 | 9 |
| **TOTAL SINGLE DX** | 709 | 1.7 | <1 | 1 | 1 | 2 | 2 | 2 | 3 | 3 |
| **TOTAL MULTIPLE DX** | 16,439 | 1.9 | 1 | 1 | 2 | 2 | 2 | 3 | 3 | 5 |
| **TOTAL** | | | | | | | | | | |
| 0–19 Years | 4 | 1.4 | <1 | 1 | 1 | 2 | 2 | 2 | 2 | 2 |
| 20–34 | 3,103 | 1.8 | <1 | 1 | 2 | 2 | 2 | 3 | 3 | 4 |
| 35–49 | 10,605 | 1.8 | <1 | 1 | 2 | 2 | 2 | 3 | 3 | 5 |
| 50–64 | 2,702 | 2.0 | 1 | 1 | 2 | 2 | 3 | 3 | 4 | 5 |
| 65+ | 734 | 2.5 | 3 | 2 | 2 | 3 | 3 | 4 | 4 | 9 |
| **GRAND TOTAL** | 17,148 | 1.9 | 1 | 1 | 2 | 2 | 2 | 3 | 3 | 5 |

## 68.59: VAGINAL HYSTERECTOMY NEC. Formerly included in operation group(s) 690.

| Type of Patients | Observed Patients | Avg. Stay | Variance | 10th | 25th | 50th | 75th | 90th | 95th | 99th |
|---|---|---|---|---|---|---|---|---|---|---|
| **1. SINGLE DX** | | | | | | | | | | |
| 0–19 Years | 1 | 1.0 | 0 | 1 | 1 | 1 | 1 | 1 | 1 | 1 |
| 20–34 | 741 | 1.7 | <1 | 1 | 1 | 2 | 2 | 2 | 3 | 3 |
| 35–49 | 1,604 | 1.7 | <1 | 1 | 1 | 2 | 2 | 3 | 3 | 5 |
| 50–64 | 629 | 2.1 | <1 | 1 | 1 | 2 | 3 | 3 | 3 | 5 |
| 65+ | 468 | 2.5 | <1 | 1 | 2 | 3 | 3 | 3 | 4 | 5 |
| **2. MULTIPLE DX** | | | | | | | | | | |
| 0–19 Years | 7 | 1.4 | <1 | 1 | 1 | 1 | 2 | 2 | 3 | 3 |
| 20–34 | 5,621 | 1.9 | <1 | 1 | 1 | 2 | 2 | 3 | 3 | 5 |
| 35–49 | 20,752 | 2.0 | 1 | 1 | 2 | 2 | 3 | 3 | 3 | 5 |
| 50–64 | 7,177 | 2.3 | 1 | 1 | 2 | 2 | 3 | 3 | 4 | 5 |
| 65+ | 5,791 | 2.8 | 2 | 2 | 2 | 3 | 3 | 4 | 5 | 7 |
| **TOTAL SINGLE DX** | 3,443 | 1.9 | <1 | 1 | 1 | 2 | 2 | 3 | 3 | 4 |
| **TOTAL MULTIPLE DX** | 39,348 | 2.2 | 1 | 1 | 2 | 2 | 3 | 3 | 4 | 6 |
| **TOTAL** | | | | | | | | | | |
| 0–19 Years | 8 | 1.4 | <1 | 1 | 1 | 1 | 2 | 2 | 3 | 3 |
| 20–34 | 6,362 | 1.9 | <1 | 1 | 1 | 2 | 2 | 3 | 3 | 5 |
| 35–49 | 22,356 | 2.0 | <1 | 1 | 2 | 2 | 3 | 3 | 3 | 5 |
| 50–64 | 7,806 | 2.2 | <1 | 1 | 2 | 2 | 3 | 3 | 4 | 5 |
| 65+ | 6,259 | 2.8 | 2 | 2 | 2 | 3 | 3 | 4 | 5 | 7 |
| **GRAND TOTAL** | 42,791 | 2.1 | 1 | 1 | 2 | 2 | 3 | 3 | 4 | 5 |

Length of Stay by Diagnosis and Operation, United States, 2000

# United States, October 1998–September 1999 Data, by Operation

## 68.6: RADICAL ABD HYSTERECTOMY. Formerly included in operation group(s) 691.

| Type of Patients | Observed Patients | Avg. Stay | Variance | 10th | 25th | 50th | 75th | 90th | 95th | 99th |
|---|---|---|---|---|---|---|---|---|---|---|
| **1. SINGLE DX** | | | | | | | | | | |
| 0–19 Years | 0 | | | | | | | | | |
| 20–34 | 72 | 3.9 | 1 | 2 | 3 | 4 | 5 | 5 | 6 | 6 |
| 35–49 | 91 | 4.2 | 2 | 2 | 3 | 4 | 5 | 6 | 7 | 9 |
| 50–64 | 33 | 4.0 | <1 | 3 | 3 | 4 | 5 | 5 | 5 | 6 |
| 65+ | 15 | 4.3 | 2 | 3 | 3 | 4 | 6 | 6 | 6 | 6 |
| **2. MULTIPLE DX** | | | | | | | | | | |
| 0–19 Years | 2 | 6.7 | 5 | 5 | 5 | 5 | 9 | 9 | 9 | 9 |
| 20–34 | 201 | 5.2 | 10 | 3 | 4 | 5 | 6 | 7 | 10 | 20 |
| 35–49 | 603 | 6.0 | 40 | 3 | 3 | 4 | 6 | 8 | 22 | 31 |
| 50–64 | 368 | 5.2 | 12 | 3 | 3 | 5 | 6 | 8 | 11 | 18 |
| 65+ | 291 | 7.8 | 27 | 3 | 4 | 6 | 10 | 16 | 20 | 20 |
| **TOTAL SINGLE DX** | 211 | 4.1 | 2 | 2 | 3 | 4 | 5 | 6 | 6 | 9 |
| **TOTAL MULTIPLE DX** | 1,465 | 6.1 | 28 | 3 | 4 | 5 | 6 | 11 | 16 | 31 |
| **TOTAL** | | | | | | | | | | |
| 0–19 Years | 2 | 6.7 | 5 | 5 | 5 | 5 | 9 | 9 | 9 | 9 |
| 20–34 | 273 | 4.8 | 8 | 3 | 4 | 5 | 6 | 7 | 8 | 15 |
| 35–49 | 694 | 5.8 | 35 | 3 | 3 | 4 | 6 | 8 | 14 | 31 |
| 50–64 | 401 | 5.1 | 11 | 3 | 3 | 4 | 6 | 8 | 11 | 16 |
| 65+ | 306 | 7.7 | 27 | 3 | 4 | 6 | 10 | 15 | 20 | 20 |
| **GRAND TOTAL** | 1,676 | 5.8 | 25 | 3 | 3 | 4 | 6 | 9 | 14 | 31 |

## 68.7: RADICAL VAG HYSTERECTOMY. Formerly included in operation group(s) 691.

| Type of Patients | Observed Patients | Avg. Stay | Variance | 10th | 25th | 50th | 75th | 90th | 95th | 99th |
|---|---|---|---|---|---|---|---|---|---|---|
| **1. SINGLE DX** | | | | | | | | | | |
| 0–19 Years | 0 | | | | | | | | | |
| 20–34 | 7 | 2.1 | <1 | 1 | 1 | 2 | 3 | 3 | 3 | 3 |
| 35–49 | 4 | 2.6 | 1 | 1 | 2 | 3 | 3 | 4 | 4 | 4 |
| 50–64 | 0 | | | | | | | | | |
| 65+ | 3 | 3.5 | <1 | 2 | 2 | 4 | 4 | 4 | 4 | 4 |
| **2. MULTIPLE DX** | | | | | | | | | | |
| 0–19 Years | 0 | | | | | | | | | |
| 20–34 | 26 | 2.6 | <1 | 2 | 2 | 2 | 3 | 3 | 4 | 5 |
| 35–49 | 73 | 2.5 | 2 | 1 | 2 | 2 | 2 | 4 | 5 | 9 |
| 50–64 | 39 | 3.3 | 4 | 2 | 2 | 3 | 3 | 6 | 8 | 8 |
| 65+ | 23 | 3.8 | 8 | 2 | 2 | 3 | 4 | 7 | 11 | 13 |
| **TOTAL SINGLE DX** | 14 | 2.5 | 1 | 1 | 2 | 3 | 3 | 4 | 4 | 4 |
| **TOTAL MULTIPLE DX** | 161 | 2.8 | 3 | 1 | 2 | 2 | 3 | 5 | 7 | 9 |
| **TOTAL** | | | | | | | | | | |
| 0–19 Years | 0 | | | | | | | | | |
| 20–34 | 33 | 2.5 | <1 | 2 | 2 | 2 | 3 | 3 | 4 | 5 |
| 35–49 | 77 | 2.5 | 2 | 1 | 2 | 2 | 2 | 4 | 5 | 9 |
| 50–64 | 39 | 3.3 | 4 | 2 | 2 | 3 | 4 | 6 | 8 | 8 |
| 65+ | 26 | 3.8 | 7 | 2 | 2 | 3 | 4 | 7 | 11 | 13 |
| **GRAND TOTAL** | 175 | 2.8 | 3 | 1 | 2 | 2 | 3 | 5 | 7 | 9 |

## 68.8: PELVIC EVISCERATION. Formerly included in operation group(s) 691.

| Type of Patients | Observed Patients | Avg. Stay | Variance | 10th | 25th | 50th | 75th | 90th | 95th | 99th |
|---|---|---|---|---|---|---|---|---|---|---|
| **1. SINGLE DX** | | | | | | | | | | |
| 0–19 Years | 0 | | | | | | | | | |
| 20–34 | 1 | 5.0 | 0 | 5 | 5 | 5 | 5 | 5 | 5 | 5 |
| 35–49 | 5 | 5.5 | 13 | 3 | 3 | 5 | 8 | 11 | 11 | 11 |
| 50–64 | 2 | 6.3 | 1 | 5 | 5 | 7 | 7 | 7 | 7 | 7 |
| 65+ | 4 | 6.0 | <1 | 5 | 6 | 6 | 6 | 7 | 7 | 7 |
| **2. MULTIPLE DX** | | | | | | | | | | |
| 0–19 Years | 0 | | | | | | | | | |
| 20–34 | 8 | 19.6 | 175 | 10 | 10 | 13 | 29 | 29 | 54 | 54 |
| 35–49 | 49 | 18.8 | 285 | 8 | 9 | 12 | 19 | 61 | 61 | 61 |
| 50–64 | 64 | 15.5 | 82 | 6 | 10 | 12 | 22 | 25 | 39 | 41 |
| 65+ | 122 | 13.7 | 57 | 7 | 9 | 13 | 15 | 21 | 29 | 50 |
| **TOTAL SINGLE DX** | 12 | 5.7 | 8 | 3 | 3 | 6 | 8 | 11 | 11 | 11 |
| **TOTAL MULTIPLE DX** | 243 | 15.3 | 112 | 7 | 9 | 12 | 17 | 28 | 39 | 61 |
| **TOTAL** | | | | | | | | | | |
| 0–19 Years | 0 | | | | | | | | | |
| 20–34 | 9 | 19.0 | 176 | 10 | 10 | 13 | 29 | 29 | 54 | 54 |
| 35–49 | 54 | 16.7 | 266 | 6 | 8 | 11 | 18 | 61 | 61 | 61 |
| 50–64 | 66 | 15.3 | 82 | 6 | 9 | 11 | 22 | 25 | 39 | 41 |
| 65+ | 126 | 13.5 | 57 | 7 | 9 | 13 | 15 | 21 | 29 | 50 |
| **GRAND TOTAL** | 255 | 14.8 | 111 | 7 | 9 | 12 | 17 | 26 | 37 | 61 |

## 68.9: HYSTERECTOMY NEC & NOS. Formerly included in operation group(s) 689.

| Type of Patients | Observed Patients | Avg. Stay | Variance | 10th | 25th | 50th | 75th | 90th | 95th | 99th |
|---|---|---|---|---|---|---|---|---|---|---|
| **1. SINGLE DX** | | | | | | | | | | |
| 0–19 Years | 0 | | | | | | | | | |
| 20–34 | 7 | 3.0 | 2 | 2 | 2 | 2 | 4 | 4 | 4 | 9 |
| 35–49 | 17 | 2.4 | <1 | 2 | 2 | 3 | 3 | 3 | 3 | 3 |
| 50–64 | 9 | 3.0 | <1 | 2 | 2 | 3 | 4 | 4 | 4 | 4 |
| 65+ | 0 | | | | | | | | | |
| **2. MULTIPLE DX** | | | | | | | | | | |
| 0–19 Years | 5 | 2.3 | 3 | 1 | 1 | 2 | 2 | 7 | 7 | 7 |
| 20–34 | 51 | 3.8 | 8 | 2 | 2 | 3 | 4 | 7 | 8 | 19 |
| 35–49 | 253 | 3.2 | 3 | 2 | 2 | 3 | 3 | 5 | 5 | 10 |
| 50–64 | 59 | 3.0 | 4 | 1 | 2 | 3 | 3 | 4 | 5 | 13 |
| 65+ | 43 | 6.8 | 28 | 2 | 3 | 5 | 8 | 15 | 16 | 24 |
| **TOTAL SINGLE DX** | 33 | 2.7 | 1 | 2 | 2 | 3 | 3 | 4 | 4 | 9 |
| **TOTAL MULTIPLE DX** | 411 | 3.6 | 8 | 2 | 2 | 3 | 4 | 6 | 8 | 17 |
| **TOTAL** | | | | | | | | | | |
| 0–19 Years | 5 | 2.3 | 3 | 1 | 1 | 2 | 2 | 7 | 7 | 7 |
| 20–34 | 58 | 3.7 | 7 | 2 | 3 | 3 | 4 | 7 | 8 | 19 |
| 35–49 | 270 | 3.1 | 3 | 2 | 3 | 3 | 3 | 5 | 7 | 10 |
| 50–64 | 68 | 3.0 | 3 | 2 | 3 | 3 | 3 | 4 | 5 | 13 |
| 65+ | 43 | 6.8 | 28 | 2 | 3 | 5 | 8 | 15 | 16 | 24 |
| **GRAND TOTAL** | 444 | 3.5 | 7 | 2 | 2 | 3 | 4 | 5 | 8 | 16 |

Length of Stay by Diagnosis and Operation, United States, 2000

# United States, October 1998–September 1999 Data, by Operation

## 69.0: UTERINE D&C. Formerly included in operation group(s) 692, 693.

| Type of Patients | Observed Patients | Avg. Stay | Vari-ance | 10th | 25th | 50th | 75th | 90th | 95th | 99th |
|---|---|---|---|---|---|---|---|---|---|---|
| **1. SINGLE DX** | | | | | | | | | | |
| 0–19 Years | 554 | 1.2 | <1 | 1 | 1 | 1 | 1 | 2 | 2 | 4 |
| 20–34 | 2,416 | 1.3 | <1 | 1 | 1 | 1 | 1 | 2 | 2 | 4 |
| 35–49 | 660 | 1.3 | <1 | 1 | 1 | 1 | 1 | 2 | 2 | 4 |
| 50–64 | 27 | 1.5 | 4 | 1 | 1 | 1 | 1 | 2 | 3 | 13 |
| 65+ | 17 | 2.9 | 8 | 1 | 2 | 2 | 4 | 4 | 12 | 12 |
| **2. MULTIPLE DX** | | | | | | | | | | |
| 0–19 Years | 604 | 2.3 | 3 | 1 | 1 | 2 | 3 | 4 | 5 | 8 |
| 20–34 | 3,869 | 2.4 | 6 | 1 | 1 | 2 | 3 | 4 | 6 | 12 |
| 35–49 | 2,160 | 2.6 | 7 | 1 | 1 | 2 | 3 | 5 | 8 | 14 |
| 50–64 | 489 | 3.9 | 20 | 1 | 1 | 2 | 5 | 8 | 13 | 22 |
| 65+ | 710 | 6.9 | 58 | 2 | 2 | 5 | 9 | 13 | 19 | 46 |
| **TOTAL SINGLE DX** | 3,674 | 1.3 | <1 | 1 | 1 | 1 | 1 | 2 | 2 | 4 |
| **TOTAL MULTIPLE DX** | 7,832 | 2.9 | 13 | 1 | 1 | 2 | 3 | 6 | 8 | 17 |
| **TOTAL** | | | | | | | | | | |
| 0–19 Years | 1,158 | 1.7 | 2 | 1 | 1 | 1 | 2 | 3 | 4 | 6 |
| 20–34 | 6,285 | 1.9 | 5 | 1 | 1 | 1 | 2 | 3 | 5 | 10 |
| 35–49 | 2,820 | 2.3 | 6 | 1 | 1 | 2 | 3 | 4 | 6 | 12 |
| 50–64 | 516 | 3.8 | 20 | 1 | 2 | 2 | 4 | 8 | 13 | 22 |
| 65+ | 727 | 6.8 | 58 | 2 | 2 | 5 | 9 | 13 | 19 | 46 |
| **GRAND TOTAL** | 11,506 | 2.3 | 9 | 1 | 1 | 1 | 3 | 4 | 7 | 15 |

## 69.09: D&C NEC. Formerly included in operation group(s) 693.

| Type of Patients | Observed Patients | Avg. Stay | Vari-ance | 10th | 25th | 50th | 75th | 90th | 95th | 99th |
|---|---|---|---|---|---|---|---|---|---|---|
| **1. SINGLE DX** | | | | | | | | | | |
| 0–19 Years | 35 | 1.5 | <1 | 1 | 1 | 1 | 2 | 3 | 3 | 4 |
| 20–34 | 178 | 1.5 | <1 | 1 | 1 | 1 | 2 | 3 | 3 | 3 |
| 35–49 | 98 | 1.4 | <1 | 1 | 1 | 1 | 1 | 2 | 3 | 5 |
| 50–64 | 24 | 1.6 | 5 | 1 | 1 | 2 | 2 | 4 | 5 | 13 |
| 65+ | 17 | 2.9 | 8 | 1 | 1 | 2 | 4 | 4 | 12 | 12 |
| **2. MULTIPLE DX** | | | | | | | | | | |
| 0–19 Years | 106 | 2.6 | 7 | 1 | 1 | 2 | 3 | 5 | 5 | 7 |
| 20–34 | 697 | 2.5 | 6 | 1 | 1 | 2 | 3 | 5 | 7 | 11 |
| 35–49 | 1,205 | 2.8 | 8 | 1 | 1 | 2 | 3 | 5 | 9 | 12 |
| 50–64 | 488 | 3.9 | 20 | 1 | 1 | 2 | 5 | 8 | 13 | 22 |
| 65+ | 710 | 6.9 | 58 | 2 | 2 | 5 | 9 | 13 | 19 | 46 |
| **TOTAL SINGLE DX** | 352 | 1.5 | 1 | 1 | 1 | 1 | 2 | 3 | 3 | 5 |
| **TOTAL MULTIPLE DX** | 3,206 | 3.7 | 22 | 1 | 1 | 2 | 4 | 8 | 12 | 22 |
| **TOTAL** | | | | | | | | | | |
| 0–19 Years | 141 | 2.3 | 5 | 1 | 1 | 2 | 3 | 5 | 5 | 7 |
| 20–34 | 875 | 2.3 | 5 | 1 | 1 | 2 | 3 | 4 | 6 | 10 |
| 35–49 | 1,303 | 2.7 | 7 | 1 | 1 | 2 | 3 | 5 | 7 | 12 |
| 50–64 | 512 | 3.8 | 20 | 1 | 1 | 2 | 5 | 8 | 13 | 22 |
| 65+ | 727 | 6.8 | 58 | 2 | 2 | 5 | 9 | 13 | 19 | 46 |
| **GRAND TOTAL** | 3,558 | 3.5 | 21 | 1 | 1 | 2 | 4 | 8 | 11 | 21 |

## 69.02: D&C POST DEL OR AB. Formerly included in operation group(s) 693.

| Type of Patients | Observed Patients | Avg. Stay | Vari-ance | 10th | 25th | 50th | 75th | 90th | 95th | 99th |
|---|---|---|---|---|---|---|---|---|---|---|
| **1. SINGLE DX** | | | | | | | | | | |
| 0–19 Years | 503 | 1.2 | <1 | 1 | 1 | 1 | 1 | 2 | 2 | 4 |
| 20–34 | 2,180 | 1.3 | <1 | 1 | 1 | 1 | 1 | 2 | 2 | 4 |
| 35–49 | 550 | 1.2 | <1 | 1 | 1 | 1 | 1 | 2 | 2 | 4 |
| 50–64 | 3 | 1.2 | <1 | 1 | 1 | 1 | 1 | 2 | 3 | 3 |
| 65+ | 0 | | | | | | | | | |
| **2. MULTIPLE DX** | | | | | | | | | | |
| 0–19 Years | 483 | 2.2 | 3 | 1 | 1 | 2 | 3 | 3 | 4 | 8 |
| 20–34 | 3,071 | 2.3 | 6 | 1 | 1 | 2 | 3 | 4 | 6 | 11 |
| 35–49 | 909 | 2.4 | 7 | 1 | 1 | 2 | 3 | 4 | 6 | 14 |
| 50–64 | 1 | 2.0 | 0 | 2 | 2 | 2 | 2 | 2 | 2 | 2 |
| 65+ | 0 | | | | | | | | | |
| **TOTAL SINGLE DX** | 3,236 | 1.2 | <1 | 1 | 1 | 1 | 1 | 2 | 2 | 4 |
| **TOTAL MULTIPLE DX** | 4,464 | 2.4 | 6 | 1 | 1 | 2 | 3 | 4 | 6 | 12 |
| **TOTAL** | | | | | | | | | | |
| 0–19 Years | 986 | 1.7 | 2 | 1 | 1 | 1 | 2 | 3 | 3 | 6 |
| 20–34 | 5,251 | 1.9 | 4 | 1 | 1 | 1 | 2 | 3 | 5 | 9 |
| 35–49 | 1,459 | 2.0 | 5 | 1 | 1 | 1 | 2 | 3 | 5 | 12 |
| 50–64 | 4 | 1.2 | <1 | 1 | 1 | 1 | 1 | 2 | 3 | 3 |
| 65+ | 0 | | | | | | | | | |
| **GRAND TOTAL** | 7,700 | 1.9 | 4 | 1 | 1 | 1 | 2 | 3 | 4 | 9 |

## 69.1: EXC/DESTR UTER/SUPP LES. Formerly included in operation group(s) 697.

| Type of Patients | Observed Patients | Avg. Stay | Vari-ance | 10th | 25th | 50th | 75th | 90th | 95th | 99th |
|---|---|---|---|---|---|---|---|---|---|---|
| **1. SINGLE DX** | | | | | | | | | | |
| 0–19 Years | 22 | 2.3 | <1 | 2 | 2 | 2 | 2 | 4 | 4 | 4 |
| 20–34 | 28 | 2.2 | <1 | 2 | 2 | 2 | 3 | 3 | 3 | 3 |
| 35–49 | 20 | 1.9 | <1 | 1 | 1 | 2 | 2 | 3 | 3 | 1 |
| 50–64 | 0 | 1.0 | 0 | 1 | 1 | 1 | 1 | 1 | 1 | 1 |
| 65+ | | | | | | | | | | |
| **2. MULTIPLE DX** | | | | | | | | | | |
| 0–19 Years | 32 | 2.4 | 1 | 1 | 2 | 2 | 3 | 4 | 4 | 5 |
| 20–34 | 168 | 3.0 | 9 | 1 | 2 | 2 | 3 | 5 | 6 | 22 |
| 35–49 | 147 | 2.7 | 2 | 1 | 2 | 2 | 3 | 3 | 5 | 7 |
| 50–64 | 27 | 2.9 | 9 | 1 | 2 | 2 | 3 | 5 | 9 | 17 |
| 65+ | 16 | 3.8 | 4 | 2 | 3 | 3 | 6 | 6 | 9 | 9 |
| **TOTAL SINGLE DX** | 71 | 2.2 | <1 | 1 | 2 | 2 | 2 | 3 | 4 | 4 |
| **TOTAL MULTIPLE DX** | 390 | 2.8 | 5 | 1 | 2 | 2 | 3 | 5 | 6 | 9 |
| **TOTAL** | | | | | | | | | | |
| 0–19 Years | 54 | 2.3 | <1 | 1 | 2 | 2 | 3 | 4 | 4 | 4 |
| 20–34 | 196 | 2.9 | 8 | 1 | 2 | 2 | 3 | 5 | 6 | 7 |
| 35–49 | 167 | 2.6 | 2 | 1 | 2 | 2 | 3 | 4 | 5 | 7 |
| 50–64 | 28 | 2.8 | 8 | 1 | 1 | 2 | 3 | 5 | 9 | 17 |
| 65+ | 16 | 3.8 | 4 | 2 | 3 | 3 | 6 | 6 | 9 | 9 |
| **GRAND TOTAL** | 461 | 2.7 | 4 | 1 | 2 | 2 | 3 | 4 | 5 | 9 |

Length of Stay by Diagnosis and Operation, United States, 2000

# United States, October 1998–September 1999 Data, by Operation

## 69.19: EXC UTER/SUPP STRUCT NEC. Formerly included in operation group(s) 697.

| Type of Patients | Observed Patients | Avg. Stay | Variance | Percentiles | | | | | | |
|---|---|---|---|---|---|---|---|---|---|---|
| | | | | 10th | 25th | 50th | 75th | 90th | 95th | 99th |
| **1. SINGLE DX** | | | | | | | | | | |
| 0–19 Years | 22 | 2.3 | <1 | 1 | 2 | 2 | 2 | 4 | 4 | 4 |
| 20–34 | 28 | 2.2 | <1 | 1 | 2 | 2 | 2 | 3 | 3 | 3 |
| 35–49 | 20 | 1.9 | <1 | 1 | 2 | 2 | 2 | 3 | 3 | 3 |
| 50–64 | 1 | 1.0 | 0 | 1 | 1 | 1 | 1 | 1 | 1 | 1 |
| 65+ | 0 | | | | | | | | | |
| **2. MULTIPLE DX** | | | | | | | | | | |
| 0–19 Years | 32 | 2.4 | 1 | 1 | 2 | 2 | 3 | 4 | 4 | 5 |
| 20–34 | 168 | 3.0 | 9 | 1 | 2 | 2 | 3 | 5 | 6 | 22 |
| 35–49 | 147 | 2.7 | 2 | 1 | 2 | 2 | 3 | 4 | 5 | 7 |
| 50–64 | 27 | 2.9 | 9 | 1 | 1 | 2 | 3 | 5 | 9 | 17 |
| 65+ | 16 | 3.8 | 4 | 2 | 3 | 3 | 6 | 6 | 9 | 9 |
| **TOTAL SINGLE DX** | 71 | 2.2 | <1 | 1 | 2 | 2 | 2 | 3 | 4 | 4 |
| **TOTAL MULTIPLE DX** | 390 | 2.8 | 5 | 1 | 2 | 2 | 3 | 5 | 6 | 9 |
| **TOTAL** | | | | | | | | | | |
| 0–19 Years | 54 | 2.3 | <1 | 1 | 2 | 2 | 3 | 4 | 4 | 4 |
| 20–34 | 196 | 2.9 | 8 | 1 | 2 | 2 | 3 | 5 | 6 | 7 |
| 35–49 | 167 | 2.6 | 2 | 1 | 2 | 2 | 3 | 4 | 5 | 7 |
| 50–64 | 28 | 2.8 | 8 | 1 | 1 | 2 | 3 | 5 | 9 | 17 |
| 65+ | 16 | 3.8 | 4 | 2 | 3 | 3 | 6 | 6 | 9 | 9 |
| **GRAND TOTAL** | 461 | 2.7 | 4 | 1 | 2 | 2 | 3 | 4 | 5 | 9 |

## 69.2: UTERINE SUPP STRUCT REP. Formerly included in operation group(s) 696.

| Type of Patients | Observed Patients | Avg. Stay | Variance | Percentiles | | | | | | |
|---|---|---|---|---|---|---|---|---|---|---|
| | | | | 10th | 25th | 50th | 75th | 90th | 95th | 99th |
| **1. SINGLE DX** | | | | | | | | | | |
| 0–19 Years | 1 | 2.0 | 0 | 2 | 2 | 2 | 2 | 2 | 2 | 2 |
| 20–34 | 15 | 1.5 | <1 | 1 | 1 | 1 | 2 | 2 | 2 | 3 |
| 35–49 | 5 | 2.7 | <1 | 2 | 2 | 3 | 3 | 3 | 4 | 4 |
| 50–64 | 4 | 2.1 | <1 | 2 | 2 | 2 | 2 | 2 | 2 | 3 |
| 65+ | 2 | 1.5 | <1 | 1 | 1 | 2 | 2 | 2 | 2 | 2 |
| **2. MULTIPLE DX** | | | | | | | | | | |
| 0–19 Years | 5 | 4.2 | 8 | 2 | 3 | 3 | 5 | 10 | 10 | 10 |
| 20–34 | 67 | 2.3 | 3 | 1 | 1 | 2 | 3 | 3 | 4 | 14 |
| 35–49 | 49 | 2.5 | 2 | 1 | 2 | 2 | 3 | 4 | 4 | 9 |
| 50–64 | 14 | 2.0 | <1 | 1 | 1 | 2 | 3 | 3 | 3 | 3 |
| 65+ | 22 | 2.3 | 1 | 1 | 1 | 2 | 3 | 4 | 5 | 5 |
| **TOTAL SINGLE DX** | 27 | 1.8 | <1 | 1 | 1 | 2 | 2 | 3 | 3 | 4 |
| **TOTAL MULTIPLE DX** | 157 | 2.4 | 2 | 1 | 2 | 2 | 3 | 3 | 4 | 9 |
| **TOTAL** | | | | | | | | | | |
| 0–19 Years | 6 | 3.5 | 7 | 2 | 2 | 3 | 3 | 10 | 10 | 10 |
| 20–34 | 82 | 2.1 | 3 | 1 | 1 | 2 | 3 | 3 | 3 | 14 |
| 35–49 | 54 | 2.5 | 2 | 1 | 2 | 2 | 3 | 3 | 4 | 9 |
| 50–64 | 18 | 2.0 | <1 | 1 | 1 | 2 | 3 | 3 | 3 | 3 |
| 65+ | 24 | 2.3 | 1 | 1 | 2 | 2 | 3 | 4 | 5 | 5 |
| **GRAND TOTAL** | 184 | 2.3 | 2 | 1 | 2 | 2 | 3 | 3 | 4 | 9 |

## 69.3: PARACERV UTERINE DENERV. Formerly included in operation group(s) 696.

| Type of Patients | Observed Patients | Avg. Stay | Variance | Percentiles | | | | | | |
|---|---|---|---|---|---|---|---|---|---|---|
| | | | | 10th | 25th | 50th | 75th | 90th | 95th | 99th |
| **1. SINGLE DX** | | | | | | | | | | |
| 0–19 Years | 0 | | | | | | | | | |
| 20–34 | 0 | | | | | | | | | |
| 35–49 | 1 | 1.0 | 0 | 1 | 1 | 1 | 1 | 1 | 1 | 1 |
| 50–64 | 0 | | | | | | | | | |
| 65+ | 0 | | | | | | | | | |
| **2. MULTIPLE DX** | | | | | | | | | | |
| 0–19 Years | 2 | 2.8 | 4 | 2 | 2 | 2 | 4 | 4 | 4 | 4 |
| 20–34 | 4 | 1.3 | <1 | 1 | 1 | 1 | 2 | 2 | 2 | 2 |
| 35–49 | 0 | | | | | | | | | |
| 50–64 | 0 | | | | | | | | | |
| 65+ | 0 | | | | | | | | | |
| **TOTAL SINGLE DX** | 1 | 1.0 | 0 | 1 | 1 | 1 | 1 | 1 | 1 | 1 |
| **TOTAL MULTIPLE DX** | 6 | 2.0 | 1 | 1 | 1 | 2 | 2 | 4 | 4 | 4 |
| **TOTAL** | | | | | | | | | | |
| 0–19 Years | 2 | 2.8 | 1 | 2 | 2 | 2 | 4 | 4 | 4 | 4 |
| 20–34 | 4 | 1.3 | <1 | 1 | 1 | 1 | 2 | 2 | 2 | 2 |
| 35–49 | 1 | 1.0 | 0 | 1 | 1 | 1 | 1 | 1 | 1 | 1 |
| 50–64 | 0 | | | | | | | | | |
| 65+ | 0 | | | | | | | | | |
| **GRAND TOTAL** | 7 | 1.9 | 1 | 1 | 1 | 2 | 2 | 4 | 4 | 4 |

## 69.4: UTERINE REPAIR. Formerly included in operation group(s) 697.

| Type of Patients | Observed Patients | Avg. Stay | Variance | Percentiles | | | | | | |
|---|---|---|---|---|---|---|---|---|---|---|
| | | | | 10th | 25th | 50th | 75th | 90th | 95th | 99th |
| **1. SINGLE DX** | | | | | | | | | | |
| 0–19 Years | 4 | 1.9 | <1 | 2 | 2 | 2 | 2 | 2 | 2 | 2 |
| 20–34 | 7 | 3.9 | 25 | 1 | 2 | 3 | 3 | 3 | 19 | 19 |
| 35–49 | 1 | 1.0 | 0 | 1 | 1 | 1 | 1 | 1 | 1 | 1 |
| 50–64 | 0 | | | | | | | | | |
| 65+ | 0 | | | | | | | | | |
| **2. MULTIPLE DX** | | | | | | | | | | |
| 0–19 Years | 5 | 2.2 | <1 | 2 | 2 | 2 | 2 | 3 | 3 | 3 |
| 20–34 | 60 | 3.8 | 5 | 2 | 3 | 3 | 4 | 6 | 8 | 13 |
| 35–49 | 24 | 3.2 | 3 | 3 | 2 | 3 | 3 | 6 | 6 | 11 |
| 50–64 | 3 | 4.0 | <1 | 2 | 4 | 4 | 4 | 5 | 5 | 5 |
| 65+ | 4 | 2.2 | <1 | 2 | 2 | 2 | 2 | 3 | 3 | 3 |
| **TOTAL SINGLE DX** | 12 | 3.1 | 16 | 1 | 2 | 2 | 3 | 3 | 19 | 19 |
| **TOTAL MULTIPLE DX** | 96 | 3.5 | 4 | 2 | 2 | 3 | 4 | 6 | 8 | 13 |
| **TOTAL** | | | | | | | | | | |
| 0–19 Years | 9 | 2.0 | <1 | 2 | 2 | 2 | 2 | 2 | 2 | 3 |
| 20–34 | 67 | 3.8 | 8 | 2 | 2 | 3 | 4 | 6 | 8 | 19 |
| 35–49 | 25 | 3.1 | 3 | 3 | 2 | 3 | 3 | 6 | 6 | 11 |
| 50–64 | 3 | 4.0 | <1 | 3 | 4 | 4 | 4 | 5 | 5 | 5 |
| 65+ | 4 | 2.2 | <1 | 2 | 2 | 2 | 2 | 3 | 3 | 3 |
| **GRAND TOTAL** | 108 | 3.5 | 6 | 2 | 2 | 3 | 4 | 6 | 8 | 14 |

Length of Stay by Diagnosis and Operation, United States, 2000

# United States, October 1998–September 1999 Data, by Operation

## 69.5: ASP CURETTAGE UTERUS. Formerly included in operation group(s) 694, 695.

| Type of Patients | Observed Patients | Avg. Stay | Variance | 10th | 25th | 50th | 75th | 90th | 95th | 99th |
|---|---|---|---|---|---|---|---|---|---|---|
| **1. SINGLE DX** | | | | | | | | | | |
| 0–19 Years | 410 | 1.1 | <1 | 1 | 1 | 1 | 1 | 2 | 2 | 3 |
| 20–34 | 1,740 | 1.2 | <1 | 1 | 1 | 1 | 1 | 2 | 2 | 3 |
| 35–49 | 467 | 1.2 | <1 | 1 | 1 | 1 | 1 | 2 | 2 | 4 |
| 50–64 | 0 | | | | | | | | | |
| 65+ | 0 | | | | | | | | | |
| **2. MULTIPLE DX** | | | | | | | | | | |
| 0–19 Years | 285 | 1.8 | 2 | 1 | 1 | 1 | 2 | 3 | 4 | 6 |
| 20–34 | 1,654 | 2.3 | 5 | 1 | 1 | 2 | 3 | 4 | 5 | 10 |
| 35–49 | 583 | 2.3 | 7 | 1 | 1 | 1 | 3 | 4 | 6 | 12 |
| 50–64 | 27 | 8.3 | 42 | 1 | 1 | 14 | 14 | 14 | 14 | 25 |
| 65+ | 26 | 5.3 | 10 | 2 | 3 | 5 | 7 | 9 | 10 | 16 |
| **TOTAL SINGLE DX** | 2,617 | 1.2 | <1 | 1 | 1 | 1 | 1 | 2 | 2 | 3 |
| **TOTAL MULTIPLE DX** | 2,575 | 2.4 | 7 | 1 | 1 | 2 | 3 | 4 | 6 | 14 |
| **TOTAL** | | | | | | | | | | |
| 0–19 Years | 695 | 1.4 | <1 | 1 | 1 | 1 | 1 | 2 | 3 | 4 |
| 20–34 | 3,394 | 1.7 | 3 | 1 | 1 | 1 | 2 | 3 | 4 | 7 |
| 35–49 | 1,050 | 1.8 | 4 | 1 | 1 | 1 | 2 | 4 | 4 | 10 |
| 50–64 | 27 | 8.3 | 42 | 1 | 1 | 14 | 14 | 14 | 14 | 25 |
| 65+ | 26 | 5.3 | 10 | 2 | 3 | 5 | 7 | 9 | 10 | 16 |
| **GRAND TOTAL** | 5,192 | 1.8 | 4 | 1 | 1 | 1 | 2 | 3 | 4 | 12 |

## 69.51: ASP CURETTAGE-PREG TERM. Formerly included in operation group(s) 694.

| Type of Patients | Observed Patients | Avg. Stay | Variance | 10th | 25th | 50th | 75th | 90th | 95th | 99th |
|---|---|---|---|---|---|---|---|---|---|---|
| **1. SINGLE DX** | | | | | | | | | | |
| 0–19 Years | 17 | 1.5 | 1 | 1 | 1 | 1 | 2 | 2 | 5 | 5 |
| 20–34 | 62 | 1.7 | 4 | 1 | 1 | 1 | 2 | 2 | 4 | 14 |
| 35–49 | 15 | 1.1 | <1 | 1 | 1 | 1 | 1 | 1 | 1 | 3 |
| 50–64 | 0 | | | | | | | | | |
| 65+ | 0 | | | | | | | | | |
| **2. MULTIPLE DX** | | | | | | | | | | |
| 0–19 Years | 23 | 2.4 | 3 | 1 | 1 | 2 | 4 | 4 | 5 | 9 |
| 20–34 | 145 | 4.4 | 21 | 1 | 1 | 3 | 5 | 8 | 10 | 23 |
| 35–49 | 47 | 2.6 | 5 | 1 | 1 | 2 | 3 | 6 | 6 | 13 |
| 50–64 | 0 | | | | | | | | | |
| 65+ | 0 | | | | | | | | | |
| **TOTAL SINGLE DX** | 94 | 1.5 | 2 | 1 | 1 | 1 | 1 | 2 | 4 | 6 |
| **TOTAL MULTIPLE DX** | 215 | 3.7 | 16 | 1 | 1 | 3 | 5 | 6 | 10 | 22 |
| **TOTAL** | | | | | | | | | | |
| 0–19 Years | 40 | 2.0 | 2 | 1 | 1 | 1 | 2 | 4 | 5 | 9 |
| 20–34 | 207 | 3.8 | 19 | 1 | 1 | 2 | 5 | 7 | 10 | 23 |
| 35–49 | 62 | 2.2 | 4 | 1 | 1 | 1 | 3 | 5 | 6 | 13 |
| 50–64 | 0 | | | | | | | | | |
| 65+ | 0 | | | | | | | | | |
| **GRAND TOTAL** | 309 | 3.2 | 13 | 1 | 1 | 2 | 4 | 6 | 8 | 18 |

## 69.52: ASP CURETTE POST DEL/AB. Formerly included in operation group(s) 695.

| Type of Patients | Observed Patients | Avg. Stay | Variance | 10th | 25th | 50th | 75th | 90th | 95th | 99th |
|---|---|---|---|---|---|---|---|---|---|---|
| **1. SINGLE DX** | | | | | | | | | | |
| 0–19 Years | 366 | 1.1 | <1 | 1 | 1 | 1 | 1 | 1 | 2 | 3 |
| 20–34 | 1,571 | 1.2 | <1 | 1 | 1 | 1 | 1 | 2 | 2 | 3 |
| 35–49 | 423 | 1.2 | <1 | 1 | 1 | 1 | 1 | 2 | 2 | 4 |
| 50–64 | 0 | | | | | | | | | |
| 65+ | 0 | | | | | | | | | |
| **2. MULTIPLE DX** | | | | | | | | | | |
| 0–19 Years | 226 | 1.8 | 2 | 1 | 1 | 1 | 2 | 3 | 4 | 6 |
| 20–34 | 1,367 | 2.1 | 2 | 1 | 1 | 2 | 3 | 4 | 5 | 7 |
| 35–49 | 434 | 2.3 | 8 | 1 | 1 | 1 | 3 | 4 | 6 | 12 |
| 50–64 | 1 | 5.0 | 0 | 5 | 5 | 5 | 5 | 5 | 5 | 5 |
| 65+ | 0 | | | | | | | | | |
| **TOTAL SINGLE DX** | 2,360 | 1.2 | <1 | 1 | 1 | 1 | 1 | 2 | 2 | 3 |
| **TOTAL MULTIPLE DX** | 2,028 | 2.1 | 4 | 1 | 1 | 2 | 2 | 4 | 5 | 9 |
| **TOTAL** | | | | | | | | | | |
| 0–19 Years | 592 | 1.3 | <1 | 1 | 1 | 1 | 1 | 2 | 3 | 4 |
| 20–34 | 2,938 | 1.6 | 1 | 1 | 1 | 1 | 2 | 3 | 4 | 6 |
| 35–49 | 857 | 1.7 | 4 | 1 | 1 | 1 | 2 | 3 | 4 | 9 |
| 50–64 | 1 | 5.0 | 0 | 5 | 5 | 5 | 5 | 5 | 5 | 5 |
| 65+ | 0 | | | | | | | | | |
| **GRAND TOTAL** | 4,388 | 1.6 | 2 | 1 | 1 | 1 | 2 | 3 | 4 | 7 |

## 69.59: ASP CURETTAGE UTERUS NEC. Formerly included in operation group(s) 695.

| Type of Patients | Observed Patients | Avg. Stay | Variance | 10th | 25th | 50th | 75th | 90th | 95th | 99th |
|---|---|---|---|---|---|---|---|---|---|---|
| **1. SINGLE DX** | | | | | | | | | | |
| 0–19 Years | 27 | 1.5 | <1 | 1 | 1 | 1 | 2 | 2 | 3 | 4 |
| 20–34 | 107 | 1.6 | <1 | 1 | 1 | 1 | 2 | 3 | 3 | 3 |
| 35–49 | 29 | 1.8 | 7 | 1 | 1 | 1 | 2 | 2 | 2 | 18 |
| 50–64 | 0 | | | | | | | | | |
| 65+ | 0 | | | | | | | | | |
| **2. MULTIPLE DX** | | | | | | | | | | |
| 0–19 Years | 36 | 2.1 | 2 | 1 | 1 | 2 | 3 | 3 | 5 | 12 |
| 20–34 | 142 | 2.6 | 6 | 1 | 1 | 2 | 3 | 5 | 6 | 14 |
| 35–49 | 102 | 2.1 | 4 | 1 | 1 | 2 | 3 | 4 | 4 | 13 |
| 50–64 | 26 | 8.3 | 42 | 1 | 3 | 14 | 14 | 14 | 14 | 25 |
| 65+ | 26 | 5.3 | 10 | 2 | 3 | 5 | 7 | 9 | 10 | 16 |
| **TOTAL SINGLE DX** | 163 | 1.6 | 2 | 1 | 1 | 1 | 2 | 3 | 3 | 4 |
| **TOTAL MULTIPLE DX** | 332 | 3.7 | 18 | 1 | 1 | 2 | 4 | 14 | 14 | 14 |
| **TOTAL** | | | | | | | | | | |
| 0–19 Years | 63 | 1.8 | 1 | 1 | 1 | 1 | 2 | 3 | 4 | 5 |
| 20–34 | 249 | 2.2 | 4 | 1 | 1 | 1 | 2 | 3 | 5 | 14 |
| 35–49 | 131 | 2.0 | 4 | 1 | 1 | 1 | 2 | 3 | 3 | 13 |
| 50–64 | 26 | 8.3 | 42 | 1 | 3 | 14 | 14 | 14 | 14 | 25 |
| 65+ | 26 | 5.3 | 10 | 2 | 3 | 5 | 7 | 9 | 10 | 16 |
| **GRAND TOTAL** | 495 | 3.1 | 14 | 1 | 1 | 2 | 3 | 7 | 14 | 14 |

Length of Stay by Diagnosis and Operation, United States, 2000

# United States, October 1998–September 1999 Data, by Operation

## 69.6: MENSTRUAL EXTRACTION. Formerly included in operation group(s) 704.

| Type of Patients | Observed Patients | Avg. Stay | Variance | 10th | 25th | 50th | 75th | 90th | 95th | 99th |
|---|---|---|---|---|---|---|---|---|---|---|
| **1. SINGLE DX** | | | | | | | | | | |
| 0–19 Years | 0 | | | | | | | | | |
| 20–34 | 0 | | | | | | | | | |
| 35–49 | 0 | | | | | | | | | |
| 50–64 | 0 | | | | | | | | | |
| 65+ | 0 | | | | | | | | | |
| **2. MULTIPLE DX** | | | | | | | | | | |
| 0–19 Years | 2 | 6.6 | 5 | 4 | 4 | 8 | 8 | 8 | 8 | 8 |
| 20–34 | 0 | | | | | | | | | |
| 35–49 | 1 | 4.0 | 0 | 4 | 4 | 4 | 4 | 4 | 4 | 4 |
| 50–64 | 0 | | | | | | | | | |
| 65+ | 0 | | | | | | | | | |
| **TOTAL SINGLE DX** | 0 | | | | | | | | | |
| **TOTAL MULTIPLE DX** | 3 | 5.9 | 5 | 4 | 4 | 4 | 8 | 8 | 8 | 8 |
| **TOTAL** | | | | | | | | | | |
| 0–19 Years | 2 | 6.6 | 5 | 4 | 4 | 8 | 8 | 8 | 8 | 8 |
| 20–34 | 0 | | | | | | | | | |
| 35–49 | 1 | 4.0 | 0 | 4 | 4 | 4 | 4 | 4 | 4 | 4 |
| 50–64 | 0 | | | | | | | | | |
| 65+ | 0 | | | | | | | | | |
| **GRAND TOTAL** | 3 | 5.9 | 5 | 4 | 4 | 4 | 8 | 8 | 8 | 8 |

## 69.9: OTHER OPS UTERUS/ADNEXA. Formerly included in operation group(s) 697, 704.

| Type of Patients | Observed Patients | Avg. Stay | Variance | 10th | 25th | 50th | 75th | 90th | 95th | 99th |
|---|---|---|---|---|---|---|---|---|---|---|
| **1. SINGLE DX** | | | | | | | | | | |
| 0–19 Years | 20 | 1.4 | <1 | 1 | 1 | 1 | 2 | 2 | 2 | 3 |
| 20–34 | 109 | 1.6 | 10 | 1 | 1 | 1 | 2 | 2 | 3 | 4 |
| 35–49 | 46 | 1.5 | <1 | 1 | 1 | 1 | 2 | 2 | 2 | 5 |
| 50–64 | 11 | 2.0 | <1 | 1 | 2 | 2 | 2 | 3 | 3 | 3 |
| 65+ | 9 | 2.6 | <1 | 2 | 2 | 2 | 3 | 4 | 4 | 4 |
| **2. MULTIPLE DX** | | | | | | | | | | |
| 0–19 Years | 63 | 3.4 | 86 | 1 | 1 | 1 | 2 | 4 | 10 | 68 |
| 20–34 | 411 | 4.0 | 49 | 1 | 1 | 1 | 3 | 9 | 19 | 38 |
| 35–49 | 141 | 2.9 | 6 | 1 | 2 | 2 | 4 | 7 | 7 | 10 |
| 50–64 | 34 | 2.5 | 3 | 1 | 2 | 2 | 3 | 4 | 4 | 13 |
| 65+ | 22 | 2.8 | <1 | 2 | 3 | 3 | 3 | 3 | 4 | 8 |
| **TOTAL SINGLE DX** | 195 | 1.6 | 5 | 1 | 1 | 1 | 2 | 2 | 3 | 4 |
| **TOTAL MULTIPLE DX** | 671 | 3.5 | 37 | 1 | 1 | 2 | 3 | 7 | 10 | 33 |
| **TOTAL** | | | | | | | | | | |
| 0–19 Years | 83 | 2.8 | 62 | 1 | 1 | 1 | 2 | 4 | 5 | 68 |
| 20–34 | 520 | 3.5 | 42 | 1 | 1 | 2 | 3 | 6 | 14 | 38 |
| 35–49 | 187 | 2.5 | 5 | 1 | 2 | 2 | 3 | 7 | 7 | 10 |
| 50–64 | 45 | 2.4 | 3 | 1 | 2 | 2 | 3 | 4 | 4 | 13 |
| 65+ | 31 | 2.8 | <1 | 2 | 3 | 3 | 3 | 3 | 4 | 8 |
| **GRAND TOTAL** | 866 | 3.1 | 30 | 1 | 1 | 2 | 3 | 6 | 9 | 26 |

## 69.7: INSERTION OF IUD. Formerly included in operation group(s) 704.

| Type of Patients | Observed Patients | Avg. Stay | Variance | 10th | 25th | 50th | 75th | 90th | 95th | 99th |
|---|---|---|---|---|---|---|---|---|---|---|
| **1. SINGLE DX** | | | | | | | | | | |
| 0–19 Years | 0 | | | | | | | | | |
| 20–34 | 0 | | | | | | | | | |
| 35–49 | 0 | | | | | | | | | |
| 50–64 | 0 | | | | | | | | | |
| 65+ | 0 | | | | | | | | | |
| **2. MULTIPLE DX** | | | | | | | | | | |
| 0–19 Years | 0 | | | | | | | | | |
| 20–34 | 1 | 27.0 | 0 | 27 | 27 | 27 | 27 | 27 | 27 | 27 |
| 35–49 | 0 | | | | | | | | | |
| 50–64 | 0 | | | | | | | | | |
| 65+ | 0 | | | | | | | | | |
| **TOTAL SINGLE DX** | 0 | | | | | | | | | |
| **TOTAL MULTIPLE DX** | 1 | 27.0 | 0 | 27 | 27 | 27 | 27 | 27 | 27 | 27 |
| **TOTAL** | | | | | | | | | | |
| 0–19 Years | 0 | | | | | | | | | |
| 20–34 | 1 | 27.0 | 0 | 27 | 27 | 27 | 27 | 27 | 27 | 27 |
| 35–49 | 0 | | | | | | | | | |
| 50–64 | 0 | | | | | | | | | |
| 65+ | 0 | | | | | | | | | |
| **GRAND TOTAL** | 1 | 27.0 | 0 | 27 | 27 | 27 | 27 | 27 | 27 | 27 |

## 69.93: INSERTION OF LAMINARIA. Formerly included in operation group(s) 697.

| Type of Patients | Observed Patients | Avg. Stay | Variance | 10th | 25th | 50th | 75th | 90th | 95th | 99th |
|---|---|---|---|---|---|---|---|---|---|---|
| **1. SINGLE DX** | | | | | | | | | | |
| 0–19 Years | 18 | 1.4 | <1 | 1 | 1 | 1 | 2 | 2 | 2 | 3 |
| 20–34 | 61 | 1.2 | <1 | 1 | 1 | 1 | 1 | 2 | 2 | 3 |
| 35–49 | 21 | 1.3 | <1 | 1 | 1 | 1 | 1 | 2 | 2 | 3 |
| 50–64 | 0 | | | | | | | | | |
| 65+ | 0 | | | | | | | | | |
| **2. MULTIPLE DX** | | | | | | | | | | |
| 0–19 Years | 44 | 1.9 | 4 | 1 | 1 | 1 | 2 | 4 | 4 | 16 |
| 20–34 | 179 | 1.9 | 5 | 1 | 1 | 1 | 2 | 3 | 5 | 18 |
| 35–49 | 69 | 1.6 | 1 | 1 | 1 | 1 | 2 | 3 | 4 | 6 |
| 50–64 | 0 | | | | | | | | | |
| 65+ | 0 | | | | | | | | | |
| **TOTAL SINGLE DX** | 100 | 1.3 | <1 | 1 | 1 | 1 | 1 | 2 | 2 | 3 |
| **TOTAL MULTIPLE DX** | 292 | 1.8 | 4 | 1 | 1 | 1 | 2 | 3 | 5 | 16 |
| **TOTAL** | | | | | | | | | | |
| 0–19 Years | 62 | 1.7 | 3 | 1 | 1 | 1 | 2 | 3 | 4 | 16 |
| 20–34 | 240 | 1.7 | 4 | 1 | 1 | 1 | 2 | 3 | 5 | 10 |
| 35–49 | 90 | 1.5 | <1 | 1 | 1 | 1 | 2 | 3 | 4 | 5 |
| 50–64 | 0 | | | | | | | | | |
| 65+ | 0 | | | | | | | | | |
| **GRAND TOTAL** | 392 | 1.7 | 3 | 1 | 1 | 1 | 2 | 3 | 4 | 7 |

258

# United States, October 1998–September 1999 Data, by Operation

## 69.96: RMVL CERVICAL CERCLAGE. Formerly included in operation group(s) 697.

| Type of Patients | Observed Patients | Avg. Stay | Variance | 10th | 25th | 50th | 75th | 90th | 95th | 99th |
|---|---|---|---|---|---|---|---|---|---|---|
| **1. SINGLE DX** | | | | | | | | | | |
| 0–19 Years | 1 | 2.0 | 0 | 2 | 2 | 2 | 2 | 2 | 2 | 2 |
| 20–34 | 45 | 2.1 | 28 | 1 | 1 | 1 | 2 | 3 | 3 | 52 |
| 35–49 | 9 | 1.4 | 1 | 1 | 1 | 1 | 1 | 2 | 5 | 5 |
| 50–64 | 0 | | | | | | | | | |
| 65+ | 0 | | | | | | | | | |
| **2. MULTIPLE DX** | | | | | | | | | | |
| 0–19 Years | 17 | 9.8 | 383 | 1 | 1 | 2 | 5 | 12 | 68 | 68 |
| 20–34 | 209 | 6.2 | 88 | 1 | 2 | 2 | 6 | 19 | 25 | 45 |
| 35–49 | 37 | 4.3 | 9 | 1 | 2 | 3 | 7 | 7 | 7 | 10 |
| 50–64 | 0 | | | | | | | | | |
| 65+ | 0 | | | | | | | | | |
| **TOTAL SINGLE DX** | 55 | 1.9 | 20 | 1 | 1 | 1 | 2 | 3 | 3 | 5 |
| **TOTAL MULTIPLE DX** | 263 | 5.9 | 84 | 1 | 2 | 3 | 6 | 12 | 23 | 45 |
| **TOTAL** | | | | | | | | | | |
| 0–19 Years | 18 | 9.6 | 375 | 1 | 1 | 2 | 5 | 12 | 68 | 68 |
| 20–34 | 254 | 5.6 | 81 | 1 | 1 | 2 | 6 | 14 | 24 | 45 |
| 35–49 | 46 | 3.9 | 9 | 1 | 2 | 3 | 7 | 7 | 7 | 10 |
| 50–64 | 0 | | | | | | | | | |
| 65+ | 0 | | | | | | | | | |
| **GRAND TOTAL** | 318 | 5.3 | 77 | 1 | 1 | 2 | 6 | 10 | 20 | 45 |

## 70.0: CULDOCENTESIS. Formerly included in operation group(s) 700.

| Type of Patients | Observed Patients | Avg. Stay | Variance | 10th | 25th | 50th | 75th | 90th | 95th | 99th |
|---|---|---|---|---|---|---|---|---|---|---|
| **1. SINGLE DX** | | | | | | | | | | |
| 0–19 Years | 5 | 2.6 | 6 | 1 | 1 | 1 | 3 | 7 | 7 | 7 |
| 20–34 | 21 | 1.9 | 2 | 1 | 1 | 1 | 3 | 4 | 4 | 5 |
| 35–49 | 9 | 2.3 | 3 | 1 | 1 | 2 | 2 | 6 | 6 | 9 |
| 50–64 | 0 | | | | | | | | | |
| 65+ | 0 | | | | | | | | | |
| **2. MULTIPLE DX** | | | | | | | | | | |
| 0–19 Years | 18 | 3.9 | 15 | 1 | 1 | 3 | 4 | 8 | 12 | 18 |
| 20–34 | 50 | 3.4 | 5 | 1 | 2 | 3 | 5 | 7 | 7 | 9 |
| 35–49 | 36 | 4.4 | 11 | 2 | 2 | 4 | 6 | 9 | 11 | 16 |
| 50–64 | 7 | 4.5 | 2 | 3 | 4 | 5 | 6 | 5 | 6 | 6 |
| 65+ | 8 | 6.3 | 7 | 2 | 6 | 7 | 8 | 8 | 10 | 10 |
| **TOTAL SINGLE DX** | 35 | 2.1 | 3 | 1 | 1 | 1 | 3 | 4 | 6 | 7 |
| **TOTAL MULTIPLE DX** | 119 | 4.0 | 8 | 1 | 2 | 4 | 5 | 8 | 9 | 16 |
| **TOTAL** | | | | | | | | | | |
| 0–19 Years | 23 | 3.6 | 13 | 1 | 1 | 3 | 4 | 8 | 12 | 18 |
| 20–34 | 71 | 3.0 | 4 | 1 | 2 | 2 | 5 | 7 | 7 | 8 |
| 35–49 | 45 | 3.8 | 10 | 2 | 2 | 4 | 5 | 8 | 10 | 16 |
| 50–64 | 7 | 4.5 | 2 | 3 | 4 | 5 | 5 | 5 | 6 | 6 |
| 65+ | 8 | 6.3 | 7 | 2 | 6 | 7 | 8 | 8 | 10 | 10 |
| **GRAND TOTAL** | 154 | 3.5 | 8 | 1 | 1 | 3 | 5 | 7 | 8 | 12 |

## 70.1: INC VAGINA & CUL-DE-SAC. Formerly included in operation group(s) 700.

| Type of Patients | Observed Patients | Avg. Stay | Variance | 10th | 25th | 50th | 75th | 90th | 95th | 99th |
|---|---|---|---|---|---|---|---|---|---|---|
| **1. SINGLE DX** | | | | | | | | | | |
| 0–19 Years | 16 | 2.6 | 3 | 1 | 1 | 2 | 4 | 4 | 7 | 8 |
| 20–34 | 29 | 2.5 | 4 | 1 | 1 | 2 | 3 | 6 | 7 | 9 |
| 35–49 | 33 | 3.0 | 3 | 1 | 2 | 3 | 4 | 6 | 6 | 9 |
| 50–64 | 15 | 2.2 | 2 | 1 | 1 | 1 | 3 | 5 | 5 | 6 |
| 65+ | 4 | 1.4 | <1 | 1 | 1 | 1 | 1 | 3 | 3 | 3 |
| **2. MULTIPLE DX** | | | | | | | | | | |
| 0–19 Years | 68 | 3.3 | 10 | 1 | 1 | 2 | 4 | 7 | 9 | 15 |
| 20–34 | 155 | 4.5 | 14 | 1 | 2 | 4 | 6 | 9 | 13 | 17 |
| 35–49 | 209 | 5.1 | 19 | 2 | 2 | 4 | 8 | 10 | 13 | 22 |
| 50–64 | 71 | 5.9 | 48 | 1 | 2 | 5 | 7 | 12 | 14 | 41 |
| 65+ | 78 | 5.7 | 21 | 1 | 2 | 5 | 7 | 13 | 15 | 19 |
| **TOTAL SINGLE DX** | 97 | 2.6 | 3 | 1 | 1 | 2 | 3 | 5 | 6 | 8 |
| **TOTAL MULTIPLE DX** | 581 | 4.9 | 22 | 1 | 2 | 4 | 6 | 10 | 14 | 19 |
| **TOTAL** | | | | | | | | | | |
| 0–19 Years | 84 | 3.2 | 9 | 1 | 1 | 2 | 4 | 7 | 9 | 15 |
| 20–34 | 184 | 4.1 | 13 | 1 | 1 | 3 | 6 | 8 | 11 | 17 |
| 35–49 | 242 | 4.8 | 17 | 1 | 2 | 4 | 7 | 10 | 11 | 22 |
| 50–64 | 86 | 5.4 | 42 | 1 | 2 | 3 | 7 | 12 | 12 | 41 |
| 65+ | 82 | 5.5 | 21 | 1 | 2 | 5 | 7 | 13 | 15 | 19 |
| **GRAND TOTAL** | 678 | 4.5 | 19 | 1 | 2 | 3 | 6 | 10 | 13 | 19 |

## 70.12: CULDOTOMY. Formerly included in operation group(s) 700.

| Type of Patients | Observed Patients | Avg. Stay | Variance | 10th | 25th | 50th | 75th | 90th | 95th | 99th |
|---|---|---|---|---|---|---|---|---|---|---|
| **1. SINGLE DX** | | | | | | | | | | |
| 0–19 Years | 6 | 4.4 | 3 | 3 | 3 | 4 | 5 | 8 | 8 | 8 |
| 20–34 | 11 | 3.2 | 5 | 2 | 2 | 2 | 4 | 7 | 8 | 9 |
| 35–49 | 14 | 2.8 | 3 | 1 | 1 | 3 | 4 | 4 | 6 | 9 |
| 50–64 | 6 | 2.5 | 2 | 1 | 1 | 3 | 3 | 5 | 5 | 5 |
| 65+ | 0 | | | | | | | | | |
| **2. MULTIPLE DX** | | | | | | | | | | |
| 0–19 Years | 24 | 6.0 | 13 | 2 | 4 | 5 | 7 | 12 | 15 | 15 |
| 20–34 | 83 | 5.7 | 13 | 3 | 3 | 6 | 7 | 9 | 13 | 19 |
| 35–49 | 110 | 6.1 | 17 | 2 | 3 | 5 | 7 | 10 | 15 | 18 |
| 50–64 | 32 | 7.5 | 86 | 1 | 2 | 5 | 10 | 14 | 21 | 49 |
| 65+ | 35 | 8.3 | 22 | 3 | 5 | 6 | 12 | 15 | 17 | 20 |
| **TOTAL SINGLE DX** | 37 | 3.1 | 4 | 1 | 2 | 3 | 4 | 7 | 7 | 9 |
| **TOTAL MULTIPLE DX** | 284 | 6.4 | 27 | 2 | 3 | 5 | 8 | 12 | 15 | 20 |
| **TOTAL** | | | | | | | | | | |
| 0–19 Years | 30 | 5.7 | 12 | 2 | 2 | 5 | 7 | 10 | 15 | 15 |
| 20–34 | 94 | 5.2 | 12 | 2 | 2 | 5 | 7 | 8 | 12 | 19 |
| 35–49 | 124 | 5.7 | 16 | 2 | 3 | 5 | 7 | 10 | 15 | 18 |
| 50–64 | 38 | 6.5 | 74 | 1 | 1 | 3 | 8 | 12 | 18 | 49 |
| 65+ | 35 | 8.3 | 22 | 3 | 5 | 6 | 12 | 15 | 17 | 20 |
| **GRAND TOTAL** | 321 | 6.0 | 25 | 2 | 3 | 5 | 7 | 11 | 15 | 20 |

Length of Stay by Diagnosis and Operation, United States, 2000

# United States, October 1998–September 1999 Data, by Operation

## 70.14: VAGINOTOMY NEC. Formerly included in operation group(s) 700.

| Type of Patients | Observed Patients | Avg. Stay | Variance | 10th | 25th | 50th | 75th | 90th | 95th | 99th |
|---|---|---|---|---|---|---|---|---|---|---|
| **1. SINGLE DX** | | | | | | | | | | |
| 0–19 Years | 4 | 2.1 | 2 | 1 | 1 | 2 | 4 | 4 | 4 | 4 |
| 20–34 | 13 | 2.2 | 3 | 1 | 1 | 1 | 3 | 4 | 6 | 6 |
| 35–49 | 19 | 3.1 | 3 | 1 | 2 | 3 | 4 | 6 | 6 | 6 |
| 50–64 | 8 | 1.9 | 2 | 1 | 1 | 2 | 2 | 3 | 6 | 6 |
| 65+ | 4 | 1.4 | <1 | 1 | 1 | 1 | 1 | 3 | 3 | 3 |
| **2. MULTIPLE DX** | | | | | | | | | | |
| 0–19 Years | 21 | 3.1 | 5 | 1 | 1 | 2 | 4 | 5 | 9 | 9 |
| 20–34 | 68 | 3.6 | 14 | 1 | 1 | 2 | 5 | 9 | 15 | 15 |
| 35–49 | 96 | 4.1 | 19 | 1 | 2 | 3 | 5 | 7 | 11 | 30 |
| 50–64 | 34 | 5.2 | 19 | 1 | 2 | 3 | 12 | 12 | 12 | 16 |
| 65+ | 37 | 3.7 | 11 | 1 | 1 | 2 | 6 | 7 | 11 | 19 |
| **TOTAL SINGLE DX** | 48 | 2.4 | 3 | 1 | 1 | 2 | 3 | 5 | 6 | 6 |
| **TOTAL MULTIPLE DX** | 256 | 4.0 | 16 | 1 | 2 | 3 | 5 | 9 | 12 | 19 |
| **TOTAL** | | | | | | | | | | |
| 0–19 Years | 25 | 2.9 | 4 | 1 | 1 | 2 | 4 | 5 | 9 | 9 |
| 20–34 | 81 | 3.3 | 12 | 1 | 1 | 2 | 4 | 7 | 11 | 15 |
| 35–49 | 115 | 4.0 | 16 | 1 | 2 | 3 | 4 | 6 | 10 | 22 |
| 50–64 | 42 | 4.8 | 18 | 1 | 2 | 3 | 6 | 12 | 12 | 16 |
| 65+ | 41 | 3.5 | 11 | 1 | 1 | 2 | 5 | 7 | 11 | 19 |
| **GRAND TOTAL** | 304 | 3.8 | 14 | 1 | 2 | 3 | 5 | 8 | 12 | 17 |

## 70.3: LOC EXC/DESTR VAG/CUL. Formerly included in operation group(s) 700.

| Type of Patients | Observed Patients | Avg. Stay | Variance | 10th | 25th | 50th | 75th | 90th | 95th | 99th |
|---|---|---|---|---|---|---|---|---|---|---|
| **1. SINGLE DX** | | | | | | | | | | |
| 0–19 Years | 14 | 1.1 | <1 | 1 | 1 | 1 | 1 | 1 | 1 | 3 |
| 20–34 | 24 | 1.5 | <1 | 1 | 1 | 1 | 2 | 2 | 2 | 4 |
| 35–49 | 15 | 3.1 | 4 | 1 | 1 | 2 | 6 | 6 | 6 | 6 |
| 50–64 | 10 | 2.6 | <1 | 1 | 3 | 3 | 3 | 3 | 4 | 4 |
| 65+ | 5 | 1.5 | 1 | 1 | 1 | 1 | 1 | 4 | 4 | 4 |
| **2. MULTIPLE DX** | | | | | | | | | | |
| 0–19 Years | 67 | 1.9 | 1 | 1 | 1 | 1 | 2 | 4 | 4 | 7 |
| 20–34 | 313 | 2.4 | 3 | 1 | 1 | 2 | 3 | 4 | 8 | 10 |
| 35–49 | 161 | 2.5 | 10 | 1 | 1 | 2 | 3 | 7 | 6 | 10 |
| 50–64 | 82 | 3.0 | 9 | 1 | 1 | 2 | 3 | 7 | 7 | 17 |
| 65+ | 88 | 4.3 | 17 | 1 | 1 | 2 | 7 | 12 | 12 | 20 |
| **TOTAL SINGLE DX** | 68 | 1.7 | 1 | 1 | 1 | 1 | 2 | 3 | 4 | 6 |
| **TOTAL MULTIPLE DX** | 711 | 2.6 | 7 | 1 | 1 | 2 | 3 | 5 | 8 | 12 |
| **TOTAL** | | | | | | | | | | |
| 0–19 Years | 81 | 1.7 | 1 | 1 | 1 | 1 | 2 | 3 | 4 | 7 |
| 20–34 | 337 | 2.4 | 3 | 1 | 1 | 2 | 3 | 4 | 7 | 10 |
| 35–49 | 176 | 2.5 | 10 | 1 | 1 | 2 | 3 | 6 | 6 | 10 |
| 50–64 | 92 | 2.9 | 7 | 1 | 1 | 2 | 3 | 6 | 7 | 17 |
| 65+ | 93 | 4.1 | 17 | 1 | 1 | 2 | 7 | 12 | 12 | 15 |
| **GRAND TOTAL** | 779 | 2.5 | 7 | 1 | 1 | 2 | 3 | 4 | 7 | 12 |

## 70.2: VAG/CUL-DE-SAC DXTIC PX. Formerly included in operation group(s) 700, 704.

| Type of Patients | Observed Patients | Avg. Stay | Variance | 10th | 25th | 50th | 75th | 90th | 95th | 99th |
|---|---|---|---|---|---|---|---|---|---|---|
| **1. SINGLE DX** | | | | | | | | | | |
| 0–19 Years | 18 | 1.5 | <1 | 1 | 1 | 1 | 2 | 2 | 2 | 4 |
| 20–34 | 3 | 1.0 | 0 | 1 | 1 | 1 | 1 | 1 | 1 | 1 |
| 35–49 | 4 | 1.9 | <1 | 2 | 2 | 2 | 2 | 2 | 3 | 3 |
| 50–64 | 6 | 1.8 | <1 | 1 | 1 | 2 | 2 | 3 | 3 | 3 |
| 65+ | 5 | 3.0 | 1 | 2 | 2 | 4 | 4 | 4 | 4 | 4 |
| **2. MULTIPLE DX** | | | | | | | | | | |
| 0–19 Years | 30 | 6.8 | 146 | 1 | 1 | 2 | 4 | 20 | 52 | 52 |
| 20–34 | 43 | 3.9 | 8 | 1 | 2 | 3 | 6 | 6 | 10 | 12 |
| 35–49 | 67 | 3.6 | 10 | 1 | 2 | 3 | 5 | 7 | 10 | 19 |
| 50–64 | 63 | 6.4 | 36 | 2 | 3 | 4 | 8 | 14 | 20 | 34 |
| 65+ | 151 | 5.9 | 40 | 1 | 2 | 5 | 7 | 12 | 14 | 25 |
| **TOTAL SINGLE DX** | 36 | 1.7 | <1 | 1 | 1 | 2 | 2 | 3 | 4 | 4 |
| **TOTAL MULTIPLE DX** | 354 | 5.4 | 44 | 1 | 2 | 3 | 7 | 12 | 15 | 34 |
| **TOTAL** | | | | | | | | | | |
| 0–19 Years | 48 | 4.7 | 93 | 1 | 2 | 2 | 3 | 8 | 20 | 52 |
| 20–34 | 46 | 3.7 | 8 | 2 | 2 | 3 | 6 | 6 | 10 | 12 |
| 35–49 | 71 | 3.5 | 10 | 1 | 2 | 2 | 4 | 7 | 10 | 19 |
| 50–64 | 69 | 6.2 | 35 | 2 | 2 | 4 | 8 | 12 | 17 | 34 |
| 65+ | 156 | 5.8 | 38 | 2 | 2 | 4 | 7 | 12 | 14 | 25 |
| **GRAND TOTAL** | 390 | 5.0 | 40 | 1 | 2 | 3 | 6 | 11 | 14 | 34 |

## 70.33: EXC/DESTR VAG LESION. Formerly included in operation group(s) 700.

| Type of Patients | Observed Patients | Avg. Stay | Variance | 10th | 25th | 50th | 75th | 90th | 95th | 99th |
|---|---|---|---|---|---|---|---|---|---|---|
| **1. SINGLE DX** | | | | | | | | | | |
| 0–19 Years | 8 | 1.3 | <1 | 1 | 1 | 1 | 1 | 3 | 3 | 3 |
| 20–34 | 20 | 1.4 | <1 | 1 | 1 | 1 | 2 | 2 | 2 | 2 |
| 35–49 | 11 | 2.0 | 2 | 1 | 1 | 2 | 2 | 3 | 4 | 4 |
| 50–64 | 8 | 1.4 | <1 | 1 | 1 | 1 | 1 | 3 | 4 | 4 |
| 65+ | 5 | 1.5 | 1 | 1 | 1 | 1 | 1 | 4 | 4 | 4 |
| **2. MULTIPLE DX** | | | | | | | | | | |
| 0–19 Years | 43 | 2.0 | 1 | 1 | 1 | 2 | 3 | 3 | 4 | 7 |
| 20–34 | 217 | 2.2 | 2 | 1 | 1 | 2 | 2 | 3 | 5 | 8 |
| 35–49 | 123 | 2.5 | 13 | 1 | 1 | 2 | 3 | 4 | 6 | 10 |
| 50–64 | 71 | 2.9 | 9 | 1 | 1 | 2 | 3 | 6 | 7 | 17 |
| 65+ | 85 | 4.2 | 17 | 1 | 2 | 2 | 7 | 12 | 12 | 20 |
| **TOTAL SINGLE DX** | 52 | 1.5 | <1 | 1 | 1 | 1 | 2 | 2 | 3 | 6 |
| **TOTAL MULTIPLE DX** | 539 | 2.6 | 8 | 1 | 1 | 2 | 3 | 5 | 8 | 12 |
| **TOTAL** | | | | | | | | | | |
| 0–19 Years | 51 | 2.0 | 1 | 1 | 1 | 2 | 3 | 3 | 4 | 7 |
| 20–34 | 237 | 2.1 | 2 | 1 | 1 | 2 | 2 | 3 | 5 | 8 |
| 35–49 | 134 | 2.4 | 13 | 1 | 1 | 2 | 3 | 4 | 6 | 10 |
| 50–64 | 79 | 2.8 | 9 | 1 | 1 | 2 | 3 | 6 | 7 | 17 |
| 65+ | 90 | 4.0 | 16 | 1 | 2 | 2 | 7 | 12 | 12 | 20 |
| **GRAND TOTAL** | 591 | 2.5 | 7 | 1 | 1 | 2 | 3 | 4 | 8 | 12 |

Length of Stay by Diagnosis and Operation, United States, 2000

# United States, October 1998–September 1999 Data, by Operation

## 70.4: VAGINAL OBLITERATION. Formerly included in operation group(s) 700.

| Type of Patients | Observed Patients | Avg. Stay | Vari-ance | 10th | 25th | 50th | 75th | 90th | 95th | 99th |
|---|---|---|---|---|---|---|---|---|---|---|
| **1. SINGLE DX** | | | | | | | | | | |
| 0–19 Years | 0 | | | | | | | | | |
| 20–34 | 2 | 2.4 | <1 | 2 | 2 | 2 | 3 | 3 | 3 | 3 |
| 35–49 | 5 | 1.8 | 2 | 1 | 1 | 1 | 2 | 3 | 3 | 5 |
| 50–64 | 5 | 1.5 | <1 | 1 | 1 | 1 | 2 | 3 | 3 | 5 |
| 65+ | 5 | 3.1 | 7 | 1 | 1 | 2 | 4 | 8 | 8 | 8 |
| **2. MULTIPLE DX** | | | | | | | | | | |
| 0–19 Years | 0 | | | | | | | | | |
| 20–34 | 4 | 3.4 | 1 | 1 | 3 | 4 | 4 | 4 | 4 | 4 |
| 35–49 | 21 | 4.7 | 14 | 2 | 3 | 3 | 5 | 7 | 14 | 20 |
| 50–64 | 26 | 2.9 | 8 | 1 | 1 | 1 | 6 | 7 | 9 | 10 |
| 65+ | 76 | 4.2 | 13 | 1 | 2 | 3 | 6 | 9 | 10 | 20 |
| **TOTAL SINGLE DX** | 17 | 2.0 | 3 | 1 | 1 | 1 | 3 | 5 | 5 | 8 |
| **TOTAL MULTIPLE DX** | 127 | 4.1 | 12 | 1 | 2 | 3 | 6 | 8 | 10 | 20 |
| **TOTAL** | | | | | | | | | | |
| 0–19 Years | 0 | | | | | | | | | |
| 20–34 | 6 | 3.2 | 1 | 2 | 3 | 3 | 4 | 4 | 4 | 4 |
| 35–49 | 26 | 3.8 | 12 | 1 | 1 | 3 | 5 | 7 | 8 | 20 |
| 50–64 | 31 | 2.7 | 7 | 1 | 1 | 1 | 4 | 7 | 9 | 10 |
| 65+ | 81 | 4.2 | 13 | 1 | 2 | 3 | 6 | 9 | 10 | 20 |
| **GRAND TOTAL** | 144 | 3.8 | 12 | 1 | 2 | 3 | 5 | 8 | 10 | 20 |

## 70.50: REP CYSTOCELE/RECTOCELE. Formerly included in operation group(s) 698.

| Type of Patients | Observed Patients | Avg. Stay | Vari-ance | 10th | 25th | 50th | 75th | 90th | 95th | 99th |
|---|---|---|---|---|---|---|---|---|---|---|
| **1. SINGLE DX** | | | | | | | | | | |
| 0–19 Years | 0 | | | | | | | | | |
| 20–34 | 21 | 1.8 | <1 | 1 | 1 | 2 | 2 | 2 | 2 | 3 |
| 35–49 | 142 | 1.8 | <1 | 1 | 1 | 2 | 2 | 2 | 3 | 3 |
| 50–64 | 386 | 2.0 | <1 | 1 | 2 | 2 | 2 | 3 | 3 | 4 |
| 65+ | 367 | 2.1 | <1 | 1 | 2 | 2 | 2 | 3 | 4 | 5 |
| **2. MULTIPLE DX** | | | | | | | | | | |
| 0–19 Years | 0 | | | | | | | | | |
| 20–34 | 90 | 2.2 | 1 | 1 | 2 | 2 | 3 | 3 | 4 | 8 |
| 35–49 | 880 | 2.2 | <1 | 1 | 2 | 2 | 3 | 3 | 4 | 5 |
| 50–64 | 2,065 | 2.2 | 1 | 1 | 2 | 2 | 3 | 3 | 4 | 6 |
| 65+ | 2,692 | 2.6 | 2 | 1 | 2 | 2 | 3 | 4 | 5 | 8 |
| **TOTAL SINGLE DX** | 916 | 2.0 | <1 | 1 | 1 | 2 | 2 | 3 | 3 | 5 |
| **TOTAL MULTIPLE DX** | 5,727 | 2.4 | 2 | 1 | 2 | 2 | 3 | 4 | 4 | 7 |
| **TOTAL** | | | | | | | | | | |
| 0–19 Years | 0 | | | | | | | | | |
| 20–34 | 111 | 2.1 | <1 | 1 | 2 | 2 | 2 | 3 | 3 | 6 |
| 35–49 | 1,022 | 2.1 | <1 | 1 | 2 | 2 | 3 | 3 | 4 | 5 |
| 50–64 | 2,451 | 2.2 | 1 | 1 | 2 | 2 | 3 | 3 | 4 | 6 |
| 65+ | 3,059 | 2.5 | 2 | 1 | 2 | 2 | 3 | 4 | 5 | 8 |
| **GRAND TOTAL** | 6,643 | 2.3 | 2 | 1 | 2 | 2 | 3 | 3 | 4 | 7 |

## 70.5: CYSTOCELE/RECTOCELE REP. Formerly included in operation group(s) 698.

| Type of Patients | Observed Patients | Avg. Stay | Vari-ance | 10th | 25th | 50th | 75th | 90th | 95th | 99th |
|---|---|---|---|---|---|---|---|---|---|---|
| **1. SINGLE DX** | | | | | | | | | | |
| 0–19 Years | 0 | | | | | | | | | |
| 20–34 | 60 | 1.7 | <1 | 1 | 1 | 2 | 2 | 3 | 3 | 3 |
| 35–49 | 321 | 1.7 | <1 | 1 | 1 | 2 | 2 | 3 | 3 | 4 |
| 50–64 | 796 | 1.7 | <1 | 1 | 1 | 2 | 2 | 3 | 3 | 4 |
| 65+ | 739 | 2.0 | 1 | 1 | 1 | 2 | 2 | 3 | 4 | 5 |
| **2. MULTIPLE DX** | | | | | | | | | | |
| 0–19 Years | 7 | 1.1 | <1 | 1 | 1 | 1 | 1 | 1 | 2 | 5 |
| 20–34 | 209 | 2.1 | <1 | 1 | 1 | 2 | 3 | 3 | 3 | 5 |
| 35–49 | 1,699 | 2.1 | 1 | 1 | 1 | 2 | 3 | 3 | 4 | 5 |
| 50–64 | 3,830 | 2.1 | 2 | 1 | 1 | 2 | 3 | 3 | 4 | 7 |
| 65+ | 5,019 | 2.4 | 2 | 1 | 2 | 2 | 3 | 4 | 5 | 8 |
| **TOTAL SINGLE DX** | 1,916 | 1.8 | <1 | 1 | 1 | 2 | 2 | 3 | 3 | 5 |
| **TOTAL MULTIPLE DX** | 10,764 | 2.2 | 2 | 1 | 2 | 2 | 3 | 3 | 4 | 7 |
| **TOTAL** | | | | | | | | | | |
| 0–19 Years | 7 | 1.1 | <1 | 1 | 1 | 1 | 1 | 1 | 2 | 5 |
| 20–34 | 269 | 2.0 | <1 | 1 | 1 | 2 | 2 | 3 | 3 | 4 |
| 35–49 | 2,020 | 2.0 | 1 | 1 | 1 | 2 | 3 | 3 | 4 | 5 |
| 50–64 | 4,626 | 2.1 | 2 | 1 | 1 | 2 | 3 | 3 | 4 | 6 |
| 65+ | 5,758 | 2.3 | 2 | 1 | 2 | 2 | 3 | 4 | 4 | 8 |
| **GRAND TOTAL** | 12,680 | 2.2 | 2 | 1 | 1 | 2 | 3 | 3 | 4 | 7 |

## 70.51: CYSTOCELE REPAIR. Formerly included in operation group(s) 698.

| Type of Patients | Observed Patients | Avg. Stay | Vari-ance | 10th | 25th | 50th | 75th | 90th | 95th | 99th |
|---|---|---|---|---|---|---|---|---|---|---|
| **1. SINGLE DX** | | | | | | | | | | |
| 0–19 Years | 0 | | | | | | | | | |
| 20–34 | 10 | 1.3 | <1 | 1 | 1 | 1 | 1 | 2 | 3 | 3 |
| 35–49 | 40 | 1.7 | <1 | 1 | 1 | 2 | 2 | 3 | 3 | 6 |
| 50–64 | 169 | 1.7 | <1 | 1 | 1 | 1 | 2 | 3 | 3 | 4 |
| 65+ | 205 | 1.8 | 1 | 1 | 1 | 1 | 2 | 3 | 3 | 8 |
| **2. MULTIPLE DX** | | | | | | | | | | |
| 0–19 Years | 3 | 1.1 | <1 | 1 | 1 | 1 | 1 | 1 | 1 | 5 |
| 20–34 | 50 | 2.0 | <1 | 1 | 1 | 2 | 2 | 3 | 3 | 5 |
| 35–49 | 414 | 2.0 | 1 | 1 | 1 | 2 | 3 | 3 | 4 | 6 |
| 50–64 | 882 | 2.1 | 4 | 1 | 1 | 2 | 3 | 3 | 4 | 8 |
| 65+ | 1,252 | 2.2 | 3 | 1 | 2 | 2 | 3 | 4 | 4 | 8 |
| **TOTAL SINGLE DX** | 424 | 1.7 | <1 | 1 | 1 | 1 | 2 | 3 | 3 | 6 |
| **TOTAL MULTIPLE DX** | 2,601 | 2.1 | 3 | 1 | 1 | 2 | 3 | 3 | 4 | 7 |
| **TOTAL** | | | | | | | | | | |
| 0–19 Years | 3 | 1.1 | <1 | 1 | 1 | 1 | 1 | 1 | 1 | 5 |
| 20–34 | 60 | 1.9 | <1 | 1 | 1 | 2 | 2 | 3 | 3 | 4 |
| 35–49 | 454 | 2.0 | 1 | 1 | 1 | 2 | 3 | 3 | 4 | 6 |
| 50–64 | 1,051 | 2.0 | 4 | 1 | 1 | 2 | 2 | 3 | 4 | 7 |
| 65+ | 1,457 | 2.1 | 3 | 1 | 1 | 2 | 3 | 3 | 4 | 8 |
| **GRAND TOTAL** | 3,025 | 2.0 | 3 | 1 | 1 | 2 | 2 | 3 | 4 | 7 |

Length of Stay by Diagnosis and Operation, United States, 2000

# United States, October 1998–September 1999 Data, by Operation

## 70.52: RECTOCELE REPAIR. Formerly included in operation group(s) 698.

| Type of Patients | Observed Patients | Avg. Stay | Vari-ance | 10th | 25th | 50th | 75th | 90th | 95th | 99th |
|---|---|---|---|---|---|---|---|---|---|---|
| **1. SINGLE DX** | | | | | | | | | | |
| 0–19 Years | 0 | | | | | | | | | |
| 20–34 | 29 | 1.7 | <1 | 1 | 1 | 2 | 2 | 3 | 3 | 3 |
| 35–49 | 139 | 1.5 | <1 | 1 | 1 | 1 | 2 | 2 | 3 | 4 |
| 50–64 | 241 | 1.4 | <1 | 1 | 1 | 1 | 2 | 2 | 2 | 3 |
| 65+ | 167 | 1.7 | <1 | 1 | 1 | 1 | 2 | 3 | 4 | 4 |
| **2. MULTIPLE DX** | | | | | | | | | | |
| 0–19 Years | 4 | 1.2 | <1 | 1 | 1 | 1 | 1 | 2 | 2 | 2 |
| 20–34 | 69 | 1.9 | <1 | 1 | 1 | 2 | 3 | 3 | 4 | 4 |
| 35–49 | 405 | 1.9 | 1 | 1 | 1 | 2 | 2 | 3 | 4 | 6 |
| 50–64 | 883 | 2.0 | 1 | 1 | 1 | 2 | 2 | 3 | 4 | 7 |
| 65+ | 1,075 | 2.1 | 2 | 1 | 1 | 2 | 3 | 3 | 4 | 7 |
| **TOTAL SINGLE DX** | 576 | 1.5 | <1 | 1 | 1 | 1 | 2 | 2 | 3 | 4 |
| **TOTAL MULTIPLE DX** | 2,436 | 2.0 | 2 | 1 | 1 | 2 | 3 | 3 | 4 | 6 |
| **TOTAL** | | | | | | | | | | |
| 0–19 Years | 4 | 1.2 | <1 | 1 | 1 | 2 | 2 | 2 | 2 | 2 |
| 20–34 | 98 | 1.9 | <1 | 1 | 1 | 2 | 2 | 3 | 3 | 4 |
| 35–49 | 544 | 1.8 | 1 | 1 | 1 | 2 | 2 | 3 | 4 | 5 |
| 50–64 | 1,124 | 1.9 | 1 | 1 | 1 | 2 | 2 | 3 | 4 | 6 |
| 65+ | 1,242 | 2.1 | 2 | 1 | 1 | 2 | 3 | 3 | 4 | 6 |
| **GRAND TOTAL** | 3,012 | 1.9 | 1 | 1 | 1 | 2 | 2 | 3 | 4 | 6 |

## 70.7: OTHER VAGINAL REPAIR. Formerly included in operation group(s) 699.

| Type of Patients | Observed Patients | Avg. Stay | Vari-ance | 10th | 25th | 50th | 75th | 90th | 95th | 99th |
|---|---|---|---|---|---|---|---|---|---|---|
| **1. SINGLE DX** | | | | | | | | | | |
| 0–19 Years | 52 | 2.3 | 4 | 1 | 1 | 1 | 3 | 6 | 6 | 6 |
| 20–34 | 109 | 1.8 | 2 | 1 | 1 | 1 | 2 | 3 | 4 | 6 |
| 35–49 | 106 | 2.0 | 1 | 1 | 1 | 2 | 2 | 3 | 5 | 6 |
| 50–64 | 105 | 2.2 | 1 | 1 | 2 | 2 | 3 | 4 | 4 | 7 |
| 65+ | 81 | 2.3 | <1 | 1 | 2 | 2 | 3 | 4 | 4 | 4 |
| **2. MULTIPLE DX** | | | | | | | | | | |
| 0–19 Years | 150 | 2.8 | 5 | 1 | 1 | 2 | 4 | 6 | 8 | 10 |
| 20–34 | 275 | 2.5 | 4 | 1 | 1 | 2 | 3 | 5 | 6 | 10 |
| 35–49 | 438 | 3.1 | 9 | 1 | 2 | 3 | 3 | 5 | 7 | 15 |
| 50–64 | 722 | 3.1 | 8 | 1 | 2 | 2 | 3 | 6 | 7 | 16 |
| 65+ | 957 | 4.4 | 30 | 2 | 2 | 3 | 4 | 8 | 10 | 27 |
| **TOTAL SINGLE DX** | 453 | 2.1 | 2 | 1 | 1 | 2 | 3 | 4 | 5 | 6 |
| **TOTAL MULTIPLE DX** | 2,542 | 3.5 | 16 | 1 | 2 | 3 | 4 | 6 | 9 | 18 |
| **TOTAL** | | | | | | | | | | |
| 0–19 Years | 202 | 2.7 | 4 | 1 | 1 | 2 | 3 | 6 | 6 | 10 |
| 20–34 | 384 | 2.3 | 4 | 1 | 1 | 2 | 3 | 4 | 6 | 8 |
| 35–49 | 544 | 2.9 | 8 | 1 | 2 | 2 | 3 | 5 | 6 | 15 |
| 50–64 | 827 | 3.0 | 7 | 1 | 2 | 2 | 3 | 5 | 7 | 15 |
| 65+ | 1,038 | 4.3 | 29 | 2 | 2 | 3 | 4 | 8 | 10 | 26 |
| **GRAND TOTAL** | 2,995 | 3.3 | 14 | 1 | 2 | 3 | 4 | 6 | 8 | 18 |

## 70.6: VAGINAL CONSTR/RECONST. Formerly included in operation group(s) 699.

| Type of Patients | Observed Patients | Avg. Stay | Vari-ance | 10th | 25th | 50th | 75th | 90th | 95th | 99th |
|---|---|---|---|---|---|---|---|---|---|---|
| **1. SINGLE DX** | | | | | | | | | | |
| 0–19 Years | 7 | 5.7 | 4 | 5 | 5 | 5 | 8 | 8 | 8 | 8 |
| 20–34 | 2 | 8.0 | 0 | 8 | 8 | 8 | 8 | 8 | 8 | 8 |
| 35–49 | 1 | 6.0 | 0 | 6 | 6 | 6 | 6 | 6 | 6 | 6 |
| 50–64 | 0 | | | | | | | | | |
| 65+ | 0 | | | | | | | | | |
| **2. MULTIPLE DX** | | | | | | | | | | |
| 0–19 Years | 29 | 6.1 | 10 | 1 | 3 | 8 | 8 | 9 | 9 | 16 |
| 20–34 | 10 | 1.5 | 3 | 1 | 1 | 1 | 1 | 2 | 6 | 10 |
| 35–49 | 12 | 6.3 | 18 | 3 | 3 | 7 | 7 | 9 | 21 | 21 |
| 50–64 | 8 | 5.8 | 19 | 2 | 2 | 3 | 10 | 12 | 12 | 12 |
| 65+ | 8 | 10.6 | 52 | 2 | 3 | 7 | 18 | 18 | 18 | 18 |
| **TOTAL SINGLE DX** | 10 | 6.0 | 3 | 5 | 5 | 6 | 8 | 8 | 8 | 8 |
| **TOTAL MULTIPLE DX** | 67 | 4.3 | 19 | 1 | 1 | 2 | 7 | 9 | 12 | 18 |
| **TOTAL** | | | | | | | | | | |
| 0–19 Years | 36 | 6.0 | 9 | 1 | 4 | 7 | 8 | 9 | 9 | 11 |
| 20–34 | 12 | 1.7 | 4 | 1 | 1 | 1 | 1 | 3 | 7 | 10 |
| 35–49 | 13 | 6.3 | 16 | 3 | 3 | 7 | 7 | 9 | 21 | 21 |
| 50–64 | 8 | 5.8 | 19 | 2 | 2 | 3 | 10 | 12 | 12 | 12 |
| 65+ | 8 | 10.6 | 52 | 2 | 3 | 7 | 18 | 18 | 18 | 18 |
| **GRAND TOTAL** | 77 | 4.4 | 18 | 1 | 1 | 3 | 7 | 9 | 12 | 18 |

## 70.71: SUTURE VAGINA LACERATION. Formerly included in operation group(s) 699.

| Type of Patients | Observed Patients | Avg. Stay | Vari-ance | 10th | 25th | 50th | 75th | 90th | 95th | 99th |
|---|---|---|---|---|---|---|---|---|---|---|
| **1. SINGLE DX** | | | | | | | | | | |
| 0–19 Years | 26 | 1.1 | <1 | 1 | 1 | 1 | 1 | 1 | 1 | 2 |
| 20–34 | 17 | 1.4 | <1 | 1 | 1 | 1 | 2 | 2 | 3 | 3 |
| 35–49 | 23 | 1.5 | <1 | 1 | 1 | 2 | 2 | 2 | 3 | 5 |
| 50–64 | 4 | 1.6 | <1 | 1 | 1 | 2 | 2 | 2 | 2 | 2 |
| 65+ | 3 | 1.7 | <1 | 1 | 1 | 2 | 2 | 2 | 2 | 2 |
| **2. MULTIPLE DX** | | | | | | | | | | |
| 0–19 Years | 62 | 1.9 | 3 | 1 | 1 | 1 | 2 | 3 | 7 | 8 |
| 20–34 | 50 | 1.8 | 2 | 1 | 1 | 1 | 2 | 3 | 4 | 8 |
| 35–49 | 61 | 2.2 | 3 | 1 | 1 | 2 | 2 | 3 | 6 | 8 |
| 50–64 | 39 | 2.2 | 3 | 1 | 1 | 2 | 3 | 3 | 4 | 8 |
| 65+ | 41 | 3.5 | 7 | 1 | 2 | 3 | 4 | 10 | 10 | 10 |
| **TOTAL SINGLE DX** | 73 | 1.2 | <1 | 1 | 1 | 1 | 1 | 2 | 2 | 5 |
| **TOTAL MULTIPLE DX** | 253 | 2.3 | 3 | 1 | 1 | 2 | 3 | 5 | 6 | 10 |
| **TOTAL** | | | | | | | | | | |
| 0–19 Years | 88 | 1.6 | 2 | 1 | 1 | 1 | 2 | 2 | 5 | 8 |
| 20–34 | 67 | 1.8 | 2 | 1 | 1 | 1 | 2 | 3 | 4 | 8 |
| 35–49 | 84 | 2.1 | 3 | 1 | 1 | 2 | 3 | 3 | 6 | 8 |
| 50–64 | 43 | 2.1 | 2 | 1 | 2 | 2 | 3 | 3 | 4 | 8 |
| 65+ | 44 | 3.4 | 7 | 1 | 2 | 3 | 4 | 10 | 10 | 10 |
| **GRAND TOTAL** | 326 | 2.0 | 3 | 1 | 1 | 1 | 2 | 4 | 6 | 10 |

Length of Stay by Diagnosis and Operation, United States, 2000

# United States, October 1998–September 1999 Data, by Operation

## 70.73: REP RECTOVAGINAL FISTULA. Formerly included in operation group(s) 699.

| Type of Patients | Observed Patients | Avg. Stay | Variance | 10th | 25th | 50th | 75th | 90th | 95th | 99th |
|---|---|---|---|---|---|---|---|---|---|---|
| **1. SINGLE DX** | | | | | | | | | | |
| 0–19 Years | 7 | 2.6 | 1 | 1 | 1 | 3 | 3 | 4 | 5 | 5 |
| 20–34 | 79 | 1.7 | 1 | 1 | 1 | 1 | 2 | 3 | 3 | 5 |
| 35–49 | 44 | 2.3 | 2 | 1 | 1 | 2 | 3 | 4 | 5 | 6 |
| 50–64 | 15 | 1.7 | 1 | 1 | 1 | 1 | 3 | 4 | 4 | 4 |
| 65+ | 2 | 1.3 | <1 | 1 | 1 | 1 | 2 | 2 | 2 | 2 |
| **2. MULTIPLE DX** | | | | | | | | | | |
| 0–19 Years | 24 | 3.4 | 1 | 2 | 3 | 4 | 4 | 4 | 4 | 7 |
| 20–34 | 158 | 2.3 | 2 | 1 | 1 | 2 | 3 | 4 | 5 | 7 |
| 35–49 | 146 | 3.0 | 3 | 1 | 2 | 3 | 6 | 6 | 7 | 12 |
| 50–64 | 69 | 4.1 | 10 | 1 | 2 | 3 | 6 | 7 | 12 | 16 |
| 65+ | 63 | 8.9 | 76 | 2 | 4 | 7 | 10 | 16 | 21 | 70 |
| **TOTAL SINGLE DX** | 147 | 2.0 | 2 | 1 | 1 | 2 | 2 | 3 | 4 | 6 |
| **TOTAL MULTIPLE DX** | 460 | 3.9 | 22 | 1 | 2 | 3 | 4 | 8 | 10 | 20 |
| **TOTAL** | | | | | | | | | | |
| 0–19 Years | 31 | 3.1 | 1 | 1 | 2 | 3 | 4 | 4 | 5 | 7 |
| 20–34 | 237 | 2.1 | 2 | 1 | 1 | 2 | 3 | 3 | 4 | 7 |
| 35–49 | 190 | 2.8 | 7 | 1 | 2 | 3 | 5 | 5 | 7 | 12 |
| 50–64 | 84 | 3.7 | 9 | 1 | 2 | 3 | 6 | 7 | 10 | 16 |
| 65+ | 65 | 8.6 | 76 | 2 | 4 | 7 | 10 | 16 | 21 | 70 |
| **GRAND TOTAL** | 607 | 3.4 | 18 | 1 | 1 | 2 | 4 | 7 | 9 | 18 |

## 70.79: VAGINAL REPAIR NEC. Formerly included in operation group(s) 699.

| Type of Patients | Observed Patients | Avg. Stay | Variance | 10th | 25th | 50th | 75th | 90th | 95th | 99th |
|---|---|---|---|---|---|---|---|---|---|---|
| **1. SINGLE DX** | | | | | | | | | | |
| 0–19 Years | 19 | 4.0 | 5 | 1 | 2 | 5 | 6 | 6 | 6 | 8 |
| 20–34 | 9 | 2.7 | 4 | 1 | 1 | 2 | 4 | 6 | 6 | 6 |
| 35–49 | 18 | 2.3 | 3 | 1 | 1 | 2 | 3 | 5 | 7 | 7 |
| 50–64 | 9 | 2.1 | 1 | 1 | 1 | 2 | 2 | 4 | 4 | 4 |
| 65+ | 4 | 2.2 | <1 | 2 | 2 | 2 | 2 | 3 | 3 | 3 |
| **2. MULTIPLE DX** | | | | | | | | | | |
| 0–19 Years | 56 | 3.4 | 6 | 1 | 2 | 3 | 5 | 6 | 10 | 10 |
| 20–34 | 47 | 2.5 | 3 | 1 | 2 | 2 | 3 | 4 | 5 | 11 |
| 35–49 | 87 | 2.8 | 2 | 1 | 1 | 3 | 3 | 5 | 6 | 8 |
| 50–64 | 95 | 2.4 | 6 | 1 | 1 | 2 | 3 | 5 | 4 | 10 |
| 65+ | 89 | 2.9 | 3 | 1 | 2 | 2 | 4 | 5 | 6 | 10 |
| **TOTAL SINGLE DX** | 59 | 3.1 | 4 | 1 | 1 | 2 | 6 | 6 | 6 | 7 |
| **TOTAL MULTIPLE DX** | 374 | 2.8 | 4 | 1 | 2 | 3 | 3 | 5 | 6 | 10 |
| **TOTAL** | | | | | | | | | | |
| 0–19 Years | 75 | 3.6 | 6 | 1 | 2 | 3 | 6 | 6 | 8 | 10 |
| 20–34 | 56 | 2.5 | 3 | 1 | 2 | 2 | 3 | 4 | 6 | 8 |
| 35–49 | 105 | 2.7 | 2 | 1 | 2 | 3 | 3 | 5 | 6 | 8 |
| 50–64 | 104 | 2.4 | 6 | 1 | 2 | 2 | 3 | 5 | 4 | 10 |
| 65+ | 93 | 2.8 | 3 | 1 | 2 | 2 | 4 | 5 | 6 | 10 |
| **GRAND TOTAL** | 433 | 2.9 | 4 | 1 | 2 | 2 | 3 | 6 | 6 | 10 |

## 70.77: VAGINAL SUSP & FIXATION. Formerly included in operation group(s) 699.

| Type of Patients | Observed Patients | Avg. Stay | Variance | 10th | 25th | 50th | 75th | 90th | 95th | 99th |
|---|---|---|---|---|---|---|---|---|---|---|
| **1. SINGLE DX** | | | | | | | | | | |
| 0–19 Years | 0 | | | | | | | | | |
| 20–34 | 4 | 2.1 | <1 | 1 | 2 | 2 | 3 | 3 | 3 | 3 |
| 35–49 | 20 | 1.8 | <1 | 1 | 1 | 2 | 2 | 3 | 3 | 3 |
| 50–64 | 74 | 2.2 | <1 | 1 | 2 | 2 | 3 | 3 | 4 | 4 |
| 65+ | 71 | 2.4 | <1 | 1 | 2 | 2 | 3 | 4 | 4 | 4 |
| **2. MULTIPLE DX** | | | | | | | | | | |
| 0–19 Years | 3 | 3.0 | 2 | 1 | 1 | 4 | 4 | 4 | 4 | 4 |
| 20–34 | 5 | 2.6 | <1 | 2 | 2 | 3 | 3 | 4 | 5 | 5 |
| 35–49 | 120 | 2.8 | 3 | 1 | 2 | 3 | 3 | 4 | 5 | 9 |
| 50–64 | 480 | 2.7 | 2 | 1 | 2 | 2 | 3 | 4 | 5 | 8 |
| 65+ | 696 | 3.2 | 5 | 2 | 2 | 3 | 4 | 5 | 6 | 11 |
| **TOTAL SINGLE DX** | 169 | 2.2 | <1 | 1 | 2 | 2 | 3 | 3 | 4 | 4 |
| **TOTAL MULTIPLE DX** | 1,304 | 3.0 | 3 | 1 | 2 | 3 | 3 | 4 | 6 | 10 |
| **TOTAL** | | | | | | | | | | |
| 0–19 Years | 3 | 3.0 | 2 | 1 | 1 | 4 | 4 | 4 | 4 | 4 |
| 20–34 | 9 | 2.3 | <1 | 1 | 2 | 2 | 3 | 3 | 3 | 3 |
| 35–49 | 140 | 2.6 | 3 | 1 | 2 | 2 | 3 | 4 | 5 | 9 |
| 50–64 | 554 | 2.6 | 2 | 1 | 2 | 2 | 3 | 4 | 5 | 8 |
| 65+ | 767 | 3.2 | 4 | 2 | 2 | 3 | 4 | 5 | 6 | 11 |
| **GRAND TOTAL** | 1,473 | 2.9 | 3 | 2 | 2 | 3 | 3 | 4 | 5 | 9 |

## 70.8: VAGINAL VAULT OBLIT. Formerly included in operation group(s) 700.

| Type of Patients | Observed Patients | Avg. Stay | Variance | 10th | 25th | 50th | 75th | 90th | 95th | 99th |
|---|---|---|---|---|---|---|---|---|---|---|
| **1. SINGLE DX** | | | | | | | | | | |
| 0–19 Years | 0 | | | | | | | | | |
| 20–34 | 2 | 1.0 | 0 | 1 | 1 | 1 | 1 | 1 | 1 | 1 |
| 35–49 | 0 | | | | | | | | | |
| 50–64 | 2 | 2.0 | 0 | 2 | 2 | 2 | 2 | 2 | 2 | 2 |
| 65+ | 40 | 1.7 | <1 | 1 | 1 | 1 | 2 | 3 | 3 | 5 |
| **2. MULTIPLE DX** | | | | | | | | | | |
| 0–19 Years | 1 | 42.0 | 0 | 42 | 42 | 42 | 42 | 42 | 42 | 42 |
| 20–34 | 4 | 1.0 | 0 | 1 | 1 | 1 | 1 | 1 | 1 | 1 |
| 35–49 | 2 | 2.0 | 0 | 2 | 2 | 2 | 2 | 2 | 2 | 2 |
| 50–64 | 16 | 2.8 | 6 | 1 | 2 | 2 | 3 | 4 | 5 | 13 |
| 65+ | 302 | 2.2 | 3 | 1 | 1 | 2 | 3 | 3 | 5 | 9 |
| **TOTAL SINGLE DX** | 44 | 1.7 | <1 | 1 | 1 | 1 | 2 | 3 | 3 | 5 |
| **TOTAL MULTIPLE DX** | 325 | 2.3 | 6 | 1 | 1 | 2 | 3 | 4 | 5 | 11 |
| **TOTAL** | | | | | | | | | | |
| 0–19 Years | 1 | 42.0 | 0 | 42 | 42 | 42 | 42 | 42 | 42 | 42 |
| 20–34 | 6 | 1.0 | 0 | 1 | 1 | 1 | 1 | 1 | 1 | 1 |
| 35–49 | 2 | 2.0 | 0 | 2 | 2 | 2 | 2 | 2 | 2 | 2 |
| 50–64 | 18 | 2.7 | 5 | 1 | 2 | 2 | 3 | 4 | 5 | 13 |
| 65+ | 342 | 2.1 | 2 | 1 | 1 | 2 | 2 | 3 | 5 | 8 |
| **GRAND TOTAL** | 369 | 2.2 | 5 | 1 | 1 | 2 | 3 | 3 | 5 | 9 |

Length of Stay by Diagnosis and Operation, United States, 2000

# United States, October 1998–September 1999 Data, by Operation

## 70.9: OTH VAG & CUL-DE-SAC OPS. Formerly included in operation group(s) 700.

| Type of Patients | Observed Patients | Avg. Stay | Variance | 10th | 25th | 50th | 75th | 90th | 95th | 99th |
|---|---|---|---|---|---|---|---|---|---|---|
| **1. SINGLE DX** | | | | | | | | | | |
| 0–19 Years | 0 | | | | | | | | | |
| 20–34 | 4 | 1.8 | <1 | 1 | 1 | 2 | 3 | 3 | 3 | 3 |
| 35–49 | 19 | 2.3 | 1 | 1 | 1 | 2 | 3 | 3 | 5 | 5 |
| 50–64 | 60 | 2.1 | <1 | 1 | 1 | 2 | 3 | 3 | 4 | 5 |
| 65+ | 61 | 2.2 | 1 | 1 | 1 | 2 | 3 | 3 | 5 | 7 |
| **2. MULTIPLE DX** | | | | | | | | | | |
| 0–19 Years | 2 | 2.7 | <1 | 2 | 2 | 3 | 3 | 3 | 3 | 3 |
| 20–34 | 66 | 2.3 | 2 | 1 | 2 | 3 | 3 | 3 | 4 | 5 |
| 35–49 | 399 | 2.3 | 1 | 1 | 2 | 2 | 3 | 3 | 4 | 7 |
| 50–64 | 1,292 | 2.4 | 2 | 1 | 2 | 2 | 3 | 4 | 4 | 6 |
| 65+ | 2,242 | 2.7 | 3 | 1 | 2 | 3 | 3 | 4 | 5 | 11 |
| **TOTAL SINGLE DX** | 144 | 2.2 | 1 | 1 | 1 | 2 | 3 | 3 | 4 | 5 |
| **TOTAL MULTIPLE DX** | 4,001 | 2.5 | 3 | 1 | 2 | 2 | 3 | 4 | 5 | 9 |
| **TOTAL** | | | | | | | | | | |
| 0–19 Years | 2 | 2.7 | <1 | 2 | 2 | 3 | 3 | 3 | 3 | 3 |
| 20–34 | 70 | 2.3 | 2 | 1 | 2 | 2 | 3 | 3 | 4 | 5 |
| 35–49 | 418 | 2.3 | 1 | 1 | 2 | 2 | 3 | 3 | 4 | 7 |
| 50–64 | 1,352 | 2.3 | 2 | 1 | 2 | 2 | 3 | 4 | 4 | 6 |
| 65+ | 2,303 | 2.7 | 3 | 1 | 2 | 2 | 3 | 4 | 5 | 10 |
| **GRAND TOTAL** | 4,145 | 2.5 | 3 | 1 | 2 | 2 | 3 | 4 | 5 | 9 |

## 71.0: INC VULVA & PERINEUM. Formerly included in operation group(s) 701.

| Type of Patients | Observed Patients | Avg. Stay | Variance | 10th | 25th | 50th | 75th | 90th | 95th | 99th |
|---|---|---|---|---|---|---|---|---|---|---|
| **1. SINGLE DX** | | | | | | | | | | |
| 0–19 Years | 46 | 1.8 | 2 | 1 | 1 | 1 | 2 | 3 | 5 | 8 |
| 20–34 | 51 | 2.3 | 3 | 1 | 1 | 2 | 3 | 4 | 5 | 8 |
| 35–49 | 29 | 2.0 | 2 | 2 | 2 | 2 | 2 | 4 | 6 | 6 |
| 50–64 | 5 | 5.4 | 33 | 2 | 3 | 3 | 3 | 15 | 15 | 15 |
| 65+ | 2 | 2.7 | <1 | 2 | 3 | 3 | 3 | 3 | 3 | 3 |
| **2. MULTIPLE DX** | | | | | | | | | | |
| 0–19 Years | 76 | 3.3 | 9 | 1 | 2 | 2 | 4 | 5 | 9 | 17 |
| 20–34 | 168 | 3.5 | 11 | 1 | 2 | 2 | 4 | 7 | 10 | 17 |
| 35–49 | 173 | 4.9 | 19 | 1 | 2 | 4 | 6 | 8 | 14 | 26 |
| 50–64 | 110 | 4.3 | 15 | 1 | 2 | 3 | 5 | 9 | 14 | 25 |
| 65+ | 86 | 9.5 | 64 | 3 | 4 | 7 | 12 | 23 | 30 | 30 |
| **TOTAL SINGLE DX** | 133 | 2.1 | 3 | 1 | 1 | 1 | 2 | 4 | 5 | 9 |
| **TOTAL MULTIPLE DX** | 613 | 5.1 | 28 | 1 | 2 | 3 | 6 | 10 | 14 | 30 |
| **TOTAL** | | | | | | | | | | |
| 0–19 Years | 122 | 2.7 | 7 | 1 | 1 | 2 | 3 | 5 | 8 | 17 |
| 20–34 | 219 | 3.3 | 9 | 1 | 2 | 2 | 4 | 6 | 9 | 17 |
| 35–49 | 202 | 4.5 | 18 | 1 | 2 | 3 | 6 | 8 | 14 | 24 |
| 50–64 | 115 | 4.3 | 15 | 1 | 2 | 3 | 5 | 9 | 14 | 25 |
| 65+ | 88 | 9.4 | 64 | 3 | 4 | 7 | 12 | 23 | 30 | 30 |
| **GRAND TOTAL** | 746 | 4.6 | 25 | 1 | 2 | 3 | 5 | 9 | 14 | 30 |

## 70.92: CUL-DE-SAC OPERATION NEC. Formerly included in operation group(s) 700.

| Type of Patients | Observed Patients | Avg. Stay | Variance | 10th | 25th | 50th | 75th | 90th | 95th | 99th |
|---|---|---|---|---|---|---|---|---|---|---|
| **1. SINGLE DX** | | | | | | | | | | |
| 0–19 Years | 0 | | | | | | | | | |
| 20–34 | 3 | 2.2 | <1 | 1 | 2 | 2 | 3 | 3 | 3 | 3 |
| 35–49 | 17 | 2.3 | 1 | 1 | 2 | 2 | 3 | 3 | 5 | 5 |
| 50–64 | 59 | 2.2 | <1 | 1 | 1 | 2 | 3 | 3 | 4 | 5 |
| 65+ | 61 | 2.2 | 1 | 1 | 1 | 2 | 3 | 3 | 5 | 7 |
| **2. MULTIPLE DX** | | | | | | | | | | |
| 0–19 Years | 0 | | | | | | | | | |
| 20–34 | 60 | 2.3 | 2 | 1 | 2 | 3 | 3 | 3 | 3 | 15 |
| 35–49 | 389 | 2.4 | 1 | 1 | 2 | 2 | 3 | 3 | 4 | 7 |
| 50–64 | 1,282 | 2.4 | 2 | 1 | 2 | 2 | 3 | 4 | 4 | 6 |
| 65+ | 2,231 | 2.7 | 3 | 1 | 2 | 2 | 3 | 4 | 5 | 10 |
| **TOTAL SINGLE DX** | 140 | 2.2 | 1 | 1 | 1 | 2 | 3 | 3 | 4 | 5 |
| **TOTAL MULTIPLE DX** | 3,962 | 2.5 | 3 | 1 | 2 | 2 | 3 | 4 | 5 | 9 |
| **TOTAL** | | | | | | | | | | |
| 0–19 Years | 0 | | | | | | | | | |
| 20–34 | 63 | 2.3 | 2 | 1 | 2 | 2 | 3 | 3 | 4 | 15 |
| 35–49 | 406 | 2.4 | 1 | 1 | 1 | 2 | 3 | 3 | 4 | 7 |
| 50–64 | 1,341 | 2.3 | 2 | 1 | 2 | 2 | 3 | 4 | 4 | 6 |
| 65+ | 2,292 | 2.6 | 3 | 1 | 2 | 2 | 3 | 4 | 5 | 10 |
| **GRAND TOTAL** | 4,102 | 2.5 | 2 | 1 | 2 | 2 | 3 | 4 | 5 | 8 |

## 71.09: INC VULVA/PERINEUM NEC. Formerly included in operation group(s) 701.

| Type of Patients | Observed Patients | Avg. Stay | Variance | 10th | 25th | 50th | 75th | 90th | 95th | 99th |
|---|---|---|---|---|---|---|---|---|---|---|
| **1. SINGLE DX** | | | | | | | | | | |
| 0–19 Years | 40 | 2.1 | 2 | 1 | 1 | 1 | 3 | 4 | 5 | 9 |
| 20–34 | 51 | 2.3 | 3 | 1 | 1 | 2 | 3 | 4 | 5 | 8 |
| 35–49 | 29 | 2.0 | 2 | 2 | 2 | 2 | 2 | 4 | 6 | 6 |
| 50–64 | 5 | 5.4 | 33 | 2 | 3 | 3 | 3 | 15 | 15 | 15 |
| 65+ | 2 | 2.7 | <1 | 2 | 3 | 3 | 3 | 3 | 3 | 3 |
| **2. MULTIPLE DX** | | | | | | | | | | |
| 0–19 Years | 74 | 3.3 | 9 | 1 | 2 | 2 | 4 | 5 | 9 | 17 |
| 20–34 | 168 | 3.5 | 11 | 1 | 2 | 2 | 4 | 7 | 10 | 17 |
| 35–49 | 172 | 4.9 | 19 | 1 | 2 | 4 | 6 | 8 | 14 | 26 |
| 50–64 | 109 | 4.3 | 15 | 1 | 2 | 3 | 5 | 9 | 14 | 25 |
| 65+ | 82 | 9.7 | 65 | 3 | 4 | 8 | 12 | 30 | 30 | 30 |
| **TOTAL SINGLE DX** | 127 | 2.2 | 3 | 1 | 1 | 2 | 3 | 4 | 5 | 9 |
| **TOTAL MULTIPLE DX** | 605 | 5.1 | 28 | 1 | 2 | 3 | 7 | 10 | 14 | 30 |
| **TOTAL** | | | | | | | | | | |
| 0–19 Years | 114 | 2.9 | 7 | 1 | 2 | 3 | 4 | 5 | 8 | 17 |
| 20–34 | 219 | 3.3 | 9 | 1 | 2 | 3 | 4 | 6 | 9 | 17 |
| 35–49 | 201 | 4.5 | 18 | 1 | 2 | 3 | 6 | 8 | 14 | 24 |
| 50–64 | 114 | 4.3 | 15 | 1 | 2 | 3 | 5 | 9 | 14 | 25 |
| 65+ | 84 | 9.6 | 64 | 3 | 4 | 8 | 12 | 23 | 30 | 30 |
| **GRAND TOTAL** | 732 | 4.7 | 25 | 1 | 2 | 3 | 5 | 9 | 14 | 30 |

Length of Stay by Diagnosis and Operation, United States, 2000

# United States, October 1998–September 1999 Data, by Operation

## 71.1: VULVAR DIAGNOSTIC PX. Formerly included in operation group(s) 701, 704.

| Type of Patients | Observed Patients | Avg. Stay | Variance | Percentiles | | | | | | |
|---|---|---|---|---|---|---|---|---|---|---|
| | | | | 10th | 25th | 50th | 75th | 90th | 95th | 99th |
| **1. SINGLE DX** | | | | | | | | | | |
| 0–19 Years | 3 | 3.6 | <1 | 2 | 4 | 4 | 4 | 4 | 4 | 4 |
| 20–34 | 0 | | | | | | | | | |
| 35–49 | 3 | 2.2 | 2 | 1 | 1 | 2 | 4 | 4 | 4 | 4 |
| 50–64 | 2 | 6.9 | 25 | 2 | 2 | 11 | 11 | 11 | 11 | 11 |
| 65+ | 5 | 1.7 | <1 | 1 | 1 | 2 | 2 | 2 | 3 | 3 |
| **2. MULTIPLE DX** | | | | | | | | | | |
| 0–19 Years | 14 | 2.8 | 3 | 2 | 2 | 2 | 3 | 4 | 9 | 9 |
| 20–34 | 44 | 2.3 | 7 | 1 | 1 | 1 | 3 | 3 | 9 | 16 |
| 35–49 | 28 | 3.9 | 35 | 1 | 2 | 2 | 3 | 11 | 13 | 36 |
| 50–64 | 33 | 5.3 | 42 | 1 | 2 | 2 | 6 | 12 | 22 | 35 |
| 65+ | 79 | 9.9 | 94 | 1 | 2 | 7 | 12 | 30 | 30 | 38 |
| **TOTAL SINGLE DX** | 13 | 3.1 | 8 | 2 | 2 | 2 | 4 | 11 | 11 | 11 |
| **TOTAL MULTIPLE DX** | 198 | 6.2 | 62 | 1 | 2 | 2 | 7 | 14 | 30 | 38 |
| **TOTAL** | | | | | | | | | | |
| 0–19 Years | 17 | 2.9 | 3 | 2 | 2 | 2 | 4 | 4 | 9 | 9 |
| 20–34 | 44 | 2.3 | 7 | 1 | 1 | 2 | 3 | 4 | 4 | 16 |
| 35–49 | 31 | 3.7 | 32 | 1 | 2 | 2 | 3 | 9 | 13 | 36 |
| 50–64 | 35 | 5.4 | 41 | 2 | 2 | 2 | 6 | 11 | 22 | 35 |
| 65+ | 84 | 9.6 | 93 | 1 | 2 | 7 | 12 | 30 | 30 | 38 |
| **GRAND TOTAL** | 211 | 6.1 | 60 | 1 | 2 | 2 | 7 | 14 | 30 | 38 |

## 71.2: BARTHOLIN'S GLAND OPS. Formerly included in operation group(s) 701.

| Type of Patients | Observed Patients | Avg. Stay | Variance | Percentiles | | | | | | |
|---|---|---|---|---|---|---|---|---|---|---|
| | | | | 10th | 25th | 50th | 75th | 90th | 95th | 99th |
| **1. SINGLE DX** | | | | | | | | | | |
| 0–19 Years | 15 | 1.2 | <1 | 1 | 1 | 1 | 1 | 2 | 2 | 2 |
| 20–34 | 62 | 1.5 | <1 | 1 | 1 | 1 | 2 | 2 | 2 | 2 |
| 35–49 | 23 | 1.3 | <1 | 1 | 1 | 1 | 1 | 3 | 3 | 4 |
| 50–64 | 5 | 1.7 | <1 | 1 | 2 | 2 | 2 | 2 | 3 | 4 |
| 65+ | 1 | 1.0 | 0 | 1 | 1 | 1 | 1 | 1 | 1 | 1 |
| **2. MULTIPLE DX** | | | | | | | | | | |
| 0–19 Years | 52 | 3.6 | 5 | 2 | 2 | 3 | 4 | 8 | 8 | 8 |
| 20–34 | 122 | 2.3 | 3 | 1 | 1 | 2 | 3 | 4 | 7 | 11 |
| 35–49 | 60 | 3.1 | 12 | 1 | 1 | 2 | 4 | 8 | 10 | 14 |
| 50–64 | 35 | 3.3 | 16 | 1 | 2 | 3 | 4 | 5 | 6 | 25 |
| 65+ | 32 | 3.5 | 4 | 2 | 2 | 3 | 5 | 6 | 6 | 12 |
| **TOTAL SINGLE DX** | 106 | 1.4 | <1 | 1 | 1 | 1 | 2 | 3 | 3 | 4 |
| **TOTAL MULTIPLE DX** | 301 | 3.0 | 7 | 1 | 1 | 2 | 3 | 6 | 8 | 12 |
| **TOTAL** | | | | | | | | | | |
| 0–19 Years | 67 | 3.1 | 5 | 1 | 1 | 3 | 3 | 8 | 8 | 8 |
| 20–34 | 184 | 1.9 | 2 | 1 | 1 | 1 | 2 | 3 | 4 | 8 |
| 35–49 | 83 | 2.5 | 9 | 1 | 1 | 1 | 2 | 5 | 10 | 14 |
| 50–64 | 40 | 3.0 | 13 | 1 | 1 | 2 | 4 | 6 | 6 | 25 |
| 65+ | 33 | 3.3 | 4 | 1 | 2 | 3 | 4 | 6 | 6 | 12 |
| **GRAND TOTAL** | 407 | 2.5 | 6 | 1 | 1 | 2 | 3 | 5 | 8 | 10 |

## 71.3: LOC VULVAR/PERI EXC NEC. Formerly included in operation group(s) 701.

| Type of Patients | Observed Patients | Avg. Stay | Variance | Percentiles | | | | | | |
|---|---|---|---|---|---|---|---|---|---|---|
| | | | | 10th | 25th | 50th | 75th | 90th | 95th | 99th |
| **1. SINGLE DX** | | | | | | | | | | |
| 0–19 Years | 11 | 1.5 | <1 | 1 | 1 | 1 | 2 | 2 | 3 | 3 |
| 20–34 | 24 | 2.2 | <1 | 1 | 2 | 2 | 3 | 3 | 4 | 6 |
| 35–49 | 17 | 2.3 | 8 | 1 | 1 | 1 | 1 | 2 | 2 | 17 |
| 50–64 | 6 | 1.6 | 2 | 1 | 1 | 1 | 1 | 4 | 4 | 4 |
| 65+ | 7 | 1.7 | <1 | 1 | 1 | 1 | 2 | 3 | 4 | 4 |
| **2. MULTIPLE DX** | | | | | | | | | | |
| 0–19 Years | 103 | 2.6 | 14 | 1 | 1 | 2 | 2 | 3 | 6 | 27 |
| 20–34 | 542 | 2.4 | 18 | 1 | 1 | 2 | 2 | 3 | 5 | 21 |
| 35–49 | 168 | 2.9 | 11 | 1 | 1 | 2 | 2 | 5 | 11 | 22 |
| 50–64 | 124 | 3.6 | 9 | 1 | 2 | 2 | 6 | 9 | 9 | 12 |
| 65+ | 119 | 5.8 | 86 | 1 | 1 | 2 | 6 | 11 | 27 | 63 |
| **TOTAL SINGLE DX** | 65 | 2.0 | 2 | 1 | 1 | 2 | 2 | 3 | 4 | 6 |
| **TOTAL MULTIPLE DX** | 1,056 | 3.0 | 23 | 1 | 1 | 2 | 3 | 6 | 9 | 27 |
| **TOTAL** | | | | | | | | | | |
| 0–19 Years | 114 | 2.5 | 12 | 1 | 1 | 2 | 2 | 3 | 5 | 27 |
| 20–34 | 566 | 2.4 | 17 | 1 | 1 | 2 | 2 | 3 | 4 | 21 |
| 35–49 | 185 | 2.8 | 11 | 1 | 1 | 2 | 2 | 5 | 11 | 22 |
| 50–64 | 130 | 3.6 | 9 | 1 | 2 | 2 | 6 | 9 | 9 | 12 |
| 65+ | 126 | 5.5 | 81 | 1 | 1 | 2 | 6 | 11 | 26 | 63 |
| **GRAND TOTAL** | 1,121 | 3.0 | 22 | 1 | 1 | 2 | 2 | 6 | 9 | 27 |

## 71.4: OPERATIONS ON CLITORIS. Formerly included in operation group(s) 701.

| Type of Patients | Observed Patients | Avg. Stay | Variance | Percentiles | | | | | | |
|---|---|---|---|---|---|---|---|---|---|---|
| | | | | 10th | 25th | 50th | 75th | 90th | 95th | 99th |
| **1. SINGLE DX** | | | | | | | | | | |
| 0–19 Years | 11 | 1.7 | <1 | 1 | 1 | 2 | 2 | 2 | 2 | 5 |
| 20–34 | 5 | 1.7 | <1 | 1 | 1 | 2 | 2 | 3 | 3 | 3 |
| 35–49 | 0 | | | | | | | | | |
| 50–64 | 0 | | | | | | | | | |
| 65+ | 0 | | | | | | | | | |
| **2. MULTIPLE DX** | | | | | | | | | | |
| 0–19 Years | 25 | 2.1 | 5 | 1 | 1 | 2 | 2 | 4 | 4 | 20 |
| 20–34 | 9 | 3.3 | 9 | 1 | 1 | 1 | 8 | 8 | 8 | 8 |
| 35–49 | 3 | 7.2 | 16 | 1 | 4 | 10 | 10 | 10 | 10 | 10 |
| 50–64 | 0 | | | | | | | | | |
| 65+ | 2 | 4.2 | 4 | 3 | 3 | 3 | 6 | 6 | 6 | 6 |
| **TOTAL SINGLE DX** | 16 | 1.7 | <1 | 1 | 1 | 2 | 2 | 2 | 3 | 5 |
| **TOTAL MULTIPLE DX** | 39 | 2.5 | 7 | 1 | 1 | 2 | 3 | 4 | 8 | 10 |
| **TOTAL** | | | | | | | | | | |
| 0–19 Years | 36 | 2.0 | 5 | 1 | 1 | 2 | 2 | 4 | 4 | 9 |
| 20–34 | 14 | 2.8 | 7 | 1 | 1 | 2 | 3 | 8 | 8 | 8 |
| 35–49 | 3 | 7.2 | 16 | 1 | 4 | 10 | 10 | 10 | 10 | 10 |
| 50–64 | 0 | | | | | | | | | |
| 65+ | 2 | 4.2 | 4 | 3 | 3 | 3 | 6 | 6 | 6 | 6 |
| **GRAND TOTAL** | 55 | 2.4 | 6 | 1 | 1 | 2 | 2 | 4 | 8 | 10 |

Length of Stay by Diagnosis and Operation, United States, 2000

**United States, October 1998–September 1999 Data, by Operation**

### 71.5: RADICAL VULVECTOMY. Formerly included in operation group(s) 702.

| Type of Patients | Observed Patients | Avg. Stay | Vari-ance | 10th | 25th | 50th | 75th | 90th | 95th | 99th |
|---|---|---|---|---|---|---|---|---|---|---|
| **1. SINGLE DX** | | | | | | | | | | |
| 0–19 Years | 0 | | | | | | | | | |
| 20–34 | 2 | 3.0 | 0 | 3 | 3 | 3 | 3 | 3 | 3 | 3 |
| 35–49 | 14 | 3.4 | 4 | 2 | 2 | 2 | 5 | 6 | 6 | 11 |
| 50–64 | 19 | 3.4 | 1 | 2 | 3 | 4 | 4 | 4 | 5 | 5 |
| 65+ | 30 | 2.8 | 4 | 1 | 1 | 2 | 3 | 5 | 8 | 8 |
| **2. MULTIPLE DX** | | | | | | | | | | |
| 0–19 Years | 0 | | | | | | | | | |
| 20–34 | 10 | 8.6 | 40 | 2 | 4 | 4 | 17 | 17 | 17 | 17 |
| 35–49 | 71 | 6.2 | 26 | 2 | 3 | 5 | 7 | 15 | 18 | 21 |
| 50–64 | 82 | 4.5 | 13 | 1 | 2 | 4 | 6 | 7 | 9 | 22 |
| 65+ | 304 | 5.4 | 14 | 2 | 3 | 4 | 7 | 10 | 14 | 20 |
| **TOTAL SINGLE DX** | 65 | 3.1 | 3 | 1 | 2 | 3 | 4 | 5 | 6 | 8 |
| **TOTAL MULTIPLE DX** | 467 | 5.4 | 16 | 2 | 3 | 4 | 7 | 10 | 14 | 21 |
| **TOTAL** | | | | | | | | | | |
| 0–19 Years | 0 | | | | | | | | | |
| 20–34 | 12 | 7.6 | 37 | 2 | 3 | 4 | 13 | 17 | 17 | 17 |
| 35–49 | 85 | 5.6 | 23 | 2 | 2 | 5 | 6 | 14 | 18 | 21 |
| 50–64 | 101 | 4.3 | 11 | 1 | 1 | 4 | 6 | 7 | 8 | 22 |
| 65+ | 334 | 5.2 | 13 | 2 | 3 | 4 | 6 | 9 | 14 | 20 |
| **GRAND TOTAL** | 532 | 5.1 | 15 | 2 | 3 | 4 | 6 | 9 | 14 | 21 |

### 71.6: OTHER VULVECTOMY. Formerly included in operation group(s) 702.

| Type of Patients | Observed Patients | Avg. Stay | Vari-ance | 10th | 25th | 50th | 75th | 90th | 95th | 99th |
|---|---|---|---|---|---|---|---|---|---|---|
| **1. SINGLE DX** | | | | | | | | | | |
| 0–19 Years | 2 | 1.8 | <1 | 1 | 2 | 2 | 2 | 2 | 2 | 2 |
| 20–34 | 10 | 2.8 | 2 | 1 | 1 | 2 | 4 | 5 | 5 | 5 |
| 35–49 | 39 | 2.2 | 3 | 1 | 1 | 2 | 2 | 4 | 8 | 8 |
| 50–64 | 21 | 1.5 | <1 | 1 | 1 | 1 | 2 | 3 | 3 | 3 |
| 65+ | 22 | 1.9 | <1 | 1 | 1 | 2 | 2 | 3 | 5 | 5 |
| **2. MULTIPLE DX** | | | | | | | | | | |
| 0–19 Years | 3 | 1.1 | <1 | 1 | 1 | 1 | 1 | 1 | 2 | 2 |
| 20–34 | 26 | 2.9 | 5 | 1 | 1 | 2 | 4 | 7 | 7 | 8 |
| 35–49 | 86 | 3.0 | 8 | 1 | 1 | 2 | 3 | 6 | 9 | 16 |
| 50–64 | 73 | 4.3 | 13 | 1 | 2 | 3 | 5 | 12 | 13 | 14 |
| 65+ | 178 | 3.7 | 7 | 1 | 2 | 3 | 5 | 7 | 9 | 12 |
| **TOTAL SINGLE DX** | 94 | 2.0 | 2 | 1 | 1 | 2 | 2 | 3 | 5 | 8 |
| **TOTAL MULTIPLE DX** | 366 | 3.6 | 8 | 1 | 2 | 3 | 5 | 7 | 9 | 14 |
| **TOTAL** | | | | | | | | | | |
| 0–19 Years | 5 | 1.4 | <1 | 1 | 1 | 1 | 2 | 2 | 2 | 2 |
| 20–34 | 36 | 2.9 | 4 | 1 | 1 | 2 | 4 | 7 | 7 | 8 |
| 35–49 | 125 | 2.7 | 7 | 1 | 1 | 2 | 3 | 6 | 8 | 14 |
| 50–64 | 94 | 3.7 | 11 | 1 | 2 | 3 | 4 | 9 | 13 | 14 |
| 65+ | 200 | 3.4 | 6 | 1 | 2 | 3 | 5 | 7 | 9 | 12 |
| **GRAND TOTAL** | 460 | 3.3 | 7 | 1 | 1 | 2 | 4 | 7 | 9 | 13 |

### 71.61: UNILATERAL VULVECTOMY. Formerly included in operation group(s) 702.

| Type of Patients | Observed Patients | Avg. Stay | Vari-ance | 10th | 25th | 50th | 75th | 90th | 95th | 99th |
|---|---|---|---|---|---|---|---|---|---|---|
| **1. SINGLE DX** | | | | | | | | | | |
| 0–19 Years | 0 | | | | | | | | | |
| 20–34 | 5 | 1.9 | 1 | 1 | 1 | 1 | 2 | 4 | 4 | 4 |
| 35–49 | 24 | 1.6 | <1 | 1 | 1 | 1 | 2 | 2 | 3 | 3 |
| 50–64 | 17 | 1.3 | <1 | 1 | 1 | 1 | 1 | 2 | 3 | 3 |
| 65+ | 16 | 1.9 | 1 | 1 | 2 | 2 | 2 | 3 | 5 | 5 |
| **2. MULTIPLE DX** | | | | | | | | | | |
| 0–19 Years | 2 | 1.2 | <1 | 1 | 1 | 1 | 1 | 2 | 2 | 2 |
| 20–34 | 17 | 2.8 | 6 | 1 | 1 | 3 | 3 | 7 | 7 | 8 |
| 35–49 | 61 | 2.9 | 7 | 1 | 2 | 3 | 5 | 7 | 8 | 14 |
| 50–64 | 57 | 4.5 | 16 | 1 | 2 | 3 | 5 | 13 | 13 | 14 |
| 65+ | 125 | 3.8 | 7 | 1 | 3 | 3 | 6 | 8 | 8 | 13 |
| **TOTAL SINGLE DX** | 62 | 1.7 | <1 | 1 | 1 | 1 | 2 | 3 | 3 | 5 |
| **TOTAL MULTIPLE DX** | 262 | 3.7 | 9 | 1 | 1 | 3 | 5 | 8 | 10 | 14 |
| **TOTAL** | | | | | | | | | | |
| 0–19 Years | 2 | 1.2 | <1 | 1 | 1 | 1 | 1 | 2 | 2 | 2 |
| 20–34 | 22 | 2.5 | 5 | 1 | 1 | 1 | 3 | 7 | 7 | 8 |
| 35–49 | 85 | 2.5 | 6 | 1 | 2 | 2 | 3 | 6 | 7 | 11 |
| 50–64 | 74 | 3.7 | 14 | 1 | 2 | 3 | 5 | 12 | 13 | 14 |
| 65+ | 141 | 3.5 | 7 | 1 | 1 | 3 | 5 | 7 | 8 | 12 |
| **GRAND TOTAL** | 324 | 3.3 | 8 | 1 | 1 | 2 | 5 | 7 | 9 | 13 |

### 71.7: VULVAR & PERINEAL REPAIR. Formerly included in operation group(s) 703.

| Type of Patients | Observed Patients | Avg. Stay | Vari-ance | 10th | 25th | 50th | 75th | 90th | 95th | 99th |
|---|---|---|---|---|---|---|---|---|---|---|
| **1. SINGLE DX** | | | | | | | | | | |
| 0–19 Years | 50 | 1.3 | <1 | 1 | 1 | 1 | 1 | 2 | 3 | 6 |
| 20–34 | 34 | 2.5 | 2 | 1 | 1 | 2 | 4 | 4 | 5 | 7 |
| 35–49 | 24 | 1.4 | <1 | 1 | 1 | 1 | 2 | 2 | 2 | 3 |
| 50–64 | 25 | 1.3 | <1 | 1 | 1 | 1 | 2 | 2 | 3 | 5 |
| 65+ | 14 | 3.0 | 2 | 1 | 2 | 3 | 5 | 5 | 5 | 5 |
| **2. MULTIPLE DX** | | | | | | | | | | |
| 0–19 Years | 68 | 2.5 | 5 | 1 | 1 | 2 | 3 | 4 | 9 | 11 |
| 20–34 | 138 | 2.2 | 3 | 1 | 1 | 2 | 2 | 3 | 4 | 12 |
| 35–49 | 112 | 2.4 | 10 | 1 | 1 | 2 | 2 | 3 | 5 | 21 |
| 50–64 | 182 | 2.2 | 1 | 1 | 2 | 2 | 3 | 3 | 6 | 8 |
| 65+ | 223 | 2.8 | 4 | 1 | 2 | 2 | 3 | 5 | 6 | 12 |
| **TOTAL SINGLE DX** | 147 | 1.8 | 2 | 1 | 1 | 1 | 2 | 4 | 5 | 6 |
| **TOTAL MULTIPLE DX** | 723 | 2.4 | 4 | 1 | 1 | 2 | 3 | 4 | 5 | 12 |
| **TOTAL** | | | | | | | | | | |
| 0–19 Years | 118 | 2.1 | 4 | 1 | 1 | 1 | 3 | 4 | 5 | 11 |
| 20–34 | 172 | 2.3 | 3 | 1 | 1 | 2 | 2 | 4 | 5 | 12 |
| 35–49 | 136 | 2.2 | 9 | 1 | 1 | 2 | 3 | 3 | 4 | 15 |
| 50–64 | 207 | 2.1 | 1 | 1 | 2 | 2 | 3 | 3 | 4 | 8 |
| 65+ | 237 | 2.8 | 4 | 1 | 2 | 2 | 3 | 5 | 6 | 12 |
| **GRAND TOTAL** | 870 | 2.3 | 4 | 1 | 1 | 2 | 3 | 4 | 5 | 12 |

Length of Stay by Diagnosis and Operation, United States, 2000

# United States, October 1998–September 1999 Data, by Operation

## 71.71: SUTURE VULVAR/PERI LAC. Formerly included in operation group(s) 703.

| Type of Patients | Observed Patients | Avg. Stay | Variance | 10th | 25th | 50th | 75th | 90th | 95th | 99th |
|---|---|---|---|---|---|---|---|---|---|---|
| **1. SINGLE DX** | | | | | | | | | | |
| 0–19 Years | 41 | 1.2 | <1 | 1 | 1 | 1 | 1 | 2 | 2 | 3 |
| 20–34 | 18 | 2.5 | 2 | 1 | 1 | 2 | 4 | 4 | 4 | 4 |
| 35–49 | 14 | 1.3 | <1 | 1 | 1 | 1 | 2 | 2 | 2 | 2 |
| 50–64 | 13 | 1.2 | <1 | 1 | 1 | 1 | 2 | 2 | 2 | 2 |
| 65+ | 8 | 2.2 | 1 | 1 | 2 | 2 | 2 | 4 | 5 | 5 |
| **2. MULTIPLE DX** | | | | | | | | | | |
| 0–19 Years | 56 | 2.5 | 5 | 1 | 1 | 2 | 3 | 4 | 5 | 11 |
| 20–34 | 59 | 2.0 | 3 | 1 | 1 | 2 | 2 | 3 | 3 | 14 |
| 35–49 | 41 | 1.8 | <1 | 1 | 1 | 2 | 2 | 3 | 4 | 5 |
| 50–64 | 73 | 2.1 | 1 | 1 | 1 | 2 | 3 | 3 | 4 | 5 |
| 65+ | 104 | 3.1 | 5 | 2 | 2 | 3 | 3 | 5 | 9 | 12 |
| **TOTAL SINGLE DX** | 94 | 1.6 | 1 | 1 | 1 | 1 | 2 | 4 | 4 | 4 |
| **TOTAL MULTIPLE DX** | 333 | 2.4 | 3 | 1 | 1 | 2 | 3 | 4 | 4 | 12 |
| **TOTAL** | | | | | | | | | | |
| 0–19 Years | 97 | 2.0 | 3 | 1 | 1 | 1 | 3 | 4 | 4 | 11 |
| 20–34 | 77 | 2.2 | 3 | 1 | 1 | 2 | 2 | 4 | 4 | 13 |
| 35–49 | 55 | 1.8 | <1 | 1 | 1 | 2 | 2 | 3 | 4 | 5 |
| 50–64 | 86 | 1.9 | 1 | 1 | 1 | 2 | 3 | 3 | 4 | 5 |
| 65+ | 112 | 3.0 | 5 | 2 | 2 | 3 | 3 | 5 | 7 | 12 |
| **GRAND TOTAL** | 427 | 2.2 | 3 | 1 | 1 | 2 | 3 | 4 | 4 | 11 |

## 71.8: OTHER VULVAR OPERATIONS. Formerly included in operation group(s) 703.

| Type of Patients | Observed Patients | Avg. Stay | Variance | 10th | 25th | 50th | 75th | 90th | 95th | 99th |
|---|---|---|---|---|---|---|---|---|---|---|
| **1. SINGLE DX** | | | | | | | | | | |
| 0–19 Years | 0 | | | | | | | | | |
| 20–34 | 0 | | | | | | | | | |
| 35–49 | 0 | | | | | | | | | |
| 50–64 | 0 | | | | | | | | | |
| 65+ | 0 | | | | | | | | | |
| **2. MULTIPLE DX** | | | | | | | | | | |
| 0–19 Years | 1 | 1.0 | 0 | 1 | 1 | 1 | 1 | 1 | 1 | 1 |
| 20–34 | 1 | 1.0 | 0 | 1 | 1 | 1 | 1 | 1 | 1 | 1 |
| 35–49 | 0 | | | | | | | | | |
| 50–64 | 3 | 1.0 | 0 | 1 | 1 | 1 | 1 | 1 | 1 | 1 |
| 65+ | 0 | | | | | | | | | |
| **TOTAL SINGLE DX** | 0 | | | | | | | | | |
| **TOTAL MULTIPLE DX** | 5 | 1.0 | 0 | 1 | 1 | 1 | 1 | 1 | 1 | 1 |
| **TOTAL** | | | | | | | | | | |
| 0–19 Years | 1 | 1.0 | 0 | 1 | 1 | 1 | 1 | 1 | 1 | 1 |
| 20–34 | 1 | 1.0 | 0 | 1 | 1 | 1 | 1 | 1 | 1 | 1 |
| 35–49 | 0 | | | | | | | | | |
| 50–64 | 3 | 1.0 | 0 | 1 | 1 | 1 | 1 | 1 | 1 | 1 |
| 65+ | 0 | | | | | | | | | |
| **GRAND TOTAL** | 5 | 1.0 | 0 | 1 | 1 | 1 | 1 | 1 | 1 | 1 |

## 71.79: VULVAR/PERINEUM REP NEC. Formerly included in operation group(s) 703.

| Type of Patients | Observed Patients | Avg. Stay | Variance | 10th | 25th | 50th | 75th | 90th | 95th | 99th |
|---|---|---|---|---|---|---|---|---|---|---|
| **1. SINGLE DX** | | | | | | | | | | |
| 0–19 Years | 8 | 3.1 | 5 | 1 | 1 | 2 | 6 | 6 | 6 | 6 |
| 20–34 | 15 | 2.5 | 3 | 1 | 1 | 2 | 3 | 5 | 5 | 7 |
| 35–49 | 9 | 1.3 | <1 | 1 | 1 | 1 | 1 | 2 | 3 | 3 |
| 50–64 | 12 | 1.6 | <1 | 1 | 1 | 1 | 2 | 3 | 3 | 3 |
| 65+ | 6 | 3.7 | 2 | 2 | 2 | 4 | 5 | 5 | 5 | 5 |
| **2. MULTIPLE DX** | | | | | | | | | | |
| 0–19 Years | 11 | 2.4 | 6 | 1 | 1 | 2 | 3 | 5 | 10 | 10 |
| 20–34 | 73 | 2.4 | 3 | 1 | 1 | 2 | 2 | 3 | 4 | 12 |
| 35–49 | 66 | 2.1 | 7 | 1 | 1 | 2 | 2 | 3 | 4 | 21 |
| 50–64 | 109 | 2.3 | 2 | 1 | 2 | 2 | 3 | 3 | 4 | 8 |
| 65+ | 117 | 2.5 | 2 | 1 | 2 | 2 | 3 | 3 | 6 | 7 |
| **TOTAL SINGLE DX** | 50 | 2.3 | 3 | 1 | 1 | 2 | 3 | 5 | 5 | 7 |
| **TOTAL MULTIPLE DX** | 376 | 2.3 | 4 | 1 | 1 | 2 | 3 | 4 | 5 | 10 |
| **TOTAL** | | | | | | | | | | |
| 0–19 Years | 19 | 2.5 | 5 | 1 | 1 | 2 | 3 | 6 | 10 | 10 |
| 20–34 | 88 | 2.4 | 3 | 1 | 1 | 2 | 3 | 5 | 5 | 11 |
| 35–49 | 75 | 2.0 | 7 | 1 | 1 | 2 | 2 | 3 | 4 | 5 |
| 50–64 | 121 | 2.2 | 2 | 1 | 2 | 2 | 3 | 3 | 4 | 8 |
| 65+ | 123 | 2.6 | 2 | 1 | 2 | 2 | 3 | 5 | 6 | 7 |
| **GRAND TOTAL** | 426 | 2.3 | 3 | 1 | 1 | 2 | 3 | 4 | 5 | 10 |

## 71.9: OTHER FEMALE GENITAL OPS. Formerly included in operation group(s) 703.

| Type of Patients | Observed Patients | Avg. Stay | Variance | 10th | 25th | 50th | 75th | 90th | 95th | 99th |
|---|---|---|---|---|---|---|---|---|---|---|
| **1. SINGLE DX** | | | | | | | | | | |
| 0–19 Years | 1 | 2.0 | 0 | 2 | 2 | 2 | 2 | 2 | 2 | 2 |
| 20–34 | 0 | | | | | | | | | |
| 35–49 | 1 | 9.0 | 0 | 9 | 9 | 9 | 9 | 9 | 9 | 9 |
| 50–64 | 0 | | | | | | | | | |
| 65+ | 0 | | | | | | | | | |
| **2. MULTIPLE DX** | | | | | | | | | | |
| 0–19 Years | 0 | | | | | | | | | |
| 20–34 | 2 | 4.2 | 4 | 3 | 3 | 3 | 3 | 5 | 7 | 7 |
| 35–49 | 2 | 10.0 | 1 | 9 | 9 | 11 | 11 | 11 | 11 | 11 |
| 50–64 | 0 | | | | | | | | | |
| 65+ | 0 | | | | | | | | | |
| **TOTAL SINGLE DX** | 2 | 6.6 | 0 | 2 | 2 | 9 | 9 | 9 | 9 | 9 |
| **TOTAL MULTIPLE DX** | 4 | 6.4 | 11 | 3 | 3 | 7 | 7 | 11 | 11 | 11 |
| **TOTAL** | | | | | | | | | | |
| 0–19 Years | 1 | 2.0 | 0 | 2 | 2 | 2 | 2 | 2 | 2 | 2 |
| 20–34 | 2 | 4.2 | 4 | 3 | 3 | 3 | 3 | 5 | 7 | 7 |
| 35–49 | 3 | 9.9 | 1 | 9 | 9 | 9 | 11 | 11 | 11 | 11 |
| 50–64 | 0 | | | | | | | | | |
| 65+ | 0 | | | | | | | | | |
| **GRAND TOTAL** | 6 | 6.4 | 11 | 3 | 3 | 7 | 9 | 11 | 11 | 11 |

Length of Stay by Diagnosis and Operation, United States, 2000

# United States, October 1998–September 1999 Data, by Operation

## 72.0: LOW FORCEPS OPERATION. Formerly included in operation group(s) 705.

| Type of Patients | Observed Patients | Avg. Stay | Variance | 10th | 25th | 50th | 75th | 90th | 95th | 99th |
|---|---|---|---|---|---|---|---|---|---|---|
| **1. SINGLE DX** | | | | | | | | | | |
| 0–19 Years | 139 | 1.9 | <1 | 1 | 1 | 2 | 2 | 3 | 3 | 3 |
| 20–34 | 469 | 1.8 | <1 | 1 | 1 | 2 | 2 | 3 | 3 | 3 |
| 35–49 | 62 | 1.9 | <1 | 1 | 2 | 2 | 2 | 3 | 3 | 3 |
| 50–64 | 0 | | | | | | | | | |
| 65+ | 0 | | | | | | | | | |
| **2. MULTIPLE DX** | | | | | | | | | | |
| 0–19 Years | 974 | 2.3 | 1 | 1 | 2 | 3 | 3 | 3 | 4 | 7 |
| 20–34 | 4,491 | 2.3 | 4 | 1 | 2 | 3 | 3 | 3 | 3 | 7 |
| 35–49 | 748 | 2.5 | 5 | 1 | 2 | 3 | 3 | 3 | 4 | 8 |
| 50–64 | 1 | 5.0 | 0 | 5 | 5 | 5 | 5 | 5 | 5 | 5 |
| 65+ | 0 | | | | | | | | | |
| **TOTAL SINGLE DX** | 670 | 1.8 | <1 | 1 | 1 | 2 | 2 | 3 | 3 | 3 |
| **TOTAL MULTIPLE DX** | 6,214 | 2.3 | 4 | 1 | 2 | 2 | 3 | 3 | 4 | 7 |
| **TOTAL** | | | | | | | | | | |
| 0–19 Years | 1,113 | 2.3 | 1 | 1 | 2 | 2 | 3 | 3 | 3 | 6 |
| 20–34 | 4,960 | 2.3 | 4 | 1 | 2 | 2 | 2 | 3 | 3 | 7 |
| 35–49 | 810 | 2.4 | 5 | 1 | 2 | 2 | 3 | 3 | 4 | 7 |
| 50–64 | 1 | 5.0 | 0 | 5 | 5 | 5 | 5 | 5 | 5 | 5 |
| 65+ | 0 | | | | | | | | | |
| **GRAND TOTAL** | 6,884 | 2.3 | 4 | 1 | 2 | 2 | 3 | 3 | 3 | 7 |

## 72.1: LOW FORCEPS OPERATION W EPISIOTOMY. Formerly included in operation group(s) 705.

| Type of Patients | Observed Patients | Avg. Stay | Variance | 10th | 25th | 50th | 75th | 90th | 95th | 99th |
|---|---|---|---|---|---|---|---|---|---|---|
| **1. SINGLE DX** | | | | | | | | | | |
| 0–19 Years | 1,008 | 2.0 | <1 | 1 | 2 | 2 | 2 | 3 | 3 | 4 |
| 20–34 | 4,136 | 2.0 | <1 | 1 | 2 | 2 | 2 | 3 | 3 | 3 |
| 35–49 | 426 | 2.1 | <1 | 1 | 2 | 2 | 2 | 3 | 3 | 3 |
| 50–64 | 0 | | | | | | | | | |
| 65+ | 0 | | | | | | | | | |
| **2. MULTIPLE DX** | | | | | | | | | | |
| 0–19 Years | 2,657 | 2.3 | <1 | 1 | 2 | 2 | 3 | 3 | 4 | 6 |
| 20–34 | 13,891 | 2.3 | 1 | 2 | 2 | 2 | 3 | 3 | 4 | 5 |
| 35–49 | 2,249 | 2.4 | 1 | 2 | 2 | 2 | 3 | 3 | 4 | 6 |
| 50–64 | 1 | 7.0 | 0 | 7 | 7 | 7 | 7 | 7 | 7 | 7 |
| 65+ | 0 | | | | | | | | | |
| **TOTAL SINGLE DX** | 5,570 | 2.0 | <1 | 1 | 2 | 2 | 2 | 3 | 3 | 3 |
| **TOTAL MULTIPLE DX** | 18,798 | 2.3 | 1 | 2 | 2 | 2 | 3 | 3 | 4 | 5 |
| **TOTAL** | | | | | | | | | | |
| 0–19 Years | 3,665 | 2.2 | <1 | 1 | 2 | 2 | 3 | 3 | 3 | 5 |
| 20–34 | 18,027 | 2.3 | 1 | 1 | 2 | 2 | 3 | 3 | 4 | 5 |
| 35–49 | 2,675 | 2.4 | 1 | 2 | 2 | 3 | 3 | 3 | 4 | 7 |
| 50–64 | 1 | 7.0 | 0 | 7 | 7 | 7 | 7 | 7 | 7 | 7 |
| 65+ | 0 | | | | | | | | | |
| **GRAND TOTAL** | 24,368 | 2.3 | 1 | 2 | 2 | 3 | 3 | 3 | 3 | 5 |

## 72.2: MID FORCEPS OPERATION. Formerly included in operation group(s) 707.

| Type of Patients | Observed Patients | Avg. Stay | Variance | 10th | 25th | 50th | 75th | 90th | 95th | 99th |
|---|---|---|---|---|---|---|---|---|---|---|
| **1. SINGLE DX** | | | | | | | | | | |
| 0–19 Years | 43 | 2.1 | <1 | 1 | 1 | 2 | 3 | 3 | 3 | 3 |
| 20–34 | 201 | 2.2 | <1 | 1 | 2 | 2 | 3 | 3 | 3 | 4 |
| 35–49 | 24 | 2.2 | <1 | 2 | 2 | 2 | 2 | 3 | 3 | 3 |
| 50–64 | 0 | | | | | | | | | |
| 65+ | 0 | | | | | | | | | |
| **2. MULTIPLE DX** | | | | | | | | | | |
| 0–19 Years | 150 | 2.3 | <1 | 1 | 2 | 2 | 3 | 3 | 3 | 6 |
| 20–34 | 873 | 2.3 | <1 | 1 | 2 | 2 | 3 | 3 | 4 | 5 |
| 35–49 | 172 | 2.6 | 19 | 1 | 2 | 2 | 2 | 3 | 3 | 5 |
| 50–64 | 0 | | | | | | | | | |
| 65+ | 0 | | | | | | | | | |
| **TOTAL SINGLE DX** | 268 | 2.2 | <1 | 1 | 2 | 2 | 3 | 3 | 3 | 4 |
| **TOTAL MULTIPLE DX** | 1,195 | 2.3 | 4 | 1 | 2 | 2 | 3 | 3 | 4 | 5 |
| **TOTAL** | | | | | | | | | | |
| 0–19 Years | 193 | 2.3 | <1 | 1 | 2 | 2 | 3 | 3 | 3 | 5 |
| 20–34 | 1,074 | 2.3 | <1 | 1 | 2 | 2 | 3 | 3 | 3 | 5 |
| 35–49 | 196 | 2.5 | 17 | 1 | 2 | 2 | 2 | 3 | 3 | 5 |
| 50–64 | 0 | | | | | | | | | |
| 65+ | 0 | | | | | | | | | |
| **GRAND TOTAL** | 1,463 | 2.3 | 3 | 1 | 2 | 2 | 3 | 3 | 4 | 5 |

## 72.21: MID FORCEPS W EPISIOTOMY. Formerly included in operation group(s) 707.

| Type of Patients | Observed Patients | Avg. Stay | Variance | 10th | 25th | 50th | 75th | 90th | 95th | 99th |
|---|---|---|---|---|---|---|---|---|---|---|
| **1. SINGLE DX** | | | | | | | | | | |
| 0–19 Years | 35 | 2.1 | <1 | 1 | 1 | 2 | 3 | 3 | 3 | 3 |
| 20–34 | 173 | 2.2 | <1 | 1 | 2 | 2 | 3 | 3 | 3 | 4 |
| 35–49 | 21 | 2.3 | <1 | 2 | 2 | 2 | 3 | 3 | 3 | 3 |
| 50–64 | 0 | | | | | | | | | |
| 65+ | 0 | | | | | | | | | |
| **2. MULTIPLE DX** | | | | | | | | | | |
| 0–19 Years | 126 | 2.3 | <1 | 1 | 2 | 2 | 3 | 3 | 3 | 6 |
| 20–34 | 677 | 2.3 | <1 | 1 | 2 | 2 | 3 | 3 | 4 | 5 |
| 35–49 | 130 | 2.5 | 13 | 1 | 2 | 2 | 2 | 3 | 3 | 5 |
| 50–64 | 0 | | | | | | | | | |
| 65+ | 0 | | | | | | | | | |
| **TOTAL SINGLE DX** | 229 | 2.2 | <1 | 1 | 2 | 2 | 3 | 3 | 3 | 4 |
| **TOTAL MULTIPLE DX** | 933 | 2.3 | 2 | 1 | 2 | 2 | 3 | 3 | 4 | 5 |
| **TOTAL** | | | | | | | | | | |
| 0–19 Years | 161 | 2.3 | <1 | 1 | 2 | 2 | 3 | 3 | 3 | 5 |
| 20–34 | 850 | 2.3 | <1 | 1 | 2 | 2 | 3 | 3 | 4 | 4 |
| 35–49 | 151 | 2.4 | 11 | 1 | 2 | 2 | 2 | 3 | 3 | 5 |
| 50–64 | 0 | | | | | | | | | |
| 65+ | 0 | | | | | | | | | |
| **GRAND TOTAL** | 1,162 | 2.3 | 2 | 1 | 2 | 2 | 3 | 3 | 4 | 5 |

# United States, October 1998–September 1999 Data, by Operation

## 72.29: MID FORCEPS OP NEC. Formerly included in operation group(s) 707.

| Type of Patients | Observed Patients | Avg. Stay | Variance | 10th | 25th | 50th | 75th | 90th | 95th | 99th |
|---|---|---|---|---|---|---|---|---|---|---|
| **1. SINGLE DX** | | | | | | | | | | |
| 0–19 Years | 8 | 2.3 | <1 | 1 | 2 | 2 | 3 | 3 | 3 | 3 |
| 20–34 | 28 | 1.8 | <1 | 1 | 1 | 2 | 2 | 3 | 3 | 3 |
| 35–49 | 3 | 2.0 | 0 | 2 | 2 | 2 | 2 | 2 | 2 | 2 |
| 50–64 | 0 | | | | | | | | | |
| 65+ | 0 | | | | | | | | | |
| **2. MULTIPLE DX** | | | | | | | | | | |
| 0–19 Years | 24 | 2.1 | <1 | 1 | 2 | 2 | 2 | 3 | 4 | 4 |
| 20–34 | 196 | 2.2 | 2 | 1 | 2 | 2 | 3 | 3 | 4 | 6 |
| 35–49 | 42 | 2.9 | 38 | 2 | 2 | 2 | 2 | 3 | 4 | 51 |
| 50–64 | 0 | | | | | | | | | |
| 65+ | 0 | | | | | | | | | |
| **TOTAL SINGLE DX** | 39 | 1.9 | <1 | 1 | 2 | 2 | 2 | 2 | 3 | 3 |
| **TOTAL MULTIPLE DX** | 262 | 2.3 | 9 | 1 | 2 | 2 | 3 | 3 | 4 | 6 |
| **TOTAL** | | | | | | | | | | |
| 0–19 Years | 32 | 2.2 | <1 | 1 | 2 | 2 | 3 | 3 | 4 | 4 |
| 20–34 | 224 | 2.2 | 2 | 1 | 2 | 2 | 3 | 3 | 4 | 6 |
| 35–49 | 45 | 2.7 | 32 | 2 | 2 | 2 | 2 | 3 | 4 | 51 |
| 50–64 | 0 | | | | | | | | | |
| 65+ | 0 | | | | | | | | | |
| **GRAND TOTAL** | 301 | 2.3 | 8 | 1 | 2 | 2 | 2 | 3 | 3 | 6 |

## 72.3: HIGH FORCEPS OPERATION. Formerly included in operation group(s) 707.

| Type of Patients | Observed Patients | Avg. Stay | Variance | 10th | 25th | 50th | 75th | 90th | 95th | 99th |
|---|---|---|---|---|---|---|---|---|---|---|
| **1. SINGLE DX** | | | | | | | | | | |
| 0–19 Years | 0 | | | | | | | | | |
| 20–34 | 9 | 1.8 | <1 | 1 | 1 | 2 | 2 | 3 | 3 | 3 |
| 35–49 | 0 | | | | | | | | | |
| 50–64 | 0 | | | | | | | | | |
| 65+ | 0 | | | | | | | | | |
| **2. MULTIPLE DX** | | | | | | | | | | |
| 0–19 Years | 3 | 1.8 | <1 | 1 | 1 | 2 | 2 | 3 | 3 | 3 |
| 20–34 | 17 | 2.7 | 2 | 1 | 2 | 3 | 3 | 4 | 4 | 9 |
| 35–49 | 4 | 5.5 | 34 | 1 | 3 | 3 | 5 | 17 | 17 | 17 |
| 50–64 | 0 | | | | | | | | | |
| 65+ | 0 | | | | | | | | | |
| **TOTAL SINGLE DX** | 9 | 1.8 | <1 | 1 | 1 | 2 | 2 | 3 | 3 | 3 |
| **TOTAL MULTIPLE DX** | 24 | 2.8 | 4 | 1 | 2 | 3 | 3 | 4 | 4 | 17 |
| **TOTAL** | | | | | | | | | | |
| 0–19 Years | 3 | 1.8 | <1 | 1 | 1 | 2 | 2 | 3 | 3 | 3 |
| 20–34 | 26 | 2.4 | 1 | 1 | 2 | 2 | 3 | 4 | 4 | 9 |
| 35–49 | 4 | 5.5 | 34 | 1 | 3 | 3 | 5 | 17 | 17 | 17 |
| 50–64 | 0 | | | | | | | | | |
| 65+ | 0 | | | | | | | | | |
| **GRAND TOTAL** | 33 | 2.5 | 4 | 2 | 2 | 2 | 3 | 4 | 4 | 17 |

## 72.4: FORCEPS ROT FETAL HEAD. Formerly included in operation group(s) 707.

| Type of Patients | Observed Patients | Avg. Stay | Variance | 10th | 25th | 50th | 75th | 90th | 95th | 99th |
|---|---|---|---|---|---|---|---|---|---|---|
| **1. SINGLE DX** | | | | | | | | | | |
| 0–19 Years | 9 | 2.0 | <1 | 1 | 2 | 2 | 2 | 3 | 3 | 3 |
| 20–34 | 24 | 2.1 | <1 | 1 | 1 | 2 | 3 | 3 | 4 | 4 |
| 35–49 | 2 | 2.0 | 0 | 2 | 2 | 2 | 2 | 2 | 2 | 2 |
| 50–64 | 0 | | | | | | | | | |
| 65+ | 0 | | | | | | | | | |
| **2. MULTIPLE DX** | | | | | | | | | | |
| 0–19 Years | 34 | 2.1 | <1 | 2 | 2 | 2 | 2 | 3 | 3 | 3 |
| 20–34 | 169 | 2.2 | 1 | 1 | 2 | 2 | 3 | 3 | 3 | 4 |
| 35–49 | 24 | 2.1 | <1 | 1 | 2 | 2 | 3 | 3 | 3 | 4 |
| 50–64 | 0 | | | | | | | | | |
| 65+ | 0 | | | | | | | | | |
| **TOTAL SINGLE DX** | 35 | 2.0 | <1 | 1 | 2 | 2 | 2 | 3 | 4 | 4 |
| **TOTAL MULTIPLE DX** | 227 | 2.2 | <1 | 1 | 2 | 2 | 3 | 3 | 3 | 4 |
| **TOTAL** | | | | | | | | | | |
| 0–19 Years | 43 | 2.1 | <1 | 2 | 2 | 2 | 2 | 3 | 3 | 3 |
| 20–34 | 193 | 2.2 | 1 | 1 | 2 | 2 | 3 | 3 | 3 | 4 |
| 35–49 | 26 | 2.1 | <1 | 1 | 2 | 2 | 3 | 3 | 3 | 4 |
| 50–64 | 0 | | | | | | | | | |
| 65+ | 0 | | | | | | | | | |
| **GRAND TOTAL** | 262 | 2.2 | <1 | 1 | 2 | 2 | 3 | 3 | 3 | 4 |

## 72.5: BREECH EXTRACTION. Formerly included in operation group(s) 706.

| Type of Patients | Observed Patients | Avg. Stay | Variance | 10th | 25th | 50th | 75th | 90th | 95th | 99th |
|---|---|---|---|---|---|---|---|---|---|---|
| **1. SINGLE DX** | | | | | | | | | | |
| 0–19 Years | 24 | 1.8 | 1 | 1 | 2 | 2 | 2 | 2 | 3 | 6 |
| 20–34 | 114 | 1.8 | <1 | 1 | 1 | 2 | 2 | 2 | 3 | 3 |
| 35–49 | 15 | 1.3 | <1 | 1 | 1 | 1 | 1 | 2 | 2 | 3 |
| 50–64 | 0 | | | | | | | | | |
| 65+ | 0 | | | | | | | | | |
| **2. MULTIPLE DX** | | | | | | | | | | |
| 0–19 Years | 150 | 2.0 | 5 | 1 | 1 | 2 | 2 | 3 | 4 | 12 |
| 20–34 | 867 | 3.0 | 23 | 1 | 2 | 2 | 3 | 4 | 9 | 24 |
| 35–49 | 208 | 2.4 | 6 | 1 | 2 | 2 | 2 | 2 | 6 | 18 |
| 50–64 | 2 | 2.0 | 0 | 2 | 2 | 2 | 2 | 2 | 2 | 2 |
| 65+ | 0 | | | | | | | | | |
| **TOTAL SINGLE DX** | 153 | 1.7 | <1 | 1 | 1 | 2 | 2 | 2 | 3 | 4 |
| **TOTAL MULTIPLE DX** | 1,227 | 2.8 | 17 | 1 | 1 | 2 | 3 | 4 | 7 | 24 |
| **TOTAL** | | | | | | | | | | |
| 0–19 Years | 174 | 2.0 | 4 | 1 | 2 | 2 | 2 | 3 | 4 | 10 |
| 20–34 | 981 | 2.9 | 20 | 1 | 2 | 2 | 3 | 4 | 8 | 24 |
| 35–49 | 223 | 2.3 | 6 | 1 | 1 | 2 | 2 | 3 | 5 | 17 |
| 50–64 | 2 | 2.0 | 0 | 2 | 2 | 2 | 2 | 2 | 2 | 2 |
| 65+ | 0 | | | | | | | | | |
| **GRAND TOTAL** | 1,380 | 2.6 | 16 | 1 | 1 | 2 | 2 | 4 | 6 | 24 |

Length of Stay by Diagnosis and Operation, United States, 2000

# United States, October 1998–September 1999 Data, by Operation

## 72.6: FORCEPS-AFTERCOMING HEAD. Formerly included in operation group(s) 706.

| Type of Patients | Observed Patients | Avg. Stay | Variance | Percentiles | | | | | | |
|---|---|---|---|---|---|---|---|---|---|---|
| | | | | 10th | 25th | 50th | 75th | 90th | 95th | 99th |
| **1. SINGLE DX** | | | | | | | | | | |
| 0–19 Years | 3 | 2.0 | 0 | 2 | 2 | 2 | 2 | 2 | 2 | 2 |
| 20–34 | 13 | 2.1 | <1 | 2 | 2 | 2 | 2 | 3 | 3 | 3 |
| 35–49 | 1 | 2.0 | 0 | 2 | 2 | 2 | 2 | 2 | 2 | 2 |
| 50–64 | 0 | | | | | | | | | |
| 65+ | 0 | | | | | | | | | |
| **2. MULTIPLE DX** | | | | | | | | | | |
| 0–19 Years | 2 | 2.6 | <1 | 2 | 2 | 3 | 3 | 3 | 3 | 3 |
| 20–34 | 38 | 1.9 | <1 | 1 | 1 | 2 | 2 | 3 | 3 | 3 |
| 35–49 | 6 | 1.8 | <1 | 1 | 1 | 2 | 2 | 2 | 3 | 3 |
| 50–64 | 0 | | | | | | | | | |
| 65+ | 0 | | | | | | | | | |
| **TOTAL SINGLE DX** | 17 | 2.1 | <1 | 2 | 2 | 2 | 2 | 3 | 3 | 3 |
| **TOTAL MULTIPLE DX** | 46 | 1.9 | <1 | 1 | 1 | 2 | 2 | 3 | 3 | 3 |
| **TOTAL** | | | | | | | | | | |
| 0–19 Years | 5 | 2.2 | <1 | 2 | 2 | 2 | 2 | 3 | 3 | 3 |
| 20–34 | 51 | 2.0 | <1 | 1 | 1 | 2 | 2 | 3 | 3 | 3 |
| 35–49 | 7 | 1.8 | <1 | 1 | 1 | 2 | 2 | 2 | 3 | 3 |
| 50–64 | 0 | | | | | | | | | |
| 65+ | 0 | | | | | | | | | |
| **GRAND TOTAL** | 63 | 2.0 | <1 | 1 | 2 | 2 | 2 | 3 | 3 | 3 |

## 72.7: VACUUM EXTRACTION DEL. Formerly included in operation group(s) 707.

| Type of Patients | Observed Patients | Avg. Stay | Variance | Percentiles | | | | | | |
|---|---|---|---|---|---|---|---|---|---|---|
| | | | | 10th | 25th | 50th | 75th | 90th | 95th | 99th |
| **1. SINGLE DX** | | | | | | | | | | |
| 0–19 Years | 3,215 | 1.9 | <1 | 1 | 1 | 2 | 2 | 3 | 3 | 4 |
| 20–34 | 11,993 | 1.9 | <1 | 1 | 1 | 2 | 2 | 3 | 3 | 3 |
| 35–49 | 1,166 | 1.9 | <1 | 1 | 2 | 2 | 2 | 3 | 3 | 4 |
| 50–64 | 0 | | | | | | | | | |
| 65+ | 0 | | | | | | | | | |
| **2. MULTIPLE DX** | | | | | | | | | | |
| 0–19 Years | 8,583 | 2.2 | <1 | 1 | 2 | 2 | 3 | 3 | 3 | 5 |
| 20–34 | 40,474 | 2.1 | <1 | 1 | 2 | 2 | 2 | 3 | 3 | 5 |
| 35–49 | 6,561 | 2.2 | 2 | 1 | 2 | 2 | 2 | 3 | 3 | 5 |
| 50–64 | 0 | | | | | | | | | |
| 65+ | 0 | | | | | | | | | |
| **TOTAL SINGLE DX** | 16,374 | 1.9 | <1 | 1 | 1 | 2 | 2 | 3 | 3 | 3 |
| **TOTAL MULTIPLE DX** | 55,618 | 2.1 | 1 | 1 | 2 | 2 | 2 | 3 | 3 | 5 |
| **TOTAL** | | | | | | | | | | |
| 0–19 Years | 11,798 | 2.1 | <1 | 1 | 2 | 2 | 2 | 3 | 3 | 4 |
| 20–34 | 52,467 | 2.1 | <1 | 1 | 2 | 2 | 2 | 3 | 3 | 4 |
| 35–49 | 7,727 | 2.1 | 1 | 1 | 2 | 2 | 2 | 3 | 3 | 5 |
| 50–64 | 0 | | | | | | | | | |
| 65+ | 0 | | | | | | | | | |
| **GRAND TOTAL** | 71,992 | 2.1 | <1 | 1 | 2 | 2 | 2 | 3 | 3 | 5 |

## 72.52: PART BREECH EXTRACT NEC. Formerly included in operation group(s) 706.

| Type of Patients | Observed Patients | Avg. Stay | Variance | Percentiles | | | | | | |
|---|---|---|---|---|---|---|---|---|---|---|
| | | | | 10th | 25th | 50th | 75th | 90th | 95th | 99th |
| **1. SINGLE DX** | | | | | | | | | | |
| 0–19 Years | 10 | 1.5 | <1 | 1 | 1 | 2 | 2 | 2 | 2 | 2 |
| 20–34 | 39 | 1.8 | <1 | 1 | 2 | 2 | 2 | 2 | 2 | 3 |
| 35–49 | 6 | 1.4 | <1 | 1 | 1 | 1 | 2 | 2 | 3 | 3 |
| 50–64 | 0 | | | | | | | | | |
| 65+ | 0 | | | | | | | | | |
| **2. MULTIPLE DX** | | | | | | | | | | |
| 0–19 Years | 51 | 1.9 | 1 | 1 | 1 | 2 | 2 | 3 | 4 | 6 |
| 20–34 | 308 | 2.6 | 15 | 1 | 1 | 2 | 2 | 4 | 6 | 24 |
| 35–49 | 87 | 2.5 | 8 | 1 | 1 | 2 | 3 | 3 | 6 | 18 |
| 50–64 | 2 | 2.0 | 0 | 2 | 2 | 2 | 2 | 2 | 2 | 2 |
| 65+ | 0 | | | | | | | | | |
| **TOTAL SINGLE DX** | 55 | 1.7 | <1 | 1 | 1 | 2 | 2 | 2 | 2 | 3 |
| **TOTAL MULTIPLE DX** | 448 | 2.5 | 12 | 1 | 1 | 2 | 2 | 4 | 6 | 19 |
| **TOTAL** | | | | | | | | | | |
| 0–19 Years | 61 | 1.8 | <1 | 1 | 1 | 2 | 2 | 3 | 3 | 6 |
| 20–34 | 347 | 2.5 | 13 | 1 | 1 | 2 | 2 | 4 | 5 | 24 |
| 35–49 | 93 | 2.5 | 8 | 1 | 2 | 2 | 3 | 3 | 6 | 18 |
| 50–64 | 2 | 2.0 | 0 | 2 | 2 | 2 | 2 | 2 | 2 | 2 |
| 65+ | 0 | | | | | | | | | |
| **GRAND TOTAL** | 503 | 2.4 | 11 | 1 | 1 | 2 | 2 | 3 | 5 | 19 |

## 72.54: TOT BREECH EXTRACT NEC. Formerly included in operation group(s) 706.

| Type of Patients | Observed Patients | Avg. Stay | Variance | Percentiles | | | | | | |
|---|---|---|---|---|---|---|---|---|---|---|
| | | | | 10th | 25th | 50th | 75th | 90th | 95th | 99th |
| **1. SINGLE DX** | | | | | | | | | | |
| 0–19 Years | 11 | 1.5 | <1 | 1 | 1 | 2 | 2 | 2 | 2 | 2 |
| 20–34 | 60 | 1.8 | <1 | 1 | 1 | 2 | 2 | 3 | 3 | 4 |
| 35–49 | 5 | 1.2 | <1 | 1 | 1 | 1 | 1 | 2 | 2 | 2 |
| 50–64 | 0 | | | | | | | | | |
| 65+ | 0 | | | | | | | | | |
| **2. MULTIPLE DX** | | | | | | | | | | |
| 0–19 Years | 81 | 2.1 | 7 | 1 | 1 | 2 | 2 | 3 | 5 | 19 |
| 20–34 | 459 | 3.4 | 33 | 1 | 2 | 2 | 3 | 5 | 10 | 26 |
| 35–49 | 99 | 2.4 | 5 | 1 | 2 | 2 | 3 | 4 | 5 | 17 |
| 50–64 | 0 | | | | | | | | | |
| 65+ | 0 | | | | | | | | | |
| **TOTAL SINGLE DX** | 76 | 1.7 | <1 | 1 | 1 | 2 | 2 | 2 | 3 | 3 |
| **TOTAL MULTIPLE DX** | 639 | 3.0 | 25 | 1 | 1 | 2 | 2 | 4 | 9 | 24 |
| **TOTAL** | | | | | | | | | | |
| 0–19 Years | 92 | 2.1 | 6 | 1 | 1 | 2 | 2 | 3 | 4 | 19 |
| 20–34 | 519 | 3.2 | 29 | 1 | 1 | 2 | 3 | 4 | 9 | 25 |
| 35–49 | 104 | 2.3 | 5 | 1 | 1 | 2 | 2 | 4 | 5 | 17 |
| 50–64 | 0 | | | | | | | | | |
| 65+ | 0 | | | | | | | | | |
| **GRAND TOTAL** | 715 | 2.9 | 22 | 1 | 1 | 2 | 2 | 4 | 7 | 24 |

Length of Stay by Diagnosis and Operation, United States, 2000

# United States, October 1998–September 1999 Data, by Operation

## 72.71: VED W EPISIOTOMY. Formerly included in operation group(s) 707.

| Type of Patients | Observed Patients | Avg. Stay | Vari-ance | Percentiles | | | | | | |
|---|---|---|---|---|---|---|---|---|---|---|
| | | | | 10th | 25th | 50th | 75th | 90th | 95th | 99th |
| **1. SINGLE DX** | | | | | | | | | | |
| 0–19 Years | 2,600 | 1.9 | <1 | 1 | 1 | 2 | 2 | 3 | 3 | 4 |
| 20–34 | 9,249 | 1.9 | <1 | 1 | 2 | 2 | 2 | 3 | 3 | 3 |
| 35–49 | 887 | 2.0 | <1 | 1 | 2 | 2 | 2 | 3 | 3 | 4 |
| 50–64 | 0 | | | | | | | | | |
| 65+ | 0 | | | | | | | | | |
| **2. MULTIPLE DX** | | | | | | | | | | |
| 0–19 Years | 5,567 | 2.2 | <1 | 1 | 2 | 2 | 3 | 3 | 4 | 5 |
| 20–34 | 24,941 | 2.2 | <1 | 1 | 2 | 2 | 3 | 3 | 3 | 5 |
| 35–49 | 3,882 | 2.2 | 2 | 1 | 2 | 2 | 3 | 3 | 3 | 6 |
| 50–64 | 0 | | | | | | | | | |
| 65+ | 0 | | | | | | | | | |
| **TOTAL SINGLE DX** | 12,736 | 1.9 | <1 | 1 | 2 | 2 | 2 | 3 | 3 | 3 |
| **TOTAL MULTIPLE DX** | 34,390 | 2.2 | <1 | 1 | 2 | 2 | 3 | 3 | 3 | 5 |
| **TOTAL** | | | | | | | | | | |
| 0–19 Years | 8,167 | 2.1 | <1 | 1 | 2 | 2 | 2 | 3 | 3 | 5 |
| 20–34 | 34,190 | 2.1 | <1 | 1 | 2 | 2 | 2 | 3 | 3 | 4 |
| 35–49 | 4,769 | 2.2 | 1 | 1 | 2 | 2 | 2 | 3 | 3 | 5 |
| 50–64 | 0 | | | | | | | | | |
| 65+ | 0 | | | | | | | | | |
| **GRAND TOTAL** | 47,126 | 2.1 | <1 | 1 | 2 | 2 | 2 | 3 | 3 | 5 |

## 72.79: VACUUM EXTRACT DEL NEC. Formerly included in operation group(s) 707.

| Type of Patients | Observed Patients | Avg. Stay | Vari-ance | Percentiles | | | | | | |
|---|---|---|---|---|---|---|---|---|---|---|
| | | | | 10th | 25th | 50th | 75th | 90th | 95th | 99th |
| **1. SINGLE DX** | | | | | | | | | | |
| 0–19 Years | 615 | 1.8 | <1 | 1 | 1 | 2 | 2 | 3 | 3 | 4 |
| 20–34 | 2,744 | 1.7 | <1 | 1 | 2 | 2 | 2 | 3 | 3 | 3 |
| 35–49 | 279 | 1.8 | <1 | 1 | 2 | 2 | 2 | 2 | 3 | 3 |
| 50–64 | 0 | | | | | | | | | |
| 65+ | 0 | | | | | | | | | |
| **2. MULTIPLE DX** | | | | | | | | | | |
| 0–19 Years | 3,016 | 2.1 | <1 | 1 | 2 | 2 | 3 | 3 | 4 | 5 |
| 20–34 | 15,533 | 2.0 | 1 | 1 | 1 | 2 | 3 | 3 | 3 | 5 |
| 35–49 | 2,679 | 2.1 | 2 | 1 | 1 | 2 | 3 | 3 | 3 | 5 |
| 50–64 | 0 | | | | | | | | | |
| 65+ | 0 | | | | | | | | | |
| **TOTAL SINGLE DX** | 3,638 | 1.8 | <1 | 1 | 1 | 2 | 2 | 3 | 3 | 3 |
| **TOTAL MULTIPLE DX** | 21,228 | 2.0 | 1 | 1 | 1 | 2 | 3 | 3 | 3 | 5 |
| **TOTAL** | | | | | | | | | | |
| 0–19 Years | 3,631 | 2.0 | <1 | 1 | 1 | 2 | 2 | 3 | 3 | 4 |
| 20–34 | 18,277 | 2.0 | 1 | 1 | 1 | 2 | 2 | 3 | 3 | 5 |
| 35–49 | 2,958 | 2.0 | 2 | 1 | 1 | 2 | 2 | 3 | 3 | 5 |
| 50–64 | 0 | | | | | | | | | |
| 65+ | 0 | | | | | | | | | |
| **GRAND TOTAL** | 24,866 | 2.0 | <1 | 1 | 1 | 2 | 2 | 3 | 3 | 5 |

## 72.8: INSTRUMENTAL DEL NEC. Formerly included in operation group(s) 707.

| Type of Patients | Observed Patients | Avg. Stay | Vari-ance | Percentiles | | | | | | |
|---|---|---|---|---|---|---|---|---|---|---|
| | | | | 10th | 25th | 50th | 75th | 90th | 95th | 99th |
| **1. SINGLE DX** | | | | | | | | | | |
| 0–19 Years | 1 | 2.0 | 0 | 2 | 2 | 2 | 2 | 2 | 2 | 2 |
| 20–34 | 1 | 1.0 | 0 | 1 | 1 | 1 | 1 | 1 | 1 | 1 |
| 35–49 | 0 | | | | | | | | | |
| 50–64 | 0 | | | | | | | | | |
| 65+ | 0 | | | | | | | | | |
| **2. MULTIPLE DX** | | | | | | | | | | |
| 0–19 Years | 4 | 2.7 | <1 | 2 | 2 | 3 | 3 | 3 | 3 | 3 |
| 20–34 | 18 | 2.2 | 1 | 2 | 2 | 2 | 3 | 3 | 5 | 5 |
| 35–49 | 1 | 11.0 | 0 | 11 | 11 | 11 | 11 | 11 | 11 | 11 |
| 50–64 | 0 | | | | | | | | | |
| 65+ | 0 | | | | | | | | | |
| **TOTAL SINGLE DX** | 2 | 1.8 | <1 | 1 | 2 | 2 | 2 | 2 | 2 | 2 |
| **TOTAL MULTIPLE DX** | 23 | 2.8 | 5 | 1 | 2 | 2 | 3 | 3 | 11 | 11 |
| **TOTAL** | | | | | | | | | | |
| 0–19 Years | 5 | 2.5 | <1 | 2 | 2 | 2 | 3 | 3 | 3 | 3 |
| 20–34 | 19 | 2.2 | 1 | 1 | 1 | 2 | 3 | 3 | 5 | 5 |
| 35–49 | 1 | 11.0 | 0 | 11 | 11 | 11 | 11 | 11 | 11 | 11 |
| 50–64 | 0 | | | | | | | | | |
| 65+ | 0 | | | | | | | | | |
| **GRAND TOTAL** | 25 | 2.7 | 4 | 2 | 2 | 2 | 3 | 3 | 5 | 11 |

## 72.9: INSTRUMENTAL DEL NOS. Formerly included in operation group(s) 707.

| Type of Patients | Observed Patients | Avg. Stay | Vari-ance | Percentiles | | | | | | |
|---|---|---|---|---|---|---|---|---|---|---|
| | | | | 10th | 25th | 50th | 75th | 90th | 95th | 99th |
| **1. SINGLE DX** | | | | | | | | | | |
| 0–19 Years | 12 | 2.1 | <1 | 2 | 2 | 2 | 2 | 3 | 3 | 3 |
| 20–34 | 33 | 1.8 | <1 | 1 | 1 | 2 | 2 | 3 | 3 | 4 |
| 35–49 | 3 | 2.4 | <1 | 2 | 2 | 2 | 3 | 3 | 3 | 3 |
| 50–64 | 0 | | | | | | | | | |
| 65+ | 0 | | | | | | | | | |
| **2. MULTIPLE DX** | | | | | | | | | | |
| 0–19 Years | 28 | 1.9 | <1 | 1 | 1 | 2 | 2 | 3 | 3 | 3 |
| 20–34 | 129 | 2.2 | 1 | 1 | 2 | 2 | 3 | 3 | 4 | 5 |
| 35–49 | 23 | 2.5 | 5 | 1 | 1 | 2 | 3 | 6 | 8 | 10 |
| 50–64 | 0 | | | | | | | | | |
| 65+ | 0 | | | | | | | | | |
| **TOTAL SINGLE DX** | 48 | 1.9 | <1 | 1 | 2 | 2 | 2 | 3 | 3 | 4 |
| **TOTAL MULTIPLE DX** | 180 | 2.2 | 2 | 1 | 1 | 2 | 3 | 3 | 4 | 8 |
| **TOTAL** | | | | | | | | | | |
| 0–19 Years | 40 | 2.0 | <1 | 1 | 2 | 2 | 2 | 3 | 3 | 3 |
| 20–34 | 162 | 2.2 | 1 | 1 | 1 | 2 | 3 | 3 | 4 | 4 |
| 35–49 | 26 | 2.5 | 5 | 1 | 2 | 2 | 3 | 6 | 8 | 10 |
| 50–64 | 0 | | | | | | | | | |
| 65+ | 0 | | | | | | | | | |
| **GRAND TOTAL** | 228 | 2.2 | 1 | 1 | 2 | 2 | 3 | 3 | 4 | 7 |

© 2000 by HCIA-Sachs, L.L.C.

Length of Stay by Diagnosis and Operation, United States, 2000

# United States, October 1998–September 1999 Data, by Operation

## 73.0: ARTIFICIAL RUPT MEMBRANE. Formerly included in operation group(s) 708.

| Type of Patients | Observed Patients | Avg. Stay | Variance | Percentiles | | | | | | |
|---|---|---|---|---|---|---|---|---|---|---|
| | | | | 10th | 25th | 50th | 75th | 90th | 95th | 99th |
| **1. SINGLE DX** | | | | | | | | | | |
| 0–19 Years | 1,653 | 1.9 | 4 | 1 | 1 | 2 | 2 | 3 | 3 | 4 |
| 20–34 | 8,571 | 1.7 | <1 | 1 | 1 | 2 | 2 | 2 | 3 | 3 |
| 35–49 | 727 | 1.8 | 2 | 1 | 1 | 2 | 2 | 2 | 3 | 3 |
| 50–64 | 0 | | | | | | | | | |
| 65+ | 0 | | | | | | | | | |
| **2. MULTIPLE DX** | | | | | | | | | | |
| 0–19 Years | 1,814 | 2.2 | 3 | 1 | 1 | 2 | 2 | 3 | 3 | 15 |
| 20–34 | 9,721 | 2.0 | 2 | 1 | 1 | 2 | 2 | 3 | 3 | 5 |
| 35–49 | 1,409 | 1.9 | 1 | 1 | 1 | 2 | 2 | 3 | 3 | 5 |
| 50–64 | 0 | | | | | | | | | |
| 65+ | 0 | | | | | | | | | |
| **TOTAL SINGLE DX** | 10,951 | 1.7 | 1 | 1 | 1 | 2 | 2 | 2 | 3 | 3 |
| **TOTAL MULTIPLE DX** | 12,944 | 2.0 | 2 | 1 | 1 | 2 | 2 | 3 | 3 | 5 |
| **TOTAL** | | | | | | | | | | |
| 0–19 Years | 3,467 | 2.1 | 3 | 1 | 1 | 2 | 2 | 3 | 3 | 7 |
| 20–34 | 18,292 | 1.8 | 1 | 1 | 1 | 2 | 2 | 3 | 3 | 4 |
| 35–49 | 2,136 | 1.9 | 1 | 1 | 1 | 2 | 2 | 3 | 3 | 5 |
| 50–64 | 0 | | | | | | | | | |
| 65+ | 0 | | | | | | | | | |
| **GRAND TOTAL** | 23,895 | 1.9 | 2 | 1 | 1 | 2 | 2 | 3 | 3 | 4 |

## 73.09: ARTIF RUPT MEMBRANES NEC. Formerly included in operation group(s) 708.

| Type of Patients | Observed Patients | Avg. Stay | Variance | Percentiles | | | | | | |
|---|---|---|---|---|---|---|---|---|---|---|
| | | | | 10th | 25th | 50th | 75th | 90th | 95th | 99th |
| **1. SINGLE DX** | | | | | | | | | | |
| 0–19 Years | 1,504 | 1.9 | 4 | 1 | 1 | 2 | 2 | 3 | 3 | 4 |
| 20–34 | 7,422 | 1.7 | <1 | 1 | 1 | 2 | 2 | 2 | 3 | 3 |
| 35–49 | 606 | 1.8 | 2 | 1 | 1 | 2 | 2 | 2 | 3 | 4 |
| 50–64 | 0 | | | | | | | | | |
| 65+ | 0 | | | | | | | | | |
| **2. MULTIPLE DX** | | | | | | | | | | |
| 0–19 Years | 1,600 | 2.2 | 3 | 1 | 1 | 2 | 2 | 3 | 3 | 15 |
| 20–34 | 8,001 | 1.9 | 2 | 1 | 1 | 2 | 2 | 3 | 3 | 5 |
| 35–49 | 1,100 | 1.9 | 1 | 1 | 1 | 2 | 2 | 3 | 3 | 5 |
| 50–64 | 0 | | | | | | | | | |
| 65+ | 0 | | | | | | | | | |
| **TOTAL SINGLE DX** | 9,532 | 1.8 | 1 | 1 | 1 | 2 | 2 | 2 | 3 | 3 |
| **TOTAL MULTIPLE DX** | 10,701 | 2.0 | 2 | 1 | 1 | 2 | 2 | 3 | 3 | 5 |
| **TOTAL** | | | | | | | | | | |
| 0–19 Years | 3,104 | 2.1 | 4 | 1 | 1 | 2 | 2 | 3 | 3 | 7 |
| 20–34 | 15,423 | 1.8 | 1 | 1 | 1 | 2 | 2 | 3 | 3 | 4 |
| 35–49 | 1,706 | 1.9 | 1 | 1 | 1 | 2 | 2 | 3 | 3 | 5 |
| 50–64 | 0 | | | | | | | | | |
| 65+ | 0 | | | | | | | | | |
| **GRAND TOTAL** | 20,233 | 1.9 | 2 | 1 | 1 | 2 | 2 | 3 | 3 | 4 |

## 73.01: INDUCTION LABOR BY AROM. Formerly included in operation group(s) 708.

| Type of Patients | Observed Patients | Avg. Stay | Variance | Percentiles | | | | | | |
|---|---|---|---|---|---|---|---|---|---|---|
| | | | | 10th | 25th | 50th | 75th | 90th | 95th | 99th |
| **1. SINGLE DX** | | | | | | | | | | |
| 0–19 Years | 149 | 1.7 | <1 | 1 | 1 | 2 | 2 | 3 | 3 | 3 |
| 20–34 | 1,149 | 1.7 | <1 | 1 | 1 | 2 | 2 | 2 | 3 | 3 |
| 35–49 | 121 | 1.7 | <1 | 1 | 1 | 2 | 2 | 2 | 3 | 3 |
| 50–64 | 0 | | | | | | | | | |
| 65+ | 0 | | | | | | | | | |
| **2. MULTIPLE DX** | | | | | | | | | | |
| 0–19 Years | 214 | 2.1 | <1 | 1 | 2 | 2 | 2 | 3 | 3 | 4 |
| 20–34 | 1,720 | 2.0 | 2 | 1 | 2 | 2 | 2 | 3 | 3 | 5 |
| 35–49 | 309 | 2.0 | <1 | 1 | 2 | 2 | 2 | 3 | 3 | 5 |
| 50–64 | 0 | | | | | | | | | |
| 65+ | 0 | | | | | | | | | |
| **TOTAL SINGLE DX** | 1,419 | 1.7 | <1 | 1 | 1 | 2 | 2 | 2 | 3 | 3 |
| **TOTAL MULTIPLE DX** | 2,243 | 2.0 | 2 | 1 | 2 | 2 | 2 | 3 | 3 | 5 |
| **TOTAL** | | | | | | | | | | |
| 0–19 Years | 363 | 2.0 | <1 | 1 | 1 | 2 | 2 | 3 | 3 | 4 |
| 20–34 | 2,869 | 1.9 | 2 | 1 | 1 | 2 | 2 | 3 | 3 | 4 |
| 35–49 | 430 | 1.9 | <1 | 1 | 1 | 2 | 2 | 3 | 3 | 5 |
| 50–64 | 0 | | | | | | | | | |
| 65+ | 0 | | | | | | | | | |
| **GRAND TOTAL** | 3,662 | 1.9 | 1 | 1 | 1 | 2 | 2 | 3 | 3 | 4 |

## 73.1: SURG INDUCTION LABOR NEC. Formerly included in operation group(s) 708.

| Type of Patients | Observed Patients | Avg. Stay | Variance | Percentiles | | | | | | |
|---|---|---|---|---|---|---|---|---|---|---|
| | | | | 10th | 25th | 50th | 75th | 90th | 95th | 99th |
| **1. SINGLE DX** | | | | | | | | | | |
| 0–19 Years | 13 | 2.1 | 1 | 1 | 1 | 2 | 3 | 4 | 4 | 4 |
| 20–34 | 91 | 2.0 | <1 | 1 | 1 | 2 | 2 | 3 | 3 | 5 |
| 35–49 | 8 | 2.0 | <1 | 2 | 2 | 2 | 2 | 2 | 2 | 3 |
| 50–64 | 0 | | | | | | | | | |
| 65+ | 0 | | | | | | | | | |
| **2. MULTIPLE DX** | | | | | | | | | | |
| 0–19 Years | 37 | 2.3 | 1 | 1 | 2 | 2 | 3 | 3 | 3 | 7 |
| 20–34 | 186 | 2.5 | 2 | 1 | 1 | 2 | 3 | 4 | 4 | 10 |
| 35–49 | 23 | 2.7 | <1 | 2 | 2 | 3 | 3 | 3 | 4 | 5 |
| 50–64 | 0 | | | | | | | | | |
| 65+ | 0 | | | | | | | | | |
| **TOTAL SINGLE DX** | 112 | 2.0 | <1 | 1 | 1 | 2 | 2 | 3 | 3 | 5 |
| **TOTAL MULTIPLE DX** | 246 | 2.5 | 2 | 1 | 1 | 2 | 3 | 4 | 4 | 7 |
| **TOTAL** | | | | | | | | | | |
| 0–19 Years | 50 | 2.3 | 1 | 1 | 2 | 2 | 3 | 3 | 4 | 7 |
| 20–34 | 277 | 2.3 | 2 | 1 | 1 | 2 | 3 | 4 | 4 | 7 |
| 35–49 | 31 | 2.4 | <1 | 2 | 2 | 2 | 3 | 3 | 4 | 4 |
| 50–64 | 0 | | | | | | | | | |
| 65+ | 0 | | | | | | | | | |
| **GRAND TOTAL** | 358 | 2.3 | 2 | 1 | 1 | 2 | 3 | 4 | 4 | 7 |

Length of Stay by Diagnosis and Operation, United States, 2000

# United States, October 1998–September 1999 Data, by Operation

## 73.2: INT/COMB VERSION/EXTRACT. Formerly included in operation group(s) 707.

| Type of Patients | Observed Patients | Avg. Stay | Variance | Percentiles | | | | | | |
|---|---|---|---|---|---|---|---|---|---|---|
| | | | | 10th | 25th | 50th | 75th | 90th | 95th | 99th |
| **1. SINGLE DX** | | | | | | | | | | |
| 0–19 Years | 3 | 1.0 | 0 | 1 | 1 | 1 | 1 | 1 | 1 | 1 |
| 20–34 | 15 | 1.3 | <1 | 1 | 1 | 1 | 2 | 2 | 2 | 2 |
| 35–49 | 7 | 1.5 | <1 | 1 | 1 | 1 | 2 | 2 | 3 | 3 |
| 50–64 | 0 | | | | | | | | | |
| 65+ | 0 | | | | | | | | | |
| **2. MULTIPLE DX** | | | | | | | | | | |
| 0–19 Years | 5 | 3.7 | 2 | 2 | 3 | 4 | 5 | 5 | 5 | 5 |
| 20–34 | 40 | 2.4 | <1 | 2 | 2 | 2 | 3 | 4 | 4 | 4 |
| 35–49 | 13 | 2.2 | <1 | 1 | 2 | 2 | 3 | 3 | 3 | 3 |
| 50–64 | 0 | | | | | | | | | |
| 65+ | 0 | | | | | | | | | |
| **TOTAL SINGLE DX** | 25 | 1.3 | <1 | 1 | 1 | 1 | 2 | 2 | 2 | 3 |
| **TOTAL MULTIPLE DX** | 58 | 2.4 | <1 | 2 | 2 | 2 | 3 | 4 | 4 | 5 |
| **TOTAL** | | | | | | | | | | |
| 0–19 Years | 8 | 2.9 | 3 | 1 | 1 | 3 | 4 | 5 | 5 | 5 |
| 20–34 | 55 | 2.1 | <1 | 1 | 2 | 2 | 2 | 3 | 3 | 4 |
| 35–49 | 20 | 2.1 | <1 | 1 | 2 | 2 | 2 | 3 | 3 | 3 |
| 50–64 | 0 | | | | | | | | | |
| 65+ | 0 | | | | | | | | | |
| **GRAND TOTAL** | 83 | 2.2 | <1 | 1 | 2 | 2 | 3 | 4 | 4 | 5 |

## 73.3: FAILED FORCEPS. Formerly included in operation group(s) 708.

| Type of Patients | Observed Patients | Avg. Stay | Variance | Percentiles | | | | | | |
|---|---|---|---|---|---|---|---|---|---|---|
| | | | | 10th | 25th | 50th | 75th | 90th | 95th | 99th |
| **1. SINGLE DX** | | | | | | | | | | |
| 0–19 Years | 0 | | | | | | | | | |
| 20–34 | 2 | 2.0 | 0 | 2 | 2 | 2 | 2 | 2 | 2 | 2 |
| 35–49 | 0 | | | | | | | | | |
| 50–64 | 0 | | | | | | | | | |
| 65+ | 0 | | | | | | | | | |
| **2. MULTIPLE DX** | | | | | | | | | | |
| 0–19 Years | 3 | 2.0 | 0 | 2 | 2 | 2 | 2 | 2 | 2 | 2 |
| 20–34 | 10 | 3.1 | 1 | 2 | 2 | 3 | 4 | 4 | 5 | 5 |
| 35–49 | 0 | | | | | | | | | |
| 50–64 | 0 | | | | | | | | | |
| 65+ | 0 | | | | | | | | | |
| **TOTAL SINGLE DX** | 2 | 2.0 | 0 | 2 | 2 | 2 | 2 | 2 | 2 | 2 |
| **TOTAL MULTIPLE DX** | 13 | 2.7 | 1 | 2 | 2 | 2 | 4 | 4 | 4 | 5 |
| **TOTAL** | | | | | | | | | | |
| 0–19 Years | 3 | 2.0 | 0 | 2 | 2 | 2 | 2 | 2 | 2 | 2 |
| 20–34 | 12 | 2.9 | 1 | 2 | 2 | 3 | 4 | 4 | 5 | 5 |
| 35–49 | 0 | | | | | | | | | |
| 50–64 | 0 | | | | | | | | | |
| 65+ | 0 | | | | | | | | | |
| **GRAND TOTAL** | 15 | 2.6 | 1 | 2 | 2 | 2 | 3 | 4 | 4 | 5 |

## 73.4: MEDICAL INDUCTION LABOR. Formerly included in operation group(s) 708.

| Type of Patients | Observed Patients | Avg. Stay | Variance | Percentiles | | | | | | |
|---|---|---|---|---|---|---|---|---|---|---|
| | | | | 10th | 25th | 50th | 75th | 90th | 95th | 99th |
| **1. SINGLE DX** | | | | | | | | | | |
| 0–19 Years | 741 | 1.9 | <1 | 1 | 1 | 2 | 2 | 3 | 3 | 4 |
| 20–34 | 4,565 | 1.7 | <1 | 1 | 1 | 2 | 2 | 3 | 3 | 4 |
| 35–49 | 516 | 1.8 | <1 | 1 | 1 | 2 | 2 | 3 | 3 | 4 |
| 50–64 | 0 | | | | | | | | | |
| 65+ | 0 | | | | | | | | | |
| **2. MULTIPLE DX** | | | | | | | | | | |
| 0–19 Years | 1,631 | 2.5 | 4 | 1 | 2 | 2 | 3 | 4 | 4 | 8 |
| 20–34 | 10,458 | 2.2 | 3 | 1 | 1 | 2 | 3 | 3 | 4 | 7 |
| 35–49 | 1,922 | 2.2 | 3 | 1 | 1 | 2 | 3 | 3 | 4 | 8 |
| 50–64 | 1 | 1.0 | 0 | 1 | 1 | 1 | 1 | 1 | 1 | 1 |
| 65+ | 0 | | | | | | | | | |
| **TOTAL SINGLE DX** | 5,822 | 1.8 | <1 | 1 | 1 | 2 | 2 | 3 | 3 | 4 |
| **TOTAL MULTIPLE DX** | 14,012 | 2.2 | 3 | 1 | 1 | 2 | 3 | 3 | 4 | 7 |
| **TOTAL** | | | | | | | | | | |
| 0–19 Years | 2,372 | 2.3 | 3 | 1 | 1 | 2 | 3 | 4 | 4 | 7 |
| 20–34 | 15,023 | 2.1 | 2 | 1 | 1 | 2 | 2 | 3 | 4 | 6 |
| 35–49 | 2,438 | 2.1 | 2 | 1 | 1 | 2 | 2 | 3 | 4 | 7 |
| 50–64 | 1 | 1.0 | 0 | 1 | 1 | 1 | 1 | 1 | 1 | 1 |
| 65+ | 0 | | | | | | | | | |
| **GRAND TOTAL** | 19,834 | 2.1 | 2 | 1 | 1 | 2 | 2 | 3 | 4 | 6 |

## 73.5: MANUALLY ASSISTED DEL. Formerly included in operation group(s) 708.

| Type of Patients | Observed Patients | Avg. Stay | Variance | Percentiles | | | | | | |
|---|---|---|---|---|---|---|---|---|---|---|
| | | | | 10th | 25th | 50th | 75th | 90th | 95th | 99th |
| **1. SINGLE DX** | | | | | | | | | | |
| 0–19 Years | 24,797 | 1.8 | <1 | 1 | 1 | 2 | 2 | 3 | 3 | 4 |
| 20–34 | 118,306 | 1.7 | <1 | 1 | 1 | 2 | 2 | 3 | 3 | 3 |
| 35–49 | 11,331 | 1.8 | <1 | 1 | 1 | 2 | 2 | 3 | 3 | 3 |
| 50–64 | 0 | | | | | | | | | |
| 65+ | 0 | | | | | | | | | |
| **2. MULTIPLE DX** | | | | | | | | | | |
| 0–19 Years | 29,395 | 2.3 | 5 | 1 | 2 | 2 | 2 | 3 | 4 | 9 |
| 20–34 | 148,491 | 2.1 | 3 | 1 | 1 | 2 | 2 | 3 | 3 | 7 |
| 35–49 | 24,403 | 2.1 | 4 | 1 | 1 | 2 | 2 | 3 | 3 | 7 |
| 50–64 | 5 | 4.6 | 10 | 2 | 2 | 3 | 5 | 11 | 11 | 11 |
| 65+ | 0 | | | | | | | | | |
| **TOTAL SINGLE DX** | 154,434 | 1.7 | <1 | 1 | 1 | 2 | 2 | 3 | 3 | 3 |
| **TOTAL MULTIPLE DX** | 202,294 | 2.1 | 4 | 1 | 1 | 2 | 2 | 3 | 3 | 7 |
| **TOTAL** | | | | | | | | | | |
| 0–19 Years | 54,192 | 2.1 | 3 | 1 | 1 | 2 | 2 | 3 | 3 | 7 |
| 20–34 | 266,797 | 1.9 | 2 | 1 | 1 | 2 | 2 | 3 | 3 | 5 |
| 35–49 | 35,734 | 2.0 | 3 | 1 | 1 | 2 | 2 | 3 | 3 | 6 |
| 50–64 | 5 | 4.6 | 10 | 2 | 2 | 3 | 5 | 11 | 11 | 11 |
| 65+ | 0 | | | | | | | | | |
| **GRAND TOTAL** | 356,728 | 1.9 | 2 | 1 | 1 | 2 | 2 | 3 | 3 | 5 |

# United States, October 1998–September 1999 Data, by Operation

## 73.51: MANUAL ROT FETAL HEAD. Formerly included in operation group(s) 708.

| Type of Patients | Observed Patients | Avg. Stay | Vari-ance | Percentiles | | | | | | |
|---|---|---|---|---|---|---|---|---|---|---|
| | | | | 10th | 25th | 50th | 75th | 90th | 95th | 99th |
| **1. SINGLE DX** | | | | | | | | | | |
| 0–19 Years | 13 | 2.0 | <1 | 2 | 2 | 2 | 2 | 2 | 3 | 3 |
| 20–34 | 79 | 1.7 | <1 | 1 | 1 | 2 | 2 | 3 | 3 | 3 |
| 35–49 | 8 | 1.8 | <1 | 1 | 1 | 2 | 2 | 3 | 3 | 3 |
| 50–64 | 0 | | | | | | | | | |
| 65+ | 0 | | | | | | | | | |
| **2. MULTIPLE DX** | | | | | | | | | | |
| 0–19 Years | 45 | 2.2 | <1 | 1 | 2 | 2 | 3 | 3 | 4 | 4 |
| 20–34 | 292 | 1.8 | <1 | 1 | 1 | 2 | 2 | 3 | 3 | 3 |
| 35–49 | 49 | 2.0 | <1 | 1 | 2 | 2 | 2 | 3 | 3 | 5 |
| 50–64 | 1 | 3.0 | 0 | 3 | 3 | 3 | 3 | 3 | 3 | 3 |
| 65+ | 0 | | | | | | | | | |
| **TOTAL SINGLE DX** | 100 | 1.7 | <1 | 1 | 1 | 2 | 2 | 3 | 3 | 3 |
| **TOTAL MULTIPLE DX** | 387 | 1.9 | <1 | 1 | 1 | 2 | 2 | 3 | 3 | 4 |
| **TOTAL** | | | | | | | | | | |
| 0–19 Years | 58 | 2.2 | <1 | 2 | 2 | 2 | 2 | 3 | 4 | 4 |
| 20–34 | 371 | 1.8 | <1 | 1 | 1 | 2 | 2 | 3 | 3 | 3 |
| 35–49 | 57 | 2.0 | <1 | 1 | 2 | 2 | 2 | 3 | 3 | 5 |
| 50–64 | 1 | 3.0 | 0 | 3 | 3 | 3 | 3 | 3 | 3 | 3 |
| 65+ | 0 | | | | | | | | | |
| **GRAND TOTAL** | 487 | 1.9 | <1 | 1 | 1 | 2 | 2 | 3 | 3 | 4 |

## 73.6: EPISIOTOMY. Formerly included in operation group(s) 708.

| Type of Patients | Observed Patients | Avg. Stay | Vari-ance | Percentiles | | | | | | |
|---|---|---|---|---|---|---|---|---|---|---|
| | | | | 10th | 25th | 50th | 75th | 90th | 95th | 99th |
| **1. SINGLE DX** | | | | | | | | | | |
| 0–19 Years | 16,884 | 1.9 | <1 | 1 | 1 | 2 | 2 | 3 | 3 | 4 |
| 20–34 | 74,087 | 1.9 | <1 | 1 | 1 | 2 | 2 | 3 | 3 | 3 |
| 35–49 | 8,643 | 1.9 | <1 | 1 | 2 | 2 | 2 | 3 | 3 | 3 |
| 50–64 | 1 | 2.0 | 0 | 2 | 2 | 2 | 2 | 2 | 2 | 2 |
| 65+ | 0 | | | | | | | | | |
| **2. MULTIPLE DX** | | | | | | | | | | |
| 0–19 Years | 12,379 | 2.3 | 2 | 1 | 2 | 2 | 3 | 3 | 4 | 6 |
| 20–34 | 56,190 | 2.2 | 2 | 1 | 2 | 2 | 3 | 3 | 3 | 6 |
| 35–49 | 10,717 | 2.2 | 2 | 1 | 2 | 2 | 2 | 3 | 3 | 6 |
| 50–64 | 0 | | | | | | | | | |
| 65+ | 0 | | | | | | | | | |
| **TOTAL SINGLE DX** | 99,615 | 1.9 | <1 | 1 | 1 | 2 | 2 | 3 | 3 | 3 |
| **TOTAL MULTIPLE DX** | 79,286 | 2.2 | 2 | 1 | 2 | 2 | 2 | 3 | 3 | 6 |
| **TOTAL** | | | | | | | | | | |
| 0–19 Years | 29,263 | 2.0 | 1 | 1 | 2 | 2 | 2 | 3 | 3 | 5 |
| 20–34 | 130,277 | 2.0 | 1 | 1 | 2 | 2 | 2 | 3 | 3 | 4 |
| 35–49 | 19,360 | 2.1 | 1 | 1 | 2 | 2 | 2 | 3 | 3 | 4 |
| 50–64 | 1 | 2.0 | 0 | 2 | 2 | 2 | 2 | 2 | 2 | 2 |
| 65+ | 0 | | | | | | | | | |
| **GRAND TOTAL** | 178,901 | 2.0 | 1 | 1 | 2 | 2 | 2 | 3 | 3 | 4 |

## 73.59: MANUAL ASSISTED DEL NEC. Formerly included in operation group(s) 708.

| Type of Patients | Observed Patients | Avg. Stay | Vari-ance | Percentiles | | | | | | |
|---|---|---|---|---|---|---|---|---|---|---|
| | | | | 10th | 25th | 50th | 75th | 90th | 95th | 99th |
| **1. SINGLE DX** | | | | | | | | | | |
| 0–19 Years | 24,784 | 1.8 | <1 | 1 | 1 | 2 | 2 | 3 | 3 | 4 |
| 20–34 | 118,227 | 1.7 | <1 | 1 | 1 | 2 | 2 | 2 | 3 | 3 |
| 35–49 | 11,323 | 1.8 | <1 | 1 | 1 | 2 | 2 | 3 | 3 | 3 |
| 50–64 | 0 | | | | | | | | | |
| 65+ | 0 | | | | | | | | | |
| **2. MULTIPLE DX** | | | | | | | | | | |
| 0–19 Years | 29,350 | 2.3 | 5 | 1 | 2 | 2 | 2 | 3 | 4 | 9 |
| 20–34 | 148,199 | 2.1 | 3 | 1 | 1 | 2 | 2 | 3 | 3 | 7 |
| 35–49 | 24,354 | 2.1 | 4 | 1 | 1 | 2 | 2 | 3 | 3 | 7 |
| 50–64 | 4 | 5.1 | 13 | 2 | 2 | 5 | 5 | 11 | 11 | 11 |
| 65+ | 0 | | | | | | | | | |
| **TOTAL SINGLE DX** | 154,334 | 1.7 | <1 | 1 | 1 | 2 | 2 | 2 | 3 | 3 |
| **TOTAL MULTIPLE DX** | 201,907 | 2.1 | 4 | 1 | 1 | 2 | 2 | 3 | 3 | 7 |
| **TOTAL** | | | | | | | | | | |
| 0–19 Years | 54,134 | 2.1 | 3 | 1 | 1 | 2 | 2 | 3 | 3 | 7 |
| 20–34 | 266,426 | 1.9 | 2 | 1 | 1 | 2 | 2 | 3 | 3 | 5 |
| 35–49 | 35,677 | 2.0 | 3 | 1 | 1 | 2 | 2 | 3 | 3 | 6 |
| 50–64 | 4 | 5.1 | 13 | 2 | 2 | 5 | 5 | 11 | 11 | 11 |
| 65+ | 0 | | | | | | | | | |
| **GRAND TOTAL** | 356,241 | 1.9 | 2 | 1 | 1 | 2 | 2 | 3 | 3 | 5 |

## 73.8: FETAL OPS-FACILITATE DEL. Formerly included in operation group(s) 716.

| Type of Patients | Observed Patients | Avg. Stay | Vari-ance | Percentiles | | | | | | |
|---|---|---|---|---|---|---|---|---|---|---|
| | | | | 10th | 25th | 50th | 75th | 90th | 95th | 99th |
| **1. SINGLE DX** | | | | | | | | | | |
| 0–19 Years | 0 | | | | | | | | | |
| 20–34 | 1 | 2.0 | 0 | 2 | 2 | 2 | 2 | 2 | 2 | 2 |
| 35–49 | 0 | | | | | | | | | |
| 50–64 | 0 | | | | | | | | | |
| 65+ | 0 | | | | | | | | | |
| **2. MULTIPLE DX** | | | | | | | | | | |
| 0–19 Years | 0 | | | | | | | | | |
| 20–34 | 2 | 5.3 | 16 | 2 | 2 | 8 | 8 | 8 | 8 | 8 |
| 35–49 | 0 | | | | | | | | | |
| 50–64 | 0 | | | | | | | | | |
| 65+ | 0 | | | | | | | | | |
| **TOTAL SINGLE DX** | 1 | 2.0 | 0 | 2 | 2 | 2 | 2 | 2 | 2 | 2 |
| **TOTAL MULTIPLE DX** | 2 | 5.3 | 16 | 2 | 2 | 8 | 8 | 8 | 8 | 8 |
| **TOTAL** | | | | | | | | | | |
| 0–19 Years | 0 | | | | | | | | | |
| 20–34 | 3 | 3.0 | 6 | 2 | 2 | 2 | 2 | 8 | 8 | 8 |
| 35–49 | 0 | | | | | | | | | |
| 50–64 | 0 | | | | | | | | | |
| 65+ | 0 | | | | | | | | | |
| **GRAND TOTAL** | 3 | 3.0 | 6 | 2 | 2 | 2 | 2 | 8 | 8 | 8 |

Length of Stay by Diagnosis and Operation, United States, 2000

# United States, October 1998–September 1999 Data, by Operation

## 73.9: OTH OPS ASSISTING DEL. Formerly included in operation group(s) 708, 716.

| Type of Patients | Observed Patients | Avg. Stay | Variance | 10th | 25th | 50th | 75th | 90th | 95th | 99th |
|---|---|---|---|---|---|---|---|---|---|---|
| **1. SINGLE DX** | | | | | | | | | | |
| 0–19 Years | 10 | 1.7 | <1 | 1 | 1 | 2 | 2 | 3 | 3 | 3 |
| 20–34 | 59 | 1.3 | <1 | 1 | 1 | 1 | 1 | 2 | 3 | 3 |
| 35–49 | 8 | 1.1 | <1 | 1 | 1 | 1 | 1 | 1 | 3 | 3 |
| 50–64 | 0 | | | | | | | | | |
| 65+ | 0 | | | | | | | | | |
| **2. MULTIPLE DX** | | | | | | | | | | |
| 0–19 Years | 24 | 2.6 | 3 | 1 | 1 | 2 | 3 | 4 | 4 | 10 |
| 20–34 | 221 | 2.0 | 1 | 1 | 1 | 2 | 3 | 3 | 4 | 5 |
| 35–49 | 55 | 2.2 | 4 | 1 | 1 | 2 | 2 | 3 | 5 | 12 |
| 50–64 | 0 | | | | | | | | | |
| 65+ | 0 | | | | | | | | | |
| **TOTAL SINGLE DX** | 77 | 1.3 | <1 | 1 | 1 | 1 | 1 | 3 | 3 | 3 |
| **TOTAL MULTIPLE DX** | 300 | 2.1 | 2 | 1 | 1 | 2 | 3 | 3 | 4 | 7 |
| **TOTAL** | | | | | | | | | | |
| 0–19 Years | 34 | 2.3 | 2 | 1 | 1 | 2 | 3 | 4 | 4 | 10 |
| 20–34 | 280 | 1.9 | 1 | 1 | 1 | 2 | 2 | 3 | 4 | 4 |
| 35–49 | 63 | 2.0 | 4 | 1 | 1 | 2 | 2 | 3 | 5 | 12 |
| 50–64 | 0 | | | | | | | | | |
| 65+ | 0 | | | | | | | | | |
| **GRAND TOTAL** | 377 | 1.9 | 2 | 1 | 1 | 2 | 2 | 3 | 4 | 6 |

## 74.1: LOW CERVICAL CD. Formerly included in operation group(s) 709.

| Type of Patients | Observed Patients | Avg. Stay | Variance | 10th | 25th | 50th | 75th | 90th | 95th | 99th |
|---|---|---|---|---|---|---|---|---|---|---|
| **1. SINGLE DX** | | | | | | | | | | |
| 0–19 Years | 3,747 | 3.0 | <1 | 2 | 2 | 3 | 3 | 4 | 4 | 5 |
| 20–34 | 29,295 | 3.0 | <1 | 2 | 2 | 3 | 3 | 4 | 4 | 5 |
| 35–49 | 4,071 | 3.2 | <1 | 2 | 3 | 3 | 4 | 4 | 4 | 5 |
| 50–64 | 0 | | | | | | | | | |
| 65+ | 0 | | | | | | | | | |
| **2. MULTIPLE DX** | | | | | | | | | | |
| 0–19 Years | 20,185 | 3.9 | 7 | 2 | 3 | 3 | 4 | 5 | 7 | 13 |
| 20–34 | 162,364 | 3.6 | 7 | 2 | 3 | 3 | 4 | 5 | 6 | 12 |
| 35–49 | 40,446 | 3.8 | 10 | 2 | 3 | 3 | 4 | 5 | 6 | 16 |
| 50–64 | 19 | 9.8 | 64 | 4 | 4 | 5 | 22 | 22 | 22 | 22 |
| 65+ | 0 | | | | | | | | | |
| **TOTAL SINGLE DX** | 37,113 | 3.0 | <1 | 2 | 2 | 3 | 3 | 4 | 4 | 5 |
| **TOTAL MULTIPLE DX** | 223,014 | 3.7 | 7 | 2 | 3 | 3 | 4 | 5 | 6 | 13 |
| **TOTAL** | | | | | | | | | | |
| 0–19 Years | 23,932 | 3.7 | 6 | 2 | 3 | 3 | 4 | 5 | 6 | 12 |
| 20–34 | 191,659 | 3.5 | 6 | 2 | 3 | 3 | 4 | 5 | 6 | 11 |
| 35–49 | 44,517 | 3.7 | 9 | 2 | 3 | 3 | 4 | 5 | 6 | 15 |
| 50–64 | 19 | 9.8 | 64 | 4 | 4 | 5 | 22 | 22 | 22 | 22 |
| 65+ | 0 | | | | | | | | | |
| **GRAND TOTAL** | 260,127 | 3.6 | 6 | 2 | 3 | 3 | 4 | 5 | 5 | 12 |

## 74.0: CLASSICAL CD. Formerly included in operation group(s) 710.

| Type of Patients | Observed Patients | Avg. Stay | Variance | 10th | 25th | 50th | 75th | 90th | 95th | 99th |
|---|---|---|---|---|---|---|---|---|---|---|
| **1. SINGLE DX** | | | | | | | | | | |
| 0–19 Years | 10 | 3.2 | <1 | 3 | 3 | 3 | 4 | 4 | 4 | 4 |
| 20–34 | 148 | 3.0 | <1 | 2 | 3 | 3 | 3 | 3 | 4 | 4 |
| 35–49 | 32 | 3.3 | <1 | 2 | 3 | 3 | 4 | 5 | 5 | 5 |
| 50–64 | 0 | | | | | | | | | |
| 65+ | 0 | | | | | | | | | |
| **2. MULTIPLE DX** | | | | | | | | | | |
| 0–19 Years | 327 | 5.0 | 24 | 2 | 3 | 3 | 5 | 9 | 14 | 24 |
| 20–34 | 2,473 | 6.0 | 47 | 3 | 3 | 4 | 6 | 12 | 18 | 35 |
| 35–49 | 717 | 7.0 | 115 | 3 | 3 | 5 | 7 | 14 | 20 | 79 |
| 50–64 | 1 | 44.0 | 0 | 44 | 44 | 44 | 44 | 44 | 44 | 44 |
| 65+ | 0 | | | | | | | | | |
| **TOTAL SINGLE DX** | 190 | 3.0 | <1 | 2 | 3 | 3 | 3 | 4 | 4 | 5 |
| **TOTAL MULTIPLE DX** | 3,518 | 6.1 | 60 | 2 | 3 | 4 | 6 | 12 | 18 | 42 |
| **TOTAL** | | | | | | | | | | |
| 0–19 Years | 337 | 4.9 | 24 | 2 | 3 | 3 | 5 | 9 | 14 | 24 |
| 20–34 | 2,621 | 5.8 | 45 | 2 | 3 | 4 | 6 | 11 | 18 | 35 |
| 35–49 | 749 | 6.8 | 111 | 3 | 3 | 4 | 5 | 14 | 20 | 79 |
| 50–64 | 1 | 44.0 | 0 | 44 | 44 | 44 | 44 | 44 | 44 | 44 |
| 65+ | 0 | | | | | | | | | |
| **GRAND TOTAL** | 3,708 | 6.0 | 58 | 2 | 3 | 4 | 5 | 11 | 18 | 41 |

## 74.2: EXTRAPERITONEAL CD. Formerly included in operation group(s) 711.

| Type of Patients | Observed Patients | Avg. Stay | Variance | 10th | 25th | 50th | 75th | 90th | 95th | 99th |
|---|---|---|---|---|---|---|---|---|---|---|
| **1. SINGLE DX** | | | | | | | | | | |
| 0–19 Years | 0 | | | | | | | | | |
| 20–34 | 3 | 3.0 | 1 | 2 | 2 | 3 | 4 | 4 | 4 | 4 |
| 35–49 | 1 | 2.0 | 0 | 2 | 2 | 2 | 2 | 2 | 2 | 2 |
| 50–64 | 0 | | | | | | | | | |
| 65+ | 0 | | | | | | | | | |
| **2. MULTIPLE DX** | | | | | | | | | | |
| 0–19 Years | 0 | | | | | | | | | |
| 20–34 | 32 | 3.0 | <1 | 2 | 3 | 3 | 4 | 4 | 4 | 5 |
| 35–49 | 10 | 3.6 | <1 | 3 | 3 | 4 | 4 | 4 | 4 | 4 |
| 50–64 | 0 | | | | | | | | | |
| 65+ | 0 | | | | | | | | | |
| **TOTAL SINGLE DX** | 4 | 2.7 | <1 | 2 | 2 | 2 | 4 | 4 | 4 | 4 |
| **TOTAL MULTIPLE DX** | 42 | 3.1 | <1 | 2 | 3 | 3 | 4 | 4 | 4 | 5 |
| **TOTAL** | | | | | | | | | | |
| 0–19 Years | 0 | | | | | | | | | |
| 20–34 | 35 | 3.0 | <1 | 2 | 2 | 3 | 4 | 4 | 4 | 5 |
| 35–49 | 11 | 3.5 | <1 | 2 | 3 | 4 | 4 | 4 | 4 | 4 |
| 50–64 | 0 | | | | | | | | | |
| 65+ | 0 | | | | | | | | | |
| **GRAND TOTAL** | 46 | 3.1 | <1 | 2 | 2 | 3 | 4 | 4 | 4 | 5 |

Length of Stay by Diagnosis and Operation, United States, 2000

# United States, October 1998–September 1999 Data, by Operation

## 74.3: RMVL EXTRATUBAL PREG. Formerly included in operation group(s) 712.

| Type of Patients | Observed Patients | Avg. Stay | Variance | Percentiles | | | | | | |
|---|---|---|---|---|---|---|---|---|---|---|
| | | | | 10th | 25th | 50th | 75th | 90th | 95th | 99th |
| **1. SINGLE DX** | | | | | | | | | | |
| 0–19 Years | 9 | 2.6 | <1 | 2 | 2 | 3 | 3 | 3 | 3 | 4 |
| 20–34 | 66 | 2.4 | 2 | 1 | 1 | 3 | 3 | 3 | 6 | 6 |
| 35–49 | 13 | 2.3 | 1 | 1 | 1 | 2 | 3 | 4 | 4 | 4 |
| 50–64 | 0 | | | | | | | | | |
| 65+ | 0 | | | | | | | | | |
| **2. MULTIPLE DX** | | | | | | | | | | |
| 0–19 Years | 13 | 3.0 | 10 | 1 | 1 | 2 | 3 | 4 | 12 | 12 |
| 20–34 | 153 | 3.0 | 9 | 1 | 2 | 2 | 3 | 4 | 6 | 23 |
| 35–49 | 56 | 2.9 | 2 | 1 | 2 | 3 | 4 | 4 | 5 | 5 |
| 50–64 | 0 | | | | | | | | | |
| 65+ | 0 | | | | | | | | | |
| **TOTAL SINGLE DX** | 88 | 2.4 | 2 | 1 | 2 | 2 | 3 | 4 | 6 | 6 |
| **TOTAL MULTIPLE DX** | 222 | 3.0 | 7 | 1 | 2 | 3 | 3 | 4 | 6 | 12 |
| **TOTAL** | | | | | | | | | | |
| 0–19 Years | 22 | 2.8 | 6 | 1 | 2 | 2 | 3 | 4 | 12 | 12 |
| 20–34 | 219 | 2.8 | 7 | 1 | 2 | 2 | 3 | 4 | 6 | 23 |
| 35–49 | 69 | 2.8 | 2 | 1 | 2 | 3 | 3 | 4 | 5 | 5 |
| 50–64 | 0 | | | | | | | | | |
| 65+ | 0 | | | | | | | | | |
| **GRAND TOTAL** | 310 | 2.8 | 5 | 1 | 2 | 3 | 3 | 4 | 6 | 12 |

## 74.4: CESAREAN SECTION NEC. Formerly included in operation group(s) 711.

| Type of Patients | Observed Patients | Avg. Stay | Variance | Percentiles | | | | | | |
|---|---|---|---|---|---|---|---|---|---|---|
| | | | | 10th | 25th | 50th | 75th | 90th | 95th | 99th |
| **1. SINGLE DX** | | | | | | | | | | |
| 0–19 Years | 3 | 2.9 | <1 | 2 | 2 | 3 | 4 | 4 | 4 | 4 |
| 20–34 | 46 | 3.2 | 5 | 2 | 2 | 3 | 3 | 4 | 6 | 14 |
| 35–49 | 6 | 2.7 | <1 | 2 | 2 | 3 | 3 | 4 | 4 | 4 |
| 50–64 | 0 | | | | | | | | | |
| 65+ | 0 | | | | | | | | | |
| **2. MULTIPLE DX** | | | | | | | | | | |
| 0–19 Years | 48 | 5.3 | 9 | 2 | 3 | 4 | 8 | 8 | 8 | 16 |
| 20–34 | 371 | 6.4 | 78 | 2 | 3 | 3 | 5 | 12 | 30 | 40 |
| 35–49 | 112 | 4.3 | 13 | 3 | 3 | 3 | 5 | 6 | 10 | 16 |
| 50–64 | 0 | | | | | | | | | |
| 65+ | 0 | | | | | | | | | |
| **TOTAL SINGLE DX** | 55 | 3.2 | 5 | 2 | 2 | 3 | 3 | 4 | 6 | 14 |
| **TOTAL MULTIPLE DX** | 531 | 5.9 | 57 | 2 | 3 | 3 | 5 | 9 | 27 | 37 |
| **TOTAL** | | | | | | | | | | |
| 0–19 Years | 51 | 5.3 | 9 | 2 | 3 | 4 | 8 | 8 | 8 | 16 |
| 20–34 | 417 | 6.0 | 70 | 2 | 3 | 3 | 5 | 11 | 27 | 40 |
| 35–49 | 118 | 4.3 | 13 | 2 | 3 | 3 | 4 | 6 | 8 | 16 |
| 50–64 | 0 | | | | | | | | | |
| 65+ | 0 | | | | | | | | | |
| **GRAND TOTAL** | 586 | 5.6 | 53 | 2 | 3 | 3 | 5 | 8 | 27 | 37 |

## 74.9: CESAREAN SECTION NOS. Formerly included in operation group(s) 711, 712.

| Type of Patients | Observed Patients | Avg. Stay | Variance | Percentiles | | | | | | |
|---|---|---|---|---|---|---|---|---|---|---|
| | | | | 10th | 25th | 50th | 75th | 90th | 95th | 99th |
| **1. SINGLE DX** | | | | | | | | | | |
| 0–19 Years | 21 | 2.8 | 2 | 2 | 2 | 2 | 3 | 4 | 4 | 8 |
| 20–34 | 102 | 2.9 | <1 | 2 | 2 | 3 | 3 | 4 | 4 | 4 |
| 35–49 | 13 | 2.9 | <1 | 2 | 3 | 3 | 3 | 3 | 4 | 4 |
| 50–64 | 0 | | | | | | | | | |
| 65+ | 0 | | | | | | | | | |
| **2. MULTIPLE DX** | | | | | | | | | | |
| 0–19 Years | 54 | 3.5 | 3 | 2 | 2 | 3 | 4 | 5 | 6 | 15 |
| 20–34 | 346 | 3.7 | 9 | 2 | 2 | 3 | 4 | 5 | 8 | 14 |
| 35–49 | 80 | 3.8 | 4 | 2 | 3 | 3 | 4 | 5 | 5 | 13 |
| 50–64 | 0 | | | | | | | | | |
| 65+ | 0 | | | | | | | | | |
| **TOTAL SINGLE DX** | 136 | 2.9 | <1 | 2 | 2 | 3 | 3 | 4 | 4 | 5 |
| **TOTAL MULTIPLE DX** | 480 | 3.7 | 7 | 2 | 3 | 3 | 4 | 5 | 7 | 14 |
| **TOTAL** | | | | | | | | | | |
| 0–19 Years | 75 | 3.3 | 3 | 2 | 2 | 3 | 4 | 5 | 6 | 11 |
| 20–34 | 448 | 3.5 | 7 | 2 | 2 | 3 | 4 | 5 | 6 | 13 |
| 35–49 | 93 | 3.7 | 4 | 2 | 3 | 3 | 4 | 5 | 5 | 13 |
| 50–64 | 0 | | | | | | | | | |
| 65+ | 0 | | | | | | | | | |
| **GRAND TOTAL** | 616 | 3.5 | 6 | 2 | 3 | 3 | 4 | 5 | 6 | 13 |

## 74.99: OTHER CD TYPE NOS. Formerly included in operation group(s) 711.

| Type of Patients | Observed Patients | Avg. Stay | Variance | Percentiles | | | | | | |
|---|---|---|---|---|---|---|---|---|---|---|
| | | | | 10th | 25th | 50th | 75th | 90th | 95th | 99th |
| **1. SINGLE DX** | | | | | | | | | | |
| 0–19 Years | 21 | 2.8 | 2 | 2 | 2 | 2 | 3 | 4 | 4 | 8 |
| 20–34 | 101 | 2.9 | <1 | 2 | 2 | 3 | 3 | 4 | 4 | 4 |
| 35–49 | 13 | 2.9 | <1 | 2 | 3 | 3 | 3 | 3 | 4 | 4 |
| 50–64 | 0 | | | | | | | | | |
| 65+ | 0 | | | | | | | | | |
| **2. MULTIPLE DX** | | | | | | | | | | |
| 0–19 Years | 53 | 3.4 | 3 | 2 | 2 | 3 | 4 | 5 | 5 | 15 |
| 20–34 | 328 | 3.5 | 8 | 2 | 2 | 3 | 4 | 5 | 6 | 13 |
| 35–49 | 74 | 3.7 | 3 | 3 | 3 | 3 | 4 | 5 | 5 | 12 |
| 50–64 | 0 | | | | | | | | | |
| 65+ | 0 | | | | | | | | | |
| **TOTAL SINGLE DX** | 135 | 2.9 | <1 | 2 | 2 | 3 | 3 | 4 | 4 | 5 |
| **TOTAL MULTIPLE DX** | 455 | 3.5 | 7 | 2 | 3 | 3 | 4 | 5 | 6 | 12 |
| **TOTAL** | | | | | | | | | | |
| 0–19 Years | 74 | 3.3 | 3 | 2 | 2 | 3 | 4 | 5 | 5 | 11 |
| 20–34 | 429 | 3.4 | 7 | 2 | 2 | 3 | 4 | 5 | 6 | 12 |
| 35–49 | 87 | 3.6 | 3 | 2 | 3 | 3 | 4 | 5 | 5 | 11 |
| 50–64 | 0 | | | | | | | | | |
| 65+ | 0 | | | | | | | | | |
| **GRAND TOTAL** | 590 | 3.4 | 5 | 2 | 3 | 3 | 4 | 5 | 5 | 12 |

Length of Stay by Diagnosis and Operation, United States, 2000

# United States, October 1998–September 1999 Data, by Operation

## 75.0: INTRA-AMNIO INJECT-AB. Formerly included in operation group(s) 713.

| Type of Patients | Observed Patients | Avg. Stay | Vari-ance | Percentiles 10th | 25th | 50th | 75th | 90th | 95th | 99th |
|---|---|---|---|---|---|---|---|---|---|---|
| **1. SINGLE DX** | | | | | | | | | | |
| 0–19 Years | 49 | 1.3 | <1 | 1 | 1 | 1 | 2 | 2 | 2 | 2 |
| 20–34 | 114 | 1.3 | <1 | 1 | 1 | 1 | 2 | 2 | 2 | 3 |
| 35–49 | 12 | 1.7 | <1 | 1 | 1 | 2 | 2 | 2 | 3 | 4 |
| 50–64 | 0 | | | | | | | | | |
| 65+ | 0 | | | | | | | | | |
| **2. MULTIPLE DX** | | | | | | | | | | |
| 0–19 Years | 9 | 2.3 | <1 | 1 | 2 | 2 | 3 | 3 | 3 | 3 |
| 20–34 | 67 | 1.7 | 2 | 1 | 1 | 1 | 2 | 4 | 5 | 5 |
| 35–49 | 21 | 2.2 | 6 | 1 | 1 | 1 | 2 | 5 | 10 | 10 |
| 50–64 | 0 | | | | | | | | | |
| 65+ | 0 | | | | | | | | | |
| **TOTAL SINGLE DX** | 175 | 1.3 | <1 | 1 | 1 | 1 | 2 | 2 | 2 | 3 |
| **TOTAL MULTIPLE DX** | 97 | 1.8 | 2 | 1 | 1 | 1 | 2 | 4 | 5 | 8 |
| **TOTAL** | | | | | | | | | | |
| 0–19 Years | 58 | 1.5 | <1 | 1 | 1 | 1 | 2 | 2 | 3 | 3 |
| 20–34 | 181 | 1.5 | <1 | 1 | 1 | 1 | 2 | 2 | 3 | 5 |
| 35–49 | 33 | 2.1 | 4 | 1 | 1 | 1 | 2 | 4 | 8 | 10 |
| 50–64 | 0 | | | | | | | | | |
| 65+ | 0 | | | | | | | | | |
| **GRAND TOTAL** | 272 | 1.6 | 1 | 1 | 1 | 1 | 2 | 2 | 3 | 5 |

## 75.1: DIAGNOSTIC AMNIOCENTESIS. Formerly included in operation group(s) 714.

| Type of Patients | Observed Patients | Avg. Stay | Vari-ance | Percentiles 10th | 25th | 50th | 75th | 90th | 95th | 99th |
|---|---|---|---|---|---|---|---|---|---|---|
| **1. SINGLE DX** | | | | | | | | | | |
| 0–19 Years | 73 | 5.0 | 81 | 1 | 2 | 2 | 3 | 7 | 37 | 37 |
| 20–34 | 278 | 3.4 | 16 | 1 | 2 | 2 | 3 | 7 | 11 | 21 |
| 35–49 | 18 | 2.8 | 6 | 1 | 1 | 2 | 4 | 6 | 6 | 12 |
| 50–64 | 0 | | | | | | | | | |
| 65+ | 0 | | | | | | | | | |
| **2. MULTIPLE DX** | | | | | | | | | | |
| 0–19 Years | 182 | 6.5 | 59 | 1 | 2 | 3 | 8 | 16 | 26 | 30 |
| 20–34 | 790 | 5.4 | 43 | 1 | 2 | 3 | 5 | 13 | 19 | 27 |
| 35–49 | 164 | 5.4 | 55 | 1 | 2 | 3 | 5 | 11 | 18 | 27 |
| 50–64 | 0 | | | | | | | | | |
| 65+ | 0 | | | | | | | | | |
| **TOTAL SINGLE DX** | 369 | 3.6 | 25 | 1 | 1 | 2 | 3 | 7 | 11 | 37 |
| **TOTAL MULTIPLE DX** | 1,136 | 5.5 | 47 | 1 | 2 | 3 | 5 | 13 | 20 | 27 |
| **TOTAL** | | | | | | | | | | |
| 0–19 Years | 255 | 6.0 | 66 | 1 | 2 | 3 | 7 | 16 | 26 | 37 |
| 20–34 | 1,068 | 4.7 | 35 | 1 | 2 | 3 | 5 | 10 | 17 | 27 |
| 35–49 | 182 | 5.1 | 51 | 1 | 2 | 3 | 5 | 11 | 18 | 27 |
| 50–64 | 0 | | | | | | | | | |
| 65+ | 0 | | | | | | | | | |
| **GRAND TOTAL** | 1,505 | 4.9 | 41 | 1 | 2 | 3 | 5 | 11 | 18 | 30 |

## 75.2: INTRAUTERINE TRANSFUSION. Formerly included in operation group(s) 715.

| Type of Patients | Observed Patients | Avg. Stay | Vari-ance | Percentiles 10th | 25th | 50th | 75th | 90th | 95th | 99th |
|---|---|---|---|---|---|---|---|---|---|---|
| **1. SINGLE DX** | | | | | | | | | | |
| 0–19 Years | 0 | | | | | | | | | |
| 20–34 | 4 | 2.2 | 2 | 1 | 1 | 1 | 4 | 4 | 4 | 4 |
| 35–49 | 2 | 1.0 | 0 | 1 | 1 | 1 | 1 | 1 | 1 | 1 |
| 50–64 | 0 | | | | | | | | | |
| 65+ | 0 | | | | | | | | | |
| **2. MULTIPLE DX** | | | | | | | | | | |
| 0–19 Years | 2 | 1.4 | 1 | 1 | 1 | 1 | 1 | 4 | 4 | 4 |
| 20–34 | 9 | 2.2 | <1 | 1 | 2 | 2 | 3 | 3 | 3 | 3 |
| 35–49 | 1 | 2.0 | 0 | 2 | 2 | 2 | 2 | 2 | 2 | 2 |
| 50–64 | 0 | | | | | | | | | |
| 65+ | 0 | | | | | | | | | |
| **TOTAL SINGLE DX** | 6 | 1.9 | 2 | 1 | 1 | 1 | 4 | 4 | 4 | 4 |
| **TOTAL MULTIPLE DX** | 12 | 1.9 | <1 | 1 | 1 | 2 | 3 | 3 | 3 | 4 |
| **TOTAL** | | | | | | | | | | |
| 0–19 Years | 2 | 1.4 | 1 | 1 | 1 | 1 | 1 | 4 | 4 | 4 |
| 20–34 | 13 | 2.2 | 1 | 1 | 2 | 2 | 3 | 4 | 4 | 4 |
| 35–49 | 3 | 1.4 | <1 | 1 | 2 | 2 | 2 | 2 | 2 | 2 |
| 50–64 | 0 | | | | | | | | | |
| 65+ | 0 | | | | | | | | | |
| **GRAND TOTAL** | 18 | 1.9 | 1 | 1 | 1 | 2 | 3 | 4 | 4 | 4 |

## 75.3: IU OPS FETUS & AMNIO NEC. Formerly included in operation group(s) 715.

| Type of Patients | Observed Patients | Avg. Stay | Vari-ance | Percentiles 10th | 25th | 50th | 75th | 90th | 95th | 99th |
|---|---|---|---|---|---|---|---|---|---|---|
| **1. SINGLE DX** | | | | | | | | | | |
| 0–19 Years | 1,023 | 1.8 | 1 | 1 | 1 | 2 | 2 | 3 | 3 | 6 |
| 20–34 | 5,416 | 1.9 | 4 | 1 | 1 | 2 | 2 | 3 | 3 | 8 |
| 35–49 | 700 | 1.7 | 3 | 1 | 1 | 1 | 2 | 3 | 3 | 6 |
| 50–64 | 1 | 2.0 | 0 | 2 | 2 | 2 | 2 | 2 | 2 | 2 |
| 65+ | 0 | | | | | | | | | |
| **2. MULTIPLE DX** | | | | | | | | | | |
| 0–19 Years | 1,611 | 2.9 | 15 | 1 | 1 | 2 | 3 | 5 | 7 | 30 |
| 20–34 | 7,970 | 2.7 | 15 | 1 | 1 | 2 | 3 | 4 | 6 | 17 |
| 35–49 | 1,525 | 2.9 | 16 | 1 | 1 | 2 | 3 | 5 | 7 | 21 |
| 50–64 | 4 | 2.3 | 7 | 1 | 1 | 1 | 1 | 7 | 7 | 7 |
| 65+ | 0 | | | | | | | | | |
| **TOTAL SINGLE DX** | 7,140 | 1.8 | 4 | 1 | 1 | 2 | 2 | 3 | 3 | 8 |
| **TOTAL MULTIPLE DX** | 11,110 | 2.8 | 15 | 1 | 1 | 2 | 3 | 4 | 6 | 19 |
| **TOTAL** | | | | | | | | | | |
| 0–19 Years | 2,634 | 2.4 | 10 | 1 | 1 | 2 | 2 | 4 | 5 | 15 |
| 20–34 | 13,386 | 2.3 | 11 | 1 | 1 | 2 | 2 | 4 | 5 | 13 |
| 35–49 | 2,225 | 2.4 | 11 | 1 | 1 | 2 | 2 | 4 | 5 | 18 |
| 50–64 | 5 | 2.3 | 6 | 1 | 1 | 1 | 2 | 7 | 7 | 7 |
| 65+ | 0 | | | | | | | | | |
| **GRAND TOTAL** | 18,250 | 2.3 | 10 | 1 | 1 | 2 | 2 | 4 | 5 | 14 |

Length of Stay by Diagnosis and Operation, United States, 2000

# United States, October 1998–September 1999 Data, by Operation

## 75.32: FETAL EKG (SCALP). Formerly included in operation group(s) 715.

| Type of Patients | Observed Patients | Avg. Stay | Variance | 10th | 25th | 50th | 75th | 90th | 95th | 99th |
|---|---|---|---|---|---|---|---|---|---|---|
| **1. SINGLE DX** | | | | | | | | | | |
| 0–19 Years | 133 | 1.9 | <1 | 1 | 1 | 2 | 2 | 3 | 3 | 3 |
| 20–34 | 549 | 1.9 | <1 | 1 | 1 | 2 | 2 | 3 | 3 | 4 |
| 35–49 | 52 | 1.6 | <1 | 1 | 1 | 2 | 2 | 3 | 3 | 3 |
| 50–64 | 0 | | | | | | | | | |
| 65+ | 0 | | | | | | | | | |
| **2. MULTIPLE DX** | | | | | | | | | | |
| 0–19 Years | 153 | 2.3 | <1 | 1 | 2 | 2 | 3 | 3 | 3 | 5 |
| 20–34 | 699 | 2.4 | 3 | 1 | 2 | 2 | 3 | 3 | 4 | 8 |
| 35–49 | 99 | 2.3 | 1 | 1 | 2 | 2 | 3 | 3 | 3 | 8 |
| 50–64 | 0 | | | | | | | | | |
| 65+ | 0 | | | | | | | | | |
| **TOTAL SINGLE DX** | 734 | 1.9 | <1 | 1 | 1 | 2 | 2 | 3 | 3 | 4 |
| **TOTAL MULTIPLE DX** | 951 | 2.3 | 3 | 1 | 2 | 2 | 3 | 3 | 4 | 8 |
| **TOTAL** | | | | | | | | | | |
| 0–19 Years | 286 | 2.1 | <1 | 1 | 2 | 2 | 2 | 3 | 3 | 5 |
| 20–34 | 1,248 | 2.2 | 2 | 1 | 2 | 2 | 3 | 3 | 3 | 6 |
| 35–49 | 151 | 2.0 | 1 | 1 | 1 | 2 | 3 | 3 | 3 | 6 |
| 50–64 | 0 | | | | | | | | | |
| 65+ | 0 | | | | | | | | | |
| **GRAND TOTAL** | 1,685 | 2.1 | 2 | 1 | 1 | 2 | 2 | 3 | 3 | 6 |

## 75.35: DXTIC PX FETUS/AMNIO NEC. Formerly included in operation group(s) 715.

| Type of Patients | Observed Patients | Avg. Stay | Variance | 10th | 25th | 50th | 75th | 90th | 95th | 99th |
|---|---|---|---|---|---|---|---|---|---|---|
| **1. SINGLE DX** | | | | | | | | | | |
| 0–19 Years | 99 | 1.5 | 2 | 1 | 1 | 1 | 1 | 2 | 4 | 11 |
| 20–34 | 525 | 1.3 | 1 | 1 | 1 | 1 | 1 | 2 | 3 | 6 |
| 35–49 | 102 | 1.3 | <1 | 1 | 1 | 1 | 1 | 2 | 2 | 5 |
| 50–64 | 0 | | | | | | | | | |
| 65+ | 0 | | | | | | | | | |
| **2. MULTIPLE DX** | | | | | | | | | | |
| 0–19 Years | 222 | 2.0 | 3 | 1 | 1 | 2 | 2 | 4 | 5 | 8 |
| 20–34 | 880 | 2.3 | 6 | 1 | 1 | 2 | 3 | 4 | 6 | 11 |
| 35–49 | 140 | 2.6 | 9 | 1 | 1 | 1 | 3 | 5 | 8 | 19 |
| 50–64 | 0 | | | | | | | | | |
| 65+ | 0 | | | | | | | | | |
| **TOTAL SINGLE DX** | 726 | 1.3 | 1 | 1 | 1 | 1 | 1 | 2 | 3 | 6 |
| **TOTAL MULTIPLE DX** | 1,242 | 2.3 | 6 | 1 | 1 | 2 | 3 | 4 | 6 | 11 |
| **TOTAL** | | | | | | | | | | |
| 0–19 Years | 321 | 1.8 | 3 | 1 | 1 | 1 | 2 | 3 | 5 | 8 |
| 20–34 | 1,405 | 1.8 | 4 | 1 | 1 | 1 | 2 | 3 | 5 | 10 |
| 35–49 | 242 | 1.8 | 5 | 1 | 1 | 1 | 2 | 3 | 5 | 13 |
| 50–64 | 0 | | | | | | | | | |
| 65+ | 0 | | | | | | | | | |
| **GRAND TOTAL** | 1,968 | 1.8 | 4 | 1 | 1 | 1 | 2 | 3 | 5 | 10 |

## 75.34: FETAL MONITORING NOS. Formerly included in operation group(s) 715.

| Type of Patients | Observed Patients | Avg. Stay | Variance | 10th | 25th | 50th | 75th | 90th | 95th | 99th |
|---|---|---|---|---|---|---|---|---|---|---|
| **1. SINGLE DX** | | | | | | | | | | |
| 0–19 Years | 784 | 1.8 | 1 | 1 | 1 | 2 | 2 | 3 | 3 | 6 |
| 20–34 | 4,299 | 2.0 | 5 | 1 | 1 | 2 | 2 | 3 | 4 | 9 |
| 35–49 | 545 | 1.9 | 4 | 1 | 1 | 2 | 2 | 3 | 4 | 7 |
| 50–64 | 1 | 2.0 | 0 | 2 | 2 | 2 | 2 | 2 | 2 | 2 |
| 65+ | 0 | | | | | | | | | |
| **2. MULTIPLE DX** | | | | | | | | | | |
| 0–19 Years | 1,205 | 3.2 | 20 | 1 | 1 | 2 | 3 | 5 | 8 | 30 |
| 20–34 | 6,215 | 2.8 | 19 | 1 | 1 | 2 | 3 | 4 | 7 | 21 |
| 35–49 | 1,251 | 3.0 | 19 | 1 | 1 | 2 | 3 | 5 | 7 | 27 |
| 50–64 | 3 | 2.8 | 8 | 1 | 1 | 1 | 7 | 7 | 7 | 7 |
| 65+ | 0 | | | | | | | | | |
| **TOTAL SINGLE DX** | 5,629 | 1.9 | 5 | 1 | 1 | 2 | 2 | 3 | 4 | 8 |
| **TOTAL MULTIPLE DX** | 8,674 | 2.9 | 19 | 1 | 1 | 2 | 3 | 5 | 7 | 25 |
| **TOTAL** | | | | | | | | | | |
| 0–19 Years | 1,989 | 2.6 | 12 | 1 | 1 | 2 | 3 | 4 | 6 | 30 |
| 20–34 | 10,514 | 2.4 | 13 | 1 | 1 | 2 | 3 | 4 | 5 | 15 |
| 35–49 | 1,796 | 2.6 | 14 | 1 | 1 | 2 | 3 | 4 | 6 | 21 |
| 50–64 | 4 | 2.6 | 7 | 1 | 1 | 1 | 2 | 7 | 7 | 7 |
| 65+ | 0 | | | | | | | | | |
| **GRAND TOTAL** | 14,303 | 2.5 | 13 | 1 | 1 | 2 | 3 | 4 | 5 | 16 |

## 75.4: MAN RMVL OF RET PLACENTA. Formerly included in operation group(s) 716.

| Type of Patients | Observed Patients | Avg. Stay | Variance | 10th | 25th | 50th | 75th | 90th | 95th | 99th |
|---|---|---|---|---|---|---|---|---|---|---|
| **1. SINGLE DX** | | | | | | | | | | |
| 0–19 Years | 60 | 1.5 | <1 | 1 | 1 | 1 | 2 | 2 | 2 | 3 |
| 20–34 | 343 | 1.6 | <1 | 1 | 1 | 2 | 2 | 2 | 3 | 3 |
| 35–49 | 60 | 1.5 | <1 | 1 | 1 | 1 | 2 | 2 | 3 | 3 |
| 50–64 | 1 | 2.0 | 0 | 2 | 2 | 2 | 2 | 2 | 2 | 2 |
| 65+ | 0 | | | | | | | | | |
| **2. MULTIPLE DX** | | | | | | | | | | |
| 0–19 Years | 130 | 2.1 | 2 | 1 | 1 | 2 | 3 | 3 | 4 | 7 |
| 20–34 | 857 | 2.1 | 5 | 1 | 1 | 2 | 2 | 3 | 4 | 7 |
| 35–49 | 149 | 2.6 | 8 | 1 | 2 | 2 | 3 | 4 | 6 | 18 |
| 50–64 | 0 | | | | | | | | | |
| 65+ | 0 | | | | | | | | | |
| **TOTAL SINGLE DX** | 464 | 1.6 | <1 | 1 | 1 | 2 | 2 | 2 | 3 | 3 |
| **TOTAL MULTIPLE DX** | 1,136 | 2.2 | 5 | 1 | 1 | 2 | 3 | 3 | 4 | 7 |
| **TOTAL** | | | | | | | | | | |
| 0–19 Years | 190 | 2.0 | 2 | 1 | 1 | 2 | 2 | 3 | 4 | 6 |
| 20–34 | 1,200 | 2.0 | 4 | 1 | 1 | 2 | 2 | 3 | 4 | 6 |
| 35–49 | 209 | 2.2 | 6 | 1 | 1 | 2 | 2 | 3 | 4 | 12 |
| 50–64 | 1 | 2.0 | 0 | 2 | 2 | 2 | 2 | 2 | 2 | 2 |
| 65+ | 0 | | | | | | | | | |
| **GRAND TOTAL** | 1,600 | 2.0 | 4 | 1 | 1 | 2 | 2 | 3 | 4 | 7 |

Length of Stay by Diagnosis and Operation, United States, 2000

## United States, October 1998–September 1999 Data, by Operation

### 75.5: REP CURRENT OB LAC UTER. Formerly included in operation group(s) 716.

| Type of Patients | Observed Patients | Avg. Stay | Vari-ance | Percentiles | | | | | | |
|---|---|---|---|---|---|---|---|---|---|---|
| | | | | 10th | 25th | 50th | 75th | 90th | 95th | 99th |
| **1. SINGLE DX** | | | | | | | | | | |
| 0–19 Years | 28 | 2.0 | <1 | 1 | 1 | 2 | 2 | 2 | 3 | 3 |
| 20–34 | 116 | 1.9 | <1 | 1 | 1 | 2 | 2 | 2 | 3 | 3 |
| 35–49 | 10 | 2.1 | <1 | 1 | 2 | 2 | 3 | 3 | 3 | 3 |
| 50–64 | 0 | | | | | | | | | |
| 65+ | 0 | | | | | | | | | |
| **2. MULTIPLE DX** | | | | | | | | | | |
| 0–19 Years | 182 | 2.2 | 3 | 1 | 2 | 2 | 2 | 3 | 4 | 5 |
| 20–34 | 846 | 2.3 | 2 | 1 | 2 | 2 | 3 | 3 | 4 | 7 |
| 35–49 | 134 | 2.6 | 6 | 1 | 2 | 2 | 3 | 4 | 5 | 10 |
| 50–64 | 0 | | | | | | | | | |
| 65+ | 0 | | | | | | | | | |
| **TOTAL SINGLE DX** | 154 | 1.9 | <1 | 1 | 2 | 2 | 2 | 3 | 3 | 3 |
| **TOTAL MULTIPLE DX** | 1,162 | 2.4 | 3 | 1 | 2 | 2 | 3 | 3 | 4 | 8 |
| **TOTAL** | | | | | | | | | | |
| 0–19 Years | 210 | 2.2 | 3 | 1 | 2 | 2 | 2 | 3 | 4 | 5 |
| 20–34 | 962 | 2.3 | 2 | 1 | 2 | 2 | 3 | 3 | 4 | 7 |
| 35–49 | 144 | 2.6 | 5 | 1 | 2 | 2 | 3 | 4 | 5 | 10 |
| 50–64 | 0 | | | | | | | | | |
| 65+ | 0 | | | | | | | | | |
| **GRAND TOTAL** | 1,316 | 2.3 | 3 | 1 | 2 | 2 | 3 | 3 | 4 | 7 |

### 75.51: REP CURRENT OB LAC CERV. Formerly included in operation group(s) 716.

| Type of Patients | Observed Patients | Avg. Stay | Vari-ance | Percentiles | | | | | | |
|---|---|---|---|---|---|---|---|---|---|---|
| | | | | 10th | 25th | 50th | 75th | 90th | 95th | 99th |
| **1. SINGLE DX** | | | | | | | | | | |
| 0–19 Years | 28 | 2.0 | <1 | 1 | 1 | 2 | 2 | 3 | 3 | 3 |
| 20–34 | 113 | 1.9 | <1 | 1 | 2 | 2 | 2 | 2 | 3 | 3 |
| 35–49 | 10 | 2.1 | <1 | 1 | 2 | 2 | 3 | 3 | 3 | 3 |
| 50–64 | 0 | | | | | | | | | |
| 65+ | 0 | | | | | | | | | |
| **2. MULTIPLE DX** | | | | | | | | | | |
| 0–19 Years | 178 | 2.3 | 3 | 1 | 2 | 2 | 2 | 3 | 4 | 5 |
| 20–34 | 832 | 2.3 | 3 | 1 | 2 | 2 | 3 | 3 | 4 | 7 |
| 35–49 | 129 | 2.5 | 5 | 1 | 2 | 2 | 3 | 4 | 5 | 10 |
| 50–64 | 0 | | | | | | | | | |
| 65+ | 0 | | | | | | | | | |
| **TOTAL SINGLE DX** | 151 | 1.9 | <1 | 1 | 2 | 2 | 2 | 3 | 3 | 3 |
| **TOTAL MULTIPLE DX** | 1,139 | 2.3 | 2 | 1 | 2 | 2 | 3 | 3 | 4 | 7 |
| **TOTAL** | | | | | | | | | | |
| 0–19 Years | 206 | 2.2 | 3 | 1 | 2 | 2 | 2 | 3 | 4 | 5 |
| 20–34 | 945 | 2.3 | 2 | 1 | 2 | 2 | 3 | 3 | 4 | 7 |
| 35–49 | 139 | 2.5 | 5 | 1 | 2 | 2 | 3 | 4 | 5 | 10 |
| 50–64 | 0 | | | | | | | | | |
| 65+ | 0 | | | | | | | | | |
| **GRAND TOTAL** | 1,290 | 2.3 | 2 | 1 | 2 | 2 | 3 | 3 | 4 | 7 |

### 75.6: REP OTH CURRENT OB LAC. Formerly included in operation group(s) 716.

| Type of Patients | Observed Patients | Avg. Stay | Vari-ance | Percentiles | | | | | | |
|---|---|---|---|---|---|---|---|---|---|---|
| | | | | 10th | 25th | 50th | 75th | 90th | 95th | 99th |
| **1. SINGLE DX** | | | | | | | | | | |
| 0–19 Years | 8,044 | 1.8 | <1 | 1 | 1 | 2 | 2 | 2 | 3 | 3 |
| 20–34 | 41,568 | 1.7 | <1 | 1 | 1 | 2 | 2 | 2 | 3 | 3 |
| 35–49 | 4,613 | 1.8 | <1 | 1 | 1 | 2 | 2 | 2 | 3 | 3 |
| 50–64 | 0 | 2.0 | 0 | 2 | 2 | 2 | 2 | 2 | 2 | 2 |
| 65+ | 0 | | | | | | | | | |
| **2. MULTIPLE DX** | | | | | | | | | | |
| 0–19 Years | 16,759 | 2.1 | 2 | 1 | 2 | 2 | 2 | 2 | 3 | 5 |
| 20–34 | 87,874 | 2.0 | 2 | 1 | 1 | 2 | 2 | 3 | 3 | 5 |
| 35–49 | 15,740 | 2.0 | 2 | 1 | 2 | 2 | 2 | 3 | 3 | 5 |
| 50–64 | 1 | 4.0 | 0 | 4 | 4 | 4 | 4 | 4 | 4 | 4 |
| 65+ | 0 | | | | | | | | | |
| **TOTAL SINGLE DX** | 54,226 | 1.7 | <1 | 1 | 1 | 2 | 2 | 2 | 3 | 3 |
| **TOTAL MULTIPLE DX** | 120,374 | 2.0 | 2 | 1 | 1 | 2 | 2 | 3 | 3 | 5 |
| **TOTAL** | | | | | | | | | | |
| 0–19 Years | 24,803 | 2.0 | 1 | 1 | 1 | 2 | 2 | 2 | 3 | 5 |
| 20–34 | 129,442 | 1.9 | 1 | 1 | 1 | 2 | 2 | 2 | 3 | 4 |
| 35–49 | 20,353 | 2.0 | 2 | 1 | 1 | 2 | 2 | 3 | 4 | 4 |
| 50–64 | 2 | 3.9 | <1 | 4 | 4 | 4 | 4 | 4 | 4 | 4 |
| 65+ | 0 | | | | | | | | | |
| **GRAND TOTAL** | 174,600 | 1.9 | 1 | 1 | 1 | 2 | 2 | 2 | 3 | 4 |

### 75.61: REP OB LAC BLAD/URETHRA. Formerly included in operation group(s) 716.

| Type of Patients | Observed Patients | Avg. Stay | Vari-ance | Percentiles | | | | | | |
|---|---|---|---|---|---|---|---|---|---|---|
| | | | | 10th | 25th | 50th | 75th | 90th | 95th | 99th |
| **1. SINGLE DX** | | | | | | | | | | |
| 0–19 Years | 276 | 1.7 | <1 | 1 | 1 | 2 | 2 | 2 | 3 | 3 |
| 20–34 | 1,156 | 1.7 | <1 | 1 | 1 | 2 | 2 | 2 | 3 | 3 |
| 35–49 | 76 | 1.7 | <1 | 1 | 1 | 2 | 2 | 2 | 3 | 3 |
| 50–64 | 0 | | | | | | | | | |
| 65+ | 0 | | | | | | | | | |
| **2. MULTIPLE DX** | | | | | | | | | | |
| 0–19 Years | 1,141 | 2.0 | 2 | 1 | 1 | 2 | 2 | 3 | 3 | 7 |
| 20–34 | 4,597 | 2.1 | 4 | 1 | 1 | 2 | 2 | 3 | 3 | 6 |
| 35–49 | 508 | 2.0 | 1 | 1 | 2 | 2 | 2 | 3 | 3 | 5 |
| 50–64 | 0 | | | | | | | | | |
| 65+ | 0 | | | | | | | | | |
| **TOTAL SINGLE DX** | 1,508 | 1.7 | <1 | 1 | 1 | 2 | 2 | 2 | 3 | 3 |
| **TOTAL MULTIPLE DX** | 6,246 | 2.1 | 3 | 1 | 1 | 2 | 2 | 3 | 3 | 6 |
| **TOTAL** | | | | | | | | | | |
| 0–19 Years | 1,417 | 2.0 | 2 | 1 | 1 | 2 | 2 | 3 | 3 | 6 |
| 20–34 | 5,753 | 2.0 | 3 | 1 | 1 | 2 | 2 | 3 | 3 | 7 |
| 35–49 | 584 | 2.0 | <1 | 1 | 1 | 2 | 2 | 3 | 3 | 5 |
| 50–64 | 0 | | | | | | | | | |
| 65+ | 0 | | | | | | | | | |
| **GRAND TOTAL** | 7,754 | 2.0 | 3 | 1 | 1 | 2 | 2 | 3 | 3 | 5 |

Length of Stay by Diagnosis and Operation, United States, 2000

# United States, October 1998–September 1999 Data, by Operation

## 75.7: PP MANUAL EXPLOR UTERUS. Formerly included in operation group(s) 716.

| Type of Patients | Observed Patients | Avg. Stay | Vari-ance | Percentiles | | | | | | |
|---|---|---|---|---|---|---|---|---|---|---|
| | | | | 10th | 25th | 50th | 75th | 90th | 95th | 99th |
| **1. SINGLE DX** | | | | | | | | | | |
| 0–19 Years | 27 | 2.1 | <1 | 1 | 2 | 2 | 2 | 3 | 3 | 3 |
| 20–34 | 133 | 1.8 | <1 | 1 | 1 | 2 | 2 | 3 | 3 | 4 |
| 35–49 | 25 | 2.9 | 13 | 1 | 1 | 2 | 2 | 3 | 15 | 15 |
| 50–64 | 0 | | | | | | | | | |
| 65+ | 0 | | | | | | | | | |
| **2. MULTIPLE DX** | | | | | | | | | | |
| 0–19 Years | 37 | 2.3 | <1 | 2 | 2 | 2 | 3 | 3 | 3 | 5 |
| 20–34 | 201 | 2.3 | 2 | 1 | 2 | 2 | 3 | 3 | 4 | 8 |
| 35–49 | 34 | 1.9 | 1 | 1 | 1 | 2 | 2 | 3 | 4 | 6 |
| 50–64 | 0 | | | | | | | | | |
| 65+ | 0 | | | | | | | | | |
| **TOTAL SINGLE DX** | 185 | 2.0 | 2 | 1 | 1 | 2 | 2 | 3 | 3 | 15 |
| **TOTAL MULTIPLE DX** | 272 | 2.2 | 1 | 1 | 2 | 2 | 3 | 3 | 4 | 8 |
| **TOTAL** | | | | | | | | | | |
| 0–19 Years | 64 | 2.2 | <1 | 2 | 2 | 2 | 3 | 3 | 3 | 5 |
| 20–34 | 334 | 2.1 | 1 | 1 | 2 | 2 | 2 | 3 | 3 | 8 |
| 35–49 | 59 | 2.2 | 6 | 1 | 1 | 2 | 2 | 3 | 5 | 15 |
| 50–64 | 0 | | | | | | | | | |
| 65+ | 0 | | | | | | | | | |
| **GRAND TOTAL** | 457 | 2.1 | 2 | 1 | 2 | 2 | 2 | 3 | 3 | 8 |

## 75.8: OB TAMPONADE UTERUS/VAG. Formerly included in operation group(s) 716.

| Type of Patients | Observed Patients | Avg. Stay | Vari-ance | Percentiles | | | | | | |
|---|---|---|---|---|---|---|---|---|---|---|
| | | | | 10th | 25th | 50th | 75th | 90th | 95th | 99th |
| **1. SINGLE DX** | | | | | | | | | | |
| 0–19 Years | 0 | | | | | | | | | |
| 20–34 | 1 | 2.0 | 0 | 2 | 2 | 2 | 2 | 2 | 2 | 2 |
| 35–49 | 0 | | | | | | | | | |
| 50–64 | 0 | | | | | | | | | |
| 65+ | 0 | | | | | | | | | |
| **2. MULTIPLE DX** | | | | | | | | | | |
| 0–19 Years | 1 | 2.0 | 0 | 2 | 2 | 2 | 2 | 2 | 2 | 2 |
| 20–34 | 2 | 2.0 | 1 | 1 | 1 | 2 | 3 | 3 | 3 | 3 |
| 35–49 | 1 | 2.0 | 0 | 2 | 2 | 2 | 2 | 2 | 2 | 2 |
| 50–64 | 0 | | | | | | | | | |
| 65+ | 0 | | | | | | | | | |
| **TOTAL SINGLE DX** | 1 | 2.0 | 0 | 2 | 2 | 2 | 2 | 2 | 2 | 2 |
| **TOTAL MULTIPLE DX** | 4 | 2.0 | <1 | 1 | 1 | 2 | 2 | 3 | 3 | 3 |
| **TOTAL** | | | | | | | | | | |
| 0–19 Years | 1 | 2.0 | 0 | 2 | 2 | 2 | 2 | 2 | 2 | 2 |
| 20–34 | 3 | 2.0 | <1 | 1 | 1 | 2 | 2 | 3 | 3 | 3 |
| 35–49 | 1 | 2.0 | 0 | 2 | 2 | 2 | 2 | 2 | 2 | 2 |
| 50–64 | 0 | | | | | | | | | |
| 65+ | 0 | | | | | | | | | |
| **GRAND TOTAL** | 5 | 2.0 | <1 | 1 | 2 | 2 | 2 | 3 | 3 | 3 |

## 75.62: REP OB LAC RECTUM/ANUS. Formerly included in operation group(s) 716.

| Type of Patients | Observed Patients | Avg. Stay | Vari-ance | Percentiles | | | | | | |
|---|---|---|---|---|---|---|---|---|---|---|
| | | | | 10th | 25th | 50th | 75th | 90th | 95th | 99th |
| **1. SINGLE DX** | | | | | | | | | | |
| 0–19 Years | 685 | 1.9 | <1 | 1 | 1 | 2 | 2 | 3 | 3 | 3 |
| 20–34 | 2,974 | 1.9 | <1 | 1 | 2 | 2 | 2 | 3 | 3 | 3 |
| 35–49 | 232 | 2.0 | <1 | 1 | 2 | 2 | 2 | 3 | 3 | 3 |
| 50–64 | 0 | | | | | | | | | |
| 65+ | 0 | | | | | | | | | |
| **2. MULTIPLE DX** | | | | | | | | | | |
| 0–19 Years | 1,767 | 2.1 | <1 | 1 | 2 | 2 | 3 | 3 | 3 | 5 |
| 20–34 | 8,771 | 2.2 | 1 | 1 | 2 | 2 | 3 | 3 | 3 | 5 |
| 35–49 | 1,184 | 2.2 | 2 | 1 | 2 | 2 | 3 | 3 | 3 | 4 |
| 50–64 | 0 | | | | | | | | | |
| 65+ | 0 | | | | | | | | | |
| **TOTAL SINGLE DX** | 3,891 | 1.9 | <1 | 1 | 2 | 2 | 2 | 3 | 3 | 3 |
| **TOTAL MULTIPLE DX** | 11,722 | 2.2 | 1 | 1 | 2 | 2 | 3 | 3 | 3 | 5 |
| **TOTAL** | | | | | | | | | | |
| 0–19 Years | 2,452 | 2.1 | <1 | 1 | 2 | 2 | 2 | 3 | 3 | 5 |
| 20–34 | 11,745 | 2.1 | <1 | 1 | 2 | 2 | 2 | 3 | 3 | 4 |
| 35–49 | 1,416 | 2.2 | 1 | 1 | 2 | 2 | 2 | 3 | 3 | 4 |
| 50–64 | 0 | | | | | | | | | |
| 65+ | 0 | | | | | | | | | |
| **GRAND TOTAL** | 15,613 | 2.1 | <1 | 1 | 2 | 2 | 2 | 3 | 3 | 4 |

## 75.69: REP CURRENT OB LAC NEC. Formerly included in operation group(s) 716.

| Type of Patients | Observed Patients | Avg. Stay | Vari-ance | Percentiles | | | | | | |
|---|---|---|---|---|---|---|---|---|---|---|
| | | | | 10th | 25th | 50th | 75th | 90th | 95th | 99th |
| **1. SINGLE DX** | | | | | | | | | | |
| 0–19 Years | 7,083 | 1.7 | <1 | 1 | 1 | 2 | 2 | 2 | 3 | 3 |
| 20–34 | 37,438 | 1.7 | <1 | 1 | 1 | 2 | 2 | 2 | 3 | 3 |
| 35–49 | 4,305 | 1.8 | <1 | 1 | 1 | 2 | 2 | 2 | 3 | 3 |
| 50–64 | 1 | 2.0 | 0 | 2 | 2 | 2 | 2 | 2 | 2 | 2 |
| 65+ | 0 | | | | | | | | | |
| **2. MULTIPLE DX** | | | | | | | | | | |
| 0–19 Years | 13,851 | 2.1 | 2 | 1 | 2 | 2 | 2 | 3 | 3 | 5 |
| 20–34 | 74,506 | 2.0 | 2 | 1 | 1 | 2 | 2 | 3 | 3 | 5 |
| 35–49 | 14,048 | 2.0 | 3 | 1 | 2 | 2 | 2 | 3 | 3 | 5 |
| 50–64 | 1 | 4.0 | 0 | 4 | 4 | 4 | 4 | 4 | 4 | 4 |
| 65+ | 0 | | | | | | | | | |
| **TOTAL SINGLE DX** | 48,827 | 1.7 | <1 | 1 | 1 | 2 | 2 | 2 | 3 | 3 |
| **TOTAL MULTIPLE DX** | 102,406 | 2.0 | 2 | 1 | 1 | 2 | 2 | 3 | 3 | 5 |
| **TOTAL** | | | | | | | | | | |
| 0–19 Years | 20,934 | 2.0 | 1 | 1 | 1 | 2 | 2 | 3 | 3 | 5 |
| 20–34 | 111,944 | 1.9 | 1 | 1 | 1 | 2 | 2 | 3 | 3 | 4 |
| 35–49 | 18,353 | 2.0 | 2 | 1 | 1 | 2 | 2 | 3 | 3 | 4 |
| 50–64 | 2 | 3.9 | <1 | 4 | 4 | 4 | 4 | 4 | 4 | 4 |
| 65+ | 0 | | | | | | | | | |
| **GRAND TOTAL** | 151,233 | 1.9 | 1 | 1 | 1 | 2 | 2 | 3 | 3 | 4 |

Length of Stay by Diagnosis and Operation, United States, 2000

# United States, October 1998–September 1999 Data, by Operation

## 75.9: OTHER OBSTETRICAL OPS. Formerly included in operation group(s) 716.

| Type of Patients | Observed Patients | Avg. Stay | Variance | 10th | 25th | 50th | 75th | 90th | 95th | 99th |
|---|---|---|---|---|---|---|---|---|---|---|
| **1. SINGLE DX** | | | | | | | | | | |
| 0–19 Years | 10 | 2.6 | 2 | 1 | 2 | 2 | 4 | 5 | 5 | 5 |
| 20–34 | 26 | 2.3 | 2 | 1 | 2 | 2 | 3 | 5 | 5 | 5 |
| 35–49 | 6 | 1.8 | 3 | 1 | 1 | 1 | 2 | 2 | 2 | 9 |
| 50–64 | 1 | | | | | | | | | |
| 65+ | 0 | | | | | | | | | |
| **2. MULTIPLE DX** | | | | | | | | | | |
| 0–19 Years | 23 | 2.9 | 2 | 2 | 2 | 2 | 3 | 5 | 6 | 6 |
| 20–34 | 119 | 3.2 | 10 | 2 | 2 | 3 | 3 | 5 | 6 | 12 |
| 35–49 | 14 | 2.1 | 1 | 1 | 1 | 2 | 3 | 3 | 5 | 5 |
| 50–64 | 0 | | | | | | | | | |
| 65+ | 0 | | | | | | | | | |
| **TOTAL SINGLE DX** | 42 | 2.2 | 2 | 1 | 1 | 2 | 2 | 4 | 5 | 9 |
| **TOTAL MULTIPLE DX** | 156 | 3.1 | 8 | 2 | 2 | 3 | 3 | 5 | 6 | 12 |
| **TOTAL** | | | | | | | | | | |
| 0–19 | 33 | 2.8 | 2 | 1 | 2 | 2 | 3 | 5 | 6 | 6 |
| 20–34 | 145 | 3.1 | 9 | 2 | 2 | 3 | 3 | 5 | 6 | 12 |
| 35–49 | 20 | 2.0 | 2 | 1 | 1 | 2 | 2 | 3 | 5 | 9 |
| 50–64 | 0 | | | | | | | | | |
| 65+ | 0 | | | | | | | | | |
| **GRAND TOTAL** | 198 | 2.9 | 7 | 1 | 2 | 2 | 3 | 5 | 5 | 12 |

## 76.1: DXTIC PX FACIAL BONE/JT. Formerly included in operation group(s) 717, 767.

| Type of Patients | Observed Patients | Avg. Stay | Variance | 10th | 25th | 50th | 75th | 90th | 95th | 99th |
|---|---|---|---|---|---|---|---|---|---|---|
| **1. SINGLE DX** | | | | | | | | | | |
| 0–19 Years | 4 | 1.5 | 2 | 1 | 1 | 1 | 1 | 5 | 5 | 5 |
| 20–34 | 1 | 1.0 | 0 | 1 | 1 | 1 | 1 | 1 | 1 | 1 |
| 35–49 | 2 | 3.4 | 1 | 2 | 2 | 4 | 4 | 4 | 4 | 4 |
| 50–64 | 3 | 1.3 | <1 | 1 | 1 | 2 | 2 | 2 | 2 | 2 |
| 65+ | 1 | 2.0 | 0 | 2 | 2 | 2 | 2 | 2 | 2 | 2 |
| **2. MULTIPLE DX** | | | | | | | | | | |
| 0–19 Years | 5 | 10.3 | 75 | 1 | 1 | 10 | 13 | 23 | 23 | 23 |
| 20–34 | 4 | 3.5 | 8 | 1 | 1 | 4 | 4 | 9 | 8 | 9 |
| 35–49 | 11 | 3.2 | 6 | 2 | 2 | 2 | 4 | 8 | 8 | 10 |
| 50–64 | 7 | 10.5 | 50 | 5 | 6 | 7 | 22 | 22 | 22 | 22 |
| 65+ | 16 | 5.6 | 20 | 3 | 3 | 3 | 7 | 10 | 10 | 22 |
| **TOTAL SINGLE DX** | 11 | 1.8 | 2 | 1 | 1 | 1 | 2 | 4 | 5 | 5 |
| **TOTAL MULTIPLE DX** | 43 | 5.8 | 32 | 1 | 2 | 4 | 8 | 10 | 22 | 23 |
| **TOTAL** | | | | | | | | | | |
| 0–19 | 9 | 6.5 | 62 | 1 | 1 | 1 | 10 | 23 | 23 | 23 |
| 20–34 | 5 | 3.3 | 8 | 1 | 1 | 4 | 4 | 8 | 8 | 9 |
| 35–49 | 13 | 3.2 | 5 | 1 | 2 | 2 | 4 | 8 | 8 | 10 |
| 50–64 | 10 | 7.9 | 53 | 1 | 2 | 6 | 8 | 22 | 22 | 22 |
| 65+ | 17 | 5.4 | 20 | 2 | 3 | 3 | 7 | 10 | 10 | 22 |
| **GRAND TOTAL** | 54 | 5.1 | 29 | 1 | 2 | 3 | 6 | 10 | 22 | 23 |

## 76.0: FACIAL BONE INCISION. Formerly included in operation group(s) 721.

| Type of Patients | Observed Patients | Avg. Stay | Variance | 10th | 25th | 50th | 75th | 90th | 95th | 99th |
|---|---|---|---|---|---|---|---|---|---|---|
| **1. SINGLE DX** | | | | | | | | | | |
| 0–19 Years | 5 | 3.1 | 6 | 1 | 1 | 2 | 6 | 6 | 7 | 7 |
| 20–34 | 3 | 2.1 | <1 | 2 | 2 | 2 | 2 | 3 | 3 | 3 |
| 35–49 | 6 | 2.0 | 1 | 1 | 1 | 2 | 2 | 4 | 4 | 4 |
| 50–64 | 1 | 2.0 | 0 | 2 | 2 | 2 | 2 | 2 | 2 | 2 |
| 65+ | 0 | | | | | | | | | |
| **2. MULTIPLE DX** | | | | | | | | | | |
| 0–19 Years | 11 | 4.9 | 12 | 2 | 3 | 3 | 6 | 10 | 10 | 18 |
| 20–34 | 11 | 3.9 | 2 | 2 | 2 | 5 | 5 | 5 | 5 | 5 |
| 35–49 | 21 | 3.3 | 15 | 1 | 2 | 2 | 3 | 6 | 14 | 21 |
| 50–64 | 9 | 6.1 | 13 | 2 | 3 | 6 | 10 | 11 | 13 | 13 |
| 65+ | 12 | 6.1 | 12 | 1 | 3 | 6 | 9 | 11 | 12 | 12 |
| **TOTAL SINGLE DX** | 15 | 2.3 | 2 | 1 | 2 | 2 | 2 | 4 | 6 | 7 |
| **TOTAL MULTIPLE DX** | 64 | 4.3 | 12 | 1 | 2 | 3 | 5 | 7 | 11 | 21 |
| **TOTAL** | | | | | | | | | | |
| 0–19 | 16 | 4.2 | 10 | 1 | 2 | 3 | 6 | 6 | 10 | 18 |
| 20–34 | 14 | 3.2 | 2 | 2 | 2 | 2 | 5 | 5 | 5 | 5 |
| 35–49 | 27 | 3.1 | 13 | 1 | 1 | 2 | 3 | 6 | 7 | 21 |
| 50–64 | 10 | 5.8 | 13 | 2 | 3 | 4 | 7 | 11 | 13 | 13 |
| 65+ | 12 | 6.1 | 12 | 1 | 3 | 6 | 9 | 11 | 12 | 12 |
| **GRAND TOTAL** | 79 | 3.8 | 10 | 1 | 2 | 2 | 5 | 7 | 10 | 18 |

## 76.2: DESTR FACIAL BONE LES. Formerly included in operation group(s) 717.

| Type of Patients | Observed Patients | Avg. Stay | Variance | 10th | 25th | 50th | 75th | 90th | 95th | 99th |
|---|---|---|---|---|---|---|---|---|---|---|
| **1. SINGLE DX** | | | | | | | | | | |
| 0–19 Years | 23 | 2.0 | 1 | 1 | 1 | 2 | 3 | 3 | 4 | 4 |
| 20–34 | 14 | 1.6 | <1 | 1 | 1 | 1 | 2 | 3 | 4 | 2 |
| 35–49 | 16 | 1.8 | 2 | 1 | 1 | 2 | 2 | 4 | 5 | 6 |
| 50–64 | 7 | 2.2 | 2 | 1 | 1 | 2 | 3 | 5 | 5 | 5 |
| 65+ | 2 | 1.0 | 0 | 1 | 1 | 1 | 1 | 1 | 1 | 1 |
| **2. MULTIPLE DX** | | | | | | | | | | |
| 0–19 Years | 43 | 7.0 | 216 | 1 | 2 | 6 | 6 | 6 | 15 | 90 |
| 20–34 | 51 | 6.1 | 66 | 1 | 2 | 4 | 7 | 8 | 15 | 42 |
| 35–49 | 85 | 5.8 | 36 | 1 | 2 | 4 | 7 | 13 | 21 | 28 |
| 50–64 | 53 | 4.8 | 13 | 1 | 1 | 4 | 9 | 10 | 10 | 10 |
| 65+ | 67 | 4.0 | 22 | 1 | 3 | 3 | 4 | 8 | 18 | 23 |
| **TOTAL SINGLE DX** | 62 | 1.8 | 1 | 1 | 1 | 1 | 2 | 3 | 4 | 5 |
| **TOTAL MULTIPLE DX** | 299 | 5.6 | 72 | 1 | 2 | 4 | 6 | 10 | 15 | 42 |
| **TOTAL** | | | | | | | | | | |
| 0–19 | 66 | 5.8 | 169 | 1 | 1 | 3 | 6 | 6 | 12 | 90 |
| 20–34 | 65 | 4.6 | 50 | 1 | 1 | 2 | 6 | 8 | 9 | 42 |
| 35–49 | 101 | 5.1 | 33 | 1 | 1 | 3 | 6 | 12 | 21 | 28 |
| 50–64 | 60 | 4.6 | 12 | 1 | 1 | 3 | 9 | 10 | 10 | 10 |
| 65+ | 69 | 3.9 | 21 | 1 | 1 | 3 | 4 | 8 | 14 | 23 |
| **GRAND TOTAL** | 361 | 4.9 | 62 | 1 | 3 | 3 | 6 | 9 | 12 | 42 |

Length of Stay by Diagnosis and Operation, United States, 2000

## United States, October 1998–September 1999 Data, by Operation

### 76.3: PARTIAL FACIAL OSTEOTOMY. Formerly included in operation group(s) 717.

| Type of Patients | Observed Patients | Avg. Stay | Vari-ance | 10th | 25th | 50th | 75th | 90th | 95th | 99th |
|---|---|---|---|---|---|---|---|---|---|---|
| **1. SINGLE DX** | | | | | | | | | | |
| 0–19 Years | 19 | 4.7 | 11 | 1 | 2 | 7 | 7 | 7 | 9 | 19 |
| 20–34 | 17 | 2.1 | 2 | 1 | 1 | 1 | 3 | 5 | 5 | 5 |
| 35–49 | 17 | 3.1 | 4 | 1 | 2 | 2 | 4 | 7 | 7 | 8 |
| 50–64 | 11 | 3.4 | 7 | 1 | 2 | 2 | 5 | 6 | 11 | 11 |
| 65+ | 7 | 3.0 | 1 | 2 | 2 | 2 | 4 | 5 | 5 | 5 |
| **2. MULTIPLE DX** | | | | | | | | | | |
| 0–19 Years | 35 | 4.0 | 14 | 1 | 2 | 3 | 6 | 6 | 11 | 21 |
| 20–34 | 43 | 3.3 | 15 | 1 | 1 | 2 | 5 | 6 | 9 | 19 |
| 35–49 | 61 | 4.8 | 14 | 2 | 2 | 3 | 7 | 9 | 13 | 18 |
| 50–64 | 85 | 4.8 | 33 | 1 | 2 | 3 | 7 | 10 | 12 | 31 |
| 65+ | 179 | 6.1 | 47 | 2 | 2 | 6 | 7 | 9 | 13 | 41 |
| **TOTAL SINGLE DX** | 71 | 3.4 | 7 | 1 | 2 | 2 | 5 | 7 | 7 | 11 |
| **TOTAL MULTIPLE DX** | 403 | 5.1 | 33 | 1 | 2 | 3 | 7 | 9 | 12 | 29 |
| **TOTAL** | | | | | | | | | | |
| 0–19 Years | 54 | 4.2 | 13 | 1 | 2 | 3 | 6 | 7 | 9 | 21 |
| 20–34 | 60 | 3.1 | 12 | 1 | 1 | 2 | 5 | 5 | 8 | 19 |
| 35–49 | 78 | 4.5 | 13 | 1 | 2 | 3 | 7 | 9 | 13 | 18 |
| 50–64 | 96 | 4.6 | 30 | 2 | 2 | 3 | 6 | 9 | 12 | 31 |
| 65+ | 186 | 6.0 | 46 | 2 | 2 | 6 | 7 | 9 | 12 | 41 |
| **GRAND TOTAL** | 474 | 4.9 | 30 | 1 | 2 | 3 | 7 | 9 | 12 | 22 |

### 76.31: PARTIAL MANDIBULECTOMY. Formerly included in operation group(s) 717.

| Type of Patients | Observed Patients | Avg. Stay | Vari-ance | 10th | 25th | 50th | 75th | 90th | 95th | 99th |
|---|---|---|---|---|---|---|---|---|---|---|
| **1. SINGLE DX** | | | | | | | | | | |
| 0–19 Years | 12 | 5.2 | 12 | 1 | 1 | 7 | 7 | 9 | 9 | 19 |
| 20–34 | 9 | 2.2 | 3 | 1 | 1 | 1 | 4 | 5 | 5 | 5 |
| 35–49 | 9 | 3.5 | 6 | 1 | 2 | 3 | 7 | 7 | 8 | 8 |
| 50–64 | 9 | 3.2 | 9 | 1 | 2 | 2 | 2 | 6 | 11 | 11 |
| 65+ | 4 | 2.8 | <1 | 2 | 2 | 2 | 4 | 4 | 4 | 4 |
| **2. MULTIPLE DX** | | | | | | | | | | |
| 0–19 Years | 26 | 3.7 | 6 | 1 | 2 | 3 | 6 | 6 | 7 | 11 |
| 20–34 | 37 | 3.3 | 15 | 1 | 1 | 2 | 5 | 6 | 10 | 19 |
| 35–49 | 44 | 5.4 | 16 | 2 | 2 | 4 | 8 | 11 | 13 | 18 |
| 50–64 | 69 | 5.0 | 36 | 2 | 2 | 3 | 7 | 10 | 12 | 31 |
| 65+ | 131 | 6.5 | 53 | 2 | 3 | 6 | 7 | 10 | 14 | 41 |
| **TOTAL SINGLE DX** | 43 | 3.7 | 8 | 1 | 1 | 2 | 7 | 7 | 9 | 11 |
| **TOTAL MULTIPLE DX** | 307 | 5.3 | 36 | 1 | 2 | 4 | 7 | 9 | 13 | 29 |
| **TOTAL** | | | | | | | | | | |
| 0–19 Years | 38 | 4.3 | 9 | 1 | 2 | 4 | 7 | 7 | 9 | 11 |
| 20–34 | 46 | 3.1 | 13 | 1 | 1 | 2 | 5 | 5 | 9 | 19 |
| 35–49 | 53 | 5.2 | 15 | 2 | 2 | 3 | 8 | 9 | 13 | 18 |
| 50–64 | 78 | 4.8 | 34 | 1 | 2 | 3 | 6 | 10 | 12 | 31 |
| 65+ | 135 | 6.3 | 51 | 2 | 3 | 6 | 7 | 9 | 13 | 41 |
| **GRAND TOTAL** | 350 | 5.1 | 33 | 1 | 2 | 3 | 7 | 9 | 12 | 29 |

### 76.4: FACIAL BONE EXC/RECONST. Formerly included in operation group(s) 718.

| Type of Patients | Observed Patients | Avg. Stay | Vari-ance | 10th | 25th | 50th | 75th | 90th | 95th | 99th |
|---|---|---|---|---|---|---|---|---|---|---|
| **1. SINGLE DX** | | | | | | | | | | |
| 0–19 Years | 30 | 3.0 | 2 | 2 | 2 | 2 | 4 | 5 | 5 | 7 |
| 20–34 | 17 | 2.3 | <1 | 1 | 2 | 3 | 3 | 3 | 3 | 3 |
| 35–49 | 11 | 1.9 | 1 | 1 | 1 | 2 | 2 | 3 | 4 | 5 |
| 50–64 | 8 | 3.2 | 22 | 1 | 2 | 2 | 2 | 16 | 16 | 16 |
| 65+ | 0 | | | | | | | | | |
| **2. MULTIPLE DX** | | | | | | | | | | |
| 0–19 Years | 111 | 3.3 | 9 | 1 | 2 | 3 | 4 | 5 | 7 | 19 |
| 20–34 | 46 | 4.6 | 21 | 1 | 2 | 3 | 8 | 8 | 19 | 20 |
| 35–49 | 51 | 4.0 | 19 | 1 | 2 | 2 | 4 | 15 | 15 | 15 |
| 50–64 | 33 | 4.2 | 52 | 1 | 1 | 2 | 4 | 8 | 18 | 51 |
| 65+ | 36 | 7.4 | 66 | 2 | 2 | 3 | 9 | 19 | 24 | 34 |
| **TOTAL SINGLE DX** | 66 | 2.7 | 4 | 1 | 2 | 2 | 3 | 5 | 5 | 16 |
| **TOTAL MULTIPLE DX** | 277 | 4.2 | 27 | 1 | 2 | 3 | 4 | 8 | 15 | 24 |
| **TOTAL** | | | | | | | | | | |
| 0–19 Years | 141 | 3.2 | 7 | 1 | 2 | 3 | 4 | 5 | 6 | 11 |
| 20–34 | 63 | 4.1 | 17 | 1 | 2 | 3 | 5 | 8 | 15 | 20 |
| 35–49 | 62 | 3.6 | 16 | 1 | 1 | 2 | 3 | 11 | 15 | 15 |
| 50–64 | 41 | 4.1 | 48 | 1 | 2 | 3 | 4 | 8 | 16 | 51 |
| 65+ | 36 | 7.4 | 66 | 2 | 2 | 3 | 9 | 19 | 24 | 34 |
| **GRAND TOTAL** | 343 | 3.9 | 22 | 1 | 2 | 2 | 4 | 8 | 15 | 20 |

### 76.5: TMJ ARTHROPLASTY. Formerly included in operation group(s) 718.

| Type of Patients | Observed Patients | Avg. Stay | Vari-ance | 10th | 25th | 50th | 75th | 90th | 95th | 99th |
|---|---|---|---|---|---|---|---|---|---|---|
| **1. SINGLE DX** | | | | | | | | | | |
| 0–19 Years | 18 | 1.5 | <1 | 1 | 1 | 1 | 2 | 3 | 3 | 3 |
| 20–34 | 76 | 1.4 | <1 | 1 | 1 | 1 | 2 | 2 | 2 | 3 |
| 35–49 | 105 | 1.9 | 2 | 1 | 1 | 1 | 2 | 3 | 6 | 7 |
| 50–64 | 36 | 1.8 | 2 | 1 | 1 | 2 | 2 | 2 | 3 | 9 |
| 65+ | 2 | 1.6 | <1 | 1 | 1 | 2 | 2 | 2 | 2 | 2 |
| **2. MULTIPLE DX** | | | | | | | | | | |
| 0–19 Years | 43 | 3.0 | 4 | 1 | 1 | 2 | 5 | 5 | 8 | 8 |
| 20–34 | 123 | 1.9 | 2 | 1 | 1 | 2 | 2 | 4 | 4 | 11 |
| 35–49 | 196 | 2.0 | 3 | 1 | 1 | 2 | 2 | 4 | 4 | 8 |
| 50–64 | 54 | 2.2 | 2 | 1 | 1 | 2 | 3 | 4 | 4 | 6 |
| 65+ | 20 | 5.1 | 54 | 1 | 1 | 2 | 3 | 21 | 21 | 21 |
| **TOTAL SINGLE DX** | 237 | 1.7 | 2 | 1 | 1 | 1 | 2 | 3 | 4 | 7 |
| **TOTAL MULTIPLE DX** | 436 | 2.2 | 5 | 1 | 1 | 2 | 2 | 4 | 5 | 11 |
| **TOTAL** | | | | | | | | | | |
| 0–19 Years | 61 | 2.6 | 4 | 1 | 1 | 2 | 2 | 5 | 7 | 8 |
| 20–34 | 199 | 1.7 | 2 | 1 | 1 | 1 | 2 | 3 | 4 | 7 |
| 35–49 | 301 | 1.9 | 3 | 1 | 1 | 1 | 2 | 4 | 4 | 8 |
| 50–64 | 90 | 2.1 | 2 | 1 | 1 | 2 | 3 | 4 | 4 | 6 |
| 65+ | 22 | 4.7 | 49 | 1 | 1 | 2 | 3 | 21 | 21 | 21 |
| **GRAND TOTAL** | 673 | 2.0 | 4 | 1 | 1 | 1 | 2 | 4 | 5 | 8 |

Length of Stay by Diagnosis and Operation, United States, 2000

# United States, October 1998–September 1999 Data, by Operation

## 76.6: OTHER FACIAL BONE REPAIR. Formerly included in operation group(s) 718.

| Type of Patients | Observed Patients | Avg. Stay | Vari-ance | 10th | 25th | 50th | 75th | 90th | 95th | 99th |
|---|---|---|---|---|---|---|---|---|---|---|
| **1. SINGLE DX** | | | | | | | | | | |
| 0–19 Years | 375 | 1.7 | <1 | 1 | 1 | 1 | 2 | 2 | 3 | 5 |
| 20–34 | 233 | 1.5 | <1 | 1 | 1 | 1 | 2 | 2 | 3 | 5 |
| 35–49 | 146 | 1.6 | <1 | 1 | 1 | 1 | 2 | 2 | 3 | 5 |
| 50–64 | 25 | 1.8 | <1 | 1 | 1 | 2 | 2 | 3 | 5 | 5 |
| 65+ | 1 | 1.0 | 0 | 1 | 1 | 1 | 1 | 1 | 1 | 1 |
| **2. MULTIPLE DX** | | | | | | | | | | |
| 0–19 Years | 1,297 | 2.2 | 3 | 1 | 1 | 2 | 3 | 4 | 4 | 8 |
| 20–34 | 736 | 1.9 | 2 | 1 | 1 | 2 | 2 | 3 | 4 | 5 |
| 35–49 | 476 | 2.2 | 5 | 1 | 1 | 2 | 2 | 3 | 4 | 12 |
| 50–64 | 120 | 2.1 | 3 | 1 | 1 | 2 | 2 | 3 | 4 | 14 |
| 65+ | 13 | 3.2 | 5 | 1 | 1 | 3 | 4 | 8 | 8 | 9 |
| **TOTAL SINGLE DX** | 780 | 1.6 | <1 | 1 | 1 | 1 | 2 | 2 | 3 | 5 |
| **TOTAL MULTIPLE DX** | 2,642 | 2.1 | 3 | 1 | 1 | 2 | 2 | 3 | 4 | 9 |
| **TOTAL** | | | | | | | | | | |
| 0–19 Years | 1,672 | 2.0 | 3 | 1 | 1 | 2 | 2 | 3 | 4 | 7 |
| 20–34 | 969 | 1.8 | 2 | 1 | 1 | 2 | 2 | 3 | 4 | 5 |
| 35–49 | 622 | 2.1 | 4 | 1 | 1 | 2 | 2 | 3 | 4 | 12 |
| 50–64 | 145 | 2.1 | 3 | 1 | 1 | 2 | 2 | 3 | 4 | 14 |
| 65+ | 14 | 3.0 | 5 | 1 | 1 | 3 | 4 | 8 | 8 | 9 |
| **GRAND TOTAL** | 3,422 | 2.0 | 3 | 1 | 1 | 2 | 2 | 3 | 4 | 7 |

## 76.62: OPN OSTY MAND RAMUS. Formerly included in operation group(s) 718.

| Type of Patients | Observed Patients | Avg. Stay | Vari-ance | 10th | 25th | 50th | 75th | 90th | 95th | 99th |
|---|---|---|---|---|---|---|---|---|---|---|
| **1. SINGLE DX** | | | | | | | | | | |
| 0–19 Years | 91 | 1.4 | <1 | 1 | 1 | 1 | 2 | 2 | 2 | 3 |
| 20–34 | 49 | 1.4 | <1 | 1 | 1 | 1 | 2 | 2 | 2 | 3 |
| 35–49 | 36 | 1.3 | <1 | 1 | 1 | 1 | 2 | 2 | 2 | 3 |
| 50–64 | 6 | 1.8 | <1 | 1 | 2 | 2 | 2 | 2 | 2 | 2 |
| 65+ | 0 | | | | | | | | | |
| **2. MULTIPLE DX** | | | | | | | | | | |
| 0–19 Years | 198 | 1.7 | 2 | 1 | 1 | 1 | 2 | 3 | 3 | 6 |
| 20–34 | 95 | 2.3 | 3 | 1 | 1 | 2 | 3 | 5 | 5 | 5 |
| 35–49 | 102 | 1.6 | <1 | 1 | 1 | 2 | 2 | 2 | 3 | 5 |
| 50–64 | 19 | 1.4 | 1 | 1 | 1 | 1 | 1 | 3 | 3 | 6 |
| 65+ | 2 | 3.5 | 15 | 1 | 2 | 3 | 8 | 8 | 8 | 8 |
| **TOTAL SINGLE DX** | 182 | 1.4 | <1 | 1 | 1 | 1 | 2 | 2 | 2 | 3 |
| **TOTAL MULTIPLE DX** | 416 | 1.8 | 2 | 1 | 1 | 1 | 2 | 3 | 5 | 6 |
| **TOTAL** | | | | | | | | | | |
| 0–19 Years | 289 | 1.6 | 1 | 1 | 1 | 1 | 2 | 3 | 3 | 5 |
| 20–34 | 144 | 2.0 | 2 | 1 | 1 | 2 | 2 | 5 | 5 | 5 |
| 35–49 | 138 | 1.6 | 1 | 1 | 1 | 2 | 2 | 2 | 3 | 4 |
| 50–64 | 25 | 1.5 | <1 | 1 | 1 | 1 | 2 | 2 | 3 | 6 |
| 65+ | 2 | 3.5 | 15 | 1 | 2 | 3 | 8 | 8 | 8 | 8 |
| **GRAND TOTAL** | 598 | 1.7 | 1 | 1 | 1 | 1 | 2 | 3 | 4 | 5 |

## 76.64: MAND ORTHOGNATHIC OP NEC. Formerly included in operation group(s) 718.

| Type of Patients | Observed Patients | Avg. Stay | Vari-ance | 10th | 25th | 50th | 75th | 90th | 95th | 99th |
|---|---|---|---|---|---|---|---|---|---|---|
| **1. SINGLE DX** | | | | | | | | | | |
| 0–19 Years | 84 | 1.5 | <1 | 1 | 1 | 1 | 2 | 2 | 3 | 4 |
| 20–34 | 56 | 1.6 | <1 | 1 | 1 | 2 | 2 | 2 | 3 | 3 |
| 35–49 | 41 | 1.7 | <1 | 1 | 1 | 1 | 2 | 2 | 3 | 6 |
| 50–64 | 5 | 1.6 | <1 | 1 | 1 | 2 | 2 | 2 | 2 | 2 |
| 65+ | 0 | | | | | | | | | |
| **2. MULTIPLE DX** | | | | | | | | | | |
| 0–19 Years | 189 | 2.6 | 12 | 1 | 1 | 2 | 3 | 4 | 5 | 23 |
| 20–34 | 100 | 1.8 | <1 | 1 | 1 | 2 | 2 | 2 | 3 | 6 |
| 35–49 | 77 | 1.7 | 1 | 1 | 1 | 1 | 2 | 2 | 3 | 8 |
| 50–64 | 27 | 2.7 | 5 | 2 | 2 | 3 | 3 | 3 | 5 | 15 |
| 65+ | 3 | 3.1 | 5 | 1 | 1 | 3 | 3 | 8 | 8 | 8 |
| **TOTAL SINGLE DX** | 186 | 1.5 | <1 | 1 | 1 | 1 | 2 | 2 | 3 | 4 |
| **TOTAL MULTIPLE DX** | 396 | 2.2 | 7 | 1 | 1 | 2 | 2 | 3 | 4 | 23 |
| **TOTAL** | | | | | | | | | | |
| 0–19 Years | 273 | 2.3 | 9 | 1 | 1 | 2 | 2 | 4 | 4 | 23 |
| 20–34 | 156 | 1.7 | <1 | 1 | 1 | 1 | 2 | 2 | 3 | 4 |
| 35–49 | 118 | 1.7 | 1 | 1 | 1 | 2 | 2 | 3 | 3 | 6 |
| 50–64 | 32 | 2.6 | 5 | 1 | 2 | 3 | 3 | 3 | 5 | 15 |
| 65+ | 3 | 3.1 | 5 | 1 | 1 | 3 | 3 | 8 | 8 | 8 |
| **GRAND TOTAL** | 582 | 2.0 | 5 | 1 | 1 | 2 | 2 | 3 | 4 | 15 |

## 76.65: SEG OSTEOPLASTY MAXILLA. Formerly included in operation group(s) 718.

| Type of Patients | Observed Patients | Avg. Stay | Vari-ance | 10th | 25th | 50th | 75th | 90th | 95th | 99th |
|---|---|---|---|---|---|---|---|---|---|---|
| **1. SINGLE DX** | | | | | | | | | | |
| 0–19 Years | 105 | 1.7 | <1 | 1 | 1 | 2 | 2 | 2 | 3 | 4 |
| 20–34 | 71 | 1.4 | <1 | 1 | 1 | 1 | 2 | 2 | 3 | 3 |
| 35–49 | 36 | 1.5 | <1 | 1 | 1 | 1 | 2 | 2 | 3 | 3 |
| 50–64 | 9 | 2.1 | 2 | 1 | 1 | 1 | 3 | 5 | 5 | 5 |
| 65+ | 1 | 1.0 | 0 | 1 | 1 | 2 | 2 | 1 | 1 | 1 |
| **2. MULTIPLE DX** | | | | | | | | | | |
| 0–19 Years | 585 | 2.1 | 1 | 1 | 1 | 2 | 2 | 3 | 4 | 5 |
| 20–34 | 372 | 1.9 | 1 | 1 | 1 | 2 | 2 | 3 | 3 | 5 |
| 35–49 | 196 | 2.1 | 1 | 1 | 2 | 2 | 2 | 3 | 3 | 6 |
| 50–64 | 50 | 2.1 | 4 | 1 | 1 | 2 | 2 | 4 | 4 | 14 |
| 65+ | 5 | 3.7 | 4 | 1 | 2 | 4 | 4 | 4 | 9 | 9 |
| **TOTAL SINGLE DX** | 222 | 1.6 | <1 | 1 | 1 | 1 | 2 | 2 | 3 | 4 |
| **TOTAL MULTIPLE DX** | 1,208 | 2.0 | 2 | 1 | 1 | 2 | 2 | 3 | 4 | 6 |
| **TOTAL** | | | | | | | | | | |
| 0–19 Years | 690 | 2.0 | 1 | 1 | 1 | 2 | 2 | 3 | 4 | 5 |
| 20–34 | 443 | 1.8 | 1 | 1 | 1 | 2 | 2 | 3 | 3 | 5 |
| 35–49 | 232 | 2.0 | <1 | 1 | 1 | 2 | 2 | 3 | 3 | 5 |
| 50–64 | 59 | 2.1 | 4 | 1 | 2 | 2 | 2 | 4 | 4 | 14 |
| 65+ | 6 | 3.2 | 4 | 1 | 1 | 4 | 4 | 4 | 9 | 9 |
| **GRAND TOTAL** | 1,430 | 2.0 | 1 | 1 | 1 | 2 | 2 | 3 | 4 | 5 |

## United States, October 1998–September 1999 Data, by Operation

### 76.66: TOT OSTEOPLASTY MAXILLA. Formerly included in operation group(s) 718.

| Type of Patients | Observed Patients | Avg. Stay | Variance | 10th | 25th | 50th | 75th | 90th | 95th | 99th |
|---|---|---|---|---|---|---|---|---|---|---|
| **1. SINGLE DX** | | | | | | | | | | |
| 0–19 Years | 38 | 2.3 | 2 | 1 | 1 | 2 | 3 | 5 | 5 | 5 |
| 20–34 | 24 | 2.0 | 2 | 1 | 1 | 2 | 3 | 5 | 5 | 5 |
| 35–49 | 10 | 2.0 | 3 | 1 | 2 | 2 | 2 | 3 | 3 | 3 |
| 50–64 | 1 | 2.0 | <1 | 2 | 2 | 2 | 2 | 2 | 3 | 3 |
| 65+ | 0 | 2.0 | 0 | 2 | 2 | 2 | 2 | 2 | 2 | 2 |
| **2. MULTIPLE DX** | | | | | | | | | | |
| 0–19 Years | 171 | 2.2 | 1 | 1 | 2 | 2 | 3 | 3 | 4 | 8 |
| 20–34 | 90 | 1.7 | 6 | 1 | 1 | 1 | 2 | 2 | 3 | 5 |
| 35–49 | 45 | 1.6 | <1 | 1 | 1 | 2 | 2 | 2 | 3 | 4 |
| 50–64 | 5 | 2.0 | <1 | 1 | 2 | 2 | 2 | 3 | 3 | 3 |
| 65+ | 0 | | | | | | | | | |
| **TOTAL SINGLE DX** | 73 | 2.2 | 2 | 1 | 1 | 2 | 3 | 5 | 5 | 5 |
| **TOTAL MULTIPLE DX** | 311 | 2.0 | 3 | 1 | 1 | 2 | 2 | 3 | 3 | 8 |
| **TOTAL** | | | | | | | | | | |
| 0–19 Years | 209 | 2.2 | 2 | 1 | 1 | 2 | 3 | 3 | 5 | 8 |
| 20–34 | 114 | 1.7 | 5 | 1 | 1 | 1 | 2 | 3 | 4 | 5 |
| 35–49 | 55 | 1.7 | <1 | 1 | 1 | 2 | 2 | 3 | 3 | 4 |
| 50–64 | 6 | 2.0 | <1 | 2 | 2 | 2 | 2 | 3 | 3 | 3 |
| 65+ | 0 | | | | | | | | | |
| **GRAND TOTAL** | 384 | 2.0 | 3 | 1 | 1 | 2 | 2 | 3 | 4 | 8 |

### 76.72: OPEN RED MALAR/ZMC FX. Formerly included in operation group(s) 720.

| Type of Patients | Observed Patients | Avg. Stay | Variance | 10th | 25th | 50th | 75th | 90th | 95th | 99th |
|---|---|---|---|---|---|---|---|---|---|---|
| **1. SINGLE DX** | | | | | | | | | | |
| 0–19 Years | 24 | 1.4 | <1 | 1 | 1 | 1 | 1 | 3 | 3 | 4 |
| 20–34 | 58 | 1.7 | <1 | 1 | 1 | 1 | 2 | 3 | 4 | 6 |
| 35–49 | 46 | 1.5 | <1 | 1 | 1 | 1 | 1 | 3 | 5 | 7 |
| 50–64 | 13 | 1.3 | <1 | 1 | 1 | 1 | 2 | 2 | 2 | 3 |
| 65+ | 2 | 6.7 | 7 | 2 | 8 | 8 | 8 | 8 | 8 | 8 |
| **2. MULTIPLE DX** | | | | | | | | | | |
| 0–19 Years | 115 | 4.5 | 48 | 1 | 1 | 2 | 5 | 9 | 15 | 44 |
| 20–34 | 269 | 3.1 | 8 | 1 | 1 | 2 | 4 | 6 | 9 | 13 |
| 35–49 | 272 | 4.2 | 17 | 1 | 2 | 3 | 5 | 9 | 11 | 18 |
| 50–64 | 95 | 4.5 | 16 | 1 | 2 | 4 | 6 | 10 | 16 | 18 |
| 65+ | 58 | 5.7 | 23 | 2 | 2 | 6 | 6 | 10 | 15 | 25 |
| **TOTAL SINGLE DX** | 143 | 1.6 | 1 | 1 | 1 | 1 | 2 | 3 | 4 | 7 |
| **TOTAL MULTIPLE DX** | 809 | 4.0 | 18 | 1 | 2 | 3 | 5 | 9 | 11 | 20 |
| **TOTAL** | | | | | | | | | | |
| 0–19 Years | 139 | 4.1 | 43 | 1 | 1 | 2 | 5 | 7 | 14 | 44 |
| 20–34 | 327 | 2.9 | 7 | 1 | 1 | 2 | 3 | 5 | 8 | 13 |
| 35–49 | 318 | 3.7 | 15 | 1 | 2 | 3 | 4 | 9 | 10 | 18 |
| 50–64 | 108 | 4.2 | 15 | 1 | 2 | 4 | 5 | 9 | 13 | 17 |
| 65+ | 60 | 5.7 | 22 | 2 | 2 | 6 | 6 | 10 | 15 | 25 |
| **GRAND TOTAL** | 952 | 3.6 | 16 | 1 | 1 | 2 | 4 | 8 | 10 | 19 |

### 76.7: REDUCTION OF FACIAL FX. Formerly included in operation group(s) 719, 720.

| Type of Patients | Observed Patients | Avg. Stay | Variance | 10th | 25th | 50th | 75th | 90th | 95th | 99th |
|---|---|---|---|---|---|---|---|---|---|---|
| **1. SINGLE DX** | | | | | | | | | | |
| 0–19 Years | 306 | 2.0 | 2 | 1 | 1 | 2 | 2 | 3 | 5 | 7 |
| 20–34 | 481 | 2.1 | 2 | 1 | 1 | 2 | 3 | 4 | 5 | 7 |
| 35–49 | 236 | 2.1 | 3 | 1 | 1 | 2 | 3 | 4 | 5 | 8 |
| 50–64 | 39 | 1.9 | 3 | 1 | 1 | 1 | 2 | 3 | 6 | 8 |
| 65+ | 9 | 3.3 | 9 | 1 | 1 | 2 | 8 | 8 | 8 | 8 |
| **2. MULTIPLE DX** | | | | | | | | | | |
| 0–19 Years | 1,216 | 3.6 | 18 | 1 | 1 | 2 | 4 | 7 | 10 | 19 |
| 20–34 | 2,005 | 3.6 | 14 | 1 | 2 | 3 | 4 | 7 | 9 | 17 |
| 35–49 | 1,599 | 4.0 | 18 | 1 | 2 | 3 | 5 | 8 | 11 | 20 |
| 50–64 | 414 | 5.4 | 30 | 1 | 2 | 4 | 7 | 11 | 16 | 24 |
| 65+ | 338 | 5.6 | 22 | 2 | 2 | 4 | 7 | 12 | 15 | 22 |
| **TOTAL SINGLE DX** | 1,071 | 2.1 | 2 | 1 | 1 | 2 | 3 | 4 | 5 | 8 |
| **TOTAL MULTIPLE DX** | 5,572 | 3.9 | 18 | 1 | 2 | 3 | 5 | 8 | 11 | 19 |
| **TOTAL** | | | | | | | | | | |
| 0–19 Years | 1,522 | 3.3 | 15 | 1 | 1 | 2 | 4 | 7 | 9 | 17 |
| 20–34 | 2,486 | 3.3 | 12 | 1 | 1 | 2 | 4 | 7 | 9 | 16 |
| 35–49 | 1,835 | 3.7 | 17 | 1 | 1 | 3 | 6 | 7 | 10 | 19 |
| 50–64 | 453 | 5.2 | 29 | 1 | 2 | 4 | 6 | 11 | 16 | 20 |
| 65+ | 347 | 5.5 | 22 | 2 | 2 | 4 | 7 | 12 | 15 | 22 |
| **GRAND TOTAL** | 6,643 | 3.6 | 16 | 1 | 1 | 2 | 4 | 7 | 10 | 18 |

### 76.74: OPEN RED MAXILLARY FX. Formerly included in operation group(s) 720.

| Type of Patients | Observed Patients | Avg. Stay | Variance | 10th | 25th | 50th | 75th | 90th | 95th | 99th |
|---|---|---|---|---|---|---|---|---|---|---|
| **1. SINGLE DX** | | | | | | | | | | |
| 0–19 Years | 8 | 3.1 | 10 | 1 | 1 | 1 | 7 | 9 | 9 | 9 |
| 20–34 | 16 | 1.2 | <1 | 1 | 1 | 1 | 1 | 2 | 3 | 4 |
| 35–49 | 9 | 1.6 | 4 | 1 | 1 | 1 | 1 | 3 | 3 | 10 |
| 50–64 | 2 | 1.7 | <1 | 1 | 1 | 2 | 2 | 2 | 2 | 2 |
| 65+ | 0 | | | | | | | | | |
| **2. MULTIPLE DX** | | | | | | | | | | |
| 0–19 Years | 70 | 3.9 | 18 | 1 | 2 | 3 | 5 | 7 | 9 | 14 |
| 20–34 | 121 | 4.6 | 15 | 1 | 2 | 3 | 8 | 9 | 12 | 18 |
| 35–49 | 119 | 4.7 | 22 | 1 | 3 | 3 | 7 | 11 | 12 | 22 |
| 50–64 | 42 | 7.7 | 32 | 3 | 3 | 8 | 16 | 16 | 16 | 16 |
| 65+ | 34 | 9.8 | 46 | 2 | 4 | 8 | 14 | 22 | 22 | 22 |
| **TOTAL SINGLE DX** | 35 | 1.8 | 4 | 1 | 1 | 1 | 1 | 3 | 7 | 9 |
| **TOTAL MULTIPLE DX** | 386 | 5.4 | 25 | 1 | 2 | 3 | 8 | 12 | 16 | 22 |
| **TOTAL** | | | | | | | | | | |
| 0–19 Years | 78 | 3.8 | 16 | 1 | 1 | 2 | 5 | 9 | 9 | 14 |
| 20–34 | 137 | 3.9 | 14 | 1 | 3 | 3 | 5 | 9 | 10 | 18 |
| 35–49 | 128 | 4.3 | 21 | 1 | 2 | 3 | 6 | 11 | 11 | 22 |
| 50–64 | 44 | 7.6 | 33 | 3 | 4 | 8 | 16 | 16 | 16 | 16 |
| 65+ | 34 | 9.8 | 46 | 2 | 4 | 8 | 14 | 22 | 22 | 22 |
| **GRAND TOTAL** | 421 | 4.9 | 24 | 1 | 1 | 3 | 8 | 11 | 16 | 22 |

# United States, October 1998–September 1999 Data, by Operation

## 76.75: CLSD RED MANDIBULAR FX. Formerly included in operation group(s) 719.

| Type of Patients | Observed Patients | Avg. Stay | Variance | Percentiles | | | | | | |
|---|---|---|---|---|---|---|---|---|---|---|
| | | | | 10th | 25th | 50th | 75th | 90th | 95th | 99th |
| **1. SINGLE DX** | | | | | | | | | | |
| 0–19 Years | 97 | 2.0 | <1 | 1 | 1 | 2 | 2 | 3 | 4 | 5 |
| 20–34 | 117 | 2.3 | 1 | 1 | 1 | 2 | 3 | 4 | 5 | 8 |
| 35–49 | 38 | 2.4 | 2 | 1 | 1 | 2 | 3 | 5 | 5 | 6 |
| 50–64 | 2 | 1.0 | 0 | 1 | 1 | 1 | 1 | 1 | 1 | 1 |
| 65+ | 1 | 1.0 | 0 | 1 | 1 | 1 | 1 | 1 | 1 | 1 |
| **2. MULTIPLE DX** | | | | | | | | | | |
| 0–19 Years | 239 | 2.7 | 7 | 1 | 1 | 2 | 3 | 6 | 9 | 14 |
| 20–34 | 256 | 3.3 | 27 | 1 | 1 | 2 | 4 | 6 | 9 | 14 |
| 35–49 | 170 | 3.3 | 11 | 1 | 1 | 2 | 4 | 7 | 14 | 16 |
| 50–64 | 32 | 5.2 | 27 | 1 | 4 | 4 | 5 | 5 | 25 | 25 |
| 65+ | 32 | 6.5 | 39 | 1 | 2 | 4 | 8 | 20 | 21 | 21 |
| **TOTAL SINGLE DX** | 255 | 2.2 | 2 | 1 | 1 | 2 | 3 | 4 | 5 | 6 |
| **TOTAL MULTIPLE DX** | 729 | 3.3 | 18 | 1 | 1 | 2 | 4 | 6 | 9 | 17 |
| **TOTAL** | | | | | | | | | | |
| 0–19 Years | 336 | 2.5 | 5 | 1 | 1 | 2 | 3 | 4 | 7 | 11 |
| 20–34 | 373 | 3.1 | 21 | 1 | 1 | 2 | 4 | 4 | 5 | 9 |
| 35–49 | 208 | 3.2 | 10 | 1 | 1 | 2 | 4 | 5 | 10 | 16 |
| 50–64 | 34 | 5.1 | 27 | 1 | 3 | 4 | 5 | 5 | 25 | 25 |
| 65+ | 33 | 6.4 | 38 | 1 | 2 | 3 | 8 | 20 | 21 | 21 |
| **GRAND TOTAL** | 984 | 3.1 | 14 | 1 | 1 | 2 | 4 | 6 | 9 | 14 |

## 76.76: OPEN RED MANDIBULAR FX. Formerly included in operation group(s) 720.

| Type of Patients | Observed Patients | Avg. Stay | Variance | Percentiles | | | | | | |
|---|---|---|---|---|---|---|---|---|---|---|
| | | | | 10th | 25th | 50th | 75th | 90th | 95th | 99th |
| **1. SINGLE DX** | | | | | | | | | | |
| 0–19 Years | 134 | 2.3 | 2 | 1 | 1 | 2 | 3 | 4 | 5 | 7 |
| 20–34 | 230 | 2.5 | 2 | 1 | 2 | 2 | 3 | 4 | 6 | 7 |
| 35–49 | 116 | 3.0 | 3 | 1 | 2 | 3 | 4 | 5 | 6 | 8 |
| 50–64 | 17 | 2.5 | 3 | 1 | 1 | 3 | 3 | 3 | 8 | 8 |
| 65+ | 4 | 1.8 | <1 | 1 | 1 | 2 | 2 | 3 | 3 | 3 |
| **2. MULTIPLE DX** | | | | | | | | | | |
| 0–19 Years | 591 | 3.7 | 17 | 1 | 2 | 2 | 4 | 7 | 11 | 20 |
| 20–34 | 1,078 | 3.5 | 11 | 1 | 2 | 3 | 4 | 7 | 10 | 17 |
| 35–49 | 776 | 4.0 | 20 | 1 | 2 | 3 | 5 | 7 | 10 | 26 |
| 50–64 | 156 | 4.7 | 37 | 1 | 2 | 3 | 5 | 8 | 17 | 17 |
| 65+ | 140 | 5.1 | 15 | 2 | 3 | 4 | 6 | 10 | 14 | 18 |
| **TOTAL SINGLE DX** | 501 | 2.5 | 2 | 1 | 2 | 2 | 3 | 4 | 5 | 8 |
| **TOTAL MULTIPLE DX** | 2,741 | 3.8 | 16 | 1 | 2 | 3 | 4 | 7 | 10 | 18 |
| **TOTAL** | | | | | | | | | | |
| 0–19 Years | 725 | 3.5 | 15 | 1 | 2 | 2 | 4 | 6 | 10 | 17 |
| 20–34 | 1,308 | 3.3 | 9 | 1 | 2 | 3 | 4 | 7 | 8 | 17 |
| 35–49 | 892 | 3.9 | 18 | 1 | 2 | 3 | 4 | 6 | 9 | 23 |
| 50–64 | 173 | 4.5 | 35 | 1 | 2 | 3 | 6 | 8 | 17 | 17 |
| 65+ | 144 | 5.1 | 15 | 2 | 3 | 4 | 6 | 10 | 14 | 18 |
| **GRAND TOTAL** | 3,242 | 3.6 | 15 | 1 | 2 | 3 | 4 | 7 | 10 | 18 |

## 76.79: OPEN RED FACIAL FX NEC. Formerly included in operation group(s) 720.

| Type of Patients | Observed Patients | Avg. Stay | Variance | Percentiles | | | | | | |
|---|---|---|---|---|---|---|---|---|---|---|
| | | | | 10th | 25th | 50th | 75th | 90th | 95th | 99th |
| **1. SINGLE DX** | | | | | | | | | | |
| 0–19 Years | 27 | 1.2 | <1 | 1 | 1 | 1 | 1 | 1 | 2 | 7 |
| 20–34 | 46 | 1.6 | 2 | 1 | 1 | 1 | 2 | 3 | 5 | 8 |
| 35–49 | 14 | 1.0 | <1 | 1 | 1 | 1 | 1 | 1 | 1 | 2 |
| 50–64 | 4 | 2.0 | 3 | 1 | 1 | 1 | 4 | 6 | 6 | 6 |
| 65+ | 2 | 1.0 | 0 | 1 | 1 | 1 | 1 | 1 | 1 | 1 |
| **2. MULTIPLE DX** | | | | | | | | | | |
| 0–19 Years | 143 | 3.6 | 11 | 1 | 1 | 2 | 5 | 8 | 11 | 17 |
| 20–34 | 215 | 4.0 | 16 | 1 | 1 | 3 | 5 | 9 | 10 | 15 |
| 35–49 | 213 | 4.1 | 19 | 1 | 1 | 3 | 5 | 8 | 13 | 19 |
| 50–64 | 74 | 6.3 | 30 | 1 | 2 | 5 | 11 | 11 | 13 | 34 |
| 65+ | 65 | 4.5 | 13 | 1 | 2 | 4 | 5 | 11 | 12 | 14 |
| **TOTAL SINGLE DX** | 93 | 1.4 | 1 | 1 | 1 | 1 | 1 | 2 | 4 | 7 |
| **TOTAL MULTIPLE DX** | 710 | 4.1 | 17 | 1 | 1 | 3 | 5 | 9 | 11 | 19 |
| **TOTAL** | | | | | | | | | | |
| 0–19 Years | 170 | 3.2 | 10 | 1 | 1 | 2 | 4 | 8 | 10 | 17 |
| 20–34 | 261 | 3.5 | 14 | 1 | 1 | 2 | 4 | 8 | 9 | 15 |
| 35–49 | 227 | 3.6 | 17 | 1 | 1 | 2 | 4 | 8 | 11 | 19 |
| 50–64 | 78 | 5.9 | 29 | 1 | 2 | 5 | 9 | 11 | 12 | 34 |
| 65+ | 67 | 4.5 | 13 | 1 | 2 | 4 | 5 | 11 | 12 | 14 |
| **GRAND TOTAL** | 803 | 3.7 | 15 | 1 | 1 | 2 | 5 | 9 | 11 | 19 |

## 76.9: OTH OPS FACIAL BONE/JT. Formerly included in operation group(s) 721, 729, 767.

| Type of Patients | Observed Patients | Avg. Stay | Variance | Percentiles | | | | | | |
|---|---|---|---|---|---|---|---|---|---|---|
| | | | | 10th | 25th | 50th | 75th | 90th | 95th | 99th |
| **1. SINGLE DX** | | | | | | | | | | |
| 0–19 Years | 59 | 1.8 | <1 | 1 | 1 | 2 | 2 | 3 | 4 | 5 |
| 20–34 | 50 | 2.0 | 3 | 1 | 1 | 1 | 3 | 4 | 5 | 8 |
| 35–49 | 40 | 3.7 | 10 | 1 | 2 | 3 | 4 | 7 | 14 | 14 |
| 50–64 | 16 | 1.8 | 2 | 1 | 1 | 1 | 1 | 2 | 2 | 2 |
| 65+ | 4 | 1.1 | <1 | 1 | 1 | 1 | 1 | 2 | 2 | 2 |
| **2. MULTIPLE DX** | | | | | | | | | | |
| 0–19 Years | 137 | 2.8 | 23 | 1 | 1 | 2 | 3 | 4 | 5 | 7 |
| 20–34 | 115 | 4.7 | 57 | 1 | 1 | 3 | 3 | 14 | 16 | 48 |
| 35–49 | 156 | 3.6 | 24 | 1 | 1 | 2 | 5 | 6 | 10 | 29 |
| 50–64 | 78 | 3.8 | 14 | 1 | 1 | 2 | 4 | 10 | 10 | 12 |
| 65+ | 74 | 4.7 | 33 | 1 | 2 | 2 | 6 | 8 | 14 | 31 |
| **TOTAL SINGLE DX** | 169 | 2.4 | 5 | 1 | 1 | 2 | 3 | 4 | 7 | 14 |
| **TOTAL MULTIPLE DX** | 560 | 3.7 | 30 | 1 | 1 | 2 | 4 | 6 | 10 | 29 |
| **TOTAL** | | | | | | | | | | |
| 0–19 Years | 196 | 2.6 | 18 | 1 | 1 | 2 | 3 | 4 | 5 | 7 |
| 20–34 | 165 | 4.0 | 45 | 1 | 1 | 2 | 4 | 6 | 16 | 48 |
| 35–49 | 196 | 3.6 | 22 | 1 | 1 | 2 | 4 | 7 | 10 | 29 |
| 50–64 | 94 | 3.3 | 12 | 1 | 1 | 2 | 4 | 8 | 10 | 12 |
| 65+ | 78 | 4.5 | 32 | 1 | 2 | 2 | 6 | 8 | 14 | 31 |
| **GRAND TOTAL** | 729 | 3.4 | 25 | 1 | 1 | 2 | 4 | 6 | 10 | 29 |

Length of Stay by Diagnosis and Operation, United States, 2000

# United States, October 1998–September 1999 Data, by Operation

## 77.0: SEQUESTRECTOMY. Formerly included in operation group(s) 722, 723.

| Type of Patients | Observed Patients | Avg. Stay | Variance | 10th | 25th | 50th | 75th | 90th | 95th | 99th |
|---|---|---|---|---|---|---|---|---|---|---|
| **1. SINGLE DX** | | | | | | | | | | |
| 0–19 Years | 4 | 5.3 | 7 | 1 | 2 | 7 | 7 | 7 | 7 | 7 |
| 20–34 | 2 | 6.1 | 2 | 4 | 4 | 7 | 7 | 7 | 7 | 7 |
| 35–49 | 6 | 2.7 | 1 | 2 | 2 | 2 | 4 | 4 | 4 | 6 |
| 50–64 | 2 | 4.8 | 7 | 2 | 2 | 2 | 7 | 7 | 7 | 7 |
| 65+ | 0 | | | | | | | | | |
| **2. MULTIPLE DX** | | | | | | | | | | |
| 0–19 Years | 11 | 8.1 | 92 | 1 | 3 | 6 | 6 | 18 | 38 | 38 |
| 20–34 | 24 | 6.6 | 78 | 2 | 3 | 4 | 8 | 9 | 10 | 46 |
| 35–49 | 41 | 11.8 | 129 | 2 | 5 | 6 | 17 | 32 | 32 | 32 |
| 50–64 | 35 | 6.4 | 62 | 2 | 3 | 6 | 6 | 10 | 36 | 39 |
| 65+ | 31 | 7.4 | 31 | 2 | 4 | 5 | 12 | 13 | 20 | 25 |
| **TOTAL SINGLE DX** | 14 | 3.8 | 5 | 2 | 2 | 3 | 7 | 7 | 7 | 7 |
| **TOTAL MULTIPLE DX** | 142 | 9.0 | 94 | 2 | 3 | 5 | 11 | 32 | 32 | 39 |
| **TOTAL** | | | | | | | | | | |
| 0–19 Years | 15 | 7.2 | 67 | 3 | 3 | 6 | 7 | 18 | 18 | 38 |
| 20–34 | 26 | 6.6 | 69 | 2 | 3 | 5 | 7 | 9 | 10 | 46 |
| 35–49 | 47 | 10.3 | 119 | 2 | 3 | 5 | 12 | 32 | 32 | 32 |
| 50–64 | 37 | 6.3 | 59 | 2 | 3 | 5 | 6 | 10 | 36 | 39 |
| 65+ | 31 | 7.4 | 31 | 2 | 4 | 5 | 12 | 13 | 20 | 25 |
| **GRAND TOTAL** | 156 | 8.4 | 86 | 2 | 3 | 5 | 8 | 25 | 32 | 39 |

## 77.1: OTHER BONE INC W/O DIV. Formerly included in operation group(s) 722, 723.

| Type of Patients | Observed Patients | Avg. Stay | Variance | 10th | 25th | 50th | 75th | 90th | 95th | 99th |
|---|---|---|---|---|---|---|---|---|---|---|
| **1. SINGLE DX** | | | | | | | | | | |
| 0–19 Years | 70 | 2.4 | 2 | 1 | 2 | 2 | 3 | 5 | 5 | 8 |
| 20–34 | 40 | 1.8 | 4 | 1 | 1 | 1 | 2 | 3 | 4 | 11 |
| 35–49 | 29 | 2.6 | 3 | 1 | 1 | 2 | 3 | 5 | 6 | 7 |
| 50–64 | 16 | 5.2 | 10 | 1 | 2 | 5 | 7 | 7 | 13 | 13 |
| 65+ | 1 | 5.0 | 0 | 5 | 5 | 5 | 5 | 5 | 5 | 5 |
| **2. MULTIPLE DX** | | | | | | | | | | |
| 0–19 Years | 154 | 5.8 | 80 | 2 | 2 | 4 | 7 | 9 | 13 | 44 |
| 20–34 | 57 | 4.7 | 23 | 2 | 2 | 4 | 5 | 8 | 11 | 17 |
| 35–49 | 87 | 4.1 | 26 | 1 | 2 | 2 | 4 | 9 | 17 | 24 |
| 50–64 | 73 | 5.1 | 50 | 2 | 3 | 3 | 6 | 13 | 14 | 59 |
| 65+ | 73 | 9.1 | 78 | 2 | 3 | 7 | 10 | 22 | 32 | 39 |
| **TOTAL SINGLE DX** | 156 | 2.5 | 4 | 1 | 1 | 2 | 3 | 5 | 7 | 11 |
| **TOTAL MULTIPLE DX** | 444 | 5.6 | 57 | 1 | 2 | 3 | 7 | 11 | 16 | 36 |
| **TOTAL** | | | | | | | | | | |
| 0–19 Years | 224 | 4.4 | 51 | 1 | 1 | 2 | 5 | 8 | 10 | 36 |
| 20–34 | 97 | 3.3 | 16 | 1 | 1 | 2 | 4 | 7 | 8 | 17 |
| 35–49 | 116 | 3.9 | 23 | 1 | 2 | 2 | 4 | 6 | 14 | 24 |
| 50–64 | 89 | 5.1 | 42 | 1 | 2 | 3 | 7 | 13 | 14 | 19 |
| 65+ | 74 | 9.1 | 77 | 2 | 3 | 7 | 10 | 21 | 32 | 39 |
| **GRAND TOTAL** | 600 | 4.8 | 44 | 1 | 2 | 3 | 6 | 10 | 14 | 32 |

## 77.2: WEDGE OSTEOTOMY. Formerly included in operation group(s) 722, 723.

| Type of Patients | Observed Patients | Avg. Stay | Variance | 10th | 25th | 50th | 75th | 90th | 95th | 99th |
|---|---|---|---|---|---|---|---|---|---|---|
| **1. SINGLE DX** | | | | | | | | | | |
| 0–19 Years | 148 | 2.0 | 1 | 1 | 1 | 2 | 2 | 3 | 4 | 7 |
| 20–34 | 18 | 2.9 | 2 | 1 | 2 | 2 | 2 | 4 | 4 | 6 |
| 35–49 | 61 | 2.3 | <1 | 1 | 2 | 2 | 3 | 3 | 3 | 5 |
| 50–64 | 27 | 2.9 | 3 | 1 | 1 | 2 | 5 | 5 | 5 | 5 |
| 65+ | 2 | 1.0 | 0 | 1 | 1 | 1 | 1 | 1 | 1 | 1 |
| **2. MULTIPLE DX** | | | | | | | | | | |
| 0–19 Years | 384 | 3.1 | 18 | 1 | 2 | 3 | 3 | 5 | 7 | 17 |
| 20–34 | 66 | 2.7 | 2 | 1 | 1 | 3 | 3 | 5 | 6 | 9 |
| 35–49 | 163 | 2.7 | 2 | 1 | 2 | 2 | 4 | 4 | 5 | 9 |
| 50–64 | 136 | 2.7 | 3 | 2 | 2 | 3 | 3 | 5 | 7 | 7 |
| 65+ | 28 | 4.9 | 17 | 2 | 2 | 3 | 7 | 11 | 14 | 19 |
| **TOTAL SINGLE DX** | 256 | 2.2 | 2 | 1 | 1 | 2 | 3 | 4 | 5 | 6 |
| **TOTAL MULTIPLE DX** | 777 | 2.9 | 9 | 1 | 2 | 3 | 3 | 5 | 7 | 14 |
| **TOTAL** | | | | | | | | | | |
| 0–19 Years | 532 | 2.8 | 13 | 1 | 2 | 3 | 3 | 4 | 6 | 17 |
| 20–34 | 84 | 2.7 | 2 | 1 | 2 | 3 | 3 | 4 | 6 | 6 |
| 35–49 | 224 | 2.6 | 2 | 1 | 2 | 3 | 3 | 5 | 5 | 8 |
| 50–64 | 163 | 2.8 | 3 | 1 | 2 | 3 | 3 | 5 | 7 | 7 |
| 65+ | 30 | 4.8 | 17 | 1 | 2 | 3 | 7 | 11 | 14 | 19 |
| **GRAND TOTAL** | 1,033 | 2.8 | 8 | 1 | 2 | 2 | 3 | 4 | 6 | 11 |

## 77.25: FEMORAL WEDGE OSTEOTOMY. Formerly included in operation group(s) 722, 723.

| Type of Patients | Observed Patients | Avg. Stay | Variance | 10th | 25th | 50th | 75th | 90th | 95th | 99th |
|---|---|---|---|---|---|---|---|---|---|---|
| **1. SINGLE DX** | | | | | | | | | | |
| 0–19 Years | 51 | 2.5 | 1 | 1 | 2 | 2 | 3 | 3 | 4 | 9 |
| 20–34 | 6 | 4.0 | <1 | 4 | 4 | 4 | 4 | 3 | 6 | 6 |
| 35–49 | 6 | 2.6 | <1 | 2 | 2 | 3 | 3 | 3 | 3 | 3 |
| 50–64 | 0 | | | | | | | | | |
| 65+ | 0 | | | | | | | | | |
| **2. MULTIPLE DX** | | | | | | | | | | |
| 0–19 Years | 203 | 3.6 | 11 | 2 | 2 | 3 | 4 | 5 | 8 | 17 |
| 20–34 | 28 | 3.3 | 2 | 1 | 3 | 3 | 4 | 5 | 6 | 6 |
| 35–49 | 34 | 3.6 | 2 | 2 | 3 | 4 | 4 | 5 | 8 | 8 |
| 50–64 | 11 | 4.8 | 8 | 1 | 1 | 7 | 7 | 7 | 11 | 11 |
| 65+ | 7 | 6.9 | 9 | 3 | 4 | 8 | 8 | 8 | 14 | 14 |
| **TOTAL SINGLE DX** | 63 | 2.7 | 1 | 1 | 2 | 2 | 3 | 4 | 4 | 6 |
| **TOTAL MULTIPLE DX** | 283 | 3.6 | 7 | 2 | 2 | 3 | 4 | 6 | 7 | 17 |
| **TOTAL** | | | | | | | | | | |
| 0–19 Years | 254 | 3.3 | 9 | 2 | 2 | 3 | 4 | 5 | 7 | 17 |
| 20–34 | 34 | 3.3 | 2 | 2 | 3 | 3 | 4 | 5 | 6 | 6 |
| 35–49 | 40 | 3.5 | 2 | 2 | 4 | 4 | 7 | 7 | 5 | 8 |
| 50–64 | 11 | 4.8 | 8 | 1 | 1 | 7 | 7 | 8 | 14 | 11 |
| 65+ | 7 | 6.9 | 9 | 3 | 4 | 8 | 8 | 8 | 14 | 14 |
| **GRAND TOTAL** | 346 | 3.5 | 6 | 2 | 2 | 3 | 4 | 6 | 7 | 17 |

© 2000 by HCIA-Sachs, L.L.C.

Length of Stay by Diagnosis and Operation, United States, 2000

# United States, October 1998–September 1999 Data, by Operation

## 77.27: TIB & FIB WEDGE OSTY. Formerly included in operation group(s) 723.

| Type of Patients | Observed Patients | Avg. Stay | Variance | 10th | 25th | 50th | 75th | 90th | 95th | 99th |
|---|---|---|---|---|---|---|---|---|---|---|
| **1. SINGLE DX** | | | | | | | | | | |
| 0–19 Years | 38 | 2.0 | 2 | 1 | 1 | 2 | 2 | 3 | 4 | 7 |
| 20–34 | 7 | 2.1 | <1 | 1 | 2 | 2 | 2 | 3 | 4 | 4 |
| 35–49 | 51 | 2.2 | <1 | 1 | 2 | 2 | 2 | 4 | 4 | 6 |
| 50–64 | 24 | 3.0 | 3 | 1 | 1 | 2 | 5 | 5 | 5 | 5 |
| 65+ | 1 | 1.0 | 0 | 1 | 1 | 1 | 1 | 1 | 1 | 1 |
| **2. MULTIPLE DX** | | | | | | | | | | |
| 0–19 Years | 87 | 3.0 | 40 | 1 | 1 | 2 | 3 | 4 | 4 | 63 |
| 20–34 | 33 | 1.9 | 1 | 1 | 1 | 2 | 3 | 3 | 3 | 6 |
| 35–49 | 108 | 2.4 | 2 | 1 | 2 | 2 | 3 | 3 | 4 | 9 |
| 50–64 | 112 | 2.5 | 1 | 1 | 2 | 2 | 3 | 4 | 4 | 7 |
| 65+ | 15 | 2.8 | 2 | 1 | 2 | 2 | 4 | 5 | 5 | 6 |
| **TOTAL SINGLE DX** | 121 | 2.3 | 2 | 1 | 1 | 2 | 3 | 5 | 5 | 5 |
| **TOTAL MULTIPLE DX** | 355 | 2.5 | 12 | 1 | 1 | 2 | 3 | 4 | 4 | 8 |
| **TOTAL** | | | | | | | | | | |
| 0–19 Years | 125 | 2.7 | 31 | 1 | 1 | 2 | 3 | 4 | 4 | 22 |
| 20–34 | 40 | 1.9 | 1 | 1 | 1 | 2 | 3 | 3 | 4 | 6 |
| 35–49 | 159 | 2.4 | 2 | 1 | 1 | 2 | 3 | 3 | 5 | 8 |
| 50–64 | 136 | 2.6 | 2 | 2 | 2 | 2 | 3 | 5 | 5 | 7 |
| 65+ | 16 | 2.7 | 2 | 2 | 2 | 2 | 4 | 5 | 5 | 6 |
| **GRAND TOTAL** | 476 | 2.5 | 9 | 1 | 1 | 2 | 3 | 4 | 5 | 8 |

## 77.3: OTHER DIVISION OF BONE. Formerly included in operation group(s) 722, 723.

| Type of Patients | Observed Patients | Avg. Stay | Variance | 10th | 25th | 50th | 75th | 90th | 95th | 99th |
|---|---|---|---|---|---|---|---|---|---|---|
| **1. SINGLE DX** | | | | | | | | | | |
| 0–19 Years | 609 | 2.6 | 2 | 1 | 2 | 2 | 3 | 4 | 5 | 8 |
| 20–34 | 55 | 2.5 | 2 | 1 | 1 | 2 | 3 | 4 | 5 | 7 |
| 35–49 | 117 | 2.2 | 1 | 1 | 1 | 2 | 3 | 4 | 4 | 5 |
| 50–64 | 66 | 2.1 | 1 | 1 | 1 | 2 | 3 | 4 | 4 | 5 |
| 65+ | 8 | 2.3 | <1 | 2 | 2 | 2 | 3 | 3 | 3 | 3 |
| **2. MULTIPLE DX** | | | | | | | | | | |
| 0–19 Years | 1,292 | 3.0 | 7 | 1 | 2 | 3 | 3 | 5 | 6 | 14 |
| 20–34 | 171 | 2.6 | 5 | 1 | 1 | 2 | 3 | 5 | 6 | 9 |
| 35–49 | 332 | 4.8 | 102 | 1 | 2 | 2 | 3 | 6 | 15 | 48 |
| 50–64 | 214 | 4.8 | 26 | 2 | 2 | 3 | 5 | 15 | 15 | 18 |
| 65+ | 83 | 5.5 | 24 | 2 | 3 | 3 | 7 | 14 | 15 | 28 |
| **TOTAL SINGLE DX** | 855 | 2.5 | 2 | 1 | 2 | 2 | 3 | 4 | 5 | 8 |
| **TOTAL MULTIPLE DX** | 2,092 | 3.5 | 27 | 1 | 2 | 2 | 3 | 5 | 8 | 29 |
| **TOTAL** | | | | | | | | | | |
| 0–19 Years | 1,901 | 2.8 | 5 | 1 | 2 | 2 | 3 | 5 | 6 | 11 |
| 20–34 | 226 | 2.6 | 4 | 1 | 1 | 2 | 3 | 4 | 6 | 9 |
| 35–49 | 449 | 4.2 | 79 | 1 | 1 | 2 | 3 | 5 | 13 | 48 |
| 50–64 | 280 | 4.2 | 22 | 2 | 2 | 3 | 4 | 12 | 15 | 18 |
| 65+ | 91 | 5.4 | 23 | 2 | 3 | 3 | 7 | 14 | 14 | 28 |
| **GRAND TOTAL** | 2,947 | 3.2 | 20 | 1 | 2 | 2 | 3 | 5 | 7 | 18 |

## 77.35: FEMORAL DIVISION NEC. Formerly included in operation group(s) 722.

| Type of Patients | Observed Patients | Avg. Stay | Variance | 10th | 25th | 50th | 75th | 90th | 95th | 99th |
|---|---|---|---|---|---|---|---|---|---|---|
| **1. SINGLE DX** | | | | | | | | | | |
| 0–19 Years | 221 | 3.0 | 3 | 1 | 2 | 3 | 3 | 6 | 8 | 9 |
| 20–34 | 9 | 3.0 | 2 | 1 | 2 | 3 | 5 | 5 | 5 | 5 |
| 35–49 | 14 | 2.6 | <1 | 2 | 2 | 2 | 3 | 4 | 4 | 6 |
| 50–64 | 6 | 2.6 | <1 | 2 | 3 | 3 | 3 | 4 | 4 | 4 |
| 65+ | 1 | 3.0 | 0 | 3 | 3 | 3 | 3 | 3 | 3 | 3 |
| **2. MULTIPLE DX** | | | | | | | | | | |
| 0–19 Years | 700 | 3.3 | 5 | 2 | 2 | 3 | 4 | 5 | 7 | 10 |
| 20–34 | 45 | 3.9 | 3 | 2 | 3 | 3 | 5 | 6 | 8 | 9 |
| 35–49 | 46 | 4.6 | 13 | 2 | 3 | 3 | 4 | 13 | 15 | 15 |
| 50–64 | 30 | 3.4 | 2 | 2 | 3 | 3 | 4 | 4 | 7 | 9 |
| 65+ | 24 | 6.4 | 35 | 3 | 3 | 5 | 5 | 14 | 21 | 28 |
| **TOTAL SINGLE DX** | 251 | 3.0 | 3 | 1 | 2 | 3 | 3 | 5 | 7 | 9 |
| **TOTAL MULTIPLE DX** | 845 | 3.5 | 6 | 2 | 2 | 3 | 4 | 5 | 7 | 15 |
| **TOTAL** | | | | | | | | | | |
| 0–19 Years | 921 | 3.2 | 4 | 2 | 2 | 3 | 4 | 5 | 7 | 9 |
| 20–34 | 54 | 3.7 | 3 | 2 | 3 | 3 | 5 | 6 | 6 | 9 |
| 35–49 | 60 | 3.9 | 10 | 2 | 2 | 3 | 4 | 6 | 13 | 15 |
| 50–64 | 36 | 3.3 | 2 | 2 | 3 | 3 | 4 | 4 | 7 | 9 |
| 65+ | 25 | 6.3 | 34 | 3 | 3 | 5 | 5 | 14 | 21 | 28 |
| **GRAND TOTAL** | 1,096 | 3.4 | 5 | 2 | 2 | 3 | 4 | 5 | 7 | 13 |

## 77.37: TIBIA/FIBULA DIV NEC. Formerly included in operation group(s) 723.

| Type of Patients | Observed Patients | Avg. Stay | Variance | 10th | 25th | 50th | 75th | 90th | 95th | 99th |
|---|---|---|---|---|---|---|---|---|---|---|
| **1. SINGLE DX** | | | | | | | | | | |
| 0–19 Years | 207 | 2.3 | 2 | 1 | 2 | 2 | 3 | 4 | 4 | 6 |
| 20–34 | 26 | 2.3 | <1 | 1 | 2 | 2 | 3 | 4 | 5 | 6 |
| 35–49 | 84 | 2.2 | 1 | 1 | 2 | 2 | 3 | 3 | 4 | 5 |
| 50–64 | 49 | 2.0 | 1 | 1 | 2 | 2 | 3 | 4 | 4 | 5 |
| 65+ | 4 | 2.3 | <1 | 3 | 3 | 3 | 3 | 3 | 3 | 3 |
| **2. MULTIPLE DX** | | | | | | | | | | |
| 0–19 Years | 354 | 2.6 | 13 | 1 | 2 | 2 | 3 | 4 | 5 | 14 |
| 20–34 | 82 | 2.4 | 2 | 1 | 2 | 2 | 3 | 3 | 4 | 8 |
| 35–49 | 222 | 2.2 | 2 | 1 | 2 | 2 | 3 | 3 | 4 | 7 |
| 50–64 | 114 | 4.6 | 19 | 1 | 3 | 3 | 5 | 15 | 15 | 15 |
| 65+ | 23 | 4.7 | 16 | 3 | 3 | 3 | 7 | 14 | 14 | 14 |
| **TOTAL SINGLE DX** | 370 | 2.2 | 1 | 1 | 2 | 2 | 3 | 4 | 4 | 5 |
| **TOTAL MULTIPLE DX** | 795 | 2.7 | 10 | 1 | 2 | 2 | 3 | 4 | 7 | 15 |
| **TOTAL** | | | | | | | | | | |
| 0–19 Years | 561 | 2.5 | 9 | 1 | 2 | 2 | 3 | 4 | 5 | 14 |
| 20–34 | 108 | 2.4 | 2 | 1 | 2 | 2 | 3 | 3 | 4 | 6 |
| 35–49 | 306 | 2.2 | 2 | 1 | 2 | 2 | 3 | 4 | 4 | 7 |
| 50–64 | 163 | 3.9 | 16 | 1 | 2 | 3 | 4 | 12 | 15 | 15 |
| 65+ | 27 | 4.5 | 15 | 2 | 2 | 3 | 5 | 13 | 14 | 14 |
| **GRAND TOTAL** | 1,165 | 2.6 | 7 | 1 | 2 | 2 | 3 | 4 | 6 | 15 |

Length of Stay by Diagnosis and Operation, United States, 2000

# United States, October 1998–September 1999 Data, by Operation

## 77.39: BONE DIVISION NEC. Formerly included in operation group(s) 723.

| Type of Patients | Observed Patients | Avg. Stay | Vari-ance | 10th | 25th | 50th | 75th | 90th | 95th | 99th |
|---|---|---|---|---|---|---|---|---|---|---|
| **1. SINGLE DX** | | | | | | | | | | |
| 0–19 Years | 128 | 2.4 | 1 | 1 | 2 | 2 | 3 | 4 | 4 | 7 |
| 20–34 | 7 | 3.6 | 3 | 3 | 3 | 3 | 3 | 6 | 7 | 10 |
| 35–49 | 5 | 2.2 | 2 | 1 | 1 | 3 | 2 | 5 | 5 | 5 |
| 50–64 | 1 | 1.0 | 0 | 1 | 1 | 1 | 1 | 1 | 1 | 1 |
| 65+ | 0 | | | | | | | | | |
| **2. MULTIPLE DX** | | | | | | | | | | |
| 0–19 Years | 129 | 3.1 | 3 | 1 | 2 | 3 | 4 | 5 | 7 | 9 |
| 20–34 | 14 | 6.1 | 13 | 1 | 3 | 6 | 7 | 10 | 16 | 16 |
| 35–49 | 14 | 4.2 | 13 | 1 | 2 | 2 | 5 | 10 | 13 | 13 |
| 50–64 | 15 | 6.6 | 53 | 2 | 2 | 2 | 14 | 15 | 16 | 29 |
| 65+ | 5 | 5.7 | 32 | 1 | 1 | 3 | 11 | 15 | 15 | 15 |
| **TOTAL SINGLE DX** | 141 | 2.5 | 2 | 1 | 2 | 2 | 3 | 4 | 4 | 7 |
| **TOTAL MULTIPLE DX** | 177 | 3.7 | 11 | 1 | 2 | 3 | 4 | 7 | 10 | 16 |
| **TOTAL** | | | | | | | | | | |
| 0–19 Years | 257 | 2.8 | 2 | 1 | 2 | 3 | 3 | 4 | 6 | 8 |
| 20–34 | 21 | 4.5 | 8 | 3 | 3 | 3 | 6 | 8 | 10 | 16 |
| 35–49 | 19 | 3.6 | 11 | 1 | 2 | 2 | 5 | 10 | 10 | 13 |
| 50–64 | 16 | 6.4 | 52 | 2 | 2 | 2 | 14 | 15 | 16 | 29 |
| 65+ | 5 | 5.7 | 32 | 1 | 1 | 3 | 11 | 15 | 15 | 15 |
| **GRAND TOTAL** | 318 | 3.2 | 7 | 1 | 2 | 3 | 4 | 5 | 7 | 15 |

## 77.41: CHEST CAGE BONE BIOPSY. Formerly included in operation group(s) 726.

| Type of Patients | Observed Patients | Avg. Stay | Vari-ance | 10th | 25th | 50th | 75th | 90th | 95th | 99th |
|---|---|---|---|---|---|---|---|---|---|---|
| **1. SINGLE DX** | | | | | | | | | | |
| 0–19 Years | 20 | 2.4 | 16 | 1 | 1 | 1 | 2 | 5 | 7 | 24 |
| 20–34 | 3 | 2.5 | 9 | 1 | 1 | 1 | 2 | 5 | 9 | 9 |
| 35–49 | 4 | 2.6 | 9 | 1 | 1 | 1 | 2 | 8 | 8 | 8 |
| 50–64 | 4 | 1.4 | <1 | 1 | 1 | 1 | 2 | 3 | 3 | 3 |
| 65+ | 3 | 1.9 | 3 | 1 | 1 | 1 | 1 | 5 | 5 | 5 |
| **2. MULTIPLE DX** | | | | | | | | | | |
| 0–19 Years | 19 | 4.8 | 26 | 1 | 1 | 5 | 5 | 10 | 22 | 22 |
| 20–34 | 4 | 5.1 | 25 | 2 | 2 | 3 | 10 | 13 | 13 | 13 |
| 35–49 | 41 | 5.5 | 38 | 1 | 2 | 3 | 6 | 16 | 18 | 32 |
| 50–64 | 76 | 7.6 | 49 | 2 | 1 | 5 | 13 | 16 | 24 | 30 |
| 65+ | 150 | 8.6 | 33 | 3 | 4 | 7 | 11 | 17 | 21 | 27 |
| **TOTAL SINGLE DX** | 34 | 2.4 | 12 | 1 | 1 | 1 | 2 | 5 | 8 | 24 |
| **TOTAL MULTIPLE DX** | 290 | 7.6 | 39 | 1 | 3 | 6 | 10 | 16 | 21 | 28 |
| **TOTAL** | | | | | | | | | | |
| 0–19 Years | 39 | 3.6 | 22 | 1 | 1 | 2 | 5 | 6 | 13 | 24 |
| 20–34 | 7 | 4.0 | 19 | 1 | 2 | 2 | 2 | 13 | 13 | 13 |
| 35–49 | 45 | 5.1 | 35 | 1 | 2 | 3 | 6 | 13 | 18 | 32 |
| 50–64 | 80 | 7.4 | 49 | 1 | 1 | 5 | 13 | 15 | 24 | 30 |
| 65+ | 153 | 8.5 | 33 | 2 | 4 | 7 | 11 | 16 | 21 | 27 |
| **GRAND TOTAL** | 324 | 6.9 | 39 | 1 | 2 | 5 | 10 | 15 | 21 | 27 |

## 77.4: BIOPSY OF BONE. Formerly included in operation group(s) 725, 726.

| Type of Patients | Observed Patients | Avg. Stay | Vari-ance | 10th | 25th | 50th | 75th | 90th | 95th | 99th |
|---|---|---|---|---|---|---|---|---|---|---|
| **1. SINGLE DX** | | | | | | | | | | |
| 0–19 Years | 269 | 3.0 | 9 | 1 | 1 | 2 | 4 | 7 | 9 | 13 |
| 20–34 | 52 | 3.5 | 8 | 1 | 2 | 2 | 5 | 8 | 11 | 11 |
| 35–49 | 73 | 2.4 | 4 | 1 | 1 | 2 | 3 | 6 | 7 | 8 |
| 50–64 | 50 | 3.9 | 24 | 1 | 1 | 2 | 6 | 7 | 9 | 35 |
| 65+ | 41 | 3.7 | 9 | 1 | 1 | 2 | 6 | 8 | 10 | 11 |
| **2. MULTIPLE DX** | | | | | | | | | | |
| 0–19 Years | 351 | 7.8 | 89 | 2 | 3 | 5 | 10 | 14 | 19 | 60 |
| 20–34 | 153 | 9.4 | 112 | 2 | 3 | 6 | 13 | 15 | 28 | 57 |
| 35–49 | 536 | 8.3 | 75 | 2 | 3 | 6 | 10 | 17 | 24 | 49 |
| 50–64 | 858 | 8.7 | 65 | 2 | 3 | 7 | 12 | 18 | 24 | 40 |
| 65+ | 1,827 | 9.9 | 57 | 3 | 5 | 8 | 13 | 19 | 25 | 39 |
| **TOTAL SINGLE DX** | 485 | 3.1 | 9 | 1 | 1 | 2 | 4 | 7 | 9 | 12 |
| **TOTAL MULTIPLE DX** | 3,725 | 9.1 | 67 | 2 | 4 | 7 | 12 | 18 | 24 | 42 |
| **TOTAL** | | | | | | | | | | |
| 0–19 Years | 620 | 5.7 | 59 | 1 | 2 | 3 | 7 | 13 | 16 | 34 |
| 20–34 | 205 | 7.8 | 90 | 1 | 2 | 5 | 11 | 15 | 22 | 53 |
| 35–49 | 609 | 7.6 | 70 | 1 | 3 | 5 | 9 | 16 | 24 | 46 |
| 50–64 | 908 | 8.5 | 64 | 1 | 3 | 6 | 11 | 18 | 23 | 40 |
| 65+ | 1,868 | 9.8 | 57 | 3 | 5 | 8 | 13 | 19 | 25 | 39 |
| **GRAND TOTAL** | 4,210 | 8.4 | 64 | 1 | 3 | 6 | 11 | 17 | 23 | 40 |

## 77.45: FEMORAL BIOPSY. Formerly included in operation group(s) 725.

| Type of Patients | Observed Patients | Avg. Stay | Vari-ance | 10th | 25th | 50th | 75th | 90th | 95th | 99th |
|---|---|---|---|---|---|---|---|---|---|---|
| **1. SINGLE DX** | | | | | | | | | | |
| 0–19 Years | 88 | 2.9 | 8 | 1 | 1 | 2 | 3 | 5 | 7 | 15 |
| 20–34 | 18 | 3.1 | 8 | 1 | 1 | 2 | 3 | 8 | 10 | 12 |
| 35–49 | 27 | 1.9 | 2 | 1 | 1 | 2 | 2 | 3 | 5 | 8 |
| 50–64 | 7 | 2.7 | 4 | 1 | 2 | 2 | 3 | 6 | 6 | 6 |
| 65+ | 9 | 2.6 | 2 | 1 | 2 | 2 | 4 | 5 | 6 | 6 |
| **2. MULTIPLE DX** | | | | | | | | | | |
| 0–19 Years | 124 | 8.5 | 92 | 2 | 3 | 7 | 11 | 14 | 21 | 60 |
| 20–34 | 26 | 6.9 | 56 | 1 | 2 | 5 | 8 | 14 | 20 | 42 |
| 35–49 | 74 | 8.6 | 60 | 2 | 4 | 7 | 12 | 15 | 31 | 36 |
| 50–64 | 135 | 8.8 | 52 | 2 | 4 | 6 | 12 | 21 | 21 | 31 |
| 65+ | 319 | 8.0 | 46 | 3 | 4 | 6 | 9 | 16 | 21 | 40 |
| **TOTAL SINGLE DX** | 149 | 2.7 | 7 | 1 | 1 | 2 | 3 | 5 | 6 | 15 |
| **TOTAL MULTIPLE DX** | 678 | 8.3 | 59 | 2 | 4 | 6 | 10 | 16 | 21 | 40 |
| **TOTAL** | | | | | | | | | | |
| 0–19 Years | 212 | 6.2 | 66 | 1 | 2 | 4 | 8 | 14 | 14 | 60 |
| 20–34 | 44 | 5.2 | 38 | 1 | 1 | 3 | 7 | 11 | 20 | 42 |
| 35–49 | 101 | 7.1 | 55 | 2 | 2 | 5 | 10 | 15 | 23 | 36 |
| 50–64 | 142 | 8.6 | 52 | 2 | 3 | 6 | 11 | 21 | 21 | 31 |
| 65+ | 328 | 7.9 | 45 | 2 | 4 | 6 | 9 | 16 | 21 | 40 |
| **GRAND TOTAL** | 827 | 7.3 | 54 | 1 | 3 | 5 | 9 | 15 | 21 | 37 |

Length of Stay by Diagnosis and Operation, United States, 2000

# United States, October 1998–September 1999 Data, by Operation

## 77.47: TIBIA & FIBULA BIOPSY. Formerly included in operation group(s) 726.

| Type of Patients | Observed Patients | Avg. Stay | Variance | 10th | 25th | 50th | 75th | 90th | 95th | 99th |
|---|---|---|---|---|---|---|---|---|---|---|
| **1. SINGLE DX** | | | | | | | | | | |
| 0–19 Years | 72 | 3.1 | 7 | 1 | 1 | 2 | 4 | 8 | 8 | 10 |
| 20–34 | 9 | 2.3 | 1 | 1 | 2 | 2 | 2 | 4 | 8 | 5 |
| 35–49 | 8 | 2.8 | 3 | 1 | 1 | 2 | 3 | 6 | 5 | 6 |
| 50–64 | 5 | 2.1 | <1 | 1 | 2 | 2 | 3 | 3 | 3 | 3 |
| 65+ | 2 | 2.9 | 8 | 1 | 1 | 1 | 5 | 5 | 5 | 5 |
| **2. MULTIPLE DX** | | | | | | | | | | |
| 0–19 Years | 65 | 8.2 | 183 | 1 | 2 | 5 | 10 | 13 | 18 | 92 |
| 20–34 | 19 | 6.2 | 20 | 2 | 3 | 7 | 10 | 11 | 12 | 22 |
| 35–49 | 58 | 7.8 | 66 | 3 | 5 | 5 | 9 | 15 | 22 | 37 |
| 50–64 | 42 | 10.7 | 142 | 2 | 3 | 6 | 11 | 31 | 40 | 48 |
| 65+ | 55 | 9.2 | 60 | 2 | 4 | 7 | 13 | 18 | 26 | 35 |
| **TOTAL SINGLE DX** | 96 | 2.9 | 5 | 1 | 1 | 2 | 4 | 8 | 8 | 9 |
| **TOTAL MULTIPLE DX** | 239 | 8.5 | 107 | 2 | 3 | 5 | 10 | 16 | 26 | 48 |
| **TOTAL** | | | | | | | | | | |
| 0–19 Years | 137 | 5.5 | 94 | 1 | 1 | 3 | 7 | 11 | 13 | 59 |
| 20–34 | 28 | 4.7 | 17 | 1 | 2 | 3 | 7 | 11 | 12 | 22 |
| 35–49 | 66 | 6.8 | 58 | 2 | 3 | 4 | 9 | 14 | 19 | 37 |
| 50–64 | 47 | 10.1 | 136 | 2 | 3 | 6 | 11 | 31 | 40 | 48 |
| 65+ | 57 | 9.1 | 60 | 2 | 4 | 7 | 13 | 18 | 26 | 35 |
| **GRAND TOTAL** | 335 | 6.8 | 82 | 1 | 2 | 4 | 8 | 13 | 22 | 46 |

## 77.49: BONE BIOPSY NEC. Formerly included in operation group(s) 726.

| Type of Patients | Observed Patients | Avg. Stay | Variance | 10th | 25th | 50th | 75th | 90th | 95th | 99th |
|---|---|---|---|---|---|---|---|---|---|---|
| **1. SINGLE DX** | | | | | | | | | | |
| 0–19 Years | 40 | 3.5 | 10 | 1 | 1 | 1 | 5 | 9 | 11 | 11 |
| 20–34 | 14 | 4.7 | 10 | 1 | 2 | 5 | 5 | 11 | 11 | 11 |
| 35–49 | 25 | 2.8 | 4 | 1 | 1 | 2 | 4 | 5 | 8 | 8 |
| 50–64 | 26 | 3.8 | 33 | 1 | 1 | 2 | 4 | 9 | 11 | 35 |
| 65+ | 25 | 4.5 | 12 | 1 | 1 | 3 | 8 | 10 | 10 | 11 |
| **2. MULTIPLE DX** | | | | | | | | | | |
| 0–19 Years | 90 | 8.3 | 74 | 2 | 3 | 6 | 11 | 19 | 19 | 34 |
| 20–34 | 76 | 11.2 | 136 | 3 | 4 | 7 | 13 | 16 | 31 | 73 |
| 35–49 | 278 | 9.1 | 91 | 2 | 3 | 6 | 11 | 23 | 29 | 65 |
| 50–64 | 521 | 8.4 | 69 | 1 | 3 | 6 | 11 | 18 | 24 | 50 |
| 65+ | 1,153 | 10.7 | 59 | 3 | 5 | 9 | 14 | 20 | 26 | 37 |
| **TOTAL SINGLE DX** | 130 | 3.7 | 12 | 1 | 1 | 2 | 5 | 9 | 11 | 11 |
| **TOTAL MULTIPLE DX** | 2,118 | 9.9 | 70 | 2 | 4 | 8 | 13 | 19 | 25 | 45 |
| **TOTAL** | | | | | | | | | | |
| 0–19 Years | 130 | 6.5 | 55 | 1 | 2 | 4 | 9 | 13 | 19 | 34 |
| 20–34 | 90 | 10.0 | 118 | 2 | 4 | 7 | 13 | 15 | 28 | 73 |
| 35–49 | 303 | 8.6 | 88 | 1 | 3 | 6 | 10 | 21 | 29 | 65 |
| 50–64 | 547 | 8.2 | 69 | 1 | 3 | 6 | 11 | 18 | 24 | 50 |
| 65+ | 1,178 | 10.6 | 59 | 3 | 5 | 9 | 14 | 20 | 26 | 37 |
| **GRAND TOTAL** | 2,248 | 9.5 | 69 | 2 | 4 | 8 | 13 | 19 | 24 | 42 |

## 77.5: TOE DEFORMITY EXC/REP. Formerly included in operation group(s) 724.

| Type of Patients | Observed Patients | Avg. Stay | Variance | 10th | 25th | 50th | 75th | 90th | 95th | 99th |
|---|---|---|---|---|---|---|---|---|---|---|
| **1. SINGLE DX** | | | | | | | | | | |
| 0–19 Years | 38 | 1.6 | <1 | 1 | 1 | 1 | 2 | 3 | 4 | 4 |
| 20–34 | 21 | 1.6 | <1 | 1 | 1 | 1 | 2 | 3 | 3 | 3 |
| 35–49 | 42 | 1.4 | <1 | 1 | 1 | 1 | 2 | 2 | 2 | 2 |
| 50–64 | 35 | 1.5 | <1 | 1 | 1 | 1 | 2 | 2 | 2 | 3 |
| 65+ | 17 | 1.3 | <1 | 1 | 1 | 1 | 2 | 2 | 2 | 3 |
| **2. MULTIPLE DX** | | | | | | | | | | |
| 0–19 Years | 66 | 1.6 | <1 | 1 | 1 | 1 | 2 | 3 | 4 | 4 |
| 20–34 | 39 | 1.7 | 5 | 1 | 1 | 1 | 2 | 3 | 3 | 4 |
| 35–49 | 111 | 2.4 | 5 | 1 | 1 | 2 | 3 | 4 | 10 | 11 |
| 50–64 | 245 | 2.4 | 4 | 1 | 1 | 2 | 3 | 3 | 7 | 9 |
| 65+ | 340 | 3.0 | 10 | 1 | 1 | 2 | 3 | 5 | 8 | 18 |
| **TOTAL SINGLE DX** | 153 | 1.5 | <1 | 1 | 1 | 1 | 2 | 2 | 3 | 4 |
| **TOTAL MULTIPLE DX** | 801 | 2.5 | 6 | 1 | 1 | 2 | 3 | 4 | 7 | 13 |
| **TOTAL** | | | | | | | | | | |
| 0–19 Years | 104 | 1.6 | <1 | 1 | 1 | 1 | 2 | 3 | 4 | 4 |
| 20–34 | 60 | 1.6 | 3 | 1 | 1 | 1 | 2 | 3 | 3 | 4 |
| 35–49 | 153 | 2.2 | 4 | 1 | 1 | 2 | 2 | 4 | 7 | 11 |
| 50–64 | 280 | 2.3 | 3 | 1 | 1 | 2 | 3 | 3 | 6 | 9 |
| 65+ | 357 | 2.9 | 10 | 1 | 1 | 2 | 3 | 5 | 8 | 18 |
| **GRAND TOTAL** | 954 | 2.3 | 5 | 1 | 1 | 2 | 3 | 4 | 6 | 13 |

## 77.51: BUNIONECT/STC/OSTY. Formerly included in operation group(s) 724.

| Type of Patients | Observed Patients | Avg. Stay | Variance | 10th | 25th | 50th | 75th | 90th | 95th | 99th |
|---|---|---|---|---|---|---|---|---|---|---|
| **1. SINGLE DX** | | | | | | | | | | |
| 0–19 Years | 22 | 1.2 | <1 | 1 | 1 | 1 | 1 | 2 | 2 | 2 |
| 20–34 | 14 | 1.2 | <1 | 1 | 1 | 1 | 1 | 2 | 2 | 2 |
| 35–49 | 32 | 1.4 | <1 | 1 | 1 | 1 | 2 | 2 | 2 | 2 |
| 50–64 | 23 | 1.4 | <1 | 1 | 1 | 1 | 2 | 2 | 2 | 3 |
| 65+ | 12 | 1.3 | <1 | 1 | 1 | 2 | 2 | 2 | 3 | 3 |
| **2. MULTIPLE DX** | | | | | | | | | | |
| 0–19 Years | 30 | 1.6 | 1 | 1 | 1 | 1 | 2 | 3 | 3 | 7 |
| 20–34 | 18 | 2.0 | 1 | 1 | 2 | 2 | 2 | 3 | 4 | 4 |
| 35–49 | 41 | 2.4 | 7 | 1 | 2 | 2 | 2 | 4 | 10 | 10 |
| 50–64 | 99 | 2.0 | 2 | 1 | 1 | 2 | 3 | 3 | 4 | 5 |
| 65+ | 101 | 3.1 | 20 | 1 | 1 | 2 | 2 | 8 | 17 | 20 |
| **TOTAL SINGLE DX** | 103 | 1.4 | <1 | 1 | 1 | 1 | 2 | 2 | 2 | 3 |
| **TOTAL MULTIPLE DX** | 289 | 2.3 | 8 | 1 | 1 | 2 | 2 | 4 | 6 | 17 |
| **TOTAL** | | | | | | | | | | |
| 0–19 Years | 52 | 1.5 | <1 | 1 | 1 | 1 | 2 | 3 | 3 | 4 |
| 20–34 | 32 | 1.7 | <1 | 1 | 1 | 1 | 2 | 3 | 4 | 4 |
| 35–49 | 73 | 2.0 | 4 | 1 | 1 | 1 | 2 | 3 | 10 | 10 |
| 50–64 | 122 | 1.9 | 2 | 1 | 1 | 2 | 2 | 3 | 4 | 5 |
| 65+ | 113 | 3.0 | 19 | 1 | 1 | 2 | 2 | 6 | 17 | 18 |
| **GRAND TOTAL** | 392 | 2.1 | 6 | 1 | 1 | 2 | 2 | 3 | 4 | 17 |

Length of Stay by Diagnosis and Operation, United States, 2000

# United States, October 1998–September 1999 Data, by Operation

## 77.6: LOC EXC BONE LESION. Formerly included in operation group(s) 725, 726.

| Type of Patients | Observed Patients | Avg. Stay | Vari-ance | Percentiles | | | | | | |
|---|---|---|---|---|---|---|---|---|---|---|
| | | | | 10th | 25th | 50th | 75th | 90th | 95th | 99th |
| **1. SINGLE DX** | | | | | | | | | | |
| 0–19 Years | 477 | 1.8 | 3 | 1 | 1 | 1 | 2 | 3 | 6 | 8 |
| 20–34 | 145 | 2.6 | 5 | 1 | 1 | 2 | 3 | 4 | 7 | 13 |
| 35–49 | 153 | 2.3 | 2 | 1 | 1 | 2 | 3 | 4 | 5 | 7 |
| 50–64 | 73 | 3.0 | 8 | 1 | 1 | 2 | 4 | 8 | 8 | 8 |
| 65+ | 20 | 2.0 | 2 | 1 | 1 | 2 | 2 | 4 | 5 | 6 |
| **2. MULTIPLE DX** | | | | | | | | | | |
| 0–19 Years | 444 | 5.9 | 66 | 1 | 1 | 3 | 8 | 13 | 20 | 76 |
| 20–34 | 376 | 6.2 | 77 | 1 | 2 | 3 | 6 | 12 | 24 | 45 |
| 35–49 | 855 | 6.7 | 56 | 1 | 2 | 4 | 9 | 15 | 18 | 43 |
| 50–64 | 896 | 8.2 | 104 | 1 | 2 | 4 | 10 | 18 | 40 | 40 |
| 65+ | 957 | 8.1 | 65 | 2 | 2 | 6 | 11 | 16 | 25 | 41 |
| **TOTAL SINGLE DX** | 868 | 2.1 | 4 | 1 | 1 | 1 | 2 | 4 | 6 | 9 |
| **TOTAL MULTIPLE DX** | 3,528 | 7.3 | 76 | 1 | 2 | 4 | 9 | 15 | 24 | 43 |
| **TOTAL** | | | | | | | | | | |
| 0–19 Years | 921 | 3.6 | 35 | 1 | 1 | 2 | 4 | 8 | 12 | 34 |
| 20–34 | 521 | 5.3 | 61 | 1 | 2 | 3 | 5 | 10 | 18 | 45 |
| 35–49 | 1,008 | 6.1 | 51 | 1 | 2 | 4 | 9 | 15 | 16 | 40 |
| 50–64 | 969 | 7.9 | 100 | 1 | 2 | 4 | 10 | 17 | 40 | 40 |
| 65+ | 977 | 8.0 | 65 | 2 | 2 | 6 | 10 | 16 | 25 | 41 |
| **GRAND TOTAL** | 4,396 | 6.2 | 65 | 1 | 2 | 3 | 8 | 14 | 20 | 40 |

## 77.65: LOC EXC BONE LES FEMUR. Formerly included in operation group(s) 725.

| Type of Patients | Observed Patients | Avg. Stay | Vari-ance | Percentiles | | | | | | |
|---|---|---|---|---|---|---|---|---|---|---|
| | | | | 10th | 25th | 50th | 75th | 90th | 95th | 99th |
| **1. SINGLE DX** | | | | | | | | | | |
| 0–19 Years | 118 | 1.7 | 2 | 1 | 1 | 1 | 2 | 3 | 6 | 7 |
| 20–34 | 47 | 2.4 | 2 | 1 | 1 | 2 | 3 | 4 | 5 | 9 |
| 35–49 | 54 | 1.8 | 1 | 1 | 1 | 1 | 2 | 3 | 4 | 5 |
| 50–64 | 18 | 1.4 | <1 | 1 | 1 | 1 | 2 | 2 | 3 | 3 |
| 65+ | 3 | 2.0 | 0 | 2 | 2 | 2 | 2 | 2 | 2 | 2 |
| **2. MULTIPLE DX** | | | | | | | | | | |
| 0–19 Years | 109 | 6.0 | 26 | 1 | 2 | 5 | 9 | 12 | 20 | >99 |
| 20–34 | 79 | 4.2 | 48 | 1 | 2 | 3 | 4 | 7 | 9 | 51 |
| 35–49 | 155 | 4.3 | 48 | 1 | 2 | 3 | 4 | 9 | 15 | 57 |
| 50–64 | 73 | 3.0 | 15 | 1 | 2 | 2 | 3 | 5 | 6 | 34 |
| 65+ | 95 | 7.4 | 29 | 1 | 4 | 7 | 9 | 14 | 17 | 25 |
| **TOTAL SINGLE DX** | 240 | 1.8 | 2 | 1 | 1 | 1 | 2 | 4 | 5 | 7 |
| **TOTAL MULTIPLE DX** | 511 | 5.0 | 36 | 1 | 2 | 3 | 7 | 11 | 15 | 51 |
| **TOTAL** | | | | | | | | | | |
| 0–19 Years | 227 | 3.6 | 17 | 1 | 2 | 2 | 5 | 9 | 12 | >99 |
| 20–34 | 126 | 3.6 | 34 | 1 | 2 | 2 | 4 | 5 | 7 | 24 |
| 35–49 | 209 | 3.7 | 38 | 1 | 2 | 2 | 3 | 7 | 11 | 45 |
| 50–64 | 91 | 2.8 | 14 | 1 | 2 | 2 | 3 | 5 | 6 | 34 |
| 65+ | 98 | 7.3 | 29 | 1 | 4 | 7 | 9 | 14 | 17 | 25 |
| **GRAND TOTAL** | 751 | 4.0 | 27 | 1 | 1 | 2 | 5 | 9 | 12 | 37 |

## 77.61: EXC CHEST CAGE BONE LES. Formerly included in operation group(s) 726.

| Type of Patients | Observed Patients | Avg. Stay | Vari-ance | Percentiles | | | | | | |
|---|---|---|---|---|---|---|---|---|---|---|
| | | | | 10th | 25th | 50th | 75th | 90th | 95th | 99th |
| **1. SINGLE DX** | | | | | | | | | | |
| 0–19 Years | 24 | 1.6 | 3 | 1 | 1 | 1 | 1 | 4 | 4 | 10 |
| 20–34 | 7 | 1.9 | <1 | 1 | 2 | 2 | 2 | 3 | 3 | 3 |
| 35–49 | 7 | 1.6 | <1 | 1 | 1 | 1 | 1 | 3 | 8 | 8 |
| 50–64 | 7 | 3.4 | 33 | 1 | 1 | 1 | 3 | 4 | 22 | 22 |
| 65+ | 4 | 1.3 | <1 | 1 | 1 | 1 | 2 | 2 | 2 | 2 |
| **2. MULTIPLE DX** | | | | | | | | | | |
| 0–19 Years | 22 | 12.1 | 373 | 1 | 2 | 5 | 18 | 18 | 76 | 76 |
| 20–34 | 15 | 9.2 | 91 | 1 | 2 | 3 | 19 | 28 | 28 | 28 |
| 35–49 | 79 | 8.8 | 155 | 1 | 1 | 3 | 16 | 19 | 22 | 72 |
| 50–64 | 155 | 10.3 | 94 | 2 | 3 | 8 | 15 | 19 | 25 | 43 |
| 65+ | 199 | 12.0 | 139 | 1 | 4 | 8 | 16 | 30 | 40 | 48 |
| **TOTAL SINGLE DX** | 49 | 1.8 | 6 | 1 | 1 | 1 | 2 | 3 | 4 | 10 |
| **TOTAL MULTIPLE DX** | 470 | 10.7 | 139 | 1 | 3 | 7 | 15 | 21 | 33 | 69 |
| **TOTAL** | | | | | | | | | | |
| 0–19 Years | 46 | 6.0 | 182 | 1 | 1 | 1 | 4 | 18 | 18 | 76 |
| 20–34 | 22 | 6.6 | 70 | 1 | 2 | 2 | 7 | 19 | 28 | 28 |
| 35–49 | 86 | 8.2 | 146 | 1 | 1 | 3 | 12 | 19 | 20 | 72 |
| 50–64 | 162 | 10.0 | 93 | 1 | 3 | 8 | 14 | 19 | 25 | 43 |
| 65+ | 203 | 11.9 | 138 | 1 | 4 | 8 | 15 | 29 | 40 | 48 |
| **GRAND TOTAL** | 519 | 9.7 | 132 | 1 | 2 | 6 | 14 | 20 | 33 | 54 |

## 77.67: LOC EXC LES TIBIA/FIBULA. Formerly included in operation group(s) 726.

| Type of Patients | Observed Patients | Avg. Stay | Vari-ance | Percentiles | | | | | | |
|---|---|---|---|---|---|---|---|---|---|---|
| | | | | 10th | 25th | 50th | 75th | 90th | 95th | 99th |
| **1. SINGLE DX** | | | | | | | | | | |
| 0–19 Years | 139 | 1.7 | 6 | 1 | 1 | 1 | 2 | 3 | 5 | 7 |
| 20–34 | 29 | 2.8 | 10 | 1 | 2 | 2 | 3 | 4 | 5 | 18 |
| 35–49 | 18 | 2.5 | 3 | 1 | 2 | 2 | 4 | 4 | 7 | 7 |
| 50–64 | 9 | 5.4 | 10 | 1 | 1 | 8 | 8 | 8 | 8 | 8 |
| 65+ | 3 | 4.4 | <1 | 4 | 4 | 4 | 5 | 5 | 5 | 5 |
| **2. MULTIPLE DX** | | | | | | | | | | |
| 0–19 Years | 115 | 3.9 | 29 | 1 | 2 | 2 | 5 | 10 | 10 | 22 |
| 20–34 | 72 | 5.5 | 14 | 2 | 3 | 5 | 8 | 9 | 10 | 22 |
| 35–49 | 127 | 7.2 | 89 | 1 | 2 | 4 | 7 | 13 | 27 | 43 |
| 50–64 | 91 | 5.6 | 39 | 1 | 2 | 4 | 7 | 11 | 15 | 25 |
| 65+ | 85 | 8.6 | 41 | 2 | 4 | 7 | 11 | 18 | 23 | 27 |
| **TOTAL SINGLE DX** | 198 | 2.1 | 7 | 1 | 1 | 1 | 2 | 4 | 7 | 8 |
| **TOTAL MULTIPLE DX** | 490 | 6.0 | 45 | 1 | 2 | 4 | 8 | 12 | 16 | 34 |
| **TOTAL** | | | | | | | | | | |
| 0–19 Years | 254 | 2.6 | 16 | 1 | 1 | 1 | 2 | 6 | 10 | 13 |
| 20–34 | 101 | 5.0 | 14 | 1 | 2 | 4 | 7 | 9 | 10 | 22 |
| 35–49 | 145 | 6.4 | 77 | 1 | 2 | 4 | 7 | 13 | 21 | 43 |
| 50–64 | 100 | 5.6 | 35 | 1 | 2 | 4 | 8 | 11 | 14 | 25 |
| 65+ | 88 | 8.5 | 40 | 2 | 4 | 6 | 10 | 18 | 23 | 27 |
| **GRAND TOTAL** | 688 | 4.7 | 36 | 1 | 1 | 3 | 6 | 10 | 13 | 28 |

Length of Stay by Diagnosis and Operation, United States, 2000

## United States, October 1998–September 1999 Data, by Operation

### 77.68: LOC EXC LES MT/TARSAL. Formerly included in operation group(s) 726.

| Type of Patients | Observed Patients | Avg. Stay | Variance | Percentiles | | | | | | |
|---|---|---|---|---|---|---|---|---|---|---|
| | | | | 10th | 25th | 50th | 75th | 90th | 95th | 99th |
| **1. SINGLE DX** | | | | | | | | | | |
| 0–19 Years | 24 | 2.3 | 3 | 1 | 1 | 2 | 3 | 3 | 5 | 8 |
| 20–34 | 8 | 1.9 | <1 | 1 | 1 | 2 | 2 | 3 | 3 | 3 |
| 35–49 | 8 | 2.3 | <1 | 1 | 1 | 2 | 3 | 3 | 3 | 3 |
| 50–64 | 4 | 3.3 | <1 | 2 | 3 | 3 | 4 | 4 | 4 | 4 |
| 65+ | 1 | 2.0 | 0 | 2 | 2 | 2 | 2 | 2 | 2 | 2 |
| **2. MULTIPLE DX** | | | | | | | | | | |
| 0–19 Years | 27 | 6.6 | 49 | 2 | 2 | 4 | 11 | 14 | 14 | 42 |
| 20–34 | 40 | 6.1 | 33 | 3 | 3 | 4 | 7 | 11 | 18 | 32 |
| 35–49 | 118 | 8.8 | 22 | 2 | 4 | 9 | 11 | 15 | 15 | 16 |
| 50–64 | 204 | 13.2 | 207 | 2 | 3 | 7 | 16 | 40 | 40 | 40 |
| 65+ | 199 | 8.3 | 46 | 2 | 3 | 6 | 12 | 16 | 18 | 41 |
| **TOTAL SINGLE DX** | 45 | 2.3 | 2 | 1 | 1 | 2 | 3 | 4 | 5 | 8 |
| **TOTAL MULTIPLE DX** | 588 | 10.1 | 100 | 2 | 3 | 8 | 12 | 17 | 40 | 40 |
| **TOTAL** | | | | | | | | | | |
| 0–19 | 51 | 4.5 | 32 | 1 | 1 | 3 | 4 | 14 | 14 | 14 |
| 20–34 | 48 | 5.6 | 31 | 1 | 2 | 4 | 6 | 10 | 18 | 32 |
| 35–49 | 126 | 8.7 | 22 | 2 | 4 | 9 | 11 | 15 | 15 | 16 |
| 50–64 | 208 | 13.0 | 205 | 2 | 3 | 7 | 16 | 40 | 40 | 40 |
| 65+ | 200 | 8.3 | 46 | 2 | 3 | 6 | 12 | 16 | 18 | 41 |
| **GRAND TOTAL** | 633 | 9.7 | 98 | 1 | 3 | 7 | 11 | 17 | 40 | 40 |

### 77.7: EXC BONE FOR GRAFT. Formerly included in operation group(s) 725, 726.

| Type of Patients | Observed Patients | Avg. Stay | Variance | Percentiles | | | | | | |
|---|---|---|---|---|---|---|---|---|---|---|
| | | | | 10th | 25th | 50th | 75th | 90th | 95th | 99th |
| **1. SINGLE DX** | | | | | | | | | | |
| 0–19 Years | 83 | 1.8 | 3 | 1 | 1 | 1 | 2 | 3 | 4 | 11 |
| 20–34 | 96 | 1.9 | 1 | 1 | 1 | 1 | 2 | 3 | 4 | 7 |
| 35–49 | 169 | 2.2 | 3 | 1 | 1 | 2 | 2 | 3 | 4 | 9 |
| 50–64 | 67 | 2.6 | 2 | 1 | 1 | 2 | 3 | 4 | 5 | 9 |
| 65+ | 18 | 1.8 | <1 | 1 | 1 | 1 | 2 | 3 | 4 | 4 |
| **2. MULTIPLE DX** | | | | | | | | | | |
| 0–19 Years | 151 | 2.4 | 5 | 1 | 1 | 2 | 3 | 4 | 5 | 12 |
| 20–34 | 210 | 2.4 | 7 | 1 | 2 | 2 | 3 | 4 | 5 | 12 |
| 35–49 | 374 | 2.3 | 4 | 1 | 2 | 2 | 3 | 4 | 5 | 9 |
| 50–64 | 313 | 2.9 | 34 | 1 | 2 | 2 | 4 | 4 | 6 | 20 |
| 65+ | 153 | 2.8 | 4 | 1 | 2 | 2 | 3 | 4 | 6 | 10 |
| **TOTAL SINGLE DX** | 433 | 2.1 | 3 | 1 | 1 | 2 | 3 | 4 | 4 | 9 |
| **TOTAL MULTIPLE DX** | 1,201 | 2.5 | 12 | 1 | 2 | 2 | 4 | 4 | 6 | 11 |
| **TOTAL** | | | | | | | | | | |
| 0–19 | 234 | 2.2 | 4 | 1 | 1 | 2 | 2 | 4 | 4 | 11 |
| 20–34 | 306 | 2.3 | 6 | 1 | 1 | 2 | 3 | 4 | 5 | 8 |
| 35–49 | 543 | 2.3 | 3 | 1 | 1 | 2 | 3 | 4 | 5 | 9 |
| 50–64 | 380 | 2.8 | 28 | 1 | 2 | 2 | 4 | 4 | 6 | 17 |
| 65+ | 171 | 2.7 | 4 | 1 | 2 | 2 | 3 | 4 | 6 | 10 |
| **GRAND TOTAL** | 1,634 | 2.4 | 10 | 1 | 1 | 2 | 3 | 4 | 5 | 11 |

### 77.69: LOC EXC BONE LESION NEC. Formerly included in operation group(s) 726.

| Type of Patients | Observed Patients | Avg. Stay | Variance | Percentiles | | | | | | |
|---|---|---|---|---|---|---|---|---|---|---|
| | | | | 10th | 25th | 50th | 75th | 90th | 95th | 99th |
| **1. SINGLE DX** | | | | | | | | | | |
| 0–19 Years | 80 | 2.3 | 4 | 1 | 1 | 2 | 3 | 3 | 5 | 7 |
| 20–34 | 32 | 3.5 | 8 | 1 | 2 | 2 | 5 | 6 | 7 | 11 |
| 35–49 | 37 | 3.0 | 2 | 1 | 2 | 3 | 4 | 5 | 10 | 11 |
| 50–64 | 26 | 2.3 | 2 | 1 | 2 | 3 | 4 | 4 | 4 | 7 |
| 65+ | 7 | 1.7 | 2 | 1 | 1 | 1 | 2 | 2 | 6 | 6 |
| **2. MULTIPLE DX** | | | | | | | | | | |
| 0–19 Years | 99 | 8.5 | 103 | 2 | 2 | 6 | 8 | 26 | 34 | 44 |
| 20–34 | 99 | 10.1 | 200 | 1 | 2 | 4 | 11 | 42 | 45 | 45 |
| 35–49 | 248 | 6.4 | 62 | 1 | 2 | 4 | 9 | 13 | 18 | 35 |
| 50–64 | 285 | 6.9 | 40 | 2 | 3 | 5 | 10 | 13 | 17 | 29 |
| 65+ | 274 | 8.6 | 66 | 3 | 3 | 6 | 12 | 16 | 29 | 41 |
| **TOTAL SINGLE DX** | 182 | 2.6 | 4 | 1 | 1 | 2 | 3 | 6 | 7 | 10 |
| **TOTAL MULTIPLE DX** | 1,005 | 7.7 | 76 | 1 | 3 | 5 | 10 | 16 | 27 | 45 |
| **TOTAL** | | | | | | | | | | |
| 0–19 | 179 | 5.5 | 63 | 1 | 1 | 3 | 6 | 11 | 26 | 36 |
| 20–34 | 131 | 8.6 | 162 | 1 | 3 | 4 | 7 | 29 | 45 | 45 |
| 35–49 | 285 | 6.0 | 55 | 2 | 2 | 4 | 7 | 12 | 18 | 35 |
| 50–64 | 311 | 6.6 | 39 | 2 | 3 | 4 | 9 | 13 | 17 | 29 |
| 65+ | 281 | 8.5 | 65 | 3 | 3 | 6 | 11 | 16 | 27 | 41 |
| **GRAND TOTAL** | 1,187 | 6.9 | 68 | 1 | 2 | 4 | 8 | 14 | 24 | 45 |

### 77.79: EXC BONE FOR GRAFT NEC. Formerly included in operation group(s) 726.

| Type of Patients | Observed Patients | Avg. Stay | Variance | Percentiles | | | | | | |
|---|---|---|---|---|---|---|---|---|---|---|
| | | | | 10th | 25th | 50th | 75th | 90th | 95th | 99th |
| **1. SINGLE DX** | | | | | | | | | | |
| 0–19 Years | 66 | 1.6 | 2 | 1 | 1 | 1 | 2 | 3 | 3 | 8 |
| 20–34 | 83 | 1.8 | 1 | 1 | 1 | 1 | 2 | 3 | 4 | 5 |
| 35–49 | 152 | 2.2 | 3 | 1 | 1 | 2 | 2 | 3 | 4 | 9 |
| 50–64 | 60 | 2.6 | 2 | 1 | 2 | 2 | 3 | 4 | 5 | 9 |
| 65+ | 15 | 1.7 | <1 | 1 | 1 | 1 | 2 | 3 | 4 | 4 |
| **2. MULTIPLE DX** | | | | | | | | | | |
| 0–19 Years | 118 | 2.3 | 3 | 1 | 1 | 2 | 2 | 4 | 4 | 10 |
| 20–34 | 172 | 2.2 | 8 | 1 | 1 | 2 | 2 | 4 | 4 | 11 |
| 35–49 | 335 | 2.2 | 3 | 1 | 1 | 2 | 3 | 5 | 5 | 9 |
| 50–64 | 270 | 2.9 | 37 | 1 | 2 | 2 | 3 | 4 | 6 | 21 |
| 65+ | 127 | 2.8 | 3 | 2 | 2 | 2 | 3 | 4 | 6 | 9 |
| **TOTAL SINGLE DX** | 376 | 2.0 | 2 | 1 | 1 | 2 | 2 | 3 | 4 | 9 |
| **TOTAL MULTIPLE DX** | 1,022 | 2.4 | 13 | 1 | 1 | 2 | 3 | 4 | 5 | 10 |
| **TOTAL** | | | | | | | | | | |
| 0–19 | 184 | 2.0 | 2 | 1 | 1 | 2 | 2 | 4 | 4 | 8 |
| 20–34 | 255 | 2.1 | 6 | 1 | 1 | 2 | 3 | 4 | 4 | 8 |
| 35–49 | 487 | 2.2 | 3 | 1 | 1 | 2 | 3 | 5 | 5 | 9 |
| 50–64 | 330 | 2.9 | 31 | 1 | 2 | 2 | 3 | 4 | 6 | 11 |
| 65+ | 142 | 2.7 | 2 | 1 | 2 | 2 | 3 | 4 | 6 | 9 |
| **GRAND TOTAL** | 1,398 | 2.3 | 10 | 1 | 1 | 2 | 3 | 4 | 5 | 9 |

Length of Stay by Diagnosis and Operation, United States, 2000

# United States, October 1998–September 1999 Data, by Operation

## 77.8: OTHER PARTIAL OSTECTOMY. Formerly included in operation group(s) 725, 726.

| Type of Patients | Observed Patients | Avg. Stay | Vari-ance | Percentiles | | | | | | |
|---|---|---|---|---|---|---|---|---|---|---|
| | | | | 10th | 25th | 50th | 75th | 90th | 95th | 99th |
| **1. SINGLE DX** | | | | | | | | | | |
| 0-19 Years | 187 | 2.1 | 3 | 1 | 1 | 1 | 2 | 5 | 7 | 8 |
| 20-34 | 104 | 2.2 | 4 | 1 | 1 | 2 | 3 | 5 | 5 | 13 |
| 35-49 | 177 | 3.2 | 9 | 1 | 1 | 2 | 4 | 9 | 9 | 9 |
| 50-64 | 196 | 2.3 | 4 | 1 | 1 | 2 | 3 | 4 | 5 | 16 |
| 65+ | 38 | 2.5 | 3 | 1 | 1 | 2 | 4 | 4 | 4 | 11 |
| **2. MULTIPLE DX** | | | | | | | | | | |
| 0-19 Years | 259 | 5.1 | 40 | 1 | 1 | 3 | 6 | 10 | 14 | 43 |
| 20-34 | 274 | 5.6 | 39 | 1 | 2 | 4 | 5 | 11 | 19 | 32 |
| 35-49 | 693 | 5.1 | 31 | 1 | 2 | 3 | 7 | 10 | 15 | 33 |
| 50-64 | 808 | 4.8 | 38 | 1 | 2 | 3 | 6 | 10 | 15 | 34 |
| 65+ | 1,030 | 6.1 | 40 | 1 | 2 | 4 | 8 | 14 | 20 | 30 |
| **TOTAL SINGLE DX** | 612 | 2.5 | 6 | 1 | 1 | 2 | 3 | 7 | 7 | 9 |
| **TOTAL MULTIPLE DX** | 3,064 | 5.4 | 37 | 1 | 2 | 3 | 7 | 11 | 17 | 33 |
| **TOTAL** | | | | | | | | | | |
| 0-19 Years | 446 | 3.8 | 26 | 1 | 1 | 2 | 5 | 8 | 11 | 36 |
| 20-34 | 378 | 4.8 | 33 | 1 | 2 | 3 | 5 | 10 | 16 | 31 |
| 35-49 | 870 | 4.7 | 27 | 1 | 2 | 3 | 6 | 9 | 13 | 28 |
| 50-64 | 914 | 4.6 | 35 | 1 | 2 | 3 | 5 | 9 | 14 | 34 |
| 65+ | 1,068 | 6.0 | 39 | 1 | 2 | 4 | 8 | 14 | 20 | 30 |
| **GRAND TOTAL** | 3,676 | 4.9 | 33 | 1 | 2 | 3 | 6 | 10 | 15 | 31 |

## 77.85: PART OSTECTOMY-FEMUR. Formerly included in operation group(s) 725.

| Type of Patients | Observed Patients | Avg. Stay | Vari-ance | Percentiles | | | | | | |
|---|---|---|---|---|---|---|---|---|---|---|
| | | | | 10th | 25th | 50th | 75th | 90th | 95th | 99th |
| **1. SINGLE DX** | | | | | | | | | | |
| 0-19 Years | 38 | 3.0 | 6 | 1 | 1 | 2 | 4 | 8 | 8 | 11 |
| 20-34 | 12 | 4.1 | 5 | 1 | 2 | 5 | 5 | 7 | 7 | 8 |
| 35-49 | 17 | 2.5 | 5 | 1 | 1 | 2 | 4 | 4 | 4 | 13 |
| 50-64 | 2 | 3.1 | 5 | 1 | 1 | 5 | 5 | 5 | 5 | 5 |
| 65+ | 2 | 3.6 | <1 | 2 | 4 | 4 | 4 | 4 | 4 | 4 |
| **2. MULTIPLE DX** | | | | | | | | | | |
| 0-19 Years | 105 | 6.2 | 57 | 1 | 3 | 5 | 7 | 10 | 20 | 43 |
| 20-34 | 68 | 8.1 | 70 | 3 | 3 | 4 | 10 | 22 | 27 | 37 |
| 35-49 | 71 | 10.9 | 92 | 3 | 3 | 7 | 20 | 27 | 37 | >99 |
| 50-64 | 58 | 13.1 | 199 | 5 | 5 | 7 | 15 | 33 | 49 | 70 |
| 65+ | 150 | 9.8 | 80 | 3 | 4 | 7 | 12 | 20 | 23 | 54 |
| **TOTAL SINGLE DX** | 71 | 3.0 | 6 | 1 | 1 | 2 | 4 | 7 | 8 | 11 |
| **TOTAL MULTIPLE DX** | 452 | 9.1 | 90 | 2 | 3 | 6 | 11 | 21 | 28 | 54 |
| **TOTAL** | | | | | | | | | | |
| 0-19 Years | 143 | 5.4 | 46 | 1 | 2 | 4 | 6 | 8 | 11 | 43 |
| 20-34 | 80 | 7.6 | 64 | 2 | 3 | 4 | 10 | 21 | 24 | 37 |
| 35-49 | 88 | 9.4 | 86 | 2 | 3 | 5 | 13 | 22 | 33 | >99 |
| 50-64 | 60 | 12.7 | 195 | 4 | 4 | 7 | 15 | 33 | 49 | 70 |
| 65+ | 152 | 9.7 | 80 | 3 | 4 | 7 | 12 | 20 | 23 | 54 |
| **GRAND TOTAL** | 523 | 8.3 | 83 | 1 | 3 | 5 | 10 | 20 | 28 | 49 |

## 77.81: OTH CHEST CAGE OSTECTOMY. Formerly included in operation group(s) 726.

| Type of Patients | Observed Patients | Avg. Stay | Vari-ance | Percentiles | | | | | | |
|---|---|---|---|---|---|---|---|---|---|---|
| | | | | 10th | 25th | 50th | 75th | 90th | 95th | 99th |
| **1. SINGLE DX** | | | | | | | | | | |
| 0-19 Years | 15 | 1.4 | 2 | 1 | 1 | 1 | 1 | 2 | 3 | 8 |
| 20-34 | 30 | 1.9 | 1 | 1 | 1 | 2 | 2 | 3 | 3 | 9 |
| 35-49 | 49 | 1.2 | <1 | 1 | 1 | 1 | 1 | 2 | 3 | 3 |
| 50-64 | 23 | 1.5 | <1 | 1 | 1 | 2 | 2 | 2 | 2 | 4 |
| 65+ | 5 | 1.8 | <1 | 1 | 2 | 2 | 2 | 2 | 2 | 2 |
| **2. MULTIPLE DX** | | | | | | | | | | |
| 0-19 Years | 19 | 5.8 | 16 | 1 | 3 | 5 | 8 | 12 | 12 | 13 |
| 20-34 | 38 | 3.6 | 6 | 1 | 1 | 4 | 5 | 5 | 5 | 15 |
| 35-49 | 151 | 2.9 | 9 | 1 | 1 | 2 | 3 | 8 | 10 | 13 |
| 50-64 | 138 | 3.7 | 39 | 1 | 1 | 2 | 3 | 8 | 14 | 36 |
| 65+ | 119 | 4.2 | 39 | 1 | 1 | 2 | 4 | 8 | 14 | 33 |
| **TOTAL SINGLE DX** | 122 | 1.4 | <1 | 1 | 1 | 1 | 2 | 2 | 3 | 4 |
| **TOTAL MULTIPLE DX** | 465 | 3.6 | 25 | 1 | 1 | 2 | 4 | 8 | 12 | 31 |
| **TOTAL** | | | | | | | | | | |
| 0-19 Years | 34 | 4.3 | 15 | 1 | 1 | 3 | 7 | 12 | 12 | 13 |
| 20-34 | 68 | 3.0 | 5 | 1 | 1 | 2 | 5 | 5 | 5 | 15 |
| 35-49 | 200 | 2.5 | 8 | 1 | 1 | 1 | 2 | 6 | 10 | 13 |
| 50-64 | 161 | 3.4 | 34 | 1 | 1 | 2 | 4 | 6 | 13 | 36 |
| 65+ | 124 | 4.1 | 38 | 1 | 2 | 2 | 4 | 8 | 14 | 33 |
| **GRAND TOTAL** | 587 | 3.2 | 21 | 1 | 1 | 2 | 3 | 7 | 11 | 28 |

## 77.86: PARTIAL PATELLECTOMY. Formerly included in operation group(s) 726.

| Type of Patients | Observed Patients | Avg. Stay | Vari-ance | Percentiles | | | | | | |
|---|---|---|---|---|---|---|---|---|---|---|
| | | | | 10th | 25th | 50th | 75th | 90th | 95th | 99th |
| **1. SINGLE DX** | | | | | | | | | | |
| 0-19 Years | 4 | 2.7 | <1 | 2 | 2 | 3 | 3 | 3 | 3 | 3 |
| 20-34 | 11 | 1.6 | <1 | 1 | 1 | 1 | 2 | 3 | 3 | 3 |
| 35-49 | 28 | 4.4 | 6 | 1 | 2 | 4 | 7 | 7 | 7 | 7 |
| 50-64 | 30 | 2.4 | 2 | 1 | 1 | 2 | 3 | 4 | 5 | 7 |
| 65+ | 18 | 3.2 | 3 | 2 | 2 | 3 | 4 | 4 | 4 | 11 |
| **2. MULTIPLE DX** | | | | | | | | | | |
| 0-19 Years | 10 | 3.0 | 2 | 1 | 2 | 3 | 4 | 4 | 4 | 6 |
| 20-34 | 43 | 5.6 | 34 | 1 | 2 | 3 | 10 | 10 | 10 | 18 |
| 35-49 | 76 | 4.5 | 11 | 1 | 2 | 3 | 6 | 7 | 9 | 18 |
| 50-64 | 107 | 3.9 | 13 | 1 | 2 | 4 | 6 | 8 | 9 | 20 |
| 65+ | 197 | 4.5 | 11 | 2 | 3 | 4 | 6 | 9 | 11 | 19 |
| **TOTAL SINGLE DX** | 91 | 3.3 | 5 | 1 | 2 | 3 | 4 | 7 | 7 | 7 |
| **TOTAL MULTIPLE DX** | 433 | 4.4 | 14 | 2 | 2 | 3 | 6 | 9 | 10 | 18 |
| **TOTAL** | | | | | | | | | | |
| 0-19 Years | 14 | 3.0 | 1 | 1 | 2 | 3 | 4 | 4 | 4 | 6 |
| 20-34 | 54 | 4.6 | 29 | 1 | 3 | 3 | 7 | 10 | 10 | 18 |
| 35-49 | 104 | 4.4 | 9 | 1 | 3 | 3 | 6 | 7 | 8 | 18 |
| 50-64 | 137 | 3.6 | 11 | 1 | 2 | 3 | 4 | 7 | 9 | 17 |
| 65+ | 215 | 4.5 | 11 | 2 | 3 | 4 | 5 | 9 | 11 | 14 |
| **GRAND TOTAL** | 524 | 4.2 | 12 | 1 | 2 | 3 | 5 | 8 | 10 | 18 |

# United States, October 1998–September 1999 Data, by Operation

## 77.88: PART OSTECTOMY-MT/TARSAL. Formerly included in operation group(s) 726.

| Type of Patients | Observed Patients | Avg. Stay | Variance | 10th | 25th | 50th | 75th | 90th | 95th | 99th |
|---|---|---|---|---|---|---|---|---|---|---|
| **1. SINGLE DX** | | | | | | | | | | |
| 0–19 Years | 46 | 1.1 | <1 | 1 | 1 | 1 | 1 | 2 | 2 | 2 |
| 20–34 | 3 | 5.8 | 42 | 1 | 1 | 1 | 13 | 13 | 13 | 13 |
| 35–49 | 6 | 1.9 | <1 | 1 | 1 | 1 | 3 | 3 | 3 | 3 |
| 50–64 | 5 | 2.7 | 4 | 1 | 1 | 2 | 3 | 7 | 7 | 7 |
| 65+ | 2 | 1.0 | 0 | 1 | 1 | 1 | 1 | 1 | 1 | 1 |
| **2. MULTIPLE DX** | | | | | | | | | | |
| 0–19 Years | 16 | 1.7 | <1 | 1 | 1 | 1 | 2 | 4 | 4 | 4 |
| 20–34 | 23 | 4.7 | 10 | 1 | 1 | 4 | 5 | 7 | 11 | 16 |
| 35–49 | 131 | 5.8 | 12 | 1 | 2 | 5 | 8 | 10 | 11 | 17 |
| 50–64 | 216 | 5.1 | 20 | 1 | 1 | 4 | 7 | 10 | 13 | 22 |
| 65+ | 225 | 7.1 | 35 | 2 | 3 | 5 | 9 | 14 | 18 | 31 |
| **TOTAL SINGLE DX** | 62 | 1.3 | 2 | 1 | 1 | 1 | 1 | 2 | 3 | 7 |
| **TOTAL MULTIPLE DX** | 611 | 5.7 | 22 | 1 | 3 | 4 | 8 | 11 | 14 | 23 |
| **TOTAL** | | | | | | | | | | |
| 0–19 Years | 62 | 1.2 | <1 | 1 | 1 | 1 | 1 | 2 | 2 | 4 |
| 20–34 | 26 | 4.7 | 11 | 1 | 2 | 4 | 5 | 7 | 13 | 16 |
| 35–49 | 137 | 5.7 | 12 | 1 | 2 | 5 | 8 | 10 | 11 | 17 |
| 50–64 | 221 | 5.1 | 20 | 1 | 2 | 4 | 7 | 10 | 13 | 22 |
| 65+ | 227 | 7.0 | 35 | 2 | 3 | 5 | 9 | 14 | 18 | 31 |
| **GRAND TOTAL** | 673 | 5.3 | 22 | 1 | 2 | 4 | 8 | 11 | 13 | 22 |

## 77.9: TOTAL OSTECTOMY. Formerly included in operation group(s) 725, 726.

| Type of Patients | Observed Patients | Avg. Stay | Variance | 10th | 25th | 50th | 75th | 90th | 95th | 99th |
|---|---|---|---|---|---|---|---|---|---|---|
| **1. SINGLE DX** | | | | | | | | | | |
| 0–19 Years | 39 | 1.7 | <1 | 1 | 1 | 1 | 2 | 3 | 4 | 4 |
| 20–34 | 100 | 1.8 | <1 | 1 | 1 | 2 | 2 | 3 | 4 | 4 |
| 35–49 | 131 | 2.4 | 2 | 1 | 1 | 2 | 3 | 4 | 5 | 5 |
| 50–64 | 35 | 2.2 | 1 | 1 | 1 | 2 | 3 | 4 | 4 | 6 |
| 65+ | 9 | 5.1 | 37 | 1 | 1 | 4 | 5 | 8 | 24 | 24 |
| **2. MULTIPLE DX** | | | | | | | | | | |
| 0–19 Years | 62 | 2.8 | 8 | 1 | 2 | 2 | 2 | 5 | 7 | 17 |
| 20–34 | 153 | 3.7 | 13 | 1 | 1 | 3 | 5 | 7 | 8 | 12 |
| 35–49 | 308 | 2.9 | 11 | 1 | 1 | 2 | 3 | 6 | 7 | 16 |
| 50–64 | 192 | 5.5 | 31 | 1 | 2 | 3 | 6 | 14 | 14 | 35 |
| 65+ | 208 | 6.8 | 46 | 2 | 3 | 4 | 8 | 16 | 19 | 42 |
| **TOTAL SINGLE DX** | 314 | 2.2 | 2 | 1 | 1 | 2 | 3 | 4 | 5 | 5 |
| **TOTAL MULTIPLE DX** | 923 | 4.4 | 24 | 1 | 2 | 3 | 5 | 9 | 14 | 23 |
| **TOTAL** | | | | | | | | | | |
| 0–19 Years | 101 | 2.5 | 6 | 1 | 1 | 2 | 2 | 5 | 7 | 17 |
| 20–34 | 253 | 2.9 | 8 | 1 | 1 | 2 | 4 | 5 | 6 | 10 |
| 35–49 | 439 | 2.8 | 8 | 1 | 2 | 2 | 3 | 5 | 6 | 13 |
| 50–64 | 227 | 5.0 | 29 | 1 | 2 | 3 | 6 | 14 | 14 | 21 |
| 65+ | 217 | 6.8 | 46 | 2 | 3 | 4 | 8 | 16 | 19 | 33 |
| **GRAND TOTAL** | 1,237 | 3.7 | 19 | 1 | 1 | 2 | 4 | 7 | 13 | 20 |

## 77.89: PARTIAL OSTECTOMY NEC. Formerly included in operation group(s) 726.

| Type of Patients | Observed Patients | Avg. Stay | Variance | 10th | 25th | 50th | 75th | 90th | 95th | 99th |
|---|---|---|---|---|---|---|---|---|---|---|
| **1. SINGLE DX** | | | | | | | | | | |
| 0–19 Years | 27 | 3.1 | 6 | 1 | 1 | 2 | 6 | 7 | 7 | 7 |
| 20–34 | 22 | 2.2 | 6 | 1 | 1 | 1 | 3 | 3 | 6 | 17 |
| 35–49 | 38 | 5.0 | 12 | 1 | 2 | 3 | 9 | 9 | 9 | 9 |
| 50–64 | 27 | 2.6 | 12 | 1 | 1 | 1 | 3 | 4 | 16 | 16 |
| 65+ | 5 | 1.9 | <1 | 1 | 1 | 2 | 3 | 3 | 3 | 3 |
| **2. MULTIPLE DX** | | | | | | | | | | |
| 0–19 Years | 39 | 6.3 | 20 | 1 | 2 | 5 | 10 | 14 | 15 | 15 |
| 20–34 | 54 | 8.0 | 69 | 1 | 2 | 5 | 11 | 21 | 21 | 37 |
| 35–49 | 155 | 5.9 | 58 | 1 | 2 | 5 | 7 | 11 | 20 | 42 |
| 50–64 | 185 | 6.0 | 51 | 1 | 2 | 4 | 7 | 11 | 21 | 43 |
| 65+ | 221 | 5.5 | 31 | 1 | 1 | 4 | 8 | 13 | 17 | 39 |
| **TOTAL SINGLE DX** | 119 | 3.6 | 10 | 1 | 1 | 2 | 6 | 9 | 9 | 16 |
| **TOTAL MULTIPLE DX** | 654 | 5.9 | 44 | 1 | 2 | 4 | 7 | 13 | 20 | 42 |
| **TOTAL** | | | | | | | | | | |
| 0–19 Years | 66 | 4.7 | 15 | 1 | 1 | 3 | 7 | 10 | 14 | 15 |
| 20–34 | 76 | 6.3 | 58 | 1 | 1 | 3 | 7 | 19 | 21 | 37 |
| 35–49 | 193 | 5.6 | 45 | 1 | 2 | 4 | 8 | 10 | 14 | 40 |
| 50–64 | 212 | 5.7 | 48 | 1 | 2 | 4 | 7 | 11 | 20 | 43 |
| 65+ | 226 | 5.4 | 30 | 1 | 1 | 4 | 8 | 13 | 17 | 39 |
| **GRAND TOTAL** | 773 | 5.5 | 39 | 1 | 2 | 4 | 7 | 12 | 16 | 39 |

## 77.91,91: TOT CHEST CAGE OSTECTOMY. Formerly included in operation group(s) 726.

| Type of Patients | Observed Patients | Avg. Stay | Variance | 10th | 25th | 50th | 75th | 90th | 95th | 99th |
|---|---|---|---|---|---|---|---|---|---|---|
| **1. SINGLE DX** | | | | | | | | | | |
| 0–19 Years | 29 | 1.8 | 1 | 1 | 1 | 1 | 2 | 3 | 4 | 4 |
| 20–34 | 87 | 1.8 | <1 | 1 | 1 | 2 | 2 | 3 | 4 | 4 |
| 35–49 | 107 | 2.2 | 1 | 1 | 1 | 2 | 2 | 3 | 4 | 5 |
| 50–64 | 20 | 2.1 | 1 | 1 | 1 | 2 | 3 | 3 | 3 | 6 |
| 65+ | 1 | 3.0 | 0 | 3 | 3 | 3 | 3 | 3 | 3 | 3 |
| **2. MULTIPLE DX** | | | | | | | | | | |
| 0–19 Years | 33 | 2.5 | 4 | 1 | 1 | 2 | 3 | 5 | 9 | 10 |
| 20–34 | 107 | 3.0 | 4 | 1 | 2 | 2 | 4 | 5 | 8 | 10 |
| 35–49 | 213 | 2.8 | 12 | 1 | 2 | 2 | 3 | 6 | 8 | 16 |
| 50–64 | 65 | 6.7 | 46 | 2 | 4 | 8 | 14 | 14 | 16 | 38 |
| 65+ | 45 | 9.1 | 37 | 4 | 4 | 8 | 13 | 16 | 17 | 24 |
| **TOTAL SINGLE DX** | 244 | 2.0 | 1 | 1 | 1 | 2 | 2 | 3 | 4 | 5 |
| **TOTAL MULTIPLE DX** | 463 | 4.1 | 22 | 1 | 1 | 2 | 4 | 12 | 14 | 21 |
| **TOTAL** | | | | | | | | | | |
| 0–19 Years | 62 | 2.1 | 3 | 1 | 1 | 2 | 3 | 4 | 5 | 9 |
| 20–34 | 194 | 2.4 | 3 | 1 | 1 | 2 | 3 | 4 | 6 | 8 |
| 35–49 | 320 | 2.6 | 7 | 1 | 1 | 2 | 3 | 4 | 5 | 13 |
| 50–64 | 85 | 5.8 | 40 | 1 | 2 | 3 | 10 | 14 | 14 | 38 |
| 65+ | 46 | 9.0 | 37 | 1 | 4 | 7 | 13 | 16 | 17 | 24 |
| **GRAND TOTAL** | 707 | 3.2 | 15 | 1 | 1 | 2 | 3 | 6 | 13 | 17 |

Length of Stay by Diagnosis and Operation, United States, 2000

## United States, October 1998–September 1999 Data, by Operation

### 78.0: BONE GRAFT. Formerly included in operation group(s) 727, 728.

| Type of Patients | Observed Patients | Avg. Stay | Variance | Percentiles | | | | | | |
|---|---|---|---|---|---|---|---|---|---|---|
| | | | | 10th | 25th | 50th | 75th | 90th | 95th | 99th |
| **1. SINGLE DX** | | | | | | | | | | |
| 0–19 Years | 150 | 2.2 | 2 | 1 | 1 | 2 | 3 | 4 | 4 | 12 |
| 20–34 | 142 | 2.0 | 2 | 1 | 1 | 2 | 2 | 4 | 5 | 5 |
| 35–49 | 148 | 2.5 | 2 | 1 | 1 | 2 | 3 | 4 | 5 | 7 |
| 50–64 | 38 | 2.7 | 4 | 1 | 1 | 2 | 3 | 7 | 7 | 8 |
| 65+ | 20 | 2.3 | <1 | 1 | 2 | 2 | 3 | 3 | 4 | 4 |
| **2. MULTIPLE DX** | | | | | | | | | | |
| 0–19 Years | 169 | 2.8 | 6 | 1 | 1 | 2 | 4 | 5 | 6 | 14 |
| 20–34 | 287 | 2.9 | 4 | 1 | 2 | 3 | 4 | 5 | 6 | 9 |
| 35–49 | 469 | 3.4 | 11 | 1 | 2 | 3 | 4 | 6 | 8 | 18 |
| 50–64 | 246 | 3.8 | 25 | 1 | 2 | 3 | 4 | 7 | 9 | 23 |
| 65+ | 138 | 4.4 | 16 | 1 | 2 | 3 | 5 | 9 | 9 | 21 |
| **TOTAL SINGLE DX** | 498 | 2.3 | 2 | 1 | 1 | 2 | 3 | 4 | 5 | 8 |
| **TOTAL MULTIPLE DX** | 1,309 | 3.4 | 12 | 1 | 2 | 3 | 4 | 6 | 8 | 19 |
| **TOTAL** | | | | | | | | | | |
| 0–19 Years | 319 | 2.5 | 4 | 1 | 1 | 2 | 3 | 4 | 5 | 12 |
| 20–34 | 429 | 2.5 | 3 | 1 | 1 | 2 | 3 | 5 | 5 | 9 |
| 35–49 | 617 | 3.1 | 9 | 2 | 2 | 3 | 4 | 5 | 7 | 12 |
| 50–64 | 284 | 3.7 | 22 | 1 | 2 | 3 | 4 | 7 | 9 | 22 |
| 65+ | 158 | 4.2 | 15 | 1 | 2 | 3 | 5 | 8 | 9 | 21 |
| **GRAND TOTAL** | 1,807 | 3.0 | 10 | 1 | 1 | 2 | 3 | 5 | 7 | 15 |

### 78.05: BONE GRAFT TO FEMUR. Formerly included in operation group(s) 727.

| Type of Patients | Observed Patients | Avg. Stay | Variance | Percentiles | | | | | | |
|---|---|---|---|---|---|---|---|---|---|---|
| | | | | 10th | 25th | 50th | 75th | 90th | 95th | 99th |
| **1. SINGLE DX** | | | | | | | | | | |
| 0–19 Years | 69 | 2.5 | 3 | 1 | 2 | 2 | 3 | 4 | 5 | 12 |
| 20–34 | 59 | 3.1 | 4 | 2 | 2 | 3 | 4 | 5 | 5 | 14 |
| 35–49 | 64 | 2.3 | 3 | 1 | 1 | 2 | 3 | 4 | 8 | 8 |
| 50–64 | 12 | 3.9 | 7 | 1 | 1 | 2 | 7 | 7 | 8 | 8 |
| 65+ | 6 | 2.3 | <1 | 1 | 2 | 2 | 3 | 3 | 3 | 3 |
| **2. MULTIPLE DX** | | | | | | | | | | |
| 0–19 Years | 68 | 3.6 | 10 | 1 | 2 | 3 | 5 | 6 | 7 | 16 |
| 20–34 | 105 | 3.7 | 6 | 2 | 3 | 3 | 4 | 5 | 6 | 19 |
| 35–49 | 193 | 4.3 | 14 | 1 | 2 | 3 | 5 | 7 | 9 | 23 |
| 50–64 | 82 | 3.4 | 6 | 1 | 2 | 3 | 4 | 6 | 7 | 13 |
| 65+ | 59 | 4.5 | 15 | 1 | 3 | 3 | 5 | 7 | 14 | 21 |
| **TOTAL SINGLE DX** | 210 | 2.6 | 4 | 1 | 1 | 2 | 3 | 5 | 7 | 12 |
| **TOTAL MULTIPLE DX** | 507 | 4.0 | 11 | 1 | 2 | 3 | 5 | 7 | 8 | 20 |
| **TOTAL** | | | | | | | | | | |
| 0–19 Years | 137 | 3.0 | 7 | 1 | 2 | 2 | 4 | 5 | 6 | 14 |
| 20–34 | 164 | 3.4 | 5 | 2 | 2 | 3 | 4 | 5 | 6 | 14 |
| 35–49 | 257 | 3.8 | 12 | 1 | 2 | 3 | 5 | 7 | 8 | 20 |
| 50–64 | 94 | 3.4 | 6 | 1 | 2 | 3 | 4 | 7 | 7 | 13 |
| 65+ | 65 | 4.4 | 14 | 1 | 3 | 3 | 5 | 7 | 10 | 21 |
| **GRAND TOTAL** | 717 | 3.5 | 9 | 1 | 2 | 3 | 4 | 6 | 7 | 18 |

### 78.07: BONE GRAFT TIBIA/FIBULA. Formerly included in operation group(s) 728.

| Type of Patients | Observed Patients | Avg. Stay | Variance | Percentiles | | | | | | |
|---|---|---|---|---|---|---|---|---|---|---|
| | | | | 10th | 25th | 50th | 75th | 90th | 95th | 99th |
| **1. SINGLE DX** | | | | | | | | | | |
| 0–19 Years | 51 | 1.8 | 1 | 1 | 1 | 1 | 2 | 4 | 4 | 5 |
| 20–34 | 56 | 1.7 | <1 | 1 | 1 | 3 | 3 | 2 | 3 | 5 |
| 35–49 | 67 | 2.7 | 1 | 2 | 2 | 3 | 3 | 3 | 4 | 7 |
| 50–64 | 18 | 2.2 | 2 | 1 | 2 | 3 | 3 | 3 | 4 | 9 |
| 65+ | 7 | 2.5 | <1 | 1 | 2 | 3 | 3 | 4 | 4 | 4 |
| **2. MULTIPLE DX** | | | | | | | | | | |
| 0–19 Years | 68 | 2.6 | 1 | 1 | 2 | 3 | 3 | 4 | 4 | 6 |
| 20–34 | 128 | 3.1 | 3 | 1 | 2 | 3 | 4 | 5 | 7 | 9 |
| 35–49 | 184 | 2.7 | 7 | 2 | 2 | 2 | 3 | 4 | 5 | 9 |
| 50–64 | 106 | 4.3 | 38 | 1 | 2 | 3 | 4 | 7 | 14 | 29 |
| 65+ | 44 | 3.9 | 8 | 1 | 2 | 3 | 4 | 8 | 8 | 17 |
| **TOTAL SINGLE DX** | 199 | 2.2 | 1 | 1 | 1 | 2 | 3 | 3 | 4 | 7 |
| **TOTAL MULTIPLE DX** | 530 | 3.2 | 13 | 1 | 2 | 3 | 3 | 5 | 7 | 22 |
| **TOTAL** | | | | | | | | | | |
| 0–19 Years | 119 | 2.3 | 2 | 1 | 1 | 2 | 3 | 4 | 4 | 6 |
| 20–34 | 184 | 2.5 | 3 | 1 | 1 | 2 | 3 | 5 | 5 | 9 |
| 35–49 | 251 | 2.7 | 5 | 1 | 2 | 3 | 3 | 4 | 5 | 8 |
| 50–64 | 124 | 4.1 | 34 | 1 | 2 | 3 | 3 | 7 | 10 | 23 |
| 65+ | 51 | 3.7 | 7 | 1 | 2 | 3 | 4 | 7 | 8 | 17 |
| **GRAND TOTAL** | 729 | 2.9 | 10 | 1 | 2 | 2 | 3 | 4 | 7 | 14 |

### 78.1: APPL EXT FIXATION DEVICE. Formerly included in operation group(s) 727, 728.

| Type of Patients | Observed Patients | Avg. Stay | Variance | Percentiles | | | | | | |
|---|---|---|---|---|---|---|---|---|---|---|
| | | | | 10th | 25th | 50th | 75th | 90th | 95th | 99th |
| **1. SINGLE DX** | | | | | | | | | | |
| 0–19 Years | 237 | 4.1 | 29 | 1 | 1 | 3 | 4 | 7 | 18 | 31 |
| 20–34 | 97 | 3.4 | 6 | 1 | 1 | 3 | 4 | 7 | 7 | 13 |
| 35–49 | 116 | 2.4 | 5 | 1 | 1 | 1 | 3 | 5 | 6 | 12 |
| 50–64 | 76 | 2.2 | 2 | 1 | 1 | 2 | 3 | 4 | 5 | 7 |
| 65+ | 49 | 1.7 | 1 | 1 | 1 | 1 | 2 | 3 | 5 | 5 |
| **2. MULTIPLE DX** | | | | | | | | | | |
| 0–19 Years | 273 | 9.3 | 158 | 1 | 3 | 4 | 10 | 31 | 42 | >99 |
| 20–34 | 214 | 7.1 | 46 | 1 | 2 | 5 | 8 | 19 | 19 | 33 |
| 35–49 | 358 | 6.1 | 42 | 1 | 2 | 4 | 8 | 13 | 16 | 41 |
| 50–64 | 267 | 5.5 | 35 | 1 | 2 | 3 | 6 | 15 | 19 | 28 |
| 65+ | 473 | 5.4 | 46 | 1 | 2 | 3 | 6 | 13 | 20 | 49 |
| **TOTAL SINGLE DX** | 575 | 3.2 | 15 | 1 | 1 | 2 | 4 | 6 | 7 | 22 |
| **TOTAL MULTIPLE DX** | 1,585 | 6.5 | 64 | 1 | 2 | 4 | 7 | 15 | 20 | 47 |
| **TOTAL** | | | | | | | | | | |
| 0–19 Years | 510 | 6.9 | 104 | 1 | 2 | 3 | 6 | 18 | 39 | 60 |
| 20–34 | 311 | 5.8 | 35 | 1 | 2 | 4 | 7 | 14 | 19 | 30 |
| 35–49 | 474 | 5.1 | 35 | 1 | 1 | 3 | 6 | 11 | 15 | 34 |
| 50–64 | 343 | 4.9 | 30 | 1 | 2 | 3 | 5 | 12 | 19 | 27 |
| 65+ | 522 | 5.1 | 44 | 1 | 2 | 3 | 6 | 11 | 20 | 38 |
| **GRAND TOTAL** | 2,160 | 5.6 | 53 | 1 | 2 | 3 | 6 | 13 | 19 | 42 |

© 2000 by HCIA-Sachs, L.L.C.

Length of Stay by Diagnosis and Operation, United States, 2000

# United States, October 1998–September 1999 Data, by Operation

## 78.13: APPL EXT FIX RAD/ULNA. Formerly included in operation group(s) 728.

| Type of Patients | Observed Patients | Avg. Stay | Variance | Percentiles | | | | | | |
|---|---|---|---|---|---|---|---|---|---|---|
| | | | | 10th | 25th | 50th | 75th | 90th | 95th | 99th |
| **1. SINGLE DX** | | | | | | | | | | |
| 0–19 Years | 11 | 1.8 | 1 | 1 | 1 | 2 | 2 | 2 | 5 | 5 |
| 20–34 | 42 | 2.0 | 1 | 1 | 1 | 2 | 3 | 3 | 5 | 4 |
| 35–49 | 54 | 1.3 | <1 | 1 | 1 | 1 | 1 | 2 | 4 | 4 |
| 50–64 | 47 | 1.5 | <1 | 1 | 1 | 1 | 2 | 2 | 3 | 5 |
| 65+ | 41 | 1.5 | <1 | 1 | 1 | 1 | 2 | 2 | 3 | 5 |
| **2. MULTIPLE DX** | | | | | | | | | | |
| 0–19 Years | 19 | 2.8 | 9 | 1 | 1 | 1 | 3 | 9 | 11 | 11 |
| 20–34 | 51 | 3.9 | 21 | 1 | 1 | 3 | 4 | 8 | 19 | >99 |
| 35–49 | 106 | 3.1 | 7 | 1 | 2 | 2 | 4 | 6 | 9 | 11 |
| 50–64 | 108 | 3.7 | 15 | 1 | 1 | 2 | 4 | 9 | 13 | 17 |
| 65+ | 293 | 3.0 | 7 | 1 | 1 | 2 | 4 | 6 | 8 | 15 |
| **TOTAL SINGLE DX** | 195 | 1.6 | <1 | 1 | 1 | 1 | 2 | 3 | 3 | 5 |
| **TOTAL MULTIPLE DX** | 577 | 3.3 | 10 | 1 | 1 | 2 | 4 | 7 | 10 | 17 |
| **TOTAL** | | | | | | | | | | |
| 0–19 Years | 30 | 2.4 | 6 | 1 | 1 | 1 | 3 | 5 | 9 | 11 |
| 20–34 | 93 | 3.0 | 12 | 1 | 1 | 2 | 3 | 4 | 8 | 25 |
| 35–49 | 160 | 2.5 | 5 | 1 | 1 | 2 | 3 | 6 | 7 | 11 |
| 50–64 | 155 | 3.1 | 12 | 1 | 1 | 2 | 4 | 6 | 11 | 17 |
| 65+ | 334 | 2.9 | 7 | 1 | 1 | 2 | 3 | 6 | 8 | 15 |
| **GRAND TOTAL** | 772 | 2.8 | 8 | 1 | 1 | 2 | 3 | 6 | 8 | 17 |

## 78.15: APPL EXT FIX DEV FEMUR. Formerly included in operation group(s) 727.

| Type of Patients | Observed Patients | Avg. Stay | Variance | Percentiles | | | | | | |
|---|---|---|---|---|---|---|---|---|---|---|
| | | | | 10th | 25th | 50th | 75th | 90th | 95th | 99th |
| **1. SINGLE DX** | | | | | | | | | | |
| 0–19 Years | 154 | 5.2 | 38 | 1 | 2 | 3 | 5 | 14 | 18 | 33 |
| 20–34 | 1 | 4.0 | 0 | 4 | 4 | 4 | 4 | 4 | 4 | 4 |
| 35–49 | 1 | 9.0 | 0 | 9 | 9 | 9 | 9 | 9 | 9 | 9 |
| 50–64 | 3 | 3.6 | <1 | 3 | 3 | 3 | 4 | 5 | 5 | 5 |
| 65+ | 1 | 5.0 | 0 | 5 | 5 | 5 | 5 | 5 | 5 | 5 |
| **2. MULTIPLE DX** | | | | | | | | | | |
| 0–19 Years | 167 | 9.9 | 132 | 2 | 3 | 5 | 13 | 31 | 42 | >99 |
| 20–34 | 23 | 10.4 | 63 | 4 | 6 | 6 | 13 | 20 | 33 | 33 |
| 35–49 | 27 | 9.2 | 83 | 2 | 5 | 9 | 19 | 23 | 34 | 45 |
| 50–64 | 24 | 13.1 | 84 | 3 | 5 | 12 | 19 | 19 | 29 | 45 |
| 65+ | 53 | 14.2 | 160 | 4 | 5 | 8 | 20 | 31 | 49 | 49 |
| **TOTAL SINGLE DX** | 160 | 5.2 | 37 | 1 | 2 | 3 | 5 | 14 | 18 | 33 |
| **TOTAL MULTIPLE DX** | 294 | 11.1 | 125 | 2 | 4 | 6 | 18 | 26 | 42 | >99 |
| **TOTAL** | | | | | | | | | | |
| 0–19 Years | 321 | 7.6 | 92 | 1 | 3 | 4 | 8 | 22 | 35 | >99 |
| 20–34 | 24 | 10.3 | 62 | 4 | 6 | 6 | 13 | 20 | 33 | 33 |
| 35–49 | 28 | 9.2 | 81 | 2 | 5 | 5 | 9 | 23 | 34 | 46 |
| 50–64 | 27 | 12.3 | 84 | 3 | 5 | 9 | 19 | 19 | 29 | 38 |
| 65+ | 54 | 14.2 | 159 | 4 | 5 | 8 | 20 | 31 | 49 | 49 |
| **GRAND TOTAL** | 454 | 9.1 | 103 | 2 | 3 | 5 | 12 | 21 | 34 | 49 |

## 78.17: APPL EXT FIX DEV TIB/FIB. Formerly included in operation group(s) 728.

| Type of Patients | Observed Patients | Avg. Stay | Variance | Percentiles | | | | | | |
|---|---|---|---|---|---|---|---|---|---|---|
| | | | | 10th | 25th | 50th | 75th | 90th | 95th | 99th |
| **1. SINGLE DX** | | | | | | | | | | |
| 0–19 Years | 49 | 2.6 | 13 | 1 | 1 | 1 | 3 | 5 | 7 | 25 |
| 20–34 | 47 | 4.4 | 7 | 1 | 2 | 4 | 7 | 7 | 7 | 14 |
| 35–49 | 55 | 3.6 | 8 | 1 | 1 | 3 | 5 | 6 | 8 | 14 |
| 50–64 | 25 | 3.4 | 3 | 2 | 3 | 3 | 4 | 5 | 6 | 10 |
| 65+ | 5 | 3.6 | 2 | 2 | 2 | 4 | 5 | 5 | 5 | 5 |
| **2. MULTIPLE DX** | | | | | | | | | | |
| 0–19 Years | 56 | 9.7 | 203 | 2 | 3 | 3 | 7 | 42 | 45 | 50 |
| 20–34 | 112 | 7.4 | 43 | 1 | 2 | 6 | 9 | 19 | 19 | 30 |
| 35–49 | 168 | 7.4 | 38 | 2 | 3 | 5 | 11 | 15 | 17 | 28 |
| 50–64 | 102 | 5.9 | 23 | 2 | 3 | 4 | 8 | 13 | 17 | 19 |
| 65+ | 88 | 6.8 | 20 | 2 | 4 | 5 | 9 | 14 | 15 | 20 |
| **TOTAL SINGLE DX** | 181 | 3.5 | 9 | 1 | 1 | 3 | 5 | 7 | 7 | 14 |
| **TOTAL MULTIPLE DX** | 526 | 7.3 | 57 | 2 | 3 | 5 | 9 | 15 | 19 | 44 |
| **TOTAL** | | | | | | | | | | |
| 0–19 Years | 105 | 6.5 | 128 | 1 | 1 | 3 | 5 | 11 | 42 | 50 |
| 20–34 | 159 | 6.3 | 32 | 1 | 2 | 4 | 8 | 17 | 19 | 27 |
| 35–49 | 223 | 6.4 | 32 | 1 | 3 | 5 | 8 | 13 | 15 | 28 |
| 50–64 | 127 | 5.4 | 19 | 2 | 3 | 4 | 6 | 12 | 16 | 18 |
| 65+ | 93 | 6.7 | 20 | 2 | 4 | 5 | 9 | 14 | 15 | 20 |
| **GRAND TOTAL** | 707 | 6.2 | 46 | 1 | 3 | 4 | 7 | 14 | 19 | 42 |

## 78.2: LIMB SHORTENING PX. Formerly included in operation group(s) 727, 728.

| Type of Patients | Observed Patients | Avg. Stay | Variance | Percentiles | | | | | | |
|---|---|---|---|---|---|---|---|---|---|---|
| | | | | 10th | 25th | 50th | 75th | 90th | 95th | 99th |
| **1. SINGLE DX** | | | | | | | | | | |
| 0–19 Years | 162 | 1.9 | <1 | 1 | 1 | 2 | 2 | 3 | 4 | 5 |
| 20–34 | 9 | 2.5 | 2 | 1 | 1 | 3 | 3 | 3 | 4 | 4 |
| 35–49 | 9 | 1.8 | 2 | 1 | 1 | 1 | 1 | 5 | 5 | 4 |
| 50–64 | 1 | 4.0 | 0 | 4 | 4 | 4 | 4 | 4 | 4 | 4 |
| 65+ | 0 | | | | | | | | | |
| **2. MULTIPLE DX** | | | | | | | | | | |
| 0–19 Years | 290 | 2.3 | 3 | 1 | 1 | 2 | 2 | 4 | 5 | 9 |
| 20–34 | 15 | 7.0 | 332 | 2 | 2 | 3 | 5 | 6 | 12 | 94 |
| 35–49 | 12 | 2.7 | <1 | 1 | 2 | 3 | 3 | 4 | 3 | 4 |
| 50–64 | 11 | 4.5 | 247 | 1 | 1 | 1 | 1 | 3 | 7 | 83 |
| 65+ | 2 | 3.0 | 0 | 3 | 3 | 3 | 3 | 3 | 3 | 3 |
| **TOTAL SINGLE DX** | 181 | 1.9 | 1 | 1 | 1 | 2 | 2 | 3 | 4 | 5 |
| **TOTAL MULTIPLE DX** | 330 | 2.6 | 28 | 1 | 1 | 2 | 3 | 4 | 5 | 10 |
| **TOTAL** | | | | | | | | | | |
| 0–19 Years | 452 | 2.1 | 2 | 1 | 1 | 2 | 3 | 4 | 5 | 9 |
| 20–34 | 24 | 5.8 | 245 | 1 | 2 | 3 | 4 | 6 | 12 | 94 |
| 35–49 | 21 | 2.5 | 1 | 1 | 2 | 3 | 3 | 4 | 4 | 5 |
| 50–64 | 12 | 4.5 | 244 | 1 | 1 | 3 | 1 | 3 | 7 | 83 |
| 65+ | 2 | 3.0 | 0 | 3 | 3 | 3 | 3 | 3 | 3 | 3 |
| **GRAND TOTAL** | 511 | 2.3 | 18 | 1 | 1 | 2 | 3 | 4 | 5 | 9 |

Length of Stay by Diagnosis and Operation, United States, 2000

# United States, October 1998–September 1999 Data, by Operation

## 78.25: LIMB SHORT PX FEMUR. Formerly included in operation group(s) 727.

| Type of Patients | Observed Patients | Avg. Stay | Variance | Percentiles 10th | 25th | 50th | 75th | 90th | 95th | 99th |
|---|---|---|---|---|---|---|---|---|---|---|
| **1. SINGLE DX** | | | | | | | | | | |
| 0–19 Years | 104 | 1.9 | <1 | 1 | 1 | 2 | 3 | 3 | 3 | 5 |
| 20–34 | 3 | 3.7 | <1 | 3 | 3 | 4 | 4 | 4 | 4 | 4 |
| 35–49 | 1 | 3.0 | 0 | 3 | 3 | 3 | 3 | 3 | 3 | 3 |
| 50–64 | 1 | 4.0 | 0 | 4 | 4 | 4 | 4 | 4 | 4 | 4 |
| 65+ | 0 | | | | | | | | | |
| **2. MULTIPLE DX** | | | | | | | | | | |
| 0–19 Years | 182 | 2.4 | 4 | 1 | 1 | 2 | 3 | 4 | 8 | 10 |
| 20–34 | 10 | 10.4 | 550 | 3 | 2 | 3 | 6 | 12 | 94 | 94 |
| 35–49 | 5 | 2.9 | <1 | 3 | 2 | 3 | 3 | 4 | 4 | 4 |
| 50–64 | 4 | 34.5 | >999 | 2 | 2 | 4 | 83 | 83 | 83 | 83 |
| 65+ | 0 | | | | | | | | | |
| **TOTAL SINGLE DX** | 109 | 1.9 | <1 | 1 | 1 | 2 | 3 | 3 | 3 | 5 |
| **TOTAL MULTIPLE DX** | 201 | 3.0 | 44 | 1 | 1 | 2 | 3 | 4 | 8 | 13 |
| **TOTAL** | | | | | | | | | | |
| 0–19 Years | 286 | 2.2 | 3 | 1 | 1 | 2 | 3 | 4 | 5 | 9 |
| 20–34 | 13 | 9.3 | 460 | 2 | 2 | 4 | 6 | 12 | 94 | 94 |
| 35–49 | 6 | 2.9 | <1 | 2 | 2 | 3 | 3 | 4 | 4 | 4 |
| 50–64 | 5 | 30.5 | >999 | 2 | 3 | 4 | 83 | 83 | 83 | 83 |
| 65+ | 0 | | | | | | | | | |
| **GRAND TOTAL** | 310 | 2.6 | 28 | 1 | 1 | 2 | 3 | 4 | 5 | 10 |

## 78.3: LIMB LENGTHENING PX. Formerly included in operation group(s) 727, 728.

| Type of Patients | Observed Patients | Avg. Stay | Variance | Percentiles 10th | 25th | 50th | 75th | 90th | 95th | 99th |
|---|---|---|---|---|---|---|---|---|---|---|
| **1. SINGLE DX** | | | | | | | | | | |
| 0–19 Years | 86 | 2.2 | 3 | 1 | 1 | 2 | 2 | 3 | 5 | 12 |
| 20–34 | 4 | 2.0 | 1 | 1 | 1 | 2 | 3 | 3 | 3 | 3 |
| 35–49 | 6 | 2.4 | <1 | 2 | 2 | 2 | 3 | 3 | 3 | 3 |
| 50–64 | 0 | | | | | | | | | |
| 65+ | 1 | 4.0 | 0 | 4 | 4 | 4 | 4 | 4 | 4 | 4 |
| **2. MULTIPLE DX** | | | | | | | | | | |
| 0–19 Years | 160 | 2.4 | 2 | 1 | 2 | 2 | 3 | 4 | 5 | 6 |
| 20–34 | 27 | 2.3 | 1 | 2 | 2 | 2 | 2 | 4 | 5 | 6 |
| 35–49 | 25 | 8.0 | 53 | 2 | 2 | 3 | 17 | 17 | 17 | 17 |
| 50–64 | 14 | 4.0 | 6 | 2 | 2 | 3 | 6 | 8 | 8 | 8 |
| 65+ | 7 | 5.7 | 54 | 2 | 3 | 3 | 4 | 24 | 24 | 24 |
| **TOTAL SINGLE DX** | 97 | 2.2 | 3 | 1 | 1 | 2 | 3 | 3 | 5 | 12 |
| **TOTAL MULTIPLE DX** | 233 | 3.2 | 13 | 1 | 2 | 2 | 3 | 5 | 17 | 17 |
| **TOTAL** | | | | | | | | | | |
| 0–19 Years | 246 | 2.3 | 2 | 1 | 2 | 2 | 3 | 4 | 5 | 7 |
| 20–34 | 31 | 2.3 | 1 | 2 | 2 | 3 | 3 | 4 | 5 | 6 |
| 35–49 | 31 | 7.5 | 51 | 1 | 2 | 3 | 17 | 17 | 17 | 17 |
| 50–64 | 14 | 4.0 | 6 | 2 | 2 | 3 | 6 | 8 | 8 | 8 |
| 65+ | 8 | 5.6 | 50 | 2 | 2 | 3 | 4 | 24 | 24 | 24 |
| **GRAND TOTAL** | 330 | 3.0 | 11 | 1 | 2 | 2 | 3 | 5 | 8 | 17 |

## 78.4: OTHER BONE REPAIR. Formerly included in operation group(s) 727, 728.

| Type of Patients | Observed Patients | Avg. Stay | Variance | Percentiles 10th | 25th | 50th | 75th | 90th | 95th | 99th |
|---|---|---|---|---|---|---|---|---|---|---|
| **1. SINGLE DX** | | | | | | | | | | |
| 0–19 Years | 40 | 2.1 | 6 | 1 | 1 | 1 | 2 | 7 | 7 | 14 |
| 20–34 | 30 | 2.2 | 3 | 1 | 1 | 2 | 3 | 3 | 4 | 12 |
| 35–49 | 30 | 1.8 | 2 | 1 | 1 | 1 | 2 | 4 | 4 | 5 |
| 50–64 | 6 | 1.6 | <1 | 1 | 1 | 1 | 2 | 3 | 3 | 3 |
| 65+ | 6 | 2.7 | <1 | 2 | 3 | 3 | 3 | 3 | 3 | 3 |
| **2. MULTIPLE DX** | | | | | | | | | | |
| 0–19 Years | 169 | 4.7 | 63 | 1 | 1 | 2 | 4 | 7 | 35 | 35 |
| 20–34 | 56 | 2.9 | 13 | 1 | 1 | 2 | 3 | 6 | 8 | 22 |
| 35–49 | 102 | 2.6 | 8 | 1 | 1 | 2 | 3 | 6 | 6 | 10 |
| 50–64 | 90 | 4.4 | 10 | 1 | 2 | 4 | 5 | 8 | 11 | 14 |
| 65+ | 133 | 5.5 | 25 | 1 | 2 | 4 | 7 | 12 | 17 | 28 |
| **TOTAL SINGLE DX** | 112 | 2.0 | 3 | 1 | 1 | 1 | 2 | 4 | 5 | 12 |
| **TOTAL MULTIPLE DX** | 550 | 4.0 | 25 | 1 | 2 | 3 | 4 | 7 | 11 | 35 |
| **TOTAL** | | | | | | | | | | |
| 0–19 Years | 209 | 3.9 | 47 | 1 | 1 | 2 | 3 | 7 | 14 | 35 |
| 20–34 | 86 | 2.7 | 10 | 1 | 1 | 2 | 3 | 5 | 8 | 22 |
| 35–49 | 132 | 2.4 | 7 | 1 | 2 | 2 | 3 | 4 | 5 | 8 |
| 50–64 | 96 | 4.2 | 10 | 1 | 2 | 3 | 5 | 7 | 11 | 14 |
| 65+ | 139 | 5.4 | 24 | 1 | 2 | 4 | 7 | 11 | 16 | 28 |
| **GRAND TOTAL** | 662 | 3.6 | 21 | 1 | 1 | 2 | 4 | 7 | 10 | 31 |

## 78.5: INT FIX W/O FX REDUCTION. Formerly included in operation group(s) 727, 728.

| Type of Patients | Observed Patients | Avg. Stay | Variance | Percentiles 10th | 25th | 50th | 75th | 90th | 95th | 99th |
|---|---|---|---|---|---|---|---|---|---|---|
| **1. SINGLE DX** | | | | | | | | | | |
| 0–19 Years | 814 | 2.8 | 19 | 1 | 1 | 2 | 2 | 4 | 7 | 25 |
| 20–34 | 280 | 2.5 | 2 | 1 | 2 | 2 | 3 | 4 | 5 | 7 |
| 35–49 | 238 | 2.7 | 3 | 1 | 2 | 3 | 4 | 5 | 5 | 9 |
| 50–64 | 148 | 2.7 | 3 | 1 | 2 | 3 | 4 | 4 | 5 | 6 |
| 65+ | 199 | 4.0 | 3 | 2 | 3 | 4 | 5 | 6 | 7 | 8 |
| **2. MULTIPLE DX** | | | | | | | | | | |
| 0–19 Years | 699 | 5.5 | 39 | 1 | 2 | 3 | 7 | 12 | 19 | 34 |
| 20–34 | 639 | 5.5 | 39 | 1 | 2 | 3 | 7 | 11 | 17 | 28 |
| 35–49 | 899 | 4.6 | 34 | 1 | 2 | 4 | 5 | 8 | 12 | 29 |
| 50–64 | 1,003 | 5.5 | 27 | 2 | 3 | 4 | 7 | 10 | 14 | 30 |
| 65+ | 4,933 | 6.1 | 28 | 3 | 4 | 5 | 7 | 10 | 13 | 26 |
| **TOTAL SINGLE DX** | 1,679 | 2.9 | 11 | 1 | 1 | 2 | 3 | 5 | 6 | 23 |
| **TOTAL MULTIPLE DX** | 8,173 | 5.8 | 30 | 2 | 3 | 4 | 7 | 10 | 14 | 27 |
| **TOTAL** | | | | | | | | | | |
| 0–19 Years | 1,513 | 4.0 | 29 | 1 | 2 | 3 | 4 | 8 | 16 | 27 |
| 20–34 | 919 | 4.7 | 30 | 1 | 2 | 3 | 5 | 11 | 13 | 25 |
| 35–49 | 1,137 | 4.2 | 28 | 1 | 2 | 3 | 5 | 8 | 11 | 25 |
| 50–64 | 1,151 | 5.1 | 24 | 2 | 3 | 4 | 6 | 9 | 12 | 26 |
| 65+ | 5,132 | 6.0 | 27 | 3 | 4 | 5 | 7 | 10 | 13 | 26 |
| **GRAND TOTAL** | 9,852 | 5.2 | 28 | 1 | 3 | 4 | 6 | 9 | 13 | 26 |

Length of Stay by Diagnosis and Operation, United States, 2000

# United States, October 1998–September 1999 Data, by Operation

## 78.52: INT FIX W/O RED HUMERUS. Formerly included in operation group(s) 728.

| Type of Patients | Observed Patients | Avg. Stay | Variance | 10th | 25th | 50th | 75th | 90th | 95th | 99th |
|---|---|---|---|---|---|---|---|---|---|---|
| **1. SINGLE DX** | | | | | | | | | | |
| 0–19 Years | 37 | 1.4 | <1 | 1 | 1 | 1 | 2 | 2 | 3 | 3 |
| 20–34 | 16 | 2.1 | 2 | 1 | 1 | 2 | 3 | 3 | 3 | 9 |
| 35–49 | 14 | 3.2 | 2 | 1 | 2 | 4 | 4 | 4 | 6 | 6 |
| 50–64 | 9 | 3.4 | 2 | 2 | 2 | 4 | 5 | 5 | 6 | 6 |
| 65+ | 8 | 2.2 | <1 | 1 | 2 | 2 | 3 | 3 | 3 | 3 |
| **2. MULTIPLE DX** | | | | | | | | | | |
| 0–19 Years | 14 | 1.8 | <1 | 1 | 1 | 2 | 3 | 3 | 3 | 5 |
| 20–34 | 34 | 3.0 | 4 | 1 | 2 | 3 | 4 | 5 | 6 | 13 |
| 35–49 | 73 | 4.6 | 41 | 1 | 2 | 2 | 4 | 8 | 21 | 30 |
| 50–64 | 108 | 4.1 | 19 | 1 | 2 | 2 | 5 | 10 | 12 | 23 |
| 65+ | 232 | 5.4 | 29 | 2 | 2 | 4 | 7 | 11 | 14 | 29 |
| **TOTAL SINGLE DX** | 84 | 2.1 | 2 | 1 | 1 | 2 | 3 | 4 | 4 | 6 |
| **TOTAL MULTIPLE DX** | 461 | 4.6 | 26 | 1 | 2 | 3 | 5 | 10 | 14 | 30 |
| **TOTAL** | | | | | | | | | | |
| 0–19 Years | 51 | 1.6 | <1 | 1 | 1 | 1 | 2 | 3 | 3 | 3 |
| 20–34 | 50 | 2.7 | 3 | 1 | 2 | 2 | 3 | 5 | 6 | 9 |
| 35–49 | 87 | 4.4 | 36 | 1 | 2 | 2 | 4 | 7 | 15 | 30 |
| 50–64 | 117 | 4.1 | 18 | 1 | 2 | 2 | 5 | 10 | 12 | 23 |
| 65+ | 240 | 5.3 | 28 | 2 | 2 | 4 | 7 | 11 | 14 | 29 |
| **GRAND TOTAL** | 545 | 4.2 | 23 | 1 | 2 | 3 | 5 | 10 | 13 | 29 |

## 78.55: INT FIX W/O RED FEMUR. Formerly included in operation group(s) 727.

| Type of Patients | Observed Patients | Avg. Stay | Variance | 10th | 25th | 50th | 75th | 90th | 95th | 99th |
|---|---|---|---|---|---|---|---|---|---|---|
| **1. SINGLE DX** | | | | | | | | | | |
| 0–19 Years | 637 | 2.9 | 22 | 1 | 1 | 2 | 2 | 4 | 11 | 25 |
| 20–34 | 97 | 3.1 | 2 | 2 | 2 | 3 | 4 | 5 | 6 | 7 |
| 35–49 | 65 | 3.3 | 4 | 1 | 2 | 3 | 4 | 6 | 6 | 9 |
| 50–64 | 73 | 2.9 | 2 | 1 | 2 | 3 | 4 | 4 | 5 | 7 |
| 65+ | 170 | 4.1 | 3 | 2 | 3 | 4 | 5 | 7 | 7 | 8 |
| **2. MULTIPLE DX** | | | | | | | | | | |
| 0–19 Years | 486 | 5.9 | 46 | 1 | 2 | 3 | 7 | 14 | 20 | 35 |
| 20–34 | 323 | 6.6 | 48 | 2 | 3 | 5 | 8 | 13 | 18 | 32 |
| 35–49 | 433 | 5.7 | 50 | 2 | 3 | 4 | 6 | 10 | 14 | 31 |
| 50–64 | 634 | 6.2 | 28 | 2 | 3 | 5 | 7 | 11 | 14 | 30 |
| 65+ | 4,413 | 6.1 | 27 | 3 | 4 | 5 | 7 | 10 | 13 | 26 |
| **TOTAL SINGLE DX** | 1,042 | 3.1 | 16 | 1 | 1 | 2 | 4 | 5 | 7 | 24 |
| **TOTAL MULTIPLE DX** | 6,289 | 6.1 | 31 | 3 | 4 | 5 | 7 | 10 | 14 | 28 |
| **TOTAL** | | | | | | | | | | |
| 0–19 Years | 1,123 | 4.1 | 34 | 1 | 2 | 2 | 4 | 9 | 19 | 27 |
| 20–34 | 420 | 5.8 | 40 | 2 | 2 | 4 | 7 | 11 | 17 | 32 |
| 35–49 | 498 | 5.4 | 45 | 2 | 3 | 4 | 6 | 9 | 13 | 30 |
| 50–64 | 707 | 5.8 | 27 | 2 | 3 | 5 | 7 | 10 | 14 | 30 |
| 65+ | 4,583 | 6.1 | 26 | 3 | 4 | 5 | 7 | 10 | 13 | 26 |
| **GRAND TOTAL** | 7,331 | 5.7 | 30 | 3 | 3 | 4 | 6 | 10 | 14 | 27 |

## 78.57: INT FIX W/O RED TIB/FIB. Formerly included in operation group(s) 728.

| Type of Patients | Observed Patients | Avg. Stay | Variance | 10th | 25th | 50th | 75th | 90th | 95th | 99th |
|---|---|---|---|---|---|---|---|---|---|---|
| **1. SINGLE DX** | | | | | | | | | | |
| 0–19 Years | 94 | 2.8 | 9 | 1 | 1 | 2 | 4 | 4 | 6 | 23 |
| 20–34 | 137 | 2.4 | 1 | 1 | 2 | 2 | 3 | 4 | 5 | 5 |
| 35–49 | 127 | 2.5 | 2 | 1 | 2 | 2 | 3 | 4 | 4 | 9 |
| 50–64 | 48 | 2.4 | 1 | 1 | 2 | 2 | 3 | 4 | 4 | 6 |
| 65+ | 18 | 4.0 | 4 | 1 | 2 | 4 | 6 | 6 | 6 | 6 |
| **2. MULTIPLE DX** | | | | | | | | | | |
| 0–19 Years | 112 | 4.3 | 16 | 1 | 2 | 4 | 4 | 8 | 15 | 16 |
| 20–34 | 193 | 4.8 | 39 | 1 | 2 | 3 | 5 | 11 | 25 | 25 |
| 35–49 | 293 | 4.1 | 16 | 1 | 2 | 2 | 4 | 7 | 9 | 18 |
| 50–64 | 181 | 3.9 | 16 | 1 | 2 | 3 | 5 | 7 | 9 | 18 |
| 65+ | 167 | 6.0 | 59 | 2 | 2 | 4 | 7 | 10 | 14 | 34 |
| **TOTAL SINGLE DX** | 424 | 2.6 | 3 | 1 | 2 | 2 | 3 | 4 | 6 | 7 |
| **TOTAL MULTIPLE DX** | 946 | 4.5 | 28 | 1 | 2 | 3 | 5 | 8 | 12 | 25 |
| **TOTAL** | | | | | | | | | | |
| 0–19 Years | 206 | 3.6 | 13 | 1 | 2 | 3 | 4 | 6 | 9 | 17 |
| 20–34 | 330 | 3.9 | 26 | 1 | 2 | 3 | 3 | 7 | 11 | 25 |
| 35–49 | 420 | 3.5 | 12 | 1 | 2 | 3 | 4 | 6 | 8 | 17 |
| 50–64 | 229 | 3.6 | 13 | 1 | 2 | 3 | 4 | 6 | 8 | 14 |
| 65+ | 185 | 5.6 | 50 | 2 | 2 | 4 | 6 | 10 | 14 | 34 |
| **GRAND TOTAL** | 1,370 | 3.9 | 21 | 1 | 2 | 3 | 4 | 7 | 10 | 25 |

## 78.59: INT FIX W/O FX RED NEC. Formerly included in operation group(s) 728.

| Type of Patients | Observed Patients | Avg. Stay | Variance | 10th | 25th | 50th | 75th | 90th | 95th | 99th |
|---|---|---|---|---|---|---|---|---|---|---|
| **1. SINGLE DX** | | | | | | | | | | |
| 0–19 Years | 29 | 2.5 | 1 | 1 | 1 | 3 | 3 | 4 | 4 | 4 |
| 20–34 | 17 | 2.4 | 2 | 1 | 1 | 3 | 3 | 3 | 3 | 8 |
| 35–49 | 20 | 1.7 | 2 | 1 | 1 | 2 | 2 | 3 | 3 | 4 |
| 50–64 | 5 | 2.2 | 1 | 1 | 1 | 2 | 3 | 4 | 4 | 4 |
| 65+ | 1 | 8.0 | 0 | 8 | 8 | 8 | 8 | 8 | 8 | 8 |
| **2. MULTIPLE DX** | | | | | | | | | | |
| 0–19 Years | 62 | 5.2 | 32 | 1 | 2 | 4 | 7 | 9 | 11 | 21 |
| 20–34 | 49 | 6.7 | 22 | 1 | 1 | 6 | 8 | 12 | 12 | 16 |
| 35–49 | 38 | 4.1 | 13 | 1 | 2 | 4 | 8 | 10 | 11 | 13 |
| 50–64 | 28 | 10.7 | 95 | 2 | 4 | 7 | 17 | 24 | 37 | 37 |
| 65+ | 55 | 8.2 | 50 | 1 | 4 | 6 | 11 | 18 | 21 | 31 |
| **TOTAL SINGLE DX** | 72 | 2.2 | 2 | 1 | 1 | 2 | 3 | 3 | 4 | 8 |
| **TOTAL MULTIPLE DX** | 232 | 6.4 | 37 | 1 | 2 | 5 | 11 | 12 | 15 | 31 |
| **TOTAL** | | | | | | | | | | |
| 0–19 Years | 91 | 4.3 | 23 | 1 | 1 | 3 | 5 | 8 | 11 | 11 |
| 20–34 | 66 | 5.7 | 21 | 1 | 1 | 4 | 7 | 12 | 12 | 12 |
| 35–49 | 58 | 3.2 | 10 | 1 | 1 | 2 | 3 | 8 | 11 | 13 |
| 50–64 | 33 | 9.6 | 91 | 2 | 3 | 5 | 15 | 24 | 37 | 37 |
| 65+ | 56 | 8.2 | 50 | 1 | 4 | 6 | 11 | 17 | 21 | 31 |
| **GRAND TOTAL** | 304 | 5.4 | 32 | 1 | 2 | 3 | 8 | 11 | 13 | 28 |

Length of Stay by Diagnosis and Operation, United States, 2000

# United States, October 1998–September 1999 Data, by Operation

## 78.6: RMVL IMPL DEV FROM BONE. Formerly included in operation group(s) 729.

| Type of Patients | Observed Patients | Avg. Stay | Vari- ance | Percentiles | | | | | | |
|---|---|---|---|---|---|---|---|---|---|---|
| | | | | 10th | 25th | 50th | 75th | 90th | 95th | 99th |
| 1. SINGLE DX | | | | | | | | | | |
| 0–19 Years | 293 | 2.5 | 18 | 1 | 1 | 1 | 2 | 3 | 12 | 22 |
| 20–34 | 286 | 2.2 | 3 | 1 | 1 | 2 | 3 | 5 | 6 | 7 |
| 35–49 | 371 | 1.9 | 1 | 1 | 1 | 2 | 2 | 4 | 4 | 5 |
| 50–64 | 179 | 2.0 | 4 | 1 | 1 | 2 | 2 | 3 | 5 | 10 |
| 65+ | 127 | 2.0 | 2 | 1 | 1 | 2 | 2 | 4 | 5 | 7 |
| 2. MULTIPLE DX | | | | | | | | | | |
| 0–19 Years | 826 | 3.0 | 27 | 1 | 1 | 1 | 3 | 5 | 9 | 29 |
| 20–34 | 673 | 3.5 | 18 | 1 | 1 | 1 | 4 | 6 | 10 | 19 |
| 35–49 | 1,216 | 3.7 | 29 | 1 | 1 | 2 | 4 | 7 | 11 | 27 |
| 50–64 | 991 | 4.5 | 31 | 1 | 2 | 3 | 5 | 9 | 14 | 29 |
| 65+ | 1,285 | 5.4 | 39 | 1 | 2 | 4 | 6 | 10 | 15 | 39 |
| TOTAL SINGLE DX | 1,256 | 2.2 | 7 | 1 | 1 | 1 | 2 | 4 | 5 | 20 |
| TOTAL MULTIPLE DX | 4,991 | 4.1 | 30 | 1 | 1 | 3 | 4 | 8 | 12 | 29 |
| TOTAL | | | | | | | | | | |
| 0–19 Years | 1,119 | 2.9 | 24 | 1 | 1 | 1 | 3 | 5 | 9 | 24 |
| 20–34 | 959 | 3.1 | 14 | 1 | 1 | 2 | 3 | 6 | 8 | 19 |
| 35–49 | 1,587 | 3.3 | 23 | 1 | 1 | 2 | 4 | 6 | 10 | 23 |
| 50–64 | 1,170 | 4.1 | 27 | 1 | 1 | 2 | 4 | 8 | 14 | 28 |
| 65+ | 1,412 | 5.2 | 37 | 1 | 2 | 4 | 6 | 10 | 14 | 39 |
| GRAND TOTAL | 6,247 | 3.7 | 26 | 1 | 1 | 2 | 4 | 7 | 11 | 27 |

## 78.65: RMVL IMPL DEV FEMUR. Formerly included in operation group(s) 729.

| Type of Patients | Observed Patients | Avg. Stay | Vari- ance | Percentiles | | | | | | |
|---|---|---|---|---|---|---|---|---|---|---|
| | | | | 10th | 25th | 50th | 75th | 90th | 95th | 99th |
| 1. SINGLE DX | | | | | | | | | | |
| 0–19 Years | 145 | 2.8 | 30 | 1 | 1 | 1 | 1 | 3 | 21 | 24 |
| 20–34 | 60 | 1.6 | 1 | 1 | 1 | 1 | 2 | 3 | 6 | 6 |
| 35–49 | 34 | 2.2 | 1 | 1 | 1 | 2 | 3 | 3 | 4 | 7 |
| 50–64 | 24 | 3.3 | 19 | 1 | 1 | 2 | 3 | 4 | 7 | 22 |
| 65+ | 61 | 2.5 | 3 | 1 | 1 | 2 | 4 | 4 | 6 | 8 |
| 2. MULTIPLE DX | | | | | | | | | | |
| 0–19 Years | 331 | 2.9 | 34 | 1 | 1 | 1 | 3 | 5 | 10 | 37 |
| 20–34 | 108 | 4.3 | 40 | 1 | 1 | 3 | 4 | 11 | 19 | 19 |
| 35–49 | 160 | 4.8 | 41 | 1 | 3 | 4 | 5 | 11 | 15 | 30 |
| 50–64 | 135 | 5.5 | 37 | 1 | 4 | 4 | 7 | 14 | 17 | 28 |
| 65+ | 570 | 5.5 | 36 | 1 | 4 | 4 | 7 | 10 | 15 | 32 |
| TOTAL SINGLE DX | 324 | 2.6 | 19 | 1 | 1 | 1 | 2 | 4 | 8 | 22 |
| TOTAL MULTIPLE DX | 1,304 | 4.6 | 38 | 1 | 3 | 3 | 5 | 9 | 15 | 31 |
| TOTAL | | | | | | | | | | |
| 0–19 Years | 476 | 2.9 | 33 | 1 | 1 | 1 | 2 | 5 | 14 | 29 |
| 20–34 | 168 | 3.5 | 29 | 1 | 1 | 2 | 3 | 8 | 19 | 19 |
| 35–49 | 194 | 4.5 | 36 | 1 | 2 | 3 | 5 | 10 | 14 | 30 |
| 50–64 | 159 | 5.2 | 35 | 1 | 2 | 3 | 5 | 11 | 17 | 28 |
| 65+ | 631 | 5.3 | 34 | 1 | 2 | 4 | 6 | 10 | 14 | 32 |
| GRAND TOTAL | 1,628 | 4.2 | 35 | 1 | 1 | 2 | 5 | 8 | 15 | 29 |

## 78.63: RMVL IMPL DEV RAD/ULNA. Formerly included in operation group(s) 729.

| Type of Patients | Observed Patients | Avg. Stay | Vari- ance | Percentiles | | | | | | |
|---|---|---|---|---|---|---|---|---|---|---|
| | | | | 10th | 25th | 50th | 75th | 90th | 95th | 99th |
| 1. SINGLE DX | | | | | | | | | | |
| 0–19 Years | 19 | 2.4 | 22 | 1 | 1 | 1 | 2 | 3 | 5 | 24 |
| 20–34 | 25 | 1.7 | 3 | 1 | 1 | 1 | 2 | 3 | 5 | 11 |
| 35–49 | 13 | 2.6 | 2 | 1 | 1 | 3 | 4 | 4 | 4 | 4 |
| 50–64 | 9 | 3.9 | 10 | 1 | 2 | 2 | 6 | 10 | 10 | 10 |
| 65+ | 3 | 1.0 | 0 | 1 | 1 | 1 | 1 | 1 | 1 | 1 |
| 2. MULTIPLE DX | | | | | | | | | | |
| 0–19 Years | 49 | 1.5 | 4 | 1 | 1 | 1 | 2 | 2 | 3 | 4 |
| 20–34 | 54 | 2.2 | 20 | 1 | 1 | 1 | 2 | 4 | 6 | 41 |
| 35–49 | 60 | 2.9 | 11 | 1 | 2 | 2 | 3 | 3 | 7 | 12 |
| 50–64 | 73 | 5.9 | 41 | 1 | 2 | 4 | 8 | 9 | 16 | 30 |
| 65+ | 75 | 6.8 | 101 | 1 | 2 | 4 | 7 | 10 | 42 | 42 |
| TOTAL SINGLE DX | 69 | 2.1 | 7 | 1 | 1 | 1 | 2 | 4 | 5 | 11 |
| TOTAL MULTIPLE DX | 311 | 3.6 | 36 | 1 | 1 | 2 | 3 | 8 | 9 | 42 |
| TOTAL | | | | | | | | | | |
| 0–19 Years | 68 | 1.7 | 7 | 1 | 1 | 1 | 2 | 2 | 3 | 20 |
| 20–34 | 79 | 2.1 | 16 | 1 | 1 | 1 | 2 | 4 | 6 | 11 |
| 35–49 | 73 | 2.9 | 10 | 1 | 2 | 2 | 4 | 8 | 7 | 12 |
| 50–64 | 82 | 5.8 | 39 | 1 | 2 | 4 | 8 | 9 | 13 | 30 |
| 65+ | 78 | 6.6 | 99 | 1 | 2 | 3 | 7 | 10 | 42 | 42 |
| GRAND TOTAL | 380 | 3.4 | 32 | 1 | 1 | 2 | 3 | 7 | 9 | 42 |

## 78.67: RMVL IMPL DEV TIB & FIB. Formerly included in operation group(s) 729.

| Type of Patients | Observed Patients | Avg. Stay | Vari- ance | Percentiles | | | | | | |
|---|---|---|---|---|---|---|---|---|---|---|
| | | | | 10th | 25th | 50th | 75th | 90th | 95th | 99th |
| 1. SINGLE DX | | | | | | | | | | |
| 0–19 Years | 35 | 2.5 | 11 | 1 | 1 | 1 | 2 | 2 | 12 | 12 |
| 20–34 | 58 | 2.2 | 4 | 1 | 1 | 1 | 2 | 6 | 7 | 8 |
| 35–49 | 65 | 2.0 | 1 | 1 | 1 | 2 | 2 | 3 | 5 | 5 |
| 50–64 | 32 | 1.7 | 2 | 1 | 1 | 1 | 2 | 2 | 4 | 6 |
| 65+ | 11 | 1.7 | <1 | 1 | 1 | 1 | 2 | 2 | 4 | 4 |
| 2. MULTIPLE DX | | | | | | | | | | |
| 0–19 Years | 109 | 2.4 | 12 | 1 | 1 | 1 | 3 | 5 | 5 | 19 |
| 20–34 | 155 | 4.0 | 12 | 1 | 2 | 3 | 5 | 7 | 10 | 18 |
| 35–49 | 259 | 5.1 | 58 | 1 | 2 | 3 | 5 | 10 | 17 | 51 |
| 50–64 | 207 | 5.0 | 51 | 1 | 3 | 3 | 5 | 10 | 17 | 45 |
| 65+ | 184 | 5.6 | 33 | 1 | 3 | 4 | 7 | 10 | 14 | 36 |
| TOTAL SINGLE DX | 201 | 2.0 | 4 | 1 | 1 | 1 | 2 | 4 | 6 | 12 |
| TOTAL MULTIPLE DX | 914 | 4.5 | 38 | 1 | 1 | 3 | 5 | 8 | 12 | 41 |
| TOTAL | | | | | | | | | | |
| 0–19 Years | 144 | 2.4 | 11 | 1 | 1 | 1 | 3 | 5 | 5 | 19 |
| 20–34 | 213 | 3.6 | 10 | 1 | 1 | 3 | 4 | 7 | 10 | 16 |
| 35–49 | 324 | 4.3 | 45 | 1 | 1 | 2 | 4 | 8 | 12 | 44 |
| 50–64 | 239 | 4.3 | 43 | 1 | 1 | 2 | 4 | 8 | 14 | 42 |
| 65+ | 195 | 5.4 | 32 | 1 | 3 | 4 | 7 | 10 | 12 | 28 |
| GRAND TOTAL | 1,115 | 4.0 | 31 | 1 | 1 | 2 | 4 | 8 | 12 | 36 |

Length of Stay by Diagnosis and Operation, United States, 2000

# United States, October 1998–September 1999 Data, by Operation

## 78.69: RMVL IMPL DEV SITE NEC. Formerly included in operation group(s) 729.

| Type of Patients | Observed Patients | Avg. Stay | Variance | Percentiles | | | | | | |
|---|---|---|---|---|---|---|---|---|---|---|
| | | | | 10th | 25th | 50th | 75th | 90th | 95th | 99th |
| **1. SINGLE DX** | | | | | | | | | | |
| 0–19 Years | 72 | 1.9 | 3 | 1 | 1 | 2 | 2 | 2 | 4 | 7 |
| 20–34 | 110 | 2.1 | 1 | 1 | 1 | 2 | 3 | 3 | 5 | 5 |
| 35–49 | 225 | 1.7 | 1 | 1 | 1 | 1 | 2 | 3 | 5 | 5 |
| 50–64 | 95 | 1.9 | 1 | 1 | 1 | 2 | 2 | 3 | 4 | 5 |
| 65+ | 38 | 1.8 | 2 | 1 | 1 | 1 | 2 | 3 | 5 | 6 |
| **2. MULTIPLE DX** | | | | | | | | | | |
| 0–19 Years | 255 | 4.0 | 32 | 1 | 2 | 3 | 5 | 8 | 9 | 29 |
| 20–34 | 259 | 3.4 | 16 | 1 | 2 | 2 | 4 | 6 | 8 | 29 |
| 35–49 | 567 | 3.1 | 20 | 1 | 2 | 2 | 3 | 6 | 8 | 20 |
| 50–64 | 416 | 3.9 | 21 | 1 | 2 | 2 | 4 | 9 | 14 | 23 |
| 65+ | 277 | 4.7 | 30 | 1 | 2 | 3 | 5 | 10 | 14 | 35 |
| **TOTAL SINGLE DX** | 540 | 1.9 | 2 | 1 | 1 | 2 | 2 | 3 | 4 | 6 |
| **TOTAL MULTIPLE DX** | 1,774 | 3.7 | 23 | 1 | 2 | 2 | 4 | 7 | 11 | 23 |
| **TOTAL** | | | | | | | | | | |
| 0–19 Years | 327 | 3.5 | 26 | 1 | 1 | 2 | 4 | 7 | 9 | 18 |
| 20–34 | 369 | 2.9 | 11 | 1 | 1 | 2 | 3 | 5 | 7 | 22 |
| 35–49 | 792 | 2.7 | 15 | 1 | 1 | 2 | 3 | 5 | 7 | 16 |
| 50–64 | 511 | 3.4 | 17 | 1 | 2 | 3 | 4 | 7 | 13 | 20 |
| 65+ | 315 | 4.3 | 27 | 1 | 2 | 3 | 5 | 8 | 13 | 27 |
| **GRAND TOTAL** | 2,314 | 3.2 | 18 | 1 | 1 | 2 | 3 | 6 | 9 | 21 |

## 78.7: OSTEOCLASIS. Formerly included in operation group(s) 727, 728.

| Type of Patients | Observed Patients | Avg. Stay | Variance | Percentiles | | | | | | |
|---|---|---|---|---|---|---|---|---|---|---|
| | | | | 10th | 25th | 50th | 75th | 90th | 95th | 99th |
| **1. SINGLE DX** | | | | | | | | | | |
| 0–19 Years | 10 | 3.8 | 31 | 1 | 1 | 1 | 4 | 17 | 17 | 17 |
| 20–34 | 0 | | | | | | | | | |
| 35–49 | 1 | 3.0 | 0 | 3 | 3 | 3 | 3 | 3 | 3 | 3 |
| 50–64 | 1 | 4.0 | 0 | 4 | 4 | 4 | 4 | 4 | 4 | 4 |
| 65+ | 0 | | | | | | | | | |
| **2. MULTIPLE DX** | | | | | | | | | | |
| 0–19 Years | 15 | 6.0 | 70 | 1 | 2 | 2 | 4 | 24 | 24 | 24 |
| 20–34 | 2 | 10.0 | 184 | 4 | 4 | 4 | 4 | 37 | 37 | 37 |
| 35–49 | 6 | 5.4 | 13 | 1 | 3 | 6 | 6 | 14 | 14 | 14 |
| 50–64 | 2 | 1.5 | <1 | 1 | 1 | 1 | 2 | 2 | 2 | 2 |
| 65+ | 6 | 5.2 | 14 | 1 | 3 | 4 | 6 | 12 | 12 | 12 |
| **TOTAL SINGLE DX** | 12 | 3.8 | 19 | 1 | 1 | 3 | 4 | 4 | 17 | 17 |
| **TOTAL MULTIPLE DX** | 31 | 6.0 | 59 | 1 | 2 | 4 | 6 | 21 | 24 | 37 |
| **TOTAL** | | | | | | | | | | |
| 0–19 Years | 25 | 4.9 | 50 | 1 | 1 | 2 | 4 | 17 | 24 | 24 |
| 20–34 | 2 | 10.0 | 184 | 4 | 4 | 4 | 4 | 37 | 37 | 37 |
| 35–49 | 7 | 4.9 | 11 | 2 | 3 | 4 | 6 | 6 | 14 | 14 |
| 50–64 | 3 | 3.4 | 1 | 2 | 4 | 4 | 4 | 4 | 4 | 4 |
| 65+ | 6 | 5.2 | 14 | 1 | 3 | 4 | 6 | 12 | 12 | 12 |
| **GRAND TOTAL** | 43 | 5.1 | 43 | 1 | 1 | 4 | 4 | 14 | 21 | 37 |

## 78.8: OTHER BONE DIAGNOSTIC PX. Formerly included in operation group(s) 727, 728.

| Type of Patients | Observed Patients | Avg. Stay | Variance | Percentiles | | | | | | |
|---|---|---|---|---|---|---|---|---|---|---|
| | | | | 10th | 25th | 50th | 75th | 90th | 95th | 99th |
| **1. SINGLE DX** | | | | | | | | | | |
| 0–19 Years | 3 | 2.7 | 2 | 2 | 2 | 2 | 2 | 5 | 5 | 5 |
| 20–34 | 0 | | | | | | | | | |
| 35–49 | 0 | | | | | | | | | |
| 50–64 | 0 | | | | | | | | | |
| 65+ | 0 | | | | | | | | | |
| **2. MULTIPLE DX** | | | | | | | | | | |
| 0–19 Years | 10 | 5.7 | 6 | 3 | 4 | 6 | 6 | 10 | 10 | 10 |
| 20–34 | 0 | | | | | | | | | |
| 35–49 | 0 | | | | | | | | | |
| 50–64 | 2 | 7.7 | 32 | 4 | 4 | 4 | 14 | 14 | 14 | 14 |
| 65+ | 0 | | | | | | | | | |
| **TOTAL SINGLE DX** | 3 | 2.7 | 2 | 2 | 2 | 2 | 2 | 5 | 5 | 5 |
| **TOTAL MULTIPLE DX** | 12 | 5.9 | 9 | 3 | 4 | 6 | 6 | 10 | 10 | 14 |
| **TOTAL** | | | | | | | | | | |
| 0–19 Years | 13 | 4.4 | 6 | 2 | 2 | 4 | 6 | 7 | 10 | 10 |
| 20–34 | 0 | | | | | | | | | |
| 35–49 | 0 | | | | | | | | | |
| 50–64 | 2 | 7.7 | 32 | 4 | 4 | 4 | 14 | 14 | 14 | 14 |
| 65+ | 0 | | | | | | | | | |
| **GRAND TOTAL** | 15 | 4.6 | 8 | 2 | 2 | 4 | 6 | 10 | 10 | 14 |

## 78.9: INSERT BONE GROWTH STIM. Formerly included in operation group(s) 727, 728.

| Type of Patients | Observed Patients | Avg. Stay | Variance | Percentiles | | | | | | |
|---|---|---|---|---|---|---|---|---|---|---|
| | | | | 10th | 25th | 50th | 75th | 90th | 95th | 99th |
| **1. SINGLE DX** | | | | | | | | | | |
| 0–19 Years | 2 | 1.0 | 0 | 1 | 1 | 1 | 1 | 1 | 1 | 1 |
| 20–34 | 4 | 1.4 | <1 | 1 | 1 | 1 | 2 | 2 | 2 | 2 |
| 35–49 | 5 | 2.3 | 6 | 1 | 1 | 1 | 4 | 8 | 8 | 8 |
| 50–64 | 3 | 3.2 | <1 | 2 | 2 | 3 | 4 | 4 | 4 | 4 |
| 65+ | 2 | 2.5 | <1 | 1 | 1 | 3 | 3 | 3 | 3 | 3 |
| **2. MULTIPLE DX** | | | | | | | | | | |
| 0–19 Years | 5 | 1.7 | <1 | 1 | 1 | 2 | 2 | 2 | 2 | 2 |
| 20–34 | 7 | 3.6 | 9 | 2 | 2 | 3 | 3 | 4 | 10 | 10 |
| 35–49 | 12 | 2.7 | 2 | 1 | 1 | 2 | 4 | 4 | 5 | 5 |
| 50–64 | 11 | 2.6 | 3 | 1 | 1 | 2 | 3 | 5 | 5 | 7 |
| 65+ | 8 | 5.6 | 17 | 3 | 4 | 4 | 6 | 12 | 15 | 15 |
| **TOTAL SINGLE DX** | 16 | 2.2 | 3 | 1 | 1 | 1 | 3 | 4 | 4 | 8 |
| **TOTAL MULTIPLE DX** | 43 | 3.8 | 10 | 1 | 1 | 3 | 4 | 7 | 15 | 15 |
| **TOTAL** | | | | | | | | | | |
| 0–19 Years | 7 | 1.5 | <1 | 1 | 1 | 2 | 2 | 2 | 2 | 2 |
| 20–34 | 11 | 2.6 | 6 | 1 | 1 | 2 | 3 | 3 | 10 | 10 |
| 35–49 | 17 | 2.5 | 4 | 1 | 1 | 2 | 4 | 4 | 8 | 8 |
| 50–64 | 14 | 2.8 | 2 | 2 | 1 | 2 | 4 | 4 | 5 | 7 |
| 65+ | 10 | 5.1 | 15 | 3 | 3 | 4 | 6 | 12 | 15 | 15 |
| **GRAND TOTAL** | 59 | 3.3 | 9 | 1 | 1 | 3 | 4 | 5 | 10 | 15 |

Length of Stay by Diagnosis and Operation, United States, 2000

## United States, October 1998–September 1999 Data, by Operation

### 79.0: CLSD FX RED W/O INT FIX. Formerly included in operation group(s) 732, 735.

| Type of Patients | Observed Patients | Avg. Stay | Variance | 10th | 25th | 50th | 75th | 90th | 95th | 99th |
|---|---|---|---|---|---|---|---|---|---|---|
| **1. SINGLE DX** | | | | | | | | | | |
| 0–19 Years | 3,197 | 1.9 | 8 | 1 | 1 | 1 | 2 | 3 | 4 | 18 |
| 20–34 | 338 | 1.8 | 9 | 1 | 1 | 1 | 2 | 3 | 4 | 6 |
| 35–49 | 347 | 1.8 | 2 | 1 | 1 | 1 | 2 | 3 | 4 | 7 |
| 50–64 | 192 | 1.9 | 2 | 1 | 1 | 1 | 2 | 4 | 5 | 6 |
| 65+ | 165 | 2.2 | 3 | 1 | 1 | 2 | 3 | 5 | 6 | 7 |
| **2. MULTIPLE DX** | | | | | | | | | | |
| 0–19 Years | 1,418 | 3.4 | 23 | 1 | 1 | 2 | 3 | 8 | 12 | 23 |
| 20–34 | 613 | 2.9 | 14 | 1 | 1 | 2 | 3 | 8 | 8 | 14 |
| 35–49 | 880 | 3.6 | 15 | 1 | 1 | 2 | 4 | 8 | 10 | 18 |
| 50–64 | 852 | 4.6 | 25 | 1 | 2 | 3 | 5 | 11 | 14 | 20 |
| 65+ | 2,960 | 4.9 | 27 | 1 | 2 | 4 | 6 | 9 | 12 | 29 |
| **TOTAL SINGLE DX** | 4,239 | 1.9 | 7 | 1 | 1 | 1 | 2 | 3 | 4 | 14 |
| **TOTAL MULTIPLE DX** | 6,723 | 4.1 | 24 | 1 | 2 | 3 | 5 | 8 | 12 | 25 |
| **TOTAL** | | | | | | | | | | |
| 0–19 Years | 4,615 | 2.4 | 13 | 1 | 1 | 2 | 2 | 4 | 7 | 22 |
| 20–34 | 951 | 2.5 | 12 | 1 | 1 | 2 | 3 | 5 | 6 | 12 |
| 35–49 | 1,227 | 3.0 | 11 | 1 | 1 | 2 | 3 | 6 | 8 | 14 |
| 50–64 | 1,044 | 4.0 | 22 | 1 | 1 | 3 | 5 | 10 | 14 | 19 |
| 65+ | 3,125 | 4.7 | 26 | 1 | 2 | 4 | 6 | 8 | 11 | 27 |
| **GRAND TOTAL** | 10,962 | 3.2 | 18 | 1 | 1 | 2 | 4 | 6 | 10 | 22 |

### 79.01: CLSD FX RED HUMERUS. Formerly included in operation group(s) 735.

| Type of Patients | Observed Patients | Avg. Stay | Variance | 10th | 25th | 50th | 75th | 90th | 95th | 99th |
|---|---|---|---|---|---|---|---|---|---|---|
| **1. SINGLE DX** | | | | | | | | | | |
| 0–19 Years | 325 | 1.4 | 3 | 1 | 1 | 1 | 2 | 2 | 4 | 6 |
| 20–34 | 29 | 1.2 | <1 | 1 | 1 | 1 | 1 | 2 | 2 | 2 |
| 35–49 | 16 | 1.8 | 2 | 1 | 1 | 2 | 2 | 5 | 5 | 5 |
| 50–64 | 28 | 1.5 | <1 | 1 | 1 | 1 | 2 | 3 | 3 | 3 |
| 65+ | 40 | 2.0 | 2 | 1 | 1 | 2 | 3 | 4 | 4 | 5 |
| **2. MULTIPLE DX** | | | | | | | | | | |
| 0–19 Years | 120 | 2.7 | 14 | 1 | 1 | 1 | 2 | 6 | 8 | 21 |
| 20–34 | 85 | 1.9 | 4 | 1 | 1 | 1 | 2 | 4 | 5 | 7 |
| 35–49 | 92 | 4.5 | 25 | 1 | 2 | 4 | 6 | 9 | 14 | 17 |
| 50–64 | 89 | 4.4 | 18 | 1 | 2 | 3 | 6 | 11 | 13 | 17 |
| 65+ | 521 | 5.1 | 50 | 1 | 2 | 4 | 5 | 8 | 14 | 44 |
| **TOTAL SINGLE DX** | 438 | 1.4 | 3 | 1 | 1 | 1 | 1 | 2 | 3 | 6 |
| **TOTAL MULTIPLE DX** | 907 | 4.3 | 36 | 1 | 2 | 3 | 5 | 8 | 12 | 44 |
| **TOTAL** | | | | | | | | | | |
| 0–19 Years | 445 | 1.7 | 7 | 1 | 1 | 1 | 2 | 2 | 4 | 21 |
| 20–34 | 114 | 1.6 | 2 | 1 | 1 | 1 | 2 | 3 | 5 | 7 |
| 35–49 | 108 | 3.9 | 21 | 1 | 1 | 2 | 5 | 7 | 14 | 17 |
| 50–64 | 117 | 3.5 | 14 | 1 | 1 | 2 | 5 | 8 | 13 | 17 |
| 65+ | 561 | 4.9 | 48 | 1 | 2 | 3 | 5 | 8 | 14 | 44 |
| **GRAND TOTAL** | 1,345 | 3.2 | 26 | 1 | 1 | 2 | 4 | 6 | 9 | 39 |

### 79.02: CLSD RED FX RADIUS/ULNA. Formerly included in operation group(s) 735.

| Type of Patients | Observed Patients | Avg. Stay | Variance | 10th | 25th | 50th | 75th | 90th | 95th | 99th |
|---|---|---|---|---|---|---|---|---|---|---|
| **1. SINGLE DX** | | | | | | | | | | |
| 0–19 Years | 1,028 | 1.3 | <1 | 1 | 1 | 1 | 1 | 2 | 3 | 4 |
| 20–34 | 59 | 2.1 | 48 | 1 | 1 | 1 | 1 | 2 | 3 | 57 |
| 35–49 | 83 | 1.2 | <1 | 1 | 1 | 1 | 1 | 2 | 2 | 3 |
| 50–64 | 48 | 1.3 | <1 | 1 | 1 | 1 | 1 | 2 | 3 | 4 |
| 65+ | 47 | 1.6 | 2 | 1 | 1 | 1 | 2 | 3 | 4 | 9 |
| **2. MULTIPLE DX** | | | | | | | | | | |
| 0–19 Years | 329 | 1.8 | 4 | 1 | 1 | 1 | 2 | 3 | 4 | 9 |
| 20–34 | 150 | 2.7 | 6 | 1 | 1 | 2 | 3 | 5 | 6 | 16 |
| 35–49 | 230 | 2.8 | 9 | 1 | 1 | 2 | 3 | 6 | 9 | 18 |
| 50–64 | 241 | 3.3 | 11 | 1 | 2 | 2 | 4 | 6 | 9 | 20 |
| 65+ | 1,082 | 4.5 | 20 | 1 | 2 | 3 | 6 | 8 | 11 | 27 |
| **TOTAL SINGLE DX** | 1,265 | 1.3 | 3 | 1 | 1 | 1 | 1 | 2 | 3 | 4 |
| **TOTAL MULTIPLE DX** | 2,032 | 3.5 | 15 | 1 | 1 | 2 | 4 | 7 | 10 | 22 |
| **TOTAL** | | | | | | | | | | |
| 0–19 Years | 1,357 | 1.4 | 1 | 1 | 1 | 1 | 1 | 2 | 3 | 5 |
| 20–34 | 209 | 2.5 | 17 | 1 | 1 | 1 | 3 | 5 | 6 | 16 |
| 35–49 | 313 | 2.3 | 7 | 1 | 1 | 2 | 3 | 4 | 7 | 18 |
| 50–64 | 289 | 2.9 | 10 | 1 | 1 | 2 | 3 | 6 | 8 | 17 |
| 65+ | 1,129 | 4.4 | 20 | 1 | 2 | 3 | 6 | 8 | 11 | 27 |
| **GRAND TOTAL** | 3,297 | 2.6 | 11 | 1 | 1 | 1 | 3 | 6 | 7 | 17 |

### 79.05: CLSD FX RED FEMUR. Formerly included in operation group(s) 732.

| Type of Patients | Observed Patients | Avg. Stay | Variance | 10th | 25th | 50th | 75th | 90th | 95th | 99th |
|---|---|---|---|---|---|---|---|---|---|---|
| **1. SINGLE DX** | | | | | | | | | | |
| 0–19 Years | 947 | 3.0 | 21 | 1 | 1 | 2 | 2 | 6 | 13 | 27 |
| 20–34 | 8 | 2.6 | 3 | 1 | 1 | 3 | 4 | 6 | 6 | 6 |
| 35–49 | 7 | 3.0 | 1 | 1 | 2 | 3 | 4 | 4 | 5 | 5 |
| 50–64 | 8 | 1.8 | <1 | 1 | 1 | 1 | 3 | 3 | 3 | 3 |
| 65+ | 11 | 3.2 | 3 | 1 | 3 | 3 | 3 | 7 | 7 | 7 |
| **2. MULTIPLE DX** | | | | | | | | | | |
| 0–19 Years | 514 | 4.9 | 41 | 1 | 1 | 3 | 5 | 12 | 20 | 27 |
| 20–34 | 45 | 4.8 | 10 | 2 | 2 | 4 | 6 | 9 | 12 | 14 |
| 35–49 | 41 | 5.3 | 19 | 2 | 3 | 4 | 8 | 8 | 11 | 28 |
| 50–64 | 48 | 5.8 | 61 | 2 | 2 | 5 | 6 | 11 | 16 | 57 |
| 65+ | 307 | 6.2 | 23 | 2 | 3 | 5 | 8 | 11 | 15 | 22 |
| **TOTAL SINGLE DX** | 981 | 3.0 | 21 | 1 | 1 | 2 | 3 | 6 | 13 | 27 |
| **TOTAL MULTIPLE DX** | 955 | 5.3 | 35 | 1 | 2 | 3 | 7 | 12 | 17 | 27 |
| **TOTAL** | | | | | | | | | | |
| 0–19 Years | 1,461 | 3.7 | 29 | 1 | 1 | 2 | 3 | 10 | 16 | 27 |
| 20–34 | 53 | 4.6 | 10 | 2 | 2 | 4 | 6 | 7 | 12 | 14 |
| 35–49 | 48 | 5.1 | 18 | 2 | 3 | 4 | 8 | 8 | 9 | 28 |
| 50–64 | 56 | 5.5 | 56 | 2 | 2 | 5 | 5 | 11 | 14 | 57 |
| 65+ | 318 | 6.1 | 23 | 2 | 3 | 5 | 8 | 11 | 15 | 22 |
| **GRAND TOTAL** | 1,936 | 4.2 | 29 | 1 | 1 | 2 | 4 | 10 | 15 | 27 |

Length of Stay by Diagnosis and Operation, United States, 2000

# United States, October 1998–September 1999 Data, by Operation

## 79.06: CLSD FX RED TIBIA/FIBULA. Formerly included in operation group(s) 735.

| Type of Patients | Observed Patients | Avg. Stay | Variance | Percentiles | | | | | | |
|---|---|---|---|---|---|---|---|---|---|---|
| | | | | 10th | 25th | 50th | 75th | 90th | 95th | 99th |
| **1. SINGLE DX** | | | | | | | | | | |
| 0–19 Years | 843 | 1.7 | 2 | 1 | 1 | 1 | 2 | 3 | 3 | 5 |
| 20–34 | 207 | 1.9 | 1 | 1 | 1 | 1 | 2 | 3 | 3 | 6 |
| 35–49 | 208 | 1.8 | 1 | 1 | 1 | 1 | 2 | 3 | 4 | 9 |
| 50–64 | 96 | 2.5 | 2 | 1 | 2 | 2 | 4 | 5 | 6 | 6 |
| 65+ | 59 | 2.5 | 3 | 1 | 1 | 2 | 3 | 6 | 6 | 6 |
| **2. MULTIPLE DX** | | | | | | | | | | |
| 0–19 Years | 375 | 3.0 | 14 | 1 | 1 | 2 | 3 | 6 | 8 | 21 |
| 20–34 | 214 | 3.2 | 10 | 1 | 1 | 2 | 4 | 7 | 10 | 13 |
| 35–49 | 403 | 3.9 | 12 | 1 | 2 | 3 | 5 | 8 | 11 | 18 |
| 50–64 | 390 | 5.4 | 30 | 1 | 2 | 3 | 6 | 14 | 14 | 21 |
| 65+ | 912 | 4.7 | 21 | 2 | 2 | 4 | 5 | 8 | 10 | 26 |
| **TOTAL SINGLE DX** | 1,413 | 1.8 | 2 | 1 | 1 | 1 | 2 | 3 | 4 | 6 |
| **TOTAL MULTIPLE DX** | 2,294 | 4.2 | 20 | 1 | 2 | 3 | 5 | 8 | 12 | 19 |
| **TOTAL** | | | | | | | | | | |
| 0–19 Years | 1,218 | 2.1 | 6 | 1 | 1 | 1 | 2 | 3 | 5 | 12 |
| 20–34 | 421 | 2.5 | 6 | 1 | 1 | 2 | 3 | 5 | 7 | 11 |
| 35–49 | 611 | 3.0 | 9 | 1 | 1 | 2 | 4 | 6 | 9 | 13 |
| 50–64 | 486 | 4.8 | 26 | 1 | 2 | 3 | 5 | 14 | 14 | 19 |
| 65+ | 971 | 4.6 | 21 | 2 | 2 | 3 | 5 | 8 | 10 | 26 |
| **GRAND TOTAL** | 3,707 | 3.2 | 14 | 1 | 1 | 2 | 4 | 7 | 9 | 15 |

## 79.11: CRIF HUMERUS. Formerly included in operation group(s) 733.

| Type of Patients | Observed Patients | Avg. Stay | Variance | Percentiles | | | | | | |
|---|---|---|---|---|---|---|---|---|---|---|
| | | | | 10th | 25th | 50th | 75th | 90th | 95th | 99th |
| **1. SINGLE DX** | | | | | | | | | | |
| 0–19 Years | 2,044 | 1.2 | <1 | 1 | 1 | 1 | 1 | 2 | 2 | 3 |
| 20–34 | 25 | 2.0 | 1 | 1 | 2 | 2 | 3 | 3 | 4 | 6 |
| 35–49 | 16 | 1.7 | 1 | 1 | 1 | 2 | 3 | 3 | 5 | 6 |
| 50–64 | 18 | 2.1 | <1 | 2 | 2 | 2 | 2 | 2 | 3 | 5 |
| 65+ | 30 | 2.2 | 1 | 1 | 1 | 2 | 3 | 4 | 4 | 6 |
| **2. MULTIPLE DX** | | | | | | | | | | |
| 0–19 Years | 421 | 2.0 | 5 | 1 | 1 | 2 | 2 | 4 | 5 | 13 |
| 20–34 | 47 | 4.8 | 16 | 1 | 3 | 3 | 5 | 13 | 13 | 18 |
| 35–49 | 61 | 5.3 | 26 | 1 | 2 | 3 | 7 | 13 | 19 | 19 |
| 50–64 | 102 | 5.2 | 25 | 1 | 3 | 3 | 7 | 11 | 19 | 19 |
| 65+ | 390 | 5.2 | 35 | 1 | 2 | 4 | 6 | 10 | 17 | 23 |
| **TOTAL SINGLE DX** | 2,133 | 1.2 | <1 | 1 | 1 | 1 | 1 | 2 | 2 | 3 |
| **TOTAL MULTIPLE DX** | 1,021 | 3.7 | 21 | 1 | 1 | 2 | 4 | 8 | 12 | 19 |
| **TOTAL** | | | | | | | | | | |
| 0–19 Years | 2,465 | 1.3 | 2 | 1 | 1 | 1 | 2 | 2 | 2 | 5 |
| 20–34 | 72 | 4.1 | 14 | 1 | 2 | 3 | 5 | 10 | 13 | 18 |
| 35–49 | 77 | 4.5 | 23 | 1 | 1 | 2 | 6 | 10 | 19 | 19 |
| 50–64 | 120 | 4.3 | 20 | 1 | 2 | 2 | 5 | 10 | 15 | 19 |
| 65+ | 420 | 5.0 | 34 | 1 | 2 | 3 | 6 | 9 | 15 | 22 |
| **GRAND TOTAL** | 3,154 | 2.0 | 8 | 1 | 1 | 1 | 2 | 3 | 6 | 15 |

## 79.1: CLSD FX RED W INT FIX. Formerly included in operation group(s) 730, 733.

| Type of Patients | Observed Patients | Avg. Stay | Variance | Percentiles | | | | | | |
|---|---|---|---|---|---|---|---|---|---|---|
| | | | | 10th | 25th | 50th | 75th | 90th | 95th | 99th |
| **1. SINGLE DX** | | | | | | | | | | |
| 0–19 Years | 3,101 | 1.6 | 3 | 1 | 1 | 1 | 2 | 3 | 3 | 7 |
| 20–34 | 559 | 2.3 | 2 | 1 | 1 | 2 | 3 | 4 | 5 | 6 |
| 35–49 | 542 | 2.6 | 2 | 1 | 2 | 2 | 3 | 5 | 6 | 7 |
| 50–64 | 342 | 2.6 | 2 | 1 | 2 | 2 | 3 | 4 | 5 | 7 |
| 65+ | 309 | 3.2 | 3 | 1 | 2 | 3 | 4 | 5 | 6 | 7 |
| **2. MULTIPLE DX** | | | | | | | | | | |
| 0–19 Years | 1,400 | 4.5 | 37 | 1 | 2 | 3 | 5 | 9 | 17 | 28 |
| 20–34 | 1,191 | 4.8 | 17 | 1 | 2 | 4 | 6 | 9 | 11 | 21 |
| 35–49 | 1,288 | 5.1 | 22 | 1 | 2 | 4 | 6 | 10 | 13 | 24 |
| 50–64 | 1,330 | 5.4 | 21 | 1 | 3 | 4 | 7 | 10 | 14 | 21 |
| 65+ | 7,369 | 5.9 | 17 | 3 | 4 | 5 | 7 | 10 | 14 | 22 |
| **TOTAL SINGLE DX** | 4,853 | 1.9 | 3 | 1 | 1 | 1 | 2 | 4 | 5 | 7 |
| **TOTAL MULTIPLE DX** | 12,578 | 5.5 | 21 | 2 | 3 | 4 | 6 | 10 | 13 | 23 |
| **TOTAL** | | | | | | | | | | |
| 0–19 Years | 4,501 | 2.4 | 15 | 1 | 1 | 2 | 2 | 5 | 7 | 23 |
| 20–34 | 1,750 | 4.0 | 13 | 1 | 2 | 3 | 5 | 7 | 10 | 17 |
| 35–49 | 1,830 | 4.3 | 17 | 1 | 2 | 3 | 5 | 8 | 12 | 19 |
| 50–64 | 1,672 | 4.7 | 19 | 1 | 3 | 4 | 6 | 9 | 12 | 20 |
| 65+ | 7,678 | 5.8 | 17 | 3 | 4 | 5 | 7 | 10 | 13 | 21 |
| **GRAND TOTAL** | 17,431 | 4.4 | 18 | 1 | 2 | 3 | 5 | 8 | 12 | 21 |

## 79.12: CRIF RADIUS/ULNA. Formerly included in operation group(s) 733.

| Type of Patients | Observed Patients | Avg. Stay | Variance | Percentiles | | | | | | |
|---|---|---|---|---|---|---|---|---|---|---|
| | | | | 10th | 25th | 50th | 75th | 90th | 95th | 99th |
| **1. SINGLE DX** | | | | | | | | | | |
| 0–19 Years | 215 | 1.2 | <1 | 1 | 1 | 1 | 1 | 2 | 2 | 3 |
| 20–34 | 80 | 1.4 | <1 | 1 | 1 | 1 | 2 | 2 | 3 | 4 |
| 35–49 | 95 | 1.5 | <1 | 1 | 1 | 1 | 2 | 3 | 3 | 4 |
| 50–64 | 90 | 1.5 | <1 | 1 | 1 | 1 | 2 | 2 | 3 | 4 |
| 65+ | 75 | 1.4 | <1 | 1 | 1 | 1 | 2 | 2 | 3 | 4 |
| **2. MULTIPLE DX** | | | | | | | | | | |
| 0–19 Years | 80 | 2.7 | 6 | 1 | 1 | 2 | 4 | 7 | 8 | 9 |
| 20–34 | 130 | 3.3 | 17 | 1 | 1 | 2 | 4 | 7 | 10 | 16 |
| 35–49 | 185 | 3.1 | 11 | 1 | 1 | 2 | 3 | 6 | 10 | 17 |
| 50–64 | 187 | 3.8 | 17 | 1 | 2 | 2 | 5 | 10 | 10 | 20 |
| 65+ | 533 | 3.5 | 12 | 1 | 2 | 2 | 4 | 8 | 11 | 15 |
| **TOTAL SINGLE DX** | 555 | 1.3 | <1 | 1 | 1 | 1 | 2 | 2 | 3 | 4 |
| **TOTAL MULTIPLE DX** | 1,115 | 3.4 | 13 | 1 | 1 | 2 | 4 | 8 | 10 | 16 |
| **TOTAL** | | | | | | | | | | |
| 0–19 Years | 295 | 1.6 | 2 | 1 | 1 | 1 | 3 | 3 | 4 | 8 |
| 20–34 | 210 | 2.7 | 12 | 1 | 1 | 2 | 3 | 5 | 8 | 16 |
| 35–49 | 280 | 2.6 | 8 | 1 | 1 | 2 | 3 | 4 | 7 | 13 |
| 50–64 | 277 | 3.1 | 13 | 1 | 1 | 2 | 3 | 7 | 10 | 17 |
| 65+ | 608 | 3.2 | 11 | 1 | 1 | 2 | 4 | 7 | 10 | 15 |
| **GRAND TOTAL** | 1,670 | 2.7 | 10 | 1 | 1 | 2 | 3 | 6 | 8 | 15 |

Length of Stay by Diagnosis and Operation, United States, 2000

# United States, October 1998–September 1999 Data, by Operation

## 79.15: CRIF FEMUR. Formerly included in operation group(s) 730.

| Type of Patients | Observed Patients | Avg. Stay | Variance | Percentiles | | | | | | |
|---|---|---|---|---|---|---|---|---|---|---|
| | | | | 10th | 25th | 50th | 75th | 90th | 95th | 99th |
| **1. SINGLE DX** | | | | | | | | | | |
| 0-19 Years | 534 | 3.0 | 11 | 1 | 1 | 2 | 3 | 5 | 7 | 23 |
| 20-34 | 142 | 3.2 | 1 | 2 | 2 | 3 | 4 | 5 | 5 | 8 |
| 35-49 | 138 | 3.5 | 3 | 2 | 2 | 3 | 5 | 6 | 6 | 8 |
| 50-64 | 114 | 3.3 | 1 | 2 | 3 | 3 | 4 | 5 | 6 | 7 |
| 65+ | 175 | 3.9 | 2 | 3 | 3 | 4 | 5 | 6 | 6 | 8 |
| **2. MULTIPLE DX** | | | | | | | | | | |
| 0-19 Years | 652 | 6.7 | 49 | 2 | 3 | 4 | 7 | 16 | 23 | 32 |
| 20-34 | 555 | 5.8 | 15 | 3 | 4 | 5 | 7 | 10 | 12 | 22 |
| 35-49 | 491 | 6.2 | 24 | 2 | 3 | 5 | 7 | 12 | 14 | 30 |
| 50-64 | 667 | 6.2 | 21 | 3 | 4 | 5 | 7 | 11 | 14 | 24 |
| 65+ | 6,115 | 6.2 | 16 | 3 | 4 | 5 | 7 | 10 | 14 | 22 |
| **TOTAL SINGLE DX** | 1,103 | 3.2 | 7 | 2 | 2 | 3 | 4 | 5 | 6 | 13 |
| **TOTAL MULTIPLE DX** | 8,480 | 6.2 | 20 | 3 | 4 | 5 | 7 | 10 | 14 | 24 |
| **TOTAL** | | | | | | | | | | |
| 0-19 Years | 1,186 | 4.9 | 35 | 2 | 2 | 3 | 5 | 10 | 19 | 28 |
| 20-34 | 697 | 5.2 | 13 | 2 | 3 | 4 | 6 | 9 | 11 | 21 |
| 35-49 | 629 | 5.6 | 20 | 2 | 3 | 5 | 6 | 10 | 14 | 24 |
| 50-64 | 781 | 5.7 | 19 | 3 | 3 | 4 | 7 | 10 | 13 | 24 |
| 65+ | 6,290 | 6.1 | 16 | 3 | 4 | 5 | 7 | 10 | 14 | 22 |
| **GRAND TOTAL** | 9,583 | 5.8 | 19 | 3 | 3 | 5 | 7 | 10 | 14 | 23 |

## 79.2: OPEN FRACTURE REDUCTION. Formerly included in operation group(s) 732, 735.

| Type of Patients | Observed Patients | Avg. Stay | Variance | Percentiles | | | | | | |
|---|---|---|---|---|---|---|---|---|---|---|
| | | | | 10th | 25th | 50th | 75th | 90th | 95th | 99th |
| **1. SINGLE DX** | | | | | | | | | | |
| 0-19 Years | 184 | 2.3 | 2 | 1 | 1 | 2 | 3 | 4 | 5 | 8 |
| 20-34 | 70 | 2.3 | 3 | 1 | 1 | 2 | 3 | 4 | 6 | 9 |
| 35-49 | 65 | 3.1 | 10 | 1 | 2 | 2 | 3 | 8 | 12 | 12 |
| 50-64 | 36 | 2.2 | 3 | 1 | 1 | 2 | 3 | 5 | 6 | 7 |
| 65+ | 14 | 2.6 | 3 | 1 | 1 | 2 | 4 | 5 | 5 | 5 |
| **2. MULTIPLE DX** | | | | | | | | | | |
| 0-19 Years | 174 | 4.3 | 14 | 1 | 2 | 3 | 5 | 9 | 11 | 20 |
| 20-34 | 151 | 5.6 | 40 | 1 | 2 | 3 | 7 | 11 | 13 | 34 |
| 35-49 | 192 | 5.2 | 55 | 1 | 2 | 3 | 6 | 9 | 14 | 58 |
| 50-64 | 131 | 4.7 | 17 | 1 | 2 | 4 | 6 | 9 | 13 | 17 |
| 65+ | 240 | 5.9 | 17 | 2 | 3 | 5 | 7 | 10 | 15 | 21 |
| **TOTAL SINGLE DX** | 369 | 2.4 | 4 | 1 | 1 | 2 | 3 | 5 | 6 | 12 |
| **TOTAL MULTIPLE DX** | 888 | 5.2 | 28 | 1 | 2 | 4 | 7 | 11 | 13 | 25 |
| **TOTAL** | | | | | | | | | | |
| 0-19 Years | 358 | 3.2 | 9 | 1 | 1 | 2 | 4 | 7 | 9 | 14 |
| 20-34 | 221 | 4.5 | 30 | 1 | 1 | 3 | 5 | 11 | 12 | 30 |
| 35-49 | 257 | 4.7 | 44 | 1 | 2 | 3 | 6 | 9 | 12 | 40 |
| 50-64 | 167 | 4.2 | 15 | 1 | 2 | 3 | 5 | 9 | 11 | 17 |
| 65+ | 254 | 5.8 | 17 | 2 | 3 | 5 | 7 | 10 | 15 | 21 |
| **GRAND TOTAL** | 1,257 | 4.3 | 22 | 1 | 2 | 3 | 5 | 9 | 12 | 21 |

## 79.16: CRIF TIBIA & FIBULA. Formerly included in operation group(s) 733.

| Type of Patients | Observed Patients | Avg. Stay | Variance | Percentiles | | | | | | |
|---|---|---|---|---|---|---|---|---|---|---|
| | | | | 10th | 25th | 50th | 75th | 90th | 95th | 99th |
| **1. SINGLE DX** | | | | | | | | | | |
| 0-19 Years | 237 | 2.0 | 1 | 1 | 1 | 2 | 3 | 3 | 4 | 5 |
| 20-34 | 220 | 2.7 | 2 | 1 | 2 | 2 | 4 | 5 | 5 | 6 |
| 35-49 | 232 | 2.9 | 2 | 1 | 2 | 3 | 3 | 5 | 6 | 7 |
| 50-64 | 102 | 2.8 | 2 | 1 | 2 | 3 | 4 | 5 | 6 | 7 |
| 65+ | 22 | 3.0 | 2 | 1 | 2 | 3 | 3 | 6 | 6 | 7 |
| **2. MULTIPLE DX** | | | | | | | | | | |
| 0-19 Years | 158 | 5.2 | 67 | 1 | 2 | 3 | 5 | 9 | 16 | 65 |
| 20-34 | 302 | 4.3 | 20 | 2 | 2 | 3 | 5 | 7 | 10 | 25 |
| 35-49 | 404 | 4.7 | 17 | 2 | 2 | 3 | 6 | 10 | 13 | 23 |
| 50-64 | 278 | 4.4 | 13 | 1 | 3 | 3 | 5 | 9 | 11 | 18 |
| 65+ | 243 | 5.4 | 20 | 2 | 3 | 4 | 6 | 12 | 12 | 20 |
| **TOTAL SINGLE DX** | 813 | 2.6 | 2 | 1 | 2 | 2 | 3 | 4 | 5 | 6 |
| **TOTAL MULTIPLE DX** | 1,385 | 4.7 | 23 | 2 | 2 | 3 | 6 | 9 | 12 | 23 |
| **TOTAL** | | | | | | | | | | |
| 0-19 Years | 395 | 3.1 | 27 | 1 | 2 | 2 | 3 | 5 | 8 | 23 |
| 20-34 | 522 | 3.7 | 13 | 2 | 2 | 3 | 4 | 6 | 7 | 17 |
| 35-49 | 636 | 3.9 | 12 | 2 | 2 | 3 | 5 | 7 | 11 | 14 |
| 50-64 | 380 | 3.9 | 10 | 2 | 3 | 3 | 5 | 7 | 10 | 17 |
| 65+ | 265 | 5.3 | 20 | 2 | 3 | 4 | 6 | 12 | 12 | 20 |
| **GRAND TOTAL** | 2,198 | 3.8 | 16 | 1 | 2 | 3 | 4 | 7 | 10 | 18 |

## 79.26: OPEN RED TIBIA/FIB FX. Formerly included in operation group(s) 735.

| Type of Patients | Observed Patients | Avg. Stay | Variance | Percentiles | | | | | | |
|---|---|---|---|---|---|---|---|---|---|---|
| | | | | 10th | 25th | 50th | 75th | 90th | 95th | 99th |
| **1. SINGLE DX** | | | | | | | | | | |
| 0-19 Years | 67 | 2.6 | 2 | 1 | 2 | 2 | 3 | 4 | 5 | 9 |
| 20-34 | 34 | 2.4 | 3 | 1 | 1 | 2 | 3 | 5 | 6 | 6 |
| 35-49 | 29 | 4.4 | 15 | 2 | 2 | 3 | 7 | 12 | 12 | 12 |
| 50-64 | 16 | 3.2 | 3 | 2 | 2 | 3 | 4 | 7 | 7 | 7 |
| 65+ | 4 | 4.2 | <1 | 4 | 4 | 4 | 4 | 5 | 5 | 5 |
| **2. MULTIPLE DX** | | | | | | | | | | |
| 0-19 Years | 81 | 4.8 | 13 | 2 | 2 | 4 | 7 | 11 | 11 | 19 |
| 20-34 | 62 | 6.2 | 41 | 2 | 3 | 4 | 7 | 11 | 13 | 34 |
| 35-49 | 79 | 6.5 | 100 | 2 | 4 | 4 | 6 | 10 | 17 | 58 |
| 50-64 | 66 | 5.8 | 22 | 2 | 4 | 4 | 7 | 10 | 17 | 28 |
| 65+ | 57 | 6.8 | 26 | 3 | 3 | 5 | 7 | 17 | 19 | 21 |
| **TOTAL SINGLE DX** | 150 | 3.0 | 5 | 1 | 2 | 2 | 4 | 5 | 7 | 12 |
| **TOTAL MULTIPLE DX** | 345 | 5.9 | 37 | 2 | 3 | 4 | 7 | 11 | 17 | 28 |
| **TOTAL** | | | | | | | | | | |
| 0-19 Years | 148 | 3.8 | 9 | 1 | 2 | 3 | 5 | 7 | 11 | 13 |
| 20-34 | 96 | 4.8 | 29 | 1 | 2 | 3 | 6 | 9 | 12 | 34 |
| 35-49 | 108 | 5.9 | 75 | 2 | 3 | 4 | 6 | 11 | 14 | 58 |
| 50-64 | 82 | 5.4 | 20 | 2 | 3 | 4 | 6 | 10 | 17 | 28 |
| 65+ | 61 | 6.7 | 25 | 3 | 3 | 5 | 7 | 14 | 19 | 21 |
| **GRAND TOTAL** | 495 | 5.0 | 29 | 1 | 2 | 4 | 6 | 10 | 12 | 26 |

# United States, October 1998–September 1999 Data, by Operation

## 79.3: OPEN FX REDUCT W INT FIX. Formerly included in operation group(s) 731, 734.

| Type of Patients | Observed Patients | Avg. Stay | Variance | 10th | 25th | 50th | 75th | 90th | 95th | 99th |
|---|---|---|---|---|---|---|---|---|---|---|
| **1. SINGLE DX** | | | | | | | | | | |
| 0–19 Years | 4,679 | 1.9 | 2 | 1 | 1 | 2 | 2 | 3 | 4 | 7 |
| 20–34 | 4,974 | 2.3 | 3 | 1 | 1 | 2 | 3 | 4 | 6 | 9 |
| 35–49 | 5,584 | 2.4 | 3 | 1 | 1 | 2 | 3 | 4 | 5 | 9 |
| 50–64 | 3,283 | 2.7 | 3 | 1 | 1 | 2 | 3 | 5 | 6 | 9 |
| 65+ | 1,980 | 3.3 | 5 | 1 | 2 | 3 | 4 | 6 | 7 | 10 |
| **2. MULTIPLE DX** | | | | | | | | | | |
| 0–19 Years | 4,019 | 4.4 | 27 | 1 | 2 | 3 | 5 | 8 | 13 | 25 |
| 20–34 | 8,138 | 4.8 | 26 | 1 | 2 | 3 | 6 | 10 | 13 | 26 |
| 35–49 | 11,289 | 5.1 | 32 | 1 | 2 | 3 | 6 | 11 | 14 | 35 |
| 50–64 | 11,616 | 5.2 | 27 | 1 | 2 | 4 | 6 | 10 | 14 | 26 |
| 65+ | 47,276 | 6.1 | 21 | 3 | 4 | 5 | 7 | 10 | 13 | 23 |
| **TOTAL SINGLE DX** | 20,500 | 2.4 | 3 | 1 | 1 | 2 | 3 | 4 | 6 | 9 |
| **TOTAL MULTIPLE DX** | 82,338 | 5.6 | 25 | 2 | 3 | 4 | 7 | 10 | 13 | 25 |
| **TOTAL** | | | | | | | | | | |
| 0–19 Years | 8,698 | 3.0 | 15 | 1 | 1 | 2 | 3 | 6 | 8 | 17 |
| 20–34 | 13,112 | 3.8 | 18 | 1 | 2 | 3 | 4 | 8 | 11 | 21 |
| 35–49 | 16,873 | 4.1 | 23 | 1 | 2 | 3 | 5 | 8 | 12 | 26 |
| 50–64 | 14,899 | 4.6 | 23 | 1 | 2 | 3 | 5 | 9 | 12 | 24 |
| 65+ | 49,256 | 6.0 | 21 | 3 | 4 | 5 | 7 | 10 | 13 | 23 |
| **GRAND TOTAL** | 102,838 | 4.9 | 22 | 1 | 2 | 4 | 6 | 9 | 12 | 23 |

## 79.31: ORIF HUMERUS. Formerly included in operation group(s) 734.

| Type of Patients | Observed Patients | Avg. Stay | Variance | 10th | 25th | 50th | 75th | 90th | 95th | 99th |
|---|---|---|---|---|---|---|---|---|---|---|
| **1. SINGLE DX** | | | | | | | | | | |
| 0–19 Years | 1,073 | 1.5 | <1 | 1 | 1 | 1 | 2 | 3 | 3 | 4 |
| 20–34 | 242 | 2.0 | 2 | 1 | 1 | 2 | 2 | 4 | 6 | 6 |
| 35–49 | 247 | 2.0 | 1 | 1 | 1 | 2 | 2 | 3 | 4 | 6 |
| 50–64 | 186 | 3.1 | 6 | 1 | 1 | 2 | 3 | 7 | 9 | 9 |
| 65+ | 173 | 2.5 | 2 | 1 | 2 | 3 | 3 | 4 | 5 | 7 |
| **2. MULTIPLE DX** | | | | | | | | | | |
| 0–19 Years | 520 | 2.8 | 8 | 1 | 1 | 3 | 3 | 6 | 8 | 14 |
| 20–34 | 575 | 4.7 | 22 | 1 | 2 | 3 | 6 | 9 | 15 | 18 |
| 35–49 | 711 | 3.9 | 15 | 1 | 2 | 3 | 4 | 8 | 10 | 20 |
| 50–64 | 954 | 4.2 | 21 | 1 | 2 | 3 | 5 | 8 | 11 | 25 |
| 65+ | 2,206 | 4.7 | 20 | 1 | 3 | 3 | 6 | 9 | 13 | 20 |
| **TOTAL SINGLE DX** | 1,921 | 1.9 | 2 | 1 | 1 | 1 | 2 | 3 | 4 | 7 |
| **TOTAL MULTIPLE DX** | 4,966 | 4.2 | 19 | 1 | 2 | 3 | 5 | 8 | 11 | 21 |
| **TOTAL** | | | | | | | | | | |
| 0–19 Years | 1,593 | 1.9 | 3 | 1 | 1 | 1 | 2 | 3 | 5 | 9 |
| 20–34 | 817 | 3.9 | 17 | 1 | 2 | 3 | 5 | 8 | 11 | 16 |
| 35–49 | 958 | 3.4 | 12 | 1 | 2 | 2 | 4 | 7 | 9 | 17 |
| 50–64 | 1,140 | 4.1 | 19 | 1 | 2 | 3 | 5 | 8 | 10 | 24 |
| 65+ | 2,379 | 4.5 | 19 | 1 | 2 | 3 | 6 | 9 | 12 | 19 |
| **GRAND TOTAL** | 6,887 | 3.6 | 15 | 1 | 1 | 2 | 4 | 7 | 10 | 18 |

## 79.32: ORIF RADIUS/ULNA. Formerly included in operation group(s) 734.

| Type of Patients | Observed Patients | Avg. Stay | Variance | 10th | 25th | 50th | 75th | 90th | 95th | 99th |
|---|---|---|---|---|---|---|---|---|---|---|
| **1. SINGLE DX** | | | | | | | | | | |
| 0–19 Years | 1,039 | 1.6 | <1 | 1 | 1 | 1 | 2 | 3 | 3 | 4 |
| 20–34 | 623 | 1.9 | 2 | 1 | 1 | 2 | 2 | 3 | 5 | 7 |
| 35–49 | 506 | 1.8 | 1 | 1 | 1 | 2 | 2 | 3 | 4 | 6 |
| 50–64 | 293 | 1.9 | 1 | 1 | 1 | 2 | 2 | 3 | 4 | 6 |
| 65+ | 192 | 1.9 | 1 | 1 | 1 | 2 | 3 | 3 | 3 | 5 |
| **2. MULTIPLE DX** | | | | | | | | | | |
| 0–19 Years | 526 | 2.8 | 13 | 1 | 1 | 2 | 3 | 5 | 7 | 18 |
| 20–34 | 1,037 | 3.5 | 12 | 1 | 2 | 3 | 4 | 7 | 10 | 16 |
| 35–49 | 1,140 | 3.4 | 14 | 1 | 1 | 2 | 4 | 7 | 9 | 17 |
| 50–64 | 898 | 3.7 | 13 | 1 | 2 | 3 | 4 | 7 | 10 | 20 |
| 65+ | 1,588 | 3.7 | 14 | 1 | 2 | 3 | 4 | 7 | 10 | 22 |
| **TOTAL SINGLE DX** | 2,653 | 1.8 | 1 | 1 | 1 | 2 | 2 | 3 | 4 | 6 |
| **TOTAL MULTIPLE DX** | 5,189 | 3.5 | 13 | 1 | 2 | 3 | 4 | 7 | 10 | 19 |
| **TOTAL** | | | | | | | | | | |
| 0–19 Years | 1,565 | 2.0 | 5 | 1 | 1 | 2 | 3 | 3 | 5 | 9 |
| 20–34 | 1,660 | 2.9 | 8 | 1 | 2 | 2 | 3 | 5 | 8 | 13 |
| 35–49 | 1,646 | 2.8 | 10 | 1 | 2 | 2 | 3 | 6 | 8 | 17 |
| 50–64 | 1,191 | 3.1 | 10 | 1 | 2 | 3 | 3 | 6 | 9 | 20 |
| 65+ | 1,780 | 3.5 | 13 | 1 | 2 | 3 | 4 | 7 | 10 | 20 |
| **GRAND TOTAL** | 7,842 | 2.8 | 9 | 1 | 1 | 2 | 3 | 5 | 8 | 16 |

## 79.33: ORIF CARPALS/METACARPALS. Formerly included in operation group(s) 734.

| Type of Patients | Observed Patients | Avg. Stay | Variance | 10th | 25th | 50th | 75th | 90th | 95th | 99th |
|---|---|---|---|---|---|---|---|---|---|---|
| **1. SINGLE DX** | | | | | | | | | | |
| 0–19 Years | 41 | 1.5 | 2 | 1 | 1 | 1 | 2 | 3 | 3 | 4 |
| 20–34 | 97 | 1.6 | 2 | 1 | 1 | 1 | 2 | 3 | 3 | 9 |
| 35–49 | 60 | 1.4 | <1 | 1 | 1 | 1 | 2 | 2 | 3 | 4 |
| 50–64 | 13 | 1.7 | <1 | 1 | 1 | 1 | 2 | 3 | 3 | 3 |
| 65+ | 10 | 1.1 | <1 | 1 | 1 | 1 | 1 | 1 | 1 | 2 |
| **2. MULTIPLE DX** | | | | | | | | | | |
| 0–19 Years | 86 | 2.6 | 5 | 1 | 1 | 2 | 3 | 4 | 7 | 13 |
| 20–34 | 203 | 3.6 | 15 | 1 | 1 | 2 | 5 | 7 | 10 | 19 |
| 35–49 | 144 | 3.2 | 8 | 1 | 2 | 2 | 4 | 7 | 10 | 16 |
| 50–64 | 63 | 3.3 | 12 | 1 | 2 | 2 | 4 | 6 | 9 | 25 |
| 65+ | 50 | 3.6 | 14 | 1 | 2 | 2 | 3 | 10 | 14 | 16 |
| **TOTAL SINGLE DX** | 221 | 1.5 | 1 | 1 | 1 | 1 | 2 | 2 | 3 | 5 |
| **TOTAL MULTIPLE DX** | 546 | 3.3 | 11 | 1 | 2 | 2 | 4 | 7 | 10 | 16 |
| **TOTAL** | | | | | | | | | | |
| 0–19 Years | 127 | 2.3 | 5 | 1 | 1 | 1 | 3 | 4 | 5 | 13 |
| 20–34 | 300 | 3.0 | 12 | 1 | 1 | 2 | 3 | 7 | 9 | 15 |
| 35–49 | 204 | 2.7 | 7 | 1 | 2 | 2 | 3 | 6 | 8 | 14 |
| 50–64 | 76 | 3.1 | 11 | 1 | 2 | 2 | 4 | 5 | 7 | 25 |
| 65+ | 60 | 2.9 | 11 | 1 | 2 | 2 | 3 | 7 | 11 | 16 |
| **GRAND TOTAL** | 767 | 2.8 | 9 | 1 | 1 | 2 | 3 | 6 | 9 | 15 |

Length of Stay by Diagnosis and Operation, United States, 2000

## 79.34: ORIF FINGER. Formerly included in operation group(s) 734.

| Type of Patients | Observed Patients | Avg. Stay | Vari-ance | Percentiles | | | | | | |
|---|---|---|---|---|---|---|---|---|---|---|
| | | | | 10th | 25th | 50th | 75th | 90th | 95th | 99th |
| **1. SINGLE DX** | | | | | | | | | | |
| 0–19 Years | 71 | 1.7 | 2 | 1 | 1 | 1 | 2 | 2 | 7 | 8 |
| 20–34 | 91 | 1.5 | 4 | 1 | 1 | 1 | 2 | 3 | 3 | 5 |
| 35–49 | 97 | 1.4 | <1 | 1 | 1 | 1 | 1 | 2 | 3 | 8 |
| 50–64 | 39 | 1.5 | <1 | 1 | 1 | 1 | 2 | 2 | 3 | 3 |
| 65+ | 15 | 1.0 | <1 | 1 | 1 | 1 | 1 | 1 | 1 | 2 |
| **2. MULTIPLE DX** | | | | | | | | | | |
| 0–19 Years | 157 | 2.1 | 3 | 1 | 1 | 2 | 3 | 4 | 6 | 9 |
| 20–34 | 277 | 2.2 | 3 | 1 | 1 | 2 | 3 | 4 | 6 | 10 |
| 35–49 | 274 | 2.3 | 3 | 1 | 1 | 2 | 3 | 5 | 7 | 7 |
| 50–64 | 132 | 3.6 | 7 | 1 | 1 | 3 | 6 | 8 | 9 | 9 |
| 65+ | 94 | 2.7 | 17 | 1 | 1 | 2 | 2 | 4 | 7 | 12 |
| **TOTAL SINGLE DX** | 313 | 1.4 | 1 | 1 | 1 | 1 | 1 | 2 | 3 | 7 |
| **TOTAL MULTIPLE DX** | 934 | 2.5 | 5 | 1 | 1 | 2 | 3 | 5 | 7 | 9 |
| **TOTAL** | | | | | | | | | | |
| 0–19 Years | 228 | 2.0 | 3 | 1 | 1 | 1 | 2 | 4 | 6 | 8 |
| 20–34 | 368 | 2.1 | 3 | 1 | 1 | 1 | 3 | 4 | 5 | 10 |
| 35–49 | 371 | 2.1 | 3 | 1 | 1 | 1 | 3 | 5 | 7 | 8 |
| 50–64 | 171 | 3.2 | 7 | 1 | 1 | 2 | 3 | 8 | 8 | 9 |
| 65+ | 109 | 2.0 | 10 | 1 | 1 | 1 | 2 | 3 | 5 | 12 |
| **GRAND TOTAL** | 1,247 | 2.2 | 5 | 1 | 1 | 1 | 2 | 5 | 7 | 9 |

## 79.35: ORIF FEMUR. Formerly included in operation group(s) 731.

| Type of Patients | Observed Patients | Avg. Stay | Vari-ance | Percentiles | | | | | | |
|---|---|---|---|---|---|---|---|---|---|---|
| | | | | 10th | 25th | 50th | 75th | 90th | 95th | 99th |
| **1. SINGLE DX** | | | | | | | | | | |
| 0–19 Years | 572 | 3.3 | 7 | 1 | 2 | 3 | 4 | 5 | 7 | 10 |
| 20–34 | 334 | 3.9 | 4 | 2 | 3 | 4 | 5 | 6 | 7 | 12 |
| 35–49 | 360 | 3.7 | 3 | 2 | 2 | 4 | 4 | 6 | 6 | 9 |
| 50–64 | 304 | 4.3 | 5 | 2 | 3 | 4 | 5 | 7 | 8 | 11 |
| 65+ | 729 | 4.9 | 6 | 3 | 3 | 4 | 6 | 7 | 9 | 14 |
| **2. MULTIPLE DX** | | | | | | | | | | |
| 0–19 Years | 1,154 | 6.6 | 53 | 2 | 3 | 5 | 7 | 14 | 17 | 44 |
| 20–34 | 1,612 | 7.5 | 32 | 3 | 4 | 6 | 9 | 13 | 19 | 32 |
| 35–49 | 2,155 | 8.5 | 64 | 3 | 4 | 6 | 10 | 17 | 28 | 36 |
| 50–64 | 3,452 | 7.5 | 40 | 3 | 4 | 6 | 8 | 14 | 18 | 36 |
| 65+ | 36,583 | 6.6 | 21 | 3 | 4 | 6 | 7 | 10 | 13 | 24 |
| **TOTAL SINGLE DX** | 2,299 | 4.0 | 6 | 2 | 3 | 4 | 5 | 6 | 8 | 12 |
| **TOTAL MULTIPLE DX** | 44,956 | 6.8 | 27 | 3 | 4 | 6 | 8 | 11 | 14 | 30 |
| **TOTAL** | | | | | | | | | | |
| 0–19 Years | 1,726 | 5.6 | 41 | 2 | 3 | 4 | 6 | 11 | 14 | 44 |
| 20–34 | 1,946 | 6.7 | 28 | 2 | 4 | 5 | 8 | 12 | 17 | 28 |
| 35–49 | 2,515 | 7.9 | 59 | 2 | 4 | 5 | 9 | 15 | 24 | 36 |
| 50–64 | 3,756 | 7.2 | 38 | 3 | 4 | 5 | 8 | 13 | 18 | 35 |
| 65+ | 37,312 | 6.5 | 21 | 3 | 4 | 6 | 7 | 10 | 13 | 24 |
| **GRAND TOTAL** | 47,255 | 6.7 | 26 | 3 | 4 | 5 | 7 | 11 | 14 | 28 |

## 79.36: ORIF TIBIA & FIBULA. Formerly included in operation group(s) 734.

| Type of Patients | Observed Patients | Avg. Stay | Vari-ance | Percentiles | | | | | | |
|---|---|---|---|---|---|---|---|---|---|---|
| | | | | 10th | 25th | 50th | 75th | 90th | 95th | 99th |
| **1. SINGLE DX** | | | | | | | | | | |
| 0–19 Years | 1,690 | 1.9 | 1 | 1 | 1 | 2 | 2 | 3 | 4 | 6 |
| 20–34 | 3,142 | 2.3 | 3 | 1 | 1 | 2 | 3 | 4 | 5 | 9 |
| 35–49 | 3,742 | 2.4 | 2 | 1 | 1 | 2 | 3 | 4 | 5 | 9 |
| 50–64 | 2,181 | 2.5 | 3 | 1 | 2 | 2 | 3 | 4 | 5 | 9 |
| 65+ | 815 | 2.7 | 2 | 1 | 2 | 2 | 3 | 5 | 6 | 8 |
| **2. MULTIPLE DX** | | | | | | | | | | |
| 0–19 Years | 1,259 | 3.5 | 12 | 1 | 2 | 2 | 4 | 7 | 10 | 16 |
| 20–34 | 3,531 | 4.1 | 23 | 1 | 2 | 3 | 5 | 8 | 11 | 26 |
| 35–49 | 5,762 | 4.1 | 18 | 1 | 2 | 3 | 5 | 8 | 13 | 19 |
| 50–64 | 5,444 | 4.0 | 16 | 1 | 2 | 3 | 5 | 7 | 10 | 20 |
| 65+ | 6,354 | 4.6 | 15 | 2 | 3 | 4 | 5 | 8 | 11 | 20 |
| **TOTAL SINGLE DX** | 11,570 | 2.3 | 2 | 1 | 1 | 2 | 3 | 4 | 5 | 9 |
| **TOTAL MULTIPLE DX** | 22,350 | 4.2 | 18 | 1 | 2 | 3 | 5 | 8 | 11 | 21 |
| **TOTAL** | | | | | | | | | | |
| 0–19 Years | 2,949 | 2.5 | 6 | 1 | 1 | 2 | 3 | 5 | 7 | 12 |
| 20–34 | 6,673 | 3.2 | 14 | 1 | 2 | 3 | 4 | 6 | 8 | 19 |
| 35–49 | 9,504 | 3.4 | 12 | 1 | 2 | 3 | 4 | 7 | 9 | 18 |
| 50–64 | 7,625 | 3.6 | 13 | 1 | 2 | 3 | 4 | 7 | 9 | 17 |
| 65+ | 7,169 | 4.4 | 14 | 2 | 3 | 4 | 5 | 8 | 10 | 19 |
| **GRAND TOTAL** | 33,920 | 3.5 | 13 | 1 | 2 | 3 | 4 | 7 | 9 | 18 |

## 79.37: ORIF METATARSAL/TARSAL. Formerly included in operation group(s) 734.

| Type of Patients | Observed Patients | Avg. Stay | Vari-ance | Percentiles | | | | | | |
|---|---|---|---|---|---|---|---|---|---|---|
| | | | | 10th | 25th | 50th | 75th | 90th | 95th | 99th |
| **1. SINGLE DX** | | | | | | | | | | |
| 0–19 Years | 110 | 2.6 | 3 | 1 | 2 | 2 | 4 | 5 | 5 | 9 |
| 20–34 | 309 | 2.7 | 4 | 1 | 1 | 2 | 4 | 5 | 6 | 9 |
| 35–49 | 428 | 2.8 | 5 | 1 | 1 | 3 | 3 | 6 | 7 | 10 |
| 50–64 | 191 | 3.0 | 3 | 1 | 2 | 3 | 4 | 6 | 8 | 8 |
| 65+ | 28 | 3.0 | 2 | 1 | 2 | 3 | 4 | 5 | 5 | 5 |
| **2. MULTIPLE DX** | | | | | | | | | | |
| 0–19 Years | 106 | 4.3 | 8 | 1 | 3 | 4 | 5 | 5 | 11 | 15 |
| 20–34 | 405 | 4.2 | 21 | 1 | 2 | 3 | 5 | 9 | 12 | 20 |
| 35–49 | 523 | 4.6 | 19 | 1 | 2 | 3 | 6 | 10 | 16 | 19 |
| 50–64 | 327 | 4.6 | 17 | 2 | 2 | 3 | 6 | 10 | 14 | 19 |
| 65+ | 163 | 5.4 | 12 | 2 | 3 | 4 | 8 | 10 | 11 | 15 |
| **TOTAL SINGLE DX** | 1,066 | 2.8 | 4 | 1 | 2 | 2 | 4 | 5 | 6 | 9 |
| **TOTAL MULTIPLE DX** | 1,524 | 4.5 | 17 | 1 | 2 | 3 | 5 | 9 | 13 | 20 |
| **TOTAL** | | | | | | | | | | |
| 0–19 Years | 216 | 3.4 | 6 | 1 | 2 | 3 | 4 | 5 | 8 | 15 |
| 20–34 | 714 | 3.6 | 14 | 1 | 2 | 3 | 4 | 6 | 10 | 20 |
| 35–49 | 951 | 3.7 | 13 | 1 | 2 | 3 | 5 | 7 | 11 | 19 |
| 50–64 | 518 | 4.0 | 12 | 1 | 2 | 3 | 5 | 8 | 11 | 16 |
| 65+ | 191 | 4.8 | 11 | 2 | 2 | 4 | 7 | 10 | 10 | 14 |
| **GRAND TOTAL** | 2,590 | 3.7 | 12 | 1 | 2 | 3 | 4 | 7 | 10 | 19 |

## United States, October 1998–September 1999 Data, by Operation

### 79.39: ORIF BONE NEC X FACIAL. Formerly included in operation group(s) 734.

| Type of Patients | Observed Patients | Avg. Stay | Variance | 10th | 25th | 50th | 75th | 90th | 95th | 99th |
|---|---|---|---|---|---|---|---|---|---|---|
| **1. SINGLE DX** | | | | | | | | | | |
| 0–19 Years | 58 | 2.3 | 3 | 1 | 1 | 2 | 3 | 5 | 7 | 7 |
| 20–34 | 114 | 3.0 | 9 | 1 | 1 | 1 | 5 | 7 | 8 | 11 |
| 35–49 | 121 | 4.4 | 17 | 1 | 1 | 3 | 7 | 11 | 11 | 18 |
| 50–64 | 64 | 3.0 | 5 | 1 | 2 | 2 | 4 | 5 | 7 | 10 |
| 65+ | 18 | 3.4 | 8 | 1 | 2 | 2 | 4 | 7 | 12 | 12 |
| **2. MULTIPLE DX** | | | | | | | | | | |
| 0–19 Years | 187 | 7.2 | 43 | 1 | 2 | 6 | 9 | 15 | 19 | 33 |
| 20–34 | 472 | 8.0 | 43 | 2 | 3 | 7 | 10 | 16 | 19 | 32 |
| 35–49 | 550 | 8.0 | 51 | 1 | 3 | 7 | 11 | 15 | 24 | 33 |
| 50–64 | 325 | 8.9 | 53 | 2 | 4 | 7 | 12 | 17 | 20 | 37 |
| 65+ | 222 | 8.5 | 46 | 2 | 3 | 6 | 12 | 16 | 21 | 26 |
| **TOTAL SINGLE DX** | 375 | 3.4 | 11 | 1 | 1 | 2 | 5 | 7 | 11 | 13 |
| **TOTAL MULTIPLE DX** | 1,756 | 8.1 | 48 | 2 | 3 | 7 | 11 | 16 | 21 | 33 |
| **TOTAL** | | | | | | | | | | |
| 0–19 Years | 245 | 6.3 | 39 | 1 | 2 | 5 | 8 | 14 | 17 | 32 |
| 20–34 | 586 | 6.7 | 38 | 1 | 2 | 5 | 9 | 13 | 18 | 30 |
| 35–49 | 671 | 7.3 | 46 | 1 | 3 | 6 | 10 | 14 | 21 | 32 |
| 50–64 | 389 | 7.8 | 50 | 1 | 3 | 6 | 11 | 16 | 20 | 37 |
| 65+ | 240 | 8.2 | 45 | 2 | 3 | 6 | 12 | 16 | 21 | 26 |
| **GRAND TOTAL** | 2,131 | 7.2 | 44 | 1 | 2 | 6 | 10 | 15 | 20 | 32 |

### 79.5: OPEN RED SEP EPIPHYSIS. Formerly included in operation group(s) 731, 734.

| Type of Patients | Observed Patients | Avg. Stay | Variance | 10th | 25th | 50th | 75th | 90th | 95th | 99th |
|---|---|---|---|---|---|---|---|---|---|---|
| **1. SINGLE DX** | | | | | | | | | | |
| 0–19 Years | 152 | 1.7 | <1 | 1 | 1 | 1 | 2 | 3 | 4 | 4 |
| 20–34 | 16 | 2.5 | 4 | 1 | 1 | 2 | 3 | 4 | 8 | 9 |
| 35–49 | 16 | 1.9 | <1 | 1 | 1 | 2 | 3 | 3 | 3 | 3 |
| 50–64 | 7 | 2.6 | 3 | 1 | 1 | 3 | 3 | 3 | 8 | 8 |
| 65+ | 5 | 3.5 | 4 | 1 | 2 | 4 | 5 | 6 | 6 | 6 |
| **2. MULTIPLE DX** | | | | | | | | | | |
| 0–19 Years | 53 | 3.0 | 4 | 1 | 2 | 2 | 3 | 6 | 7 | 12 |
| 20–34 | 29 | 4.9 | 18 | 2 | 3 | 4 | 5 | 7 | 18 | 21 |
| 35–49 | 38 | 4.8 | 12 | 2 | 3 | 4 | 6 | 11 | 11 | 13 |
| 50–64 | 28 | 5.2 | 16 | 2 | 3 | 5 | 6 | 11 | 15 | 20 |
| 65+ | 48 | 6.6 | 10 | 3 | 4 | 6 | 8 | 10 | 12 | 18 |
| **TOTAL SINGLE DX** | 196 | 1.9 | 1 | 1 | 1 | 2 | 2 | 4 | 4 | 6 |
| **TOTAL MULTIPLE DX** | 196 | 4.6 | 12 | 2 | 2 | 3 | 6 | 10 | 12 | 20 |
| **TOTAL** | | | | | | | | | | |
| 0–19 Years | 205 | 2.1 | 2 | 1 | 1 | 2 | 2 | 4 | 4 | 7 |
| 20–34 | 45 | 4.2 | 15 | 1 | 2 | 4 | 4 | 7 | 12 | 21 |
| 35–49 | 54 | 3.9 | 10 | 1 | 2 | 3 | 4 | 11 | 11 | 13 |
| 50–64 | 35 | 4.4 | 13 | 1 | 3 | 3 | 6 | 8 | 12 | 20 |
| 65+ | 53 | 6.4 | 10 | 3 | 4 | 6 | 8 | 10 | 12 | 18 |
| **GRAND TOTAL** | 392 | 3.2 | 8 | 1 | 1 | 2 | 4 | 6 | 10 | 15 |

### 79.4: CR SEP EPIPHYSIS. Formerly included in operation group(s) 732, 735.

| Type of Patients | Observed Patients | Avg. Stay | Variance | 10th | 25th | 50th | 75th | 90th | 95th | 99th |
|---|---|---|---|---|---|---|---|---|---|---|
| **1. SINGLE DX** | | | | | | | | | | |
| 0–19 Years | 250 | 1.6 | 1 | 1 | 1 | 1 | 2 | 3 | 3 | 4 |
| 20–34 | 8 | 3.1 | 8 | 1 | 1 | 2 | 5 | 10 | 10 | 10 |
| 35–49 | 6 | 3.5 | 7 | 1 | 2 | 2 | 4 | 10 | 10 | 10 |
| 50–64 | 5 | 2.3 | <1 | 2 | 2 | 2 | 3 | 3 | 3 | 3 |
| 65+ | 4 | 2.4 | <1 | 1 | 1 | 3 | 3 | 3 | 3 | 3 |
| **2. MULTIPLE DX** | | | | | | | | | | |
| 0–19 Years | 88 | 2.9 | 4 | 1 | 2 | 2 | 2 | 6 | 6 | 8 |
| 20–34 | 12 | 3.2 | 7 | 1 | 2 | 3 | 5 | 6 | 11 | 11 |
| 35–49 | 15 | 4.3 | 3 | 2 | 3 | 5 | 6 | 6 | 7 | 7 |
| 50–64 | 11 | 2.4 | 4 | 1 | 1 | 2 | 3 | 5 | 6 | 9 |
| 65+ | 18 | 3.5 | 6 | 1 | 2 | 3 | 3 | 8 | 10 | 10 |
| **TOTAL SINGLE DX** | 273 | 1.7 | 2 | 1 | 1 | 1 | 2 | 3 | 3 | 7 |
| **TOTAL MULTIPLE DX** | 144 | 3.0 | 4 | 1 | 2 | 2 | 4 | 6 | 7 | 10 |
| **TOTAL** | | | | | | | | | | |
| 0–19 Years | 338 | 1.9 | 2 | 1 | 1 | 1 | 2 | 3 | 4 | 7 |
| 20–34 | 20 | 3.2 | 7 | 1 | 2 | 2 | 4 | 5 | 10 | 11 |
| 35–49 | 21 | 4.1 | 4 | 1 | 2 | 4 | 6 | 7 | 8 | 8 |
| 50–64 | 16 | 2.4 | 3 | 1 | 1 | 3 | 3 | 5 | 6 | 9 |
| 65+ | 22 | 3.3 | 5 | 1 | 2 | 3 | 3 | 7 | 8 | 10 |
| **GRAND TOTAL** | 417 | 2.0 | 3 | 1 | 1 | 1 | 2 | 4 | 5 | 8 |

### 79.6: OPEN FX SITE DEBRIDEMENT. Formerly included in operation group(s) 725, 726.

| Type of Patients | Observed Patients | Avg. Stay | Variance | 10th | 25th | 50th | 75th | 90th | 95th | 99th |
|---|---|---|---|---|---|---|---|---|---|---|
| **1. SINGLE DX** | | | | | | | | | | |
| 0–19 Years | 364 | 2.5 | 3 | 1 | 1 | 2 | 3 | 4 | 5 | 8 |
| 20–34 | 252 | 2.9 | 9 | 1 | 1 | 2 | 3 | 5 | 8 | 10 |
| 35–49 | 205 | 3.1 | 8 | 1 | 1 | 2 | 4 | 6 | 12 | 12 |
| 50–64 | 81 | 2.1 | 3 | 1 | 1 | 1 | 3 | 4 | 6 | 12 |
| 65+ | 35 | 2.6 | 5 | 1 | 2 | 2 | 3 | 5 | 7 | 12 |
| **2. MULTIPLE DX** | | | | | | | | | | |
| 0–19 Years | 472 | 7.2 | 128 | 1 | 2 | 3 | 7 | 15 | 23 | 65 |
| 20–34 | 808 | 5.8 | 39 | 1 | 2 | 4 | 7 | 12 | 18 | 28 |
| 35–49 | 716 | 6.1 | 63 | 1 | 2 | 4 | 8 | 13 | 18 | 40 |
| 50–64 | 384 | 6.0 | 60 | 1 | 2 | 4 | 7 | 12 | 17 | 47 |
| 65+ | 381 | 6.2 | 57 | 1 | 2 | 4 | 7 | 13 | 20 | 42 |
| **TOTAL SINGLE DX** | 937 | 2.7 | 6 | 1 | 1 | 2 | 3 | 5 | 6 | 12 |
| **TOTAL MULTIPLE DX** | 2,761 | 6.2 | 69 | 1 | 2 | 4 | 7 | 13 | 19 | 48 |
| **TOTAL** | | | | | | | | | | |
| 0–19 Years | 836 | 5.3 | 82 | 1 | 2 | 3 | 5 | 12 | 18 | 65 |
| 20–34 | 1,060 | 5.1 | 34 | 1 | 2 | 3 | 6 | 11 | 15 | 28 |
| 35–49 | 921 | 5.3 | 50 | 1 | 2 | 3 | 6 | 12 | 16 | 35 |
| 50–64 | 465 | 4.9 | 48 | 1 | 2 | 3 | 6 | 10 | 15 | 37 |
| 65+ | 416 | 6.0 | 54 | 1 | 2 | 4 | 7 | 13 | 20 | 37 |
| **GRAND TOTAL** | 3,698 | 5.3 | 54 | 1 | 2 | 3 | 6 | 11 | 16 | 37 |

Length of Stay by Diagnosis and Operation, United States, 2000

## United States, October 1998–September 1999 Data, by Operation

### 79.62: DEBRIDE OPEN FX RAD/ULNA. Formerly included in operation group(s) 726.

| Type of Patients | Observed Patients | Avg. Stay | Vari-ance | Percentiles | | | | | | |
|---|---|---|---|---|---|---|---|---|---|---|
| | | | | 10th | 25th | 50th | 75th | 90th | 95th | 99th |
| **1. SINGLE DX** | | | | | | | | | | |
| 0–19 Years | 125 | 2.2 | 2 | 1 | 1 | 2 | 3 | 4 | 5 | 8 |
| 20–34 | 24 | 2.4 | 1 | 1 | 2 | 2 | 3 | 3 | 5 | 6 |
| 35–49 | 29 | 2.3 | 3 | 1 | 1 | 2 | 3 | 3 | 8 | 10 |
| 50–64 | 19 | 2.9 | 3 | 1 | 2 | 2 | 4 | 6 | 6 | 6 |
| 65+ | 12 | 1.8 | 2 | 1 | 1 | 1 | 2 | 3 | 6 | 6 |
| **2. MULTIPLE DX** | | | | | | | | | | |
| 0–19 Years | 65 | 4.0 | 18 | 1 | 2 | 3 | 4 | 8 | 15 | 20 |
| 20–34 | 87 | 4.9 | 42 | 1 | 2 | 3 | 5 | 9 | 14 | 44 |
| 35–49 | 77 | 4.0 | 16 | 1 | 2 | 2 | 5 | 9 | 12 | 27 |
| 50–64 | 53 | 6.7 | 97 | 2 | 2 | 4 | 7 | 11 | 31 | 58 |
| 65+ | 117 | 3.3 | 4 | 1 | 2 | 3 | 4 | 7 | 7 | 9 |
| **TOTAL SINGLE DX** | 209 | 2.3 | 2 | 1 | 1 | 2 | 3 | 4 | 5 | 8 |
| **TOTAL MULTIPLE DX** | 399 | 4.3 | 28 | 1 | 2 | 3 | 5 | 8 | 12 | 27 |
| **TOTAL** | | | | | | | | | | |
| 0–19 Years | 190 | 2.8 | 8 | 1 | 1 | 2 | 3 | 5 | 7 | 20 |
| 20–34 | 111 | 4.4 | 34 | 1 | 2 | 3 | 5 | 8 | 12 | 44 |
| 35–49 | 106 | 3.5 | 13 | 1 | 2 | 2 | 4 | 7 | 12 | 17 |
| 50–64 | 72 | 5.2 | 63 | 1 | 2 | 3 | 6 | 10 | 17 | 47 |
| 65+ | 129 | 3.2 | 4 | 1 | 2 | 3 | 4 | 7 | 7 | 9 |
| **GRAND TOTAL** | 608 | 3.5 | 19 | 1 | 2 | 2 | 4 | 7 | 9 | 22 |

### 79.64: DEBRIDE OPEN FX FINGER. Formerly included in operation group(s) 726.

| Type of Patients | Observed Patients | Avg. Stay | Vari-ance | Percentiles | | | | | | |
|---|---|---|---|---|---|---|---|---|---|---|
| | | | | 10th | 25th | 50th | 75th | 90th | 95th | 99th |
| **1. SINGLE DX** | | | | | | | | | | |
| 0–19 Years | 32 | 1.6 | 1 | 1 | 1 | 1 | 2 | 3 | 4 | 6 |
| 20–34 | 34 | 1.8 | 1 | 1 | 1 | 1 | 3 | 3 | 3 | 5 |
| 35–49 | 35 | 1.5 | 1 | 1 | 1 | 1 | 1 | 3 | 4 | 6 |
| 50–64 | 8 | 1.1 | <1 | 1 | 1 | 1 | 1 | 1 | 3 | 3 |
| 65+ | 4 | 1.5 | <1 | 1 | 1 | 1 | 3 | 3 | 3 | 3 |
| **2. MULTIPLE DX** | | | | | | | | | | |
| 0–19 Years | 50 | 4.3 | 21 | 1 | 1 | 2 | 9 | 12 | 12 | 12 |
| 20–34 | 98 | 2.3 | 2 | 1 | 1 | 2 | 3 | 4 | 6 | 7 |
| 35–49 | 84 | 2.1 | 10 | 1 | 1 | 1 | 2 | 4 | 8 | 14 |
| 50–64 | 45 | 2.1 | 4 | 1 | 1 | 1 | 3 | 3 | 4 | 9 |
| 65+ | 42 | 2.6 | 5 | 1 | 1 | 2 | 3 | 4 | 6 | 13 |
| **TOTAL SINGLE DX** | 113 | 1.5 | <1 | 1 | 1 | 1 | 1 | 3 | 3 | 6 |
| **TOTAL MULTIPLE DX** | 319 | 2.7 | 9 | 1 | 1 | 2 | 3 | 6 | 12 | 12 |
| **TOTAL** | | | | | | | | | | |
| 0–19 Years | 82 | 3.4 | 16 | 1 | 1 | 1 | 3 | 12 | 12 | 12 |
| 20–34 | 132 | 2.1 | 2 | 1 | 1 | 2 | 3 | 4 | 5 | 7 |
| 35–49 | 119 | 1.9 | 7 | 1 | 1 | 1 | 2 | 3 | 4 | 12 |
| 50–64 | 53 | 1.6 | 1 | 1 | 1 | 1 | 1 | 3 | 4 | 8 |
| 65+ | 46 | 2.6 | 5 | 1 | 1 | 2 | 3 | 4 | 6 | 13 |
| **GRAND TOTAL** | 432 | 2.2 | 7 | 1 | 1 | 1 | 2 | 4 | 7 | 12 |

### 79.66: DEBRIDE OPN FX TIBIA/FIB. Formerly included in operation group(s) 726.

| Type of Patients | Observed Patients | Avg. Stay | Vari-ance | Percentiles | | | | | | |
|---|---|---|---|---|---|---|---|---|---|---|
| | | | | 10th | 25th | 50th | 75th | 90th | 95th | 99th |
| **1. SINGLE DX** | | | | | | | | | | |
| 0–19 Years | 141 | 3.0 | 3 | 2 | 2 | 2 | 4 | 5 | 5 | 7 |
| 20–34 | 114 | 2.8 | 3 | 1 | 2 | 3 | 4 | 5 | 7 | 9 |
| 35–49 | 88 | 4.4 | 12 | 2 | 2 | 3 | 4 | 12 | 12 | 15 |
| 50–64 | 36 | 3.3 | 3 | 2 | 2 | 3 | 4 | 5 | 7 | 12 |
| 65+ | 12 | 4.6 | 7 | 3 | 3 | 3 | 5 | 8 | 12 | 12 |
| **2. MULTIPLE DX** | | | | | | | | | | |
| 0–19 Years | 185 | 6.5 | 48 | 1 | 2 | 4 | 8 | 18 | 19 | 27 |
| 20–34 | 347 | 6.6 | 38 | 2 | 3 | 5 | 8 | 14 | 17 | 30 |
| 35–49 | 330 | 7.5 | 78 | 2 | 3 | 5 | 9 | 14 | 19 | 49 |
| 50–64 | 162 | 7.5 | 78 | 2 | 4 | 5 | 8 | 13 | 17 | 51 |
| 65+ | 127 | 10.0 | 105 | 3 | 4 | 6 | 13 | 24 | 31 | 47 |
| **TOTAL SINGLE DX** | 391 | 3.4 | 6 | 2 | 2 | 3 | 4 | 5 | 8 | 12 |
| **TOTAL MULTIPLE DX** | 1,151 | 7.3 | 63 | 2 | 3 | 5 | 9 | 15 | 20 | 42 |
| **TOTAL** | | | | | | | | | | |
| 0–19 Years | 326 | 5.2 | 34 | 1 | 2 | 3 | 6 | 12 | 18 | 27 |
| 20–34 | 461 | 5.7 | 32 | 2 | 3 | 4 | 7 | 11 | 15 | 28 |
| 35–49 | 418 | 6.6 | 61 | 2 | 3 | 4 | 8 | 12 | 17 | 38 |
| 50–64 | 198 | 6.7 | 67 | 2 | 3 | 5 | 7 | 12 | 16 | 51 |
| 65+ | 139 | 9.7 | 101 | 3 | 3 | 6 | 13 | 23 | 31 | 47 |
| **GRAND TOTAL** | 1,542 | 6.2 | 50 | 2 | 2 | 4 | 7 | 13 | 18 | 33 |

### 79.7: CLOSED RED DISLOCATION. Formerly included in operation group(s) 736, 737.

| Type of Patients | Observed Patients | Avg. Stay | Vari-ance | Percentiles | | | | | | |
|---|---|---|---|---|---|---|---|---|---|---|
| | | | | 10th | 25th | 50th | 75th | 90th | 95th | 99th |
| **1. SINGLE DX** | | | | | | | | | | |
| 0–19 Years | 237 | 2.0 | 5 | 1 | 1 | 1 | 2 | 4 | 6 | 9 |
| 20–34 | 138 | 1.9 | 1 | 1 | 1 | 2 | 2 | 3 | 3 | 7 |
| 35–49 | 176 | 1.5 | 2 | 1 | 1 | 1 | 1 | 3 | 4 | 8 |
| 50–64 | 161 | 1.7 | 1 | 1 | 1 | 1 | 2 | 4 | 4 | 5 |
| 65+ | 377 | 1.7 | 2 | 1 | 1 | 1 | 2 | 3 | 3 | 6 |
| **2. MULTIPLE DX** | | | | | | | | | | |
| 0–19 Years | 228 | 3.9 | 100 | 1 | 1 | 2 | 3 | 6 | 10 | 62 |
| 20–34 | 379 | 3.0 | 15 | 1 | 2 | 2 | 4 | 5 | 6 | 11 |
| 35–49 | 514 | 3.8 | 47 | 1 | 2 | 2 | 4 | 6 | 10 | 48 |
| 50–64 | 614 | 2.8 | 12 | 1 | 2 | 2 | 3 | 6 | 9 | 14 |
| 65+ | 2,221 | 3.8 | 17 | 1 | 2 | 2 | 4 | 9 | 10 | 22 |
| **TOTAL SINGLE DX** | 1,089 | 1.7 | 2 | 1 | 1 | 1 | 2 | 3 | 4 | 9 |
| **TOTAL MULTIPLE DX** | 3,956 | 3.5 | 26 | 1 | 1 | 2 | 4 | 7 | 10 | 25 |
| **TOTAL** | | | | | | | | | | |
| 0–19 Years | 465 | 3.1 | 64 | 1 | 1 | 1 | 2 | 5 | 8 | 62 |
| 20–34 | 517 | 2.6 | 11 | 1 | 1 | 2 | 3 | 6 | 6 | 10 |
| 35–49 | 690 | 3.2 | 35 | 1 | 1 | 2 | 3 | 6 | 8 | 48 |
| 50–64 | 775 | 2.5 | 10 | 1 | 1 | 2 | 3 | 5 | 7 | 14 |
| 65+ | 2,598 | 3.5 | 16 | 1 | 1 | 2 | 4 | 8 | 10 | 20 |
| **GRAND TOTAL** | 5,045 | 3.2 | 21 | 1 | 1 | 2 | 3 | 6 | 10 | 21 |

Length of Stay by Diagnosis and Operation, United States, 2000

### 79.71: CLSD RED DISLOC SHOULDER. Formerly included in operation group(s) 737.

| Type of Patients | Observed Patients | Avg. Stay | Variance | Percentiles | | | | | | |
|---|---|---|---|---|---|---|---|---|---|---|
| | | | | 10th | 25th | 50th | 75th | 90th | 95th | 99th |
| **1. SINGLE DX** | | | | | | | | | | |
| 0–19 Years | 8 | 1.1 | <1 | 1 | 1 | 1 | 1 | 1 | 2 | 2 |
| 20–34 | 31 | 1.0 | <1 | 1 | 1 | 1 | 1 | 1 | 1 | 2 |
| 35–49 | 20 | 1.1 | <1 | 1 | 1 | 1 | 1 | 1 | 2 | 2 |
| 50–64 | 10 | 1.1 | <1 | 1 | 1 | 1 | 1 | 1 | 2 | 3 |
| 65+ | 17 | 1.7 | <1 | 1 | 1 | 1 | 2 | 3 | 3 | 3 |
| **2. MULTIPLE DX** | | | | | | | | | | |
| 0–19 Years | 18 | 1.7 | 2 | 1 | 1 | 1 | 2 | 3 | 7 | 7 |
| 20–34 | 77 | 2.3 | 2 | 1 | 1 | 2 | 3 | 4 | 6 | 6 |
| 35–49 | 79 | 6.9 | 163 | 1 | 1 | 3 | 5 | 13 | 48 | 48 |
| 50–64 | 78 | 2.4 | 5 | 1 | 1 | 2 | 3 | 4 | 7 | 9 |
| 65+ | 327 | 5.4 | 16 | 1 | 2 | 4 | 10 | 10 | 12 | 15 |
| **TOTAL SINGLE DX** | **86** | **1.2** | **<1** | **1** | **1** | **1** | **1** | **2** | **2** | **3** |
| **TOTAL MULTIPLE DX** | **579** | **4.7** | **32** | **1** | **1** | **3** | **6** | **10** | **11** | **29** |
| **TOTAL** | | | | | | | | | | |
| 0–19 Years | 26 | 1.5 | 1 | 1 | 1 | 1 | 2 | 2 | 3 | 7 |
| 20–34 | 108 | 2.0 | 2 | 1 | 1 | 1 | 3 | 4 | 5 | 6 |
| 35–49 | 99 | 5.7 | 137 | 1 | 1 | 2 | 4 | 8 | 48 | 48 |
| 50–64 | 88 | 2.2 | 5 | 1 | 1 | 2 | 3 | 4 | 6 | 9 |
| 65+ | 344 | 5.3 | 16 | 1 | 2 | 4 | 10 | 10 | 12 | 15 |
| **GRAND TOTAL** | **665** | **4.3** | **30** | **1** | **1** | **3** | **6** | **10** | **10** | **27** |

### 79.75: CLSD RED DISLOC HIP. Formerly included in operation group(s) 736.

| Type of Patients | Observed Patients | Avg. Stay | Variance | Percentiles | | | | | | |
|---|---|---|---|---|---|---|---|---|---|---|
| | | | | 10th | 25th | 50th | 75th | 90th | 95th | 99th |
| **1. SINGLE DX** | | | | | | | | | | |
| 0–19 Years | 99 | 2.5 | 7 | 1 | 1 | 2 | 2 | 6 | 9 | 14 |
| 20–34 | 55 | 2.0 | 1 | 1 | 2 | 2 | 2 | 2 | 3 | 7 |
| 35–49 | 110 | 1.5 | 1 | 1 | 1 | 1 | 2 | 2 | 4 | 8 |
| 50–64 | 137 | 1.7 | 1 | 1 | 1 | 1 | 2 | 4 | 4 | 5 |
| 65+ | 343 | 1.7 | 2 | 1 | 1 | 1 | 2 | 3 | 3 | 6 |
| **2. MULTIPLE DX** | | | | | | | | | | |
| 0–19 Years | 136 | 3.5 | 57 | 1 | 1 | 2 | 3 | 6 | 7 | 62 |
| 20–34 | 176 | 3.0 | 9 | 1 | 1 | 2 | 4 | 5 | 5 | 18 |
| 35–49 | 299 | 3.0 | 14 | 1 | 1 | 2 | 4 | 6 | 8 | 27 |
| 50–64 | 444 | 2.9 | 15 | 1 | 1 | 2 | 3 | 6 | 10 | 15 |
| 65+ | 1,747 | 3.4 | 17 | 1 | 1 | 2 | 4 | 7 | 10 | 24 |
| **TOTAL SINGLE DX** | **744** | **1.8** | **2** | **1** | **1** | **1** | **2** | **3** | **4** | **9** |
| **TOTAL MULTIPLE DX** | **2,802** | **3.3** | **19** | **1** | **1** | **2** | **4** | **6** | **9** | **25** |
| **TOTAL** | | | | | | | | | | |
| 0–19 Years | 235 | 3.2 | 41 | 1 | 1 | 2 | 3 | 6 | 9 | 22 |
| 20–34 | 231 | 2.6 | 6 | 1 | 1 | 2 | 3 | 5 | 5 | 11 |
| 35–49 | 409 | 2.6 | 11 | 1 | 1 | 2 | 3 | 6 | 7 | 17 |
| 50–64 | 581 | 2.6 | 11 | 1 | 1 | 1 | 3 | 5 | 8 | 14 |
| 65+ | 2,090 | 3.2 | 15 | 1 | 1 | 2 | 4 | 6 | 9 | 23 |
| **GRAND TOTAL** | **3,546** | **3.0** | **16** | **1** | **1** | **2** | **3** | **6** | **9** | **20** |

### 79.8: OPEN RED DISLOCATION. Formerly included in operation group(s) 736, 737.

| Type of Patients | Observed Patients | Avg. Stay | Variance | Percentiles | | | | | | |
|---|---|---|---|---|---|---|---|---|---|---|
| | | | | 10th | 25th | 50th | 75th | 90th | 95th | 99th |
| **1. SINGLE DX** | | | | | | | | | | |
| 0–19 Years | 197 | 1.9 | 2 | 1 | 1 | 1 | 2 | 3 | 4 | 7 |
| 20–34 | 62 | 1.7 | <1 | 1 | 1 | 1 | 2 | 3 | 4 | 6 |
| 35–49 | 34 | 2.6 | 2 | 1 | 2 | 3 | 3 | 3 | 5 | 8 |
| 50–64 | 29 | 1.6 | 3 | 1 | 1 | 1 | 1 | 3 | 5 | 10 |
| 65+ | 8 | 3.7 | 12 | 1 | 2 | 2 | 4 | 10 | 10 | 10 |
| **2. MULTIPLE DX** | | | | | | | | | | |
| 0–19 Years | 244 | 3.5 | 11 | 1 | 2 | 3 | 4 | 6 | 9 | 21 |
| 20–34 | 102 | 4.5 | 17 | 1 | 2 | 3 | 5 | 8 | 10 | 19 |
| 35–49 | 134 | 4.4 | 26 | 1 | 1 | 2 | 5 | 13 | 17 | 18 |
| 50–64 | 97 | 3.3 | 9 | 1 | 1 | 2 | 6 | 7 | 7 | 12 |
| 65+ | 234 | 6.5 | 23 | 2 | 3 | 6 | 8 | 11 | 15 | 21 |
| **TOTAL SINGLE DX** | **330** | **2.0** | **2** | **1** | **1** | **1** | **2** | **3** | **5** | **8** |
| **TOTAL MULTIPLE DX** | **811** | **4.5** | **19** | **1** | **2** | **3** | **6** | **9** | **13** | **21** |
| **TOTAL** | | | | | | | | | | |
| 0–19 Years | 441 | 2.8 | 8 | 1 | 1 | 2 | 3 | 5 | 7 | 21 |
| 20–34 | 164 | 3.6 | 13 | 1 | 1 | 2 | 4 | 8 | 9 | 16 |
| 35–49 | 168 | 4.0 | 20 | 1 | 1 | 3 | 4 | 9 | 17 | 18 |
| 50–64 | 126 | 2.9 | 8 | 1 | 1 | 1 | 4 | 7 | 7 | 11 |
| 65+ | 242 | 6.4 | 23 | 2 | 3 | 6 | 8 | 11 | 15 | 19 |
| **GRAND TOTAL** | **1,141** | **3.8** | **15** | **1** | **1** | **3** | **5** | **8** | **11** | **19** |

### 79.85: OPEN RED DISLOC HIP. Formerly included in operation group(s) 736.

| Type of Patients | Observed Patients | Avg. Stay | Variance | Percentiles | | | | | | |
|---|---|---|---|---|---|---|---|---|---|---|
| | | | | 10th | 25th | 50th | 75th | 90th | 95th | 99th |
| **1. SINGLE DX** | | | | | | | | | | |
| 0–19 Years | 134 | 2.2 | 3 | 1 | 1 | 2 | 2 | 4 | 5 | 8 |
| 20–34 | 2 | 2.5 | 3 | 1 | 1 | 4 | 4 | 4 | 4 | 4 |
| 35–49 | 3 | 5.9 | 5 | 2 | 5 | 5 | 8 | 8 | 8 | 8 |
| 50–64 | 3 | 7.1 | 13 | 3 | 4 | 10 | 10 | 10 | 10 | 10 |
| 65+ | 3 | 4.7 | 15 | 1 | 1 | 4 | 10 | 10 | 10 | 10 |
| **2. MULTIPLE DX** | | | | | | | | | | |
| 0–19 Years | 199 | 3.7 | 12 | 1 | 2 | 3 | 4 | 6 | 9 | 21 |
| 20–34 | 9 | 4.6 | 9 | 2 | 2 | 5 | 5 | 8 | 10 | 16 |
| 35–49 | 17 | 10.7 | 45 | 3 | 3 | 17 | 17 | 17 | 17 | 18 |
| 50–64 | 27 | 4.9 | 12 | 2 | 3 | 4 | 6 | 9 | 9 | 21 |
| 65+ | 149 | 7.5 | 27 | 3 | 4 | 7 | 9 | 12 | 15 | 24 |
| **TOTAL SINGLE DX** | **145** | **2.4** | **4** | **1** | **1** | **2** | **3** | **4** | **7** | **10** |
| **TOTAL MULTIPLE DX** | **401** | **5.7** | **24** | **2** | **3** | **4** | **7** | **11** | **17** | **21** |
| **TOTAL** | | | | | | | | | | |
| 0–19 Years | 333 | 3.1 | 9 | 1 | 2 | 2 | 3 | 6 | 7 | 21 |
| 20–34 | 11 | 4.5 | 9 | 2 | 2 | 4 | 5 | 8 | 10 | 16 |
| 35–49 | 20 | 10.1 | 43 | 3 | 3 | 8 | 17 | 17 | 17 | 18 |
| 50–64 | 30 | 5.0 | 12 | 2 | 3 | 4 | 7 | 9 | 10 | 21 |
| 65+ | 152 | 7.5 | 27 | 3 | 4 | 7 | 9 | 12 | 15 | 24 |
| **GRAND TOTAL** | **546** | **4.9** | **21** | **1** | **2** | **3** | **6** | **9** | **16** | **21** |

## United States, October 1998–September 1999 Data, by Operation

### 79.9: BONE INJURY OP NOS. Formerly included in operation group(s) 727, 728.

| Type of Patients | Observed Patients | Avg. Stay | Vari-ance | 10th | 25th | 50th | 75th | 90th | 95th | 99th |
|---|---|---|---|---|---|---|---|---|---|---|
| **1. SINGLE DX** | | | | | | | | | | |
| 0–19 Years | 1 | 1.0 | 0 | 1 | 1 | 1 | 1 | 1 | 1 | 1 |
| 20–34 | 0 | | | | | | | | | |
| 35–49 | 0 | | | | | | | | | |
| 50–64 | 1 | 1.0 | 0 | 1 | 1 | 1 | 1 | 1 | 1 | 1 |
| 65+ | 0 | | | | | | | | | |
| **2. MULTIPLE DX** | | | | | | | | | | |
| 0–19 Years | 0 | | | | | | | | | |
| 20–34 | 0 | | | | | | | | | |
| 35–49 | 0 | | | | | | | | | |
| 50–64 | 0 | | | | | | | | | |
| 65+ | 1 | 6.0 | | 6 | 6 | 6 | 6 | 6 | 6 | 6 |
| **TOTAL SINGLE DX** | 2 | 1.0 | 0 | 1 | 1 | 1 | 1 | 1 | 1 | 1 |
| **TOTAL MULTIPLE DX** | 1 | 6.0 | 0 | 6 | 6 | 6 | 6 | 6 | 6 | 6 |
| **TOTAL** | | | | | | | | | | |
| 0–19 Years | 1 | 1.0 | 0 | 1 | 1 | 1 | 1 | 1 | 1 | 1 |
| 20–34 | 0 | | | | | | | | | |
| 35–49 | 0 | | | | | | | | | |
| 50–64 | 1 | 1.0 | 0 | 1 | 1 | 1 | 1 | 1 | 1 | 1 |
| 65+ | 1 | 6.0 | 0 | 6 | 6 | 6 | 6 | 6 | 6 | 6 |
| **GRAND TOTAL** | 3 | 2.8 | 7 | 1 | 1 | 1 | 6 | 6 | 6 | 6 |

### 80.05: RMVL PROSTH HIP INC. Formerly included in operation group(s) 738.

| Type of Patients | Observed Patients | Avg. Stay | Vari-ance | 10th | 25th | 50th | 75th | 90th | 95th | 99th |
|---|---|---|---|---|---|---|---|---|---|---|
| **1. SINGLE DX** | | | | | | | | | | |
| 0–19 Years | 1 | 1.0 | 0 | 1 | 1 | 1 | 1 | 1 | 1 | 1 |
| 20–34 | 1 | 4.0 | 0 | 4 | 4 | 4 | 4 | 4 | 4 | 4 |
| 35–49 | 4 | 3.5 | 2 | 2 | 3 | 3 | 4 | 5 | 5 | 5 |
| 50–64 | 4 | 5.4 | 8 | 3 | 3 | 3 | 7 | 9 | 9 | 9 |
| 65+ | 3 | 4.6 | 7 | 1 | 4 | 4 | 7 | 7 | 7 | 7 |
| **2. MULTIPLE DX** | | | | | | | | | | |
| 0–19 Years | 5 | 3.3 | 6 | 1 | 1 | 2 | 6 | 6 | 6 | 6 |
| 20–34 | 13 | 9.1 | 145 | 3 | 3 | 3 | 8 | 40 | 40 | 40 |
| 35–49 | 66 | 43.7 | >999 | 4 | 7 | 22 | 83 | 83 | 83 | 83 |
| 50–64 | 102 | 10.1 | 41 | 4 | 6 | 8 | 12 | 21 | 24 | 28 |
| 65+ | 357 | 10.9 | 92 | 4 | 5 | 8 | 13 | 21 | 28 | 56 |
| **TOTAL SINGLE DX** | 13 | 4.5 | 7 | 1 | 3 | 4 | 7 | 9 | 9 | 9 |
| **TOTAL MULTIPLE DX** | 543 | 17.6 | 541 | 4 | 5 | 8 | 16 | 67 | 83 | 83 |
| **TOTAL** | | | | | | | | | | |
| 0–19 Years | 6 | 3.0 | 6 | 1 | 1 | 1 | 6 | 6 | 6 | 6 |
| 20–34 | 14 | 9.0 | 143 | 3 | 3 | 3 | 8 | 40 | 40 | 40 |
| 35–49 | 70 | 43.2 | >999 | 4 | 7 | 20 | 83 | 83 | 83 | 83 |
| 50–64 | 106 | 9.9 | 41 | 4 | 6 | 8 | 11 | 20 | 24 | 28 |
| 65+ | 360 | 10.9 | 91 | 4 | 5 | 7 | 13 | 21 | 28 | 56 |
| **GRAND TOTAL** | 556 | 17.4 | 536 | 3 | 5 | 8 | 16 | 57 | 83 | 83 |

### 80.0: ARTHROTOMY RMVL PROSTH. Formerly included in operation group(s) 738.

| Type of Patients | Observed Patients | Avg. Stay | Vari-ance | 10th | 25th | 50th | 75th | 90th | 95th | 99th |
|---|---|---|---|---|---|---|---|---|---|---|
| **1. SINGLE DX** | | | | | | | | | | |
| 0–19 Years | 3 | 2.3 | 5 | 1 | 1 | 1 | 5 | 5 | 5 | 5 |
| 20–34 | 6 | 2.8 | 1 | 1 | 2 | 3 | 4 | 4 | 4 | 4 |
| 35–49 | 15 | 2.1 | 2 | 1 | 1 | 1 | 3 | 4 | 5 | 6 |
| 50–64 | 27 | 4.3 | 3 | 1 | 4 | 4 | 5 | 6 | 9 | 9 |
| 65+ | 20 | 4.9 | 26 | 1 | 1 | 3 | 6 | 10 | 16 | 23 |
| **2. MULTIPLE DX** | | | | | | | | | | |
| 0–19 Years | 13 | 4.0 | 12 | 1 | 1 | 3 | 6 | 8 | 12 | 13 |
| 20–34 | 31 | 8.3 | 126 | 1 | 3 | 3 | 8 | 31 | 40 | 43 |
| 35–49 | 147 | 26.5 | >999 | 2 | 5 | 7 | 83 | 83 | 83 | 83 |
| 50–64 | 295 | 8.4 | 43 | 3 | 4 | 6 | 10 | 16 | 22 | 36 |
| 65+ | 859 | 9.6 | 82 | 3 | 4 | 7 | 11 | 18 | 23 | 48 |
| **TOTAL SINGLE DX** | 71 | 3.8 | 10 | 1 | 2 | 4 | 5 | 6 | 9 | 23 |
| **TOTAL MULTIPLE DX** | 1,345 | 12.0 | 285 | 3 | 4 | 7 | 11 | 21 | 44 | 83 |
| **TOTAL** | | | | | | | | | | |
| 0–19 Years | 16 | 3.8 | 12 | 1 | 3 | 3 | 6 | 8 | 12 | 13 |
| 20–34 | 37 | 7.8 | 117 | 1 | 3 | 3 | 8 | 18 | 40 | 43 |
| 35–49 | 162 | 25.1 | >999 | 2 | 5 | 7 | 28 | 83 | 83 | 83 |
| 50–64 | 322 | 8.0 | 41 | 2 | 4 | 6 | 10 | 16 | 22 | 36 |
| 65+ | 879 | 9.5 | 81 | 3 | 4 | 7 | 11 | 18 | 23 | 46 |
| **GRAND TOTAL** | 1,416 | 11.7 | 276 | 3 | 4 | 7 | 11 | 20 | 43 | 83 |

### 80.06: RMVL PROSTH KNEE INC. Formerly included in operation group(s) 738.

| Type of Patients | Observed Patients | Avg. Stay | Vari-ance | 10th | 25th | 50th | 75th | 90th | 95th | 99th |
|---|---|---|---|---|---|---|---|---|---|---|
| **1. SINGLE DX** | | | | | | | | | | |
| 0–19 Years | 1 | 5.0 | 0 | 5 | 5 | 5 | 5 | 5 | 5 | 5 |
| 20–34 | 0 | | | | | | | | | |
| 35–49 | 6 | 4.0 | <1 | 3 | 3 | 4 | 4 | 6 | 6 | 6 |
| 50–64 | 16 | 4.3 | 1 | 3 | 4 | 4 | 5 | 6 | 6 | 6 |
| 65+ | 13 | 5.1 | 36 | 1 | 1 | 3 | 5 | 16 | 23 | 23 |
| **2. MULTIPLE DX** | | | | | | | | | | |
| 0–19 Years | 4 | 8.6 | 5 | 6 | 8 | 8 | 8 | 13 | 13 | 13 |
| 20–34 | 8 | 11.6 | 177 | 4 | 4 | 8 | 8 | 43 | 43 | 43 |
| 35–49 | 51 | 7.0 | 16 | 4 | 5 | 5 | 8 | 12 | 12 | 30 |
| 50–64 | 159 | 7.9 | 37 | 3 | 4 | 6 | 9 | 15 | 20 | 36 |
| 65+ | 450 | 9.1 | 79 | 3 | 4 | 7 | 11 | 16 | 21 | 43 |
| **TOTAL SINGLE DX** | 36 | 4.5 | 14 | 1 | 3 | 4 | 5 | 6 | 10 | 23 |
| **TOTAL MULTIPLE DX** | 672 | 8.7 | 65 | 3 | 4 | 7 | 10 | 15 | 19 | 43 |
| **TOTAL** | | | | | | | | | | |
| 0–19 Years | 5 | 7.9 | 7 | 5 | 6 | 8 | 8 | 13 | 13 | 13 |
| 20–34 | 8 | 11.6 | 177 | 4 | 4 | 8 | 8 | 43 | 43 | 43 |
| 35–49 | 57 | 6.9 | 15 | 3 | 4 | 6 | 8 | 12 | 12 | 30 |
| 50–64 | 175 | 7.5 | 34 | 3 | 4 | 6 | 9 | 14 | 17 | 36 |
| 65+ | 463 | 9.0 | 79 | 3 | 4 | 7 | 11 | 16 | 21 | 43 |
| **GRAND TOTAL** | 708 | 8.5 | 64 | 3 | 4 | 6 | 10 | 15 | 19 | 43 |

# United States, October 1998–September 1999 Data, by Operation

## 80.1: OTHER ARTHROTOMY. Formerly included in operation group(s) 738.

| Type of Patients | Observed Patients | Avg. Stay | Variance | Percentiles | | | | | | |
|---|---|---|---|---|---|---|---|---|---|---|
| | | | | 10th | 25th | 50th | 75th | 90th | 95th | 99th |
| **1. SINGLE DX** | | | | | | | | | | |
| 0–19 Years | 343 | 3.8 | 8 | 1 | 2 | 3 | 5 | 7 | 9 | 13 |
| 20–34 | 176 | 2.7 | 4 | 1 | 1 | 2 | 3 | 5 | 6 | 11 |
| 35–49 | 153 | 3.0 | 5 | 1 | 2 | 3 | 3 | 5 | 6 | 11 |
| 50–64 | 76 | 3.4 | 4 | 1 | 1 | 3 | 5 | 6 | 7 | 10 |
| 65+ | 43 | 3.0 | 6 | 1 | 1 | 3 | 4 | 8 | 9 | 9 |
| **2. MULTIPLE DX** | | | | | | | | | | |
| 0–19 Years | 656 | 6.0 | 34 | 2 | 3 | 5 | 7 | 11 | 15 | 26 |
| 20–34 | 536 | 4.6 | 24 | 1 | 2 | 3 | 6 | 8 | 12 | 24 |
| 35–49 | 889 | 5.9 | 37 | 2 | 2 | 4 | 8 | 12 | 18 | 31 |
| 50–64 | 784 | 7.4 | 50 | 1 | 3 | 5 | 10 | 14 | 19 | 32 |
| 65+ | 1,118 | 8.1 | 44 | 2 | 4 | 6 | 10 | 16 | 20 | 31 |
| **TOTAL SINGLE DX** | 791 | 3.3 | 6 | 1 | 2 | 3 | 4 | 6 | 8 | 12 |
| **TOTAL MULTIPLE DX** | 3,983 | 6.5 | 40 | 2 | 3 | 5 | 8 | 14 | 18 | 31 |
| **TOTAL** | | | | | | | | | | |
| 0–19 Years | 999 | 5.2 | 26 | 1 | 2 | 4 | 7 | 10 | 13 | 22 |
| 20–34 | 712 | 4.2 | 21 | 1 | 2 | 3 | 5 | 7 | 11 | 23 |
| 35–49 | 1,042 | 5.4 | 33 | 1 | 2 | 3 | 7 | 10 | 16 | 30 |
| 50–64 | 860 | 7.0 | 47 | 1 | 3 | 5 | 9 | 14 | 19 | 32 |
| 65+ | 1,161 | 7.9 | 44 | 2 | 4 | 6 | 10 | 16 | 20 | 31 |
| **GRAND TOTAL** | 4,774 | 6.0 | 36 | 1 | 2 | 4 | 7 | 12 | 16 | 30 |

## 80.11: OTH ARTHROTOMY SHOULDER. Formerly included in operation group(s) 738.

| Type of Patients | Observed Patients | Avg. Stay | Variance | Percentiles | | | | | | |
|---|---|---|---|---|---|---|---|---|---|---|
| | | | | 10th | 25th | 50th | 75th | 90th | 95th | 99th |
| **1. SINGLE DX** | | | | | | | | | | |
| 0–19 Years | 10 | 3.9 | 10 | 1 | 1 | 4 | 6 | 9 | 9 | 9 |
| 20–34 | 7 | 1.6 | <1 | 1 | 1 | 1 | 2 | 2 | 3 | 3 |
| 35–49 | 5 | 1.1 | <1 | 1 | 1 | 1 | 1 | 1 | 2 | 2 |
| 50–64 | 9 | 2.8 | 4 | 1 | 1 | 1 | 5 | 5 | 7 | 7 |
| 65+ | 4 | 3.3 | 6 | 1 | 2 | 3 | 3 | 7 | 7 | 7 |
| **2. MULTIPLE DX** | | | | | | | | | | |
| 0–19 Years | 25 | 7.0 | 102 | 1 | 3 | 5 | 8 | 17 | 17 | 82 |
| 20–34 | 26 | 4.1 | 29 | 1 | 1 | 3 | 5 | 9 | 21 | 22 |
| 35–49 | 56 | 9.4 | 109 | 1 | 2 | 6 | 10 | 25 | 25 | 58 |
| 50–64 | 53 | 6.2 | 46 | 1 | 2 | 4 | 6 | 14 | 15 | 36 |
| 65+ | 107 | 8.3 | 46 | 3 | 4 | 7 | 11 | 14 | 17 | 34 |
| **TOTAL SINGLE DX** | 35 | 2.7 | 5 | 1 | 1 | 1 | 4 | 6 | 9 | 9 |
| **TOTAL MULTIPLE DX** | 267 | 7.5 | 66 | 1 | 3 | 5 | 10 | 16 | 22 | 36 |
| **TOTAL** | | | | | | | | | | |
| 0–19 Years | 35 | 6.3 | 83 | 1 | 1 | 4 | 7 | 17 | 17 | 82 |
| 20–34 | 33 | 3.7 | 26 | 1 | 1 | 1 | 4 | 9 | 21 | 22 |
| 35–49 | 61 | 8.8 | 106 | 1 | 2 | 4 | 10 | 25 | 25 | 58 |
| 50–64 | 62 | 5.6 | 40 | 1 | 2 | 4 | 6 | 14 | 15 | 36 |
| 65+ | 111 | 8.2 | 46 | 3 | 4 | 7 | 11 | 14 | 17 | 34 |
| **GRAND TOTAL** | 302 | 7.0 | 61 | 1 | 2 | 5 | 10 | 14 | 21 | 36 |

## 80.12: OTH ARTHROTOMY ELBOW. Formerly included in operation group(s) 738.

| Type of Patients | Observed Patients | Avg. Stay | Variance | Percentiles | | | | | | |
|---|---|---|---|---|---|---|---|---|---|---|
| | | | | 10th | 25th | 50th | 75th | 90th | 95th | 99th |
| **1. SINGLE DX** | | | | | | | | | | |
| 0–19 Years | 24 | 1.9 | 4 | 1 | 1 | 1 | 2 | 2 | 6 | 9 |
| 20–34 | 13 | 1.8 | <1 | 1 | 1 | 2 | 4 | 4 | 4 | 4 |
| 35–49 | 14 | 2.8 | 4 | 1 | 2 | 2 | 2 | 3 | 7 | 19 |
| 50–64 | 6 | 1.6 | 2 | 1 | 1 | 2 | 2 | 2 | 7 | 7 |
| 65+ | 4 | 2.6 | <1 | 2 | 2 | 3 | 3 | 3 | 3 | 3 |
| **2. MULTIPLE DX** | | | | | | | | | | |
| 0–19 Years | 42 | 6.4 | 38 | 3 | 3 | 6 | 9 | 11 | 11 | 57 |
| 20–34 | 33 | 3.8 | 6 | 1 | 2 | 4 | 6 | 8 | 8 | 12 |
| 35–49 | 78 | 3.7 | 17 | 1 | 2 | 2 | 5 | 7 | 8 | 19 |
| 50–64 | 58 | 3.1 | 13 | 1 | 1 | 2 | 6 | 6 | 10 | 22 |
| 65+ | 95 | 6.1 | 9 | 2 | 3 | 6 | 10 | 10 | 11 | 12 |
| **TOTAL SINGLE DX** | 61 | 2.0 | 3 | 1 | 1 | 1 | 2 | 2 | 6 | 9 |
| **TOTAL MULTIPLE DX** | 306 | 4.6 | 17 | 1 | 2 | 4 | 7 | 8 | 11 | 19 |
| **TOTAL** | | | | | | | | | | |
| 0–19 Years | 66 | 4.2 | 26 | 1 | 1 | 3 | 7 | 8 | 9 | 14 |
| 20–34 | 46 | 3.3 | 5 | 1 | 2 | 3 | 5 | 7 | 8 | 12 |
| 35–49 | 92 | 3.6 | 15 | 1 | 2 | 2 | 6 | 7 | 8 | 19 |
| 50–64 | 64 | 2.9 | 12 | 1 | 1 | 2 | 6 | 6 | 7 | 22 |
| 65+ | 99 | 6.0 | 9 | 2 | 3 | 6 | 10 | 10 | 11 | 12 |
| **GRAND TOTAL** | 367 | 4.1 | 15 | 1 | 2 | 3 | 6 | 8 | 10 | 14 |

## 80.14: OTH ARTHROTOMY HAND. Formerly included in operation group(s) 738.

| Type of Patients | Observed Patients | Avg. Stay | Variance | Percentiles | | | | | | |
|---|---|---|---|---|---|---|---|---|---|---|
| | | | | 10th | 25th | 50th | 75th | 90th | 95th | 99th |
| **1. SINGLE DX** | | | | | | | | | | |
| 0–19 Years | 17 | 3.3 | 8 | 1 | 2 | 2 | 3 | 3 | 10 | 10 |
| 20–34 | 30 | 4.0 | 5 | 1 | 3 | 3 | 6 | 5 | 7 | 11 |
| 35–49 | 22 | 2.6 | 3 | 1 | 2 | 2 | 2 | 5 | 7 | 8 |
| 50–64 | 6 | 2.2 | 2 | 1 | 2 | 2 | 2 | 7 | 7 | 7 |
| 65+ | 8 | 1.6 | 2 | 1 | 1 | 1 | 2 | 4 | 4 | 6 |
| **2. MULTIPLE DX** | | | | | | | | | | |
| 0–19 Years | 30 | 3.1 | 3 | 1 | 3 | 3 | 3 | 5 | 7 | 8 |
| 20–34 | 106 | 3.4 | 4 | 2 | 2 | 3 | 5 | 5 | 6 | 12 |
| 35–49 | 127 | 3.6 | 8 | 1 | 2 | 3 | 4 | 6 | 8 | 15 |
| 50–64 | 61 | 4.0 | 8 | 2 | 3 | 3 | 5 | 8 | 11 | 12 |
| 65+ | 51 | 5.9 | 14 | 3 | 3 | 4 | 8 | 9 | 12 | 23 |
| **TOTAL SINGLE DX** | 83 | 3.2 | 5 | 1 | 2 | 2 | 4 | 7 | 7 | 11 |
| **TOTAL MULTIPLE DX** | 375 | 3.8 | 8 | 2 | 3 | 3 | 5 | 9 | 9 | 14 |
| **TOTAL** | | | | | | | | | | |
| 0–19 Years | 47 | 3.2 | 5 | 1 | 2 | 3 | 3 | 6 | 10 | 10 |
| 20–34 | 136 | 3.6 | 5 | 2 | 2 | 3 | 5 | 6 | 7 | 12 |
| 35–49 | 149 | 3.4 | 8 | 1 | 2 | 3 | 4 | 6 | 8 | 14 |
| 50–64 | 67 | 3.9 | 8 | 1 | 2 | 3 | 5 | 8 | 11 | 12 |
| 65+ | 59 | 5.1 | 14 | 3 | 4 | 4 | 8 | 9 | 12 | 17 |
| **GRAND TOTAL** | 458 | 3.7 | 7 | 1 | 2 | 3 | 5 | 9 | 9 | 12 |

Length of Stay by Diagnosis and Operation, United States, 2000

# United States, October 1998–September 1999 Data, by Operation

## 80.2: ARTHROSCOPY. Formerly included in operation group(s) 742.

| Type of Patients | Observed Patients | Avg. Stay | Variance | Percentiles | | | | | | |
|---|---|---|---|---|---|---|---|---|---|---|
| | | | | 10th | 25th | 50th | 75th | 90th | 95th | 99th |
| **1. SINGLE DX** | | | | | | | | | | |
| 0–19 Years | 74 | 1.9 | 2 | 1 | 1 | 1 | 2 | 3 | 5 | 11 |
| 20–34 | 79 | 1.5 | <1 | 1 | 1 | 1 | 2 | 2 | 4 | 4 |
| 35–49 | 77 | 1.7 | <1 | 1 | 1 | 1 | 2 | 3 | 4 | 6 |
| 50–64 | 39 | 1.8 | <1 | 1 | 1 | 2 | 2 | 3 | 4 | 4 |
| 65+ | 21 | 1.3 | <1 | 1 | 1 | 1 | 1 | 2 | 4 | 4 |
| **2. MULTIPLE DX** | | | | | | | | | | |
| 0–19 Years | 71 | 2.8 | 9 | 1 | 1 | 2 | 3 | 6 | 9 | 15 |
| 20–34 | 104 | 3.4 | 13 | 1 | 1 | 2 | 3 | 9 | 13 | 13 |
| 35–49 | 208 | 2.9 | 14 | 1 | 1 | 1 | 3 | 7 | 11 | 18 |
| 50–64 | 172 | 4.1 | 41 | 1 | 2 | 2 | 5 | 9 | 20 | 30 |
| 65+ | 188 | 4.8 | 41 | 1 | 2 | 2 | 6 | 14 | 15 | 36 |
| **TOTAL SINGLE DX** | 290 | 1.7 | 1 | 1 | 1 | 1 | 2 | 3 | 4 | 6 |
| **TOTAL MULTIPLE DX** | 743 | 3.7 | 25 | 1 | 1 | 2 | 4 | 9 | 13 | 22 |
| **TOTAL** | | | | | | | | | | |
| 0–19 Years | 145 | 2.4 | 6 | 1 | 1 | 2 | 3 | 5 | 6 | 11 |
| 20–34 | 183 | 2.8 | 9 | 1 | 1 | 2 | 3 | 6 | 13 | 13 |
| 35–49 | 285 | 2.7 | 12 | 1 | 1 | 1 | 2 | 7 | 10 | 16 |
| 50–64 | 211 | 3.8 | 36 | 1 | 1 | 2 | 4 | 9 | 20 | 23 |
| 65+ | 209 | 4.6 | 39 | 1 | 2 | 2 | 6 | 14 | 14 | 32 |
| **GRAND TOTAL** | 1,033 | 3.2 | 20 | 1 | 1 | 2 | 3 | 8 | 13 | 20 |

## 80.21: SHOULDER ARTHROSCOPY. Formerly included in operation group(s) 742.

| Type of Patients | Observed Patients | Avg. Stay | Variance | Percentiles | | | | | | |
|---|---|---|---|---|---|---|---|---|---|---|
| | | | | 10th | 25th | 50th | 75th | 90th | 95th | 99th |
| **1. SINGLE DX** | | | | | | | | | | |
| 0–19 Years | 13 | 1.6 | 1 | 1 | 1 | 1 | 1 | 4 | 4 | 4 |
| 20–34 | 33 | 1.3 | <1 | 1 | 1 | 1 | 1 | 2 | 2 | 5 |
| 35–49 | 38 | 1.4 | <1 | 1 | 1 | 1 | 2 | 2 | 3 | 4 |
| 50–64 | 25 | 1.5 | <1 | 1 | 1 | 1 | 2 | 2 | 3 | 4 |
| 65+ | 18 | 1.2 | <1 | 1 | 1 | 1 | 1 | 2 | 2 | 4 |
| **2. MULTIPLE DX** | | | | | | | | | | |
| 0–19 Years | 10 | 4.2 | 55 | 1 | 1 | 2 | 2 | 24 | 24 | 24 |
| 20–34 | 21 | 1.9 | 2 | 1 | 1 | 1 | 2 | 3 | 5 | 9 |
| 35–49 | 62 | 2.3 | 7 | 1 | 1 | 1 | 2 | 7 | 7 | 13 |
| 50–64 | 72 | 3.6 | 38 | 1 | 1 | 2 | 2 | 17 | 20 | 23 |
| 65+ | 77 | 2.4 | 7 | 1 | 1 | 2 | 2 | 5 | 8 | 12 |
| **TOTAL SINGLE DX** | 127 | 1.4 | <1 | 1 | 1 | 1 | 2 | 2 | 3 | 4 |
| **TOTAL MULTIPLE DX** | 242 | 2.9 | 21 | 1 | 1 | 1 | 2 | 5 | 14 | 20 |
| **TOTAL** | | | | | | | | | | |
| 0–19 Years | 23 | 2.5 | 20 | 1 | 1 | 1 | 2 | 4 | 4 | 24 |
| 20–34 | 54 | 1.5 | 1 | 1 | 1 | 1 | 2 | 3 | 4 | 5 |
| 35–49 | 100 | 2.0 | 5 | 1 | 1 | 1 | 2 | 3 | 7 | 13 |
| 50–64 | 97 | 3.3 | 33 | 1 | 1 | 1 | 2 | 9 | 20 | 23 |
| 65+ | 95 | 2.2 | 6 | 1 | 1 | 1 | 2 | 4 | 8 | 12 |
| **GRAND TOTAL** | 369 | 2.4 | 15 | 1 | 1 | 1 | 2 | 4 | 8 | 20 |

## 80.15: OTH ARTHROTOMY HIP. Formerly included in operation group(s) 738.

| Type of Patients | Observed Patients | Avg. Stay | Variance | Percentiles | | | | | | |
|---|---|---|---|---|---|---|---|---|---|---|
| | | | | 10th | 25th | 50th | 75th | 90th | 95th | 99th |
| **1. SINGLE DX** | | | | | | | | | | |
| 0–19 Years | 112 | 4.6 | 8 | 2 | 3 | 4 | 6 | 8 | 9 | 11 |
| 20–34 | 8 | 4.0 | 3 | 2 | 3 | 4 | 5 | 6 | 8 | 8 |
| 35–49 | 18 | 5.9 | 58 | 1 | 2 | 3 | 5 | 23 | 23 | 23 |
| 50–64 | 10 | 4.8 | 5 | 2 | 3 | 4 | 6 | 9 | 9 | 9 |
| 65+ | 11 | 3.4 | 4 | 1 | 3 | 3 | 4 | 8 | 8 | 8 |
| **2. MULTIPLE DX** | | | | | | | | | | |
| 0–19 Years | 229 | 7.2 | 33 | 2 | 4 | 6 | 8 | 13 | 18 | 28 |
| 20–34 | 84 | 7.9 | 62 | 2 | 4 | 7 | 9 | 14 | 22 | 50 |
| 35–49 | 100 | 10.4 | 61 | 3 | 4 | 9 | 14 | 18 | 22 | 43 |
| 50–64 | 96 | 9.2 | 62 | 2 | 5 | 6 | 11 | 21 | 24 | 41 |
| 65+ | 208 | 10.0 | 56 | 2 | 5 | 7 | 15 | 20 | 22 | 29 |
| **TOTAL SINGLE DX** | 159 | 4.7 | 12 | 2 | 3 | 4 | 6 | 8 | 9 | 23 |
| **TOTAL MULTIPLE DX** | 717 | 8.7 | 52 | 2 | 4 | 7 | 11 | 18 | 21 | 42 |
| **TOTAL** | | | | | | | | | | |
| 0–19 Years | 341 | 6.4 | 27 | 2 | 3 | 5 | 8 | 12 | 15 | 24 |
| 20–34 | 92 | 7.6 | 58 | 2 | 4 | 7 | 9 | 14 | 19 | 50 |
| 35–49 | 118 | 9.9 | 62 | 2 | 4 | 8 | 13 | 18 | 23 | 43 |
| 50–64 | 106 | 8.8 | 60 | 2 | 4 | 6 | 11 | 21 | 24 | 41 |
| 65+ | 219 | 9.7 | 56 | 2 | 4 | 7 | 15 | 20 | 22 | 29 |
| **GRAND TOTAL** | 876 | 8.0 | 47 | 2 | 4 | 6 | 10 | 18 | 21 | 39 |

## 80.16: OTH ARTHROTOMY KNEE. Formerly included in operation group(s) 738.

| Type of Patients | Observed Patients | Avg. Stay | Variance | Percentiles | | | | | | |
|---|---|---|---|---|---|---|---|---|---|---|
| | | | | 10th | 25th | 50th | 75th | 90th | 95th | 99th |
| **1. SINGLE DX** | | | | | | | | | | |
| 0–19 Years | 135 | 3.8 | 9 | 1 | 2 | 3 | 5 | 7 | 8 | 21 |
| 20–34 | 96 | 2.4 | 4 | 1 | 1 | 3 | 3 | 5 | 5 | 16 |
| 35–49 | 79 | 2.8 | <1 | 2 | 3 | 3 | 3 | 3 | 4 | 7 |
| 50–64 | 35 | 3.0 | 5 | 1 | 2 | 3 | 4 | 6 | 6 | 11 |
| 65+ | 15 | 3.8 | 8 | 1 | 1 | 3 | 4 | 9 | 9 | 10 |
| **2. MULTIPLE DX** | | | | | | | | | | |
| 0–19 Years | 226 | 4.8 | 21 | 1 | 2 | 3 | 6 | 10 | 15 | 26 |
| 20–34 | 223 | 4.4 | 21 | 1 | 2 | 3 | 6 | 7 | 10 | 24 |
| 35–49 | 393 | 5.4 | 25 | 2 | 2 | 4 | 8 | 10 | 12 | 30 |
| 50–64 | 408 | 8.6 | 60 | 2 | 4 | 6 | 13 | 15 | 20 | 32 |
| 65+ | 531 | 8.2 | 47 | 3 | 4 | 6 | 10 | 14 | 21 | 39 |
| **TOTAL SINGLE DX** | 360 | 3.1 | 5 | 1 | 2 | 3 | 3 | 5 | 7 | 13 |
| **TOTAL MULTIPLE DX** | 1,781 | 6.6 | 40 | 2 | 2 | 5 | 9 | 14 | 17 | 31 |
| **TOTAL** | | | | | | | | | | |
| 0–19 Years | 361 | 4.4 | 16 | 2 | 2 | 3 | 5 | 8 | 12 | 21 |
| 20–34 | 319 | 3.9 | 17 | 1 | 2 | 3 | 5 | 7 | 9 | 23 |
| 35–49 | 472 | 4.8 | 21 | 2 | 2 | 3 | 7 | 10 | 11 | 30 |
| 50–64 | 443 | 8.2 | 58 | 2 | 3 | 6 | 12 | 14 | 20 | 32 |
| 65+ | 546 | 8.1 | 47 | 2 | 4 | 6 | 10 | 14 | 21 | 39 |
| **GRAND TOTAL** | 2,141 | 5.9 | 35 | 2 | 2 | 4 | 8 | 12 | 15 | 30 |

Length of Stay by Diagnosis and Operation, United States, 2000

## United States, October 1998–September 1999 Data, by Operation

### 80.26: KNEE ARTHROSCOPY. Formerly included in operation group(s) 742.

| Type of Patients | Observed Patients | Avg. Stay | Vari-ance | Percentiles | | | | | | |
|---|---|---|---|---|---|---|---|---|---|---|
| | | | | 10th | 25th | 50th | 75th | 90th | 95th | 99th |
| **1. SINGLE DX** | | | | | | | | | | |
| 0–19 Years | 56 | 2.0 | 3 | 1 | 1 | 2 | 2 | 3 | 5 | 11 |
| 20–34 | 44 | 1.5 | <1 | 1 | 1 | 1 | 2 | 2 | 3 | 4 |
| 35–49 | 36 | 1.9 | 1 | 1 | 1 | 2 | 2 | 4 | 3 | 6 |
| 50–64 | 10 | 2.3 | <1 | 1 | 2 | 2 | 3 | 4 | 4 | 4 |
| 65+ | 3 | 1.5 | 1 | 1 | 1 | 1 | 1 | 4 | 4 | 4 |
| **2. MULTIPLE DX** | | | | | | | | | | |
| 0–19 Years | 56 | 2.7 | 6 | 1 | 1 | 2 | 3 | 6 | 9 | 15 |
| 20–34 | 78 | 3.7 | 14 | 1 | 1 | 2 | 4 | 13 | 13 | 13 |
| 35–49 | 129 | 3.1 | 17 | 1 | 1 | 1 | 3 | 8 | 11 | 22 |
| 50–64 | 92 | 4.8 | 48 | 1 | 2 | 3 | 6 | 9 | 11 | 45 |
| 65+ | 105 | 5.7 | 51 | 1 | 1 | 3 | 8 | 14 | 15 | 43 |
| **TOTAL SINGLE DX** | 149 | 1.9 | 2 | 1 | 1 | 1 | 2 | 3 | 4 | 6 |
| **TOTAL MULTIPLE DX** | 460 | 4.0 | 28 | 1 | 1 | 2 | 5 | 10 | 14 | 24 |
| **TOTAL** | | | | | | | | | | |
| 0–19 Years | 112 | 2.4 | 5 | 1 | 1 | 2 | 3 | 5 | 8 | 11 |
| 20–34 | 122 | 3.1 | 11 | 1 | 1 | 2 | 3 | 8 | 13 | 13 |
| 35–49 | 165 | 2.9 | 15 | 1 | 1 | 1 | 3 | 7 | 11 | 18 |
| 50–64 | 102 | 4.6 | 44 | 1 | 2 | 3 | 5 | 9 | 11 | 45 |
| 65+ | 108 | 5.6 | 50 | 1 | 1 | 3 | 8 | 14 | 15 | 43 |
| **GRAND TOTAL** | 609 | 3.5 | 23 | 1 | 1 | 2 | 4 | 9 | 13 | 18 |

### 80.4: JT CAPSULE/LIG/CART DIV. Formerly included in operation group(s) 738.

| Type of Patients | Observed Patients | Avg. Stay | Vari-ance | Percentiles | | | | | | |
|---|---|---|---|---|---|---|---|---|---|---|
| | | | | 10th | 25th | 50th | 75th | 90th | 95th | 99th |
| **1. SINGLE DX** | | | | | | | | | | |
| 0–19 Years | 287 | 1.6 | 1 | 1 | 1 | 1 | 2 | 3 | 4 | 7 |
| 20–34 | 65 | 1.9 | <1 | 1 | 1 | 2 | 2 | 3 | 3 | 4 |
| 35–49 | 67 | 1.8 | <1 | 1 | 1 | 2 | 2 | 3 | 3 | 4 |
| 50–64 | 26 | 2.4 | <1 | 1 | 2 | 2 | 3 | 4 | 5 | 5 |
| 65+ | 9 | 3.5 | 4 | 1 | 2 | 4 | 4 | 8 | 8 | 8 |
| **2. MULTIPLE DX** | | | | | | | | | | |
| 0–19 Years | 297 | 2.3 | 8 | 1 | 1 | 2 | 3 | 4 | 5 | 8 |
| 20–34 | 135 | 3.4 | 20 | 1 | 2 | 3 | 4 | 7 | 7 | 7 |
| 35–49 | 233 | 2.4 | 8 | 1 | 1 | 2 | 4 | 6 | 6 | 22 |
| 50–64 | 158 | 3.7 | 9 | 1 | 2 | 3 | 6 | 6 | 6 | 10 |
| 65+ | 164 | 3.8 | 9 | 1 | 2 | 3 | 4 | 6 | 9 | 20 |
| **TOTAL SINGLE DX** | 454 | 1.7 | 1 | 1 | 1 | 1 | 2 | 3 | 4 | 7 |
| **TOTAL MULTIPLE DX** | 987 | 2.9 | 10 | 1 | 1 | 2 | 3 | 6 | 7 | 14 |
| **TOTAL** | | | | | | | | | | |
| 0–19 Years | 584 | 1.9 | 5 | 1 | 1 | 1 | 2 | 3 | 5 | 7 |
| 20–34 | 200 | 2.9 | 13 | 1 | 2 | 2 | 3 | 6 | 7 | 7 |
| 35–49 | 300 | 2.2 | 6 | 1 | 1 | 2 | 3 | 3 | 5 | 14 |
| 50–64 | 184 | 3.6 | 9 | 1 | 2 | 3 | 5 | 6 | 6 | 10 |
| 65+ | 173 | 3.8 | 9 | 1 | 2 | 3 | 4 | 6 | 9 | 20 |
| **GRAND TOTAL** | 1,441 | 2.5 | 8 | 1 | 1 | 2 | 3 | 5 | 6 | 10 |

### 80.3: BIOPSY JOINT STRUCTURE. Formerly included in operation group(s) 743.

| Type of Patients | Observed Patients | Avg. Stay | Vari-ance | Percentiles | | | | | | |
|---|---|---|---|---|---|---|---|---|---|---|
| | | | | 10th | 25th | 50th | 75th | 90th | 95th | 99th |
| **1. SINGLE DX** | | | | | | | | | | |
| 0–19 Years | 13 | 4.0 | 6 | 1 | 1 | 5 | 6 | 6 | 8 | 8 |
| 20–34 | 4 | 3.4 | 1 | 1 | 2 | 4 | 4 | 6 | 5 | 5 |
| 35–49 | 6 | 4.2 | 3 | 2 | 3 | 4 | 5 | 7 | 7 | 7 |
| 50–64 | 4 | 3.2 | 3 | 1 | 1 | 4 | 4 | 5 | 5 | 5 |
| 65+ | 2 | 1.2 | <1 | 1 | 1 | 1 | 1 | 2 | 2 | 2 |
| **2. MULTIPLE DX** | | | | | | | | | | |
| 0–19 Years | 47 | 6.7 | 28 | 1 | 4 | 5 | 7 | 15 | 20 | 22 |
| 20–34 | 26 | 5.2 | 28 | 1 | 3 | 3 | 6 | 14 | 16 | 27 |
| 35–49 | 43 | 7.8 | 44 | 2 | 4 | 8 | 9 | 11 | 17 | 36 |
| 50–64 | 68 | 8.5 | 26 | 3 | 5 | 8 | 9 | 13 | 22 | 29 |
| 65+ | 150 | 7.7 | 51 | 2 | 3 | 6 | 9 | 15 | 25 | 36 |
| **TOTAL SINGLE DX** | 29 | 3.6 | 4 | 1 | 2 | 4 | 5 | 6 | 7 | 8 |
| **TOTAL MULTIPLE DX** | 334 | 7.6 | 41 | 2 | 4 | 6 | 9 | 15 | 22 | 34 |
| **TOTAL** | | | | | | | | | | |
| 0–19 Years | 60 | 6.4 | 26 | 1 | 1 | 5 | 7 | 15 | 18 | 22 |
| 20–34 | 30 | 4.9 | 23 | 2 | 2 | 4 | 5 | 14 | 14 | 27 |
| 35–49 | 49 | 7.4 | 41 | 1 | 4 | 8 | 9 | 10 | 15 | 36 |
| 50–64 | 72 | 8.2 | 26 | 2 | 5 | 8 | 9 | 13 | 22 | 29 |
| 65+ | 152 | 7.6 | 51 | 2 | 3 | 6 | 9 | 15 | 25 | 36 |
| **GRAND TOTAL** | 363 | 7.3 | 39 | 2 | 4 | 6 | 9 | 13 | 21 | 34 |

### 80.46: KNEE STRUCTURE DIVISION. Formerly included in operation group(s) 738.

| Type of Patients | Observed Patients | Avg. Stay | Vari-ance | Percentiles | | | | | | |
|---|---|---|---|---|---|---|---|---|---|---|
| | | | | 10th | 25th | 50th | 75th | 90th | 95th | 99th |
| **1. SINGLE DX** | | | | | | | | | | |
| 0–19 Years | 62 | 2.3 | 2 | 1 | 1 | 2 | 3 | 4 | 4 | 6 |
| 20–34 | 56 | 1.9 | <1 | 1 | 1 | 2 | 2 | 3 | 3 | 6 |
| 35–49 | 40 | 1.7 | 1 | 1 | 1 | 2 | 3 | 3 | 3 | 7 |
| 50–64 | 18 | 2.6 | 1 | 1 | 2 | 2 | 3 | 4 | 5 | 5 |
| 65+ | 7 | 3.0 | 2 | 1 | 2 | 4 | 4 | 4 | 5 | 5 |
| **2. MULTIPLE DX** | | | | | | | | | | |
| 0–19 Years | 97 | 2.4 | 3 | 1 | 1 | 2 | 3 | 4 | 5 | 8 |
| 20–34 | 90 | 2.8 | 3 | 1 | 1 | 2 | 3 | 4 | 7 | 7 |
| 35–49 | 150 | 2.5 | 5 | 1 | 2 | 2 | 3 | 6 | 6 | 14 |
| 50–64 | 98 | 4.2 | 5 | 2 | 2 | 4 | 6 | 6 | 6 | 9 |
| 65+ | 122 | 4.0 | 8 | 2 | 3 | 3 | 4 | 6 | 11 | 20 |
| **TOTAL SINGLE DX** | 183 | 2.0 | 1 | 1 | 2 | 2 | 2 | 4 | 4 | 6 |
| **TOTAL MULTIPLE DX** | 557 | 3.1 | 6 | 1 | 3 | 3 | 4 | 6 | 7 | 11 |
| **TOTAL** | | | | | | | | | | |
| 0–19 Years | 159 | 2.4 | 2 | 1 | 1 | 2 | 3 | 4 | 5 | 8 |
| 20–34 | 146 | 2.4 | 2 | 1 | 1 | 2 | 3 | 4 | 6 | 7 |
| 35–49 | 190 | 2.3 | 4 | 1 | 2 | 2 | 3 | 4 | 5 | 7 |
| 50–64 | 116 | 4.1 | 4 | 2 | 2 | 3 | 6 | 6 | 6 | 9 |
| 65+ | 129 | 3.9 | 8 | 2 | 2 | 3 | 4 | 6 | 7 | 20 |
| **GRAND TOTAL** | 740 | 2.8 | 5 | 1 | 2 | 3 | 3 | 6 | 6 | 11 |

Length of Stay by Diagnosis and Operation, United States, 2000

# United States, October 1998–September 1999 Data, by Operation

## 80.5: IV DISC EXC/DESTRUCTION. Formerly included in operation group(s) 739, 740.

| Type of Patients | Observed Patients | Avg. Stay | Variance | 10th | 25th | 50th | 75th | 90th | 95th | 99th |
|---|---|---|---|---|---|---|---|---|---|---|
| **1. SINGLE DX** | | | | | | | | | | |
| 0–19 Years | 329 | 1.8 | 3 | 1 | 1 | 1 | 2 | 3 | 4 | 11 |
| 20–34 | 6,068 | 1.6 | 1 | 1 | 1 | 1 | 2 | 3 | 3 | 5 |
| 35–49 | 13,346 | 1.6 | 1 | 1 | 1 | 1 | 2 | 3 | 3 | 6 |
| 50–64 | 5,332 | 1.7 | 2 | 1 | 1 | 1 | 2 | 3 | 4 | 7 |
| 65+ | 1,413 | 2.1 | 2 | 1 | 1 | 2 | 3 | 4 | 4 | 6 |
| **2. MULTIPLE DX** | | | | | | | | | | |
| 0–19 Years | 210 | 4.4 | 42 | 1 | 1 | 2 | 6 | 9 | 16 | 33 |
| 20–34 | 4,171 | 2.4 | 7 | 1 | 1 | 2 | 3 | 4 | 6 | 12 |
| 35–49 | 14,838 | 2.4 | 6 | 1 | 1 | 2 | 3 | 4 | 6 | 11 |
| 50–64 | 11,868 | 2.6 | 7 | 1 | 1 | 2 | 3 | 5 | 7 | 13 |
| 65+ | 8,723 | 3.7 | 14 | 1 | 2 | 3 | 4 | 7 | 10 | 19 |
| **TOTAL SINGLE DX** | 26,488 | 1.7 | 1 | 1 | 1 | 1 | 2 | 3 | 4 | 6 |
| **TOTAL MULTIPLE DX** | 39,810 | 2.7 | 8 | 1 | 2 | 2 | 3 | 5 | 7 | 14 |
| **TOTAL** | | | | | | | | | | |
| 0–19 Years | 539 | 2.8 | 19 | 1 | 1 | 2 | 3 | 6 | 9 | 18 |
| 20–34 | 10,239 | 1.9 | 3 | 1 | 1 | 1 | 2 | 3 | 5 | 9 |
| 35–49 | 28,184 | 2.0 | 4 | 1 | 1 | 1 | 2 | 4 | 5 | 9 |
| 50–64 | 17,200 | 2.3 | 6 | 1 | 1 | 2 | 3 | 5 | 7 | 11 |
| 65+ | 10,136 | 3.5 | 13 | 1 | 2 | 3 | 4 | 7 | 9 | 18 |
| **GRAND TOTAL** | 66,298 | 2.3 | 6 | 1 | 1 | 2 | 3 | 4 | 6 | 12 |

## 80.51: IV DISC EXCISION. Formerly included in operation group(s) 740.

| Type of Patients | Observed Patients | Avg. Stay | Variance | 10th | 25th | 50th | 75th | 90th | 95th | 99th |
|---|---|---|---|---|---|---|---|---|---|---|
| **1. SINGLE DX** | | | | | | | | | | |
| 0–19 Years | 326 | 1.8 | 3 | 1 | 1 | 1 | 2 | 3 | 4 | 11 |
| 20–34 | 6,049 | 1.6 | 1 | 1 | 1 | 1 | 2 | 3 | 3 | 5 |
| 35–49 | 13,304 | 1.6 | 1 | 1 | 1 | 1 | 2 | 3 | 3 | 6 |
| 50–64 | 5,315 | 1.7 | 2 | 1 | 1 | 1 | 2 | 3 | 4 | 7 |
| 65+ | 1,406 | 2.1 | 2 | 1 | 1 | 2 | 3 | 4 | 4 | 6 |
| **2. MULTIPLE DX** | | | | | | | | | | |
| 0–19 Years | 210 | 4.4 | 42 | 1 | 1 | 2 | 6 | 9 | 16 | 33 |
| 20–34 | 4,160 | 2.4 | 7 | 1 | 1 | 2 | 3 | 4 | 6 | 12 |
| 35–49 | 14,788 | 2.4 | 6 | 1 | 1 | 2 | 3 | 4 | 6 | 11 |
| 50–64 | 11,830 | 2.6 | 7 | 1 | 1 | 2 | 3 | 5 | 7 | 13 |
| 65+ | 8,694 | 3.7 | 14 | 1 | 2 | 3 | 4 | 7 | 10 | 19 |
| **TOTAL SINGLE DX** | 26,400 | 1.7 | 1 | 1 | 1 | 1 | 2 | 3 | 4 | 6 |
| **TOTAL MULTIPLE DX** | 39,682 | 2.7 | 8 | 1 | 2 | 2 | 3 | 5 | 7 | 14 |
| **TOTAL** | | | | | | | | | | |
| 0–19 Years | 536 | 2.8 | 19 | 1 | 1 | 2 | 3 | 6 | 9 | 18 |
| 20–34 | 10,209 | 1.9 | 3 | 1 | 1 | 1 | 2 | 3 | 5 | 9 |
| 35–49 | 28,092 | 2.0 | 4 | 1 | 1 | 1 | 2 | 4 | 5 | 9 |
| 50–64 | 17,145 | 2.3 | 6 | 1 | 1 | 2 | 3 | 5 | 7 | 11 |
| 65+ | 10,100 | 3.5 | 13 | 1 | 2 | 3 | 4 | 7 | 9 | 18 |
| **GRAND TOTAL** | 66,082 | 2.3 | 6 | 1 | 1 | 2 | 3 | 4 | 6 | 12 |

## 80.6: EXC KNEE SEMILUNAR CART. Formerly included in operation group(s) 741.

| Type of Patients | Observed Patients | Avg. Stay | Variance | 10th | 25th | 50th | 75th | 90th | 95th | 99th |
|---|---|---|---|---|---|---|---|---|---|---|
| **1. SINGLE DX** | | | | | | | | | | |
| 0–19 Years | 23 | 1.1 | <1 | 1 | 1 | 1 | 1 | 1 | 2 | 3 |
| 20–34 | 39 | 1.3 | <1 | 1 | 1 | 1 | 2 | 3 | 3 | 3 |
| 35–49 | 47 | 1.4 | <1 | 1 | 1 | 1 | 2 | 3 | 3 | 3 |
| 50–64 | 23 | 1.9 | <1 | 1 | 2 | 2 | 2 | 4 | 4 | 4 |
| 65+ | 16 | 1.8 | 2 | 1 | 1 | 2 | 2 | 4 | 5 | 5 |
| **2. MULTIPLE DX** | | | | | | | | | | |
| 0–19 Years | 137 | 1.6 | 1 | 1 | 1 | 1 | 2 | 2 | 3 | 5 |
| 20–34 | 325 | 1.7 | 2 | 1 | 1 | 1 | 2 | 3 | 4 | 7 |
| 35–49 | 526 | 2.2 | 4 | 1 | 2 | 2 | 3 | 4 | 5 | 10 |
| 50–64 | 417 | 3.5 | 14 | 1 | 2 | 2 | 4 | 7 | 15 | 15 |
| 65+ | 399 | 4.0 | 26 | 1 | 2 | 2 | 4 | 9 | 12 | 32 |
| **TOTAL SINGLE DX** | 148 | 1.4 | <1 | 1 | 1 | 1 | 2 | 3 | 3 | 4 |
| **TOTAL MULTIPLE DX** | 1,804 | 2.7 | 10 | 1 | 1 | 2 | 3 | 5 | 8 | 15 |
| **TOTAL** | | | | | | | | | | |
| 0–19 Years | 160 | 1.5 | <1 | 1 | 1 | 1 | 2 | 2 | 3 | 5 |
| 20–34 | 364 | 1.7 | 2 | 1 | 1 | 1 | 2 | 3 | 4 | 7 |
| 35–49 | 573 | 2.1 | 4 | 1 | 2 | 2 | 3 | 4 | 5 | 9 |
| 50–64 | 440 | 3.4 | 14 | 1 | 2 | 2 | 4 | 7 | 15 | 15 |
| 65+ | 415 | 4.0 | 26 | 1 | 2 | 2 | 4 | 9 | 12 | 32 |
| **GRAND TOTAL** | 1,952 | 2.6 | 10 | 1 | 1 | 2 | 3 | 5 | 8 | 15 |

## 80.7: SYNOVECTOMY. Formerly included in operation group(s) 743.

| Type of Patients | Observed Patients | Avg. Stay | Variance | 10th | 25th | 50th | 75th | 90th | 95th | 99th |
|---|---|---|---|---|---|---|---|---|---|---|
| **1. SINGLE DX** | | | | | | | | | | |
| 0–19 Years | 33 | 2.1 | 2 | 1 | 1 | 2 | 3 | 4 | 5 | 6 |
| 20–34 | 25 | 3.0 | 3 | 1 | 2 | 2 | 4 | 6 | 6 | 8 |
| 35–49 | 46 | 2.5 | 3 | 1 | 2 | 2 | 3 | 4 | 5 | 14 |
| 50–64 | 20 | 2.1 | 10 | 1 | 1 | 1 | 1 | 4 | 5 | 19 |
| 65+ | 12 | 2.4 | 3 | 1 | 1 | 3 | 3 | 4 | 8 | 8 |
| **2. MULTIPLE DX** | | | | | | | | | | |
| 0–19 Years | 76 | 4.8 | 40 | 1 | 2 | 4 | 5 | 9 | 15 | 28 |
| 20–34 | 126 | 3.9 | 18 | 1 | 2 | 2 | 4 | 11 | 11 | 26 |
| 35–49 | 256 | 4.5 | 33 | 1 | 3 | 3 | 5 | 8 | 12 | 38 |
| 50–64 | 256 | 5.5 | 38 | 1 | 4 | 4 | 7 | 13 | 16 | 26 |
| 65+ | 361 | 7.8 | 63 | 1 | 3 | 5 | 9 | 17 | 20 | 31 |
| **TOTAL SINGLE DX** | 136 | 2.4 | 5 | 1 | 1 | 2 | 3 | 4 | 5 | 14 |
| **TOTAL MULTIPLE DX** | 1,075 | 5.5 | 42 | 1 | 2 | 4 | 7 | 12 | 17 | 29 |
| **TOTAL** | | | | | | | | | | |
| 0–19 Years | 109 | 4.0 | 31 | 1 | 1 | 3 | 4 | 9 | 9 | 28 |
| 20–34 | 151 | 3.8 | 16 | 1 | 2 | 2 | 4 | 11 | 11 | 26 |
| 35–49 | 302 | 4.3 | 30 | 1 | 1 | 3 | 5 | 8 | 12 | 34 |
| 50–64 | 276 | 4.9 | 35 | 1 | 2 | 3 | 6 | 11 | 16 | 26 |
| 65+ | 373 | 7.6 | 62 | 1 | 3 | 5 | 9 | 17 | 19 | 30 |
| **GRAND TOTAL** | 1,211 | 5.2 | 39 | 1 | 2 | 3 | 6 | 11 | 16 | 28 |

Length of Stay by Diagnosis and Operation, United States, 2000

## United States, October 1998–September 1999 Data, by Operation

### 80.76: KNEE SYNOVECTOMY. Formerly included in operation group(s) 743.

| Type of Patients | Observed Patients | Avg. Stay | Variance | 10th | 25th | 50th | 75th | 90th | 95th | 99th |
|---|---|---|---|---|---|---|---|---|---|---|
| **1. SINGLE DX** | | | | | | | | | | |
| 0–19 Years | 28 | 2.1 | 2 | 1 | 1 | 2 | 3 | 4 | 5 | 6 |
| 20–34 | 20 | 3.1 | 3 | 1 | 2 | 2 | 5 | 6 | 6 | 8 |
| 35–49 | 33 | 2.8 | 4 | 1 | 2 | 2 | 5 | 6 | 6 | 14 |
| 50–64 | 16 | 2.1 | 11 | 1 | 1 | 1 | 1 | 4 | 5 | 19 |
| 65+ | 10 | 2.1 | 1 | 1 | 1 | 2 | 3 | 4 | 4 | 4 |
| **2. MULTIPLE DX** | | | | | | | | | | |
| 0–19 Years | 45 | 4.3 | 24 | 1 | 2 | 3 | 5 | 7 | 16 | 28 |
| 20–34 | 108 | 3.9 | 18 | 1 | 2 | 3 | 4 | 11 | 11 | 26 |
| 35–49 | 210 | 4.2 | 17 | 1 | 2 | 3 | 5 | 8 | 12 | 19 |
| 50–64 | 198 | 5.8 | 42 | 2 | 2 | 4 | 7 | 14 | 16 | 26 |
| 65+ | 302 | 7.9 | 62 | 2 | 3 | 6 | 10 | 16 | 19 | 33 |
| **TOTAL SINGLE DX** | 107 | 2.4 | 6 | 1 | 1 | 2 | 3 | 4 | 5 | 19 |
| **TOTAL MULTIPLE DX** | 863 | 5.5 | 38 | 1 | 2 | 4 | 7 | 12 | 16 | 26 |
| **TOTAL** | | | | | | | | | | |
| 0–19 Years | 73 | 3.5 | 17 | 1 | 1 | 2 | 4 | 6 | 9 | 28 |
| 20–34 | 128 | 3.8 | 17 | 1 | 2 | 2 | 4 | 11 | 11 | 26 |
| 35–49 | 243 | 4.1 | 16 | 1 | 2 | 3 | 5 | 8 | 12 | 19 |
| 50–64 | 214 | 5.1 | 38 | 1 | 2 | 4 | 6 | 11 | 16 | 26 |
| 65+ | 312 | 7.7 | 61 | 2 | 3 | 6 | 9 | 16 | 19 | 33 |
| **GRAND TOTAL** | 970 | 5.1 | 35 | 1 | 2 | 4 | 6 | 11 | 16 | 26 |

### 80.81: DESTR SHOULDER LES NEC. Formerly included in operation group(s) 743.

| Type of Patients | Observed Patients | Avg. Stay | Variance | 10th | 25th | 50th | 75th | 90th | 95th | 99th |
|---|---|---|---|---|---|---|---|---|---|---|
| **1. SINGLE DX** | | | | | | | | | | |
| 0–19 Years | 8 | 2.3 | 3 | 1 | 1 | 1 | 4 | 5 | 5 | 5 |
| 20–34 | 10 | 1.1 | <1 | 1 | 1 | 1 | 1 | 2 | 3 | 2 |
| 35–49 | 35 | 1.4 | <1 | 1 | 1 | 2 | 2 | 2 | 3 | 4 |
| 50–64 | 31 | 2.0 | <1 | 1 | 1 | 2 | 2 | 4 | 4 | 4 |
| 65+ | 27 | 2.0 | 2 | 1 | 1 | 2 | 2 | 4 | 4 | 7 |
| **2. MULTIPLE DX** | | | | | | | | | | |
| 0–19 Years | 20 | 2.7 | 6 | 1 | 1 | 2 | 2 | 6 | 7 | 14 |
| 20–34 | 66 | 2.2 | 5 | 1 | 1 | 2 | 2 | 6 | 8 | 12 |
| 35–49 | 241 | 2.9 | 22 | 1 | 1 | 1 | 2 | 9 | 11 | 17 |
| 50–64 | 360 | 2.7 | 15 | 1 | 1 | 1 | 2 | 6 | 9 | 24 |
| 65+ | 397 | 4.7 | 43 | 1 | 2 | 2 | 5 | 11 | 15 | 29 |
| **TOTAL SINGLE DX** | 111 | 1.8 | 1 | 1 | 1 | 1 | 2 | 4 | 4 | 6 |
| **TOTAL MULTIPLE DX** | 1,084 | 3.3 | 24 | 1 | 2 | 2 | 3 | 8 | 12 | 24 |
| **TOTAL** | | | | | | | | | | |
| 0–19 Years | 28 | 2.5 | 4 | 1 | 2 | 2 | 4 | 5 | 6 | 7 |
| 20–34 | 76 | 2.1 | 5 | 1 | 1 | 1 | 2 | 4 | 4 | 12 |
| 35–49 | 276 | 2.7 | 20 | 1 | 1 | 1 | 2 | 8 | 10 | 17 |
| 50–64 | 391 | 2.7 | 14 | 1 | 1 | 1 | 2 | 5 | 8 | 23 |
| 65+ | 424 | 4.5 | 41 | 1 | 2 | 2 | 5 | 11 | 15 | 29 |
| **GRAND TOTAL** | 1,195 | 3.1 | 22 | 1 | 2 | 2 | 3 | 7 | 12 | 23 |

### 80.8: OTH EXC/DESTR JOINT LES. Formerly included in operation group(s) 743.

| Type of Patients | Observed Patients | Avg. Stay | Variance | 10th | 25th | 50th | 75th | 90th | 95th | 99th |
|---|---|---|---|---|---|---|---|---|---|---|
| **1. SINGLE DX** | | | | | | | | | | |
| 0–19 Years | 119 | 3.2 | 8 | 1 | 1 | 2 | 3 | 4 | 5 | 6 |
| 20–34 | 107 | 4.2 | 22 | 1 | 2 | 2 | 5 | 6 | 6 | 8 |
| 35–49 | 134 | 2.6 | 6 | 1 | 1 | 2 | 2 | 5 | 6 | 14 |
| 50–64 | 96 | 2.8 | 6 | 1 | 1 | 1 | 3 | 4 | 5 | 19 |
| 65+ | 48 | 2.6 | 6 | 1 | 1 | 2 | 3 | 4 | 4 | 4 |
| **2. MULTIPLE DX** | | | | | | | | | | |
| 0–19 Years | 296 | 5.5 | 44 | 1 | 2 | 3 | 5 | 7 | 16 | 28 |
| 20–34 | 429 | 3.9 | 21 | 1 | 2 | 2 | 4 | 11 | 11 | 26 |
| 35–49 | 869 | 4.3 | 42 | 1 | 1 | 3 | 5 | 9 | 12 | 26 |
| 50–64 | 934 | 5.0 | 27 | 1 | 1 | 3 | 5 | 11 | 15 | 24 |
| 65+ | 1,110 | 6.8 | 59 | 1 | 2 | 6 | 8 | 14 | 19 | 33 |
| **TOTAL SINGLE DX** | 504 | 3.1 | 10 | 1 | 1 | 2 | 4 | 6 | 12 | 19 |
| **TOTAL MULTIPLE DX** | 3,638 | 5.1 | 41 | 1 | 2 | 3 | 6 | 11 | 15 | 30 |
| **TOTAL** | | | | | | | | | | |
| 0–19 Years | 415 | 4.8 | 35 | 1 | 2 | 3 | 5 | 9 | 15 | 22 |
| 20–34 | 536 | 4.0 | 21 | 1 | 2 | 3 | 4 | 9 | 14 | 21 |
| 35–49 | 1,003 | 4.1 | 38 | 1 | 1 | 3 | 5 | 8 | 12 | 25 |
| 50–64 | 1,030 | 4.7 | 25 | 1 | 2 | 4 | 6 | 11 | 14 | 24 |
| 65+ | 1,158 | 6.6 | 57 | 1 | 2 | 6 | 8 | 14 | 19 | 41 |
| **GRAND TOTAL** | 4,142 | 4.9 | 37 | 1 | 2 | 3 | 6 | 11 | 15 | 29 |

### 80.85: DESTR HIP LESION NEC. Formerly included in operation group(s) 743.

| Type of Patients | Observed Patients | Avg. Stay | Variance | 10th | 25th | 50th | 75th | 90th | 95th | 99th |
|---|---|---|---|---|---|---|---|---|---|---|
| **1. SINGLE DX** | | | | | | | | | | |
| 0–19 Years | 20 | 5.0 | 18 | 2 | 2 | 4 | 5 | 15 | 15 | 15 |
| 20–34 | 12 | 3.0 | 2 | 1 | 1 | 3 | 4 | 6 | 6 | 15 |
| 35–49 | 16 | 3.9 | 10 | 1 | 1 | 4 | 6 | 6 | 8 | 11 |
| 50–64 | 8 | 1.3 | <1 | 1 | 1 | 1 | 1 | 2 | 4 | 4 |
| 65+ | 4 | 7.3 | 31 | 3 | 3 | 4 | 14 | 14 | 14 | 14 |
| **2. MULTIPLE DX** | | | | | | | | | | |
| 0–19 Years | 47 | 6.1 | 19 | 3 | 4 | 5 | 7 | 10 | 11 | 25 |
| 20–34 | 38 | 8.1 | 138 | 1 | 2 | 4 | 9 | 21 | 30 | 64 |
| 35–49 | 80 | 7.0 | 199 | 1 | 1 | 5 | 6 | 11 | 17 | 98 |
| 50–64 | 68 | 6.7 | 24 | 2 | 3 | 6 | 10 | 11 | 12 | 26 |
| 65+ | 114 | 8.6 | 44 | 2 | 4 | 6 | 13 | 18 | 19 | 36 |
| **TOTAL SINGLE DX** | 60 | 3.9 | 13 | 1 | 1 | 3 | 5 | 6 | 12 | 15 |
| **TOTAL MULTIPLE DX** | 347 | 7.3 | 86 | 1 | 3 | 5 | 9 | 14 | 18 | 51 |
| **TOTAL** | | | | | | | | | | |
| 0–19 Years | 67 | 5.8 | 19 | 2 | 3 | 5 | 7 | 11 | 15 | 20 |
| 20–34 | 50 | 6.7 | 104 | 1 | 2 | 3 | 6 | 20 | 30 | 55 |
| 35–49 | 96 | 6.7 | 181 | 1 | 1 | 5 | 6 | 10 | 17 | 98 |
| 50–64 | 76 | 6.2 | 24 | 2 | 2 | 5 | 10 | 11 | 12 | 26 |
| 65+ | 118 | 8.6 | 44 | 2 | 4 | 6 | 13 | 16 | 19 | 36 |
| **GRAND TOTAL** | 407 | 6.9 | 78 | 1 | 3 | 5 | 8 | 14 | 18 | 43 |

Length of Stay by Diagnosis and Operation, United States, 2000

**United States, October 1998–September 1999 Data, by Operation**

### 80.86: DESTR KNEE LESION NEC. Formerly included in operation group(s) 743.

| Type of Patients | Observed Patients | Avg. Stay | Variance | 10th | 25th | 50th | 75th | 90th | 95th | 99th |
|---|---|---|---|---|---|---|---|---|---|---|
| **1. SINGLE DX** | | | | | | | | | | |
| 0–19 Years | 61 | 2.9 | 5 | 1 | 1 | 2 | 3 | 6 | 9 | 11 |
| 20–34 | 53 | 2.9 | 4 | 1 | 2 | 2 | 3 | 5 | 7 | 10 |
| 35–49 | 41 | 3.3 | 10 | 1 | 1 | 2 | 4 | 11 | 11 | 11 |
| 50–64 | 32 | 2.4 | 1 | 1 | 2 | 2 | 3 | 4 | 5 | 5 |
| 65+ | 8 | 3.3 | 9 | 1 | 1 | 2 | 6 | 10 | 10 | 10 |
| **2. MULTIPLE DX** | | | | | | | | | | |
| 0–19 Years | 139 | 5.8 | 77 | 1 | 2 | 4 | 6 | 11 | 15 | 49 |
| 20–34 | 182 | 4.3 | 18 | 1 | 2 | 3 | 5 | 9 | 10 | 19 |
| 35–49 | 323 | 4.8 | 21 | 1 | 3 | 3 | 5 | 9 | 14 | 28 |
| 50–64 | 320 | 6.3 | 32 | 2 | 2 | 5 | 8 | 13 | 15 | 34 |
| 65+ | 381 | 8.3 | 68 | 2 | 4 | 6 | 10 | 15 | 21 | 47 |
| **TOTAL SINGLE DX** | 195 | 2.9 | 5 | 1 | 2 | 2 | 3 | 5 | 6 | 11 |
| **TOTAL MULTIPLE DX** | 1,345 | 6.0 | 41 | 1 | 3 | 4 | 7 | 12 | 16 | 37 |
| **TOTAL** | | | | | | | | | | |
| 0–19 Years | 200 | 4.9 | 56 | 1 | 2 | 3 | 5 | 9 | 12 | 41 |
| 20–34 | 235 | 4.1 | 16 | 1 | 2 | 3 | 4 | 9 | 10 | 17 |
| 35–49 | 364 | 4.6 | 21 | 1 | 2 | 3 | 5 | 9 | 14 | 25 |
| 50–64 | 352 | 5.8 | 30 | 1 | 2 | 4 | 7 | 12 | 15 | 29 |
| 65+ | 389 | 8.2 | 67 | 2 | 3 | 6 | 10 | 15 | 21 | 47 |
| **GRAND TOTAL** | 1,540 | 5.6 | 37 | 1 | 2 | 4 | 7 | 11 | 15 | 34 |

### 81.0: SPINAL FUSION. Formerly included in operation group(s) 744.

| Type of Patients | Observed Patients | Avg. Stay | Variance | 10th | 25th | 50th | 75th | 90th | 95th | 99th |
|---|---|---|---|---|---|---|---|---|---|---|
| **1. SINGLE DX** | | | | | | | | | | |
| 0–19 Years | 1,264 | 5.1 | 3 | 3 | 4 | 5 | 6 | 7 | 8 | 11 |
| 20–34 | 2,057 | 2.7 | 4 | 1 | 1 | 2 | 4 | 5 | 6 | 11 |
| 35–49 | 7,782 | 2.3 | 2 | 1 | 1 | 2 | 3 | 4 | 5 | 8 |
| 50–64 | 3,292 | 2.5 | 4 | 1 | 1 | 2 | 3 | 5 | 6 | 9 |
| 65+ | 577 | 2.8 | 4 | 1 | 2 | 2 | 4 | 5 | 6 | 8 |
| **2. MULTIPLE DX** | | | | | | | | | | |
| 0–19 Years | 2,907 | 7.9 | 50 | 4 | 5 | 6 | 8 | 13 | 21 | 35 |
| 20–34 | 3,973 | 4.4 | 18 | 1 | 2 | 3 | 5 | 8 | 11 | 22 |
| 35–49 | 17,717 | 3.6 | 15 | 1 | 2 | 3 | 4 | 6 | 8 | 18 |
| 50–64 | 14,643 | 4.1 | 19 | 1 | 2 | 3 | 5 | 8 | 11 | 21 |
| 65+ | 9,165 | 6.0 | 36 | 2 | 3 | 4 | 7 | 12 | 16 | 33 |
| **TOTAL SINGLE DX** | 14,972 | 2.7 | 4 | 1 | 1 | 2 | 4 | 5 | 6 | 9 |
| **TOTAL MULTIPLE DX** | 48,405 | 4.5 | 24 | 1 | 2 | 3 | 5 | 8 | 12 | 24 |
| **TOTAL** | | | | | | | | | | |
| 0–19 Years | 4,171 | 7.0 | 37 | 4 | 4 | 6 | 7 | 11 | 16 | 33 |
| 20–34 | 6,030 | 3.8 | 13 | 1 | 2 | 3 | 4 | 7 | 10 | 18 |
| 35–49 | 25,499 | 3.2 | 11 | 1 | 2 | 3 | 4 | 6 | 7 | 16 |
| 50–64 | 17,935 | 3.8 | 16 | 1 | 3 | 4 | 5 | 7 | 10 | 19 |
| 65+ | 9,742 | 5.8 | 35 | 2 | 3 | 4 | 7 | 11 | 16 | 33 |
| **GRAND TOTAL** | 63,377 | 4.0 | 19 | 1 | 2 | 3 | 5 | 7 | 10 | 21 |

### 80.9: OTHER JOINT EXCISION. Formerly included in operation group(s) 743.

| Type of Patients | Observed Patients | Avg. Stay | Variance | 10th | 25th | 50th | 75th | 90th | 95th | 99th |
|---|---|---|---|---|---|---|---|---|---|---|
| **1. SINGLE DX** | | | | | | | | | | |
| 0–19 Years | 18 | 2.1 | 1 | 1 | 1 | 2 | 3 | 3 | 4 | 7 |
| 20–34 | 8 | 1.2 | <1 | 1 | 1 | 1 | 1 | 2 | 2 | 2 |
| 35–49 | 13 | 2.1 | 1 | 1 | 1 | 2 | 3 | 4 | 4 | 4 |
| 50–64 | 6 | 2.0 | <1 | 1 | 1 | 2 | 3 | 3 | 3 | 3 |
| 65+ | 2 | 2.3 | 3 | 1 | 1 | 1 | 4 | 4 | 4 | 4 |
| **2. MULTIPLE DX** | | | | | | | | | | |
| 0–19 Years | 26 | 2.7 | 20 | 1 | 1 | 2 | 2 | 5 | 7 | 30 |
| 20–34 | 26 | 5.2 | 66 | 1 | 2 | 3 | 5 | 9 | 24 | 45 |
| 35–49 | 73 | 3.2 | 13 | 1 | 1 | 2 | 3 | 9 | 12 | 20 |
| 50–64 | 58 | 4.0 | 21 | 1 | 1 | 2 | 6 | 10 | 11 | 15 |
| 65+ | 89 | 8.2 | 90 | 2 | 3 | 6 | 8 | 16 | 29 | 44 |
| **TOTAL SINGLE DX** | 47 | 1.9 | 1 | 1 | 1 | 2 | 3 | 3 | 4 | 4 |
| **TOTAL MULTIPLE DX** | 272 | 4.9 | 45 | 1 | 1 | 2 | 6 | 10 | 14 | 44 |
| **TOTAL** | | | | | | | | | | |
| 0–19 Years | 44 | 2.4 | 12 | 1 | 1 | 2 | 3 | 4 | 5 | 20 |
| 20–34 | 34 | 3.5 | 42 | 1 | 1 | 2 | 3 | 9 | 9 | 45 |
| 35–49 | 86 | 3.1 | 12 | 1 | 1 | 2 | 3 | 9 | 12 | 20 |
| 50–64 | 64 | 3.8 | 20 | 1 | 1 | 2 | 6 | 10 | 11 | 15 |
| 65+ | 91 | 8.1 | 89 | 2 | 3 | 6 | 8 | 14 | 29 | 44 |
| **GRAND TOTAL** | 319 | 4.4 | 39 | 1 | 1 | 2 | 5 | 9 | 14 | 44 |

### 81.01: ATLAS-AXIS SP FUSION. Formerly included in operation group(s) 744.

| Type of Patients | Observed Patients | Avg. Stay | Variance | 10th | 25th | 50th | 75th | 90th | 95th | 99th |
|---|---|---|---|---|---|---|---|---|---|---|
| **1. SINGLE DX** | | | | | | | | | | |
| 0–19 Years | 16 | 3.6 | 2 | 2 | 2 | 3 | 5 | 6 | 6 | 6 |
| 20–34 | 13 | 2.8 | 7 | 1 | 1 | 1 | 5 | 8 | 8 | 13 |
| 35–49 | 23 | 2.2 | 3 | 1 | 1 | 1 | 3 | 5 | 5 | 10 |
| 50–64 | 17 | 1.7 | <1 | 1 | 1 | 2 | 2 | 3 | 3 | 4 |
| 65+ | 8 | 2.7 | 2 | 1 | 2 | 2 | 4 | 5 | 5 | 5 |
| **2. MULTIPLE DX** | | | | | | | | | | |
| 0–19 Years | 70 | 8.2 | 106 | 3 | 4 | 5 | 8 | 17 | 28 | 69 |
| 20–34 | 42 | 5.4 | 43 | 1 | 1 | 3 | 6 | 14 | 18 | 30 |
| 35–49 | 88 | 6.3 | 59 | 2 | 3 | 4 | 7 | 11 | 15 | 48 |
| 50–64 | 116 | 6.7 | 45 | 3 | 3 | 5 | 7 | 17 | 18 | 33 |
| 65+ | 198 | 10.1 | 71 | 3 | 4 | 7 | 13 | 18 | 25 | 43 |
| **TOTAL SINGLE DX** | 77 | 2.6 | 4 | 1 | 1 | 2 | 4 | 5 | 6 | 8 |
| **TOTAL MULTIPLE DX** | 514 | 8.0 | 70 | 2 | 3 | 6 | 10 | 18 | 21 | 43 |
| **TOTAL** | | | | | | | | | | |
| 0–19 Years | 86 | 7.2 | 87 | 2 | 3 | 4 | 7 | 16 | 17 | 69 |
| 20–34 | 55 | 4.7 | 35 | 1 | 1 | 2 | 6 | 11 | 18 | 30 |
| 35–49 | 111 | 5.2 | 49 | 2 | 2 | 4 | 6 | 9 | 12 | 48 |
| 50–64 | 133 | 6.0 | 42 | 2 | 2 | 4 | 7 | 15 | 17 | 33 |
| 65+ | 206 | 9.9 | 71 | 3 | 4 | 7 | 13 | 18 | 25 | 43 |
| **GRAND TOTAL** | 591 | 7.2 | 64 | 1 | 3 | 5 | 8 | 17 | 18 | 43 |

# United States, October 1998–September 1999 Data, by Operation

## 81.02: ANTERIOR CERV FUSION NEC. Formerly included in operation group(s) 744.

| Type of Patients | Observed Patients | Avg. Stay | Variance | 10th | 25th | 50th | 75th | 90th | 95th | 99th |
|---|---|---|---|---|---|---|---|---|---|---|
| **1. SINGLE DX** | | | | | | | | | | |
| 0–19 Years | 27 | 4.4 | 9 | 1 | 2 | 4 | 6 | 8 | 9 | 13 |
| 20–34 | 982 | 1.7 | 2 | 1 | 1 | 1 | 2 | 3 | 3 | 10 |
| 35–49 | 5,024 | 1.5 | <1 | 1 | 1 | 1 | 2 | 2 | 3 | 5 |
| 50–64 | 2,156 | 1.7 | 1 | 1 | 1 | 1 | 2 | 3 | 3 | 8 |
| 65+ | 324 | 2.0 | 2 | 2 | 1 | 2 | 2 | 3 | 4 | 7 |
| **2. MULTIPLE DX** | | | | | | | | | | |
| 0–19 Years | 87 | 6.9 | 63 | 2 | 3 | 4 | 9 | 13 | 16 | 58 |
| 20–34 | 1,011 | 2.8 | 18 | 1 | 2 | 2 | 3 | 5 | 5 | 18 |
| 35–49 | 7,881 | 2.2 | 10 | 1 | 1 | 2 | 3 | 3 | 5 | 12 |
| 50–64 | 6,045 | 2.4 | 8 | 1 | 1 | 2 | 2 | 4 | 6 | 13 |
| 65+ | 2,330 | 4.4 | 40 | 1 | 2 | 2 | 5 | 9 | 14 | 33 |
| **TOTAL SINGLE DX** | 8,513 | 1.6 | 1 | 1 | 1 | 1 | 2 | 3 | 3 | 7 |
| **TOTAL MULTIPLE DX** | 17,354 | 2.5 | 14 | 1 | 1 | 2 | 3 | 4 | 7 | 16 |
| **TOTAL** | | | | | | | | | | |
| 0–19 Years | 114 | 6.5 | 55 | 2 | 3 | 4 | 9 | 12 | 16 | 58 |
| 20–34 | 1,993 | 2.2 | 10 | 1 | 1 | 2 | 2 | 4 | 6 | 13 |
| 35–49 | 12,905 | 1.9 | 7 | 1 | 1 | 1 | 2 | 3 | 4 | 9 |
| 50–64 | 8,201 | 2.2 | 6 | 1 | 1 | 2 | 2 | 4 | 6 | 13 |
| 65+ | 2,654 | 4.1 | 36 | 1 | 1 | 2 | 4 | 9 | 13 | 31 |
| **GRAND TOTAL** | 25,867 | 2.2 | 10 | 1 | 1 | 2 | 2 | 4 | 6 | 14 |

## 81.03: POST CERVICAL FUSION NEC. Formerly included in operation group(s) 744.

| Type of Patients | Observed Patients | Avg. Stay | Variance | 10th | 25th | 50th | 75th | 90th | 95th | 99th |
|---|---|---|---|---|---|---|---|---|---|---|
| **1. SINGLE DX** | | | | | | | | | | |
| 0–19 Years | 28 | 3.9 | 3 | 2 | 4 | 4 | 4 | 5 | 5 | 13 |
| 20–34 | 53 | 3.0 | 4 | 1 | 2 | 3 | 4 | 5 | 8 | 9 |
| 35–49 | 124 | 3.1 | 3 | 1 | 2 | 3 | 4 | 5 | 6 | 8 |
| 50–64 | 61 | 3.1 | 3 | 1 | 2 | 3 | 5 | 5 | 5 | 11 |
| 65+ | 18 | 3.1 | <1 | 2 | 2 | 3 | 4 | 5 | 5 | 5 |
| **2. MULTIPLE DX** | | | | | | | | | | |
| 0–19 Years | 113 | 7.5 | 128 | 2 | 3 | 5 | 9 | 12 | 19 | 86 |
| 20–34 | 158 | 6.5 | 28 | 2 | 3 | 5 | 8 | 15 | 17 | 29 |
| 35–49 | 356 | 5.6 | 76 | 1 | 2 | 3 | 6 | 12 | 18 | 49 |
| 50–64 | 407 | 5.0 | 29 | 2 | 3 | 4 | 6 | 9 | 14 | 30 |
| 65+ | 372 | 6.9 | 35 | 2 | 3 | 5 | 9 | 14 | 18 | 33 |
| **TOTAL SINGLE DX** | 284 | 3.2 | 3 | 1 | 2 | 3 | 4 | 5 | 6 | 11 |
| **TOTAL MULTIPLE DX** | 1,406 | 6.0 | 54 | 2 | 3 | 4 | 7 | 13 | 16 | 33 |
| **TOTAL** | | | | | | | | | | |
| 0–19 Years | 141 | 6.8 | 104 | 2 | 4 | 4 | 7 | 10 | 13 | 86 |
| 20–34 | 211 | 5.1 | 21 | 1 | 2 | 4 | 6 | 10 | 15 | 24 |
| 35–49 | 480 | 4.9 | 58 | 1 | 2 | 3 | 5 | 9 | 15 | 38 |
| 50–64 | 468 | 4.7 | 25 | 2 | 3 | 4 | 6 | 8 | 13 | 30 |
| 65+ | 390 | 6.8 | 34 | 2 | 3 | 4 | 9 | 14 | 18 | 33 |
| **GRAND TOTAL** | 1,690 | 5.5 | 45 | 1 | 2 | 4 | 6 | 11 | 15 | 32 |

## 81.04: ANTERIOR DORSAL FUSION. Formerly included in operation group(s) 744.

| Type of Patients | Observed Patients | Avg. Stay | Variance | 10th | 25th | 50th | 75th | 90th | 95th | 99th |
|---|---|---|---|---|---|---|---|---|---|---|
| **1. SINGLE DX** | | | | | | | | | | |
| 0–19 Years | 127 | 5.7 | 7 | 4 | 4 | 5 | 6 | 7 | 8 | 20 |
| 20–34 | 7 | 5.4 | 7 | 2 | 4 | 6 | 7 | 11 | 11 | 11 |
| 35–49 | 22 | 5.5 | 13 | 1 | 3 | 4 | 7 | 13 | 13 | 13 |
| 50–64 | 10 | 5.4 | 4 | 2 | 5 | 5 | 6 | 7 | 11 | 11 |
| 65+ | 2 | 6.4 | 10 | 4 | 4 | 4 | 9 | 9 | 9 | 9 |
| **2. MULTIPLE DX** | | | | | | | | | | |
| 0–19 Years | 410 | 9.9 | 70 | 4 | 6 | 7 | 10 | 18 | 28 | 44 |
| 20–34 | 97 | 8.8 | 25 | 4 | 6 | 8 | 10 | 15 | 17 | 29 |
| 35–49 | 181 | 8.9 | 63 | 3 | 5 | 7 | 10 | 15 | 23 | 60 |
| 50–64 | 151 | 11.3 | 62 | 5 | 7 | 10 | 13 | 17 | 23 | 56 |
| 65+ | 111 | 13.9 | 77 | 5 | 7 | 13 | 18 | 25 | 37 | 37 |
| **TOTAL SINGLE DX** | 168 | 5.7 | 8 | 4 | 4 | 5 | 6 | 8 | 11 | 15 |
| **TOTAL MULTIPLE DX** | 950 | 10.2 | 66 | 4 | 6 | 8 | 12 | 18 | 27 | 40 |
| **TOTAL** | | | | | | | | | | |
| 0–19 Years | 537 | 9.1 | 61 | 4 | 6 | 7 | 9 | 16 | 24 | 40 |
| 20–34 | 104 | 8.7 | 25 | 4 | 6 | 7 | 10 | 15 | 17 | 29 |
| 35–49 | 203 | 8.6 | 59 | 3 | 5 | 7 | 10 | 15 | 23 | 60 |
| 50–64 | 161 | 11.0 | 61 | 5 | 7 | 9 | 13 | 16 | 22 | 38 |
| 65+ | 113 | 13.8 | 77 | 5 | 7 | 13 | 17 | 25 | 37 | 37 |
| **GRAND TOTAL** | 1,118 | 9.6 | 61 | 4 | 5 | 7 | 11 | 17 | 24 | 39 |

## 81.05: POSTERIOR DORSAL FUSION. Formerly included in operation group(s) 744.

| Type of Patients | Observed Patients | Avg. Stay | Variance | 10th | 25th | 50th | 75th | 90th | 95th | 99th |
|---|---|---|---|---|---|---|---|---|---|---|
| **1. SINGLE DX** | | | | | | | | | | |
| 0–19 Years | 851 | 5.3 | 2 | 4 | 4 | 5 | 6 | 7 | 8 | 10 |
| 20–34 | 55 | 7.1 | 12 | 4 | 5 | 6 | 10 | 13 | 13 | 14 |
| 35–49 | 45 | 5.0 | 3 | 2 | 3 | 6 | 6 | 8 | 8 | 8 |
| 50–64 | 17 | 6.6 | 8 | 3 | 3 | 7 | 9 | 9 | 9 | 14 |
| 65+ | 3 | 4.9 | <1 | 5 | 5 | 5 | 5 | 5 | 5 | 5 |
| **2. MULTIPLE DX** | | | | | | | | | | |
| 0–19 Years | 1,710 | 7.9 | 39 | 4 | 5 | 6 | 8 | 12 | 21 | 34 |
| 20–34 | 258 | 9.9 | 52 | 4 | 5 | 8 | 11 | 17 | 29 | 39 |
| 35–49 | 376 | 8.7 | 48 | 4 | 5 | 7 | 10 | 16 | 20 | 34 |
| 50–64 | 262 | 9.9 | 46 | 3 | 5 | 8 | 15 | 18 | 18 | 34 |
| 65+ | 280 | 11.9 | 103 | 4 | 6 | 9 | 15 | 20 | 32 | 46 |
| **TOTAL SINGLE DX** | 971 | 5.4 | 3 | 4 | 4 | 5 | 6 | 7 | 9 | 13 |
| **TOTAL MULTIPLE DX** | 2,886 | 8.7 | 49 | 4 | 5 | 7 | 10 | 15 | 22 | 39 |
| **TOTAL** | | | | | | | | | | |
| 0–19 Years | 2,561 | 7.0 | 28 | 4 | 5 | 6 | 7 | 11 | 14 | 33 |
| 20–34 | 313 | 9.4 | 46 | 4 | 5 | 8 | 11 | 17 | 24 | 38 |
| 35–49 | 421 | 8.2 | 43 | 3 | 5 | 7 | 9 | 15 | 20 | 34 |
| 50–64 | 279 | 9.6 | 43 | 3 | 5 | 8 | 15 | 18 | 18 | 34 |
| 65+ | 283 | 11.7 | 101 | 4 | 5 | 8 | 15 | 20 | 31 | 46 |
| **GRAND TOTAL** | 3,857 | 7.8 | 39 | 4 | 5 | 6 | 8 | 14 | 19 | 34 |

Length of Stay by Diagnosis and Operation, United States, 2000

# United States, October 1998–September 1999 Data, by Operation

## 81.08: POSTERIOR LUMBAR FUSION. Formerly included in operation group(s) 744.

| Type of Patients | Observed Patients | Avg. Stay | Variance | Percentiles 10th | 25th | 50th | 75th | 90th | 95th | 99th |
|---|---|---|---|---|---|---|---|---|---|---|
| **1. SINGLE DX** | | | | | | | | | | |
| 0–19 Years | 144 | 4.7 | 3 | 3 | 4 | 4 | 6 | 7 | 8 | 11 |
| 20–34 | 522 | 3.7 | 3 | 2 | 3 | 3 | 4 | 5 | 6 | 10 |
| 35–49 | 1,242 | 3.6 | 2 | 2 | 3 | 3 | 4 | 5 | 6 | 9 |
| 50–64 | 547 | 4.1 | 3 | 2 | 4 | 4 | 5 | 6 | 8 | 10 |
| 65+ | 147 | 3.9 | 4 | 2 | 3 | 4 | 4 | 6 | 7 | 8 |
| **2. MULTIPLE DX** | | | | | | | | | | |
| 0–19 Years | 289 | 6.4 | 35 | 3 | 4 | 5 | 7 | 9 | 14 | 31 |
| 20–34 | 1,258 | 4.5 | 10 | 2 | 3 | 4 | 5 | 7 | 11 | 19 |
| 35–49 | 4,603 | 4.4 | 8 | 2 | 3 | 4 | 5 | 7 | 8 | 15 |
| 50–64 | 4,523 | 4.9 | 12 | 2 | 3 | 4 | 6 | 8 | 10 | 17 |
| 65+ | 3,862 | 5.7 | 19 | 3 | 4 | 5 | 6 | 9 | 13 | 26 |
| **TOTAL SINGLE DX** | 2,602 | 3.8 | 3 | 2 | 3 | 4 | 5 | 6 | 7 | 10 |
| **TOTAL MULTIPLE DX** | 14,535 | 4.9 | 13 | 2 | 3 | 4 | 6 | 8 | 10 | 19 |
| **TOTAL** | | | | | | | | | | |
| 0–19 Years | 433 | 5.8 | 26 | 3 | 4 | 5 | 7 | 8 | 11 | 24 |
| 20–34 | 1,780 | 4.2 | 8 | 2 | 3 | 4 | 5 | 7 | 9 | 16 |
| 35–49 | 5,845 | 4.2 | 7 | 2 | 3 | 4 | 5 | 7 | 9 | 15 |
| 50–64 | 5,070 | 4.8 | 11 | 2 | 3 | 4 | 6 | 8 | 10 | 17 |
| 65+ | 4,009 | 5.6 | 18 | 3 | 4 | 5 | 6 | 9 | 13 | 25 |
| **GRAND TOTAL** | 17,137 | 4.7 | 11 | 2 | 3 | 4 | 5 | 7 | 9 | 18 |

## 81.09: REFUSION OF SPINE. Formerly included in operation group(s) 744.

| Type of Patients | Observed Patients | Avg. Stay | Variance | Percentiles 10th | 25th | 50th | 75th | 90th | 95th | 99th |
|---|---|---|---|---|---|---|---|---|---|---|
| **1. SINGLE DX** | | | | | | | | | | |
| 0–19 Years | 17 | 4.5 | 2 | 3 | 3 | 4 | 6 | 6 | 6 | 9 |
| 20–34 | 63 | 3.3 | 1 | 2 | 3 | 3 | 4 | 4 | 4 | 5 |
| 35–49 | 216 | 3.1 | 3 | 1 | 2 | 3 | 4 | 6 | 7 | 8 |
| 50–64 | 107 | 3.1 | 2 | 1 | 2 | 3 | 4 | 5 | 5 | 6 |
| 65+ | 9 | 3.6 | 3 | 1 | 2 | 5 | 5 | 5 | 5 | 5 |
| **2. MULTIPLE DX** | | | | | | | | | | |
| 0–19 Years | 115 | 6.3 | 23 | 3 | 3 | 5 | 8 | 11 | 15 | 24 |
| 20–34 | 257 | 3.7 | 5 | 2 | 3 | 3 | 5 | 6 | 7 | 12 |
| 35–49 | 1,173 | 4.2 | 14 | 1 | 3 | 4 | 5 | 7 | 8 | 18 |
| 50–64 | 885 | 4.9 | 18 | 2 | 3 | 4 | 6 | 10 | 13 | 21 |
| 65+ | 415 | 6.9 | 45 | 2 | 4 | 5 | 7 | 12 | 26 | 33 |
| **TOTAL SINGLE DX** | 412 | 3.3 | 3 | 1 | 2 | 3 | 4 | 5 | 6 | 8 |
| **TOTAL MULTIPLE DX** | 2,845 | 4.8 | 20 | 2 | 3 | 4 | 5 | 8 | 12 | 24 |
| **TOTAL** | | | | | | | | | | |
| 0–19 Years | 132 | 5.8 | 19 | 3 | 3 | 5 | 6 | 10 | 12 | 24 |
| 20–34 | 320 | 3.6 | 4 | 2 | 3 | 3 | 4 | 5 | 6 | 11 |
| 35–49 | 1,389 | 4.0 | 13 | 1 | 2 | 4 | 5 | 7 | 9 | 18 |
| 50–64 | 992 | 4.8 | 17 | 1 | 2 | 4 | 5 | 10 | 13 | 21 |
| 65+ | 424 | 6.8 | 44 | 2 | 3 | 5 | 7 | 12 | 26 | 33 |
| **GRAND TOTAL** | 3,257 | 4.6 | 18 | 2 | 2 | 4 | 5 | 8 | 11 | 24 |

## 81.06: ANTERIOR LUMBAR FUSION. Formerly included in operation group(s) 744.

| Type of Patients | Observed Patients | Avg. Stay | Variance | Percentiles 10th | 25th | 50th | 75th | 90th | 95th | 99th |
|---|---|---|---|---|---|---|---|---|---|---|
| **1. SINGLE DX** | | | | | | | | | | |
| 0–19 Years | 22 | 5.6 | 7 | 3 | 4 | 5 | 6 | 11 | 11 | 11 |
| 20–34 | 276 | 3.0 | 2 | 1 | 2 | 3 | 4 | 5 | 5 | 9 |
| 35–49 | 812 | 3.3 | 2 | 2 | 2 | 3 | 4 | 5 | 5 | 12 |
| 50–64 | 223 | 4.1 | 11 | 2 | 2 | 3 | 4 | 6 | 16 | 16 |
| 65+ | 26 | 3.4 | 2 | 2 | 3 | 3 | 5 | 5 | 6 | 7 |
| **2. MULTIPLE DX** | | | | | | | | | | |
| 0–19 Years | 72 | 7.3 | 32 | 4 | 4 | 6 | 8 | 12 | 17 | 28 |
| 20–34 | 679 | 3.7 | 5 | 2 | 2 | 3 | 5 | 6 | 7 | 12 |
| 35–49 | 2,254 | 4.2 | 9 | 2 | 3 | 3 | 5 | 7 | 9 | 18 |
| 50–64 | 1,228 | 5.6 | 46 | 2 | 3 | 4 | 6 | 9 | 13 | 42 |
| 65+ | 449 | 7.0 | 48 | 3 | 4 | 5 | 7 | 13 | 17 | 51 |
| **TOTAL SINGLE DX** | 1,359 | 3.4 | 4 | 2 | 2 | 3 | 4 | 5 | 6 | 12 |
| **TOTAL MULTIPLE DX** | 4,682 | 4.8 | 21 | 2 | 3 | 4 | 5 | 8 | 11 | 22 |
| **TOTAL** | | | | | | | | | | |
| 0–19 Years | 94 | 7.0 | 28 | 3 | 4 | 6 | 7 | 11 | 17 | 28 |
| 20–34 | 955 | 3.5 | 4 | 2 | 3 | 3 | 4 | 6 | 7 | 11 |
| 35–49 | 3,066 | 3.9 | 7 | 2 | 3 | 3 | 5 | 6 | 8 | 15 |
| 50–64 | 1,451 | 5.4 | 40 | 2 | 3 | 4 | 5 | 9 | 13 | 42 |
| 65+ | 475 | 6.9 | 47 | 3 | 4 | 5 | 7 | 13 | 17 | 51 |
| **GRAND TOTAL** | 6,041 | 4.4 | 17 | 2 | 3 | 4 | 5 | 7 | 10 | 19 |

## 81.07: LAT TRANS LUMBAR FUSION. Formerly included in operation group(s) 744.

| Type of Patients | Observed Patients | Avg. Stay | Variance | Percentiles 10th | 25th | 50th | 75th | 90th | 95th | 99th |
|---|---|---|---|---|---|---|---|---|---|---|
| **1. SINGLE DX** | | | | | | | | | | |
| 0–19 Years | 23 | 3.0 | 2 | 2 | 2 | 2 | 4 | 5 | 5 | 7 |
| 20–34 | 83 | 3.6 | 2 | 2 | 3 | 3 | 4 | 5 | 5 | 7 |
| 35–49 | 261 | 3.5 | 3 | 2 | 2 | 3 | 4 | 6 | 7 | 9 |
| 50–64 | 150 | 3.9 | 3 | 2 | 2 | 4 | 5 | 6 | 9 | 9 |
| 65+ | 36 | 4.4 | 6 | 1 | 3 | 4 | 6 | 7 | 10 | 10 |
| **2. MULTIPLE DX** | | | | | | | | | | |
| 0–19 Years | 25 | 8.7 | 137 | 2 | 3 | 6 | 9 | 12 | 20 | 65 |
| 20–34 | 207 | 4.8 | 14 | 2 | 3 | 4 | 5 | 9 | 12 | 17 |
| 35–49 | 780 | 4.2 | 9 | 2 | 3 | 4 | 5 | 6 | 8 | 18 |
| 50–64 | 1,004 | 4.9 | 15 | 2 | 3 | 4 | 6 | 8 | 9 | 19 |
| 65+ | 1,124 | 5.5 | 17 | 3 | 3 | 5 | 6 | 9 | 12 | 21 |
| **TOTAL SINGLE DX** | 553 | 3.6 | 3 | 2 | 2 | 3 | 4 | 6 | 7 | 9 |
| **TOTAL MULTIPLE DX** | 3,140 | 4.9 | 15 | 2 | 3 | 4 | 6 | 8 | 10 | 19 |
| **TOTAL** | | | | | | | | | | |
| 0–19 Years | 48 | 5.0 | 56 | 2 | 2 | 3 | 5 | 8 | 11 | 65 |
| 20–34 | 290 | 4.5 | 11 | 2 | 3 | 4 | 5 | 7 | 11 | 17 |
| 35–49 | 1,041 | 4.0 | 7 | 2 | 3 | 4 | 5 | 6 | 8 | 15 |
| 50–64 | 1,154 | 4.8 | 14 | 2 | 3 | 4 | 6 | 8 | 9 | 19 |
| 65+ | 1,160 | 5.5 | 16 | 3 | 3 | 4 | 6 | 9 | 12 | 21 |
| **GRAND TOTAL** | 3,693 | 4.7 | 13 | 2 | 3 | 4 | 6 | 8 | 10 | 18 |

# United States, October 1998–September 1999 Data, by Operation

## 81.1: FOOT & ANKLE ARTHRODESIS. Formerly included in operation group(s) 745.

| Type of Patients | Observed Patients | Avg. Stay | Variance | 10th | 25th | 50th | 75th | 90th | 95th | 99th |
|---|---|---|---|---|---|---|---|---|---|---|
| **1. SINGLE DX** | | | | | | | | | | |
| 0–19 Years | 45 | 1.8 | <1 | 1 | 1 | 2 | 2 | 3 | 3 | 4 |
| 20–34 | 100 | 2.2 | 1 | 1 | 1 | 2 | 3 | 3 | 5 | 6 |
| 35–49 | 245 | 1.9 | <1 | 1 | 1 | 2 | 2 | 3 | 3 | 6 |
| 50–64 | 186 | 1.8 | <1 | 1 | 1 | 2 | 2 | 3 | 3 | 5 |
| 65+ | 81 | 2.1 | 1 | 1 | 1 | 2 | 3 | 4 | 4 | 5 |
| **2. MULTIPLE DX** | | | | | | | | | | |
| 0–19 Years | 180 | 2.2 | 2 | 1 | 1 | 2 | 3 | 4 | 7 | 7 |
| 20–34 | 270 | 2.4 | 4 | 1 | 1 | 2 | 3 | 4 | 5 | 13 |
| 35–49 | 812 | 2.6 | 6 | 1 | 2 | 2 | 3 | 4 | 5 | 12 |
| 50–64 | 906 | 2.9 | 4 | 1 | 2 | 2 | 3 | 4 | 7 | 9 |
| 65+ | 767 | 3.3 | 7 | 1 | 2 | 3 | 4 | 5 | 8 | 13 |
| **TOTAL SINGLE DX** | 657 | 1.9 | 1 | 1 | 1 | 2 | 2 | 3 | 4 | 6 |
| **TOTAL MULTIPLE DX** | 2,935 | 2.8 | 5 | 1 | 2 | 2 | 3 | 5 | 6 | 12 |
| **TOTAL** | | | | | | | | | | |
| 0–19 | 225 | 2.2 | 2 | 1 | 1 | 2 | 2 | 4 | 5 | 7 |
| 20–34 | 370 | 2.4 | 3 | 1 | 1 | 2 | 3 | 3 | 5 | 13 |
| 35–49 | 1,057 | 2.4 | 5 | 1 | 1 | 2 | 3 | 4 | 5 | 12 |
| 50–64 | 1,092 | 2.7 | 3 | 2 | 2 | 2 | 3 | 4 | 7 | 8 |
| 65+ | 848 | 3.2 | 6 | 1 | 2 | 3 | 4 | 5 | 7 | 13 |
| **GRAND TOTAL** | 3,592 | 2.6 | 4 | 1 | 2 | 2 | 3 | 4 | 6 | 11 |

## 81.11: ANKLE FUSION. Formerly included in operation group(s) 745.

| Type of Patients | Observed Patients | Avg. Stay | Variance | 10th | 25th | 50th | 75th | 90th | 95th | 99th |
|---|---|---|---|---|---|---|---|---|---|---|
| **1. SINGLE DX** | | | | | | | | | | |
| 0–19 Years | 8 | 2.3 | <1 | 1 | 2 | 2 | 3 | 3 | 4 | 4 |
| 20–34 | 39 | 2.4 | 1 | 1 | 2 | 2 | 3 | 4 | 5 | 6 |
| 35–49 | 122 | 1.8 | 1 | 1 | 1 | 2 | 2 | 3 | 4 | 6 |
| 50–64 | 90 | 1.7 | 1 | 1 | 1 | 1 | 2 | 3 | 3 | 6 |
| 65+ | 33 | 2.5 | 1 | 1 | 2 | 3 | 3 | 4 | 4 | 5 |
| **2. MULTIPLE DX** | | | | | | | | | | |
| 0–19 Years | 17 | 2.2 | <1 | 1 | 2 | 2 | 3 | 5 | 4 | 4 |
| 20–34 | 142 | 2.9 | 6 | 1 | 2 | 2 | 3 | 5 | 7 | 13 |
| 35–49 | 409 | 2.7 | 10 | 1 | 2 | 2 | 3 | 4 | 6 | 15 |
| 50–64 | 423 | 3.0 | 5 | 1 | 2 | 2 | 3 | 6 | 8 | 11 |
| 65+ | 367 | 3.3 | 10 | 1 | 2 | 3 | 4 | 5 | 7 | 22 |
| **TOTAL SINGLE DX** | 292 | 1.9 | 1 | 1 | 2 | 2 | 2 | 3 | 4 | 6 |
| **TOTAL MULTIPLE DX** | 1,358 | 3.0 | 8 | 1 | 2 | 2 | 3 | 5 | 7 | 14 |
| **TOTAL** | | | | | | | | | | |
| 0–19 | 25 | 2.3 | <1 | 1 | 2 | 2 | 3 | 3 | 4 | 4 |
| 20–34 | 181 | 2.8 | 5 | 1 | 2 | 2 | 3 | 5 | 5 | 13 |
| 35–49 | 531 | 2.4 | 7 | 1 | 1 | 2 | 3 | 4 | 5 | 9 |
| 50–64 | 513 | 2.7 | 4 | 1 | 2 | 2 | 3 | 4 | 7 | 10 |
| 65+ | 400 | 3.2 | 9 | 1 | 2 | 3 | 4 | 5 | 7 | 17 |
| **GRAND TOTAL** | 1,650 | 2.7 | 6 | 2 | 2 | 2 | 3 | 5 | 6 | 13 |

## 81.12: TRIPLE ARTHRODESIS. Formerly included in operation group(s) 745.

| Type of Patients | Observed Patients | Avg. Stay | Variance | 10th | 25th | 50th | 75th | 90th | 95th | 99th |
|---|---|---|---|---|---|---|---|---|---|---|
| **1. SINGLE DX** | | | | | | | | | | |
| 0–19 Years | 29 | 1.8 | <1 | 1 | 1 | 2 | 2 | 3 | 3 | 4 |
| 20–34 | 24 | 3.0 | 2 | 1 | 3 | 3 | 3 | 6 | 6 | 6 |
| 35–49 | 36 | 2.0 | <1 | 1 | 1 | 3 | 3 | 3 | 3 | 6 |
| 50–64 | 30 | 2.3 | <1 | 1 | 1 | 3 | 3 | 3 | 3 | 3 |
| 65+ | 17 | 2.4 | 1 | 1 | 1 | 2 | 3 | 4 | 4 | 4 |
| **2. MULTIPLE DX** | | | | | | | | | | |
| 0–19 Years | 102 | 2.6 | 3 | 1 | 2 | 2 | 3 | 5 | 7 | 7 |
| 20–34 | 54 | 2.3 | <1 | 1 | 1 | 3 | 3 | 3 | 4 | 6 |
| 35–49 | 161 | 2.7 | 5 | 1 | 2 | 3 | 3 | 5 | 6 | 14 |
| 50–64 | 229 | 2.9 | 3 | 2 | 2 | 3 | 3 | 4 | 7 | 8 |
| 65+ | 192 | 3.2 | 3 | 2 | 2 | 3 | 4 | 5 | 8 | 9 |
| **TOTAL SINGLE DX** | 136 | 2.3 | 1 | 1 | 1 | 2 | 3 | 3 | 4 | 6 |
| **TOTAL MULTIPLE DX** | 738 | 2.8 | 3 | 1 | 2 | 2 | 3 | 4 | 7 | 9 |
| **TOTAL** | | | | | | | | | | |
| 0–19 | 131 | 2.4 | 3 | 1 | 2 | 2 | 3 | 5 | 7 | 7 |
| 20–34 | 78 | 2.5 | 1 | 1 | 2 | 3 | 3 | 3 | 4 | 13 |
| 35–49 | 197 | 2.6 | 4 | 1 | 2 | 3 | 3 | 4 | 5 | 12 |
| 50–64 | 259 | 2.9 | 3 | 1 | 2 | 3 | 3 | 4 | 7 | 8 |
| 65+ | 209 | 3.2 | 3 | 1 | 2 | 3 | 4 | 5 | 6 | 9 |
| **GRAND TOTAL** | 874 | 2.8 | 3 | 1 | 2 | 2 | 3 | 4 | 6 | 9 |

## 81.13: SUBTALAR FUSION. Formerly included in operation group(s) 745.

| Type of Patients | Observed Patients | Avg. Stay | Variance | 10th | 25th | 50th | 75th | 90th | 95th | 99th |
|---|---|---|---|---|---|---|---|---|---|---|
| **1. SINGLE DX** | | | | | | | | | | |
| 0–19 Years | 5 | 1.1 | <1 | 1 | 1 | 1 | 1 | 2 | 2 | 2 |
| 20–34 | 22 | 1.5 | <1 | 1 | 1 | 1 | 2 | 3 | 3 | 7 |
| 35–49 | 54 | 1.8 | <1 | 1 | 1 | 2 | 2 | 3 | 3 | 3 |
| 50–64 | 34 | 1.7 | <1 | 1 | 2 | 2 | 2 | 3 | 2 | 4 |
| 65+ | 14 | 1.5 | <1 | 1 | 1 | 1 | 2 | 3 | 3 | 4 |
| **2. MULTIPLE DX** | | | | | | | | | | |
| 0–19 Years | 47 | 1.7 | <1 | 1 | 1 | 1 | 2 | 3 | 4 | 5 |
| 20–34 | 36 | 2.0 | <1 | 1 | 2 | 2 | 2 | 3 | 7 | 7 |
| 35–49 | 124 | 2.2 | 4 | 1 | 1 | 2 | 2 | 3 | 6 | 12 |
| 50–64 | 106 | 2.2 | 2 | 1 | 2 | 2 | 2 | 3 | 4 | 10 |
| 65+ | 63 | 3.0 | 4 | 1 | 3 | 3 | 4 | 6 | 6 | 8 |
| **TOTAL SINGLE DX** | 129 | 1.6 | <1 | 1 | 1 | 2 | 2 | 2 | 3 | 4 |
| **TOTAL MULTIPLE DX** | 376 | 2.2 | 3 | 1 | 2 | 2 | 2 | 4 | 5 | 10 |
| **TOTAL** | | | | | | | | | | |
| 0–19 | 52 | 1.7 | <1 | 1 | 1 | 2 | 2 | 3 | 4 | 5 |
| 20–34 | 58 | 1.7 | <1 | 1 | 1 | 2 | 2 | 3 | 3 | 4 |
| 35–49 | 178 | 2.1 | 3 | 1 | 1 | 2 | 2 | 3 | 4 | 12 |
| 50–64 | 140 | 2.0 | 1 | 1 | 2 | 2 | 2 | 3 | 4 | 10 |
| 65+ | 77 | 2.7 | 4 | 1 | 2 | 3 | 4 | 6 | 6 | 8 |
| **GRAND TOTAL** | 505 | 2.1 | 2 | 1 | 1 | 2 | 2 | 3 | 4 | 8 |

Length of Stay by Diagnosis and Operation, United States, 2000

# United States, October 1998–September 1999 Data, by Operation

## 81.2: ARTHRODESIS OF OTH JOINT. Formerly included in operation group(s) 745.

| Type of Patients | Observed Patients | Avg. Stay | Vari-ance | 10th | 25th | 50th | 75th | 90th | 95th | 99th |
|---|---|---|---|---|---|---|---|---|---|---|
| **1. SINGLE DX** | | | | | | | | | | |
| 0–19 Years | 20 | 3.7 | 6 | 1 | 2 | 3 | 7 | 7 | 7 | 7 |
| 20–34 | 36 | 1.5 | <1 | 1 | 1 | 1 | 2 | 2 | 3 | 4 |
| 35–49 | 56 | 2.2 | <1 | 1 | 2 | 2 | 3 | 3 | 4 | 4 |
| 50–64 | 30 | 1.9 | 1 | 1 | 1 | 2 | 2 | 3 | 5 | 6 |
| 65+ | 14 | 2.4 | 8 | 1 | 1 | 1 | 2 | 9 | 10 | 10 |
| **2. MULTIPLE DX** | | | | | | | | | | |
| 0–19 Years | 37 | 8.6 | 126 | 1 | 2 | 4 | 7 | 32 | 32 | 32 |
| 20–34 | 94 | 2.9 | 27 | 1 | 1 | 2 | 3 | 6 | 7 | 45 |
| 35–49 | 146 | 3.6 | 27 | 1 | 2 | 3 | 4 | 5 | 8 | 22 |
| 50–64 | 150 | 5.0 | 23 | 1 | 2 | 3 | 7 | 11 | 11 | 23 |
| 65+ | 171 | 5.2 | 20 | 1 | 3 | 4 | 7 | 10 | 13 | 23 |
| **TOTAL SINGLE DX** | 156 | 2.3 | 2 | 1 | 1 | 2 | 3 | 4 | 7 | 7 |
| **TOTAL MULTIPLE DX** | 598 | 4.6 | 34 | 1 | 2 | 3 | 5 | 9 | 11 | 32 |
| **TOTAL** | | | | | | | | | | |
| 0–19 Years | 57 | 6.6 | 83 | 1 | 2 | 4 | 7 | 32 | 32 | 32 |
| 20–34 | 130 | 2.5 | 21 | 1 | 1 | 2 | 2 | 5 | 6 | 18 |
| 35–49 | 202 | 3.1 | 18 | 1 | 2 | 2 | 3 | 5 | 6 | 22 |
| 50–64 | 180 | 4.2 | 19 | 1 | 2 | 3 | 5 | 11 | 11 | 23 |
| 65+ | 185 | 5.0 | 19 | 1 | 2 | 4 | 7 | 10 | 12 | 23 |
| **GRAND TOTAL** | 754 | 4.0 | 27 | 1 | 1 | 2 | 4 | 8 | 11 | 32 |

## 81.40: REPAIR OF HIP NEC. Formerly included in operation group(s) 747.

| Type of Patients | Observed Patients | Avg. Stay | Vari-ance | 10th | 25th | 50th | 75th | 90th | 95th | 99th |
|---|---|---|---|---|---|---|---|---|---|---|
| **1. SINGLE DX** | | | | | | | | | | |
| 0–19 Years | 70 | 2.8 | 4 | 2 | 2 | 2 | 3 | 3 | 4 | 16 |
| 20–34 | 2 | 6.1 | 11 | 2 | 2 | 8 | 8 | 8 | 8 | 8 |
| 35–49 | 9 | 5.1 | 6 | 2 | 3 | 6 | 8 | 8 | 8 | 8 |
| 50–64 | 3 | 4.3 | <1 | 4 | 4 | 4 | 5 | 5 | 5 | 5 |
| 65+ | 3 | 4.0 | 0 | 4 | 4 | 4 | 4 | 4 | 4 | 4 |
| **2. MULTIPLE DX** | | | | | | | | | | |
| 0–19 Years | 129 | 3.4 | 3 | 2 | 2 | 3 | 4 | 5 | 6 | 13 |
| 20–34 | 11 | 4.8 | 15 | 1 | 2 | 3 | 7 | 12 | 12 | 15 |
| 35–49 | 21 | 4.9 | 4 | 3 | 4 | 4 | 6 | 9 | 9 | 10 |
| 50–64 | 22 | 6.4 | 16 | 4 | 4 | 5 | 10 | 11 | 13 | 22 |
| 65+ | 87 | 9.3 | 59 | 4 | 4 | 6 | 12 | 19 | 26 | 36 |
| **TOTAL SINGLE DX** | 87 | 3.0 | 5 | 2 | 2 | 3 | 3 | 4 | 6 | 16 |
| **TOTAL MULTIPLE DX** | 270 | 5.0 | 23 | 2 | 3 | 4 | 5 | 10 | 13 | 27 |
| **TOTAL** | | | | | | | | | | |
| 0–19 Years | 199 | 3.2 | 4 | 2 | 2 | 3 | 4 | 5 | 5 | 13 |
| 20–34 | 13 | 5.0 | 14 | 1 | 3 | 4 | 7 | 9 | 12 | 15 |
| 35–49 | 30 | 4.9 | 4 | 3 | 4 | 4 | 7 | 8 | 9 | 10 |
| 50–64 | 25 | 6.0 | 13 | 2 | 4 | 5 | 8 | 11 | 11 | 22 |
| 65+ | 90 | 9.1 | 58 | 4 | 4 | 6 | 12 | 18 | 26 | 36 |
| **GRAND TOTAL** | 357 | 4.5 | 19 | 2 | 2 | 3 | 5 | 8 | 13 | 24 |

## 81.4: LOW LIMB JOINT REP NEC. Formerly included in operation group(s) 747, 749, 751.

| Type of Patients | Observed Patients | Avg. Stay | Vari-ance | 10th | 25th | 50th | 75th | 90th | 95th | 99th |
|---|---|---|---|---|---|---|---|---|---|---|
| **1. SINGLE DX** | | | | | | | | | | |
| 0–19 Years | 694 | 1.6 | 1 | 1 | 1 | 1 | 2 | 3 | 3 | 4 |
| 20–34 | 737 | 1.4 | <1 | 1 | 1 | 1 | 2 | 2 | 3 | 4 |
| 35–49 | 474 | 1.6 | 1 | 1 | 1 | 1 | 2 | 3 | 4 | 6 |
| 50–64 | 81 | 2.9 | 4 | 1 | 1 | 3 | 4 | 5 | 6 | 10 |
| 65+ | 45 | 3.3 | 3 | 1 | 2 | 3 | 4 | 5 | 6 | 10 |
| **2. MULTIPLE DX** | | | | | | | | | | |
| 0–19 Years | 1,024 | 1.8 | 2 | 1 | 1 | 1 | 2 | 3 | 5 | 7 |
| 20–34 | 1,591 | 2.0 | 5 | 1 | 1 | 1 | 2 | 3 | 6 | 12 |
| 35–49 | 1,375 | 2.4 | 6 | 1 | 2 | 2 | 3 | 4 | 7 | 12 |
| 50–64 | 447 | 4.8 | 22 | 1 | 2 | 3 | 5 | 14 | 17 | 17 |
| 65+ | 382 | 5.2 | 22 | 2 | 3 | 4 | 6 | 9 | 13 | 28 |
| **TOTAL SINGLE DX** | 2,031 | 1.6 | 1 | 1 | 1 | 1 | 2 | 3 | 3 | 5 |
| **TOTAL MULTIPLE DX** | 4,819 | 2.5 | 8 | 1 | 1 | 2 | 3 | 5 | 8 | 17 |
| **TOTAL** | | | | | | | | | | |
| 0–19 Years | 1,718 | 1.7 | 2 | 1 | 1 | 1 | 2 | 3 | 4 | 6 |
| 20–34 | 2,328 | 1.8 | 3 | 1 | 1 | 1 | 2 | 3 | 4 | 11 |
| 35–49 | 1,849 | 2.2 | 4 | 1 | 1 | 2 | 3 | 4 | 6 | 12 |
| 50–64 | 528 | 4.5 | 20 | 2 | 2 | 3 | 5 | 12 | 17 | 17 |
| 65+ | 427 | 5.1 | 21 | 2 | 3 | 4 | 6 | 9 | 13 | 28 |
| **GRAND TOTAL** | 6,850 | 2.3 | 6 | 1 | 1 | 1 | 2 | 4 | 6 | 14 |

## 81.44: PATELLAR STABILIZATION. Formerly included in operation group(s) 749.

| Type of Patients | Observed Patients | Avg. Stay | Vari-ance | 10th | 25th | 50th | 75th | 90th | 95th | 99th |
|---|---|---|---|---|---|---|---|---|---|---|
| **1. SINGLE DX** | | | | | | | | | | |
| 0–19 Years | 79 | 1.6 | <1 | 1 | 1 | 1 | 2 | 3 | 3 | 4 |
| 20–34 | 49 | 1.7 | <1 | 1 | 1 | 2 | 2 | 3 | 3 | 5 |
| 35–49 | 27 | 1.9 | 1 | 1 | 2 | 2 | 3 | 3 | 4 | 5 |
| 50–64 | 9 | 2.1 | 1 | 1 | 1 | 2 | 3 | 4 | 4 | 4 |
| 65+ | 6 | 3.4 | 1 | 2 | 3 | 3 | 3 | 6 | 6 | 6 |
| **2. MULTIPLE DX** | | | | | | | | | | |
| 0–19 Years | 73 | 1.7 | 1 | 1 | 1 | 1 | 2 | 2 | 5 | 5 |
| 20–34 | 72 | 2.4 | 3 | 1 | 1 | 2 | 3 | 4 | 5 | 12 |
| 35–49 | 61 | 2.8 | 3 | 1 | 2 | 3 | 3 | 4 | 4 | 14 |
| 50–64 | 22 | 2.6 | 2 | 1 | 2 | 3 | 3 | 4 | 4 | 6 |
| 65+ | 32 | 3.8 | 19 | 2 | 3 | 3 | 4 | 6 | 9 | 29 |
| **TOTAL SINGLE DX** | 170 | 1.8 | <1 | 1 | 1 | 2 | 2 | 3 | 4 | 5 |
| **TOTAL MULTIPLE DX** | 260 | 2.3 | 4 | 1 | 1 | 2 | 3 | 4 | 5 | 10 |
| **TOTAL** | | | | | | | | | | |
| 0–19 Years | 152 | 1.7 | <1 | 1 | 1 | 1 | 2 | 3 | 3 | 5 |
| 20–34 | 121 | 2.2 | 2 | 1 | 1 | 2 | 3 | 4 | 4 | 12 |
| 35–49 | 88 | 2.6 | 3 | 1 | 2 | 3 | 3 | 4 | 4 | 10 |
| 50–64 | 31 | 2.5 | 2 | 1 | 1 | 3 | 3 | 4 | 4 | 6 |
| 65+ | 38 | 3.7 | 16 | 2 | 2 | 3 | 4 | 6 | 7 | 29 |
| **GRAND TOTAL** | 430 | 2.1 | 3 | 1 | 1 | 2 | 3 | 4 | 4 | 7 |

Length of Stay by Diagnosis and Operation, United States, 2000

# United States, October 1998–September 1999 Data, by Operation

## 81.45: CRUCIATE LIG REPAIR NEC. Formerly included in operation group(s) 749.

| Type of Patients | Observed Patients | Avg. Stay | Variance | 10th | 25th | 50th | 75th | 90th | 95th | 99th |
|---|---|---|---|---|---|---|---|---|---|---|
| **1. SINGLE DX** | | | | | | | | | | |
| 0–19 Years | 458 | 1.4 | <1 | 1 | 1 | 1 | 2 | 2 | 2 | 4 |
| 20–34 | 560 | 1.3 | <1 | 1 | 1 | 1 | 1 | 2 | 2 | 4 |
| 35–49 | 278 | 1.3 | <1 | 1 | 1 | 1 | 1 | 2 | 2 | 4 |
| 50–64 | 17 | 1.4 | <1 | 1 | 1 | 1 | 2 | 2 | 3 | 3 |
| 65+ | 0 | | | | | | | | | |
| **2. MULTIPLE DX** | | | | | | | | | | |
| 0–19 Years | 657 | 1.4 | <1 | 1 | 1 | 1 | 2 | 2 | 3 | 4 |
| 20–34 | 1,162 | 1.7 | 2 | 1 | 1 | 1 | 2 | 2 | 4 | 9 |
| 35–49 | 805 | 1.9 | 3 | 1 | 1 | 1 | 2 | 3 | 4 | 11 |
| 50–64 | 112 | 3.3 | 12 | 1 | 1 | 2 | 3 | 8 | 14 | 14 |
| 65+ | 9 | 3.1 | 4 | 1 | 2 | 2 | 3 | 7 | 7 | 7 |
| **TOTAL SINGLE DX** | 1,313 | 1.3 | <1 | 1 | 1 | 1 | 2 | 2 | 2 | 4 |
| **TOTAL MULTIPLE DX** | 2,745 | 1.7 | 3 | 1 | 1 | 1 | 2 | 3 | 4 | 11 |
| **TOTAL** | | | | | | | | | | |
| 0–19 Years | 1,115 | 1.4 | <1 | 1 | 1 | 1 | 2 | 2 | 3 | 4 |
| 20–34 | 1,722 | 1.5 | 2 | 1 | 1 | 1 | 2 | 2 | 4 | 9 |
| 35–49 | 1,083 | 1.7 | 3 | 1 | 1 | 1 | 2 | 3 | 4 | 11 |
| 50–64 | 129 | 3.0 | 11 | 1 | 2 | 2 | 3 | 8 | 14 | 14 |
| 65+ | 9 | 3.1 | 4 | 1 | 2 | 2 | 3 | 7 | 7 | 7 |
| **GRAND TOTAL** | 4,058 | 1.6 | 2 | 1 | 1 | 1 | 2 | 2 | 3 | 9 |

## 81.5: JOINT REPL LOWER EXT. Formerly included in operation group(s) 746, 747, 748, 749, 750.

| Type of Patients | Observed Patients | Avg. Stay | Variance | 10th | 25th | 50th | 75th | 90th | 95th | 99th |
|---|---|---|---|---|---|---|---|---|---|---|
| **1. SINGLE DX** | | | | | | | | | | |
| 0–19 Years | 29 | 3.6 | 4 | 1 | 3 | 3 | 4 | 5 | 6 | 12 |
| 20–34 | 298 | 3.9 | 1 | 3 | 3 | 4 | 4 | 5 | 6 | 8 |
| 35–49 | 2,157 | 3.9 | 2 | 3 | 3 | 4 | 4 | 5 | 6 | 8 |
| 50–64 | 5,354 | 4.0 | 2 | 3 | 3 | 4 | 5 | 5 | 6 | 8 |
| 65+ | 8,266 | 4.1 | 2 | 3 | 3 | 4 | 5 | 6 | 7 | 8 |
| **2. MULTIPLE DX** | | | | | | | | | | |
| 0–19 Years | 133 | 5.2 | 15 | 3 | 3 | 4 | 6 | 9 | 10 | 22 |
| 20–34 | 1,206 | 4.7 | 13 | 3 | 3 | 4 | 5 | 7 | 8 | 16 |
| 35–49 | 8,365 | 4.6 | 10 | 3 | 3 | 4 | 5 | 7 | 8 | 16 |
| 50–64 | 30,525 | 4.6 | 6 | 3 | 3 | 4 | 5 | 7 | 8 | 14 |
| 65+ | 100,251 | 5.2 | 11 | 3 | 4 | 4 | 6 | 8 | 10 | 18 |
| **TOTAL SINGLE DX** | 16,104 | 4.0 | 2 | 3 | 3 | 4 | 5 | 6 | 7 | 8 |
| **TOTAL MULTIPLE DX** | 140,480 | 5.0 | 10 | 3 | 3 | 4 | 6 | 7 | 9 | 17 |
| **TOTAL** | | | | | | | | | | |
| 0–19 Years | 162 | 4.9 | 13 | 3 | 3 | 4 | 5 | 9 | 10 | 17 |
| 20–34 | 1,504 | 4.5 | 11 | 3 | 3 | 4 | 5 | 7 | 8 | 15 |
| 35–49 | 10,522 | 4.5 | 9 | 3 | 3 | 4 | 5 | 6 | 8 | 14 |
| 50–64 | 35,879 | 4.5 | 6 | 3 | 3 | 4 | 5 | 6 | 8 | 13 |
| 65+ | 108,517 | 5.1 | 10 | 3 | 4 | 4 | 6 | 8 | 10 | 18 |
| **GRAND TOTAL** | 156,584 | 4.9 | 9 | 3 | 3 | 4 | 5 | 7 | 9 | 16 |

## 81.47: OTHER REPAIR OF KNEE. Formerly included in operation group(s) 749.

| Type of Patients | Observed Patients | Avg. Stay | Variance | 10th | 25th | 50th | 75th | 90th | 95th | 99th |
|---|---|---|---|---|---|---|---|---|---|---|
| **1. SINGLE DX** | | | | | | | | | | |
| 0–19 Years | 53 | 1.4 | <1 | 1 | 1 | 1 | 2 | 2 | 2 | 4 |
| 20–34 | 86 | 1.8 | <1 | 1 | 1 | 2 | 2 | 3 | 3 | 5 |
| 35–49 | 133 | 2.0 | 1 | 1 | 1 | 2 | 3 | 3 | 3 | 6 |
| 50–64 | 49 | 3.5 | 4 | 1 | 2 | 3 | 5 | 6 | 6 | 10 |
| 65+ | 33 | 3.4 | 4 | 2 | 2 | 3 | 4 | 5 | 7 | 10 |
| **2. MULTIPLE DX** | | | | | | | | | | |
| 0–19 Years | 112 | 1.9 | 2 | 1 | 1 | 1 | 2 | 3 | 4 | 7 |
| 20–34 | 229 | 3.0 | 9 | 1 | 2 | 2 | 3 | 7 | 7 | 11 |
| 35–49 | 373 | 3.1 | 9 | 1 | 2 | 4 | 4 | 7 | 11 | 12 |
| 50–64 | 232 | 6.1 | 31 | 2 | 3 | 4 | 7 | 17 | 17 | 17 |
| 65+ | 224 | 4.3 | 8 | 2 | 3 | 3 | 5 | 8 | 9 | 13 |
| **TOTAL SINGLE DX** | 354 | 2.1 | 2 | 1 | 1 | 2 | 2 | 3 | 5 | 6 |
| **TOTAL MULTIPLE DX** | 1,170 | 3.7 | 14 | 1 | 2 | 2 | 4 | 8 | 12 | 17 |
| **TOTAL** | | | | | | | | | | |
| 0–19 Years | 165 | 1.7 | 2 | 1 | 1 | 1 | 2 | 3 | 3 | 7 |
| 20–34 | 315 | 2.5 | 5 | 1 | 2 | 2 | 3 | 5 | 7 | 11 |
| 35–49 | 506 | 2.8 | 8 | 1 | 2 | 3 | 4 | 6 | 11 | 12 |
| 50–64 | 281 | 5.6 | 27 | 2 | 3 | 4 | 6 | 17 | 17 | 17 |
| 65+ | 257 | 4.2 | 8 | 2 | 3 | 3 | 5 | 7 | 9 | 13 |
| **GRAND TOTAL** | 1,524 | 3.2 | 11 | 1 | 2 | 2 | 3 | 7 | 11 | 17 |

## 81.51: TOTAL HIP REPLACEMENT. Formerly included in operation group(s) 746.

| Type of Patients | Observed Patients | Avg. Stay | Variance | 10th | 25th | 50th | 75th | 90th | 95th | 99th |
|---|---|---|---|---|---|---|---|---|---|---|
| **1. SINGLE DX** | | | | | | | | | | |
| 0–19 Years | 12 | 4.4 | 1 | 3 | 4 | 4 | 5 | 5 | 7 | 7 |
| 20–34 | 175 | 3.9 | 1 | 3 | 3 | 4 | 4 | 5 | 6 | 8 |
| 35–49 | 1,023 | 4.1 | 2 | 3 | 3 | 4 | 5 | 5 | 7 | 12 |
| 50–64 | 1,699 | 4.0 | 2 | 3 | 3 | 4 | 5 | 5 | 6 | 7 |
| 65+ | 2,078 | 4.0 | 2 | 3 | 3 | 4 | 5 | 6 | 7 | 8 |
| **2. MULTIPLE DX** | | | | | | | | | | |
| 0–19 Years | 59 | 5.6 | 11 | 3 | 3 | 4 | 5 | 6 | 12 | 22 |
| 20–34 | 784 | 4.8 | 12 | 3 | 3 | 4 | 5 | 7 | 8 | 16 |
| 35–49 | 3,858 | 4.6 | 9 | 3 | 3 | 4 | 5 | 6 | 8 | 13 |
| 50–64 | 9,054 | 4.4 | 4 | 3 | 3 | 4 | 5 | 6 | 7 | 12 |
| 65+ | 23,334 | 4.8 | 8 | 3 | 3 | 4 | 5 | 7 | 8 | 16 |
| **TOTAL SINGLE DX** | 4,987 | 4.0 | 2 | 3 | 3 | 4 | 5 | 5 | 6 | 8 |
| **TOTAL MULTIPLE DX** | 37,089 | 4.7 | 7 | 3 | 3 | 4 | 5 | 7 | 8 | 15 |
| **TOTAL** | | | | | | | | | | |
| 0–19 Years | 71 | 5.4 | 10 | 3 | 4 | 4 | 6 | 8 | 12 | 22 |
| 20–34 | 959 | 4.6 | 10 | 3 | 3 | 4 | 5 | 7 | 7 | 15 |
| 35–49 | 4,881 | 4.5 | 7 | 3 | 3 | 4 | 5 | 6 | 7 | 12 |
| 50–64 | 10,753 | 4.3 | 4 | 3 | 3 | 4 | 5 | 6 | 7 | 11 |
| 65+ | 25,412 | 4.7 | 7 | 3 | 3 | 4 | 5 | 7 | 8 | 15 |
| **GRAND TOTAL** | 42,076 | 4.6 | 6 | 3 | 3 | 4 | 5 | 7 | 8 | 14 |

Length of Stay by Diagnosis and Operation, United States, 2000

# United States, October 1998–September 1999 Data, by Operation

## 81.54: TOTAL KNEE REPLACEMENT. Formerly included in operation group(s) 748.

| Type of Patients | Observed Patients | Avg. Stay | Vari-ance | Percentiles | | | | | | |
|---|---|---|---|---|---|---|---|---|---|---|
| | | | | 10th | 25th | 50th | 75th | 90th | 95th | 99th |
| **1. SINGLE DX** | | | | | | | | | | |
| 0–19 Years | 7 | 4.8 | 14 | 1 | 1 | 4 | 5 | 12 | 12 | 12 |
| 20–34 | 57 | 3.7 | 2 | 1 | 3 | 4 | 4 | 5 | 6 | 8 |
| 35–49 | 787 | 3.8 | 1 | 3 | 3 | 4 | 4 | 5 | 6 | 7 |
| 50–64 | 3,123 | 3.9 | 2 | 3 | 3 | 4 | 5 | 5 | 6 | 8 |
| 65+ | 4,749 | 4.0 | 2 | 3 | 3 | 4 | 5 | 5 | 6 | 8 |
| **2. MULTIPLE DX** | | | | | | | | | | |
| 0–19 Years | 22 | 6.9 | 46 | 4 | 4 | 5 | 6 | 8 | 10 | 36 |
| 20–34 | 148 | 4.3 | 4 | 3 | 3 | 4 | 5 | 7 | 8 | 13 |
| 35–49 | 2,740 | 4.4 | 5 | 3 | 3 | 4 | 5 | 6 | 7 | 12 |
| 50–64 | 16,742 | 4.4 | 4 | 3 | 3 | 4 | 5 | 6 | 8 | 11 |
| 65+ | 42,794 | 4.5 | 4 | 3 | 3 | 4 | 5 | 6 | 8 | 13 |
| **TOTAL SINGLE DX** | 8,723 | 3.9 | 2 | 3 | 3 | 4 | 5 | 5 | 6 | 8 |
| **TOTAL MULTIPLE DX** | 62,446 | 4.5 | 4 | 3 | 3 | 4 | 5 | 6 | 8 | 12 |
| **TOTAL** | | | | | | | | | | |
| 0–19 Years | 29 | 6.4 | 38 | 4 | 4 | 5 | 6 | 10 | 12 | 36 |
| 20–34 | 205 | 4.1 | 4 | 3 | 3 | 4 | 5 | 6 | 7 | 12 |
| 35–49 | 3,527 | 4.3 | 4 | 3 | 3 | 4 | 5 | 6 | 7 | 11 |
| 50–64 | 19,865 | 4.3 | 3 | 3 | 3 | 4 | 5 | 6 | 8 | 11 |
| 65+ | 47,543 | 4.5 | 4 | 3 | 3 | 4 | 5 | 6 | 8 | 13 |
| **GRAND TOTAL** | 71,169 | 4.4 | 4 | 3 | 3 | 4 | 5 | 6 | 7 | 12 |

## 81.55: KNEE REPLACEMENT REV. Formerly included in operation group(s) 749.

| Type of Patients | Observed Patients | Avg. Stay | Vari-ance | Percentiles | | | | | | |
|---|---|---|---|---|---|---|---|---|---|---|
| | | | | 10th | 25th | 50th | 75th | 90th | 95th | 99th |
| **1. SINGLE DX** | | | | | | | | | | |
| 0–19 Years | 1 | 3.0 | 0 | 3 | 3 | 3 | 3 | 3 | 3 | 3 |
| 20–34 | 4 | 3.8 | <1 | 3 | 3 | 3 | 4 | 4 | 4 | 4 |
| 35–49 | 71 | 3.4 | 3 | 1 | 2 | 3 | 5 | 5 | 5 | 7 |
| 50–64 | 186 | 3.9 | 4 | 2 | 3 | 4 | 5 | 6 | 6 | 12 |
| 65+ | 295 | 4.1 | 2 | 3 | 3 | 4 | 5 | 6 | 7 | 10 |
| **2. MULTIPLE DX** | | | | | | | | | | |
| 0–19 Years | 15 | 5.0 | 3 | 3 | 4 | 4 | 7 | 7 | 7 | 12 |
| 20–34 | 38 | 3.5 | 4 | 2 | 3 | 3 | 4 | 6 | 6 | 12 |
| 35–49 | 410 | 4.5 | 5 | 3 | 3 | 4 | 5 | 6 | 8 | 12 |
| 50–64 | 1,474 | 4.8 | 10 | 3 | 3 | 4 | 5 | 7 | 10 | 17 |
| 65+ | 3,995 | 5.0 | 14 | 3 | 3 | 4 | 5 | 7 | 9 | 19 |
| **TOTAL SINGLE DX** | 557 | 3.9 | 3 | 2 | 3 | 4 | 5 | 6 | 6 | 11 |
| **TOTAL MULTIPLE DX** | 5,932 | 4.9 | 12 | 3 | 3 | 4 | 5 | 7 | 9 | 17 |
| **TOTAL** | | | | | | | | | | |
| 0–19 Years | 16 | 3.9 | 2 | 3 | 3 | 3 | 4 | 7 | 7 | 8 |
| 20–34 | 42 | 3.5 | 4 | 2 | 3 | 3 | 4 | 6 | 6 | 12 |
| 35–49 | 481 | 4.3 | 5 | 3 | 3 | 4 | 5 | 7 | 8 | 12 |
| 50–64 | 1,660 | 4.7 | 10 | 3 | 3 | 4 | 5 | 7 | 9 | 16 |
| 65+ | 4,290 | 4.9 | 13 | 3 | 3 | 4 | 5 | 7 | 9 | 17 |
| **GRAND TOTAL** | 6,489 | 4.8 | 11 | 3 | 3 | 4 | 5 | 7 | 9 | 16 |

## 81.52: PARTIAL HIP REPLACEMENT. Formerly included in operation group(s) 747.

| Type of Patients | Observed Patients | Avg. Stay | Vari-ance | Percentiles | | | | | | |
|---|---|---|---|---|---|---|---|---|---|---|
| | | | | 10th | 25th | 50th | 75th | 90th | 95th | 99th |
| **1. SINGLE DX** | | | | | | | | | | |
| 0–19 Years | 5 | 3.7 | 3 | 2 | 2 | 4 | 4 | 4 | 5 | 11 |
| 20–34 | 23 | 3.9 | 2 | 2 | 3 | 4 | 4 | 6 | 8 | 8 |
| 35–49 | 62 | 4.3 | 3 | 3 | 3 | 4 | 5 | 6 | 7 | 10 |
| 50–64 | 95 | 5.0 | 4 | 3 | 4 | 4 | 6 | 7 | 8 | 15 |
| 65+ | 797 | 5.0 | 4 | 3 | 4 | 5 | 6 | 7 | 8 | 11 |
| **2. MULTIPLE DX** | | | | | | | | | | |
| 0–19 Years | 29 | 5.3 | 10 | 3 | 3 | 4 | 9 | 9 | 9 | 17 |
| 20–34 | 72 | 6.0 | 28 | 3 | 3 | 4 | 7 | 14 | 14 | 19 |
| 35–49 | 370 | 6.9 | 50 | 3 | 4 | 5 | 7 | 13 | 19 | 28 |
| 50–64 | 1,535 | 7.1 | 32 | 3 | 4 | 6 | 8 | 11 | 15 | 34 |
| 65+ | 25,007 | 6.6 | 18 | 4 | 4 | 6 | 7 | 11 | 14 | 24 |
| **TOTAL SINGLE DX** | 982 | 4.9 | 4 | 3 | 4 | 4 | 6 | 7 | 8 | 12 |
| **TOTAL MULTIPLE DX** | 27,013 | 6.7 | 20 | 3 | 4 | 6 | 8 | 11 | 14 | 25 |
| **TOTAL** | | | | | | | | | | |
| 0–19 Years | 34 | 5.1 | 9 | 2 | 3 | 4 | 9 | 9 | 9 | 17 |
| 20–34 | 95 | 5.5 | 23 | 3 | 3 | 4 | 6 | 11 | 14 | 16 |
| 35–49 | 432 | 6.5 | 43 | 3 | 4 | 5 | 7 | 12 | 17 | 28 |
| 50–64 | 1,630 | 7.0 | 31 | 3 | 4 | 6 | 8 | 11 | 14 | 34 |
| 65+ | 25,804 | 6.6 | 18 | 4 | 4 | 5 | 7 | 11 | 14 | 24 |
| **GRAND TOTAL** | 27,995 | 6.6 | 19 | 3 | 4 | 5 | 7 | 11 | 14 | 24 |

## 81.53: HIP REPLACEMENT REVISION. Formerly included in operation group(s) 747.

| Type of Patients | Observed Patients | Avg. Stay | Vari-ance | Percentiles | | | | | | |
|---|---|---|---|---|---|---|---|---|---|---|
| | | | | 10th | 25th | 50th | 75th | 90th | 95th | 99th |
| **1. SINGLE DX** | | | | | | | | | | |
| 0–19 Years | 1 | 4.0 | 0 | 4 | 4 | 4 | 4 | 4 | 4 | 4 |
| 20–34 | 37 | 3.7 | 1 | 3 | 3 | 3 | 4 | 5 | 6 | 8 |
| 35–49 | 198 | 4.0 | 3 | 3 | 3 | 4 | 5 | 6 | 7 | 8 |
| 50–64 | 235 | 3.8 | 3 | 3 | 3 | 3 | 4 | 6 | 7 | 9 |
| 65+ | 334 | 4.4 | 3 | 3 | 3 | 4 | 5 | 7 | 8 | 9 |
| **2. MULTIPLE DX** | | | | | | | | | | |
| 0–19 Years | 6 | 3.8 | 7 | 3 | 3 | 3 | 3 | 5 | 9 | 15 |
| 20–34 | 150 | 5.1 | 25 | 3 | 3 | 4 | 6 | 8 | 10 | 31 |
| 35–49 | 939 | 4.9 | 18 | 3 | 3 | 5 | 5 | 7 | 10 | 22 |
| 50–64 | 1,628 | 5.5 | 11 | 3 | 4 | 5 | 6 | 8 | 12 | 19 |
| 65+ | 5,026 | 5.8 | 23 | 3 | 4 | 5 | 6 | 9 | 13 | 21 |
| **TOTAL SINGLE DX** | 805 | 4.1 | 3 | 3 | 3 | 4 | 5 | 6 | 7 | 9 |
| **TOTAL MULTIPLE DX** | 7,749 | 5.6 | 20 | 3 | 4 | 4 | 6 | 9 | 12 | 21 |
| **TOTAL** | | | | | | | | | | |
| 0–19 Years | 7 | 3.8 | 6 | 3 | 3 | 3 | 3 | 5 | 9 | 15 |
| 20–34 | 187 | 4.8 | 20 | 3 | 3 | 4 | 5 | 8 | 9 | 31 |
| 35–49 | 1,137 | 4.7 | 16 | 3 | 3 | 4 | 6 | 7 | 9 | 22 |
| 50–64 | 1,863 | 5.2 | 11 | 3 | 3 | 4 | 6 | 8 | 11 | 18 |
| 65+ | 5,360 | 5.7 | 21 | 3 | 4 | 5 | 6 | 9 | 12 | 21 |
| **GRAND TOTAL** | 8,554 | 5.5 | 18 | 3 | 3 | 4 | 6 | 9 | 12 | 20 |

Length of Stay by Diagnosis and Operation, United States, 2000

# United States, October 1998–September 1999 Data, by Operation

## 81.7: HAND/FINGER ARTHROPLASTY. Formerly included in operation group(s) 750, 751.

| Type of Patients | Observed Patients | Avg. Stay | Variance | 10th | 25th | 50th | 75th | 90th | 95th | 99th |
|---|---|---|---|---|---|---|---|---|---|---|
| **1. SINGLE DX** | | | | | | | | | | |
| 0–19 Years | 10 | 1.1 | <1 | 1 | 1 | 1 | 1 | 2 | 2 | 2 |
| 20–34 | 14 | 1.5 | 2 | 1 | 1 | 1 | 1 | 2 | 2 | 7 |
| 35–49 | 29 | 1.7 | <1 | 1 | 1 | 2 | 2 | 2 | 2 | 5 |
| 50–64 | 51 | 1.3 | <1 | 1 | 1 | 1 | 1 | 2 | 2 | 4 |
| 65+ | 46 | 1.3 | <1 | 1 | 1 | 1 | 2 | 2 | 2 | 2 |
| **2. MULTIPLE DX** | | | | | | | | | | |
| 0–19 Years | 20 | 1.6 | 3 | 1 | 1 | 1 | 2 | 2 | 2 | 9 |
| 20–34 | 39 | 1.9 | 2 | 1 | 1 | 1 | 2 | 4 | 4 | 8 |
| 35–49 | 78 | 1.8 | 2 | 1 | 1 | 2 | 2 | 2 | 3 | 7 |
| 50–64 | 148 | 1.8 | 1 | 1 | 1 | 1 | 2 | 2 | 3 | 5 |
| 65+ | 195 | 1.9 | 3 | 1 | 1 | 1 | 2 | 3 | 5 | 9 |
| **TOTAL SINGLE DX** | 150 | 1.4 | <1 | 1 | 1 | 1 | 2 | 2 | 2 | 5 |
| **TOTAL MULTIPLE DX** | 480 | 1.8 | 2 | 1 | 1 | 1 | 2 | 3 | 4 | 8 |
| **TOTAL** | | | | | | | | | | |
| 0–19 Years | 30 | 1.4 | 2 | 1 | 1 | 1 | 1 | 2 | 2 | 9 |
| 20–34 | 53 | 1.8 | 2 | 1 | 1 | 1 | 2 | 4 | 4 | 9 |
| 35–49 | 107 | 1.8 | 2 | 1 | 1 | 2 | 2 | 2 | 3 | 6 |
| 50–64 | 199 | 1.7 | <1 | 1 | 1 | 1 | 2 | 3 | 3 | 5 |
| 65+ | 241 | 1.8 | 2 | 1 | 1 | 1 | 2 | 3 | 5 | 9 |
| **GRAND TOTAL** | 630 | 1.7 | 2 | 1 | 1 | 1 | 2 | 3 | 4 | 8 |

## 81.8: SHOULD/ELB ARTHROPLASTY. Formerly included in operation group(s) 750, 751.

| Type of Patients | Observed Patients | Avg. Stay | Variance | 10th | 25th | 50th | 75th | 90th | 95th | 99th |
|---|---|---|---|---|---|---|---|---|---|---|
| **1. SINGLE DX** | | | | | | | | | | |
| 0–19 Years | 183 | 1.4 | <1 | 1 | 1 | 1 | 2 | 2 | 2 | 4 |
| 20–34 | 387 | 1.4 | 2 | 1 | 1 | 1 | 1 | 2 | 2 | 5 |
| 35–49 | 560 | 1.5 | <1 | 1 | 1 | 1 | 2 | 2 | 3 | 4 |
| 50–64 | 670 | 1.8 | 1 | 1 | 1 | 2 | 2 | 3 | 4 | 6 |
| 65+ | 679 | 2.1 | 1 | 1 | 2 | 2 | 3 | 3 | 4 | 6 |
| **2. MULTIPLE DX** | | | | | | | | | | |
| 0–19 Years | 107 | 2.0 | 7 | 1 | 1 | 1 | 2 | 4 | 5 | 17 |
| 20–34 | 434 | 2.0 | 3 | 1 | 1 | 1 | 2 | 3 | 5 | 8 |
| 35–49 | 1,464 | 1.8 | 3 | 1 | 1 | 1 | 2 | 3 | 4 | 8 |
| 50–64 | 2,924 | 2.1 | 5 | 1 | 1 | 2 | 2 | 3 | 4 | 11 |
| 65+ | 5,507 | 2.9 | 6 | 1 | 2 | 2 | 3 | 5 | 7 | 14 |
| **TOTAL SINGLE DX** | 2,479 | 1.7 | 1 | 1 | 1 | 1 | 2 | 3 | 3 | 5 |
| **TOTAL MULTIPLE DX** | 10,436 | 2.4 | 6 | 1 | 1 | 2 | 3 | 4 | 6 | 12 |
| **TOTAL** | | | | | | | | | | |
| 0–19 Years | 290 | 1.6 | 3 | 1 | 1 | 1 | 2 | 2 | 3 | 8 |
| 20–34 | 821 | 1.7 | 2 | 1 | 1 | 1 | 2 | 3 | 4 | 6 |
| 35–49 | 2,024 | 1.7 | 2 | 1 | 1 | 1 | 2 | 3 | 4 | 7 |
| 50–64 | 3,594 | 2.0 | 5 | 1 | 1 | 2 | 2 | 3 | 4 | 9 |
| 65+ | 6,186 | 2.8 | 6 | 1 | 1 | 2 | 3 | 5 | 7 | 14 |
| **GRAND TOTAL** | 12,915 | 2.3 | 5 | 1 | 1 | 2 | 3 | 4 | 5 | 11 |

## 81.80: TOTAL SHOULDER REPL. Formerly included in operation group(s) 750.

| Type of Patients | Observed Patients | Avg. Stay | Variance | 10th | 25th | 50th | 75th | 90th | 95th | 99th |
|---|---|---|---|---|---|---|---|---|---|---|
| **1. SINGLE DX** | | | | | | | | | | |
| 0–19 Years | 0 | | | | | | | | | |
| 20–34 | 7 | 2.9 | <1 | 2 | 3 | 3 | 3 | 3 | 3 | 3 |
| 35–49 | 38 | 2.3 | <1 | 2 | 2 | 2 | 3 | 3 | 3 | 4 |
| 50–64 | 125 | 2.1 | <1 | 1 | 2 | 2 | 2 | 3 | 3 | 9 |
| 65+ | 166 | 2.5 | <1 | 1 | 2 | 2 | 3 | 4 | 5 | 5 |
| **2. MULTIPLE DX** | | | | | | | | | | |
| 0–19 Years | 0 | | | | | | | | | |
| 20–34 | 13 | 3.4 | 2 | 2 | 2 | 3 | 5 | 5 | 5 | 5 |
| 35–49 | 121 | 3.0 | 9 | 1 | 2 | 2 | 3 | 5 | 6 | 14 |
| 50–64 | 441 | 2.6 | 3 | 1 | 2 | 2 | 3 | 4 | 5 | 12 |
| 65+ | 1,313 | 3.1 | 4 | 2 | 2 | 3 | 3 | 5 | 6 | 10 |
| **TOTAL SINGLE DX** | 336 | 2.3 | 1 | 1 | 2 | 2 | 3 | 3 | 4 | 5 |
| **TOTAL MULTIPLE DX** | 1,888 | 3.0 | 4 | 1 | 2 | 3 | 3 | 5 | 6 | 10 |
| **TOTAL** | | | | | | | | | | |
| 0–19 Years | 0 | | | | | | | | | |
| 20–34 | 20 | 3.1 | 1 | 2 | 3 | 3 | 3 | 5 | 5 | 5 |
| 35–49 | 159 | 2.8 | 7 | 1 | 2 | 2 | 3 | 5 | 5 | 14 |
| 50–64 | 566 | 2.5 | 3 | 1 | 2 | 2 | 3 | 3 | 5 | 10 |
| 65+ | 1,479 | 3.0 | 3 | 2 | 3 | 3 | 3 | 5 | 6 | 10 |
| **GRAND TOTAL** | 2,224 | 2.9 | 3 | 2 | 2 | 3 | 3 | 5 | 5 | 10 |

## 81.81: PARTIAL SHOULDER REPL. Formerly included in operation group(s) 750.

| Type of Patients | Observed Patients | Avg. Stay | Variance | 10th | 25th | 50th | 75th | 90th | 95th | 99th |
|---|---|---|---|---|---|---|---|---|---|---|
| **1. SINGLE DX** | | | | | | | | | | |
| 0–19 Years | 4 | 3.1 | 1 | 2 | 2 | 4 | 4 | 4 | 4 | 4 |
| 20–34 | 10 | 2.1 | <1 | 1 | 1 | 2 | 3 | 4 | 4 | 5 |
| 35–49 | 43 | 2.5 | 1 | 1 | 2 | 2 | 3 | 5 | 5 | 5 |
| 50–64 | 108 | 2.5 | 1 | 2 | 2 | 2 | 3 | 4 | 4 | 7 |
| 65+ | 174 | 2.6 | 2 | 1 | 2 | 2 | 3 | 4 | 5 | 6 |
| **2. MULTIPLE DX** | | | | | | | | | | |
| 0–19 Years | 7 | 3.1 | 3 | 1 | 1 | 3 | 4 | 4 | 6 | 6 |
| 20–34 | 48 | 3.0 | 8 | 1 | 2 | 2 | 3 | 6 | 6 | 24 |
| 35–49 | 166 | 3.4 | 8 | 1 | 2 | 2 | 4 | 6 | 9 | 15 |
| 50–64 | 489 | 3.5 | 16 | 1 | 2 | 2 | 4 | 6 | 9 | 26 |
| 65+ | 1,666 | 3.9 | 11 | 2 | 3 | 3 | 4 | 7 | 10 | 17 |
| **TOTAL SINGLE DX** | 339 | 2.5 | 1 | 1 | 2 | 2 | 3 | 4 | 5 | 7 |
| **TOTAL MULTIPLE DX** | 2,376 | 3.8 | 12 | 1 | 2 | 3 | 4 | 7 | 9 | 18 |
| **TOTAL** | | | | | | | | | | |
| 0–19 Years | 11 | 3.1 | 2 | 1 | 2 | 3 | 4 | 4 | 6 | 6 |
| 20–34 | 58 | 2.9 | 7 | 1 | 2 | 3 | 3 | 5 | 5 | 24 |
| 35–49 | 209 | 3.2 | 7 | 1 | 2 | 2 | 3 | 5 | 8 | 15 |
| 50–64 | 597 | 3.3 | 13 | 2 | 2 | 3 | 4 | 6 | 8 | 25 |
| 65+ | 1,840 | 3.8 | 10 | 2 | 3 | 3 | 4 | 7 | 9 | 17 |
| **GRAND TOTAL** | 2,715 | 3.6 | 11 | 1 | 2 | 3 | 4 | 6 | 9 | 17 |

Length of Stay by Diagnosis and Operation, United States, 2000

## United States, October 1998–September 1999 Data, by Operation

### 81.84: TOTAL ELBOW REPLACEMENT. Formerly included in operation group(s) 750.

| Type of Patients | Observed Patients | Avg. Stay | Vari-ance | 10th | 25th | 50th | 75th | 90th | 95th | 99th |
|---|---|---|---|---|---|---|---|---|---|---|
| **1. SINGLE DX** | | | | | | | | | | |
| 0–19 Years | 3 | 3.0 | 2 | 1 | 2 | 4 | 4 | 4 | 4 | 4 |
| 20–34 | 8 | 2.0 | <1 | 1 | 1 | 2 | 3 | 3 | 3 | 3 |
| 35–49 | 19 | 1.7 | <1 | 1 | 2 | 2 | 2 | 3 | 3 | 3 |
| 50–64 | 20 | 2.8 | 2 | 1 | 2 | 3 | 4 | 4 | 4 | 4 |
| 65+ | 9 | 1.7 | <1 | 1 | 1 | 1 | 3 | 3 | 3 | 3 |
| **2. MULTIPLE DX** | | | | | | | | | | |
| 0–19 Years | 1 | 17.0 | 0 | 17 | 17 | 17 | 17 | 17 | 17 | 17 |
| 20–34 | 25 | 3.3 | 3 | 2 | 2 | 3 | 3 | 6 | 7 | 8 |
| 35–49 | 59 | 2.7 | 3 | 1 | 2 | 2 | 3 | 5 | 6 | 9 |
| 50–64 | 92 | 2.5 | 3 | 1 | 2 | 2 | 3 | 4 | 4 | 10 |
| 65+ | 150 | 3.2 | 6 | 1 | 2 | 3 | 4 | 6 | 6 | 12 |
| **TOTAL SINGLE DX** | 59 | 2.2 | 1 | 1 | 1 | 2 | 3 | 4 | 4 | 4 |
| **TOTAL MULTIPLE DX** | 327 | 3.1 | 6 | 1 | 2 | 2 | 3 | 5 | 7 | 17 |
| **TOTAL** | | | | | | | | | | |
| 0–19 Years | 4 | 10.3 | 52 | 1 | 4 | 17 | 17 | 17 | 17 | 17 |
| 20–34 | 33 | 3.0 | 3 | 1 | 2 | 3 | 3 | 5 | 7 | 8 |
| 35–49 | 78 | 2.5 | 3 | 1 | 1 | 2 | 3 | 4 | 5 | 9 |
| 50–64 | 112 | 2.6 | 3 | 1 | 2 | 2 | 3 | 4 | 6 | 10 |
| 65+ | 159 | 3.1 | 6 | 1 | 2 | 3 | 4 | 6 | 6 | 12 |
| **GRAND TOTAL** | 386 | 2.9 | 5 | 1 | 2 | 3 | 3 | 5 | 6 | 17 |

### 81.9: OTHER JOINT STRUCTURE OP. Formerly included in operation group(s) 750, 751, 767.

| Type of Patients | Observed Patients | Avg. Stay | Vari-ance | 10th | 25th | 50th | 75th | 90th | 95th | 99th |
|---|---|---|---|---|---|---|---|---|---|---|
| **1. SINGLE DX** | | | | | | | | | | |
| 0–19 Years | 400 | 2.8 | 4 | 1 | 2 | 2 | 4 | 6 | 7 | 9 |
| 20–34 | 135 | 2.7 | 3 | 1 | 2 | 2 | 4 | 4 | 6 | 9 |
| 35–49 | 143 | 2.8 | 3 | 1 | 3 | 3 | 3 | 6 | 7 | 9 |
| 50–64 | 71 | 2.1 | 2 | 1 | 1 | 2 | 2 | 4 | 5 | 7 |
| 65+ | 78 | 3.1 | 4 | 1 | 2 | 3 | 4 | 5 | 7 | 11 |
| **2. MULTIPLE DX** | | | | | | | | | | |
| 0–19 Years | 624 | 4.0 | 12 | 1 | 2 | 3 | 5 | 8 | 11 | 20 |
| 20–34 | 578 | 4.8 | 20 | 1 | 2 | 4 | 6 | 8 | 13 | 28 |
| 35–49 | 1,269 | 5.4 | 32 | 2 | 3 | 4 | 6 | 11 | 15 | 30 |
| 50–64 | 1,754 | 5.5 | 28 | 2 | 3 | 5 | 7 | 10 | 15 | 27 |
| 65+ | 5,806 | 6.4 | 29 | 2 | 3 | 5 | 8 | 13 | 16 | 27 |
| **TOTAL SINGLE DX** | 827 | 2.8 | 3 | 1 | 1 | 2 | 4 | 5 | 6 | 9 |
| **TOTAL MULTIPLE DX** | 10,031 | 5.9 | 28 | 2 | 3 | 4 | 7 | 11 | 15 | 27 |
| **TOTAL** | | | | | | | | | | |
| 0–19 Years | 1,024 | 3.6 | 10 | 1 | 2 | 3 | 4 | 7 | 10 | 14 |
| 20–34 | 713 | 4.4 | 18 | 1 | 2 | 3 | 6 | 8 | 11 | 27 |
| 35–49 | 1,412 | 5.2 | 30 | 1 | 2 | 4 | 6 | 10 | 14 | 26 |
| 50–64 | 1,825 | 5.4 | 28 | 2 | 2 | 4 | 7 | 10 | 14 | 26 |
| 65+ | 5,884 | 6.4 | 29 | 2 | 3 | 5 | 8 | 13 | 16 | 27 |
| **GRAND TOTAL** | 10,858 | 5.6 | 27 | 2 | 3 | 4 | 7 | 11 | 15 | 26 |

### 81.82: REP RECUR SHOULD DISLOC. Formerly included in operation group(s) 751.

| Type of Patients | Observed Patients | Avg. Stay | Vari-ance | 10th | 25th | 50th | 75th | 90th | 95th | 99th |
|---|---|---|---|---|---|---|---|---|---|---|
| **1. SINGLE DX** | | | | | | | | | | |
| 0–19 Years | 123 | 1.2 | <1 | 1 | 1 | 1 | 1 | 2 | 2 | 3 |
| 20–34 | 241 | 1.3 | <1 | 1 | 1 | 1 | 1 | 2 | 2 | 3 |
| 35–49 | 94 | 1.2 | <1 | 1 | 1 | 1 | 1 | 2 | 2 | 3 |
| 50–64 | 18 | 1.8 | <1 | 1 | 1 | 1 | 2 | 4 | 4 | 4 |
| 65+ | 4 | 5.5 | 18 | 1 | 2 | 2 | 10 | 10 | 10 | 10 |
| **2. MULTIPLE DX** | | | | | | | | | | |
| 0–19 Years | 60 | 1.2 | <1 | 1 | 1 | 1 | 1 | 2 | 2 | 2 |
| 20–34 | 152 | 1.6 | <1 | 1 | 1 | 1 | 2 | 3 | 3 | 4 |
| 35–49 | 116 | 1.5 | <1 | 1 | 1 | 1 | 2 | 2 | 3 | 5 |
| 50–64 | 44 | 1.9 | 3 | 1 | 1 | 1 | 2 | 3 | 3 | 10 |
| 65+ | 54 | 3.7 | 21 | 1 | 2 | 3 | 4 | 5 | 8 | 42 |
| **TOTAL SINGLE DX** | 480 | 1.3 | 2 | 1 | 1 | 1 | 1 | 2 | 2 | 4 |
| **TOTAL MULTIPLE DX** | 426 | 1.8 | 3 | 1 | 1 | 1 | 2 | 3 | 4 | 6 |
| **TOTAL** | | | | | | | | | | |
| 0–19 Years | 183 | 1.2 | <1 | 1 | 1 | 1 | 1 | 2 | 2 | 3 |
| 20–34 | 393 | 1.4 | 2 | 1 | 1 | 1 | 2 | 2 | 3 | 4 |
| 35–49 | 210 | 1.4 | <1 | 1 | 1 | 1 | 2 | 2 | 3 | 3 |
| 50–64 | 62 | 1.9 | 3 | 1 | 1 | 1 | 2 | 3 | 4 | 10 |
| 65+ | 58 | 3.9 | 21 | 1 | 2 | 3 | 4 | 5 | 8 | 42 |
| **GRAND TOTAL** | 906 | 1.5 | 3 | 1 | 1 | 1 | 2 | 2 | 3 | 5 |

### 81.83: SHOULD ARTHROPLASTY NEC. Formerly included in operation group(s) 751.

| Type of Patients | Observed Patients | Avg. Stay | Vari-ance | 10th | 25th | 50th | 75th | 90th | 95th | 99th |
|---|---|---|---|---|---|---|---|---|---|---|
| **1. SINGLE DX** | | | | | | | | | | |
| 0–19 Years | 48 | 1.4 | <1 | 1 | 1 | 1 | 2 | 2 | 2 | 3 |
| 20–34 | 111 | 1.4 | <1 | 1 | 1 | 1 | 2 | 2 | 3 | 5 |
| 35–49 | 359 | 1.4 | <1 | 1 | 1 | 1 | 2 | 2 | 2 | 4 |
| 50–64 | 395 | 1.5 | <1 | 1 | 1 | 1 | 2 | 2 | 3 | 4 |
| 65+ | 319 | 1.6 | <1 | 1 | 1 | 1 | 2 | 3 | 3 | 4 |
| **2. MULTIPLE DX** | | | | | | | | | | |
| 0–19 Years | 29 | 1.7 | 1 | 1 | 1 | 1 | 2 | 4 | 4 | 4 |
| 20–34 | 176 | 1.7 | 3 | 1 | 1 | 1 | 2 | 4 | 5 | 9 |
| 35–49 | 977 | 1.5 | 2 | 1 | 1 | 1 | 2 | 2 | 3 | 5 |
| 50–64 | 1,831 | 1.6 | 2 | 1 | 1 | 1 | 2 | 2 | 3 | 7 |
| 65+ | 2,302 | 2.0 | 2 | 1 | 1 | 2 | 2 | 3 | 4 | 9 |
| **TOTAL SINGLE DX** | 1,232 | 1.5 | <1 | 1 | 1 | 1 | 2 | 2 | 3 | 5 |
| **TOTAL MULTIPLE DX** | 5,315 | 1.7 | 2 | 1 | 1 | 1 | 2 | 3 | 4 | 7 |
| **TOTAL** | | | | | | | | | | |
| 0–19 Years | 77 | 1.5 | <1 | 1 | 1 | 1 | 2 | 2 | 3 | 4 |
| 20–34 | 287 | 1.6 | 2 | 1 | 1 | 1 | 2 | 2 | 4 | 5 |
| 35–49 | 1,336 | 1.5 | 1 | 1 | 1 | 1 | 2 | 2 | 3 | 4 |
| 50–64 | 2,226 | 1.6 | 1 | 1 | 1 | 1 | 2 | 2 | 3 | 6 |
| 65+ | 2,621 | 1.9 | 2 | 1 | 1 | 2 | 2 | 3 | 4 | 8 |
| **GRAND TOTAL** | 6,547 | 1.7 | 2 | 1 | 1 | 1 | 2 | 3 | 3 | 7 |

Length of Stay by Diagnosis and Operation, United States, 2000

# United States, October 1998–September 1999 Data, by Operation

## 82.0: INC HAND SOFT TISSUE. Formerly included in operation group(s) 752.

| Type of Patients | Observed Patients | Avg. Stay | Variance | Percentiles | | | | | | |
|---|---|---|---|---|---|---|---|---|---|---|
| | | | | 10th | 25th | 50th | 75th | 90th | 95th | 99th |
| **1. SINGLE DX** | | | | | | | | | | |
| 0–19 Years | 46 | 1.5 | 2 | 1 | 1 | 1 | 2 | 2 | 4 | 10 |
| 20–34 | 64 | 3.0 | 2 | 1 | 2 | 3 | 4 | 4 | 5 | 6 |
| 35–49 | 72 | 2.9 | 3 | 1 | 1 | 3 | 4 | 5 | 7 | 7 |
| 50–64 | 29 | 1.9 | 2 | 1 | 1 | 1 | 3 | 3 | 4 | 12 |
| 65+ | 10 | 2.3 | <1 | 1 | 1 | 2 | 3 | 3 | 4 | 4 |
| **2. MULTIPLE DX** | | | | | | | | | | |
| 0–19 Years | 85 | 3.3 | 4 | 1 | 2 | 3 | 4 | 6 | 7 | 12 |
| 20–34 | 211 | 3.5 | 5 | 1 | 2 | 3 | 4 | 6 | 7 | 12 |
| 35–49 | 290 | 3.7 | 5 | 2 | 2 | 3 | 5 | 6 | 8 | 13 |
| 50–64 | 151 | 4.9 | 11 | 2 | 3 | 4 | 6 | 10 | 10 | 14 |
| 65+ | 148 | 6.3 | 38 | 2 | 3 | 4 | 8 | 10 | 16 | 34 |
| **TOTAL SINGLE DX** | 221 | 2.4 | 2 | 1 | 1 | 2 | 3 | 4 | 5 | 7 |
| **TOTAL MULTIPLE DX** | 885 | 4.1 | 10 | 2 | 2 | 3 | 5 | 7 | 10 | 15 |
| **TOTAL** | | | | | | | | | | |
| 0–19 | 131 | 2.6 | 4 | 1 | 1 | 2 | 3 | 6 | 6 | 11 |
| 20–34 | 275 | 3.3 | 4 | 1 | 2 | 3 | 4 | 5 | 7 | 9 |
| 35–49 | 362 | 3.6 | 5 | 1 | 2 | 3 | 5 | 6 | 8 | 13 |
| 50–64 | 180 | 4.2 | 10 | 1 | 2 | 3 | 6 | 9 | 10 | 14 |
| 65+ | 158 | 6.0 | 36 | 2 | 3 | 4 | 8 | 10 | 16 | 34 |
| **GRAND TOTAL** | 1,106 | 3.7 | 9 | 1 | 2 | 3 | 5 | 7 | 9 | 14 |

## 82.01: EXPLOR TEND SHEATH HAND. Formerly included in operation group(s) 752.

| Type of Patients | Observed Patients | Avg. Stay | Variance | Percentiles | | | | | | |
|---|---|---|---|---|---|---|---|---|---|---|
| | | | | 10th | 25th | 50th | 75th | 90th | 95th | 99th |
| **1. SINGLE DX** | | | | | | | | | | |
| 0–19 Years | 26 | 1.5 | 1 | 1 | 1 | 1 | 2 | 2 | 4 | 6 |
| 20–34 | 32 | 3.0 | 2 | 1 | 2 | 3 | 4 | 4 | 4 | 6 |
| 35–49 | 53 | 3.1 | 3 | 1 | 2 | 3 | 4 | 5 | 7 | 7 |
| 50–64 | 18 | 1.8 | 1 | 1 | 1 | 1 | 2 | 3 | 4 | 12 |
| 65+ | 9 | 2.4 | <1 | 1 | 2 | 2 | 3 | 3 | 4 | 4 |
| **2. MULTIPLE DX** | | | | | | | | | | |
| 0–19 Years | 32 | 3.2 | 2 | 2 | 2 | 3 | 3 | 4 | 7 | 7 |
| 20–34 | 119 | 3.4 | 4 | 1 | 2 | 3 | 4 | 6 | 7 | 12 |
| 35–49 | 168 | 3.5 | 4 | 2 | 2 | 3 | 5 | 6 | 8 | 10 |
| 50–64 | 74 | 4.6 | 8 | 2 | 2 | 4 | 7 | 9 | 10 | 10 |
| 65+ | 82 | 4.9 | 16 | 2 | 2 | 4 | 6 | 9 | 10 | 28 |
| **TOTAL SINGLE DX** | 138 | 2.4 | 2 | 1 | 1 | 2 | 3 | 4 | 5 | 7 |
| **TOTAL MULTIPLE DX** | 475 | 3.8 | 7 | 2 | 2 | 3 | 5 | 7 | 9 | 12 |
| **TOTAL** | | | | | | | | | | |
| 0–19 | 58 | 2.2 | 2 | 1 | 2 | 2 | 3 | 4 | 6 | 7 |
| 20–34 | 151 | 3.2 | 3 | 1 | 2 | 3 | 4 | 5 | 7 | 8 |
| 35–49 | 221 | 3.4 | 4 | 1 | 2 | 3 | 5 | 6 | 7 | 10 |
| 50–64 | 92 | 3.8 | 8 | 1 | 2 | 3 | 5 | 8 | 10 | 10 |
| 65+ | 91 | 4.6 | 15 | 2 | 2 | 4 | 5 | 9 | 10 | 22 |
| **GRAND TOTAL** | 613 | 3.4 | 6 | 1 | 2 | 3 | 4 | 6 | 8 | 10 |

## 81.91: ARTHROCENTESIS. Formerly included in operation group(s) 767.

| Type of Patients | Observed Patients | Avg. Stay | Variance | Percentiles | | | | | | |
|---|---|---|---|---|---|---|---|---|---|---|
| | | | | 10th | 25th | 50th | 75th | 90th | 95th | 99th |
| **1. SINGLE DX** | | | | | | | | | | |
| 0–19 Years | 355 | 3.0 | 4 | 1 | 2 | 2 | 4 | 6 | 7 | 9 |
| 20–34 | 82 | 3.0 | 3 | 1 | 1 | 3 | 4 | 6 | 6 | 9 |
| 35–49 | 98 | 3.0 | 4 | 1 | 2 | 3 | 3 | 6 | 7 | 9 |
| 50–64 | 48 | 2.4 | 2 | 1 | 1 | 2 | 3 | 4 | 6 | 7 |
| 65+ | 41 | 3.2 | 6 | 1 | 2 | 3 | 4 | 5 | 11 | 11 |
| **2. MULTIPLE DX** | | | | | | | | | | |
| 0–19 Years | 577 | 4.1 | 12 | 1 | 2 | 3 | 5 | 8 | 11 | 19 |
| 20–34 | 439 | 4.9 | 23 | 2 | 2 | 4 | 6 | 9 | 14 | 29 |
| 35–49 | 991 | 5.4 | 31 | 1 | 3 | 4 | 6 | 11 | 15 | 30 |
| 50–64 | 1,263 | 5.6 | 26 | 2 | 3 | 4 | 7 | 10 | 14 | 26 |
| 65+ | 3,649 | 6.4 | 28 | 2 | 3 | 5 | 8 | 12 | 15 | 27 |
| **TOTAL SINGLE DX** | 624 | 3.0 | 4 | 1 | 2 | 2 | 4 | 6 | 7 | 9 |
| **TOTAL MULTIPLE DX** | 6,919 | 5.8 | 27 | 2 | 3 | 4 | 7 | 11 | 15 | 26 |
| **TOTAL** | | | | | | | | | | |
| 0–19 | 932 | 3.7 | 9 | 1 | 2 | 3 | 4 | 7 | 10 | 14 |
| 20–34 | 521 | 4.6 | 21 | 1 | 2 | 4 | 6 | 8 | 13 | 29 |
| 35–49 | 1,089 | 5.2 | 29 | 1 | 3 | 4 | 6 | 10 | 15 | 30 |
| 50–64 | 1,311 | 5.5 | 26 | 2 | 3 | 4 | 7 | 10 | 14 | 26 |
| 65+ | 3,690 | 6.4 | 28 | 2 | 3 | 5 | 8 | 12 | 15 | 27 |
| **GRAND TOTAL** | 7,543 | 5.5 | 25 | 2 | 3 | 4 | 7 | 11 | 14 | 26 |

## 81.92: INJECTION INTO JOINT. Formerly included in operation group(s) 767.

| Type of Patients | Observed Patients | Avg. Stay | Variance | Percentiles | | | | | | |
|---|---|---|---|---|---|---|---|---|---|---|
| | | | | 10th | 25th | 50th | 75th | 90th | 95th | 99th |
| **1. SINGLE DX** | | | | | | | | | | |
| 0–19 Years | 9 | 1.4 | 1 | 1 | 1 | 1 | 1 | 1 | 4 | 6 |
| 20–34 | 8 | 3.2 | 1 | 2 | 3 | 3 | 4 | 4 | 4 | 4 |
| 35–49 | 11 | 2.6 | 4 | 1 | 1 | 2 | 4 | 5 | 7 | 7 |
| 50–64 | 7 | 1.6 | 1 | 1 | 1 | 1 | 1 | 4 | 4 | 5 |
| 65+ | 21 | 3.1 | 3 | 1 | 1 | 3 | 4 | 5 | 7 | 7 |
| **2. MULTIPLE DX** | | | | | | | | | | |
| 0–19 Years | 15 | 6.5 | 52 | 1 | 3 | 4 | 5 | 24 | 24 | 24 |
| 20–34 | 73 | 5.4 | 11 | 1 | 3 | 5 | 7 | 9 | 14 | 15 |
| 35–49 | 196 | 6.4 | 44 | 2 | 3 | 5 | 8 | 11 | 15 | 23 |
| 50–64 | 404 | 5.9 | 38 | 1 | 3 | 4 | 7 | 12 | 17 | 37 |
| 65+ | 2,006 | 6.8 | 32 | 2 | 3 | 5 | 8 | 14 | 17 | 30 |
| **TOTAL SINGLE DX** | 56 | 2.4 | 3 | 1 | 1 | 1 | 4 | 5 | 6 | 7 |
| **TOTAL MULTIPLE DX** | 2,694 | 6.6 | 34 | 2 | 3 | 5 | 8 | 13 | 17 | 30 |
| **TOTAL** | | | | | | | | | | |
| 0–19 | 24 | 3.7 | 30 | 1 | 1 | 1 | 4 | 5 | 21 | 24 |
| 20–34 | 81 | 5.3 | 11 | 1 | 3 | 5 | 7 | 9 | 14 | 15 |
| 35–49 | 207 | 6.2 | 43 | 1 | 3 | 5 | 8 | 11 | 15 | 23 |
| 50–64 | 411 | 5.8 | 37 | 1 | 3 | 4 | 7 | 12 | 17 | 37 |
| 65+ | 2,027 | 6.8 | 32 | 2 | 3 | 5 | 8 | 14 | 17 | 28 |
| **GRAND TOTAL** | 2,750 | 6.5 | 33 | 2 | 3 | 5 | 8 | 13 | 16 | 30 |

Length of Stay by Diagnosis and Operation, United States, 2000

# United States, October 1998–September 1999 Data, by Operation

## 82.09: INC SOFT TISSUE HAND NEC. Formerly included in operation group(s) 752.

| Type of Patients | Observed Patients | Avg. Stay | Variance | Percentiles | | | | | | |
|---|---|---|---|---|---|---|---|---|---|---|
| | | | | 10th | 25th | 50th | 75th | 90th | 95th | 99th |
| **1. SINGLE DX** | | | | | | | | | | |
| 0–19 Years | 16 | 1.7 | 4 | 1 | 1 | 1 | 1 | 3 | 6 | 10 |
| 20–34 | 27 | 2.6 | 4 | 1 | 1 | 2 | 4 | 5 | 5 | 11 |
| 35–49 | 15 | 2.1 | 3 | 1 | 1 | 1 | 3 | 6 | 6 | 6 |
| 50–64 | 8 | 2.1 | <1 | 1 | 2 | 2 | 2 | 3 | 3 | 3 |
| 65+ | 1 | 1.0 | 0 | 1 | 1 | 1 | 1 | 1 | 1 | 1 |
| **2. MULTIPLE DX** | | | | | | | | | | |
| 0–19 Years | 37 | 3.3 | 5 | 1 | 2 | 3 | 4 | 6 | 6 | 12 |
| 20–34 | 74 | 3.5 | 4 | 1 | 2 | 3 | 5 | 6 | 8 | 9 |
| 35–49 | 102 | 3.9 | 6 | 2 | 2 | 3 | 5 | 7 | 8 | 13 |
| 50–64 | 66 | 5.5 | 17 | 2 | 3 | 4 | 7 | 12 | 14 | 22 |
| 65+ | 56 | 8.2 | 63 | 2 | 3 | 5 | 10 | 16 | 34 | 35 |
| **TOTAL SINGLE DX** | 67 | 2.1 | 3 | 1 | 1 | 1 | 2 | 5 | 6 | 10 |
| **TOTAL MULTIPLE DX** | 335 | 4.5 | 16 | 2 | 2 | 3 | 5 | 8 | 12 | 22 |
| **TOTAL** | | | | | | | | | | |
| 0–19 Years | 53 | 2.9 | 5 | 1 | 1 | 2 | 3 | 6 | 6 | 12 |
| 20–34 | 101 | 3.3 | 4 | 1 | 2 | 3 | 4 | 6 | 8 | 9 |
| 35–49 | 117 | 3.8 | 6 | 2 | 2 | 3 | 5 | 7 | 8 | 13 |
| 50–64 | 74 | 5.3 | 16 | 2 | 3 | 4 | 6 | 12 | 14 | 22 |
| 65+ | 57 | 8.1 | 63 | 2 | 3 | 5 | 10 | 16 | 34 | 35 |
| **GRAND TOTAL** | 402 | 4.2 | 15 | 1 | 2 | 3 | 5 | 8 | 11 | 21 |

## 82.2: EXC LES HAND SOFT TISSUE. Formerly included in operation group(s) 753.

| Type of Patients | Observed Patients | Avg. Stay | Variance | Percentiles | | | | | | |
|---|---|---|---|---|---|---|---|---|---|---|
| | | | | 10th | 25th | 50th | 75th | 90th | 95th | 99th |
| **1. SINGLE DX** | | | | | | | | | | |
| 0–19 Years | 19 | 1.6 | 2 | 1 | 1 | 1 | 2 | 2 | 6 | 6 |
| 20–34 | 2 | 2.0 | 2 | 1 | 1 | 2 | 3 | 3 | 3 | 3 |
| 35–49 | 6 | 1.0 | 0 | 1 | 1 | 1 | 1 | 1 | 1 | 1 |
| 50–64 | 1 | 1.0 | 0 | 1 | 1 | 1 | 1 | 1 | 1 | 1 |
| 65+ | 0 | | | | | | | | | |
| **2. MULTIPLE DX** | | | | | | | | | | |
| 0–19 Years | 5 | 2.3 | 1 | 1 | 1 | 3 | 3 | 3 | 3 | 5 |
| 20–34 | 14 | 4.5 | 30 | 1 | 2 | 5 | 5 | 8 | 24 | 24 |
| 35–49 | 29 | 3.8 | 7 | 1 | 2 | 4 | 5 | 5 | 7 | 15 |
| 50–64 | 19 | 7.0 | 185 | 2 | 2 | 3 | 5 | 17 | 17 | 94 |
| 65+ | 16 | 2.9 | 14 | 1 | 2 | 3 | 5 | 7 | 12 | 15 |
| **TOTAL SINGLE DX** | 28 | 1.4 | 1 | 1 | 1 | 1 | 1 | 2 | 3 | 6 |
| **TOTAL MULTIPLE DX** | 83 | 4.2 | 55 | 1 | 2 | 3 | 5 | 7 | 15 | 24 |
| **TOTAL** | | | | | | | | | | |
| 0–19 Years | 24 | 2.0 | 1 | 1 | 1 | 2 | 3 | 3 | 3 | 6 |
| 20–34 | 16 | 4.3 | 28 | 1 | 2 | 2 | 5 | 8 | 24 | 24 |
| 35–49 | 35 | 3.5 | 7 | 1 | 2 | 3 | 5 | 5 | 7 | 15 |
| 50–64 | 20 | 6.7 | 180 | 1 | 2 | 3 | 5 | 17 | 17 | 94 |
| 65+ | 16 | 2.9 | 14 | 1 | 1 | 3 | 3 | 7 | 12 | 15 |
| **GRAND TOTAL** | 111 | 3.8 | 48 | 1 | 1 | 2 | 4 | 6 | 15 | 17 |

## 82.1: DIV HAND MUSC/TEND/FASC. Formerly included in operation group(s) 754.

| Type of Patients | Observed Patients | Avg. Stay | Variance | Percentiles | | | | | | |
|---|---|---|---|---|---|---|---|---|---|---|
| | | | | 10th | 25th | 50th | 75th | 90th | 95th | 99th |
| **1. SINGLE DX** | | | | | | | | | | |
| 0–19 Years | 5 | 2.0 | <1 | 1 | 1 | 2 | 3 | 3 | 3 | 3 |
| 20–34 | 16 | 3.3 | 3 | 2 | 2 | 3 | 5 | 5 | 6 | 6 |
| 35–49 | 13 | 3.7 | 4 | 2 | 2 | 3 | 4 | 7 | 7 | 7 |
| 50–64 | 5 | 2.5 | 1 | 1 | 2 | 2 | 4 | 4 | 4 | 4 |
| 65+ | 0 | | | | | | | | | |
| **2. MULTIPLE DX** | | | | | | | | | | |
| 0–19 Years | 24 | 3.8 | 50 | 1 | 1 | 3 | 4 | 6 | 6 | 58 |
| 20–34 | 40 | 5.3 | 16 | 2 | 3 | 3 | 6 | 13 | 13 | 17 |
| 35–49 | 39 | 4.2 | 17 | 1 | 2 | 3 | 5 | 8 | 16 | 16 |
| 50–64 | 18 | 7.3 | 68 | 2 | 3 | 4 | 7 | 16 | 31 | 32 |
| 65+ | 25 | 5.1 | 14 | 2 | 3 | 5 | 8 | 12 | 12 | 13 |
| **TOTAL SINGLE DX** | 39 | 3.2 | 3 | 1 | 2 | 3 | 4 | 6 | 7 | 7 |
| **TOTAL MULTIPLE DX** | 146 | 5.0 | 28 | 1 | 2 | 3 | 6 | 13 | 14 | 27 |
| **TOTAL** | | | | | | | | | | |
| 0–19 Years | 29 | 3.6 | 44 | 1 | 2 | 3 | 3 | 6 | 13 | 27 |
| 20–34 | 56 | 4.9 | 14 | 2 | 3 | 3 | 6 | 13 | 13 | 17 |
| 35–49 | 52 | 4.1 | 13 | 1 | 2 | 3 | 5 | 8 | 15 | 16 |
| 50–64 | 23 | 6.0 | 54 | 2 | 2 | 4 | 6 | 16 | 31 | 32 |
| 65+ | 25 | 5.1 | 14 | 2 | 2 | 4 | 8 | 12 | 12 | 13 |
| **GRAND TOTAL** | 185 | 4.6 | 23 | 1 | 2 | 3 | 6 | 11 | 13 | 27 |

## 82.3: OTH EXC HAND SOFT TISS. Formerly included in operation group(s) 754.

| Type of Patients | Observed Patients | Avg. Stay | Variance | Percentiles | | | | | | |
|---|---|---|---|---|---|---|---|---|---|---|
| | | | | 10th | 25th | 50th | 75th | 90th | 95th | 99th |
| **1. SINGLE DX** | | | | | | | | | | |
| 0–19 Years | 5 | 4.4 | 7 | 1 | 3 | 5 | 5 | 5 | 12 | 12 |
| 20–34 | 3 | 1.2 | <1 | 1 | 1 | 1 | 1 | 2 | 2 | 8 |
| 35–49 | 11 | 2.3 | 3 | 1 | 1 | 1 | 3 | 4 | 8 | 8 |
| 50–64 | 9 | 1.1 | <1 | 1 | 1 | 1 | 1 | 2 | 2 | 2 |
| 65+ | 7 | 1.0 | 0 | 1 | 1 | 1 | 1 | 1 | 1 | 1 |
| **2. MULTIPLE DX** | | | | | | | | | | |
| 0–19 Years | 13 | 3.4 | 23 | 1 | 1 | 2 | 3 | 5 | 18 | 18 |
| 20–34 | 18 | 7.0 | 62 | 1 | 3 | 4 | 7 | 25 | 28 | 28 |
| 35–49 | 35 | 4.8 | 15 | 2 | 2 | 4 | 6 | 10 | 11 | 22 |
| 50–64 | 32 | 4.0 | 28 | 1 | 1 | 3 | 3 | 13 | 14 | 24 |
| 65+ | 45 | 2.6 | 15 | 1 | 1 | 1 | 2 | 6 | 8 | 19 |
| **TOTAL SINGLE DX** | 35 | 2.0 | 4 | 1 | 1 | 1 | 2 | 5 | 5 | 12 |
| **TOTAL MULTIPLE DX** | 143 | 4.0 | 25 | 1 | 1 | 2 | 4 | 9 | 14 | 28 |
| **TOTAL** | | | | | | | | | | |
| 0–19 Years | 18 | 3.9 | 15 | 1 | 2 | 3 | 5 | 5 | 16 | 18 |
| 20–34 | 21 | 4.2 | 41 | 1 | 1 | 2 | 4 | 8 | 25 | 28 |
| 35–49 | 46 | 4.3 | 14 | 1 | 2 | 3 | 5 | 9 | 11 | 22 |
| 50–64 | 41 | 3.3 | 23 | 1 | 1 | 1 | 3 | 9 | 13 | 24 |
| 65+ | 52 | 2.5 | 14 | 1 | 1 | 1 | 2 | 5 | 8 | 19 |
| **GRAND TOTAL** | 178 | 3.5 | 20 | 1 | 1 | 2 | 4 | 7 | 12 | 25 |

Length of Stay by Diagnosis and Operation, United States, 2000

**United States, October 1998–September 1999 Data, by Operation**

### 82.45: SUTURE HAND TENDON NEC. Formerly included in operation group(s) 755.

| Type of Patients | Observed Patients | Avg. Stay | Vari-ance | 10th | 25th | 50th | 75th | 90th | 95th | 99th |
|---|---|---|---|---|---|---|---|---|---|---|
| **1. SINGLE DX** | | | | | | | | | | |
| 0–19 Years | 27 | 1.3 | <1 | 1 | 1 | 1 | 1 | 2 | 2 | 4 |
| 20–34 | 47 | 1.4 | <1 | 1 | 1 | 1 | 2 | 2 | 2 | 3 |
| 35–49 | 38 | 1.2 | <1 | 1 | 1 | 1 | 1 | 2 | 2 | 2 |
| 50–64 | 8 | 1.1 | <1 | 1 | 1 | 1 | 1 | 2 | 2 | 2 |
| 65+ | 2 | 1.0 | 0 | 1 | 1 | 1 | 1 | 1 | 1 | 1 |
| **2. MULTIPLE DX** | | | | | | | | | | |
| 0–19 Years | 49 | 3.0 | 60 | 1 | 1 | 2 | 3 | 4 | 5 | 73 |
| 20–34 | 105 | 2.0 | 2 | 1 | 1 | 1 | 2 | 3 | 5 | 10 |
| 35–49 | 79 | 2.4 | 4 | 1 | 1 | 1 | 3 | 6 | 7 | 7 |
| 50–64 | 42 | 2.4 | 5 | 1 | 1 | 2 | 3 | 4 | 6 | 13 |
| 65+ | 28 | 2.3 | 9 | 1 | 1 | 1 | 2 | 6 | 8 | 14 |
| **TOTAL SINGLE DX** | 122 | 1.3 | <1 | 1 | 1 | 1 | 2 | 2 | 2 | 3 |
| **TOTAL MULTIPLE DX** | 303 | 2.4 | 13 | 1 | 1 | 2 | 3 | 5 | 6 | 13 |
| **TOTAL** | | | | | | | | | | |
| 0–19 | 76 | 2.5 | 43 | 1 | 1 | 1 | 3 | 3 | 5 | 7 |
| 20–34 | 152 | 1.8 | 2 | 1 | 1 | 1 | 2 | 3 | 4 | 7 |
| 35–49 | 117 | 2.2 | 3 | 1 | 1 | 1 | 3 | 5 | 7 | 7 |
| 50–64 | 50 | 2.2 | 5 | 1 | 1 | 2 | 2 | 4 | 6 | 13 |
| 65+ | 30 | 2.3 | 9 | 1 | 1 | 1 | 2 | 6 | 8 | 14 |
| **GRAND TOTAL** | 425 | 2.1 | 10 | 1 | 1 | 1 | 2 | 4 | 6 | 10 |

### 82.5: HAND MUSC/TEND TRANSPL. Formerly included in operation group(s) 755.

| Type of Patients | Observed Patients | Avg. Stay | Vari-ance | 10th | 25th | 50th | 75th | 90th | 95th | 99th |
|---|---|---|---|---|---|---|---|---|---|---|
| **1. SINGLE DX** | | | | | | | | | | |
| 0–19 Years | 5 | 1.0 | 0 | 1 | 1 | 1 | 1 | 1 | 1 | 1 |
| 20–34 | 3 | 1.0 | 0 | 1 | 1 | 1 | 1 | 1 | 1 | 1 |
| 35–49 | 1 | 4.0 | 0 | 4 | 4 | 4 | 4 | 4 | 4 | 4 |
| 50–64 | 0 | | | | | | | | | |
| 65+ | 3 | 1.0 | 0 | 1 | 1 | 1 | 1 | 1 | 1 | 1 |
| **2. MULTIPLE DX** | | | | | | | | | | |
| 0–19 Years | 19 | 1.3 | <1 | 1 | 1 | 1 | 1 | 3 | 3 | 3 |
| 20–34 | 6 | 2.1 | 3 | 1 | 1 | 1 | 3 | 5 | 6 | 6 |
| 35–49 | 13 | 13.3 | 69 | 1 | 2 | 19 | 19 | 19 | 19 | 19 |
| 50–64 | 7 | 1.9 | 1 | 1 | 1 | 1 | 3 | 3 | 4 | 4 |
| 65+ | 18 | 2.4 | 3 | 1 | 1 | 1 | 4 | 4 | 5 | 9 |
| **TOTAL SINGLE DX** | 12 | 1.0 | <1 | 1 | 1 | 1 | 1 | 1 | 1 | 1 |
| **TOTAL MULTIPLE DX** | 63 | 4.6 | 44 | 1 | 1 | 1 | 3 | 19 | 19 | 19 |
| **TOTAL** | | | | | | | | | | |
| 0–19 | 24 | 1.3 | <1 | 1 | 1 | 1 | 1 | 3 | 3 | 3 |
| 20–34 | 9 | 1.9 | 3 | 1 | 1 | 1 | 2 | 5 | 5 | 6 |
| 35–49 | 14 | 13.0 | 69 | 1 | 2 | 19 | 19 | 19 | 19 | 19 |
| 50–64 | 7 | 1.9 | 1 | 1 | 1 | 1 | 3 | 3 | 4 | 4 |
| 65+ | 21 | 1.2 | <1 | 1 | 1 | 1 | 1 | 5 | 5 | 5 |
| **GRAND TOTAL** | 75 | 3.0 | 27 | 1 | 1 | 1 | 1 | 5 | 19 | 19 |

### 82.4: SUTURE HAND SOFT TISSUE. Formerly included in operation group(s) 755.

| Type of Patients | Observed Patients | Avg. Stay | Vari-ance | 10th | 25th | 50th | 75th | 90th | 95th | 99th |
|---|---|---|---|---|---|---|---|---|---|---|
| **1. SINGLE DX** | | | | | | | | | | |
| 0–19 Years | 66 | 1.4 | <1 | 1 | 1 | 1 | 2 | 2 | 2 | 4 |
| 20–34 | 93 | 1.4 | <1 | 1 | 1 | 1 | 2 | 2 | 2 | 3 |
| 35–49 | 70 | 1.3 | <1 | 1 | 1 | 1 | 1 | 2 | 2 | 4 |
| 50–64 | 13 | 1.2 | <1 | 1 | 1 | 1 | 1 | 2 | 2 | 2 |
| 65+ | 3 | 1.0 | 0 | 1 | 1 | 1 | 1 | 1 | 1 | 1 |
| **2. MULTIPLE DX** | | | | | | | | | | |
| 0–19 Years | 129 | 1.9 | 23 | 1 | 1 | 1 | 2 | 3 | 4 | 7 |
| 20–34 | 242 | 2.3 | 5 | 1 | 1 | 2 | 2 | 4 | 6 | 13 |
| 35–49 | 187 | 2.4 | 4 | 1 | 1 | 1 | 3 | 5 | 7 | 10 |
| 50–64 | 79 | 2.3 | 4 | 1 | 1 | 2 | 2 | 4 | 5 | 13 |
| 65+ | 55 | 2.5 | 8 | 1 | 1 | 1 | 2 | 6 | 8 | 14 |
| **TOTAL SINGLE DX** | 245 | 1.3 | <1 | 1 | 1 | 1 | 2 | 2 | 2 | 4 |
| **TOTAL MULTIPLE DX** | 692 | 2.3 | 8 | 1 | 1 | 2 | 2 | 4 | 6 | 13 |
| **TOTAL** | | | | | | | | | | |
| 0–19 | 195 | 1.8 | 16 | 1 | 1 | 1 | 2 | 3 | 3 | 5 |
| 20–34 | 335 | 2.1 | 4 | 1 | 1 | 2 | 2 | 4 | 5 | 13 |
| 35–49 | 257 | 2.2 | 4 | 1 | 1 | 1 | 3 | 5 | 7 | 10 |
| 50–64 | 92 | 2.1 | 3 | 1 | 1 | 2 | 2 | 4 | 5 | 13 |
| 65+ | 58 | 2.4 | 8 | 1 | 1 | 1 | 2 | 6 | 8 | 14 |
| **GRAND TOTAL** | 937 | 2.1 | 7 | 1 | 1 | 1 | 2 | 4 | 5 | 13 |

### 82.44: SUT FLEXOR TEND HAND NEC. Formerly included in operation group(s) 755.

| Type of Patients | Observed Patients | Avg. Stay | Vari-ance | 10th | 25th | 50th | 75th | 90th | 95th | 99th |
|---|---|---|---|---|---|---|---|---|---|---|
| **1. SINGLE DX** | | | | | | | | | | |
| 0–19 Years | 29 | 1.5 | <1 | 1 | 1 | 1 | 2 | 2 | 3 | 4 |
| 20–34 | 32 | 1.3 | <1 | 1 | 1 | 1 | 1 | 2 | 2 | 3 |
| 35–49 | 25 | 1.4 | <1 | 1 | 1 | 1 | 2 | 2 | 3 | 4 |
| 50–64 | 3 | 1.1 | <1 | 1 | 1 | 1 | 1 | 1 | 2 | 2 |
| 65+ | 0 | | | | | | | | | |
| **2. MULTIPLE DX** | | | | | | | | | | |
| 0–19 Years | 59 | 1.3 | <1 | 1 | 1 | 1 | 1 | 2 | 3 | 4 |
| 20–34 | 106 | 2.5 | 7 | 1 | 1 | 2 | 3 | 4 | 6 | 13 |
| 35–49 | 84 | 2.5 | 6 | 1 | 2 | 2 | 3 | 6 | 10 | 13 |
| 50–64 | 23 | 2.1 | 2 | 1 | 2 | 1 | 2 | 2 | 5 | 5 |
| 65+ | 20 | 2.0 | 2 | 1 | 1 | 1 | 3 | 5 | 5 | 5 |
| **TOTAL SINGLE DX** | 89 | 1.4 | <1 | 1 | 1 | 1 | 2 | 2 | 3 | 4 |
| **TOTAL MULTIPLE DX** | 292 | 2.2 | 5 | 1 | 1 | 2 | 2 | 4 | 6 | 13 |
| **TOTAL** | | | | | | | | | | |
| 0–19 | 88 | 1.4 | <1 | 1 | 1 | 1 | 1 | 2 | 3 | 4 |
| 20–34 | 138 | 2.4 | 6 | 1 | 1 | 2 | 2 | 4 | 6 | 13 |
| 35–49 | 109 | 2.3 | 5 | 1 | 1 | 2 | 2 | 5 | 8 | 13 |
| 50–64 | 26 | 2.0 | 2 | 1 | 2 | 1 | 2 | 2 | 5 | 10 |
| 65+ | 20 | 2.0 | 2 | 1 | 1 | 1 | 3 | 5 | 5 | 5 |
| **GRAND TOTAL** | 381 | 2.0 | 4 | 1 | 1 | 1 | 2 | 3 | 5 | 13 |

Length of Stay by Diagnosis and Operation, United States, 2000

# United States, October 1998–September 1999 Data, by Operation

## 82.6: RECONSTRUCTION OF THUMB. Formerly included in operation group(s) 755.

| Type of Patients | Observed Patients | Avg. Stay | Variance | 10th | 25th | 50th | 75th | 90th | 95th | 99th |
|---|---|---|---|---|---|---|---|---|---|---|
| **1. SINGLE DX** | | | | | | | | | | |
| 0–19 Years | 13 | 1.4 | <1 | 1 | 1 | 1 | 1 | 2 | 4 | 4 |
| 20–34 | 0 | | | | | | | | | |
| 35–49 | 1 | 5.0 | 0 | 5 | 5 | 5 | 5 | 5 | 5 | 5 |
| 50–64 | 2 | 1.3 | <1 | 1 | 1 | 1 | 2 | 2 | 2 | 2 |
| 65+ | 0 | | | | | | | | | |
| **2. MULTIPLE DX** | | | | | | | | | | |
| 0–19 Years | 14 | 2.4 | 5 | 1 | 1 | 2 | 3 | 4 | 4 | 14 |
| 20–34 | 7 | 4.1 | 14 | 2 | 2 | 2 | 4 | 13 | 13 | 13 |
| 35–49 | 7 | 7.4 | 93 | 2 | 3 | 4 | 7 | 33 | 33 | 33 |
| 50–64 | 3 | 1.7 | 4 | 1 | 1 | 1 | 1 | 7 | 7 | 7 |
| 65+ | 1 | 1.0 | 0 | 1 | 1 | 1 | 1 | 1 | 1 | 1 |
| **TOTAL SINGLE DX** | 16 | 1.4 | <1 | 1 | 1 | 1 | 2 | 2 | 4 | 5 |
| **TOTAL MULTIPLE DX** | 32 | 3.3 | 21 | 1 | 1 | 2 | 4 | 6 | 13 | 33 |
| **TOTAL** | | | | | | | | | | |
| 0–19 Years | 27 | 1.9 | 3 | 1 | 1 | 1 | 2 | 4 | 4 | 14 |
| 20–34 | 7 | 4.1 | 14 | 2 | 2 | 2 | 4 | 13 | 13 | 13 |
| 35–49 | 8 | 7.2 | 86 | 2 | 3 | 4 | 7 | 33 | 33 | 33 |
| 50–64 | 5 | 1.6 | 3 | 1 | 1 | 1 | 1 | 1 | 7 | 7 |
| 65+ | 1 | 1.0 | 0 | 1 | 1 | 1 | 1 | 1 | 1 | 1 |
| **GRAND TOTAL** | 48 | 2.6 | 14 | 1 | 1 | 2 | 2 | 4 | 7 | 33 |

## 82.7: PLASTIC OP HND GRFT/IMPL. Formerly included in operation group(s) 755.

| Type of Patients | Observed Patients | Avg. Stay | Variance | 10th | 25th | 50th | 75th | 90th | 95th | 99th |
|---|---|---|---|---|---|---|---|---|---|---|
| **1. SINGLE DX** | | | | | | | | | | |
| 0–19 Years | 2 | 1.0 | 0 | 1 | 1 | 1 | 1 | 1 | 1 | 1 |
| 20–34 | 4 | 1.0 | 0 | 1 | 1 | 1 | 1 | 1 | 1 | 1 |
| 35–49 | 4 | 1.0 | 0 | 1 | 1 | 1 | 1 | 1 | 1 | 1 |
| 50–64 | 1 | 1.0 | | 1 | 1 | 1 | 1 | 1 | 1 | 1 |
| 65+ | 0 | | | | | | | | | |
| **2. MULTIPLE DX** | | | | | | | | | | |
| 0–19 Years | 4 | 1.0 | 0 | 1 | 1 | 1 | 1 | 1 | 1 | 1 |
| 20–34 | 7 | 3.0 | 7 | 1 | 1 | 2 | 3 | 4 | 10 | 10 |
| 35–49 | 10 | 2.7 | 11 | 1 | 1 | 2 | 3 | 4 | 14 | 14 |
| 50–64 | 5 | 1.7 | 1 | 1 | 1 | 1 | 2 | 4 | 4 | 4 |
| 65+ | 2 | 1.0 | 0 | 1 | 1 | 1 | 1 | 1 | 1 | 1 |
| **TOTAL SINGLE DX** | 11 | 1.0 | 0 | 1 | 1 | 1 | 1 | 1 | 1 | 1 |
| **TOTAL MULTIPLE DX** | 28 | 2.2 | 6 | 1 | 1 | 1 | 3 | 3 | 4 | 14 |
| **TOTAL** | | | | | | | | | | |
| 0–19 Years | 6 | 1.0 | 0 | 1 | 1 | 1 | 1 | 1 | 1 | 1 |
| 20–34 | 11 | 1.9 | 4 | 1 | 1 | 1 | 2 | 4 | 4 | 10 |
| 35–49 | 14 | 1.6 | 4 | 1 | 1 | 1 | 2 | 3 | 4 | 14 |
| 50–64 | 6 | 1.7 | 1 | 1 | 1 | 1 | 2 | 4 | 4 | 14 |
| 65+ | 2 | 1.0 | 0 | 1 | 1 | 1 | 1 | 1 | 1 | 1 |
| **GRAND TOTAL** | 39 | 1.6 | 3 | 1 | 1 | 1 | 1 | 3 | 4 | 14 |

## 82.8: OTHER PLASTIC OPS HAND. Formerly included in operation group(s) 755.

| Type of Patients | Observed Patients | Avg. Stay | Variance | 10th | 25th | 50th | 75th | 90th | 95th | 99th |
|---|---|---|---|---|---|---|---|---|---|---|
| **1. SINGLE DX** | | | | | | | | | | |
| 0–19 Years | 13 | 1.4 | <1 | 1 | 1 | 1 | 2 | 2 | 2 | 4 |
| 20–34 | 18 | 1.8 | 2 | 1 | 1 | 1 | 2 | 5 | 5 | 5 |
| 35–49 | 4 | 2.0 | 2 | 1 | 1 | 1 | 2 | 5 | 5 | 5 |
| 50–64 | 1 | 1.0 | 0 | 1 | 1 | 1 | 1 | 1 | 1 | 1 |
| 65+ | 0 | | | | | | | | | |
| **2. MULTIPLE DX** | | | | | | | | | | |
| 0–19 Years | 23 | 2.0 | 2 | 1 | 1 | 2 | 2 | 3 | 6 | 6 |
| 20–34 | 31 | 1.9 | 4 | 1 | 1 | 2 | 2 | 3 | 6 | 13 |
| 35–49 | 24 | 2.5 | 4 | 2 | 2 | 2 | 3 | 5 | 5 | 12 |
| 50–64 | 15 | 2.4 | 4 | 1 | 1 | 2 | 3 | 6 | 6 | 9 |
| 65+ | 11 | 1.7 | 1 | 1 | 1 | 2 | 2 | 4 | 4 | 4 |
| **TOTAL SINGLE DX** | 36 | 1.7 | 1 | 1 | 1 | 1 | 2 | 4 | 5 | 5 |
| **TOTAL MULTIPLE DX** | 104 | 2.1 | 3 | 1 | 1 | 2 | 2 | 4 | 6 | 9 |
| **TOTAL** | | | | | | | | | | |
| 0–19 Years | 36 | 1.8 | 1 | 1 | 1 | 1 | 2 | 3 | 6 | 6 |
| 20–34 | 49 | 1.9 | 3 | 1 | 1 | 1 | 2 | 4 | 5 | 13 |
| 35–49 | 28 | 2.5 | 4 | 1 | 2 | 2 | 3 | 5 | 6 | 12 |
| 50–64 | 16 | 2.3 | 4 | 1 | 1 | 2 | 3 | 6 | 6 | 9 |
| 65+ | 11 | 1.7 | 1 | 1 | 1 | 2 | 2 | 4 | 4 | 4 |
| **GRAND TOTAL** | 140 | 2.0 | 3 | 1 | 1 | 1 | 2 | 4 | 6 | 9 |

## 82.9: OTH HAND SOFT TISSUE OPS. Formerly included in operation group(s) 755, 767.

| Type of Patients | Observed Patients | Avg. Stay | Variance | 10th | 25th | 50th | 75th | 90th | 95th | 99th |
|---|---|---|---|---|---|---|---|---|---|---|
| **1. SINGLE DX** | | | | | | | | | | |
| 0–19 Years | 2 | 1.2 | <1 | 1 | 1 | 1 | 1 | 1 | 5 | 5 |
| 20–34 | 0 | | | | | | | | | |
| 35–49 | 1 | 1.0 | 0 | 1 | 1 | 1 | 1 | 1 | 1 | 1 |
| 50–64 | 3 | 1.5 | 1 | 1 | 1 | 1 | 1 | 3 | 3 | 3 |
| 65+ | 0 | | | | | | | | | |
| **2. MULTIPLE DX** | | | | | | | | | | |
| 0–19 Years | 2 | 1.6 | <1 | 1 | 1 | 2 | 2 | 2 | 2 | 2 |
| 20–34 | 16 | 1.6 | 2 | 1 | 1 | 1 | 2 | 2 | 5 | 10 |
| 35–49 | 13 | 2.7 | 1 | 2 | 3 | 3 | 3 | 14 | 14 | 7 |
| 50–64 | 7 | 4.8 | 22 | 2 | 2 | 2 | 5 | 14 | 14 | 14 |
| 65+ | 18 | 6.4 | 23 | 3 | 3 | 6 | 7 | 7 | 12 | 30 |
| **TOTAL SINGLE DX** | 6 | 1.2 | <1 | 1 | 1 | 1 | 1 | 1 | 5 | 5 |
| **TOTAL MULTIPLE DX** | 56 | 3.6 | 14 | 1 | 1 | 2 | 4 | 7 | 12 | 14 |
| **TOTAL** | | | | | | | | | | |
| 0–19 Years | 4 | 1.3 | <1 | 1 | 1 | 1 | 1 | 2 | 5 | 5 |
| 20–34 | 16 | 1.6 | 2 | 1 | 1 | 1 | 2 | 2 | 5 | 10 |
| 35–49 | 14 | 2.7 | 1 | 3 | 3 | 3 | 5 | 14 | 4 | 7 |
| 50–64 | 10 | 4.7 | 21 | 2 | 2 | 2 | 5 | 14 | 14 | 14 |
| 65+ | 18 | 6.4 | 23 | 3 | 3 | 6 | 7 | 7 | 12 | 30 |
| **GRAND TOTAL** | 62 | 2.8 | 11 | 1 | 1 | 2 | 3 | 7 | 9 | 14 |

Length of Stay by Diagnosis and Operation, United States, 2000

# United States, October 1998–September 1999 Data, by Operation

## 83.0: INC MUSC/TEND/FASC/BURSA. Formerly included in operation group(s) 752.

| Type of Patients | Observed Patients | Variance | Avg. Stay | 10th | 25th | 50th | 75th | 90th | 95th | 99th |
|---|---|---|---|---|---|---|---|---|---|---|
| **1. SINGLE DX** | | | | | | | | | | |
| 0–19 Years | 108 | 4 | 2.8 | 1 | 1 | 2 | 2 | 6 | 7 | 8 |
| 20–34 | 84 | 4 | 2.4 | 1 | 1 | 2 | 3 | 6 | 7 | 7 |
| 35–49 | 83 | 5 | 2.7 | 1 | 1 | 2 | 4 | 7 | 7 | 9 |
| 50–64 | 26 | 4 | 1.5 | 1 | 1 | 1 | 1 | 2 | 3 | 7 |
| 65+ | 9 | 6 | 2.4 | 1 | 1 | 1 | 3 | 7 | 8 | 8 |
| **2. MULTIPLE DX** | | | | | | | | | | |
| 0–19 Years | 253 | 19 | 4.7 | 1 | 2 | 3 | 6 | 10 | 12 | 21 |
| 20–34 | 374 | 33 | 5.4 | 1 | 2 | 3 | 6 | 12 | 23 | 23 |
| 35–49 | 618 | 38 | 6.2 | 2 | 3 | 4 | 7 | 12 | 17 | 34 |
| 50–64 | 500 | 22 | 5.7 | 1 | 3 | 4 | 8 | 12 | 17 | >99 |
| 65+ | 561 | 71 | 7.5 | 2 | 3 | 5 | 9 | 14 | 20 | 58 |
| **TOTAL SINGLE DX** | 310 | 4 | 2.4 | 1 | 1 | 2 | 3 | 6 | 7 | 9 |
| **TOTAL MULTIPLE DX** | 2,306 | 38 | 6.0 | 2 | 3 | 4 | 7 | 12 | 18 | 42 |
| **TOTAL** | | | | | | | | | | |
| 0–19 Years | 361 | 15 | 4.1 | 1 | 2 | 3 | 6 | 9 | 11 | 16 |
| 20–34 | 458 | 29 | 4.9 | 1 | 2 | 3 | 6 | 11 | 21 | 23 |
| 35–49 | 701 | 36 | 5.9 | 2 | 3 | 4 | 7 | 12 | 16 | 34 |
| 50–64 | 526 | 22 | 5.1 | 1 | 2 | 4 | 7 | 11 | 17 | >99 |
| 65+ | 570 | 71 | 7.5 | 2 | 3 | 5 | 9 | 14 | 20 | 58 |
| **GRAND TOTAL** | 2,616 | 35 | 5.5 | 1 | 2 | 4 | 7 | 11 | 16 | 35 |

## 83.03: BURSOTOMY. Formerly included in operation group(s) 752.

| Type of Patients | Observed Patients | Variance | Avg. Stay | 10th | 25th | 50th | 75th | 90th | 95th | 99th |
|---|---|---|---|---|---|---|---|---|---|---|
| **1. SINGLE DX** | | | | | | | | | | |
| 0–19 Years | 6 | <1 | 2.9 | 2 | 3 | 3 | 3 | 3 | 3 | 3 |
| 20–34 | 12 | 2 | 2.8 | 2 | 2 | 2 | 4 | 5 | 5 | 7 |
| 35–49 | 23 | 2 | 2.5 | 1 | 1 | 2 | 2 | 4 | 4 | 5 |
| 50–64 | 4 | 1 | 2.3 | 1 | 2 | 2 | 3 | 5 | 5 | 5 |
| 65+ | 3 | <1 | 2.0 | 1 | 1 | 2 | 3 | 3 | 3 | 3 |
| **2. MULTIPLE DX** | | | | | | | | | | |
| 0–19 Years | 29 | 5 | 3.4 | 2 | 2 | 3 | 4 | 7 | 10 | 10 |
| 20–34 | 75 | 6 | 4.3 | 2 | 3 | 4 | 6 | 6 | 11 | 12 |
| 35–49 | 157 | 9 | 4.5 | 2 | 3 | 4 | 6 | 7 | 8 | 14 |
| 50–64 | 149 | 7 | 4.5 | 1 | 3 | 4 | 6 | 8 | 8 | 12 |
| 65+ | 150 | 167 | 8.5 | 2 | 3 | 4 | 7 | 12 | 58 | 58 |
| **TOTAL SINGLE DX** | 48 | 1 | 2.6 | 1 | 2 | 2 | 3 | 4 | 5 | 5 |
| **TOTAL MULTIPLE DX** | 560 | 44 | 5.3 | 2 | 3 | 4 | 6 | 8 | 11 | 58 |
| **TOTAL** | | | | | | | | | | |
| 0–19 Years | 35 | 4 | 3.3 | 2 | 2 | 3 | 3 | 6 | 9 | 10 |
| 20–34 | 87 | 6 | 3.9 | 2 | 2 | 3 | 5 | 6 | 8 | 10 |
| 35–49 | 180 | 8 | 4.3 | 2 | 3 | 4 | 5 | 7 | 8 | 14 |
| 50–64 | 153 | 7 | 4.4 | 1 | 2 | 4 | 6 | 8 | 8 | 12 |
| 65+ | 153 | 166 | 8.5 | 2 | 3 | 4 | 7 | 12 | 58 | 58 |
| **GRAND TOTAL** | 608 | 41 | 5.1 | 2 | 2 | 4 | 6 | 8 | 11 | 58 |

## 83.02: MYOTOMY. Formerly included in operation group(s) 752.

| Type of Patients | Observed Patients | Variance | Avg. Stay | 10th | 25th | 50th | 75th | 90th | 95th | 99th |
|---|---|---|---|---|---|---|---|---|---|---|
| **1. SINGLE DX** | | | | | | | | | | |
| 0–19 Years | 16 | 3 | 2.5 | 1 | 1 | 2 | 2 | 5 | 7 | 7 |
| 20–34 | 8 | <1 | 1.1 | 1 | 1 | 1 | 1 | 1 | 1 | 2 |
| 35–49 | 8 | <1 | 1.4 | 1 | 1 | 1 | 2 | 2 | 4 | 4 |
| 50–64 | 2 | 3 | 3.5 | 2 | 2 | 2 | 5 | 5 | 5 | 5 |
| 65+ | 1 | 0 | 7.0 | 7 | 7 | 7 | 7 | 7 | 7 | 7 |
| **2. MULTIPLE DX** | | | | | | | | | | |
| 0–19 Years | 43 | 40 | 6.3 | 1 | 2 | 6 | 7 | 10 | 14 | 42 |
| 20–34 | 64 | 19 | 4.9 | 2 | 2 | 3 | 6 | 10 | 13 | 23 |
| 35–49 | 103 | 48 | 6.6 | 1 | 3 | 4 | 8 | 12 | 28 | 29 |
| 50–64 | 63 | 39 | 9.4 | 3 | 6 | 11 | 17 | >99 | >99 | >99 |
| 65+ | 75 | 32 | 6.8 | 2 | 3 | 5 | 8 | 15 | 21 | 30 |
| **TOTAL SINGLE DX** | 35 | 3 | 2.3 | 1 | 1 | 2 | 2 | 5 | 7 | 7 |
| **TOTAL MULTIPLE DX** | 348 | 37 | 6.6 | 2 | 3 | 5 | 8 | 17 | 28 | >99 |
| **TOTAL** | | | | | | | | | | |
| 0–19 Years | 59 | 26 | 4.5 | 1 | 2 | 3 | 6 | 8 | 10 | 25 |
| 20–34 | 72 | 19 | 4.8 | 1 | 3 | 3 | 5 | 10 | 13 | 23 |
| 35–49 | 111 | 47 | 6.3 | 1 | 2 | 4 | 8 | 12 | 28 | 29 |
| 50–64 | 65 | 39 | 9.2 | 3 | 5 | 11 | 17 | >99 | >99 | >99 |
| 65+ | 76 | 32 | 6.8 | 2 | 3 | 5 | 8 | 15 | 21 | 30 |
| **GRAND TOTAL** | 383 | 35 | 6.1 | 1 | 2 | 4 | 8 | 15 | 28 | >99 |

## 83.09: SOFT TISSUE INCISION NEC. Formerly included in operation group(s) 752.

| Type of Patients | Observed Patients | Variance | Avg. Stay | 10th | 25th | 50th | 75th | 90th | 95th | 99th |
|---|---|---|---|---|---|---|---|---|---|---|
| **1. SINGLE DX** | | | | | | | | | | |
| 0–19 Years | 80 | 5 | 3.1 | 1 | 1 | 2 | 2 | 6 | 8 | 9 |
| 20–34 | 54 | 3 | 2.2 | 1 | 1 | 1 | 2 | 4 | 7 | 7 |
| 35–49 | 47 | 7 | 2.9 | 1 | 1 | 2 | 2 | 6 | 9 | 9 |
| 50–64 | 15 | 5 | 1.4 | 1 | 1 | 1 | 1 | 2 | 2 | 7 |
| 65+ | 5 | 7 | 1.9 | 1 | 1 | 1 | 1 | 8 | 8 | 8 |
| **2. MULTIPLE DX** | | | | | | | | | | |
| 0–19 Years | 168 | 16 | 4.7 | 1 | 2 | 4 | 7 | 10 | 12 | 18 |
| 20–34 | 217 | 45 | 6.0 | 1 | 3 | 4 | 5 | 17 | 23 | 23 |
| 35–49 | 338 | 49 | 7.2 | 2 | 3 | 5 | 8 | 13 | 20 | 34 |
| 50–64 | 275 | 26 | 6.0 | 1 | 3 | 4 | 8 | 11 | 16 | 24 |
| 65+ | 313 | 33 | 7.4 | 2 | 4 | 6 | 9 | 14 | 18 | 28 |
| **TOTAL SINGLE DX** | 201 | 5 | 2.4 | 1 | 1 | 1 | 3 | 6 | 7 | 9 |
| **TOTAL MULTIPLE DX** | 1,311 | 37 | 6.4 | 1 | 3 | 4 | 8 | 13 | 19 | 34 |
| **TOTAL** | | | | | | | | | | |
| 0–19 Years | 248 | 13 | 4.2 | 1 | 1 | 3 | 6 | 10 | 11 | 15 |
| 20–34 | 271 | 38 | 5.2 | 1 | 1 | 3 | 6 | 14 | 23 | 23 |
| 35–49 | 385 | 46 | 6.7 | 1 | 3 | 5 | 8 | 13 | 18 | 34 |
| 50–64 | 290 | 25 | 5.0 | 1 | 1 | 4 | 7 | 10 | 15 | 24 |
| 65+ | 318 | 33 | 7.3 | 2 | 4 | 6 | 9 | 14 | 18 | 28 |
| **GRAND TOTAL** | 1,512 | 34 | 5.7 | 1 | 2 | 4 | 7 | 12 | 17 | 32 |

Length of Stay by Diagnosis and Operation, United States, 2000

# United States, October 1998–September 1999 Data, by Operation

## 83.1: MUSC/TEND/FASC DIVISION. Formerly included in operation group(s) 752.

| Type of Patients | Observed Patients | Avg. Stay | Vari-ance | 10th | 25th | 50th | 75th | 90th | 95th | 99th |
|---|---|---|---|---|---|---|---|---|---|---|
| **1. SINGLE DX** | | | | | | | | | | |
| 0–19 Years | 220 | 1.9 | 4 | 1 | 1 | 1 | 2 | 3 | 5 | 8 |
| 20–34 | 61 | 3.6 | 7 | 1 | 1 | 3 | 5 | 7 | 7 | 13 |
| 35–49 | 50 | 2.3 | 2 | 1 | 1 | 3 | 2 | 5 | 5 | 7 |
| 50–64 | 12 | 2.2 | 3 | 1 | 1 | 1 | 2 | 5 | 5 | 5 |
| 65+ | 7 | 4.3 | 12 | 1 | 1 | 3 | 8 | 9 | 9 | 9 |
| **2. MULTIPLE DX** | | | | | | | | | | |
| 0–19 Years | 1,079 | 3.1 | 25 | 1 | 1 | 2 | 3 | 5 | 8 | 19 |
| 20–34 | 258 | 5.8 | 34 | 2 | 2 | 4 | 7 | 11 | 17 | 28 |
| 35–49 | 309 | 6.2 | 66 | 1 | 2 | 4 | 7 | 12 | 19 | 39 |
| 50–64 | 170 | 6.3 | 55 | 1 | 2 | 3 | 8 | 14 | 26 | 36 |
| 65+ | 215 | 5.3 | 28 | 1 | 2 | 4 | 7 | 11 | 16 | 28 |
| **TOTAL SINGLE DX** | 350 | 2.5 | 5 | 1 | 1 | 2 | 3 | 5 | 7 | 10 |
| **TOTAL MULTIPLE DX** | 2,031 | 4.4 | 38 | 1 | 1 | 3 | 5 | 9 | 14 | 33 |
| **TOTAL** | | | | | | | | | | |
| 0–19 Years | 1,299 | 2.9 | 22 | 1 | 1 | 2 | 3 | 5 | 8 | 19 |
| 20–34 | 319 | 5.2 | 28 | 1 | 2 | 4 | 7 | 10 | 15 | 28 |
| 35–49 | 359 | 5.8 | 60 | 1 | 2 | 4 | 7 | 11 | 18 | 38 |
| 50–64 | 182 | 6.1 | 54 | 1 | 2 | 3 | 7 | 14 | 26 | 36 |
| 65+ | 222 | 5.3 | 28 | 1 | 2 | 4 | 7 | 11 | 16 | 28 |
| **GRAND TOTAL** | 2,381 | 4.1 | 33 | 1 | 1 | 2 | 5 | 8 | 12 | 29 |

## 83.12: ADDUCTOR TENOTOMY OF HIP. Formerly included in operation group(s) 752.

| Type of Patients | Observed Patients | Avg. Stay | Vari-ance | 10th | 25th | 50th | 75th | 90th | 95th | 99th |
|---|---|---|---|---|---|---|---|---|---|---|
| **1. SINGLE DX** | | | | | | | | | | |
| 0–19 Years | 63 | 2.4 | 12 | 1 | 1 | 1 | 2 | 4 | 5 | 22 |
| 20–34 | 0 | | | | | | | | | |
| 35–49 | 2 | 2.0 | 0 | 2 | 2 | 2 | 2 | 2 | 2 | 2 |
| 50–64 | 0 | | | | | | | | | |
| 65+ | 1 | 3.0 | 0 | 3 | 3 | 3 | 3 | 3 | 3 | 3 |
| **2. MULTIPLE DX** | | | | | | | | | | |
| 0–19 Years | 408 | 3.2 | 34 | 1 | 1 | 2 | 3 | 5 | 7 | 44 |
| 20–34 | 10 | 4.2 | 10 | 2 | 2 | 3 | 5 | 7 | 15 | 15 |
| 35–49 | 9 | 3.7 | 6 | 3 | 2 | 3 | 5 | 7 | 8 | 8 |
| 50–64 | 6 | 6.9 | 112 | 2 | 3 | 3 | 5 | 37 | 37 | >99 |
| 65+ | 20 | 7.3 | 20 | 2 | 4 | 8 | 8 | 11 | 15 | 24 |
| **TOTAL SINGLE DX** | 66 | 2.4 | 11 | 1 | 1 | 1 | 2 | 4 | 5 | 22 |
| **TOTAL MULTIPLE DX** | 453 | 3.4 | 35 | 1 | 1 | 2 | 3 | 6 | 8 | 44 |
| **TOTAL** | | | | | | | | | | |
| 0–19 Years | 471 | 3.1 | 32 | 1 | 1 | 2 | 3 | 5 | 7 | 24 |
| 20–34 | 10 | 4.2 | 10 | 2 | 2 | 3 | 5 | 7 | 15 | 15 |
| 35–49 | 11 | 2.8 | 4 | 2 | 2 | 3 | 3 | 7 | 7 | 8 |
| 50–64 | 6 | 6.9 | 112 | 2 | 3 | 3 | 5 | 37 | 37 | >99 |
| 65+ | 21 | 7.3 | 20 | 3 | 4 | 8 | 8 | 11 | 15 | 24 |
| **GRAND TOTAL** | 519 | 3.3 | 33 | 1 | 1 | 2 | 3 | 5 | 8 | 37 |

## 83.13: OTHER TENOTOMY. Formerly included in operation group(s) 752.

| Type of Patients | Observed Patients | Avg. Stay | Vari-ance | 10th | 25th | 50th | 75th | 90th | 95th | 99th |
|---|---|---|---|---|---|---|---|---|---|---|
| **1. SINGLE DX** | | | | | | | | | | |
| 0–19 Years | 55 | 1.6 | 1 | 1 | 1 | 1 | 2 | 3 | 3 | 5 |
| 20–34 | 6 | 2.3 | <1 | 1 | 2 | 2 | 3 | 3 | 3 | 3 |
| 35–49 | 7 | 1.4 | <1 | 1 | 1 | 1 | 2 | 2 | 2 | 2 |
| 50–64 | 2 | 1.0 | 0 | 1 | 1 | 1 | 1 | 1 | 1 | 1 |
| 65+ | 1 | 8.0 | 0 | 8 | 8 | 8 | 8 | 8 | 8 | 8 |
| **2. MULTIPLE DX** | | | | | | | | | | |
| 0–19 Years | 356 | 2.3 | 10 | 1 | 1 | 2 | 3 | 4 | 5 | 8 |
| 20–34 | 32 | 2.8 | 5 | 1 | 1 | 2 | 4 | 4 | 9 | 10 |
| 35–49 | 40 | 3.2 | 8 | 1 | 2 | 2 | 4 | 6 | 9 | 16 |
| 50–64 | 39 | 2.6 | 2 | 1 | 2 | 3 | 3 | 4 | 4 | 8 |
| 65+ | 72 | 4.0 | 16 | 1 | 2 | 3 | 4 | 7 | 8 | 22 |
| **TOTAL SINGLE DX** | 71 | 1.7 | 1 | 1 | 1 | 1 | 2 | 3 | 3 | 5 |
| **TOTAL MULTIPLE DX** | 539 | 2.7 | 10 | 1 | 1 | 2 | 3 | 4 | 7 | 12 |
| **TOTAL** | | | | | | | | | | |
| 0–19 Years | 411 | 2.2 | 9 | 1 | 1 | 2 | 3 | 4 | 5 | 8 |
| 20–34 | 38 | 2.7 | 4 | 1 | 1 | 2 | 4 | 4 | 9 | 10 |
| 35–49 | 47 | 3.1 | 8 | 1 | 2 | 2 | 3 | 6 | 9 | 16 |
| 50–64 | 41 | 2.6 | 2 | 1 | 2 | 3 | 3 | 4 | 4 | 8 |
| 65+ | 73 | 4.0 | 16 | 1 | 2 | 3 | 4 | 7 | 8 | 22 |
| **GRAND TOTAL** | 610 | 2.6 | 9 | 1 | 1 | 2 | 3 | 4 | 6 | 12 |

## 83.14: FASCIOTOMY. Formerly included in operation group(s) 752.

| Type of Patients | Observed Patients | Avg. Stay | Vari-ance | 10th | 25th | 50th | 75th | 90th | 95th | 99th |
|---|---|---|---|---|---|---|---|---|---|---|
| **1. SINGLE DX** | | | | | | | | | | |
| 0–19 Years | 57 | 2.2 | 2 | 1 | 1 | 2 | 3 | 4 | 5 | 7 |
| 20–34 | 39 | 4.7 | 7 | 1 | 2 | 5 | 7 | 7 | 7 | 13 |
| 35–49 | 28 | 2.9 | 3 | 1 | 1 | 2 | 4 | 5 | 6 | 7 |
| 50–64 | 6 | 2.7 | 3 | 1 | 1 | 2 | 5 | 5 | 5 | 5 |
| 65+ | 5 | 3.8 | 12 | 1 | 1 | 2 | 6 | 9 | 9 | 9 |
| **2. MULTIPLE DX** | | | | | | | | | | |
| 0–19 Years | 206 | 4.7 | 35 | 1 | 2 | 4 | 5 | 8 | 12 | 20 |
| 20–34 | 179 | 7.4 | 43 | 2 | 3 | 5 | 10 | 15 | 23 | 28 |
| 35–49 | 206 | 7.5 | 83 | 2 | 3 | 5 | 8 | 14 | 22 | 46 |
| 50–64 | 105 | 8.2 | 65 | 1 | 3 | 5 | 11 | 18 | 29 | 36 |
| 65+ | 97 | 6.1 | 38 | 1 | 2 | 4 | 8 | 13 | 18 | 28 |
| **TOTAL SINGLE DX** | 135 | 3.4 | 6 | 1 | 1 | 3 | 5 | 7 | 7 | 10 |
| **TOTAL MULTIPLE DX** | 793 | 6.8 | 57 | 2 | 3 | 5 | 8 | 14 | 19 | 35 |
| **TOTAL** | | | | | | | | | | |
| 0–19 Years | 263 | 4.0 | 28 | 1 | 1 | 3 | 5 | 8 | 11 | 20 |
| 20–34 | 218 | 6.7 | 35 | 2 | 3 | 5 | 8 | 12 | 17 | 28 |
| 35–49 | 234 | 7.2 | 78 | 2 | 3 | 5 | 7 | 13 | 21 | 46 |
| 50–64 | 111 | 8.1 | 64 | 2 | 3 | 5 | 11 | 18 | 29 | 36 |
| 65+ | 102 | 6.1 | 37 | 1 | 2 | 4 | 8 | 13 | 17 | 28 |
| **GRAND TOTAL** | 928 | 6.2 | 50 | 1 | 2 | 4 | 7 | 12 | 18 | 34 |

Length of Stay by Diagnosis and Operation, United States, 2000

# United States, October 1998–September 1999 Data, by Operation

## 83.2: SOFT TISSUE DXTIC PX. Formerly included in operation group(s) 753, 767.

| Type of Patients | Observed Patients | Avg. Stay | Vari-ance | Percentiles | | | | | | |
|---|---|---|---|---|---|---|---|---|---|---|
| | | | | 10th | 25th | 50th | 75th | 90th | 95th | 99th |
| **1. SINGLE DX** | | | | | | | | | | |
| 0–19 Years | 111 | 2.2 | 4 | 1 | 1 | 1 | 3 | 5 | 6 | 10 |
| 20–34 | 113 | 2.0 | 4 | 1 | 1 | 1 | 5 | 4 | 6 | 11 |
| 35–49 | 25 | 3.1 | 9 | 1 | 1 | 2 | 5 | 5 | 9 | 14 |
| 50–64 | 24 | 4.1 | 29 | 1 | 1 | 2 | 3 | 9 | 16 | 22 |
| 65+ | 17 | 3.2 | 16 | 1 | 1 | 2 | 2 | 7 | 14 | 15 |
| **2. MULTIPLE DX** | | | | | | | | | | |
| 0–19 Years | 259 | 9.2 | 117 | 1 | 2 | 6 | 10 | 21 | 32 | 60 |
| 20–34 | 146 | 9.9 | 92 | 2 | 3 | 8 | 14 | 19 | 30 | 53 |
| 35–49 | 337 | 9.1 | 87 | 2 | 3 | 7 | 12 | 18 | 30 | 46 |
| 50–64 | 451 | 9.1 | 47 | 2 | 5 | 8 | 12 | 17 | 23 | 36 |
| 65+ | 796 | 10.5 | 58 | 3 | 5 | 9 | 13 | 20 | 23 | 40 |
| **TOTAL SINGLE DX** | 290 | 2.4 | 7 | 1 | 1 | 1 | 3 | 5 | 8 | 14 |
| **TOTAL MULTIPLE DX** | 1,989 | 9.7 | 73 | 2 | 4 | 8 | 12 | 19 | 26 | 43 |
| **TOTAL** | | | | | | | | | | |
| 0–19 Years | 370 | 6.8 | 89 | 1 | 2 | 3 | 8 | 18 | 27 | 60 |
| 20–34 | 259 | 7.6 | 80 | 1 | 2 | 4 | 12 | 14 | 25 | 53 |
| 35–49 | 362 | 8.8 | 84 | 2 | 3 | 6 | 11 | 16 | 30 | 44 |
| 50–64 | 475 | 8.9 | 47 | 2 | 5 | 8 | 11 | 16 | 22 | 35 |
| 65+ | 813 | 10.4 | 59 | 3 | 5 | 9 | 13 | 20 | 23 | 40 |
| **GRAND TOTAL** | 2,279 | 8.9 | 70 | 1 | 3 | 7 | 12 | 18 | 24 | 41 |

## 83.3: EXC LES SOFT TISSUE. Formerly included in operation group(s) 753.

| Type of Patients | Observed Patients | Avg. Stay | Vari-ance | Percentiles | | | | | | |
|---|---|---|---|---|---|---|---|---|---|---|
| | | | | 10th | 25th | 50th | 75th | 90th | 95th | 99th |
| **1. SINGLE DX** | | | | | | | | | | |
| 0–19 Years | 164 | 2.4 | 5 | 1 | 1 | 2 | 2 | 6 | 7 | 11 |
| 20–34 | 89 | 2.0 | 2 | 1 | 1 | 1 | 2 | 4 | 6 | 7 |
| 35–49 | 115 | 2.0 | 4 | 1 | 1 | 1 | 2 | 5 | 6 | 8 |
| 50–64 | 88 | 2.1 | 4 | 1 | 1 | 2 | 2 | 4 | 6 | 14 |
| 65+ | 50 | 2.7 | 5 | 1 | 1 | 2 | 3 | 6 | 7 | 11 |
| **2. MULTIPLE DX** | | | | | | | | | | |
| 0–19 Years | 139 | 4.6 | 58 | 1 | 1 | 2 | 5 | 10 | 12 | 46 |
| 20–34 | 118 | 4.6 | 18 | 1 | 2 | 4 | 5 | 9 | 15 | 22 |
| 35–49 | 336 | 4.0 | 22 | 1 | 1 | 2 | 4 | 9 | 15 | 23 |
| 50–64 | 373 | 4.1 | 22 | 1 | 1 | 3 | 5 | 10 | 14 | 18 |
| 65+ | 524 | 5.8 | 58 | 1 | 2 | 3 | 7 | 12 | 16 | 47 |
| **TOTAL SINGLE DX** | 506 | 2.2 | 4 | 1 | 1 | 1 | 2 | 5 | 7 | 10 |
| **TOTAL MULTIPLE DX** | 1,490 | 4.7 | 37 | 1 | 1 | 3 | 5 | 10 | 15 | 41 |
| **TOTAL** | | | | | | | | | | |
| 0–19 Years | 303 | 3.3 | 28 | 1 | 1 | 2 | 3 | 7 | 10 | 43 |
| 20–34 | 207 | 3.6 | 13 | 1 | 1 | 2 | 4 | 8 | 11 | 16 |
| 35–49 | 451 | 3.3 | 17 | 1 | 1 | 2 | 4 | 7 | 11 | 20 |
| 50–64 | 461 | 3.7 | 20 | 1 | 1 | 3 | 5 | 8 | 14 | 17 |
| 65+ | 574 | 5.4 | 53 | 2 | 2 | 3 | 7 | 12 | 16 | 47 |
| **GRAND TOTAL** | 1,996 | 3.9 | 28 | 1 | 1 | 2 | 4 | 8 | 13 | 27 |

## 83.21: SOFT TISSUE BIOPSY. Formerly included in operation group(s) 753.

| Type of Patients | Observed Patients | Avg. Stay | Vari-ance | Percentiles | | | | | | |
|---|---|---|---|---|---|---|---|---|---|---|
| | | | | 10th | 25th | 50th | 75th | 90th | 95th | 99th |
| **1. SINGLE DX** | | | | | | | | | | |
| 0–19 Years | 111 | 2.2 | 4 | 1 | 1 | 1 | 3 | 5 | 6 | 10 |
| 20–34 | 113 | 2.0 | 4 | 1 | 1 | 1 | 5 | 4 | 6 | 11 |
| 35–49 | 25 | 3.1 | 9 | 1 | 1 | 2 | 5 | 5 | 9 | 14 |
| 50–64 | 24 | 4.1 | 29 | 1 | 1 | 2 | 3 | 9 | 16 | 22 |
| 65+ | 17 | 3.2 | 16 | 1 | 1 | 2 | 2 | 7 | 14 | 15 |
| **2. MULTIPLE DX** | | | | | | | | | | |
| 0–19 Years | 259 | 9.2 | 117 | 1 | 2 | 6 | 10 | 21 | 32 | 60 |
| 20–34 | 146 | 9.9 | 92 | 2 | 3 | 8 | 14 | 19 | 30 | 53 |
| 35–49 | 337 | 9.1 | 87 | 2 | 3 | 7 | 12 | 18 | 30 | 46 |
| 50–64 | 451 | 9.1 | 47 | 2 | 5 | 8 | 12 | 17 | 23 | 36 |
| 65+ | 796 | 10.5 | 58 | 3 | 5 | 9 | 13 | 20 | 23 | 40 |
| **TOTAL SINGLE DX** | 290 | 2.4 | 7 | 1 | 1 | 1 | 3 | 5 | 8 | 14 |
| **TOTAL MULTIPLE DX** | 1,989 | 9.7 | 73 | 2 | 4 | 8 | 12 | 19 | 26 | 43 |
| **TOTAL** | | | | | | | | | | |
| 0–19 Years | 370 | 6.8 | 89 | 1 | 2 | 3 | 8 | 18 | 27 | 60 |
| 20–34 | 259 | 7.6 | 80 | 1 | 2 | 4 | 12 | 14 | 25 | 53 |
| 35–49 | 362 | 8.8 | 84 | 2 | 3 | 6 | 11 | 16 | 30 | 44 |
| 50–64 | 475 | 8.9 | 47 | 2 | 5 | 8 | 11 | 16 | 22 | 35 |
| 65+ | 813 | 10.4 | 59 | 3 | 5 | 9 | 13 | 20 | 23 | 40 |
| **GRAND TOTAL** | 2,279 | 8.9 | 70 | 1 | 3 | 7 | 12 | 18 | 24 | 41 |

## 83.32: EXC LESION OF MUSCLE. Formerly included in operation group(s) 753.

| Type of Patients | Observed Patients | Avg. Stay | Vari-ance | Percentiles | | | | | | |
|---|---|---|---|---|---|---|---|---|---|---|
| | | | | 10th | 25th | 50th | 75th | 90th | 95th | 99th |
| **1. SINGLE DX** | | | | | | | | | | |
| 0–19 Years | 41 | 2.2 | 2 | 1 | 1 | 2 | 3 | 4 | 4 | 4 |
| 20–34 | 25 | 2.0 | 2 | 1 | 1 | 1 | 3 | 3 | 6 | 6 |
| 35–49 | 24 | 3.5 | 8 | 2 | 2 | 2 | 3 | 5 | 8 | 9 |
| 50–64 | 24 | 2.7 | 6 | 1 | 1 | 2 | 3 | 5 | 6 | 14 |
| 65+ | 9 | 3.3 | 5 | 2 | 2 | 2 | 6 | 6 | 9 | 9 |
| **2. MULTIPLE DX** | | | | | | | | | | |
| 0–19 Years | 42 | 6.5 | 150 | 1 | 1 | 1 | 4 | 21 | 46 | 46 |
| 20–34 | 27 | 3.9 | 14 | 1 | 2 | 3 | 3 | 6 | 15 | 21 |
| 35–49 | 72 | 4.8 | 33 | 1 | 2 | 3 | 5 | 10 | 20 | 31 |
| 50–64 | 71 | 3.9 | 13 | 1 | 2 | 3 | 4 | 8 | 11 | 16 |
| 65+ | 123 | 4.7 | 18 | 2 | 2 | 3 | 6 | 11 | 13 | 22 |
| **TOTAL SINGLE DX** | 123 | 2.6 | 4 | 1 | 1 | 2 | 3 | 5 | 8 | 9 |
| **TOTAL MULTIPLE DX** | 335 | 4.7 | 38 | 1 | 2 | 3 | 5 | 10 | 15 | 43 |
| **TOTAL** | | | | | | | | | | |
| 0–19 Years | 83 | 4.1 | 72 | 1 | 1 | 2 | 4 | 5 | 9 | 46 |
| 20–34 | 52 | 2.9 | 9 | 1 | 1 | 2 | 4 | 5 | 6 | 15 |
| 35–49 | 96 | 4.4 | 26 | 1 | 2 | 2 | 5 | 9 | 15 | 31 |
| 50–64 | 95 | 3.6 | 11 | 1 | 2 | 3 | 4 | 8 | 10 | 16 |
| 65+ | 132 | 4.6 | 17 | 2 | 3 | 3 | 6 | 11 | 13 | 22 |
| **GRAND TOTAL** | 458 | 4.0 | 28 | 1 | 1 | 2 | 4 | 8 | 13 | 31 |

Length of Stay by Diagnosis and Operation, United States, 2000

# United States, October 1998–September 1999 Data, by Operation

## 83.39: EXC LES SOFT TISSUE NEC. Formerly included in operation group(s) 753.

| Type of Patients | Observed Patients | Avg. Stay | Vari-ance | 10th | 25th | 50th | 75th | 90th | 95th | 99th |
|---|---|---|---|---|---|---|---|---|---|---|
| **1. SINGLE DX** | | | | | | | | | | |
| 0-19 Years | 117 | 2.6 | 7 | 1 | 1 | 2 | 2 | 7 | 9 | 14 |
| 20-34 | 61 | 2.0 | 4 | 1 | 1 | 2 | 2 | 4 | 9 | 7 |
| 35-49 | 85 | 1.7 | 2 | 1 | 1 | 1 | 2 | 4 | 6 | 8 |
| 50-64 | 62 | 1.9 | 3 | 1 | 1 | 1 | 2 | 4 | 5 | 9 |
| 65+ | 41 | 2.6 | 5 | 1 | 1 | 2 | 3 | 5 | 7 | 11 |
| **2. MULTIPLE DX** | | | | | | | | | | |
| 0-19 Years | 96 | 3.9 | 20 | 1 | 1 | 2 | 5 | 9 | 10 | 20 |
| 20-34 | 87 | 4.9 | 19 | 1 | 2 | 4 | 7 | 10 | 15 | 22 |
| 35-49 | 249 | 4.0 | 21 | 1 | 2 | 2 | 4 | 9 | 15 | 19 |
| 50-64 | 284 | 4.2 | 25 | 1 | 2 | 3 | 5 | 10 | 14 | 18 |
| 65+ | 387 | 6.1 | 70 | 1 | 2 | 3 | 8 | 13 | 21 | 47 |
| **TOTAL SINGLE DX** | 366 | 2.1 | 4 | 1 | 1 | 1 | 2 | 5 | 7 | 11 |
| **TOTAL MULTIPLE DX** | 1,103 | 4.8 | 37 | 1 | 1 | 3 | 5 | 11 | 15 | 41 |
| **TOTAL** | | | | | | | | | | |
| 0-19 Years | 213 | 3.1 | 13 | 1 | 1 | 2 | 4 | 7 | 10 | 14 |
| 20-34 | 148 | 3.9 | 15 | 1 | 1 | 3 | 4 | 8 | 11 | 16 |
| 35-49 | 334 | 3.2 | 16 | 1 | 1 | 2 | 4 | 7 | 11 | 19 |
| 50-64 | 346 | 3.8 | 22 | 1 | 1 | 3 | 5 | 8 | 14 | 18 |
| 65+ | 428 | 5.7 | 63 | 1 | 2 | 3 | 7 | 12 | 18 | 47 |
| **GRAND TOTAL** | 1,469 | 4.0 | 29 | 1 | 1 | 2 | 5 | 9 | 14 | 26 |

## 83.45: OTHER MYECTOMY. Formerly included in operation group(s) 756.

| Type of Patients | Observed Patients | Avg. Stay | Vari-ance | 10th | 25th | 50th | 75th | 90th | 95th | 99th |
|---|---|---|---|---|---|---|---|---|---|---|
| **1. SINGLE DX** | | | | | | | | | | |
| 0-19 Years | 12 | 3.3 | 8 | 2 | 2 | 2 | 3 | 9 | 9 | 13 |
| 20-34 | 30 | 2.5 | 5 | 1 | 1 | 2 | 3 | 4 | 7 | 15 |
| 35-49 | 25 | 2.3 | 2 | 1 | 1 | 2 | 2 | 4 | 7 | 7 |
| 50-64 | 10 | 2.5 | 4 | 2 | 2 | 2 | 2 | 2 | 4 | 11 |
| 65+ | 3 | 10.4 | 36 | 1 | 14 | 14 | 14 | 14 | 14 | 14 |
| **2. MULTIPLE DX** | | | | | | | | | | |
| 0-19 Years | 49 | 6.4 | 37 | 1 | 1 | 5 | 9 | 16 | 21 | 26 |
| 20-34 | 116 | 7.1 | 93 | 1 | 2 | 5 | 7 | 16 | 27 | 56 |
| 35-49 | 165 | 7.5 | 80 | 1 | 2 | 5 | 9 | 16 | 21 | 49 |
| 50-64 | 143 | 14.0 | 226 | 2 | 4 | 9 | 17 | 35 | 56 | 56 |
| 65+ | 279 | 10.6 | 108 | 2 | 3 | 7 | 15 | 21 | 35 | 45 |
| **TOTAL SINGLE DX** | 80 | 2.7 | 7 | 1 | 2 | 2 | 2 | 4 | 9 | 14 |
| **TOTAL MULTIPLE DX** | 752 | 9.7 | 125 | 1 | 3 | 6 | 13 | 20 | 32 | 56 |
| **TOTAL** | | | | | | | | | | |
| 0-19 Years | 61 | 6.0 | 34 | 1 | 2 | 5 | 9 | 13 | 21 | 22 |
| 20-34 | 146 | 6.1 | 77 | 1 | 2 | 4 | 6 | 15 | 21 | 41 |
| 35-49 | 190 | 6.7 | 72 | 1 | 2 | 4 | 8 | 14 | 21 | 49 |
| 50-64 | 153 | 11.7 | 203 | 2 | 2 | 6 | 17 | 24 | 56 | 56 |
| 65+ | 282 | 10.6 | 107 | 2 | 3 | 7 | 15 | 21 | 35 | 45 |
| **GRAND TOTAL** | 832 | 8.9 | 116 | 1 | 2 | 5 | 12 | 20 | 29 | 56 |

## 83.4: OTHER EXC MUSC/TEND/FASC. Formerly included in operation group(s) 756.

| Type of Patients | Observed Patients | Avg. Stay | Vari-ance | 10th | 25th | 50th | 75th | 90th | 95th | 99th |
|---|---|---|---|---|---|---|---|---|---|---|
| **1. SINGLE DX** | | | | | | | | | | |
| 0-19 Years | 30 | 1.9 | 4 | 1 | 1 | 1 | 2 | 3 | 4 | 13 |
| 20-34 | 41 | 2.6 | 4 | 1 | 2 | 2 | 3 | 4 | 5 | 15 |
| 35-49 | 53 | 1.9 | 2 | 1 | 1 | 1 | 2 | 4 | 5 | 7 |
| 50-64 | 30 | 2.3 | 3 | 1 | 2 | 2 | 2 | 4 | 5 | 11 |
| 65+ | 13 | 6.6 | 15 | 1 | 4 | 7 | 7 | 14 | 14 | 14 |
| **2. MULTIPLE DX** | | | | | | | | | | |
| 0-19 Years | 81 | 5.5 | 32 | 1 | 4 | 4 | 7 | 13 | 21 | 24 |
| 20-34 | 161 | 6.5 | 69 | 1 | 3 | 5 | 6 | 13 | 23 | 36 |
| 35-49 | 255 | 7.5 | 76 | 1 | 2 | 4 | 9 | 16 | 23 | 44 |
| 50-64 | 245 | 9.8 | 153 | 1 | 5 | 5 | 13 | 20 | 41 | 56 |
| 65+ | 403 | 9.4 | 99 | 1 | 3 | 6 | 13 | 20 | 29 | 45 |
| **TOTAL SINGLE DX** | 167 | 2.4 | 5 | 1 | 1 | 2 | 2 | 3 | 4 | 14 |
| **TOTAL MULTIPLE DX** | 1,145 | 8.3 | 99 | 1 | 2 | 5 | 10 | 19 | 26 | 56 |
| **TOTAL** | | | | | | | | | | |
| 0-19 Years | 111 | 4.7 | 28 | 1 | 2 | 2 | 5 | 11 | 19 | 22 |
| 20-34 | 202 | 5.9 | 60 | 1 | 2 | 4 | 5 | 11 | 19 | 36 |
| 35-49 | 308 | 6.1 | 63 | 1 | 1 | 4 | 8 | 13 | 20 | 44 |
| 50-64 | 275 | 8.6 | 136 | 1 | 2 | 4 | 10 | 20 | 30 | 56 |
| 65+ | 416 | 9.3 | 96 | 1 | 3 | 6 | 13 | 20 | 28 | 45 |
| **GRAND TOTAL** | 1,312 | 7.4 | 89 | 1 | 2 | 4 | 9 | 18 | 23 | 56 |

## 83.5: BURSECTOMY. Formerly included in operation group(s) 756.

| Type of Patients | Observed Patients | Avg. Stay | Vari-ance | 10th | 25th | 50th | 75th | 90th | 95th | 99th |
|---|---|---|---|---|---|---|---|---|---|---|
| **1. SINGLE DX** | | | | | | | | | | |
| 0-19 Years | 1 | 3.0 | 0 | 3 | 3 | 3 | 3 | 3 | 3 | 3 |
| 20-34 | 11 | 2.6 | 2 | 1 | 1 | 3 | 4 | 4 | 4 | 6 |
| 35-49 | 37 | 2.0 | 1 | 1 | 1 | 2 | 2 | 3 | 5 | 5 |
| 50-64 | 40 | 2.5 | <1 | 1 | 2 | 2 | 3 | 3 | 5 | 5 |
| 65+ | 12 | 3.3 | 48 | 1 | 1 | 3 | 3 | 3 | 30 | 30 |
| **2. MULTIPLE DX** | | | | | | | | | | |
| 0-19 Years | 15 | 3.1 | 3 | 1 | 2 | 3 | 4 | 5 | 8 | 8 |
| 20-34 | 56 | 3.6 | 4 | 1 | 2 | 3 | 4 | 6 | 7 | 11 |
| 35-49 | 182 | 3.3 | 7 | 1 | 1 | 2 | 5 | 8 | 7 | 14 |
| 50-64 | 220 | 3.5 | 9 | 1 | 2 | 2 | 4 | 8 | 10 | 16 |
| 65+ | 241 | 4.8 | 23 | 1 | 2 | 3 | 7 | 10 | 13 | 18 |
| **TOTAL SINGLE DX** | 101 | 2.5 | 4 | 1 | 1 | 2 | 3 | 3 | 4 | 6 |
| **TOTAL MULTIPLE DX** | 714 | 3.9 | 13 | 1 | 2 | 3 | 5 | 8 | 10 | 17 |
| **TOTAL** | | | | | | | | | | |
| 0-19 Years | 16 | 3.1 | 3 | 1 | 2 | 3 | 4 | 5 | 8 | 8 |
| 20-34 | 67 | 3.4 | 4 | 1 | 2 | 3 | 4 | 6 | 7 | 11 |
| 35-49 | 219 | 3.1 | 6 | 1 | 1 | 2 | 4 | 6 | 9 | 14 |
| 50-64 | 260 | 3.2 | 7 | 1 | 2 | 3 | 4 | 7 | 9 | 15 |
| 65+ | 253 | 4.7 | 24 | 1 | 2 | 3 | 7 | 9 | 13 | 18 |
| **GRAND TOTAL** | 815 | 3.6 | 11 | 1 | 2 | 3 | 4 | 7 | 9 | 16 |

# United States, October 1998–September 1999 Data, by Operation

## 83.6: SUTURE MUSC/TENDON/FASC. Formerly included in operation group(s) 756.

| Type of Patients | Observed Patients | Avg. Stay | Vari- ance | Percentiles | | | | | | |
|---|---|---|---|---|---|---|---|---|---|---|
| | | | | 10th | 25th | 50th | 75th | 90th | 95th | 99th |
| **1. SINGLE DX** | | | | | | | | | | |
| 0–19 Years | 136 | 1.3 | <1 | 1 | 1 | 1 | 1 | 2 | 2 | 4 |
| 20–34 | 312 | 1.4 | <1 | 1 | 1 | 1 | 2 | 2 | 3 | 4 |
| 35–49 | 551 | 1.4 | <1 | 1 | 1 | 1 | 2 | 2 | 3 | 5 |
| 50–64 | 517 | 1.5 | <1 | 1 | 1 | 1 | 2 | 3 | 3 | 6 |
| 65+ | 364 | 1.6 | 3 | 1 | 1 | 1 | 2 | 3 | 3 | 5 |
| **2. MULTIPLE DX** | | | | | | | | | | |
| 0–19 Years | 249 | 2.4 | 3 | 1 | 1 | 2 | 3 | 4 | 6 | 9 |
| 20–34 | 521 | 2.5 | 22 | 1 | 1 | 1 | 2 | 5 | 5 | 29 |
| 35–49 | 1,032 | 2.2 | 6 | 1 | 1 | 2 | 3 | 5 | 5 | 10 |
| 50–64 | 1,694 | 1.9 | 3 | 1 | 1 | 1 | 2 | 3 | 5 | 9 |
| 65+ | 2,254 | 2.4 | 6 | 1 | 1 | 2 | 3 | 4 | 6 | 16 |
| **TOTAL SINGLE DX** | 1,880 | 1.4 | <1 | 1 | 1 | 1 | 2 | 2 | 3 | 5 |
| **TOTAL MULTIPLE DX** | 5,750 | 2.2 | 7 | 1 | 1 | 2 | 2 | 4 | 5 | 11 |
| **TOTAL** | | | | | | | | | | |
| 0–19 Years | 385 | 1.8 | 2 | 1 | 1 | 1 | 2 | 3 | 4 | 9 |
| 20–34 | 833 | 2.1 | 14 | 1 | 1 | 1 | 2 | 4 | 5 | 11 |
| 35–49 | 1,583 | 1.9 | 4 | 1 | 1 | 1 | 2 | 3 | 4 | 8 |
| 50–64 | 2,211 | 1.8 | 3 | 1 | 1 | 1 | 2 | 3 | 4 | 9 |
| 65+ | 2,618 | 2.3 | 6 | 1 | 1 | 2 | 2 | 4 | 6 | 14 |
| **GRAND TOTAL** | 7,630 | 2.0 | 5 | 1 | 1 | 1 | 2 | 3 | 5 | 9 |

## 83.64: OTHER SUTURE OF TENDON. Formerly included in operation group(s) 756.

| Type of Patients | Observed Patients | Avg. Stay | Vari- ance | Percentiles | | | | | | |
|---|---|---|---|---|---|---|---|---|---|---|
| | | | | 10th | 25th | 50th | 75th | 90th | 95th | 99th |
| **1. SINGLE DX** | | | | | | | | | | |
| 0–19 Years | 80 | 1.2 | <1 | 1 | 1 | 1 | 1 | 2 | 2 | 4 |
| 20–34 | 199 | 1.5 | <1 | 1 | 1 | 1 | 2 | 3 | 3 | 4 |
| 35–49 | 256 | 1.5 | <1 | 1 | 1 | 1 | 2 | 2 | 3 | 5 |
| 50–64 | 68 | 1.8 | 2 | 1 | 1 | 1 | 2 | 3 | 3 | 7 |
| 65+ | 33 | 1.9 | 1 | 1 | 2 | 2 | 2 | 3 | 5 | 6 |
| **2. MULTIPLE DX** | | | | | | | | | | |
| 0–19 Years | 140 | 2.3 | 3 | 1 | 1 | 2 | 3 | 4 | 5 | 9 |
| 20–34 | 255 | 2.7 | 30 | 1 | 1 | 1 | 3 | 5 | 5 | 46 |
| 35–49 | 271 | 3.0 | 13 | 1 | 1 | 2 | 3 | 4 | 7 | 19 |
| 50–64 | 188 | 2.8 | 12 | 1 | 1 | 2 | 4 | 6 | 8 | 11 |
| 65+ | 214 | 4.9 | 18 | 2 | 2 | 3 | 7 | 12 | 16 | 16 |
| **TOTAL SINGLE DX** | 636 | 1.5 | <1 | 1 | 1 | 1 | 2 | 2 | 3 | 5 |
| **TOTAL MULTIPLE DX** | 1,068 | 3.1 | 18 | 1 | 1 | 2 | 3 | 5 | 8 | 16 |
| **TOTAL** | | | | | | | | | | |
| 0–19 Years | 220 | 1.7 | 2 | 1 | 1 | 1 | 2 | 3 | 4 | 9 |
| 20–34 | 454 | 2.2 | 18 | 1 | 1 | 1 | 2 | 4 | 5 | 12 |
| 35–49 | 527 | 2.2 | 7 | 1 | 1 | 1 | 3 | 3 | 5 | 16 |
| 50–64 | 256 | 2.5 | 10 | 1 | 1 | 2 | 3 | 4 | 7 | 11 |
| 65+ | 247 | 4.5 | 17 | 1 | 2 | 3 | 5 | 11 | 16 | 16 |
| **GRAND TOTAL** | 1,704 | 2.4 | 11 | 1 | 1 | 1 | 3 | 4 | 6 | 16 |

## 83.63: ROTATOR CUFF REPAIR. Formerly included in operation group(s) 756.

| Type of Patients | Observed Patients | Avg. Stay | Vari- ance | Percentiles | | | | | | |
|---|---|---|---|---|---|---|---|---|---|---|
| | | | | 10th | 25th | 50th | 75th | 90th | 95th | 99th |
| **1. SINGLE DX** | | | | | | | | | | |
| 0–19 Years | 2 | 1.0 | 0 | 1 | 1 | 1 | 1 | 1 | 1 | 1 |
| 20–34 | 33 | 1.1 | <1 | 1 | 1 | 1 | 1 | 2 | 2 | 2 |
| 35–49 | 218 | 1.3 | <1 | 1 | 1 | 1 | 2 | 2 | 2 | 3 |
| 50–64 | 422 | 1.4 | <1 | 1 | 1 | 1 | 2 | 2 | 3 | 3 |
| 65+ | 321 | 1.5 | 3 | 1 | 1 | 1 | 2 | 2 | 2 | 4 |
| **2. MULTIPLE DX** | | | | | | | | | | |
| 0–19 Years | 0 | | | | | | | | | |
| 20–34 | 46 | 2.2 | 12 | 1 | 1 | 2 | 3 | 3 | 3 | 31 |
| 35–49 | 519 | 1.6 | 2 | 1 | 1 | 1 | 2 | 3 | 3 | 7 |
| 50–64 | 1,379 | 1.7 | 2 | 1 | 1 | 1 | 2 | 3 | 3 | 9 |
| 65+ | 1,911 | 2.0 | 3 | 1 | 1 | 2 | 2 | 3 | 4 | 7 |
| **TOTAL SINGLE DX** | 996 | 1.4 | 1 | 1 | 1 | 1 | 2 | 2 | 3 | 3 |
| **TOTAL MULTIPLE DX** | 3,855 | 1.8 | 2 | 1 | 1 | 1 | 2 | 3 | 4 | 8 |
| **TOTAL** | | | | | | | | | | |
| 0–19 Years | 2 | 1.0 | 0 | 1 | 1 | 1 | 1 | 1 | 1 | 1 |
| 20–34 | 79 | 1.7 | 7 | 1 | 1 | 2 | 2 | 3 | 3 | 11 |
| 35–49 | 737 | 1.5 | 2 | 1 | 1 | 1 | 2 | 3 | 3 | 5 |
| 50–64 | 1,801 | 1.6 | 1 | 1 | 1 | 1 | 2 | 3 | 3 | 8 |
| 65+ | 2,232 | 1.9 | 3 | 1 | 1 | 2 | 2 | 3 | 4 | 7 |
| **GRAND TOTAL** | 4,851 | 1.7 | 2 | 1 | 1 | 1 | 2 | 3 | 3 | 7 |

## 83.65: OTHER MUSCLE/FASC SUTURE. Formerly included in operation group(s) 756.

| Type of Patients | Observed Patients | Avg. Stay | Vari- ance | Percentiles | | | | | | |
|---|---|---|---|---|---|---|---|---|---|---|
| | | | | 10th | 25th | 50th | 75th | 90th | 95th | 99th |
| **1. SINGLE DX** | | | | | | | | | | |
| 0–19 Years | 41 | 1.6 | 1 | 1 | 1 | 1 | 2 | 3 | 4 | 6 |
| 20–34 | 46 | 1.4 | <1 | 1 | 1 | 1 | 2 | 2 | 3 | 5 |
| 35–49 | 41 | 1.5 | <1 | 1 | 1 | 1 | 2 | 3 | 3 | 5 |
| 50–64 | 10 | 3.2 | 4 | 1 | 2 | 2 | 6 | 6 | 6 | 6 |
| 65+ | 1 | 1.0 | 0 | 1 | 1 | 1 | 1 | 1 | 1 | 1 |
| **2. MULTIPLE DX** | | | | | | | | | | |
| 0–19 Years | 92 | 2.4 | 4 | 1 | 1 | 2 | 3 | 6 | 6 | 10 |
| 20–34 | 176 | 2.2 | 12 | 1 | 1 | 1 | 3 | 5 | 6 | 9 |
| 35–49 | 185 | 2.4 | 5 | 1 | 1 | 2 | 3 | 6 | 6 | 10 |
| 50–64 | 80 | 2.9 | 6 | 1 | 2 | 2 | 3 | 5 | 7 | 14 |
| 65+ | 76 | 4.6 | 25 | 1 | 2 | 3 | 6 | 8 | 11 | 25 |
| **TOTAL SINGLE DX** | 139 | 1.6 | 1 | 1 | 1 | 1 | 2 | 3 | 4 | 6 |
| **TOTAL MULTIPLE DX** | 609 | 2.5 | 9 | 1 | 1 | 2 | 3 | 5 | 7 | 11 |
| **TOTAL** | | | | | | | | | | |
| 0–19 Years | 133 | 2.1 | 3 | 1 | 1 | 1 | 2 | 4 | 6 | 10 |
| 20–34 | 222 | 2.1 | 10 | 1 | 1 | 1 | 2 | 3 | 5 | 8 |
| 35–49 | 226 | 2.2 | 4 | 1 | 1 | 2 | 3 | 5 | 6 | 8 |
| 50–64 | 90 | 2.9 | 6 | 1 | 2 | 2 | 4 | 6 | 7 | 14 |
| 65+ | 77 | 4.5 | 25 | 1 | 2 | 3 | 6 | 8 | 11 | 25 |
| **GRAND TOTAL** | 748 | 2.4 | 8 | 1 | 1 | 2 | 3 | 5 | 6 | 10 |

Length of Stay by Diagnosis and Operation, United States, 2000

# United States, October 1998–September 1999 Data, by Operation

## 83.7: MUSCLE/TENDON RECONST. Formerly included in operation group(s) 757.

| Type of Patients | Observed Patients | Avg. Stay | Vari-ance | 10th | 25th | 50th | 75th | 90th | 95th | 99th |
|---|---|---|---|---|---|---|---|---|---|---|
| **1. SINGLE DX** | | | | | | | | | | |
| 0–19 Years | 101 | 1.9 | 1 | 1 | 1 | 2 | 2 | 3 | 5 | 6 |
| 20–34 | 30 | 2.2 | 1 | 1 | 1 | 2 | 3 | 3 | 5 | 6 |
| 35–49 | 31 | 1.3 | <1 | 1 | 1 | 1 | 1 | 2 | 3 | 5 |
| 50–64 | 23 | 1.5 | <1 | 1 | 1 | 1 | 2 | 3 | 3 | 6 |
| 65+ | 12 | 1.7 | <1 | 1 | 1 | 1 | 2 | 3 | 3 | 3 |
| **2. MULTIPLE DX** | | | | | | | | | | |
| 0–19 Years | 396 | 2.0 | 5 | 1 | 1 | 1 | 2 | 3 | 5 | 14 |
| 20–34 | 82 | 2.5 | 3 | 1 | 2 | 2 | 3 | 4 | 6 | 10 |
| 35–49 | 127 | 3.2 | 13 | 1 | 2 | 3 | 3 | 4 | 5 | 29 |
| 50–64 | 152 | 2.6 | 5 | 1 | 2 | 2 | 3 | 3 | 4 | 16 |
| 65+ | 124 | 3.2 | 6 | 1 | 2 | 3 | 4 | 6 | 6 | 16 |
| **TOTAL SINGLE DX** | 197 | 1.7 | 1 | 1 | 1 | 1 | 2 | 3 | 3 | 6 |
| **TOTAL MULTIPLE DX** | 881 | 2.6 | 7 | 1 | 1 | 2 | 3 | 4 | 6 | 14 |
| **TOTAL** | | | | | | | | | | |
| 0–19 Years | 497 | 2.0 | 4 | 1 | 1 | 1 | 2 | 3 | 5 | 14 |
| 20–34 | 112 | 2.4 | 2 | 1 | 2 | 2 | 3 | 4 | 6 | 10 |
| 35–49 | 158 | 2.9 | 12 | 1 | 1 | 2 | 3 | 4 | 5 | 29 |
| 50–64 | 175 | 2.5 | 5 | 1 | 1 | 2 | 3 | 3 | 4 | 16 |
| 65+ | 136 | 3.1 | 6 | 1 | 2 | 3 | 4 | 6 | 6 | 16 |
| **GRAND TOTAL** | 1,078 | 2.5 | 6 | 1 | 1 | 2 | 3 | 4 | 6 | 14 |

## 83.8: MUSC/TEND/FASC OP NEC. Formerly included in operation group(s) 757.

| Type of Patients | Observed Patients | Avg. Stay | Vari-ance | 10th | 25th | 50th | 75th | 90th | 95th | 99th |
|---|---|---|---|---|---|---|---|---|---|---|
| **1. SINGLE DX** | | | | | | | | | | |
| 0–19 Years | 669 | 1.4 | <1 | 1 | 1 | 1 | 1 | 2 | 3 | 5 |
| 20–34 | 154 | 2.3 | 3 | 1 | 1 | 2 | 4 | 4 | 4 | 6 |
| 35–49 | 226 | 1.5 | <1 | 1 | 1 | 1 | 2 | 2 | 3 | 4 |
| 50–64 | 98 | 1.7 | 1 | 1 | 1 | 1 | 2 | 3 | 4 | 6 |
| 65+ | 49 | 2.7 | 2 | 1 | 2 | 3 | 4 | 5 | 5 | 6 |
| **2. MULTIPLE DX** | | | | | | | | | | |
| 0–19 Years | 1,112 | 2.2 | 12 | 1 | 1 | 2 | 2 | 3 | 4 | 10 |
| 20–34 | 233 | 4.2 | 35 | 1 | 1 | 4 | 4 | 8 | 20 | 27 |
| 35–49 | 358 | 4.3 | 38 | 1 | 2 | 2 | 4 | 9 | 13 | 29 |
| 50–64 | 436 | 3.3 | 15 | 1 | 2 | 2 | 3 | 7 | 8 | 22 |
| 65+ | 530 | 4.2 | 35 | 1 | 2 | 3 | 5 | 8 | 12 | 22 |
| **TOTAL SINGLE DX** | 1,196 | 1.6 | 1 | 1 | 1 | 1 | 2 | 3 | 4 | 5 |
| **TOTAL MULTIPLE DX** | 2,669 | 3.2 | 23 | 1 | 1 | 2 | 3 | 6 | 9 | 26 |
| **TOTAL** | | | | | | | | | | |
| 0–19 Years | 1,781 | 1.9 | 8 | 1 | 1 | 1 | 2 | 3 | 4 | 7 |
| 20–34 | 387 | 3.2 | 19 | 1 | 1 | 2 | 4 | 4 | 8 | 27 |
| 35–49 | 584 | 2.8 | 20 | 1 | 1 | 2 | 3 | 5 | 8 | 16 |
| 50–64 | 534 | 3.0 | 13 | 1 | 1 | 2 | 3 | 6 | 8 | 21 |
| 65+ | 579 | 4.1 | 33 | 1 | 2 | 3 | 5 | 8 | 11 | 22 |
| **GRAND TOTAL** | 3,865 | 2.6 | 16 | 1 | 1 | 2 | 3 | 4 | 7 | 19 |

## 83.75: TENDON TRANSF/TRANSPL. Formerly included in operation group(s) 757.

| Type of Patients | Observed Patients | Avg. Stay | Vari-ance | 10th | 25th | 50th | 75th | 90th | 95th | 99th |
|---|---|---|---|---|---|---|---|---|---|---|
| **1. SINGLE DX** | | | | | | | | | | |
| 0–19 Years | 69 | 1.7 | <1 | 1 | 1 | 1 | 2 | 3 | 3 | 6 |
| 20–34 | 16 | 2.6 | <1 | 2 | 2 | 3 | 3 | 3 | 3 | 3 |
| 35–49 | 9 | 1.2 | <1 | 1 | 1 | 1 | 1 | 2 | 3 | 3 |
| 50–64 | 13 | 1.4 | <1 | 1 | 1 | 1 | 2 | 2 | 3 | 6 |
| 65+ | 7 | 1.1 | <1 | 1 | 1 | 1 | 1 | 2 | 2 | 2 |
| **2. MULTIPLE DX** | | | | | | | | | | |
| 0–19 Years | 228 | 1.7 | 1 | 1 | 1 | 2 | 2 | 3 | 3 | 7 |
| 20–34 | 48 | 2.0 | <1 | 1 | 2 | 2 | 2 | 3 | 3 | 4 |
| 35–49 | 54 | 2.9 | 2 | 1 | 2 | 3 | 4 | 4 | 4 | 5 |
| 50–64 | 80 | 2.3 | 2 | 1 | 2 | 2 | 3 | 3 | 4 | 7 |
| 65+ | 61 | 3.0 | 3 | 1 | 2 | 3 | 4 | 4 | 6 | 8 |
| **TOTAL SINGLE DX** | 114 | 1.6 | <1 | 1 | 1 | 1 | 2 | 3 | 3 | 4 |
| **TOTAL MULTIPLE DX** | 471 | 2.2 | 2 | 1 | 1 | 2 | 3 | 4 | 4 | 7 |
| **TOTAL** | | | | | | | | | | |
| 0–19 Years | 297 | 1.7 | 1 | 1 | 1 | 1 | 2 | 3 | 3 | 7 |
| 20–34 | 64 | 2.1 | <1 | 1 | 2 | 2 | 3 | 3 | 3 | 4 |
| 35–49 | 63 | 2.4 | 2 | 1 | 2 | 2 | 3 | 4 | 4 | 5 |
| 50–64 | 93 | 2.2 | 2 | 1 | 1 | 2 | 3 | 3 | 4 | 7 |
| 65+ | 68 | 2.8 | 3 | 1 | 2 | 3 | 4 | 4 | 5 | 8 |
| **GRAND TOTAL** | 585 | 2.1 | 2 | 1 | 1 | 2 | 3 | 3 | 4 | 7 |

## 83.84: CLUBFOOT RELEASE NEC. Formerly included in operation group(s) 757.

| Type of Patients | Observed Patients | Avg. Stay | Vari-ance | 10th | 25th | 50th | 75th | 90th | 95th | 99th |
|---|---|---|---|---|---|---|---|---|---|---|
| **1. SINGLE DX** | | | | | | | | | | |
| 0–19 Years | 456 | 1.4 | <1 | 1 | 1 | 1 | 1 | 2 | 3 | 7 |
| 20–34 | 1 | 2.0 | 0 | 2 | 2 | 2 | 2 | 2 | 2 | 2 |
| 35–49 | 4 | 1.6 | <1 | 1 | 1 | 1 | 2 | 3 | 3 | 3 |
| 50–64 | 0 | | | | | | | | | |
| 65+ | 0 | | | | | | | | | |
| **2. MULTIPLE DX** | | | | | | | | | | |
| 0–19 Years | 157 | 1.9 | 3 | 1 | 1 | 1 | 2 | 4 | 7 | 9 |
| 20–34 | 2 | 1.4 | <1 | 1 | 1 | 1 | 2 | 2 | 2 | 2 |
| 35–49 | 2 | 4.2 | 2 | 2 | 2 | 5 | 5 | 5 | 5 | 5 |
| 50–64 | 1 | 2.0 | 0 | 2 | 2 | 2 | 2 | 2 | 2 | 2 |
| 65+ | 0 | | | | | | | | | |
| **TOTAL SINGLE DX** | 461 | 1.4 | <1 | 1 | 1 | 1 | 1 | 2 | 3 | 7 |
| **TOTAL MULTIPLE DX** | 162 | 1.9 | 3 | 1 | 1 | 1 | 2 | 4 | 7 | 9 |
| **TOTAL** | | | | | | | | | | |
| 0–19 Years | 613 | 1.5 | 1 | 1 | 1 | 1 | 2 | 2 | 4 | 7 |
| 20–34 | 3 | 1.6 | <1 | 1 | 1 | 2 | 2 | 2 | 2 | 2 |
| 35–49 | 6 | 2.6 | 3 | 2 | 2 | 2 | 5 | 5 | 5 | 5 |
| 50–64 | 1 | 2.0 | 0 | 2 | 2 | 2 | 2 | 2 | 2 | 2 |
| 65+ | 0 | | | | | | | | | |
| **GRAND TOTAL** | 623 | 1.5 | 2 | 1 | 1 | 1 | 2 | 2 | 4 | 7 |

Length of Stay by Diagnosis and Operation, United States, 2000

## United States, October 1998–September 1999 Data, by Operation

### 83.85: CHANGE IN M/T LENGTH NEC. Formerly included in operation group(s) 757.

| Type of Patients | Observed Patients | Avg. Stay | Variance | 10th | 25th | 50th | 75th | 90th | 95th | 99th |
|---|---|---|---|---|---|---|---|---|---|---|
| **1. SINGLE DX** | | | | | | | | | | |
| 0–19 Years | 177 | 1.3 | <1 | 1 | 1 | 1 | 1 | 2 | 3 | 3 |
| 20–34 | 11 | 1.4 | <1 | 1 | 1 | 1 | 1 | 3 | 3 | 3 |
| 35–49 | 8 | 2.5 | 2 | 1 | 2 | 2 | 2 | 5 | 5 | 6 |
| 50–64 | 4 | 1.6 | <1 | 1 | 1 | 2 | 2 | 2 | 2 | 2 |
| 65+ | 3 | 2.5 | <1 | 2 | 2 | 3 | 3 | 3 | 3 | 3 |
| **2. MULTIPLE DX** | | | | | | | | | | |
| 0–19 Years | 874 | 2.1 | 12 | 1 | 1 | 2 | 2 | 3 | 4 | 7 |
| 20–34 | 67 | 2.9 | 6 | 1 | 2 | 2 | 4 | 4 | 4 | 18 |
| 35–49 | 81 | 4.3 | 16 | 1 | 2 | 3 | 4 | 13 | 13 | 13 |
| 50–64 | 93 | 2.6 | 5 | 1 | 1 | 2 | 3 | 5 | 8 | 13 |
| 65+ | 64 | 2.9 | 6 | 1 | 2 | 2 | 3 | 6 | 9 | 14 |
| **TOTAL SINGLE DX** | 203 | 1.4 | <1 | 1 | 1 | 1 | 2 | 3 | 3 | 5 |
| **TOTAL MULTIPLE DX** | 1,179 | 2.4 | 12 | 1 | 1 | 2 | 3 | 4 | 5 | 13 |
| **TOTAL** | | | | | | | | | | |
| 0–19 Years | 1,051 | 1.9 | 10 | 1 | 1 | 1 | 2 | 3 | 3 | 7 |
| 20–34 | 78 | 2.6 | 5 | 1 | 1 | 2 | 4 | 4 | 4 | 11 |
| 35–49 | 89 | 4.2 | 15 | 1 | 2 | 3 | 4 | 13 | 13 | 13 |
| 50–64 | 97 | 2.6 | 5 | 1 | 1 | 2 | 3 | 5 | 7 | 13 |
| 65+ | 67 | 2.9 | 6 | 2 | 2 | 2 | 3 | 6 | 9 | 14 |
| **GRAND TOTAL** | 1,382 | 2.3 | 10 | 1 | 1 | 2 | 3 | 4 | 4 | 13 |

### 83.88: OTHER PLASTIC OPS TENDON. Formerly included in operation group(s) 757.

| Type of Patients | Observed Patients | Avg. Stay | Variance | 10th | 25th | 50th | 75th | 90th | 95th | 99th |
|---|---|---|---|---|---|---|---|---|---|---|
| **1. SINGLE DX** | | | | | | | | | | |
| 0–19 Years | 16 | 1.5 | <1 | 1 | 1 | 1 | 1 | 3 | 4 | 4 |
| 20–34 | 111 | 2.4 | 2 | 1 | 1 | 2 | 4 | 4 | 4 | 5 |
| 35–49 | 171 | 1.4 | <1 | 1 | 1 | 1 | 2 | 2 | 3 | 3 |
| 50–64 | 54 | 1.5 | <1 | 1 | 1 | 1 | 2 | 2 | 2 | 4 |
| 65+ | 26 | 2.7 | 2 | 1 | 2 | 2 | 4 | 4 | 5 | 5 |
| **2. MULTIPLE DX** | | | | | | | | | | |
| 0–19 Years | 31 | 2.1 | 14 | 1 | 1 | 1 | 2 | 3 | 5 | 31 |
| 20–34 | 94 | 2.3 | 4 | 1 | 2 | 2 | 3 | 5 | 6 | 9 |
| 35–49 | 172 | 3.1 | 32 | 1 | 2 | 2 | 3 | 5 | 7 | 16 |
| 50–64 | 199 | 2.5 | 4 | 1 | 2 | 2 | 3 | 5 | 7 | 8 |
| 65+ | 261 | 3.1 | 5 | 1 | 2 | 3 | 4 | 6 | 7 | 10 |
| **TOTAL SINGLE DX** | 378 | 1.8 | 1 | 1 | 1 | 1 | 2 | 4 | 4 | 4 |
| **TOTAL MULTIPLE DX** | 757 | 2.8 | 12 | 1 | 1 | 2 | 3 | 6 | 7 | 12 |
| **TOTAL** | | | | | | | | | | |
| 0–19 Years | 47 | 2.0 | 11 | 1 | 1 | 1 | 2 | 3 | 4 | 31 |
| 20–34 | 205 | 2.4 | 3 | 1 | 1 | 2 | 4 | 4 | 4 | 6 |
| 35–49 | 343 | 2.0 | 12 | 1 | 1 | 1 | 2 | 3 | 4 | 9 |
| 50–64 | 253 | 2.2 | 4 | 1 | 1 | 1 | 3 | 5 | 7 | 8 |
| 65+ | 287 | 3.1 | 5 | 1 | 1 | 3 | 4 | 6 | 7 | 10 |
| **GRAND TOTAL** | 1,135 | 2.3 | 7 | 1 | 1 | 2 | 3 | 4 | 6 | 9 |

### 83.9: OTHER CONN TISSUE OPS. Formerly included in operation group(s) 757, 767.

| Type of Patients | Observed Patients | Avg. Stay | Variance | 10th | 25th | 50th | 75th | 90th | 95th | 99th |
|---|---|---|---|---|---|---|---|---|---|---|
| **1. SINGLE DX** | | | | | | | | | | |
| 0–19 Years | 18 | 2.3 | 2 | 1 | 1 | 2 | 3 | 5 | 5 | 7 |
| 20–34 | 8 | 3.0 | 2 | 1 | 2 | 3 | 5 | 5 | 5 | 5 |
| 35–49 | 14 | 2.9 | 9 | 1 | 2 | 2 | 3 | 3 | 5 | 15 |
| 50–64 | 17 | 2.7 | 3 | 1 | 2 | 2 | 3 | 5 | 5 | 7 |
| 65+ | 10 | 2.7 | <1 | 2 | 3 | 3 | 3 | 4 | 4 | 4 |
| **2. MULTIPLE DX** | | | | | | | | | | |
| 0–19 Years | 63 | 5.4 | 89 | 1 | 3 | 4 | 4 | 7 | 14 | 67 |
| 20–34 | 95 | 5.9 | 28 | 2 | 3 | 4 | 8 | 12 | 20 | 27 |
| 35–49 | 242 | 6.2 | 38 | 2 | 2 | 5 | 8 | 12 | 22 | 27 |
| 50–64 | 293 | 6.6 | 31 | 2 | 3 | 5 | 8 | 15 | 17 | 26 |
| 65+ | 552 | 7.5 | 48 | 2 | 3 | 5 | 8 | 16 | 22 | 36 |
| **TOTAL SINGLE DX** | 67 | 2.6 | 4 | 1 | 1 | 2 | 3 | 5 | 5 | 15 |
| **TOTAL MULTIPLE DX** | 1,245 | 6.7 | 44 | 2 | 3 | 5 | 8 | 14 | 19 | 33 |
| **TOTAL** | | | | | | | | | | |
| 0–19 Years | 81 | 4.8 | 73 | 1 | 2 | 3 | 4 | 7 | 14 | 67 |
| 20–34 | 103 | 5.7 | 27 | 1 | 3 | 4 | 8 | 12 | 20 | 27 |
| 35–49 | 256 | 6.0 | 37 | 2 | 2 | 4 | 7 | 12 | 22 | 27 |
| 50–64 | 310 | 6.5 | 30 | 2 | 3 | 5 | 8 | 14 | 17 | 26 |
| 65+ | 562 | 7.4 | 48 | 2 | 3 | 5 | 8 | 16 | 22 | 36 |
| **GRAND TOTAL** | 1,312 | 6.6 | 42 | 2 | 3 | 5 | 8 | 14 | 18 | 33 |

### 83.94: ASPIRATION OF BURSA. Formerly included in operation group(s) 767.

| Type of Patients | Observed Patients | Avg. Stay | Variance | 10th | 25th | 50th | 75th | 90th | 95th | 99th |
|---|---|---|---|---|---|---|---|---|---|---|
| **1. SINGLE DX** | | | | | | | | | | |
| 0–19 Years | 1 | 1.0 | 0 | 1 | 1 | 1 | 1 | 1 | 1 | 1 |
| 20–34 | 0 | | | | | | | | | |
| 35–49 | 3 | 7.2 | 38 | 3 | 3 | 3 | 15 | 15 | 15 | 15 |
| 50–64 | 0 | | | | | | | | | |
| 65+ | 1 | 3.0 | 0 | 3 | 3 | 3 | 3 | 3 | 3 | 3 |
| **2. MULTIPLE DX** | | | | | | | | | | |
| 0–19 Years | 13 | 4.7 | 6 | 2 | 2 | 6 | 6 | 7 | 7 | 11 |
| 20–34 | 21 | 3.8 | 6 | 1 | 2 | 3 | 5 | 5 | 8 | 9 |
| 35–49 | 86 | 3.6 | 8 | 2 | 2 | 3 | 4 | 5 | 7 | 25 |
| 50–64 | 72 | 5.5 | 30 | 2 | 3 | 4 | 6 | 8 | 12 | 31 |
| 65+ | 119 | 5.5 | 35 | 2 | 2 | 4 | 7 | 9 | 12 | 40 |
| **TOTAL SINGLE DX** | 5 | 5.1 | 31 | 1 | 1 | 3 | 3 | 15 | 15 | 15 |
| **TOTAL MULTIPLE DX** | 311 | 4.8 | 24 | 2 | 2 | 4 | 6 | 8 | 11 | 31 |
| **TOTAL** | | | | | | | | | | |
| 0–19 Years | 14 | 4.5 | 7 | 2 | 2 | 5 | 7 | 7 | 7 | 11 |
| 20–34 | 21 | 3.8 | 6 | 1 | 2 | 3 | 5 | 8 | 8 | 9 |
| 35–49 | 89 | 3.7 | 9 | 2 | 2 | 3 | 4 | 5 | 7 | 25 |
| 50–64 | 72 | 5.5 | 30 | 2 | 3 | 4 | 6 | 9 | 12 | 31 |
| 65+ | 120 | 5.5 | 35 | 2 | 2 | 4 | 7 | 9 | 12 | 40 |
| **GRAND TOTAL** | 316 | 4.8 | 24 | 2 | 2 | 4 | 6 | 8 | 12 | 31 |

Length of Stay by Diagnosis and Operation, United States, 2000

## 83.95: SOFT TISSUE ASP NEC. Formerly included in operation group(s) 767.

| Type of Patients | Observed Patients | Avg. Stay | Vari-ance | 10th | 25th | 50th | 75th | 90th | 95th | 99th |
|---|---|---|---|---|---|---|---|---|---|---|
| **1. SINGLE DX** | | | | | | | | | | |
| 0–19 Years | 14 | 2.5 | 2 | 1 | 2 | 2 | 3 | 5 | 5 | 7 |
| 20–34 | 6 | 3.7 | 2 | 2 | 2 | 3 | 5 | 5 | 5 | 5 |
| 35–49 | 7 | 2.1 | <1 | 1 | 2 | 2 | 3 | 3 | 3 | 5 |
| 50–64 | 7 | 3.4 | 2 | 2 | 2 | 3 | 5 | 5 | 5 | 5 |
| 65+ | 2 | 3.2 | 1 | 2 | 2 | 4 | 4 | 4 | 4 | 4 |
| **2. MULTIPLE DX** | | | | | | | | | | |
| 0–19 Years | 39 | 4.8 | 21 | 2 | 3 | 4 | 4 | 8 | 14 | 29 |
| 20–34 | 45 | 7.5 | 35 | 3 | 3 | 6 | 8 | 20 | 20 | 23 |
| 35–49 | 87 | 8.6 | 49 | 2 | 5 | 6 | 11 | 18 | 24 | 33 |
| 50–64 | 110 | 8.7 | 29 | 2 | 4 | 8 | 13 | 17 | 17 | 19 |
| 65+ | 156 | 9.3 | 62 | 3 | 5 | 7 | 10 | 18 | 32 | 36 |
| **TOTAL SINGLE DX** | 36 | 2.6 | 2 | 1 | 2 | 2 | 3 | 5 | 5 | 7 |
| **TOTAL MULTIPLE DX** | 437 | 8.3 | 44 | 2 | 4 | 6 | 11 | 17 | 20 | 33 |
| **TOTAL** | | | | | | | | | | |
| 0–19 Years | 53 | 4.2 | 17 | 2 | 2 | 4 | 4 | 5 | 14 | 29 |
| 20–34 | 51 | 7.2 | 34 | 3 | 3 | 6 | 8 | 14 | 20 | 23 |
| 35–49 | 94 | 7.9 | 48 | 2 | 3 | 6 | 11 | 18 | 24 | 33 |
| 50–64 | 117 | 8.5 | 29 | 2 | 3 | 7 | 13 | 17 | 17 | 19 |
| 65+ | 158 | 9.2 | 62 | 3 | 5 | 7 | 10 | 18 | 32 | 36 |
| **GRAND TOTAL** | 473 | 7.8 | 43 | 2 | 3 | 6 | 10 | 17 | 20 | 33 |

## 84.01: FINGER AMPUTATION. Formerly included in operation group(s) 758.

| Type of Patients | Observed Patients | Avg. Stay | Vari-ance | 10th | 25th | 50th | 75th | 90th | 95th | 99th |
|---|---|---|---|---|---|---|---|---|---|---|
| **1. SINGLE DX** | | | | | | | | | | |
| 0–19 Years | 47 | 2.5 | 5 | 1 | 1 | 1 | 2 | 7 | 7 | 7 |
| 20–34 | 104 | 1.6 | 1 | 1 | 1 | 1 | 2 | 3 | 4 | 8 |
| 35–49 | 77 | 1.6 | 1 | 1 | 1 | 1 | 2 | 3 | 4 | 5 |
| 50–64 | 38 | 1.9 | 3 | 1 | 1 | 1 | 2 | 7 | 7 | 7 |
| 65+ | 12 | 2.0 | 1 | 1 | 2 | 2 | 2 | 2 | 3 | 7 |
| **2. MULTIPLE DX** | | | | | | | | | | |
| 0–19 Years | 63 | 2.9 | 10 | 1 | 1 | 2 | 3 | 8 | 10 | 15 |
| 20–34 | 160 | 3.7 | 37 | 1 | 1 | 3 | 3 | 9 | 13 | 44 |
| 35–49 | 315 | 5.1 | 30 | 1 | 1 | 4 | 7 | 10 | 15 | 34 |
| 50–64 | 286 | 5.7 | 62 | 1 | 3 | 3 | 6 | 15 | 20 | 43 |
| 65+ | 280 | 6.4 | 51 | 1 | 2 | 5 | 8 | 14 | 16 | 36 |
| **TOTAL SINGLE DX** | 278 | 1.9 | 3 | 1 | 1 | 1 | 2 | 4 | 7 | 7 |
| **TOTAL MULTIPLE DX** | 1,104 | 5.2 | 44 | 1 | 1 | 3 | 6 | 11 | 16 | 39 |
| **TOTAL** | | | | | | | | | | |
| 0–19 Years | 110 | 2.7 | 8 | 1 | 1 | 2 | 3 | 7 | 8 | 10 |
| 20–34 | 264 | 2.9 | 24 | 1 | 1 | 1 | 3 | 7 | 9 | 36 |
| 35–49 | 392 | 4.5 | 27 | 1 | 1 | 3 | 6 | 10 | 13 | 29 |
| 50–64 | 324 | 5.4 | 58 | 1 | 1 | 4 | 6 | 14 | 20 | 43 |
| 65+ | 292 | 6.0 | 48 | 1 | 2 | 5 | 7 | 14 | 16 | 36 |
| **GRAND TOTAL** | 1,382 | 4.5 | 37 | 1 | 1 | 3 | 6 | 10 | 15 | 36 |

## 84.0: AMPUTATION OF UPPER LIMB. Formerly included in operation group(s) 758, 759.

| Type of Patients | Observed Patients | Avg. Stay | Vari-ance | 10th | 25th | 50th | 75th | 90th | 95th | 99th |
|---|---|---|---|---|---|---|---|---|---|---|
| **1. SINGLE DX** | | | | | | | | | | |
| 0–19 Years | 54 | 2.5 | 5 | 1 | 1 | 1 | 2 | 5 | 5 | 7 |
| 20–34 | 128 | 1.8 | 3 | 1 | 1 | 1 | 2 | 5 | 5 | 5 |
| 35–49 | 104 | 3.1 | 15 | 1 | 1 | 1 | 3 | 13 | 13 | 13 |
| 50–64 | 45 | 1.8 | 3 | 1 | 1 | 1 | 2 | 3 | 3 | 7 |
| 65+ | 20 | 1.9 | 1 | 1 | 1 | 2 | 2 | 2 | 4 | 7 |
| **2. MULTIPLE DX** | | | | | | | | | | |
| 0–19 Years | 90 | 3.8 | 31 | 1 | 1 | 2 | 4 | 8 | 10 | 34 |
| 20–34 | 215 | 5.9 | 71 | 1 | 1 | 2 | 7 | 14 | 28 | 37 |
| 35–49 | 403 | 5.7 | 38 | 1 | 1 | 4 | 8 | 12 | 16 | 34 |
| 50–64 | 370 | 6.1 | 66 | 1 | 1 | 3 | 7 | 15 | 22 | 45 |
| 65+ | 378 | 6.8 | 59 | 1 | 2 | 5 | 7 | 14 | 20 | 44 |
| **TOTAL SINGLE DX** | 351 | 2.3 | 7 | 1 | 1 | 1 | 2 | 5 | 7 | 13 |
| **TOTAL MULTIPLE DX** | 1,456 | 5.9 | 55 | 1 | 1 | 3 | 7 | 14 | 19 | 39 |
| **TOTAL** | | | | | | | | | | |
| 0–19 Years | 144 | 3.2 | 20 | 1 | 1 | 2 | 3 | 7 | 10 | 22 |
| 20–34 | 343 | 4.5 | 52 | 1 | 1 | 2 | 4 | 14 | 16 | 36 |
| 35–49 | 507 | 5.2 | 35 | 1 | 1 | 3 | 7 | 12 | 16 | 34 |
| 50–64 | 415 | 5.7 | 61 | 1 | 1 | 3 | 6 | 14 | 20 | 43 |
| 65+ | 398 | 6.4 | 56 | 1 | 2 | 5 | 7 | 14 | 19 | 44 |
| **GRAND TOTAL** | 1,807 | 5.2 | 48 | 1 | 1 | 3 | 6 | 13 | 17 | 36 |

## 84.1: AMPUTATION OF LOWER LIMB. Formerly included in operation group(s) 760, 761, 762, 763.

| Type of Patients | Observed Patients | Avg. Stay | Vari-ance | 10th | 25th | 50th | 75th | 90th | 95th | 99th |
|---|---|---|---|---|---|---|---|---|---|---|
| **1. SINGLE DX** | | | | | | | | | | |
| 0–19 Years | 63 | 3.8 | 11 | 1 | 3 | 3 | 4 | 7 | 15 | 15 |
| 20–34 | 54 | 4.8 | 15 | 1 | 2 | 3 | 9 | 9 | 10 | 17 |
| 35–49 | 75 | 4.4 | 9 | 1 | 2 | 4 | 6 | 9 | 10 | 14 |
| 50–64 | 75 | 5.1 | 38 | 1 | 2 | 3 | 6 | 12 | 13 | 50 |
| 65+ | 124 | 4.1 | 9 | 1 | 2 | 3 | 5 | 8 | 9 | 15 |
| **2. MULTIPLE DX** | | | | | | | | | | |
| 0–19 Years | 166 | 9.6 | 215 | 2 | 2 | 4 | 10 | 29 | 47 | >99 |
| 20–34 | 586 | 9.0 | 89 | 2 | 4 | 7 | 10 | 19 | 28 | 52 |
| 35–49 | 3,571 | 10.2 | 76 | 3 | 5 | 8 | 13 | 20 | 27 | 41 |
| 50–64 | 8,794 | 10.8 | 79 | 3 | 5 | 8 | 14 | 21 | 27 | 48 |
| 65+ | 19,682 | 10.6 | 84 | 3 | 5 | 8 | 13 | 21 | 28 | 47 |
| **TOTAL SINGLE DX** | 391 | 4.4 | 16 | 1 | 2 | 3 | 5 | 9 | 12 | 16 |
| **TOTAL MULTIPLE DX** | 32,799 | 10.6 | 82 | 3 | 5 | 8 | 13 | 21 | 27 | 47 |
| **TOTAL** | | | | | | | | | | |
| 0–19 Years | 229 | 7.3 | 141 | 1 | 2 | 3 | 7 | 15 | 31 | >99 |
| 20–34 | 640 | 8.6 | 84 | 2 | 4 | 6 | 10 | 17 | 27 | 46 |
| 35–49 | 3,646 | 10.1 | 75 | 3 | 4 | 8 | 13 | 20 | 27 | 41 |
| 50–64 | 8,869 | 10.8 | 79 | 3 | 5 | 8 | 14 | 21 | 27 | 48 |
| 65+ | 19,806 | 10.5 | 84 | 3 | 5 | 8 | 13 | 21 | 27 | 47 |
| **GRAND TOTAL** | 33,190 | 10.5 | 82 | 3 | 5 | 8 | 13 | 21 | 27 | 47 |

# United States, October 1998–September 1999 Data, by Operation

## 84.11: TOE AMPUTATION. Formerly included in operation group(s) 760.

| Type of Patients | Observed Patients | Avg. Stay | Variance | 10th | 25th | 50th | 75th | 90th | 95th | 99th |
|---|---|---|---|---|---|---|---|---|---|---|
| **1. SINGLE DX** | | | | | | | | | | |
| 0–19 Years | 22 | 2.7 | <1 | 1 | 3 | 3 | 3 | 3 | 3 | 7 |
| 20–34 | 25 | 4.6 | 13 | 1 | 1 | 3 | 9 | 9 | 9 | 10 |
| 35–49 | 35 | 3.8 | 9 | 1 | 2 | 3 | 6 | 10 | 10 | 11 |
| 50–64 | 27 | 3.2 | 10 | 1 | 1 | 3 | 3 | 6 | 10 | 16 |
| 65+ | 28 | 2.9 | 7 | 1 | 2 | 2 | 4 | 6 | 7 | 11 |
| **2. MULTIPLE DX** | | | | | | | | | | |
| 0–19 Years | 53 | 8.5 | 141 | 1 | 2 | 3 | 8 | 29 | 33 | 54 |
| 20–34 | 239 | 6.5 | 45 | 1 | 3 | 4 | 8 | 13 | 20 | 31 |
| 35–49 | 1,563 | 8.1 | 40 | 2 | 4 | 7 | 11 | 15 | 19 | 32 |
| 50–64 | 3,175 | 9.0 | 50 | 2 | 4 | 7 | 12 | 16 | 23 | 39 |
| 65+ | 4,267 | 8.9 | 52 | 2 | 4 | 7 | 12 | 18 | 22 | 34 |
| **TOTAL SINGLE DX** | 137 | 3.4 | 7 | 1 | 1 | 3 | 3 | 9 | 9 | 11 |
| **TOTAL MULTIPLE DX** | 9,297 | 8.7 | 50 | 2 | 4 | 7 | 11 | 17 | 22 | 35 |
| **TOTAL** | | | | | | | | | | |
| 0–19 Years | 75 | 5.2 | 68 | 1 | 2 | 3 | 3 | 9 | 29 | 54 |
| 20–34 | 264 | 6.3 | 42 | 1 | 3 | 4 | 8 | 12 | 18 | 31 |
| 35–49 | 1,598 | 8.0 | 40 | 2 | 4 | 7 | 11 | 15 | 19 | 32 |
| 50–64 | 3,202 | 8.9 | 50 | 2 | 4 | 7 | 12 | 16 | 23 | 39 |
| 65+ | 4,295 | 8.9 | 52 | 2 | 4 | 7 | 12 | 18 | 22 | 34 |
| **GRAND TOTAL** | 9,434 | 8.6 | 49 | 2 | 4 | 7 | 11 | 17 | 21 | 35 |

## 84.15: BK AMPUTATION NEC. Formerly included in operation group(s) 761.

| Type of Patients | Observed Patients | Avg. Stay | Variance | 10th | 25th | 50th | 75th | 90th | 95th | 99th |
|---|---|---|---|---|---|---|---|---|---|---|
| **1. SINGLE DX** | | | | | | | | | | |
| 0–19 Years | 11 | 7.7 | 28 | 3 | 3 | 4 | 15 | 15 | 15 | 15 |
| 20–34 | 12 | 5.5 | 7 | 2 | 4 | 5 | 8 | 10 | 10 | 10 |
| 35–49 | 23 | 5.3 | 10 | 2 | 2 | 4 | 7 | 10 | 14 | 14 |
| 50–64 | 23 | 6.7 | 85 | 2 | 2 | 4 | 5 | 13 | 14 | 50 |
| 65+ | 48 | 4.9 | 12 | 2 | 2 | 4 | 5 | 9 | 15 | 15 |
| **2. MULTIPLE DX** | | | | | | | | | | |
| 0–19 Years | 29 | 20.4 | 653 | 3 | 4 | 12 | 24 | 54 | 97 | >99 |
| 20–34 | 184 | 9.9 | 89 | 3 | 5 | 8 | 12 | 20 | 27 | 46 |
| 35–49 | 1,034 | 11.7 | 94 | 3 | 5 | 8 | 16 | 26 | 30 | 51 |
| 50–64 | 2,777 | 11.7 | 83 | 3 | 5 | 9 | 15 | 22 | 28 | 49 |
| 65+ | 5,898 | 11.9 | 107 | 3 | 5 | 9 | 15 | 24 | 30 | 55 |
| **TOTAL SINGLE DX** | 117 | 5.9 | 32 | 2 | 3 | 4 | 8 | 14 | 15 | 15 |
| **TOTAL MULTIPLE DX** | 9,922 | 11.8 | 100 | 3 | 5 | 9 | 15 | 24 | 30 | 53 |
| **TOTAL** | | | | | | | | | | |
| 0–19 Years | 40 | 14.9 | 421 | 3 | 5 | 9 | 15 | 39 | 87 | 97 |
| 20–34 | 196 | 9.8 | 87 | 3 | 5 | 8 | 12 | 18 | 27 | 46 |
| 35–49 | 1,057 | 11.6 | 93 | 3 | 5 | 9 | 15 | 25 | 30 | 51 |
| 50–64 | 2,800 | 11.7 | 83 | 3 | 5 | 9 | 15 | 22 | 28 | 49 |
| 65+ | 5,946 | 11.8 | 107 | 3 | 5 | 9 | 15 | 24 | 30 | 55 |
| **GRAND TOTAL** | 10,039 | 11.7 | 99 | 3 | 5 | 9 | 15 | 23 | 30 | 53 |

## 84.12: AMPUTATION THROUGH FOOT. Formerly included in operation group(s) 763.

| Type of Patients | Observed Patients | Avg. Stay | Variance | 10th | 25th | 50th | 75th | 90th | 95th | 99th |
|---|---|---|---|---|---|---|---|---|---|---|
| **1. SINGLE DX** | | | | | | | | | | |
| 0–19 Years | 8 | 2.8 | 11 | 1 | 1 | 2 | 2 | 3 | 3 | 14 |
| 20–34 | 5 | 3.4 | 10 | 2 | 3 | 3 | 3 | 9 | 9 | 20 |
| 35–49 | 6 | 4.7 | 13 | 2 | 2 | 3 | 6 | 10 | 10 | 10 |
| 50–64 | 3 | 4.3 | 3 | 3 | 3 | 4 | 6 | 6 | 6 | 6 |
| 65+ | 3 | 4.6 | 5 | 3 | 3 | 4 | 8 | 8 | 8 | 8 |
| **2. MULTIPLE DX** | | | | | | | | | | |
| 0–19 Years | 12 | 6.3 | 32 | 1 | 2 | 6 | 8 | 19 | 19 | 22 |
| 20–34 | 77 | 10.6 | 131 | 3 | 5 | 7 | 13 | 28 | 33 | >99 |
| 35–49 | 546 | 10.8 | 69 | 3 | 5 | 9 | 13 | 22 | 25 | 42 |
| 50–64 | 1,370 | 11.9 | 90 | 3 | 5 | 9 | 16 | 23 | 30 | 47 |
| 65+ | 1,880 | 11.7 | 91 | 3 | 6 | 10 | 15 | 22 | 29 | 49 |
| **TOTAL SINGLE DX** | 25 | 3.7 | 10 | 2 | 2 | 3 | 3 | 8 | 10 | 20 |
| **TOTAL MULTIPLE DX** | 3,885 | 11.6 | 88 | 3 | 5 | 9 | 15 | 22 | 29 | 48 |
| **TOTAL** | | | | | | | | | | |
| 0–19 Years | 20 | 5.2 | 27 | 1 | 2 | 2 | 6 | 12 | 19 | 22 |
| 20–34 | 82 | 9.7 | 122 | 3 | 3 | 7 | 11 | 28 | 29 | >99 |
| 35–49 | 552 | 10.7 | 69 | 2 | 5 | 9 | 13 | 22 | 25 | 42 |
| 50–64 | 1,373 | 11.9 | 90 | 3 | 5 | 9 | 16 | 23 | 30 | 47 |
| 65+ | 1,883 | 11.7 | 90 | 3 | 6 | 10 | 15 | 22 | 29 | 49 |
| **GRAND TOTAL** | 3,910 | 11.5 | 88 | 3 | 5 | 9 | 15 | 22 | 29 | 48 |

## 84.17: ABOVE KNEE AMPUTATION. Formerly included in operation group(s) 762.

| Type of Patients | Observed Patients | Avg. Stay | Variance | 10th | 25th | 50th | 75th | 90th | 95th | 99th |
|---|---|---|---|---|---|---|---|---|---|---|
| **1. SINGLE DX** | | | | | | | | | | |
| 0–19 Years | 7 | 5.3 | 8 | 2 | 3 | 5 | 7 | 10 | 10 | 10 |
| 20–34 | 8 | 9.0 | 40 | 2 | 4 | 6 | 17 | 17 | 17 | 17 |
| 35–49 | 9 | 4.5 | 3 | 2 | 3 | 4 | 6 | 8 | 8 | 9 |
| 50–64 | 18 | 5.3 | 8 | 2 | 3 | 5 | 6 | 8 | 8 | 16 |
| 65+ | 43 | 4.0 | 6 | 1 | 2 | 3 | 5 | 8 | 8 | 11 |
| **2. MULTIPLE DX** | | | | | | | | | | |
| 0–19 Years | 21 | 8.5 | 159 | 2 | 3 | 3 | 6 | 19 | 56 | 56 |
| 20–34 | 56 | 11.4 | 84 | 4 | 6 | 6 | 14 | 26 | 29 | 46 |
| 35–49 | 329 | 12.1 | 117 | 3 | 6 | 6 | 16 | 22 | 29 | 54 |
| 50–64 | 1,339 | 12.6 | 118 | 3 | 6 | 9 | 15 | 27 | 34 | 55 |
| 65+ | 7,363 | 10.2 | 80 | 3 | 5 | 8 | 12 | 20 | 28 | 44 |
| **TOTAL SINGLE DX** | 85 | 4.9 | 10 | 2 | 3 | 4 | 6 | 8 | 10 | 17 |
| **TOTAL MULTIPLE DX** | 9,108 | 10.7 | 89 | 3 | 5 | 8 | 13 | 21 | 29 | 47 |
| **TOTAL** | | | | | | | | | | |
| 0–19 Years | 28 | 8.1 | 139 | 2 | 3 | 4 | 6 | 12 | 22 | 56 |
| 20–34 | 64 | 11.2 | 81 | 4 | 6 | 8 | 14 | 24 | 29 | 46 |
| 35–49 | 338 | 12.0 | 116 | 3 | 6 | 8 | 16 | 22 | 29 | 54 |
| 50–64 | 1,357 | 12.5 | 118 | 3 | 6 | 9 | 15 | 27 | 34 | 55 |
| 65+ | 7,406 | 10.2 | 80 | 3 | 5 | 8 | 12 | 20 | 28 | 44 |
| **GRAND TOTAL** | 9,193 | 10.6 | 89 | 3 | 5 | 8 | 13 | 21 | 29 | 47 |

Length of Stay by Diagnosis and Operation, United States, 2000

# United States, October 1998–September 1999 Data, by Operation

## 84.2: EXTREMITY REATTACHMENT. Formerly included in operation group(s) 764.

| Type of Patients | Observed Patients | Avg. Stay | Variance | 10th | 25th | 50th | 75th | 90th | 95th | 99th |
|---|---|---|---|---|---|---|---|---|---|---|
| **1. SINGLE DX** | | | | | | | | | | |
| 0–19 Years | 42 | 4.3 | 7 | 1 | 3 | 3 | 7 | 7 | 10 | 11 |
| 20–34 | 40 | 5.9 | 9 | 2 | 3 | 7 | 8 | 10 | 10 | 10 |
| 35–49 | 34 | 6.0 | 10 | 2 | 4 | 6 | 7 | 12 | 12 | 12 |
| 50–64 | 10 | 5.1 | 3 | 2 | 4 | 6 | 6 | 6 | 6 | 7 |
| 65+ | 1 | 8.0 | 0 | 8 | 8 | 8 | 8 | 8 | 8 | 8 |
| **2. MULTIPLE DX** | | | | | | | | | | |
| 0–19 Years | 54 | 7.0 | 43 | 1 | 2 | 6 | 8 | 15 | 24 | 35 |
| 20–34 | 61 | 8.0 | 13 | 3 | 5 | 7 | 11 | 13 | 13 | 15 |
| 35–49 | 54 | 6.1 | 20 | 2 | 3 | 6 | 8 | 11 | 11 | 26 |
| 50–64 | 51 | 6.1 | 15 | 2 | 4 | 5 | 8 | 11 | 13 | 21 |
| 65+ | 8 | 9.8 | 96 | 1 | 2 | 10 | 10 | 15 | 35 | 35 |
| **TOTAL SINGLE DX** | 127 | 5.4 | 9 | 2 | 3 | 6 | 7 | 10 | 10 | 12 |
| **TOTAL MULTIPLE DX** | 228 | 7.1 | 25 | 2 | 4 | 7 | 9 | 13 | 14 | 26 |
| **TOTAL** | | | | | | | | | | |
| 0–19 Years | 96 | 5.8 | 29 | 1 | 2 | 5 | 7 | 10 | 15 | 24 |
| 20–34 | 101 | 7.2 | 13 | 2 | 5 | 7 | 10 | 13 | 13 | 15 |
| 35–49 | 88 | 6.1 | 15 | 2 | 3 | 6 | 7 | 11 | 12 | 26 |
| 50–64 | 61 | 5.8 | 11 | 2 | 4 | 6 | 7 | 9 | 11 | 18 |
| 65+ | 9 | 9.5 | 79 | 1 | 5 | 8 | 10 | 15 | 35 | 35 |
| **GRAND TOTAL** | 355 | 6.4 | 19 | 2 | 3 | 6 | 8 | 11 | 13 | 24 |

## 84.4: IMPL OR FIT PROSTH LIMB. Formerly included in operation group(s) 766, 767.

| Type of Patients | Observed Patients | Avg. Stay | Variance | 10th | 25th | 50th | 75th | 90th | 95th | 99th |
|---|---|---|---|---|---|---|---|---|---|---|
| **1. SINGLE DX** | | | | | | | | | | |
| 0–19 Years | 2 | 4.9 | 3 | 4 | 4 | 4 | 4 | 8 | 8 | 8 |
| 20–34 | 1 | 2.0 | 0 | 2 | 2 | 2 | 2 | 2 | 2 | 2 |
| 35–49 | 0 | | | | | | | | | |
| 50–64 | 2 | 1.8 | 1 | 1 | 1 | 1 | 3 | 3 | 3 | 3 |
| 65+ | 1 | 2.0 | 0 | 2 | 2 | 2 | 2 | 2 | 2 | 2 |
| **2. MULTIPLE DX** | | | | | | | | | | |
| 0–19 Years | 1 | 39.0 | 0 | 39 | 39 | 39 | 39 | 39 | 39 | 39 |
| 20–34 | 2 | 5.0 | 0 | 2 | 2 | 2 | 2 | 2 | 2 | 2 |
| 35–49 | 1 | 5.0 | 0 | 5 | 5 | 5 | 5 | 5 | 5 | 5 |
| 50–64 | 6 | 6.9 | 98 | 2 | 2 | 4 | 4 | 27 | 27 | 27 |
| 65+ | 3 | 7.1 | 31 | 2 | 2 | 5 | 14 | 14 | 14 | 14 |
| **TOTAL SINGLE DX** | 6 | 4.3 | 4 | 2 | 4 | 4 | 4 | 8 | 8 | 8 |
| **TOTAL MULTIPLE DX** | 13 | 7.8 | 104 | 2 | 2 | 4 | 5 | 27 | 27 | 39 |
| **TOTAL** | | | | | | | | | | |
| 0–19 Years | 3 | 6.5 | 56 | 4 | 4 | 4 | 8 | 8 | 8 | 39 |
| 20–34 | 3 | 2.0 | 0 | 2 | 2 | 2 | 2 | 2 | 2 | 2 |
| 35–49 | 1 | 5.0 | 0 | 5 | 5 | 5 | 5 | 5 | 5 | 5 |
| 50–64 | 8 | 5.8 | 79 | 2 | 2 | 4 | 4 | 27 | 27 | 27 |
| 65+ | 4 | 6.2 | 29 | 2 | 2 | 5 | 14 | 14 | 14 | 14 |
| **GRAND TOTAL** | 19 | 5.9 | 51 | 2 | 2 | 4 | 5 | 14 | 27 | 39 |

## 84.3: AMPUTATION STUMP REV. Formerly included in operation group(s) 765.

| Type of Patients | Observed Patients | Avg. Stay | Variance | 10th | 25th | 50th | 75th | 90th | 95th | 99th |
|---|---|---|---|---|---|---|---|---|---|---|
| **1. SINGLE DX** | | | | | | | | | | |
| 0–19 Years | 16 | 2.0 | 1 | 1 | 1 | 2 | 3 | 3 | 3 | 6 |
| 20–34 | 19 | 4.4 | 12 | 1 | 1 | 3 | 8 | 8 | 10 | 14 |
| 35–49 | 34 | 2.8 | 5 | 1 | 1 | 3 | 3 | 5 | 8 | 12 |
| 50–64 | 28 | 3.7 | 11 | 1 | 1 | 3 | 4 | 10 | 13 | 13 |
| 65+ | 19 | 4.7 | 11 | 1 | 1 | 4 | 7 | 8 | 12 | 13 |
| **2. MULTIPLE DX** | | | | | | | | | | |
| 0–19 Years | 43 | 5.8 | 39 | 1 | 2 | 2 | 10 | 18 | 18 | 34 |
| 20–34 | 92 | 4.6 | 18 | 1 | 2 | 4 | 6 | 8 | 11 | 17 |
| 35–49 | 417 | 7.3 | 52 | 2 | 2 | 6 | 10 | 14 | 19 | 38 |
| 50–64 | 795 | 9.8 | 196 | 2 | 3 | 6 | 11 | 19 | 32 | 81 |
| 65+ | 1,286 | 8.5 | 65 | 2 | 4 | 7 | 10 | 18 | 22 | 38 |
| **TOTAL SINGLE DX** | 116 | 3.4 | 8 | 1 | 1 | 3 | 4 | 8 | 9 | 13 |
| **TOTAL MULTIPLE DX** | 2,633 | 8.5 | 103 | 2 | 3 | 6 | 10 | 17 | 22 | 64 |
| **TOTAL** | | | | | | | | | | |
| 0–19 Years | 59 | 5.0 | 34 | 1 | 2 | 2 | 6 | 18 | 18 | 18 |
| 20–34 | 111 | 4.5 | 17 | 1 | 2 | 4 | 6 | 8 | 11 | 17 |
| 35–49 | 451 | 6.9 | 49 | 2 | 3 | 5 | 10 | 14 | 18 | 38 |
| 50–64 | 823 | 9.6 | 192 | 2 | 3 | 6 | 10 | 19 | 32 | 81 |
| 65+ | 1,305 | 8.5 | 65 | 2 | 4 | 7 | 10 | 18 | 22 | 38 |
| **GRAND TOTAL** | 2,749 | 8.3 | 100 | 2 | 3 | 6 | 10 | 17 | 22 | 63 |

## 84.9: OTHER MUSCULOSKELETAL OP. Formerly included in operation group(s) 766.

| Type of Patients | Observed Patients | Avg. Stay | Variance | 10th | 25th | 50th | 75th | 90th | 95th | 99th |
|---|---|---|---|---|---|---|---|---|---|---|
| **1. SINGLE DX** | | | | | | | | | | |
| 0–19 Years | 1 | 6.0 | 0 | 6 | 6 | 6 | 6 | 6 | 6 | 6 |
| 20–34 | 0 | | | | | | | | | |
| 35–49 | 0 | | | | | | | | | |
| 50–64 | 0 | | | | | | | | | |
| **2. MULTIPLE DX** | | | | | | | | | | |
| 0–19 Years | 14 | 14.5 | 105 | 1 | 10 | 12 | 18 | 35 | 35 | 38 |
| 20–34 | 0 | | | | | | | | | |
| 35–49 | 1 | 3.0 | 0 | 3 | 3 | 3 | 3 | 3 | 3 | 3 |
| 50–64 | 0 | | | | | | | | | |
| 65+ | 0 | | | | | | | | | |
| **TOTAL SINGLE DX** | 1 | 6.0 | 0 | 6 | 6 | 6 | 6 | 6 | 6 | 6 |
| **TOTAL MULTIPLE DX** | 15 | 13.9 | 107 | 1 | 3 | 12 | 18 | 23 | 35 | 38 |
| **TOTAL** | | | | | | | | | | |
| 0–19 Years | 15 | 13.9 | 103 | 1 | 6 | 12 | 18 | 23 | 35 | 38 |
| 20–34 | 0 | | | | | | | | | |
| 35–49 | 1 | 3.0 | 0 | 3 | 3 | 3 | 3 | 3 | 3 | 3 |
| 50–64 | 0 | | | | | | | | | |
| 65+ | 0 | | | | | | | | | |
| **GRAND TOTAL** | 16 | 13.4 | 103 | 1 | 4 | 12 | 18 | 23 | 35 | 38 |

Length of Stay by Diagnosis and Operation, United States, 2000

# United States, October 1998–September 1999 Data, by Operation

## 85.0: MASTOTOMY. Formerly included in operation group(s) 771.

| Type of Patients | Observed Patients | Avg. Stay | Variance | Percentiles 10th | 25th | 50th | 75th | 90th | 95th | 99th |
|---|---|---|---|---|---|---|---|---|---|---|
| **1. SINGLE DX** | | | | | | | | | | |
| 0–19 Years | 37 | 2.8 | 3 | 1 | 1 | 3 | 4 | 4 | 5 | 9 |
| 20–34 | 140 | 3.3 | 6 | 1 | 2 | 2 | 4 | 4 | 5 | 9 |
| 35–49 | 96 | 2.5 | 2 | 1 | 1 | 2 | 4 | 4 | 5 | 6 |
| 50–64 | 26 | 2.2 | 1 | 1 | 1 | 2 | 3 | 4 | 5 | 5 |
| 65+ | 8 | 1.7 | 5 | 1 | 1 | 1 | 1 | 1 | 10 | 10 |
| **2. MULTIPLE DX** | | | | | | | | | | |
| 0–19 Years | 51 | 4.0 | 7 | 2 | 2 | 3 | 5 | 8 | 12 | 12 |
| 20–34 | 160 | 3.1 | 5 | 2 | 2 | 2 | 3 | 6 | 9 | 9 |
| 35–49 | 222 | 3.3 | 11 | 1 | 1 | 2 | 3 | 7 | 9 | 16 |
| 50–64 | 167 | 4.6 | 10 | 2 | 2 | 2 | 4 | 6 | 10 | 12 |
| 65+ | 119 | 5.8 | 40 | 1 | 2 | 4 | 7 | 12 | 16 | 33 |
| **TOTAL SINGLE DX** | 307 | 2.9 | 4 | 1 | 1 | 2 | 4 | 4 | 8 | 9 |
| **TOTAL MULTIPLE DX** | 719 | 3.9 | 13 | 1 | 2 | 3 | 4 | 8 | 10 | 17 |
| **TOTAL** | | | | | | | | | | |
| 0–19 Years | 88 | 3.4 | 5 | 1 | 2 | 3 | 4 | 6 | 8 | 12 |
| 20–34 | 300 | 3.2 | 5 | 1 | 2 | 2 | 4 | 8 | 8 | 9 |
| 35–49 | 318 | 3.1 | 9 | 1 | 1 | 2 | 4 | 6 | 8 | 14 |
| 50–64 | 193 | 4.3 | 10 | 1 | 2 | 3 | 5 | 9 | 10 | 12 |
| 65+ | 127 | 5.4 | 38 | 1 | 2 | 3 | 7 | 11 | 16 | 33 |
| **GRAND TOTAL** | 1,026 | 3.6 | 11 | 1 | 2 | 3 | 4 | 8 | 9 | 16 |

## 85.1: BREAST DIAGNOSTIC PX. Formerly included in operation group(s) 768, 780.

| Type of Patients | Observed Patients | Avg. Stay | Variance | Percentiles 10th | 25th | 50th | 75th | 90th | 95th | 99th |
|---|---|---|---|---|---|---|---|---|---|---|
| **1. SINGLE DX** | | | | | | | | | | |
| 0–19 Years | 5 | 1.4 | <1 | 1 | 1 | 1 | 1 | 1 | 3 | 3 |
| 20–34 | 18 | 2.5 | 2 | 1 | 2 | 2 | 3 | 4 | 4 | 7 |
| 35–49 | 44 | 2.2 | 5 | 1 | 1 | 1 | 2 | 4 | 7 | 14 |
| 50–64 | 25 | 2.1 | 3 | 1 | 1 | 1 | 3 | 4 | 5 | 11 |
| 65+ | 13 | 3.1 | 2 | 1 | 4 | 4 | 4 | 4 | 4 | 6 |
| **2. MULTIPLE DX** | | | | | | | | | | |
| 0–19 Years | 8 | 2.9 | 14 | 1 | 3 | 3 | 5 | 6 | 15 | 15 |
| 20–34 | 38 | 6.5 | 23 | 2 | 3 | 5 | 10 | 14 | 14 | 24 |
| 35–49 | 209 | 5.7 | 28 | 1 | 2 | 4 | 8 | 10 | 14 | 27 |
| 50–64 | 335 | 6.4 | 29 | 1 | 3 | 5 | 8 | 12 | 15 | 28 |
| 65+ | 600 | 7.5 | 70 | 2 | 3 | 6 | 9 | 15 | 20 | 63 |
| **TOTAL SINGLE DX** | 105 | 2.4 | 4 | 1 | 1 | 2 | 3 | 4 | 6 | 11 |
| **TOTAL MULTIPLE DX** | 1,190 | 6.8 | 50 | 1 | 3 | 5 | 8 | 13 | 18 | 33 |
| **TOTAL** | | | | | | | | | | |
| 0–19 Years | 13 | 2.7 | 12 | 1 | 2 | 2 | 4 | 6 | 15 | 15 |
| 20–34 | 56 | 5.6 | 21 | 1 | 3 | 4 | 9 | 13 | 14 | 17 |
| 35–49 | 253 | 4.9 | 26 | 1 | 2 | 3 | 7 | 10 | 14 | 21 |
| 50–64 | 360 | 6.1 | 28 | 1 | 3 | 5 | 8 | 12 | 15 | 24 |
| 65+ | 613 | 7.3 | 68 | 1 | 3 | 5 | 8 | 14 | 20 | 63 |
| **GRAND TOTAL** | 1,295 | 6.4 | 47 | 1 | 2 | 5 | 8 | 13 | 17 | 30 |

## 85.11: PERC BREAST BIOPSY. Formerly included in operation group(s) 768.

| Type of Patients | Observed Patients | Avg. Stay | Variance | Percentiles 10th | 25th | 50th | 75th | 90th | 95th | 99th |
|---|---|---|---|---|---|---|---|---|---|---|
| **1. SINGLE DX** | | | | | | | | | | |
| 0–19 Years | 0 | | | | | | | | | |
| 20–34 | 5 | 2.4 | 2 | 1 | 1 | 3 | 4 | 4 | 4 | 4 |
| 35–49 | 10 | 3.1 | 7 | 1 | 1 | 2 | 4 | 7 | 10 | 10 |
| 50–64 | 7 | 4.5 | 6 | 3 | 3 | 4 | 5 | 6 | 11 | 11 |
| 65+ | 3 | 3.6 | 5 | 1 | 1 | 3 | 6 | 6 | 6 | 6 |
| **2. MULTIPLE DX** | | | | | | | | | | |
| 0–19 Years | 2 | 2.0 | 0 | 2 | 2 | 2 | 2 | 2 | 2 | 2 |
| 20–34 | 12 | 9.3 | 15 | 5 | 5 | 10 | 10 | 14 | 17 | 17 |
| 35–49 | 89 | 6.8 | 22 | 2 | 3 | 6 | 10 | 11 | 18 | 19 |
| 50–64 | 175 | 7.3 | 36 | 2 | 4 | 7 | 9 | 15 | 21 | 29 |
| 65+ | 339 | 7.1 | 36 | 2 | 3 | 6 | 9 | 14 | 19 | 30 |
| **TOTAL SINGLE DX** | 25 | 3.5 | 6 | 1 | 1 | 3 | 4 | 6 | 10 | 11 |
| **TOTAL MULTIPLE DX** | 617 | 7.1 | 34 | 2 | 3 | 6 | 9 | 14 | 19 | 28 |
| **TOTAL** | | | | | | | | | | |
| 0–19 Years | 2 | 2.0 | 0 | 2 | 2 | 2 | 2 | 2 | 2 | 2 |
| 20–34 | 17 | 8.3 | 19 | 3 | 5 | 9 | 10 | 14 | 17 | 17 |
| 35–49 | 99 | 6.4 | 22 | 1 | 3 | 5 | 10 | 11 | 18 | 19 |
| 50–64 | 182 | 7.2 | 36 | 2 | 4 | 7 | 9 | 14 | 21 | 28 |
| 65+ | 342 | 7.1 | 36 | 2 | 3 | 6 | 9 | 14 | 19 | 30 |
| **GRAND TOTAL** | 642 | 7.0 | 33 | 2 | 3 | 6 | 9 | 13 | 19 | 28 |

## 85.12: OPEN BIOPSY OF BREAST. Formerly included in operation group(s) 768.

| Type of Patients | Observed Patients | Avg. Stay | Variance | Percentiles 10th | 25th | 50th | 75th | 90th | 95th | 99th |
|---|---|---|---|---|---|---|---|---|---|---|
| **1. SINGLE DX** | | | | | | | | | | |
| 0–19 Years | 5 | 1.4 | <1 | 1 | 1 | 1 | 1 | 1 | 3 | 3 |
| 20–34 | 13 | 2.6 | 2 | 1 | 2 | 2 | 3 | 4 | 7 | 7 |
| 35–49 | 33 | 1.6 | <1 | 1 | 1 | 1 | 2 | 2 | 7 | 7 |
| 50–64 | 18 | 1.4 | <1 | 1 | 1 | 1 | 2 | 2 | 3 | 3 |
| 65+ | 10 | 3.1 | 2 | 1 | 2 | 4 | 4 | 4 | 4 | 4 |
| **2. MULTIPLE DX** | | | | | | | | | | |
| 0–19 Years | 6 | 3.1 | 17 | 1 | 1 | 1 | 4 | 4 | 15 | 15 |
| 20–34 | 26 | 4.8 | 21 | 1 | 2 | 3 | 6 | 13 | 13 | 24 |
| 35–49 | 120 | 4.7 | 31 | 1 | 2 | 4 | 6 | 9 | 12 | 30 |
| 50–64 | 160 | 5.2 | 18 | 1 | 2 | 4 | 7 | 12 | 12 | 20 |
| 65+ | 259 | 8.0 | 106 | 1 | 2 | 6 | 9 | 15 | 20 | 63 |
| **TOTAL SINGLE DX** | 79 | 2.0 | 2 | 1 | 1 | 2 | 3 | 3 | 4 | 7 |
| **TOTAL MULTIPLE DX** | 571 | 6.5 | 66 | 1 | 2 | 4 | 8 | 13 | 16 | 63 |
| **TOTAL** | | | | | | | | | | |
| 0–19 Years | 11 | 2.8 | 15 | 1 | 2 | 1 | 3 | 3 | 15 | 15 |
| 20–34 | 39 | 4.1 | 16 | 1 | 1 | 3 | 4 | 11 | 13 | 24 |
| 35–49 | 153 | 3.9 | 25 | 1 | 2 | 2 | 5 | 8 | 10 | 30 |
| 50–64 | 178 | 4.9 | 17 | 1 | 2 | 4 | 7 | 11 | 12 | 20 |
| 65+ | 269 | 7.6 | 100 | 1 | 2 | 5 | 8 | 15 | 20 | 63 |
| **GRAND TOTAL** | 650 | 5.9 | 60 | 1 | 2 | 4 | 7 | 12 | 15 | 63 |

Length of Stay by Diagnosis and Operation, United States, 2000

## United States, October 1998–September 1999 Data, by Operation

### 85.2: EXC/DESTR BREAST TISS. Formerly included in operation group(s) 768, 771.

| Type of Patients | Observed Patients | Avg. Stay | Variance | 10th | 25th | 50th | 75th | 90th | 95th | 99th |
|---|---|---|---|---|---|---|---|---|---|---|
| **1. SINGLE DX** | | | | | | | | | | |
| 0–19 Years | 22 | 1.4 | <1 | 1 | 1 | 1 | 1 | 3 | 3 | 4 |
| 20–34 | 66 | 1.9 | 1 | 1 | 1 | 1 | 3 | 3 | 3 | 5 |
| 35–49 | 502 | 1.5 | 1 | 1 | 1 | 2 | 2 | 2 | 3 | 6 |
| 50–64 | 594 | 1.4 | <1 | 1 | 1 | 1 | 2 | 2 | 3 | 4 |
| 65+ | 440 | 1.3 | <1 | 1 | 1 | 1 | 1 | 2 | 2 | 4 |
| **2. MULTIPLE DX** | | | | | | | | | | |
| 0–19 Years | 11 | 2.9 | 25 | 1 | 1 | 1 | 2 | 4 | 11 | 29 |
| 20–34 | 147 | 2.9 | 16 | 1 | 1 | 1 | 3 | 7 | 11 | 20 |
| 35–49 | 1,013 | 2.4 | 9 | 1 | 1 | 1 | 2 | 6 | 9 | 15 |
| 50–64 | 1,604 | 2.2 | 8 | 1 | 1 | 1 | 2 | 5 | 7 | 14 |
| 65+ | 2,366 | 2.8 | 18 | 1 | 1 | 2 | 2 | 7 | 11 | 23 |
| **TOTAL SINGLE DX** | 1,624 | 1.4 | <1 | 1 | 1 | 1 | 2 | 2 | 3 | 6 |
| **TOTAL MULTIPLE DX** | 5,141 | 2.5 | 13 | 1 | 1 | 1 | 2 | 5 | 9 | 19 |
| **TOTAL** | | | | | | | | | | |
| 0–19 Years | 33 | 2.0 | 11 | 1 | 1 | 1 | 2 | 3 | 4 | 29 |
| 20–34 | 213 | 2.6 | 12 | 1 | 1 | 1 | 3 | 5 | 9 | 20 |
| 35–49 | 1,515 | 2.2 | 7 | 1 | 1 | 1 | 2 | 4 | 9 | 11 |
| 50–64 | 2,198 | 2.0 | 6 | 1 | 1 | 1 | 2 | 4 | 6 | 13 |
| 65+ | 2,806 | 2.6 | 16 | 1 | 1 | 1 | 2 | 6 | 10 | 21 |
| **GRAND TOTAL** | 6,765 | 2.3 | 10 | 1 | 1 | 1 | 2 | 4 | 8 | 16 |

### 85.21: LOCAL EXC BREAST LESION. Formerly included in operation group(s) 768.

| Type of Patients | Observed Patients | Avg. Stay | Variance | 10th | 25th | 50th | 75th | 90th | 95th | 99th |
|---|---|---|---|---|---|---|---|---|---|---|
| **1. SINGLE DX** | | | | | | | | | | |
| 0–19 Years | 20 | 1.5 | <1 | 1 | 1 | 1 | 1 | 3 | 4 | 4 |
| 20–34 | 38 | 2.3 | 1 | 1 | 1 | 2 | 3 | 3 | 3 | 5 |
| 35–49 | 278 | 1.6 | 2 | 1 | 1 | 1 | 2 | 3 | 6 | 6 |
| 50–64 | 334 | 1.3 | <1 | 1 | 1 | 1 | 1 | 2 | 2 | 4 |
| 65+ | 220 | 1.3 | <1 | 1 | 1 | 1 | 1 | 2 | 3 | 4 |
| **2. MULTIPLE DX** | | | | | | | | | | |
| 0–19 Years | 6 | 3.0 | 11 | 1 | 1 | 1 | 2 | 11 | 11 | 11 |
| 20–34 | 112 | 3.1 | 18 | 1 | 1 | 1 | 4 | 9 | 11 | 20 |
| 35–49 | 664 | 2.8 | 13 | 1 | 1 | 1 | 3 | 9 | 11 | 19 |
| 50–64 | 995 | 2.4 | 8 | 1 | 1 | 1 | 2 | 5 | 7 | 14 |
| 65+ | 1,429 | 3.3 | 24 | 1 | 1 | 1 | 3 | 8 | 13 | 27 |
| **TOTAL SINGLE DX** | 890 | 1.4 | <1 | 1 | 1 | 1 | 2 | 2 | 3 | 6 |
| **TOTAL MULTIPLE DX** | 3,206 | 2.9 | 16 | 1 | 1 | 1 | 3 | 7 | 11 | 20 |
| **TOTAL** | | | | | | | | | | |
| 0–19 Years | 26 | 1.9 | 4 | 1 | 1 | 1 | 2 | 4 | 4 | 11 |
| 20–34 | 150 | 2.9 | 14 | 1 | 1 | 1 | 3 | 7 | 10 | 20 |
| 35–49 | 942 | 2.5 | 10 | 1 | 1 | 1 | 2 | 6 | 9 | 16 |
| 50–64 | 1,329 | 2.1 | 6 | 1 | 1 | 1 | 2 | 5 | 7 | 13 |
| 65+ | 1,649 | 3.0 | 22 | 1 | 1 | 1 | 3 | 7 | 12 | 27 |
| **GRAND TOTAL** | 4,096 | 2.6 | 14 | 1 | 1 | 1 | 2 | 6 | 9 | 19 |

### 85.22: QUADRANT RESECT BREAST. Formerly included in operation group(s) 768.

| Type of Patients | Observed Patients | Avg. Stay | Variance | 10th | 25th | 50th | 75th | 90th | 95th | 99th |
|---|---|---|---|---|---|---|---|---|---|---|
| **1. SINGLE DX** | | | | | | | | | | |
| 0–19 Years | 0 | | | | | | | | | |
| 20–34 | 5 | 1.0 | 0 | 1 | 1 | 1 | 1 | 1 | | 1 |
| 35–49 | 53 | 1.5 | <1 | 1 | 1 | 1 | 2 | 2 | 2 | 4 |
| 50–64 | 53 | 1.4 | <1 | 1 | 1 | 1 | 2 | 2 | 2 | 3 |
| 65+ | 39 | 1.3 | <1 | 1 | 1 | 1 | 2 | 2 | 2 | 3 |
| **2. MULTIPLE DX** | | | | | | | | | | |
| 0–19 Years | 0 | | | | | | | | | |
| 20–34 | 5 | 4.8 | 24 | 1 | 1 | 3 | 6 | 13 | 13 | 13 |
| 35–49 | 78 | 1.3 | <1 | 1 | 1 | 1 | 1 | 2 | 3 | 5 |
| 50–64 | 117 | 1.8 | 3 | 1 | 1 | 1 | 2 | 4 | 4 | 7 |
| 65+ | 174 | 2.3 | 11 | 1 | 1 | 1 | 2 | 4 | 7 | 21 |
| **TOTAL SINGLE DX** | 150 | 1.4 | <1 | 1 | 1 | 1 | 2 | 2 | 2 | 3 |
| **TOTAL MULTIPLE DX** | 374 | 1.8 | 5 | 1 | 1 | 1 | 2 | 3 | 4 | 13 |
| **TOTAL** | | | | | | | | | | |
| 0–19 Years | 0 | | | | | | | | | |
| 20–34 | 10 | 2.8 | 14 | 1 | 1 | 1 | 1 | 6 | 13 | 13 |
| 35–49 | 131 | 1.4 | <1 | 1 | 1 | 1 | 2 | 2 | 3 | 4 |
| 50–64 | 170 | 1.7 | 2 | 1 | 1 | 1 | 2 | 3 | 4 | 6 |
| 65+ | 213 | 2.1 | 9 | 1 | 1 | 1 | 2 | 3 | 6 | 21 |
| **GRAND TOTAL** | 524 | 1.7 | 4 | 1 | 1 | 1 | 2 | 3 | 4 | 8 |

### 85.23: SUBTOTAL MASTECTOMY. Formerly included in operation group(s) 768.

| Type of Patients | Observed Patients | Avg. Stay | Variance | 10th | 25th | 50th | 75th | 90th | 95th | 99th |
|---|---|---|---|---|---|---|---|---|---|---|
| **1. SINGLE DX** | | | | | | | | | | |
| 0–19 Years | 2 | 1.0 | 0 | 1 | 1 | 1 | 1 | 1 | 1 | 1 |
| 20–34 | 21 | 1.1 | <1 | 1 | 1 | 1 | 1 | 1 | 2 | 3 |
| 35–49 | 168 | 1.2 | <1 | 1 | 1 | 1 | 1 | 2 | 2 | 3 |
| 50–64 | 203 | 1.4 | <1 | 1 | 1 | 1 | 2 | 3 | 3 | 4 |
| 65+ | 178 | 1.3 | <1 | 1 | 1 | 1 | 2 | 2 | 3 | 2 |
| **2. MULTIPLE DX** | | | | | | | | | | |
| 0–19 Years | 3 | 2.8 | 49 | 1 | 1 | 1 | 2 | 2 | 29 | 29 |
| 20–34 | 25 | 1.5 | 4 | 1 | 1 | 1 | 2 | 2 | 4 | 17 |
| 35–49 | 261 | 1.7 | 3 | 1 | 1 | 1 | 2 | 2 | 5 | 10 |
| 50–64 | 480 | 1.7 | 5 | 1 | 1 | 1 | 2 | 3 | 4 | 13 |
| 65+ | 745 | 2.0 | 6 | 1 | 1 | 1 | 2 | 3 | 6 | 15 |
| **TOTAL SINGLE DX** | 572 | 1.3 | <1 | 1 | 1 | 1 | 1 | 2 | 3 | 3 |
| **TOTAL MULTIPLE DX** | 1,514 | 1.9 | 5 | 1 | 1 | 1 | 2 | 3 | 5 | 14 |
| **TOTAL** | | | | | | | | | | |
| 0–19 Years | 5 | 2.4 | 37 | 1 | 1 | 1 | 1 | 1 | 2 | 29 |
| 20–34 | 46 | 1.3 | 2 | 1 | 1 | 1 | 2 | 2 | 3 | 5 |
| 35–49 | 429 | 1.6 | 2 | 1 | 1 | 1 | 2 | 2 | 3 | 10 |
| 50–64 | 683 | 1.6 | 3 | 1 | 1 | 1 | 2 | 3 | 3 | 13 |
| 65+ | 923 | 1.9 | 5 | 1 | 1 | 1 | 2 | 3 | 4 | 15 |
| **GRAND TOTAL** | 2,086 | 1.7 | 4 | 1 | 1 | 1 | 2 | 2 | 4 | 13 |

Length of Stay by Diagnosis and Operation, United States, 2000

# United States, October 1998–September 1999 Data, by Operation

## 85.3: RED MAMMOPLASTY/ECTOMY. Formerly included in operation group(s) 771.

| Type of Patients | Observed Patients | Avg. Stay | Vari-ance | Percentiles | | | | | | |
|---|---|---|---|---|---|---|---|---|---|---|
| | | | | 10th | 25th | 50th | 75th | 90th | 95th | 99th |
| **1. SINGLE DX** | | | | | | | | | | |
| 0–19 Years | 124 | 1.1 | <1 | 1 | 1 | 1 | 1 | 2 | 2 | 2 |
| 20–34 | 470 | 1.2 | <1 | 1 | 1 | 1 | 1 | 2 | 2 | 3 |
| 35–49 | 330 | 1.4 | <1 | 1 | 1 | 1 | 2 | 2 | 2 | 4 |
| 50–64 | 145 | 1.3 | <1 | 1 | 1 | 1 | 1 | 2 | 3 | 6 |
| 65+ | 21 | 1.2 | <1 | 1 | 1 | 1 | 1 | 2 | 2 | 2 |
| **2. MULTIPLE DX** | | | | | | | | | | |
| 0–19 Years | 100 | 1.3 | <1 | 1 | 1 | 1 | 1 | 2 | 3 | 6 |
| 20–34 | 496 | 1.4 | <1 | 1 | 1 | 1 | 2 | 2 | 3 | 4 |
| 35–49 | 687 | 1.5 | 1 | 1 | 1 | 1 | 2 | 2 | 3 | 6 |
| 50–64 | 398 | 1.6 | 1 | 1 | 1 | 1 | 2 | 3 | 4 | 6 |
| 65+ | 132 | 2.1 | 10 | 1 | 1 | 1 | 2 | 3 | 6 | 14 |
| **TOTAL SINGLE DX** | 1,090 | 1.3 | <1 | 1 | 1 | 1 | 1 | 2 | 2 | 4 |
| **TOTAL MULTIPLE DX** | 1,813 | 1.5 | 2 | 1 | 1 | 1 | 2 | 2 | 3 | 6 |
| **TOTAL** | | | | | | | | | | |
| 0–19 Years | 224 | 1.2 | <1 | 1 | 1 | 1 | 1 | 2 | 2 | 3 |
| 20–34 | 966 | 1.3 | <1 | 1 | 1 | 1 | 2 | 2 | 2 | 4 |
| 35–49 | 1,017 | 1.5 | <1 | 1 | 1 | 1 | 2 | 2 | 3 | 6 |
| 50–64 | 543 | 1.5 | <1 | 1 | 1 | 1 | 2 | 3 | 4 | 6 |
| 65+ | 153 | 2.0 | 9 | 1 | 1 | 1 | 2 | 3 | 6 | 10 |
| **GRAND TOTAL** | 2,903 | 1.4 | 1 | 1 | 1 | 1 | 2 | 2 | 3 | 6 |

## 85.32: BILAT RED MAMMOPLASTY. Formerly included in operation group(s) 771.

| Type of Patients | Observed Patients | Avg. Stay | Vari-ance | Percentiles | | | | | | |
|---|---|---|---|---|---|---|---|---|---|---|
| | | | | 10th | 25th | 50th | 75th | 90th | 95th | 99th |
| **1. SINGLE DX** | | | | | | | | | | |
| 0–19 Years | 110 | 1.1 | <1 | 1 | 1 | 1 | 1 | 2 | 2 | 2 |
| 20–34 | 456 | 1.2 | <1 | 1 | 1 | 1 | 1 | 2 | 2 | 3 |
| 35–49 | 290 | 1.3 | <1 | 1 | 1 | 1 | 2 | 2 | 2 | 3 |
| 50–64 | 121 | 1.1 | <1 | 1 | 1 | 1 | 1 | 1 | 2 | 2 |
| 65+ | 19 | 1.3 | <1 | 1 | 1 | 1 | 2 | 2 | 2 | 2 |
| **2. MULTIPLE DX** | | | | | | | | | | |
| 0–19 Years | 89 | 1.3 | <1 | 1 | 1 | 1 | 1 | 2 | 2 | 6 |
| 20–34 | 458 | 1.4 | <1 | 1 | 1 | 1 | 2 | 2 | 2 | 4 |
| 35–49 | 529 | 1.4 | <1 | 1 | 1 | 1 | 2 | 2 | 3 | 4 |
| 50–64 | 285 | 1.4 | <1 | 1 | 1 | 1 | 2 | 2 | 3 | 5 |
| 65+ | 89 | 1.5 | <1 | 1 | 1 | 1 | 2 | 2 | 3 | 5 |
| **TOTAL SINGLE DX** | 996 | 1.2 | <1 | 1 | 1 | 1 | 1 | 2 | 2 | 3 |
| **TOTAL MULTIPLE DX** | 1,450 | 1.4 | <1 | 1 | 1 | 1 | 2 | 2 | 3 | 4 |
| **TOTAL** | | | | | | | | | | |
| 0–19 Years | 199 | 1.2 | <1 | 1 | 1 | 1 | 1 | 2 | 2 | 3 |
| 20–34 | 914 | 1.3 | <1 | 1 | 1 | 1 | 2 | 2 | 2 | 3 |
| 35–49 | 819 | 1.4 | <1 | 1 | 1 | 1 | 2 | 2 | 2 | 4 |
| 50–64 | 406 | 1.3 | <1 | 1 | 1 | 1 | 2 | 2 | 2 | 4 |
| 65+ | 108 | 1.5 | <1 | 1 | 1 | 1 | 2 | 2 | 3 | 5 |
| **GRAND TOTAL** | 2,446 | 1.3 | <1 | 1 | 1 | 1 | 2 | 2 | 2 | 4 |

## 85.4: MASTECTOMY. Formerly included in operation group(s) 769, 770.

| Type of Patients | Observed Patients | Avg. Stay | Vari-ance | Percentiles | | | | | | |
|---|---|---|---|---|---|---|---|---|---|---|
| | | | | 10th | 25th | 50th | 75th | 90th | 95th | 99th |
| **1. SINGLE DX** | | | | | | | | | | |
| 0–19 Years | 9 | 1.2 | <1 | 1 | 1 | 1 | 1 | 1 | 3 | 5 |
| 20–34 | 132 | 2.0 | 2 | 1 | 1 | 2 | 3 | 3 | 4 | 6 |
| 35–49 | 1,537 | 2.2 | 2 | 1 | 1 | 2 | 2 | 3 | 4 | 6 |
| 50–64 | 1,807 | 2.0 | 1 | 1 | 1 | 2 | 3 | 3 | 4 | 6 |
| 65+ | 1,539 | 1.8 | 1 | 1 | 1 | 2 | 2 | 2 | 3 | 5 |
| **2. MULTIPLE DX** | | | | | | | | | | |
| 0–19 Years | 7 | 2.0 | <1 | 2 | 2 | 2 | 2 | 2 | 2 | 5 |
| 20–34 | 393 | 2.6 | 4 | 2 | 2 | 2 | 3 | 3 | 4 | 9 |
| 35–49 | 3,862 | 2.7 | 4 | 1 | 1 | 2 | 3 | 4 | 5 | 12 |
| 50–64 | 5,972 | 2.5 | 4 | 1 | 1 | 2 | 3 | 4 | 6 | 11 |
| 65+ | 9,423 | 2.6 | 6 | 1 | 1 | 2 | 3 | 4 | 7 | 12 |
| **TOTAL SINGLE DX** | 5,024 | 2.0 | 1 | 1 | 1 | 2 | 2 | 3 | 4 | 6 |
| **TOTAL MULTIPLE DX** | 19,657 | 2.6 | 5 | 1 | 1 | 2 | 3 | 4 | 6 | 12 |
| **TOTAL** | | | | | | | | | | |
| 0–19 Years | 16 | 1.6 | <1 | 1 | 1 | 1 | 2 | 2 | 2 | 5 |
| 20–34 | 525 | 2.4 | 3 | 1 | 2 | 2 | 3 | 4 | 5 | 8 |
| 35–49 | 5,399 | 2.6 | 4 | 1 | 1 | 2 | 3 | 4 | 6 | 12 |
| 50–64 | 7,779 | 2.4 | 4 | 1 | 1 | 2 | 3 | 4 | 5 | 9 |
| 65+ | 10,962 | 2.5 | 6 | 1 | 1 | 2 | 3 | 4 | 6 | 12 |
| **GRAND TOTAL** | 24,681 | 2.5 | 5 | 1 | 1 | 2 | 3 | 4 | 6 | 11 |

## 85.41: UNILAT SIMPLE MASTECTOMY. Formerly included in operation group(s) 769.

| Type of Patients | Observed Patients | Avg. Stay | Vari-ance | Percentiles | | | | | | |
|---|---|---|---|---|---|---|---|---|---|---|
| | | | | 10th | 25th | 50th | 75th | 90th | 95th | 99th |
| **1. SINGLE DX** | | | | | | | | | | |
| 0–19 Years | 5 | 1.2 | <1 | 1 | 1 | 1 | 1 | 2 | 3 | 3 |
| 20–34 | 19 | 2.1 | 1 | 1 | 1 | 2 | 3 | 4 | 4 | 5 |
| 35–49 | 312 | 2.2 | 2 | 1 | 1 | 2 | 2 | 3 | 5 | 6 |
| 50–64 | 300 | 2.0 | 2 | 1 | 1 | 2 | 2 | 3 | 5 | 6 |
| 65+ | 225 | 1.7 | 3 | 1 | 1 | 1 | 2 | 2 | 3 | 6 |
| **2. MULTIPLE DX** | | | | | | | | | | |
| 0–19 Years | 5 | 2.0 | <1 | 2 | 2 | 2 | 2 | 2 | 2 | 5 |
| 20–34 | 51 | 2.7 | 4 | 2 | 2 | 2 | 4 | 4 | 6 | 8 |
| 35–49 | 597 | 2.9 | 6 | 1 | 1 | 2 | 3 | 4 | 7 | 12 |
| 50–64 | 820 | 2.4 | 5 | 1 | 1 | 2 | 3 | 4 | 6 | 11 |
| 65+ | 1,296 | 3.0 | 12 | 1 | 1 | 2 | 3 | 8 | 10 | 18 |
| **TOTAL SINGLE DX** | 861 | 2.0 | 2 | 1 | 1 | 2 | 2 | 3 | 5 | 6 |
| **TOTAL MULTIPLE DX** | 2,769 | 2.8 | 8 | 1 | 1 | 2 | 3 | 4 | 8 | 13 |
| **TOTAL** | | | | | | | | | | |
| 0–19 Years | 10 | 1.7 | <1 | 1 | 1 | 1 | 2 | 2 | 2 | 3 |
| 20–34 | 70 | 2.4 | 4 | 1 | 1 | 2 | 3 | 3 | 5 | 7 |
| 35–49 | 909 | 2.6 | 5 | 1 | 1 | 2 | 3 | 3 | 6 | 12 |
| 50–64 | 1,120 | 2.3 | 4 | 1 | 1 | 2 | 3 | 4 | 5 | 11 |
| 65+ | 1,521 | 2.8 | 11 | 1 | 1 | 2 | 3 | 8 | 10 | 17 |
| **GRAND TOTAL** | 3,630 | 2.6 | 7 | 1 | 1 | 2 | 3 | 5 | 8 | 12 |

Length of Stay by Diagnosis and Operation, United States, 2000

# United States, October 1998–September 1999 Data, by Operation

## 85.42: BILAT SIMPLE MASTECTOMY. Formerly included in operation group(s) 769.

| Type of Patients | Observed Patients | Avg. Stay | Variance | 10th | 25th | 50th | 75th | 90th | 95th | 99th |
|---|---|---|---|---|---|---|---|---|---|---|
| **1. SINGLE DX** | | | | | | | | | | |
| 0–19 Years | 2 | 1.0 | 0 | 1 | 1 | 1 | 1 | 1 | 1 | 1 |
| 20–34 | 9 | 1.3 | <1 | 1 | 1 | 1 | 1 | 2 | 3 | 5 |
| 35–49 | 65 | 2.2 | 2 | 1 | 1 | 2 | 3 | 4 | 5 | 5 |
| 50–64 | 51 | 2.6 | 2 | 1 | 2 | 2 | 3 | 5 | 5 | 6 |
| 65+ | 15 | 2.0 | <1 | 1 | 2 | 2 | 2 | 3 | 3 | 3 |
| **2. MULTIPLE DX** | | | | | | | | | | |
| 0–19 Years | 1 | 1.0 | 0 | 1 | 1 | 1 | 1 | 1 | 1 | 1 |
| 20–34 | 34 | 2.0 | 3 | 1 | 1 | 2 | 2 | 3 | 5 | 9 |
| 35–49 | 225 | 2.6 | 3 | 1 | 1 | 2 | 3 | 5 | 6 | 8 |
| 50–64 | 213 | 3.0 | 4 | 1 | 2 | 2 | 4 | 6 | 7 | 11 |
| 65+ | 96 | 3.0 | 16 | 1 | 1 | 2 | 3 | 5 | 8 | 35 |
| **TOTAL SINGLE DX** | 142 | 2.2 | 2 | 1 | 1 | 2 | 3 | 4 | 5 | 6 |
| **TOTAL MULTIPLE DX** | 569 | 2.8 | 6 | 1 | 1 | 2 | 3 | 6 | 6 | 9 |
| **TOTAL** | | | | | | | | | | |
| 0–19 Years | 3 | 1.0 | 0 | 1 | 1 | 1 | 1 | 1 | 1 | 1 |
| 20–34 | 43 | 1.8 | 2 | 1 | 1 | 1 | 2 | 3 | 4 | 9 |
| 35–49 | 290 | 2.5 | 3 | 1 | 1 | 2 | 3 | 5 | 6 | 8 |
| 50–64 | 264 | 3.0 | 4 | 1 | 2 | 2 | 4 | 6 | 7 | 10 |
| 65+ | 111 | 2.9 | 15 | 1 | 1 | 2 | 3 | 5 | 8 | 35 |
| **GRAND TOTAL** | 711 | 2.7 | 5 | 1 | 1 | 2 | 3 | 5 | 6 | 9 |

## 85.43: UNILAT EXTEN SMP MAST. Formerly included in operation group(s) 770.

| Type of Patients | Observed Patients | Avg. Stay | Variance | 10th | 25th | 50th | 75th | 90th | 95th | 99th |
|---|---|---|---|---|---|---|---|---|---|---|
| **1. SINGLE DX** | | | | | | | | | | |
| 0–19 Years | 2 | 1.2 | <1 | 1 | 1 | 1 | 1 | 1 | 1 | 5 |
| 20–34 | 96 | 2.1 | 2 | 1 | 1 | 2 | 3 | 4 | 5 | 6 |
| 35–49 | 1,108 | 2.2 | 2 | 1 | 1 | 2 | 3 | 4 | 5 | 6 |
| 50–64 | 1,403 | 2.0 | 1 | 1 | 1 | 2 | 3 | 3 | 4 | 6 |
| 65+ | 1,262 | 1.8 | <1 | 1 | 1 | 2 | 2 | 3 | 3 | 5 |
| **2. MULTIPLE DX** | | | | | | | | | | |
| 0–19 Years | 1 | 3.0 | 0 | 3 | 3 | 3 | 3 | 3 | 3 | 3 |
| 20–34 | 285 | 2.6 | 5 | 1 | 2 | 2 | 3 | 4 | 5 | 7 |
| 35–49 | 2,872 | 2.7 | 4 | 1 | 2 | 2 | 3 | 5 | 6 | 12 |
| 50–64 | 4,671 | 2.4 | 4 | 1 | 1 | 2 | 3 | 4 | 5 | 9 |
| 65+ | 7,722 | 2.5 | 5 | 1 | 1 | 2 | 3 | 4 | 6 | 11 |
| **TOTAL SINGLE DX** | 3,871 | 2.0 | 1 | 1 | 1 | 2 | 2 | 3 | 4 | 6 |
| **TOTAL MULTIPLE DX** | 15,551 | 2.5 | 4 | 1 | 1 | 2 | 3 | 4 | 6 | 11 |
| **TOTAL** | | | | | | | | | | |
| 0–19 Years | 3 | 1.2 | <1 | 1 | 1 | 1 | 1 | 1 | 3 | 5 |
| 20–34 | 381 | 2.5 | 4 | 1 | 2 | 2 | 3 | 4 | 5 | 7 |
| 35–49 | 3,980 | 2.6 | 3 | 1 | 1 | 2 | 3 | 5 | 5 | 11 |
| 50–64 | 6,074 | 2.3 | 3 | 1 | 1 | 2 | 3 | 4 | 5 | 8 |
| 65+ | 8,984 | 2.4 | 5 | 1 | 1 | 2 | 3 | 4 | 5 | 10 |
| **GRAND TOTAL** | 19,422 | 2.4 | 4 | 1 | 1 | 2 | 3 | 4 | 5 | 10 |

## 85.44: BILAT EXTEN SMP MAST. Formerly included in operation group(s) 770.

| Type of Patients | Observed Patients | Avg. Stay | Variance | 10th | 25th | 50th | 75th | 90th | 95th | 99th |
|---|---|---|---|---|---|---|---|---|---|---|
| **1. SINGLE DX** | | | | | | | | | | |
| 0–19 Years | 0 | | | | | | | | | |
| 20–34 | 3 | 2.2 | <1 | 2 | 2 | 2 | 2 | 3 | 3 | 3 |
| 35–49 | 25 | 2.4 | 2 | 1 | 2 | 2 | 3 | 5 | 5 | 6 |
| 50–64 | 29 | 2.7 | 1 | 2 | 2 | 3 | 3 | 4 | 5 | 5 |
| 65+ | 16 | 1.9 | <1 | 1 | 1 | 2 | 3 | 3 | 3 | 5 |
| **2. MULTIPLE DX** | | | | | | | | | | |
| 0–19 Years | 0 | | | | | | | | | |
| 20–34 | 14 | 3.9 | 7 | 2 | 2 | 4 | 4 | 7 | 13 | 13 |
| 35–49 | 105 | 2.9 | 1 | 1 | 2 | 3 | 4 | 4 | 5 | 7 |
| 50–64 | 164 | 2.6 | 4 | 1 | 2 | 2 | 3 | 4 | 5 | 14 |
| 65+ | 154 | 3.1 | 6 | 2 | 2 | 3 | 3 | 6 | 6 | 18 |
| **TOTAL SINGLE DX** | 73 | 2.4 | 1 | 1 | 2 | 2 | 3 | 4 | 5 | 6 |
| **TOTAL MULTIPLE DX** | 437 | 2.9 | 4 | 1 | 2 | 3 | 3 | 4 | 6 | 13 |
| **TOTAL** | | | | | | | | | | |
| 0–19 Years | 0 | | | | | | | | | |
| 20–34 | 17 | 3.7 | 6 | 2 | 2 | 3 | 4 | 7 | 7 | 13 |
| 35–49 | 130 | 2.9 | 2 | 1 | 2 | 3 | 4 | 4 | 5 | 6 |
| 50–64 | 193 | 2.6 | 4 | 1 | 2 | 2 | 3 | 4 | 5 | 8 |
| 65+ | 170 | 3.0 | 6 | 1 | 2 | 3 | 3 | 6 | 6 | 18 |
| **GRAND TOTAL** | 510 | 2.8 | 4 | 1 | 2 | 2 | 3 | 4 | 6 | 9 |

## 85.45: UNILAT RAD MASTECTOMY. Formerly included in operation group(s) 770.

| Type of Patients | Observed Patients | Avg. Stay | Variance | 10th | 25th | 50th | 75th | 90th | 95th | 99th |
|---|---|---|---|---|---|---|---|---|---|---|
| **1. SINGLE DX** | | | | | | | | | | |
| 0–19 Years | 0 | | | | | | | | | |
| 20–34 | 5 | 4.3 | 9 | 1 | 1 | 4 | 8 | 8 | 8 | 8 |
| 35–49 | 24 | 2.1 | <1 | 1 | 2 | 2 | 2 | 4 | 4 | 4 |
| 50–64 | 21 | 2.2 | 3 | 1 | 2 | 2 | 3 | 3 | 4 | 10 |
| 65+ | 19 | 2.1 | <1 | 1 | 2 | 2 | 3 | 3 | 3 | 4 |
| **2. MULTIPLE DX** | | | | | | | | | | |
| 0–19 Years | 0 | | | | | | | | | |
| 20–34 | 9 | 2.4 | <1 | 2 | 2 | 2 | 2 | 4 | 5 | 5 |
| 35–49 | 54 | 2.7 | 8 | 1 | 1 | 3 | 3 | 4 | 5 | 14 |
| 50–64 | 82 | 4.8 | 23 | 1 | 2 | 3 | 6 | 12 | 17 | 17 |
| 65+ | 132 | 3.1 | 7 | 1 | 2 | 3 | 4 | 7 | 8 | 15 |
| **TOTAL SINGLE DX** | 69 | 2.3 | 2 | 1 | 1 | 2 | 3 | 4 | 4 | 9 |
| **TOTAL MULTIPLE DX** | 277 | 3.4 | 12 | 1 | 2 | 2 | 4 | 7 | 11 | 17 |
| **TOTAL** | | | | | | | | | | |
| 0–19 Years | 0 | | | | | | | | | |
| 20–34 | 14 | 3.1 | 4 | 1 | 2 | 2 | 4 | 8 | 8 | 8 |
| 35–49 | 78 | 2.6 | 6 | 1 | 2 | 2 | 3 | 4 | 5 | 14 |
| 50–64 | 103 | 4.1 | 18 | 1 | 2 | 2 | 4 | 11 | 17 | 17 |
| 65+ | 151 | 3.0 | 6 | 1 | 2 | 2 | 3 | 6 | 8 | 15 |
| **GRAND TOTAL** | 346 | 3.1 | 10 | 1 | 2 | 2 | 3 | 6 | 11 | 17 |

Length of Stay by Diagnosis and Operation, United States, 2000

## United States, October 1998–September 1999 Data, by Operation

### 85.5: AUGMENTATION MAMMOPLASTY. Formerly included in operation group(s) 771.

| Type of Patients | Observed Patients | Avg. Stay | Variance | 10th | 25th | 50th | 75th | 90th | 95th | 99th |
|---|---|---|---|---|---|---|---|---|---|---|
| **1. SINGLE DX** | | | | | | | | | | |
| 0–19 Years | 5 | 1.2 | <1 | 1 | 1 | 1 | 1 | 1 | 3 | 3 |
| 20–34 | 32 | 1.0 | 0 | 1 | 1 | 1 | 1 | 1 |  | 1 |
| 35–49 | 19 | 1.1 | <1 | 1 | 1 | 1 | 1 | 1 | 2 | 1 |
| 50–64 | 7 | 1.5 | <1 | 1 | 1 | 2 | 2 | 2 | 4 | 4 |
| 65+ | 1 | 2.0 | 0 | 2 | 2 | 2 | 2 | 2 | 2 | 2 |
| **2. MULTIPLE DX** | | | | | | | | | | |
| 0–19 Years | 3 | 1.0 | 0 | 1 | 1 | 1 | 1 | 1 |  | 1 |
| 20–34 | 31 | 1.2 | <1 | 1 | 1 | 1 | 1 | 2 | 3 | 3 |
| 35–49 | 43 | 1.2 | <1 | 1 | 1 | 1 | 2 | 2 | 2 | 3 |
| 50–64 | 34 | 1.9 | 1 | 1 | 1 | 2 | 3 | 4 | 4 | 7 |
| 65+ | 13 | 1.1 | <1 | 1 | 1 | 2 | 2 | 2 | 2 | 2 |
| **TOTAL SINGLE DX** | 64 | 1.1 | <1 | 1 | 1 | 1 | 1 | 1 | 2 | 3 |
| **TOTAL MULTIPLE DX** | 124 | 1.4 | <1 | 1 | 1 | 1 | 2 | 2 | 3 | 4 |
| **TOTAL** | | | | | | | | | | |
| 0–19 Years | 8 | 1.1 | <1 | 1 | 1 | 1 | 1 | 1 | 3 | 3 |
| 20–34 | 63 | 1.1 | <1 | 1 | 1 | 1 | 1 | 1 | 3 | 3 |
| 35–49 | 62 | 1.2 | <1 | 1 | 1 | 1 | 1 | 2 | 2 | 3 |
| 50–64 | 41 | 1.9 | 1 | 1 | 1 | 2 | 3 | 4 | 4 | 7 |
| 65+ | 14 | 1.1 | <1 | 2 | 2 | 2 | 2 | 2 | 2 | 2 |
| **GRAND TOTAL** | 188 | 1.3 | <1 | 1 | 1 | 1 | 2 | 2 | 3 | 4 |

### 85.6: MASTOPEXY. Formerly included in operation group(s) 771.

| Type of Patients | Observed Patients | Avg. Stay | Variance | 10th | 25th | 50th | 75th | 90th | 95th | 99th |
|---|---|---|---|---|---|---|---|---|---|---|
| **1. SINGLE DX** | | | | | | | | | | |
| 0–19 Years | 3 | 1.6 | <1 | 1 | 1 | 1 | 3 | 3 | 3 | 3 |
| 20–34 | 3 | 1.0 | 0 | 1 | 1 | 1 | 1 | 1 | 1 | 1 |
| 35–49 | 8 | 1.2 | <1 | 1 | 1 | 1 | 1 | 1 | 2 | 2 |
| 50–64 | 3 | 1.0 | 0 | 1 | 1 | 1 | 1 | 1 | 1 | 1 |
| 65+ | 0 | | | | | | | | | |
| **2. MULTIPLE DX** | | | | | | | | | | |
| 0–19 Years | 3 | 1.7 | <1 | 1 | 1 | 2 | 2 | 2 | 2 | 2 |
| 20–34 | 11 | 1.2 | <1 | 1 | 1 | 1 | 1 | 1 | 2 | 3 |
| 35–49 | 30 | 1.6 | <1 | 1 | 1 | 2 | 2 | 2 | 2 | 4 |
| 50–64 | 16 | 1.5 | <1 | 1 | 1 | 1 | 2 | 2 | 3 | 3 |
| 65+ | 6 | 1.2 | <1 | 1 | 1 | 1 | 1 | 1 | 2 | 2 |
| **TOTAL SINGLE DX** | 17 | 1.2 | <1 | 1 | 1 | 1 | 1 | 1 | 2 | 3 |
| **TOTAL MULTIPLE DX** | 66 | 1.4 | <1 | 1 | 1 | 1 | 2 | 2 | 3 | 4 |
| **TOTAL** | | | | | | | | | | |
| 0–19 Years | 6 | 1.6 | <1 | 1 | 1 | 1 | 2 | 2 | 3 | 3 |
| 20–34 | 14 | 1.2 | <1 | 1 | 1 | 1 | 1 | 1 | 2 | 3 |
| 35–49 | 38 | 1.6 | <1 | 1 | 1 | 2 | 2 | 2 | 3 | 4 |
| 50–64 | 19 | 1.4 | <1 | 1 | 1 | 1 | 2 | 2 | 3 | 3 |
| 65+ | 6 | 1.2 | <1 | 1 | 1 | 1 | 1 | 1 | 2 | 2 |
| **GRAND TOTAL** | 83 | 1.4 | <1 | 1 | 1 | 1 | 2 | 2 | 3 | 4 |

### 85.7: TOTAL BREAST RECONST. Formerly included in operation group(s) 771.

| Type of Patients | Observed Patients | Avg. Stay | Variance | 10th | 25th | 50th | 75th | 90th | 95th | 99th |
|---|---|---|---|---|---|---|---|---|---|---|
| **1. SINGLE DX** | | | | | | | | | | |
| 0–19 Years | 3 | 3.0 | 2 | 1 | 1 | 4 | 4 | 4 | 4 | 4 |
| 20–34 | 3 | 3.5 | 1 | 3 | 3 | 3 | 3 | 3 | 6 | 6 |
| 35–49 | 36 | 3.7 | 3 | 2 | 3 | 3 | 4 | 5 | 6 | 16 |
| 50–64 | 29 | 3.9 | 1 | 3 | 3 | 4 | 5 | 6 | 6 | 6 |
| 65+ | 0 | | | | | | | | | |
| **2. MULTIPLE DX** | | | | | | | | | | |
| 0–19 Years | 0 | | | | | | | | | |
| 20–34 | 51 | 3.5 | 2 | 2 | 2 | 4 | 4 | 5 | 5 | 8 |
| 35–49 | 598 | 3.8 | 2 | 2 | 3 | 4 | 5 | 5 | 6 | 9 |
| 50–64 | 582 | 4.0 | 4 | 2 | 3 | 4 | 5 | 6 | 7 | 11 |
| 65+ | 82 | 3.5 | 6 | 1 | 2 | 3 | 5 | 7 | 7 | 10 |
| **TOTAL SINGLE DX** | 71 | 3.7 | 2 | 3 | 3 | 3 | 4 | 6 | 6 | 7 |
| **TOTAL MULTIPLE DX** | 1,313 | 3.9 | 3 | 2 | 3 | 4 | 5 | 6 | 7 | 10 |
| **TOTAL** | | | | | | | | | | |
| 0–19 Years | 3 | 3.0 | 2 | 1 | 1 | 4 | 4 | 4 | 4 | 4 |
| 20–34 | 54 | 3.5 | 2 | 2 | 2 | 3 | 4 | 5 | 6 | 6 |
| 35–49 | 634 | 3.8 | 3 | 2 | 3 | 4 | 4 | 5 | 6 | 9 |
| 50–64 | 611 | 4.0 | 4 | 2 | 3 | 4 | 5 | 6 | 7 | 11 |
| 65+ | 82 | 3.5 | 6 | 1 | 2 | 3 | 5 | 7 | 7 | 10 |
| **GRAND TOTAL** | 1,384 | 3.9 | 3 | 2 | 3 | 4 | 5 | 6 | 7 | 10 |

### 85.8: OTHER BREAST REPAIR. Formerly included in operation group(s) 771.

| Type of Patients | Observed Patients | Avg. Stay | Variance | 10th | 25th | 50th | 75th | 90th | 95th | 99th |
|---|---|---|---|---|---|---|---|---|---|---|
| **1. SINGLE DX** | | | | | | | | | | |
| 0–19 Years | 3 | 1.2 | <1 | 1 | 1 | 1 | 1 | 1 | 2 | 2 |
| 20–34 | 15 | 2.1 | 2 | 1 | 1 | 3 | 3 | 4 | 4 | 5 |
| 35–49 | 52 | 2.9 | 1 | 2 | 2 | 3 | 4 | 4 | 4 | 6 |
| 50–64 | 39 | 2.7 | 2 | 1 | 1 | 2 | 3 | 5 | 6 | 6 |
| 65+ | 8 | 1.6 | <1 | 1 | 1 | 1 | 2 | 3 | 3 | 3 |
| **2. MULTIPLE DX** | | | | | | | | | | |
| 0–19 Years | 10 | 2.6 | 4 | 1 | 1 | 2 | 3 | 3 | 4 | 11 |
| 20–34 | 56 | 3.1 | 9 | 1 | 1 | 2 | 4 | 5 | 9 | 17 |
| 35–49 | 300 | 3.6 | 26 | 1 | 2 | 3 | 5 | 5 | 7 | 35 |
| 50–64 | 328 | 2.9 | 7 | 1 | 1 | 2 | 3 | 5 | 7 | 14 |
| 65+ | 106 | 4.1 | 27 | 1 | 2 | 3 | 4 | 8 | 14 | 35 |
| **TOTAL SINGLE DX** | 117 | 2.6 | 2 | 1 | 2 | 2 | 4 | 4 | 5 | 6 |
| **TOTAL MULTIPLE DX** | 800 | 3.3 | 16 | 1 | 2 | 3 | 4 | 5 | 8 | 19 |
| **TOTAL** | | | | | | | | | | |
| 0–19 Years | 13 | 2.4 | 4 | 1 | 2 | 2 | 3 | 3 | 4 | 11 |
| 20–34 | 71 | 2.8 | 7 | 1 | 2 | 2 | 4 | 5 | 9 | 12 |
| 35–49 | 352 | 3.5 | 22 | 1 | 2 | 3 | 5 | 5 | 6 | 28 |
| 50–64 | 367 | 2.9 | 6 | 1 | 2 | 2 | 3 | 5 | 7 | 14 |
| 65+ | 114 | 4.0 | 26 | 1 | 2 | 3 | 4 | 8 | 14 | 35 |
| **GRAND TOTAL** | 917 | 3.2 | 14 | 1 | 2 | 3 | 4 | 5 | 7 | 16 |

341

Length of Stay by Diagnosis and Operation, United States, 2000

# United States, October 1998–September 1999 Data, by Operation

## 85.85: BREAST MUSCLE FLAP GRAFT. Formerly included in operation group(s) 771.

| Type of Patients | Observed Patients | Avg. Stay | Variance | Percentiles | | | | | | |
|---|---|---|---|---|---|---|---|---|---|---|
| | | | | 10th | 25th | 50th | 75th | 90th | 95th | 99th |
| **1. SINGLE DX** | | | | | | | | | | |
| 0–19 Years | 1 | 2.0 | 0 | 2 | 2 | 2 | 2 | 2 | 2 | 2 |
| 20–34 | 5 | 3.2 | 1 | 1 | 3 | 4 | 4 | 4 | 4 | 4 |
| 35–49 | 38 | 3.1 | 1 | 2 | 2 | 3 | 4 | 4 | 4 | 7 |
| 50–64 | 23 | 3.0 | 1 | 2 | 2 | 3 | 3 | 4 | 5 | 6 |
| 65+ | 4 | 1.8 | <1 | 1 | 1 | 2 | 3 | 3 | 3 | 3 |
| **2. MULTIPLE DX** | | | | | | | | | | |
| 0–19 Years | 4 | 3.2 | <1 | 3 | 3 | 3 | 4 | 4 | 4 | 4 |
| 20–34 | 24 | 2.9 | 1 | 2 | 2 | 3 | 4 | 4 | 4 | 7 |
| 35–49 | 190 | 3.2 | 6 | 2 | 2 | 3 | 4 | 5 | 6 | 10 |
| 50–64 | 196 | 3.1 | 4 | 1 | 2 | 3 | 4 | 4 | 6 | 11 |
| 65+ | 56 | 3.7 | 3 | 2 | 3 | 3 | 4 | 5 | 9 | 9 |
| **TOTAL SINGLE DX** | 71 | 3.0 | 1 | 2 | 2 | 3 | 4 | 4 | 4 | 6 |
| **TOTAL MULTIPLE DX** | 470 | 3.2 | 5 | 2 | 2 | 3 | 4 | 5 | 6 | 11 |
| **TOTAL** | | | | | | | | | | |
| 0–19 Years | 5 | 3.1 | <1 | 3 | 3 | 3 | 3 | 4 | 4 | 4 |
| 20–34 | 29 | 3.0 | 1 | 2 | 2 | 3 | 4 | 4 | 4 | 7 |
| 35–49 | 228 | 3.2 | 5 | 2 | 2 | 3 | 4 | 5 | 6 | 9 |
| 50–64 | 219 | 3.0 | 4 | 1 | 2 | 3 | 4 | 4 | 6 | 11 |
| 65+ | 60 | 3.6 | 3 | 2 | 3 | 3 | 4 | 5 | 9 | 9 |
| **GRAND TOTAL** | 541 | 3.2 | 4 | 2 | 2 | 3 | 4 | 5 | 6 | 10 |

## 85.9: OTHER BREAST OPERATIONS. Formerly included in operation group(s) 771, 780.

| Type of Patients | Observed Patients | Avg. Stay | Variance | Percentiles | | | | | | |
|---|---|---|---|---|---|---|---|---|---|---|
| | | | | 10th | 25th | 50th | 75th | 90th | 95th | 99th |
| **1. SINGLE DX** | | | | | | | | | | |
| 0–19 Years | 11 | 2.2 | <1 | 1 | 2 | 2 | 3 | 3 | 4 | 4 |
| 20–34 | 11 | 2.2 | 2 | 1 | 1 | 1 | 4 | 4 | 5 | 5 |
| 35–49 | 45 | 2.0 | 1 | 1 | 1 | 2 | 3 | 3 | 5 | 5 |
| 50–64 | 34 | 1.9 | 2 | 2 | 1 | 1 | 3 | 3 | 5 | 6 |
| 65+ | 6 | 2.3 | 6 | 1 | 1 | 1 | 2 | 7 | 7 | 7 |
| **2. MULTIPLE DX** | | | | | | | | | | |
| 0–19 Years | 7 | 2.0 | <1 | 2 | 2 | 2 | 2 | 2 | 2 | 3 |
| 20–34 | 57 | 2.6 | 3 | 1 | 1 | 2 | 4 | 5 | 5 | 7 |
| 35–49 | 304 | 3.6 | 19 | 1 | 1 | 2 | 4 | 8 | 9 | 30 |
| 50–64 | 361 | 4.1 | 21 | 1 | 1 | 3 | 4 | 7 | 12 | 23 |
| 65+ | 175 | 4.0 | 12 | 1 | 2 | 3 | 6 | 8 | 10 | 16 |
| **TOTAL SINGLE DX** | 107 | 2.0 | 2 | 1 | 1 | 2 | 3 | 4 | 5 | 7 |
| **TOTAL MULTIPLE DX** | 904 | 3.8 | 18 | 1 | 1 | 3 | 5 | 7 | 10 | 23 |
| **TOTAL** | | | | | | | | | | |
| 0–19 Years | 18 | 2.1 | <1 | 1 | 2 | 2 | 2 | 3 | 3 | 4 |
| 20–34 | 68 | 2.5 | 3 | 1 | 1 | 2 | 4 | 5 | 5 | 7 |
| 35–49 | 349 | 3.4 | 17 | 1 | 1 | 2 | 4 | 6 | 8 | 30 |
| 50–64 | 395 | 4.0 | 20 | 1 | 1 | 3 | 4 | 7 | 12 | 23 |
| 65+ | 181 | 4.0 | 12 | 1 | 1 | 3 | 6 | 8 | 10 | 16 |
| **GRAND TOTAL** | 1,011 | 3.6 | 16 | 1 | 1 | 2 | 4 | 7 | 9 | 23 |

## 85.94: BREAST IMPLANT REMOVAL. Formerly included in operation group(s) 771.

| Type of Patients | Observed Patients | Avg. Stay | Variance | Percentiles | | | | | | |
|---|---|---|---|---|---|---|---|---|---|---|
| | | | | 10th | 25th | 50th | 75th | 90th | 95th | 99th |
| **1. SINGLE DX** | | | | | | | | | | |
| 0–19 Years | 0 | | | | | | | | | |
| 20–34 | 5 | 1.9 | 3 | 1 | 1 | 1 | 1 | 5 | 5 | 5 |
| 35–49 | 28 | 1.7 | 1 | 1 | 1 | 1 | 2 | 3 | 4 | 5 |
| 50–64 | 17 | 1.9 | 1 | 1 | 2 | 2 | 2 | 4 | 5 | 5 |
| 65+ | 4 | 1.0 | 0 | 1 | 1 | 1 | 1 | 1 | 1 | 1 |
| **2. MULTIPLE DX** | | | | | | | | | | |
| 0–19 Years | 0 | | | | | | | | | |
| 20–34 | 20 | 1.6 | 2 | 1 | 1 | 1 | 2 | 3 | 5 | 7 |
| 35–49 | 145 | 4.1 | 29 | 1 | 2 | 3 | 4 | 7 | 10 | 30 |
| 50–64 | 167 | 4.1 | 15 | 1 | 2 | 3 | 4 | 7 | 10 | 20 |
| 65+ | 63 | 3.0 | 8 | 1 | 1 | 2 | 4 | 7 | 7 | 16 |
| **TOTAL SINGLE DX** | 54 | 1.8 | 1 | 1 | 1 | 1 | 2 | 4 | 5 | 5 |
| **TOTAL MULTIPLE DX** | 395 | 3.7 | 18 | 1 | 1 | 3 | 4 | 7 | 8 | 30 |
| **TOTAL** | | | | | | | | | | |
| 0–19 Years | 0 | | | | | | | | | |
| 20–34 | 25 | 1.7 | 2 | 1 | 1 | 1 | 2 | 4 | 5 | 7 |
| 35–49 | 173 | 3.7 | 26 | 1 | 2 | 3 | 4 | 6 | 9 | 30 |
| 50–64 | 184 | 3.9 | 14 | 1 | 2 | 3 | 4 | 6 | 8 | 20 |
| 65+ | 67 | 2.9 | 8 | 1 | 1 | 2 | 3 | 7 | 7 | 16 |
| **GRAND TOTAL** | 449 | 3.6 | 17 | 1 | 1 | 3 | 4 | 6 | 8 | 30 |

## 86.0: INCISION SKIN & SUBCU. Formerly included in operation group(s) 772, 775, 776, 779, 780.

| Type of Patients | Observed Patients | Avg. Stay | Variance | Percentiles | | | | | | |
|---|---|---|---|---|---|---|---|---|---|---|
| | | | | 10th | 25th | 50th | 75th | 90th | 95th | 99th |
| **1. SINGLE DX** | | | | | | | | | | |
| 0–19 Years | 1,738 | 3.1 | 6 | 1 | 1 | 2 | 4 | 6 | 7 | 16 |
| 20–34 | 892 | 2.8 | 4 | 1 | 1 | 2 | 3 | 5 | 6 | 10 |
| 35–49 | 867 | 2.8 | 4 | 1 | 2 | 2 | 4 | 5 | 7 | 10 |
| 50–64 | 438 | 3.6 | 7 | 1 | 2 | 3 | 5 | 7 | 8 | 14 |
| 65+ | 218 | 3.1 | 9 | 1 | 1 | 2 | 4 | 7 | 8 | 11 |
| **2. MULTIPLE DX** | | | | | | | | | | |
| 0–19 Years | 5,188 | 6.6 | 67 | 1 | 2 | 4 | 7 | 14 | 21 | 47 |
| 20–34 | 4,898 | 6.1 | 63 | 1 | 2 | 4 | 7 | 12 | 17 | 40 |
| 35–49 | 10,170 | 6.2 | 38 | 2 | 3 | 4 | 7 | 12 | 17 | 31 |
| 50–64 | 9,772 | 7.3 | 58 | 2 | 3 | 5 | 9 | 15 | 21 | 46 |
| 65+ | 11,864 | 8.2 | 59 | 2 | 4 | 6 | 10 | 17 | 23 | 40 |
| **TOTAL SINGLE DX** | 4,153 | 3.0 | 6 | 1 | 1 | 2 | 4 | 6 | 7 | 12 |
| **TOTAL MULTIPLE DX** | 41,892 | 7.0 | 56 | 2 | 3 | 5 | 8 | 14 | 20 | 39 |
| **TOTAL** | | | | | | | | | | |
| 0–19 Years | 6,926 | 5.7 | 54 | 1 | 2 | 4 | 6 | 11 | 19 | 41 |
| 20–34 | 5,790 | 5.6 | 55 | 1 | 2 | 4 | 6 | 11 | 15 | 38 |
| 35–49 | 11,037 | 5.9 | 37 | 2 | 3 | 4 | 7 | 12 | 17 | 31 |
| 50–64 | 10,210 | 7.1 | 57 | 2 | 3 | 5 | 8 | 14 | 21 | 44 |
| 65+ | 12,082 | 8.2 | 59 | 2 | 3 | 6 | 10 | 16 | 22 | 40 |
| **GRAND TOTAL** | 46,045 | 6.6 | 52 | 1 | 3 | 5 | 8 | 14 | 19 | 37 |

Length of Stay by Diagnosis and Operation, United States, 2000

# United States, October 1998–September 1999 Data, by Operation

## 86.01: ASPIRATION SKIN & SUBCU. Formerly included in operation group(s) 780.

| Type of Patients | Observed Patients | Avg. Stay | Variance | 10th | 25th | 50th | 75th | 90th | 95th | 99th |
|---|---|---|---|---|---|---|---|---|---|---|
| **1. SINGLE DX** | | | | | | | | | | |
| 0–19 Years | 59 | 3.4 | 4 | 1 | 2 | 3 | 5 | 6 | 6 | 11 |
| 20–34 | 30 | 2.6 | 5 | 1 | 1 | 2 | 3 | 5 | 6 | 12 |
| 35–49 | 29 | 4.0 | 5 | 2 | 2 | 3 | 6 | 7 | 7 | 10 |
| 50–64 | 17 | 4.4 | 4 | 2 | 4 | 5 | 5 | 7 | 7 | 11 |
| 65+ | 9 | 5.2 | 11 | 1 | 3 | 4 | 9 | 9 | 9 | 9 |
| **2. MULTIPLE DX** | | | | | | | | | | |
| 0–19 Years | 171 | 4.4 | 10 | 1 | 2 | 4 | 6 | 9 | 10 | 16 |
| 20–34 | 159 | 5.5 | 66 | 1 | 2 | 3 | 6 | 10 | 14 | 29 |
| 35–49 | 377 | 6.3 | 32 | 2 | 3 | 4 | 8 | 12 | 19 | 27 |
| 50–64 | 335 | 6.2 | 31 | 2 | 3 | 5 | 8 | 11 | 16 | 29 |
| 65+ | 571 | 6.8 | 30 | 2 | 4 | 5 | 8 | 12 | 17 | 28 |
| **TOTAL SINGLE DX** | 144 | 3.6 | 5 | 1 | 2 | 3 | 5 | 7 | 7 | 11 |
| **TOTAL MULTIPLE DX** | 1,613 | 6.2 | 32 | 2 | 3 | 5 | 8 | 11 | 16 | 28 |
| **TOTAL** | | | | | | | | | | |
| 0–19 Years | 230 | 4.2 | 8 | 1 | 2 | 3 | 6 | 9 | 9 | 16 |
| 20–34 | 189 | 5.1 | 58 | 1 | 2 | 3 | 6 | 9 | 13 | 29 |
| 35–49 | 406 | 6.2 | 31 | 2 | 3 | 4 | 8 | 11 | 19 | 25 |
| 50–64 | 352 | 6.1 | 29 | 2 | 3 | 5 | 8 | 11 | 15 | 29 |
| 65+ | 580 | 6.8 | 30 | 2 | 4 | 5 | 8 | 12 | 17 | 28 |
| **GRAND TOTAL** | 1,757 | 5.9 | 31 | 2 | 3 | 5 | 7 | 11 | 15 | 27 |

## 86.04: OTHER SKIN & SUBCU I&D. Formerly included in operation group(s) 775.

| Type of Patients | Observed Patients | Avg. Stay | Variance | 10th | 25th | 50th | 75th | 90th | 95th | 99th |
|---|---|---|---|---|---|---|---|---|---|---|
| **1. SINGLE DX** | | | | | | | | | | |
| 0–19 Years | 862 | 3.0 | 3 | 1 | 2 | 3 | 4 | 5 | 7 | 9 |
| 20–34 | 546 | 2.5 | 3 | 1 | 2 | 2 | 3 | 5 | 6 | 8 |
| 35–49 | 538 | 2.9 | 3 | 1 | 2 | 2 | 4 | 5 | 6 | 9 |
| 50–64 | 211 | 3.9 | 8 | 1 | 2 | 3 | 5 | 7 | 8 | 14 |
| 65+ | 107 | 3.3 | 11 | 1 | 2 | 2 | 4 | 7 | 7 | 11 |
| **2. MULTIPLE DX** | | | | | | | | | | |
| 0–19 Years | 1,874 | 4.5 | 26 | 1 | 2 | 3 | 5 | 8 | 11 | 21 |
| 20–34 | 2,435 | 4.4 | 14 | 1 | 2 | 3 | 5 | 8 | 11 | 19 |
| 35–49 | 4,941 | 4.9 | 17 | 2 | 2 | 4 | 6 | 9 | 12 | 21 |
| 50–64 | 3,574 | 6.4 | 54 | 2 | 3 | 5 | 7 | 11 | 16 | 49 |
| 65+ | 3,885 | 6.6 | 28 | 2 | 3 | 5 | 8 | 13 | 17 | 25 |
| **TOTAL SINGLE DX** | 2,264 | 2.9 | 4 | 1 | 2 | 2 | 4 | 5 | 7 | 9 |
| **TOTAL MULTIPLE DX** | 16,709 | 5.5 | 28 | 2 | 3 | 4 | 7 | 10 | 14 | 26 |
| **TOTAL** | | | | | | | | | | |
| 0–19 Years | 2,736 | 4.0 | 19 | 1 | 2 | 3 | 5 | 7 | 9 | 21 |
| 20–34 | 2,981 | 4.1 | 12 | 1 | 2 | 3 | 6 | 8 | 10 | 18 |
| 35–49 | 5,479 | 4.7 | 16 | 1 | 2 | 4 | 6 | 9 | 11 | 21 |
| 50–64 | 3,785 | 6.2 | 52 | 2 | 3 | 5 | 7 | 11 | 16 | 49 |
| 65+ | 3,992 | 6.6 | 28 | 2 | 3 | 5 | 8 | 13 | 16 | 25 |
| **GRAND TOTAL** | 18,973 | 5.2 | 26 | 1 | 2 | 4 | 6 | 10 | 13 | 24 |

## 86.03: INCISION PILONIDAL SINUS. Formerly included in operation group(s) 772.

| Type of Patients | Observed Patients | Avg. Stay | Variance | 10th | 25th | 50th | 75th | 90th | 95th | 99th |
|---|---|---|---|---|---|---|---|---|---|---|
| **1. SINGLE DX** | | | | | | | | | | |
| 0–19 Years | 134 | 2.0 | 2 | 1 | 1 | 2 | 2 | 4 | 5 | 6 |
| 20–34 | 83 | 1.5 | <1 | 1 | 1 | 1 | 3 | 3 | 4 | 5 |
| 35–49 | 16 | 2.0 | 1 | 1 | 2 | 2 | 3 | 4 | 4 | 5 |
| 50–64 | 2 | 3.4 | 1 | 2 | 2 | 4 | 4 | 4 | 4 | 4 |
| 65+ | 0 | | | | | | | | | |
| **2. MULTIPLE DX** | | | | | | | | | | |
| 0–19 Years | 69 | 2.7 | 11 | 1 | 1 | 2 | 3 | 4 | 4 | 18 |
| 20–34 | 73 | 3.0 | 8 | 1 | 1 | 2 | 4 | 5 | 6 | 21 |
| 35–49 | 39 | 3.0 | 4 | 1 | 2 | 3 | 4 | 5 | 6 | 13 |
| 50–64 | 18 | 5.1 | 10 | 2 | 3 | 4 | 7 | 10 | 12 | 12 |
| 65+ | 7 | 4.3 | 12 | 1 | 2 | 2 | 6 | 8 | 12 | 12 |
| **TOTAL SINGLE DX** | 235 | 1.9 | 1 | 1 | 1 | 1 | 2 | 4 | 5 | 6 |
| **TOTAL MULTIPLE DX** | 206 | 3.1 | 9 | 1 | 1 | 2 | 4 | 6 | 9 | 18 |
| **TOTAL** | | | | | | | | | | |
| 0–19 Years | 203 | 2.3 | 5 | 1 | 1 | 2 | 3 | 4 | 5 | 18 |
| 20–34 | 156 | 2.1 | 4 | 1 | 1 | 2 | 2 | 4 | 5 | 8 |
| 35–49 | 55 | 2.5 | 3 | 1 | 2 | 2 | 3 | 5 | 5 | 10 |
| 50–64 | 20 | 5.0 | 10 | 2 | 3 | 4 | 7 | 10 | 12 | 12 |
| 65+ | 7 | 4.3 | 12 | 1 | 2 | 2 | 6 | 8 | 12 | 12 |
| **GRAND TOTAL** | 441 | 2.4 | 5 | 1 | 1 | 2 | 3 | 4 | 6 | 12 |

## 86.05: INC W RMVL FB SKIN/SUBCU. Formerly included in operation group(s) 775.

| Type of Patients | Observed Patients | Avg. Stay | Variance | 10th | 25th | 50th | 75th | 90th | 95th | 99th |
|---|---|---|---|---|---|---|---|---|---|---|
| **1. SINGLE DX** | | | | | | | | | | |
| 0–19 Years | 161 | 1.4 | <1 | 1 | 1 | 1 | 2 | 2 | 3 | 4 |
| 20–34 | 67 | 2.5 | 6 | 1 | 1 | 2 | 3 | 3 | 3 | 6 |
| 35–49 | 56 | 1.4 | <1 | 1 | 1 | 1 | 2 | 3 | 3 | 6 |
| 50–64 | 21 | 2.4 | 4 | 1 | 1 | 2 | 3 | 3 | 4 | 10 |
| 65+ | 11 | 1.9 | 2 | 1 | 1 | 1 | 2 | 2 | 5 | 5 |
| **2. MULTIPLE DX** | | | | | | | | | | |
| 0–19 Years | 880 | 7.0 | 66 | 1 | 2 | 4 | 9 | 16 | 22 | 38 |
| 20–34 | 580 | 7.2 | 53 | 1 | 3 | 5 | 8 | 16 | 19 | 33 |
| 35–49 | 1,124 | 7.1 | 42 | 2 | 3 | 6 | 8 | 15 | 18 | 33 |
| 50–64 | 1,164 | 7.7 | 46 | 2 | 3 | 6 | 9 | 15 | 21 | 36 |
| 65+ | 1,154 | 8.0 | 43 | 2 | 4 | 6 | 10 | 16 | 20 | 33 |
| **TOTAL SINGLE DX** | 316 | 1.7 | 2 | 1 | 1 | 1 | 2 | 2 | 4 | 5 |
| **TOTAL MULTIPLE DX** | 4,902 | 7.4 | 49 | 2 | 3 | 6 | 9 | 16 | 20 | 36 |
| **TOTAL** | | | | | | | | | | |
| 0–19 Years | 1,041 | 6.1 | 59 | 1 | 1 | 3 | 7 | 15 | 20 | 36 |
| 20–34 | 647 | 6.5 | 49 | 1 | 2 | 4 | 9 | 14 | 19 | 32 |
| 35–49 | 1,180 | 6.7 | 41 | 1 | 3 | 5 | 8 | 14 | 18 | 33 |
| 50–64 | 1,185 | 7.7 | 46 | 2 | 3 | 6 | 9 | 15 | 21 | 36 |
| 65+ | 1,165 | 7.9 | 43 | 2 | 4 | 6 | 10 | 16 | 20 | 32 |
| **GRAND TOTAL** | 5,218 | 7.0 | 48 | 1 | 2 | 5 | 9 | 15 | 19 | 35 |

Length of Stay by Diagnosis and Operation, United States, 2000

# United States, October 1998–September 1999 Data, by Operation

## 86.06: INSERTION INFUSION PUMP. Formerly included in operation group(s) 775.

| Type of Patients | Observed Patients | Avg. Stay | Vari-ance | Percentiles | | | | | | |
|---|---|---|---|---|---|---|---|---|---|---|
| | | | | 10th | 25th | 50th | 75th | 90th | 95th | 99th |
| **1. SINGLE DX** | | | | | | | | | | |
| 0–19 Years | 88 | 3.1 | 3 | 1 | 1 | 3 | 5 | 5 | 7 | 7 |
| 20–34 | 36 | 4.2 | 3 | 1 | 3 | 5 | 5 | 5 | 5 | 11 |
| 35–49 | 89 | 2.3 | 3 | 1 | 1 | 2 | 3 | 5 | 7 | 10 |
| 50–64 | 70 | 2.3 | 2 | 1 | 1 | 2 | 3 | 4 | 5 | 7 |
| 65+ | 28 | 2.5 | 3 | 1 | 1 | 2 | 4 | 5 | 6 | 7 |
| **2. MULTIPLE DX** | | | | | | | | | | |
| 0–19 Years | 262 | 4.3 | 13 | 2 | 2 | 3 | 5 | 8 | 9 | 22 |
| 20–34 | 180 | 6.9 | 186 | 2 | 2 | 3 | 5 | 11 | 27 | 67 |
| 35–49 | 532 | 5.9 | 118 | 1 | 2 | 3 | 6 | 11 | 19 | 83 |
| 50–64 | 510 | 6.0 | 54 | 1 | 2 | 3 | 7 | 14 | 22 | 41 |
| 65+ | 437 | 6.8 | 58 | 1 | 2 | 4 | 8 | 17 | 23 | 34 |
| **TOTAL SINGLE DX** | 311 | 3.0 | 4 | 1 | 1 | 3 | 5 | 5 | 6 | 7 |
| **TOTAL MULTIPLE DX** | 1,921 | 5.9 | 83 | 1 | 2 | 3 | 6 | 14 | 20 | 58 |
| **TOTAL** | | | | | | | | | | |
| 0–19 Years | 350 | 4.0 | 12 | 1 | 2 | 3 | 5 | 7 | 8 | 18 |
| 20–34 | 216 | 6.4 | 148 | 1 | 2 | 3 | 5 | 7 | 20 | 67 |
| 35–49 | 621 | 5.6 | 107 | 1 | 2 | 3 | 5 | 11 | 17 | 83 |
| 50–64 | 580 | 5.6 | 51 | 1 | 2 | 3 | 6 | 14 | 22 | 39 |
| 65+ | 465 | 6.6 | 57 | 1 | 2 | 4 | 8 | 17 | 23 | 34 |
| **GRAND TOTAL** | 2,232 | 5.6 | 74 | 1 | 2 | 3 | 6 | 12 | 19 | 44 |

## 86.09: SKIN/SUBCU INCISION NEC. Formerly included in operation group(s) 775.

| Type of Patients | Observed Patients | Avg. Stay | Vari-ance | Percentiles | | | | | | |
|---|---|---|---|---|---|---|---|---|---|---|
| | | | | 10th | 25th | 50th | 75th | 90th | 95th | 99th |
| **1. SINGLE DX** | | | | | | | | | | |
| 0–19 Years | 121 | 2.9 | 3 | 1 | 1 | 2 | 4 | 6 | 6 | 7 |
| 20–34 | 50 | 2.6 | 2 | 1 | 2 | 2 | 3 | 4 | 5 | 8 |
| 35–49 | 70 | 2.8 | 5 | 1 | 2 | 2 | 3 | 7 | 7 | 11 |
| 50–64 | 26 | 2.9 | 4 | 1 | 2 | 2 | 3 | 6 | 7 | 11 |
| 65+ | 13 | 2.6 | 2 | 1 | 1 | 3 | 4 | 4 | 5 | 5 |
| **2. MULTIPLE DX** | | | | | | | | | | |
| 0–19 Years | 423 | 5.4 | 35 | 1 | 1 | 3 | 7 | 13 | 20 | 27 |
| 20–34 | 364 | 5.2 | 39 | 1 | 2 | 3 | 7 | 10 | 13 | 38 |
| 35–49 | 732 | 5.2 | 28 | 1 | 2 | 4 | 6 | 9 | 12 | 28 |
| 50–64 | 738 | 6.2 | 22 | 2 | 3 | 5 | 8 | 13 | 15 | 24 |
| 65+ | 750 | 7.7 | 46 | 2 | 3 | 6 | 9 | 15 | 21 | 33 |
| **TOTAL SINGLE DX** | 280 | 2.8 | 4 | 1 | 1 | 2 | 4 | 6 | 6 | 9 |
| **TOTAL MULTIPLE DX** | 3,007 | 6.0 | 34 | 1 | 2 | 5 | 7 | 12 | 17 | 32 |
| **TOTAL** | | | | | | | | | | |
| 0–19 Years | 544 | 4.7 | 27 | 1 | 1 | 3 | 6 | 10 | 19 | 25 |
| 20–34 | 414 | 4.9 | 35 | 1 | 2 | 3 | 6 | 10 | 13 | 38 |
| 35–49 | 802 | 5.1 | 27 | 1 | 2 | 4 | 6 | 9 | 12 | 26 |
| 50–64 | 764 | 6.2 | 22 | 2 | 3 | 5 | 7 | 13 | 15 | 24 |
| 65+ | 763 | 7.6 | 46 | 2 | 3 | 6 | 9 | 15 | 21 | 33 |
| **GRAND TOTAL** | 3,287 | 5.7 | 32 | 1 | 2 | 4 | 7 | 12 | 16 | 31 |

## 86.07: VAD INSERTION. Formerly included in operation group(s) 776.

| Type of Patients | Observed Patients | Avg. Stay | Vari-ance | Percentiles | | | | | | |
|---|---|---|---|---|---|---|---|---|---|---|
| | | | | 10th | 25th | 50th | 75th | 90th | 95th | 99th |
| **1. SINGLE DX** | | | | | | | | | | |
| 0–19 Years | 304 | 4.9 | 17 | 1 | 2 | 4 | 6 | 10 | 16 | 17 |
| 20–34 | 80 | 5.7 | 14 | 1 | 3 | 6 | 7 | 9 | 14 | 21 |
| 35–49 | 69 | 4.2 | 8 | 1 | 2 | 4 | 6 | 7 | 12 | 14 |
| 50–64 | 91 | 3.3 | 7 | 1 | 1 | 3 | 4 | 6 | 7 | 15 |
| 65+ | 50 | 3.1 | 10 | 1 | 1 | 2 | 4 | 7 | 7 | 18 |
| **2. MULTIPLE DX** | | | | | | | | | | |
| 0–19 Years | 1,507 | 9.9 | 127 | 2 | 4 | 6 | 12 | 23 | 32 | 72 |
| 20–34 | 1,105 | 10.1 | 144 | 2 | 4 | 7 | 12 | 19 | 28 | 76 |
| 35–49 | 2,423 | 9.2 | 64 | 3 | 4 | 7 | 11 | 18 | 26 | 41 |
| 50–64 | 3,432 | 8.7 | 76 | 2 | 3 | 6 | 11 | 18 | 25 | 45 |
| 65+ | 5,058 | 9.9 | 87 | 2 | 4 | 7 | 12 | 21 | 30 | 44 |
| **TOTAL SINGLE DX** | 594 | 4.7 | 15 | 1 | 2 | 4 | 6 | 9 | 15 | 17 |
| **TOTAL MULTIPLE DX** | 13,525 | 9.5 | 91 | 2 | 4 | 7 | 12 | 20 | 28 | 50 |
| **TOTAL** | | | | | | | | | | |
| 0–19 Years | 1,811 | 9.0 | 111 | 1 | 3 | 6 | 11 | 20 | 28 | 71 |
| 20–34 | 1,185 | 9.9 | 137 | 2 | 4 | 6 | 11 | 18 | 27 | 76 |
| 35–49 | 2,492 | 9.1 | 63 | 2 | 4 | 7 | 11 | 18 | 26 | 41 |
| 50–64 | 3,523 | 8.6 | 75 | 2 | 3 | 6 | 11 | 18 | 25 | 45 |
| 65+ | 5,108 | 9.9 | 87 | 2 | 4 | 7 | 12 | 21 | 30 | 44 |
| **GRAND TOTAL** | 14,119 | 9.3 | 88 | 2 | 4 | 7 | 11 | 19 | 28 | 49 |

## 86.1: SKIN & SUBCU DXTIC PX. Formerly included in operation group(s) 773, 780.

| Type of Patients | Observed Patients | Avg. Stay | Vari-ance | Percentiles | | | | | | |
|---|---|---|---|---|---|---|---|---|---|---|
| | | | | 10th | 25th | 50th | 75th | 90th | 95th | 99th |
| **1. SINGLE DX** | | | | | | | | | | |
| 0–19 Years | 63 | 4.0 | 11 | 1 | 2 | 3 | 4 | 9 | 10 | 15 |
| 20–34 | 21 | 4.4 | 5 | 1 | 2 | 5 | 6 | 7 | 7 | 8 |
| 35–49 | 22 | 4.0 | 8 | 2 | 3 | 4 | 4 | 6 | 8 | 16 |
| 50–64 | 18 | 3.7 | 7 | 1 | 3 | 3 | 5 | 7 | 7 | 12 |
| 65+ | 15 | 4.1 | 5 | 1 | 2 | 4 | 5 | 6 | 10 | 10 |
| **2. MULTIPLE DX** | | | | | | | | | | |
| 0–19 Years | 340 | 8.3 | 99 | 2 | 3 | 5 | 9 | 18 | 29 | 58 |
| 20–34 | 325 | 12.4 | 205 | 2 | 3 | 6 | 13 | 44 | 44 | 45 |
| 35–49 | 711 | 7.7 | 64 | 2 | 3 | 6 | 9 | 14 | 21 | 40 |
| 50–64 | 670 | 7.2 | 45 | 2 | 3 | 5 | 9 | 14 | 20 | 39 |
| 65+ | 1,268 | 7.7 | 41 | 3 | 4 | 6 | 9 | 15 | 21 | 35 |
| **TOTAL SINGLE DX** | 139 | 4.0 | 9 | 1 | 2 | 3 | 5 | 7 | 9 | 16 |
| **TOTAL MULTIPLE DX** | 3,314 | 8.2 | 73 | 2 | 3 | 6 | 9 | 16 | 24 | 44 |
| **TOTAL** | | | | | | | | | | |
| 0–19 Years | 403 | 7.7 | 89 | 2 | 3 | 4 | 8 | 17 | 29 | 58 |
| 20–34 | 346 | 12.1 | 200 | 2 | 3 | 6 | 13 | 44 | 44 | 45 |
| 35–49 | 733 | 7.6 | 62 | 2 | 3 | 6 | 9 | 14 | 21 | 40 |
| 50–64 | 688 | 7.2 | 45 | 2 | 3 | 5 | 9 | 14 | 20 | 39 |
| 65+ | 1,283 | 7.7 | 41 | 3 | 4 | 6 | 9 | 15 | 21 | 34 |
| **GRAND TOTAL** | 3,453 | 8.0 | 72 | 2 | 3 | 6 | 9 | 16 | 23 | 44 |

Length of Stay by Diagnosis and Operation, United States, 2000

# United States, October 1998–September 1999 Data, by Operation

## 86.11: SKIN & SUBCU BIOPSY. Formerly included in operation group(s) 773.

| Type of Patients | Observed Patients | Avg. Stay | Variance | 10th | 25th | 50th | 75th | 90th | 95th | 99th |
|---|---|---|---|---|---|---|---|---|---|---|
| **1. SINGLE DX** | | | | | | | | | | |
| 0–19 Years | 63 | 4.0 | 11 | 1 | 2 | 3 | 4 | 9 | 10 | 15 |
| 20–34 | 21 | 4.4 | 5 | 1 | 2 | 5 | 6 | 7 | 7 | 8 |
| 35–49 | 22 | 4.0 | 8 | 2 | 2 | 4 | 4 | 6 | 8 | 16 |
| 50–64 | 18 | 3.7 | 7 | 1 | 3 | 3 | 5 | 7 | 7 | 12 |
| 65+ | 15 | 4.1 | 5 | 1 | 2 | 4 | 5 | 6 | 10 | 10 |
| **2. MULTIPLE DX** | | | | | | | | | | |
| 0–19 Years | 335 | 8.4 | 100 | 2 | 3 | 5 | 9 | 18 | 29 | 58 |
| 20–34 | 323 | 12.4 | 206 | 2 | 3 | 6 | 13 | 44 | 44 | 45 |
| 35–49 | 709 | 7.7 | 64 | 2 | 3 | 6 | 9 | 14 | 21 | 40 |
| 50–64 | 667 | 7.2 | 45 | 2 | 3 | 5 | 9 | 14 | 20 | 39 |
| 65+ | 1,262 | 7.7 | 42 | 3 | 4 | 6 | 9 | 15 | 21 | 35 |
| **TOTAL SINGLE DX** | 139 | 4.0 | 9 | 1 | 2 | 3 | 5 | 7 | 9 | 16 |
| **TOTAL MULTIPLE DX** | 3,296 | 8.2 | 74 | 2 | 3 | 6 | 9 | 16 | 24 | 44 |
| **TOTAL** | | | | | | | | | | |
| 0–19 Years | 398 | 7.8 | 90 | 2 | 3 | 4 | 8 | 17 | 29 | 58 |
| 20–34 | 344 | 12.1 | 201 | 2 | 3 | 6 | 13 | 44 | 44 | 45 |
| 35–49 | 731 | 7.6 | 62 | 2 | 3 | 6 | 9 | 14 | 21 | 40 |
| 50–64 | 685 | 7.2 | 45 | 2 | 3 | 5 | 9 | 14 | 20 | 39 |
| 65+ | 1,277 | 7.7 | 41 | 3 | 4 | 6 | 9 | 15 | 21 | 34 |
| **GRAND TOTAL** | 3,435 | 8.1 | 72 | 2 | 3 | 6 | 9 | 16 | 23 | 44 |

## 86.21: EXCISION OF PILONID CYST. Formerly included in operation group(s) 772.

| Type of Patients | Observed Patients | Avg. Stay | Variance | 10th | 25th | 50th | 75th | 90th | 95th | 99th |
|---|---|---|---|---|---|---|---|---|---|---|
| **1. SINGLE DX** | | | | | | | | | | |
| 0–19 Years | 139 | 2.1 | 5 | 1 | 1 | 1 | 2 | 5 | 8 | 9 |
| 20–34 | 81 | 1.6 | 1 | 1 | 1 | 1 | 2 | 3 | 4 | 6 |
| 35–49 | 23 | 2.6 | 3 | 1 | 2 | 2 | 3 | 6 | 6 | 7 |
| 50–64 | 6 | 1.5 | <1 | 1 | 1 | 1 | 2 | 2 | 2 | 2 |
| 65+ | 0 | | | | | | | | | |
| **2. MULTIPLE DX** | | | | | | | | | | |
| 0–19 Years | 75 | 2.6 | 6 | 1 | 1 | 2 | 3 | 4 | 6 | 12 |
| 20–34 | 68 | 2.3 | 15 | 1 | 1 | 2 | 3 | 4 | 4 | 6 |
| 35–49 | 38 | 4.3 | 8 | 1 | 2 | 4 | 7 | 7 | 8 | 19 |
| 50–64 | 19 | 3.0 | 9 | 1 | 2 | 2 | 2 | 9 | 12 | 14 |
| 65+ | 6 | 6.1 | 8 | 1 | 5 | 7 | 7 | 7 | 12 | 12 |
| **TOTAL SINGLE DX** | 249 | 1.9 | 3 | 1 | 1 | 1 | 2 | 4 | 6 | 8 |
| **TOTAL MULTIPLE DX** | 206 | 3.0 | 11 | 1 | 1 | 2 | 3 | 7 | 8 | 13 |
| **TOTAL** | | | | | | | | | | |
| 0–19 Years | 214 | 2.2 | 5 | 1 | 1 | 1 | 2 | 4 | 4 | 11 |
| 20–34 | 149 | 1.9 | 7 | 1 | 1 | 1 | 2 | 4 | 4 | 6 |
| 35–49 | 61 | 3.7 | 7 | 1 | 2 | 3 | 6 | 7 | 8 | 8 |
| 50–64 | 25 | 2.9 | 9 | 1 | 2 | 2 | 2 | 4 | 12 | 13 |
| 65+ | 6 | 6.1 | 8 | 1 | 5 | 7 | 7 | 7 | 12 | 12 |
| **GRAND TOTAL** | 455 | 2.4 | 7 | 1 | 1 | 2 | 3 | 5 | 7 | 11 |

## 86.2: EXC/DESTR SKIN LESION. Formerly included in operation group(s) 772, 774, 779, 780.

| Type of Patients | Observed Patients | Avg. Stay | Variance | 10th | 25th | 50th | 75th | 90th | 95th | 99th |
|---|---|---|---|---|---|---|---|---|---|---|
| **1. SINGLE DX** | | | | | | | | | | |
| 0–19 Years | 1,034 | 2.8 | 8 | 1 | 1 | 2 | 3 | 6 | 8 | 14 |
| 20–34 | 950 | 3.2 | 11 | 1 | 1 | 2 | 4 | 7 | 9 | 15 |
| 35–49 | 847 | 3.4 | 11 | 1 | 1 | 2 | 4 | 6 | 10 | 17 |
| 50–64 | 336 | 4.2 | 18 | 1 | 2 | 3 | 5 | 9 | 13 | 19 |
| 65+ | 243 | 4.1 | 15 | 1 | 2 | 3 | 5 | 8 | 12 | 17 |
| **2. MULTIPLE DX** | | | | | | | | | | |
| 0–19 Years | 5,049 | 5.8 | 65 | 2 | 2 | 3 | 6 | 14 | 21 | 43 |
| 20–34 | 5,837 | 7.4 | 77 | 1 | 3 | 5 | 9 | 16 | 22 | 51 |
| 35–49 | 11,301 | 9.3 | 111 | 2 | 3 | 6 | 11 | 20 | 30 | 65 |
| 50–64 | 12,988 | 10.2 | 101 | 2 | 4 | 7 | 13 | 21 | 29 | 53 |
| 65+ | 24,481 | 10.8 | 105 | 3 | 5 | 8 | 13 | 21 | 30 | 55 |
| **TOTAL SINGLE DX** | 3,410 | 3.3 | 11 | 1 | 1 | 2 | 4 | 7 | 9 | 17 |
| **TOTAL MULTIPLE DX** | 59,656 | 9.6 | 102 | 2 | 4 | 7 | 12 | 20 | 28 | 55 |
| **TOTAL** | | | | | | | | | | |
| 0–19 Years | 6,083 | 5.2 | 55 | 1 | 2 | 3 | 5 | 12 | 19 | 39 |
| 20–34 | 6,787 | 6.8 | 70 | 1 | 2 | 4 | 8 | 15 | 21 | 47 |
| 35–49 | 12,148 | 8.9 | 106 | 2 | 3 | 6 | 11 | 19 | 29 | 64 |
| 50–64 | 13,324 | 10.0 | 100 | 2 | 4 | 7 | 13 | 21 | 28 | 53 |
| 65+ | 24,724 | 10.7 | 105 | 3 | 5 | 8 | 13 | 21 | 30 | 55 |
| **GRAND TOTAL** | 63,066 | 9.3 | 99 | 2 | 3 | 6 | 11 | 20 | 28 | 54 |

## 86.22: EXC DEBRIDE WND/INFECT. Formerly included in operation group(s) 774.

| Type of Patients | Observed Patients | Avg. Stay | Variance | 10th | 25th | 50th | 75th | 90th | 95th | 99th |
|---|---|---|---|---|---|---|---|---|---|---|
| **1. SINGLE DX** | | | | | | | | | | |
| 0–19 Years | 714 | 3.1 | 8 | 1 | 2 | 2 | 4 | 6 | 7 | 13 |
| 20–34 | 793 | 3.5 | 13 | 1 | 1 | 2 | 4 | 7 | 10 | 15 |
| 35–49 | 761 | 3.5 | 12 | 1 | 1 | 2 | 4 | 6 | 11 | 17 |
| 50–64 | 311 | 4.2 | 18 | 1 | 2 | 3 | 5 | 9 | 13 | 19 |
| 65+ | 217 | 4.1 | 15 | 1 | 2 | 3 | 5 | 8 | 12 | 16 |
| **2. MULTIPLE DX** | | | | | | | | | | |
| 0–19 Years | 2,893 | 7.6 | 88 | 1 | 2 | 4 | 9 | 18 | 27 | 47 |
| 20–34 | 5,176 | 7.7 | 83 | 2 | 3 | 5 | 10 | 16 | 23 | 57 |
| 35–49 | 9,969 | 9.6 | 119 | 2 | 3 | 6 | 12 | 21 | 32 | 65 |
| 50–64 | 11,200 | 10.5 | 107 | 2 | 4 | 7 | 13 | 22 | 29 | 56 |
| 65+ | 18,989 | 11.2 | 117 | 3 | 5 | 8 | 14 | 22 | 31 | 59 |
| **TOTAL SINGLE DX** | 2,796 | 3.5 | 12 | 1 | 2 | 3 | 4 | 7 | 10 | 17 |
| **TOTAL MULTIPLE DX** | 48,227 | 10.1 | 111 | 2 | 4 | 7 | 13 | 21 | 30 | 60 |
| **TOTAL** | | | | | | | | | | |
| 0–19 Years | 3,607 | 6.6 | 74 | 1 | 2 | 4 | 7 | 16 | 23 | 46 |
| 20–34 | 5,969 | 7.2 | 75 | 1 | 2 | 4 | 9 | 16 | 22 | 50 |
| 35–49 | 10,730 | 9.2 | 114 | 2 | 3 | 6 | 11 | 20 | 30 | 65 |
| 50–64 | 11,511 | 10.3 | 106 | 3 | 4 | 7 | 13 | 22 | 30 | 55 |
| 65+ | 19,206 | 11.1 | 116 | 3 | 5 | 8 | 14 | 22 | 31 | 59 |
| **GRAND TOTAL** | 51,023 | 9.7 | 108 | 2 | 3 | 7 | 12 | 21 | 29 | 58 |

Length of Stay by Diagnosis and Operation, United States, 2000

# United States, October 1998–September 1999 Data, by Operation

## 86.23: NAIL REMOVAL. Formerly included in operation group(s) 779.

| Type of Patients | Observed Patients | Avg. Stay | Variance | 10th | 25th | 50th | 75th | 90th | 95th | 99th |
|---|---|---|---|---|---|---|---|---|---|---|
| **1. SINGLE DX** | | | | | | | | | | |
| 0–19 Years | 17 | 2.0 | 4 | 1 | 1 | 1 | 2 | 3 | 8 | 8 |
| 20–34 | 0 | | | | | | | | | |
| 35–49 | 4 | 2.8 | 2 | 1 | 1 | 3 | 4 | 4 | 4 | 4 |
| 50–64 | 1 | 2.0 | 0 | 2 | 2 | 2 | 2 | 2 | 2 | 2 |
| 65+ | 2 | 1.0 | 0 | 1 | 1 | 1 | 1 | 1 | 1 | 1 |
| **2. MULTIPLE DX** | | | | | | | | | | |
| 0–19 Years | 44 | 4.3 | 90 | 1 | 1 | 2 | 4 | 8 | 10 | 17 |
| 20–34 | 43 | 4.7 | 24 | 1 | 2 | 3 | 6 | 12 | 14 | 28 |
| 35–49 | 81 | 9.0 | 84 | 2 | 5 | 7 | 14 | 14 | 14 | 87 |
| 50–64 | 120 | 7.7 | 50 | 2 | 3 | 5 | 12 | 15 | 20 | 42 |
| 65+ | 327 | 8.8 | 59 | 2 | 4 | 6 | 11 | 21 | 27 | 32 |
| **TOTAL SINGLE DX** | 24 | 2.0 | 3 | 1 | 1 | 1 | 2 | 3 | 8 | 8 |
| **TOTAL MULTIPLE DX** | 615 | 8.1 | 64 | 2 | 3 | 6 | 10 | 16 | 27 | 33 |
| **TOTAL** | | | | | | | | | | |
| 0–19 Years | 61 | 3.6 | 67 | 1 | 1 | 2 | 4 | 8 | 8 | 17 |
| 20–34 | 43 | 4.7 | 24 | 1 | 2 | 3 | 6 | 12 | 14 | 28 |
| 35–49 | 85 | 8.9 | 84 | 2 | 4 | 5 | 14 | 14 | 14 | 87 |
| 50–64 | 121 | 7.6 | 50 | 2 | 3 | 6 | 10 | 14 | 20 | 42 |
| 65+ | 329 | 8.8 | 59 | 2 | 4 | 6 | 11 | 21 | 27 | 32 |
| **GRAND TOTAL** | 639 | 7.9 | 63 | 1 | 3 | 5 | 10 | 15 | 26 | 33 |

## 86.26: LIG DERMAL APPENDAGE. Formerly included in operation group(s) 780.

| Type of Patients | Observed Patients | Avg. Stay | Variance | 10th | 25th | 50th | 75th | 90th | 95th | 99th |
|---|---|---|---|---|---|---|---|---|---|---|
| **1. SINGLE DX** | | | | | | | | | | |
| 0–19 Years | 26 | 1.1 | <1 | 1 | 1 | 1 | 1 | 1 | 1 | 2 |
| 20–34 | 0 | | | | | | | | | |
| 35–49 | 0 | | | | | | | | | |
| 50–64 | 0 | | | | | | | | | |
| 65+ | | | | | | | | | | |
| **2. MULTIPLE DX** | | | | | | | | | | |
| 0–19 Years | 1,421 | 2.5 | 13 | 1 | 1 | 2 | 3 | 3 | 5 | 17 |
| 20–34 | 0 | | | | | | | | | |
| 35–49 | 1 | 1.0 | 0 | 1 | 1 | 1 | 1 | 1 | 1 | 1 |
| 50–64 | 2 | 5.0 | 0 | 5 | 5 | 5 | 5 | 5 | 5 | 5 |
| 65+ | 1 | 11.0 | 0 | 11 | 11 | 11 | 11 | 11 | 11 | 11 |
| **TOTAL SINGLE DX** | 26 | 1.1 | <1 | 1 | 1 | 1 | 1 | 1 | 1 | 2 |
| **TOTAL MULTIPLE DX** | 1,425 | 2.5 | 13 | 1 | 1 | 2 | 3 | 3 | 5 | 17 |
| **TOTAL** | | | | | | | | | | |
| 0–19 Years | 1,447 | 2.5 | 13 | 1 | 1 | 2 | 3 | 3 | 5 | 17 |
| 20–34 | 0 | | | | | | | | | |
| 35–49 | 1 | 1.0 | 0 | 1 | 1 | 1 | 1 | 1 | 1 | 1 |
| 50–64 | 2 | 5.0 | 0 | 5 | 5 | 5 | 5 | 5 | 5 | 5 |
| 65+ | 1 | 11.0 | 0 | 11 | 11 | 11 | 11 | 11 | 11 | 11 |
| **GRAND TOTAL** | 1,451 | 2.5 | 13 | 1 | 1 | 2 | 3 | 3 | 5 | 17 |

## 86.27: DEBRIDEMENT OF NAIL. Formerly included in operation group(s) 780.

| Type of Patients | Observed Patients | Avg. Stay | Variance | 10th | 25th | 50th | 75th | 90th | 95th | 99th |
|---|---|---|---|---|---|---|---|---|---|---|
| **1. SINGLE DX** | | | | | | | | | | |
| 0–19 Years | 7 | 1.1 | <1 | 1 | 1 | 1 | 1 | 1 | 2 | 2 |
| 20–34 | 0 | | | | | | | | | |
| 35–49 | 2 | 3.6 | 1 | | | | | | | |
| 50–64 | 1 | 20.0 | 0 | 20 | 20 | 20 | 20 | 20 | 20 | 20 |
| 65+ | 4 | 4.6 | 8 | 2 | 2 | 3 | 6 | 9 | 9 | 9 |
| **2. MULTIPLE DX** | | | | | | | | | | |
| 0–19 Years | 11 | 10.0 | 74 | 1 | 1 | 12 | 20 | 20 | 20 | >99 |
| 20–34 | 46 | 13.0 | 68 | 4 | 8 | 14 | 15 | 20 | 25 | 58 |
| 35–49 | 230 | 11.2 | 57 | 5 | 7 | 9 | 13 | 18 | 25 | 43 |
| 50–64 | 478 | 11.5 | 93 | 3 | 5 | 9 | 15 | 24 | 31 | 55 |
| 65+ | 2,654 | 10.4 | 75 | 3 | 5 | 8 | 13 | 20 | 25 | 50 |
| **TOTAL SINGLE DX** | 14 | 2.0 | 10 | 1 | 1 | 1 | 2 | 4 | 6 | 20 |
| **TOTAL MULTIPLE DX** | 3,419 | 10.7 | 76 | 3 | 5 | 8 | 14 | 21 | 26 | 51 |
| **TOTAL** | | | | | | | | | | |
| 0–19 Years | 18 | 4.3 | 45 | 1 | 1 | 2 | 2 | 20 | 20 | >99 |
| 20–34 | 46 | 13.0 | 68 | 4 | 8 | 14 | 15 | 20 | 25 | 58 |
| 35–49 | 232 | 11.1 | 57 | 5 | 7 | 9 | 13 | 18 | 25 | 43 |
| 50–64 | 479 | 11.6 | 93 | 3 | 5 | 9 | 15 | 24 | 31 | 55 |
| 65+ | 2,658 | 10.4 | 75 | 3 | 5 | 8 | 13 | 20 | 25 | 50 |
| **GRAND TOTAL** | 3,433 | 10.6 | 76 | 3 | 5 | 8 | 14 | 20 | 26 | 51 |

## 86.28: NONEXC DEBRIDEMENT WOUND. Formerly included in operation group(s) 779.

| Type of Patients | Observed Patients | Avg. Stay | Variance | 10th | 25th | 50th | 75th | 90th | 95th | 99th |
|---|---|---|---|---|---|---|---|---|---|---|
| **1. SINGLE DX** | | | | | | | | | | |
| 0–19 Years | 130 | 2.8 | 8 | 1 | 1 | 2 | 3 | 7 | 8 | 14 |
| 20–34 | 75 | 3.3 | 7 | 1 | 2 | 3 | 4 | 6 | 7 | 21 |
| 35–49 | 57 | 2.3 | 3 | 1 | 2 | 3 | 3 | 5 | 5 | 11 |
| 50–64 | 14 | 3.8 | 5 | 1 | 3 | 3 | 6 | 7 | 7 | 7 |
| 65+ | 20 | 4.9 | 14 | 1 | 3 | 5 | 7 | 7 | 14 | 19 |
| **2. MULTIPLE DX** | | | | | | | | | | |
| 0–19 Years | 601 | 4.6 | 35 | 1 | 1 | 3 | 5 | 10 | 13 | 28 |
| 20–34 | 504 | 5.2 | 31 | 1 | 2 | 4 | 6 | 9 | 13 | 29 |
| 35–49 | 981 | 5.9 | 34 | 2 | 3 | 4 | 7 | 12 | 15 | 31 |
| 50–64 | 1,162 | 7.1 | 35 | 2 | 3 | 6 | 9 | 13 | 17 | 29 |
| 65+ | 2,495 | 8.7 | 60 | 3 | 4 | 7 | 10 | 16 | 27 | 42 |
| **TOTAL SINGLE DX** | 296 | 3.0 | 7 | 1 | 1 | 2 | 4 | 6 | 8 | 14 |
| **TOTAL MULTIPLE DX** | 5,743 | 7.1 | 47 | 2 | 3 | 5 | 9 | 14 | 20 | 35 |
| **TOTAL** | | | | | | | | | | |
| 0–19 Years | 731 | 4.2 | 30 | 1 | 1 | 2 | 5 | 9 | 13 | 27 |
| 20–34 | 579 | 5.0 | 29 | 1 | 2 | 4 | 6 | 8 | 13 | 24 |
| 35–49 | 1,038 | 5.7 | 33 | 2 | 3 | 6 | 7 | 12 | 15 | 31 |
| 50–64 | 1,176 | 7.1 | 35 | 2 | 3 | 6 | 9 | 13 | 17 | 29 |
| 65+ | 2,515 | 8.7 | 60 | 3 | 4 | 7 | 10 | 16 | 27 | 42 |
| **GRAND TOTAL** | 6,039 | 6.9 | 46 | 2 | 3 | 5 | 8 | 13 | 19 | 34 |

Length of Stay by Diagnosis and Operation, United States, 2000

## United States, October 1998–September 1999 Data, by Operation

### 86.3: OTH LOC EXC/DESTR SKIN. Formerly included in operation group(s) 773.

| Type of Patients | Observed Patients | Avg. Stay | Variance | 10th | 25th | 50th | 75th | 90th | 95th | 99th |
|---|---|---|---|---|---|---|---|---|---|---|
| **1. SINGLE DX** | | | | | | | | | | |
| 0–19 Years | 336 | 1.3 | 1 | 1 | 1 | 1 | 1 | 2 | 3 | 5 |
| 20–34 | 86 | 2.0 | 5 | 1 | 1 | 1 | 2 | 5 | 5 | 14 |
| 35–49 | 125 | 2.4 | 5 | 1 | 1 | 1 | 3 | 5 | 5 | 13 |
| 50–64 | 60 | 2.1 | 3 | 1 | 1 | 1 | 3 | 3 | 6 | 8 |
| 65+ | 43 | 2.5 | 3 | 1 | 1 | 2 | 3 | 5 | 5 | 8 |
| **2. MULTIPLE DX** | | | | | | | | | | |
| 0–19 Years | 362 | 3.6 | 41 | 1 | 1 | 2 | 3 | 6 | 13 | 31 |
| 20–34 | 254 | 4.7 | 52 | 1 | 1 | 2 | 5 | 13 | 16 | 44 |
| 35–49 | 567 | 5.4 | 40 | 1 | 2 | 3 | 7 | 11 | 15 | 35 |
| 50–64 | 581 | 5.4 | 42 | 1 | 2 | 3 | 7 | 11 | 16 | 35 |
| 65+ | 1,256 | 7.0 | 58 | 1 | 3 | 5 | 8 | 13 | 18 | 38 |
| **TOTAL SINGLE DX** | 650 | 1.6 | 3 | 1 | 1 | 1 | 1 | 3 | 4 | 8 |
| **TOTAL MULTIPLE DX** | 3,020 | 5.7 | 49 | 1 | 2 | 3 | 7 | 13 | 16 | 35 |
| **TOTAL** | | | | | | | | | | |
| 0–19 Years | 698 | 2.3 | 20 | 1 | 1 | 1 | 2 | 5 | 6 | 23 |
| 20–34 | 340 | 4.1 | 41 | 1 | 1 | 2 | 4 | 10 | 16 | 33 |
| 35–49 | 692 | 5.0 | 36 | 1 | 2 | 3 | 6 | 10 | 14 | 28 |
| 50–64 | 641 | 5.1 | 39 | 1 | 2 | 3 | 6 | 11 | 15 | 35 |
| 65+ | 1,299 | 6.8 | 57 | 1 | 3 | 5 | 8 | 13 | 17 | 38 |
| **GRAND TOTAL** | 3,670 | 4.8 | 42 | 1 | 1 | 3 | 6 | 11 | 15 | 32 |

### 86.5: SKIN & SUBCU SUTURE. Formerly included in operation group(s) 775.

| Type of Patients | Observed Patients | Avg. Stay | Variance | 10th | 25th | 50th | 75th | 90th | 95th | 99th |
|---|---|---|---|---|---|---|---|---|---|---|
| **1. SINGLE DX** | | | | | | | | | | |
| 0–19 Years | 1,267 | 1.4 | 1 | 1 | 1 | 1 | 1 | 3 | 3 | 6 |
| 20–34 | 219 | 1.8 | 3 | 1 | 1 | 1 | 2 | 3 | 4 | 13 |
| 35–49 | 114 | 1.8 | 2 | 1 | 1 | 1 | 2 | 3 | 5 | 8 |
| 50–64 | 38 | 1.6 | <1 | 1 | 1 | 1 | 2 | 3 | 3 | 4 |
| 65+ | 55 | 2.2 | 3 | 1 | 1 | 1 | 3 | 5 | 6 | 6 |
| **2. MULTIPLE DX** | | | | | | | | | | |
| 0–19 Years | 2,401 | 3.0 | 22 | 1 | 1 | 2 | 3 | 6 | 8 | 26 |
| 20–34 | 3,416 | 3.2 | 17 | 1 | 1 | 2 | 4 | 7 | 9 | 23 |
| 35–49 | 3,159 | 3.1 | 15 | 1 | 1 | 2 | 4 | 6 | 8 | 19 |
| 50–64 | 1,815 | 3.7 | 17 | 1 | 2 | 3 | 5 | 7 | 10 | 20 |
| 65+ | 5,602 | 4.8 | 26 | 1 | 2 | 3 | 6 | 9 | 13 | 26 |
| **TOTAL SINGLE DX** | 1,693 | 1.6 | 2 | 1 | 1 | 1 | 2 | 3 | 4 | 7 |
| **TOTAL MULTIPLE DX** | 16,393 | 3.7 | 21 | 1 | 1 | 2 | 4 | 7 | 10 | 24 |
| **TOTAL** | | | | | | | | | | |
| 0–19 Years | 3,668 | 2.8 | 19 | 1 | 1 | 2 | 3 | 5 | 7 | 26 |
| 20–34 | 3,635 | 3.1 | 16 | 1 | 1 | 2 | 3 | 6 | 9 | 23 |
| 35–49 | 3,273 | 3.1 | 14 | 1 | 1 | 2 | 3 | 6 | 8 | 19 |
| 50–64 | 1,853 | 3.6 | 17 | 1 | 1 | 3 | 5 | 7 | 9 | 19 |
| 65+ | 5,657 | 4.7 | 26 | 1 | 2 | 3 | 6 | 9 | 13 | 26 |
| **GRAND TOTAL** | 18,086 | 3.6 | 20 | 1 | 1 | 2 | 4 | 7 | 10 | 24 |

### 86.4: RAD EXCISION SKIN LESION. Formerly included in operation group(s) 775.

| Type of Patients | Observed Patients | Avg. Stay | Variance | 10th | 25th | 50th | 75th | 90th | 95th | 99th |
|---|---|---|---|---|---|---|---|---|---|---|
| **1. SINGLE DX** | | | | | | | | | | |
| 0–19 Years | 80 | 1.6 | 2 | 1 | 1 | 1 | 1 | 2 | 5 | 8 |
| 20–34 | 55 | 2.6 | 19 | 1 | 1 | 1 | 2 | 5 | 9 | 41 |
| 35–49 | 73 | 2.1 | 3 | 1 | 1 | 2 | 3 | 4 | 5 | 9 |
| 50–64 | 78 | 2.3 | 5 | 1 | 1 | 1 | 2 | 6 | 8 | 13 |
| 65+ | 116 | 2.5 | 6 | 1 | 1 | 2 | 3 | 5 | 7 | 14 |
| **2. MULTIPLE DX** | | | | | | | | | | |
| 0–19 Years | 96 | 7.1 | 84 | 1 | 3 | 3 | 9 | 21 | 28 | 31 |
| 20–34 | 146 | 7.6 | 54 | 1 | 3 | 6 | 9 | 15 | 22 | 36 |
| 35–49 | 322 | 7.9 | 117 | 1 | 2 | 4 | 8 | 20 | 27 | 59 |
| 50–64 | 401 | 6.2 | 80 | 1 | 2 | 3 | 7 | 13 | 19 | 62 |
| 65+ | 1,022 | 6.2 | 56 | 1 | 2 | 4 | 7 | 15 | 23 | 35 |
| **TOTAL SINGLE DX** | 402 | 2.2 | 6 | 1 | 1 | 1 | 2 | 4 | 7 | 10 |
| **TOTAL MULTIPLE DX** | 1,987 | 6.6 | 72 | 1 | 2 | 4 | 8 | 16 | 23 | 40 |
| **TOTAL** | | | | | | | | | | |
| 0–19 Years | 176 | 4.0 | 45 | 1 | 1 | 3 | 3 | 9 | 20 | 31 |
| 20–34 | 201 | 6.3 | 50 | 1 | 4 | 4 | 8 | 13 | 21 | 36 |
| 35–49 | 395 | 6.9 | 103 | 1 | 3 | 3 | 7 | 19 | 24 | 58 |
| 50–64 | 479 | 5.5 | 69 | 1 | 1 | 3 | 6 | 12 | 16 | 48 |
| 65+ | 1,138 | 5.8 | 52 | 1 | 3 | 3 | 7 | 15 | 21 | 33 |
| **GRAND TOTAL** | 2,389 | 5.8 | 63 | 1 | 3 | 3 | 7 | 14 | 21 | 38 |

### 86.59: SKIN SUTURE NEC. Formerly included in operation group(s) 775.

| Type of Patients | Observed Patients | Avg. Stay | Variance | 10th | 25th | 50th | 75th | 90th | 95th | 99th |
|---|---|---|---|---|---|---|---|---|---|---|
| **1. SINGLE DX** | | | | | | | | | | |
| 0–19 Years | 1,266 | 1.4 | 1 | 1 | 1 | 1 | 1 | 3 | 3 | 6 |
| 20–34 | 219 | 1.8 | 3 | 1 | 1 | 1 | 2 | 3 | 4 | 13 |
| 35–49 | 112 | 1.8 | 2 | 1 | 1 | 1 | 2 | 3 | 5 | 8 |
| 50–64 | 38 | 1.6 | <1 | 1 | 1 | 1 | 2 | 3 | 3 | 4 |
| 65+ | 53 | 2.2 | 3 | 1 | 1 | 1 | 3 | 5 | 6 | 6 |
| **2. MULTIPLE DX** | | | | | | | | | | |
| 0–19 Years | 2,394 | 3.0 | 22 | 1 | 1 | 2 | 3 | 6 | 8 | 26 |
| 20–34 | 3,412 | 3.2 | 17 | 1 | 1 | 2 | 4 | 7 | 9 | 23 |
| 35–49 | 3,154 | 3.1 | 15 | 1 | 1 | 2 | 4 | 6 | 8 | 19 |
| 50–64 | 1,810 | 3.7 | 17 | 1 | 2 | 3 | 5 | 7 | 10 | 20 |
| 65+ | 5,596 | 4.8 | 26 | 1 | 2 | 3 | 6 | 9 | 13 | 26 |
| **TOTAL SINGLE DX** | 1,688 | 1.6 | 2 | 1 | 1 | 1 | 2 | 3 | 4 | 7 |
| **TOTAL MULTIPLE DX** | 16,366 | 3.7 | 21 | 1 | 1 | 2 | 4 | 7 | 10 | 24 |
| **TOTAL** | | | | | | | | | | |
| 0–19 Years | 3,660 | 2.8 | 19 | 1 | 1 | 2 | 3 | 5 | 7 | 26 |
| 20–34 | 3,631 | 3.1 | 16 | 1 | 1 | 2 | 3 | 6 | 9 | 23 |
| 35–49 | 3,266 | 3.1 | 14 | 1 | 1 | 2 | 3 | 6 | 8 | 19 |
| 50–64 | 1,848 | 3.6 | 17 | 1 | 1 | 3 | 5 | 7 | 9 | 20 |
| 65+ | 5,649 | 4.7 | 26 | 1 | 2 | 3 | 6 | 9 | 13 | 26 |
| **GRAND TOTAL** | 18,054 | 3.6 | 20 | 1 | 1 | 2 | 4 | 7 | 10 | 24 |

Length of Stay by Diagnosis and Operation, United States, 2000

## United States, October 1998–September 1999 Data, by Operation

### 86.6: FREE SKIN GRAFT. Formerly included in operation group(s) 777.

| Type of Patients | Observed Patients | Avg. Stay | Vari-ance | Percentiles | | | | | | |
|---|---|---|---|---|---|---|---|---|---|---|
| | | | | 10th | 25th | 50th | 75th | 90th | 95th | 99th |
| **1. SINGLE DX** | | | | | | | | | | |
| 0–19 Years | 170 | 5.5 | 36 | 1 | 1 | 3 | 8 | 12 | 21 | 25 |
| 20–34 | 154 | 5.3 | 24 | 1 | 1 | 4 | 6 | 14 | 14 | 18 |
| 35–49 | 154 | 4.3 | 15 | 1 | 2 | 3 | 6 | 8 | 11 | 18 |
| 50–64 | 104 | 4.8 | 15 | 1 | 1 | 4 | 6 | 10 | 12 | 16 |
| 65+ | 88 | 3.9 | 7 | 1 | 2 | 3 | 5 | 7 | 10 | 12 |
| **2. MULTIPLE DX** | | | | | | | | | | |
| 0–19 Years | 1,007 | 12.4 | 128 | 1 | 4 | 10 | 17 | 26 | 34 | 66 |
| 20–34 | 1,022 | 10.9 | 91 | 2 | 4 | 9 | 15 | 22 | 28 | 50 |
| 35–49 | 1,549 | 12.1 | 121 | 2 | 4 | 9 | 16 | 26 | 39 | 47 |
| 50–64 | 1,213 | 11.4 | 168 | 1 | 4 | 7 | 12 | 29 | 35 | 72 |
| 65+ | 1,839 | 10.4 | 111 | 2 | 4 | 7 | 13 | 25 | 33 | 48 |
| **TOTAL SINGLE DX** | 670 | 4.9 | 23 | 1 | 1 | 3 | 6 | 11 | 14 | 21 |
| **TOTAL MULTIPLE DX** | 6,630 | 11.4 | 123 | 2 | 4 | 8 | 15 | 25 | 34 | 55 |
| **TOTAL** | | | | | | | | | | |
| 0–19 Years | 1,177 | 11.3 | 120 | 1 | 3 | 8 | 17 | 25 | 32 | 66 |
| 20–34 | 1,176 | 10.2 | 87 | 1 | 4 | 8 | 14 | 22 | 28 | 47 |
| 35–49 | 1,703 | 11.4 | 116 | 2 | 4 | 8 | 16 | 25 | 37 | 46 |
| 50–64 | 1,317 | 11.0 | 161 | 1 | 3 | 7 | 12 | 28 | 35 | 72 |
| 65+ | 1,927 | 10.2 | 109 | 2 | 3 | 7 | 13 | 24 | 33 | 48 |
| **GRAND TOTAL** | 7,300 | 10.8 | 118 | 1 | 4 | 7 | 14 | 25 | 33 | 52 |

### 86.62: HAND SKIN GRAFT NEC. Formerly included in operation group(s) 777.

| Type of Patients | Observed Patients | Avg. Stay | Vari-ance | Percentiles | | | | | | |
|---|---|---|---|---|---|---|---|---|---|---|
| | | | | 10th | 25th | 50th | 75th | 90th | 95th | 99th |
| **1. SINGLE DX** | | | | | | | | | | |
| 0–19 Years | 10 | 3.8 | 15 | 1 | 1 | 2 | 3 | 11 | 13 | 13 |
| 20–34 | 6 | 1.5 | <1 | 1 | 1 | 1 | 2 | 2 | 3 | 3 |
| 35–49 | 5 | 3.8 | 16 | 1 | 1 | 2 | 6 | 11 | 11 | 11 |
| 50–64 | 5 | 1.6 | 2 | 1 | 1 | 1 | 1 | 5 | 5 | 5 |
| 65+ | 0 | | | | | | | | | |
| **2. MULTIPLE DX** | | | | | | | | | | |
| 0–19 Years | 68 | 15.5 | 394 | 1 | 2 | 8 | 17 | 66 | 66 | 66 |
| 20–34 | 88 | 8.4 | 97 | 1 | 2 | 5 | 11 | 19 | 22 | 57 |
| 35–49 | 94 | 13.0 | 96 | 3 | 3 | 12 | 19 | 24 | 30 | 44 |
| 50–64 | 26 | 9.8 | 113 | 2 | 3 | 6 | 12 | 35 | 35 | 46 |
| 65+ | 38 | 9.8 | 74 | 3 | 4 | 6 | 12 | 27 | 29 | 33 |
| **TOTAL SINGLE DX** | 26 | 2.7 | 9 | 1 | 1 | 2 | 2 | 7 | 11 | 13 |
| **TOTAL MULTIPLE DX** | 314 | 11.7 | 157 | 1 | 3 | 7 | 17 | 24 | 34 | 66 |
| **TOTAL** | | | | | | | | | | |
| 0–19 Years | 78 | 14.5 | 372 | 1 | 2 | 7 | 17 | 56 | 66 | 66 |
| 20–34 | 94 | 8.1 | 95 | 1 | 1 | 5 | 11 | 19 | 22 | 57 |
| 35–49 | 99 | 12.8 | 96 | 3 | 3 | 12 | 18 | 24 | 30 | 44 |
| 50–64 | 31 | 8.6 | 104 | 3 | 2 | 6 | 12 | 15 | 35 | 46 |
| 65+ | 38 | 9.8 | 74 | 3 | 4 | 6 | 12 | 27 | 29 | 33 |
| **GRAND TOTAL** | 340 | 11.2 | 153 | 1 | 3 | 7 | 17 | 24 | 34 | 66 |

### 86.63: FTHICK SKIN GRAFT NEC. Formerly included in operation group(s) 777.

| Type of Patients | Observed Patients | Avg. Stay | Vari-ance | Percentiles | | | | | | |
|---|---|---|---|---|---|---|---|---|---|---|
| | | | | 10th | 25th | 50th | 75th | 90th | 95th | 99th |
| **1. SINGLE DX** | | | | | | | | | | |
| 0–19 Years | 11 | 7.6 | 15 | 1 | 5 | 10 | 10 | 10 | 10 | 10 |
| 20–34 | 8 | 2.8 | 15 | 1 | 1 | 1 | 3 | 6 | 14 | 17 |
| 35–49 | 6 | 3.0 | <1 | 2 | 2 | 3 | 4 | 4 | 4 | 4 |
| 50–64 | 6 | 2.6 | 4 | 1 | 1 | 1 | 3 | 6 | 6 | 6 |
| 65+ | 2 | 1.5 | <1 | 1 | 1 | 2 | 2 | 2 | 2 | 2 |
| **2. MULTIPLE DX** | | | | | | | | | | |
| 0–19 Years | 56 | 4.2 | 31 | 1 | 1 | 2 | 4 | 12 | 18 | 25 |
| 20–34 | 34 | 7.3 | 22 | 1 | 3 | 5 | 13 | 13 | 13 | 13 |
| 35–49 | 49 | 10.0 | 57 | 1 | 4 | 8 | 14 | 21 | 25 | 32 |
| 50–64 | 50 | 6.9 | 76 | 1 | 2 | 3 | 8 | 17 | 24 | 39 |
| 65+ | 119 | 8.0 | 89 | 1 | 2 | 4 | 12 | 15 | 26 | 48 |
| **TOTAL SINGLE DX** | 33 | 4.1 | 15 | 1 | 1 | 3 | 6 | 10 | 10 | 17 |
| **TOTAL MULTIPLE DX** | 308 | 7.3 | 64 | 1 | 2 | 4 | 12 | 15 | 24 | 39 |
| **TOTAL** | | | | | | | | | | |
| 0–19 Years | 67 | 4.8 | 30 | 1 | 1 | 2 | 8 | 10 | 18 | 25 |
| 20–34 | 42 | 5.9 | 24 | 1 | 1 | 4 | 13 | 13 | 13 | 17 |
| 35–49 | 55 | 8.7 | 54 | 1 | 3 | 5 | 14 | 16 | 25 | 32 |
| 50–64 | 56 | 6.7 | 73 | 1 | 2 | 3 | 8 | 17 | 24 | 39 |
| 65+ | 121 | 7.9 | 88 | 1 | 2 | 4 | 12 | 15 | 26 | 48 |
| **GRAND TOTAL** | 341 | 6.9 | 59 | 1 | 2 | 4 | 10 | 14 | 22 | 39 |

### 86.69: FREE SKIN GRAFT NEC. Formerly included in operation group(s) 777.

| Type of Patients | Observed Patients | Avg. Stay | Vari-ance | Percentiles | | | | | | |
|---|---|---|---|---|---|---|---|---|---|---|
| | | | | 10th | 25th | 50th | 75th | 90th | 95th | 99th |
| **1. SINGLE DX** | | | | | | | | | | |
| 0–19 Years | 137 | 5.5 | 37 | 1 | 1 | 3 | 8 | 14 | 21 | 21 |
| 20–34 | 129 | 6.0 | 25 | 1 | 2 | 5 | 7 | 14 | 14 | 23 |
| 35–49 | 128 | 4.6 | 17 | 1 | 2 | 4 | 7 | 9 | 11 | 20 |
| 50–64 | 90 | 5.2 | 15 | 1 | 2 | 4 | 7 | 10 | 13 | 16 |
| 65+ | 79 | 4.1 | 7 | 1 | 2 | 4 | 6 | 8 | 10 | 12 |
| **2. MULTIPLE DX** | | | | | | | | | | |
| 0–19 Years | 714 | 12.9 | 104 | 2 | 6 | 11 | 18 | 25 | 30 | 50 |
| 20–34 | 773 | 11.3 | 82 | 2 | 5 | 10 | 16 | 22 | 28 | 45 |
| 35–49 | 1,248 | 11.3 | 110 | 2 | 4 | 7 | 16 | 23 | 35 | 46 |
| 50–64 | 1,042 | 10.9 | 121 | 2 | 4 | 7 | 12 | 28 | 34 | 53 |
| 65+ | 1,574 | 10.4 | 112 | 2 | 4 | 7 | 13 | 25 | 33 | 48 |
| **TOTAL SINGLE DX** | 563 | 5.2 | 24 | 1 | 2 | 4 | 7 | 12 | 15 | 21 |
| **TOTAL MULTIPLE DX** | 5,351 | 11.2 | 108 | 2 | 4 | 8 | 15 | 25 | 32 | 48 |
| **TOTAL** | | | | | | | | | | |
| 0–19 Years | 851 | 11.6 | 100 | 1 | 4 | 10 | 17 | 25 | 28 | 49 |
| 20–34 | 902 | 10.6 | 78 | 2 | 4 | 9 | 15 | 22 | 28 | 44 |
| 35–49 | 1,376 | 10.7 | 105 | 2 | 4 | 7 | 16 | 23 | 32 | 44 |
| 50–64 | 1,132 | 10.6 | 117 | 2 | 4 | 7 | 12 | 25 | 34 | 50 |
| 65+ | 1,653 | 10.2 | 110 | 2 | 4 | 7 | 13 | 25 | 33 | 48 |
| **GRAND TOTAL** | 5,914 | 10.7 | 103 | 2 | 4 | 7 | 14 | 24 | 31 | 47 |

Length of Stay by Diagnosis and Operation, United States, 2000

# United States, October 1998–September 1999 Data, by Operation

## 86.7: PEDICLE GRAFTS OR FLAPS. Formerly included in operation group(s) 778.

| Type of Patients | Observed Patients | Avg. Stay | Variance | 10th | 25th | 50th | 75th | 90th | 95th | 99th |
|---|---|---|---|---|---|---|---|---|---|---|
| **1. SINGLE DX** | | | | | | | | | | |
| 0–19 Years | 85 | 2.5 | 16 | 1 | 1 | 1 | 3 | 5 | 8 | 12 |
| 20–34 | 88 | 3.4 | 14 | 1 | 1 | 2 | 5 | 8 | 11 | 14 |
| 35–49 | 84 | 3.4 | 9 | 1 | 1 | 2 | 5 | 8 | 11 | 14 |
| 50–64 | 45 | 4.0 | 9 | 1 | 2 | 3 | 7 | 7 | 8 | 14 |
| 65+ | 41 | 3.8 | 31 | 1 | 1 | 1 | 5 | 9 | 20 | 24 |
| **2. MULTIPLE DX** | | | | | | | | | | |
| 0–19 Years | 278 | 7.8 | 136 | 1 | 2 | 4 | 8 | 21 | 30 | 71 |
| 20–34 | 392 | 8.8 | 118 | 1 | 2 | 5 | 11 | 22 | 30 | 51 |
| 35–49 | 680 | 11.6 | 200 | 1 | 3 | 6 | 15 | 35 | 42 | >99 |
| 50–64 | 616 | 10.6 | 190 | 1 | 3 | 6 | 12 | 23 | 37 | 71 |
| 65+ | 812 | 10.8 | 128 | 1 | 3 | 7 | 14 | 25 | 35 | 50 |
| **TOTAL SINGLE DX** | 343 | 3.2 | 15 | 1 | 1 | 2 | 5 | 7 | 9 | 20 |
| **TOTAL MULTIPLE DX** | 2,778 | 10.3 | 158 | 1 | 3 | 6 | 13 | 26 | 38 | 71 |
| **TOTAL** | | | | | | | | | | |
| 0–19 Years | 363 | 5.9 | 101 | 1 | 1 | 3 | 6 | 13 | 27 | 48 |
| 20–34 | 480 | 7.9 | 104 | 1 | 2 | 5 | 9 | 20 | 30 | 50 |
| 35–49 | 764 | 10.3 | 178 | 1 | 2 | 5 | 13 | 32 | 42 | >99 |
| 50–64 | 661 | 10.0 | 177 | 1 | 3 | 6 | 11 | 22 | 35 | 71 |
| 65+ | 853 | 10.2 | 124 | 1 | 3 | 6 | 13 | 24 | 35 | 50 |
| **GRAND TOTAL** | 3,121 | 9.2 | 143 | 1 | 2 | 5 | 11 | 23 | 35 | 71 |

## 86.74: ATTACH PEDICLE GRAFT NEC. Formerly included in operation group(s) 778.

| Type of Patients | Observed Patients | Avg. Stay | Variance | 10th | 25th | 50th | 75th | 90th | 95th | 99th |
|---|---|---|---|---|---|---|---|---|---|---|
| **1. SINGLE DX** | | | | | | | | | | |
| 0–19 Years | 46 | 2.5 | 8 | 1 | 1 | 1 | 3 | 5 | 9 | 15 |
| 20–34 | 29 | 3.4 | 9 | 1 | 1 | 2 | 5 | 7 | 10 | 14 |
| 35–49 | 38 | 4.3 | 11 | 1 | 1 | 4 | 6 | 8 | 8 | 18 |
| 50–64 | 21 | 4.9 | 6 | 2 | 3 | 5 | 7 | 7 | 8 | 8 |
| 65+ | 31 | 3.9 | 38 | 1 | 1 | 1 | 3 | 10 | 24 | 24 |
| **2. MULTIPLE DX** | | | | | | | | | | |
| 0–19 Years | 151 | 8.7 | 143 | 1 | 2 | 4 | 11 | 25 | 30 | 48 |
| 20–34 | 251 | 10.5 | 137 | 1 | 3 | 7 | 14 | 28 | 37 | 51 |
| 35–49 | 402 | 12.8 | 191 | 2 | 4 | 7 | 18 | 42 | 43 | >99 |
| 50–64 | 377 | 12.8 | 267 | 1 | 3 | 7 | 14 | 28 | 66 | 71 |
| 65+ | 564 | 10.7 | 119 | 1 | 4 | 7 | 14 | 26 | 34 | 55 |
| **TOTAL SINGLE DX** | 165 | 3.8 | 16 | 1 | 1 | 2 | 5 | 7 | 9 | 24 |
| **TOTAL MULTIPLE DX** | 1,745 | 11.4 | 173 | 1 | 3 | 7 | 14 | 29 | 42 | 71 |
| **TOTAL** | | | | | | | | | | |
| 0–19 Years | 197 | 7.3 | 119 | 1 | 1 | 4 | 7 | 13 | 30 | 48 |
| 20–34 | 280 | 9.7 | 128 | 1 | 2 | 6 | 13 | 20 | 34 | 50 |
| 35–49 | 440 | 11.5 | 174 | 1 | 2 | 7 | 15 | 32 | 42 | >99 |
| 50–64 | 398 | 12.2 | 250 | 1 | 3 | 7 | 14 | 27 | 62 | 71 |
| 65+ | 595 | 10.1 | 115 | 1 | 3 | 7 | 13 | 24 | 34 | 55 |
| **GRAND TOTAL** | 1,910 | 10.5 | 161 | 1 | 3 | 6 | 13 | 27 | 39 | 71 |

## 86.72: PEDICLE GRAFT ADV. Formerly included in operation group(s) 778.

| Type of Patients | Observed Patients | Avg. Stay | Variance | 10th | 25th | 50th | 75th | 90th | 95th | 99th |
|---|---|---|---|---|---|---|---|---|---|---|
| **1. SINGLE DX** | | | | | | | | | | |
| 0–19 Years | 10 | 1.8 | 2 | 1 | 1 | 1 | 2 | 3 | 5 | 5 |
| 20–34 | 12 | 3.7 | 7 | 1 | 1 | 3 | 7 | 8 | 8 | 8 |
| 35–49 | 9 | 4.1 | 15 | 1 | 1 | 2 | 5 | 12 | 12 | 12 |
| 50–64 | 5 | 2.8 | 3 | 1 | 2 | 4 | 4 | 5 | 5 | 5 |
| 65+ | 2 | 4.3 | 3 | 1 | 5 | 5 | 5 | 5 | 5 | 5 |
| **2. MULTIPLE DX** | | | | | | | | | | |
| 0–19 Years | 48 | 6.5 | 178 | 1 | 1 | 2 | 4 | 15 | 23 | 85 |
| 20–34 | 35 | 5.8 | 44 | 1 | 2 | 3 | 6 | 13 | 22 | 31 |
| 35–49 | 64 | 8.9 | 277 | 1 | 2 | 4 | 8 | 23 | 28 | 87 |
| 50–64 | 62 | 8.3 | 48 | 1 | 4 | 6 | 11 | 14 | 22 | 32 |
| 65+ | 63 | 16.7 | 306 | 1 | 5 | 7 | 26 | 47 | 47 | 47 |
| **TOTAL SINGLE DX** | 38 | 3.3 | 8 | 1 | 1 | 2 | 5 | 7 | 8 | 12 |
| **TOTAL MULTIPLE DX** | 272 | 9.4 | 182 | 1 | 2 | 5 | 10 | 23 | 47 | 77 |
| **TOTAL** | | | | | | | | | | |
| 0–19 Years | 58 | 5.8 | 156 | 1 | 1 | 2 | 3 | 13 | 23 | 82 |
| 20–34 | 47 | 5.5 | 39 | 1 | 2 | 3 | 6 | 13 | 22 | 31 |
| 35–49 | 73 | 8.3 | 247 | 1 | 2 | 3 | 8 | 21 | 26 | 87 |
| 50–64 | 67 | 8.1 | 48 | 1 | 3 | 6 | 11 | 14 | 22 | 32 |
| 65+ | 65 | 16.2 | 299 | 1 | 5 | 7 | 22 | 47 | 47 | 47 |
| **GRAND TOTAL** | 310 | 8.8 | 168 | 1 | 2 | 5 | 9 | 22 | 47 | 53 |

## 86.75: REV PEDICLE/FLAP GRAFT. Formerly included in operation group(s) 778.

| Type of Patients | Observed Patients | Avg. Stay | Variance | 10th | 25th | 50th | 75th | 90th | 95th | 99th |
|---|---|---|---|---|---|---|---|---|---|---|
| **1. SINGLE DX** | | | | | | | | | | |
| 0–19 Years | 11 | 4.0 | 47 | 1 | 3 | 3 | 5 | 5 | 8 | 8 |
| 20–34 | 16 | 2.7 | 5 | 1 | 2 | 2 | 3 | 5 | 5 | 5 |
| 35–49 | 15 | 2.6 | 3 | 1 | 2 | 2 | 4 | 5 | 5 | 7 |
| 50–64 | 5 | 6.6 | 24 | 1 | 4 | 4 | 12 | 12 | 12 | 12 |
| 65+ | 2 | 2.8 | 3 | 1 | 4 | 4 | 4 | 4 | 4 | 4 |
| **2. MULTIPLE DX** | | | | | | | | | | |
| 0–19 Years | 39 | 5.7 | 81 | 1 | 3 | 3 | 7 | 12 | 24 | 29 |
| 20–34 | 56 | 10.4 | 210 | 2 | 4 | 4 | 14 | 30 | 36 | >99 |
| 35–49 | 121 | 10.2 | 169 | 1 | 3 | 5 | 13 | 23 | 35 | 63 |
| 50–64 | 104 | 7.1 | 81 | 1 | 2 | 5 | 7 | 18 | 27 | >99 |
| 65+ | 103 | 8.5 | 65 | 2 | 3 | 6 | 11 | 18 | 22 | 43 |
| **TOTAL SINGLE DX** | 49 | 3.6 | 27 | 1 | 2 | 2 | 5 | 5 | 8 | 12 |
| **TOTAL MULTIPLE DX** | 423 | 8.6 | 121 | 1 | 2 | 5 | 11 | 21 | 30 | 76 |
| **TOTAL** | | | | | | | | | | |
| 0–19 Years | 50 | 4.8 | 63 | 1 | 2 | 3 | 5 | 8 | 12 | 29 |
| 20–34 | 72 | 8.2 | 164 | 1 | 3 | 5 | 10 | 30 | 30 | >99 |
| 35–49 | 136 | 9.4 | 156 | 1 | 2 | 5 | 11 | 27 | 35 | 63 |
| 50–64 | 109 | 7.0 | 78 | 1 | 2 | 5 | 8 | 17 | 25 | >99 |
| 65+ | 105 | 8.4 | 65 | 2 | 3 | 6 | 11 | 18 | 22 | 43 |
| **GRAND TOTAL** | 472 | 7.8 | 109 | 1 | 2 | 4 | 8 | 18 | 30 | 68 |

Length of Stay by Diagnosis and Operation, United States, 2000

# United States, October 1998–September 1999 Data, by Operation

## 86.8: OTHER SKIN & SUBCU REP. Formerly included in operation group(s) 779.

| Type of Patients | Observed Patients | Avg. Stay | Variance | 10th | 25th | 50th | 75th | 90th | 95th | 99th |
|---|---|---|---|---|---|---|---|---|---|---|
| **1. SINGLE DX** | | | | | | | | | | |
| 0–19 Years | 122 | 1.2 | 1 | 1 | 1 | 1 | 1 | 2 | 2 | 4 |
| 20–34 | 112 | 2.1 | 3 | 1 | 1 | 1 | 3 | 4 | 4 | 6 |
| 35–49 | 210 | 1.4 | <1 | 1 | 1 | 1 | 2 | 2 | 2 | 4 |
| 50–64 | 139 | 1.8 | 5 | 1 | 1 | 1 | 1 | 3 | 10 | 10 |
| 65+ | 37 | 1.7 | <1 | 1 | 1 | 1 | 2 | 2 | 3 | 6 |
| **2. MULTIPLE DX** | | | | | | | | | | |
| 0–19 Years | 219 | 2.8 | 61 | 1 | 1 | 2 | 2 | 4 | 8 | 18 |
| 20–34 | 364 | 2.4 | 4 | 1 | 1 | 2 | 3 | 4 | 5 | 8 |
| 35–49 | 964 | 2.6 | 10 | 1 | 1 | 2 | 3 | 4 | 8 | 18 |
| 50–64 | 850 | 3.2 | 35 | 1 | 1 | 2 | 3 | 6 | 9 | 48 |
| 65+ | 296 | 3.9 | 42 | 1 | 1 | 2 | 4 | 9 | 15 | 43 |
| **TOTAL SINGLE DX** | 620 | 1.6 | 2 | 1 | 1 | 1 | 2 | 2 | 4 | 10 |
| **TOTAL MULTIPLE DX** | 2,693 | 2.9 | 25 | 1 | 1 | 2 | 3 | 5 | 8 | 24 |
| **TOTAL** | | | | | | | | | | |
| 0–19 Years | 341 | 2.1 | 36 | 1 | 1 | 1 | 2 | 3 | 6 | 18 |
| 20–34 | 476 | 2.3 | 4 | 1 | 1 | 2 | 3 | 4 | 5 | 8 |
| 35–49 | 1,174 | 2.4 | 8 | 1 | 1 | 2 | 3 | 4 | 6 | 14 |
| 50–64 | 989 | 3.0 | 30 | 1 | 1 | 2 | 3 | 6 | 10 | 48 |
| 65+ | 333 | 3.7 | 39 | 1 | 1 | 2 | 3 | 8 | 14 | 43 |
| **GRAND TOTAL** | 3,313 | 2.6 | 21 | 1 | 1 | 2 | 3 | 4 | 8 | 18 |

## 86.83: SIZE RED PLASTIC OP. Formerly included in operation group(s) 779.

| Type of Patients | Observed Patients | Avg. Stay | Variance | 10th | 25th | 50th | 75th | 90th | 95th | 99th |
|---|---|---|---|---|---|---|---|---|---|---|
| **1. SINGLE DX** | | | | | | | | | | |
| 0–19 Years | 3 | 1.1 | <1 | 1 | 1 | 1 | 1 | 2 | 2 | 2 |
| 20–34 | 90 | 1.8 | 1 | 1 | 1 | 1 | 2 | 4 | 4 | 4 |
| 35–49 | 177 | 1.4 | <1 | 1 | 1 | 1 | 2 | 2 | 2 | 4 |
| 50–64 | 79 | 2.3 | 8 | 1 | 1 | 2 | 2 | 10 | 10 | 10 |
| 65+ | 16 | 2.2 | 2 | 1 | 2 | 2 | 2 | 3 | 6 | 6 |
| **2. MULTIPLE DX** | | | | | | | | | | |
| 0–19 Years | 15 | 2.2 | 1 | 1 | 1 | 2 | 3 | 4 | 4 | 4 |
| 20–34 | 257 | 2.3 | 3 | 1 | 1 | 2 | 3 | 4 | 5 | 6 |
| 35–49 | 775 | 2.6 | 9 | 1 | 1 | 2 | 3 | 4 | 7 | 13 |
| 50–64 | 538 | 4.3 | 57 | 1 | 1 | 2 | 4 | 8 | 17 | 48 |
| 65+ | 105 | 6.0 | 85 | 1 | 2 | 3 | 5 | 11 | 20 | 43 |
| **TOTAL SINGLE DX** | 365 | 1.7 | 3 | 1 | 1 | 1 | 2 | 3 | 4 | 10 |
| **TOTAL MULTIPLE DX** | 1,690 | 3.3 | 28 | 1 | 1 | 2 | 3 | 5 | 8 | 33 |
| **TOTAL** | | | | | | | | | | |
| 0–19 Years | 18 | 1.7 | 1 | 1 | 1 | 1 | 2 | 4 | 4 | 4 |
| 20–34 | 347 | 2.2 | 3 | 1 | 1 | 2 | 3 | 4 | 6 | 6 |
| 35–49 | 952 | 2.3 | 7 | 1 | 1 | 2 | 3 | 4 | 6 | 11 |
| 50–64 | 617 | 4.0 | 49 | 1 | 1 | 2 | 3 | 8 | 13 | 48 |
| 65+ | 121 | 5.5 | 76 | 1 | 2 | 3 | 5 | 9 | 18 | 43 |
| **GRAND TOTAL** | 2,055 | 2.9 | 23 | 1 | 1 | 2 | 3 | 5 | 8 | 28 |

## 86.82: FACIAL RHYTIDECTOMY. Formerly included in operation group(s) 779.

| Type of Patients | Observed Patients | Avg. Stay | Variance | 10th | 25th | 50th | 75th | 90th | 95th | 99th |
|---|---|---|---|---|---|---|---|---|---|---|
| **1. SINGLE DX** | | | | | | | | | | |
| 0–19 Years | 0 | | | | | | | | | |
| 20–34 | 0 | | | | | | | | | |
| 35–49 | 17 | 1.1 | <1 | 1 | 1 | 1 | 1 | 1 | 1 | 2 |
| 50–64 | 47 | 1.1 | <1 | 1 | 1 | 1 | 1 | 1 | 1 | 2 |
| 65+ | 15 | 1.2 | <1 | 1 | 1 | 1 | 1 | 2 | 2 | 3 |
| **2. MULTIPLE DX** | | | | | | | | | | |
| 0–19 Years | 2 | 1.0 | 0 | 1 | 1 | 1 | 1 | 1 | 1 | 1 |
| 20–34 | 0 | | | | | | | | | |
| 35–49 | 59 | 1.2 | <1 | 1 | 1 | 1 | 2 | 2 | 2 | 3 |
| 50–64 | 223 | 1.5 | <1 | 1 | 1 | 1 | 2 | 2 | 2 | 6 |
| 65+ | 104 | 1.6 | 2 | 1 | 1 | 1 | 3 | 3 | 3 | 9 |
| **TOTAL SINGLE DX** | 79 | 1.1 | <1 | 1 | 1 | 1 | 1 | 1 | 2 | 3 |
| **TOTAL MULTIPLE DX** | 388 | 1.5 | <1 | 1 | 1 | 1 | 2 | 2 | 2 | 6 |
| **TOTAL** | | | | | | | | | | |
| 0–19 Years | 2 | 1.0 | 0 | 1 | 1 | 1 | 1 | 1 | 1 | 1 |
| 20–34 | 0 | | | | | | | | | |
| 35–49 | 76 | 1.1 | <1 | 1 | 1 | 1 | 2 | 1 | 1 | 3 |
| 50–64 | 270 | 1.4 | <1 | 1 | 1 | 1 | 1 | 2 | 2 | 6 |
| 65+ | 119 | 1.5 | 2 | 1 | 1 | 1 | 3 | 3 | 3 | 9 |
| **GRAND TOTAL** | 467 | 1.4 | <1 | 1 | 1 | 1 | 2 | 2 | 2 | 6 |

## 86.89: SKIN REP & RECONST NEC. Formerly included in operation group(s) 779.

| Type of Patients | Observed Patients | Avg. Stay | Variance | 10th | 25th | 50th | 75th | 90th | 95th | 99th |
|---|---|---|---|---|---|---|---|---|---|---|
| **1. SINGLE DX** | | | | | | | | | | |
| 0–19 Years | 36 | 1.4 | <1 | 1 | 1 | 1 | 2 | 2 | 3 | 3 |
| 20–34 | 15 | 2.6 | 2 | 1 | 3 | 3 | 4 | 4 | 4 | 4 |
| 35–49 | 8 | 1.4 | <1 | 1 | 1 | 1 | 2 | 5 | 5 | 5 |
| 50–64 | 7 | 2.4 | 2 | 1 | 2 | 2 | 3 | 5 | 5 | 5 |
| 65+ | 3 | 1.8 | <1 | 1 | 2 | 2 | 2 | 2 | 2 | 2 |
| **2. MULTIPLE DX** | | | | | | | | | | |
| 0–19 Years | 92 | 3.1 | 13 | 1 | 1 | 2 | 3 | 8 | 11 | 18 |
| 20–34 | 75 | 2.8 | 6 | 1 | 1 | 2 | 3 | 7 | 8 | 12 |
| 35–49 | 78 | 4.7 | 25 | 2 | 2 | 3 | 5 | 12 | 13 | 26 |
| 50–64 | 59 | 4.9 | 36 | 1 | 1 | 3 | 7 | 14 | 14 | 27 |
| 65+ | 69 | 5.7 | 44 | 1 | 1 | 3 | 7 | 17 | 23 | 29 |
| **TOTAL SINGLE DX** | 69 | 1.8 | 1 | 1 | 1 | 1 | 2 | 3 | 4 | 4 |
| **TOTAL MULTIPLE DX** | 373 | 4.0 | 23 | 1 | 2 | 2 | 4 | 9 | 14 | 24 |
| **TOTAL** | | | | | | | | | | |
| 0–19 Years | 128 | 2.6 | 10 | 1 | 1 | 2 | 3 | 6 | 10 | 18 |
| 20–34 | 90 | 2.7 | 5 | 1 | 1 | 2 | 3 | 5 | 8 | 12 |
| 35–49 | 86 | 4.4 | 24 | 1 | 2 | 3 | 5 | 12 | 13 | 26 |
| 50–64 | 66 | 4.8 | 35 | 1 | 1 | 3 | 5 | 14 | 14 | 27 |
| 65+ | 72 | 5.5 | 42 | 1 | 1 | 3 | 6 | 15 | 23 | 29 |
| **GRAND TOTAL** | 442 | 3.7 | 21 | 1 | 1 | 2 | 4 | 8 | 13 | 23 |

Length of Stay by Diagnosis and Operation, United States, 2000

# United States, October 1998–September 1999 Data, by Operation

## 86.9: OTHER SKIN & SUBCU OPS. Formerly included in operation group(s) 777, 779, 780.

| Type of Patients | Observed Patients | Avg. Stay | Variance | 10th | 25th | 50th | 75th | 90th | 95th | 99th |
|---|---|---|---|---|---|---|---|---|---|---|
| **1. SINGLE DX** | | | | | | | | | | |
| 0–19 Years | 30 | 1.2 | <1 | 1 | 1 | 1 | 1 | 2 | 3 | 4 |
| 20–34 | 2 | 1.0 | 0 | 1 | 1 | 1 | 1 | 1 | 1 | 1 |
| 35–49 | 2 | 1.9 | 1 | 1 | 1 | 1 | 3 | 3 | 3 | 3 |
| 50–64 | 1 | 4.0 | 0 | 4 | 4 | 4 | 4 | 4 | 4 | 4 |
| 65+ | 2 | 1.6 | <1 | 1 | 1 | 2 | 2 | 2 | 2 | 2 |
| **2. MULTIPLE DX** | | | | | | | | | | |
| 0–19 Years | 64 | 3.0 | 16 | 1 | 1 | 2 | 3 | 5 | 8 | 22 |
| 20–34 | 22 | 2.4 | 13 | 1 | 1 | 1 | 2 | 5 | 10 | 20 |
| 35–49 | 21 | 2.8 | 21 | 1 | 2 | 1 | 2 | 7 | 7 | 22 |
| 50–64 | 12 | 5.4 | 72 | 2 | 3 | 3 | 4 | 11 | 11 | 48 |
| 65+ | 13 | 4.6 | 7 | 2 | 3 | 5 | 5 | 11 | 11 | 11 |
| **TOTAL SINGLE DX** | 37 | 1.3 | <1 | 1 | 1 | 1 | 1 | 2 | 3 | 4 |
| **TOTAL MULTIPLE DX** | 132 | 3.2 | 20 | 1 | 1 | 2 | 3 | 7 | 11 | 22 |
| **TOTAL** | | | | | | | | | | |
| 0–19 Years | 94 | 2.3 | 11 | 1 | 1 | 1 | 2 | 4 | 8 | 22 |
| 20–34 | 24 | 2.3 | 12 | 1 | 1 | 1 | 2 | 5 | 10 | 20 |
| 35–49 | 23 | 2.8 | 20 | 1 | 1 | 2 | 2 | 7 | 7 | 22 |
| 50–64 | 13 | 5.3 | 67 | 2 | 3 | 3 | 4 | 11 | 11 | 48 |
| 65+ | 15 | 4.5 | 7 | 1 | 3 | 5 | 5 | 5 | 11 | 11 |
| **GRAND TOTAL** | 169 | 2.8 | 16 | 1 | 1 | 3 | 3 | 5 | 9 | 22 |

## 87.03: CAT SCAN HEAD. Formerly included in operation group(s) 786.

| Type of Patients | Observed Patients | Avg. Stay | Variance | 10th | 25th | 50th | 75th | 90th | 95th | 99th |
|---|---|---|---|---|---|---|---|---|---|---|
| **1. SINGLE DX** | | | | | | | | | | |
| 0–19 Years | 1,213 | 2.0 | 7 | 1 | 1 | 1 | 2 | 4 | 5 | 10 |
| 20–34 | 456 | 3.3 | 12 | 1 | 1 | 2 | 3 | 8 | 10 | 14 |
| 35–49 | 402 | 4.8 | 44 | 1 | 1 | 2 | 3 | 15 | 20 | 33 |
| 50–64 | 299 | 3.3 | 18 | 1 | 1 | 2 | 3 | 7 | 10 | 20 |
| 65+ | 347 | 3.1 | 7 | 1 | 2 | 2 | 4 | 5 | 7 | 20 |
| **2. MULTIPLE DX** | | | | | | | | | | |
| 0–19 Years | 3,488 | 3.8 | 29 | 1 | 2 | 2 | 4 | 8 | 12 | 30 |
| 20–34 | 2,443 | 4.6 | 30 | 1 | 3 | 3 | 6 | 10 | 15 | 26 |
| 35–49 | 4,967 | 4.8 | 31 | 1 | 2 | 4 | 6 | 10 | 14 | 31 |
| 50–64 | 7,001 | 5.5 | 57 | 1 | 3 | 4 | 6 | 10 | 15 | 42 |
| 65+ | 26,069 | 5.4 | 23 | 2 | 3 | 4 | 7 | 10 | 14 | 23 |
| **TOTAL SINGLE DX** | 2,717 | 3.1 | 16 | 1 | 1 | 2 | 3 | 6 | 10 | 20 |
| **TOTAL MULTIPLE DX** | 43,968 | 5.2 | 31 | 1 | 2 | 4 | 6 | 10 | 14 | 29 |
| **TOTAL** | | | | | | | | | | |
| 0–19 Years | 4,701 | 3.3 | 23 | 1 | 2 | 3 | 3 | 6 | 10 | 25 |
| 20–34 | 2,899 | 4.4 | 27 | 1 | 2 | 3 | 5 | 10 | 14 | 23 |
| 35–49 | 5,369 | 4.8 | 32 | 1 | 2 | 3 | 5 | 10 | 15 | 33 |
| 50–64 | 7,300 | 5.4 | 55 | 1 | 3 | 4 | 6 | 10 | 14 | 42 |
| 65+ | 26,416 | 5.3 | 23 | 2 | 3 | 4 | 6 | 10 | 13 | 23 |
| **GRAND TOTAL** | 46,685 | 5.0 | 30 | 1 | 2 | 4 | 6 | 10 | 14 | 29 |

## 87.0: HEAD/NECK SFT TISS X-RAY. Formerly included in operation group(s) 781, 786, 787.

| Type of Patients | Observed Patients | Avg. Stay | Variance | 10th | 25th | 50th | 75th | 90th | 95th | 99th |
|---|---|---|---|---|---|---|---|---|---|---|
| **1. SINGLE DX** | | | | | | | | | | |
| 0–19 Years | 1,228 | 2.0 | 7 | 1 | 1 | 1 | 1 | 2 | 3 | 10 |
| 20–34 | 461 | 3.3 | 12 | 1 | 1 | 1 | 3 | 5 | 10 | 14 |
| 35–49 | 407 | 4.7 | 43 | 1 | 1 | 2 | 5 | 15 | 20 | 33 |
| 50–64 | 302 | 3.4 | 19 | 1 | 1 | 2 | 3 | 7 | 10 | 20 |
| 65+ | 352 | 3.1 | 7 | 2 | 2 | 2 | 4 | 5 | 7 | 20 |
| **2. MULTIPLE DX** | | | | | | | | | | |
| 0–19 Years | 3,550 | 3.8 | 29 | 1 | 1 | 2 | 4 | 8 | 12 | 30 |
| 20–34 | 2,466 | 4.6 | 30 | 1 | 3 | 3 | 6 | 10 | 15 | 28 |
| 35–49 | 5,008 | 4.8 | 31 | 2 | 3 | 3 | 6 | 10 | 14 | 31 |
| 50–64 | 7,043 | 5.5 | 57 | 2 | 4 | 4 | 6 | 10 | 15 | 42 |
| 65+ | 26,226 | 5.4 | 23 | 3 | 4 | 4 | 7 | 10 | 14 | 23 |
| **TOTAL SINGLE DX** | 2,750 | 3.1 | 16 | 1 | 1 | 2 | 3 | 6 | 10 | 20 |
| **TOTAL MULTIPLE DX** | 44,293 | 5.2 | 31 | 2 | 2 | 4 | 6 | 10 | 14 | 29 |
| **TOTAL** | | | | | | | | | | |
| 0–19 Years | 4,778 | 3.3 | 23 | 1 | 2 | 2 | 3 | 6 | 10 | 25 |
| 20–34 | 2,927 | 4.4 | 28 | 1 | 3 | 3 | 5 | 10 | 14 | 24 |
| 35–49 | 5,415 | 4.8 | 32 | 2 | 3 | 3 | 5 | 10 | 15 | 33 |
| 50–64 | 7,345 | 5.4 | 55 | 1 | 3 | 4 | 6 | 10 | 14 | 42 |
| 65+ | 26,578 | 5.3 | 23 | 3 | 4 | 4 | 6 | 10 | 13 | 23 |
| **GRAND TOTAL** | 47,043 | 5.0 | 30 | 1 | 2 | 4 | 6 | 10 | 14 | 29 |

## 87.1: OTHER HEAD/NECK X-RAY. Formerly included in operation group(s) 787.

| Type of Patients | Observed Patients | Avg. Stay | Variance | 10th | 25th | 50th | 75th | 90th | 95th | 99th |
|---|---|---|---|---|---|---|---|---|---|---|
| **1. SINGLE DX** | | | | | | | | | | |
| 0–19 Years | 6 | 1.9 | 2 | 1 | 1 | 1 | 4 | 4 | 4 | 4 |
| 20–34 | 0 | | | | | | | | | |
| 35–49 | 2 | 4.0 | 0 | 4 | 4 | 4 | 4 | 4 | 4 | 4 |
| 50–64 | 1 | 2.0 | 0 | 2 | 2 | 2 | 2 | 2 | 2 | 2 |
| 65+ | 0 | | | | | | | | | |
| **2. MULTIPLE DX** | | | | | | | | | | |
| 0–19 Years | 16 | 2.3 | 4 | 1 | 1 | 2 | 2 | 4 | 8 | 9 |
| 20–34 | 6 | 3.5 | 8 | 2 | 2 | 2 | 6 | 9 | 9 | 9 |
| 35–49 | 8 | 6.1 | 56 | 2 | 4 | 4 | 5 | 20 | 27 | 27 |
| 50–64 | 8 | 4.8 | 15 | 3 | 3 | 3 | 7 | 12 | 12 | 12 |
| 65+ | 15 | 9.5 | 32 | 3 | 5 | 5 | 10 | 15 | 20 | 26 |
| **TOTAL SINGLE DX** | 9 | 2.3 | 2 | 1 | 1 | 2 | 4 | 4 | 4 | 4 |
| **TOTAL MULTIPLE DX** | 53 | 5.7 | 30 | 1 | 2 | 3 | 10 | 10 | 15 | 26 |
| **TOTAL** | | | | | | | | | | |
| 0–19 Years | 22 | 2.3 | 4 | 1 | 2 | 2 | 2 | 4 | 7 | 9 |
| 20–34 | 6 | 3.5 | 8 | 2 | 2 | 2 | 6 | 9 | 9 | 9 |
| 35–49 | 10 | 5.8 | 48 | 2 | 4 | 4 | 5 | 20 | 27 | 27 |
| 50–64 | 9 | 4.6 | 14 | 2 | 5 | 5 | 7 | 12 | 12 | 12 |
| 65+ | 15 | 9.5 | 32 | 3 | 5 | 5 | 10 | 15 | 20 | 26 |
| **GRAND TOTAL** | 62 | 5.5 | 28 | 1 | 2 | 3 | 10 | 10 | 15 | 26 |

Length of Stay by Diagnosis and Operation, United States, 2000

# United States, October 1998–September 1999 Data, by Operation

## 87.2: X-RAY OF SPINE. Formerly included in operation group(s) 782, 787.

| Type of Patients | Observed Patients | Avg. Stay | Variance | 10th | 25th | 50th | 75th | 90th | 95th | 99th |
|---|---|---|---|---|---|---|---|---|---|---|
| **1. SINGLE DX** | | | | | | | | | | |
| 0–19 Years | 13 | 2.6 | 2 | 1 | 1 | 3 | 4 | 5 | 5 | 5 |
| 20–34 | 70 | 3.3 | 4 | 1 | 2 | 3 | 4 | 5 | 7 | 9 |
| 35–49 | 162 | 4.4 | 7 | 1 | 2 | 4 | 7 | 7 | 7 | 8 |
| 50–64 | 103 | 2.5 | 4 | 1 | 1 | 2 | 3 | 6 | 7 | 9 |
| 65+ | 55 | 1.3 | 1 | 1 | 1 | 1 | 1 | 2 | 3 | 6 |
| **2. MULTIPLE DX** | | | | | | | | | | |
| 0–19 Years | 32 | 3.5 | 7 | 1 | 1 | 3 | 6 | 7 | 7 | 14 |
| 20–34 | 159 | 3.9 | 10 | 1 | 1 | 3 | 6 | 8 | 12 | 12 |
| 35–49 | 540 | 3.8 | 13 | 1 | 1 | 3 | 5 | 8 | 10 | 18 |
| 50–64 | 512 | 4.6 | 12 | 1 | 2 | 4 | 6 | 9 | 10 | 16 |
| 65+ | 818 | 6.2 | 35 | 2 | 3 | 5 | 8 | 12 | 13 | 30 |
| **TOTAL SINGLE DX** | 403 | 3.2 | 6 | 1 | 1 | 2 | 5 | 7 | 7 | 9 |
| **TOTAL MULTIPLE DX** | 2,061 | 4.8 | 21 | 1 | 2 | 4 | 6 | 9 | 12 | 23 |
| **TOTAL** | | | | | | | | | | |
| 0–19 Years | 45 | 3.3 | 6 | 1 | 1 | 3 | 5 | 6 | 7 | 10 |
| 20–34 | 229 | 3.7 | 8 | 1 | 1 | 3 | 5 | 8 | 10 | 12 |
| 35–49 | 702 | 4.0 | 11 | 1 | 1 | 3 | 7 | 7 | 9 | 13 |
| 50–64 | 615 | 4.3 | 12 | 1 | 2 | 4 | 5 | 8 | 10 | 15 |
| 65+ | 873 | 5.4 | 33 | 2 | 3 | 5 | 7 | 11 | 13 | 28 |
| **GRAND TOTAL** | 2,464 | 4.4 | 18 | 1 | 2 | 4 | 6 | 8 | 11 | 20 |

## 87.21: CONTRAST MYELOGRAM. Formerly included in operation group(s) 782.

| Type of Patients | Observed Patients | Avg. Stay | Variance | 10th | 25th | 50th | 75th | 90th | 95th | 99th |
|---|---|---|---|---|---|---|---|---|---|---|
| **1. SINGLE DX** | | | | | | | | | | |
| 0–19 Years | 6 | 3.0 | 2 | 1 | 2 | 3 | 4 | 5 | 5 | 5 |
| 20–34 | 56 | 3.5 | 4 | 1 | 2 | 4 | 4 | 6 | 7 | 9 |
| 35–49 | 154 | 4.4 | 7 | 1 | 2 | 5 | 7 | 7 | 7 | 8 |
| 50–64 | 102 | 2.5 | 4 | 1 | 1 | 2 | 3 | 6 | 7 | 9 |
| 65+ | 54 | 1.3 | 1 | 1 | 1 | 1 | 1 | 2 | 3 | 6 |
| **2. MULTIPLE DX** | | | | | | | | | | |
| 0–19 Years | 16 | 4.3 | 8 | 1 | 2 | 4 | 6 | 7 | 8 | 14 |
| 20–34 | 141 | 4.0 | 11 | 1 | 1 | 3 | 6 | 9 | 12 | 12 |
| 35–49 | 507 | 3.8 | 14 | 1 | 2 | 3 | 5 | 8 | 10 | 19 |
| 50–64 | 499 | 4.6 | 12 | 1 | 2 | 4 | 6 | 9 | 10 | 15 |
| 65+ | 751 | 6.3 | 36 | 2 | 3 | 5 | 8 | 12 | 13 | 30 |
| **TOTAL SINGLE DX** | 372 | 3.3 | 6 | 1 | 1 | 2 | 5 | 7 | 7 | 9 |
| **TOTAL MULTIPLE DX** | 1,914 | 4.9 | 22 | 1 | 2 | 4 | 6 | 9 | 12 | 25 |
| **TOTAL** | | | | | | | | | | |
| 0–19 Years | 22 | 4.0 | 7 | 1 | 2 | 3 | 6 | 6 | 8 | 14 |
| 20–34 | 197 | 3.9 | 9 | 1 | 1 | 3 | 5 | 8 | 9 | 12 |
| 35–49 | 661 | 4.0 | 11 | 1 | 1 | 3 | 7 | 7 | 9 | 13 |
| 50–64 | 601 | 4.3 | 11 | 1 | 2 | 4 | 5 | 8 | 10 | 14 |
| 65+ | 805 | 5.4 | 34 | 2 | 3 | 4 | 7 | 11 | 13 | 28 |
| **GRAND TOTAL** | 2,286 | 4.5 | 18 | 1 | 2 | 4 | 6 | 9 | 11 | 20 |

## 87.3: THORAX SOFT TISSUE X-RAY. Formerly included in operation group(s) 787.

| Type of Patients | Observed Patients | Avg. Stay | Variance | 10th | 25th | 50th | 75th | 90th | 95th | 99th |
|---|---|---|---|---|---|---|---|---|---|---|
| **1. SINGLE DX** | | | | | | | | | | |
| 0–19 Years | 9 | 1.0 | <1 | 1 | 1 | 1 | 1 | 1 | 1 | 2 |
| 20–34 | 3 | 3.8 | 7 | 1 | 3 | 3 | 7 | 7 | 7 | 7 |
| 35–49 | 10 | 4.8 | 7 | 2 | 2 | 4 | 8 | 8 | 8 | 8 |
| 50–64 | 0 | | | | | | | | | |
| 65+ | 0 | | | | | | | | | |
| **2. MULTIPLE DX** | | | | | | | | | | |
| 0–19 Years | 49 | 9.3 | 87 | 2 | 2 | 5 | 18 | 22 | 26 | 37 |
| 20–34 | 9 | 7.1 | 77 | 1 | 1 | 8 | 8 | 11 | 11 | 57 |
| 35–49 | 42 | 6.5 | 8 | 2 | 3 | 7 | 9 | 9 | 10 | 11 |
| 50–64 | 52 | 4.8 | 8 | 2 | 3 | 4 | 6 | 9 | 10 | 16 |
| 65+ | 95 | 5.1 | 11 | 2 | 3 | 4 | 6 | 9 | 10 | 15 |
| **TOTAL SINGLE DX** | 22 | 3.3 | 8 | 1 | 1 | 2 | 4 | 8 | 8 | 8 |
| **TOTAL MULTIPLE DX** | 247 | 6.0 | 23 | 2 | 3 | 5 | 8 | 10 | 11 | 25 |
| **TOTAL** | | | | | | | | | | |
| 0–19 Years | 58 | 8.2 | 83 | 1 | 2 | 4 | 12 | 22 | 26 | 37 |
| 20–34 | 12 | 6.8 | 70 | 1 | 1 | 7 | 8 | 9 | 11 | 57 |
| 35–49 | 52 | 6.4 | 9 | 2 | 3 | 7 | 9 | 9 | 10 | 11 |
| 50–64 | 52 | 4.8 | 8 | 2 | 3 | 4 | 6 | 9 | 10 | 16 |
| 65+ | 95 | 5.1 | 11 | 2 | 3 | 4 | 6 | 9 | 10 | 15 |
| **GRAND TOTAL** | 269 | 5.9 | 22 | 2 | 3 | 5 | 8 | 9 | 11 | 25 |

## 87.4: OTHER X-RAY OF THORAX. Formerly included in operation group(s) 786, 787.

| Type of Patients | Observed Patients | Avg. Stay | Variance | 10th | 25th | 50th | 75th | 90th | 95th | 99th |
|---|---|---|---|---|---|---|---|---|---|---|
| **1. SINGLE DX** | | | | | | | | | | |
| 0–19 Years | 206 | 3.0 | 14 | 1 | 1 | 2 | 4 | 5 | 6 | 11 |
| 20–34 | 83 | 3.9 | 32 | 1 | 2 | 2 | 4 | 7 | 12 | 38 |
| 35–49 | 114 | 4.0 | 53 | 1 | 2 | 2 | 5 | 7 | 8 | 44 |
| 50–64 | 93 | 3.4 | 26 | 1 | 1 | 3 | 4 | 7 | 10 | 20 |
| 65+ | 61 | 3.8 | 7 | 1 | 2 | 3 | 5 | 7 | 8 | 14 |
| **2. MULTIPLE DX** | | | | | | | | | | |
| 0–19 Years | 758 | 4.3 | 29 | 1 | 2 | 3 | 5 | 8 | 12 | 28 |
| 20–34 | 455 | 4.6 | 17 | 1 | 2 | 3 | 6 | 10 | 11 | 19 |
| 35–49 | 1,199 | 5.7 | 31 | 1 | 2 | 4 | 7 | 12 | 15 | 23 |
| 50–64 | 1,790 | 5.2 | 24 | 1 | 2 | 4 | 7 | 10 | 13 | 27 |
| 65+ | 4,827 | 5.8 | 19 | 2 | 3 | 5 | 7 | 11 | 13 | 22 |
| **TOTAL SINGLE DX** | 557 | 3.4 | 24 | 1 | 1 | 2 | 4 | 6 | 8 | 18 |
| **TOTAL MULTIPLE DX** | 9,029 | 5.5 | 22 | 2 | 3 | 4 | 7 | 11 | 13 | 23 |
| **TOTAL** | | | | | | | | | | |
| 0–19 Years | 964 | 4.0 | 26 | 1 | 2 | 3 | 5 | 7 | 11 | 26 |
| 20–34 | 538 | 4.5 | 18 | 1 | 2 | 3 | 6 | 9 | 11 | 20 |
| 35–49 | 1,313 | 5.6 | 32 | 1 | 2 | 4 | 7 | 11 | 14 | 23 |
| 50–64 | 1,883 | 5.2 | 24 | 1 | 2 | 4 | 6 | 10 | 13 | 27 |
| 65+ | 4,888 | 5.8 | 19 | 2 | 3 | 5 | 7 | 11 | 13 | 22 |
| **GRAND TOTAL** | 9,586 | 5.4 | 22 | 1 | 2 | 4 | 7 | 11 | 13 | 23 |

Length of Stay by Diagnosis and Operation, United States, 2000

## United States, October 1998–September 1999 Data, by Operation

### 87.41: CAT SCAN THORAX. Formerly included in operation group(s) 786.

| Type of Patients | Observed Patients | Avg. Stay | Variance | Percentiles | | | | | | |
|---|---|---|---|---|---|---|---|---|---|---|
| | | | | 10th | 25th | 50th | 75th | 90th | 95th | 99th |
| **1. SINGLE DX** | | | | | | | | | | |
| 0–19 Years | 45 | 3.6 | 8 | 1 | 1 | 3 | 5 | 8 | 10 | 11 |
| 20–34 | 39 | 4.0 | 30 | 1 | 2 | 2 | 7 | 7 | 11 | 38 |
| 35–49 | 54 | 4.5 | 20 | 1 | 2 | 4 | 6 | 10 | 10 | 31 |
| 50–64 | 49 | 3.2 | 9 | 1 | 1 | 2 | 4 | 6 | 9 | 20 |
| 65+ | 33 | 3.4 | 3 | 2 | 2 | 4 | 4 | 5 | 7 | 8 |
| **2. MULTIPLE DX** | | | | | | | | | | |
| 0–19 Years | 200 | 6.1 | 36 | 1 | 2 | 6 | 7 | 11 | 14 | 28 |
| 20–34 | 287 | 4.9 | 17 | 1 | 2 | 4 | 6 | 11 | 11 | 17 |
| 35–49 | 806 | 6.2 | 28 | 1 | 3 | 5 | 8 | 12 | 19 | 23 |
| 50–64 | 1,247 | 5.7 | 26 | 2 | 3 | 4 | 7 | 11 | 13 | 28 |
| 65+ | 3,142 | 6.1 | 18 | 2 | 3 | 5 | 8 | 11 | 13 | 22 |
| **TOTAL SINGLE DX** | 220 | 3.7 | 14 | 1 | 2 | 3 | 5 | 7 | 9 | 20 |
| **TOTAL MULTIPLE DX** | 5,682 | 5.9 | 22 | 2 | 3 | 5 | 8 | 11 | 13 | 23 |
| **TOTAL** | | | | | | | | | | |
| 0–19 Years | 245 | 5.7 | 33 | 1 | 2 | 5 | 7 | 11 | 14 | 28 |
| 20–34 | 326 | 4.8 | 18 | 2 | 2 | 4 | 6 | 11 | 11 | 20 |
| 35–49 | 860 | 6.2 | 27 | 1 | 3 | 5 | 8 | 12 | 19 | 23 |
| 50–64 | 1,296 | 5.6 | 26 | 2 | 3 | 4 | 7 | 11 | 13 | 28 |
| 65+ | 3,175 | 6.1 | 18 | 2 | 3 | 5 | 8 | 11 | 13 | 22 |
| **GRAND TOTAL** | 5,902 | 5.9 | 22 | 2 | 3 | 5 | 7 | 11 | 13 | 23 |

### 87.44: ROUTINE CHEST X-RAY. Formerly included in operation group(s) 787.

| Type of Patients | Observed Patients | Avg. Stay | Variance | Percentiles | | | | | | |
|---|---|---|---|---|---|---|---|---|---|---|
| | | | | 10th | 25th | 50th | 75th | 90th | 95th | 99th |
| **1. SINGLE DX** | | | | | | | | | | |
| 0–19 Years | 110 | 3.0 | 21 | 1 | 2 | 2 | 4 | 5 | 5 | 14 |
| 20–34 | 32 | 4.4 | 48 | 1 | 1 | 2 | 4 | 11 | 18 | 41 |
| 35–49 | 49 | 3.7 | 122 | 1 | 1 | 1 | 2 | 4 | 6 | 70 |
| 50–64 | 36 | 4.5 | 68 | 1 | 1 | 2 | 6 | 9 | 10 | 32 |
| 65+ | 22 | 4.8 | 16 | 1 | 2 | 3 | 8 | 12 | 14 | 14 |
| **2. MULTIPLE DX** | | | | | | | | | | |
| 0–19 Years | 327 | 3.9 | 36 | 1 | 2 | 3 | 4 | 6 | 10 | 31 |
| 20–34 | 110 | 3.7 | 12 | 1 | 2 | 3 | 4 | 6 | 8 | 21 |
| 35–49 | 279 | 4.2 | 42 | 2 | 2 | 3 | 5 | 7 | 11 | 21 |
| 50–64 | 341 | 3.3 | 15 | 1 | 1 | 2 | 4 | 6 | 8 | 14 |
| 65+ | 1,081 | 4.7 | 20 | 1 | 2 | 4 | 6 | 9 | 12 | 24 |
| **TOTAL SINGLE DX** | 249 | 3.6 | 44 | 1 | 1 | 2 | 4 | 6 | 9 | 25 |
| **TOTAL MULTIPLE DX** | 2,138 | 4.2 | 25 | 1 | 2 | 3 | 5 | 7 | 11 | 24 |
| **TOTAL** | | | | | | | | | | |
| 0–19 Years | 437 | 3.7 | 32 | 1 | 2 | 2 | 4 | 6 | 10 | 31 |
| 20–34 | 142 | 3.8 | 17 | 1 | 2 | 3 | 4 | 6 | 9 | 24 |
| 35–49 | 328 | 4.1 | 50 | 1 | 1 | 3 | 5 | 7 | 11 | 37 |
| 50–64 | 377 | 3.4 | 19 | 1 | 1 | 2 | 6 | 7 | 8 | 14 |
| 65+ | 1,103 | 4.7 | 20 | 1 | 2 | 4 | 6 | 9 | 12 | 24 |
| **GRAND TOTAL** | 2,387 | 4.1 | 27 | 1 | 2 | 3 | 5 | 7 | 11 | 24 |

### 87.49: CHEST X-RAY NEC. Formerly included in operation group(s) 787.

| Type of Patients | Observed Patients | Avg. Stay | Variance | Percentiles | | | | | | |
|---|---|---|---|---|---|---|---|---|---|---|
| | | | | 10th | 25th | 50th | 75th | 90th | 95th | 99th |
| **1. SINGLE DX** | | | | | | | | | | |
| 0–19 Years | 51 | 2.3 | 1 | 1 | 1 | 2 | 3 | 4 | 4 | 4 |
| 20–34 | 11 | 3.1 | 8 | 1 | 2 | 2 | 3 | 7 | 7 | 14 |
| 35–49 | 10 | 2.1 | 2 | 1 | 1 | 2 | 4 | 5 | 11 | 18 |
| 50–64 | 8 | 2.1 | 2 | 1 | 1 | 1 | 4 | 4 | 4 | 4 |
| 65+ | 6 | 3.2 | <1 | 2 | 3 | 3 | 4 | 5 | 5 | 5 |
| **2. MULTIPLE DX** | | | | | | | | | | |
| 0–19 Years | 220 | 3.2 | 7 | 1 | 2 | 4 | 4 | 5 | 7 | 20 |
| 20–34 | 53 | 3.8 | 22 | 1 | 2 | 3 | 4 | 5 | 8 | 15 |
| 35–49 | 104 | 3.8 | 20 | 1 | 3 | 4 | 4 | 6 | 11 | 14 |
| 50–64 | 197 | 3.7 | 5 | 1 | 2 | 3 | 5 | 6 | 7 | 18 |
| 65+ | 582 | 4.3 | 11 | 1 | 2 | 3 | 5 | 8 | 10 | 16 |
| **TOTAL SINGLE DX** | 86 | 2.4 | 2 | 1 | 1 | 2 | 3 | 4 | 4 | 7 |
| **TOTAL MULTIPLE DX** | 1,156 | 3.8 | 11 | 1 | 2 | 3 | 5 | 7 | 9 | 16 |
| **TOTAL** | | | | | | | | | | |
| 0–19 Years | 271 | 3.0 | 6 | 1 | 2 | 2 | 3 | 5 | 7 | 16 |
| 20–34 | 64 | 3.7 | 20 | 1 | 2 | 3 | 4 | 6 | 8 | 15 |
| 35–49 | 114 | 3.7 | 19 | 1 | 2 | 3 | 4 | 6 | 11 | 18 |
| 50–64 | 205 | 3.6 | 5 | 1 | 2 | 3 | 5 | 6 | 7 | 12 |
| 65+ | 588 | 4.3 | 11 | 1 | 2 | 3 | 5 | 8 | 10 | 16 |
| **GRAND TOTAL** | 1,242 | 3.7 | 10 | 1 | 2 | 3 | 4 | 7 | 8 | 16 |

### 87.5: BILIARY TRACT X-RAY. Formerly included in operation group(s) 787.

| Type of Patients | Observed Patients | Avg. Stay | Variance | Percentiles | | | | | | |
|---|---|---|---|---|---|---|---|---|---|---|
| | | | | 10th | 25th | 50th | 75th | 90th | 95th | 99th |
| **1. SINGLE DX** | | | | | | | | | | |
| 0–19 Years | 6 | 2.5 | 2 | 1 | 1 | 2 | 4 | 4 | 6 | 6 |
| 20–34 | 10 | 1.7 | <1 | 1 | 1 | 1 | 2 | 2 | 2 | 2 |
| 35–49 | 13 | 10.7 | 46 | 1 | 16 | 16 | 16 | 16 | 16 | 16 |
| 50–64 | 18 | 4.0 | 13 | 1 | 1 | 3 | 8 | 8 | 13 | 13 |
| 65+ | 5 | 2.9 | 5 | 1 | 1 | 2 | 5 | 7 | 7 | 7 |
| **2. MULTIPLE DX** | | | | | | | | | | |
| 0–19 Years | 50 | 7.2 | 157 | 1 | 1 | 4 | 7 | 19 | 51 | 55 |
| 20–34 | 79 | 5.0 | 18 | 1 | 2 | 4 | 7 | 9 | 14 | 24 |
| 35–49 | 137 | 6.1 | 33 | 1 | 2 | 5 | 8 | 12 | 16 | 28 |
| 50–64 | 225 | 5.2 | 18 | 2 | 2 | 4 | 7 | 11 | 12 | 22 |
| 65+ | 404 | 6.1 | 29 | 2 | 3 | 4 | 8 | 13 | 17 | 30 |
| **TOTAL SINGLE DX** | 52 | 6.3 | 38 | 1 | 1 | 3 | 16 | 16 | 16 | 16 |
| **TOTAL MULTIPLE DX** | 895 | 5.9 | 37 | 2 | 2 | 4 | 7 | 12 | 16 | 30 |
| **TOTAL** | | | | | | | | | | |
| 0–19 Years | 56 | 6.8 | 146 | 1 | 2 | 4 | 5 | 19 | 51 | 55 |
| 20–34 | 89 | 4.5 | 17 | 1 | 2 | 3 | 7 | 9 | 14 | 24 |
| 35–49 | 150 | 6.8 | 38 | 1 | 2 | 5 | 9 | 16 | 16 | 28 |
| 50–64 | 243 | 5.1 | 18 | 1 | 3 | 4 | 7 | 11 | 13 | 19 |
| 65+ | 409 | 6.1 | 29 | 2 | 3 | 4 | 8 | 13 | 16 | 30 |
| **GRAND TOTAL** | 947 | 5.9 | 37 | 1 | 2 | 4 | 7 | 13 | 16 | 30 |

Length of Stay by Diagnosis and Operation, United States, 2000

# United States, October 1998–September 1999 Data, by Operation

## 87.51: PERC HEPAT CHOLANGIOGRAM. Formerly included in operation group(s) 787.

| Type of Patients | Observed Patients | Avg. Stay | Variance | 10th | 25th | 50th | 75th | 90th | 95th | 99th |
|---|---|---|---|---|---|---|---|---|---|---|
| **1. SINGLE DX** | | | | | | | | | | |
| 0–19 Years | 1 | 4.0 | 0 | 4 | 4 | 4 | 4 | 4 | 4 | 4 |
| 20–34 | 2 | 2.0 | 0 | 2 | 2 | 2 | 2 | 2 | 2 | 2 |
| 35–49 | 5 | 14.8 | 14 | 16 | 16 | 16 | 16 | 16 | 16 | 16 |
| 50–64 | 10 | 5.1 | 14 | 1 | 2 | 3 | 8 | 8 | 13 | 13 |
| 65+ | 4 | 2.4 | 3 | 1 | 1 | 2 | 5 | 5 | 5 | 5 |
| **2. MULTIPLE DX** | | | | | | | | | | |
| 0–19 Years | 19 | 4.1 | 16 | 2 | 2 | 3 | 4 | 9 | 11 | 19 |
| 20–34 | 29 | 7.6 | 42 | 2 | 2 | 3 | 11 | 15 | 24 | 26 |
| 35–49 | 61 | 7.3 | 61 | 2 | 3 | 5 | 8 | 14 | 19 | 44 |
| 50–64 | 109 | 5.4 | 19 | 1 | 2 | 4 | 8 | 12 | 14 | 22 |
| 65+ | 210 | 7.3 | 38 | 2 | 3 | 5 | 10 | 15 | 21 | 30 |
| **TOTAL SINGLE DX** | 22 | 9.6 | 40 | 1 | 3 | 8 | 16 | 16 | 16 | 16 |
| **TOTAL MULTIPLE DX** | 428 | 6.6 | 36 | 2 | 3 | 5 | 8 | 14 | 17 | 30 |
| **TOTAL** | | | | | | | | | | |
| 0–19 Years | 20 | 4.1 | 16 | 2 | 2 | 3 | 4 | 9 | 11 | 19 |
| 20–34 | 31 | 7.2 | 41 | 2 | 2 | 4 | 10 | 15 | 24 | 26 |
| 35–49 | 66 | 9.5 | 59 | 2 | 3 | 7 | 16 | 16 | 16 | 44 |
| 50–64 | 119 | 5.4 | 18 | 1 | 2 | 4 | 8 | 12 | 13 | 22 |
| 65+ | 214 | 7.3 | 38 | 2 | 3 | 5 | 9 | 15 | 21 | 30 |
| **GRAND TOTAL** | 450 | 6.9 | 37 | 2 | 3 | 5 | 9 | 16 | 17 | 30 |

## 87.61: BARIUM SWALLOW. Formerly included in operation group(s) 787.

| Type of Patients | Observed Patients | Avg. Stay | Variance | 10th | 25th | 50th | 75th | 90th | 95th | 99th |
|---|---|---|---|---|---|---|---|---|---|---|
| **1. SINGLE DX** | | | | | | | | | | |
| 0–19 Years | 8 | 1.3 | <1 | 1 | 1 | 1 | 1 | 3 | 3 | 3 |
| 20–34 | 2 | 3.7 | 13 | 1 | 1 | 4 | 7 | 7 | 7 | 7 |
| 35–49 | 4 | 1.0 | <1 | 1 | 1 | 1 | 1 | 1 | 1 | 2 |
| 50–64 | 1 | 5.0 | 0 | 5 | 5 | 5 | 5 | 5 | 5 | 5 |
| 65+ | 2 | 1.4 | <1 | 1 | 1 | 1 | 3 | 3 | 3 | 3 |
| **2. MULTIPLE DX** | | | | | | | | | | |
| 0–19 Years | 73 | 5.2 | 36 | 1 | 2 | 3 | 6 | 11 | 16 | 38 |
| 20–34 | 29 | 4.9 | 13 | 1 | 2 | 4 | 6 | 11 | 15 | 15 |
| 35–49 | 37 | 6.6 | 54 | 2 | 3 | 4 | 9 | 11 | 20 | 53 |
| 50–64 | 83 | 5.8 | 33 | 3 | 4 | 4 | 6 | 13 | 20 | 25 |
| 65+ | 355 | 7.7 | 49 | 3 | 5 | 6 | 9 | 12 | 16 | 38 |
| **TOTAL SINGLE DX** | 17 | 1.4 | 1 | 1 | 1 | 1 | 1 | 3 | 3 | 7 |
| **TOTAL MULTIPLE DX** | 577 | 6.9 | 44 | 2 | 3 | 6 | 8 | 12 | 16 | 33 |
| **TOTAL** | | | | | | | | | | |
| 0–19 Years | 81 | 4.7 | 33 | 1 | 1 | 3 | 6 | 10 | 15 | 38 |
| 20–34 | 31 | 4.8 | 13 | 1 | 2 | 4 | 6 | 9 | 15 | 15 |
| 35–49 | 41 | 5.5 | 48 | 1 | 2 | 3 | 7 | 9 | 16 | 53 |
| 50–64 | 84 | 5.8 | 33 | 2 | 2 | 4 | 6 | 13 | 20 | 25 |
| 65+ | 357 | 7.6 | 49 | 3 | 5 | 6 | 9 | 12 | 16 | 38 |
| **GRAND TOTAL** | 594 | 6.7 | 44 | 2 | 3 | 6 | 8 | 12 | 16 | 33 |

## 87.6: OTH DIGESTIVE SYST X-RAY. Formerly included in operation group(s) 787.

| Type of Patients | Observed Patients | Avg. Stay | Variance | 10th | 25th | 50th | 75th | 90th | 95th | 99th |
|---|---|---|---|---|---|---|---|---|---|---|
| **1. SINGLE DX** | | | | | | | | | | |
| 0–19 Years | 234 | 2.3 | 3 | 1 | 1 | 2 | 3 | 4 | 6 | 9 |
| 20–34 | 18 | 2.2 | 4 | 1 | 1 | 2 | 2 | 4 | 7 | 10 |
| 35–49 | 39 | 2.7 | 1 | 1 | 2 | 3 | 3 | 4 | 4 | 8 |
| 50–64 | 20 | 3.1 | 2 | 2 | 2 | 3 | 5 | 5 | 5 | 5 |
| 65+ | 16 | 2.3 | 2 | 1 | 1 | 2 | 3 | 4 | 6 | 6 |
| **2. MULTIPLE DX** | | | | | | | | | | |
| 0–19 Years | 813 | 4.6 | 31 | 1 | 2 | 3 | 5 | 9 | 13 | 32 |
| 20–34 | 141 | 4.0 | 8 | 1 | 2 | 3 | 6 | 8 | 11 | 15 |
| 35–49 | 344 | 5.0 | 20 | 2 | 2 | 4 | 6 | 9 | 10 | 27 |
| 50–64 | 421 | 4.8 | 23 | 2 | 2 | 3 | 6 | 10 | 15 | 25 |
| 65+ | 1,142 | 5.6 | 27 | 2 | 2 | 5 | 7 | 10 | 13 | 23 |
| **TOTAL SINGLE DX** | 327 | 2.4 | 3 | 1 | 1 | 2 | 3 | 4 | 6 | 9 |
| **TOTAL MULTIPLE DX** | 2,861 | 5.1 | 26 | 2 | 2 | 4 | 6 | 10 | 13 | 25 |
| **TOTAL** | | | | | | | | | | |
| 0–19 Years | 1,047 | 4.1 | 26 | 1 | 2 | 3 | 5 | 9 | 12 | 30 |
| 20–34 | 159 | 3.8 | 8 | 1 | 2 | 3 | 5 | 8 | 10 | 11 |
| 35–49 | 383 | 4.5 | 17 | 1 | 2 | 4 | 5 | 8 | 9 | 20 |
| 50–64 | 441 | 4.8 | 23 | 1 | 2 | 4 | 6 | 10 | 15 | 25 |
| 65+ | 1,158 | 5.6 | 27 | 2 | 2 | 5 | 7 | 10 | 13 | 23 |
| **GRAND TOTAL** | 3,188 | 4.8 | 24 | 1 | 2 | 3 | 6 | 9 | 12 | 24 |

## 87.62: UPPER GI SERIES. Formerly included in operation group(s) 787.

| Type of Patients | Observed Patients | Avg. Stay | Variance | 10th | 25th | 50th | 75th | 90th | 95th | 99th |
|---|---|---|---|---|---|---|---|---|---|---|
| **1. SINGLE DX** | | | | | | | | | | |
| 0–19 Years | 153 | 2.7 | 4 | 1 | 1 | 2 | 4 | 5 | 7 | 9 |
| 20–34 | 7 | 2.4 | 1 | 1 | 2 | 2 | 3 | 4 | 4 | 4 |
| 35–49 | 18 | 2.4 | 2 | 1 | 2 | 2 | 4 | 5 | 5 | 5 |
| 50–64 | 10 | 3.1 | 2 | 2 | 2 | 3 | 5 | 6 | 6 | 6 |
| 65+ | 6 | 3.5 | 3 | 1 | 3 | 3 | 6 | 6 | 6 | 6 |
| **2. MULTIPLE DX** | | | | | | | | | | |
| 0–19 Years | 608 | 4.8 | 35 | 1 | 2 | 3 | 5 | 10 | 13 | 32 |
| 20–34 | 78 | 3.8 | 7 | 1 | 2 | 3 | 5 | 8 | 11 | 11 |
| 35–49 | 209 | 4.8 | 23 | 1 | 2 | 4 | 5 | 9 | 11 | 34 |
| 50–64 | 218 | 3.7 | 9 | 1 | 2 | 3 | 5 | 7 | 11 | 13 |
| 65+ | 445 | 4.6 | 14 | 2 | 2 | 4 | 6 | 9 | 11 | 20 |
| **TOTAL SINGLE DX** | 194 | 2.7 | 4 | 1 | 1 | 2 | 4 | 5 | 6 | 9 |
| **TOTAL MULTIPLE DX** | 1,558 | 4.5 | 22 | 1 | 2 | 3 | 5 | 9 | 11 | 24 |
| **TOTAL** | | | | | | | | | | |
| 0–19 Years | 761 | 4.4 | 30 | 1 | 2 | 3 | 5 | 9 | 12 | 30 |
| 20–34 | 85 | 3.7 | 7 | 1 | 2 | 3 | 4 | 8 | 11 | 11 |
| 35–49 | 227 | 4.7 | 22 | 1 | 2 | 4 | 5 | 8 | 10 | 27 |
| 50–64 | 228 | 3.7 | 8 | 1 | 2 | 3 | 5 | 7 | 15 | 13 |
| 65+ | 451 | 4.6 | 14 | 2 | 2 | 4 | 6 | 9 | 11 | 20 |
| **GRAND TOTAL** | 1,752 | 4.4 | 21 | 1 | 2 | 3 | 5 | 9 | 11 | 23 |

Length of Stay by Diagnosis and Operation, United States, 2000

# United States, October 1998–September 1999 Data, by Operation

## 87.64: LOWER GI SERIES. Formerly included in operation group(s) 787.

| Type of Patients | Observed Patients | Avg. Stay | Variance | 10th | 25th | 50th | 75th | 90th | 95th | 99th |
|---|---|---|---|---|---|---|---|---|---|---|
| **1. SINGLE DX** | | | | | | | | | | |
| 0–19 Years | 59 | 1.5 | <1 | 1 | 1 | 1 | 2 | 3 | 3 | 4 |
| 20–34 | 6 | 2.9 | 6 | 2 | 2 | 2 | 2 | 6 | 10 | 10 |
| 35–49 | 7 | 3.4 | 4 | 2 | 2 | 3 | 3 | 7 | 8 | 8 |
| 50–64 | 6 | 3.2 | 3 | 1 | 1 | 3 | 5 | 5 | 5 | 5 |
| 65+ | 5 | 2.1 | 1 | 1 | 1 | 2 | 3 | 4 | 4 | 4 |
| **2. MULTIPLE DX** | | | | | | | | | | |
| 0–19 Years | 90 | 2.7 | 5 | 1 | 1 | 2 | 3 | 5 | 7 | 11 |
| 20–34 | 9 | 3.6 | 3 | 1 | 2 | 3 | 5 | 6 | 6 | 6 |
| 35–49 | 43 | 4.1 | 5 | 1 | 2 | 3 | 5 | 6 | 9 | 11 |
| 50–64 | 64 | 4.0 | 8 | 2 | 2 | 3 | 5 | 8 | 8 | 18 |
| 65+ | 213 | 4.5 | 13 | 2 | 2 | 3 | 6 | 8 | 10 | 23 |
| **TOTAL SINGLE DX** | 83 | 2.0 | 3 | 1 | 1 | 2 | 2 | 3 | 5 | 10 |
| **TOTAL MULTIPLE DX** | 419 | 4.1 | 10 | 1 | 2 | 3 | 5 | 8 | 9 | 18 |
| **TOTAL** | | | | | | | | | | |
| 0–19 Years | 149 | 2.3 | 4 | 1 | 1 | 2 | 3 | 4 | 6 | 11 |
| 20–34 | 15 | 3.1 | 5 | 2 | 2 | 2 | 4 | 6 | 10 | 10 |
| 35–49 | 50 | 4.0 | 5 | 1 | 2 | 4 | 5 | 7 | 8 | 11 |
| 50–64 | 70 | 4.0 | 8 | 2 | 2 | 3 | 5 | 8 | 8 | 18 |
| 65+ | 218 | 4.5 | 13 | 2 | 2 | 3 | 6 | 8 | 10 | 23 |
| **GRAND TOTAL** | 502 | 3.8 | 9 | 1 | 2 | 3 | 5 | 7 | 9 | 18 |

## 87.73: IV PYELOGRAM. Formerly included in operation group(s) 787.

| Type of Patients | Observed Patients | Avg. Stay | Variance | 10th | 25th | 50th | 75th | 90th | 95th | 99th |
|---|---|---|---|---|---|---|---|---|---|---|
| **1. SINGLE DX** | | | | | | | | | | |
| 0–19 Years | 70 | 2.2 | 2 | 1 | 1 | 2 | 3 | 4 | 5 | 5 |
| 20–34 | 277 | 1.6 | 1 | 1 | 1 | 1 | 2 | 3 | 4 | 6 |
| 35–49 | 383 | 1.5 | 1 | 1 | 1 | 1 | 2 | 2 | 3 | 6 |
| 50–64 | 152 | 1.4 | <1 | 1 | 1 | 1 | 2 | 2 | 3 | 7 |
| 65+ | 55 | 2.5 | 8 | 1 | 2 | 2 | 3 | 4 | 4 | 19 |
| **2. MULTIPLE DX** | | | | | | | | | | |
| 0–19 Years | 191 | 2.8 | 16 | 1 | 1 | 2 | 3 | 5 | 5 | 11 |
| 20–34 | 818 | 2.5 | 3 | 1 | 1 | 2 | 3 | 5 | 6 | 8 |
| 35–49 | 1,039 | 2.5 | 4 | 1 | 1 | 2 | 3 | 5 | 6 | 10 |
| 50–64 | 823 | 2.9 | 8 | 1 | 1 | 2 | 4 | 6 | 8 | 12 |
| 65+ | 967 | 3.8 | 10 | 1 | 2 | 3 | 5 | 7 | 10 | 15 |
| **TOTAL SINGLE DX** | 937 | 1.6 | 1 | 1 | 1 | 1 | 2 | 3 | 3 | 6 |
| **TOTAL MULTIPLE DX** | 3,838 | 2.9 | 7 | 1 | 1 | 2 | 4 | 6 | 7 | 13 |
| **TOTAL** | | | | | | | | | | |
| 0–19 Years | 261 | 2.7 | 12 | 1 | 2 | 2 | 3 | 5 | 5 | 9 |
| 20–34 | 1,095 | 2.2 | 3 | 1 | 1 | 2 | 3 | 4 | 5 | 8 |
| 35–49 | 1,422 | 2.2 | 3 | 1 | 1 | 2 | 3 | 4 | 6 | 9 |
| 50–64 | 975 | 2.6 | 7 | 1 | 1 | 2 | 3 | 5 | 8 | 12 |
| 65+ | 1,022 | 3.8 | 10 | 1 | 2 | 3 | 5 | 7 | 10 | 15 |
| **GRAND TOTAL** | 4,775 | 2.6 | 6 | 1 | 1 | 2 | 3 | 5 | 7 | 12 |

## 87.7: X-RAY OF URINARY SYSTEM. Formerly included in operation group(s) 786, 787.

| Type of Patients | Observed Patients | Avg. Stay | Variance | 10th | 25th | 50th | 75th | 90th | 95th | 99th |
|---|---|---|---|---|---|---|---|---|---|---|
| **1. SINGLE DX** | | | | | | | | | | |
| 0–19 Years | 273 | 2.3 | 2 | 1 | 1 | 2 | 3 | 4 | 5 | 8 |
| 20–34 | 515 | 1.8 | 1 | 1 | 1 | 1 | 2 | 3 | 4 | 6 |
| 35–49 | 705 | 1.7 | 1 | 1 | 1 | 1 | 2 | 3 | 4 | 5 |
| 50–64 | 298 | 1.7 | 1 | 1 | 1 | 1 | 2 | 3 | 4 | 6 |
| 65+ | 96 | 2.2 | 5 | 1 | 2 | 2 | 3 | 4 | 4 | 19 |
| **2. MULTIPLE DX** | | | | | | | | | | |
| 0–19 Years | 1,379 | 4.2 | 17 | 1 | 2 | 3 | 5 | 8 | 11 | 17 |
| 20–34 | 1,785 | 2.8 | 5 | 1 | 1 | 2 | 4 | 5 | 7 | 11 |
| 35–49 | 2,582 | 3.2 | 9 | 1 | 1 | 2 | 4 | 6 | 8 | 16 |
| 50–64 | 2,375 | 3.8 | 16 | 1 | 1 | 3 | 5 | 8 | 10 | 19 |
| 65+ | 3,715 | 5.5 | 22 | 1 | 2 | 4 | 7 | 11 | 14 | 23 |
| **TOTAL SINGLE DX** | 1,887 | 1.8 | 2 | 1 | 1 | 1 | 2 | 3 | 4 | 6 |
| **TOTAL MULTIPLE DX** | 11,836 | 4.0 | 16 | 1 | 2 | 3 | 5 | 8 | 11 | 19 |
| **TOTAL** | | | | | | | | | | |
| 0–19 Years | 1,652 | 3.8 | 15 | 1 | 2 | 3 | 5 | 7 | 10 | 17 |
| 20–34 | 2,300 | 2.6 | 4 | 1 | 1 | 2 | 3 | 5 | 6 | 10 |
| 35–49 | 3,287 | 2.9 | 8 | 1 | 1 | 2 | 3 | 6 | 8 | 15 |
| 50–64 | 2,673 | 3.5 | 15 | 1 | 1 | 4 | 4 | 8 | 10 | 18 |
| 65+ | 3,811 | 5.4 | 22 | 1 | 2 | 4 | 7 | 11 | 14 | 23 |
| **GRAND TOTAL** | 13,723 | 3.7 | 14 | 1 | 1 | 3 | 5 | 8 | 10 | 18 |

## 87.74: RETROGRADE PYELOGRAM. Formerly included in operation group(s) 787.

| Type of Patients | Observed Patients | Avg. Stay | Variance | 10th | 25th | 50th | 75th | 90th | 95th | 99th |
|---|---|---|---|---|---|---|---|---|---|---|
| **1. SINGLE DX** | | | | | | | | | | |
| 0–19 Years | 59 | 2.1 | 2 | 1 | 2 | 2 | 3 | 3 | 5 | 8 |
| 20–34 | 206 | 2.0 | 2 | 1 | 1 | 1 | 2 | 3 | 4 | 6 |
| 35–49 | 287 | 1.8 | 1 | 1 | 1 | 1 | 2 | 2 | 3 | 5 |
| 50–64 | 130 | 1.9 | 1 | 1 | 1 | 2 | 2 | 3 | 4 | 5 |
| 65+ | 37 | 1.8 | 1 | 1 | 1 | 1 | 2 | 2 | 4 | 5 |
| **2. MULTIPLE DX** | | | | | | | | | | |
| 0–19 Years | 164 | 2.9 | 6 | 1 | 1 | 2 | 4 | 6 | 8 | 12 |
| 20–34 | 797 | 3.0 | 6 | 1 | 1 | 2 | 4 | 5 | 7 | 11 |
| 35–49 | 1,305 | 3.7 | 13 | 1 | 2 | 3 | 4 | 7 | 10 | 17 |
| 50–64 | 1,277 | 4.2 | 21 | 1 | 2 | 3 | 5 | 9 | 12 | 19 |
| 65+ | 2,147 | 6.1 | 22 | 2 | 3 | 5 | 8 | 12 | 14 | 23 |
| **TOTAL SINGLE DX** | 719 | 1.9 | 1 | 1 | 1 | 2 | 2 | 4 | 5 | 6 |
| **TOTAL MULTIPLE DX** | 5,690 | 4.5 | 18 | 1 | 2 | 3 | 6 | 9 | 12 | 20 |
| **TOTAL** | | | | | | | | | | |
| 0–19 Years | 223 | 2.6 | 5 | 1 | 1 | 2 | 3 | 5 | 7 | 11 |
| 20–34 | 1,003 | 2.8 | 5 | 1 | 1 | 2 | 4 | 4 | 7 | 11 |
| 35–49 | 1,592 | 3.3 | 11 | 1 | 2 | 3 | 4 | 7 | 9 | 16 |
| 50–64 | 1,407 | 4.0 | 19 | 1 | 3 | 3 | 5 | 9 | 11 | 18 |
| 65+ | 2,184 | 6.0 | 22 | 2 | 3 | 5 | 8 | 12 | 14 | 23 |
| **GRAND TOTAL** | 6,409 | 4.2 | 17 | 1 | 2 | 3 | 5 | 9 | 12 | 19 |

Length of Stay by Diagnosis and Operation, United States, 2000

# United States, October 1998–September 1999 Data, by Operation

## 87.76: RETRO CYSTOURETHROGRAM. Formerly included in operation group(s) 787.

| Type of Patients | Observed Patients | Avg. Stay | Variance | Percentiles | | | | | | |
|---|---|---|---|---|---|---|---|---|---|---|
| | | | | 10th | 25th | 50th | 75th | 90th | 95th | 99th |
| **1. SINGLE DX** | | | | | | | | | | |
| 0–19 Years | 89 | 3.1 | 4 | 1 | 1 | 3 | 4 | 5 | 6 | 10 |
| 20–34 | 4 | 2.1 | <1 | 1 | 2 | 2 | 3 | 3 | 3 | 3 |
| 35–49 | 2 | 1.0 | 0 | 1 | 1 | 1 | 1 | 1 | 1 | 1 |
| 50–64 | 0 | | | | | | | | | |
| 65+ | 0 | | | | | | | | | |
| **2. MULTIPLE DX** | | | | | | | | | | |
| 0–19 Years | 737 | 5.1 | 21 | 2 | 3 | 4 | 6 | 9 | 11 | 20 |
| 20–34 | 17 | 4.3 | 6 | 3 | 3 | 4 | 4 | 6 | 9 | 18 |
| 35–49 | 37 | 3.9 | 11 | 2 | 2 | 4 | 5 | 7 | 8 | 10 |
| 50–64 | 44 | 7.5 | 35 | 2 | 4 | 6 | 8 | 19 | 21 | 28 |
| 65+ | 70 | 6.8 | 38 | 2 | 3 | 6 | 7 | 12 | 17 | 31 |
| **TOTAL SINGLE DX** | 95 | 3.0 | 4 | 1 | 1 | 3 | 4 | 5 | 6 | 10 |
| **TOTAL MULTIPLE DX** | 905 | 5.3 | 23 | 2 | 3 | 4 | 7 | 9 | 12 | 24 |
| **TOTAL** | | | | | | | | | | |
| 0–19 Years | 826 | 5.0 | 20 | 2 | 3 | 4 | 6 | 9 | 11 | 20 |
| 20–34 | 21 | 4.0 | 6 | 2 | 3 | 4 | 4 | 6 | 9 | 18 |
| 35–49 | 39 | 3.8 | 11 | 2 | 2 | 4 | 5 | 7 | 8 | 10 |
| 50–64 | 44 | 7.5 | 35 | 2 | 4 | 6 | 8 | 19 | 21 | 28 |
| 65+ | 70 | 6.8 | 38 | 2 | 3 | 6 | 7 | 12 | 17 | 31 |
| **GRAND TOTAL** | 1,000 | 5.2 | 22 | 2 | 3 | 4 | 6 | 9 | 11 | 24 |

## 87.79: URINARY SYSTEM X-RAY NEC. Formerly included in operation group(s) 787.

| Type of Patients | Observed Patients | Avg. Stay | Variance | Percentiles | | | | | | |
|---|---|---|---|---|---|---|---|---|---|---|
| | | | | 10th | 25th | 50th | 75th | 90th | 95th | 99th |
| **1. SINGLE DX** | | | | | | | | | | |
| 0–19 Years | 32 | 1.8 | 1 | 1 | 1 | 1 | 2 | 3 | 4 | 7 |
| 20–34 | 17 | 2.8 | 3 | 1 | 1 | 2 | 4 | 6 | 6 | 6 |
| 35–49 | 21 | 1.9 | 3 | 1 | 1 | 2 | 3 | 4 | 6 | 8 |
| 50–64 | 10 | 2.5 | <1 | 2 | 2 | 3 | 3 | 4 | 4 | 5 |
| 65+ | 1 | 3.0 | 0 | 3 | 3 | 3 | 3 | 3 | 3 | 3 |
| **2. MULTIPLE DX** | | | | | | | | | | |
| 0–19 Years | 162 | 4.0 | 12 | 1 | 2 | 3 | 5 | 8 | 11 | 17 |
| 20–34 | 57 | 3.5 | 9 | 1 | 2 | 3 | 5 | 8 | 9 | 18 |
| 35–49 | 86 | 4.1 | 20 | 1 | 2 | 3 | 5 | 8 | 9 | 25 |
| 50–64 | 100 | 4.0 | 18 | 1 | 3 | 3 | 5 | 6 | 14 | 22 |
| 65+ | 202 | 6.2 | 34 | 2 | 3 | 5 | 8 | 12 | 16 | 29 |
| **TOTAL SINGLE DX** | 81 | 2.1 | 2 | 1 | 1 | 2 | 3 | 4 | 4 | 7 |
| **TOTAL MULTIPLE DX** | 607 | 4.8 | 23 | 1 | 2 | 3 | 6 | 9 | 14 | 24 |
| **TOTAL** | | | | | | | | | | |
| 0–19 Years | 194 | 3.7 | 11 | 1 | 2 | 3 | 4 | 7 | 11 | 17 |
| 20–34 | 74 | 3.4 | 8 | 1 | 2 | 3 | 5 | 7 | 9 | 18 |
| 35–49 | 107 | 3.7 | 17 | 1 | 2 | 3 | 5 | 7 | 14 | 25 |
| 50–64 | 110 | 3.8 | 15 | 2 | 3 | 5 | 5 | 6 | 16 | 22 |
| 65+ | 203 | 6.2 | 34 | 2 | 3 | 5 | 8 | 12 | 16 | 29 |
| **GRAND TOTAL** | 688 | 4.5 | 21 | 1 | 2 | 3 | 5 | 9 | 12 | 24 |

## 87.77: CYSTOGRAM NEC. Formerly included in operation group(s) 787.

| Type of Patients | Observed Patients | Avg. Stay | Variance | Percentiles | | | | | | |
|---|---|---|---|---|---|---|---|---|---|---|
| | | | | 10th | 25th | 50th | 75th | 90th | 95th | 99th |
| **1. SINGLE DX** | | | | | | | | | | |
| 0–19 Years | 12 | 2.5 | 3 | 1 | 1 | 1 | 4 | 5 | 5 | 7 |
| 20–34 | 4 | 2.6 | <1 | 1 | 3 | 3 | 3 | 3 | 3 | 3 |
| 35–49 | 4 | 1.9 | <1 | 2 | 2 | 2 | 3 | 3 | 3 | 3 |
| 50–64 | 2 | 2.0 | 0 | 1 | 1 | 2 | 3 | 3 | 3 | 3 |
| 65+ | 2 | 2.0 | 4 | 1 | 1 | 1 | 1 | 6 | 6 | 6 |
| **2. MULTIPLE DX** | | | | | | | | | | |
| 0–19 Years | 90 | 4.5 | 13 | 1 | 3 | 4 | 5 | 8 | 13 | 19 |
| 20–34 | 48 | 5.1 | 14 | 2 | 2 | 4 | 8 | 9 | 11 | 18 |
| 35–49 | 52 | 5.3 | 11 | 1 | 2 | 5 | 7 | 9 | 10 | 17 |
| 50–64 | 55 | 5.1 | 12 | 1 | 2 | 5 | 7 | 11 | 12 | 16 |
| 65+ | 184 | 7.4 | 37 | 2 | 3 | 6 | 9 | 14 | 17 | 32 |
| **TOTAL SINGLE DX** | 24 | 2.3 | 2 | 1 | 1 | 2 | 3 | 5 | 5 | 7 |
| **TOTAL MULTIPLE DX** | 429 | 5.9 | 23 | 2 | 3 | 5 | 8 | 12 | 14 | 28 |
| **TOTAL** | | | | | | | | | | |
| 0–19 Years | 102 | 4.3 | 13 | 1 | 2 | 4 | 5 | 7 | 13 | 17 |
| 20–34 | 52 | 5.0 | 14 | 2 | 2 | 4 | 8 | 9 | 11 | 18 |
| 35–49 | 56 | 5.0 | 11 | 1 | 2 | 5 | 7 | 9 | 10 | 17 |
| 50–64 | 57 | 5.1 | 12 | 1 | 2 | 5 | 7 | 11 | 12 | 16 |
| 65+ | 186 | 7.3 | 37 | 2 | 3 | 6 | 9 | 14 | 17 | 32 |
| **GRAND TOTAL** | 453 | 5.7 | 23 | 1 | 3 | 4 | 7 | 11 | 14 | 28 |

## 87.8: FEMALE GENITAL X-RAY. Formerly included in operation group(s) 787.

| Type of Patients | Observed Patients | Avg. Stay | Variance | Percentiles | | | | | | |
|---|---|---|---|---|---|---|---|---|---|---|
| | | | | 10th | 25th | 50th | 75th | 90th | 95th | 99th |
| **1. SINGLE DX** | | | | | | | | | | |
| 0–19 Years | 1 | 2.0 | 0 | 2 | 2 | 2 | 2 | 2 | 2 | 2 |
| 20–34 | 0 | | | | | | | | | |
| 35–49 | 0 | | | | | | | | | |
| 50–64 | 0 | | | | | | | | | |
| 65+ | 0 | | | | | | | | | |
| **2. MULTIPLE DX** | | | | | | | | | | |
| 0–19 Years | 0 | | | | | | | | | |
| 20–34 | 2 | 3.0 | 0 | 3 | 3 | 3 | 3 | 3 | 3 | 3 |
| 35–49 | 3 | 2.1 | <1 | 1 | 1 | 2 | 3 | 3 | 3 | 3 |
| 50–64 | 0 | | | | | | | | | |
| 65+ | 1 | 6.0 | 0 | 6 | 6 | 6 | 6 | 6 | 6 | 6 |
| **TOTAL SINGLE DX** | 1 | 2.0 | 0 | 2 | 2 | 2 | 2 | 2 | 2 | 2 |
| **TOTAL MULTIPLE DX** | 6 | 2.7 | 2 | 1 | 2 | 3 | 3 | 6 | 6 | 6 |
| **TOTAL** | | | | | | | | | | |
| 0–19 Years | 1 | 2.0 | 0 | 2 | 2 | 2 | 2 | 2 | 2 | 2 |
| 20–34 | 2 | 3.0 | 0 | 3 | 3 | 3 | 3 | 3 | 3 | 3 |
| 35–49 | 3 | 2.1 | <1 | 1 | 1 | 2 | 3 | 3 | 3 | 3 |
| 50–64 | 0 | | | | | | | | | |
| 65+ | 1 | 6.0 | 0 | 6 | 6 | 6 | 6 | 6 | 6 | 6 |
| **GRAND TOTAL** | 7 | 2.7 | 2 | 1 | 2 | 3 | 3 | 6 | 6 | 6 |

Length of Stay by Diagnosis and Operation, United States, 2000

# United States, October 1998–September 1999 Data, by Operation

## 87.9: MALE GENITAL X-RAY. Formerly included in operation group(s) 787.

| Type of Patients | Observed Patients | Avg. Stay | Variance | 10th | 25th | 50th | 75th | 90th | 95th | 99th |
|---|---|---|---|---|---|---|---|---|---|---|
| **1. SINGLE DX** | | | | | | | | | | |
| 0–19 Years | 0 | | | | | | | | | |
| 20–34 | 0 | | | | | | | | | |
| 35–49 | 0 | | | | | | | | | |
| 50–64 | 0 | | | | | | | | | |
| 65+ | 0 | | | | | | | | | |
| **2. MULTIPLE DX** | | | | | | | | | | |
| 0–19 Years | 0 | | | | | | | | | |
| 20–34 | 0 | | | | | | | | | |
| 35–49 | 2 | 10.1 | 3 | 8 | 8 | 11 | 11 | 11 | 11 | 11 |
| 50–64 | 1 | 3.0 | 0 | 3 | 3 | 3 | 3 | 3 | 3 | 3 |
| 65+ | 1 | 1.0 | 0 | 1 | 1 | 1 | 1 | 1 | 1 | 1 |
| **TOTAL SINGLE DX** | 0 | | | | | | | | | |
| **TOTAL MULTIPLE DX** | 4 | 3.6 | 5 | 3 | 3 | 3 | 3 | 3 | 11 | 11 |
| **TOTAL** | | | | | | | | | | |
| 0–19 Years | 0 | | | | | | | | | |
| 20–34 | 0 | | | | | | | | | |
| 35–49 | 2 | 10.1 | 3 | 8 | 8 | 11 | 11 | 11 | 11 | 11 |
| 50–64 | 1 | 3.0 | 0 | 3 | 3 | 3 | 3 | 3 | 3 | 3 |
| 65+ | 1 | 1.0 | 0 | 1 | 1 | 1 | 1 | 1 | 1 | 1 |
| **GRAND TOTAL** | 4 | 3.6 | 5 | 3 | 3 | 3 | 3 | 3 | 11 | 11 |

## 88.01: CAT SCAN OF ABDOMEN. Formerly included in operation group(s) 786.

| Type of Patients | Observed Patients | Avg. Stay | Variance | 10th | 25th | 50th | 75th | 90th | 95th | 99th |
|---|---|---|---|---|---|---|---|---|---|---|
| **1. SINGLE DX** | | | | | | | | | | |
| 0–19 Years | 493 | 2.0 | 2 | 1 | 1 | 1 | 2 | 4 | 5 | 7 |
| 20–34 | 521 | 2.3 | 4 | 1 | 1 | 2 | 3 | 4 | 5 | 7 |
| 35–49 | 541 | 2.6 | 4 | 1 | 1 | 2 | 3 | 5 | 5 | 8 |
| 50–64 | 278 | 3.2 | 3 | 1 | 2 | 3 | 4 | 5 | 6 | 8 |
| 65+ | 161 | 3.1 | 3 | 1 | 1 | 3 | 4 | 5 | 6 | 8 |
| **2. MULTIPLE DX** | | | | | | | | | | |
| 0–19 Years | 1,142 | 3.3 | 16 | 1 | 1 | 2 | 4 | 7 | 9 | 16 |
| 20–34 | 1,754 | 3.7 | 10 | 1 | 1 | 3 | 5 | 8 | 9 | 14 |
| 35–49 | 3,339 | 4.4 | 12 | 1 | 2 | 3 | 6 | 8 | 11 | 19 |
| 50–64 | 3,233 | 4.6 | 21 | 1 | 2 | 4 | 6 | 8 | 12 | 19 |
| 65+ | 6,483 | 5.4 | 20 | 2 | 3 | 4 | 7 | 11 | 13 | 21 |
| **TOTAL SINGLE DX** | 1,994 | 2.5 | 4 | 1 | 1 | 2 | 3 | 5 | 6 | 8 |
| **TOTAL MULTIPLE DX** | 15,951 | 4.7 | 17 | 1 | 2 | 4 | 6 | 9 | 12 | 21 |
| **TOTAL** | | | | | | | | | | |
| 0–19 Years | 1,635 | 2.8 | 11 | 1 | 1 | 2 | 3 | 6 | 8 | 15 |
| 20–34 | 2,275 | 3.3 | 8 | 1 | 2 | 3 | 4 | 7 | 8 | 14 |
| 35–49 | 3,880 | 4.1 | 11 | 1 | 2 | 3 | 5 | 8 | 11 | 18 |
| 50–64 | 3,511 | 4.5 | 19 | 2 | 2 | 4 | 6 | 8 | 11 | 19 |
| 65+ | 6,644 | 5.3 | 19 | 3 | 3 | 4 | 7 | 10 | 13 | 21 |
| **GRAND TOTAL** | 17,945 | 4.4 | 16 | 1 | 2 | 3 | 6 | 8 | 11 | 20 |

## 88.0: SOFT TISSUE X-RAY ABD. Formerly included in operation group(s) 786, 787.

| Type of Patients | Observed Patients | Avg. Stay | Variance | 10th | 25th | 50th | 75th | 90th | 95th | 99th |
|---|---|---|---|---|---|---|---|---|---|---|
| **1. SINGLE DX** | | | | | | | | | | |
| 0–19 Years | 498 | 2.0 | 2 | 1 | 1 | 1 | 2 | 4 | 5 | 7 |
| 20–34 | 524 | 2.3 | 4 | 1 | 1 | 2 | 3 | 4 | 5 | 7 |
| 35–49 | 545 | 2.6 | 4 | 1 | 1 | 2 | 3 | 5 | 8 | 8 |
| 50–64 | 281 | 3.2 | 3 | 2 | 2 | 3 | 4 | 5 | 6 | 8 |
| 65+ | 163 | 3.1 | 3 | 1 | 1 | 3 | 4 | 5 | 6 | 8 |
| **2. MULTIPLE DX** | | | | | | | | | | |
| 0–19 Years | 1,159 | 3.3 | 15 | 1 | 1 | 2 | 4 | 7 | 9 | 16 |
| 20–34 | 1,770 | 3.7 | 10 | 1 | 2 | 3 | 5 | 8 | 9 | 14 |
| 35–49 | 3,377 | 4.4 | 12 | 1 | 2 | 3 | 6 | 8 | 11 | 19 |
| 50–64 | 3,271 | 4.6 | 21 | 1 | 2 | 4 | 6 | 8 | 12 | 19 |
| 65+ | 6,569 | 5.4 | 20 | 2 | 3 | 4 | 7 | 11 | 13 | 21 |
| **TOTAL SINGLE DX** | 2,011 | 2.5 | 4 | 1 | 1 | 2 | 3 | 5 | 6 | 8 |
| **TOTAL MULTIPLE DX** | 16,146 | 4.7 | 17 | 1 | 2 | 4 | 6 | 9 | 12 | 21 |
| **TOTAL** | | | | | | | | | | |
| 0–19 Years | 1,657 | 2.8 | 11 | 1 | 2 | 2 | 3 | 6 | 8 | 15 |
| 20–34 | 2,294 | 3.3 | 9 | 1 | 1 | 2 | 4 | 7 | 8 | 14 |
| 35–49 | 3,922 | 4.1 | 11 | 1 | 2 | 3 | 5 | 8 | 11 | 18 |
| 50–64 | 3,552 | 4.5 | 19 | 2 | 2 | 3 | 6 | 8 | 11 | 19 |
| 65+ | 6,732 | 5.3 | 20 | 2 | 3 | 4 | 7 | 10 | 13 | 21 |
| **GRAND TOTAL** | 18,157 | 4.4 | 16 | 1 | 2 | 3 | 6 | 8 | 11 | 20 |

## 88.1: OTHER X-RAY OF ABDOMEN. Formerly included in operation group(s) 787.

| Type of Patients | Observed Patients | Avg. Stay | Variance | 10th | 25th | 50th | 75th | 90th | 95th | 99th |
|---|---|---|---|---|---|---|---|---|---|---|
| **1. SINGLE DX** | | | | | | | | | | |
| 0–19 Years | 17 | 2.4 | 2 | 1 | 1 | 1 | 4 | 5 | 5 | 5 |
| 20–34 | 13 | 2.3 | 3 | 1 | 1 | 1 | 3 | 4 | 5 | 5 |
| 35–49 | 6 | 2.9 | 10 | 1 | 1 | 2 | 4 | 5 | 12 | 12 |
| 50–64 | 3 | 2.2 | <1 | 2 | 2 | 2 | 2 | 3 | 3 | 3 |
| 65+ | 1 | 3.0 | 0 | 3 | 3 | 3 | 3 | 3 | 3 | 3 |
| **2. MULTIPLE DX** | | | | | | | | | | |
| 0–19 Years | 49 | 2.7 | 4 | 1 | 2 | 2 | 3 | 4 | 7 | 14 |
| 20–34 | 45 | 2.9 | 6 | 1 | 1 | 3 | 4 | 6 | 7 | 13 |
| 35–49 | 74 | 5.0 | 61 | 1 | 1 | 3 | 5 | 13 | 14 | 38 |
| 50–64 | 77 | 5.5 | 18 | 2 | 2 | 4 | 10 | 11 | 11 | 19 |
| 65+ | 191 | 3.9 | 7 | 1 | 3 | 3 | 5 | 7 | 9 | 14 |
| **TOTAL SINGLE DX** | 40 | 2.4 | 3 | 1 | 1 | 2 | 3 | 5 | 5 | 12 |
| **TOTAL MULTIPLE DX** | 436 | 4.1 | 16 | 1 | 2 | 3 | 5 | 9 | 11 | 16 |
| **TOTAL** | | | | | | | | | | |
| 0–19 Years | 66 | 2.6 | 4 | 1 | 1 | 2 | 3 | 5 | 5 | 14 |
| 20–34 | 58 | 2.8 | 5 | 1 | 1 | 2 | 4 | 6 | 7 | 13 |
| 35–49 | 80 | 4.8 | 57 | 1 | 1 | 3 | 5 | 12 | 14 | 38 |
| 50–64 | 80 | 5.3 | 17 | 1 | 2 | 3 | 10 | 11 | 11 | 16 |
| 65+ | 192 | 3.9 | 7 | 1 | 2 | 3 | 5 | 7 | 9 | 14 |
| **GRAND TOTAL** | 476 | 4.0 | 15 | 1 | 2 | 3 | 5 | 9 | 11 | 16 |

Length of Stay by Diagnosis and Operation, United States, 2000

**United States, October 1998–September 1999 Data, by Operation**

### 88.19: ABDOMINAL X-RAY NEC. Formerly included in operation group(s) 787.

| Type of Patients | Observed Patients | Avg. Stay | Vari-ance | 10th | 25th | 50th | 75th | 90th | 95th | 99th |
|---|---|---|---|---|---|---|---|---|---|---|
| **1. SINGLE DX** | | | | | | | | | | |
| 0–19 Years | 15 | 2.4 | 2 | 1 | 1 | 2 | 4 | 5 | 5 | 5 |
| 20–34 | 10 | 2.1 | 2 | 1 | 1 | 1 | 3 | 5 | 5 | 5 |
| 35–49 | 4 | 1.5 | <1 | 1 | 1 | 1 | 2 | 3 | 3 | 3 |
| 50–64 | 2 | 2.3 | <1 | 2 | 2 | 2 | 3 | 3 | 3 | 3 |
| 65+ | 1 | 3.0 | 0 | 3 | 3 | 3 | 3 | 3 | 3 | 3 |
| **2. MULTIPLE DX** | | | | | | | | | | |
| 0–19 Years | 41 | 2.5 | 4 | 1 | 1 | 2 | 3 | 3 | 5 | 14 |
| 20–34 | 23 | 2.2 | 3 | 1 | 1 | 1 | 3 | 5 | 6 | 7 |
| 35–49 | 51 | 3.7 | 56 | 1 | 1 | 2 | 4 | 5 | 8 | 28 |
| 50–64 | 56 | 4.4 | 12 | 2 | 2 | 3 | 5 | 10 | 11 | 16 |
| 65+ | 167 | 3.7 | 7 | 2 | 2 | 3 | 5 | 7 | 8 | 14 |
| **TOTAL SINGLE DX** | 32 | 2.2 | 2 | 1 | 1 | 2 | 3 | 5 | 5 | 5 |
| **TOTAL MULTIPLE DX** | 338 | 3.6 | 13 | 1 | 2 | 3 | 4 | 7 | 9 | 14 |
| **TOTAL** | | | | | | | | | | |
| 0–19 Years | 56 | 2.5 | 4 | 1 | 1 | 2 | 3 | 4 | 5 | 14 |
| 20–34 | 33 | 2.2 | 3 | 1 | 1 | 1 | 3 | 5 | 5 | 7 |
| 35–49 | 55 | 3.5 | 51 | 1 | 1 | 2 | 4 | 5 | 8 | 28 |
| 50–64 | 58 | 4.3 | 11 | 2 | 2 | 3 | 5 | 10 | 11 | 16 |
| 65+ | 168 | 3.7 | 7 | 1 | 2 | 3 | 5 | 7 | 8 | 14 |
| **GRAND TOTAL** | 370 | 3.5 | 12 | 1 | 2 | 3 | 4 | 7 | 9 | 14 |

### 88.3: OTHER X-RAY. Formerly included in operation group(s) 786, 787.

| Type of Patients | Observed Patients | Avg. Stay | Vari-ance | 10th | 25th | 50th | 75th | 90th | 95th | 99th |
|---|---|---|---|---|---|---|---|---|---|---|
| **1. SINGLE DX** | | | | | | | | | | |
| 0–19 Years | 194 | 2.6 | 8 | 1 | 1 | 2 | 3 | 5 | 6 | 9 |
| 20–34 | 90 | 2.6 | 2 | 1 | 2 | 3 | 3 | 4 | 5 | 7 |
| 35–49 | 96 | 2.6 | 3 | 1 | 2 | 3 | 3 | 5 | 6 | 7 |
| 50–64 | 57 | 3.6 | 5 | 2 | 4 | 4 | 4 | 5 | 7 | 10 |
| 65+ | 36 | 5.0 | 6 | 3 | 3 | 7 | 7 | 7 | 7 | 9 |
| **2. MULTIPLE DX** | | | | | | | | | | |
| 0–19 Years | 439 | 3.7 | 15 | 1 | 2 | 3 | 4 | 7 | 10 | 18 |
| 20–34 | 293 | 4.0 | 16 | 1 | 2 | 3 | 4 | 7 | 11 | 18 |
| 35–49 | 536 | 4.7 | 22 | 1 | 2 | 4 | 6 | 8 | 13 | 19 |
| 50–64 | 564 | 5.4 | 23 | 2 | 3 | 4 | 7 | 9 | 14 | 21 |
| 65+ | 1,322 | 5.8 | 17 | 2 | 3 | 5 | 8 | 11 | 14 | 20 |
| **TOTAL SINGLE DX** | 473 | 3.1 | 6 | 1 | 1 | 2 | 4 | 7 | 7 | 9 |
| **TOTAL MULTIPLE DX** | 3,154 | 5.1 | 20 | 1 | 3 | 4 | 6 | 9 | 12 | 20 |
| **TOTAL** | | | | | | | | | | |
| 0–19 Years | 633 | 3.4 | 13 | 1 | 2 | 3 | 4 | 6 | 9 | 17 |
| 20–34 | 383 | 3.6 | 13 | 1 | 2 | 3 | 4 | 6 | 10 | 15 |
| 35–49 | 632 | 4.4 | 20 | 1 | 2 | 4 | 5 | 8 | 11 | 17 |
| 50–64 | 621 | 5.2 | 22 | 2 | 3 | 4 | 7 | 9 | 14 | 21 |
| 65+ | 1,358 | 5.8 | 16 | 2 | 3 | 5 | 7 | 10 | 13 | 20 |
| **GRAND TOTAL** | 3,627 | 4.8 | 18 | 1 | 2 | 4 | 6 | 9 | 11 | 20 |

### 88.2: SKEL X-RAY-EXT & PELVIS. Formerly included in operation group(s) 787.

| Type of Patients | Observed Patients | Avg. Stay | Vari-ance | 10th | 25th | 50th | 75th | 90th | 95th | 99th |
|---|---|---|---|---|---|---|---|---|---|---|
| **1. SINGLE DX** | | | | | | | | | | |
| 0–19 Years | 14 | 3.2 | 17 | 1 | 1 | 2 | 3 | 9 | 18 | 18 |
| 20–34 | 6 | 1.7 | 1 | 1 | 1 | 1 | 3 | 4 | 4 | 4 |
| 35–49 | 6 | 1.5 | 1 | 1 | 1 | 1 | 1 | 4 | 4 | 4 |
| 50–64 | 4 | 1.0 | 0 | 1 | 1 | 1 | 1 | 1 | 1 | 1 |
| 65+ | 3 | 4.0 | 2 | 3 | 3 | 3 | 6 | 6 | 6 | 6 |
| **2. MULTIPLE DX** | | | | | | | | | | |
| 0–19 Years | 51 | 2.5 | 8 | 1 | 1 | 2 | 3 | 5 | 8 | 8 |
| 20–34 | 28 | 5.2 | 24 | 1 | 2 | 3 | 7 | 11 | 12 | 26 |
| 35–49 | 38 | 5.4 | 40 | 1 | 2 | 3 | 8 | 10 | 14 | 31 |
| 50–64 | 27 | 4.9 | 22 | 1 | 2 | 3 | 7 | 12 | 18 | 18 |
| 65+ | 111 | 7.3 | 104 | 1 | 2 | 5 | 7 | 14 | 29 | 67 |
| **TOTAL SINGLE DX** | 33 | 2.4 | 10 | 1 | 1 | 1 | 3 | 4 | 9 | 18 |
| **TOTAL MULTIPLE DX** | 255 | 5.4 | 58 | 2 | 2 | 3 | 7 | 11 | 18 | 41 |
| **TOTAL** | | | | | | | | | | |
| 0–19 Years | 65 | 2.7 | 10 | 1 | 1 | 2 | 3 | 5 | 8 | 18 |
| 20–34 | 34 | 4.8 | 23 | 1 | 2 | 3 | 7 | 11 | 12 | 26 |
| 35–49 | 44 | 4.6 | 34 | 1 | 2 | 2 | 5 | 10 | 13 | 31 |
| 50–64 | 31 | 4.6 | 22 | 1 | 2 | 2 | 7 | 12 | 14 | 18 |
| 65+ | 114 | 7.3 | 102 | 1 | 2 | 5 | 7 | 14 | 29 | 67 |
| **GRAND TOTAL** | 288 | 5.1 | 53 | 1 | 2 | 3 | 6 | 11 | 16 | 39 |

### 88.38: OTHER C.A.T. SCAN. Formerly included in operation group(s) 786.

| Type of Patients | Observed Patients | Avg. Stay | Vari-ance | 10th | 25th | 50th | 75th | 90th | 95th | 99th |
|---|---|---|---|---|---|---|---|---|---|---|
| **1. SINGLE DX** | | | | | | | | | | |
| 0–19 Years | 137 | 2.7 | 9 | 1 | 1 | 2 | 3 | 5 | 7 | 9 |
| 20–34 | 90 | 2.6 | 2 | 1 | 2 | 3 | 3 | 4 | 5 | 7 |
| 35–49 | 94 | 2.6 | 5 | 1 | 2 | 3 | 3 | 5 | 6 | 7 |
| 50–64 | 56 | 3.6 | 5 | 1 | 2 | 4 | 4 | 5 | 7 | 10 |
| 65+ | 35 | 5.1 | 6 | 1 | 3 | 7 | 7 | 7 | 7 | 9 |
| **2. MULTIPLE DX** | | | | | | | | | | |
| 0–19 Years | 357 | 3.6 | 14 | 1 | 2 | 3 | 4 | 6 | 9 | 17 |
| 20–34 | 284 | 3.8 | 16 | 1 | 2 | 3 | 4 | 8 | 9 | 25 |
| 35–49 | 514 | 4.7 | 22 | 2 | 2 | 4 | 6 | 9 | 13 | 19 |
| 50–64 | 540 | 5.4 | 23 | 2 | 3 | 4 | 7 | 9 | 14 | 21 |
| 65+ | 1,262 | 5.8 | 17 | 2 | 3 | 5 | 8 | 11 | 14 | 20 |
| **TOTAL SINGLE DX** | 412 | 3.1 | 6 | 1 | 1 | 3 | 4 | 7 | 7 | 9 |
| **TOTAL MULTIPLE DX** | 2,957 | 5.1 | 19 | 2 | 3 | 4 | 6 | 9 | 12 | 20 |
| **TOTAL** | | | | | | | | | | |
| 0–19 Years | 494 | 3.4 | 13 | 1 | 2 | 3 | 4 | 6 | 8 | 16 |
| 20–34 | 374 | 3.5 | 13 | 1 | 2 | 3 | 4 | 6 | 9 | 15 |
| 35–49 | 608 | 4.4 | 20 | 1 | 2 | 3 | 5 | 8 | 11 | 17 |
| 50–64 | 596 | 5.2 | 22 | 2 | 3 | 4 | 7 | 9 | 14 | 21 |
| 65+ | 1,297 | 5.8 | 16 | 2 | 3 | 5 | 7 | 10 | 13 | 20 |
| **GRAND TOTAL** | 3,369 | 4.8 | 18 | 1 | 2 | 4 | 6 | 9 | 11 | 20 |

Length of Stay by Diagnosis and Operation, United States, 2000

# United States, October 1998–September 1999 Data, by Operation

## 88.4: CONTRAST ARTERIOGRAPHY. Formerly included in operation group(s) 783, 785.

| Type of Patients | Observed Patients | Avg. Stay | Vari-ance | 10th | 25th | 50th | 75th | 90th | 95th | 99th |
|---|---|---|---|---|---|---|---|---|---|---|
| **1. SINGLE DX** | | | | | | | | | | |
| 0–19 Years | 145 | 2.1 | 4 | 1 | 1 | 1 | 3 | 4 | 7 | 11 |
| 20–34 | 340 | 2.6 | 4 | 1 | 1 | 1 | 3 | 6 | 7 | 10 |
| 35–49 | 484 | 3.2 | 8 | 1 | 2 | 2 | 4 | 7 | 7 | 11 |
| 50–64 | 404 | 2.9 | 7 | 1 | 1 | 2 | 3 | 7 | 8 | 12 |
| 65+ | 382 | 2.6 | 11 | 1 | 1 | 1 | 3 | 6 | 7 | 14 |
| **2. MULTIPLE DX** | | | | | | | | | | |
| 0–19 Years | 391 | 5.1 | 57 | 1 | 2 | 3 | 6 | 10 | 15 | 40 |
| 20–34 | 1,340 | 4.7 | 17 | 1 | 2 | 4 | 6 | 10 | 11 | 19 |
| 35–49 | 3,542 | 4.9 | 17 | 1 | 2 | 4 | 6 | 9 | 12 | 19 |
| 50–64 | 6,016 | 5.3 | 22 | 1 | 2 | 4 | 7 | 10 | 13 | 20 |
| 65+ | 12,279 | 5.5 | 22 | 1 | 2 | 4 | 7 | 11 | 13 | 23 |
| **TOTAL SINGLE DX** | 1,755 | 2.8 | 7 | 1 | 1 | 2 | 3 | 6 | 8 | 12 |
| **TOTAL MULTIPLE DX** | 23,568 | 5.3 | 22 | 1 | 2 | 4 | 7 | 10 | 13 | 22 |
| **TOTAL** | | | | | | | | | | |
| 0–19 Years | 536 | 4.4 | 45 | 1 | 2 | 2 | 5 | 9 | 14 | 40 |
| 20–34 | 1,680 | 4.2 | 15 | 1 | 2 | 3 | 6 | 9 | 11 | 17 |
| 35–49 | 4,026 | 4.7 | 16 | 1 | 2 | 4 | 6 | 9 | 12 | 18 |
| 50–64 | 6,420 | 5.1 | 21 | 1 | 2 | 4 | 7 | 10 | 12 | 19 |
| 65+ | 12,661 | 5.4 | 22 | 1 | 2 | 4 | 7 | 10 | 13 | 23 |
| **GRAND TOTAL** | 25,323 | 5.1 | 21 | 1 | 2 | 4 | 7 | 10 | 13 | 22 |

## 88.41: CEREBRAL ARTERIOGRAM. Formerly included in operation group(s) 783.

| Type of Patients | Observed Patients | Avg. Stay | Vari-ance | 10th | 25th | 50th | 75th | 90th | 95th | 99th |
|---|---|---|---|---|---|---|---|---|---|---|
| **1. SINGLE DX** | | | | | | | | | | |
| 0–19 Years | 77 | 2.5 | 6 | 1 | 1 | 1 | 3 | 6 | 10 | 11 |
| 20–34 | 166 | 2.8 | 5 | 1 | 1 | 2 | 3 | 6 | 8 | 8 |
| 35–49 | 288 | 3.8 | 10 | 1 | 2 | 2 | 5 | 10 | 11 | 13 |
| 50–64 | 205 | 3.0 | 8 | 1 | 1 | 2 | 4 | 7 | 9 | 12 |
| 65+ | 181 | 3.1 | 9 | 1 | 1 | 2 | 4 | 7 | 11 | 17 |
| **2. MULTIPLE DX** | | | | | | | | | | |
| 0–19 Years | 186 | 4.7 | 54 | 1 | 3 | 3 | 6 | 10 | 13 | 34 |
| 20–34 | 530 | 5.7 | 24 | 1 | 3 | 4 | 8 | 11 | 15 | 24 |
| 35–49 | 1,646 | 5.2 | 19 | 1 | 2 | 4 | 7 | 10 | 13 | 22 |
| 50–64 | 2,573 | 5.5 | 19 | 1 | 3 | 4 | 7 | 10 | 13 | 21 |
| 65+ | 4,922 | 5.6 | 22 | 1 | 3 | 5 | 7 | 10 | 13 | 26 |
| **TOTAL SINGLE DX** | 917 | 3.2 | 8 | 1 | 1 | 2 | 4 | 7 | 11 | 13 |
| **TOTAL MULTIPLE DX** | 9,857 | 5.5 | 22 | 1 | 3 | 4 | 7 | 10 | 13 | 24 |
| **TOTAL** | | | | | | | | | | |
| 0–19 Years | 263 | 4.0 | 41 | 1 | 2 | 2 | 5 | 9 | 11 | 22 |
| 20–34 | 696 | 4.9 | 21 | 1 | 2 | 3 | 7 | 10 | 12 | 22 |
| 35–49 | 1,934 | 4.9 | 18 | 1 | 2 | 4 | 7 | 10 | 13 | 20 |
| 50–64 | 2,778 | 5.3 | 19 | 1 | 2 | 4 | 7 | 10 | 13 | 21 |
| 65+ | 5,103 | 5.5 | 22 | 1 | 3 | 4 | 7 | 10 | 12 | 26 |
| **GRAND TOTAL** | 10,774 | 5.3 | 21 | 1 | 2 | 4 | 7 | 10 | 12 | 23 |

## 88.42: CONTRAST AORTOGRAM. Formerly included in operation group(s) 785.

| Type of Patients | Observed Patients | Avg. Stay | Vari-ance | 10th | 25th | 50th | 75th | 90th | 95th | 99th |
|---|---|---|---|---|---|---|---|---|---|---|
| **1. SINGLE DX** | | | | | | | | | | |
| 0–19 Years | 13 | 1.9 | 2 | 1 | 1 | 1 | 2 | 4 | 6 | 6 |
| 20–34 | 30 | 2.1 | 2 | 1 | 1 | 2 | 2 | 4 | 6 | 6 |
| 35–49 | 52 | 2.1 | 2 | 1 | 1 | 2 | 2 | 4 | 5 | 7 |
| 50–64 | 50 | 2.0 | 4 | 1 | 1 | 1 | 2 | 4 | 6 | 14 |
| 65+ | 86 | 2.2 | 27 | 1 | 1 | 1 | 2 | 4 | 6 | 6 |
| **2. MULTIPLE DX** | | | | | | | | | | |
| 0–19 Years | 52 | 6.6 | 81 | 1 | 2 | 4 | 7 | 14 | 18 | 47 |
| 20–34 | 148 | 4.4 | 11 | 1 | 2 | 4 | 5 | 10 | 10 | 17 |
| 35–49 | 452 | 4.9 | 17 | 1 | 3 | 4 | 6 | 9 | 12 | 16 |
| 50–64 | 1,105 | 5.3 | 17 | 1 | 2 | 4 | 7 | 10 | 13 | 21 |
| 65+ | 2,733 | 5.3 | 21 | 1 | 2 | 4 | 7 | 11 | 13 | 20 |
| **TOTAL SINGLE DX** | 231 | 2.1 | 9 | 1 | 1 | 1 | 2 | 4 | 5 | 7 |
| **TOTAL MULTIPLE DX** | 4,490 | 5.2 | 20 | 1 | 2 | 4 | 7 | 10 | 13 | 20 |
| **TOTAL** | | | | | | | | | | |
| 0–19 Years | 65 | 5.9 | 72 | 1 | 2 | 3 | 7 | 11 | 15 | 47 |
| 20–34 | 178 | 4.0 | 10 | 1 | 2 | 3 | 5 | 8 | 10 | 17 |
| 35–49 | 504 | 4.5 | 11 | 1 | 2 | 4 | 6 | 8 | 11 | 16 |
| 50–64 | 1,155 | 5.2 | 17 | 1 | 2 | 4 | 7 | 9 | 12 | 21 |
| 65+ | 2,819 | 5.2 | 22 | 1 | 2 | 4 | 7 | 11 | 13 | 20 |
| **GRAND TOTAL** | 4,721 | 5.1 | 20 | 1 | 2 | 4 | 7 | 10 | 13 | 20 |

## 88.43: PULMONARY ARTERIOGRAM. Formerly included in operation group(s) 785.

| Type of Patients | Observed Patients | Avg. Stay | Vari-ance | 10th | 25th | 50th | 75th | 90th | 95th | 99th |
|---|---|---|---|---|---|---|---|---|---|---|
| **1. SINGLE DX** | | | | | | | | | | |
| 0–19 Years | 2 | 4.0 | 10 | 2 | 2 | 2 | 7 | 7 | 7 | 7 |
| 20–34 | 53 | 3.3 | 4 | 2 | 2 | 2 | 4 | 7 | 7 | 8 |
| 35–49 | 56 | 2.5 | 5 | 1 | 1 | 1 | 4 | 6 | 7 | 9 |
| 50–64 | 35 | 3.9 | 9 | 1 | 2 | 2 | 7 | 8 | 10 | 10 |
| 65+ | 17 | 3.3 | 4 | 1 | 2 | 2 | 6 | 6 | 6 | 7 |
| **2. MULTIPLE DX** | | | | | | | | | | |
| 0–19 Years | 32 | 3.9 | 7 | 2 | 2 | 3 | 5 | 7 | 9 | 12 |
| 20–34 | 333 | 4.0 | 8 | 1 | 2 | 3 | 6 | 7 | 9 | 11 |
| 35–49 | 664 | 4.4 | 16 | 1 | 2 | 3 | 6 | 8 | 10 | 15 |
| 50–64 | 788 | 4.7 | 12 | 1 | 2 | 4 | 6 | 9 | 10 | 16 |
| 65+ | 1,037 | 5.5 | 17 | 1 | 3 | 5 | 7 | 10 | 12 | 20 |
| **TOTAL SINGLE DX** | 163 | 3.2 | 6 | 1 | 1 | 2 | 5 | 7 | 8 | 10 |
| **TOTAL MULTIPLE DX** | 2,854 | 4.8 | 15 | 1 | 2 | 4 | 6 | 9 | 11 | 16 |
| **TOTAL** | | | | | | | | | | |
| 0–19 Years | 34 | 3.9 | 8 | 2 | 2 | 3 | 5 | 7 | 9 | 12 |
| 20–34 | 386 | 3.9 | 8 | 1 | 2 | 3 | 6 | 7 | 9 | 11 |
| 35–49 | 720 | 4.2 | 16 | 1 | 2 | 3 | 6 | 8 | 10 | 15 |
| 50–64 | 823 | 4.6 | 12 | 1 | 2 | 4 | 6 | 9 | 10 | 16 |
| 65+ | 1,054 | 5.5 | 17 | 1 | 3 | 5 | 7 | 10 | 12 | 20 |
| **GRAND TOTAL** | 3,017 | 4.7 | 14 | 1 | 2 | 4 | 6 | 9 | 11 | 16 |

Length of Stay by Diagnosis and Operation, United States, 2000

# United States, October 1998–September 1999 Data, by Operation

## 88.45: RENAL ARTERIOGRAM. Formerly included in operation group(s) 785.

| Type of Patients | Observed Patients | Avg. Stay | Vari-ance | 10th | 25th | 50th | 75th | 90th | 95th | 99th |
|---|---|---|---|---|---|---|---|---|---|---|
| **1. SINGLE DX** | | | | | | | | | | |
| 0–19 Years | 4 | 2.1 | 4 | 1 | 1 | 1 | 5 | 5 | 5 | 5 |
| 20–34 | 14 | 2.7 | 4 | 1 | 1 | 2 | 4 | 6 | 6 | 6 |
| 35–49 | 23 | 2.2 | 2 | 1 | 1 | 2 | 4 | 4 | 5 | 9 |
| 50–64 | 21 | 3.3 | 7 | 1 | 1 | 2 | 4 | 8 | 8 | 8 |
| 65+ | 11 | 2.1 | 3 | 1 | 1 | 1 | 2 | 4 | 7 | 7 |
| **2. MULTIPLE DX** | | | | | | | | | | |
| 0–19 Years | 26 | 8.4 | 123 | 2 | 4 | 5 | 6 | 40 | 40 | 40 |
| 20–34 | 58 | 4.7 | 11 | 2 | 3 | 4 | 6 | 9 | 11 | 12 |
| 35–49 | 178 | 5.3 | 12 | 2 | 3 | 5 | 7 | 9 | 12 | 18 |
| 50–64 | 282 | 7.1 | 107 | 1 | 3 | 5 | 8 | 13 | 15 | 77 |
| 65+ | 551 | 6.0 | 31 | 1 | 2 | 5 | 8 | 12 | 16 | 27 |
| **TOTAL SINGLE DX** | 73 | 2.6 | 4 | 1 | 1 | 2 | 3 | 6 | 8 | 8 |
| **TOTAL MULTIPLE DX** | 1,095 | 6.3 | 54 | 1 | 2 | 5 | 8 | 12 | 15 | 40 |
| **TOTAL** | | | | | | | | | | |
| 0–19 Years | 30 | 8.2 | 120 | 1 | 4 | 5 | 6 | 18 | 40 | 40 |
| 20–34 | 72 | 4.3 | 10 | 1 | 2 | 3 | 6 | 9 | 11 | 12 |
| 35–49 | 201 | 4.9 | 11 | 2 | 2 | 5 | 6 | 9 | 12 | 18 |
| 50–64 | 303 | 6.9 | 102 | 1 | 2 | 5 | 8 | 13 | 15 | 77 |
| 65+ | 562 | 6.0 | 30 | 1 | 2 | 5 | 8 | 12 | 16 | 27 |
| **GRAND TOTAL** | 1,168 | 6.1 | 52 | 1 | 2 | 5 | 7 | 12 | 15 | 40 |

## 88.47: ABD ARTERIOGRAM NEC. Formerly included in operation group(s) 785.

| Type of Patients | Observed Patients | Avg. Stay | Vari-ance | 10th | 25th | 50th | 75th | 90th | 95th | 99th |
|---|---|---|---|---|---|---|---|---|---|---|
| **1. SINGLE DX** | | | | | | | | | | |
| 0–19 Years | 1 | 1.0 | 0 | 1 | 1 | 1 | 1 | 1 | 1 | 1 |
| 20–34 | 9 | 2.0 | 3 | 1 | 1 | 1 | 2 | 5 | 5 | 5 |
| 35–49 | 6 | 2.1 | 2 | 1 | 1 | 2 | 2 | 6 | 6 | 6 |
| 50–64 | 13 | 3.7 | 9 | 1 | 1 | 2 | 8 | 8 | 8 | 8 |
| 65+ | 15 | 2.7 | 4 | 1 | 1 | 2 | 4 | 7 | 7 | 7 |
| **2. MULTIPLE DX** | | | | | | | | | | |
| 0–19 Years | 20 | 3.3 | 20 | 1 | 1 | 1 | 5 | 7 | 15 | 22 |
| 20–34 | 42 | 6.1 | 11 | 2 | 3 | 6 | 9 | 9 | 10 | 22 |
| 35–49 | 133 | 5.1 | 29 | 1 | 2 | 3 | 6 | 9 | 16 | 35 |
| 50–64 | 256 | 4.9 | 11 | 1 | 3 | 4 | 6 | 9 | 12 | 15 |
| 65+ | 551 | 6.1 | 27 | 1 | 3 | 4 | 8 | 12 | 18 | 24 |
| **TOTAL SINGLE DX** | 44 | 3.0 | 7 | 1 | 1 | 2 | 5 | 8 | 8 | 8 |
| **TOTAL MULTIPLE DX** | 1,002 | 5.6 | 23 | 1 | 2 | 4 | 7 | 11 | 15 | 24 |
| **TOTAL** | | | | | | | | | | |
| 0–19 Years | 21 | 3.3 | 20 | 1 | 1 | 1 | 5 | 7 | 15 | 22 |
| 20–34 | 51 | 5.3 | 12 | 1 | 3 | 5 | 9 | 9 | 9 | 22 |
| 35–49 | 139 | 5.0 | 29 | 1 | 2 | 3 | 6 | 9 | 16 | 35 |
| 50–64 | 269 | 4.8 | 11 | 1 | 3 | 4 | 7 | 9 | 11 | 15 |
| 65+ | 566 | 6.0 | 27 | 1 | 3 | 4 | 8 | 12 | 18 | 24 |
| **GRAND TOTAL** | 1,046 | 5.5 | 23 | 1 | 2 | 4 | 7 | 10 | 14 | 24 |

## 88.48: CONTRAST ARTERIOGRAM-LEG. Formerly included in operation group(s) 785.

| Type of Patients | Observed Patients | Avg. Stay | Vari-ance | 10th | 25th | 50th | 75th | 90th | 95th | 99th |
|---|---|---|---|---|---|---|---|---|---|---|
| **1. SINGLE DX** | | | | | | | | | | |
| 0–19 Years | 31 | 1.3 | <1 | 1 | 1 | 1 | 1 | 2 | 3 | 6 |
| 20–34 | 42 | 1.7 | 2 | 1 | 1 | 1 | 2 | 3 | 4 | 7 |
| 35–49 | 31 | 2.4 | 6 | 1 | 1 | 1 | 2 | 7 | 8 | 13 |
| 50–64 | 55 | 2.5 | 3 | 1 | 2 | 2 | 3 | 4 | 6 | 10 |
| 65+ | 57 | 1.9 | 6 | 1 | 1 | 1 | 2 | 3 | 5 | 15 |
| **2. MULTIPLE DX** | | | | | | | | | | |
| 0–19 Years | 39 | 2.9 | 18 | 1 | 1 | 2 | 4 | 6 | 8 | 9 |
| 20–34 | 117 | 3.4 | 11 | 1 | 1 | 2 | 4 | 8 | 12 | 13 |
| 35–49 | 257 | 4.7 | 14 | 1 | 2 | 4 | 6 | 9 | 11 | 15 |
| 50–64 | 774 | 4.9 | 14 | 1 | 2 | 5 | 6 | 10 | 12 | 17 |
| 65+ | 2,101 | 5.3 | 20 | 1 | 2 | 4 | 7 | 11 | 13 | 22 |
| **TOTAL SINGLE DX** | 216 | 2.0 | 4 | 1 | 1 | 1 | 3 | 4 | 6 | 11 |
| **TOTAL MULTIPLE DX** | 3,288 | 5.1 | 18 | 1 | 2 | 4 | 7 | 10 | 13 | 20 |
| **TOTAL** | | | | | | | | | | |
| 0–19 Years | 70 | 2.1 | 10 | 1 | 1 | 1 | 2 | 4 | 6 | 9 |
| 20–34 | 159 | 3.0 | 9 | 1 | 1 | 2 | 3 | 7 | 12 | 13 |
| 35–49 | 288 | 4.5 | 14 | 1 | 2 | 4 | 6 | 9 | 11 | 15 |
| 50–64 | 829 | 4.8 | 13 | 1 | 2 | 4 | 6 | 10 | 12 | 17 |
| 65+ | 2,158 | 5.2 | 20 | 1 | 2 | 4 | 7 | 11 | 13 | 22 |
| **GRAND TOTAL** | 3,504 | 4.9 | 18 | 1 | 2 | 4 | 7 | 10 | 13 | 20 |

## 88.49: CONTRAST ARTERIOGRAM NEC. Formerly included in operation group(s) 785.

| Type of Patients | Observed Patients | Avg. Stay | Vari-ance | 10th | 25th | 50th | 75th | 90th | 95th | 99th |
|---|---|---|---|---|---|---|---|---|---|---|
| **1. SINGLE DX** | | | | | | | | | | |
| 0–19 Years | 14 | 1.3 | <1 | 1 | 1 | 1 | 1 | 2 | 3 | 4 |
| 20–34 | 23 | 1.7 | 2 | 1 | 1 | 1 | 3 | 5 | 5 | 5 |
| 35–49 | 27 | 2.0 | 1 | 1 | 2 | 2 | 3 | 4 | 4 | 5 |
| 50–64 | 24 | 1.8 | 2 | 1 | 1 | 1 | 2 | 4 | 6 | 6 |
| 65+ | 9 | 1.6 | 1 | 1 | 1 | 1 | 2 | 4 | 4 | 4 |
| **2. MULTIPLE DX** | | | | | | | | | | |
| 0–19 Years | 28 | 4.0 | 30 | 1 | 1 | 2 | 5 | 9 | 22 | 22 |
| 20–34 | 87 | 4.1 | 24 | 1 | 2 | 5 | 5 | 10 | 13 | 19 |
| 35–49 | 179 | 4.6 | 16 | 2 | 3 | 6 | 6 | 11 | 13 | 18 |
| 50–64 | 194 | 4.3 | 17 | 1 | 4 | 4 | 5 | 8 | 9 | 17 |
| 65+ | 301 | 5.5 | 31 | 1 | 2 | 4 | 8 | 10 | 14 | 25 |
| **TOTAL SINGLE DX** | 97 | 1.7 | 1 | 1 | 1 | 1 | 2 | 4 | 4 | 6 |
| **TOTAL MULTIPLE DX** | 789 | 4.8 | 23 | 1 | 2 | 3 | 6 | 10 | 13 | 22 |
| **TOTAL** | | | | | | | | | | |
| 0–19 Years | 42 | 3.0 | 20 | 1 | 1 | 1 | 3 | 6 | 13 | 22 |
| 20–34 | 110 | 3.5 | 19 | 1 | 1 | 2 | 4 | 8 | 13 | 19 |
| 35–49 | 206 | 4.3 | 15 | 1 | 2 | 3 | 6 | 11 | 11 | 15 |
| 50–64 | 218 | 4.0 | 16 | 1 | 2 | 3 | 5 | 8 | 8 | 17 |
| 65+ | 310 | 5.4 | 30 | 1 | 2 | 4 | 7 | 10 | 13 | 25 |
| **GRAND TOTAL** | 886 | 4.5 | 22 | 1 | 3 | 3 | 6 | 9 | 12 | 22 |

Length of Stay by Diagnosis and Operation, United States, 2000

# United States, October 1998–September 1999 Data, by Operation

## 88.5: CONTRAST ANGIOCARDIOGRAM. Formerly included in operation group(s) 784, 785.

| Type of Patients | Observed Patients | Avg. Stay | Variance | 10th | 25th | 50th | 75th | 90th | 95th | 99th |
|---|---|---|---|---|---|---|---|---|---|---|
| **1. SINGLE DX** | | | | | | | | | | |
| 0–19 Years | 6 | 2.1 | <1 | 1 | 1 | 2 | 2 | 4 | 4 | 4 |
| 20–34 | 11 | 3.7 | 8 | 1 | 1 | 2 | 7 | 7 | 7 | 7 |
| 35–49 | 29 | 1.9 | <1 | 1 | 1 | 2 | 2 | 3 | 3 | 3 |
| 50–64 | 37 | 1.5 | <1 | 1 | 1 | 1 | 2 | 2 | 3 | 3 |
| 65+ | 40 | 1.4 | <1 | 1 | 1 | 1 | 2 | 2 | 3 | 4 |
| **2. MULTIPLE DX** | | | | | | | | | | |
| 0–19 Years | 74 | 4.1 | 32 | 1 | 1 | 1 | 5 | 11 | 15 | 29 |
| 20–34 | 55 | 4.0 | 15 | 1 | 2 | 2 | 4 | 9 | 13 | 15 |
| 35–49 | 411 | 3.0 | 8 | 1 | 1 | 2 | 4 | 7 | 8 | 12 |
| 50–64 | 989 | 2.9 | 9 | 1 | 1 | 2 | 4 | 6 | 8 | 16 |
| 65+ | 1,408 | 3.6 | 14 | 1 | 1 | 2 | 5 | 8 | 11 | 19 |
| **TOTAL SINGLE DX** | 123 | 2.0 | 3 | 1 | 1 | 1 | 2 | 4 | 7 | 7 |
| **TOTAL MULTIPLE DX** | 2,937 | 3.3 | 12 | 1 | 1 | 2 | 4 | 7 | 9 | 18 |
| **TOTAL** | | | | | | | | | | |
| 0–19 Years | 80 | 3.8 | 29 | 1 | 1 | 1 | 4 | 11 | 15 | 29 |
| 20–34 | 66 | 4.0 | 13 | 1 | 2 | 2 | 6 | 8 | 13 | 15 |
| 35–49 | 440 | 2.9 | 8 | 1 | 1 | 2 | 4 | 6 | 8 | 11 |
| 50–64 | 1,026 | 2.8 | 9 | 1 | 1 | 2 | 4 | 6 | 7 | 16 |
| 65+ | 1,448 | 3.6 | 14 | 1 | 1 | 2 | 5 | 8 | 10 | 19 |
| **GRAND TOTAL** | 3,060 | 3.2 | 12 | 1 | 1 | 2 | 4 | 7 | 9 | 17 |

## 88.51: VC ANGIOCARDIOGRAM. Formerly included in operation group(s) 785.

| Type of Patients | Observed Patients | Avg. Stay | Variance | 10th | 25th | 50th | 75th | 90th | 95th | 99th |
|---|---|---|---|---|---|---|---|---|---|---|
| **1. SINGLE DX** | | | | | | | | | | |
| 0–19 Years | 0 | | | | | | | | | |
| 20–34 | 0 | | | | | | | | | |
| 35–49 | 2 | 1.9 | 2 | 1 | 1 | 1 | 2 | 3 | 3 | 3 |
| 50–64 | 1 | 1.0 | 0 | 1 | 1 | 1 | 1 | 1 | 1 | 1 |
| 65+ | 0 | | | | | | | | | |
| **2. MULTIPLE DX** | | | | | | | | | | |
| 0–19 Years | 13 | 7.8 | 20 | 1 | 5 | 8 | 11 | 14 | 15 | 15 |
| 20–34 | 27 | 8.0 | 29 | 1 | 5 | 8 | 12 | 13 | 15 | 28 |
| 35–49 | 67 | 6.8 | 29 | 1 | 4 | 7 | 9 | 11 | 13 | 32 |
| 50–64 | 95 | 6.3 | 25 | 2 | 3 | 5 | 7 | 11 | 17 | 26 |
| 65+ | 115 | 7.7 | 36 | 2 | 3 | 6 | 9 | 19 | 21 | 29 |
| **TOTAL SINGLE DX** | 3 | 1.6 | 1 | 1 | 1 | 1 | 3 | 3 | 3 | 3 |
| **TOTAL MULTIPLE DX** | 317 | 7.1 | 30 | 2 | 3 | 6 | 9 | 14 | 19 | 28 |
| **TOTAL** | | | | | | | | | | |
| 0–19 Years | 13 | 7.8 | 20 | 1 | 5 | 8 | 11 | 14 | 15 | 15 |
| 20–34 | 27 | 8.0 | 29 | 1 | 5 | 8 | 12 | 13 | 15 | 28 |
| 35–49 | 69 | 6.7 | 29 | 1 | 3 | 7 | 9 | 11 | 13 | 32 |
| 50–64 | 96 | 6.3 | 25 | 2 | 3 | 5 | 7 | 11 | 17 | 26 |
| 65+ | 115 | 7.7 | 36 | 2 | 3 | 6 | 9 | 19 | 21 | 29 |
| **GRAND TOTAL** | 320 | 7.1 | 30 | 2 | 3 | 6 | 8 | 13 | 19 | 28 |

## 88.56: COR ARTERIOGRAM-2 CATH. Formerly included in operation group(s) 784.

| Type of Patients | Observed Patients | Avg. Stay | Variance | 10th | 25th | 50th | 75th | 90th | 95th | 99th |
|---|---|---|---|---|---|---|---|---|---|---|
| **1. SINGLE DX** | | | | | | | | | | |
| 0–19 Years | 1 | 2.0 | 0 | 2 | 2 | 2 | 2 | 2 | 2 | 2 |
| 20–34 | 9 | 4.0 | 9 | 1 | 1 | 4 | 7 | 7 | 7 | 7 |
| 35–49 | 21 | 1.8 | <1 | 1 | 1 | 2 | 2 | 3 | 3 | 3 |
| 50–64 | 23 | 1.4 | <1 | 1 | 1 | 1 | 2 | 2 | 4 | 5 |
| 65+ | 34 | 1.3 | <1 | 1 | 1 | 1 | 2 | 2 | 3 | 4 |
| **2. MULTIPLE DX** | | | | | | | | | | |
| 0–19 Years | 5 | 6.1 | 55 | 1 | 2 | 2 | 5 | 11 | 18 | 18 |
| 20–34 | 20 | 2.7 | 2 | 2 | 3 | 2 | 4 | 4 | 5 | 5 |
| 35–49 | 266 | 2.6 | 4 | 1 | 1 | 2 | 4 | 5 | 7 | 9 |
| 50–64 | 689 | 2.6 | 8 | 1 | 1 | 2 | 3 | 5 | 6 | 13 |
| 65+ | 1,047 | 3.2 | 11 | 1 | 2 | 2 | 4 | 7 | 9 | 15 |
| **TOTAL SINGLE DX** | 88 | 2.1 | 3 | 1 | 1 | 1 | 2 | 4 | 7 | 7 |
| **TOTAL MULTIPLE DX** | 2,027 | 2.9 | 9 | 1 | 1 | 2 | 4 | 6 | 8 | 14 |
| **TOTAL** | | | | | | | | | | |
| 0–19 Years | 6 | 4.2 | 34 | 1 | 2 | 2 | 4 | 11 | 18 | 18 |
| 20–34 | 29 | 3.1 | 5 | 1 | 2 | 2 | 4 | 7 | 7 | 7 |
| 35–49 | 287 | 2.6 | 4 | 1 | 1 | 2 | 3 | 5 | 7 | 9 |
| 50–64 | 712 | 2.5 | 8 | 1 | 1 | 2 | 3 | 5 | 6 | 12 |
| 65+ | 1,081 | 3.2 | 10 | 1 | 2 | 2 | 4 | 7 | 9 | 15 |
| **GRAND TOTAL** | 2,115 | 2.9 | 8 | 1 | 1 | 2 | 4 | 6 | 8 | 14 |

## 88.6: PHLEBOGRAPHY. Formerly included in operation group(s) 785.

| Type of Patients | Observed Patients | Avg. Stay | Variance | 10th | 25th | 50th | 75th | 90th | 95th | 99th |
|---|---|---|---|---|---|---|---|---|---|---|
| **1. SINGLE DX** | | | | | | | | | | |
| 0–19 Years | 14 | 2.4 | 4 | 1 | 1 | 2 | 2 | 4 | 6 | 9 |
| 20–34 | 30 | 2.7 | 4 | 1 | 1 | 2 | 4 | 6 | 7 | 9 |
| 35–49 | 47 | 4.5 | 8 | 1 | 4 | 4 | 5 | 10 | 10 | 13 |
| 50–64 | 20 | 3.9 | 7 | 1 | 3 | 4 | 4 | 5 | 11 | 14 |
| 65+ | 15 | 4.8 | 6 | 1 | 3 | 4 | 7 | 8 | 8 | 9 |
| **2. MULTIPLE DX** | | | | | | | | | | |
| 0–19 Years | 51 | 4.8 | 17 | 1 | 2 | 4 | 6 | 9 | 17 | 21 |
| 20–34 | 136 | 5.8 | 18 | 1 | 3 | 6 | 7 | 11 | 14 | 21 |
| 35–49 | 351 | 5.4 | 16 | 2 | 3 | 5 | 7 | 10 | 13 | 20 |
| 50–64 | 367 | 5.1 | 21 | 1 | 2 | 4 | 7 | 9 | 12 | 23 |
| 65+ | 544 | 6.4 | 25 | 2 | 3 | 5 | 8 | 13 | 15 | 22 |
| **TOTAL SINGLE DX** | 126 | 3.8 | 7 | 1 | 2 | 4 | 5 | 7 | 8 | 13 |
| **TOTAL MULTIPLE DX** | 1,449 | 5.7 | 21 | 1 | 3 | 5 | 7 | 11 | 14 | 22 |
| **TOTAL** | | | | | | | | | | |
| 0–19 Years | 65 | 4.4 | 16 | 1 | 2 | 3 | 6 | 8 | 13 | 19 |
| 20–34 | 166 | 5.2 | 17 | 1 | 3 | 4 | 6 | 10 | 12 | 20 |
| 35–49 | 398 | 5.2 | 15 | 1 | 3 | 4 | 7 | 10 | 13 | 20 |
| 50–64 | 387 | 5.0 | 20 | 1 | 2 | 4 | 7 | 9 | 12 | 23 |
| 65+ | 559 | 6.4 | 24 | 2 | 3 | 5 | 8 | 13 | 14 | 22 |
| **GRAND TOTAL** | 1,575 | 5.6 | 20 | 1 | 3 | 5 | 7 | 11 | 14 | 21 |

Length of Stay by Diagnosis and Operation, United States, 2000

# United States, October 1998–September 1999 Data, by Operation

## 88.7: DIAGNOSTIC ULTRASOUND. Formerly included in operation group(s) 787.

| Type of Patients | Observed Patients | Avg. Stay | Variance | 10th | 25th | 50th | 75th | 90th | 95th | 99th |
|---|---|---|---|---|---|---|---|---|---|---|
| **1. SINGLE DX** | | | | | | | | | | |
| 0–19 Years | 1,306 | 2.5 | 4 | 1 | 1 | 2 | 3 | 4 | 5 | 9 |
| 20–34 | 1,281 | 2.2 | 4 | 1 | 1 | 2 | 3 | 4 | 5 | 8 |
| 35–49 | 909 | 2.4 | 4 | 1 | 1 | 2 | 3 | 5 | 6 | 9 |
| 50–64 | 533 | 2.6 | 7 | 1 | 1 | 2 | 3 | 5 | 6 | 10 |
| 65+ | 435 | 2.5 | 4 | 1 | 1 | 2 | 3 | 6 | 6 | 9 |
| **2. MULTIPLE DX** | | | | | | | | | | |
| 0–19 Years | 6,163 | 5.3 | 52 | 1 | 2 | 3 | 6 | 10 | 17 | 39 |
| 20–34 | 5,988 | 4.0 | 22 | 1 | 2 | 3 | 5 | 8 | 11 | 25 |
| 35–49 | 11,197 | 4.4 | 19 | 1 | 2 | 3 | 5 | 9 | 11 | 21 |
| 50–64 | 17,136 | 4.6 | 18 | 1 | 2 | 4 | 6 | 9 | 11 | 20 |
| 65+ | 44,412 | 5.3 | 19 | 2 | 3 | 4 | 7 | 10 | 12 | 21 |
| **TOTAL SINGLE DX** | 4,464 | 2.4 | 5 | 1 | 1 | 2 | 3 | 5 | 6 | 9 |
| **TOTAL MULTIPLE DX** | 84,896 | 5.0 | 22 | 1 | 2 | 4 | 6 | 9 | 12 | 22 |
| **TOTAL** | | | | | | | | | | |
| 0–19 Years | 7,469 | 4.8 | 45 | 1 | 2 | 3 | 5 | 9 | 15 | 36 |
| 20–34 | 7,269 | 3.6 | 18 | 1 | 1 | 2 | 4 | 7 | 10 | 21 |
| 35–49 | 12,106 | 4.2 | 18 | 1 | 2 | 3 | 5 | 8 | 11 | 21 |
| 50–64 | 17,669 | 4.5 | 18 | 1 | 2 | 3 | 6 | 8 | 11 | 20 |
| 65+ | 44,847 | 5.3 | 19 | 2 | 3 | 4 | 7 | 10 | 12 | 21 |
| **GRAND TOTAL** | 89,360 | 4.8 | 21 | 1 | 2 | 4 | 6 | 9 | 12 | 22 |

## 88.71: DXTIC US-HEAD/NECK. Formerly included in operation group(s) 787.

| Type of Patients | Observed Patients | Avg. Stay | Variance | 10th | 25th | 50th | 75th | 90th | 95th | 99th |
|---|---|---|---|---|---|---|---|---|---|---|
| **1. SINGLE DX** | | | | | | | | | | |
| 0–19 Years | 45 | 2.8 | 3 | 1 | 2 | 3 | 3 | 4 | 4 | 12 |
| 20–34 | 1 | 1.0 | 0 | 1 | 1 | 1 | 1 | 1 | 1 | 1 |
| 35–49 | 20 | 2.5 | 3 | 2 | 2 | 2 | 3 | 4 | 5 | 10 |
| 50–64 | 36 | 2.8 | <1 | 2 | 2 | 3 | 3 | 3 | 5 | 5 |
| 65+ | 61 | 3.0 | 5 | 1 | 1 | 1 | 6 | 6 | 6 | 6 |
| **2. MULTIPLE DX** | | | | | | | | | | |
| 0–19 Years | 579 | 14.9 | 184 | 2 | 5 | 11 | 21 | 33 | 43 | 58 |
| 20–34 | 44 | 3.8 | 16 | 1 | 2 | 2 | 4 | 7 | 12 | 19 |
| 35–49 | 307 | 4.5 | 17 | 1 | 2 | 3 | 5 | 12 | 12 | 14 |
| 50–64 | 896 | 4.0 | 31 | 1 | 2 | 3 | 5 | 8 | 9 | 20 |
| 65+ | 3,341 | 4.4 | 14 | 1 | 2 | 3 | 6 | 8 | 11 | 16 |
| **TOTAL SINGLE DX** | 163 | 2.9 | 4 | 1 | 1 | 3 | 4 | 6 | 6 | 6 |
| **TOTAL MULTIPLE DX** | 5,167 | 5.3 | 41 | 1 | 2 | 3 | 6 | 11 | 14 | 35 |
| **TOTAL** | | | | | | | | | | |
| 0–19 Years | 624 | 12.6 | 172 | 2 | 3 | 7 | 18 | 31 | 40 | 56 |
| 20–34 | 45 | 3.7 | 16 | 1 | 2 | 2 | 4 | 7 | 12 | 19 |
| 35–49 | 327 | 4.4 | 17 | 1 | 2 | 3 | 5 | 12 | 12 | 14 |
| 50–64 | 932 | 3.9 | 29 | 1 | 2 | 3 | 4 | 6 | 9 | 14 |
| 65+ | 3,402 | 4.4 | 14 | 1 | 2 | 3 | 6 | 8 | 11 | 16 |
| **GRAND TOTAL** | 5,330 | 5.1 | 39 | 1 | 2 | 3 | 6 | 10 | 14 | 34 |

## 88.66: CONTRAST PHLEBOGRAM-LEG. Formerly included in operation group(s) 785.

| Type of Patients | Observed Patients | Avg. Stay | Variance | 10th | 25th | 50th | 75th | 90th | 95th | 99th |
|---|---|---|---|---|---|---|---|---|---|---|
| **1. SINGLE DX** | | | | | | | | | | |
| 0–19 Years | 3 | 3.0 | 9 | 1 | 1 | 1 | 6 | 6 | 6 | 6 |
| 20–34 | 14 | 2.3 | 4 | 1 | 2 | 3 | 3 | 5 | 6 | 8 |
| 35–49 | 27 | 5.1 | 8 | 1 | 3 | 5 | 6 | 9 | 11 | 13 |
| 50–64 | 16 | 4.4 | 13 | 1 | 3 | 4 | 5 | 11 | 11 | 14 |
| 65+ | 12 | 4.7 | 5 | 2 | 3 | 4 | 7 | 8 | 8 | 9 |
| **2. MULTIPLE DX** | | | | | | | | | | |
| 0–19 Years | 13 | 4.3 | 7 | 1 | 2 | 4 | 6 | 7 | 10 | 10 |
| 20–34 | 65 | 5.2 | 11 | 2 | 3 | 6 | 6 | 8 | 10 | 19 |
| 35–49 | 173 | 5.0 | 13 | 1 | 3 | 5 | 6 | 10 | 12 | 19 |
| 50–64 | 181 | 4.6 | 14 | 1 | 2 | 4 | 7 | 9 | 11 | 16 |
| 65+ | 303 | 5.9 | 14 | 2 | 3 | 5 | 8 | 12 | 13 | 18 |
| **TOTAL SINGLE DX** | 72 | 4.1 | 9 | 1 | 1 | 4 | 5 | 8 | 10 | 13 |
| **TOTAL MULTIPLE DX** | 735 | 5.3 | 14 | 1 | 3 | 5 | 7 | 10 | 12 | 18 |
| **TOTAL** | | | | | | | | | | |
| 0–19 Years | 16 | 4.2 | 7 | 1 | 2 | 4 | 6 | 7 | 10 | 10 |
| 20–34 | 79 | 4.6 | 11 | 1 | 2 | 4 | 6 | 7 | 10 | 19 |
| 35–49 | 200 | 5.0 | 12 | 1 | 3 | 5 | 6 | 9 | 12 | 16 |
| 50–64 | 197 | 4.6 | 14 | 1 | 2 | 4 | 7 | 9 | 11 | 16 |
| 65+ | 315 | 5.9 | 14 | 2 | 3 | 5 | 8 | 12 | 13 | 18 |
| **GRAND TOTAL** | 807 | 5.2 | 13 | 1 | 3 | 5 | 7 | 10 | 12 | 17 |

## 88.67: CONTRAST PHLEBOGRAM NEC. Formerly included in operation group(s) 785.

| Type of Patients | Observed Patients | Avg. Stay | Variance | 10th | 25th | 50th | 75th | 90th | 95th | 99th |
|---|---|---|---|---|---|---|---|---|---|---|
| **1. SINGLE DX** | | | | | | | | | | |
| 0–19 Years | 7 | 2.7 | 5 | 1 | 1 | 2 | 4 | 4 | 9 | 9 |
| 20–34 | 13 | 3.2 | 2 | 1 | 2 | 3 | 4 | 6 | 6 | 7 |
| 35–49 | 16 | 3.9 | 2 | 2 | 4 | 4 | 4 | 5 | 5 | 13 |
| 50–64 | 3 | 3.8 | <1 | 3 | 4 | 4 | 4 | 4 | 4 | 4 |
| 65+ | 3 | 5.5 | 10 | 1 | 5 | 5 | 8 | 8 | 8 | 8 |
| **2. MULTIPLE DX** | | | | | | | | | | |
| 0–19 Years | 29 | 4.9 | 21 | 1 | 2 | 4 | 6 | 9 | 18 | 21 |
| 20–34 | 58 | 7.1 | 29 | 3 | 3 | 5 | 10 | 14 | 20 | 21 |
| 35–49 | 139 | 6.1 | 21 | 2 | 3 | 5 | 8 | 13 | 16 | 22 |
| 50–64 | 136 | 5.6 | 25 | 2 | 3 | 5 | 6 | 10 | 14 | 20 |
| 65+ | 188 | 7.2 | 40 | 2 | 3 | 5 | 9 | 14 | 17 | 32 |
| **TOTAL SINGLE DX** | 42 | 3.7 | 3 | 2 | 3 | 4 | 4 | 5 | 6 | 9 |
| **TOTAL MULTIPLE DX** | 550 | 6.4 | 30 | 2 | 3 | 5 | 8 | 13 | 16 | 30 |
| **TOTAL** | | | | | | | | | | |
| 0–19 Years | 36 | 4.6 | 19 | 1 | 1 | 4 | 6 | 9 | 18 | 21 |
| 20–34 | 71 | 6.3 | 26 | 2 | 3 | 4 | 9 | 12 | 18 | 21 |
| 35–49 | 155 | 5.7 | 18 | 2 | 3 | 4 | 7 | 11 | 16 | 20 |
| 50–64 | 139 | 5.4 | 24 | 2 | 3 | 4 | 6 | 10 | 13 | 20 |
| 65+ | 191 | 7.1 | 40 | 2 | 3 | 5 | 9 | 14 | 17 | 32 |
| **GRAND TOTAL** | 592 | 6.1 | 28 | 2 | 3 | 5 | 7 | 12 | 15 | 25 |

Length of Stay by Diagnosis and Operation, United States, 2000

# United States, October 1998–September 1999 Data, by Operation

## 88.72: DXTIC ULTRASOUND-HEART. Formerly included in operation group(s) 787.

| Type of Patients | Observed Patients | Avg. Stay | Variance | 10th | 25th | 50th | 75th | 90th | 95th | 99th |
|---|---|---|---|---|---|---|---|---|---|---|
| **1. SINGLE DX** | | | | | | | | | | |
| 0–19 Years | 326 | 2.6 | 3 | 1 | 1 | 2 | 3 | 5 | 6 | 10 |
| 20–34 | 166 | 1.6 | 2 | 1 | 1 | 1 | 2 | 3 | 4 | 8 |
| 35–49 | 359 | 1.9 | 4 | 1 | 1 | 1 | 2 | 3 | 5 | 8 |
| 50–64 | 302 | 2.6 | 13 | 1 | 1 | 2 | 3 | 5 | 5 | 32 |
| 65+ | 242 | 2.1 | 4 | 1 | 1 | 1 | 2 | 5 | 6 | 9 |
| **2. MULTIPLE DX** | | | | | | | | | | |
| 0–19 Years | 2,215 | 5.7 | 59 | 1 | 2 | 3 | 6 | 11 | 17 | 39 |
| 20–34 | 1,775 | 5.6 | 35 | 1 | 2 | 4 | 6 | 13 | 16 | 33 |
| 35–49 | 6,512 | 4.4 | 18 | 1 | 2 | 3 | 5 | 9 | 11 | 22 |
| 50–64 | 11,897 | 4.6 | 17 | 1 | 2 | 4 | 6 | 9 | 11 | 20 |
| 65+ | 32,249 | 5.4 | 20 | 2 | 3 | 4 | 7 | 10 | 13 | 22 |
| **TOTAL SINGLE DX** | 1,395 | 2.2 | 5 | 1 | 1 | 2 | 3 | 4 | 5 | 9 |
| **TOTAL MULTIPLE DX** | 54,648 | 5.1 | 21 | 1 | 2 | 4 | 6 | 9 | 13 | 22 |
| **TOTAL** | | | | | | | | | | |
| 0–19 Years | 2,541 | 5.3 | 52 | 1 | 2 | 3 | 6 | 10 | 16 | 37 |
| 20–34 | 1,941 | 5.1 | 33 | 1 | 2 | 3 | 6 | 11 | 15 | 30 |
| 35–49 | 6,871 | 4.3 | 18 | 1 | 2 | 3 | 5 | 9 | 11 | 21 |
| 50–64 | 12,199 | 4.5 | 17 | 1 | 2 | 4 | 6 | 8 | 11 | 20 |
| 65+ | 32,491 | 5.3 | 20 | 2 | 3 | 4 | 7 | 10 | 13 | 22 |
| **GRAND TOTAL** | 56,043 | 5.0 | 21 | 1 | 2 | 4 | 6 | 9 | 12 | 22 |

## 88.74: DXTIC ULTRASOUND-DIGEST. Formerly included in operation group(s) 787.

| Type of Patients | Observed Patients | Avg. Stay | Variance | 10th | 25th | 50th | 75th | 90th | 95th | 99th |
|---|---|---|---|---|---|---|---|---|---|---|
| **1. SINGLE DX** | | | | | | | | | | |
| 0–19 Years | 36 | 2.1 | <1 | 1 | 2 | 2 | 3 | 3 | 4 | 5 |
| 20–34 | 43 | 2.5 | 2 | 1 | 1 | 2 | 3 | 5 | 6 | 7 |
| 35–49 | 37 | 1.9 | 3 | 1 | 1 | 1 | 2 | 3 | 5 | 6 |
| 50–64 | 25 | 1.3 | <1 | 1 | 1 | 1 | 2 | 2 | 4 | 4 |
| 65+ | 9 | 3.6 | 9 | 1 | 2 | 2 | 5 | 10 | 10 | 10 |
| **2. MULTIPLE DX** | | | | | | | | | | |
| 0–19 Years | 83 | 3.5 | 10 | 1 | 2 | 2 | 4 | 6 | 11 | 15 |
| 20–34 | 176 | 3.2 | 10 | 1 | 2 | 2 | 3 | 6 | 11 | 14 |
| 35–49 | 309 | 3.4 | 7 | 1 | 2 | 3 | 4 | 7 | 8 | 16 |
| 50–64 | 288 | 4.1 | 10 | 1 | 2 | 3 | 5 | 8 | 10 | 16 |
| 65+ | 484 | 4.5 | 10 | 2 | 2 | 3 | 6 | 10 | 10 | 17 |
| **TOTAL SINGLE DX** | 150 | 2.0 | 2 | 1 | 1 | 1 | 2 | 5 | 5 | 6 |
| **TOTAL MULTIPLE DX** | 1,340 | 4.0 | 10 | 1 | 2 | 3 | 5 | 8 | 10 | 16 |
| **TOTAL** | | | | | | | | | | |
| 0–19 Years | 119 | 3.1 | 8 | 1 | 2 | 2 | 3 | 5 | 7 | 15 |
| 20–34 | 219 | 3.0 | 8 | 1 | 2 | 2 | 3 | 5 | 8 | 14 |
| 35–49 | 346 | 3.3 | 7 | 1 | 2 | 3 | 4 | 7 | 7 | 16 |
| 50–64 | 313 | 3.6 | 10 | 1 | 2 | 3 | 5 | 8 | 9 | 16 |
| 65+ | 493 | 4.4 | 10 | 2 | 2 | 3 | 6 | 10 | 10 | 17 |
| **GRAND TOTAL** | 1,490 | 3.8 | 9 | 1 | 2 | 3 | 5 | 8 | 10 | 16 |

## 88.75: DXTIC ULTRASOUND-URINARY. Formerly included in operation group(s) 787.

| Type of Patients | Observed Patients | Avg. Stay | Variance | 10th | 25th | 50th | 75th | 90th | 95th | 99th |
|---|---|---|---|---|---|---|---|---|---|---|
| **1. SINGLE DX** | | | | | | | | | | |
| 0–19 Years | 268 | 2.6 | 8 | 1 | 2 | 2 | 3 | 4 | 5 | 9 |
| 20–34 | 59 | 2.5 | 1 | 2 | 2 | 2 | 3 | 4 | 5 | 6 |
| 35–49 | 40 | 1.9 | 2 | 1 | 1 | 2 | 3 | 4 | 6 | 7 |
| 50–64 | 22 | 2.6 | <1 | 1 | 2 | 3 | 3 | 4 | 5 | 6 |
| 65+ | 11 | 3.3 | 2 | 1 | 2 | 4 | 4 | 4 | 5 | 7 |
| **2. MULTIPLE DX** | | | | | | | | | | |
| 0–19 Years | 1,530 | 3.6 | 9 | 2 | 2 | 3 | 4 | 6 | 8 | 16 |
| 20–34 | 583 | 3.2 | 7 | 2 | 2 | 3 | 4 | 6 | 7 | 12 |
| 35–49 | 588 | 4.5 | 19 | 1 | 2 | 3 | 5 | 8 | 10 | 21 |
| 50–64 | 756 | 4.5 | 13 | 2 | 3 | 4 | 5 | 8 | 11 | 19 |
| 65+ | 1,644 | 5.9 | 21 | 2 | 3 | 5 | 7 | 10 | 13 | 21 |
| **TOTAL SINGLE DX** | 400 | 2.6 | 5 | 1 | 2 | 2 | 3 | 4 | 4 | 7 |
| **TOTAL MULTIPLE DX** | 5,101 | 4.7 | 16 | 2 | 2 | 4 | 6 | 9 | 11 | 19 |
| **TOTAL** | | | | | | | | | | |
| 0–19 Years | 1,798 | 3.5 | 9 | 1 | 2 | 3 | 4 | 6 | 8 | 15 |
| 20–34 | 642 | 3.1 | 6 | 2 | 2 | 3 | 4 | 5 | 7 | 12 |
| 35–49 | 628 | 4.4 | 18 | 1 | 2 | 3 | 5 | 8 | 10 | 21 |
| 50–64 | 778 | 4.4 | 12 | 2 | 3 | 4 | 5 | 8 | 11 | 19 |
| 65+ | 1,655 | 5.9 | 21 | 2 | 3 | 5 | 7 | 10 | 13 | 21 |
| **GRAND TOTAL** | 5,501 | 4.5 | 16 | 2 | 2 | 4 | 6 | 8 | 11 | 19 |

## 88.76: DXTIC ULTRASOUND-ABD. Formerly included in operation group(s) 787.

| Type of Patients | Observed Patients | Avg. Stay | Variance | 10th | 25th | 50th | 75th | 90th | 95th | 99th |
|---|---|---|---|---|---|---|---|---|---|---|
| **1. SINGLE DX** | | | | | | | | | | |
| 0–19 Years | 413 | 2.3 | 2 | 1 | 1 | 2 | 3 | 4 | 5 | 7 |
| 20–34 | 292 | 2.1 | 2 | 1 | 1 | 2 | 3 | 4 | 4 | 8 |
| 35–49 | 202 | 2.5 | 3 | 1 | 1 | 2 | 5 | 5 | 6 | 7 |
| 50–64 | 57 | 2.2 | 2 | 1 | 1 | 3 | 5 | 5 | 6 | 6 |
| 65+ | 49 | 1.9 | 2 | 1 | 1 | 2 | 4 | 4 | 4 | 7 |
| **2. MULTIPLE DX** | | | | | | | | | | |
| 0–19 Years | 1,051 | 3.9 | 21 | 1 | 2 | 3 | 4 | 7 | 10 | 21 |
| 20–34 | 1,296 | 3.5 | 17 | 1 | 2 | 3 | 5 | 8 | 10 | 13 |
| 35–49 | 1,834 | 3.9 | 13 | 1 | 2 | 3 | 5 | 8 | 10 | 15 |
| 50–64 | 1,455 | 4.5 | 14 | 1 | 2 | 4 | 6 | 9 | 11 | 16 |
| 65+ | 2,690 | 5.1 | 16 | 2 | 2 | 4 | 6 | 10 | 12 | 20 |
| **TOTAL SINGLE DX** | 1,013 | 2.2 | 2 | 1 | 1 | 2 | 3 | 4 | 5 | 7 |
| **TOTAL MULTIPLE DX** | 8,326 | 4.3 | 16 | 1 | 2 | 3 | 5 | 8 | 12 | 18 |
| **TOTAL** | | | | | | | | | | |
| 0–19 Years | 1,464 | 3.4 | 17 | 1 | 2 | 2 | 4 | 7 | 9 | 20 |
| 20–34 | 1,588 | 3.3 | 15 | 1 | 2 | 3 | 4 | 6 | 8 | 13 |
| 35–49 | 2,036 | 3.8 | 12 | 1 | 2 | 3 | 5 | 7 | 9 | 15 |
| 50–64 | 1,512 | 4.4 | 13 | 1 | 2 | 3 | 6 | 9 | 11 | 16 |
| 65+ | 2,739 | 5.0 | 16 | 2 | 2 | 4 | 6 | 10 | 12 | 19 |
| **GRAND TOTAL** | 9,339 | 4.1 | 15 | 1 | 2 | 3 | 5 | 8 | 11 | 17 |

Length of Stay by Diagnosis and Operation, United States, 2000

# United States, October 1998–September 1999 Data, by Operation

## 88.77: DXTIC ULTRASOUND-VASC. Formerly included in operation group(s) 787.

| Type of Patients | Observed Patients | Avg. Stay | Vari-ance | Percentiles | | | | | | |
|---|---|---|---|---|---|---|---|---|---|---|
| | | | | 10th | 25th | 50th | 75th | 90th | 95th | 99th |
| **1. SINGLE DX** | | | | | | | | | | |
| 0–19 Years | 19 | 3.9 | 6 | 1 | 2 | 4 | 6 | 6 | 8 | 11 |
| 20–34 | 85 | 4.0 | 5 | 1 | 2 | 4 | 5 | 8 | 8 | 12 |
| 35–49 | 116 | 3.3 | 5 | 1 | 1 | 4 | 6 | 6 | 6 | 9 |
| 50–64 | 77 | 4.1 | 5 | 1 | 3 | 3 | 6 | 7 | 9 | 10 |
| 65+ | 56 | 3.2 | 2 | 1 | 3 | 3 | 3 | 4 | 5 | 10 |
| **2. MULTIPLE DX** | | | | | | | | | | |
| 0–19 Years | 93 | 4.7 | 8 | 2 | 2 | 4 | 6 | 8 | 10 | 14 |
| 20–34 | 455 | 5.0 | 14 | 1 | 3 | 4 | 6 | 8 | 11 | 18 |
| 35–49 | 1,087 | 5.5 | 18 | 2 | 3 | 4 | 7 | 11 | 13 | 28 |
| 50–64 | 1,647 | 5.3 | 27 | 1 | 3 | 4 | 6 | 10 | 13 | 24 |
| 65+ | 3,647 | 5.7 | 17 | 2 | 3 | 5 | 7 | 10 | 13 | 22 |
| **TOTAL SINGLE DX** | 353 | 3.6 | 5 | 1 | 2 | 3 | 5 | 6 | 8 | 10 |
| **TOTAL MULTIPLE DX** | 6,929 | 5.5 | 20 | 2 | 3 | 5 | 7 | 10 | 13 | 23 |
| **TOTAL** | | | | | | | | | | |
| 0–19 Years | 112 | 4.6 | 8 | 2 | 2 | 4 | 6 | 8 | 10 | 14 |
| 20–34 | 540 | 4.8 | 12 | 1 | 3 | 4 | 6 | 9 | 11 | 16 |
| 35–49 | 1,203 | 5.2 | 18 | 1 | 2 | 4 | 6 | 10 | 12 | 29 |
| 50–64 | 1,724 | 5.3 | 26 | 1 | 3 | 4 | 6 | 9 | 12 | 24 |
| 65+ | 3,703 | 5.7 | 17 | 2 | 3 | 5 | 7 | 10 | 13 | 22 |
| **GRAND TOTAL** | 7,282 | 5.4 | 19 | 2 | 3 | 4 | 7 | 10 | 12 | 23 |

## 88.78: DXTIC US-GRAVID UTERUS. Formerly included in operation group(s) 787.

| Type of Patients | Observed Patients | Avg. Stay | Vari-ance | Percentiles | | | | | | |
|---|---|---|---|---|---|---|---|---|---|---|
| | | | | 10th | 25th | 50th | 75th | 90th | 95th | 99th |
| **1. SINGLE DX** | | | | | | | | | | |
| 0–19 Years | 106 | 2.4 | 13 | 1 | 1 | 2 | 3 | 3 | 5 | 17 |
| 20–34 | 509 | 2.1 | 5 | 1 | 1 | 1 | 2 | 4 | 5 | 11 |
| 35–49 | 66 | 2.0 | 3 | 1 | 1 | 1 | 2 | 4 | 4 | 9 |
| 50–64 | 0 | | | | | | | | | |
| 65+ | 0 | | | | | | | | | |
| **2. MULTIPLE DX** | | | | | | | | | | |
| 0–19 Years | 348 | 3.7 | 24 | 1 | 1 | 3 | 4 | 6 | 10 | 15 |
| 20–34 | 1,359 | 3.1 | 16 | 1 | 1 | 2 | 3 | 6 | 9 | 19 |
| 35–49 | 284 | 4.3 | 73 | 1 | 1 | 2 | 4 | 7 | 10 | 65 |
| 50–64 | 2 | 5.0 | 0 | 5 | 5 | 5 | 5 | 5 | 5 | 5 |
| 65+ | 0 | | | | | | | | | |
| **TOTAL SINGLE DX** | 681 | 2.1 | 5 | 1 | 1 | 1 | 2 | 4 | 5 | 11 |
| **TOTAL MULTIPLE DX** | 1,993 | 3.4 | 25 | 1 | 2 | 2 | 4 | 6 | 9 | 21 |
| **TOTAL** | | | | | | | | | | |
| 0–19 Years | 454 | 3.4 | 22 | 1 | 1 | 2 | 4 | 6 | 8 | 15 |
| 20–34 | 1,868 | 2.8 | 13 | 1 | 1 | 2 | 3 | 5 | 7 | 17 |
| 35–49 | 350 | 3.7 | 58 | 1 | 1 | 2 | 3 | 7 | 9 | 40 |
| 50–64 | 2 | 5.0 | 0 | 5 | 5 | 5 | 5 | 5 | 5 | 5 |
| 65+ | 0 | | | | | | | | | |
| **GRAND TOTAL** | 2,674 | 3.0 | 20 | 1 | 1 | 2 | 3 | 6 | 8 | 18 |

## 88.79: DXTIC ULTRASOUND NEC. Formerly included in operation group(s) 787.

| Type of Patients | Observed Patients | Avg. Stay | Vari-ance | Percentiles | | | | | | |
|---|---|---|---|---|---|---|---|---|---|---|
| | | | | 10th | 25th | 50th | 75th | 90th | 95th | 99th |
| **1. SINGLE DX** | | | | | | | | | | |
| 0–19 Years | 89 | 2.1 | 3 | 1 | 1 | 2 | 2 | 4 | 5 | 10 |
| 20–34 | 123 | 1.9 | 4 | 1 | 1 | 2 | 2 | 3 | 3 | 8 |
| 35–49 | 64 | 2.3 | 2 | 1 | 1 | 2 | 3 | 4 | 5 | 7 |
| 50–64 | 13 | 4.3 | 3 | 2 | 4 | 4 | 4 | 7 | 7 | 10 |
| 65+ | 6 | 2.1 | 10 | 1 | 1 | 1 | 1 | 4 | 8 | 19 |
| **2. MULTIPLE DX** | | | | | | | | | | |
| 0–19 Years | 250 | 3.1 | 7 | 1 | 2 | 2 | 3 | 5 | 8 | 15 |
| 20–34 | 284 | 3.0 | 15 | 1 | 2 | 2 | 3 | 5 | 6 | 19 |
| 35–49 | 247 | 4.2 | 46 | 1 | 2 | 3 | 4 | 8 | 10 | 19 |
| 50–64 | 172 | 5.1 | 19 | 2 | 3 | 4 | 6 | 10 | 15 | 22 |
| 65+ | 266 | 5.2 | 30 | 1 | 2 | 4 | 6 | 10 | 13 | 24 |
| **TOTAL SINGLE DX** | 295 | 2.2 | 4 | 1 | 1 | 2 | 3 | 4 | 5 | 9 |
| **TOTAL MULTIPLE DX** | 1,219 | 4.0 | 25 | 1 | 2 | 3 | 4 | 8 | 10 | 19 |
| **TOTAL** | | | | | | | | | | |
| 0–19 Years | 339 | 2.9 | 6 | 1 | 2 | 2 | 3 | 5 | 7 | 14 |
| 20–34 | 407 | 2.7 | 13 | 1 | 1 | 2 | 3 | 5 | 6 | 16 |
| 35–49 | 311 | 3.9 | 39 | 1 | 2 | 3 | 4 | 8 | 10 | 16 |
| 50–64 | 185 | 5.1 | 18 | 2 | 3 | 4 | 6 | 10 | 15 | 22 |
| 65+ | 272 | 5.1 | 30 | 1 | 2 | 4 | 6 | 10 | 13 | 24 |
| **GRAND TOTAL** | 1,514 | 3.7 | 21 | 1 | 2 | 3 | 4 | 7 | 10 | 19 |

## 88.8: THERMOGRAPHY. Formerly included in operation group(s) 787.

| Type of Patients | Observed Patients | Avg. Stay | Vari-ance | Percentiles | | | | | | |
|---|---|---|---|---|---|---|---|---|---|---|
| | | | | 10th | 25th | 50th | 75th | 90th | 95th | 99th |
| **1. SINGLE DX** | | | | | | | | | | |
| 0–19 Years | 0 | | | | | | | | | |
| 20–34 | 0 | | | | | | | | | |
| 35–49 | 0 | | | | | | | | | |
| 50–64 | 0 | | | | | | | | | |
| 65+ | 0 | | | | | | | | | |
| **2. MULTIPLE DX** | | | | | | | | | | |
| 0–19 Years | 0 | | | | | | | | | |
| 20–34 | 2 | 3.2 | 1 | 2 | 2 | 4 | 4 | 4 | 4 | 4 |
| 35–49 | 2 | 3.8 | 4 | 1 | 1 | 5 | 5 | 5 | 5 | 5 |
| 50–64 | 0 | | | | | | | | | |
| 65+ | 3 | 9.3 | 56 | 2 | 2 | 16 | 16 | 16 | 16 | 16 |
| **TOTAL SINGLE DX** | 0 | | | | | | | | | |
| **TOTAL MULTIPLE DX** | 7 | 5.7 | 30 | 2 | 2 | 4 | 5 | 16 | 16 | 16 |
| **TOTAL** | | | | | | | | | | |
| 0–19 Years | 0 | | | | | | | | | |
| 20–34 | 2 | 3.2 | 1 | 2 | 2 | 4 | 4 | 4 | 4 | 4 |
| 35–49 | 2 | 3.8 | 4 | 1 | 1 | 5 | 5 | 5 | 5 | 5 |
| 50–64 | 0 | | | | | | | | | |
| 65+ | 3 | 9.3 | 56 | 2 | 2 | 16 | 16 | 16 | 16 | 16 |
| **GRAND TOTAL** | 7 | 5.7 | 30 | 2 | 2 | 4 | 5 | 16 | 16 | 16 |

Length of Stay by Diagnosis and Operation, United States, 2000

# United States, October 1998–September 1999 Data, by Operation

## 88.9: OTHER DIAGNOSTIC IMAGING. Formerly included in operation group(s) 787.

| Type of Patients | Observed Patients | Avg. Stay | Variance | Percentiles | | | | | | |
|---|---|---|---|---|---|---|---|---|---|---|
| | | | | 10th | 25th | 50th | 75th | 90th | 95th | 99th |
| **1. SINGLE DX** | | | | | | | | | | |
| 0–19 Years | 763 | 3.2 | 8 | 1 | 1 | 2 | 4 | 7 | 8 | 14 |
| 20–34 | 282 | 2.6 | 4 | 1 | 2 | 3 | 3 | 4 | 6 | 14 |
| 35–49 | 396 | 3.8 | 12 | 1 | 2 | 4 | 4 | 9 | 13 | 14 |
| 50–64 | 223 | 2.6 | 3 | 1 | 2 | 2 | 3 | 5 | 7 | 8 |
| 65+ | 143 | 3.8 | 3 | 1 | 3 | 5 | 5 | 5 | 6 | 10 |
| **2. MULTIPLE DX** | | | | | | | | | | |
| 0–19 Years | 2,291 | 6.1 | 47 | 1 | 2 | 4 | 7 | 13 | 18 | 29 |
| 20–34 | 1,361 | 4.3 | 19 | 1 | 2 | 3 | 5 | 9 | 12 | 23 |
| 35–49 | 3,104 | 5.1 | 23 | 2 | 2 | 4 | 6 | 10 | 13 | 30 |
| 50–64 | 4,334 | 5.1 | 21 | 2 | 2 | 4 | 6 | 9 | 13 | 23 |
| 65+ | 9,372 | 5.9 | 23 | 2 | 3 | 5 | 7 | 11 | 14 | 22 |
| **TOTAL SINGLE DX** | 1,807 | 3.2 | 7 | 1 | 2 | 2 | 4 | 6 | 8 | 14 |
| **TOTAL MULTIPLE DX** | 20,462 | 5.5 | 25 | 2 | 3 | 4 | 7 | 10 | 14 | 25 |
| **TOTAL** | | | | | | | | | | |
| 0–19 Years | 3,054 | 5.3 | 39 | 1 | 2 | 3 | 6 | 11 | 16 | 28 |
| 20–34 | 1,643 | 4.0 | 17 | 1 | 2 | 3 | 5 | 8 | 11 | 21 |
| 35–49 | 3,500 | 4.9 | 22 | 2 | 2 | 4 | 6 | 10 | 13 | 29 |
| 50–64 | 4,557 | 4.9 | 20 | 2 | 2 | 4 | 6 | 9 | 13 | 22 |
| 65+ | 9,515 | 5.8 | 22 | 2 | 3 | 5 | 7 | 11 | 14 | 22 |
| **GRAND TOTAL** | 22,269 | 5.3 | 24 | 2 | 2 | 4 | 6 | 10 | 14 | 24 |

## 88.91: MRI-BRAIN & BRAIN STEM. Formerly included in operation group(s) 787.

| Type of Patients | Observed Patients | Avg. Stay | Variance | Percentiles | | | | | | |
|---|---|---|---|---|---|---|---|---|---|---|
| | | | | 10th | 25th | 50th | 75th | 90th | 95th | 99th |
| **1. SINGLE DX** | | | | | | | | | | |
| 0–19 Years | 538 | 3.1 | 8 | 1 | 1 | 2 | 4 | 6 | 8 | 15 |
| 20–34 | 149 | 2.7 | 4 | 1 | 2 | 3 | 3 | 4 | 6 | 13 |
| 35–49 | 194 | 4.3 | 17 | 1 | 2 | 3 | 5 | 13 | 14 | 14 |
| 50–64 | 119 | 2.6 | 3 | 1 | 2 | 2 | 3 | 5 | 8 | 8 |
| 65+ | 91 | 3.7 | 3 | 1 | 3 | 4 | 5 | 5 | 5 | 6 |
| **2. MULTIPLE DX** | | | | | | | | | | |
| 0–19 Years | 1,693 | 6.0 | 43 | 1 | 2 | 4 | 7 | 13 | 18 | 29 |
| 20–34 | 823 | 4.5 | 18 | 1 | 2 | 3 | 6 | 9 | 12 | 22 |
| 35–49 | 1,946 | 4.7 | 19 | 2 | 2 | 4 | 5 | 9 | 12 | 21 |
| 50–64 | 3,016 | 4.9 | 19 | 2 | 2 | 4 | 6 | 9 | 11 | 23 |
| 65+ | 6,743 | 5.7 | 23 | 2 | 3 | 4 | 7 | 10 | 13 | 23 |
| **TOTAL SINGLE DX** | 1,091 | 3.3 | 8 | 1 | 2 | 2 | 4 | 6 | 8 | 14 |
| **TOTAL MULTIPLE DX** | 14,221 | 5.3 | 24 | 2 | 3 | 4 | 6 | 10 | 13 | 24 |
| **TOTAL** | | | | | | | | | | |
| 0–19 Years | 2,231 | 5.3 | 36 | 1 | 2 | 3 | 6 | 11 | 16 | 28 |
| 20–34 | 972 | 4.1 | 16 | 1 | 2 | 3 | 5 | 8 | 11 | 20 |
| 35–49 | 2,140 | 4.6 | 19 | 1 | 2 | 3 | 5 | 9 | 13 | 20 |
| 50–64 | 3,135 | 4.7 | 18 | 2 | 2 | 4 | 6 | 8 | 11 | 23 |
| 65+ | 6,834 | 5.6 | 22 | 2 | 3 | 4 | 7 | 10 | 13 | 22 |
| **GRAND TOTAL** | 15,312 | 5.2 | 23 | 2 | 2 | 4 | 6 | 10 | 13 | 24 |

## 88.93: MRI-SPINAL CANAL. Formerly included in operation group(s) 787.

| Type of Patients | Observed Patients | Avg. Stay | Variance | Percentiles | | | | | | |
|---|---|---|---|---|---|---|---|---|---|---|
| | | | | 10th | 25th | 50th | 75th | 90th | 95th | 99th |
| **1. SINGLE DX** | | | | | | | | | | |
| 0–19 Years | 86 | 2.7 | 5 | 1 | 1 | 2 | 3 | 5 | 5 | 11 |
| 20–34 | 93 | 2.3 | 2 | 1 | 2 | 2 | 3 | 4 | 4 | 9 |
| 35–49 | 164 | 3.1 | 2 | 1 | 2 | 3 | 4 | 5 | 5 | 9 |
| 50–64 | 76 | 2.5 | 2 | 2 | 2 | 3 | 3 | 4 | 5 | 8 |
| 65+ | 33 | 3.8 | 4 | 3 | 3 | 3 | 4 | 7 | 8 | 12 |
| **2. MULTIPLE DX** | | | | | | | | | | |
| 0–19 Years | 206 | 5.9 | 67 | 1 | 1 | 4 | 6 | 13 | 18 | 60 |
| 20–34 | 314 | 3.8 | 20 | 1 | 2 | 4 | 4 | 7 | 11 | 30 |
| 35–49 | 714 | 5.3 | 17 | 2 | 3 | 4 | 7 | 10 | 13 | 20 |
| 50–64 | 786 | 5.3 | 22 | 2 | 3 | 4 | 6 | 12 | 13 | 20 |
| 65+ | 1,494 | 6.5 | 20 | 3 | 4 | 5 | 8 | 12 | 14 | 25 |
| **TOTAL SINGLE DX** | 452 | 2.8 | 3 | 1 | 2 | 2 | 3 | 5 | 5 | 10 |
| **TOTAL MULTIPLE DX** | 3,514 | 5.6 | 23 | 2 | 3 | 4 | 7 | 11 | 14 | 23 |
| **TOTAL** | | | | | | | | | | |
| 0–19 Years | 292 | 4.6 | 46 | 1 | 1 | 3 | 5 | 9 | 14 | 28 |
| 20–34 | 407 | 3.5 | 16 | 1 | 1 | 2 | 4 | 7 | 11 | 30 |
| 35–49 | 878 | 4.9 | 15 | 2 | 2 | 4 | 6 | 9 | 12 | 18 |
| 50–64 | 862 | 5.0 | 21 | 2 | 2 | 4 | 5 | 8 | 13 | 19 |
| 65+ | 1,527 | 6.4 | 20 | 2 | 4 | 5 | 8 | 12 | 14 | 25 |
| **GRAND TOTAL** | 3,966 | 5.3 | 21 | 1 | 2 | 4 | 7 | 10 | 13 | 22 |

## 88.94: MRI-MUSCULOSKELETAL. Formerly included in operation group(s) 787.

| Type of Patients | Observed Patients | Avg. Stay | Variance | Percentiles | | | | | | |
|---|---|---|---|---|---|---|---|---|---|---|
| | | | | 10th | 25th | 50th | 75th | 90th | 95th | 99th |
| **1. SINGLE DX** | | | | | | | | | | |
| 0–19 Years | 42 | 4.4 | 8 | 1 | 2 | 4 | 7 | 7 | 7 | 14 |
| 20–34 | 10 | 2.0 | 8 | 1 | 1 | 1 | 2 | 2 | 14 | 14 |
| 35–49 | 11 | 7.5 | 79 | 1 | 1 | 5 | 7 | 26 | 26 | 26 |
| 50–64 | 10 | 2.6 | 8 | 1 | 1 | 1 | 5 | 5 | 10 | 10 |
| 65+ | 7 | 3.3 | 3 | 2 | 3 | 3 | 3 | 7 | 7 | 7 |
| **2. MULTIPLE DX** | | | | | | | | | | |
| 0–19 Years | 96 | 6.6 | 107 | 1 | 2 | 4 | 7 | 13 | 18 | 62 |
| 20–34 | 84 | 5.3 | 28 | 2 | 2 | 5 | 6 | 9 | 11 | 16 |
| 35–49 | 170 | 5.5 | 16 | 2 | 3 | 4 | 7 | 11 | 11 | 16 |
| 50–64 | 166 | 5.8 | 21 | 2 | 3 | 4 | 7 | 12 | 20 | 21 |
| 65+ | 390 | 7.5 | 32 | 2 | 3 | 5 | 9 | 19 | 19 | 19 |
| **TOTAL SINGLE DX** | 80 | 3.6 | 14 | 1 | 1 | 2 | 5 | 7 | 9 | 14 |
| **TOTAL MULTIPLE DX** | 906 | 6.5 | 33 | 2 | 3 | 5 | 8 | 14 | 19 | 21 |
| **TOTAL** | | | | | | | | | | |
| 0–19 Years | 138 | 5.8 | 73 | 1 | 2 | 4 | 7 | 9 | 14 | 62 |
| 20–34 | 94 | 4.5 | 26 | 2 | 2 | 4 | 6 | 9 | 11 | 16 |
| 35–49 | 181 | 5.6 | 18 | 2 | 3 | 4 | 7 | 11 | 11 | 18 |
| 50–64 | 176 | 5.6 | 21 | 2 | 3 | 4 | 6 | 12 | 17 | 21 |
| 65+ | 397 | 7.4 | 32 | 2 | 3 | 5 | 9 | 19 | 19 | 19 |
| **GRAND TOTAL** | 986 | 6.3 | 32 | 2 | 3 | 5 | 8 | 14 | 19 | 21 |

Length of Stay by Diagnosis and Operation, United States, 2000

**United States, October 1998–September 1999 Data, by Operation**

### 88.97: MRI SITE NEC&NOS. Formerly included in operation group(s) 787.

| Type of Patients | Observed Patients | Avg. Stay | Vari-ance | 10th | 25th | 50th | 75th | 90th | 95th | 99th |
|---|---|---|---|---|---|---|---|---|---|---|
| **1. SINGLE DX** | | | | | | | | | | |
| 0–19 Years | 81 | 3.7 | 10 | 1 | 1 | 2 | 5 | 8 | 11 | 13 |
| 20–34 | 26 | 3.8 | 7 | 1 | 2 | 3 | 6 | 9 | 9 | 10 |
| 35–49 | 22 | 2.5 | 2 | 1 | 2 | 2 | 3 | 4 | 5 | 7 |
| 50–64 | 17 | 3.1 | 4 | 1 | 1 | 3 | 5 | 6 | 7 | 7 |
| 65+ | 10 | 4.6 | 9 | 1 | 2 | 5 | 7 | 9 | 9 | 9 |
| **2. MULTIPLE DX** | | | | | | | | | | |
| 0–19 Years | 239 | 6.6 | 49 | 2 | 2 | 4 | 9 | 14 | 19 | 47 |
| 20–34 | 109 | 4.0 | 11 | 2 | 2 | 3 | 5 | 9 | 11 | 16 |
| 35–49 | 227 | 8.1 | 90 | 1 | 3 | 4 | 8 | 30 | 30 | 30 |
| 50–64 | 312 | 6.0 | 46 | 2 | 3 | 4 | 7 | 11 | 18 | 32 |
| 65+ | 630 | 5.7 | 16 | 2 | 3 | 5 | 7 | 11 | 14 | 21 |
| **TOTAL SINGLE DX** | 156 | 3.6 | 9 | 1 | 1 | 2 | 5 | 8 | 9 | 13 |
| **TOTAL MULTIPLE DX** | 1,517 | 6.1 | 38 | 2 | 3 | 4 | 7 | 12 | 17 | 30 |
| **TOTAL** | | | | | | | | | | |
| 0–19 Years | 320 | 6.0 | 42 | 2 | 2 | 4 | 7 | 14 | 16 | 28 |
| 20–34 | 135 | 4.0 | 10 | 1 | 2 | 3 | 5 | 9 | 11 | 15 |
| 35–49 | 249 | 7.7 | 86 | 1 | 2 | 4 | 8 | 30 | 30 | 30 |
| 50–64 | 329 | 5.9 | 45 | 2 | 3 | 4 | 7 | 11 | 16 | 32 |
| 65+ | 640 | 5.7 | 16 | 2 | 3 | 5 | 7 | 11 | 14 | 21 |
| **GRAND TOTAL** | 1,673 | 5.9 | 36 | 2 | 3 | 4 | 7 | 12 | 16 | 30 |

### 89.04: INTERVIEW & EVAL NEC. Formerly included in operation group(s) 796.

| Type of Patients | Observed Patients | Avg. Stay | Vari-ance | 10th | 25th | 50th | 75th | 90th | 95th | 99th |
|---|---|---|---|---|---|---|---|---|---|---|
| **1. SINGLE DX** | | | | | | | | | | |
| 0–19 Years | 22 | 1.8 | 1 | 1 | 1 | 1 | 2 | 3 | 4 | 5 |
| 20–34 | 14 | 3.1 | 8 | 1 | 1 | 1 | 3 | 10 | 10 | 10 |
| 35–49 | 12 | 4.2 | 37 | 1 | 2 | 2 | 3 | 5 | 23 | 23 |
| 50–64 | 5 | 1.7 | 1 | 1 | 1 | 1 | 2 | 4 | 4 | 4 |
| 65+ | 0 | | | | | | | | | |
| **2. MULTIPLE DX** | | | | | | | | | | |
| 0–19 Years | 45 | 3.2 | 14 | 1 | 2 | 2 | 3 | 5 | 7 | 21 |
| 20–34 | 52 | 5.3 | 51 | 1 | 2 | 2 | 6 | 15 | 18 | 48 |
| 35–49 | 94 | 5.3 | 23 | 1 | 3 | 4 | 7 | 8 | 18 | 26 |
| 50–64 | 71 | 5.4 | 54 | 1 | 2 | 3 | 6 | 12 | 14 | 56 |
| 65+ | 68 | 5.2 | 18 | 1 | 2 | 4 | 6 | 12 | 16 | 17 |
| **TOTAL SINGLE DX** | 53 | 2.5 | 9 | 1 | 1 | 2 | 3 | 4 | 5 | 23 |
| **TOTAL MULTIPLE DX** | 330 | 4.9 | 33 | 1 | 2 | 3 | 6 | 10 | 15 | 23 |
| **TOTAL** | | | | | | | | | | |
| 0–19 Years | 67 | 2.7 | 10 | 1 | 1 | 2 | 3 | 4 | 6 | 21 |
| 20–34 | 66 | 4.9 | 44 | 1 | 2 | 3 | 4 | 15 | 18 | 48 |
| 35–49 | 106 | 5.2 | 24 | 1 | 2 | 4 | 7 | 8 | 18 | 26 |
| 50–64 | 76 | 5.2 | 52 | 1 | 2 | 3 | 6 | 12 | 14 | 56 |
| 65+ | 68 | 5.2 | 18 | 1 | 2 | 4 | 6 | 12 | 16 | 17 |
| **GRAND TOTAL** | 383 | 4.6 | 30 | 1 | 2 | 3 | 5 | 9 | 15 | 23 |

### 89.0: DX INTERVIEW/CONSUL/EXAM. Formerly included in operation group(s) 796.

| Type of Patients | Observed Patients | Avg. Stay | Vari-ance | 10th | 25th | 50th | 75th | 90th | 95th | 99th |
|---|---|---|---|---|---|---|---|---|---|---|
| **1. SINGLE DX** | | | | | | | | | | |
| 0–19 Years | 51 | 2.3 | 3 | 1 | 1 | 2 | 3 | 4 | 5 | 11 |
| 20–34 | 44 | 2.5 | 11 | 1 | 1 | 2 | 3 | 4 | 10 | 11 |
| 35–49 | 46 | 2.9 | 12 | 1 | 1 | 2 | 3 | 7 | 7 | 23 |
| 50–64 | 30 | 2.0 | 1 | 1 | 1 | 2 | 3 | 4 | 5 | 6 |
| 65+ | 8 | 2.5 | 1 | 2 | 2 | 2 | 3 | 4 | 5 | 5 |
| **2. MULTIPLE DX** | | | | | | | | | | |
| 0–19 Years | 156 | 3.1 | 8 | 1 | 2 | 3 | 4 | 5 | 6 | 21 |
| 20–34 | 152 | 5.1 | 36 | 1 | 2 | 3 | 6 | 12 | 18 | 33 |
| 35–49 | 311 | 4.8 | 20 | 1 | 2 | 4 | 6 | 9 | 12 | 23 |
| 50–64 | 359 | 4.6 | 24 | 2 | 3 | 4 | 6 | 9 | 12 | 26 |
| 65+ | 870 | 5.1 | 16 | 2 | 3 | 4 | 6 | 9 | 12 | 19 |
| **TOTAL SINGLE DX** | 179 | 2.5 | 6 | 1 | 1 | 2 | 3 | 5 | 6 | 11 |
| **TOTAL MULTIPLE DX** | 1,848 | 4.7 | 20 | 1 | 2 | 4 | 6 | 9 | 12 | 21 |
| **TOTAL** | | | | | | | | | | |
| 0–19 Years | 207 | 2.9 | 7 | 1 | 1 | 2 | 3 | 5 | 6 | 15 |
| 20–34 | 196 | 4.5 | 32 | 1 | 2 | 2 | 4 | 10 | 17 | 33 |
| 35–49 | 357 | 4.6 | 19 | 1 | 2 | 4 | 6 | 8 | 11 | 23 |
| 50–64 | 389 | 4.4 | 23 | 1 | 3 | 3 | 6 | 8 | 12 | 20 |
| 65+ | 878 | 5.1 | 16 | 2 | 3 | 4 | 6 | 9 | 12 | 19 |
| **GRAND TOTAL** | 2,027 | 4.5 | 19 | 1 | 2 | 3 | 6 | 8 | 12 | 20 |

### 89.09: CONSULTATION NOS. Formerly included in operation group(s) 796.

| Type of Patients | Observed Patients | Avg. Stay | Vari-ance | 10th | 25th | 50th | 75th | 90th | 95th | 99th |
|---|---|---|---|---|---|---|---|---|---|---|
| **1. SINGLE DX** | | | | | | | | | | |
| 0–19 Years | 9 | 3.6 | 3 | 1 | 2 | 3 | 5 | 6 | 7 | 7 |
| 20–34 | 7 | 3.1 | 3 | 1 | 1 | 3 | 4 | 6 | 6 | 6 |
| 35–49 | 8 | 2.6 | 4 | 1 | 1 | 2 | 5 | 6 | 6 | 6 |
| 50–64 | 7 | 3.7 | 3 | 1 | 2 | 3 | 5 | 6 | 6 | 6 |
| 65+ | 4 | 2.9 | 3 | 1 | 2 | 2 | 5 | 5 | 5 | 5 |
| **2. MULTIPLE DX** | | | | | | | | | | |
| 0–19 Years | 53 | 4.1 | 7 | 1 | 2 | 4 | 5 | 6 | 9 | 15 |
| 20–34 | 68 | 5.8 | 33 | 2 | 2 | 4 | 7 | 12 | 16 | 33 |
| 35–49 | 157 | 5.1 | 10 | 2 | 3 | 4 | 6 | 9 | 12 | 16 |
| 50–64 | 237 | 5.0 | 17 | 2 | 3 | 4 | 6 | 10 | 12 | 29 |
| 65+ | 655 | 5.6 | 15 | 2 | 3 | 5 | 7 | 10 | 13 | 19 |
| **TOTAL SINGLE DX** | 35 | 3.3 | 3 | 1 | 2 | 3 | 5 | 6 | 6 | 7 |
| **TOTAL MULTIPLE DX** | 1,170 | 5.3 | 16 | 2 | 3 | 4 | 7 | 10 | 12 | 19 |
| **TOTAL** | | | | | | | | | | |
| 0–19 Years | 62 | 4.1 | 7 | 1 | 2 | 4 | 5 | 6 | 8 | 15 |
| 20–34 | 75 | 5.6 | 31 | 2 | 2 | 4 | 7 | 10 | 16 | 33 |
| 35–49 | 165 | 4.9 | 10 | 2 | 3 | 4 | 6 | 9 | 11 | 16 |
| 50–64 | 244 | 5.0 | 17 | 2 | 3 | 4 | 6 | 10 | 12 | 29 |
| 65+ | 659 | 5.6 | 15 | 2 | 3 | 5 | 7 | 10 | 12 | 19 |
| **GRAND TOTAL** | 1,205 | 5.3 | 15 | 2 | 3 | 4 | 7 | 10 | 12 | 19 |

Length of Stay by Diagnosis and Operation, United States, 2000

# United States, October 1998–September 1999 Data, by Operation

## 89.1: NERVOUS SYSTEM EXAMS. Formerly included in operation group(s) 796.

| Type of Patients | Observed Patients | Avg. Stay | Variance | 10th | 25th | 50th | 75th | 90th | 95th | 99th |
|---|---|---|---|---|---|---|---|---|---|---|
| **1. SINGLE DX** | | | | | | | | | | |
| 0–19 Years | 1,664 | 2.2 | 5 | 1 | 1 | 2 | 3 | 4 | 6 | 10 |
| 20–34 | 280 | 3.7 | 6 | 1 | 2 | 3 | 5 | 7 | 9 | 11 |
| 35–49 | 233 | 4.1 | 12 | 1 | 2 | 3 | 5 | 8 | 9 | 15 |
| 50–64 | 102 | 2.9 | 11 | 1 | 1 | 2 | 2 | 6 | 9 | 18 |
| 65+ | 38 | 3.8 | 20 | 1 | 1 | 2 | 4 | 8 | 17 | 17 |
| **2. MULTIPLE DX** | | | | | | | | | | |
| 0–19 Years | 3,217 | 4.4 | 37 | 1 | 1 | 2 | 5 | 9 | 14 | 29 |
| 20–34 | 810 | 5.1 | 23 | 1 | 2 | 4 | 6 | 10 | 15 | 25 |
| 35–49 | 1,116 | 5.1 | 23 | 1 | 2 | 4 | 6 | 10 | 12 | 26 |
| 50–64 | 830 | 6.3 | 32 | 2 | 2 | 5 | 7 | 11 | 14 | 41 |
| 65+ | 2,069 | 7.7 | 42 | 2 | 3 | 6 | 10 | 15 | 17 | 40 |
| **TOTAL SINGLE DX** | 2,317 | 2.5 | 6 | 1 | 1 | 2 | 3 | 5 | 7 | 12 |
| **TOTAL MULTIPLE DX** | 8,042 | 5.5 | 37 | 1 | 2 | 4 | 7 | 11 | 16 | 30 |
| **TOTAL** | | | | | | | | | | |
| 0–19 Years | 4,881 | 3.6 | 27 | 1 | 1 | 2 | 4 | 7 | 11 | 24 |
| 20–34 | 1,090 | 4.9 | 20 | 1 | 2 | 4 | 6 | 9 | 14 | 25 |
| 35–49 | 1,349 | 5.0 | 22 | 1 | 2 | 4 | 6 | 10 | 12 | 26 |
| 50–64 | 932 | 5.9 | 31 | 2 | 3 | 5 | 7 | 11 | 14 | 31 |
| 65+ | 2,107 | 7.6 | 42 | 2 | 3 | 6 | 10 | 15 | 17 | 40 |
| **GRAND TOTAL** | 10,359 | 4.8 | 31 | 1 | 2 | 3 | 6 | 10 | 15 | 26 |

## 89.14: ELECTROENCEPHALOGRAM. Formerly included in operation group(s) 796.

| Type of Patients | Observed Patients | Avg. Stay | Variance | 10th | 25th | 50th | 75th | 90th | 95th | 99th |
|---|---|---|---|---|---|---|---|---|---|---|
| **1. SINGLE DX** | | | | | | | | | | |
| 0–19 Years | 593 | 2.4 | 9 | 1 | 1 | 2 | 3 | 4 | 6 | 13 |
| 20–34 | 77 | 3.0 | 5 | 1 | 2 | 3 | 5 | 6 | 8 | 11 |
| 35–49 | 54 | 4.0 | 16 | 1 | 2 | 2 | 5 | 8 | 8 | 15 |
| 50–64 | 33 | 3.3 | 17 | 1 | 2 | 2 | 2 | 6 | 18 | 18 |
| 65+ | 17 | 6.2 | 29 | 1 | 2 | 4 | 7 | 17 | 17 | 17 |
| **2. MULTIPLE DX** | | | | | | | | | | |
| 0–19 Years | 1,445 | 4.9 | 51 | 2 | 2 | 3 | 6 | 11 | 16 | 35 |
| 20–34 | 358 | 5.6 | 31 | 1 | 2 | 4 | 6 | 13 | 20 | 25 |
| 35–49 | 620 | 5.3 | 28 | 1 | 2 | 4 | 6 | 10 | 14 | 26 |
| 50–64 | 635 | 6.2 | 23 | 2 | 3 | 5 | 8 | 12 | 13 | 22 |
| 65+ | 1,954 | 7.6 | 41 | 2 | 3 | 6 | 10 | 15 | 17 | 37 |
| **TOTAL SINGLE DX** | 774 | 2.7 | 10 | 1 | 1 | 2 | 3 | 5 | 8 | 15 |
| **TOTAL MULTIPLE DX** | 5,012 | 6.1 | 40 | 1 | 2 | 4 | 8 | 13 | 17 | 31 |
| **TOTAL** | | | | | | | | | | |
| 0–19 Years | 2,038 | 4.2 | 39 | 1 | 2 | 2 | 4 | 9 | 14 | 31 |
| 20–34 | 435 | 5.3 | 29 | 1 | 2 | 4 | 6 | 11 | 17 | 25 |
| 35–49 | 674 | 5.1 | 26 | 1 | 2 | 4 | 6 | 10 | 13 | 26 |
| 50–64 | 668 | 5.9 | 23 | 2 | 3 | 5 | 7 | 11 | 14 | 22 |
| 65+ | 1,971 | 7.6 | 40 | 2 | 3 | 6 | 10 | 15 | 17 | 37 |
| **GRAND TOTAL** | 5,786 | 5.6 | 37 | 1 | 2 | 4 | 7 | 12 | 17 | 29 |

## 89.17: POLYSOMNOGRAM. Formerly included in operation group(s) 796.

| Type of Patients | Observed Patients | Avg. Stay | Variance | 10th | 25th | 50th | 75th | 90th | 95th | 99th |
|---|---|---|---|---|---|---|---|---|---|---|
| **1. SINGLE DX** | | | | | | | | | | |
| 0–19 Years | 117 | 2.0 | 2 | 1 | 1 | 2 | 2 | 4 | 5 | 6 |
| 20–34 | 6 | 1.2 | <1 | 1 | 1 | 1 | 1 | 2 | 2 | 2 |
| 35–49 | 11 | 1.0 | 0 | 1 | 1 | 1 | 1 | 1 | 1 | 1 |
| 50–64 | 26 | 1.1 | <1 | 1 | 1 | 1 | 1 | 1 | 1 | 2 |
| 65+ | 8 | 1.0 | 0 | 1 | 1 | 1 | 1 | 1 | 1 | 1 |
| **2. MULTIPLE DX** | | | | | | | | | | |
| 0–19 Years | 293 | 6.2 | 52 | 1 | 2 | 4 | 7 | 14 | 19 | 35 |
| 20–34 | 27 | 3.5 | 7 | 1 | 1 | 3 | 6 | 6 | 6 | 14 |
| 35–49 | 30 | 5.6 | 20 | 1 | 2 | 3 | 10 | 13 | 15 | 15 |
| 50–64 | 29 | 13.1 | 186 | 3 | 5 | 6 | 22 | 41 | 41 | 41 |
| 65+ | 30 | 11.9 | 137 | 1 | 5 | 9 | 16 | 40 | 40 | 40 |
| **TOTAL SINGLE DX** | 168 | 1.9 | 2 | 1 | 1 | 1 | 2 | 3 | 5 | 6 |
| **TOTAL MULTIPLE DX** | 409 | 6.9 | 67 | 1 | 2 | 4 | 8 | 16 | 22 | 41 |
| **TOTAL** | | | | | | | | | | |
| 0–19 Years | 410 | 4.8 | 39 | 1 | 1 | 3 | 6 | 10 | 17 | 29 |
| 20–34 | 33 | 3.1 | 7 | 1 | 1 | 1 | 6 | 6 | 6 | 14 |
| 35–49 | 41 | 4.9 | 19 | 1 | 1 | 3 | 9 | 11 | 15 | 15 |
| 50–64 | 55 | 9.6 | 162 | 1 | 2 | 5 | 7 | 41 | 41 | 41 |
| 65+ | 38 | 10.2 | 131 | 1 | 2 | 6 | 16 | 40 | 40 | 40 |
| **GRAND TOTAL** | 577 | 5.3 | 52 | 1 | 2 | 3 | 6 | 11 | 18 | 41 |

## 89.19: VIDEO/TELEMETRIC EEG MON. Formerly included in operation group(s) 796.

| Type of Patients | Observed Patients | Avg. Stay | Variance | 10th | 25th | 50th | 75th | 90th | 95th | 99th |
|---|---|---|---|---|---|---|---|---|---|---|
| **1. SINGLE DX** | | | | | | | | | | |
| 0–19 Years | 918 | 2.1 | 3 | 1 | 2 | 2 | 3 | 4 | 6 | 8 |
| 20–34 | 180 | 4.4 | 6 | 1 | 3 | 4 | 6 | 7 | 9 | 12 |
| 35–49 | 151 | 4.4 | 7 | 2 | 3 | 4 | 6 | 8 | 9 | 15 |
| 50–64 | 37 | 4.5 | 6 | 2 | 3 | 4 | 5 | 8 | 11 | 11 |
| 65+ | 8 | 3.3 | 5 | 1 | 2 | 2 | 4 | 8 | 8 | 8 |
| **2. MULTIPLE DX** | | | | | | | | | | |
| 0–19 Years | 1,392 | 3.1 | 16 | 1 | 1 | 2 | 4 | 6 | 8 | 14 |
| 20–34 | 399 | 4.4 | 9 | 1 | 2 | 4 | 6 | 8 | 8 | 15 |
| 35–49 | 435 | 4.6 | 9 | 1 | 2 | 4 | 7 | 8 | 10 | 13 |
| 50–64 | 141 | 4.0 | 4 | 2 | 3 | 4 | 5 | 7 | 8 | 11 |
| 65+ | 50 | 5.0 | 20 | 2 | 2 | 4 | 7 | 8 | 12 | 26 |
| **TOTAL SINGLE DX** | 1,294 | 2.5 | 4 | 1 | 1 | 2 | 3 | 5 | 7 | 10 |
| **TOTAL MULTIPLE DX** | 2,417 | 3.5 | 14 | 1 | 1 | 2 | 4 | 7 | 9 | 14 |
| **TOTAL** | | | | | | | | | | |
| 0–19 Years | 2,310 | 2.7 | 11 | 1 | 2 | 2 | 3 | 5 | 7 | 12 |
| 20–34 | 579 | 4.4 | 8 | 1 | 2 | 4 | 6 | 8 | 9 | 14 |
| 35–49 | 586 | 4.5 | 9 | 2 | 2 | 4 | 6 | 8 | 10 | 13 |
| 50–64 | 178 | 4.0 | 5 | 2 | 3 | 4 | 5 | 7 | 8 | 11 |
| 65+ | 58 | 4.8 | 19 | 2 | 2 | 4 | 7 | 8 | 12 | 26 |
| **GRAND TOTAL** | 3,711 | 3.1 | 11 | 1 | 2 | 2 | 4 | 7 | 8 | 13 |

Length of Stay by Diagnosis and Operation, United States, 2000

# United States, October 1998–September 1999 Data, by Operation

## 89.2: GU SYSTEM-EXAMINATION. Formerly included in operation group(s) 796.

| Type of Patients | Observed Patients | Avg. Stay | Variance | 10th | 25th | 50th | 75th | 90th | 95th | 99th |
|---|---|---|---|---|---|---|---|---|---|---|
| **1. SINGLE DX** | | | | | | | | | | |
| 0-19 Years | 37 | 1.6 | <1 | 1 | 1 | 1 | 2 | 3 | 3 | 6 |
| 20-34 | 23 | 1.9 | 2 | 1 | 1 | 1 | 2 | 4 | 6 | 6 |
| 35-49 | 4 | 1.0 | 0 | 1 | 1 | 1 | 1 | 1 | 1 | 1 |
| 50-64 | 1 | 2.0 | 0 | 2 | 2 | 2 | 2 | 2 | 2 | 2 |
| 65+ | 1 | 1.0 | 0 | 1 | 1 | 1 | 1 | 1 | 1 | 1 |
| **2. MULTIPLE DX** | | | | | | | | | | |
| 0-19 Years | 107 | 4.0 | 20 | 1 | 1 | 3 | 5 | 8 | 12 | 23 |
| 20-34 | 95 | 6.2 | 57 | 1 | 2 | 4 | 9 | 11 | 12 | 45 |
| 35-49 | 145 | 6.8 | 36 | 1 | 3 | 5 | 10 | 14 | 17 | 22 |
| 50-64 | 144 | 7.7 | 66 | 2 | 3 | 5 | 8 | 14 | 26 | 46 |
| 65+ | 558 | 9.0 | 46 | 3 | 4 | 7 | 11 | 18 | 24 | 37 |
| **TOTAL SINGLE DX** | 66 | 1.7 | 1 | 1 | 1 | 1 | 2 | 3 | 3 | 6 |
| **TOTAL MULTIPLE DX** | 1,049 | 7.5 | 47 | 2 | 3 | 6 | 10 | 15 | 21 | 37 |
| **TOTAL** | | | | | | | | | | |
| 0-19 Years | 144 | 3.3 | 16 | 1 | 1 | 2 | 4 | 8 | 9 | 23 |
| 20-34 | 118 | 5.6 | 51 | 1 | 1 | 3 | 8 | 10 | 12 | 45 |
| 35-49 | 149 | 6.7 | 57 | 1 | 3 | 5 | 10 | 14 | 17 | 22 |
| 50-64 | 145 | 7.6 | 65 | 2 | 3 | 5 | 8 | 14 | 23 | 46 |
| 65+ | 559 | 8.9 | 46 | 3 | 4 | 7 | 11 | 18 | 24 | 37 |
| **GRAND TOTAL** | 1,115 | 7.1 | 46 | 1 | 3 | 5 | 9 | 14 | 20 | 37 |

## 89.26: GYNECOLOGIC EXAMINATION. Formerly included in operation group(s) 796.

| Type of Patients | Observed Patients | Avg. Stay | Variance | 10th | 25th | 50th | 75th | 90th | 95th | 99th |
|---|---|---|---|---|---|---|---|---|---|---|
| **1. SINGLE DX** | | | | | | | | | | |
| 0-19 Years | 34 | 1.6 | <1 | 1 | 1 | 1 | 2 | 3 | 3 | 6 |
| 20-34 | 18 | 1.6 | 1 | 1 | 1 | 1 | 2 | 3 | 4 | 6 |
| 35-49 | 4 | 1.0 | 0 | 1 | 1 | 1 | 1 | 1 | 1 | 1 |
| 50-64 | 0 | | | | | | | | | |
| 65+ | 1 | 1.0 | 0 | 1 | 1 | 1 | 1 | 1 | 1 | 1 |
| **2. MULTIPLE DX** | | | | | | | | | | |
| 0-19 Years | 76 | 3.8 | 15 | 2 | 2 | 3 | 5 | 6 | 12 | 23 |
| 20-34 | 54 | 6.0 | 43 | 1 | 2 | 5 | 10 | 10 | 12 | 45 |
| 35-49 | 64 | 6.0 | 22 | 1 | 2 | 5 | 7 | 14 | 15 | 18 |
| 50-64 | 17 | 4.2 | 4 | 1 | 2 | 5 | 5 | 5 | 5 | 9 |
| 65+ | 53 | 6.5 | 24 | 2 | 2 | 7 | 9 | 10 | 12 | 31 |
| **TOTAL SINGLE DX** | 57 | 1.6 | <1 | 1 | 1 | 1 | 2 | 3 | 3 | 6 |
| **TOTAL MULTIPLE DX** | 264 | 5.3 | 24 | 1 | 2 | 4 | 7 | 10 | 14 | 23 |
| **TOTAL** | | | | | | | | | | |
| 0-19 Years | 110 | 3.0 | 11 | 1 | 1 | 2 | 3 | 6 | 10 | 18 |
| 20-34 | 72 | 5.2 | 38 | 1 | 1 | 3 | 8 | 10 | 12 | 45 |
| 35-49 | 68 | 5.8 | 22 | 1 | 2 | 5 | 7 | 14 | 15 | 18 |
| 50-64 | 17 | 4.2 | 4 | 1 | 2 | 5 | 5 | 5 | 5 | 9 |
| 65+ | 54 | 6.5 | 24 | 2 | 2 | 7 | 9 | 10 | 12 | 31 |
| **GRAND TOTAL** | 321 | 4.7 | 22 | 1 | 2 | 3 | 6 | 10 | 14 | 21 |

## 89.22: CYSTOMETROGRAM. Formerly included in operation group(s) 796.

| Type of Patients | Observed Patients | Avg. Stay | Variance | 10th | 25th | 50th | 75th | 90th | 95th | 99th |
|---|---|---|---|---|---|---|---|---|---|---|
| **1. SINGLE DX** | | | | | | | | | | |
| 0-19 Years | 1 | 1.0 | 0 | 1 | 1 | 1 | 1 | 1 | 1 | 1 |
| 20-34 | 2 | 4.4 | <1 | 4 | 4 | 4 | 4 | 6 | 6 | 6 |
| 35-49 | 0 | | | | | | | | | |
| 50-64 | 1 | 2.0 | 0 | 2 | 2 | 2 | 2 | 2 | 2 | 2 |
| 65+ | 0 | | | | | | | | | |
| **2. MULTIPLE DX** | | | | | | | | | | |
| 0-19 Years | 9 | 8.0 | 14 | 6 | 8 | 8 | 8 | 8 | 9 | 25 |
| 20-34 | 29 | 8.6 | 111 | 2 | 4 | 5 | 9 | 22 | 22 | 59 |
| 35-49 | 64 | 9.5 | 57 | 3 | 4 | 5 | 13 | 20 | 20 | 48 |
| 50-64 | 96 | 9.1 | 94 | 3 | 3 | 7 | 10 | 22 | 32 | 47 |
| 65+ | 412 | 9.4 | 49 | 4 | 5 | 7 | 11 | 19 | 24 | 37 |
| **TOTAL SINGLE DX** | 4 | 3.0 | 3 | 1 | 2 | 2 | 4 | 6 | 6 | 6 |
| **TOTAL MULTIPLE DX** | 610 | 9.3 | 57 | 3 | 5 | 7 | 11 | 19 | 24 | 37 |
| **TOTAL** | | | | | | | | | | |
| 0-19 Years | 10 | 7.7 | 16 | 2 | 3 | 8 | 8 | 8 | 9 | 25 |
| 20-34 | 31 | 8.3 | 104 | 2 | 4 | 5 | 9 | 22 | 22 | 59 |
| 35-49 | 64 | 9.5 | 57 | 3 | 4 | 5 | 13 | 20 | 20 | 48 |
| 50-64 | 97 | 9.0 | 93 | 3 | 3 | 7 | 10 | 22 | 32 | 47 |
| 65+ | 412 | 9.4 | 49 | 4 | 5 | 7 | 11 | 19 | 24 | 37 |
| **GRAND TOTAL** | 614 | 9.3 | 57 | 3 | 4 | 7 | 11 | 19 | 24 | 37 |

## 89.3: OTHER EXAMINATIONS. Formerly included in operation group(s) 796.

| Type of Patients | Observed Patients | Avg. Stay | Variance | 10th | 25th | 50th | 75th | 90th | 95th | 99th |
|---|---|---|---|---|---|---|---|---|---|---|
| **1. SINGLE DX** | | | | | | | | | | |
| 0-19 Years | 507 | 1.7 | 2 | 1 | 1 | 1 | 2 | 3 | 4 | 9 |
| 20-34 | 18 | 2.6 | 2 | 1 | 1 | 3 | 3 | 4 | 7 | 7 |
| 35-49 | 23 | 1.8 | <1 | 1 | 2 | 2 | 2 | 4 | 4 | 4 |
| 50-64 | 17 | 2.6 | 2 | 1 | 1 | 3 | 3 | 5 | 5 | 5 |
| 65+ | 8 | 2.7 | 6 | 1 | 1 | 2 | 4 | 8 | 8 | 8 |
| **2. MULTIPLE DX** | | | | | | | | | | |
| 0-19 Years | 1,992 | 5.7 | 73 | 1 | 3 | 3 | 6 | 12 | 18 | 41 |
| 20-34 | 79 | 8.1 | 52 | 1 | 3 | 5 | 19 | 19 | 19 | 24 |
| 35-49 | 195 | 4.5 | 8 | 1 | 3 | 5 | 5 | 8 | 9 | 13 |
| 50-64 | 281 | 4.7 | 10 | 2 | 3 | 5 | 7 | 9 | 10 | 14 |
| 65+ | 428 | 5.9 | 26 | 2 | 3 | 5 | 7 | 9 | 13 | 31 |
| **TOTAL SINGLE DX** | 573 | 1.8 | 2 | 1 | 1 | 1 | 2 | 3 | 4 | 9 |
| **TOTAL MULTIPLE DX** | 2,975 | 5.6 | 53 | 1 | 2 | 4 | 6 | 11 | 17 | 38 |
| **TOTAL** | | | | | | | | | | |
| 0-19 Years | 2,499 | 4.7 | 59 | 1 | 1 | 2 | 5 | 10 | 16 | 40 |
| 20-34 | 97 | 7.2 | 47 | 1 | 2 | 4 | 9 | 19 | 19 | 24 |
| 35-49 | 218 | 4.3 | 8 | 1 | 2 | 4 | 5 | 8 | 9 | 13 |
| 50-64 | 298 | 4.6 | 10 | 2 | 3 | 4 | 5 | 8 | 9 | 14 |
| 65+ | 436 | 5.8 | 26 | 2 | 3 | 5 | 7 | 9 | 13 | 31 |
| **GRAND TOTAL** | 3,548 | 4.9 | 46 | 1 | 3 | 6 | 6 | 10 | 15 | 36 |

Length of Stay by Diagnosis and Operation, United States, 2000

# United States, October 1998–September 1999 Data, by Operation

## 89.37: VITAL CAPACITY. Formerly included in operation group(s) 796.

| Type of Patients | Observed Patients | Avg. Stay | Variance | Percentiles | | | | | | |
|---|---|---|---|---|---|---|---|---|---|---|
| | | | | 10th | 25th | 50th | 75th | 90th | 95th | 99th |
| **1. SINGLE DX** | | | | | | | | | | |
| 0–19 Years | 11 | 2.3 | 3 | 1 | 1 | 2 | 3 | 5 | 7 | 7 |
| 20–34 | 8 | 2.9 | 4 | 1 | 1 | 2 | 4 | 7 | 7 | 7 |
| 35–49 | 5 | 2.5 | <1 | 2 | 2 | 2 | 4 | 4 | 4 | 4 |
| 50–64 | 5 | 3.4 | <1 | 3 | 3 | 3 | 3 | 5 | 5 | 5 |
| 65+ | 0 | | | | | | | | | |
| **2. MULTIPLE DX** | | | | | | | | | | |
| 0–19 Years | 49 | 8.0 | 60 | 4 | 4 | 5 | 10 | 13 | 30 | 42 |
| 20–34 | 32 | 4.4 | 11 | 1 | 1 | 3 | 4 | 9 | 13 | 14 |
| 35–49 | 68 | 5.0 | 11 | 2 | 3 | 5 | 6 | 11 | 11 | 21 |
| 50–64 | 120 | 4.6 | 6 | 2 | 3 | 5 | 6 | 8 | 9 | 13 |
| 65+ | 181 | 5.5 | 19 | 3 | 3 | 6 | 7 | 8 | 9 | 14 |
| **TOTAL SINGLE DX** | 29 | 2.6 | 2 | 1 | 2 | 2 | 3 | 5 | 7 | 7 |
| **TOTAL MULTIPLE DX** | 450 | 5.3 | 17 | 2 | 3 | 5 | 6 | 9 | 10 | 18 |
| **TOTAL** | | | | | | | | | | |
| 0–19 Years | 60 | 6.1 | 48 | 2 | 2 | 4 | 6 | 13 | 16 | 42 |
| 20–34 | 40 | 4.0 | 9 | 1 | 2 | 3 | 4 | 9 | 13 | 14 |
| 35–49 | 73 | 4.7 | 10 | 2 | 3 | 4 | 6 | 8 | 11 | 21 |
| 50–64 | 125 | 4.6 | 5 | 2 | 3 | 5 | 5 | 8 | 9 | 13 |
| 65+ | 181 | 5.5 | 19 | 3 | 3 | 6 | 7 | 8 | 9 | 14 |
| **GRAND TOTAL** | 479 | 5.1 | 17 | 2 | 3 | 5 | 6 | 8 | 10 | 16 |

## 89.39: NONOPERATIVE EXAMS NEC. Formerly included in operation group(s) 796.

| Type of Patients | Observed Patients | Avg. Stay | Variance | Percentiles | | | | | | |
|---|---|---|---|---|---|---|---|---|---|---|
| | | | | 10th | 25th | 50th | 75th | 90th | 95th | 99th |
| **1. SINGLE DX** | | | | | | | | | | |
| 0–19 Years | 330 | 2.1 | 3 | 1 | 1 | 1 | 2 | 4 | 5 | 10 |
| 20–34 | 5 | 2.4 | <1 | 1 | 3 | 3 | 4 | 3 | 3 | 3 |
| 35–49 | 12 | 1.1 | <1 | 1 | 1 | 2 | 2 | 2 | 3 | 3 |
| 50–64 | 6 | 1.5 | <1 | 1 | 1 | 2 | 2 | 2 | 2 | 4 |
| 65+ | 3 | 1.4 | <1 | 1 | 1 | 2 | 2 | 2 | 2 | 2 |
| **2. MULTIPLE DX** | | | | | | | | | | |
| 0–19 Years | 1,297 | 5.0 | 61 | 1 | 3 | 3 | 5 | 9 | 13 | 40 |
| 20–34 | 24 | 6.8 | 45 | 1 | 5 | 5 | 6 | 19 | 24 | 24 |
| 35–49 | 62 | 2.8 | 6 | 1 | 1 | 2 | 3 | 6 | 8 | 12 |
| 50–64 | 78 | 3.9 | 12 | 1 | 2 | 3 | 5 | 10 | 10 | 10 |
| 65+ | 80 | 4.3 | 14 | 1 | 2 | 3 | 7 | 8 | 14 | 23 |
| **TOTAL SINGLE DX** | 356 | 2.1 | 3 | 1 | 1 | 1 | 2 | 4 | 5 | 10 |
| **TOTAL MULTIPLE DX** | 1,541 | 4.9 | 56 | 1 | 2 | 3 | 5 | 9 | 13 | 38 |
| **TOTAL** | | | | | | | | | | |
| 0–19 Years | 1,627 | 4.4 | 51 | 1 | 3 | 3 | 6 | 9 | 12 | 36 |
| 20–34 | 29 | 5.5 | 36 | 3 | 3 | 3 | 4 | 14 | 24 | 24 |
| 35–49 | 74 | 2.5 | 6 | 1 | 1 | 2 | 3 | 5 | 8 | 12 |
| 50–64 | 84 | 3.7 | 11 | 1 | 2 | 2 | 5 | 9 | 10 | 10 |
| 65+ | 83 | 4.2 | 14 | 1 | 2 | 3 | 7 | 8 | 14 | 23 |
| **GRAND TOTAL** | 1,897 | 4.3 | 47 | 1 | 1 | 3 | 5 | 5 | 12 | 34 |

## 89.38: RESPIRATORY MEASURE NEC. Formerly included in operation group(s) 796.

| Type of Patients | Observed Patients | Avg. Stay | Variance | Percentiles | | | | | | |
|---|---|---|---|---|---|---|---|---|---|---|
| | | | | 10th | 25th | 50th | 75th | 90th | 95th | 99th |
| **1. SINGLE DX** | | | | | | | | | | |
| 0–19 Years | 147 | 1.4 | <1 | 1 | 1 | 1 | 1 | 1 | 3 | 4 |
| 20–34 | 3 | 1.0 | 0 | 1 | 1 | 1 | 1 | 1 | 1 | 1 |
| 35–49 | 1 | 1.0 | 0 | 1 | 1 | 1 | 1 | 1 | 1 | 1 |
| 50–64 | 4 | 2.9 | 3 | 3 | 3 | 3 | 4 | 5 | 5 | 5 |
| 65+ | 5 | 3.2 | 7 | 1 | 1 | 2 | 4 | 8 | 8 | 8 |
| **2. MULTIPLE DX** | | | | | | | | | | |
| 0–19 Years | 580 | 6.6 | 92 | 1 | 1 | 3 | 8 | 18 | 27 | 42 |
| 20–34 | 10 | 3.6 | 7 | 1 | 1 | 4 | 6 | 6 | 6 | 6 |
| 35–49 | 26 | 4.9 | 4 | 3 | 3 | 5 | 5 | 8 | 8 | 12 |
| 50–64 | 42 | 5.1 | 18 | 3 | 4 | 5 | 5 | 6 | 7 | 33 |
| 65+ | 86 | 5.4 | 9 | 3 | 3 | 6 | 6 | 9 | 11 | 14 |
| **TOTAL SINGLE DX** | 160 | 1.4 | <1 | 1 | 1 | 1 | 2 | 3 | 3 | 5 |
| **TOTAL MULTIPLE DX** | 744 | 6.1 | 62 | 1 | 2 | 4 | 6 | 13 | 19 | 41 |
| **TOTAL** | | | | | | | | | | |
| 0–19 Years | 727 | 5.1 | 70 | 1 | 2 | 2 | 5 | 13 | 21 | 41 |
| 20–34 | 11 | 3.5 | 7 | 1 | 1 | 2 | 6 | 6 | 6 | 9 |
| 35–49 | 29 | 4.8 | 4 | 3 | 3 | 5 | 5 | 8 | 8 | 12 |
| 50–64 | 46 | 5.1 | 18 | 3 | 4 | 5 | 5 | 6 | 8 | 33 |
| 65+ | 91 | 5.3 | 9 | 3 | 3 | 6 | 6 | 9 | 11 | 14 |
| **GRAND TOTAL** | 904 | 5.1 | 52 | 1 | 1 | 3 | 6 | 10 | 18 | 40 |

## 89.4: PACER/CARD STRESS TEST. Formerly included in operation group(s) 796.

| Type of Patients | Observed Patients | Avg. Stay | Variance | Percentiles | | | | | | |
|---|---|---|---|---|---|---|---|---|---|---|
| | | | | 10th | 25th | 50th | 75th | 90th | 95th | 99th |
| **1. SINGLE DX** | | | | | | | | | | |
| 0–19 Years | 7 | 4.2 | 32 | 1 | 2 | 2 | 2 | 16 | 16 | 16 |
| 20–34 | 94 | 1.3 | <1 | 1 | 1 | 1 | 1 | 1 | 3 | 6 |
| 35–49 | 516 | 1.5 | <1 | 1 | 1 | 1 | 2 | 3 | 3 | 4 |
| 50–64 | 358 | 1.5 | <1 | 1 | 1 | 1 | 2 | 3 | 3 | 6 |
| 65+ | 195 | 1.9 | 2 | 1 | 2 | 2 | 2 | 3 | 5 | 9 |
| **2. MULTIPLE DX** | | | | | | | | | | |
| 0–19 Years | 21 | 4.5 | 5 | 2 | 3 | 4 | 5 | 8 | 8 | 14 |
| 20–34 | 384 | 2.0 | 2 | 1 | 1 | 1 | 2 | 4 | 5 | 9 |
| 35–49 | 3,504 | 2.0 | 2 | 1 | 1 | 2 | 3 | 4 | 5 | 8 |
| 50–64 | 5,570 | 2.5 | 5 | 1 | 2 | 2 | 3 | 5 | 7 | 12 |
| 65+ | 7,953 | 3.2 | 8 | 1 | 2 | 3 | 4 | 6 | 9 | 13 |
| **TOTAL SINGLE DX** | 1,170 | 1.5 | 1 | 1 | 1 | 1 | 2 | 3 | 3 | 6 |
| **TOTAL MULTIPLE DX** | 17,432 | 2.7 | 6 | 1 | 2 | 3 | 4 | 5 | 7 | 13 |
| **TOTAL** | | | | | | | | | | |
| 0–19 Years | 28 | 4.4 | 10 | 2 | 4 | 5 | 5 | 8 | 10 | 16 |
| 20–34 | 478 | 1.8 | 2 | 1 | 1 | 2 | 2 | 4 | 4 | 8 |
| 35–49 | 4,020 | 1.9 | 2 | 1 | 1 | 2 | 2 | 4 | 5 | 7 |
| 50–64 | 5,928 | 2.4 | 5 | 1 | 2 | 2 | 3 | 5 | 6 | 12 |
| 65+ | 8,148 | 3.2 | 8 | 1 | 2 | 3 | 4 | 6 | 8 | 13 |
| **GRAND TOTAL** | 18,602 | 2.6 | 6 | 1 | 2 | 3 | 5 | 7 | 7 | 13 |

Length of Stay by Diagnosis and Operation, United States, 2000

# United States, October 1998–September 1999 Data, by Operation

## 89.41: TREADMILL STRESS TEST. Formerly included in operation group(s) 796.

| Type of Patients | Observed Patients | Avg. Stay | Vari-ance | Percentiles | | | | | | |
|---|---|---|---|---|---|---|---|---|---|---|
| | | | | 10th | 25th | 50th | 75th | 90th | 95th | 99th |
| **1. SINGLE DX** | | | | | | | | | | |
| 0–19 Years | 3 | 1.0 | 0 | 1 | 1 | 1 | 1 | 1 | | 1 |
| 20–34 | 42 | 1.2 | <1 | 1 | 1 | 1 | 1 | 2 | 2 | 6 |
| 35–49 | 171 | 1.3 | <1 | 1 | 1 | 1 | 1 | 2 | 3 | 4 |
| 50–64 | 125 | 1.3 | <1 | 1 | 1 | 1 | 1 | 2 | 3 | 6 |
| 65+ | 56 | 1.6 | <1 | 1 | 1 | 1 | 2 | 2 | 3 | 8 |
| **2. MULTIPLE DX** | | | | | | | | | | |
| 0–19 Years | 3 | 3.4 | 3 | 2 | 2 | 2 | 5 | 5 | 5 | 5 |
| 20–34 | 139 | 1.5 | <1 | 1 | 1 | 1 | 2 | 3 | 3 | 4 |
| 35–49 | 1,210 | 1.6 | 1 | 1 | 1 | 1 | 2 | 3 | 3 | 6 |
| 50–64 | 1,679 | 1.9 | 3 | 1 | 1 | 2 | 2 | 4 | 5 | 9 |
| 65+ | 1,701 | 2.5 | 5 | 1 | 1 | 2 | 3 | 5 | 6 | 12 |
| **TOTAL SINGLE DX** | 397 | 1.3 | <1 | 1 | 1 | 1 | 1 | 2 | 2 | 6 |
| **TOTAL MULTIPLE DX** | 4,732 | 2.0 | 3 | 1 | 1 | 1 | 2 | 4 | 5 | 9 |
| **TOTAL** | | | | | | | | | | |
| 0–19 Years | 6 | 2.2 | 3 | 1 | 1 | 1 | 2 | 5 | 5 | 5 |
| 20–34 | 181 | 1.4 | <1 | 1 | 1 | 1 | 1 | 2 | 3 | 6 |
| 35–49 | 1,381 | 1.5 | 1 | 1 | 1 | 1 | 2 | 3 | 3 | 6 |
| 50–64 | 1,804 | 1.9 | 3 | 1 | 1 | 2 | 2 | 4 | 5 | 9 |
| 65+ | 1,757 | 2.4 | 5 | 1 | 1 | 2 | 3 | 5 | 6 | 12 |
| **GRAND TOTAL** | 5,129 | 2.0 | 3 | 1 | 1 | 1 | 2 | 4 | 5 | 9 |

## 89.5: OTHER CARDIAC FUNCT TEST. Formerly included in operation group(s) 796.

| Type of Patients | Observed Patients | Avg. Stay | Vari-ance | Percentiles | | | | | | |
|---|---|---|---|---|---|---|---|---|---|---|
| | | | | 10th | 25th | 50th | 75th | 90th | 95th | 99th |
| **1. SINGLE DX** | | | | | | | | | | |
| 0–19 Years | 266 | 2.7 | 5 | 1 | 1 | 2 | 3 | 5 | 7 | 12 |
| 20–34 | 131 | 2.0 | 5 | 1 | 1 | 2 | 2 | 3 | 3 | 9 |
| 35–49 | 237 | 1.9 | 4 | 1 | 1 | 2 | 2 | 3 | 5 | 8 |
| 50–64 | 204 | 1.9 | 4 | 1 | 1 | 2 | 3 | 3 | 4 | 14 |
| 65+ | 149 | 2.3 | 5 | 1 | 2 | 3 | 3 | 4 | 5 | 17 |
| **2. MULTIPLE DX** | | | | | | | | | | |
| 0–19 Years | 1,104 | 4.3 | 42 | 1 | 2 | 3 | 5 | 9 | 13 | 34 |
| 20–34 | 681 | 2.5 | 7 | 1 | 1 | 2 | 3 | 5 | 6 | 11 |
| 35–49 | 2,101 | 2.7 | 7 | 1 | 1 | 2 | 3 | 5 | 7 | 13 |
| 50–64 | 3,707 | 3.0 | 8 | 1 | 1 | 3 | 4 | 6 | 8 | 13 |
| 65+ | 10,403 | 4.3 | 18 | 1 | 2 | 3 | 5 | 8 | 10 | 18 |
| **TOTAL SINGLE DX** | 987 | 2.2 | 4 | 1 | 1 | 2 | 2 | 4 | 5 | 12 |
| **TOTAL MULTIPLE DX** | 17,996 | 3.8 | 16 | 1 | 2 | 3 | 5 | 7 | 10 | 17 |
| **TOTAL** | | | | | | | | | | |
| 0–19 Years | 1,370 | 4.0 | 36 | 1 | 2 | 2 | 4 | 8 | 12 | 33 |
| 20–34 | 812 | 2.4 | 6 | 1 | 2 | 2 | 3 | 4 | 5 | 11 |
| 35–49 | 2,338 | 2.6 | 7 | 1 | 1 | 2 | 3 | 5 | 7 | 12 |
| 50–64 | 3,911 | 3.0 | 8 | 1 | 1 | 3 | 4 | 6 | 8 | 13 |
| 65+ | 10,552 | 4.3 | 18 | 1 | 2 | 3 | 5 | 8 | 10 | 18 |
| **GRAND TOTAL** | 18,983 | 3.7 | 16 | 1 | 1 | 3 | 5 | 7 | 10 | 17 |

## 89.44: CV STRESS TEST NEC. Formerly included in operation group(s) 796.

| Type of Patients | Observed Patients | Avg. Stay | Vari-ance | Percentiles | | | | | | |
|---|---|---|---|---|---|---|---|---|---|---|
| | | | | 10th | 25th | 50th | 75th | 90th | 95th | 99th |
| **1. SINGLE DX** | | | | | | | | | | |
| 0–19 Years | 4 | 5.8 | 42 | 2 | 2 | 2 | 16 | 16 | 16 | 16 |
| 20–34 | 51 | 1.5 | <1 | 1 | 1 | 1 | 1 | 3 | 3 | 4 |
| 35–49 | 342 | 1.6 | <1 | 1 | 1 | 1 | 2 | 3 | 3 | 4 |
| 50–64 | 232 | 1.6 | <1 | 1 | 1 | 1 | 2 | 3 | 3 | 6 |
| 65+ | 138 | 1.9 | 3 | 1 | 1 | 1 | 2 | 3 | 5 | 10 |
| **2. MULTIPLE DX** | | | | | | | | | | |
| 0–19 Years | 13 | 4.6 | 6 | 1 | 3 | 4 | 7 | 8 | 8 | 10 |
| 20–34 | 239 | 2.5 | 3 | 1 | 1 | 2 | 3 | 4 | 5 | 10 |
| 35–49 | 2,274 | 2.2 | 3 | 1 | 1 | 2 | 3 | 4 | 5 | 9 |
| 50–64 | 3,856 | 2.7 | 6 | 1 | 1 | 2 | 3 | 5 | 7 | 13 |
| 65+ | 6,045 | 3.4 | 8 | 1 | 2 | 3 | 4 | 7 | 9 | 13 |
| **TOTAL SINGLE DX** | 767 | 1.7 | 1 | 1 | 1 | 1 | 2 | 3 | 3 | 6 |
| **TOTAL MULTIPLE DX** | 12,427 | 3.0 | 7 | 1 | 1 | 2 | 4 | 6 | 8 | 13 |
| **TOTAL** | | | | | | | | | | |
| 0–19 Years | 17 | 4.9 | 13 | 2 | 1 | 4 | 7 | 8 | 16 | 16 |
| 20–34 | 290 | 2.3 | 3 | 1 | 1 | 2 | 3 | 4 | 5 | 9 |
| 35–49 | 2,616 | 2.1 | 3 | 1 | 1 | 2 | 3 | 4 | 5 | 8 |
| 50–64 | 4,088 | 2.7 | 6 | 1 | 1 | 2 | 3 | 5 | 7 | 13 |
| 65+ | 6,183 | 3.4 | 8 | 1 | 2 | 3 | 4 | 7 | 9 | 13 |
| **GRAND TOTAL** | 13,194 | 2.9 | 7 | 1 | 1 | 2 | 4 | 6 | 8 | 13 |

## 89.50: AMBULATORY CARD MONITOR. Formerly included in operation group(s) 796.

| Type of Patients | Observed Patients | Avg. Stay | Vari-ance | Percentiles | | | | | | |
|---|---|---|---|---|---|---|---|---|---|---|
| | | | | 10th | 25th | 50th | 75th | 90th | 95th | 99th |
| **1. SINGLE DX** | | | | | | | | | | |
| 0–19 Years | 5 | 5.2 | 23 | 2 | 2 | 2 | 12 | 12 | 12 | 12 |
| 20–34 | 5 | 3.7 | 1 | 2 | 3 | 4 | 4 | 5 | 5 | 5 |
| 35–49 | 16 | 3.5 | 7 | 1 | 1 | 3 | 4 | 8 | 8 | 8 |
| 50–64 | 7 | 1.9 | <1 | 1 | 2 | 2 | 2 | 3 | 3 | 3 |
| 65+ | 13 | 2.6 | <1 | 1 | 2 | 2 | 3 | 4 | 5 | 5 |
| **2. MULTIPLE DX** | | | | | | | | | | |
| 0–19 Years | 30 | 3.5 | 11 | 1 | 1 | 2 | 6 | 8 | 10 | 11 |
| 20–34 | 23 | 2.6 | 3 | 1 | 3 | 3 | 3 | 5 | 7 | 7 |
| 35–49 | 67 | 5.6 | 15 | 2 | 4 | 4 | 10 | 10 | 10 | 16 |
| 50–64 | 140 | 4.6 | 9 | 2 | 4 | 5 | 6 | 10 | 10 | 16 |
| 65+ | 529 | 5.2 | 14 | 3 | 3 | 5 | 7 | 9 | 12 | 19 |
| **TOTAL SINGLE DX** | 46 | 3.5 | 9 | 1 | 2 | 2 | 4 | 8 | 12 | 12 |
| **TOTAL MULTIPLE DX** | 789 | 4.9 | 13 | 1 | 2 | 4 | 6 | 10 | 11 | 19 |
| **TOTAL** | | | | | | | | | | |
| 0–19 Years | 35 | 3.8 | 13 | 1 | 2 | 3 | 6 | 10 | 12 | 12 |
| 20–34 | 28 | 2.7 | 15 | 1 | 3 | 3 | 3 | 5 | 7 | 7 |
| 35–49 | 83 | 5.3 | 15 | 1 | 2 | 4 | 10 | 10 | 10 | 16 |
| 50–64 | 147 | 4.5 | 9 | 2 | 3 | 5 | 8 | 9 | 10 | 16 |
| 65+ | 542 | 5.2 | 14 | 3 | 3 | 5 | 7 | 9 | 11 | 19 |
| **GRAND TOTAL** | 835 | 4.9 | 13 | 1 | 2 | 4 | 6 | 10 | 11 | 19 |

Length of Stay by Diagnosis and Operation, United States, 2000

# United States, October 1998–September 1999 Data, by Operation

## 89.52: ELECTROCARDIOGRAM. Formerly included in operation group(s) 796.

| Type of Patients | Observed Patients | Avg. Stay | Variance | 10th | 25th | 50th | 75th | 90th | 95th | 99th |
|---|---|---|---|---|---|---|---|---|---|---|
| **1. SINGLE DX** | | | | | | | | | | |
| 0–19 Years | 140 | 2.8 | 5 | 1 | 1 | 2 | 3 | 3 | 7 | 14 |
| 20–34 | 36 | 3.2 | 32 | 1 | 1 | 2 | 3 | 5 | 7 | 46 |
| 35–49 | 83 | 1.6 | 11 | 1 | 1 | 1 | 2 | 5 | 6 | 15 |
| 50–64 | 66 | 2.4 | 5 | 1 | 1 | 3 | 3 | 3 | 4 | 5 |
| 65+ | 25 | 2.0 | <1 | 1 | 1 | 2 | 3 | 3 | 3 | 3 |
| **2. MULTIPLE DX** | | | | | | | | | | |
| 0–19 Years | 587 | 4.4 | 42 | 1 | 2 | 2 | 5 | 9 | 13 | 34 |
| 20–34 | 210 | 2.9 | 15 | 1 | 2 | 2 | 3 | 5 | 8 | 17 |
| 35–49 | 656 | 2.8 | 12 | 1 | 1 | 2 | 3 | 5 | 7 | 17 |
| 50–64 | 1,004 | 2.9 | 6 | 1 | 1 | 2 | 4 | 6 | 7 | 13 |
| 65+ | 2,375 | 3.9 | 12 | 1 | 2 | 3 | 5 | 7 | 9 | 17 |
| **TOTAL SINGLE DX** | 350 | 2.6 | 8 | 1 | 1 | 2 | 3 | 5 | 7 | 14 |
| **TOTAL MULTIPLE DX** | 4,832 | 3.6 | 16 | 1 | 1 | 3 | 4 | 7 | 9 | 17 |
| **TOTAL** | | | | | | | | | | |
| 0–19 Years | 727 | 4.1 | 35 | 1 | 2 | 2 | 4 | 8 | 13 | 33 |
| 20–34 | 246 | 2.9 | 17 | 1 | 1 | 2 | 3 | 5 | 8 | 21 |
| 35–49 | 739 | 2.8 | 12 | 1 | 1 | 2 | 3 | 5 | 7 | 17 |
| 50–64 | 1,070 | 2.9 | 6 | 1 | 1 | 2 | 4 | 5 | 7 | 12 |
| 65+ | 2,400 | 3.8 | 12 | 1 | 2 | 3 | 5 | 7 | 9 | 17 |
| **GRAND TOTAL** | 5,182 | 3.5 | 15 | 1 | 1 | 2 | 4 | 7 | 9 | 17 |

## 89.59: NONOP CARD/VASC EXAM NEC. Formerly included in operation group(s) 796.

| Type of Patients | Observed Patients | Avg. Stay | Variance | 10th | 25th | 50th | 75th | 90th | 95th | 99th |
|---|---|---|---|---|---|---|---|---|---|---|
| **1. SINGLE DX** | | | | | | | | | | |
| 0–19 Years | 29 | 2.1 | <1 | 1 | 1 | 2 | 3 | 3 | 4 | 5 |
| 20–34 | 24 | 2.0 | <1 | 1 | 1 | 2 | 2 | 2 | 3 | 3 |
| 35–49 | 24 | 1.7 | <1 | 1 | 1 | 2 | 2 | 2 | 3 | 3 |
| 50–64 | 17 | 2.1 | <1 | 1 | 1 | 3 | 3 | 3 | 3 | 3 |
| 65+ | 22 | 3.1 | 2 | 2 | 2 | 3 | 4 | 5 | 5 | 5 |
| **2. MULTIPLE DX** | | | | | | | | | | |
| 0–19 Years | 99 | 7.2 | 171 | 1 | 2 | 3 | 7 | 13 | 24 | >99 |
| 20–34 | 110 | 2.6 | 3 | 1 | 2 | 2 | 3 | 5 | 6 | 9 |
| 35–49 | 213 | 3.2 | 5 | 1 | 2 | 3 | 3 | 5 | 8 | 13 |
| 50–64 | 328 | 3.4 | 4 | 1 | 2 | 3 | 4 | 5 | 7 | 10 |
| 65+ | 1,085 | 5.5 | 13 | 2 | 3 | 5 | 6 | 10 | 15 | 15 |
| **TOTAL SINGLE DX** | 116 | 2.0 | <1 | 1 | 1 | 2 | 2 | 3 | 4 | 5 |
| **TOTAL MULTIPLE DX** | 1,835 | 5.0 | 18 | 2 | 3 | 4 | 6 | 10 | 13 | 15 |
| **TOTAL** | | | | | | | | | | |
| 0–19 Years | 128 | 6.3 | 144 | 2 | 2 | 3 | 6 | 12 | 19 | 87 |
| 20–34 | 134 | 2.3 | 2 | 1 | 2 | 2 | 3 | 4 | 5 | 7 |
| 35–49 | 237 | 2.7 | 4 | 1 | 2 | 3 | 3 | 4 | 6 | 13 |
| 50–64 | 345 | 3.4 | 4 | 1 | 2 | 3 | 4 | 5 | 7 | 10 |
| 65+ | 1,107 | 5.5 | 13 | 2 | 3 | 5 | 6 | 10 | 15 | 15 |
| **GRAND TOTAL** | 1,951 | 4.8 | 17 | 2 | 2 | 4 | 6 | 10 | 13 | 15 |

## 89.54: ECG MONITORING. Formerly included in operation group(s) 796.

| Type of Patients | Observed Patients | Avg. Stay | Variance | 10th | 25th | 50th | 75th | 90th | 95th | 99th |
|---|---|---|---|---|---|---|---|---|---|---|
| **1. SINGLE DX** | | | | | | | | | | |
| 0–19 Years | 89 | 2.5 | 3 | 1 | 1 | 2 | 2 | 3 | 6 | 10 |
| 20–34 | 64 | 1.8 | 2 | 1 | 1 | 1 | 3 | 3 | 6 | 8 |
| 35–49 | 113 | 1.6 | 1 | 1 | 1 | 1 | 2 | 3 | 5 | 6 |
| 50–64 | 112 | 1.4 | <1 | 1 | 1 | 1 | 1 | 2 | 4 | 5 |
| 65+ | 88 | 1.9 | 2 | 1 | 1 | 2 | 2 | 4 | 5 | 8 |
| **2. MULTIPLE DX** | | | | | | | | | | |
| 0–19 Years | 348 | 3.7 | 17 | 1 | 2 | 3 | 4 | 6 | 10 | 19 |
| 20–34 | 332 | 2.3 | 4 | 1 | 1 | 2 | 3 | 4 | 5 | 10 |
| 35–49 | 1,148 | 2.4 | 4 | 1 | 2 | 2 | 3 | 5 | 6 | 9 |
| 50–64 | 2,212 | 3.0 | 9 | 1 | 2 | 3 | 4 | 6 | 9 | 13 |
| 65+ | 6,380 | 4.1 | 21 | 2 | 2 | 3 | 5 | 8 | 10 | 19 |
| **TOTAL SINGLE DX** | 466 | 1.8 | 2 | 1 | 1 | 2 | 2 | 3 | 4 | 8 |
| **TOTAL MULTIPLE DX** | 10,420 | 3.6 | 16 | 1 | 2 | 3 | 5 | 7 | 9 | 17 |
| **TOTAL** | | | | | | | | | | |
| 0–19 Years | 437 | 3.4 | 14 | 1 | 2 | 2 | 4 | 6 | 9 | 17 |
| 20–34 | 396 | 2.2 | 4 | 1 | 1 | 2 | 3 | 4 | 5 | 10 |
| 35–49 | 1,261 | 2.4 | 4 | 1 | 2 | 2 | 4 | 5 | 6 | 9 |
| 50–64 | 2,324 | 2.9 | 8 | 1 | 2 | 3 | 4 | 6 | 8 | 13 |
| 65+ | 6,468 | 4.1 | 21 | 2 | 2 | 3 | 5 | 8 | 10 | 19 |
| **GRAND TOTAL** | 10,886 | 3.5 | 15 | 1 | 2 | 3 | 4 | 7 | 9 | 17 |

## 89.6: CIRCULATORY MONITORING. Formerly included in operation group(s) 795.

| Type of Patients | Observed Patients | Avg. Stay | Variance | 10th | 25th | 50th | 75th | 90th | 95th | 99th |
|---|---|---|---|---|---|---|---|---|---|---|
| **1. SINGLE DX** | | | | | | | | | | |
| 0–19 Years | 278 | 2.5 | 5 | 1 | 2 | 2 | 3 | 3 | 5 | 11 |
| 20–34 | 73 | 2.6 | 8 | 1 | 2 | 2 | 3 | 4 | 5 | 22 |
| 35–49 | 93 | 2.8 | 4 | 2 | 2 | 2 | 3 | 6 | 7 | 11 |
| 50–64 | 65 | 3.2 | 6 | 1 | 2 | 2 | 4 | 7 | 8 | 12 |
| 65+ | 55 | 4.4 | 6 | 1 | 3 | 4 | 7 | 7 | 7 | 11 |
| **2. MULTIPLE DX** | | | | | | | | | | |
| 0–19 Years | 1,114 | 4.9 | 49 | 1 | 2 | 3 | 5 | 10 | 16 | 37 |
| 20–34 | 693 | 4.4 | 22 | 1 | 2 | 3 | 6 | 8 | 12 | 20 |
| 35–49 | 1,652 | 5.2 | 23 | 1 | 2 | 4 | 6 | 10 | 14 | 26 |
| 50–64 | 2,388 | 6.2 | 27 | 2 | 3 | 5 | 8 | 13 | 16 | 26 |
| 65+ | 6,156 | 7.3 | 35 | 2 | 3 | 6 | 9 | 14 | 18 | 28 |
| **TOTAL SINGLE DX** | 564 | 2.8 | 6 | 1 | 2 | 2 | 3 | 5 | 7 | 11 |
| **TOTAL MULTIPLE DX** | 12,003 | 6.4 | 33 | 2 | 3 | 5 | 8 | 13 | 17 | 28 |
| **TOTAL** | | | | | | | | | | |
| 0–19 Years | 1,392 | 4.4 | 40 | 1 | 2 | 2 | 4 | 8 | 13 | 35 |
| 20–34 | 766 | 4.2 | 21 | 1 | 2 | 3 | 5 | 8 | 12 | 20 |
| 35–49 | 1,745 | 5.1 | 22 | 1 | 2 | 4 | 6 | 10 | 14 | 26 |
| 50–64 | 2,453 | 6.1 | 27 | 2 | 3 | 5 | 8 | 13 | 16 | 26 |
| 65+ | 6,211 | 7.3 | 34 | 2 | 3 | 6 | 9 | 14 | 18 | 28 |
| **GRAND TOTAL** | 12,567 | 6.2 | 32 | 2 | 3 | 5 | 8 | 13 | 16 | 28 |

Length of Stay by Diagnosis and Operation, United States, 2000

# United States, October 1998–September 1999 Data, by Operation

## 89.62: CVP MONITORING. Formerly included in operation group(s) 795.

| Type of Patients | Observed Patients | Avg. Stay | Variance | 10th | 25th | 50th | 75th | 90th | 95th | 99th |
|---|---|---|---|---|---|---|---|---|---|---|
| **1. SINGLE DX** | | | | | | | | | | |
| 0–19 Years | 3 | 4.2 | 7 | 2 | 3 | 3 | 8 | 8 | 8 | 8 |
| 20–34 | 3 | 2.2 | <1 | 1 | 2 | 2 | 3 | 3 | 3 | 3 |
| 35–49 | 5 | 4.5 | 17 | 2 | 2 | 2 | 10 | 10 | 12 | 12 |
| 50–64 | 4 | 5.1 | 8 | 3 | 3 | 4 | 5 | 11 | 11 | 11 |
| 65+ | 1 | 4.0 | 0 | 4 | 4 | 4 | 4 | 4 | 4 | 4 |
| **2. MULTIPLE DX** | | | | | | | | | | |
| 0–19 Years | 31 | 12.8 | 169 | 1 | 3 | 10 | 14 | 34 | 37 | 54 |
| 20–34 | 44 | 8.3 | 29 | 2 | 4 | 8 | 12 | 16 | 16 | 30 |
| 35–49 | 93 | 8.1 | 40 | 2 | 4 | 6 | 10 | 16 | 23 | 35 |
| 50–64 | 99 | 11.4 | 74 | 3 | 5 | 9 | 17 | 23 | 29 | 43 |
| 65+ | 312 | 10.5 | 57 | 4 | 6 | 8 | 13 | 19 | 25 | 40 |
| **TOTAL SINGLE DX** | 16 | 3.9 | 9 | 2 | 2 | 3 | 4 | 10 | 11 | 12 |
| **TOTAL MULTIPLE DX** | 579 | 10.1 | 60 | 3 | 5 | 8 | 12 | 19 | 24 | 40 |
| **TOTAL** | | | | | | | | | | |
| 0–19 Years | 34 | 12.1 | 161 | 2 | 3 | 10 | 13 | 33 | 37 | 54 |
| 20–34 | 47 | 8.0 | 29 | 2 | 4 | 7 | 12 | 16 | 16 | 30 |
| 35–49 | 98 | 8.0 | 40 | 2 | 4 | 6 | 10 | 15 | 23 | 35 |
| 50–64 | 103 | 11.1 | 73 | 3 | 5 | 9 | 15 | 23 | 29 | 43 |
| 65+ | 313 | 10.5 | 57 | 4 | 6 | 8 | 13 | 19 | 25 | 40 |
| **GRAND TOTAL** | 595 | 10.0 | 60 | 3 | 5 | 8 | 12 | 19 | 24 | 40 |

## 89.65: ARTERIAL BLD GAS MEASURE. Formerly included in operation group(s) 795.

| Type of Patients | Observed Patients | Avg. Stay | Variance | 10th | 25th | 50th | 75th | 90th | 95th | 99th |
|---|---|---|---|---|---|---|---|---|---|---|
| **1. SINGLE DX** | | | | | | | | | | |
| 0–19 Years | 258 | 2.5 | 5 | 1 | 2 | 2 | 3 | 3 | 5 | 11 |
| 20–34 | 67 | 2.6 | 9 | 1 | 1 | 2 | 3 | 4 | 5 | 22 |
| 35–49 | 79 | 2.8 | 4 | 1 | 2 | 2 | 3 | 6 | 7 | 11 |
| 50–64 | 50 | 3.7 | 8 | 1 | 2 | 2 | 5 | 7 | 11 | 12 |
| 65+ | 49 | 4.5 | 5 | 1 | 3 | 4 | 7 | 7 | 7 | 9 |
| **2. MULTIPLE DX** | | | | | | | | | | |
| 0–19 Years | 983 | 4.7 | 48 | 1 | 2 | 3 | 4 | 8 | 14 | 36 |
| 20–34 | 546 | 3.4 | 15 | 1 | 1 | 2 | 4 | 6 | 7 | 13 |
| 35–49 | 1,224 | 4.2 | 11 | 1 | 2 | 3 | 6 | 8 | 10 | 18 |
| 50–64 | 1,638 | 4.8 | 13 | 1 | 2 | 4 | 6 | 8 | 11 | 18 |
| 65+ | 4,216 | 5.9 | 22 | 2 | 3 | 5 | 7 | 11 | 13 | 24 |
| **TOTAL SINGLE DX** | 503 | 2.9 | 6 | 1 | 2 | 2 | 3 | 5 | 7 | 11 |
| **TOTAL MULTIPLE DX** | 8,607 | 5.2 | 22 | 2 | 2 | 4 | 6 | 9 | 12 | 23 |
| **TOTAL** | | | | | | | | | | |
| 0–19 Years | 1,241 | 4.2 | 38 | 1 | 2 | 3 | 4 | 7 | 11 | 35 |
| 20–34 | 613 | 3.4 | 15 | 1 | 1 | 3 | 4 | 6 | 7 | 13 |
| 35–49 | 1,303 | 4.2 | 11 | 1 | 2 | 3 | 5 | 8 | 10 | 17 |
| 50–64 | 1,688 | 4.8 | 13 | 1 | 2 | 4 | 6 | 8 | 11 | 18 |
| 65+ | 4,265 | 5.9 | 22 | 2 | 3 | 5 | 7 | 11 | 13 | 24 |
| **GRAND TOTAL** | 9,110 | 5.0 | 21 | 1 | 2 | 4 | 6 | 9 | 12 | 22 |

## 89.64: PA WEDGE MONITORING. Formerly included in operation group(s) 795.

| Type of Patients | Observed Patients | Avg. Stay | Variance | 10th | 25th | 50th | 75th | 90th | 95th | 99th |
|---|---|---|---|---|---|---|---|---|---|---|
| **1. SINGLE DX** | | | | | | | | | | |
| 0–19 Years | 0 | | | | | | | | | |
| 20–34 | 2 | 1.3 | <1 | 1 | 1 | 1 | 2 | 2 | 2 | 2 |
| 35–49 | 6 | 2.2 | <1 | 2 | 2 | 2 | 2 | 4 | 4 | 4 |
| 50–64 | 9 | 2.1 | <1 | 1 | 1 | 2 | 2 | 2 | 2 | 4 |
| 65+ | 4 | 3.5 | 16 | 1 | 1 | 2 | 3 | 11 | 11 | 11 |
| **2. MULTIPLE DX** | | | | | | | | | | |
| 0–19 Years | 11 | 3.4 | 4 | 2 | 2 | 2 | 5 | 8 | 8 | 8 |
| 20–34 | 56 | 8.6 | 54 | 1 | 4 | 8 | 11 | 16 | 23 | 37 |
| 35–49 | 237 | 8.3 | 43 | 2 | 4 | 6 | 11 | 17 | 21 | 30 |
| 50–64 | 488 | 9.6 | 40 | 2 | 5 | 8 | 13 | 16 | 21 | 32 |
| 65+ | 1,253 | 10.8 | 48 | 3 | 6 | 10 | 14 | 20 | 23 | 32 |
| **TOTAL SINGLE DX** | 21 | 2.3 | 4 | 1 | 1 | 2 | 2 | 4 | 4 | 11 |
| **TOTAL MULTIPLE DX** | 2,045 | 10.2 | 47 | 3 | 5 | 9 | 13 | 18 | 23 | 32 |
| **TOTAL** | | | | | | | | | | |
| 0–19 Years | 11 | 3.4 | 4 | 2 | 2 | 2 | 5 | 8 | 8 | 8 |
| 20–34 | 58 | 8.3 | 54 | 1 | 3 | 8 | 11 | 16 | 23 | 37 |
| 35–49 | 243 | 8.2 | 43 | 2 | 4 | 6 | 11 | 17 | 21 | 30 |
| 50–64 | 497 | 9.5 | 40 | 2 | 5 | 8 | 13 | 16 | 20 | 32 |
| 65+ | 1,257 | 10.8 | 48 | 3 | 6 | 10 | 14 | 20 | 23 | 32 |
| **GRAND TOTAL** | 2,066 | 10.1 | 47 | 3 | 5 | 9 | 13 | 18 | 23 | 32 |

## 89.68: CARDIAC OUTPUT MONIT NEC. Formerly included in operation group(s) 795.

| Type of Patients | Observed Patients | Avg. Stay | Variance | 10th | 25th | 50th | 75th | 90th | 95th | 99th |
|---|---|---|---|---|---|---|---|---|---|---|
| **1. SINGLE DX** | | | | | | | | | | |
| 0–19 Years | 2 | 2.5 | <1 | 1 | 3 | 3 | 3 | 3 | 3 | 3 |
| 20–34 | 1 | 4.0 | 0 | 4 | 4 | 4 | 4 | 4 | 4 | 4 |
| 35–49 | 0 | | | | | | | | | |
| 50–64 | 1 | 2.0 | 0 | 2 | 2 | 2 | 2 | 2 | 2 | 2 |
| 65+ | 1 | 3.0 | 0 | 3 | 3 | 3 | 3 | 3 | 3 | 3 |
| **2. MULTIPLE DX** | | | | | | | | | | |
| 0–19 Years | 20 | 5.2 | 15 | 2 | 2 | 4 | 8 | 10 | 10 | 19 |
| 20–34 | 27 | 5.5 | 14 | 1 | 3 | 5 | 7 | 12 | 13 | 13 |
| 35–49 | 51 | 4.9 | 12 | 2 | 3 | 4 | 5 | 8 | 14 | 16 |
| 50–64 | 107 | 4.9 | 15 | 2 | 3 | 4 | 6 | 10 | 13 | 17 |
| 65+ | 277 | 5.1 | 13 | 2 | 3 | 4 | 7 | 11 | 12 | 18 |
| **TOTAL SINGLE DX** | 5 | 2.2 | <1 | 2 | 2 | 2 | 2 | 3 | 3 | 4 |
| **TOTAL MULTIPLE DX** | 482 | 5.1 | 14 | 2 | 3 | 4 | 6 | 10 | 13 | 18 |
| **TOTAL** | | | | | | | | | | |
| 0–19 Years | 22 | 5.1 | 15 | 2 | 2 | 3 | 8 | 10 | 10 | 19 |
| 20–34 | 28 | 5.4 | 14 | 2 | 3 | 5 | 7 | 12 | 13 | 13 |
| 35–49 | 51 | 4.9 | 12 | 2 | 3 | 4 | 5 | 8 | 14 | 16 |
| 50–64 | 108 | 4.6 | 14 | 1 | 2 | 4 | 6 | 9 | 13 | 17 |
| 65+ | 278 | 5.1 | 13 | 2 | 3 | 4 | 7 | 11 | 12 | 18 |
| **GRAND TOTAL** | 487 | 5.0 | 14 | 2 | 2 | 4 | 6 | 10 | 13 | 18 |

Length of Stay by Diagnosis and Operation, United States, 2000

# United States, October 1998–September 1999 Data, by Operation

## 89.7: GENERAL PHYSICAL EXAM. Formerly included in operation group(s) 796.

| Type of Patients | Observed Patients | Avg. Stay | Variance | 10th | 25th | 50th | 75th | 90th | 95th | 99th |
|---|---|---|---|---|---|---|---|---|---|---|
| **1. SINGLE DX** | | | | | | | | | | |
| 0–19 Years | 52 | 2.2 | <1 | 1 | 2 | 2 | 2 | 3 | 3 | 5 |
| 20–34 | 0 | | | | | | | | | |
| 35–49 | 0 | | | | | | | | | |
| 50–64 | 0 | | | | | | | | | |
| 65+ | 0 | | | | | | | | | |
| **2. MULTIPLE DX** | | | | | | | | | | |
| 0–19 Years | 4 | 4.4 | 5 | 2 | 2 | 3 | 6 | 7 | 7 | 7 |
| 20–34 | 1 | 1.0 | 0 | 1 | 1 | 1 | 1 | 1 | 1 | 1 |
| 35–49 | 0 | | | | | | | | | |
| 50–64 | 0 | | | | | | | | | |
| 65+ | 1 | 3.0 | 0 | 3 | 3 | 3 | 3 | 3 | 3 | 3 |
| **TOTAL SINGLE DX** | 52 | 2.2 | <1 | 1 | 2 | 2 | 3 | 3 | 3 | 5 |
| **TOTAL MULTIPLE DX** | 6 | 2.7 | 4 | 1 | 1 | 2 | 3 | 6 | 7 | 7 |
| **TOTAL** | | | | | | | | | | |
| 0–19 Years | 56 | 2.3 | 1 | 1 | 2 | 2 | 3 | 3 | 5 | 7 |
| 20–34 | 1 | 1.0 | 0 | 1 | 1 | 1 | 1 | 1 | 1 | 1 |
| 35–49 | 0 | | | | | | | | | |
| 50–64 | 0 | | | | | | | | | |
| 65+ | 1 | 3.0 | 0 | 3 | 3 | 3 | 3 | 3 | 3 | 3 |
| **GRAND TOTAL** | 58 | 2.3 | 1 | 1 | 1 | 2 | 3 | 3 | 4 | 7 |

## 89.8: AUTOPSY. Formerly included in operation group(s) 796.

| Type of Patients | Observed Patients | Avg. Stay | Variance | 10th | 25th | 50th | 75th | 90th | 95th | 99th |
|---|---|---|---|---|---|---|---|---|---|---|
| **1. SINGLE DX** | | | | | | | | | | |
| 0–19 Years | 0 | | | | | | | | | |
| 20–34 | 0 | | | | | | | | | |
| 35–49 | 0 | | | | | | | | | |
| 50–64 | 1 | 1.0 | 0 | 1 | 1 | 1 | 1 | 1 | 1 | 1 |
| 65+ | 0 | | | | | | | | | |
| **2. MULTIPLE DX** | | | | | | | | | | |
| 0–19 Years | 0 | | | | | | | | | |
| 20–34 | 0 | | | | | | | | | |
| 35–49 | 0 | | | | | | | | | |
| 50–64 | 0 | | | | | | | | | |
| 65+ | 0 | | | | | | | | | |
| **TOTAL SINGLE DX** | 1 | 1.0 | 0 | 1 | 1 | 1 | 1 | 1 | 1 | 1 |
| **TOTAL MULTIPLE DX** | 0 | | | | | | | | | |
| **TOTAL** | | | | | | | | | | |
| 0–19 Years | 0 | | | | | | | | | |
| 20–34 | 0 | | | | | | | | | |
| 35–49 | 0 | | | | | | | | | |
| 50–64 | 1 | 1.0 | 0 | 1 | 1 | 1 | 1 | 1 | 1 | 1 |
| 65+ | 0 | | | | | | | | | |
| **GRAND TOTAL** | 1 | 1.0 | 0 | 1 | 1 | 1 | 1 | 1 | 1 | 1 |

## 90.0: MICRO EXAM-NERVOUS SYST. Formerly included in operation group(s) 796.

| Type of Patients | Observed Patients | Avg. Stay | Variance | 10th | 25th | 50th | 75th | 90th | 95th | 99th |
|---|---|---|---|---|---|---|---|---|---|---|
| **1. SINGLE DX** | | | | | | | | | | |
| 0–19 Years | 0 | | | | | | | | | |
| 20–34 | 0 | | | | | | | | | |
| 35–49 | 0 | | | | | | | | | |
| 50–64 | 0 | | | | | | | | | |
| 65+ | 0 | | | | | | | | | |
| **2. MULTIPLE DX** | | | | | | | | | | |
| 0–19 Years | 0 | | | | | | | | | |
| 20–34 | 1 | 3.0 | 0 | 3 | 3 | 3 | 3 | 3 | 3 | 3 |
| 35–49 | 0 | | | | | | | | | |
| 50–64 | 1 | 3.0 | 0 | 3 | 3 | 3 | 3 | 3 | 3 | 3 |
| 65+ | 1 | 12.0 | 0 | 12 | 12 | 12 | 12 | 12 | 12 | 12 |
| **TOTAL SINGLE DX** | 0 | | | | | | | | | |
| **TOTAL MULTIPLE DX** | 3 | 5.0 | 18 | 3 | 3 | 3 | 3 | 12 | 12 | 12 |
| **TOTAL** | | | | | | | | | | |
| 0–19 Years | 0 | | | | | | | | | |
| 20–34 | 1 | 3.0 | 0 | 3 | 3 | 3 | 3 | 3 | 3 | 3 |
| 35–49 | 0 | | | | | | | | | |
| 50–64 | 1 | 3.0 | 0 | 3 | 3 | 3 | 3 | 3 | 3 | 3 |
| 65+ | 1 | 12.0 | 0 | 12 | 12 | 12 | 12 | 12 | 12 | 12 |
| **GRAND TOTAL** | 3 | 5.0 | 18 | 3 | 3 | 3 | 3 | 12 | 12 | 12 |

## 90.1: MICRO EXAM-ENDOCRINE. Formerly included in operation group(s) 796.

| Type of Patients | Observed Patients | Avg. Stay | Variance | 10th | 25th | 50th | 75th | 90th | 95th | 99th |
|---|---|---|---|---|---|---|---|---|---|---|
| **1. SINGLE DX** | | | | | | | | | | |
| 0–19 Years | 0 | | | | | | | | | |
| 20–34 | 0 | | | | | | | | | |
| 35–49 | 0 | | | | | | | | | |
| 50–64 | 0 | | | | | | | | | |
| 65+ | 0 | | | | | | | | | |
| **2. MULTIPLE DX** | | | | | | | | | | |
| 0–19 Years | 0 | | | | | | | | | |
| 20–34 | 0 | | | | | | | | | |
| 35–49 | 0 | | | | | | | | | |
| 50–64 | 0 | | | | | | | | | |
| 65+ | 0 | | | | | | | | | |
| **TOTAL SINGLE DX** | 0 | | | | | | | | | |
| **TOTAL MULTIPLE DX** | 0 | | | | | | | | | |
| **TOTAL** | | | | | | | | | | |
| 0–19 Years | 0 | | | | | | | | | |
| 20–34 | 0 | | | | | | | | | |
| 35–49 | 0 | | | | | | | | | |
| 50–64 | 0 | | | | | | | | | |
| 65+ | 0 | | | | | | | | | |
| **GRAND TOTAL** | 0 | | | | | | | | | |

Length of Stay by Diagnosis and Operation, United States, 2000

## United States, October 1998–September 1999 Data, by Operation

### 90.2: MICRO EXAM-EYE. Formerly included in operation group(s) 796.

| Type of Patients | Observed Patients | Avg. Stay | Variance | 10th | 25th | 50th | 75th | 90th | 95th | 99th |
|---|---|---|---|---|---|---|---|---|---|---|
| **1. SINGLE DX** | | | | | | | | | | |
| 0–19 Years | 0 | | | | | | | | | |
| 20–34 | 0 | | | | | | | | | |
| 35–49 | 1 | 2.0 | 0 | 2 | 2 | 2 | 2 | 2 | 2 | 2 |
| 50–64 | 0 | | | | | | | | | |
| 65+ | 0 | | | | | | | | | |
| **2. MULTIPLE DX** | | | | | | | | | | |
| 0–19 Years | 9 | 2.2 | 1 | 1 | 1 | 2 | 2 | 3 | 3 | 4 |
| 20–34 | 0 | | | | | | | | | |
| 35–49 | 0 | | | | | | | | | |
| 50–64 | 2 | 5.5 | 5 | 4 | 4 | 4 | 8 | 8 | 8 | 8 |
| 65+ | 1 | 9.0 | 0 | 9 | 9 | 9 | 9 | 9 | 9 | 9 |
| **TOTAL SINGLE DX** | 1 | 2.0 | 0 | 2 | 2 | 2 | 2 | 2 | 2 | 2 |
| **TOTAL MULTIPLE DX** | 12 | 3.3 | 6 | 1 | 1 | 3 | 4 | 8 | 9 | 9 |
| **TOTAL** | | | | | | | | | | |
| 0–19 Years | 9 | 2.2 | 1 | 1 | 1 | 2 | 3 | 3 | 4 | 4 |
| 20–34 | 0 | | | | | | | | | |
| 35–49 | 1 | 2.0 | 0 | 2 | 2 | 2 | 2 | 2 | 2 | 2 |
| 50–64 | 2 | 5.5 | 5 | 4 | 4 | 4 | 8 | 8 | 8 | 8 |
| 65+ | 1 | 9.0 | 0 | 9 | 9 | 9 | 9 | 9 | 9 | 9 |
| **GRAND TOTAL** | 13 | 3.2 | 6 | 1 | 2 | 3 | 4 | 8 | 9 | 9 |

### 90.3: MICRO EXAM-ENT/LARYNX. Formerly included in operation group(s) 796.

| Type of Patients | Observed Patients | Avg. Stay | Variance | 10th | 25th | 50th | 75th | 90th | 95th | 99th |
|---|---|---|---|---|---|---|---|---|---|---|
| **1. SINGLE DX** | | | | | | | | | | |
| 0–19 Years | 1 | 7.0 | 0 | 7 | 7 | 7 | 7 | 7 | 7 | 7 |
| 20–34 | 0 | | | | | | | | | |
| 35–49 | 0 | | | | | | | | | |
| 50–64 | 0 | | | | | | | | | |
| 65+ | 0 | | | | | | | | | |
| **2. MULTIPLE DX** | | | | | | | | | | |
| 0–19 Years | 7 | 2.4 | <1 | 2 | 2 | 2 | 2 | 3 | 3 | 3 |
| 20–34 | 0 | | | | | | | | | |
| 35–49 | 1 | 4.0 | 0 | 4 | 4 | 4 | 4 | 4 | 4 | 4 |
| 50–64 | 1 | 1.0 | 0 | 1 | 1 | 1 | 1 | 1 | 1 | 1 |
| 65+ | 2 | 9.5 | <1 | 9 | 9 | 10 | 10 | 10 | 10 | 10 |
| **TOTAL SINGLE DX** | 1 | 7.0 | 0 | 7 | 7 | 7 | 7 | 7 | 7 | 7 |
| **TOTAL MULTIPLE DX** | 11 | 4.1 | 13 | 1 | 1 | 2 | 9 | 10 | 10 | 10 |
| **TOTAL** | | | | | | | | | | |
| 0–19 Years | 8 | 3.6 | 5 | 2 | 2 | 2 | 7 | 7 | 7 | 7 |
| 20–34 | 0 | | | | | | | | | |
| 35–49 | 1 | 4.0 | 0 | 4 | 4 | 4 | 4 | 4 | 4 | 4 |
| 50–64 | 1 | 1.0 | 0 | 1 | 1 | 1 | 1 | 1 | 1 | 1 |
| 65+ | 2 | 9.5 | <1 | 9 | 9 | 10 | 10 | 10 | 10 | 10 |
| **GRAND TOTAL** | 12 | 4.4 | 12 | 1 | 1 | 2 | 7 | 10 | 10 | 10 |

### 90.4: MICRO EXAM-LOWER RESP. Formerly included in operation group(s) 796.

| Type of Patients | Observed Patients | Avg. Stay | Variance | 10th | 25th | 50th | 75th | 90th | 95th | 99th |
|---|---|---|---|---|---|---|---|---|---|---|
| **1. SINGLE DX** | | | | | | | | | | |
| 0–19 Years | 0 | | | | | | | | | |
| 20–34 | 0 | | | | | | | | | |
| 35–49 | 0 | | | | | | | | | |
| 50–64 | 1 | 3.0 | 0 | 3 | 3 | 3 | 3 | 3 | 3 | 3 |
| 65+ | 0 | | | | | | | | | |
| **2. MULTIPLE DX** | | | | | | | | | | |
| 0–19 Years | 1 | 14.0 | 0 | 14 | 14 | 14 | 14 | 14 | 14 | 14 |
| 20–34 | 5 | 5.8 | 38 | 2 | 2 | 3 | 4 | 19 | 19 | 19 |
| 35–49 | 7 | 3.9 | 6 | 2 | 2 | 3 | 4 | 7 | 10 | 10 |
| 50–64 | 8 | 5.9 | 10 | 3 | 3 | 5 | 7 | 11 | 13 | 13 |
| 65+ | 23 | 5.9 | 10 | 3 | 4 | 5 | 8 | 12 | 12 | 13 |
| **TOTAL SINGLE DX** | 1 | 3.0 | 0 | 3 | 3 | 3 | 3 | 3 | 3 | 3 |
| **TOTAL MULTIPLE DX** | 44 | 5.6 | 15 | 2 | 3 | 4 | 7 | 12 | 13 | 19 |
| **TOTAL** | | | | | | | | | | |
| 0–19 Years | 1 | 14.0 | 0 | 14 | 14 | 14 | 14 | 14 | 14 | 14 |
| 20–34 | 5 | 5.8 | 38 | 2 | 2 | 3 | 4 | 19 | 19 | 19 |
| 35–49 | 7 | 3.9 | 6 | 2 | 3 | 3 | 4 | 7 | 10 | 10 |
| 50–64 | 9 | 5.7 | 10 | 3 | 3 | 5 | 7 | 11 | 13 | 13 |
| 65+ | 23 | 5.9 | 10 | 3 | 4 | 5 | 8 | 12 | 12 | 13 |
| **GRAND TOTAL** | 45 | 5.6 | 15 | 2 | 3 | 4 | 7 | 12 | 13 | 19 |

### 90.5: MICRO EXAM-BLOOD. Formerly included in operation group(s) 796.

| Type of Patients | Observed Patients | Avg. Stay | Variance | 10th | 25th | 50th | 75th | 90th | 95th | 99th |
|---|---|---|---|---|---|---|---|---|---|---|
| **1. SINGLE DX** | | | | | | | | | | |
| 0–19 Years | 54 | 4.3 | 12 | 1 | 1 | 3 | 6 | 9 | 12 | 15 |
| 20–34 | 39 | 5.6 | 44 | 1 | 1 | 2 | 6 | 18 | 21 | 26 |
| 35–49 | 25 | 8.0 | 31 | 1 | 4 | 8 | 11 | 17 | 19 | 23 |
| 50–64 | 15 | 4.9 | 61 | 1 | 2 | 4 | 4 | 9 | 35 | 35 |
| 65+ | 6 | 14.2 | 62 | 1 | 6 | 17 | 21 | 22 | 22 | 22 |
| **2. MULTIPLE DX** | | | | | | | | | | |
| 0–19 Years | 266 | 3.9 | 14 | 1 | 2 | 3 | 5 | 8 | 10 | 22 |
| 20–34 | 43 | 2.9 | 9 | 1 | 1 | 2 | 3 | 8 | 10 | 14 |
| 35–49 | 31 | 4.3 | 11 | 1 | 2 | 3 | 7 | 10 | 10 | 12 |
| 50–64 | 27 | 6.9 | 42 | 1 | 2 | 6 | 10 | 14 | 20 | 31 |
| 65+ | 75 | 6.1 | 25 | 1 | 2 | 5 | 9 | 14 | 16 | 22 |
| **TOTAL SINGLE DX** | 139 | 5.5 | 31 | 1 | 2 | 4 | 7 | 12 | 18 | 23 |
| **TOTAL MULTIPLE DX** | 442 | 4.4 | 18 | 1 | 2 | 3 | 6 | 10 | 12 | 22 |
| **TOTAL** | | | | | | | | | | |
| 0–19 Years | 320 | 4.0 | 14 | 1 | 2 | 3 | 5 | 9 | 10 | 22 |
| 20–34 | 82 | 3.8 | 22 | 1 | 1 | 2 | 4 | 18 | 17 | 22 |
| 35–49 | 56 | 5.5 | 20 | 1 | 2 | 4 | 9 | 11 | 12 | 23 |
| 50–64 | 42 | 6.1 | 49 | 1 | 2 | 4 | 7 | 14 | 20 | 35 |
| 65+ | 81 | 6.7 | 32 | 1 | 2 | 5 | 10 | 16 | 18 | 22 |
| **GRAND TOTAL** | 581 | 4.7 | 22 | 1 | 2 | 3 | 6 | 10 | 14 | 22 |

374

# United States, October 1998–September 1999 Data, by Operation

## 90.59: MICRO EXAM NEC-BLOOD. Formerly included in operation group(s) 796.

| Type of Patients | Observed Patients | Avg. Stay | Variance | Percentiles | | | | | | |
|---|---|---|---|---|---|---|---|---|---|---|
| | | | | 10th | 25th | 50th | 75th | 90th | 95th | 99th |
| **1. SINGLE DX** | | | | | | | | | | |
| 0–19 Years | 46 | 4.3 | 12 | 1 | 1 | 3 | 6 | 9 | 12 | 15 |
| 20–34 | 39 | 5.6 | 44 | 1 | 1 | 2 | 6 | 18 | 21 | 26 |
| 35–49 | 25 | 8.0 | 31 | 1 | 4 | 8 | 11 | 17 | 19 | 23 |
| 50–64 | 13 | 4.8 | 69 | 1 | 2 | 2 | 4 | 8 | 35 | 35 |
| 65+ | 4 | 17.0 | 39 | 6 | 17 | 21 | 22 | 22 | 22 | 22 |
| **2. MULTIPLE DX** | | | | | | | | | | |
| 0–19 Years | 135 | 4.6 | 20 | 1 | 2 | 3 | 6 | 10 | 14 | 24 |
| 20–34 | 29 | 2.5 | 8 | 1 | 1 | 3 | 3 | 5 | 9 | 14 |
| 35–49 | 27 | 4.5 | 12 | 1 | 2 | 3 | 7 | 10 | 12 | 12 |
| 50–64 | 20 | 7.5 | 46 | 1 | 3 | 6 | 10 | 17 | 20 | 31 |
| 65+ | 43 | 7.6 | 30 | 1 | 3 | 7 | 10 | 16 | 18 | 22 |
| **TOTAL SINGLE DX** | 127 | 5.5 | 32 | 1 | 2 | 4 | 7 | 14 | 18 | 23 |
| **TOTAL MULTIPLE DX** | 254 | 5.1 | 24 | 1 | 2 | 3 | 8 | 10 | 14 | 22 |
| **TOTAL** | | | | | | | | | | |
| 0–19 Years | 181 | 4.5 | 17 | 1 | 2 | 3 | 6 | 9 | 12 | 22 |
| 20–34 | 68 | 3.9 | 26 | 1 | 1 | 2 | 4 | 10 | 17 | 17 |
| 35–49 | 52 | 5.7 | 21 | 1 | 2 | 4 | 9 | 11 | 12 | 23 |
| 50–64 | 33 | 6.4 | 56 | 1 | 3 | 4 | 8 | 14 | 20 | 35 |
| 65+ | 47 | 8.5 | 38 | 1 | 4 | 8 | 12 | 18 | 21 | 22 |
| **GRAND TOTAL** | 381 | 5.3 | 27 | 1 | 2 | 3 | 7 | 11 | 17 | 23 |

## 90.6: MICRO EXAM-SPLEEN/MARROW. Formerly included in operation group(s) 796.

| Type of Patients | Observed Patients | Avg. Stay | Variance | Percentiles | | | | | | |
|---|---|---|---|---|---|---|---|---|---|---|
| | | | | 10th | 25th | 50th | 75th | 90th | 95th | 99th |
| **1. SINGLE DX** | | | | | | | | | | |
| 0–19 Years | 0 | | | | | | | | | |
| 20–34 | 0 | | | | | | | | | |
| 35–49 | 0 | | | | | | | | | |
| 50–64 | 0 | | | | | | | | | |
| 65+ | 0 | | | | | | | | | |
| **2. MULTIPLE DX** | | | | | | | | | | |
| 0–19 Years | 0 | | | | | | | | | |
| 20–34 | 1 | 2.0 | 0 | | | | | | | |
| 35–49 | 0 | | | | | | | | | |
| 50–64 | 0 | | | | | | | | | |
| 65+ | 1 | 8.0 | 0 | | | | | | | |
| **TOTAL SINGLE DX** | 0 | | | | | | | | | |
| **TOTAL MULTIPLE DX** | 2 | 6.0 | 10 | 2 | 2 | 8 | 8 | 8 | 8 | 8 |
| **TOTAL** | | | | | | | | | | |
| 0–19 Years | 0 | | | | | | | | | |
| 20–34 | 1 | 2.0 | 0 | 2 | 2 | 2 | 2 | 2 | 2 | 2 |
| 35–49 | 0 | | | | | | | | | |
| 50–64 | 0 | | | | | | | | | |
| 65+ | 1 | 8.0 | 0 | 8 | 8 | 8 | 8 | 8 | 8 | 8 |
| **GRAND TOTAL** | 2 | 6.0 | 10 | 2 | 2 | 8 | 8 | 8 | 8 | 8 |

## 90.7: MICRO EXAM-LYMPH SYSTEM. Formerly included in operation group(s) 796.

| Type of Patients | Observed Patients | Avg. Stay | Variance | Percentiles | | | | | | |
|---|---|---|---|---|---|---|---|---|---|---|
| | | | | 10th | 25th | 50th | 75th | 90th | 95th | 99th |
| **1. SINGLE DX** | | | | | | | | | | |
| 0–19 Years | 0 | | | | | | | | | |
| 20–34 | 0 | | | | | | | | | |
| 35–49 | 0 | | | | | | | | | |
| 50–64 | 0 | | | | | | | | | |
| 65+ | 0 | | | | | | | | | |
| **2. MULTIPLE DX** | | | | | | | | | | |
| 0–19 Years | 0 | | | | | | | | | |
| 20–34 | 1 | 3.0 | 0 | 3 | 3 | 3 | 3 | 3 | 3 | 3 |
| 35–49 | 0 | | | | | | | | | |
| 50–64 | 0 | | | | | | | | | |
| 65+ | 0 | | | | | | | | | |
| **TOTAL SINGLE DX** | 0 | | | | | | | | | |
| **TOTAL MULTIPLE DX** | 1 | 3.0 | 0 | 3 | 3 | 3 | 3 | 3 | 3 | 3 |
| **TOTAL** | | | | | | | | | | |
| 0–19 Years | 0 | | | | | | | | | |
| 20–34 | 1 | 3.0 | 0 | 3 | 3 | 3 | 3 | 3 | 3 | 3 |
| 35–49 | 0 | | | | | | | | | |
| 50–64 | 0 | | | | | | | | | |
| 65+ | 0 | | | | | | | | | |
| **GRAND TOTAL** | 1 | 3.0 | 0 | 3 | 3 | 3 | 3 | 3 | 3 | 3 |

## 90.8: MICRO EXAM-UPPER GI. Formerly included in operation group(s) 796.

| Type of Patients | Observed Patients | Avg. Stay | Variance | Percentiles | | | | | | |
|---|---|---|---|---|---|---|---|---|---|---|
| | | | | 10th | 25th | 50th | 75th | 90th | 95th | 99th |
| **1. SINGLE DX** | | | | | | | | | | |
| 0–19 Years | 0 | | | | | | | | | |
| 20–34 | 0 | | | | | | | | | |
| 35–49 | 0 | | | | | | | | | |
| 50–64 | 0 | | | | | | | | | |
| 65+ | 0 | | | | | | | | | |
| **2. MULTIPLE DX** | | | | | | | | | | |
| 0–19 Years | 0 | | | | | | | | | |
| 20–34 | 1 | 5.0 | 0 | 5 | 5 | 5 | 5 | 5 | 5 | 5 |
| 35–49 | 1 | 5.0 | 0 | 5 | 5 | 5 | 5 | 5 | 5 | 5 |
| 50–64 | 0 | | | | | | | | | |
| 65+ | 5 | 7.0 | 27 | 3 | 4 | 6 | 6 | 18 | 18 | 18 |
| **TOTAL SINGLE DX** | 0 | | | | | | | | | |
| **TOTAL MULTIPLE DX** | 7 | 6.5 | 20 | 3 | 4 | 5 | 6 | 18 | 18 | 18 |
| **TOTAL** | | | | | | | | | | |
| 0–19 Years | 0 | | | | | | | | | |
| 20–34 | 1 | 5.0 | 0 | 5 | 5 | 5 | 5 | 5 | 5 | 5 |
| 35–49 | 1 | 5.0 | 0 | 5 | 5 | 5 | 5 | 5 | 5 | 5 |
| 50–64 | 0 | | | | | | | | | |
| 65+ | 5 | 7.0 | 27 | 3 | 4 | 6 | 6 | 18 | 18 | 18 |
| **GRAND TOTAL** | 7 | 6.5 | 20 | 3 | 4 | 5 | 6 | 18 | 18 | 18 |

Length of Stay by Diagnosis and Operation, United States, 2000

**United States, October 1998–September 1999 Data, by Operation**

### 90.9: MICRO EXAM-LOWER GI. Formerly included in operation group(s) 796.

| Type of Patients | Observed Patients | Avg. Stay | Vari-ance | 10th | 25th | 50th | 75th | 90th | 95th | 99th |
|---|---|---|---|---|---|---|---|---|---|---|
| **1. SINGLE DX** | | | | | | | | | | |
| 0–19 Years | 2 | 1.0 | 0 | 1 | 1 | 1 | 1 | 1 | 1 | 1 |
| 20–34 | 0 | | | | | | | | | |
| 35–49 | 0 | | | | | | | | | |
| 50–64 | 0 | | | | | | | | | |
| 65+ | 0 | | | | | | | | | |
| **2. MULTIPLE DX** | | | | | | | | | | |
| 0–19 Years | 15 | 3.3 | 3 | 1 | 2 | 2 | 5 | 6 | 6 | 7 |
| 20–34 | 4 | 2.7 | 1 | 1 | 1 | 3 | 4 | 4 | 4 | 4 |
| 35–49 | 2 | 1.5 | <1 | 1 | 1 | 1 | 1 | 3 | 3 | 3 |
| 50–64 | 2 | 7.0 | 1 | 6 | 6 | 6 | 8 | 8 | 8 | 8 |
| 65+ | 2 | 5.0 | 0 | 5 | 5 | 5 | 5 | 5 | 5 | 5 |
| **TOTAL SINGLE DX** | 2 | 1.0 | 0 | 1 | 1 | 1 | 1 | 1 | 1 | 1 |
| **TOTAL MULTIPLE DX** | 25 | 3.5 | 4 | 1 | 2 | 3 | 5 | 6 | 7 | 8 |
| **TOTAL** | | | | | | | | | | |
| 0–19 Years | 17 | 3.0 | 3 | 1 | 2 | 2 | 4 | 6 | 6 | 7 |
| 20–34 | 4 | 2.7 | 1 | 1 | 1 | 3 | 4 | 4 | 4 | 4 |
| 35–49 | 2 | 1.5 | <1 | 1 | 1 | 1 | 1 | 3 | 3 | 3 |
| 50–64 | 2 | 7.0 | 1 | 6 | 6 | 6 | 8 | 8 | 8 | 8 |
| 65+ | 2 | 5.0 | 0 | 5 | 5 | 5 | 5 | 5 | 5 | 5 |
| **GRAND TOTAL** | 27 | 3.4 | 4 | 1 | 2 | 3 | 5 | 6 | 7 | 8 |

### 91.0: MICRO EXAM-BIL/PANCREAS. Formerly included in operation group(s) 796.

| Type of Patients | Observed Patients | Avg. Stay | Vari-ance | 10th | 25th | 50th | 75th | 90th | 95th | 99th |
|---|---|---|---|---|---|---|---|---|---|---|
| **1. SINGLE DX** | | | | | | | | | | |
| 0–19 Years | 0 | | | | | | | | | |
| 20–34 | 0 | | | | | | | | | |
| 35–49 | 0 | | | | | | | | | |
| 50–64 | 0 | | | | | | | | | |
| 65+ | 0 | | | | | | | | | |
| **2. MULTIPLE DX** | | | | | | | | | | |
| 0–19 Years | 0 | | | | | | | | | |
| 20–34 | 0 | | | | | | | | | |
| 35–49 | 1 | 1.0 | 0 | 1 | 1 | 1 | 1 | 1 | 1 | 1 |
| 50–64 | 1 | 8.0 | 0 | 8 | 8 | 8 | 8 | 8 | 8 | 8 |
| 65+ | 0 | | | | | | | | | |
| **TOTAL SINGLE DX** | 0 | | | | | | | | | |
| **TOTAL MULTIPLE DX** | 2 | 5.1 | 18 | 1 | 1 | 8 | 8 | 8 | 8 | 8 |
| **TOTAL** | | | | | | | | | | |
| 0–19 Years | 0 | | | | | | | | | |
| 20–34 | 0 | | | | | | | | | |
| 35–49 | 1 | 1.0 | 0 | 1 | 1 | 1 | 1 | 1 | 1 | 1 |
| 50–64 | 1 | 8.0 | 0 | 8 | 8 | 8 | 8 | 8 | 8 | 8 |
| 65+ | 0 | | | | | | | | | |
| **GRAND TOTAL** | 2 | 5.1 | 18 | 1 | 1 | 8 | 8 | 8 | 8 | 8 |

### 91.1: MICRO EXAM-PERITONEUM. Formerly included in operation group(s) 796.

| Type of Patients | Observed Patients | Avg. Stay | Vari-ance | 10th | 25th | 50th | 75th | 90th | 95th | 99th |
|---|---|---|---|---|---|---|---|---|---|---|
| **1. SINGLE DX** | | | | | | | | | | |
| 0–19 Years | 0 | | | | | | | | | |
| 20–34 | 0 | | | | | | | | | |
| 35–49 | 0 | | | | | | | | | |
| 50–64 | 0 | | | | | | | | | |
| 65+ | 0 | | | | | | | | | |
| **2. MULTIPLE DX** | | | | | | | | | | |
| 0–19 Years | 0 | | | | | | | | | |
| 20–34 | 0 | | | | | | | | | |
| 35–49 | 0 | | | | | | | | | |
| 50–64 | 1 | 1.0 | 0 | 1 | 1 | 1 | 1 | 1 | 1 | 1 |
| 65+ | 0 | | | | | | | | | |
| **TOTAL SINGLE DX** | 0 | | | | | | | | | |
| **TOTAL MULTIPLE DX** | 1 | 1.0 | 0 | 1 | 1 | 1 | 1 | 1 | 1 | 1 |
| **TOTAL** | | | | | | | | | | |
| 0–19 Years | 0 | | | | | | | | | |
| 20–34 | 0 | | | | | | | | | |
| 35–49 | 0 | | | | | | | | | |
| 50–64 | 1 | 1.0 | 0 | 1 | 1 | 1 | 1 | 1 | 1 | 1 |
| 65+ | 0 | | | | | | | | | |
| **GRAND TOTAL** | 1 | 1.0 | 0 | 1 | 1 | 1 | 1 | 1 | 1 | 1 |

### 91.2: MICRO EXAM-UPPER URINARY. Formerly included in operation group(s) 796.

| Type of Patients | Observed Patients | Avg. Stay | Vari-ance | 10th | 25th | 50th | 75th | 90th | 95th | 99th |
|---|---|---|---|---|---|---|---|---|---|---|
| **1. SINGLE DX** | | | | | | | | | | |
| 0–19 Years | 0 | | | | | | | | | |
| 20–34 | 0 | | | | | | | | | |
| 35–49 | 1 | 2.0 | 0 | 2 | 2 | 2 | 2 | 2 | 2 | 2 |
| 50–64 | 0 | | | | | | | | | |
| 65+ | 0 | | | | | | | | | |
| **2. MULTIPLE DX** | | | | | | | | | | |
| 0–19 Years | 2 | 15.0 | 338 | 2 | 2 | 15 | 28 | 28 | 28 | 28 |
| 20–34 | 0 | | | | | | | | | |
| 35–49 | 1 | 2.0 | 0 | 2 | 2 | 2 | 2 | 2 | 2 | 2 |
| 65+ | 0 | | | | | | | | | |
| **TOTAL SINGLE DX** | 1 | 2.0 | 0 | 2 | 2 | 2 | 2 | 2 | 2 | 2 |
| **TOTAL MULTIPLE DX** | 3 | 10.7 | 225 | 2 | 2 | 2 | 28 | 28 | 28 | 28 |
| **TOTAL** | | | | | | | | | | |
| 0–19 Years | 2 | 15.0 | 338 | 2 | 2 | 15 | 28 | 28 | 28 | 28 |
| 20–34 | 0 | | | | | | | | | |
| 35–49 | 1 | 2.0 | 0 | 2 | 2 | 2 | 2 | 2 | 2 | 2 |
| 50–64 | 1 | 2.0 | 0 | 2 | 2 | 2 | 2 | 2 | 2 | 2 |
| 65+ | 0 | | | | | | | | | |
| **GRAND TOTAL** | 4 | 5.4 | 89 | 2 | 2 | 2 | 2 | 2 | 2 | 28 |

Length of Stay by Diagnosis and Operation, United States, 2000

# United States, October 1998–September 1999 Data, by Operation

## 91.3: MICRO EXAM-LOWER URINARY. Formerly included in operation group(s) 796.

| Type of Patients | Observed Patients | Avg. Stay | Variance | 10th | 25th | 50th | 75th | 90th | 95th | 99th |
|---|---|---|---|---|---|---|---|---|---|---|
| | | | | | | Percentiles | | | | |
| **1. SINGLE DX** | | | | | | | | | | |
| 0–19 Years | 7 | 3.3 | 2 | 2 | 2 | 3 | 5 | 5 | 5 | 5 |
| 20–34 | 3 | 1.4 | <1 | 1 | 1 | 1 | 2 | 2 | 2 | 2 |
| 35–49 | 0 | | | | | | | | | |
| 50–64 | 0 | | | | | | | | | |
| 65+ | 2 | 1.0 | 0 | 1 | | 1 | 1 | 1 | 1 | 1 |
| **2. MULTIPLE DX** | | | | | | | | | | |
| 0–19 Years | 20 | 6.0 | 101 | 1 | 2 | 2 | 4 | 33 | 33 | 33 |
| 20–34 | 7 | 3.3 | 24 | 1 | 1 | 2 | 3 | 6 | 21 | 21 |
| 35–49 | 8 | 4.1 | 8 | 2 | 2 | 3 | 4 | 5 | 13 | 13 |
| 50–64 | 10 | 3.3 | 10 | 1 | 2 | 2 | 3 | 8 | 8 | 17 |
| 65+ | 86 | 3.8 | 15 | 1 | 2 | 3 | 5 | 7 | 9 | 34 |
| **TOTAL SINGLE DX** | 12 | 2.2 | 2 | 1 | 1 | 2 | 3 | 5 | 5 | 5 |
| **TOTAL MULTIPLE DX** | 131 | 4.1 | 28 | 1 | 2 | 3 | 4 | 7 | 10 | 33 |
| **TOTAL** | | | | | | | | | | |
| 0–19 Years | 27 | 5.3 | 76 | 1 | 2 | 2 | 4 | 6 | 33 | 33 |
| 20–34 | 10 | 2.5 | 15 | 1 | 1 | 2 | 2 | 3 | 6 | 21 |
| 35–49 | 8 | 4.1 | 10 | 2 | 2 | 3 | 4 | 5 | 13 | 13 |
| 50–64 | 10 | 3.3 | 10 | 1 | 2 | 2 | 3 | 8 | 8 | 17 |
| 65+ | 88 | 3.7 | 14 | 1 | 2 | 3 | 5 | 7 | 9 | 14 |
| **GRAND TOTAL** | 143 | 3.9 | 26 | 1 | 2 | 3 | 4 | 7 | 9 | 33 |

## 91.4: MICRO EXAM-FEMALE GENIT. Formerly included in operation group(s) 796.

| Type of Patients | Observed Patients | Avg. Stay | Variance | 10th | 25th | 50th | 75th | 90th | 95th | 99th |
|---|---|---|---|---|---|---|---|---|---|---|
| | | | | | | Percentiles | | | | |
| **1. SINGLE DX** | | | | | | | | | | |
| 0–19 Years | 0 | | | | | | | | | |
| 20–34 | 2 | 2.0 | 1 | 1 | 1 | 3 | 3 | 3 | 3 | 3 |
| 35–49 | 0 | | | | | | | | | |
| 50–64 | 0 | | | | | | | | | |
| 65+ | 0 | | | | | | | | | |
| **2. MULTIPLE DX** | | | | | | | | | | |
| 0–19 Years | 4 | 9.6 | 73 | 6 | 6 | 9 | 9 | 9 | 9 | 48 |
| 20–34 | 18 | 6.6 | 39 | 2 | 2 | 4 | 8 | 16 | 25 | 25 |
| 35–49 | 16 | 7.2 | 8 | 3 | 5 | 7 | 10 | 10 | 11 | 14 |
| 50–64 | 19 | 6.6 | 16 | 3 | 4 | 5 | 11 | 11 | 11 | 23 |
| 65+ | 38 | 6.5 | 15 | 3 | 3 | 6 | 9 | 10 | 15 | 20 |
| **TOTAL SINGLE DX** | 2 | 2.0 | 1 | 1 | 1 | 3 | 3 | 3 | 3 | 3 |
| **TOTAL MULTIPLE DX** | 95 | 6.9 | 21 | 3 | 4 | 6 | 9 | 11 | 13 | 25 |
| **TOTAL** | | | | | | | | | | |
| 0–19 Years | 4 | 9.6 | 73 | 6 | 6 | 9 | 9 | 9 | 9 | 48 |
| 20–34 | 20 | 6.1 | 37 | 2 | 2 | 4 | 8 | 10 | 25 | 25 |
| 35–49 | 16 | 7.2 | 8 | 3 | 5 | 7 | 10 | 10 | 11 | 14 |
| 50–64 | 19 | 6.6 | 16 | 3 | 4 | 5 | 11 | 11 | 11 | 23 |
| 65+ | 38 | 6.5 | 15 | 3 | 3 | 6 | 9 | 10 | 15 | 20 |
| **GRAND TOTAL** | 97 | 6.8 | 21 | 2 | 4 | 6 | 9 | 11 | 13 | 25 |

## 91.5: MICRO EXAM-MS/JT FLUID. Formerly included in operation group(s) 796.

| Type of Patients | Observed Patients | Avg. Stay | Variance | 10th | 25th | 50th | 75th | 90th | 95th | 99th |
|---|---|---|---|---|---|---|---|---|---|---|
| | | | | | | Percentiles | | | | |
| **1. SINGLE DX** | | | | | | | | | | |
| 0–19 Years | 0 | | | | | | | | | |
| 20–34 | 0 | | | | | | | | | |
| 35–49 | 0 | | | | | | | | | |
| 50–64 | 1 | 5.0 | 0 | 5 | 5 | 5 | 5 | 5 | 5 | 5 |
| 65+ | 0 | | | | | | | | | |
| **2. MULTIPLE DX** | | | | | | | | | | |
| 0–19 Years | 0 | | | | | | | | | |
| 20–34 | 0 | | | | | | | | | |
| 35–49 | 0 | | | | | | | | | |
| 50–64 | 0 | | | | | | | | | |
| 65+ | 3 | 4.2 | 6 | 2 | 2 | 3 | 7 | 7 | 7 | 7 |
| **TOTAL SINGLE DX** | 1 | 5.0 | 0 | 5 | 5 | 5 | 5 | 5 | 5 | 5 |
| **TOTAL MULTIPLE DX** | 3 | 4.2 | 6 | 2 | 2 | 3 | 7 | 7 | 7 | 7 |
| **TOTAL** | | | | | | | | | | |
| 0–19 Years | 0 | | | | | | | | | |
| 20–34 | 0 | | | | | | | | | |
| 35–49 | 0 | | | | | | | | | |
| 50–64 | 1 | 5.0 | 0 | 5 | 5 | 5 | 5 | 5 | 5 | 5 |
| 65+ | 3 | 4.2 | 6 | 2 | 2 | 3 | 7 | 7 | 7 | 7 |
| **GRAND TOTAL** | 4 | 4.4 | 4 | 2 | 2 | 5 | 7 | 7 | 7 | 7 |

## 91.6: MICRO EXAM-INTEGUMENT. Formerly included in operation group(s) 796.

| Type of Patients | Observed Patients | Avg. Stay | Variance | 10th | 25th | 50th | 75th | 90th | 95th | 99th |
|---|---|---|---|---|---|---|---|---|---|---|
| | | | | | | Percentiles | | | | |
| **1. SINGLE DX** | | | | | | | | | | |
| 0–19 Years | 1 | 2.0 | 0 | 2 | 2 | 2 | 2 | 2 | 2 | 2 |
| 20–34 | 0 | | | | | | | | | |
| 35–49 | 0 | | | | | | | | | |
| 50–64 | 0 | | | | | | | | | |
| 65+ | 0 | | | | | | | | | |
| **2. MULTIPLE DX** | | | | | | | | | | |
| 0–19 Years | 5 | 2.6 | 1 | 1 | 2 | 3 | 3 | 4 | 4 | 4 |
| 20–34 | 1 | 8.0 | 0 | 8 | 8 | 8 | 8 | 8 | 8 | 8 |
| 35–49 | 5 | 10.0 | 313 | 1 | 2 | 3 | 3 | 48 | 48 | 48 |
| 50–64 | 2 | 4.5 | <1 | 4 | 4 | 5 | 5 | 5 | 5 | 5 |
| 65+ | 13 | 7.3 | 28 | 3 | 5 | 5 | 8 | 12 | 24 | 24 |
| **TOTAL SINGLE DX** | 1 | 2.0 | 0 | 2 | 2 | 2 | 2 | 2 | 2 | 2 |
| **TOTAL MULTIPLE DX** | 26 | 7.3 | 106 | 2 | 3 | 4 | 7 | 12 | 24 | 48 |
| **TOTAL** | | | | | | | | | | |
| 0–19 Years | 6 | 2.3 | <1 | 2 | 2 | 3 | 3 | 4 | 4 | 4 |
| 20–34 | 1 | 8.0 | 0 | 8 | 8 | 8 | 8 | 8 | 8 | 8 |
| 35–49 | 5 | 10.0 | 313 | 1 | 2 | 3 | 3 | 48 | 48 | 48 |
| 50–64 | 2 | 4.5 | <1 | 4 | 4 | 5 | 5 | 5 | 5 | 5 |
| 65+ | 13 | 7.3 | 28 | 3 | 5 | 5 | 8 | 12 | 24 | 24 |
| **GRAND TOTAL** | 27 | 6.7 | 96 | 2 | 2 | 4 | 5 | 12 | 24 | 48 |

Length of Stay by Diagnosis and Operation, United States, 2000

### 91.7: MICRO EXAM-OP WOUND. Formerly included in operation group(s) 796.

| Type of Patients | Observed Patients | Avg. Stay | Vari-ance | 10th | 25th | 50th | 75th | 90th | 95th | 99th |
|---|---|---|---|---|---|---|---|---|---|---|
| **1. SINGLE DX** | | | | | | | | | | |
| 0–19 Years | 0 | | | | | | | | | |
| 20–34 | 0 | | | | | | | | | |
| 35–49 | 0 | | | | | | | | | |
| 50–64 | 0 | | | | | | | | | |
| 65+ | 0 | | | | | | | | | |
| **2. MULTIPLE DX** | | | | | | | | | | |
| 0–19 Years | 0 | | | | | | | | | |
| 20–34 | 1 | 10.0 | 0 | 10 | 10 | 10 | 10 | 10 | 10 | 10 |
| 35–49 | 0 | | | | | | | | | |
| 50–64 | 2 | 5.1 | 1 | 4 | 4 | 6 | 6 | 6 | 6 | 6 |
| 65+ | 1 | 9.0 | 0 | 9 | 9 | 9 | 9 | 9 | 9 | 9 |
| **TOTAL SINGLE DX** | 0 | | | | | | | | | |
| **TOTAL MULTIPLE DX** | 4 | 7.1 | 6 | 4 | 6 | 6 | 9 | 10 | 10 | 10 |
| **TOTAL** | | | | | | | | | | |
| 0–19 Years | 0 | | | | | | | | | |
| 20–34 | 1 | 10.0 | 0 | 10 | 10 | 10 | 10 | 10 | 10 | 10 |
| 35–49 | 0 | | | | | | | | | |
| 50–64 | 2 | 5.1 | 1 | 4 | 4 | 6 | 6 | 6 | 6 | 6 |
| 65+ | 1 | 9.0 | 0 | 9 | 9 | 9 | 9 | 9 | 9 | 9 |
| **GRAND TOTAL** | 4 | 7.1 | 6 | 4 | 6 | 6 | 9 | 10 | 10 | 10 |

### 91.9: MICRO EXAM NOS. Formerly included in operation group(s) 796.

| Type of Patients | Observed Patients | Avg. Stay | Vari-ance | 10th | 25th | 50th | 75th | 90th | 95th | 99th |
|---|---|---|---|---|---|---|---|---|---|---|
| **1. SINGLE DX** | | | | | | | | | | |
| 0–19 Years | 1 | 1.0 | 0 | 1 | 1 | 1 | 1 | 1 | 1 | 1 |
| 20–34 | 0 | | | | | | | | | |
| 35–49 | 0 | | | | | | | | | |
| 50–64 | 0 | | | | | | | | | |
| 65+ | 0 | | | | | | | | | |
| **2. MULTIPLE DX** | | | | | | | | | | |
| 0–19 Years | 0 | | | | | | | | | |
| 20–34 | 0 | | | | | | | | | |
| 35–49 | 0 | | | | | | | | | |
| 50–64 | 0 | | | | | | | | | |
| 65+ | 0 | | | | | | | | | |
| **TOTAL SINGLE DX** | 1 | 1.0 | 0 | 1 | 1 | 1 | 1 | 1 | 1 | 1 |
| **TOTAL MULTIPLE DX** | 0 | | | | | | | | | |
| **TOTAL** | | | | | | | | | | |
| 0–19 Years | 1 | 1.0 | 0 | 1 | 1 | 1 | 1 | 1 | 1 | 1 |
| 20–34 | 0 | | | | | | | | | |
| 35–49 | 0 | | | | | | | | | |
| 50–64 | 0 | | | | | | | | | |
| 65+ | 0 | | | | | | | | | |
| **GRAND TOTAL** | 1 | 1.0 | 0 | 1 | 1 | 1 | 1 | 1 | 1 | 1 |

### 91.8: MICRO EXAM NEC. Formerly included in operation group(s) 796.

| Type of Patients | Observed Patients | Avg. Stay | Vari-ance | 10th | 25th | 50th | 75th | 90th | 95th | 99th |
|---|---|---|---|---|---|---|---|---|---|---|
| **1. SINGLE DX** | | | | | | | | | | |
| 0–19 Years | 0 | | | | | | | | | |
| 20–34 | 0 | | | | | | | | | |
| 35–49 | 0 | | | | | | | | | |
| 50–64 | 0 | | | | | | | | | |
| 65+ | 0 | | | | | | | | | |
| **2. MULTIPLE DX** | | | | | | | | | | |
| 0–19 Years | 1 | 2.0 | 0 | 2 | 2 | 2 | 2 | 2 | 2 | 2 |
| 20–34 | 1 | 4.0 | 0 | 4 | 4 | 4 | 4 | 4 | 4 | 4 |
| 35–49 | 0 | | | | | | | | | |
| 50–64 | 1 | 4.0 | 0 | 4 | 4 | 4 | 4 | 4 | 4 | 4 |
| 65+ | 1 | 5.0 | 0 | 5 | 5 | 5 | 5 | 5 | 5 | 5 |
| **TOTAL SINGLE DX** | 0 | | | | | | | | | |
| **TOTAL MULTIPLE DX** | 4 | 4.1 | 1 | 2 | 4 | 4 | 5 | 5 | 5 | 5 |
| **TOTAL** | | | | | | | | | | |
| 0–19 Years | 1 | 2.0 | 0 | 2 | 2 | 2 | 2 | 2 | 2 | 2 |
| 20–34 | 1 | 4.0 | 0 | 4 | 4 | 4 | 4 | 4 | 4 | 4 |
| 35–49 | 0 | | | | | | | | | |
| 50–64 | 1 | 4.0 | 0 | 4 | 4 | 4 | 4 | 4 | 4 | 4 |
| 65+ | 1 | 5.0 | 0 | 5 | 5 | 5 | 5 | 5 | 5 | 5 |
| **GRAND TOTAL** | 4 | 4.1 | 1 | 2 | 4 | 4 | 5 | 5 | 5 | 5 |

### 92.0: ISOTOPE SCAN & FUNCTION. Formerly included in operation group(s) 787.

| Type of Patients | Observed Patients | Avg. Stay | Vari-ance | 10th | 25th | 50th | 75th | 90th | 95th | 99th |
|---|---|---|---|---|---|---|---|---|---|---|
| **1. SINGLE DX** | | | | | | | | | | |
| 0–19 Years | 46 | 2.3 | 4 | 1 | 1 | 1 | 3 | 6 | 7 | 7 |
| 20–34 | 41 | 2.1 | 2 | 1 | 1 | 2 | 2 | 5 | 6 | 6 |
| 35–49 | 91 | 2.0 | 1 | 1 | 1 | 2 | 2 | 3 | 4 | 6 |
| 50–64 | 68 | 2.8 | 7 | 1 | 1 | 2 | 3 | 5 | 7 | 14 |
| 65+ | 45 | 2.8 | 2 | 1 | 1 | 4 | 4 | 4 | 4 | 7 |
| **2. MULTIPLE DX** | | | | | | | | | | |
| 0–19 Years | 175 | 4.2 | 9 | 2 | 3 | 3 | 5 | 7 | 8 | 21 |
| 20–34 | 201 | 6.0 | 26 | 1 | 2 | 4 | 10 | 14 | 14 | 14 |
| 35–49 | 807 | 3.5 | 11 | 1 | 2 | 2 | 5 | 6 | 9 | 14 |
| 50–64 | 1,282 | 4.0 | 12 | 1 | 2 | 3 | 5 | 7 | 11 | 15 |
| 65+ | 2,444 | 6.0 | 28 | 2 | 2 | 4 | 8 | 14 | 16 | 22 |
| **TOTAL SINGLE DX** | 291 | 2.4 | 3 | 1 | 1 | 2 | 4 | 4 | 5 | 7 |
| **TOTAL MULTIPLE DX** | 4,909 | 5.0 | 22 | 1 | 2 | 3 | 6 | 11 | 15 | 22 |
| **TOTAL** | | | | | | | | | | |
| 0–19 Years | 221 | 3.9 | 9 | 1 | 2 | 3 | 5 | 7 | 8 | 14 |
| 20–34 | 242 | 5.5 | 25 | 1 | 2 | 3 | 10 | 14 | 14 | 14 |
| 35–49 | 898 | 3.2 | 10 | 1 | 2 | 3 | 4 | 6 | 8 | 14 |
| 50–64 | 1,350 | 3.9 | 12 | 1 | 2 | 3 | 5 | 7 | 10 | 15 |
| 65+ | 2,489 | 5.8 | 27 | 2 | 2 | 4 | 7 | 14 | 15 | 22 |
| **GRAND TOTAL** | 5,200 | 4.8 | 21 | 1 | 2 | 3 | 6 | 11 | 14 | 22 |

# United States, October 1998–September 1999 Data, by Operation

## 92.02: LIVER SCAN/ISOTOPE FUNCT. Formerly included in operation group(s) 787.

| Type of Patients | Observed Patients | Avg. Stay | Vari-ance | Percentiles | | | | | | |
|---|---|---|---|---|---|---|---|---|---|---|
| | | | | 10th | 25th | 50th | 75th | 90th | 95th | 99th |
| **1. SINGLE DX** | | | | | | | | | | |
| 0–19 Years | 5 | 2.1 | <1 | 1 | 1 | 2 | 2 | 3 | 3 | 3 |
| 20–34 | 23 | 2.2 | 2 | 1 | 1 | 2 | 2 | 6 | 6 | 6 |
| 35–49 | 13 | 1.9 | 1 | 1 | 1 | 1 | 3 | 3 | 4 | 5 |
| 50–64 | 8 | 4.0 | 6 | 2 | 2 | 3 | 5 | 9 | 9 | 9 |
| 65+ | 9 | 2.7 | 3 | 1 | 2 | 2 | 3 | 4 | 7 | 7 |
| **2. MULTIPLE DX** | | | | | | | | | | |
| 0–19 Years | 18 | 4.8 | 6 | 1 | 3 | 6 | 7 | 7 | 7 | 10 |
| 20–34 | 67 | 3.4 | 6 | 1 | 1 | 3 | 4 | 6 | 10 | 11 |
| 35–49 | 113 | 4.5 | 12 | 1 | 2 | 3 | 5 | 10 | 12 | 19 |
| 50–64 | 109 | 4.5 | 25 | 1 | 2 | 3 | 6 | 9 | 15 | 26 |
| 65+ | 231 | 5.4 | 15 | 2 | 3 | 4 | 7 | 10 | 14 | 19 |
| **TOTAL SINGLE DX** | 58 | 2.4 | 3 | 1 | 1 | 2 | 3 | 5 | 6 | 9 |
| **TOTAL MULTIPLE DX** | 538 | 4.7 | 16 | 1 | 2 | 3 | 6 | 9 | 12 | 21 |
| **TOTAL** | | | | | | | | | | |
| 0–19 Years | 23 | 4.4 | 6 | 2 | 2 | 4 | 7 | 7 | 7 | 10 |
| 20–34 | 90 | 3.0 | 5 | 1 | 1 | 2 | 4 | 6 | 8 | 11 |
| 35–49 | 126 | 4.2 | 11 | 1 | 2 | 3 | 5 | 9 | 11 | 19 |
| 50–64 | 117 | 4.5 | 24 | 1 | 2 | 4 | 6 | 9 | 13 | 26 |
| 65+ | 240 | 5.4 | 15 | 2 | 3 | 4 | 7 | 10 | 14 | 19 |
| **GRAND TOTAL** | 596 | 4.5 | 15 | 1 | 2 | 3 | 6 | 9 | 11 | 19 |

## 92.03: RENAL SCAN/ISOTOPE STUDY. Formerly included in operation group(s) 787.

| Type of Patients | Observed Patients | Avg. Stay | Vari-ance | Percentiles | | | | | | |
|---|---|---|---|---|---|---|---|---|---|---|
| | | | | 10th | 25th | 50th | 75th | 90th | 95th | 99th |
| **1. SINGLE DX** | | | | | | | | | | |
| 0–19 Years | 19 | 3.7 | 5 | 1 | 2 | 3 | 7 | 7 | 7 | 7 |
| 20–34 | 4 | 2.7 | <1 | 2 | 2 | 3 | 3 | 3 | 5 | 5 |
| 35–49 | 9 | 2.5 | 2 | 2 | 2 | 2 | 3 | 3 | 5 | 5 |
| 50–64 | 2 | 8.5 | 21 | 5 | 5 | 5 | 14 | 14 | 14 | 14 |
| 65+ | 4 | 4.0 | <1 | 4 | 4 | 4 | 4 | 4 | 4 | 5 |
| **2. MULTIPLE DX** | | | | | | | | | | |
| 0–19 Years | 99 | 4.1 | 9 | 2 | 2 | 3 | 5 | 7 | 8 | 21 |
| 20–34 | 38 | 7.4 | 14 | 1 | 4 | 10 | 10 | 10 | 12 | 12 |
| 35–49 | 62 | 4.1 | 12 | 1 | 1 | 4 | 6 | 10 | 11 | 15 |
| 50–64 | 55 | 10.2 | 25 | 4 | 5 | 9 | 15 | 15 | 15 | 18 |
| 65+ | 155 | 8.5 | 15 | 3 | 7 | 7 | 10 | 14 | 14 | 17 |
| **TOTAL SINGLE DX** | 38 | 3.7 | 2 | 2 | 3 | 4 | 4 | 4 | 5 | 14 |
| **TOTAL MULTIPLE DX** | 409 | 7.6 | 20 | 2 | 4 | 7 | 10 | 14 | 15 | 16 |
| **TOTAL** | | | | | | | | | | |
| 0–19 Years | 118 | 4.1 | 9 | 3 | 3 | 3 | 5 | 7 | 8 | 21 |
| 20–34 | 42 | 7.0 | 15 | 1 | 3 | 10 | 10 | 10 | 12 | 12 |
| 35–49 | 71 | 3.6 | 8 | 1 | 2 | 3 | 4 | 7 | 10 | 15 |
| 50–64 | 57 | 10.2 | 25 | 4 | 5 | 9 | 15 | 15 | 15 | 18 |
| 65+ | 159 | 7.6 | 15 | 4 | 7 | 7 | 10 | 14 | 14 | 16 |
| **GRAND TOTAL** | 447 | 6.9 | 19 | 2 | 4 | 6 | 9 | 14 | 15 | 15 |

## 92.04: GI SCAN & ISOTOPE STUDY. Formerly included in operation group(s) 787.

| Type of Patients | Observed Patients | Avg. Stay | Vari-ance | Percentiles | | | | | | |
|---|---|---|---|---|---|---|---|---|---|---|
| | | | | 10th | 25th | 50th | 75th | 90th | 95th | 99th |
| **1. SINGLE DX** | | | | | | | | | | |
| 0–19 Years | 13 | 3.2 | 5 | 1 | 1 | 3 | 5 | 6 | 6 | 6 |
| 20–34 | 4 | 1.1 | <1 | 1 | 1 | 1 | 1 | 2 | 2 | 2 |
| 35–49 | 9 | 2.4 | 3 | 1 | 1 | 2 | 3 | 5 | 5 | 7 |
| 50–64 | 7 | 5.0 | 4 | 3 | 4 | 4 | 7 | 7 | 7 | 7 |
| 65+ | 1 | 2.0 | 0 | 2 | 2 | 2 | 2 | 2 | 2 | 2 |
| **2. MULTIPLE DX** | | | | | | | | | | |
| 0–19 Years | 45 | 4.3 | 6 | 2 | 3 | 4 | 6 | 8 | 10 | 11 |
| 20–34 | 25 | 4.3 | 13 | 2 | 3 | 3 | 6 | 10 | 13 | 13 |
| 35–49 | 57 | 4.4 | 10 | 2 | 2 | 3 | 5 | 6 | 10 | 11 |
| 50–64 | 53 | 3.7 | 5 | 1 | 2 | 3 | 5 | 6 | 8 | 15 |
| 65+ | 125 | 4.2 | 17 | 2 | 2 | 2 | 4 | 9 | 15 | 18 |
| **TOTAL SINGLE DX** | 34 | 3.5 | 5 | 1 | 1 | 3 | 5 | 7 | 7 | 7 |
| **TOTAL MULTIPLE DX** | 305 | 4.1 | 13 | 2 | 2 | 3 | 5 | 8 | 12 | 18 |
| **TOTAL** | | | | | | | | | | |
| 0–19 Years | 58 | 4.1 | 6 | 1 | 3 | 4 | 6 | 8 | 9 | 11 |
| 20–34 | 29 | 4.0 | 13 | 1 | 1 | 2 | 6 | 10 | 13 | 13 |
| 35–49 | 66 | 4.1 | 10 | 1 | 2 | 3 | 5 | 9 | 10 | 11 |
| 50–64 | 60 | 3.9 | 5 | 2 | 2 | 2 | 5 | 7 | 8 | 10 |
| 65+ | 126 | 4.2 | 17 | 2 | 2 | 2 | 4 | 9 | 15 | 18 |
| **GRAND TOTAL** | 339 | 4.1 | 12 | 2 | 2 | 3 | 5 | 8 | 11 | 18 |

## 92.05: CV SCAN/ISOTOPE STUDY. Formerly included in operation group(s) 787.

| Type of Patients | Observed Patients | Avg. Stay | Vari-ance | Percentiles | | | | | | |
|---|---|---|---|---|---|---|---|---|---|---|
| | | | | 10th | 25th | 50th | 75th | 90th | 95th | 99th |
| **1. SINGLE DX** | | | | | | | | | | |
| 0–19 Years | 5 | 1.1 | <1 | 1 | 1 | 1 | 1 | 1 | 1 | 6 |
| 20–34 | 6 | 1.9 | 3 | 1 | 1 | 1 | 2 | 5 | 5 | 5 |
| 35–49 | 56 | 1.8 | 3 | 1 | 1 | 2 | 2 | 3 | 4 | 6 |
| 50–64 | 48 | 2.0 | 3 | 1 | 1 | 1 | 2 | 3 | 3 | 14 |
| 65+ | 27 | 1.7 | 2 | 1 | 1 | 2 | 2 | 3 | 4 | 7 |
| **2. MULTIPLE DX** | | | | | | | | | | |
| 0–19 Years | 9 | 3.1 | <1 | 3 | 3 | 3 | 3 | 4 | 5 | 7 |
| 20–34 | 53 | 7.7 | 43 | 1 | 2 | 6 | 14 | 14 | 14 | 17 |
| 35–49 | 536 | 3.0 | 10 | 1 | 1 | 2 | 4 | 6 | 7 | 13 |
| 50–64 | 1,030 | 3.5 | 7 | 1 | 2 | 3 | 5 | 7 | 7 | 14 |
| 65+ | 1,880 | 5.8 | 28 | 2 | 2 | 4 | 7 | 13 | 16 | 22 |
| **TOTAL SINGLE DX** | 142 | 1.8 | 2 | 1 | 1 | 1 | 2 | 3 | 4 | 7 |
| **TOTAL MULTIPLE DX** | 3,508 | 4.7 | 21 | 1 | 2 | 3 | 6 | 11 | 15 | 22 |
| **TOTAL** | | | | | | | | | | |
| 0–19 Years | 14 | 2.3 | 2 | 1 | 1 | 3 | 3 | 3 | 3 | 7 |
| 20–34 | 59 | 7.4 | 42 | 1 | 1 | 5 | 14 | 14 | 14 | 17 |
| 35–49 | 592 | 2.9 | 9 | 1 | 1 | 2 | 4 | 6 | 6 | 13 |
| 50–64 | 1,078 | 3.4 | 7 | 1 | 2 | 3 | 5 | 7 | 7 | 14 |
| 65+ | 1,907 | 5.6 | 28 | 2 | 2 | 4 | 7 | 13 | 16 | 22 |
| **GRAND TOTAL** | 3,650 | 4.5 | 21 | 1 | 2 | 3 | 6 | 10 | 14 | 22 |

© 2000 by HCIA-Sachs, L.L.C.

Length of Stay by Diagnosis and Operation, United States, 2000

# United States, October 1998–September 1999 Data, by Operation

## 92.1: OTHER RADIOISOTOPE SCAN. Formerly included in operation group(s) 787.

| Type of Patients | Observed Patients | Avg. Stay | Variance | 10th | 25th | 50th | 75th | 90th | 95th | 99th |
|---|---|---|---|---|---|---|---|---|---|---|
| **1. SINGLE DX** | | | | | | | | | | |
| 0–19 Years | 89 | 4.0 | 13 | 1 | 2 | 3 | 5 | 10 | 14 | 15 |
| 20–34 | 60 | 2.7 | 3 | 1 | 1 | 2 | 4 | 5 | 6 | 6 |
| 35–49 | 98 | 3.5 | 7 | 1 | 2 | 3 | 5 | 7 | 8 | 11 |
| 50–64 | 61 | 3.4 | 8 | 1 | 1 | 3 | 4 | 8 | 10 | 12 |
| 65+ | 75 | 5.5 | 15 | 1 | 2 | 4 | 8 | 14 | 14 | 15 |
| **2. MULTIPLE DX** | | | | | | | | | | |
| 0–19 Years | 224 | 6.4 | 37 | 2 | 3 | 5 | 8 | 12 | 14 | 30 |
| 20–34 | 481 | 4.6 | 28 | 1 | 2 | 4 | 5 | 8 | 11 | 19 |
| 35–49 | 1,252 | 4.2 | 12 | 1 | 2 | 3 | 6 | 8 | 11 | 16 |
| 50–64 | 1,747 | 4.8 | 11 | 2 | 3 | 4 | 6 | 9 | 10 | 17 |
| 65+ | 4,556 | 5.7 | 18 | 2 | 3 | 5 | 7 | 10 | 13 | 21 |
| **TOTAL SINGLE DX** | 383 | 3.9 | 10 | 1 | 2 | 3 | 5 | 8 | 11 | 15 |
| **TOTAL MULTIPLE DX** | 8,260 | 5.3 | 17 | 2 | 3 | 4 | 7 | 9 | 12 | 19 |
| **TOTAL** | | | | | | | | | | |
| 0–19 Years | 313 | 5.8 | 32 | 1 | 2 | 5 | 8 | 11 | 14 | 29 |
| 20–34 | 541 | 4.4 | 25 | 1 | 2 | 3 | 5 | 8 | 11 | 19 |
| 35–49 | 1,350 | 4.2 | 12 | 1 | 2 | 3 | 6 | 8 | 10 | 16 |
| 50–64 | 1,808 | 4.7 | 11 | 2 | 3 | 4 | 6 | 9 | 10 | 16 |
| 65+ | 4,631 | 5.7 | 18 | 2 | 3 | 5 | 7 | 10 | 13 | 21 |
| **GRAND TOTAL** | 8,643 | 5.2 | 17 | 2 | 3 | 4 | 7 | 9 | 12 | 19 |

## 92.14: BONE SCAN. Formerly included in operation group(s) 787.

| Type of Patients | Observed Patients | Avg. Stay | Variance | 10th | 25th | 50th | 75th | 90th | 95th | 99th |
|---|---|---|---|---|---|---|---|---|---|---|
| **1. SINGLE DX** | | | | | | | | | | |
| 0–19 Years | 72 | 4.1 | 15 | 1 | 2 | 3 | 4 | 10 | 15 | 15 |
| 20–34 | 6 | 5.1 | 1 | 3 | 4 | 6 | 6 | 6 | 6 | 6 |
| 35–49 | 11 | 3.1 | 6 | 2 | 2 | 3 | 3 | 4 | 11 | 11 |
| 50–64 | 12 | 2.8 | 3 | 1 | 2 | 2 | 4 | 6 | 6 | 6 |
| 65+ | 20 | 5.3 | 9 | 4 | 4 | 4 | 6 | 9 | 14 | 14 |
| **2. MULTIPLE DX** | | | | | | | | | | |
| 0–19 Years | 138 | 6.7 | 56 | 2 | 3 | 5 | 8 | 13 | 17 | 30 |
| 20–34 | 90 | 6.1 | 50 | 2 | 3 | 5 | 7 | 13 | 15 | 19 |
| 35–49 | 243 | 5.0 | 18 | 1 | 2 | 4 | 7 | 9 | 12 | 22 |
| 50–64 | 346 | 5.2 | 14 | 2 | 3 | 4 | 7 | 9 | 11 | 21 |
| 65+ | 1,511 | 5.9 | 22 | 2 | 3 | 5 | 7 | 10 | 14 | 23 |
| **TOTAL SINGLE DX** | 121 | 4.1 | 11 | 1 | 2 | 3 | 4 | 8 | 14 | 15 |
| **TOTAL MULTIPLE DX** | 2,328 | 5.7 | 23 | 2 | 3 | 5 | 7 | 10 | 13 | 23 |
| **TOTAL** | | | | | | | | | | |
| 0–19 Years | 210 | 5.8 | 43 | 1 | 2 | 4 | 7 | 13 | 15 | 30 |
| 20–34 | 96 | 6.0 | 45 | 2 | 3 | 5 | 7 | 13 | 15 | 19 |
| 35–49 | 254 | 4.8 | 17 | 1 | 2 | 4 | 6 | 9 | 12 | 20 |
| 50–64 | 358 | 5.2 | 14 | 2 | 3 | 4 | 7 | 9 | 11 | 21 |
| 65+ | 1,531 | 5.9 | 21 | 2 | 3 | 5 | 7 | 10 | 14 | 23 |
| **GRAND TOTAL** | 2,449 | 5.7 | 22 | 2 | 3 | 4 | 7 | 10 | 13 | 23 |

## 92.15: PULMONARY SCAN. Formerly included in operation group(s) 787.

| Type of Patients | Observed Patients | Avg. Stay | Variance | 10th | 25th | 50th | 75th | 90th | 95th | 99th |
|---|---|---|---|---|---|---|---|---|---|---|
| **1. SINGLE DX** | | | | | | | | | | |
| 0–19 Years | 6 | 2.7 | 4 | 1 | 1 | 2 | 5 | 5 | 6 | 6 |
| 20–34 | 50 | 2.4 | 2 | 1 | 1 | 2 | 4 | 5 | 5 | 6 |
| 35–49 | 81 | 3.9 | 6 | 1 | 2 | 3 | 5 | 7 | 8 | 11 |
| 50–64 | 48 | 3.4 | 9 | 1 | 2 | 2 | 5 | 9 | 10 | 12 |
| 65+ | 50 | 5.9 | 19 | 1 | 2 | 5 | 8 | 14 | 14 | 15 |
| **2. MULTIPLE DX** | | | | | | | | | | |
| 0–19 Years | 40 | 6.4 | 23 | 1 | 3 | 5 | 9 | 12 | 16 | 16 |
| 20–34 | 358 | 4.2 | 22 | 1 | 2 | 4 | 5 | 7 | 10 | 19 |
| 35–49 | 951 | 4.0 | 11 | 1 | 2 | 3 | 5 | 8 | 10 | 13 |
| 50–64 | 1,342 | 4.6 | 10 | 1 | 2 | 4 | 6 | 8 | 10 | 16 |
| 65+ | 2,854 | 5.6 | 16 | 2 | 3 | 5 | 7 | 10 | 12 | 19 |
| **TOTAL SINGLE DX** | 235 | 3.9 | 10 | 1 | 1 | 3 | 5 | 8 | 11 | 14 |
| **TOTAL MULTIPLE DX** | 5,545 | 5.0 | 14 | 1 | 3 | 4 | 7 | 9 | 11 | 18 |
| **TOTAL** | | | | | | | | | | |
| 0–19 Years | 46 | 5.9 | 22 | 1 | 2 | 5 | 8 | 11 | 16 | 16 |
| 20–34 | 408 | 4.0 | 20 | 1 | 2 | 3 | 5 | 7 | 9 | 16 |
| 35–49 | 1,032 | 4.0 | 10 | 1 | 2 | 3 | 6 | 8 | 10 | 13 |
| 50–64 | 1,390 | 4.6 | 10 | 1 | 2 | 4 | 6 | 8 | 10 | 16 |
| 65+ | 2,904 | 5.6 | 16 | 2 | 3 | 5 | 7 | 10 | 12 | 19 |
| **GRAND TOTAL** | 5,780 | 5.0 | 14 | 1 | 2 | 4 | 6 | 9 | 11 | 18 |

## 92.2: THER RADIOLOGY & NU MED. Formerly included in operation group(s) 788.

| Type of Patients | Observed Patients | Avg. Stay | Variance | 10th | 25th | 50th | 75th | 90th | 95th | 99th |
|---|---|---|---|---|---|---|---|---|---|---|
| **1. SINGLE DX** | | | | | | | | | | |
| 0–19 Years | 24 | 1.8 | 1 | 1 | 1 | 2 | 2 | 2 | 3 | 6 |
| 20–34 | 367 | 1.9 | <1 | 1 | 1 | 2 | 2 | 3 | 3 | 4 |
| 35–49 | 733 | 1.9 | <1 | 1 | 1 | 2 | 2 | 3 | 3 | 5 |
| 50–64 | 650 | 2.0 | 1 | 1 | 1 | 2 | 2 | 3 | 3 | 7 |
| 65+ | 617 | 2.1 | 4 | 1 | 1 | 2 | 2 | 3 | 4 | 12 |
| **2. MULTIPLE DX** | | | | | | | | | | |
| 0–19 Years | 212 | 6.0 | 43 | 1 | 2 | 4 | 7 | 12 | 18 | 28 |
| 20–34 | 769 | 3.8 | 27 | 1 | 2 | 3 | 4 | 7 | 13 | 29 |
| 35–49 | 2,613 | 5.0 | 27 | 1 | 2 | 3 | 6 | 11 | 15 | 26 |
| 50–64 | 4,657 | 6.6 | 50 | 1 | 2 | 4 | 8 | 15 | 18 | 32 |
| 65+ | 7,850 | 6.8 | 44 | 2 | 3 | 5 | 8 | 15 | 19 | 35 |
| **TOTAL SINGLE DX** | 2,391 | 2.0 | 2 | 1 | 1 | 2 | 2 | 3 | 4 | 8 |
| **TOTAL MULTIPLE DX** | 16,101 | 6.3 | 43 | 1 | 2 | 4 | 8 | 14 | 18 | 32 |
| **TOTAL** | | | | | | | | | | |
| 0–19 Years | 236 | 5.6 | 41 | 1 | 2 | 4 | 7 | 11 | 18 | 28 |
| 20–34 | 1,136 | 3.1 | 18 | 1 | 2 | 2 | 3 | 5 | 8 | 23 |
| 35–49 | 3,346 | 4.3 | 23 | 1 | 2 | 4 | 5 | 10 | 14 | 23 |
| 50–64 | 5,307 | 6.0 | 46 | 1 | 2 | 4 | 7 | 14 | 18 | 32 |
| 65+ | 8,467 | 6.4 | 43 | 1 | 2 | 4 | 8 | 14 | 18 | 33 |
| **GRAND TOTAL** | 18,492 | 5.7 | 40 | 1 | 2 | 4 | 7 | 13 | 17 | 31 |

Length of Stay by Diagnosis and Operation, United States, 2000

# United States, October 1998–September 1999 Data, by Operation

## 92.23: ISOTOPE TELERADIOTHERAPY. Formerly included in operation group(s) 788.

| Type of Patients | Observed Patients | Avg. Stay | Vari-ance | Percentiles | | | | | | |
|---|---|---|---|---|---|---|---|---|---|---|
| | | | | 10th | 25th | 50th | 75th | 90th | 95th | 99th |
| **1. SINGLE DX** | | | | | | | | | | |
| 0–19 Years | 2 | 2.4 | <1 | 2 | 2 | 2 | 3 | 3 | 3 | 3 |
| 20–34 | 21 | 1.6 | <1 | 1 | 1 | 2 | 2 | 2 | 3 | 3 |
| 35–49 | 36 | 1.9 | <1 | 1 | 1 | 2 | 2 | 2 | 3 | 4 |
| 50–64 | 27 | 1.7 | <1 | 1 | 1 | 2 | 2 | 2 | 3 | 3 |
| 65+ | 10 | 1.8 | <1 | 1 | 1 | 2 | 2 | 3 | 3 | 3 |
| **2. MULTIPLE DX** | | | | | | | | | | |
| 0–19 Years | 12 | 3.0 | 4 | 2 | 2 | 3 | 3 | 4 | 4 | 11 |
| 20–34 | 62 | 2.9 | 14 | 1 | 1 | 2 | 2 | 5 | 12 | 12 |
| 35–49 | 177 | 5.6 | 23 | 1 | 2 | 5 | 7 | 15 | 15 | 17 |
| 50–64 | 243 | 7.8 | 29 | 2 | 4 | 7 | 14 | 15 | 15 | 22 |
| 65+ | 371 | 10.3 | 99 | 2 | 4 | 6 | 15 | 23 | 37 | 43 |
| **TOTAL SINGLE DX** | 96 | 1.7 | <1 | 1 | 1 | 2 | 2 | 2 | 3 | 3 |
| **TOTAL MULTIPLE DX** | 865 | 7.9 | 57 | 2 | 2 | 6 | 11 | 15 | 21 | 43 |
| **TOTAL** | | | | | | | | | | |
| 0–19 Years | 14 | 2.9 | 3 | 2 | 2 | 3 | 3 | 4 | 4 | 11 |
| 20–34 | 83 | 2.5 | 11 | 1 | 1 | 2 | 2 | 3 | 7 | 12 |
| 35–49 | 213 | 5.1 | 21 | 1 | 2 | 3 | 5 | 15 | 15 | 15 |
| 50–64 | 270 | 7.2 | 29 | 2 | 3 | 6 | 10 | 15 | 15 | 21 |
| 65+ | 381 | 10.0 | 98 | 2 | 3 | 6 | 15 | 23 | 32 | 43 |
| **GRAND TOTAL** | 961 | 7.2 | 55 | 1 | 2 | 5 | 10 | 15 | 20 | 43 |

## 92.24: PHOTON TELERADIOTHERAPY. Formerly included in operation group(s) 788.

| Type of Patients | Observed Patients | Avg. Stay | Vari-ance | Percentiles | | | | | | |
|---|---|---|---|---|---|---|---|---|---|---|
| | | | | 10th | 25th | 50th | 75th | 90th | 95th | 99th |
| **1. SINGLE DX** | | | | | | | | | | |
| 0–19 Years | 0 | | | | | | | | | |
| 20–34 | 1 | 1.0 | 0 | 1 | 1 | 1 | 1 | 1 | 1 | 1 |
| 35–49 | 5 | 6.0 | 12 | 2 | 2 | 7 | 8 | 10 | 10 | 10 |
| 50–64 | 8 | 6.5 | 27 | 1 | 1 | 4 | 11 | 14 | 14 | 14 |
| 65+ | 4 | 3.0 | 3 | 1 | 1 | 3 | 3 | 6 | 6 | 6 |
| **2. MULTIPLE DX** | | | | | | | | | | |
| 0–19 Years | 40 | 8.7 | 71 | 2 | 3 | 5 | 8 | 28 | 28 | 28 |
| 20–34 | 52 | 5.8 | 19 | 2 | 3 | 6 | 7 | 10 | 15 | 23 |
| 35–49 | 323 | 7.2 | 30 | 2 | 3 | 6 | 9 | 11 | 19 | 27 |
| 50–64 | 819 | 7.7 | 98 | 2 | 3 | 5 | 10 | 14 | 20 | 84 |
| 65+ | 1,467 | 7.9 | 45 | 2 | 4 | 6 | 10 | 16 | 21 | 31 |
| **TOTAL SINGLE DX** | 18 | 5.2 | 19 | 1 | 1 | 3 | 9 | 13 | 14 | 14 |
| **TOTAL MULTIPLE DX** | 2,701 | 7.7 | 58 | 2 | 3 | 6 | 9 | 15 | 20 | 33 |
| **TOTAL** | | | | | | | | | | |
| 0–19 Years | 40 | 8.7 | 71 | 2 | 3 | 5 | 8 | 28 | 28 | 28 |
| 20–34 | 53 | 5.8 | 19 | 2 | 2 | 6 | 7 | 10 | 15 | 23 |
| 35–49 | 328 | 7.2 | 30 | 1 | 3 | 6 | 9 | 11 | 19 | 27 |
| 50–64 | 827 | 7.7 | 98 | 2 | 3 | 5 | 9 | 14 | 20 | 84 |
| 65+ | 1,471 | 7.9 | 45 | 2 | 4 | 6 | 10 | 16 | 21 | 31 |
| **GRAND TOTAL** | 2,719 | 7.7 | 58 | 2 | 3 | 6 | 9 | 15 | 20 | 33 |

## 92.27: RADIOACTIVE ELEMENT IMPL. Formerly included in operation group(s) 788.

| Type of Patients | Observed Patients | Avg. Stay | Vari-ance | Percentiles | | | | | | |
|---|---|---|---|---|---|---|---|---|---|---|
| | | | | 10th | 25th | 50th | 75th | 90th | 95th | 99th |
| **1. SINGLE DX** | | | | | | | | | | |
| 0–19 Years | 2 | 1.9 | 3 | 1 | 1 | 1 | 1 | 5 | 5 | 5 |
| 20–34 | 112 | 2.1 | <1 | 2 | 2 | 2 | 2 | 3 | 3 | 3 |
| 35–49 | 359 | 1.9 | <1 | 1 | 1 | 2 | 2 | 3 | 3 | 4 |
| 50–64 | 411 | 1.9 | <1 | 1 | 1 | 2 | 2 | 3 | 3 | 4 |
| 65+ | 512 | 1.7 | <1 | 1 | 1 | 1 | 2 | 3 | 4 | 5 |
| **2. MULTIPLE DX** | | | | | | | | | | |
| 0–19 Years | 5 | 5.9 | 3 | 2 | 4 | 7 | 7 | 7 | 7 | 7 |
| 20–34 | 112 | 2.3 | 1 | 1 | 2 | 2 | 3 | 4 | 4 | 7 |
| 35–49 | 475 | 2.5 | 4 | 1 | 1 | 2 | 3 | 4 | 6 | 11 |
| 50–64 | 796 | 2.6 | 10 | 1 | 1 | 2 | 3 | 4 | 6 | 14 |
| 65+ | 1,521 | 2.4 | 7 | 1 | 1 | 2 | 3 | 4 | 5 | 14 |
| **TOTAL SINGLE DX** | 1,396 | 1.9 | <1 | 1 | 1 | 2 | 2 | 3 | 3 | 5 |
| **TOTAL MULTIPLE DX** | 2,909 | 2.5 | 7 | 1 | 1 | 2 | 3 | 4 | 5 | 14 |
| **TOTAL** | | | | | | | | | | |
| 0–19 Years | 7 | 4.8 | 6 | 1 | 2 | 6 | 7 | 7 | 7 | 7 |
| 20–34 | 224 | 2.2 | <1 | 1 | 2 | 2 | 2 | 3 | 4 | 6 |
| 35–49 | 834 | 2.2 | 2 | 1 | 1 | 2 | 2 | 3 | 4 | 10 |
| 50–64 | 1,207 | 2.3 | 7 | 1 | 1 | 2 | 3 | 3 | 5 | 12 |
| 65+ | 2,033 | 2.3 | 5 | 1 | 1 | 2 | 3 | 3 | 5 | 11 |
| **GRAND TOTAL** | 4,305 | 2.3 | 5 | 1 | 1 | 2 | 2 | 4 | 5 | 10 |

## 92.28: ISOTOPE INJECT/INSTILL. Formerly included in operation group(s) 788.

| Type of Patients | Observed Patients | Avg. Stay | Vari-ance | Percentiles | | | | | | |
|---|---|---|---|---|---|---|---|---|---|---|
| | | | | 10th | 25th | 50th | 75th | 90th | 95th | 99th |
| **1. SINGLE DX** | | | | | | | | | | |
| 0–19 Years | 4 | 1.9 | <1 | 1 | 2 | 2 | 2 | 2 | 2 | 2 |
| 20–34 | 49 | 1.8 | <1 | 1 | 2 | 2 | 2 | 2 | 3 | 3 |
| 35–49 | 63 | 2.1 | 1 | 1 | 1 | 2 | 2 | 3 | 4 | 6 |
| 50–64 | 36 | 2.4 | 3 | 1 | 1 | 2 | 3 | 4 | 5 | 10 |
| 65+ | 19 | 2.2 | <1 | 1 | 2 | 2 | 3 | 3 | 4 | 4 |
| **2. MULTIPLE DX** | | | | | | | | | | |
| 0–19 Years | 8 | 2.1 | <1 | 1 | 2 | 2 | 2 | 4 | 4 | 4 |
| 20–34 | 67 | 2.3 | 5 | 1 | 2 | 2 | 2 | 3 | 4 | 10 |
| 35–49 | 123 | 2.1 | 1 | 1 | 1 | 2 | 3 | 3 | 4 | 7 |
| 50–64 | 112 | 2.4 | 5 | 1 | 1 | 2 | 3 | 4 | 6 | 12 |
| 65+ | 94 | 4.4 | 25 | 2 | 2 | 3 | 5 | 9 | 14 | 28 |
| **TOTAL SINGLE DX** | 171 | 2.0 | 1 | 1 | 1 | 2 | 2 | 3 | 4 | 6 |
| **TOTAL MULTIPLE DX** | 404 | 2.7 | 8 | 1 | 1 | 2 | 3 | 4 | 7 | 17 |
| **TOTAL** | | | | | | | | | | |
| 0–19 Years | 12 | 2.0 | <1 | 1 | 2 | 2 | 2 | 2 | 3 | 4 |
| 20–34 | 116 | 2.1 | 3 | 1 | 2 | 2 | 2 | 3 | 3 | 7 |
| 35–49 | 186 | 2.1 | 1 | 1 | 1 | 2 | 3 | 3 | 4 | 7 |
| 50–64 | 148 | 2.4 | 4 | 1 | 1 | 2 | 3 | 4 | 6 | 12 |
| 65+ | 113 | 3.9 | 21 | 1 | 2 | 3 | 4 | 7 | 12 | 28 |
| **GRAND TOTAL** | 575 | 2.5 | 6 | 1 | 2 | 2 | 3 | 4 | 5 | 13 |

Length of Stay by Diagnosis and Operation, United States, 2000

# United States, October 1998–September 1999 Data, by Operation

## 92.29: RADIOTHERAPEUTIC PX NEC. Formerly included in operation group(s) 788.

| Type of Patients | Observed Patients | Avg. Stay | Variance | Percentiles | | | | | | |
|---|---|---|---|---|---|---|---|---|---|---|
| | | | | 10th | 25th | 50th | 75th | 90th | 95th | 99th |
| **1. SINGLE DX** | | | | | | | | | | |
| 0–19 Years | 15 | 1.6 | 1 | 1 | 1 | 1 | 2 | 2 | 2 | 6 |
| 20–34 | 184 | 1.8 | <1 | 1 | 1 | 2 | 2 | 2 | 3 | 4 |
| 35–49 | 268 | 1.8 | <1 | 1 | 1 | 2 | 2 | 2 | 3 | 5 |
| 50–64 | 166 | 2.0 | 1 | 1 | 1 | 2 | 2 | 3 | 4 | 7 |
| 65+ | 71 | 4.4 | 19 | 1 | 1 | 2 | 5 | 12 | 12 | 12 |
| **2. MULTIPLE DX** | | | | | | | | | | |
| 0–19 Years | 136 | 5.2 | 33 | 2 | 2 | 4 | 6 | 10 | 14 | 26 |
| 20–34 | 469 | 4.1 | 37 | 1 | 2 | 4 | 4 | 8 | 15 | 34 |
| 35–49 | 1,440 | 5.4 | 33 | 1 | 2 | 3 | 7 | 12 | 17 | 29 |
| 50–64 | 2,555 | 7.3 | 42 | 2 | 3 | 5 | 10 | 17 | 18 | 32 |
| 65+ | 4,149 | 7.6 | 44 | 2 | 3 | 5 | 10 | 15 | 20 | 35 |
| **TOTAL SINGLE DX** | 704 | 2.1 | 3 | 1 | 1 | 2 | 2 | 3 | 4 | 12 |
| **TOTAL MULTIPLE DX** | 8,749 | 6.9 | 42 | 2 | 3 | 5 | 9 | 15 | 19 | 32 |
| **TOTAL** | | | | | | | | | | |
| 0–19 Years | 151 | 4.8 | 31 | 1 | 2 | 3 | 6 | 9 | 14 | 26 |
| 20–34 | 653 | 3.3 | 25 | 1 | 2 | 3 | 3 | 5 | 11 | 29 |
| 35–49 | 1,708 | 4.8 | 30 | 1 | 2 | 3 | 6 | 11 | 15 | 28 |
| 50–64 | 2,721 | 6.9 | 41 | 2 | 3 | 5 | 9 | 16 | 18 | 32 |
| 65+ | 4,220 | 7.5 | 44 | 2 | 3 | 5 | 10 | 15 | 20 | 35 |
| **GRAND TOTAL** | 9,453 | 6.6 | 41 | 2 | 2 | 4 | 8 | 15 | 18 | 32 |

## 92.3: STEREOTACTIC RADIOSURG. Formerly included in operation group(s) 505.

| Type of Patients | Observed Patients | Avg. Stay | Variance | Percentiles | | | | | | |
|---|---|---|---|---|---|---|---|---|---|---|
| | | | | 10th | 25th | 50th | 75th | 90th | 95th | 99th |
| **1. SINGLE DX** | | | | | | | | | | |
| 0–19 Years | 38 | 1.2 | <1 | 1 | 1 | 1 | 1 | 2 | 2 | 4 |
| 20–34 | 28 | 1.2 | <1 | 1 | 1 | 1 | 1 | 2 | 2 | 8 |
| 35–49 | 55 | 1.5 | 1 | 1 | 1 | 1 | 1 | 2 | 4 | 6 |
| 50–64 | 64 | 1.6 | 5 | 1 | 1 | 1 | 1 | 3 | 4 | 6 |
| 65+ | 54 | 1.8 | 12 | 1 | 1 | 1 | 2 | 3 | 4 | 11 |
| **2. MULTIPLE DX** | | | | | | | | | | |
| 0–19 Years | 36 | 2.3 | 4 | 1 | 1 | 2 | 3 | 4 | 6 | 13 |
| 20–34 | 57 | 4.4 | 52 | 1 | 1 | 1 | 2 | 22 | 22 | 22 |
| 35–49 | 187 | 5.2 | 136 | 1 | 1 | 1 | 3 | 11 | 44 | 44 |
| 50–64 | 282 | 2.9 | 17 | 1 | 1 | 1 | 3 | 8 | 13 | 13 |
| 65+ | 260 | 2.8 | 25 | 1 | 1 | 1 | 2 | 8 | 11 | 18 |
| **TOTAL SINGLE DX** | 239 | 1.5 | 4 | 1 | 1 | 1 | 1 | 2 | 3 | 6 |
| **TOTAL MULTIPLE DX** | 822 | 3.5 | 51 | 1 | 1 | 1 | 2 | 8 | 13 | 44 |
| **TOTAL** | | | | | | | | | | |
| 0–19 Years | 74 | 1.8 | 2 | 1 | 1 | 2 | 2 | 3 | 4 | 6 |
| 20–34 | 85 | 3.3 | 36 | 1 | 1 | 1 | 2 | 11 | 22 | 22 |
| 35–49 | 242 | 4.5 | 113 | 1 | 1 | 1 | 2 | 7 | 44 | 44 |
| 50–64 | 346 | 2.8 | 16 | 1 | 1 | 1 | 2 | 8 | 13 | 13 |
| 65+ | 314 | 2.7 | 24 | 1 | 1 | 1 | 2 | 7 | 11 | 18 |
| **GRAND TOTAL** | 1,061 | 3.1 | 43 | 1 | 1 | 1 | 2 | 8 | 13 | 44 |

## 92.32: MULTI-SOURCE PHOTON SURG. Formerly included in operation group(s) 505.

| Type of Patients | Observed Patients | Avg. Stay | Variance | Percentiles | | | | | | |
|---|---|---|---|---|---|---|---|---|---|---|
| | | | | 10th | 25th | 50th | 75th | 90th | 95th | 99th |
| **1. SINGLE DX** | | | | | | | | | | |
| 0–19 Years | 19 | 1.1 | <1 | 1 | 1 | 1 | 1 | 2 | 2 | 2 |
| 20–34 | 11 | 1.2 | <1 | 1 | 1 | 1 | 1 | 2 | 2 | 2 |
| 35–49 | 32 | 1.1 | <1 | 1 | 1 | 1 | 1 | 2 | 2 | 2 |
| 50–64 | 27 | 1.6 | 11 | 1 | 1 | 1 | 1 | 2 | 2 | 26 |
| 65+ | 24 | 1.8 | 20 | 1 | 1 | 1 | 1 | 2 | 2 | 36 |
| **2. MULTIPLE DX** | | | | | | | | | | |
| 0–19 Years | 13 | 1.5 | <1 | 1 | 1 | 1 | 2 | 2 | 2 | 2 |
| 20–34 | 34 | 1.6 | 3 | 1 | 1 | 1 | 2 | 2 | 3 | 11 |
| 35–49 | 106 | 1.5 | 5 | 1 | 1 | 1 | 1 | 2 | 2 | 18 |
| 50–64 | 154 | 1.5 | 10 | 1 | 1 | 1 | 1 | 2 | 2 | 13 |
| 65+ | 134 | 2.1 | 10 | 1 | 1 | 1 | 2 | 3 | 10 | 17 |
| **TOTAL SINGLE DX** | 113 | 1.4 | 6 | 1 | 1 | 1 | 1 | 2 | 2 | 6 |
| **TOTAL MULTIPLE DX** | 441 | 1.7 | 8 | 1 | 1 | 1 | 1 | 2 | 4 | 17 |
| **TOTAL** | | | | | | | | | | |
| 0–19 Years | 32 | 1.3 | <1 | 1 | 1 | 1 | 1 | 2 | 2 | 2 |
| 20–34 | 45 | 1.5 | 2 | 1 | 1 | 1 | 1 | 2 | 2 | 11 |
| 35–49 | 138 | 1.4 | 4 | 1 | 1 | 1 | 1 | 2 | 2 | 18 |
| 50–64 | 181 | 1.5 | 10 | 1 | 1 | 1 | 1 | 2 | 2 | 13 |
| 65+ | 158 | 2.1 | 11 | 1 | 1 | 1 | 2 | 2 | 10 | 17 |
| **GRAND TOTAL** | 554 | 1.6 | 8 | 1 | 1 | 1 | 1 | 2 | 3 | 17 |

## 93.0: DXTIC PHYSICAL TX. Formerly included in operation group(s) 791.

| Type of Patients | Observed Patients | Avg. Stay | Variance | Percentiles | | | | | | |
|---|---|---|---|---|---|---|---|---|---|---|
| | | | | 10th | 25th | 50th | 75th | 90th | 95th | 99th |
| **1. SINGLE DX** | | | | | | | | | | |
| 0–19 Years | 20 | 6.9 | 16 | 1 | 3 | 8 | 11 | 11 | 11 | 11 |
| 20–34 | 9 | 4.5 | 6 | 2 | 3 | 4 | 8 | 8 | 8 | 8 |
| 35–49 | 15 | 3.3 | 4 | 1 | 2 | 3 | 5 | 7 | 7 | 7 |
| 50–64 | 11 | 3.2 | 5 | 1 | 1 | 2 | 6 | 6 | 7 | 7 |
| 65+ | 8 | 4.2 | 32 | 1 | 2 | 3 | 4 | 4 | 24 | 24 |
| **2. MULTIPLE DX** | | | | | | | | | | |
| 0–19 Years | 61 | 12.5 | 235 | 3 | 5 | 8 | 12 | 29 | 61 | 75 |
| 20–34 | 68 | 8.8 | 127 | 2 | 4 | 5 | 8 | 17 | 35 | 70 |
| 35–49 | 141 | 6.2 | 33 | 2 | 2 | 4 | 8 | 11 | 20 | 28 |
| 50–64 | 223 | 6.7 | 51 | 2 | 3 | 5 | 8 | 13 | 21 | 32 |
| 65+ | 973 | 8.7 | 72 | 3 | 3 | 6 | 11 | 19 | 23 | 40 |
| **TOTAL SINGLE DX** | 63 | 5.2 | 16 | 1 | 2 | 4 | 8 | 11 | 11 | 11 |
| **TOTAL MULTIPLE DX** | 1,466 | 8.3 | 74 | 2 | 3 | 5 | 10 | 18 | 23 | 41 |
| **TOTAL** | | | | | | | | | | |
| 0–19 Years | 81 | 10.6 | 169 | 2 | 4 | 8 | 11 | 16 | 36 | 75 |
| 20–34 | 77 | 8.4 | 118 | 2 | 4 | 5 | 8 | 17 | 35 | 70 |
| 35–49 | 156 | 6.0 | 32 | 2 | 2 | 4 | 7 | 11 | 17 | 27 |
| 50–64 | 234 | 6.6 | 50 | 2 | 3 | 5 | 8 | 13 | 19 | 32 |
| 65+ | 981 | 8.7 | 72 | 3 | 3 | 6 | 11 | 19 | 23 | 40 |
| **GRAND TOTAL** | 1,529 | 8.2 | 73 | 2 | 3 | 5 | 10 | 18 | 23 | 41 |

Length of Stay by Diagnosis and Operation, United States, 2000

# United States, October 1998–September 1999 Data, by Operation

## 93.01: FUNCTIONAL PT EVALUATION. Formerly included in operation group(s) 791.

| Type of Patients | Observed Patients | Avg. Stay | Variance | 10th | 25th | 50th | 75th | 90th | 95th | 99th |
|---|---|---|---|---|---|---|---|---|---|---|
| **1. SINGLE DX** | | | | | | | | | | |
| 0–19 Years | 3 | 4.3 | 4 | 3 | 3 | 3 | 7 | 7 | 7 | 7 |
| 20–34 | 0 | | | | | | | | | |
| 35–49 | 6 | 4.0 | 6 | 1 | 2 | 4 | 7 | 7 | 7 | 7 |
| 50–64 | 3 | 3.7 | 8 | 1 | 2 | 2 | 7 | 7 | 7 | 7 |
| 65+ | 4 | 3.0 | <1 | 2 | 3 | 3 | 3 | 4 | 4 | 4 |
| **2. MULTIPLE DX** | | | | | | | | | | |
| 0–19 Years | 27 | 22.0 | 495 | 3 | 6 | 12 | 30 | 61 | 75 | 77 |
| 20–34 | 32 | 8.9 | 101 | 1 | 3 | 6 | 8 | 19 | 35 | 57 |
| 35–49 | 78 | 6.6 | 41 | 2 | 2 | 4 | 8 | 17 | 22 | 28 |
| 50–64 | 144 | 6.8 | 64 | 2 | 3 | 4 | 8 | 12 | 23 | 40 |
| 65+ | 817 | 8.9 | 78 | 3 | 3 | 6 | 11 | 19 | 25 | 43 |
| **TOTAL SINGLE DX** | 16 | 3.6 | 4 | 1 | 2 | 3 | 4 | 7 | 7 | 7 |
| **TOTAL MULTIPLE DX** | 1,098 | 8.7 | 84 | 2 | 3 | 6 | 10 | 19 | 25 | 44 |
| **TOTAL** | | | | | | | | | | |
| 0–19 Years | 30 | 20.6 | 479 | 3 | 6 | 12 | 30 | 61 | 63 | 77 |
| 20–34 | 32 | 8.9 | 101 | 1 | 3 | 6 | 8 | 19 | 35 | 57 |
| 35–49 | 84 | 6.5 | 40 | 2 | 2 | 4 | 8 | 17 | 22 | 28 |
| 50–64 | 147 | 6.8 | 64 | 2 | 3 | 4 | 8 | 12 | 23 | 40 |
| 65+ | 821 | 8.9 | 77 | 3 | 3 | 6 | 11 | 19 | 25 | 43 |
| **GRAND TOTAL** | 1,114 | 8.7 | 83 | 2 | 3 | 6 | 10 | 19 | 25 | 44 |

## 93.08: ELECTROMYOGRAPHY. Formerly included in operation group(s) 791.

| Type of Patients | Observed Patients | Avg. Stay | Variance | 10th | 25th | 50th | 75th | 90th | 95th | 99th |
|---|---|---|---|---|---|---|---|---|---|---|
| **1. SINGLE DX** | | | | | | | | | | |
| 0–19 Years | 16 | 7.2 | 16 | 1 | 4 | 9 | 11 | 11 | 11 | 11 |
| 20–34 | 6 | 3.1 | 2 | 1 | 2 | 3 | 4 | 5 | 5 | 5 |
| 35–49 | 5 | 2.7 | 5 | 1 | 1 | 2 | 4 | 7 | 7 | 7 |
| 50–64 | 3 | 3.9 | 4 | 1 | 1 | 2 | 6 | 6 | 6 | 6 |
| 65+ | 3 | 8.0 | 120 | 1 | 1 | 1 | 24 | 24 | 24 | 24 |
| **2. MULTIPLE DX** | | | | | | | | | | |
| 0–19 Years | 27 | 7.3 | 12 | 2 | 5 | 7 | 9 | 12 | 15 | 16 |
| 20–34 | 32 | 7.5 | 81 | 2 | 4 | 5 | 6 | 17 | 24 | 72 |
| 35–49 | 55 | 6.0 | 24 | 1 | 3 | 4 | 10 | 11 | 12 | 27 |
| 50–64 | 68 | 6.5 | 25 | 2 | 3 | 6 | 7 | 13 | 21 | 22 |
| 65+ | 116 | 6.9 | 22 | 2 | 4 | 5 | 10 | 15 | 19 | 20 |
| **TOTAL SINGLE DX** | 33 | 6.1 | 18 | 1 | 2 | 5 | 10 | 11 | 11 | 24 |
| **TOTAL MULTIPLE DX** | 298 | 6.7 | 27 | 2 | 3 | 5 | 9 | 13 | 17 | 23 |
| **TOTAL** | | | | | | | | | | |
| 0–19 Years | 43 | 7.2 | 14 | 2 | 5 | 7 | 10 | 11 | 12 | 16 |
| 20–34 | 38 | 6.9 | 72 | 2 | 4 | 5 | 6 | 16 | 17 | 72 |
| 35–49 | 60 | 5.9 | 24 | 1 | 3 | 4 | 9 | 11 | 12 | 27 |
| 50–64 | 71 | 6.4 | 24 | 2 | 3 | 6 | 7 | 13 | 18 | 22 |
| 65+ | 119 | 6.9 | 23 | 2 | 4 | 5 | 10 | 16 | 19 | 20 |
| **GRAND TOTAL** | 331 | 6.6 | 26 | 2 | 3 | 5 | 9 | 12 | 16 | 23 |

## 93.1: PT EXERCISES. Formerly included in operation group(s) 791.

| Type of Patients | Observed Patients | Avg. Stay | Variance | 10th | 25th | 50th | 75th | 90th | 95th | 99th |
|---|---|---|---|---|---|---|---|---|---|---|
| **1. SINGLE DX** | | | | | | | | | | |
| 0–19 Years | 6 | 7.7 | 82 | 2 | 2 | 5 | 10 | 31 | 31 | 31 |
| 20–34 | 7 | 5.7 | 66 | 1 | 3 | 3 | 4 | 28 | 28 | 28 |
| 35–49 | 17 | 2.9 | <1 | 1 | 2 | 2 | 3 | 4 | 4 | 5 |
| 50–64 | 12 | 2.3 | <1 | 1 | 2 | 2 | 3 | 4 | 4 | 4 |
| 65+ | 5 | 1.8 | 1 | 1 | 1 | 1 | 3 | 3 | 3 | 3 |
| **2. MULTIPLE DX** | | | | | | | | | | |
| 0–19 Years | 29 | 20.7 | 399 | 3 | 4 | 11 | 28 | 61 | 61 | 61 |
| 20–34 | 36 | 10.0 | 105 | 3 | 3 | 7 | 9 | 27 | 36 | 39 |
| 35–49 | 88 | 5.9 | 56 | 1 | 2 | 4 | 7 | 14 | 20 | 22 |
| 50–64 | 173 | 8.3 | 56 | 2 | 3 | 5 | 12 | 18 | 21 | 35 |
| 65+ | 529 | 9.9 | 61 | 3 | 4 | 8 | 13 | 19 | 24 | 40 |
| **TOTAL SINGLE DX** | 47 | 3.6 | 23 | 1 | 2 | 3 | 4 | 4 | 6 | 31 |
| **TOTAL MULTIPLE DX** | 855 | 9.5 | 71 | 2 | 4 | 7 | 13 | 19 | 24 | 40 |
| **TOTAL** | | | | | | | | | | |
| 0–19 Years | 35 | 18.7 | 370 | 2 | 4 | 9 | 28 | 61 | 61 | 61 |
| 20–34 | 43 | 9.1 | 100 | 2 | 3 | 9 | 9 | 27 | 36 | 39 |
| 35–49 | 105 | 5.5 | 25 | 1 | 2 | 3 | 7 | 13 | 17 | 22 |
| 50–64 | 185 | 7.9 | 55 | 3 | 3 | 5 | 11 | 18 | 21 | 35 |
| 65+ | 534 | 9.8 | 61 | 3 | 4 | 8 | 13 | 19 | 24 | 40 |
| **GRAND TOTAL** | 902 | 9.3 | 70 | 2 | 4 | 7 | 13 | 19 | 24 | 40 |

## 93.11: ASSISTING EXERCISE. Formerly included in operation group(s) 791.

| Type of Patients | Observed Patients | Avg. Stay | Variance | 10th | 25th | 50th | 75th | 90th | 95th | 99th |
|---|---|---|---|---|---|---|---|---|---|---|
| **1. SINGLE DX** | | | | | | | | | | |
| 0–19 Years | 2 | 19.3 | 148 | 10 | 10 | 10 | 10 | 31 | 31 | 31 |
| 20–34 | 2 | 13.5 | 165 | 4 | 4 | 4 | 28 | 28 | 28 | 28 |
| 35–49 | 7 | 3.4 | <1 | 3 | 3 | 3 | 4 | 4 | 4 | 5 |
| 50–64 | 4 | 3.1 | <1 | 2 | 3 | 3 | 4 | 4 | 4 | 4 |
| 65+ | 1 | 3.0 | 0 | 3 | 3 | 3 | 3 | 3 | 3 | 3 |
| **2. MULTIPLE DX** | | | | | | | | | | |
| 0–19 Years | 17 | 25.3 | 465 | 3 | 7 | 24 | 45 | 61 | 61 | 61 |
| 20–34 | 20 | 12.8 | 125 | 3 | 5 | 8 | 18 | 27 | 39 | 39 |
| 35–49 | 49 | 7.1 | 26 | 2 | 3 | 6 | 9 | 14 | 19 | 22 |
| 50–64 | 106 | 9.4 | 45 | 2 | 4 | 8 | 13 | 18 | 21 | 35 |
| 65+ | 342 | 10.0 | 52 | 3 | 5 | 8 | 14 | 19 | 23 | 40 |
| **TOTAL SINGLE DX** | 16 | 5.4 | 46 | 3 | 3 | 3 | 4 | 10 | 28 | 31 |
| **TOTAL MULTIPLE DX** | 534 | 10.1 | 65 | 3 | 5 | 8 | 14 | 19 | 24 | 42 |
| **TOTAL** | | | | | | | | | | |
| 0–19 Years | 19 | 24.9 | 442 | 4 | 4 | 24 | 33 | 61 | 61 | 61 |
| 20–34 | 22 | 12.8 | 126 | 2 | 4 | 8 | 23 | 28 | 39 | 39 |
| 35–49 | 56 | 6.5 | 24 | 3 | 3 | 5 | 9 | 14 | 17 | 22 |
| 50–64 | 110 | 9.1 | 44 | 3 | 4 | 7 | 13 | 18 | 21 | 35 |
| 65+ | 343 | 10.0 | 52 | 3 | 5 | 8 | 14 | 19 | 23 | 40 |
| **GRAND TOTAL** | 550 | 10.0 | 65 | 3 | 4 | 8 | 14 | 19 | 24 | 42 |

Length of Stay by Diagnosis and Operation, United States, 2000

# United States, October 1998–September 1999 Data, by Operation

## 93.2: OTH PT MS MANIPULATION. Formerly included in operation group(s) 791.

| Type of Patients | Observed Patients | Avg. Stay | Variance | 10th | 25th | 50th | 75th | 90th | 95th | 99th |
|---|---|---|---|---|---|---|---|---|---|---|
| **1. SINGLE DX** | | | | | | | | | | |
| 0–19 Years | 31 | 3.3 | 5 | 1 | 1 | 3 | 5 | 7 | 7 | 7 |
| 20–34 | 18 | 2.3 | 9 | 1 | 1 | 2 | 3 | 4 | 5 | 7 |
| 35–49 | 44 | 2.5 | 2 | 1 | 2 | 2 | 3 | 4 | 5 | 6 |
| 50–64 | 40 | 2.0 | 2 | 1 | 1 | 2 | 2 | 3 | 4 | 9 |
| 65+ | 29 | 2.2 | 8 | 1 | 1 | 1 | 2 | 3 | 4 | 21 |
| **2. MULTIPLE DX** | | | | | | | | | | |
| 0–19 Years | 93 | 6.9 | 139 | 1 | 2 | 3 | 9 | 15 | 27 | 78 |
| 20–34 | 61 | 9.7 | 141 | 2 | 2 | 4 | 11 | 37 | 37 | 40 |
| 35–49 | 195 | 6.2 | 66 | 1 | 2 | 4 | 7 | 13 | 16 | 50 |
| 50–64 | 472 | 8.5 | 128 | 2 | 3 | 5 | 10 | 17 | 23 | 78 |
| 65+ | 2,047 | 9.0 | 75 | 2 | 4 | 7 | 11 | 18 | 24 | 43 |
| **TOTAL SINGLE DX** | 162 | 2.4 | 4 | 1 | 1 | 2 | 3 | 4 | 5 | 10 |
| **TOTAL MULTIPLE DX** | 2,868 | 8.7 | 88 | 2 | 3 | 6 | 11 | 17 | 25 | 45 |
| **TOTAL** | | | | | | | | | | |
| 0–19 Years | 124 | 6.4 | 118 | 1 | 2 | 3 | 7 | 10 | 26 | 78 |
| 20–34 | 79 | 8.7 | 127 | 1 | 2 | 4 | 9 | 37 | 37 | 40 |
| 35–49 | 239 | 5.3 | 53 | 1 | 2 | 3 | 6 | 11 | 15 | 50 |
| 50–64 | 512 | 8.0 | 121 | 1 | 2 | 4 | 9 | 16 | 23 | 78 |
| 65+ | 2,076 | 8.9 | 75 | 2 | 4 | 7 | 11 | 18 | 24 | 43 |
| **GRAND TOTAL** | 3,030 | 8.3 | 85 | 2 | 3 | 5 | 10 | 17 | 24 | 45 |

## 93.26: MANUAL RUPT JOINT ADHES. Formerly included in operation group(s) 791.

| Type of Patients | Observed Patients | Avg. Stay | Variance | 10th | 25th | 50th | 75th | 90th | 95th | 99th |
|---|---|---|---|---|---|---|---|---|---|---|
| **1. SINGLE DX** | | | | | | | | | | |
| 0–19 Years | 5 | 2.2 | <1 | 2 | 2 | 2 | 2 | 3 | 3 | 3 |
| 20–34 | 8 | 2.8 | <1 | 2 | 2 | 3 | 3 | 3 | 4 | 4 |
| 35–49 | 23 | 2.5 | 1 | 1 | 2 | 3 | 3 | 3 | 5 | 5 |
| 50–64 | 29 | 1.8 | <1 | 1 | 1 | 2 | 2 | 3 | 3 | 4 |
| 65+ | 19 | 1.9 | 5 | 1 | 1 | 3 | 2 | 3 | 4 | 13 |
| **2. MULTIPLE DX** | | | | | | | | | | |
| 0–19 Years | 5 | 2.3 | <1 | 1 | 1 | 3 | 3 | 3 | 3 | 3 |
| 20–34 | 16 | 17.9 | 295 | 1 | 2 | 4 | 37 | 37 | 37 | 37 |
| 35–49 | 61 | 3.0 | 12 | 1 | 2 | 2 | 3 | 4 | 6 | 15 |
| 50–64 | 115 | 3.5 | 19 | 1 | 2 | 3 | 3 | 6 | 13 | 23 |
| 65+ | 131 | 3.1 | 8 | 1 | 1 | 3 | 4 | 4 | 8 | 15 |
| **TOTAL SINGLE DX** | 84 | 2.2 | 2 | 1 | 1 | 2 | 3 | 3 | 4 | 5 |
| **TOTAL MULTIPLE DX** | 328 | 4.3 | 48 | 1 | 2 | 3 | 4 | 6 | 19 | 37 |
| **TOTAL** | | | | | | | | | | |
| 0–19 Years | 10 | 2.3 | <1 | 1 | 2 | 2 | 3 | 3 | 3 | 3 |
| 20–34 | 24 | 14.7 | 270 | 1 | 2 | 3 | 37 | 37 | 37 | 37 |
| 35–49 | 84 | 2.8 | 8 | 1 | 2 | 3 | 3 | 4 | 6 | 7 |
| 50–64 | 144 | 3.2 | 17 | 1 | 1 | 2 | 3 | 5 | 7 | 23 |
| 65+ | 150 | 2.8 | 8 | 1 | 1 | 3 | 4 | 4 | 8 | 15 |
| **GRAND TOTAL** | 412 | 3.8 | 38 | 1 | 1 | 2 | 3 | 5 | 13 | 37 |

## 93.22: AMB & GAIT TRAINING. Formerly included in operation group(s) 791.

| Type of Patients | Observed Patients | Avg. Stay | Variance | 10th | 25th | 50th | 75th | 90th | 95th | 99th |
|---|---|---|---|---|---|---|---|---|---|---|
| **1. SINGLE DX** | | | | | | | | | | |
| 0–19 Years | 3 | 2.8 | 4 | 1 | 1 | 1 | 5 | 5 | 5 | 5 |
| 20–34 | 2 | 4.9 | 9 | 2 | 2 | 7 | 7 | 7 | 7 | 7 |
| 35–49 | 9 | 2.7 | 2 | 1 | 2 | 2 | 4 | 4 | 6 | 6 |
| 50–64 | 4 | 2.0 | 2 | 1 | 1 | 1 | 3 | 3 | 9 | 9 |
| 65+ | 4 | 2.4 | <1 | 2 | 2 | 2 | 3 | 4 | 4 | 4 |
| **2. MULTIPLE DX** | | | | | | | | | | |
| 0–19 Years | 28 | 12.5 | 254 | 2 | 2 | 10 | 11 | 27 | 43 | 82 |
| 20–34 | 35 | 6.7 | 54 | 2 | 2 | 4 | 9 | 11 | 18 | 40 |
| 35–49 | 105 | 8.6 | 104 | 4 | 4 | 5 | 10 | 15 | 30 | 55 |
| 50–64 | 296 | 11.4 | 174 | 3 | 5 | 8 | 12 | 19 | 30 | 80 |
| 65+ | 1,751 | 9.6 | 78 | 3 | 4 | 7 | 12 | 19 | 25 | 43 |
| **TOTAL SINGLE DX** | 22 | 2.5 | 3 | 1 | 1 | 2 | 3 | 4 | 6 | 9 |
| **TOTAL MULTIPLE DX** | 2,215 | 9.8 | 94 | 3 | 4 | 7 | 12 | 19 | 26 | 50 |
| **TOTAL** | | | | | | | | | | |
| 0–19 Years | 31 | 11.7 | 242 | 2 | 2 | 9 | 10 | 27 | 43 | 82 |
| 20–34 | 37 | 6.7 | 53 | 2 | 2 | 4 | 8 | 11 | 18 | 40 |
| 35–49 | 114 | 7.8 | 94 | 3 | 4 | 4 | 9 | 15 | 29 | 55 |
| 50–64 | 300 | 11.1 | 171 | 3 | 4 | 8 | 12 | 19 | 30 | 80 |
| 65+ | 1,755 | 9.6 | 78 | 3 | 4 | 7 | 12 | 18 | 25 | 43 |
| **GRAND TOTAL** | 2,237 | 9.7 | 93 | 3 | 4 | 7 | 12 | 18 | 26 | 50 |

## 93.3: OTHER PT THERAPEUTIC PX. Formerly included in operation group(s) 791.

| Type of Patients | Observed Patients | Avg. Stay | Variance | 10th | 25th | 50th | 75th | 90th | 95th | 99th |
|---|---|---|---|---|---|---|---|---|---|---|
| **1. SINGLE DX** | | | | | | | | | | |
| 0–19 Years | 218 | 3.2 | 9 | 1 | 1 | 2 | 4 | 6 | 8 | 18 |
| 20–34 | 54 | 3.7 | 7 | 1 | 2 | 3 | 5 | 8 | 8 | 10 |
| 35–49 | 77 | 3.4 | 7 | 2 | 2 | 3 | 4 | 5 | 7 | 18 |
| 50–64 | 46 | 4.6 | 7 | 2 | 3 | 4 | 6 | 8 | 8 | 16 |
| 65+ | 49 | 4.5 | 12 | 1 | 2 | 4 | 6 | 8 | 10 | 15 |
| **2. MULTIPLE DX** | | | | | | | | | | |
| 0–19 Years | 669 | 11.6 | 177 | 2 | 3 | 7 | 14 | 29 | 39 | 65 |
| 20–34 | 760 | 10.8 | 161 | 2 | 3 | 6 | 14 | 24 | 34 | 80 |
| 35–49 | 1,924 | 9.8 | 96 | 3 | 5 | 7 | 12 | 22 | 29 | 57 |
| 50–64 | 4,217 | 11.1 | 95 | 3 | 5 | 8 | 14 | 23 | 30 | 49 |
| 65+ | 20,216 | 10.3 | 67 | 3 | 4 | 8 | 14 | 21 | 26 | 39 |
| **TOTAL SINGLE DX** | 444 | 3.6 | 9 | 1 | 2 | 3 | 5 | 7 | 8 | 18 |
| **TOTAL MULTIPLE DX** | 27,786 | 10.4 | 78 | 3 | 4 | 8 | 14 | 21 | 27 | 43 |
| **TOTAL** | | | | | | | | | | |
| 0–19 Years | 887 | 9.6 | 150 | 1 | 2 | 5 | 11 | 25 | 35 | 62 |
| 20–34 | 814 | 10.2 | 153 | 2 | 3 | 6 | 13 | 23 | 33 | 80 |
| 35–49 | 2,001 | 9.6 | 94 | 2 | 4 | 7 | 12 | 21 | 28 | 56 |
| 50–64 | 4,263 | 11.0 | 94 | 3 | 5 | 8 | 14 | 22 | 30 | 49 |
| 65+ | 20,265 | 10.3 | 67 | 3 | 4 | 8 | 14 | 21 | 26 | 39 |
| **GRAND TOTAL** | 28,230 | 10.3 | 78 | 3 | 4 | 8 | 14 | 21 | 27 | 43 |

Length of Stay by Diagnosis and Operation, United States, 2000

# United States, October 1998–September 1999 Data, by Operation

## 93.32: WHIRLPOOL TREATMENT. Formerly included in operation group(s) 791.

| Type of Patients | Observed Patients | Avg. Stay | Variance | 10th | 25th | 50th | 75th | 90th | 95th | 99th |
|---|---|---|---|---|---|---|---|---|---|---|
| **1. SINGLE DX** | | | | | | | | | | |
| 0–19 Years | 10 | 4.7 | 9 | 2 | 2 | 3 | 7 | 10 | 10 | 10 |
| 20–34 | 6 | 2.8 | 1 | 2 | 2 | 2 | 3 | 5 | 5 | 5 |
| 35–49 | 7 | 4.1 | 2 | 3 | 3 | 4 | 4 | 5 | 5 | 8 |
| 50–64 | 3 | 3.9 | 6 | 2 | 2 | 3 | 7 | 7 | 7 | 7 |
| 65+ | 1 | 4.0 | 0 | 4 | 4 | 4 | 4 | 4 | 4 | 4 |
| **2. MULTIPLE DX** | | | | | | | | | | |
| 0–19 Years | 50 | 5.4 | 14 | 2 | 3 | 4 | 7 | 10 | 10 | 23 |
| 20–34 | 51 | 8.1 | 71 | 1 | 2 | 5 | 10 | 23 | 32 | 32 |
| 35–49 | 199 | 6.0 | 23 | 2 | 3 | 5 | 8 | 12 | 14 | 17 |
| 50–64 | 199 | 6.2 | 18 | 2 | 3 | 6 | 8 | 10 | 13 | 29 |
| 65+ | 385 | 8.3 | 83 | 3 | 4 | 6 | 9 | 15 | 24 | 47 |
| **TOTAL SINGLE DX** | 27 | 4.0 | 4 | 2 | 3 | 4 | 4 | 7 | 8 | 10 |
| **TOTAL MULTIPLE DX** | 884 | 7.1 | 51 | 2 | 3 | 6 | 8 | 13 | 17 | 37 |
| **TOTAL** | | | | | | | | | | |
| 0–19 Years | 60 | 5.3 | 13 | 2 | 3 | 4 | 7 | 10 | 10 | 23 |
| 20–34 | 57 | 7.7 | 68 | 2 | 3 | 5 | 10 | 21 | 32 | 32 |
| 35–49 | 206 | 5.9 | 22 | 2 | 3 | 5 | 8 | 11 | 14 | 17 |
| 50–64 | 202 | 6.2 | 18 | 2 | 3 | 6 | 8 | 10 | 13 | 29 |
| 65+ | 386 | 8.3 | 83 | 3 | 4 | 6 | 9 | 15 | 24 | 47 |
| **GRAND TOTAL** | 911 | 7.1 | 50 | 2 | 3 | 5 | 8 | 13 | 17 | 37 |

## 93.39: PHYSICAL THERAPY NEC. Formerly included in operation group(s) 791.

| Type of Patients | Observed Patients | Avg. Stay | Variance | 10th | 25th | 50th | 75th | 90th | 95th | 99th |
|---|---|---|---|---|---|---|---|---|---|---|
| **1. SINGLE DX** | | | | | | | | | | |
| 0–19 Years | 64 | 4.3 | 16 | 1 | 2 | 3 | 5 | 8 | 14 | 18 |
| 20–34 | 40 | 3.6 | 8 | 1 | 1 | 3 | 5 | 5 | 8 | 10 |
| 35–49 | 67 | 3.4 | 7 | 1 | 2 | 3 | 5 | 6 | 8 | 18 |
| 50–64 | 39 | 4.8 | 8 | 2 | 3 | 4 | 7 | 8 | 8 | 16 |
| 65+ | 44 | 4.6 | 10 | 1 | 3 | 5 | 6 | 7 | 8 | 12 |
| **2. MULTIPLE DX** | | | | | | | | | | |
| 0–19 Years | 502 | 12.3 | 192 | 2 | 3 | 7 | 16 | 31 | 42 | 71 |
| 20–34 | 655 | 11.2 | 169 | 2 | 3 | 7 | 14 | 24 | 36 | 80 |
| 35–49 | 1,604 | 10.5 | 103 | 3 | 4 | 9 | 14 | 23 | 31 | 62 |
| 50–64 | 3,763 | 11.5 | 96 | 3 | 5 | 9 | 14 | 23 | 31 | 49 |
| 65+ | 18,533 | 10.5 | 68 | 3 | 5 | 8 | 14 | 21 | 26 | 39 |
| **TOTAL SINGLE DX** | 254 | 4.1 | 11 | 1 | 2 | 3 | 5 | 8 | 8 | 18 |
| **TOTAL MULTIPLE DX** | 25,057 | 10.7 | 80 | 3 | 5 | 8 | 14 | 21 | 28 | 44 |
| **TOTAL** | | | | | | | | | | |
| 0–19 Years | 566 | 11.3 | 176 | 2 | 3 | 6 | 14 | 29 | 39 | 65 |
| 20–34 | 695 | 10.6 | 161 | 2 | 3 | 6 | 14 | 24 | 36 | 80 |
| 35–49 | 1,671 | 10.2 | 101 | 3 | 4 | 7 | 13 | 23 | 30 | 58 |
| 50–64 | 3,802 | 11.4 | 96 | 3 | 5 | 9 | 14 | 23 | 31 | 49 |
| 65+ | 18,577 | 10.5 | 68 | 3 | 5 | 8 | 14 | 21 | 26 | 39 |
| **GRAND TOTAL** | 25,311 | 10.6 | 79 | 3 | 4 | 8 | 14 | 21 | 27 | 44 |

## 93.38: COMBINED PT NOS. Formerly included in operation group(s) 791.

| Type of Patients | Observed Patients | Avg. Stay | Variance | 10th | 25th | 50th | 75th | 90th | 95th | 99th |
|---|---|---|---|---|---|---|---|---|---|---|
| **1. SINGLE DX** | | | | | | | | | | |
| 0–19 Years | 2 | 1.5 | 1 | 1 | 1 | 1 | 3 | 3 | 3 | 3 |
| 20–34 | 6 | 4.9 | 7 | 2 | 2 | 6 | 8 | 8 | 8 | 8 |
| 35–49 | 1 | 2.0 | 0 | 2 | 2 | 2 | 2 | 2 | 2 | 2 |
| 50–64 | 4 | 3.7 | <1 | 3 | 3 | 4 | 4 | 4 | 4 | 6 |
| 65+ | 4 | 4.1 | 24 | 1 | 1 | 1 | 3 | 15 | 15 | 15 |
| **2. MULTIPLE DX** | | | | | | | | | | |
| 0–19 Years | 33 | 18.5 | 254 | 5 | 8 | 12 | 23 | 35 | 62 | 65 |
| 20–34 | 37 | 12.3 | 245 | 1 | 3 | 8 | 16 | 26 | 36 | 91 |
| 35–49 | 94 | 8.3 | 93 | 2 | 3 | 5 | 10 | 18 | 21 | 63 |
| 50–64 | 225 | 10.8 | 125 | 2 | 4 | 8 | 13 | 22 | 28 | 59 |
| 65+ | 1,189 | 8.0 | 48 | 2 | 3 | 6 | 10 | 17 | 21 | 37 |
| **TOTAL SINGLE DX** | 17 | 4.0 | 9 | 1 | 2 | 3 | 4 | 8 | 8 | 15 |
| **TOTAL MULTIPLE DX** | 1,578 | 8.6 | 70 | 2 | 3 | 6 | 11 | 18 | 23 | 41 |
| **TOTAL** | | | | | | | | | | |
| 0–19 Years | 35 | 17.9 | 255 | 4 | 6 | 11 | 23 | 35 | 62 | 65 |
| 20–34 | 43 | 11.1 | 216 | 1 | 3 | 8 | 13 | 22 | 36 | 91 |
| 35–49 | 95 | 8.3 | 93 | 2 | 3 | 5 | 10 | 18 | 21 | 63 |
| 50–64 | 229 | 10.5 | 122 | 2 | 4 | 8 | 12 | 22 | 28 | 59 |
| 65+ | 1,193 | 8.0 | 48 | 2 | 3 | 6 | 10 | 17 | 21 | 37 |
| **GRAND TOTAL** | 1,595 | 8.6 | 70 | 2 | 3 | 6 | 11 | 18 | 23 | 41 |

## 93.4: SKELETAL & OTH TRACTION. Formerly included in operation group(s) 791.

| Type of Patients | Observed Patients | Avg. Stay | Variance | 10th | 25th | 50th | 75th | 90th | 95th | 99th |
|---|---|---|---|---|---|---|---|---|---|---|
| **1. SINGLE DX** | | | | | | | | | | |
| 0–19 Years | 177 | 13.7 | 76 | 2 | 5 | 14 | 21 | 23 | 27 | 33 |
| 20–34 | 21 | 3.8 | 3 | 2 | 3 | 3 | 5 | 7 | 7 | 7 |
| 35–49 | 13 | 6.7 | 74 | 1 | 1 | 4 | 6 | 15 | 30 | 30 |
| 50–64 | 6 | 3.1 | <1 | 3 | 3 | 3 | 3 | 4 | 5 | 5 |
| 65+ | 11 | 3.8 | 22 | 1 | 1 | 3 | 6 | 7 | 19 | 19 |
| **2. MULTIPLE DX** | | | | | | | | | | |
| 0–19 Years | 159 | 10.7 | 77 | 2 | 3 | 8 | 19 | 23 | 25 | 33 |
| 20–34 | 52 | 6.1 | 57 | 1 | 2 | 3 | 9 | 12 | 18 | 44 |
| 35–49 | 73 | 8.1 | 116 | 3 | 3 | 5 | 9 | 15 | 29 | 55 |
| 50–64 | 81 | 9.9 | 173 | 3 | 3 | 6 | 9 | 23 | 45 | 69 |
| 65+ | 337 | 8.2 | 79 | 2 | 3 | 6 | 8 | 16 | 32 | 47 |
| **TOTAL SINGLE DX** | 228 | 11.6 | 81 | 1 | 3 | 11 | 19 | 23 | 27 | 32 |
| **TOTAL MULTIPLE DX** | 702 | 9.0 | 95 | 2 | 3 | 6 | 11 | 22 | 29 | 45 |
| **TOTAL** | | | | | | | | | | |
| 0–19 Years | 336 | 12.2 | 79 | 2 | 4 | 11 | 20 | 23 | 26 | 33 |
| 20–34 | 73 | 5.4 | 42 | 1 | 2 | 4 | 7 | 11 | 15 | 44 |
| 35–49 | 86 | 7.8 | 107 | 2 | 3 | 4 | 8 | 15 | 30 | 55 |
| 50–64 | 87 | 9.4 | 163 | 3 | 3 | 5 | 9 | 21 | 45 | 69 |
| 65+ | 348 | 8.1 | 78 | 2 | 3 | 6 | 8 | 16 | 32 | 47 |
| **GRAND TOTAL** | 930 | 9.7 | 93 | 2 | 3 | 6 | 14 | 23 | 28 | 45 |

Length of Stay by Diagnosis and Operation, United States, 2000

**United States, October 1998–September 1999 Data, by Operation**

### 93.44: OTHER SKELETAL TRACTION. Formerly included in operation group(s) 791.

| Type of Patients | Observed Patients | Avg. Stay | Variance | 10th | 25th | 50th | 75th | 90th | 95th | 99th |
|---|---|---|---|---|---|---|---|---|---|---|
| **1. SINGLE DX** | | | | | | | | | | |
| 0–19 Years | 119 | 16.0 | 75 | 2 | 10 | 16 | 22 | 26 | 30 | 34 |
| 20–34 | 7 | 3.8 | 4 | 2 | 3 | 7 | 7 | 30 | 7 | 7 |
| 35–49 | 3 | 19.0 | 128 | 4 | 4 | 15 | 30 | 30 | 30 | 30 |
| 50–64 | 0 | | | | | | | | | |
| 65+ | 4 | 1.9 | 3 | 1 | 1 | 1 | 3 | 3 | 7 | 7 |
| **2. MULTIPLE DX** | | | | | | | | | | |
| 0–19 Years | 101 | 13.5 | 85 | 1 | 4 | 14 | 21 | 24 | 26 | 38 |
| 20–34 | 20 | 8.4 | 97 | 2 | 4 | 4 | 10 | 12 | 44 | 44 |
| 35–49 | 34 | 10.6 | 196 | 3 | 3 | 4 | 12 | 29 | 42 | 73 |
| 50–64 | 28 | 19.3 | 385 | 4 | 6 | 10 | 40 | 45 | 69 | 79 |
| 65+ | 72 | 12.7 | 169 | 3 | 4 | 7 | 14 | 32 | 36 | 53 |
| **TOTAL SINGLE DX** | 133 | 14.7 | 85 | 2 | 5 | 16 | 22 | 26 | 30 | 34 |
| **TOTAL MULTIPLE DX** | 255 | 13.1 | 155 | 2 | 4 | 8 | 19 | 29 | 40 | 55 |
| **TOTAL** | | | | | | | | | | |
| 0–19 Years | 220 | 14.7 | 82 | 2 | 6 | 16 | 22 | 25 | 28 | 34 |
| 20–34 | 27 | 7.0 | 72 | 2 | 3 | 4 | 9 | 12 | 21 | 44 |
| 35–49 | 37 | 11.4 | 195 | 3 | 3 | 6 | 13 | 30 | 40 | 73 |
| 50–64 | 28 | 19.3 | 385 | 4 | 6 | 10 | 40 | 45 | 69 | 79 |
| 65+ | 76 | 12.0 | 165 | 2 | 4 | 7 | 13 | 32 | 36 | 53 |
| **GRAND TOTAL** | 388 | 13.6 | 133 | 2 | 4 | 11 | 21 | 27 | 32 | 53 |

### 93.5: OTH IMMOB/PRESS/WND ATTN. Formerly included in operation group(s) 791.

| Type of Patients | Observed Patients | Avg. Stay | Variance | 10th | 25th | 50th | 75th | 90th | 95th | 99th |
|---|---|---|---|---|---|---|---|---|---|---|
| **1. SINGLE DX** | | | | | | | | | | |
| 0–19 Years | 1,116 | 3.4 | 26 | 1 | 1 | 1 | 3 | 9 | 18 | 23 |
| 20–34 | 186 | 2.1 | 7 | 1 | 1 | 1 | 2 | 4 | 5 | 13 |
| 35–49 | 169 | 1.9 | 2 | 1 | 1 | 2 | 2 | 4 | 5 | 8 |
| 50–64 | 78 | 3.0 | 25 | 1 | 1 | 2 | 3 | 4 | 9 | 32 |
| 65+ | 88 | 3.3 | 23 | 1 | 1 | 2 | 3 | 5 | 9 | 19 |
| **2. MULTIPLE DX** | | | | | | | | | | |
| 0–19 Years | 1,219 | 4.1 | 27 | 1 | 2 | 2 | 4 | 10 | 17 | 25 |
| 20–34 | 698 | 3.2 | 8 | 1 | 1 | 2 | 4 | 6 | 9 | 19 |
| 35–49 | 915 | 3.9 | 23 | 1 | 2 | 2 | 4 | 8 | 12 | 25 |
| 50–64 | 838 | 4.9 | 26 | 2 | 3 | 3 | 6 | 11 | 12 | 24 |
| 65+ | 2,938 | 5.1 | 23 | 2 | 3 | 4 | 6 | 9 | 13 | 24 |
| **TOTAL SINGLE DX** | 1,637 | 3.0 | 20 | 1 | 1 | 1 | 3 | 6 | 13 | 22 |
| **TOTAL MULTIPLE DX** | 6,608 | 4.5 | 23 | 1 | 2 | 3 | 5 | 9 | 13 | 25 |
| **TOTAL** | | | | | | | | | | |
| 0–19 Years | 2,335 | 3.9 | 27 | 1 | 1 | 2 | 4 | 10 | 17 | 24 |
| 20–34 | 884 | 3.0 | 8 | 1 | 1 | 2 | 4 | 6 | 8 | 16 |
| 35–49 | 1,084 | 3.5 | 19 | 1 | 2 | 3 | 4 | 7 | 10 | 25 |
| 50–64 | 916 | 4.7 | 26 | 1 | 3 | 4 | 6 | 11 | 12 | 25 |
| 65+ | 3,026 | 5.0 | 24 | 2 | 3 | 5 | 6 | 9 | 12 | 24 |
| **GRAND TOTAL** | 8,245 | 4.2 | 23 | 1 | 2 | 3 | 5 | 9 | 13 | 24 |

### 93.46: LIMB SKIN TRACTION NEC. Formerly included in operation group(s) 791.

| Type of Patients | Observed Patients | Avg. Stay | Variance | 10th | 25th | 50th | 75th | 90th | 95th | 99th |
|---|---|---|---|---|---|---|---|---|---|---|
| **1. SINGLE DX** | | | | | | | | | | |
| 0–19 Years | 49 | 10.1 | 52 | 2 | 3 | 7 | 16 | 20 | 23 | 29 |
| 20–34 | 5 | 4.0 | 2 | 2 | 2 | 5 | 5 | 5 | 5 | 5 |
| 35–49 | 6 | 3.2 | 8 | 1 | 1 | 2 | 4 | 10 | 10 | 10 |
| 50–64 | 3 | 3.0 | 2 | 1 | 3 | 3 | 3 | 5 | 5 | 5 |
| 65+ | 4 | 4.4 | 6 | 1 | 3 | 6 | 6 | 7 | 7 | 7 |
| **2. MULTIPLE DX** | | | | | | | | | | |
| 0–19 Years | 40 | 6.6 | 31 | 2 | 3 | 5 | 7 | 15 | 19 | 24 |
| 20–34 | 11 | 5.1 | 38 | 1 | 1 | 2 | 10 | 16 | 16 | 24 |
| 35–49 | 11 | 5.5 | 5 | 2 | 4 | 6 | 8 | 8 | 9 | 9 |
| 50–64 | 33 | 7.3 | 26 | 2 | 4 | 6 | 8 | 13 | 23 | 23 |
| 65+ | 224 | 6.7 | 42 | 2 | 3 | 5 | 7 | 13 | 19 | 41 |
| **TOTAL SINGLE DX** | 67 | 8.2 | 47 | 1 | 3 | 5 | 14 | 18 | 23 | 23 |
| **TOTAL MULTIPLE DX** | 319 | 6.7 | 37 | 2 | 3 | 5 | 8 | 14 | 18 | 29 |
| **TOTAL** | | | | | | | | | | |
| 0–19 Years | 89 | 8.4 | 45 | 2 | 3 | 5 | 14 | 18 | 23 | 29 |
| 20–34 | 16 | 4.7 | 25 | 1 | 2 | 3 | 5 | 12 | 16 | 24 |
| 35–49 | 17 | 4.2 | 8 | 2 | 2 | 4 | 6 | 8 | 10 | 10 |
| 50–64 | 36 | 6.9 | 26 | 2 | 4 | 6 | 8 | 12 | 23 | 23 |
| 65+ | 228 | 6.7 | 41 | 2 | 3 | 5 | 7 | 13 | 18 | 41 |
| **GRAND TOTAL** | 386 | 7.0 | 39 | 2 | 3 | 5 | 8 | 15 | 20 | 29 |

### 93.51: PLASTER JACKET APPL. Formerly included in operation group(s) 791.

| Type of Patients | Observed Patients | Avg. Stay | Variance | 10th | 25th | 50th | 75th | 90th | 95th | 99th |
|---|---|---|---|---|---|---|---|---|---|---|
| **1. SINGLE DX** | | | | | | | | | | |
| 0–19 Years | 181 | 5.7 | 45 | 1 | 2 | 2 | 8 | 18 | 21 | 23 |
| 20–34 | 4 | 5.1 | 7 | 2 | 3 | 4 | 8 | 8 | 8 | 8 |
| 35–49 | 1 | 4.0 | 0 | 4 | 4 | 4 | 4 | 4 | 4 | 4 |
| 50–64 | 0 | | | | | | | | | |
| 65+ | 0 | | | | | | | | | |
| **2. MULTIPLE DX** | | | | | | | | | | |
| 0–19 Years | 112 | 6.8 | 59 | 1 | 3 | 3 | 8 | 20 | 25 | 29 |
| 20–34 | 12 | 3.4 | 9 | 1 | 3 | 3 | 6 | 7 | 10 | 10 |
| 35–49 | 7 | 6.3 | 9 | 2 | 5 | 5 | 9 | 10 | 10 | 10 |
| 50–64 | 2 | 11.5 | 48 | 6 | 6 | 17 | 17 | 17 | 17 | 17 |
| 65+ | 15 | 4.5 | 6 | 1 | 3 | 5 | 5 | 6 | 11 | 11 |
| **TOTAL SINGLE DX** | 186 | 5.6 | 44 | 1 | 1 | 2 | 8 | 18 | 21 | 23 |
| **TOTAL MULTIPLE DX** | 148 | 6.3 | 50 | 1 | 1 | 3 | 8 | 18 | 24 | 29 |
| **TOTAL** | | | | | | | | | | |
| 0–19 Years | 293 | 6.0 | 50 | 1 | 2 | 2 | 8 | 19 | 22 | 28 |
| 20–34 | 16 | 3.8 | 9 | 1 | 3 | 3 | 6 | 8 | 10 | 10 |
| 35–49 | 8 | 6.1 | 8 | 4 | 4 | 5 | 9 | 10 | 10 | 10 |
| 50–64 | 2 | 11.5 | 48 | 6 | 6 | 17 | 17 | 17 | 17 | 17 |
| 65+ | 15 | 4.5 | 6 | 1 | 3 | 5 | 5 | 6 | 11 | 11 |
| **GRAND TOTAL** | 334 | 5.9 | 47 | 1 | 1 | 2 | 8 | 18 | 22 | 26 |

Length of Stay by Diagnosis and Operation, United States, 2000

# United States, October 1998–September 1999 Data, by Operation

## 93.53: OTHER CAST APPLICATION. Formerly included in operation group(s) 791.

| Type of Patients | Observed Patients | Avg. Stay | Variance | 10th | 25th | 50th | 75th | 90th | 95th | 99th |
|---|---|---|---|---|---|---|---|---|---|---|
| **1. SINGLE DX** | | | | | | | | | | |
| 0–19 Years | 371 | 3.3 | 25 | 1 | 1 | 1 | 2 | 8 | 17 | 23 |
| 20–34 | 61 | 1.7 | 1 | 1 | 1 | 1 | 2 | 3 | 3 | 5 |
| 35–49 | 71 | 1.7 | 1 | 1 | 1 | 1 | 2 | 3 | 3 | 5 |
| 50–64 | 19 | 1.8 | 1 | 1 | 1 | 1 | 3 | 3 | 4 | 6 |
| 65+ | 32 | 3.8 | 41 | 1 | 1 | 3 | 4 | 5 | 10 | 59 |
| **2. MULTIPLE DX** | | | | | | | | | | |
| 0–19 Years | 422 | 4.4 | 33 | 1 | 1 | 2 | 5 | 13 | 19 | 25 |
| 20–34 | 142 | 3.2 | 6 | 1 | 1 | 3 | 4 | 7 | 8 | 10 |
| 35–49 | 251 | 4.7 | 31 | 1 | 2 | 3 | 5 | 10 | 25 | 25 |
| 50–64 | 230 | 4.1 | 17 | 1 | 2 | 3 | 5 | 8 | 11 | 23 |
| 65+ | 894 | 4.6 | 17 | 2 | 3 | 4 | 6 | 9 | 10 | 18 |
| **TOTAL SINGLE DX** | 554 | 2.8 | 19 | 1 | 1 | 1 | 2 | 6 | 11 | 23 |
| **TOTAL MULTIPLE DX** | 1,939 | 4.4 | 22 | 1 | 2 | 3 | 5 | 9 | 13 | 25 |
| **TOTAL** | | | | | | | | | | |
| 0–19 Years | 793 | 3.9 | 30 | 1 | 1 | 2 | 3 | 10 | 18 | 25 |
| 20–34 | 203 | 2.8 | 5 | 1 | 1 | 2 | 3 | 6 | 7 | 10 |
| 35–49 | 322 | 3.9 | 25 | 1 | 1 | 2 | 4 | 8 | 13 | 25 |
| 50–64 | 249 | 3.9 | 16 | 1 | 2 | 3 | 5 | 8 | 10 | 23 |
| 65+ | 926 | 4.6 | 18 | 1 | 3 | 4 | 5 | 9 | 10 | 18 |
| **GRAND TOTAL** | 2,493 | 4.1 | 22 | 1 | 1 | 3 | 5 | 8 | 12 | 25 |

## 93.54: APPLICATION OF SPLINT. Formerly included in operation group(s) 791.

| Type of Patients | Observed Patients | Avg. Stay | Variance | 10th | 25th | 50th | 75th | 90th | 95th | 99th |
|---|---|---|---|---|---|---|---|---|---|---|
| **1. SINGLE DX** | | | | | | | | | | |
| 0–19 Years | 465 | 1.3 | <1 | 1 | 1 | 1 | 1 | 2 | 2 | 5 |
| 20–34 | 57 | 1.5 | <1 | 1 | 1 | 1 | 2 | 2 | 3 | 4 |
| 35–49 | 49 | 1.9 | 1 | 1 | 1 | 1 | 2 | 4 | 4 | 5 |
| 50–64 | 22 | 2.3 | 1 | 1 | 1 | 2 | 3 | 4 | 4 | 5 |
| 65+ | 20 | 2.3 | 3 | 1 | 1 | 2 | 2 | 4 | 5 | 11 |
| **2. MULTIPLE DX** | | | | | | | | | | |
| 0–19 Years | 273 | 2.8 | 13 | 1 | 1 | 2 | 3 | 5 | 6 | 23 |
| 20–34 | 247 | 2.7 | 5 | 1 | 1 | 2 | 3 | 4 | 6 | 14 |
| 35–49 | 286 | 3.1 | 14 | 1 | 2 | 2 | 4 | 5 | 7 | 18 |
| 50–64 | 248 | 3.5 | 12 | 1 | 2 | 2 | 4 | 8 | 10 | 19 |
| 65+ | 934 | 4.9 | 22 | 2 | 2 | 4 | 6 | 9 | 11 | 35 |
| **TOTAL SINGLE DX** | 613 | 1.6 | 1 | 1 | 1 | 1 | 2 | 3 | 4 | 5 |
| **TOTAL MULTIPLE DX** | 1,988 | 3.8 | 17 | 1 | 2 | 3 | 4 | 7 | 10 | 23 |
| **TOTAL** | | | | | | | | | | |
| 0–19 Years | 738 | 2.3 | 10 | 1 | 1 | 1 | 2 | 4 | 5 | 23 |
| 20–34 | 304 | 2.5 | 5 | 1 | 1 | 2 | 3 | 4 | 6 | 11 |
| 35–49 | 335 | 2.9 | 12 | 1 | 1 | 2 | 4 | 5 | 7 | 15 |
| 50–64 | 270 | 3.4 | 12 | 1 | 2 | 2 | 4 | 7 | 9 | 19 |
| 65+ | 954 | 4.9 | 21 | 2 | 2 | 3 | 6 | 9 | 11 | 35 |
| **GRAND TOTAL** | 2,601 | 3.6 | 15 | 1 | 1 | 2 | 4 | 7 | 10 | 22 |

## 93.57: APPL OTH WND DRESSING. Formerly included in operation group(s) 791.

| Type of Patients | Observed Patients | Avg. Stay | Variance | 10th | 25th | 50th | 75th | 90th | 95th | 99th |
|---|---|---|---|---|---|---|---|---|---|---|
| **1. SINGLE DX** | | | | | | | | | | |
| 0–19 Years | 38 | 2.5 | 13 | 1 | 1 | 1 | 2 | 4 | 8 | 18 |
| 20–34 | 17 | 2.5 | 4 | 1 | 1 | 2 | 3 | 6 | 7 | 8 |
| 35–49 | 71 | 1.7 | 1 | 1 | 1 | 1 | 2 | 3 | 4 | 4 |
| 50–64 | 8 | 1.7 | <1 | 1 | 1 | 2 | 20 | 32 | 32 | 32 |
| 65+ | 0 | 11.2 | 140 | 1 | 3 | 3 | | | | |
| **2. MULTIPLE DX** | | | | | | | | | | |
| 0–19 Years | 283 | 4.7 | 22 | 1 | 1 | 2 | 5 | 11 | 13 | 24 |
| 20–34 | 114 | 3.4 | 12 | 1 | 2 | 3 | 5 | 6 | 9 | 19 |
| 35–49 | 148 | 4.2 | 17 | 1 | 2 | 3 | 5 | 9 | 11 | 23 |
| 50–64 | 78 | 6.6 | 31 | 1 | 3 | 6 | 8 | 12 | 18 | 31 |
| 65+ | 109 | 6.8 | 69 | 1 | 3 | 5 | 8 | 14 | 15 | 37 |
| **TOTAL SINGLE DX** | 74 | 3.5 | 35 | 1 | 1 | 2 | 3 | 6 | 20 | 32 |
| **TOTAL MULTIPLE DX** | 732 | 4.8 | 27 | 1 | 2 | 3 | 6 | 11 | 14 | 24 |
| **TOTAL** | | | | | | | | | | |
| 0–19 Years | 321 | 4.5 | 22 | 1 | 1 | 3 | 6 | 11 | 13 | 24 |
| 20–34 | 131 | 3.3 | 11 | 1 | 1 | 2 | 3 | 6 | 9 | 19 |
| 35–49 | 159 | 3.9 | 16 | 1 | 2 | 2 | 5 | 9 | 11 | 23 |
| 50–64 | 86 | 7.2 | 45 | 1 | 2 | 6 | 8 | 16 | 23 | 32 |
| 65+ | 109 | 6.8 | 69 | 1 | 3 | 5 | 8 | 14 | 15 | 37 |
| **GRAND TOTAL** | 806 | 4.7 | 28 | 1 | 1 | 3 | 6 | 11 | 14 | 24 |

## 93.59: IMMOB/PRESS/WND ATTN NEC. Formerly included in operation group(s) 791.

| Type of Patients | Observed Patients | Avg. Stay | Variance | 10th | 25th | 50th | 75th | 90th | 95th | 99th |
|---|---|---|---|---|---|---|---|---|---|---|
| **1. SINGLE DX** | | | | | | | | | | |
| 0–19 Years | 39 | 2.4 | 5 | 1 | 1 | 1 | 2 | 3 | 5 | 15 |
| 20–34 | 32 | 3.9 | 27 | 1 | 1 | 2 | 5 | 5 | 13 | 37 |
| 35–49 | 31 | 2.5 | 4 | 1 | 1 | 1 | 2 | 6 | 8 | 8 |
| 50–64 | 23 | 1.8 | 3 | 1 | 1 | 1 | 2 | 3 | 7 | 9 |
| 65+ | 35 | 3.5 | 17 | 1 | 1 | 2 | 5 | 7 | 11 | 19 |
| **2. MULTIPLE DX** | | | | | | | | | | |
| 0–19 Years | 90 | 2.8 | 14 | 1 | 1 | 1 | 2 | 4 | 8 | 17 |
| 20–34 | 121 | 3.7 | 8 | 1 | 2 | 3 | 4 | 6 | 9 | 11 |
| 35–49 | 166 | 3.7 | 22 | 1 | 1 | 2 | 4 | 7 | 11 | 28 |
| 50–64 | 232 | 6.9 | 42 | 1 | 2 | 6 | 11 | 11 | 15 | 42 |
| 65+ | 880 | 5.2 | 25 | 2 | 3 | 4 | 6 | 10 | 13 | 27 |
| **TOTAL SINGLE DX** | 160 | 2.8 | 11 | 1 | 1 | 1 | 3 | 5 | 8 | 15 |
| **TOTAL MULTIPLE DX** | 1,489 | 4.9 | 26 | 1 | 2 | 4 | 6 | 11 | 13 | 28 |
| **TOTAL** | | | | | | | | | | |
| 0–19 Years | 129 | 2.8 | 12 | 1 | 1 | 1 | 3 | 4 | 8 | 17 |
| 20–34 | 153 | 3.7 | 11 | 1 | 2 | 1 | 5 | 6 | 9 | 14 |
| 35–49 | 197 | 3.5 | 19 | 1 | 1 | 2 | 4 | 7 | 10 | 28 |
| 50–64 | 255 | 6.4 | 41 | 1 | 2 | 4 | 11 | 11 | 14 | 42 |
| 65+ | 915 | 5.2 | 25 | 1 | 3 | 3 | 6 | 10 | 13 | 27 |
| **GRAND TOTAL** | 1,649 | 4.7 | 25 | 1 | 2 | 3 | 6 | 10 | 13 | 27 |

Length of Stay by Diagnosis and Operation, United States, 2000

# United States, October 1998–September 1999 Data, by Operation

## 93.6: OSTEOPATHIC MANIPULATION. Formerly included in operation group(s) 791.

| Type of Patients | Observed Patients | Avg. Stay | Vari- ance | 10th | 25th | 50th | 75th | 90th | 95th | 99th |
|---|---|---|---|---|---|---|---|---|---|---|
| **1. SINGLE DX** | | | | | | | | | | |
| 0–19 Years | 0 | | | | | | | | | |
| 20–34 | 1 | 2.0 | 0 | 2 | 2 | 2 | 2 | 2 | 2 | 2 |
| 35–49 | 2 | 2.2 | 1 | 1 | 1 | 3 | 3 | 3 | 3 | 3 |
| 50–64 | 0 | | | | | | | | | |
| 65+ | 0 | | | | | | | | | |
| **2. MULTIPLE DX** | | | | | | | | | | |
| 0–19 Years | 4 | 3.3 | 2 | 2 | 2 | 3 | 4 | 5 | 5 | 5 |
| 20–34 | 9 | 2.3 | 1 | 1 | 1 | 2 | 3 | 4 | 4 | 4 |
| 35–49 | 23 | 4.2 | 38 | 1 | 1 | 2 | 5 | 8 | 8 | 36 |
| 50–64 | 33 | 3.7 | 3 | 2 | 2 | 3 | 5 | 7 | 7 | 7 |
| 65+ | 99 | 5.4 | 9 | 2 | 3 | 5 | 7 | 9 | 12 | 13 |
| **TOTAL SINGLE DX** | 3 | 2.1 | <1 | 1 | 2 | 2 | 3 | 3 | 3 | 3 |
| **TOTAL MULTIPLE DX** | 168 | 4.6 | 14 | 1 | 2 | 4 | 6 | 8 | 9 | 16 |
| **TOTAL** | | | | | | | | | | |
| 0–19 Years | 4 | 3.3 | 2 | 2 | 2 | 3 | 4 | 5 | 5 | 5 |
| 20–34 | 10 | 2.2 | <1 | 1 | 1 | 2 | 3 | 4 | 4 | 4 |
| 35–49 | 25 | 4.1 | 37 | 1 | 1 | 2 | 5 | 8 | 8 | 36 |
| 50–64 | 33 | 3.7 | 3 | 2 | 2 | 3 | 5 | 7 | 7 | 7 |
| 65+ | 99 | 5.4 | 9 | 2 | 3 | 5 | 7 | 9 | 12 | 13 |
| **GRAND TOTAL** | 171 | 4.6 | 14 | 1 | 2 | 4 | 6 | 8 | 9 | 16 |

## 93.7: SPEECH/READ/BLIND REHAB. Formerly included in operation group(s) 791.

| Type of Patients | Observed Patients | Avg. Stay | Vari- ance | 10th | 25th | 50th | 75th | 90th | 95th | 99th |
|---|---|---|---|---|---|---|---|---|---|---|
| **1. SINGLE DX** | | | | | | | | | | |
| 0–19 Years | 3 | 3.3 | 5 | 1 | 2 | 2 | 6 | 6 | 6 | 6 |
| 20–34 | 0 | | | | | | | | | |
| 35–49 | 1 | 5.0 | 0 | 5 | 5 | 5 | 5 | 5 | 5 | 5 |
| 50–64 | 2 | 9.7 | <1 | 9 | 9 | 10 | 10 | 10 | 10 | 10 |
| 65+ | 2 | 3.3 | 7 | 2 | 2 | 2 | 2 | 8 | 8 | 8 |
| **2. MULTIPLE DX** | | | | | | | | | | |
| 0–19 Years | 48 | 10.6 | 83 | 2 | 3 | 7 | 16 | 24 | 34 | 39 |
| 20–34 | 19 | 9.0 | 63 | 1 | 3 | 7 | 14 | 20 | 20 | 35 |
| 35–49 | 43 | 7.6 | 63 | 2 | 3 | 5 | 9 | 14 | 24 | 44 |
| 50–64 | 101 | 7.6 | 54 | 2 | 3 | 5 | 10 | 17 | 20 | 42 |
| 65+ | 632 | 7.6 | 63 | 2 | 3 | 6 | 9 | 15 | 20 | 35 |
| **TOTAL SINGLE DX** | 8 | 4.7 | 9 | 2 | 2 | 5 | 6 | 10 | 10 | 10 |
| **TOTAL MULTIPLE DX** | 843 | 7.8 | 63 | 2 | 3 | 6 | 9 | 16 | 20 | 36 |
| **TOTAL** | | | | | | | | | | |
| 0–19 Years | 51 | 10.2 | 81 | 2 | 3 | 7 | 16 | 24 | 27 | 39 |
| 20–34 | 19 | 9.0 | 63 | 1 | 3 | 7 | 14 | 20 | 20 | 35 |
| 35–49 | 44 | 7.5 | 60 | 2 | 3 | 5 | 9 | 14 | 23 | 44 |
| 50–64 | 103 | 7.6 | 54 | 2 | 3 | 5 | 10 | 17 | 20 | 42 |
| 65+ | 634 | 7.6 | 63 | 2 | 3 | 6 | 9 | 15 | 20 | 35 |
| **GRAND TOTAL** | 851 | 7.7 | 62 | 2 | 3 | 6 | 9 | 15 | 20 | 36 |

## 93.75: OTHER SPEECH THERAPY. Formerly included in operation group(s) 791.

| Type of Patients | Observed Patients | Avg. Stay | Vari- ance | 10th | 25th | 50th | 75th | 90th | 95th | 99th |
|---|---|---|---|---|---|---|---|---|---|---|
| **1. SINGLE DX** | | | | | | | | | | |
| 0–19 Years | 3 | 3.3 | 5 | 1 | 2 | 2 | 6 | 6 | 6 | 6 |
| 20–34 | 0 | | | | | | | | | |
| 35–49 | 1 | 5.0 | 0 | 5 | 5 | 5 | 5 | 5 | 5 | 5 |
| 50–64 | 1 | 10.0 | 0 | 10 | 10 | 10 | 10 | 10 | 10 | 10 |
| 65+ | 2 | 3.3 | 7 | 2 | 2 | 2 | 6 | 8 | 8 | 8 |
| **2. MULTIPLE DX** | | | | | | | | | | |
| 0–19 Years | 48 | 10.6 | 83 | 2 | 3 | 7 | 16 | 24 | 34 | 39 |
| 20–34 | 17 | 8.3 | 44 | 1 | 3 | 7 | 14 | 20 | 20 | 20 |
| 35–49 | 43 | 7.6 | 63 | 2 | 3 | 5 | 9 | 14 | 24 | 44 |
| 50–64 | 93 | 7.4 | 47 | 2 | 3 | 4 | 10 | 17 | 20 | 37 |
| 65+ | 600 | 7.5 | 61 | 2 | 3 | 6 | 9 | 14 | 19 | 34 |
| **TOTAL SINGLE DX** | 7 | 4.5 | 8 | 2 | 2 | 5 | 6 | 10 | 10 | 10 |
| **TOTAL MULTIPLE DX** | 801 | 7.6 | 59 | 2 | 3 | 5 | 9 | 15 | 20 | 35 |
| **TOTAL** | | | | | | | | | | |
| 0–19 Years | 51 | 10.2 | 81 | 2 | 3 | 7 | 16 | 24 | 27 | 39 |
| 20–34 | 17 | 8.3 | 44 | 1 | 3 | 7 | 14 | 20 | 20 | 20 |
| 35–49 | 44 | 7.5 | 60 | 2 | 3 | 5 | 9 | 14 | 23 | 44 |
| 50–64 | 94 | 7.4 | 47 | 2 | 3 | 4 | 10 | 17 | 20 | 37 |
| 65+ | 602 | 7.5 | 60 | 2 | 3 | 6 | 9 | 14 | 19 | 34 |
| **GRAND TOTAL** | 808 | 7.6 | 59 | 2 | 3 | 5 | 9 | 15 | 20 | 35 |

## 93.8: OTHER REHAB THERAPY. Formerly included in operation group(s) 791.

| Type of Patients | Observed Patients | Avg. Stay | Vari- ance | 10th | 25th | 50th | 75th | 90th | 95th | 99th |
|---|---|---|---|---|---|---|---|---|---|---|
| **1. SINGLE DX** | | | | | | | | | | |
| 0–19 Years | 39 | 4.6 | 9 | 2 | 3 | 4 | 6 | 8 | 11 | 15 |
| 20–34 | 50 | 10.6 | 81 | 2 | 4 | 6 | 17 | 21 | 21 | 48 |
| 35–49 | 58 | 7.4 | 29 | 4 | 7 | 7 | 9 | 14 | 14 | 28 |
| 50–64 | 22 | 14.0 | 114 | 4 | 8 | 11 | 20 | 25 | 31 | 58 |
| 65+ | 29 | 9.2 | 52 | 2 | 5 | 7 | 14 | 17 | 22 | 31 |
| **2. MULTIPLE DX** | | | | | | | | | | |
| 0–19 Years | 420 | 11.5 | 186 | 2 | 3 | 7 | 14 | 29 | 42 | 83 |
| 20–34 | 486 | 9.5 | 94 | 2 | 4 | 7 | 13 | 21 | 28 | 47 |
| 35–49 | 921 | 12.2 | 139 | 3 | 5 | 8 | 15 | 25 | 34 | 60 |
| 50–64 | 1,371 | 12.3 | 98 | 3 | 6 | 9 | 16 | 24 | 32 | 52 |
| 65+ | 5,886 | 12.8 | 68 | 4 | 7 | 11 | 17 | 23 | 28 | 42 |
| **TOTAL SINGLE DX** | 198 | 8.7 | 58 | 2 | 4 | 7 | 11 | 20 | 22 | 43 |
| **TOTAL MULTIPLE DX** | 9,084 | 12.4 | 87 | 4 | 6 | 10 | 16 | 23 | 29 | 49 |
| **TOTAL** | | | | | | | | | | |
| 0–19 Years | 459 | 10.9 | 175 | 2 | 3 | 6 | 13 | 26 | 39 | 83 |
| 20–34 | 536 | 9.6 | 93 | 2 | 4 | 7 | 13 | 21 | 28 | 47 |
| 35–49 | 979 | 11.8 | 133 | 3 | 5 | 8 | 14 | 24 | 33 | 60 |
| 50–64 | 1,393 | 12.3 | 99 | 3 | 6 | 10 | 16 | 24 | 32 | 52 |
| 65+ | 5,915 | 12.8 | 68 | 4 | 7 | 11 | 17 | 23 | 28 | 42 |
| **GRAND TOTAL** | 9,282 | 12.3 | 86 | 3 | 6 | 10 | 16 | 23 | 28 | 48 |

Length of Stay by Diagnosis and Operation, United States, 2000

# United States, October 1998–September 1999 Data, by Operation

## 93.89: REHABILITATION NEC. Formerly included in operation group(s) 791.

| Type of Patients | Observed Patients | Avg. Stay | Variance | 10th | 25th | 50th | 75th | 90th | 95th | 99th |
|---|---|---|---|---|---|---|---|---|---|---|
| **1. SINGLE DX** | | | | | | | | | | |
| 0–19 Years | 0 | | | | | | | | | |
| 20–34 | 0 | | | | | | | | | |
| 35–49 | 2 | 13.2 | 11 | 11 | 11 | 11 | 16 | 16 | 16 | 16 |
| 50–64 | 0 | | | | | | | | | |
| 65+ | 0 | | | | | | | | | |
| **2. MULTIPLE DX** | | | | | | | | | | |
| 0–19 Years | 33 | 13.0 | 245 | 2 | 4 | 10 | 14 | 21 | 50 | 95 |
| 20–34 | 69 | 10.4 | 49 | 3 | 6 | 9 | 12 | 21 | 26 | 32 |
| 35–49 | 176 | 18.3 | 237 | 4 | 7 | 14 | 24 | 39 | 57 | 60 |
| 50–64 | 443 | 14.5 | 124 | 4 | 7 | 11 | 18 | 30 | 38 | 52 |
| 65+ | 1,871 | 14.7 | 62 | 7 | 9 | 14 | 19 | 25 | 29 | 40 |
| **TOTAL SINGLE DX** | 2 | 13.2 | 11 | 11 | 11 | 11 | 16 | 16 | 16 | 16 |
| **TOTAL MULTIPLE DX** | 2,592 | 14.9 | 91 | 6 | 8 | 13 | 19 | 26 | 30 | 54 |
| **TOTAL** | | | | | | | | | | |
| 0–19 | 33 | 13.0 | 245 | 2 | 4 | 10 | 14 | 21 | 50 | 95 |
| 20–34 | 69 | 10.4 | 49 | 3 | 6 | 9 | 12 | 21 | 26 | 32 |
| 35–49 | 178 | 18.3 | 237 | 4 | 7 | 14 | 24 | 39 | 57 | 60 |
| 50–64 | 443 | 14.5 | 124 | 4 | 7 | 11 | 18 | 30 | 38 | 52 |
| 65+ | 1,871 | 14.7 | 62 | 7 | 9 | 14 | 19 | 25 | 29 | 40 |
| **GRAND TOTAL** | 2,594 | 14.9 | 91 | 6 | 8 | 13 | 19 | 26 | 30 | 54 |

## 93.9: RESPIRATORY THERAPY. Formerly included in operation group(s) 789, 791.

| Type of Patients | Observed Patients | Avg. Stay | Variance | 10th | 25th | 50th | 75th | 90th | 95th | 99th |
|---|---|---|---|---|---|---|---|---|---|---|
| **1. SINGLE DX** | | | | | | | | | | |
| 0–19 Years | 7,616 | 2.2 | 3 | 1 | 1 | 2 | 3 | 4 | 5 | 9 |
| 20–34 | 397 | 2.4 | 4 | 1 | 1 | 2 | 3 | 4 | 5 | 8 |
| 35–49 | 426 | 2.5 | 2 | 1 | 1 | 2 | 3 | 5 | 5 | 7 |
| 50–64 | 267 | 3.0 | 5 | 1 | 2 | 2 | 4 | 5 | 6 | 14 |
| 65+ | 181 | 3.1 | 5 | 1 | 2 | 2 | 4 | 6 | 8 | 9 |
| **2. MULTIPLE DX** | | | | | | | | | | |
| 0–19 Years | 18,437 | 5.1 | 58 | 1 | 2 | 3 | 5 | 11 | 17 | 45 |
| 20–34 | 1,688 | 4.3 | 16 | 1 | 2 | 3 | 5 | 9 | 11 | 22 |
| 35–49 | 3,620 | 4.3 | 14 | 1 | 2 | 3 | 5 | 8 | 10 | 18 |
| 50–64 | 5,455 | 5.0 | 20 | 2 | 3 | 4 | 6 | 9 | 12 | 21 |
| 65+ | 12,164 | 5.6 | 20 | 2 | 3 | 4 | 7 | 11 | 14 | 21 |
| **TOTAL SINGLE DX** | 8,887 | 2.3 | 3 | 1 | 1 | 2 | 3 | 4 | 5 | 9 |
| **TOTAL MULTIPLE DX** | 41,364 | 5.1 | 39 | 1 | 2 | 3 | 6 | 10 | 15 | 34 |
| **TOTAL** | | | | | | | | | | |
| 0–19 | 26,053 | 4.3 | 44 | 1 | 2 | 3 | 4 | 8 | 14 | 39 |
| 20–34 | 2,085 | 4.0 | 14 | 1 | 2 | 3 | 5 | 8 | 10 | 21 |
| 35–49 | 4,046 | 4.1 | 13 | 1 | 2 | 3 | 5 | 8 | 10 | 17 |
| 50–64 | 5,722 | 5.0 | 19 | 1 | 3 | 4 | 6 | 9 | 12 | 21 |
| 65+ | 12,345 | 5.5 | 20 | 2 | 3 | 4 | 7 | 10 | 14 | 21 |
| **GRAND TOTAL** | 50,251 | 4.6 | 33 | 1 | 2 | 3 | 5 | 9 | 13 | 30 |

## 93.81: RECREATIONAL THERAPY. Formerly included in operation group(s) 791.

| Type of Patients | Observed Patients | Avg. Stay | Variance | 10th | 25th | 50th | 75th | 90th | 95th | 99th |
|---|---|---|---|---|---|---|---|---|---|---|
| **1. SINGLE DX** | | | | | | | | | | |
| 0–19 Years | 2 | 11.5 | 16 | 7 | 7 | 14 | 14 | 14 | 14 | 14 |
| 20–34 | 8 | 8.5 | 42 | 2 | 2 | 9 | 10 | 21 | 21 | 21 |
| 35–49 | 8 | 8.0 | 27 | 2 | 2 | 8 | 14 | 14 | 14 | 14 |
| 50–64 | 3 | 22.8 | 43 | 14 | 14 | 25 | 28 | 28 | 28 | 28 |
| 65+ | 6 | 8.5 | 13 | 5 | 5 | 8 | 13 | 14 | 14 | 14 |
| **2. MULTIPLE DX** | | | | | | | | | | |
| 0–19 Years | 84 | 14.8 | 191 | 3 | 5 | 10 | 20 | 35 | 42 | 58 |
| 20–34 | 52 | 10.6 | 71 | 3 | 5 | 8 | 14 | 21 | 26 | 51 |
| 35–49 | 84 | 11.5 | 124 | 4 | 6 | 8 | 12 | 29 | 30 | 37 |
| 50–64 | 73 | 11.0 | 67 | 4 | 6 | 8 | 15 | 21 | 29 | 45 |
| 65+ | 243 | 13.4 | 58 | 6 | 8 | 12 | 17 | 24 | 28 | 46 |
| **TOTAL SINGLE DX** | 25 | 9.5 | 39 | 2 | 5 | 8 | 14 | 14 | 25 | 28 |
| **TOTAL MULTIPLE DX** | 536 | 12.6 | 86 | 4 | 7 | 10 | 16 | 25 | 30 | 47 |
| **TOTAL** | | | | | | | | | | |
| 0–19 | 86 | 14.8 | 187 | 3 | 5 | 10 | 19 | 35 | 42 | 58 |
| 20–34 | 58 | 10.4 | 68 | 3 | 5 | 8 | 14 | 21 | 26 | 35 |
| 35–49 | 92 | 11.1 | 114 | 3 | 5 | 8 | 12 | 27 | 30 | 37 |
| 50–64 | 76 | 11.2 | 68 | 4 | 6 | 8 | 15 | 22 | 29 | 45 |
| 65+ | 249 | 13.3 | 57 | 6 | 8 | 12 | 17 | 24 | 28 | 46 |
| **GRAND TOTAL** | 561 | 12.5 | 84 | 4 | 7 | 10 | 16 | 25 | 30 | 47 |

## 93.83: OCCUPATIONAL THERAPY. Formerly included in operation group(s) 791.

| Type of Patients | Observed Patients | Avg. Stay | Variance | 10th | 25th | 50th | 75th | 90th | 95th | 99th |
|---|---|---|---|---|---|---|---|---|---|---|
| **1. SINGLE DX** | | | | | | | | | | |
| 0–19 Years | 37 | 4.3 | 7 | 2 | 2 | 3 | 6 | 8 | 10 | 15 |
| 20–34 | 44 | 10.7 | 84 | 3 | 4 | 6 | 20 | 21 | 21 | 48 |
| 35–49 | 48 | 7.2 | 29 | 2 | 4 | 7 | 8 | 11 | 14 | 28 |
| 50–64 | 18 | 12.0 | 119 | 4 | 4 | 11 | 12 | 20 | 43 | 58 |
| 65+ | 21 | 9.4 | 64 | 2 | 3 | 7 | 14 | 22 | 31 | 31 |
| **2. MULTIPLE DX** | | | | | | | | | | |
| 0–19 Years | 291 | 10.9 | 179 | 2 | 3 | 6 | 13 | 26 | 43 | 83 |
| 20–34 | 362 | 9.3 | 105 | 2 | 3 | 6 | 13 | 21 | 30 | 47 |
| 35–49 | 655 | 10.0 | 86 | 3 | 5 | 7 | 12 | 19 | 26 | 50 |
| 50–64 | 847 | 11.4 | 86 | 3 | 5 | 9 | 14 | 22 | 28 | 56 |
| 65+ | 3,709 | 11.8 | 69 | 3 | 6 | 10 | 15 | 22 | 26 | 43 |
| **TOTAL SINGLE DX** | 168 | 8.4 | 58 | 2 | 4 | 6 | 11 | 20 | 21 | 43 |
| **TOTAL MULTIPLE DX** | 5,864 | 11.3 | 81 | 3 | 5 | 9 | 15 | 22 | 27 | 47 |
| **TOTAL** | | | | | | | | | | |
| 0–19 | 328 | 10.2 | 165 | 2 | 5 | 5 | 12 | 23 | 35 | 83 |
| 20–34 | 406 | 9.5 | 103 | 3 | 6 | 6 | 13 | 21 | 30 | 47 |
| 35–49 | 703 | 9.8 | 82 | 3 | 5 | 7 | 12 | 19 | 25 | 48 |
| 50–64 | 865 | 11.4 | 86 | 3 | 6 | 9 | 14 | 22 | 28 | 56 |
| 65+ | 3,730 | 11.8 | 69 | 3 | 6 | 10 | 15 | 22 | 26 | 43 |
| **GRAND TOTAL** | 6,032 | 11.2 | 81 | 3 | 5 | 9 | 15 | 21 | 27 | 47 |

Length of Stay by Diagnosis and Operation, United States, 2000

# United States, October 1998–September 1999 Data, by Operation

## 93.90: CPAP. Formerly included in operation group(s) 789.

| Type of Patients | Observed Patients | Avg. Stay | Variance | Percentiles | | | | | | |
|---|---|---|---|---|---|---|---|---|---|---|
| | | | | 10th | 25th | 50th | 75th | 90th | 95th | 99th |
| **1. SINGLE DX** | | | | | | | | | | |
| 0–19 Years | 66 | 3.1 | 10 | 1 | 2 | 2 | 3 | 6 | 10 | 17 |
| 20–34 | 2 | 4.6 | 3 | 3 | 3 | 6 | 6 | 6 | 6 | 6 |
| 35–49 | 10 | 3.6 | 8 | 1 | 1 | 3 | 4 | 9 | 9 | 9 |
| 50–64 | 4 | 7.7 | 32 | 2 | 2 | 5 | 14 | 14 | 14 | 14 |
| 65+ | 3 | 3.2 | <1 | 2 | 3 | 3 | 3 | 5 | 5 | 5 |
| **2. MULTIPLE DX** | | | | | | | | | | |
| 0–19 Years | 3,089 | 13.8 | 205 | 2 | 4 | 9 | 17 | 35 | 47 | 74 |
| 20–34 | 175 | 6.0 | 26 | 2 | 3 | 4 | 7 | 11 | 16 | 24 |
| 35–49 | 594 | 5.8 | 22 | 2 | 3 | 5 | 8 | 10 | 13 | 25 |
| 50–64 | 1,341 | 6.6 | 33 | 2 | 4 | 5 | 8 | 12 | 16 | 28 |
| 65+ | 2,503 | 7.5 | 27 | 3 | 4 | 6 | 10 | 15 | 16 | 25 |
| **TOTAL SINGLE DX** | 85 | 3.5 | 11 | 1 | 2 | 2 | 4 | 9 | 10 | 17 |
| **TOTAL MULTIPLE DX** | 7,702 | 9.5 | 104 | 2 | 4 | 6 | 11 | 19 | 29 | 61 |
| **TOTAL** | | | | | | | | | | |
| 0–19 Years | 3,155 | 13.6 | 204 | 2 | 4 | 9 | 17 | 35 | 47 | 74 |
| 20–34 | 177 | 6.0 | 26 | 2 | 3 | 4 | 7 | 11 | 16 | 24 |
| 35–49 | 604 | 5.8 | 22 | 2 | 3 | 5 | 8 | 10 | 13 | 25 |
| 50–64 | 1,345 | 6.6 | 33 | 2 | 4 | 5 | 8 | 12 | 16 | 28 |
| 65+ | 2,506 | 7.5 | 27 | 3 | 4 | 6 | 10 | 15 | 16 | 25 |
| **GRAND TOTAL** | 7,787 | 9.4 | 104 | 2 | 4 | 6 | 11 | 19 | 29 | 61 |

## 93.91: IPPB. Formerly included in operation group(s) 789.

| Type of Patients | Observed Patients | Avg. Stay | Variance | Percentiles | | | | | | |
|---|---|---|---|---|---|---|---|---|---|---|
| | | | | 10th | 25th | 50th | 75th | 90th | 95th | 99th |
| **1. SINGLE DX** | | | | | | | | | | |
| 0–19 Years | 19 | 2.8 | 1 | 2 | 2 | 2 | 4 | 4 | 4 | 8 |
| 20–34 | 0 | | | | | | | | | |
| 35–49 | 1 | 7.0 | 0 | 7 | 7 | 7 | 7 | 7 | 7 | 7 |
| 50–64 | 1 | 2.0 | | 2 | 2 | 2 | 2 | 2 | 2 | 2 |
| 65+ | 2 | 5.1 | 13 | 1 | 1 | 8 | 8 | 8 | 8 | 8 |
| **2. MULTIPLE DX** | | | | | | | | | | |
| 0–19 Years | 99 | 6.9 | 78 | 2 | 2 | 4 | 6 | 17 | 21 | 55 |
| 20–34 | 15 | 5.4 | 17 | 3 | 3 | 3 | 7 | 9 | 18 | 19 |
| 35–49 | 24 | 6.4 | 8 | 3 | 4 | 6 | 9 | 10 | 10 | 10 |
| 50–64 | 50 | 7.3 | 14 | 3 | 4 | 7 | 10 | 12 | 13 | 17 |
| 65+ | 117 | 9.0 | 73 | 3 | 4 | 7 | 10 | 15 | 22 | 53 |
| **TOTAL SINGLE DX** | 23 | 3.1 | 3 | 2 | 2 | 2 | 4 | 4 | 8 | 8 |
| **TOTAL MULTIPLE DX** | 305 | 7.4 | 55 | 2 | 3 | 6 | 9 | 14 | 17 | 53 |
| **TOTAL** | | | | | | | | | | |
| 0–19 Years | 118 | 6.1 | 67 | 2 | 2 | 3 | 6 | 17 | 17 | 55 |
| 20–34 | 15 | 5.4 | 17 | 3 | 3 | 3 | 7 | 9 | 10 | 19 |
| 35–49 | 25 | 6.4 | 8 | 3 | 4 | 6 | 9 | 10 | 10 | 10 |
| 50–64 | 51 | 7.3 | 14 | 4 | 4 | 7 | 10 | 12 | 13 | 17 |
| 65+ | 119 | 8.8 | 72 | 3 | 4 | 7 | 10 | 15 | 21 | 53 |
| **GRAND TOTAL** | 328 | 7.0 | 52 | 3 | 3 | 5 | 9 | 13 | 17 | 53 |

## 93.93: NONMECH RESUSCITATION. Formerly included in operation group(s) 791.

| Type of Patients | Observed Patients | Avg. Stay | Variance | Percentiles | | | | | | |
|---|---|---|---|---|---|---|---|---|---|---|
| | | | | 10th | 25th | 50th | 75th | 90th | 95th | 99th |
| **1. SINGLE DX** | | | | | | | | | | |
| 0–19 Years | 141 | 1.7 | <1 | 1 | 1 | 2 | 2 | 3 | 3 | 4 |
| 20–34 | 2 | 2.0 | 0 | 2 | 2 | 2 | 2 | 2 | 2 | 2 |
| 35–49 | 0 | | | | | | | | | |
| 50–64 | 1 | 1.0 | 0 | 1 | 1 | 1 | 1 | 1 | 1 | 1 |
| 65+ | 0 | | | | | | | | | |
| **2. MULTIPLE DX** | | | | | | | | | | |
| 0–19 Years | 643 | 4.0 | 29 | 1 | 2 | 2 | 4 | 9 | 17 | 26 |
| 20–34 | 6 | 2.4 | 1 | 1 | 2 | 2 | 3 | 3 | 3 | 6 |
| 35–49 | 5 | 10.3 | 119 | 2 | 2 | 7 | 15 | 28 | 28 | 28 |
| 50–64 | 1 | 3.0 | 0 | 3 | 3 | 3 | 3 | >99 | >99 | >99 |
| 65+ | 26 | 7.6 | 67 | 1 | 4 | 5 | 9 | 23 | 31 | 37 |
| **TOTAL SINGLE DX** | 143 | 1.7 | <1 | 1 | 1 | 2 | 2 | 3 | 3 | 4 |
| **TOTAL MULTIPLE DX** | 681 | 4.1 | 30 | 1 | 2 | 2 | 4 | 9 | 17 | 26 |
| **TOTAL** | | | | | | | | | | |
| 0–19 Years | 784 | 3.6 | 24 | 1 | 2 | 2 | 3 | 7 | 15 | 26 |
| 20–34 | 7 | 2.4 | 1 | 1 | 2 | 2 | 3 | 3 | 3 | 6 |
| 35–49 | 5 | 10.3 | 119 | 2 | 2 | 7 | 15 | 28 | 28 | 28 |
| 50–64 | 2 | 3.0 | | 1 | 1 | 3 | 3 | >99 | >99 | >99 |
| 65+ | 26 | 7.6 | 67 | 1 | 4 | 5 | 9 | 23 | 31 | 37 |
| **GRAND TOTAL** | 824 | 3.7 | 25 | 1 | 1 | 2 | 3 | 7 | 16 | 26 |

## 93.94: NEBULIZER THERAPY. Formerly included in operation group(s) 791.

| Type of Patients | Observed Patients | Avg. Stay | Variance | Percentiles | | | | | | |
|---|---|---|---|---|---|---|---|---|---|---|
| | | | | 10th | 25th | 50th | 75th | 90th | 95th | 99th |
| **1. SINGLE DX** | | | | | | | | | | |
| 0–19 Years | 5,423 | 2.3 | 3 | 1 | 1 | 2 | 3 | 4 | 5 | 9 |
| 20–34 | 306 | 2.1 | 1 | 1 | 1 | 2 | 3 | 4 | 4 | 7 |
| 35–49 | 322 | 2.5 | 2 | 1 | 2 | 2 | 3 | 4 | 5 | 7 |
| 50–64 | 190 | 3.1 | 5 | 2 | 2 | 3 | 4 | 5 | 6 | 10 |
| 65+ | 116 | 3.2 | 4 | 1 | 2 | 3 | 4 | 5 | 8 | 9 |
| **2. MULTIPLE DX** | | | | | | | | | | |
| 0–19 Years | 7,899 | 3.3 | 9 | 1 | 1 | 2 | 4 | 6 | 9 | 16 |
| 20–34 | 1,032 | 3.7 | 9 | 1 | 2 | 3 | 5 | 7 | 9 | 16 |
| 35–49 | 1,975 | 3.9 | 10 | 1 | 2 | 4 | 6 | 8 | 9 | 16 |
| 50–64 | 2,342 | 4.4 | 11 | 2 | 3 | 4 | 6 | 9 | 10 | 16 |
| 65+ | 4,953 | 5.3 | 16 | 2 | 3 | 4 | 7 | 9 | 12 | 20 |
| **TOTAL SINGLE DX** | 6,357 | 2.3 | 3 | 1 | 1 | 2 | 3 | 4 | 5 | 9 |
| **TOTAL MULTIPLE DX** | 18,201 | 3.9 | 11 | 1 | 2 | 3 | 5 | 8 | 10 | 17 |
| **TOTAL** | | | | | | | | | | |
| 0–19 Years | 13,322 | 2.9 | 7 | 1 | 1 | 3 | 3 | 5 | 7 | 14 |
| 20–34 | 1,338 | 3.3 | 8 | 1 | 2 | 3 | 4 | 6 | 9 | 14 |
| 35–49 | 2,297 | 3.7 | 9 | 1 | 2 | 4 | 5 | 7 | 8 | 15 |
| 50–64 | 2,532 | 4.4 | 10 | 2 | 2 | 4 | 5 | 8 | 10 | 16 |
| 65+ | 5,069 | 5.3 | 16 | 2 | 3 | 4 | 7 | 9 | 12 | 20 |
| **GRAND TOTAL** | 24,558 | 3.5 | 10 | 1 | 2 | 3 | 4 | 7 | 9 | 15 |

Length of Stay by Diagnosis and Operation, United States, 2000

# United States, October 1998–September 1999 Data, by Operation

## 93.96: OXYGEN ENRICHMENT NEC. Formerly included in operation group(s) 791.

| Type of Patients | Observed Patients | Avg. Stay | Variance | 10th | 25th | 50th | 75th | 90th | 95th | 99th |
|---|---|---|---|---|---|---|---|---|---|---|
| **1. SINGLE DX** | | | | | | | | | | |
| 0–19 Years | 1,817 | 2.2 | 2 | 1 | 1 | 2 | 3 | 4 | 4 | 6 |
| 20–34 | 64 | 3.6 | 14 | 1 | 1 | 2 | 5 | 6 | 8 | 21 |
| 35–49 | 73 | 2.8 | 3 | 1 | 1 | 3 | 4 | 5 | 5 | 8 |
| 50–64 | 63 | 2.7 | 3 | 1 | 2 | 3 | 3 | 5 | 6 | 10 |
| 65+ | 48 | 3.3 | 6 | 1 | 2 | 3 | 4 | 6 | 7 | 17 |
| **2. MULTIPLE DX** | | | | | | | | | | |
| 0–19 Years | 6,348 | 4.5 | 40 | 1 | 2 | 3 | 5 | 9 | 14 | 35 |
| 20–34 | 326 | 4.6 | 19 | 1 | 2 | 4 | 5 | 9 | 16 | 23 |
| 35–49 | 816 | 3.8 | 10 | 1 | 2 | 3 | 5 | 8 | 10 | 14 |
| 50–64 | 1,340 | 4.1 | 14 | 1 | 2 | 3 | 5 | 7 | 9 | 16 |
| 65+ | 3,395 | 4.5 | 15 | 1 | 2 | 3 | 5 | 8 | 11 | 20 |
| **TOTAL SINGLE DX** | 2,065 | 2.3 | 2 | 1 | 1 | 2 | 3 | 4 | 5 | 8 |
| **TOTAL MULTIPLE DX** | 12,225 | 4.4 | 29 | 1 | 2 | 3 | 5 | 9 | 12 | 28 |
| **TOTAL** | | | | | | | | | | |
| 0–19 Years | 8,165 | 4.0 | 33 | 1 | 2 | 3 | 4 | 8 | 12 | 31 |
| 20–34 | 390 | 4.4 | 18 | 1 | 2 | 3 | 5 | 8 | 15 | 23 |
| 35–49 | 889 | 3.7 | 10 | 1 | 2 | 3 | 5 | 8 | 10 | 14 |
| 50–64 | 1,403 | 4.0 | 14 | 1 | 2 | 3 | 5 | 7 | 9 | 16 |
| 65+ | 3,443 | 4.5 | 14 | 1 | 2 | 3 | 5 | 8 | 11 | 19 |
| **GRAND TOTAL** | 14,290 | 4.1 | 26 | 2 | 2 | 3 | 4 | 8 | 12 | 25 |

## 93.99: OTHER RESP PROCEDURES. Formerly included in operation group(s) 791.

| Type of Patients | Observed Patients | Avg. Stay | Variance | 10th | 25th | 50th | 75th | 90th | 95th | 99th |
|---|---|---|---|---|---|---|---|---|---|---|
| **1. SINGLE DX** | | | | | | | | | | |
| 0–19 Years | 135 | 2.2 | 3 | 1 | 1 | 2 | 3 | 4 | 5 | 9 |
| 20–34 | 13 | 3.1 | 2 | 1 | 2 | 2 | 4 | 4 | 5 | 8 |
| 35–49 | 14 | 2.1 | <1 | 1 | 2 | 2 | 2 | 3 | 3 | 3 |
| 50–64 | 6 | 1.3 | <1 | 1 | 1 | 1 | 2 | 2 | 2 | 3 |
| 65+ | 8 | 2.8 | 4 | 1 | 1 | 3 | 3 | 3 | 7 | 7 |
| **2. MULTIPLE DX** | | | | | | | | | | |
| 0–19 Years | 342 | 4.2 | 31 | 1 | 2 | 2 | 4 | 9 | 14 | 20 |
| 20–34 | 102 | 5.4 | 38 | 1 | 3 | 3 | 7 | 10 | 14 | 26 |
| 35–49 | 146 | 3.9 | 12 | 1 | 2 | 3 | 5 | 8 | 12 | 15 |
| 50–64 | 320 | 5.0 | 21 | 1 | 2 | 4 | 7 | 11 | 11 | 18 |
| 65+ | 1,090 | 4.6 | 11 | 2 | 2 | 4 | 6 | 8 | 11 | 17 |
| **TOTAL SINGLE DX** | 176 | 2.2 | 2 | 1 | 1 | 2 | 3 | 4 | 5 | 8 |
| **TOTAL MULTIPLE DX** | 2,000 | 4.6 | 18 | 1 | 2 | 3 | 6 | 9 | 11 | 19 |
| **TOTAL** | | | | | | | | | | |
| 0–19 Years | 477 | 3.6 | 24 | 1 | 2 | 2 | 4 | 8 | 11 | 20 |
| 20–34 | 115 | 5.3 | 36 | 1 | 2 | 3 | 7 | 10 | 14 | 26 |
| 35–49 | 160 | 3.7 | 11 | 1 | 2 | 3 | 4 | 7 | 11 | 15 |
| 50–64 | 326 | 5.0 | 21 | 1 | 2 | 4 | 7 | 11 | 11 | 18 |
| 65+ | 1,098 | 4.6 | 11 | 2 | 2 | 4 | 6 | 8 | 11 | 17 |
| **GRAND TOTAL** | 2,176 | 4.4 | 17 | 2 | 2 | 3 | 5 | 9 | 11 | 18 |

## 94.0: PSYCH EVAL & TESTING. Formerly included in operation group(s) 792.

| Type of Patients | Observed Patients | Avg. Stay | Variance | 10th | 25th | 50th | 75th | 90th | 95th | 99th |
|---|---|---|---|---|---|---|---|---|---|---|
| **1. SINGLE DX** | | | | | | | | | | |
| 0–19 Years | 12 | 6.8 | 10 | 4 | 5 | 6 | 11 | 11 | 11 | 11 |
| 20–34 | 4 | 7.5 | 2 | 4 | 8 | 8 | 8 | 8 | 8 | 8 |
| 35–49 | 5 | 4.4 | 65 | 1 | 1 | 6 | 3 | 26 | 26 | 26 |
| 50–64 | 1 | 5.0 | 0 | 5 | 5 | 5 | 5 | 5 | 5 | 5 |
| 65+ | 0 | | | | | | | | | |
| **2. MULTIPLE DX** | | | | | | | | | | |
| 0–19 Years | 80 | 6.5 | 17 | 3 | 4 | 6 | 8 | 12 | 12 | 20 |
| 20–34 | 186 | 5.2 | 21 | 1 | 3 | 4 | 6 | 10 | 18 | 21 |
| 35–49 | 214 | 8.2 | 53 | 3 | 4 | 6 | 9 | 16 | 20 | 44 |
| 50–64 | 54 | 9.8 | 61 | 3 | 4 | 8 | 13 | 23 | 27 | 32 |
| 65+ | 25 | 13.4 | 422 | 6 | 6 | 7 | 8 | 18 | 83 | 83 |
| **TOTAL SINGLE DX** | 22 | 6.5 | 17 | 1 | 4 | 6 | 8 | 11 | 11 | 26 |
| **TOTAL MULTIPLE DX** | 559 | 7.2 | 49 | 2 | 4 | 5 | 8 | 15 | 20 | 35 |
| **TOTAL** | | | | | | | | | | |
| 0–19 Years | 92 | 6.6 | 16 | 3 | 4 | 6 | 8 | 12 | 12 | 20 |
| 20–34 | 190 | 5.2 | 21 | 1 | 3 | 4 | 6 | 10 | 18 | 21 |
| 35–49 | 219 | 8.2 | 53 | 3 | 4 | 6 | 9 | 16 | 20 | 44 |
| 50–64 | 55 | 9.8 | 61 | 3 | 4 | 8 | 13 | 23 | 27 | 32 |
| 65+ | 25 | 13.4 | 422 | 6 | 6 | 7 | 8 | 18 | 83 | 83 |
| **GRAND TOTAL** | 581 | 7.2 | 49 | 2 | 4 | 5 | 8 | 14 | 20 | 34 |

## 94.08: PSYCH EVAL & TEST NEC. Formerly included in operation group(s) 792.

| Type of Patients | Observed Patients | Avg. Stay | Variance | 10th | 25th | 50th | 75th | 90th | 95th | 99th |
|---|---|---|---|---|---|---|---|---|---|---|
| **1. SINGLE DX** | | | | | | | | | | |
| 0–19 Years | 5 | 4.9 | 1 | 4 | 4 | 4 | 5 | 6 | 8 | 8 |
| 20–34 | 1 | 4.0 | 0 | 4 | 4 | 4 | 4 | 4 | 4 | 8 |
| 35–49 | 4 | 4.4 | 68 | 1 | 1 | 3 | 3 | 26 | 26 | 26 |
| 50–64 | 1 | 5.0 | 0 | 5 | 5 | 5 | 5 | 5 | 5 | 5 |
| 65+ | 0 | | | | | | | | | |
| **2. MULTIPLE DX** | | | | | | | | | | |
| 0–19 Years | 22 | 7.1 | 16 | 2 | 2 | 4 | 7 | 12 | 12 | 13 |
| 20–34 | 162 | 5.3 | 22 | 1 | 3 | 3 | 6 | 11 | 18 | 21 |
| 35–49 | 190 | 8.3 | 55 | 3 | 3 | 4 | 6 | 17 | 24 | 44 |
| 50–64 | 47 | 9.6 | 61 | 3 | 3 | 7 | 13 | 24 | 32 | 32 |
| 65+ | 14 | 25.1 | 958 | 7 | 7 | 7 | 20 | 83 | 83 | 83 |
| **TOTAL SINGLE DX** | 11 | 4.6 | 34 | 1 | 1 | 4 | 4 | 5 | 26 | 26 |
| **TOTAL MULTIPLE DX** | 435 | 7.4 | 53 | 2 | 4 | 5 | 8 | 15 | 20 | 35 |
| **TOTAL** | | | | | | | | | | |
| 0–19 Years | 27 | 7.0 | 15 | 2 | 2 | 4 | 7 | 12 | 12 | 13 |
| 20–34 | 163 | 5.3 | 22 | 1 | 3 | 3 | 6 | 11 | 18 | 21 |
| 35–49 | 194 | 8.3 | 55 | 3 | 3 | 4 | 9 | 17 | 24 | 44 |
| 50–64 | 48 | 9.6 | 61 | 3 | 3 | 7 | 13 | 24 | 32 | 32 |
| 65+ | 14 | 25.1 | 958 | 7 | 7 | 7 | 20 | 83 | 83 | 83 |
| **GRAND TOTAL** | 446 | 7.4 | 53 | 2 | 4 | 5 | 8 | 15 | 20 | 35 |

Length of Stay by Diagnosis and Operation, United States, 2000

# United States, October 1998–September 1999 Data, by Operation

## 94.13: PSYCH COMMITMENT EVAL. Formerly included in operation group(s) 792.

| Type of Patients | Observed Patients | Avg. Stay | Vari-ance | 10th | 25th | 50th | 75th | 90th | 95th | 99th |
|---|---|---|---|---|---|---|---|---|---|---|
| **1. SINGLE DX** | | | | | | | | | | |
| 0–19 Years | 2 | 2.6 | 4 | 1 | 1 | 1 | 5 | 5 | 5 | 5 |
| 20–34 | 9 | 9.7 | 34 | 2 | 5 | 8 | 14 | 18 | 20 | 20 |
| 35–49 | 8 | 5.8 | 12 | 1 | 3 | 5 | 11 | 11 | 11 | 11 |
| 50–64 | 1 | 5.0 | 0 | 5 | 5 | 5 | 5 | 5 | 5 | 5 |
| 65+ | 3 | 15.8 | 10 | 13 | 13 | 14 | 20 | 20 | 20 | 20 |
| **2. MULTIPLE DX** | | | | | | | | | | |
| 0–19 Years | 16 | 7.1 | 66 | 1 | 1 | 4 | 10 | 22 | 28 | 28 |
| 20–34 | 66 | 6.4 | 37 | 2 | 3 | 5 | 7 | 11 | 18 | 33 |
| 35–49 | 119 | 6.7 | 31 | 2 | 3 | 5 | 8 | 13 | 18 | 28 |
| 50–64 | 57 | 10.5 | 83 | 2 | 5 | 7 | 14 | 19 | 31 | 41 |
| 65+ | 81 | 12.4 | 42 | 5 | 6 | 13 | 18 | 21 | 24 | 29 |
| **TOTAL SINGLE DX** | 23 | 8.7 | 34 | 2 | 4 | 8 | 13 | 18 | 20 | 20 |
| **TOTAL MULTIPLE DX** | 339 | 8.7 | 53 | 2 | 3 | 6 | 13 | 19 | 23 | 33 |
| **TOTAL** | | | | | | | | | | |
| 0–19 Years | 18 | 6.8 | 63 | 1 | 1 | 4 | 10 | 22 | 28 | 28 |
| 20–34 | 75 | 6.9 | 38 | 2 | 3 | 5 | 8 | 15 | 18 | 33 |
| 35–49 | 127 | 6.6 | 29 | 2 | 3 | 5 | 8 | 13 | 18 | 28 |
| 50–64 | 58 | 10.4 | 82 | 2 | 5 | 7 | 14 | 19 | 31 | 41 |
| 65+ | 84 | 12.6 | 40 | 5 | 6 | 13 | 18 | 21 | 23 | 29 |
| **GRAND TOTAL** | 362 | 8.7 | 52 | 2 | 4 | 6 | 13 | 19 | 22 | 33 |

## 94.19: PSYCH INTERVIEW/EVAL NEC. Formerly included in operation group(s) 792.

| Type of Patients | Observed Patients | Avg. Stay | Vari-ance | 10th | 25th | 50th | 75th | 90th | 95th | 99th |
|---|---|---|---|---|---|---|---|---|---|---|
| **1. SINGLE DX** | | | | | | | | | | |
| 0–19 Years | 55 | 6.5 | 36 | 2 | 3 | 5 | 7 | 12 | 23 | 28 |
| 20–34 | 48 | 3.0 | 11 | 1 | 1 | 2 | 3 | 7 | 7 | 19 |
| 35–49 | 55 | 3.1 | 60 | 1 | 1 | 2 | 2 | 4 | 6 | 62 |
| 50–64 | 9 | 4.1 | 30 | 1 | 1 | 1 | 5 | 14 | 14 | 20 |
| 65+ | 3 | 2.1 | 2 | 1 | 1 | 1 | 4 | 4 | 4 | 4 |
| **2. MULTIPLE DX** | | | | | | | | | | |
| 0–19 Years | 273 | 10.3 | 99 | 2 | 4 | 8 | 11 | 19 | 29 | 56 |
| 20–34 | 102 | 5.8 | 29 | 1 | 3 | 4 | 7 | 13 | 17 | 36 |
| 35–49 | 168 | 7.6 | 68 | 1 | 3 | 5 | 9 | 15 | 20 | 53 |
| 50–64 | 82 | 8.4 | 36 | 2 | 4 | 7 | 12 | 15 | 17 | 40 |
| 65+ | 83 | 8.5 | 104 | 1 | 2 | 6 | 10 | 16 | 27 | 52 |
| **TOTAL SINGLE DX** | 170 | 4.5 | 39 | 1 | 1 | 2 | 5 | 8 | 15 | 28 |
| **TOTAL MULTIPLE DX** | 708 | 8.5 | 76 | 2 | 3 | 6 | 10 | 16 | 23 | 53 |
| **TOTAL** | | | | | | | | | | |
| 0–19 Years | 328 | 9.5 | 88 | 2 | 4 | 7 | 11 | 18 | 28 | 56 |
| 20–34 | 150 | 5.0 | 26 | 1 | 2 | 3 | 6 | 12 | 16 | 36 |
| 35–49 | 223 | 6.7 | 70 | 1 | 2 | 5 | 8 | 14 | 20 | 53 |
| 50–64 | 91 | 8.0 | 37 | 2 | 4 | 6 | 12 | 15 | 17 | 40 |
| 65+ | 86 | 8.4 | 103 | 1 | 2 | 6 | 10 | 16 | 27 | 52 |
| **GRAND TOTAL** | 878 | 7.7 | 71 | 1 | 3 | 5 | 10 | 15 | 21 | 53 |

## 94.1: PSYCH EVAL/CONSULT. Formerly included in operation group(s) 792.

| Type of Patients | Observed Patients | Avg. Stay | Vari-ance | 10th | 25th | 50th | 75th | 90th | 95th | 99th |
|---|---|---|---|---|---|---|---|---|---|---|
| **1. SINGLE DX** | | | | | | | | | | |
| 0–19 Years | 76 | 5.9 | 36 | 1 | 2 | 4 | 7 | 12 | 23 | 28 |
| 20–34 | 90 | 7.3 | 171 | 1 | 2 | 4 | 8 | 14 | 20 | 84 |
| 35–49 | 91 | 4.4 | 50 | 1 | 1 | 2 | 5 | 11 | 12 | 62 |
| 50–64 | 16 | 4.9 | 24 | 1 | 1 | 5 | 7 | 14 | 14 | 20 |
| 65+ | 7 | 12.3 | 46 | 1 | 4 | 14 | 20 | 20 | 20 | 20 |
| **2. MULTIPLE DX** | | | | | | | | | | |
| 0–19 Years | 355 | 8.8 | 82 | 2 | 3 | 6 | 11 | 18 | 27 | 56 |
| 20–34 | 306 | 8.0 | 111 | 1 | 3 | 5 | 8 | 16 | 33 | 55 |
| 35–49 | 470 | 7.7 | 54 | 2 | 3 | 5 | 10 | 16 | 21 | 35 |
| 50–64 | 199 | 11.4 | 165 | 2 | 4 | 8 | 14 | 20 | 31 | 82 |
| 65+ | 205 | 11.6 | 85 | 2 | 5 | 10 | 16 | 23 | 27 | 52 |
| **TOTAL SINGLE DX** | 280 | 6.1 | 84 | 1 | 2 | 4 | 7 | 14 | 20 | 62 |
| **TOTAL MULTIPLE DX** | 1,535 | 9.1 | 93 | 2 | 3 | 6 | 11 | 19 | 27 | 55 |
| **TOTAL** | | | | | | | | | | |
| 0–19 Years | 431 | 8.3 | 75 | 3 | 3 | 6 | 10 | 17 | 26 | 51 |
| 20–34 | 396 | 7.8 | 123 | 1 | 3 | 5 | 8 | 16 | 28 | 66 |
| 35–49 | 561 | 7.3 | 54 | 1 | 3 | 5 | 10 | 16 | 21 | 35 |
| 50–64 | 215 | 11.0 | 160 | 2 | 4 | 7 | 13 | 20 | 31 | 82 |
| 65+ | 212 | 11.6 | 83 | 2 | 5 | 10 | 16 | 21 | 27 | 52 |
| **GRAND TOTAL** | 1,815 | 8.7 | 93 | 1 | 3 | 6 | 11 | 18 | 26 | 56 |

## 94.11: PSYCH MENTAL STATUS. Formerly included in operation group(s) 792.

| Type of Patients | Observed Patients | Avg. Stay | Vari-ance | 10th | 25th | 50th | 75th | 90th | 95th | 99th |
|---|---|---|---|---|---|---|---|---|---|---|
| **1. SINGLE DX** | | | | | | | | | | |
| 0–19 Years | 16 | 4.6 | 37 | 1 | 1 | 2 | 7 | 7 | 19 | 26 |
| 20–34 | 29 | 12.8 | 534 | 1 | 3 | 4 | 11 | 25 | 84 | 84 |
| 35–49 | 26 | 6.5 | 66 | 1 | 2 | 2 | 12 | 25 | 39 | >99 |
| 50–64 | 5 | 6.4 | 22 | 1 | 5 | 7 | 7 | 7 | 18 | 18 |
| 65+ | 1 | 1.0 | 0 | 1 | 1 | 1 | 1 | 1 | 1 | 1 |
| **2. MULTIPLE DX** | | | | | | | | | | |
| 0–19 Years | 57 | 7.4 | 53 | 2 | 3 | 5 | 8 | 15 | 20 | 38 |
| 20–34 | 94 | 11.3 | 241 | 2 | 3 | 5 | 12 | 34 | 55 | 66 |
| 35–49 | 132 | 8.6 | 59 | 2 | 3 | 6 | 11 | 21 | 25 | 35 |
| 50–64 | 45 | 17.8 | 491 | 2 | 4 | 10 | 20 | 69 | 82 | 82 |
| 65+ | 30 | 18.1 | 182 | 6 | 8 | 15 | 27 | 42 | 64 | >99 |
| **TOTAL SINGLE DX** | 77 | 8.3 | 247 | 1 | 1 | 4 | 8 | 18 | 26 | 84 |
| **TOTAL MULTIPLE DX** | 358 | 10.2 | 158 | 2 | 3 | 6 | 12 | 24 | 35 | 69 |
| **TOTAL** | | | | | | | | | | |
| 0–19 Years | 73 | 7.0 | 52 | 1 | 3 | 5 | 8 | 15 | 20 | 38 |
| 20–34 | 123 | 11.5 | 288 | 1 | 3 | 5 | 11 | 34 | 55 | 84 |
| 35–49 | 158 | 8.4 | 60 | 1 | 3 | 6 | 11 | 21 | 26 | 35 |
| 50–64 | 50 | 17.1 | 469 | 2 | 4 | 10 | 20 | 69 | 82 | 82 |
| 65+ | 31 | 17.5 | 185 | 2 | 7 | 14 | 27 | 42 | 64 | >99 |
| **GRAND TOTAL** | 435 | 10.0 | 167 | 1 | 3 | 6 | 12 | 23 | 35 | 82 |

Length of Stay by Diagnosis and Operation, United States, 2000

# United States, October 1998–September 1999 Data, by Operation

## 94.2: PSYCH SOMATOTHERAPY. Formerly included in operation group(s) 792.

| Type of Patients | Observed Patients | Avg. Stay | Vari-ance | Percentiles | | | | | | |
|---|---|---|---|---|---|---|---|---|---|---|
| | | | | 10th | 25th | 50th | 75th | 90th | 95th | 99th |
| **1. SINGLE DX** | | | | | | | | | | |
| 0–19 Years | 216 | 12.6 | 161 | 3 | 5 | 10 | 17 | 23 | 44 | >99 |
| 20–34 | 550 | 14.1 | 175 | 2 | 4 | 10 | 20 | 30 | 40 | 85 |
| 35–49 | 761 | 14.1 | 141 | 2 | 6 | 12 | 17 | 27 | 36 | 69 |
| 50–64 | 281 | 14.8 | 140 | 3 | 5 | 14 | 21 | 26 | 38 | 60 |
| 65+ | 215 | 17.8 | 129 | 4 | 11 | 16 | 21 | 31 | 38 | 65 |
| **2. MULTIPLE DX** | | | | | | | | | | |
| 0–19 Years | 1,055 | 12.1 | 172 | 3 | 5 | 8 | 15 | 29 | 53 | >99 |
| 20–34 | 2,804 | 13.1 | 151 | 3 | 5 | 9 | 18 | 27 | 35 | 70 |
| 35–49 | 4,859 | 13.7 | 147 | 3 | 6 | 10 | 18 | 29 | 36 | 62 |
| 50–64 | 2,359 | 17.1 | 220 | 4 | 7 | 13 | 22 | 35 | 45 | 80 |
| 65+ | 3,008 | 20.3 | 172 | 7 | 12 | 18 | 26 | 36 | 44 | 72 |
| **TOTAL SINGLE DX** | 2,023 | 14.5 | 152 | 3 | 6 | 13 | 20 | 29 | 39 | 71 |
| **TOTAL MULTIPLE DX** | 14,085 | 15.8 | 178 | 3 | 7 | 13 | 21 | 32 | 41 | 73 |
| **TOTAL** | | | | | | | | | | |
| 0–19 Years | 1,271 | 12.2 | 169 | 3 | 5 | 8 | 16 | 28 | 52 | >99 |
| 20–34 | 3,354 | 13.3 | 155 | 2 | 5 | 9 | 18 | 28 | 36 | 71 |
| 35–49 | 5,620 | 13.7 | 146 | 3 | 6 | 10 | 18 | 29 | 36 | 63 |
| 50–64 | 2,640 | 16.8 | 211 | 3 | 7 | 14 | 22 | 34 | 44 | 79 |
| 65+ | 3,223 | 20.2 | 169 | 7 | 12 | 18 | 26 | 36 | 44 | 70 |
| **GRAND TOTAL** | 16,108 | 15.6 | 175 | 3 | 6 | 13 | 21 | 32 | 41 | 72 |

## 94.22: LITHIUM THERAPY. Formerly included in operation group(s) 792.

| Type of Patients | Observed Patients | Avg. Stay | Vari-ance | Percentiles | | | | | | |
|---|---|---|---|---|---|---|---|---|---|---|
| | | | | 10th | 25th | 50th | 75th | 90th | 95th | 99th |
| **1. SINGLE DX** | | | | | | | | | | |
| 0–19 Years | 4 | 11.5 | 32 | 6 | 6 | 12 | 18 | 18 | 18 | 18 |
| 20–34 | 18 | 14.2 | 102 | 3 | 6 | 16 | 23 | 30 | 31 | 31 |
| 35–49 | 27 | 11.0 | 81 | 1 | 7 | 10 | 13 | 14 | 34 | 55 |
| 50–64 | 6 | 16.9 | 221 | 6 | 9 | 11 | 21 | 49 | 49 | 49 |
| 65+ | 0 | | | | | | | | | |
| **2. MULTIPLE DX** | | | | | | | | | | |
| 0–19 Years | 35 | 11.1 | 45 | 4 | 6 | 10 | 13 | 21 | 21 | 36 |
| 20–34 | 103 | 13.8 | 228 | 3 | 5 | 10 | 16 | 29 | 40 | 84 |
| 35–49 | 158 | 12.2 | 155 | 3 | 5 | 9 | 14 | 28 | 36 | 61 |
| 50–64 | 79 | 14.7 | 97 | 5 | 7 | 13 | 17 | 26 | 39 | 54 |
| 65+ | 21 | 16.2 | 141 | 6 | 7 | 12 | 26 | 35 | 43 | >99 |
| **TOTAL SINGLE DX** | 55 | 12.3 | 90 | 3 | 6 | 10 | 16 | 23 | 31 | 49 |
| **TOTAL MULTIPLE DX** | 396 | 13.2 | 157 | 3 | 6 | 10 | 16 | 28 | 39 | 71 |
| **TOTAL** | | | | | | | | | | |
| 0–19 Years | 39 | 11.2 | 42 | 4 | 6 | 11 | 13 | 21 | 21 | 36 |
| 20–34 | 121 | 13.8 | 210 | 3 | 5 | 10 | 17 | 29 | 40 | 84 |
| 35–49 | 185 | 12.0 | 142 | 3 | 5 | 9 | 14 | 24 | 35 | 61 |
| 50–64 | 85 | 14.8 | 102 | 5 | 9 | 12 | 17 | 26 | 39 | 54 |
| 65+ | 21 | 16.2 | 141 | 6 | 7 | 12 | 26 | 35 | 43 | >99 |
| **GRAND TOTAL** | 451 | 13.1 | 148 | 3 | 6 | 10 | 16 | 28 | 36 | 61 |

## 94.23: NEUROLEPTIC THERAPY. Formerly included in operation group(s) 792.

| Type of Patients | Observed Patients | Avg. Stay | Vari-ance | Percentiles | | | | | | |
|---|---|---|---|---|---|---|---|---|---|---|
| | | | | 10th | 25th | 50th | 75th | 90th | 95th | 99th |
| **1. SINGLE DX** | | | | | | | | | | |
| 0–19 Years | 53 | 12.1 | 116 | 3 | 6 | 8 | 14 | 29 | 41 | >99 |
| 20–34 | 134 | 19.1 | 318 | 2 | 7 | 14 | 24 | 39 | 58 | 92 |
| 35–49 | 152 | 18.4 | 258 | 2 | 7 | 14 | 25 | 37 | 59 | 71 |
| 50–64 | 48 | 26.3 | 456 | 6 | 11 | 20 | 38 | 42 | 71 | 98 |
| 65+ | 2 | 19.6 | 27 | 16 | 16 | 16 | 25 | 25 | 25 | 25 |
| **2. MULTIPLE DX** | | | | | | | | | | |
| 0–19 Years | 137 | 13.2 | 203 | 3 | 4 | 6 | 17 | 44 | 68 | >99 |
| 20–34 | 346 | 18.0 | 309 | 3 | 6 | 13 | 23 | 47 | 69 | 95 |
| 35–49 | 518 | 17.5 | 315 | 2 | 6 | 12 | 23 | 40 | 62 | 95 |
| 50–64 | 178 | 21.2 | 391 | 5 | 8 | 13 | 29 | 53 | 67 | 96 |
| 65+ | 62 | 27.8 | 570 | 6 | 10 | 20 | 42 | 71 | 78 | 98 |
| **TOTAL SINGLE DX** | 389 | 18.8 | 293 | 4 | 7 | 14 | 25 | 40 | 59 | 96 |
| **TOTAL MULTIPLE DX** | 1,241 | 18.5 | 341 | 3 | 6 | 12 | 24 | 47 | 67 | >99 |
| **TOTAL** | | | | | | | | | | |
| 0–19 Years | 190 | 12.9 | 179 | 3 | 5 | 8 | 16 | 41 | 56 | >99 |
| 20–34 | 480 | 18.3 | 311 | 3 | 6 | 13 | 23 | 44 | 69 | >99 |
| 35–49 | 670 | 17.7 | 301 | 2 | 6 | 13 | 24 | 39 | 62 | 95 |
| 50–64 | 226 | 22.2 | 406 | 5 | 8 | 15 | 31 | 52 | 67 | 96 |
| 65+ | 64 | 27.5 | 556 | 6 | 10 | 20 | 40 | 62 | 78 | 98 |
| **GRAND TOTAL** | 1,630 | 18.5 | 330 | 3 | 6 | 13 | 24 | 44 | 64 | >99 |

## 94.25: PSYCH DRUG THERAPY NEC. Formerly included in operation group(s) 792.

| Type of Patients | Observed Patients | Avg. Stay | Vari-ance | Percentiles | | | | | | |
|---|---|---|---|---|---|---|---|---|---|---|
| | | | | 10th | 25th | 50th | 75th | 90th | 95th | 99th |
| **1. SINGLE DX** | | | | | | | | | | |
| 0–19 Years | 143 | 12.5 | 193 | 2 | 4 | 9 | 16 | 27 | 62 | >99 |
| 20–34 | 265 | 12.7 | 174 | 2 | 4 | 9 | 16 | 30 | 40 | >99 |
| 35–49 | 313 | 14.8 | 193 | 3 | 6 | 11 | 19 | 30 | 46 | 70 |
| 50–64 | 95 | 15.0 | 149 | 3 | 4 | 13 | 20 | 32 | 45 | 60 |
| 65+ | 49 | 17.2 | 272 | 2 | 7 | 13 | 21 | 33 | 65 | 70 |
| **2. MULTIPLE DX** | | | | | | | | | | |
| 0–19 Years | 802 | 11.4 | 153 | 3 | 4 | 7 | 14 | 27 | 52 | >99 |
| 20–34 | 1,607 | 10.9 | 146 | 2 | 4 | 7 | 13 | 24 | 34 | 69 |
| 35–49 | 2,370 | 11.1 | 137 | 2 | 4 | 7 | 14 | 25 | 32 | 69 |
| 50–64 | 908 | 12.6 | 142 | 3 | 5 | 9 | 16 | 27 | 35 | 71 |
| 65+ | 613 | 14.9 | 128 | 4 | 7 | 12 | 19 | 28 | 37 | 62 |
| **TOTAL SINGLE DX** | 865 | 13.8 | 189 | 2 | 5 | 10 | 18 | 30 | 45 | >99 |
| **TOTAL MULTIPLE DX** | 6,300 | 11.8 | 143 | 2 | 5 | 8 | 15 | 26 | 35 | 74 |
| **TOTAL** | | | | | | | | | | |
| 0–19 Years | 945 | 11.6 | 163 | 3 | 4 | 8 | 14 | 27 | 52 | >99 |
| 20–34 | 1,872 | 11.1 | 151 | 2 | 4 | 7 | 14 | 25 | 36 | 71 |
| 35–49 | 2,683 | 11.5 | 145 | 2 | 4 | 8 | 14 | 25 | 34 | 70 |
| 50–64 | 1,003 | 12.9 | 144 | 3 | 5 | 9 | 16 | 27 | 35 | 70 |
| 65+ | 662 | 15.0 | 137 | 4 | 7 | 13 | 19 | 29 | 37 | 62 |
| **GRAND TOTAL** | 7,165 | 12.1 | 149 | 2 | 5 | 8 | 15 | 26 | 37 | 79 |

Length of Stay by Diagnosis and Operation, United States, 2000

# United States, October 1998–September 1999 Data, by Operation

## 94.27: ELECTROSHOCK THERAPY NEC. Formerly included in operation group(s) 792.

| Type of Patients | Observed Patients | Avg. Stay | Vari-ance | Percentiles | | | | | | |
|---|---|---|---|---|---|---|---|---|---|---|
| | | | | 10th | 25th | 50th | 75th | 90th | 95th | 99th |
| **1. SINGLE DX** | | | | | | | | | | |
| 0–19 Years | 11 | 14.1 | 27 | 4 | 10 | 17 | 17 | 21 | 21 | 25 |
| 20–34 | 127 | 14.1 | 128 | 2 | 4 | 12 | 22 | 28 | 36 | 46 |
| 35–49 | 261 | 12.7 | 72 | 3 | 7 | 12 | 15 | 23 | 31 | 40 |
| 50–64 | 130 | 13.5 | 91 | 3 | 5 | 14 | 21 | 24 | 27 | 46 |
| 65+ | 162 | 17.9 | 104 | 5 | 11 | 16 | 21 | 31 | 38 | 50 |
| **2. MULTIPLE DX** | | | | | | | | | | |
| 0–19 Years | 40 | 23.6 | 400 | 6 | 7 | 19 | 30 | 66 | 66 | >99 |
| 20–34 | 717 | 15.2 | 103 | 3 | 7 | 14 | 22 | 29 | 34 | 47 |
| 35–49 | 1,745 | 15.5 | 127 | 4 | 8 | 13 | 21 | 32 | 36 | 51 |
| 50–64 | 1,172 | 19.4 | 238 | 5 | 13 | 16 | 25 | 37 | 47 | 82 |
| 65+ | 2,303 | 21.5 | 167 | 8 | 13 | 19 | 28 | 37 | 44 | 74 |
| **TOTAL SINGLE DX** | 691 | 14.4 | 97 | 3 | 7 | 14 | 20 | 27 | 33 | 46 |
| **TOTAL MULTIPLE DX** | 5,977 | 18.5 | 171 | 5 | 9 | 16 | 24 | 35 | 42 | 72 |
| **TOTAL** | | | | | | | | | | |
| 0–19 Years | 51 | 19.2 | 248 | 6 | 10 | 17 | 21 | 55 | 66 | >99 |
| 20–34 | 844 | 15.0 | 108 | 3 | 7 | 14 | 22 | 29 | 34 | 46 |
| 35–49 | 2,006 | 15.2 | 121 | 4 | 8 | 13 | 20 | 31 | 36 | 49 |
| 50–64 | 1,302 | 18.6 | 222 | 4 | 8 | 15 | 23 | 36 | 46 | 82 |
| 65+ | 2,465 | 21.3 | 163 | 8 | 13 | 19 | 27 | 36 | 44 | 69 |
| **GRAND TOTAL** | 6,668 | 18.0 | 164 | 4 | 9 | 15 | 24 | 34 | 41 | 72 |

## 94.3: INDIVIDUAL PSYCHOTHERAPY. Formerly included in operation group(s) 792.

| Type of Patients | Observed Patients | Avg. Stay | Vari-ance | Percentiles | | | | | | |
|---|---|---|---|---|---|---|---|---|---|---|
| | | | | 10th | 25th | 50th | 75th | 90th | 95th | 99th |
| **1. SINGLE DX** | | | | | | | | | | |
| 0–19 Years | 244 | 6.1 | 12 | 2 | 4 | 6 | 7 | 10 | 12 | 17 |
| 20–34 | 208 | 7.5 | 54 | 2 | 3 | 6 | 10 | 18 | 19 | 33 |
| 35–49 | 251 | 7.8 | 40 | 2 | 4 | 6 | 10 | 16 | 21 | 26 |
| 50–64 | 86 | 8.7 | 54 | 2 | 4 | 7 | 10 | 19 | 29 | 30 |
| 65+ | 13 | 8.6 | 14 | 4 | 5 | 8 | 13 | 14 | 15 | 15 |
| **2. MULTIPLE DX** | | | | | | | | | | |
| 0–19 Years | 1,315 | 6.8 | 21 | 3 | 4 | 6 | 8 | 10 | 14 | 27 |
| 20–34 | 1,222 | 6.1 | 35 | 1 | 3 | 4 | 7 | 13 | 17 | 30 |
| 35–49 | 1,726 | 7.2 | 49 | 2 | 3 | 5 | 9 | 14 | 21 | 35 |
| 50–64 | 627 | 9.4 | 62 | 3 | 5 | 7 | 12 | 18 | 28 | 35 |
| 65+ | 1,240 | 9.8 | 60 | 3 | 5 | 7 | 12 | 19 | 26 | 35 |
| **TOTAL SINGLE DX** | 802 | 7.1 | 33 | 2 | 4 | 6 | 9 | 14 | 18 | 29 |
| **TOTAL MULTIPLE DX** | 6,130 | 7.8 | 46 | 2 | 4 | 6 | 9 | 15 | 21 | 34 |
| **TOTAL** | | | | | | | | | | |
| 0–19 Years | 1,559 | 6.7 | 20 | 3 | 4 | 6 | 8 | 10 | 14 | 24 |
| 20–34 | 1,430 | 6.3 | 37 | 1 | 3 | 5 | 8 | 14 | 18 | 30 |
| 35–49 | 1,977 | 7.3 | 48 | 2 | 4 | 6 | 9 | 15 | 21 | 33 |
| 50–64 | 713 | 9.4 | 61 | 2 | 4 | 7 | 12 | 18 | 28 | 35 |
| 65+ | 1,253 | 9.8 | 60 | 3 | 5 | 7 | 12 | 19 | 26 | 35 |
| **GRAND TOTAL** | 6,932 | 7.7 | 44 | 2 | 4 | 6 | 9 | 15 | 20 | 33 |

## 94.35: CRISIS INTERVENTION. Formerly included in operation group(s) 792.

| Type of Patients | Observed Patients | Avg. Stay | Vari-ance | Percentiles | | | | | | |
|---|---|---|---|---|---|---|---|---|---|---|
| | | | | 10th | 25th | 50th | 75th | 90th | 95th | 99th |
| **1. SINGLE DX** | | | | | | | | | | |
| 0–19 Years | 3 | 7.9 | 12 | 2 | 5 | 10 | 10 | 10 | 10 | 10 |
| 20–34 | 41 | 7.1 | 100 | 2 | 3 | 5 | 7 | 8 | 23 | 61 |
| 35–49 | 79 | 5.8 | 21 | 2 | 3 | 4 | 7 | 13 | 15 | 22 |
| 50–64 | 42 | 6.4 | 15 | 2 | 4 | 6 | 8 | 10 | 13 | 26 |
| 65+ | 0 | | | | | | | | | |
| **2. MULTIPLE DX** | | | | | | | | | | |
| 0–19 Years | 22 | 4.8 | 38 | 2 | 2 | 2 | 6 | 11 | 20 | 34 |
| 20–34 | 222 | 6.4 | 28 | 1 | 3 | 5 | 9 | 13 | 15 | 30 |
| 35–49 | 325 | 7.3 | 40 | 2 | 4 | 6 | 8 | 12 | 16 | 40 |
| 50–64 | 147 | 10.7 | 69 | 2 | 5 | 8 | 15 | 19 | 35 | 35 |
| 65+ | 675 | 9.3 | 54 | 3 | 5 | 7 | 11 | 18 | 24 | 34 |
| **TOTAL SINGLE DX** | 165 | 6.3 | 40 | 2 | 3 | 5 | 8 | 10 | 15 | 23 |
| **TOTAL MULTIPLE DX** | 1,391 | 8.7 | 52 | 2 | 4 | 7 | 11 | 17 | 23 | 35 |
| **TOTAL** | | | | | | | | | | |
| 0–19 Years | 25 | 5.6 | 33 | 2 | 2 | 2 | 10 | 10 | 15 | 34 |
| 20–34 | 263 | 6.5 | 38 | 1 | 3 | 5 | 8 | 13 | 15 | 31 |
| 35–49 | 404 | 7.0 | 37 | 2 | 3 | 6 | 8 | 12 | 16 | 35 |
| 50–64 | 189 | 10.1 | 64 | 2 | 5 | 7 | 15 | 19 | 29 | 35 |
| 65+ | 675 | 9.3 | 54 | 3 | 5 | 7 | 11 | 18 | 24 | 34 |
| **GRAND TOTAL** | 1,556 | 8.6 | 51 | 2 | 4 | 7 | 11 | 17 | 23 | 35 |

## 94.38: SUPP VERBAL PSYCHTX. Formerly included in operation group(s) 792.

| Type of Patients | Observed Patients | Avg. Stay | Vari-ance | Percentiles | | | | | | |
|---|---|---|---|---|---|---|---|---|---|---|
| | | | | 10th | 25th | 50th | 75th | 90th | 95th | 99th |
| **1. SINGLE DX** | | | | | | | | | | |
| 0–19 Years | 10 | 7.4 | 107 | 1 | 4 | 5 | 6 | 24 | 46 | 46 |
| 20–34 | 15 | 11.8 | 67 | 2 | 7 | 10 | 18 | 22 | 33 | 33 |
| 35–49 | 12 | 9.7 | 127 | 3 | 3 | 7 | 9 | 14 | 49 | 49 |
| 50–64 | 5 | 20.8 | 110 | 7 | 15 | 15 | 30 | 30 | 35 | 35 |
| 65+ | 0 | | | | | | | | | |
| **2. MULTIPLE DX** | | | | | | | | | | |
| 0–19 Years | 143 | 6.7 | 36 | 2 | 3 | 6 | 8 | 11 | 15 | 30 |
| 20–34 | 192 | 9.4 | 71 | 2 | 3 | 7 | 14 | 21 | 27 | 51 |
| 35–49 | 204 | 10.5 | 117 | 3 | 5 | 8 | 13 | 18 | 22 | 75 |
| 50–64 | 53 | 10.2 | 66 | 3 | 5 | 7 | 13 | 20 | 32 | 41 |
| 65+ | 83 | 14.6 | 102 | 4 | 7 | 13 | 18 | 33 | 33 | 40 |
| **TOTAL SINGLE DX** | 42 | 11.8 | 119 | 3 | 5 | 8 | 15 | 30 | 33 | 49 |
| **TOTAL MULTIPLE DX** | 675 | 10.2 | 91 | 3 | 4 | 7 | 14 | 20 | 28 | 58 |
| **TOTAL** | | | | | | | | | | |
| 0–19 Years | 153 | 6.8 | 39 | 2 | 3 | 6 | 8 | 11 | 15 | 32 |
| 20–34 | 207 | 9.5 | 71 | 2 | 4 | 7 | 14 | 21 | 27 | 51 |
| 35–49 | 216 | 10.4 | 117 | 3 | 5 | 8 | 13 | 18 | 22 | 75 |
| 50–64 | 58 | 11.2 | 79 | 3 | 6 | 7 | 15 | 22 | 32 | 39 |
| 65+ | 83 | 14.6 | 102 | 4 | 7 | 13 | 18 | 33 | 33 | 40 |
| **GRAND TOTAL** | 717 | 10.2 | 92 | 3 | 4 | 7 | 14 | 20 | 29 | 55 |

Length of Stay by Diagnosis and Operation, United States, 2000

# United States, October 1998–September 1999 Data, by Operation

## 94.39: INDIVIDUAL PSYCHTX NEC. Formerly included in operation group(s) 792.

| Type of Patients | Observed Patients | Avg. Stay | Vari-ance | Percentiles | | | | | | |
|---|---|---|---|---|---|---|---|---|---|---|
| | | | | 10th | 25th | 50th | 75th | 90th | 95th | 99th |
| **1. SINGLE DX** | | | | | | | | | | |
| 0–19 Years | 230 | 6.1 | 11 | 2 | 4 | 6 | 7 | 9 | 12 | 15 |
| 20–34 | 149 | 7.4 | 39 | 3 | 3 | 6 | 10 | 18 | 18 | 29 |
| 35–49 | 159 | 8.8 | 41 | 3 | 4 | 7 | 12 | 17 | 22 | 27 |
| 50–64 | 39 | 9.7 | 64 | 2 | 4 | 7 | 13 | 23 | 28 | 29 |
| 65+ | 13 | 8.6 | 14 | 4 | 5 | 8 | 13 | 14 | 15 | 15 |
| **2. MULTIPLE DX** | | | | | | | | | | |
| 0–19 Years | 1,126 | 6.8 | 19 | 3 | 4 | 6 | 8 | 10 | 14 | 23 |
| 20–34 | 796 | 5.4 | 27 | 3 | 3 | 4 | 7 | 10 | 14 | 27 |
| 35–49 | 1,190 | 6.7 | 38 | 2 | 3 | 5 | 8 | 14 | 21 | 30 |
| 50–64 | 425 | 8.6 | 55 | 2 | 4 | 7 | 11 | 17 | 23 | 29 |
| 65+ | 474 | 10.5 | 64 | 3 | 5 | 8 | 14 | 24 | 28 | 36 |
| **TOTAL SINGLE DX** | 590 | 7.1 | 27 | 2 | 4 | 6 | 9 | 14 | 18 | 28 |
| **TOTAL MULTIPLE DX** | 4,011 | 7.0 | 35 | 2 | 3 | 6 | 8 | 13 | 18 | 30 |
| **TOTAL** | | | | | | | | | | |
| 0–19 Years | 1,356 | 6.7 | 18 | 3 | 4 | 6 | 8 | 10 | 14 | 22 |
| 20–34 | 945 | 5.7 | 29 | 2 | 3 | 4 | 7 | 11 | 14 | 27 |
| 35–49 | 1,349 | 6.9 | 39 | 2 | 3 | 5 | 8 | 15 | 21 | 30 |
| 50–64 | 464 | 8.7 | 56 | 3 | 4 | 7 | 11 | 17 | 24 | 29 |
| 65+ | 487 | 10.5 | 63 | 3 | 5 | 8 | 14 | 23 | 28 | 36 |
| **GRAND TOTAL** | 4,601 | 7.0 | 34 | 2 | 4 | 6 | 8 | 13 | 18 | 30 |

## 94.44: OTHER GROUP THERAPY. Formerly included in operation group(s) 792.

| Type of Patients | Observed Patients | Avg. Stay | Vari-ance | Percentiles | | | | | | |
|---|---|---|---|---|---|---|---|---|---|---|
| | | | | 10th | 25th | 50th | 75th | 90th | 95th | 99th |
| **1. SINGLE DX** | | | | | | | | | | |
| 0–19 Years | 48 | 6.3 | 17 | 1 | 3 | 6 | 8 | 11 | 14 | 23 |
| 20–34 | 124 | 10.4 | 144 | 2 | 4 | 7 | 12 | 21 | 30 | 67 |
| 35–49 | 162 | 9.5 | 95 | 3 | 4 | 7 | 11 | 20 | 26 | 64 |
| 50–64 | 52 | 11.1 | 174 | 3 | 5 | 7 | 12 | 33 | 39 | 70 |
| 65+ | 21 | 12.5 | 67 | 2 | 7 | 8 | 19 | 26 | 28 | 29 |
| **2. MULTIPLE DX** | | | | | | | | | | |
| 0–19 Years | 417 | 9.3 | 91 | 2 | 4 | 6 | 12 | 17 | 28 | 45 |
| 20–34 | 862 | 7.0 | 59 | 2 | 3 | 5 | 8 | 13 | 17 | 44 |
| 35–49 | 1,348 | 7.5 | 44 | 2 | 4 | 6 | 9 | 14 | 19 | 40 |
| 50–64 | 577 | 9.4 | 57 | 3 | 4 | 7 | 12 | 18 | 26 | 38 |
| 65+ | 576 | 13.2 | 64 | 4 | 7 | 12 | 17 | 23 | 27 | 42 |
| **TOTAL SINGLE DX** | 407 | 9.6 | 103 | 3 | 4 | 7 | 11 | 19 | 30 | 67 |
| **TOTAL MULTIPLE DX** | 3,780 | 8.6 | 63 | 3 | 4 | 6 | 11 | 17 | 23 | 43 |
| **TOTAL** | | | | | | | | | | |
| 0–19 Years | 465 | 9.1 | 86 | 2 | 4 | 6 | 11 | 17 | 26 | 43 |
| 20–34 | 986 | 7.3 | 69 | 2 | 3 | 5 | 8 | 14 | 19 | 48 |
| 35–49 | 1,510 | 7.7 | 47 | 2 | 4 | 6 | 9 | 14 | 20 | 41 |
| 50–64 | 629 | 9.5 | 66 | 3 | 4 | 7 | 12 | 18 | 27 | 40 |
| 65+ | 597 | 13.1 | 64 | 4 | 7 | 12 | 17 | 23 | 28 | 42 |
| **GRAND TOTAL** | 4,187 | 8.7 | 66 | 3 | 4 | 6 | 11 | 17 | 23 | 44 |

## 94.4: OTH PSYCHTX/COUNSELLING. Formerly included in operation group(s) 792.

| Type of Patients | Observed Patients | Avg. Stay | Vari-ance | Percentiles | | | | | | |
|---|---|---|---|---|---|---|---|---|---|---|
| | | | | 10th | 25th | 50th | 75th | 90th | 95th | 99th |
| **1. SINGLE DX** | | | | | | | | | | |
| 0–19 Years | 63 | 6.3 | 17 | 1 | 3 | 6 | 9 | 11 | 14 | 23 |
| 20–34 | 146 | 10.1 | 133 | 2 | 4 | 7 | 12 | 19 | 30 | 67 |
| 35–49 | 183 | 10.1 | 90 | 3 | 5 | 7 | 12 | 21 | 31 | 64 |
| 50–64 | 61 | 11.6 | 168 | 3 | 5 | 8 | 12 | 29 | 39 | 70 |
| 65+ | 23 | 13.8 | 71 | 2 | 7 | 13 | 22 | 24 | 28 | 29 |
| **2. MULTIPLE DX** | | | | | | | | | | |
| 0–19 Years | 509 | 9.3 | 88 | 2 | 4 | 6 | 8 | 18 | 27 | 45 |
| 20–34 | 973 | 7.1 | 64 | 2 | 3 | 5 | 7 | 13 | 19 | 46 |
| 35–49 | 1,489 | 7.5 | 47 | 2 | 4 | 6 | 8 | 14 | 19 | 40 |
| 50–64 | 629 | 9.8 | 69 | 3 | 4 | 7 | 11 | 19 | 27 | 40 |
| 65+ | 637 | 13.5 | 67 | 4 | 7 | 13 | 18 | 24 | 28 | 44 |
| **TOTAL SINGLE DX** | 476 | 9.9 | 104 | 2 | 4 | 7 | 12 | 20 | 30 | 66 |
| **TOTAL MULTIPLE DX** | 4,237 | 8.7 | 67 | 2 | 4 | 6 | 11 | 17 | 24 | 43 |
| **TOTAL** | | | | | | | | | | |
| 0–19 Years | 572 | 9.1 | 83 | 2 | 4 | 6 | 12 | 17 | 26 | 43 |
| 20–34 | 1,119 | 7.4 | 72 | 2 | 3 | 5 | 8 | 14 | 21 | 48 |
| 35–49 | 1,672 | 7.7 | 52 | 2 | 4 | 6 | 9 | 15 | 20 | 41 |
| 50–64 | 690 | 9.9 | 77 | 3 | 4 | 7 | 12 | 19 | 29 | 42 |
| 65+ | 660 | 13.5 | 67 | 4 | 7 | 13 | 18 | 24 | 28 | 44 |
| **GRAND TOTAL** | 4,713 | 8.8 | 70 | 2 | 4 | 6 | 11 | 18 | 24 | 45 |

## 94.49: OTHER COUNSELLING. Formerly included in operation group(s) 792.

| Type of Patients | Observed Patients | Avg. Stay | Vari-ance | Percentiles | | | | | | |
|---|---|---|---|---|---|---|---|---|---|---|
| | | | | 10th | 25th | 50th | 75th | 90th | 95th | 99th |
| **1. SINGLE DX** | | | | | | | | | | |
| 0–19 Years | 6 | 6.2 | 25 | 2 | 3 | 3 | 12 | 13 | 13 | 13 |
| 20–34 | 19 | 7.2 | 41 | 1 | 2 | 7 | 11 | 13 | 14 | 32 |
| 35–49 | 18 | 19.6 | 224 | 5 | 7 | 14 | 32 | 42 | 51 | 51 |
| 50–64 | 9 | 16.7 | 79 | 11 | 11 | 15 | 15 | 29 | 41 | 41 |
| 65+ | 1 | 22.0 | 0 | 22 | 22 | 22 | 22 | 22 | 22 | 22 |
| **2. MULTIPLE DX** | | | | | | | | | | |
| 0–19 Years | 42 | 11.3 | 100 | 1 | 3 | 8 | 18 | 26 | 30 | 39 |
| 20–34 | 62 | 10.5 | 167 | 1 | 3 | 8 | 9 | 33 | 46 | 50 |
| 35–49 | 90 | 9.4 | 170 | 1 | 2 | 5 | 10 | 23 | 39 | 49 |
| 50–64 | 39 | 19.7 | 294 | 6 | 7 | 17 | 23 | 41 | 63 | 85 |
| 65+ | 59 | 18.1 | 88 | 6 | 14 | 18 | 22 | 28 | 39 | 50 |
| **TOTAL SINGLE DX** | 53 | 13.0 | 132 | 2 | 5 | 11 | 15 | 32 | 41 | 51 |
| **TOTAL MULTIPLE DX** | 292 | 13.4 | 172 | 2 | 4 | 9 | 19 | 29 | 39 | 50 |
| **TOTAL** | | | | | | | | | | |
| 0–19 Years | 48 | 10.7 | 93 | 1 | 2 | 8 | 17 | 26 | 30 | 39 |
| 20–34 | 81 | 9.6 | 134 | 1 | 3 | 6 | 10 | 29 | 46 | 49 |
| 35–49 | 108 | 11.1 | 192 | 1 | 3 | 6 | 12 | 32 | 41 | 51 |
| 50–64 | 48 | 19.1 | 251 | 6 | 10 | 15 | 23 | 41 | 42 | 85 |
| 65+ | 60 | 18.2 | 86 | 6 | 14 | 18 | 22 | 28 | 39 | 50 |
| **GRAND TOTAL** | 345 | 13.3 | 166 | 2 | 4 | 9 | 19 | 29 | 41 | 51 |

Length of Stay by Diagnosis and Operation, United States, 2000

## United States, October 1998–September 1999 Data, by Operation

### 94.5: REFFERAL PSYCH REHAB. Formerly included in operation group(s) 792.

| Type of Patients | Observed Patients | Avg. Stay | Vari-ance | 10th | 25th | 50th | 75th | 90th | 95th | 99th |
|---|---|---|---|---|---|---|---|---|---|---|
| **1. SINGLE DX** | | | | | | | | | | |
| 0–19 Years | 0 | | | | | | | | | |
| 20–34 | 0 | | | | | | | | | |
| 35–49 | 0 | | | | | | | | | |
| 50–64 | 0 | | | | | | | | | |
| 65+ | 0 | | | | | | | | | |
| **2. MULTIPLE DX** | | | | | | | | | | |
| 0–19 Years | 1 | 2.0 | 0 | 2 | 2 | 2 | 2 | 2 | 2 | 2 |
| 20–34 | 4 | 5.5 | 24 | 1 | 2 | 2 | 9 | 11 | 11 | 11 |
| 35–49 | 4 | 7.5 | 68 | 2 | 2 | 3 | 18 | 19 | 19 | 19 |
| 50–64 | 2 | 6.4 | 2 | 4 | 7 | 7 | 7 | 7 | 7 | 7 |
| 65+ | 1 | 3.0 | 0 | 3 | 3 | 3 | 3 | 3 | 3 | 3 |
| **TOTAL SINGLE DX** | 0 | | | | | | | | | |
| **TOTAL MULTIPLE DX** | 12 | 5.8 | 26 | 2 | 2 | 3 | 7 | 11 | 18 | 19 |
| **TOTAL** | | | | | | | | | | |
| 0–19 Years | 1 | 2.0 | 0 | 2 | 2 | 2 | 2 | 2 | 2 | 2 |
| 20–34 | 4 | 5.5 | 24 | 1 | 2 | 2 | 9 | 11 | 11 | 11 |
| 35–49 | 4 | 7.5 | 68 | 2 | 2 | 3 | 18 | 19 | 19 | 19 |
| 50–64 | 2 | 6.4 | 2 | 4 | 7 | 7 | 7 | 7 | 7 | 7 |
| 65+ | 1 | 3.0 | 0 | 3 | 3 | 3 | 3 | 3 | 3 | 3 |
| **GRAND TOTAL** | 12 | 5.8 | 26 | 2 | 2 | 3 | 7 | 11 | 18 | 19 |

### 94.6: ALCOHOL/DRUG REHAB/DETOX. Formerly included in operation group(s) 792.

| Type of Patients | Observed Patients | Avg. Stay | Vari-ance | 10th | 25th | 50th | 75th | 90th | 95th | 99th |
|---|---|---|---|---|---|---|---|---|---|---|
| **1. SINGLE DX** | | | | | | | | | | |
| 0–19 Years | 212 | 8.9 | 72 | 2 | 3 | 6 | 13 | 18 | 28 | 38 |
| 20–34 | 1,554 | 4.1 | 13 | 2 | 2 | 3 | 4 | 7 | 11 | 21 |
| 35–49 | 2,476 | 4.0 | 13 | 2 | 3 | 3 | 4 | 6 | 10 | 20 |
| 50–64 | 609 | 3.9 | 12 | 2 | 3 | 3 | 4 | 6 | 9 | 21 |
| 65+ | 100 | 5.4 | 18 | 2 | 3 | 4 | 7 | 10 | 14 | 28 |
| **2. MULTIPLE DX** | | | | | | | | | | |
| 0–19 Years | 1,671 | 9.3 | 74 | 2 | 3 | 6 | 13 | 22 | 30 | 41 |
| 20–34 | 18,837 | 5.6 | 28 | 2 | 3 | 4 | 6 | 12 | 17 | 28 |
| 35–49 | 38,386 | 5.4 | 22 | 2 | 3 | 4 | 6 | 11 | 15 | 25 |
| 50–64 | 11,385 | 5.5 | 20 | 2 | 3 | 4 | 6 | 10 | 14 | 22 |
| 65+ | 3,455 | 7.0 | 38 | 2 | 3 | 5 | 9 | 13 | 17 | 28 |
| **TOTAL SINGLE DX** | 4,951 | 4.3 | 16 | 2 | 2 | 3 | 4 | 7 | 12 | 22 |
| **TOTAL MULTIPLE DX** | 73,734 | 5.6 | 26 | 2 | 3 | 4 | 7 | 12 | 16 | 27 |
| **TOTAL** | | | | | | | | | | |
| 0–19 Years | 1,883 | 9.3 | 73 | 2 | 3 | 6 | 13 | 22 | 30 | 41 |
| 20–34 | 20,391 | 5.5 | 27 | 2 | 3 | 4 | 6 | 12 | 17 | 27 |
| 35–49 | 40,862 | 5.3 | 21 | 2 | 3 | 4 | 6 | 10 | 15 | 24 |
| 50–64 | 11,994 | 5.4 | 20 | 2 | 3 | 4 | 6 | 10 | 14 | 22 |
| 65+ | 3,555 | 6.9 | 38 | 2 | 3 | 5 | 9 | 13 | 17 | 28 |
| **GRAND TOTAL** | 78,685 | 5.5 | 25 | 2 | 3 | 4 | 6 | 11 | 16 | 27 |

### 94.61: ALCOHOL REHABILITATION. Formerly included in operation group(s) 792.

| Type of Patients | Observed Patients | Avg. Stay | Vari-ance | 10th | 25th | 50th | 75th | 90th | 95th | 99th |
|---|---|---|---|---|---|---|---|---|---|---|
| **1. SINGLE DX** | | | | | | | | | | |
| 0–19 Years | 6 | 19.7 | 93 | 5 | 14 | 28 | 28 | 28 | 28 | 28 |
| 20–34 | 60 | 10.7 | 74 | 3 | 6 | 8 | 11 | 24 | 28 | 43 |
| 35–49 | 139 | 14.1 | 93 | 4 | 7 | 12 | 19 | 28 | 29 | 33 |
| 50–64 | 36 | 12.7 | 104 | 5 | 5 | 9 | 16 | 28 | 28 | 53 |
| 65+ | 4 | 15.0 | 143 | 2 | 6 | 8 | 28 | 28 | 28 | 28 |
| **2. MULTIPLE DX** | | | | | | | | | | |
| 0–19 Years | 55 | 13.4 | 131 | 2 | 3 | 10 | 27 | 29 | 31 | 40 |
| 20–34 | 413 | 13.8 | 72 | 4 | 7 | 13 | 20 | 24 | 28 | 35 |
| 35–49 | 818 | 12.6 | 73 | 3 | 6 | 11 | 18 | 23 | 28 | 40 |
| 50–64 | 253 | 11.5 | 49 | 4 | 6 | 10 | 16 | 21 | 25 | 28 |
| 65+ | 99 | 12.5 | 47 | 5 | 8 | 12 | 15 | 21 | 22 | 37 |
| **TOTAL SINGLE DX** | 245 | 13.5 | 95 | 4 | 6 | 10 | 19 | 28 | 28 | 43 |
| **TOTAL MULTIPLE DX** | 1,638 | 12.7 | 71 | 3 | 6 | 11 | 18 | 24 | 28 | 37 |
| **TOTAL** | | | | | | | | | | |
| 0–19 Years | 61 | 14.2 | 130 | 2 | 4 | 11 | 28 | 29 | 31 | 40 |
| 20–34 | 473 | 13.5 | 73 | 4 | 7 | 13 | 20 | 24 | 28 | 37 |
| 35–49 | 957 | 12.7 | 75 | 3 | 6 | 11 | 18 | 25 | 28 | 40 |
| 50–64 | 289 | 11.6 | 53 | 4 | 6 | 10 | 16 | 21 | 26 | 28 |
| 65+ | 103 | 12.5 | 49 | 5 | 8 | 12 | 15 | 21 | 28 | 37 |
| **GRAND TOTAL** | 1,883 | 12.8 | 73 | 3 | 6 | 11 | 18 | 25 | 28 | 39 |

### 94.62: ALCOHOL DETOXIFICATION. Formerly included in operation group(s) 792.

| Type of Patients | Observed Patients | Avg. Stay | Vari-ance | 10th | 25th | 50th | 75th | 90th | 95th | 99th |
|---|---|---|---|---|---|---|---|---|---|---|
| **1. SINGLE DX** | | | | | | | | | | |
| 0–19 Years | 18 | 6.5 | 37 | 1 | 1 | 4 | 10 | 19 | 19 | 19 |
| 20–34 | 427 | 3.3 | 4 | 1 | 2 | 3 | 4 | 5 | 6 | 10 |
| 35–49 | 1,118 | 3.2 | 3 | 2 | 3 | 3 | 3 | 5 | 6 | 9 |
| 50–64 | 358 | 3.3 | 4 | 2 | 2 | 3 | 4 | 5 | 6 | 11 |
| 65+ | 58 | 3.7 | 6 | 2 | 2 | 4 | 5 | 6 | 7 | 15 |
| **2. MULTIPLE DX** | | | | | | | | | | |
| 0–19 Years | 145 | 3.6 | 7 | 1 | 2 | 3 | 5 | 7 | 9 | 13 |
| 20–34 | 4,097 | 3.8 | 8 | 1 | 2 | 3 | 5 | 7 | 9 | 14 |
| 35–49 | 13,776 | 4.1 | 9 | 2 | 3 | 4 | 5 | 7 | 9 | 15 |
| 50–64 | 6,249 | 4.6 | 14 | 2 | 3 | 4 | 5 | 8 | 11 | 16 |
| 65+ | 2,213 | 5.8 | 36 | 2 | 3 | 4 | 7 | 10 | 14 | 25 |
| **TOTAL SINGLE DX** | 1,979 | 3.3 | 4 | 2 | 2 | 3 | 4 | 5 | 6 | 10 |
| **TOTAL MULTIPLE DX** | 26,480 | 4.3 | 12 | 2 | 2 | 3 | 5 | 7 | 10 | 16 |
| **TOTAL** | | | | | | | | | | |
| 0–19 Years | 163 | 4.0 | 12 | 1 | 2 | 3 | 5 | 8 | 11 | 19 |
| 20–34 | 4,524 | 3.8 | 8 | 1 | 2 | 3 | 4 | 5 | 9 | 14 |
| 35–49 | 14,894 | 4.0 | 8 | 2 | 2 | 3 | 5 | 7 | 9 | 14 |
| 50–64 | 6,607 | 4.5 | 13 | 2 | 3 | 4 | 5 | 8 | 10 | 16 |
| 65+ | 2,271 | 5.7 | 35 | 2 | 3 | 4 | 7 | 10 | 14 | 25 |
| **GRAND TOTAL** | 28,459 | 4.2 | 11 | 2 | 2 | 3 | 5 | 7 | 9 | 16 |

Length of Stay by Diagnosis and Operation, United States, 2000

# United States, October 1998–September 1999 Data, by Operation

## 94.63: ALCOHOL REHAB/DETOX. Formerly included in operation group(s) 792.

| Type of Patients | Observed Patients | Avg. Stay | Variance | Percentiles | | | | | | |
|---|---|---|---|---|---|---|---|---|---|---|
| | | | | 10th | 25th | 50th | 75th | 90th | 95th | 99th |
| **1. SINGLE DX** | | | | | | | | | | |
| 0–19 Years | 6 | 5.0 | 6 | 3 | 3 | 3 | 8 | 8 | 9 | 9 |
| 20–34 | 102 | 6.3 | 36 | 3 | 3 | 4 | 7 | 14 | 23 | 26 |
| 35–49 | 278 | 6.2 | 23 | 2 | 3 | 5 | 7 | 14 | 15 | 23 |
| 50–64 | 113 | 6.6 | 27 | 2 | 3 | 5 | 7 | 15 | 18 | 22 |
| 65+ | 26 | 7.8 | 18 | 4 | 4 | 7 | 10 | 14 | 14 | 27 |
| **2. MULTIPLE DX** | | | | | | | | | | |
| 0–19 Years | 31 | 6.2 | 18 | 3 | 3 | 4 | 8 | 13 | 16 | 22 |
| 20–34 | 1,115 | 6.7 | 27 | 3 | 3 | 5 | 9 | 14 | 18 | 25 |
| 35–49 | 3,631 | 6.9 | 24 | 2 | 3 | 6 | 9 | 14 | 17 | 23 |
| 50–64 | 1,726 | 7.3 | 31 | 3 | 4 | 6 | 9 | 14 | 18 | 25 |
| 65+ | 667 | 9.7 | 37 | 4 | 6 | 8 | 13 | 17 | 21 | 32 |
| **TOTAL SINGLE DX** | 525 | 6.3 | 26 | 2 | 3 | 5 | 7 | 14 | 17 | 26 |
| **TOTAL MULTIPLE DX** | 7,170 | 7.2 | 27 | 2 | 4 | 6 | 9 | 14 | 18 | 25 |
| **TOTAL** | | | | | | | | | | |
| 0–19 Years | 37 | 5.9 | 15 | 3 | 3 | 4 | 8 | 10 | 16 | 17 |
| 20–34 | 1,217 | 6.7 | 28 | 2 | 3 | 5 | 8 | 14 | 18 | 25 |
| 35–49 | 3,909 | 6.9 | 24 | 2 | 3 | 6 | 9 | 14 | 17 | 23 |
| 50–64 | 1,839 | 7.3 | 31 | 3 | 4 | 6 | 9 | 14 | 18 | 24 |
| 65+ | 693 | 9.7 | 36 | 4 | 6 | 8 | 13 | 17 | 21 | 32 |
| **GRAND TOTAL** | 7,695 | 7.1 | 27 | 2 | 4 | 6 | 9 | 14 | 18 | 25 |

## 94.64: DRUG REHABILITATION. Formerly included in operation group(s) 792.

| Type of Patients | Observed Patients | Avg. Stay | Variance | Percentiles | | | | | | |
|---|---|---|---|---|---|---|---|---|---|---|
| | | | | 10th | 25th | 50th | 75th | 90th | 95th | 99th |
| **1. SINGLE DX** | | | | | | | | | | |
| 0–19 Years | 87 | 13.0 | 122 | 6 | 6 | 10 | 14 | 35 | 38 | 45 |
| 20–34 | 59 | 9.8 | 41 | 5 | 5 | 7 | 14 | 21 | 22 | 22 |
| 35–49 | 45 | 10.0 | 50 | 3 | 4 | 9 | 15 | 19 | 23 | 30 |
| 50–64 | 4 | 10.0 | 58 | 1 | 4 | 10 | 20 | 20 | 20 | 20 |
| 65+ | 0 | | | | | | | | | |
| **2. MULTIPLE DX** | | | | | | | | | | |
| 0–19 Years | 220 | 11.0 | 93 | 2 | 4 | 9 | 14 | 24 | 37 | 41 |
| 20–34 | 533 | 12.1 | 57 | 3 | 6 | 11 | 17 | 23 | 26 | 28 |
| 35–49 | 584 | 11.7 | 51 | 3 | 6 | 12 | 16 | 21 | 24 | 28 |
| 50–64 | 72 | 12.0 | 37 | 3 | 8 | 12 | 16 | 21 | 22 | 22 |
| 65+ | 6 | 12.4 | 28 | 5 | 6 | 12 | 14 | 20 | 21 | 21 |
| **TOTAL SINGLE DX** | 195 | 11.1 | 75 | 2 | 5 | 9 | 14 | 21 | 35 | 45 |
| **TOTAL MULTIPLE DX** | 1,415 | 11.7 | 61 | 3 | 5 | 11 | 16 | 22 | 26 | 37 |
| **TOTAL** | | | | | | | | | | |
| 0–19 Years | 307 | 11.4 | 98 | 2 | 4 | 9 | 14 | 24 | 37 | 41 |
| 20–34 | 592 | 11.8 | 55 | 3 | 6 | 11 | 17 | 22 | 26 | 28 |
| 35–49 | 629 | 11.6 | 51 | 3 | 6 | 11 | 16 | 21 | 23 | 29 |
| 50–64 | 76 | 11.9 | 37 | 3 | 8 | 12 | 16 | 21 | 22 | 22 |
| 65+ | 6 | 12.4 | 28 | 5 | 6 | 12 | 14 | 20 | 21 | 21 |
| **GRAND TOTAL** | 1,610 | 11.7 | 62 | 2 | 5 | 11 | 16 | 22 | 26 | 38 |

## 94.65: DRUG DETOXIFICATION. Formerly included in operation group(s) 792.

| Type of Patients | Observed Patients | Avg. Stay | Variance | Percentiles | | | | | | |
|---|---|---|---|---|---|---|---|---|---|---|
| | | | | 10th | 25th | 50th | 75th | 90th | 95th | 99th |
| **1. SINGLE DX** | | | | | | | | | | |
| 0–19 Years | 78 | 6.6 | 27 | 2 | 3 | 4 | 9 | 14 | 15 | 26 |
| 20–34 | 721 | 3.6 | 6 | 2 | 2 | 3 | 4 | 6 | 8 | 14 |
| 35–49 | 681 | 3.7 | 6 | 2 | 2 | 3 | 4 | 6 | 8 | 14 |
| 50–64 | 77 | 3.6 | 7 | 2 | 2 | 3 | 4 | 7 | 9 | 14 |
| 65+ | 6 | 5.5 | 15 | 3 | 3 | 6 | 6 | 14 | 14 | 14 |
| **2. MULTIPLE DX** | | | | | | | | | | |
| 0–19 Years | 380 | 4.3 | 12 | 2 | 3 | 3 | 5 | 7 | 10 | 16 |
| 20–34 | 4,956 | 3.9 | 8 | 2 | 3 | 3 | 5 | 7 | 9 | 14 |
| 35–49 | 7,713 | 4.2 | 10 | 2 | 3 | 3 | 5 | 7 | 10 | 17 |
| 50–64 | 1,465 | 4.2 | 8 | 2 | 3 | 3 | 5 | 7 | 10 | 14 |
| 65+ | 262 | 6.7 | 26 | 2 | 3 | 5 | 8 | 14 | 17 | 23 |
| **TOTAL SINGLE DX** | 1,563 | 3.8 | 7 | 2 | 2 | 3 | 4 | 7 | 9 | 14 |
| **TOTAL MULTIPLE DX** | 14,776 | 4.1 | 9 | 2 | 3 | 3 | 5 | 7 | 10 | 15 |
| **TOTAL** | | | | | | | | | | |
| 0–19 Years | 458 | 4.7 | 16 | 2 | 2 | 3 | 5 | 9 | 14 | 17 |
| 20–34 | 5,677 | 3.9 | 8 | 2 | 3 | 3 | 4 | 7 | 9 | 14 |
| 35–49 | 8,394 | 4.2 | 10 | 2 | 3 | 3 | 5 | 7 | 10 | 16 |
| 50–64 | 1,542 | 4.1 | 8 | 2 | 3 | 3 | 5 | 7 | 10 | 14 |
| 65+ | 268 | 6.6 | 26 | 2 | 3 | 5 | 8 | 14 | 16 | 23 |
| **GRAND TOTAL** | 16,339 | 4.1 | 9 | 2 | 3 | 3 | 5 | 7 | 10 | 15 |

## 94.66: DRUG REHAB/DETOX. Formerly included in operation group(s) 792.

| Type of Patients | Observed Patients | Avg. Stay | Variance | Percentiles | | | | | | |
|---|---|---|---|---|---|---|---|---|---|---|
| | | | | 10th | 25th | 50th | 75th | 90th | 95th | 99th |
| **1. SINGLE DX** | | | | | | | | | | |
| 0–19 Years | 15 | 5.2 | 13 | 2 | 3 | 3 | 3 | 7 | 13 | 18 |
| 20–34 | 140 | 5.8 | 18 | 2 | 3 | 3 | 4 | 8 | 14 | 18 |
| 35–49 | 166 | 6.4 | 28 | 2 | 3 | 5 | 5 | 8 | 19 | 27 |
| 50–64 | 15 | 3.8 | 10 | 1 | 1 | 3 | 6 | 7 | 9 | 14 |
| 65+ | 5 | 7.7 | 5 | 5 | 5 | 8 | 10 | 10 | 10 | 10 |
| **2. MULTIPLE DX** | | | | | | | | | | |
| 0–19 Years | 138 | 7.7 | 45 | 3 | 4 | 4 | 5 | 14 | 26 | 32 |
| 20–34 | 1,447 | 8.2 | 39 | 3 | 4 | 5 | 10 | 17 | 24 | 27 |
| 35–49 | 2,007 | 7.7 | 29 | 3 | 4 | 6 | 9 | 14 | 20 | 27 |
| 50–64 | 386 | 7.9 | 21 | 3 | 5 | 7 | 10 | 14 | 16 | 23 |
| 65+ | 105 | 8.1 | 15 | 3 | 5 | 8 | 10 | 13 | 14 | 19 |
| **TOTAL SINGLE DX** | 341 | 6.0 | 22 | 2 | 3 | 4 | 8 | 13 | 15 | 27 |
| **TOTAL MULTIPLE DX** | 4,083 | 7.9 | 33 | 3 | 4 | 6 | 10 | 16 | 21 | 28 |
| **TOTAL** | | | | | | | | | | |
| 0–19 Years | 153 | 7.4 | 42 | 3 | 4 | 5 | 9 | 14 | 21 | 32 |
| 20–34 | 1,587 | 8.0 | 38 | 3 | 4 | 6 | 10 | 17 | 23 | 27 |
| 35–49 | 2,173 | 7.6 | 29 | 3 | 4 | 6 | 9 | 14 | 20 | 27 |
| 50–64 | 401 | 7.7 | 21 | 3 | 5 | 7 | 10 | 14 | 16 | 23 |
| 65+ | 110 | 8.1 | 14 | 4 | 5 | 8 | 10 | 12 | 14 | 19 |
| **GRAND TOTAL** | 4,424 | 7.8 | 32 | 3 | 4 | 6 | 9 | 15 | 21 | 27 |

Length of Stay by Diagnosis and Operation, United States, 2000

# United States, October 1998–September 1999 Data, by Operation

## 94.67: ALC/DRUG REHABILITATION. Formerly included in operation group(s) 792.

| Type of Patients | Observed Patients | Avg. Stay | Variance | 10th | 25th | 50th | 75th | 90th | 95th | 99th |
|---|---|---|---|---|---|---|---|---|---|---|
| **1. SINGLE DX** | | | | | | | | | | |
| 0–19 Years | 1 | 6.0 | 0 | 6 | 6 | 6 | 6 | 6 | 6 | 6 |
| 20–34 | 1 | 16.0 | 0 | 16 | 16 | 16 | 16 | 16 | 16 | 16 |
| 35–49 | 1 | 21.0 | 0 | 21 | 21 | 21 | 21 | 21 | 21 | 21 |
| 50–64 | 0 | | | | | | | | | |
| 65+ | 0 | | | | | | | | | |
| **2. MULTIPLE DX** | | | | | | | | | | |
| 0–19 Years | 370 | 14.0 | 86 | 3 | 7 | 13 | 21 | 30 | 33 | >99 |
| 20–34 | 783 | 15.1 | 76 | 3 | 8 | 14 | 21 | 28 | 28 | 42 |
| 35–49 | 1,019 | 14.3 | 63 | 4 | 8 | 13 | 20 | 27 | 28 | 31 |
| 50–64 | 114 | 14.6 | 47 | 5 | 10 | 14 | 21 | 24 | 28 | 28 |
| 65+ | 8 | 10.5 | 28 | 5 | 6 | 11 | 13 | 14 | 25 | 25 |
| **TOTAL SINGLE DX** | 3 | 10.6 | 39 | 6 | 6 | 6 | 16 | 21 | 21 | 21 |
| **TOTAL MULTIPLE DX** | 2,294 | 14.4 | 73 | 4 | 8 | 13 | 21 | 28 | 28 | 44 |
| **TOTAL** | | | | | | | | | | |
| 0–19 Years | 371 | 14.0 | 86 | 3 | 6 | 13 | 21 | 30 | 33 | >99 |
| 20–34 | 784 | 15.1 | 76 | 3 | 8 | 14 | 21 | 28 | 28 | 42 |
| 35–49 | 1,020 | 14.3 | 63 | 4 | 8 | 13 | 20 | 27 | 28 | 31 |
| 50–64 | 114 | 14.6 | 47 | 5 | 10 | 14 | 21 | 24 | 28 | 28 |
| 65+ | 8 | 10.5 | 28 | 5 | 6 | 11 | 13 | 14 | 25 | 25 |
| **GRAND TOTAL** | 2,297 | 14.4 | 73 | 4 | 8 | 13 | 21 | 28 | 28 | 43 |

## 94.69: ALC/DRUG REHAB/DETOX. Formerly included in operation group(s) 792.

| Type of Patients | Observed Patients | Avg. Stay | Variance | 10th | 25th | 50th | 75th | 90th | 95th | 99th |
|---|---|---|---|---|---|---|---|---|---|---|
| **1. SINGLE DX** | | | | | | | | | | |
| 0–19 Years | 0 | | | | | | | | | |
| 20–34 | 14 | 4.7 | 8 | 2 | 3 | 4 | 5 | 8 | 13 | 13 |
| 35–49 | 14 | 3.5 | 3 | 1 | 3 | 3 | 4 | 7 | 7 | 7 |
| 50–64 | 3 | 4.5 | 1 | 2 | 5 | 5 | 5 | 5 | 5 | 5 |
| 65+ | 1 | 1.0 | 0 | 1 | 1 | 1 | 1 | 1 | 1 | 1 |
| **2. MULTIPLE DX** | | | | | | | | | | |
| 0–19 Years | 158 | 8.8 | 68 | 2 | 4 | 7 | 10 | 18 | 22 | 37 |
| 20–34 | 1,807 | 8.7 | 42 | 3 | 4 | 7 | 11 | 19 | 22 | 28 |
| 35–49 | 2,809 | 8.4 | 31 | 3 | 5 | 7 | 10 | 16 | 20 | 28 |
| 50–64 | 403 | 8.4 | 27 | 3 | 5 | 8 | 10 | 15 | 21 | 24 |
| 65+ | 37 | 8.4 | 20 | 3 | 5 | 6 | 12 | 15 | 17 | 17 |
| **TOTAL SINGLE DX** | 32 | 4.2 | 6 | 1 | 3 | 4 | 5 | 7 | 8 | 13 |
| **TOTAL MULTIPLE DX** | 5,214 | 8.5 | 36 | 3 | 4 | 7 | 11 | 17 | 21 | 28 |
| **TOTAL** | | | | | | | | | | |
| 0–19 Years | 158 | 8.8 | 68 | 2 | 4 | 7 | 10 | 18 | 22 | 37 |
| 20–34 | 1,821 | 8.6 | 42 | 3 | 4 | 7 | 11 | 19 | 22 | 28 |
| 35–49 | 2,823 | 8.4 | 31 | 3 | 5 | 7 | 10 | 16 | 20 | 28 |
| 50–64 | 406 | 8.3 | 27 | 3 | 5 | 8 | 10 | 15 | 21 | 24 |
| 65+ | 38 | 8.3 | 21 | 3 | 5 | 6 | 12 | 15 | 17 | 17 |
| **GRAND TOTAL** | 5,246 | 8.5 | 36 | 3 | 4 | 7 | 10 | 17 | 21 | 28 |

## 94.68: ALC/DRUG DETOXIFICATION. Formerly included in operation group(s) 792.

| Type of Patients | Observed Patients | Avg. Stay | Variance | 10th | 25th | 50th | 75th | 90th | 95th | 99th |
|---|---|---|---|---|---|---|---|---|---|---|
| **1. SINGLE DX** | | | | | | | | | | |
| 0–19 Years | 1 | 1.0 | 0 | 1 | 1 | 1 | 1 | 1 | 1 | 1 |
| 20–34 | 30 | 3.2 | <1 | 2 | 3 | 3 | 3 | 4 | 5 | 8 |
| 35–49 | 34 | 3.7 | 3 | 3 | 3 | 3 | 4 | 7 | 8 | 8 |
| 50–64 | 3 | 2.6 | <1 | 2 | 2 | 2 | 4 | 4 | 4 | 4 |
| 65+ | 0 | | | | | | | | | |
| **2. MULTIPLE DX** | | | | | | | | | | |
| 0–19 Years | 174 | 5.5 | 14 | 2 | 3 | 4 | 7 | 10 | 14 | 19 |
| 20–34 | 3,686 | 3.9 | 7 | 2 | 3 | 3 | 5 | 7 | 8 | 14 |
| 35–49 | 6,029 | 4.6 | 10 | 2 | 3 | 4 | 5 | 7 | 10 | 20 |
| 50–64 | 717 | 4.8 | 9 | 2 | 3 | 4 | 6 | 9 | 10 | 15 |
| 65+ | 58 | 5.3 | 21 | 2 | 2 | 4 | 7 | 9 | 15 | 28 |
| **TOTAL SINGLE DX** | 68 | 3.4 | 2 | 2 | 3 | 3 | 4 | 5 | 8 | 8 |
| **TOTAL MULTIPLE DX** | 10,664 | 4.4 | 9 | 2 | 3 | 3 | 5 | 7 | 10 | 17 |
| **TOTAL** | | | | | | | | | | |
| 0–19 Years | 175 | 5.5 | 14 | 2 | 3 | 4 | 7 | 10 | 14 | 19 |
| 20–34 | 3,716 | 3.9 | 7 | 2 | 3 | 3 | 5 | 7 | 8 | 14 |
| 35–49 | 6,063 | 4.6 | 10 | 2 | 3 | 4 | 5 | 7 | 10 | 20 |
| 50–64 | 720 | 4.8 | 9 | 2 | 3 | 4 | 6 | 9 | 10 | 15 |
| 65+ | 58 | 5.3 | 21 | 2 | 2 | 4 | 7 | 9 | 15 | 28 |
| **GRAND TOTAL** | 10,732 | 4.4 | 9 | 3 | 3 | 3 | 5 | 7 | 10 | 17 |

## 95.0: GEN/SUBJECTIVE EYE EXAM. Formerly included in operation group(s) 796.

| Type of Patients | Observed Patients | Avg. Stay | Variance | 10th | 25th | 50th | 75th | 90th | 95th | 99th |
|---|---|---|---|---|---|---|---|---|---|---|
| **1. SINGLE DX** | | | | | | | | | | |
| 0–19 Years | 22 | 1.5 | 1 | 1 | 1 | 1 | 1 | 3 | 4 | 6 |
| 20–34 | 1 | 6.0 | 0 | 6 | 6 | 6 | 6 | 6 | 6 | 6 |
| 35–49 | 0 | | | | | | | | | |
| 50–64 | 1 | 1.0 | 0 | 1 | 1 | 1 | 1 | 1 | 1 | 1 |
| 65+ | 1 | 1.0 | 0 | 1 | 1 | 1 | 1 | 1 | 1 | 1 |
| **2. MULTIPLE DX** | | | | | | | | | | |
| 0–19 Years | 82 | 4.2 | 63 | 1 | 1 | 1 | 4 | 10 | 17 | 50 |
| 20–34 | 4 | 2.8 | 6 | 2 | 2 | 2 | 2 | 4 | 12 | 12 |
| 35–49 | 8 | 2.9 | 5 | 3 | 3 | 3 | 3 | 6 | 6 | 10 |
| 50–64 | 2 | 3.0 | 0 | 3 | 3 | 3 | 3 | 3 | 3 | 3 |
| 65+ | 9 | 4.3 | 24 | 1 | 1 | 3 | 8 | 8 | 21 | 21 |
| **TOTAL SINGLE DX** | 25 | 1.6 | 2 | 1 | 1 | 1 | 1 | 4 | 4 | 6 |
| **TOTAL MULTIPLE DX** | 105 | 4.0 | 49 | 1 | 1 | 2 | 4 | 8 | 13 | 38 |
| **TOTAL** | | | | | | | | | | |
| 0–19 Years | 104 | 3.6 | 49 | 1 | 1 | 1 | 4 | 7 | 13 | 38 |
| 20–34 | 5 | 3.1 | 6 | 2 | 2 | 3 | 3 | 6 | 12 | 12 |
| 35–49 | 8 | 2.9 | 5 | 1 | 3 | 3 | 3 | 6 | 6 | 10 |
| 50–64 | 3 | 2.7 | <1 | 1 | 3 | 3 | 3 | 3 | 3 | 3 |
| 65+ | 10 | 4.1 | 23 | 1 | 1 | 2 | 8 | 8 | 21 | 21 |
| **GRAND TOTAL** | 130 | 3.5 | 41 | 1 | 1 | 1 | 3 | 7 | 12 | 38 |

Length of Stay by Diagnosis and Operation, United States, 2000

# United States, October 1998–September 1999 Data, by Operation

## 95.1: FORM & STRUCT EYE EXAM. Formerly included in operation group(s) 796.

| Type of Patients | Observed Patients | Avg. Stay | Vari-ance | 10th | 25th | 50th | 75th | 90th | 95th | 99th |
|---|---|---|---|---|---|---|---|---|---|---|
| **1. SINGLE DX** | | | | | | | | | | |
| 0–19 Years | 2 | 2.7 | <1 | 1 | 3 | 3 | 3 | 3 | 3 | 3 |
| 20–34 | 0 | | | | | | | | | |
| 35–49 | 0 | | | | | | | | | |
| 50–64 | 0 | | | | | | | | | |
| 65+ | 0 | | | | | | | | | |
| **2. MULTIPLE DX** | | | | | | | | | | |
| 0–19 Years | 4 | 2.3 | 2 | 1 | 1 | 2 | 4 | 4 | 4 | 4 |
| 20–34 | 4 | 3.9 | 1 | 2 | 3 | 4 | 5 | 5 | 5 | 5 |
| 35–49 | 3 | 6.7 | 34 | 1 | 3 | 3 | 13 | 13 | 13 | 13 |
| 50–64 | 3 | 8.6 | 35 | 2 | 3 | 10 | 14 | 14 | 14 | 14 |
| 65+ | 3 | 6.3 | 20 | 3 | 3 | 3 | 7 | 14 | 14 | 14 |
| **TOTAL SINGLE DX** | 2 | 2.7 | <1 | 1 | 3 | 3 | 3 | 3 | 3 | 3 |
| **TOTAL MULTIPLE DX** | 17 | 5.5 | 18 | 2 | 3 | 4 | 7 | 13 | 14 | 14 |
| **TOTAL** | | | | | | | | | | |
| 0–19 Years | 6 | 2.5 | 1 | 1 | 1 | 3 | 3 | 4 | 4 | 4 |
| 20–34 | 4 | 3.9 | 1 | 2 | 3 | 4 | 5 | 5 | 5 | 5 |
| 35–49 | 3 | 6.7 | 34 | 1 | 3 | 3 | 13 | 13 | 13 | 13 |
| 50–64 | 3 | 8.6 | 35 | 2 | 3 | 10 | 14 | 14 | 14 | 14 |
| 65+ | 3 | 6.3 | 20 | 3 | 3 | 3 | 7 | 14 | 14 | 14 |
| **GRAND TOTAL** | 19 | 5.3 | 17 | 2 | 3 | 3 | 7 | 13 | 14 | 14 |

## 95.2: OBJECTIVE FUNCT EYE TEST. Formerly included in operation group(s) 796.

| Type of Patients | Observed Patients | Avg. Stay | Vari-ance | 10th | 25th | 50th | 75th | 90th | 95th | 99th |
|---|---|---|---|---|---|---|---|---|---|---|
| **1. SINGLE DX** | | | | | | | | | | |
| 0–19 Years | 1 | 1.0 | 0 | 1 | 1 | 1 | 1 | 1 | 1 | 1 |
| 20–34 | 0 | | | | | | | | | |
| 35–49 | 0 | | | | | | | | | |
| 50–64 | 1 | 9.0 | 0 | 9 | 9 | 9 | 9 | 9 | 9 | 9 |
| 65+ | 0 | | | | | | | | | |
| **2. MULTIPLE DX** | | | | | | | | | | |
| 0–19 Years | 3 | 3.1 | 18 | 1 | 1 | 1 | 1 | 11 | 11 | 11 |
| 20–34 | 3 | 4.8 | 4 | 1 | 3 | 6 | 6 | 6 | 6 | 6 |
| 35–49 | 5 | 8.1 | 17 | 2 | 8 | 8 | 12 | 13 | 13 | 13 |
| 50–64 | 2 | 8.3 | 113 | 2 | 2 | 2 | 20 | 20 | 20 | 20 |
| 65+ | 6 | 4.4 | 1 | 3 | 3 | 5 | 5 | 5 | 6 | 6 |
| **TOTAL SINGLE DX** | 2 | 1.5 | 4 | 1 | 1 | 1 | 1 | 1 | 9 | 9 |
| **TOTAL MULTIPLE DX** | 19 | 4.6 | 7 | 1 | 3 | 5 | 6 | 6 | 11 | 13 |
| **TOTAL** | | | | | | | | | | |
| 0–19 Years | 4 | 2.1 | 10 | 1 | 1 | 1 | 1 | 11 | 11 | 11 |
| 20–34 | 3 | 4.8 | 4 | 1 | 3 | 6 | 6 | 6 | 6 | 6 |
| 35–49 | 5 | 8.1 | 17 | 2 | 8 | 9 | 12 | 13 | 13 | 13 |
| 50–64 | 3 | 8.5 | 74 | 2 | 2 | 2 | 20 | 20 | 20 | 20 |
| 65+ | 6 | 4.4 | 1 | 3 | 3 | 5 | 5 | 5 | 6 | 6 |
| **GRAND TOTAL** | 21 | 4.3 | 8 | 1 | 3 | 4 | 6 | 6 | 9 | 13 |

## 95.3: SPECIAL VISION SERVICES. Formerly included in operation group(s) 796.

| Type of Patients | Observed Patients | Avg. Stay | Vari-ance | 10th | 25th | 50th | 75th | 90th | 95th | 99th |
|---|---|---|---|---|---|---|---|---|---|---|
| **1. SINGLE DX** | | | | | | | | | | |
| 0–19 Years | 0 | | | | | | | | | |
| 20–34 | 0 | | | | | | | | | |
| 35–49 | 0 | | | | | | | | | |
| 50–64 | 0 | | | | | | | | | |
| 65+ | 0 | | | | | | | | | |
| **2. MULTIPLE DX** | | | | | | | | | | |
| 0–19 Years | 1 | 2.0 | 0 | 2 | 2 | 2 | 2 | 2 | 2 | 2 |
| 20–34 | 0 | | | | | | | | | |
| 35–49 | 0 | | | | | | | | | |
| 50–64 | 0 | | | | | | | | | |
| 65+ | 0 | | | | | | | | | |
| **TOTAL SINGLE DX** | 0 | | | | | | | | | |
| **TOTAL MULTIPLE DX** | 1 | 2.0 | 0 | 2 | 2 | 2 | 2 | 2 | 2 | 2 |
| **TOTAL** | | | | | | | | | | |
| 0–19 Years | 1 | 2.0 | 0 | 2 | 2 | 2 | 2 | 2 | 2 | 2 |
| 20–34 | 0 | | | | | | | | | |
| 35–49 | 0 | | | | | | | | | |
| 50–64 | 0 | | | | | | | | | |
| 65+ | 0 | | | | | | | | | |
| **GRAND TOTAL** | 1 | 2.0 | 0 | 2 | 2 | 2 | 2 | 2 | 2 | 2 |

## 95.4: NONOP HEARING PROCEDURE. Formerly included in operation group(s) 796.

| Type of Patients | Observed Patients | Avg. Stay | Vari-ance | 10th | 25th | 50th | 75th | 90th | 95th | 99th |
|---|---|---|---|---|---|---|---|---|---|---|
| **1. SINGLE DX** | | | | | | | | | | |
| 0–19 Years | 2,742 | 1.7 | <1 | 1 | 1 | 2 | 2 | 2 | 3 | 4 |
| 20–34 | 1 | 4.0 | 0 | 4 | 4 | 4 | 4 | 4 | 4 | 4 |
| 35–49 | 0 | | | | | | | | | |
| 50–64 | 0 | | | | | | | | | |
| 65+ | 0 | | | | | | | | | |
| **2. MULTIPLE DX** | | | | | | | | | | |
| 0–19 Years | 5,808 | 3.3 | 23 | 1 | 1 | 2 | 3 | 7 | 10 | 24 |
| 20–34 | 1 | 6.0 | 0 | 6 | 6 | 6 | 6 | 6 | 6 | 6 |
| 35–49 | 5 | 2.4 | 11 | 1 | 1 | 1 | 1 | 5 | 5 | 16 |
| 50–64 | 6 | 4.4 | 2 | 3 | 4 | 4 | 5 | 5 | 5 | 8 |
| 65+ | 20 | 5.5 | 14 | 2 | 3 | 5 | 6 | 11 | 13 | 21 |
| **TOTAL SINGLE DX** | 2,743 | 1.7 | <1 | 1 | 1 | 2 | 2 | 2 | 3 | 4 |
| **TOTAL MULTIPLE DX** | 5,840 | 3.4 | 23 | 1 | 1 | 2 | 3 | 7 | 11 | 24 |
| **TOTAL** | | | | | | | | | | |
| 0–19 Years | 8,550 | 2.8 | 17 | 1 | 1 | 2 | 3 | 5 | 8 | 22 |
| 20–34 | 2 | 5.4 | 1 | 4 | 4 | 6 | 6 | 6 | 6 | 6 |
| 35–49 | 5 | 2.4 | 11 | 1 | 1 | 1 | 1 | 5 | 5 | 16 |
| 50–64 | 6 | 4.4 | 2 | 3 | 4 | 4 | 5 | 5 | 5 | 8 |
| 65+ | 20 | 5.5 | 14 | 2 | 3 | 5 | 6 | 11 | 13 | 21 |
| **GRAND TOTAL** | 8,583 | 2.8 | 17 | 1 | 1 | 2 | 3 | 5 | 8 | 22 |

Length of Stay by Diagnosis and Operation, United States, 2000

# United States, October 1998–September 1999 Data, by Operation

## 95.41: AUDIOMETRY. Formerly included in operation group(s) 796.

| Type of Patients | Observed Patients | Avg. Stay | Variance | 10th | 25th | 50th | 75th | 90th | 95th | 99th |
|---|---|---|---|---|---|---|---|---|---|---|
| **1. SINGLE DX** | | | | | | | | | | |
| 0–19 Years | 408 | 1.8 | <1 | 1 | 1 | 2 | 2 | 2 | 3 | 4 |
| 20–34 | 1 | 4.0 | 0 | 4 | 4 | 4 | 4 | 4 | 4 | 4 |
| 35–49 | 0 | | | | | | | | | |
| 50–64 | 0 | | | | | | | | | |
| 65+ | 0 | | | | | | | | | |
| **2. MULTIPLE DX** | | | | | | | | | | |
| 0–19 Years | 546 | 7.2 | 80 | 1 | 2 | 3 | 9 | 19 | 24 | 47 |
| 20–34 | 1 | 6.0 | | 6 | 6 | 6 | 6 | 6 | 6 | 6 |
| 35–49 | 3 | 9.3 | 45 | 2 | 5 | 5 | 16 | 16 | 16 | 16 |
| 50–64 | 4 | 4.7 | 2 | 4 | 4 | 4 | 5 | 8 | 8 | 8 |
| 65+ | 8 | 4.6 | 3 | 3 | 3 | 5 | 5 | 8 | 8 | 8 |
| **TOTAL SINGLE DX** | 409 | 1.8 | <1 | 1 | 1 | 2 | 2 | 2 | 3 | 4 |
| **TOTAL MULTIPLE DX** | 562 | 7.1 | 78 | 1 | 2 | 3 | 9 | 19 | 24 | 47 |
| **TOTAL** | | | | | | | | | | |
| 0–19 Years | 954 | 5.3 | 59 | 1 | 2 | 2 | 6 | 13 | 19 | 40 |
| 20–34 | 2 | 5.4 | 1 | 4 | 4 | 6 | 6 | 6 | 6 | 6 |
| 35–49 | 3 | 9.3 | 45 | 2 | 5 | 5 | 16 | 16 | 16 | 16 |
| 50–64 | 4 | 4.7 | 2 | 4 | 4 | 4 | 5 | 8 | 8 | 8 |
| 65+ | 8 | 4.6 | 3 | 3 | 3 | 5 | 5 | 8 | 8 | 8 |
| **GRAND TOTAL** | 971 | 5.3 | 58 | 1 | 2 | 2 | 6 | 13 | 19 | 40 |

## 95.43: AUDIOLOGICAL EVALUATION. Formerly included in operation group(s) 796.

| Type of Patients | Observed Patients | Avg. Stay | Variance | 10th | 25th | 50th | 75th | 90th | 95th | 99th |
|---|---|---|---|---|---|---|---|---|---|---|
| **1. SINGLE DX** | | | | | | | | | | |
| 0–19 Years | 114 | 1.7 | <1 | 1 | 1 | 2 | 2 | 2 | 2 | 3 |
| 20–34 | 0 | | | | | | | | | |
| 35–49 | 0 | | | | | | | | | |
| 50–64 | 0 | | | | | | | | | |
| 65+ | 0 | | | | | | | | | |
| **2. MULTIPLE DX** | | | | | | | | | | |
| 0–19 Years | 676 | 2.4 | 10 | 1 | 1 | 2 | 2 | 4 | 6 | 21 |
| 20–34 | 1 | 5.0 | 0 | 5 | 5 | 5 | 5 | 5 | 5 | 5 |
| 35–49 | 0 | | | | | | | | | |
| 50–64 | 0 | | | | | | | | | |
| 65+ | 5 | 4.9 | 10 | 2 | 3 | 3 | 6 | 6 | 13 | 18 |
| **TOTAL SINGLE DX** | 114 | 1.7 | <1 | 1 | 1 | 2 | 2 | 2 | 2 | 3 |
| **TOTAL MULTIPLE DX** | 682 | 2.5 | 10 | 1 | 1 | 2 | 2 | 4 | 7 | 20 |
| **TOTAL** | | | | | | | | | | |
| 0–19 Years | 790 | 2.4 | 9 | 1 | 1 | 2 | 2 | 4 | 5 | 20 |
| 20–34 | 0 | | | | | | | | | |
| 35–49 | 1 | 5.0 | 0 | 5 | 5 | 5 | 5 | 5 | 5 | 5 |
| 50–64 | 0 | | | | | | | | | |
| 65+ | 5 | 4.9 | 10 | 2 | 3 | 3 | 6 | 6 | 13 | 18 |
| **GRAND TOTAL** | 796 | 2.4 | 9 | 1 | 1 | 2 | 2 | 4 | 6 | 20 |

## 95.46: AUDITORY & VEST TEST NEC. Formerly included in operation group(s) 796.

| Type of Patients | Observed Patients | Avg. Stay | Variance | 10th | 25th | 50th | 75th | 90th | 95th | 99th |
|---|---|---|---|---|---|---|---|---|---|---|
| **1. SINGLE DX** | | | | | | | | | | |
| 0–19 Years | 665 | 1.7 | <1 | 1 | 1 | 2 | 2 | 3 | 3 | 4 |
| 20–34 | 0 | | | | | | | | | |
| 35–49 | 0 | | | | | | | | | |
| 50–64 | 0 | | | | | | | | | |
| 65+ | 0 | | | | | | | | | |
| **2. MULTIPLE DX** | | | | | | | | | | |
| 0–19 Years | 2,464 | 3.3 | 18 | 1 | 2 | 2 | 3 | 6 | 10 | 21 |
| 20–34 | 0 | | | | | | | | | |
| 35–49 | 1 | 1.0 | 0 | 1 | 1 | 1 | 1 | 1 | 1 | 1 |
| 50–64 | 1 | 3.0 | 0 | 3 | 3 | 3 | 3 | 3 | 3 | 3 |
| 65+ | 4 | 5.5 | 11 | 1 | 4 | 4 | 5 | 11 | 11 | 11 |
| **TOTAL SINGLE DX** | 665 | 1.7 | <1 | 1 | 1 | 2 | 2 | 3 | 3 | 4 |
| **TOTAL MULTIPLE DX** | 2,470 | 3.3 | 18 | 1 | 2 | 2 | 3 | 6 | 10 | 21 |
| **TOTAL** | | | | | | | | | | |
| 0–19 Years | 3,129 | 3.0 | 15 | 1 | 2 | 2 | 3 | 5 | 8 | 20 |
| 20–34 | 0 | | | | | | | | | |
| 35–49 | 1 | 1.0 | 0 | 1 | 1 | 1 | 1 | 1 | 1 | 1 |
| 50–64 | 1 | 3.0 | 0 | 3 | 3 | 3 | 3 | 3 | 3 | 3 |
| 65+ | 4 | 5.5 | 11 | 1 | 4 | 4 | 5 | 11 | 11 | 11 |
| **GRAND TOTAL** | 3,135 | 3.0 | 15 | 1 | 2 | 2 | 3 | 5 | 8 | 20 |

## 95.47: HEARING EXAMINATION NOS. Formerly included in operation group(s) 796.

| Type of Patients | Observed Patients | Avg. Stay | Variance | 10th | 25th | 50th | 75th | 90th | 95th | 99th |
|---|---|---|---|---|---|---|---|---|---|---|
| **1. SINGLE DX** | | | | | | | | | | |
| 0–19 Years | 1,543 | 1.6 | <1 | 1 | 1 | 2 | 2 | 2 | 3 | 4 |
| 20–34 | 0 | | | | | | | | | |
| 35–49 | 0 | | | | | | | | | |
| 50–64 | 0 | | | | | | | | | |
| 65+ | 0 | | | | | | | | | |
| **2. MULTIPLE DX** | | | | | | | | | | |
| 0–19 Years | 2,110 | 2.8 | 15 | 1 | 1 | 2 | 3 | 4 | 7 | 23 |
| 20–34 | 0 | | | | | | | | | |
| 35–49 | 0 | | | | | | | | | |
| 50–64 | 1 | 4.0 | 0 | 4 | 4 | 4 | 4 | 4 | 4 | 4 |
| 65+ | 1 | 3.0 | 0 | 3 | 3 | 3 | 3 | 3 | 3 | 3 |
| **TOTAL SINGLE DX** | 1,543 | 1.6 | <1 | 1 | 1 | 2 | 2 | 2 | 3 | 4 |
| **TOTAL MULTIPLE DX** | 2,112 | 2.8 | 15 | 1 | 1 | 2 | 3 | 4 | 7 | 23 |
| **TOTAL** | | | | | | | | | | |
| 0–19 Years | 3,653 | 2.3 | 9 | 1 | 1 | 2 | 2 | 3 | 5 | 16 |
| 20–34 | 0 | | | | | | | | | |
| 35–49 | 0 | | | | | | | | | |
| 50–64 | 1 | 4.0 | 0 | 4 | 4 | 4 | 4 | 4 | 4 | 4 |
| 65+ | 1 | 3.0 | 0 | 3 | 3 | 3 | 3 | 3 | 3 | 3 |
| **GRAND TOTAL** | 3,655 | 2.3 | 9 | 1 | 1 | 2 | 2 | 3 | 5 | 16 |

Length of Stay by Diagnosis and Operation, United States, 2000

## United States, October 1998–September 1999 Data, by Operation

### 96.0: NONOP GI & RESP INTUB. Formerly included in operation group(s) 796.

| Type of Patients | Observed Patients | Avg. Stay | Vari-ance | Percentiles | | | | | | |
|---|---|---|---|---|---|---|---|---|---|---|
| | | | | 10th | 25th | 50th | 75th | 90th | 95th | 99th |
| **1. SINGLE DX** | | | | | | | | | | |
| 0–19 Years | 1,370 | 2.1 | 2 | 1 | 1 | 2 | 2 | 3 | 4 | 9 |
| 20–34 | 107 | 2.3 | 2 | 1 | 1 | 2 | 3 | 5 | 6 | 6 |
| 35–49 | 118 | 2.9 | 6 | 1 | 1 | 2 | 4 | 6 | 6 | 16 |
| 50–64 | 93 | 2.4 | 7 | 1 | 1 | 2 | 3 | 5 | 6 | 17 |
| 65+ | 102 | 3.3 | 5 | 1 | 1 | 3 | 5 | 6 | 7 | 11 |
| **2. MULTIPLE DX** | | | | | | | | | | |
| 0–19 Years | 13,785 | 14.6 | 428 | 1 | 2 | 5 | 18 | 50 | 72 | >99 |
| 20–34 | 2,254 | 5.1 | 43 | 1 | 2 | 3 | 6 | 12 | 18 | 31 |
| 35–49 | 3,867 | 6.5 | 53 | 1 | 2 | 4 | 8 | 15 | 21 | 35 |
| 50–64 | 4,472 | 8.1 | 58 | 2 | 3 | 6 | 10 | 18 | 24 | 37 |
| 65+ | 10,395 | 9.4 | 64 | 2 | 4 | 7 | 12 | 19 | 24 | 38 |
| **TOTAL SINGLE DX** | 1,790 | 2.3 | 3 | 1 | 1 | 2 | 3 | 4 | 5 | 9 |
| **TOTAL MULTIPLE DX** | 34,773 | 10.5 | 208 | 1 | 3 | 6 | 12 | 25 | 43 | 89 |
| **TOTAL** | | | | | | | | | | |
| 0–19 Years | 15,155 | 13.3 | 399 | 1 | 2 | 4 | 15 | 46 | 68 | >99 |
| 20–34 | 2,361 | 5.0 | 42 | 1 | 2 | 3 | 5 | 12 | 17 | 31 |
| 35–49 | 3,985 | 6.4 | 52 | 1 | 2 | 4 | 8 | 14 | 20 | 35 |
| 50–64 | 4,565 | 7.9 | 57 | 1 | 3 | 5 | 10 | 17 | 24 | 36 |
| 65+ | 10,497 | 9.3 | 63 | 2 | 4 | 7 | 12 | 19 | 24 | 38 |
| **GRAND TOTAL** | 36,563 | 10.1 | 201 | 1 | 2 | 5 | 11 | 24 | 41 | 88 |

### 96.05: RESP TRACT INTUB NEC. Formerly included in operation group(s) 796.

| Type of Patients | Observed Patients | Avg. Stay | Vari-ance | Percentiles | | | | | | |
|---|---|---|---|---|---|---|---|---|---|---|
| | | | | 10th | 25th | 50th | 75th | 90th | 95th | 99th |
| **1. SINGLE DX** | | | | | | | | | | |
| 0–19 Years | 152 | 1.7 | <1 | 1 | 1 | 2 | 2 | 2 | 3 | 4 |
| 20–34 | 2 | 1.6 | <1 | 1 | 1 | 2 | 2 | 2 | 2 | 2 |
| 35–49 | 0 | | | | | | | | | |
| 50–64 | 2 | 4.8 | <1 | 4 | 5 | 5 | 5 | 5 | 5 | 5 |
| 65+ | 1 | 2.0 | 0 | 2 | 2 | 2 | 2 | 2 | 2 | 2 |
| **2. MULTIPLE DX** | | | | | | | | | | |
| 0–19 Years | 580 | 3.6 | 40 | 1 | 1 | 3 | 3 | 7 | 11 | 42 |
| 20–34 | 35 | 4.6 | 19 | 1 | 2 | 3 | 5 | 9 | 13 | 27 |
| 35–49 | 49 | 7.7 | 28 | 2 | 3 | 8 | 11 | 13 | 15 | 19 |
| 50–64 | 85 | 9.6 | 56 | 3 | 4 | 8 | 13 | 19 | 22 | 46 |
| 65+ | 210 | 9.1 | 44 | 2 | 4 | 8 | 11 | 18 | 23 | 28 |
| **TOTAL SINGLE DX** | 157 | 1.7 | <1 | 1 | 1 | 2 | 2 | 3 | 3 | 5 |
| **TOTAL MULTIPLE DX** | 959 | 4.8 | 46 | 1 | 1 | 2 | 5 | 11 | 17 | 40 |
| **TOTAL** | | | | | | | | | | |
| 0–19 Years | 732 | 3.2 | 33 | 1 | 1 | 2 | 3 | 5 | 10 | 34 |
| 20–34 | 37 | 4.5 | 19 | 1 | 2 | 3 | 5 | 9 | 13 | 27 |
| 35–49 | 49 | 7.7 | 28 | 2 | 3 | 8 | 11 | 13 | 15 | 19 |
| 50–64 | 87 | 9.3 | 54 | 3 | 4 | 7 | 11 | 19 | 22 | 46 |
| 65+ | 211 | 9.1 | 44 | 2 | 4 | 8 | 11 | 18 | 23 | 28 |
| **GRAND TOTAL** | 1,116 | 4.3 | 40 | 1 | 2 | 2 | 4 | 10 | 15 | 34 |

### 96.04: INSERT ENDOTRACHEAL TUBE. Formerly included in operation group(s) 796.

| Type of Patients | Observed Patients | Avg. Stay | Vari-ance | Percentiles | | | | | | |
|---|---|---|---|---|---|---|---|---|---|---|
| | | | | 10th | 25th | 50th | 75th | 90th | 95th | 99th |
| **1. SINGLE DX** | | | | | | | | | | |
| 0–19 Years | 1,066 | 2.1 | 2 | 1 | 1 | 2 | 2 | 3 | 4 | 9 |
| 20–34 | 54 | 1.9 | 2 | 1 | 1 | 2 | 3 | 4 | 5 | 7 |
| 35–49 | 26 | 4.1 | 21 | 1 | 1 | 2 | 5 | 13 | 19 | 19 |
| 50–64 | 16 | 5.2 | 41 | 1 | 1 | 4 | 5 | 17 | 23 | 23 |
| 65+ | 14 | 5.3 | 4 | 3 | 5 | 5 | 6 | 7 | 11 | 11 |
| **2. MULTIPLE DX** | | | | | | | | | | |
| 0–19 Years | 12,301 | 16.2 | 466 | 1 | 2 | 7 | 21 | 54 | 76 | >99 |
| 20–34 | 1,724 | 5.6 | 52 | 1 | 2 | 4 | 6 | 14 | 19 | 34 |
| 35–49 | 2,797 | 7.4 | 67 | 1 | 2 | 5 | 10 | 18 | 24 | 41 |
| 50–64 | 3,153 | 9.8 | 71 | 2 | 4 | 7 | 13 | 21 | 26 | 40 |
| 65+ | 7,041 | 11.3 | 75 | 3 | 6 | 9 | 14 | 21 | 27 | 41 |
| **TOTAL SINGLE DX** | 1,176 | 2.2 | 3 | 1 | 1 | 2 | 2 | 4 | 5 | 10 |
| **TOTAL MULTIPLE DX** | 27,016 | 12.4 | 255 | 2 | 3 | 7 | 15 | 31 | 52 | 94 |
| **TOTAL** | | | | | | | | | | |
| 0–19 Years | 13,367 | 15.0 | 442 | 1 | 2 | 5 | 19 | 52 | 73 | >99 |
| 20–34 | 1,778 | 5.5 | 51 | 1 | 2 | 3 | 6 | 14 | 18 | 34 |
| 35–49 | 2,823 | 7.4 | 67 | 1 | 2 | 5 | 10 | 18 | 24 | 41 |
| 50–64 | 3,169 | 9.8 | 71 | 2 | 4 | 7 | 13 | 21 | 26 | 40 |
| 65+ | 7,055 | 11.3 | 75 | 3 | 6 | 9 | 14 | 21 | 27 | 41 |
| **GRAND TOTAL** | 28,192 | 12.0 | 248 | 1 | 3 | 7 | 14 | 30 | 50 | 93 |

### 96.07: INSERT GASTRIC TUBE NEC. Formerly included in operation group(s) 796.

| Type of Patients | Observed Patients | Avg. Stay | Vari-ance | Percentiles | | | | | | |
|---|---|---|---|---|---|---|---|---|---|---|
| | | | | 10th | 25th | 50th | 75th | 90th | 95th | 99th |
| **1. SINGLE DX** | | | | | | | | | | |
| 0–19 Years | 111 | 2.2 | 3 | 1 | 1 | 2 | 3 | 4 | 5 | 8 |
| 20–34 | 50 | 2.8 | 2 | 1 | 2 | 3 | 4 | 6 | 6 | 6 |
| 35–49 | 91 | 2.7 | 4 | 1 | 2 | 3 | 4 | 5 | 6 | 7 |
| 50–64 | 70 | 2.1 | 2 | 1 | 1 | 3 | 2 | 4 | 6 | 6 |
| 65+ | 82 | 2.9 | 4 | 1 | 1 | 4 | 4 | 5 | 7 | 11 |
| **2. MULTIPLE DX** | | | | | | | | | | |
| 0–19 Years | 698 | 6.5 | 177 | 1 | 3 | 3 | 5 | 13 | 28 | 97 |
| 20–34 | 464 | 3.4 | 11 | 1 | 2 | 3 | 4 | 7 | 11 | 17 |
| 35–49 | 970 | 4.3 | 15 | 1 | 2 | 4 | 6 | 9 | 12 | 18 |
| 50–64 | 1,144 | 4.5 | 11 | 1 | 2 | 4 | 6 | 8 | 11 | 17 |
| 65+ | 2,899 | 5.6 | 20 | 2 | 3 | 4 | 7 | 11 | 14 | 24 |
| **TOTAL SINGLE DX** | 404 | 2.5 | 3 | 1 | 1 | 2 | 3 | 5 | 6 | 8 |
| **TOTAL MULTIPLE DX** | 6,175 | 5.1 | 34 | 1 | 2 | 4 | 6 | 10 | 13 | 26 |
| **TOTAL** | | | | | | | | | | |
| 0–19 Years | 809 | 5.9 | 155 | 1 | 1 | 3 | 4 | 11 | 26 | 97 |
| 20–34 | 514 | 3.3 | 11 | 1 | 1 | 3 | 4 | 6 | 11 | 16 |
| 35–49 | 1,061 | 4.2 | 14 | 1 | 2 | 4 | 5 | 8 | 11 | 18 |
| 50–64 | 1,214 | 4.3 | 11 | 1 | 2 | 4 | 5 | 7 | 10 | 17 |
| 65+ | 2,981 | 5.5 | 20 | 2 | 3 | 4 | 7 | 11 | 14 | 24 |
| **GRAND TOTAL** | 6,579 | 4.9 | 32 | 1 | 2 | 4 | 6 | 9 | 12 | 25 |

Length of Stay by Diagnosis and Operation, United States, 2000

# United States, October 1998–September 1999 Data, by Operation

## 96.1: OTHER NONOP INSERTION. Formerly included in operation group(s) 796.

| Type of Patients | Observed Patients | Avg. Stay | Vari-ance | 10th | 25th | 50th | 75th | 90th | 95th | 99th |
|---|---|---|---|---|---|---|---|---|---|---|
| **1. SINGLE DX** | | | | | | | | | | |
| 0–19 Years | 0 | | | | | | | | | |
| 20–34 | 11 | 1.7 | 1 | 1 | 1 | 1 | 2 | 4 | 4 | 4 |
| 35–49 | 6 | 1.2 | <1 | 1 | 1 | 1 | 1 | 2 | 2 | 2 |
| 50–64 | 3 | 2.1 | <1 | 1 | 2 | 2 | 3 | 3 | 3 | 3 |
| 65+ | 1 | 1.0 | 0 | 1 | 1 | 1 | 1 | 1 | 1 | 1 |
| **2. MULTIPLE DX** | | | | | | | | | | |
| 0–19 Years | 7 | 1.2 | <1 | 1 | 1 | 1 | 1 | 1 | 4 | 4 |
| 20–34 | 25 | 3.2 | 22 | 1 | 1 | 2 | 3 | 6 | 8 | 32 |
| 35–49 | 27 | 4.0 | 5 | 1 | 2 | 3 | 7 | 7 | 7 | 9 |
| 50–64 | 17 | 3.2 | 4 | 1 | 2 | 3 | 3 | 5 | 8 | 10 |
| 65+ | 69 | 5.9 | 29 | 2 | 3 | 4 | 8 | 12 | 17 | 33 |
| **TOTAL SINGLE DX** | 21 | 1.6 | 1 | 1 | 1 | 1 | 2 | 3 | 4 | 4 |
| **TOTAL MULTIPLE DX** | 145 | 4.3 | 19 | 1 | 2 | 3 | 5 | 8 | 11 | 28 |
| **TOTAL** | | | | | | | | | | |
| 0–19 Years | 7 | 1.2 | <1 | 1 | 1 | 1 | 1 | 1 | 4 | 4 |
| 20–34 | 36 | 2.8 | 17 | 1 | 1 | 2 | 3 | 4 | 6 | 32 |
| 35–49 | 33 | 3.8 | 6 | 1 | 2 | 3 | 7 | 7 | 7 | 9 |
| 50–64 | 20 | 3.0 | 4 | 1 | 2 | 3 | 3 | 5 | 8 | 10 |
| 65+ | 70 | 5.9 | 29 | 2 | 3 | 4 | 7 | 12 | 17 | 33 |
| **GRAND TOTAL** | 166 | 4.1 | 18 | 1 | 1 | 3 | 5 | 8 | 11 | 28 |

## 96.2: NONOP DILATION & MANIP. Formerly included in operation group(s) 796.

| Type of Patients | Observed Patients | Avg. Stay | Vari-ance | 10th | 25th | 50th | 75th | 90th | 95th | 99th |
|---|---|---|---|---|---|---|---|---|---|---|
| **1. SINGLE DX** | | | | | | | | | | |
| 0–19 Years | 65 | 1.5 | <1 | 1 | 1 | 1 | 2 | 3 | 3 | 5 |
| 20–34 | 9 | 1.6 | <1 | 1 | 1 | 2 | 2 | 3 | 3 | 3 |
| 35–49 | 12 | 2.0 | <1 | 1 | 1 | 2 | 3 | 3 | 3 | 3 |
| 50–64 | 12 | 1.5 | <1 | 1 | 1 | 1 | 2 | 3 | 3 | 3 |
| 65+ | 11 | 1.8 | 3 | 1 | 1 | 1 | 2 | 6 | 6 | 6 |
| **2. MULTIPLE DX** | | | | | | | | | | |
| 0–19 Years | 124 | 4.0 | 42 | 1 | 1 | 2 | 5 | 7 | 12 | 47 |
| 20–34 | 26 | 4.0 | 20 | 1 | 2 | 2 | 4 | 8 | 17 | 21 |
| 35–49 | 57 | 2.8 | 7 | 1 | 1 | 2 | 3 | 7 | 8 | 12 |
| 50–64 | 69 | 4.0 | 22 | 1 | 1 | 2 | 5 | 9 | 15 | 28 |
| 65+ | 265 | 4.5 | 22 | 1 | 2 | 3 | 6 | 10 | 16 | 24 |
| **TOTAL SINGLE DX** | 109 | 1.7 | <1 | 1 | 1 | 1 | 2 | 3 | 3 | 6 |
| **TOTAL MULTIPLE DX** | 541 | 4.1 | 27 | 1 | 1 | 2 | 5 | 8 | 13 | 26 |
| **TOTAL** | | | | | | | | | | |
| 0–19 Years | 189 | 3.4 | 32 | 1 | 1 | 2 | 3 | 6 | 11 | 47 |
| 20–34 | 35 | 3.1 | 14 | 1 | 1 | 2 | 3 | 4 | 10 | 21 |
| 35–49 | 69 | 2.6 | 5 | 1 | 1 | 2 | 3 | 5 | 8 | 12 |
| 50–64 | 81 | 3.6 | 19 | 1 | 1 | 2 | 5 | 8 | 12 | 28 |
| 65+ | 276 | 4.3 | 22 | 1 | 2 | 3 | 6 | 10 | 15 | 24 |
| **GRAND TOTAL** | 650 | 3.7 | 23 | 1 | 1 | 2 | 4 | 8 | 12 | 24 |

## 96.3: NONOP GI IRRIG/INSTILL. Formerly included in operation group(s) 796.

| Type of Patients | Observed Patients | Avg. Stay | Vari-ance | 10th | 25th | 50th | 75th | 90th | 95th | 99th |
|---|---|---|---|---|---|---|---|---|---|---|
| **1. SINGLE DX** | | | | | | | | | | |
| 0–19 Years | 547 | 1.9 | 1 | 1 | 1 | 2 | 2 | 3 | 3 | 5 |
| 20–34 | 38 | 1.5 | <1 | 1 | 1 | 1 | 2 | 3 | 3 | 4 |
| 35–49 | 30 | 1.7 | 1 | 1 | 1 | 1 | 2 | 3 | 4 | 5 |
| 50–64 | 10 | 2.5 | 2 | 1 | 2 | 2 | 3 | 4 | 6 | 6 |
| 65+ | 9 | 2.2 | 3 | 1 | 1 | 1 | 4 | 5 | 5 | 5 |
| **2. MULTIPLE DX** | | | | | | | | | | |
| 0–19 Years | 1,579 | 4.7 | 44 | 1 | 2 | 2 | 5 | 12 | 17 | 30 |
| 20–34 | 1,038 | 2.9 | 13 | 1 | 1 | 2 | 3 | 7 | 10 | 15 |
| 35–49 | 1,097 | 2.5 | 6 | 1 | 2 | 2 | 3 | 5 | 9 | 11 |
| 50–64 | 362 | 3.7 | 10 | 1 | 2 | 3 | 6 | 6 | 8 | 14 |
| 65+ | 732 | 4.9 | 20 | 1 | 2 | 4 | 6 | 10 | 13 | 23 |
| **TOTAL SINGLE DX** | 634 | 1.8 | 1 | 1 | 1 | 2 | 2 | 3 | 3 | 5 |
| **TOTAL MULTIPLE DX** | 4,808 | 3.7 | 24 | 1 | 1 | 2 | 4 | 9 | 12 | 22 |
| **TOTAL** | | | | | | | | | | |
| 0–19 Years | 2,126 | 4.1 | 36 | 1 | 1 | 2 | 4 | 10 | 14 | 28 |
| 20–34 | 1,076 | 2.8 | 13 | 1 | 1 | 2 | 3 | 7 | 10 | 14 |
| 35–49 | 1,127 | 2.5 | 6 | 1 | 2 | 2 | 3 | 5 | 8 | 11 |
| 50–64 | 372 | 3.7 | 10 | 2 | 2 | 3 | 6 | 6 | 8 | 14 |
| 65+ | 741 | 4.9 | 20 | 1 | 2 | 3 | 6 | 10 | 13 | 23 |
| **GRAND TOTAL** | 5,442 | 3.5 | 22 | 1 | 1 | 2 | 4 | 8 | 12 | 21 |

## 96.33: GASTRIC LAVAGE. Formerly included in operation group(s) 796.

| Type of Patients | Observed Patients | Avg. Stay | Vari-ance | 10th | 25th | 50th | 75th | 90th | 95th | 99th |
|---|---|---|---|---|---|---|---|---|---|---|
| **1. SINGLE DX** | | | | | | | | | | |
| 0–19 Years | 463 | 1.8 | <1 | 1 | 1 | 2 | 2 | 3 | 3 | 4 |
| 20–34 | 34 | 1.5 | <1 | 1 | 1 | 1 | 2 | 3 | 3 | 4 |
| 35–49 | 21 | 1.3 | <1 | 1 | 2 | 2 | 2 | 2 | 2 | 3 |
| 50–64 | 5 | 2.2 | <1 | 2 | 2 | 2 | 3 | 3 | 4 | 4 |
| 65+ | 1 | 4.0 | 0 | 4 | 4 | 4 | 4 | 4 | 4 | 4 |
| **2. MULTIPLE DX** | | | | | | | | | | |
| 0–19 Years | 1,071 | 2.4 | 7 | 1 | 1 | 2 | 3 | 4 | 6 | 14 |
| 20–34 | 946 | 2.8 | 12 | 1 | 1 | 2 | 3 | 7 | 10 | 14 |
| 35–49 | 993 | 2.4 | 6 | 1 | 1 | 2 | 3 | 5 | 9 | 11 |
| 50–64 | 274 | 3.1 | 11 | 1 | 1 | 2 | 4 | 6 | 8 | 14 |
| 65+ | 158 | 4.0 | 14 | 1 | 1 | 3 | 5 | 7 | 12 | 20 |
| **TOTAL SINGLE DX** | 524 | 1.8 | <1 | 1 | 1 | 2 | 2 | 3 | 3 | 4 |
| **TOTAL MULTIPLE DX** | 3,442 | 2.6 | 9 | 1 | 1 | 2 | 3 | 5 | 8 | 14 |
| **TOTAL** | | | | | | | | | | |
| 0–19 Years | 1,534 | 2.3 | 6 | 1 | 1 | 2 | 3 | 4 | 5 | 10 |
| 20–34 | 980 | 2.7 | 12 | 1 | 1 | 2 | 3 | 6 | 10 | 14 |
| 35–49 | 1,014 | 2.4 | 6 | 1 | 1 | 2 | 3 | 5 | 9 | 11 |
| 50–64 | 279 | 3.1 | 11 | 1 | 1 | 2 | 4 | 5 | 8 | 14 |
| 65+ | 159 | 4.0 | 14 | 1 | 1 | 3 | 5 | 7 | 12 | 20 |
| **GRAND TOTAL** | 3,966 | 2.6 | 8 | 1 | 1 | 2 | 3 | 5 | 8 | 14 |

Length of Stay by Diagnosis and Operation, United States, 2000

# United States, October 1998–September 1999 Data, by Operation

## 96.35: GASTRIC GAVAGE. Formerly included in operation group(s) 796.

| Type of Patients | Observed Patients | Avg. Stay | Vari-ance | 10th | 25th | 50th | 75th | 90th | 95th | 99th |
|---|---|---|---|---|---|---|---|---|---|---|
| **1. SINGLE DX** | | | | | | | | | | |
| 0–19 Years | 4 | 7.2 | 8 | 2 | 5 | 9 | 9 | 9 | 9 | 9 |
| 20–34 | 0 | | | | | | | | | |
| 35–49 | 1 | 1.0 | 0 | 1 | 1 | 1 | 1 | 1 | 1 | 1 |
| 50–64 | 0 | | | | | | | | | |
| 65+ | 0 | | | | | | | | | |
| **2. MULTIPLE DX** | | | | | | | | | | |
| 0–19 Years | 289 | 11.0 | 94 | 3 | 6 | 9 | 14 | 21 | 24 | 63 |
| 20–34 | 15 | 3.5 | 61 | 1 | 1 | 1 | 2 | 4 | 34 | 34 |
| 35–49 | 10 | 1.3 | <1 | 1 | 1 | 1 | 2 | 2 | 2 | 2 |
| 50–64 | 1 | 6.0 | 0 | 6 | 6 | 6 | 6 | 6 | 6 | 6 |
| 65+ | 15 | 9.4 | 32 | 4 | 6 | 9 | 11 | 14 | 15 | 32 |
| **TOTAL SINGLE DX** | 5 | 5.8 | 14 | 1 | 2 | 9 | 9 | 9 | 9 | 9 |
| **TOTAL MULTIPLE DX** | 330 | 10.7 | 92 | 2 | 5 | 9 | 14 | 21 | 23 | 63 |
| **TOTAL** | | | | | | | | | | |
| 0–19 Years | 293 | 11.0 | 93 | 3 | 6 | 9 | 14 | 21 | 24 | 63 |
| 20–34 | 15 | 3.5 | 61 | 1 | 1 | 1 | 2 | 4 | 34 | 34 |
| 35–49 | 11 | 1.2 | <1 | 1 | 1 | 1 | 1 | 2 | 2 | 2 |
| 50–64 | 1 | 6.0 | 0 | 6 | 6 | 6 | 6 | 6 | 6 | 6 |
| 65+ | 15 | 9.4 | 32 | 4 | 6 | 9 | 11 | 14 | 15 | 32 |
| **GRAND TOTAL** | 335 | 10.6 | 92 | 2 | 5 | 9 | 14 | 20 | 23 | 63 |

## 96.4: DIGEST/GU IRRIG/INSTILL. Formerly included in operation group(s) 796.

| Type of Patients | Observed Patients | Avg. Stay | Vari-ance | 10th | 25th | 50th | 75th | 90th | 95th | 99th |
|---|---|---|---|---|---|---|---|---|---|---|
| **1. SINGLE DX** | | | | | | | | | | |
| 0–19 Years | 130 | 1.7 | <1 | 1 | 1 | 1 | 2 | 3 | 3 | 4 |
| 20–34 | 754 | 1.4 | <1 | 1 | 1 | 1 | 2 | 2 | 3 | 3 |
| 35–49 | 154 | 1.4 | <1 | 1 | 1 | 1 | 2 | 2 | 2 | 3 |
| 50–64 | 6 | 1.3 | <1 | 1 | 1 | 1 | 2 | 2 | 2 | 2 |
| 65+ | 8 | 1.5 | <1 | 1 | 1 | 2 | 2 | 2 | 2 | 2 |
| **2. MULTIPLE DX** | | | | | | | | | | |
| 0–19 Years | 219 | 2.3 | 3 | 1 | 1 | 1 | 3 | 4 | 5 | 12 |
| 20–34 | 1,170 | 2.1 | 2 | 1 | 1 | 1 | 2 | 3 | 4 | 8 |
| 35–49 | 377 | 2.4 | 8 | 1 | 1 | 1 | 3 | 5 | 7 | 21 |
| 50–64 | 88 | 3.4 | 8 | 1 | 2 | 2 | 4 | 6 | 7 | 18 |
| 65+ | 280 | 4.1 | 15 | 1 | 2 | 3 | 5 | 9 | 11 | 18 |
| **TOTAL SINGLE DX** | 1,052 | 1.4 | <1 | 1 | 1 | 1 | 2 | 2 | 3 | 4 |
| **TOTAL MULTIPLE DX** | 2,134 | 2.4 | 5 | 1 | 1 | 2 | 3 | 4 | 6 | 12 |
| **TOTAL** | | | | | | | | | | |
| 0–19 Years | 349 | 2.1 | 2 | 1 | 1 | 1 | 2 | 4 | 4 | 8 |
| 20–34 | 1,924 | 1.8 | 2 | 1 | 1 | 1 | 2 | 3 | 4 | 7 |
| 35–49 | 531 | 2.0 | 5 | 1 | 1 | 1 | 2 | 3 | 5 | 10 |
| 50–64 | 94 | 3.3 | 8 | 1 | 2 | 2 | 4 | 6 | 7 | 14 |
| 65+ | 288 | 4.1 | 15 | 1 | 2 | 3 | 5 | 9 | 11 | 16 |
| **GRAND TOTAL** | 3,186 | 2.0 | 4 | 1 | 1 | 1 | 2 | 3 | 5 | 10 |

## 96.38: IMPACTED FECES REMOVAL. Formerly included in operation group(s) 796.

| Type of Patients | Observed Patients | Avg. Stay | Vari-ance | 10th | 25th | 50th | 75th | 90th | 95th | 99th |
|---|---|---|---|---|---|---|---|---|---|---|
| **1. SINGLE DX** | | | | | | | | | | |
| 0–19 Years | 49 | 2.0 | 2 | 1 | 1 | 2 | 2 | 2 | 3 | 7 |
| 20–34 | 2 | 1.5 | <1 | 1 | 1 | 2 | 2 | 2 | 2 | 2 |
| 35–49 | 6 | 2.6 | 1 | 1 | 1 | 2 | 4 | 4 | 4 | 4 |
| 50–64 | 3 | 4.2 | 2 | 3 | 3 | 3 | 6 | 6 | 6 | 6 |
| 65+ | 5 | 1.1 | <1 | 1 | 1 | 1 | 1 | 2 | 2 | 2 |
| **2. MULTIPLE DX** | | | | | | | | | | |
| 0–19 Years | 141 | 2.7 | 5 | 1 | 1 | 2 | 3 | 6 | 7 | 9 |
| 20–34 | 36 | 5.5 | 38 | 1 | 2 | 3 | 6 | 21 | 21 | 21 |
| 35–49 | 49 | 2.9 | 2 | 1 | 2 | 2 | 4 | 4 | 6 | 8 |
| 50–64 | 60 | 5.0 | 7 | 1 | 3 | 6 | 6 | 7 | 7 | 20 |
| 65+ | 478 | 5.1 | 19 | 1 | 2 | 4 | 6 | 11 | 13 | 22 |
| **TOTAL SINGLE DX** | 65 | 2.0 | 2 | 1 | 1 | 2 | 2 | 3 | 4 | 7 |
| **TOTAL MULTIPLE DX** | 764 | 4.5 | 15 | 1 | 2 | 3 | 6 | 9 | 13 | 21 |
| **TOTAL** | | | | | | | | | | |
| 0–19 Years | 190 | 2.5 | 4 | 1 | 1 | 2 | 3 | 5 | 7 | 9 |
| 20–34 | 38 | 5.4 | 38 | 2 | 2 | 3 | 5 | 17 | 21 | 21 |
| 35–49 | 55 | 2.8 | 2 | 1 | 2 | 2 | 4 | 4 | 5 | 8 |
| 50–64 | 63 | 5.0 | 7 | 2 | 3 | 6 | 6 | 6 | 7 | 20 |
| 65+ | 483 | 5.0 | 19 | 1 | 2 | 4 | 6 | 10 | 13 | 22 |
| **GRAND TOTAL** | 829 | 4.3 | 15 | 1 | 2 | 3 | 6 | 8 | 12 | 21 |

## 96.49: OTHER GU INSTILLATION. Formerly included in operation group(s) 796.

| Type of Patients | Observed Patients | Avg. Stay | Vari-ance | 10th | 25th | 50th | 75th | 90th | 95th | 99th |
|---|---|---|---|---|---|---|---|---|---|---|
| **1. SINGLE DX** | | | | | | | | | | |
| 0–19 Years | 128 | 1.7 | <1 | 1 | 1 | 1 | 2 | 3 | 3 | 4 |
| 20–34 | 745 | 1.4 | <1 | 1 | 1 | 1 | 2 | 2 | 3 | 3 |
| 35–49 | 152 | 1.4 | <1 | 1 | 1 | 1 | 2 | 2 | 2 | 3 |
| 50–64 | 4 | 1.4 | <1 | 1 | 1 | 1 | 2 | 2 | 2 | 2 |
| 65+ | 0 | | | | | | | | | |
| **2. MULTIPLE DX** | | | | | | | | | | |
| 0–19 Years | 206 | 2.1 | 1 | 1 | 2 | 2 | 2 | 4 | 4 | 5 |
| 20–34 | 1,148 | 2.1 | 2 | 1 | 1 | 2 | 2 | 3 | 4 | 8 |
| 35–49 | 329 | 2.0 | 4 | 1 | 1 | 2 | 2 | 3 | 5 | 10 |
| 50–64 | 23 | 3.6 | 3 | 2 | 2 | 4 | 4 | 6 | 6 | 8 |
| 65+ | 104 | 4.0 | 16 | 1 | 2 | 2 | 5 | 9 | 12 | 19 |
| **TOTAL SINGLE DX** | 1,029 | 1.4 | <1 | 1 | 1 | 1 | 2 | 2 | 3 | 4 |
| **TOTAL MULTIPLE DX** | 1,810 | 2.1 | 3 | 1 | 1 | 2 | 2 | 4 | 5 | 10 |
| **TOTAL** | | | | | | | | | | |
| 0–19 Years | 334 | 1.9 | 1 | 1 | 1 | 2 | 2 | 3 | 4 | 5 |
| 20–34 | 1,893 | 1.8 | 2 | 1 | 1 | 1 | 2 | 3 | 3 | 7 |
| 35–49 | 481 | 1.7 | 3 | 1 | 1 | 2 | 2 | 3 | 5 | 10 |
| 50–64 | 27 | 3.4 | 3 | 2 | 2 | 2 | 4 | 6 | 6 | 8 |
| 65+ | 104 | 4.0 | 16 | 1 | 2 | 2 | 5 | 9 | 12 | 19 |
| **GRAND TOTAL** | 2,839 | 1.8 | 2 | 1 | 1 | 1 | 2 | 3 | 4 | 8 |

Length of Stay by Diagnosis and Operation, United States, 2000

# United States, October 1998–September 1999 Data, by Operation

## 96.5: OTHER NONOP IRRIG/CLEAN. Formerly included in operation group(s) 796.

| Type of Patients | Observed Patients | Avg. Stay | Vari-ance | 10th | 25th | 50th | 75th | 90th | 95th | 99th |
|---|---|---|---|---|---|---|---|---|---|---|
| **1. SINGLE DX** | | | | | | | | | | |
| 0–19 Years | 243 | 2.3 | 1 | 1 | 2 | 2 | 3 | 4 | 4 | 5 |
| 20–34 | 43 | 2.4 | 9 | 1 | 1 | 1 | 3 | 5 | 7 | 25 |
| 35–49 | 21 | 2.0 | 5 | 1 | 1 | 1 | 2 | 3 | 4 | 17 |
| 50–64 | 14 | 3.9 | 12 | 1 | 1 | 3 | 6 | 9 | 10 | 10 |
| 65+ | 6 | 9.8 | 60 | 1 | 3 | 7 | 16 | 20 | 20 | 20 |
| **2. MULTIPLE DX** | | | | | | | | | | |
| 0–19 Years | 523 | 4.1 | 21 | 1 | 2 | 3 | 4 | 8 | 11 | 24 |
| 20–34 | 219 | 6.5 | 77 | 1 | 1 | 4 | 8 | 16 | 21 | 61 |
| 35–49 | 381 | 6.4 | 42 | 1 | 2 | 5 | 8 | 14 | 20 | 34 |
| 50–64 | 370 | 7.8 | 45 | 2 | 3 | 7 | 10 | 15 | 19 | 51 |
| 65+ | 883 | 8.8 | 44 | 2 | 4 | 8 | 12 | 17 | 21 | 29 |
| **TOTAL SINGLE DX** | 327 | 2.4 | 3 | 1 | 2 | 2 | 3 | 4 | 4 | 9 |
| **TOTAL MULTIPLE DX** | 2,376 | 6.5 | 41 | 1 | 2 | 4 | 9 | 14 | 18 | 30 |
| **TOTAL** | | | | | | | | | | |
| 0–19 Years | 766 | 3.4 | 14 | 1 | 2 | 3 | 4 | 6 | 9 | 21 |
| 20–34 | 262 | 5.9 | 68 | 1 | 1 | 3 | 7 | 12 | 20 | 48 |
| 35–49 | 402 | 6.2 | 41 | 1 | 2 | 4 | 8 | 14 | 19 | 34 |
| 50–64 | 384 | 7.7 | 45 | 2 | 3 | 7 | 10 | 15 | 18 | 51 |
| 65+ | 889 | 8.8 | 44 | 2 | 4 | 8 | 12 | 17 | 21 | 29 |
| **GRAND TOTAL** | 2,703 | 5.7 | 37 | 1 | 2 | 4 | 7 | 13 | 17 | 29 |

## 96.56: BRONCH/TRACH LAVAGE NEC. Formerly included in operation group(s) 796.

| Type of Patients | Observed Patients | Avg. Stay | Vari-ance | 10th | 25th | 50th | 75th | 90th | 95th | 99th |
|---|---|---|---|---|---|---|---|---|---|---|
| **1. SINGLE DX** | | | | | | | | | | |
| 0–19 Years | 195 | 2.3 | 1 | 1 | 2 | 2 | 3 | 4 | 4 | 5 |
| 20–34 | 11 | 3.4 | 36 | 1 | 1 | 2 | 3 | 7 | 25 | 25 |
| 35–49 | 8 | 2.3 | 2 | 1 | 1 | 2 | 3 | 4 | 5 | 5 |
| 50–64 | 4 | 6.7 | 13 | 1 | 3 | 9 | 9 | 9 | 9 | 9 |
| 65+ | 2 | 3.0 | 0 | 3 | 3 | 3 | 3 | 3 | 3 | 3 |
| **2. MULTIPLE DX** | | | | | | | | | | |
| 0–19 Years | 383 | 4.2 | 20 | 2 | 2 | 3 | 4 | 8 | 12 | 26 |
| 20–34 | 99 | 11.1 | 137 | 3 | 4 | 7 | 12 | 23 | 34 | 65 |
| 35–49 | 211 | 8.5 | 51 | 2 | 4 | 7 | 11 | 18 | 23 | 48 |
| 50–64 | 240 | 8.7 | 44 | 3 | 5 | 7 | 10 | 16 | 19 | 51 |
| 65+ | 541 | 10.0 | 35 | 4 | 6 | 9 | 13 | 17 | 21 | 29 |
| **TOTAL SINGLE DX** | 220 | 2.3 | 2 | 1 | 2 | 2 | 3 | 4 | 4 | 7 |
| **TOTAL MULTIPLE DX** | 1,474 | 7.0 | 42 | 2 | 2 | 5 | 9 | 15 | 19 | 34 |
| **TOTAL** | | | | | | | | | | |
| 0–19 Years | 578 | 3.4 | 14 | 1 | 2 | 2 | 4 | 6 | 9 | 21 |
| 20–34 | 110 | 10.5 | 133 | 2 | 4 | 8 | 11 | 22 | 29 | 65 |
| 35–49 | 219 | 8.4 | 51 | 3 | 4 | 6 | 10 | 17 | 22 | 48 |
| 50–64 | 244 | 8.6 | 44 | 4 | 5 | 7 | 10 | 16 | 19 | 51 |
| 65+ | 543 | 10.0 | 35 | 4 | 6 | 9 | 13 | 17 | 21 | 29 |
| **GRAND TOTAL** | 1,694 | 5.8 | 36 | 2 | 2 | 4 | 8 | 13 | 17 | 29 |

## 96.52: IRRIGATION OF EAR. Formerly included in operation group(s) 796.

| Type of Patients | Observed Patients | Avg. Stay | Vari-ance | 10th | 25th | 50th | 75th | 90th | 95th | 99th |
|---|---|---|---|---|---|---|---|---|---|---|
| **1. SINGLE DX** | | | | | | | | | | |
| 0–19 Years | 4 | 3.8 | 1 | 3 | 3 | 4 | 5 | 5 | 5 | 5 |
| 20–34 | 0 | | | | | | | | | |
| 35–49 | 0 | | | | | | | | | |
| 50–64 | 1 | 3.0 | 0 | 3 | 3 | 3 | 3 | 3 | 3 | 3 |
| 65+ | 1 | 7.0 | 0 | 7 | 7 | 7 | 7 | 7 | 7 | 7 |
| **2. MULTIPLE DX** | | | | | | | | | | |
| 0–19 Years | 56 | 4.2 | 11 | 1 | 2 | 3 | 4 | 8 | 11 | 13 |
| 20–34 | 20 | 6.2 | 42 | 1 | 3 | 3 | 7 | 20 | 20 | 20 |
| 35–49 | 29 | 5.8 | 18 | 1 | 2 | 4 | 8 | 13 | 14 | >99 |
| 50–64 | 39 | 7.0 | 43 | 2 | 2 | 4 | 9 | 17 | 22 | 32 |
| 65+ | 203 | 7.9 | 53 | 2 | 4 | 6 | 10 | 17 | 21 | 35 |
| **TOTAL SINGLE DX** | 6 | 4.6 | 3 | 3 | 3 | 4 | 7 | 7 | 7 | 7 |
| **TOTAL MULTIPLE DX** | 347 | 6.9 | 42 | 2 | 3 | 5 | 9 | 14 | 20 | 28 |
| **TOTAL** | | | | | | | | | | |
| 0–19 Years | 60 | 4.2 | 11 | 1 | 3 | 3 | 6 | 10 | 10 | 13 |
| 20–34 | 20 | 6.2 | 42 | 1 | 3 | 3 | 7 | 20 | 20 | 20 |
| 35–49 | 29 | 5.8 | 18 | 1 | 2 | 4 | 8 | 13 | 14 | >99 |
| 50–64 | 40 | 6.9 | 42 | 2 | 2 | 4 | 9 | 16 | 22 | 32 |
| 65+ | 204 | 7.9 | 52 | 2 | 4 | 6 | 10 | 17 | 21 | 35 |
| **GRAND TOTAL** | 353 | 6.8 | 42 | 2 | 3 | 5 | 9 | 14 | 20 | 28 |

## 96.59: WOUND IRRIGATION NEC. Formerly included in operation group(s) 796.

| Type of Patients | Observed Patients | Avg. Stay | Vari-ance | 10th | 25th | 50th | 75th | 90th | 95th | 99th |
|---|---|---|---|---|---|---|---|---|---|---|
| **1. SINGLE DX** | | | | | | | | | | |
| 0–19 Years | 36 | 1.7 | 2 | 1 | 1 | 1 | 1 | 4 | 4 | 5 |
| 20–34 | 32 | 2.2 | 3 | 1 | 1 | 2 | 3 | 5 | 7 | 7 |
| 35–49 | 13 | 1.9 | 6 | 1 | 1 | 1 | 2 | 2 | 3 | 17 |
| 50–64 | 8 | 3.0 | 10 | 1 | 1 | 1 | 4 | 10 | 10 | 10 |
| 65+ | 2 | 13.9 | 95 | 1 | 1 | 20 | 20 | 20 | 20 | 20 |
| **2. MULTIPLE DX** | | | | | | | | | | |
| 0–19 Years | 58 | 3.5 | 38 | 1 | 1 | 2 | 4 | 6 | 13 | 16 |
| 20–34 | 68 | 3.1 | 10 | 1 | 1 | 2 | 4 | 6 | 10 | 16 |
| 35–49 | 95 | 4.5 | 32 | 1 | 2 | 2 | 5 | 10 | 15 | 26 |
| 50–64 | 51 | 6.6 | 64 | 1 | 3 | 5 | 7 | 12 | 19 | 56 |
| 65+ | 73 | 7.0 | 59 | 1 | 2 | 5 | 8 | 14 | 21 | 29 |
| **TOTAL SINGLE DX** | 91 | 2.3 | 8 | 1 | 1 | 2 | 2 | 4 | 7 | 20 |
| **TOTAL MULTIPLE DX** | 345 | 4.8 | 41 | 1 | 1 | 3 | 5 | 11 | 15 | 29 |
| **TOTAL** | | | | | | | | | | |
| 0–19 Years | 94 | 2.9 | 27 | 1 | 1 | 2 | 4 | 5 | 6 | 16 |
| 20–34 | 100 | 2.8 | 8 | 1 | 1 | 2 | 4 | 5 | 9 | 16 |
| 35–49 | 108 | 4.1 | 30 | 1 | 2 | 2 | 5 | 9 | 15 | 26 |
| 50–64 | 59 | 6.1 | 57 | 1 | 2 | 5 | 7 | 11 | 19 | 56 |
| 65+ | 75 | 7.1 | 61 | 1 | 2 | 5 | 8 | 17 | 21 | 29 |
| **GRAND TOTAL** | 436 | 4.3 | 35 | 1 | 1 | 2 | 5 | 9 | 14 | 26 |

## United States, October 1998–September 1999 Data, by Operation

### 96.6: ENTERAL NUTRITION. Formerly included in operation group(s) 796.

| Type of Patients | Observed Patients | Avg. Stay | Variance | 10th | 25th | 50th | 75th | 90th | 95th | 99th |
|---|---|---|---|---|---|---|---|---|---|---|
| **1. SINGLE DX** | | | | | | | | | | |
| 0–19 Years | 48 | 7.2 | 76 | 1 | 3 | 4 | 7 | 14 | 32 | 35 |
| 20–34 | 7 | 29.6 | 66 | 18 | 32 | 32 | 32 | 32 | 35 | 35 |
| 35–49 | 2 | 3.1 | 3 | 1 | 1 | 1 | 4 | 4 | 4 | 4 |
| 50–64 | 5 | 7.9 | 7 | 4 | 6 | 8 | 11 | 11 | 11 | 11 |
| 65+ | 4 | 3.9 | 6 | 1 | 3 | 3 | 5 | 9 | 9 | 9 |
| **2. MULTIPLE DX** | | | | | | | | | | |
| 0–19 Years | 1,554 | 11.8 | 125 | 2 | 3 | 9 | 16 | 28 | 36 | 54 |
| 20–34 | 226 | 12.9 | 238 | 2 | 5 | 7 | 14 | 30 | 69 | 69 |
| 35–49 | 361 | 12.3 | 256 | 2 | 4 | 7 | 12 | 26 | 53 | 81 |
| 50–64 | 675 | 12.2 | 112 | 3 | 4 | 8 | 15 | 33 | 35 | 37 |
| 65+ | 3,395 | 9.6 | 61 | 3 | 5 | 7 | 12 | 18 | 24 | 40 |
| **TOTAL SINGLE DX** | 66 | 15.6 | 188 | 2 | 3 | 8 | 32 | 32 | 32 | 35 |
| **TOTAL MULTIPLE DX** | 6,211 | 10.8 | 108 | 3 | 4 | 8 | 14 | 23 | 33 | 53 |
| **TOTAL** | | | | | | | | | | |
| 0–19 Years | 1,602 | 11.7 | 125 | 2 | 3 | 8 | 16 | 28 | 36 | 54 |
| 20–34 | 233 | 14.8 | 246 | 3 | 6 | 7 | 18 | 32 | 49 | 69 |
| 35–49 | 363 | 12.2 | 256 | 2 | 4 | 7 | 12 | 26 | 53 | 81 |
| 50–64 | 680 | 12.2 | 112 | 3 | 4 | 8 | 15 | 33 | 35 | 37 |
| 65+ | 3,399 | 9.6 | 61 | 3 | 5 | 7 | 12 | 18 | 24 | 40 |
| **GRAND TOTAL** | 6,277 | 10.9 | 109 | 3 | 4 | 8 | 14 | 23 | 33 | 53 |

### 96.70: CONT MECH VENT-TIME NOS. Formerly included in operation group(s) 790.

| Type of Patients | Observed Patients | Avg. Stay | Variance | 10th | 25th | 50th | 75th | 90th | 95th | 99th |
|---|---|---|---|---|---|---|---|---|---|---|
| **1. SINGLE DX** | | | | | | | | | | |
| 0–19 Years | 1 | 49.0 | 0 | 49 | 49 | 49 | 49 | 49 | 49 | 49 |
| 20–34 | 1 | 2.0 | 0 | 2 | 2 | 2 | 2 | 2 | 2 | 2 |
| 35–49 | 0 | | | | | | | | | |
| 50–64 | 1 | 14.0 | 0 | 14 | 14 | 14 | 14 | 14 | 14 | 14 |
| 65+ | 0 | | | | | | | | | |
| **2. MULTIPLE DX** | | | | | | | | | | |
| 0–19 Years | 86 | 9.1 | 147 | 1 | 2 | 7 | 10 | 22 | 37 | 89 |
| 20–34 | 21 | 5.3 | 23 | 1 | 2 | 3 | 7 | 14 | 16 | 17 |
| 35–49 | 32 | 7.3 | 28 | 2 | 3 | 4 | 12 | 15 | 17 | 19 |
| 50–64 | 61 | 10.8 | 80 | 2 | 5 | 8 | 14 | 27 | 30 | 37 |
| 65+ | 143 | 12.4 | 85 | 4 | 7 | 10 | 17 | 23 | 27 | 59 |
| **TOTAL SINGLE DX** | 3 | 19.4 | 529 | 2 | 2 | 14 | 49 | 49 | 49 | 49 |
| **TOTAL MULTIPLE DX** | 343 | 10.3 | 95 | 2 | 4 | 8 | 13 | 22 | 29 | 51 |
| **TOTAL** | | | | | | | | | | |
| 0–19 Years | 87 | 9.3 | 155 | 2 | 2 | 7 | 10 | 26 | 39 | 89 |
| 20–34 | 22 | 5.2 | 233 | 1 | 2 | 3 | 7 | 14 | 16 | 17 |
| 35–49 | 32 | 7.3 | 28 | 2 | 3 | 4 | 12 | 15 | 17 | 19 |
| 50–64 | 62 | 10.9 | 80 | 2 | 5 | 8 | 14 | 27 | 30 | 37 |
| 65+ | 143 | 12.4 | 85 | 4 | 7 | 10 | 17 | 23 | 27 | 59 |
| **GRAND TOTAL** | 346 | 10.3 | 97 | 2 | 4 | 8 | 13 | 22 | 29 | 51 |

### 96.7: CONT MECH VENT NEC. Formerly included in operation group(s) 790.

| Type of Patients | Observed Patients | Avg. Stay | Variance | 10th | 25th | 50th | 75th | 90th | 95th | 99th |
|---|---|---|---|---|---|---|---|---|---|---|
| **1. SINGLE DX** | | | | | | | | | | |
| 0–19 Years | 202 | 3.8 | 12 | 1 | 2 | 2 | 4 | 8 | 10 | 12 |
| 20–34 | 60 | 2.7 | 8 | 1 | 1 | 2 | 3 | 6 | 9 | 12 |
| 35–49 | 48 | 4.2 | 36 | 1 | 1 | 3 | 4 | 8 | 12 | 19 |
| 50–64 | 35 | 5.3 | 29 | 1 | 2 | 3 | 6 | 13 | 21 | 25 |
| 65+ | 40 | 10.9 | 268 | 2 | 5 | 5 | 14 | 14 | 17 | 88 |
| **2. MULTIPLE DX** | | | | | | | | | | |
| 0–19 Years | 10,607 | 19.5 | 473 | 2 | 5 | 11 | 27 | 61 | 81 | >99 |
| 20–34 | 2,977 | 7.3 | 69 | 1 | 2 | 4 | 9 | 17 | 23 | 46 |
| 35–49 | 5,642 | 9.6 | 100 | 2 | 3 | 6 | 13 | 21 | 29 | 52 |
| 50–64 | 9,314 | 11.1 | 84 | 3 | 5 | 9 | 14 | 22 | 28 | 53 |
| 65+ | 21,325 | 11.8 | 83 | 4 | 6 | 9 | 15 | 23 | 28 | 51 |
| **TOTAL SINGLE DX** | 385 | 4.5 | 49 | 1 | 2 | 3 | 5 | 9 | 13 | 21 |
| **TOTAL MULTIPLE DX** | 49,865 | 12.6 | 175 | 3 | 5 | 9 | 15 | 26 | 40 | 88 |
| **TOTAL** | | | | | | | | | | |
| 0–19 Years | 10,809 | 19.1 | 468 | 2 | 5 | 11 | 26 | 60 | 80 | >99 |
| 20–34 | 3,037 | 7.1 | 68 | 1 | 2 | 4 | 9 | 17 | 22 | 46 |
| 35–49 | 5,690 | 9.6 | 100 | 2 | 3 | 6 | 13 | 21 | 29 | 52 |
| 50–64 | 9,349 | 11.1 | 84 | 3 | 5 | 9 | 14 | 22 | 28 | 53 |
| 65+ | 21,365 | 11.8 | 84 | 4 | 6 | 9 | 15 | 23 | 28 | 51 |
| **GRAND TOTAL** | 50,250 | 12.5 | 174 | 2 | 5 | 9 | 15 | 26 | 40 | 88 |

### 96.71: CONT MECH VENT-<96 HOURS. Formerly included in operation group(s) 790.

| Type of Patients | Observed Patients | Avg. Stay | Variance | 10th | 25th | 50th | 75th | 90th | 95th | 99th |
|---|---|---|---|---|---|---|---|---|---|---|
| **1. SINGLE DX** | | | | | | | | | | |
| 0–19 Years | 186 | 3.2 | 4 | 1 | 2 | 2 | 4 | 6 | 7 | 10 |
| 20–34 | 58 | 2.7 | 8 | 1 | 1 | 2 | 3 | 6 | 9 | 12 |
| 35–49 | 44 | 3.0 | 4 | 1 | 3 | 3 | 4 | 7 | 8 | 9 |
| 50–64 | 26 | 2.9 | 4 | 1 | 2 | 3 | 4 | 6 | 6 | 6 |
| 65+ | 29 | 10.0 | 379 | 2 | 4 | 5 | 7 | 11 | 88 | 88 |
| **2. MULTIPLE DX** | | | | | | | | | | |
| 0–19 Years | 6,700 | 13.5 | 273 | 2 | 3 | 7 | 16 | 39 | 52 | 90 |
| 20–34 | 2,193 | 4.5 | 20 | 1 | 2 | 3 | 6 | 9 | 12 | 22 |
| 35–49 | 3,706 | 5.8 | 29 | 2 | 2 | 4 | 8 | 12 | 15 | 26 |
| 50–64 | 5,868 | 8.1 | 38 | 3 | 4 | 7 | 10 | 15 | 20 | 28 |
| 65+ | 14,152 | 9.0 | 41 | 3 | 5 | 7 | 11 | 16 | 20 | 31 |
| **TOTAL SINGLE DX** | 343 | 3.6 | 41 | 1 | 2 | 2 | 4 | 7 | 8 | 14 |
| **TOTAL MULTIPLE DX** | 32,619 | 8.9 | 87 | 2 | 4 | 7 | 11 | 17 | 25 | 53 |
| **TOTAL** | | | | | | | | | | |
| 0–19 Years | 6,886 | 13.1 | 267 | 2 | 3 | 7 | 15 | 37 | 52 | 87 |
| 20–34 | 2,251 | 4.4 | 19 | 1 | 2 | 3 | 6 | 9 | 12 | 22 |
| 35–49 | 3,750 | 5.8 | 29 | 2 | 3 | 4 | 8 | 12 | 15 | 26 |
| 50–64 | 5,894 | 8.1 | 38 | 3 | 4 | 7 | 10 | 15 | 20 | 28 |
| 65+ | 14,181 | 9.0 | 42 | 3 | 5 | 7 | 11 | 16 | 20 | 32 |
| **GRAND TOTAL** | 32,962 | 8.8 | 87 | 2 | 4 | 6 | 11 | 17 | 25 | 53 |

Length of Stay by Diagnosis and Operation, United States, 2000

405

# United States, October 1998–September 1999 Data, by Operation

## 96.72: CONT MECH VENT->95 HOURS. Formerly included in operation group(s) 790.

| Type of Patients | Observed Patients | Avg. Stay | Variance | 10th | 25th | 50th | 75th | 90th | 95th | 99th |
|---|---|---|---|---|---|---|---|---|---|---|
| **1. SINGLE DX** | | | | | | | | | | |
| 0–19 Years | 15 | 7.7 | 16 | 3 | 4 | 8 | 11 | 12 | 12 | 18 |
| 20-34 | 1 | 5.0 | 0 | 5 | 5 | 5 | 5 | 5 | 5 | 5 |
| 35-49 | 4 | 18.2 | 201 | 12 | 12 | 12 | 19 | 55 | 55 | 55 |
| 50-64 | 8 | 15.4 | 23 | 9 | 13 | 13 | 21 | 21 | 25 | 25 |
| 65+ | 11 | 12.8 | 16 | 6 | 11 | 14 | 14 | 16 | 17 | 24 |
| **2. MULTIPLE DX** | | | | | | | | | | |
| 0–19 Years | 3,821 | 30.4 | 649 | 8 | 11 | 21 | 53 | 85 | >99 | >99 |
| 20-34 | 763 | 16.1 | 127 | 7 | 9 | 13 | 19 | 31 | 43 | >99 |
| 35-49 | 1,904 | 18.4 | 154 | 7 | 10 | 15 | 22 | 36 | 48 | 84 |
| 50-64 | 3,385 | 17.2 | 123 | 7 | 10 | 14 | 21 | 31 | 38 | 83 |
| 65+ | 7,030 | 17.9 | 120 | 8 | 11 | 15 | 22 | 30 | 38 | 72 |
| **TOTAL SINGLE DX** | 39 | 11.2 | 48 | 4 | 7 | 12 | 14 | 17 | 21 | 55 |
| **TOTAL MULTIPLE DX** | 16,903 | 20.5 | 270 | 8 | 11 | 16 | 24 | 43 | 69 | >99 |
| **TOTAL** | | | | | | | | | | |
| 0–19 Years | 3,836 | 30.2 | 648 | 8 | 11 | 20 | 53 | 84 | >99 | >99 |
| 20-34 | 764 | 16.1 | 127 | 7 | 9 | 13 | 19 | 31 | 43 | >99 |
| 35-49 | 1,908 | 18.4 | 154 | 7 | 10 | 15 | 22 | 36 | 49 | 84 |
| 50-64 | 3,393 | 17.2 | 122 | 7 | 10 | 14 | 21 | 31 | 38 | 83 |
| 65+ | 7,041 | 17.8 | 119 | 8 | 11 | 15 | 22 | 30 | 38 | 72 |
| **GRAND TOTAL** | 16,942 | 20.4 | 269 | 8 | 11 | 16 | 24 | 43 | 69 | >99 |

## 97.02: REPL GASTROSTOMY TUBE. Formerly included in operation group(s) 796.

| Type of Patients | Observed Patients | Avg. Stay | Variance | 10th | 25th | 50th | 75th | 90th | 95th | 99th |
|---|---|---|---|---|---|---|---|---|---|---|
| **1. SINGLE DX** | | | | | | | | | | |
| 0–19 Years | 73 | 1.2 | <1 | 1 | 1 | 1 | 1 | 2 | 2 | 5 |
| 20-34 | 10 | 1.0 | 0 | 1 | 1 | 1 | 1 | 1 | 1 | 5 |
| 35-49 | 2 | 3.0 | 5 | 1 | 1 | 1 | 5 | 5 | 5 | 5 |
| 50-64 | 1 | 1.0 | 0 | 1 | 1 | 1 | 1 | 1 | 1 | 1 |
| 65+ | 15 | 2.4 | 4 | 2 | 2 | 2 | 2 | 2 | 4 | 12 |
| **2. MULTIPLE DX** | | | | | | | | | | |
| 0–19 Years | 412 | 5.1 | 38 | 1 | 1 | 3 | 7 | 13 | 16 | 31 |
| 20-34 | 107 | 7.7 | 72 | 1 | 3 | 5 | 10 | 14 | 28 | 38 |
| 35-49 | 175 | 7.3 | 76 | 2 | 3 | 5 | 8 | 17 | 21 | 56 |
| 50-64 | 279 | 8.4 | 88 | 2 | 4 | 6 | 9 | 15 | 23 | 64 |
| 65+ | 2,210 | 7.6 | 35 | 2 | 4 | 6 | 10 | 14 | 17 | 30 |
| **TOTAL SINGLE DX** | 101 | 2.1 | 3 | 1 | 2 | 2 | 2 | 2 | 4 | 12 |
| **TOTAL MULTIPLE DX** | 3,183 | 7.2 | 44 | 1 | 3 | 6 | 9 | 14 | 18 | 34 |
| **TOTAL** | | | | | | | | | | |
| 0–19 Years | 485 | 4.9 | 37 | 1 | 3 | 5 | 6 | 13 | 16 | 31 |
| 20-34 | 117 | 7.6 | 72 | 1 | 3 | 5 | 10 | 13 | 28 | 38 |
| 35-49 | 177 | 7.3 | 75 | 2 | 3 | 5 | 8 | 17 | 21 | 56 |
| 50-64 | 280 | 8.4 | 88 | 2 | 3 | 6 | 9 | 15 | 23 | 64 |
| 65+ | 2,225 | 7.4 | 35 | 2 | 4 | 6 | 9 | 14 | 17 | 30 |
| **GRAND TOTAL** | 3,284 | 7.0 | 44 | 1 | 3 | 5 | 9 | 14 | 17 | 34 |

## 97.0: GI APPLIANCE REPLACEMENT. Formerly included in operation group(s) 796.

| Type of Patients | Observed Patients | Avg. Stay | Variance | 10th | 25th | 50th | 75th | 90th | 95th | 99th |
|---|---|---|---|---|---|---|---|---|---|---|
| **1. SINGLE DX** | | | | | | | | | | |
| 0–19 Years | 76 | 1.2 | <1 | 1 | 1 | 1 | 1 | 2 | 2 | 5 |
| 20-34 | 12 | 1.3 | <1 | 1 | 1 | 1 | 1 | 3 | 3 | 5 |
| 35-49 | 4 | 2.4 | 3 | 1 | 1 | 2 | 5 | 5 | 5 | 5 |
| 50-64 | 7 | 2.2 | 3 | 1 | 1 | 2 | 2 | 6 | 6 | 6 |
| 65+ | 21 | 2.4 | 4 | 2 | 2 | 2 | 2 | 2 | 6 | 12 |
| **2. MULTIPLE DX** | | | | | | | | | | |
| 0–19 Years | 474 | 4.8 | 36 | 1 | 1 | 3 | 6 | 12 | 16 | 31 |
| 20-34 | 160 | 6.6 | 55 | 1 | 2 | 4 | 8 | 13 | 17 | 37 |
| 35-49 | 301 | 6.7 | 47 | 2 | 3 | 5 | 8 | 13 | 17 | 36 |
| 50-64 | 455 | 7.5 | 69 | 2 | 3 | 5 | 9 | 14 | 20 | 44 |
| 65+ | 2,556 | 7.3 | 35 | 2 | 3 | 6 | 9 | 14 | 17 | 30 |
| **TOTAL SINGLE DX** | 120 | 2.1 | 3 | 1 | 1 | 2 | 2 | 2 | 5 | 12 |
| **TOTAL MULTIPLE DX** | 3,946 | 6.8 | 41 | 1 | 3 | 5 | 9 | 14 | 17 | 31 |
| **TOTAL** | | | | | | | | | | |
| 0–19 Years | 550 | 4.7 | 35 | 1 | 1 | 2 | 6 | 12 | 15 | 31 |
| 20-34 | 172 | 6.5 | 55 | 1 | 2 | 4 | 8 | 13 | 17 | 37 |
| 35-49 | 305 | 6.6 | 47 | 2 | 3 | 5 | 8 | 13 | 17 | 36 |
| 50-64 | 462 | 7.4 | 68 | 2 | 3 | 5 | 9 | 14 | 20 | 44 |
| 65+ | 2,577 | 7.1 | 35 | 2 | 3 | 6 | 9 | 14 | 17 | 30 |
| **GRAND TOTAL** | 4,066 | 6.7 | 41 | 1 | 3 | 5 | 9 | 13 | 17 | 31 |

## 97.05: REPL PANC/BILIARY STENT. Formerly included in operation group(s) 796.

| Type of Patients | Observed Patients | Avg. Stay | Variance | 10th | 25th | 50th | 75th | 90th | 95th | 99th |
|---|---|---|---|---|---|---|---|---|---|---|
| **1. SINGLE DX** | | | | | | | | | | |
| 0–19 Years | 0 | | | | | | | | | |
| 20-34 | 2 | 1.9 | 2 | 1 | 1 | 3 | 3 | 3 | 3 | 3 |
| 35-49 | 2 | 1.7 | <1 | 1 | 1 | 2 | 2 | 2 | 2 | 2 |
| 50-64 | 5 | 2.5 | 3 | 1 | 1 | 2 | 3 | 6 | 6 | 6 |
| 65+ | 5 | 2.5 | 6 | 1 | 1 | 2 | 2 | 7 | 7 | 7 |
| **2. MULTIPLE DX** | | | | | | | | | | |
| 0–19 Years | 15 | 3.4 | 8 | 1 | 1 | 3 | 4 | 4 | 9 | 14 |
| 20-34 | 29 | 3.1 | 7 | 1 | 2 | 3 | 4 | 5 | 7 | 17 |
| 35-49 | 66 | 5.0 | 15 | 2 | 2 | 4 | 6 | 10 | 11 | 13 |
| 50-64 | 107 | 5.1 | 23 | 1 | 2 | 4 | 6 | 11 | 16 | 24 |
| 65+ | 219 | 4.3 | 15 | 1 | 2 | 3 | 6 | 10 | 11 | 19 |
| **TOTAL SINGLE DX** | 14 | 2.4 | 4 | 1 | 1 | 2 | 2 | 6 | 7 | 7 |
| **TOTAL MULTIPLE DX** | 436 | 4.4 | 16 | 1 | 2 | 3 | 5 | 10 | 11 | 21 |
| **TOTAL** | | | | | | | | | | |
| 0–19 Years | 15 | 3.4 | 8 | 1 | 1 | 2 | 4 | 4 | 9 | 14 |
| 20-34 | 31 | 3.1 | 7 | 1 | 2 | 4 | 4 | 5 | 7 | 17 |
| 35-49 | 68 | 4.9 | 15 | 2 | 2 | 5 | 6 | 10 | 11 | 13 |
| 50-64 | 112 | 5.0 | 22 | 1 | 2 | 5 | 6 | 11 | 16 | 24 |
| 65+ | 224 | 4.3 | 15 | 1 | 2 | 3 | 6 | 10 | 11 | 18 |
| **GRAND TOTAL** | 450 | 4.3 | 15 | 1 | 2 | 3 | 5 | 10 | 11 | 21 |

# United States, October 1998–September 1999 Data, by Operation

## 97.1: REPL MS APPLIANCE. Formerly included in operation group(s) 796.

| Type of Patients | Observed Patients | Avg. Stay | Variance | 10th | 25th | 50th | 75th | 90th | 95th | 99th |
|---|---|---|---|---|---|---|---|---|---|---|
| **1. SINGLE DX** | | | | | | | | | | |
| 0–19 Years | 47 | 4.1 | 38 | 1 | 1 | 1 | 3 | 9 | 23 | 23 |
| 20–34 | 3 | 3.1 | 6 | 1 | 1 | 2 | 6 | 6 | 6 | 6 |
| 35–49 | 1 | 1.0 | 0 | 1 | 1 | 1 | 1 | 1 | 1 | 1 |
| 50–64 | 1 | 4.0 | 0 | 4 | 4 | 4 | 4 | 4 | 4 | 4 |
| 65+ | 0 | | | | | | | | | |
| **2. MULTIPLE DX** | | | | | | | | | | |
| 0–19 Years | 68 | 2.5 | 9 | 1 | 1 | 1 | 3 | 6 | 10 | 11 |
| 20–34 | 7 | 3.6 | 6 | 1 | 1 | 4 | 5 | 7 | 7 | 7 |
| 35–49 | 17 | 7.8 | 29 | 1 | 3 | 9 | 13 | 13 | 16 | 22 |
| 50–64 | 16 | 5.5 | 12 | 3 | 3 | 6 | 6 | 8 | 18 | 18 |
| 65+ | 37 | 6.0 | 26 | 2 | 3 | 4 | 7 | 10 | 15 | 36 |
| **TOTAL SINGLE DX** | 52 | 3.7 | 31 | 1 | 1 | 1 | 3 | 9 | 23 | 23 |
| **TOTAL MULTIPLE DX** | 145 | 4.6 | 20 | 1 | 1 | 3 | 6 | 10 | 13 | 19 |
| **TOTAL** | | | | | | | | | | |
| 0–19 Years | 115 | 2.8 | 14 | 1 | 1 | 1 | 3 | 7 | 10 | 23 |
| 20–34 | 10 | 3.5 | 6 | 1 | 1 | 4 | 5 | 7 | 7 | 7 |
| 35–49 | 18 | 7.4 | 30 | 1 | 3 | 9 | 13 | 13 | 16 | 22 |
| 50–64 | 17 | 5.5 | 12 | 3 | 3 | 6 | 6 | 8 | 9 | 18 |
| 65+ | 37 | 6.0 | 26 | 2 | 3 | 4 | 7 | 10 | 15 | 36 |
| **GRAND TOTAL** | 197 | 4.5 | 21 | 1 | 1 | 3 | 6 | 9 | 13 | 23 |

## 97.2: OTHER NONOP REPLACEMENT. Formerly included in operation group(s) 796.

| Type of Patients | Observed Patients | Avg. Stay | Variance | 10th | 25th | 50th | 75th | 90th | 95th | 99th |
|---|---|---|---|---|---|---|---|---|---|---|
| **1. SINGLE DX** | | | | | | | | | | |
| 0–19 Years | 5 | 4.6 | 2 | 3 | 5 | 5 | 5 | 5 | 5 | 7 |
| 20–34 | 2 | 3.4 | <1 | 3 | 3 | 3 | 4 | 4 | 6 | 6 |
| 35–49 | 4 | 3.1 | 5 | 1 | 1 | 3 | 4 | 5 | 5 | 5 |
| 50–64 | 1 | 1.0 | 0 | 1 | 1 | 1 | 1 | 1 | 1 | 1 |
| 65+ | 1 | 5.0 | 0 | 5 | 5 | 5 | 5 | 5 | 5 | 5 |
| **2. MULTIPLE DX** | | | | | | | | | | |
| 0–19 Years | 87 | 4.6 | 46 | 1 | 1 | 2 | 4 | 14 | 17 | 32 |
| 20–34 | 28 | 6.6 | 81 | 1 | 4 | 4 | 7 | 23 | 36 | >99 |
| 35–49 | 81 | 6.8 | 70 | 1 | 2 | 5 | 8 | 15 | 19 | 45 |
| 50–64 | 142 | 8.3 | 57 | 1 | 2 | 6 | 12 | 18 | 26 | 29 |
| 65+ | 209 | 8.1 | 86 | 2 | 3 | 6 | 10 | 16 | 22 | 43 |
| **TOTAL SINGLE DX** | 13 | 4.2 | 3 | 4 | 5 | 5 | 5 | 5 | 5 | 7 |
| **TOTAL MULTIPLE DX** | 547 | 7.4 | 69 | 1 | 2 | 5 | 10 | 16 | 25 | 43 |
| **TOTAL** | | | | | | | | | | |
| 0–19 Years | 92 | 4.6 | 42 | 2 | 2 | 5 | 5 | 14 | 16 | 32 |
| 20–34 | 30 | 6.5 | 79 | 1 | 1 | 4 | 6 | 23 | 36 | >99 |
| 35–49 | 85 | 6.7 | 68 | 1 | 2 | 5 | 7 | 15 | 19 | 45 |
| 50–64 | 143 | 8.3 | 57 | 1 | 2 | 6 | 12 | 18 | 26 | 29 |
| 65+ | 210 | 8.1 | 86 | 2 | 3 | 6 | 10 | 16 | 22 | 43 |
| **GRAND TOTAL** | 560 | 7.3 | 68 | 1 | 2 | 5 | 10 | 16 | 24 | 43 |

## 97.23: REPL TRACH TUBE. Formerly included in operation group(s) 796.

| Type of Patients | Observed Patients | Avg. Stay | Variance | 10th | 25th | 50th | 75th | 90th | 95th | 99th |
|---|---|---|---|---|---|---|---|---|---|---|
| **1. SINGLE DX** | | | | | | | | | | |
| 0–19 Years | 3 | 4.6 | 1 | 3 | 5 | 5 | 5 | 5 | 5 | 5 |
| 20–34 | 1 | 3.0 | 0 | 3 | 3 | 3 | 3 | 3 | 3 | 3 |
| 35–49 | 2 | 1.0 | 0 | 1 | 1 | 1 | 1 | 1 | 1 | 1 |
| 50–64 | 1 | 1.0 | 0 | 1 | 1 | 1 | 1 | 1 | 1 | 1 |
| 65+ | 1 | 5.0 | 0 | 5 | 5 | 5 | 5 | 5 | 5 | 5 |
| **2. MULTIPLE DX** | | | | | | | | | | |
| 0–19 Years | 83 | 4.6 | 47 | 1 | 1 | 2 | 4 | 15 | 17 | 32 |
| 20–34 | 24 | 7.0 | 89 | 1 | 1 | 4 | 7 | 26 | 36 | >99 |
| 35–49 | 68 | 7.0 | 76 | 1 | 2 | 5 | 8 | 18 | 19 | 45 |
| 50–64 | 127 | 7.8 | 44 | 1 | 2 | 7 | 12 | 14 | 18 | 29 |
| 65+ | 185 | 8.6 | 93 | 2 | 4 | 7 | 10 | 17 | 25 | 52 |
| **TOTAL SINGLE DX** | 8 | 4.1 | 3 | 1 | 3 | 5 | 5 | 5 | 5 | 5 |
| **TOTAL MULTIPLE DX** | 487 | 7.4 | 69 | 1 | 2 | 5 | 10 | 15 | 21 | 44 |
| **TOTAL** | | | | | | | | | | |
| 0–19 Years | 86 | 4.6 | 43 | 2 | 2 | 2 | 5 | 14 | 16 | 32 |
| 20–34 | 25 | 6.9 | 87 | 1 | 1 | 4 | 7 | 26 | 36 | >99 |
| 35–49 | 70 | 6.9 | 76 | 1 | 2 | 5 | 8 | 18 | 19 | 45 |
| 50–64 | 128 | 7.8 | 44 | 1 | 2 | 7 | 12 | 14 | 18 | 29 |
| 65+ | 186 | 8.6 | 92 | 2 | 4 | 7 | 10 | 17 | 25 | 52 |
| **GRAND TOTAL** | 495 | 7.3 | 67 | 1 | 2 | 5 | 10 | 15 | 21 | 44 |

## 97.3: RMVL THER DEV-HEAD/NK. Formerly included in operation group(s) 796.

| Type of Patients | Observed Patients | Avg. Stay | Variance | 10th | 25th | 50th | 75th | 90th | 95th | 99th |
|---|---|---|---|---|---|---|---|---|---|---|
| **1. SINGLE DX** | | | | | | | | | | |
| 0–19 Years | 57 | 2.8 | 7 | 1 | 1 | 2 | 3 | 8 | 8 | 8 |
| 20–34 | 1 | 1.0 | 0 | 1 | 1 | 1 | 1 | 1 | 1 | 1 |
| 35–49 | 5 | 1.2 | <1 | 1 | 1 | 1 | 1 | 3 | 3 | 3 |
| 50–64 | 2 | 1.1 | <1 | 1 | 1 | 1 | 1 | 1 | 2 | 2 |
| 65+ | 1 | 2.0 | 0 | 2 | 2 | 2 | 2 | 2 | 2 | 2 |
| **2. MULTIPLE DX** | | | | | | | | | | |
| 0–19 Years | 108 | 3.8 | 79 | 1 | 1 | 2 | 3 | 7 | 15 | 63 |
| 20–34 | 31 | 5.5 | 28 | 1 | 2 | 4 | 7 | 11 | 19 | 22 |
| 35–49 | 66 | 5.9 | 82 | 1 | 2 | 3 | 6 | 13 | 16 | 28 |
| 50–64 | 54 | 10.6 | 178 | 2 | 4 | 6 | 13 | 16 | 56 | 56 |
| 65+ | 120 | 6.9 | 69 | 2 | 2 | 5 | 7 | 11 | 18 | 47 |
| **TOTAL SINGLE DX** | 66 | 2.6 | 6 | 1 | 1 | 2 | 2 | 2 | 8 | 8 |
| **TOTAL MULTIPLE DX** | 379 | 6.2 | 92 | 1 | 2 | 3 | 7 | 13 | 19 | 56 |
| **TOTAL** | | | | | | | | | | |
| 0–19 Years | 165 | 3.6 | 61 | 1 | 1 | 2 | 3 | 8 | 10 | 56 |
| 20–34 | 32 | 5.4 | 28 | 1 | 1 | 4 | 7 | 11 | 19 | 22 |
| 35–49 | 71 | 5.7 | 80 | 1 | 2 | 3 | 6 | 13 | 16 | 28 |
| 50–64 | 56 | 10.0 | 171 | 1 | 2 | 6 | 12 | 13 | 56 | 56 |
| 65+ | 121 | 6.9 | 69 | 2 | 3 | 5 | 7 | 11 | 18 | 47 |
| **GRAND TOTAL** | 445 | 5.8 | 83 | 1 | 3 | 4 | 7 | 12 | 16 | 56 |

Length of Stay by Diagnosis and Operation, United States, 2000

# United States, October 1998–September 1999 Data, by Operation

## 97.4: RMVL THOR THER DEVICE. Formerly included in operation group(s) 796.

| Type of Patients | Observed Patients | Avg. Stay | Variance | Percentiles | | | | | | |
|---|---|---|---|---|---|---|---|---|---|---|
| | | | | 10th | 25th | 50th | 75th | 90th | 95th | 99th |
| **1. SINGLE DX** | | | | | | | | | | |
| 0–19 Years | 8 | 1.8 | 2 | 1 | 1 | 1 | 4 | 4 | 4 | 4 |
| 20–34 | 5 | 8.8 | 65 | 2 | 3 | 4 | 20 | 20 | 20 | 20 |
| 35–49 | 2 | 3.4 | 2 | 1 | 4 | 4 | 4 | 4 | 4 | 4 |
| 50–64 | 1 | 1.0 | 0 | 1 | 1 | 1 | 1 | 1 | 1 | 1 |
| 65+ | 0 | | | | | | | | | |
| **2. MULTIPLE DX** | | | | | | | | | | |
| 0–19 Years | 137 | 9.2 | 148 | 2 | 2 | 7 | 11 | 15 | 23 | 53 |
| 20–34 | 118 | 5.5 | 25 | 2 | 3 | 4 | 6 | 12 | 16 | 28 |
| 35–49 | 233 | 6.0 | 30 | 2 | 3 | 5 | 7 | 10 | 14 | 41 |
| 50–64 | 282 | 5.9 | 21 | 2 | 3 | 5 | 7 | 11 | 15 | 20 |
| 65+ | 268 | 7.7 | 55 | 2 | 4 | 6 | 9 | 14 | 20 | 48 |
| **TOTAL SINGLE DX** | 16 | 4.0 | 26 | 1 | 1 | 3 | 4 | 6 | 20 | 20 |
| **TOTAL MULTIPLE DX** | 1,038 | 6.9 | 57 | 2 | 3 | 5 | 8 | 13 | 17 | 40 |
| **TOTAL** | | | | | | | | | | |
| 0–19 Years | 145 | 8.9 | 144 | 1 | 2 | 6 | 11 | 15 | 23 | 53 |
| 20–34 | 123 | 5.6 | 26 | 2 | 3 | 4 | 6 | 14 | 18 | 28 |
| 35–49 | 235 | 6.0 | 29 | 2 | 3 | 5 | 7 | 10 | 13 | 41 |
| 50–64 | 283 | 5.9 | 21 | 2 | 3 | 5 | 7 | 11 | 15 | 20 |
| 65+ | 268 | 7.7 | 55 | 2 | 4 | 6 | 9 | 14 | 20 | 48 |
| **GRAND TOTAL** | 1,054 | 6.9 | 57 | 2 | 3 | 5 | 8 | 13 | 17 | 40 |

## 97.5: NONOP RMVL GI THER DEV. Formerly included in operation group(s) 796.

| Type of Patients | Observed Patients | Avg. Stay | Variance | Percentiles | | | | | | |
|---|---|---|---|---|---|---|---|---|---|---|
| | | | | 10th | 25th | 50th | 75th | 90th | 95th | 99th |
| **1. SINGLE DX** | | | | | | | | | | |
| 0–19 Years | 1 | 5.0 | 0 | 5 | 5 | 5 | 5 | 5 | 5 | 5 |
| 20–34 | 1 | 1.0 | 0 | 1 | 1 | 1 | 1 | 1 | 1 | 1 |
| 35–49 | 3 | 2.6 | <1 | 3 | 3 | 3 | 3 | 3 | 3 | 3 |
| 50–64 | 2 | 1.3 | <1 | 1 | 1 | 1 | 1 | 2 | 2 | 2 |
| 65+ | 2 | 1.2 | <1 | 1 | 1 | 1 | 1 | 2 | 2 | 2 |
| **2. MULTIPLE DX** | | | | | | | | | | |
| 0–19 Years | 44 | 9.1 | 132 | 3 | 3 | 5 | 11 | 24 | 42 | 56 |
| 20–34 | 32 | 12.4 | 121 | 4 | 7 | 7 | 16 | 30 | 32 | 58 |
| 35–49 | 61 | 11.4 | 147 | 2 | 3 | 7 | 17 | 24 | 30 | 44 |
| 50–64 | 97 | 8.1 | 103 | 2 | 3 | 4 | 9 | 19 | 29 | 48 |
| 65+ | 290 | 8.5 | 101 | 2 | 3 | 5 | 9 | 20 | 29 | 43 |
| **TOTAL SINGLE DX** | 9 | 1.9 | 1 | 1 | 1 | 1 | 3 | 3 | 3 | 5 |
| **TOTAL MULTIPLE DX** | 524 | 9.1 | 112 | 2 | 3 | 5 | 10 | 22 | 30 | 51 |
| **TOTAL** | | | | | | | | | | |
| 0–19 Years | 45 | 9.1 | 131 | 1 | 3 | 5 | 11 | 24 | 42 | 56 |
| 20–34 | 33 | 12.1 | 121 | 3 | 6 | 7 | 16 | 30 | 32 | 58 |
| 35–49 | 64 | 10.8 | 142 | 2 | 3 | 7 | 15 | 24 | 30 | 44 |
| 50–64 | 99 | 8.0 | 102 | 2 | 3 | 4 | 9 | 19 | 29 | 48 |
| 65+ | 292 | 8.4 | 101 | 2 | 3 | 5 | 9 | 20 | 29 | 43 |
| **GRAND TOTAL** | 533 | 9.0 | 111 | 2 | 3 | 5 | 10 | 21 | 30 | 51 |

## 97.49: RMVL OTH DEV FROM THORAX. Formerly included in operation group(s) 796.

| Type of Patients | Observed Patients | Avg. Stay | Variance | Percentiles | | | | | | |
|---|---|---|---|---|---|---|---|---|---|---|
| | | | | 10th | 25th | 50th | 75th | 90th | 95th | 99th |
| **1. SINGLE DX** | | | | | | | | | | |
| 0–19 Years | 5 | 1.1 | <1 | 1 | 1 | 1 | 1 | 2 | 2 | 2 |
| 20–34 | 1 | 20.0 | 0 | 20 | 20 | 20 | 20 | 20 | 20 | 20 |
| 35–49 | 2 | 3.4 | 2 | 1 | 4 | 4 | 4 | 4 | 4 | 4 |
| 50–64 | 1 | 1.0 | 0 | 1 | 1 | 1 | 1 | 1 | 1 | 1 |
| 65+ | 0 | | | | | | | | | |
| **2. MULTIPLE DX** | | | | | | | | | | |
| 0–19 Years | 126 | 9.5 | 155 | 2 | 2 | 7 | 12 | 16 | 23 | 98 |
| 20–34 | 106 | 5.6 | 26 | 2 | 3 | 4 | 6 | 14 | 16 | 28 |
| 35–49 | 221 | 6.1 | 31 | 2 | 3 | 5 | 7 | 10 | 14 | 41 |
| 50–64 | 270 | 6.0 | 21 | 2 | 3 | 5 | 7 | 11 | 15 | 20 |
| 65+ | 245 | 7.7 | 56 | 2 | 4 | 6 | 9 | 14 | 20 | 48 |
| **TOTAL SINGLE DX** | 9 | 4.2 | 38 | 1 | 1 | 1 | 4 | 20 | 20 | 20 |
| **TOTAL MULTIPLE DX** | 968 | 7.1 | 60 | 2 | 3 | 5 | 8 | 13 | 17 | 41 |
| **TOTAL** | | | | | | | | | | |
| 0–19 Years | 131 | 9.3 | 152 | 1 | 2 | 7 | 11 | 15 | 23 | 98 |
| 20–34 | 107 | 5.8 | 28 | 2 | 3 | 4 | 6 | 15 | 18 | 28 |
| 35–49 | 223 | 6.1 | 31 | 2 | 3 | 5 | 7 | 10 | 14 | 41 |
| 50–64 | 271 | 5.9 | 21 | 2 | 3 | 5 | 7 | 11 | 15 | 20 |
| 65+ | 245 | 7.7 | 56 | 2 | 4 | 6 | 9 | 14 | 20 | 48 |
| **GRAND TOTAL** | 977 | 7.0 | 60 | 2 | 3 | 5 | 8 | 13 | 18 | 41 |

## 97.51: RMVL GASTROSTOMY TUBE. Formerly included in operation group(s) 796.

| Type of Patients | Observed Patients | Avg. Stay | Variance | Percentiles | | | | | | |
|---|---|---|---|---|---|---|---|---|---|---|
| | | | | 10th | 25th | 50th | 75th | 90th | 95th | 99th |
| **1. SINGLE DX** | | | | | | | | | | |
| 0–19 Years | 1 | 5.0 | 0 | 5 | 5 | 5 | 5 | 5 | 5 | 5 |
| 20–34 | 0 | | | | | | | | | |
| 35–49 | 1 | 3.0 | 0 | 3 | 3 | 3 | 3 | 3 | 3 | 3 |
| 50–64 | 1 | 1.0 | 0 | 1 | 1 | 1 | 1 | 1 | 1 | 1 |
| 65+ | 0 | | | | | | | | | |
| **2. MULTIPLE DX** | | | | | | | | | | |
| 0–19 Years | 31 | 11.9 | 166 | 2 | 3 | 7 | 13 | 37 | 43 | >99 |
| 20–34 | 21 | 16.1 | 159 | 5 | 8 | 10 | 19 | 32 | 39 | 58 |
| 35–49 | 37 | 14.2 | 212 | 3 | 5 | 11 | 16 | 30 | 30 | 99 |
| 50–64 | 71 | 9.8 | 127 | 2 | 3 | 5 | 14 | 22 | 40 | 51 |
| 65+ | 238 | 9.4 | 117 | 2 | 3 | 6 | 10 | 22 | 34 | 61 |
| **TOTAL SINGLE DX** | 3 | 2.3 | 3 | 1 | 1 | 1 | 3 | 5 | 5 | 5 |
| **TOTAL MULTIPLE DX** | 398 | 10.5 | 137 | 2 | 3 | 6 | 13 | 24 | 35 | 58 |
| **TOTAL** | | | | | | | | | | |
| 0–19 Years | 32 | 11.9 | 165 | 2 | 3 | 7 | 13 | 37 | 43 | >99 |
| 20–34 | 21 | 16.1 | 159 | 5 | 8 | 10 | 19 | 32 | 39 | 58 |
| 35–49 | 38 | 14.0 | 211 | 3 | 5 | 11 | 16 | 30 | 30 | 99 |
| 50–64 | 72 | 9.7 | 126 | 2 | 3 | 5 | 12 | 22 | 40 | 51 |
| 65+ | 238 | 9.4 | 117 | 2 | 3 | 6 | 10 | 22 | 34 | 61 |
| **GRAND TOTAL** | 401 | 10.4 | 136 | 2 | 3 | 6 | 13 | 24 | 35 | 58 |

Length of Stay by Diagnosis and Operation, United States, 2000

# United States, October 1998–September 1999 Data, by Operation

## 97.6: NONOP RMVL URIN THER DEV. Formerly included in operation group(s) 796.

| Type of Patients | Observed Patients | Avg. Stay | Variance | 10th | 25th | 50th | 75th | 90th | 95th | 99th |
|---|---|---|---|---|---|---|---|---|---|---|
| **1. SINGLE DX** | | | | | | | | | | |
| 0–19 Years | 17 | 1.1 | <1 | 1 | 1 | 1 | 1 | 1 | 1 | 4 |
| 20–34 | 18 | 1.4 | <1 | 1 | 1 | 1 | 2 | 2 | 2 | 4 |
| 35–49 | 20 | 2.0 | 1 | 1 | 1 | 2 | 2 | 4 | 4 | 4 |
| 50–64 | 2 | 2.8 | 1 | 2 | 1 | 2 | 4 | 4 | 4 | 4 |
| 65+ | 3 | 3.4 | 4 | 1 | 3 | 3 | 6 | 6 | 6 | 6 |
| **2. MULTIPLE DX** | | | | | | | | | | |
| 0–19 Years | 79 | 4.2 | 57 | 1 | 2 | 2 | 5 | 11 | 11 | 59 |
| 20–34 | 139 | 4.1 | 15 | 1 | 2 | 3 | 5 | 9 | 13 | 16 |
| 35–49 | 161 | 3.4 | 9 | 1 | 2 | 3 | 4 | 6 | 8 | 14 |
| 50–64 | 126 | 5.4 | 34 | 2 | 2 | 4 | 7 | 9 | 18 | 29 |
| 65+ | 233 | 6.0 | 43 | 1 | 3 | 4 | 7 | 12 | 23 | 37 |
| **TOTAL SINGLE DX** | 60 | 1.5 | <1 | 1 | 1 | 1 | 2 | 2 | 4 | 4 |
| **TOTAL MULTIPLE DX** | 738 | 4.7 | 31 | 1 | 2 | 3 | 5 | 10 | 13 | 29 |
| **TOTAL** | | | | | | | | | | |
| 0–19 Years | 96 | 3.5 | 45 | 1 | 1 | 1 | 4 | 11 | 11 | 30 |
| 20–34 | 157 | 3.8 | 14 | 1 | 2 | 3 | 5 | 9 | 13 | 16 |
| 35–49 | 181 | 3.3 | 8 | 1 | 2 | 3 | 4 | 6 | 8 | 14 |
| 50–64 | 128 | 5.4 | 33 | 1 | 2 | 4 | 7 | 9 | 18 | 29 |
| 65+ | 236 | 6.0 | 43 | 1 | 2 | 4 | 7 | 12 | 23 | 37 |
| **GRAND TOTAL** | 798 | 4.4 | 30 | 1 | 1 | 3 | 5 | 9 | 13 | 29 |

## 97.62: RMVL URETERAL DRAIN. Formerly included in operation group(s) 796.

| Type of Patients | Observed Patients | Avg. Stay | Variance | 10th | 25th | 50th | 75th | 90th | 95th | 99th |
|---|---|---|---|---|---|---|---|---|---|---|
| **1. SINGLE DX** | | | | | | | | | | |
| 0–19 Years | 13 | 1.1 | <1 | 1 | 1 | 1 | 1 | 1 | 2 | 2 |
| 20–34 | 16 | 1.3 | <1 | 1 | 1 | 1 | 2 | 2 | 2 | 2 |
| 35–49 | 18 | 2.0 | 1 | 1 | 1 | 1 | 2 | 4 | 4 | 4 |
| 50–64 | 2 | 2.8 | 1 | 2 | 1 | 2 | 4 | 4 | 4 | 4 |
| 65+ | 2 | 4.1 | 3 | 3 | 3 | 3 | 6 | 6 | 6 | 6 |
| **2. MULTIPLE DX** | | | | | | | | | | |
| 0–19 Years | 59 | 3.4 | 67 | 1 | 2 | 2 | 4 | 5 | 8 | 59 |
| 20–34 | 124 | 4.0 | 13 | 1 | 2 | 3 | 5 | 9 | 13 | 14 |
| 35–49 | 136 | 3.2 | 6 | 1 | 2 | 3 | 4 | 6 | 8 | 12 |
| 50–64 | 102 | 4.8 | 18 | 2 | 2 | 4 | 7 | 8 | 9 | 28 |
| 65+ | 173 | 6.4 | 52 | 1 | 2 | 4 | 8 | 12 | 23 | 37 |
| **TOTAL SINGLE DX** | 51 | 1.5 | <1 | 1 | 1 | 1 | 2 | 3 | 4 | 6 |
| **TOTAL MULTIPLE DX** | 594 | 4.5 | 31 | 1 | 1 | 3 | 5 | 9 | 13 | 30 |
| **TOTAL** | | | | | | | | | | |
| 0–19 Years | 72 | 2.9 | 54 | 1 | 1 | 1 | 3 | 5 | 7 | 59 |
| 20–34 | 140 | 3.7 | 12 | 1 | 1 | 3 | 4 | 9 | 13 | 14 |
| 35–49 | 154 | 3.1 | 6 | 1 | 1 | 3 | 4 | 6 | 8 | 12 |
| 50–64 | 104 | 4.8 | 17 | 1 | 2 | 4 | 7 | 8 | 9 | 28 |
| 65+ | 175 | 6.3 | 52 | 1 | 2 | 4 | 8 | 12 | 23 | 37 |
| **GRAND TOTAL** | 645 | 4.2 | 29 | 1 | 1 | 3 | 5 | 9 | 12 | 28 |

## 97.7: RMVL THER DEV GENIT SYST. Formerly included in operation group(s) 796.

| Type of Patients | Observed Patients | Avg. Stay | Variance | 10th | 25th | 50th | 75th | 90th | 95th | 99th |
|---|---|---|---|---|---|---|---|---|---|---|
| **1. SINGLE DX** | | | | | | | | | | |
| 0–19 Years | 1 | 2.0 | 0 | 2 | | | | 2 | 2 | 2 |
| 20–34 | 7 | 1.6 | 2 | 1 | 1 | 1 | 1 | 3 | 6 | 6 |
| 35–49 | 9 | 3.1 | 6 | 1 | 1 | 2 | 4 | 8 | 8 | 8 |
| 50–64 | 0 | | | | | | | | | |
| 65+ | 0 | | | | | | | | | |
| **2. MULTIPLE DX** | | | | | | | | | | |
| 0–19 Years | 4 | 11.2 | 507 | | | 3 | 3 | 57 | 57 | 57 |
| 20–34 | 46 | 2.6 | 1 | 1 | 2 | 2 | 3 | 3 | 4 | 7 |
| 35–49 | 30 | 7.0 | 10 | 2 | 4 | 4 | 9 | 9 | 9 | 12 |
| 50–64 | 14 | 4.3 | 9 | 3 | 4 | 4 | 8 | 8 | 8 | 8 |
| 65+ | 29 | 5.9 | 28 | 3 | 4 | 5 | 7 | 8 | 10 | 42 |
| **TOTAL SINGLE DX** | 17 | 2.3 | 5 | 1 | 1 | 1 | 3 | 6 | 8 | 8 |
| **TOTAL MULTIPLE DX** | 123 | 4.7 | 18 | 1 | 2 | 3 | 7 | 9 | 9 | 12 |
| **TOTAL** | | | | | | | | | | |
| 0–19 Years | 5 | 9.9 | 434 | 1 | 1 | 2 | 3 | 57 | 57 | 57 |
| 20–34 | 53 | 2.6 | 1 | 1 | 2 | 3 | 3 | 3 | 4 | 7 |
| 35–49 | 39 | 6.6 | 11 | 2 | 3 | 3 | 9 | 9 | 9 | 12 |
| 50–64 | 14 | 4.3 | 9 | 3 | 4 | 4 | 8 | 8 | 8 | 8 |
| 65+ | 29 | 5.9 | 28 | 3 | 4 | 5 | 7 | 8 | 10 | 42 |
| **GRAND TOTAL** | 140 | 4.5 | 17 | 2 | 3 | 3 | 7 | 9 | 9 | 12 |

## 97.8: OTH NONOP RMVL THER DEV. Formerly included in operation group(s) 796.

| Type of Patients | Observed Patients | Avg. Stay | Variance | 10th | 25th | 50th | 75th | 90th | 95th | 99th |
|---|---|---|---|---|---|---|---|---|---|---|
| **1. SINGLE DX** | | | | | | | | | | |
| 0–19 Years | 42 | 5.5 | 70 | 1 | 1 | 2 | 4 | 21 | 26 | 26 |
| 20–34 | 9 | 1.9 | <1 | 1 | 2 | 2 | 2 | 2 | 3 | 5 |
| 35–49 | 9 | 1.8 | <1 | 1 | 2 | 2 | 2 | 2 | 3 | 4 |
| 50–64 | 7 | 3.2 | 6 | 1 | 1 | 1 | 4 | 7 | 7 | 7 |
| 65+ | 1 | 1.0 | 0 | 1 | 1 | 1 | 1 | 1 | 1 | 1 |
| **2. MULTIPLE DX** | | | | | | | | | | |
| 0–19 Years | 171 | 5.0 | 48 | 1 | 1 | 3 | 5 | 10 | 20 | 34 |
| 20–34 | 89 | 7.6 | 84 | 2 | 2 | 5 | 9 | 13 | 27 | 46 |
| 35–49 | 183 | 9.3 | 235 | 2 | 3 | 5 | 9 | 16 | 56 | 76 |
| 50–64 | 167 | 9.5 | 260 | 2 | 2 | 4 | 9 | 14 | 42 | 90 |
| 65+ | 206 | 7.3 | 44 | 2 | 3 | 5 | 10 | 14 | 18 | 31 |
| **TOTAL SINGLE DX** | 68 | 3.5 | 32 | 1 | 1 | 2 | 2 | 7 | 21 | 26 |
| **TOTAL MULTIPLE DX** | 816 | 7.6 | 135 | 1 | 2 | 4 | 8 | 14 | 21 | 76 |
| **TOTAL** | | | | | | | | | | |
| 0–19 Years | 213 | 5.0 | 50 | 1 | 1 | 3 | 5 | 11 | 20 | 34 |
| 20–34 | 98 | 7.1 | 79 | 1 | 2 | 4 | 8 | 13 | 27 | 46 |
| 35–49 | 192 | 9.0 | 227 | 2 | 3 | 4 | 8 | 16 | 49 | 76 |
| 50–64 | 174 | 9.3 | 253 | 2 | 3 | 5 | 9 | 14 | 42 | 90 |
| 65+ | 207 | 7.3 | 44 | 2 | 3 | 5 | 10 | 14 | 18 | 31 |
| **GRAND TOTAL** | 884 | 7.4 | 131 | 1 | 2 | 4 | 8 | 14 | 21 | 76 |

Length of Stay by Diagnosis and Operation, United States, 2000

## 97.89: RMVL OTH THER DEV. Formerly included in operation group(s) 796.

| Type of Patients | Observed Patients | Avg. Stay | Variance | Percentiles | | | | | | |
|---|---|---|---|---|---|---|---|---|---|---|
| | | | | 10th | 25th | 50th | 75th | 90th | 95th | 99th |
| **1. SINGLE DX** | | | | | | | | | | |
| 0-19 Years | 24 | 1.7 | 1 | 1 | 1 | 1 | 2 | 4 | 4 | 4 |
| 20-34 | 5 | 1.8 | <1 | 1 | 2 | 2 | 2 | 2 | 2 | 2 |
| 35-49 | 3 | 2.0 | <1 | 1 | 2 | 2 | 2 | 2 | 3 | 3 |
| 50-64 | 4 | 3.6 | 8 | 1 | 1 | 2 | 7 | 7 | 7 | 7 |
| 65+ | 1 | 1.0 | 0 | 1 | 1 | 1 | 1 | 1 | 1 | 1 |
| **2. MULTIPLE DX** | | | | | | | | | | |
| 0-19 Years | 82 | 6.3 | 66 | 1 | 3 | 4 | 7 | 11 | 20 | 54 |
| 20-34 | 39 | 8.8 | 131 | 2 | 3 | 6 | 9 | 16 | 46 | 46 |
| 35-49 | 82 | 6.1 | 35 | 2 | 4 | 6 | 7 | 11 | 20 | 56 |
| 50-64 | 74 | 11.8 | 397 | 1 | 2 | 4 | 10 | 42 | 54 | 90 |
| 65+ | 97 | 7.8 | 42 | 2 | 4 | 6 | 10 | 14 | 17 | 25 |
| **TOTAL SINGLE DX** | 37 | 2.1 | 2 | 1 | 1 | 2 | 2 | 4 | 7 | 7 |
| **TOTAL MULTIPLE DX** | 374 | 8.0 | 137 | 1 | 3 | 5 | 8 | 14 | 21 | 72 |
| **TOTAL** | | | | | | | | | | |
| 0-19 Years | 106 | 6.0 | 64 | 1 | 3 | 4 | 6 | 11 | 20 | 54 |
| 20-34 | 44 | 8.2 | 123 | 2 | 2 | 5 | 8 | 13 | 46 | 46 |
| 35-49 | 85 | 5.9 | 34 | 2 | 3 | 4 | 7 | 11 | 20 | 56 |
| 50-64 | 78 | 11.6 | 388 | 1 | 2 | 4 | 9 | 42 | 54 | 90 |
| 65+ | 98 | 7.7 | 42 | 2 | 4 | 6 | 10 | 14 | 17 | 25 |
| **GRAND TOTAL** | 411 | 7.8 | 133 | 1 | 3 | 4 | 8 | 14 | 21 | 72 |

## 98.02: RMVL INTRALUM ESOPH FB. Formerly included in operation group(s) 793.

| Type of Patients | Observed Patients | Avg. Stay | Variance | Percentiles | | | | | | |
|---|---|---|---|---|---|---|---|---|---|---|
| | | | | 10th | 25th | 50th | 75th | 90th | 95th | 99th |
| **1. SINGLE DX** | | | | | | | | | | |
| 0-19 Years | 186 | 1.1 | <1 | 1 | 1 | 1 | 1 | 1 | 2 | 2 |
| 20-34 | 9 | 1.0 | 0 | 1 | 1 | 1 | 1 | 1 | 2 | 1 |
| 35-49 | 9 | 1.0 | 0 | 1 | 1 | 1 | 1 | 1 | 1 | 1 |
| 50-64 | 2 | 1.0 | 0 | 1 | 1 | 1 | 1 | 1 | 1 | 1 |
| 65+ | 4 | 1.8 | <1 | 2 | 2 | 2 | 2 | 2 | 2 | 2 |
| **2. MULTIPLE DX** | | | | | | | | | | |
| 0-19 Years | 65 | 2.3 | 10 | 1 | 1 | 1 | 2 | 4 | 10 | 14 |
| 20-34 | 12 | 1.0 | 0 | 1 | 1 | 1 | 1 | 1 | 1 | 1 |
| 35-49 | 23 | 1.9 | 6 | 1 | 1 | 1 | 1 | 5 | 10 | 10 |
| 50-64 | 39 | 2.2 | 5 | 1 | 1 | 1 | 3 | 4 | 9 | 12 |
| 65+ | 115 | 2.7 | 9 | 2 | 2 | 2 | 3 | 6 | 6 | 16 |
| **TOTAL SINGLE DX** | 202 | 1.1 | <1 | 1 | 1 | 1 | 1 | 1 | 2 | 2 |
| **TOTAL MULTIPLE DX** | 254 | 2.4 | 8 | 1 | 1 | 1 | 2 | 6 | 8 | 14 |
| **TOTAL** | | | | | | | | | | |
| 0-19 Years | 251 | 1.3 | 2 | 1 | 1 | 1 | 1 | 2 | 2 | 10 |
| 20-34 | 13 | 1.0 | 0 | 1 | 1 | 1 | 1 | 1 | 1 | 1 |
| 35-49 | 32 | 1.8 | 6 | 1 | 1 | 1 | 3 | 4 | 10 | 10 |
| 50-64 | 41 | 2.1 | 5 | 1 | 1 | 2 | 3 | 4 | 9 | 12 |
| 65+ | 119 | 2.7 | 9 | 1 | 1 | 2 | 3 | 6 | 6 | 16 |
| **GRAND TOTAL** | 456 | 1.8 | 5 | 1 | 1 | 1 | 1 | 3 | 6 | 12 |

## 98.0: RMVL INTRALUM GI FB. Formerly included in operation group(s) 793.

| Type of Patients | Observed Patients | Avg. Stay | Variance | Percentiles | | | | | | |
|---|---|---|---|---|---|---|---|---|---|---|
| | | | | 10th | 25th | 50th | 75th | 90th | 95th | 99th |
| **1. SINGLE DX** | | | | | | | | | | |
| 0-19 Years | 197 | 1.1 | <1 | 1 | 1 | 1 | 1 | 2 | 2 | 2 |
| 20-34 | 19 | 1.6 | 1 | 1 | 1 | 2 | 1 | 4 | 5 | 5 |
| 35-49 | 27 | 1.3 | <1 | 1 | 1 | 1 | 2 | 2 | 2 | 4 |
| 50-64 | 5 | 1.0 | 0 | 1 | 1 | 1 | 1 | 1 | 1 | 1 |
| 65+ | 6 | 1.6 | <1 | 1 | 1 | 2 | 2 | 2 | 2 | 2 |
| **2. MULTIPLE DX** | | | | | | | | | | |
| 0-19 Years | 79 | 2.5 | 10 | 1 | 1 | 1 | 2 | 6 | 13 | 14 |
| 20-34 | 25 | 2.3 | 10 | 1 | 2 | 2 | 2 | 4 | 6 | 20 |
| 35-49 | 51 | 2.2 | 7 | 1 | 2 | 3 | 3 | 7 | 10 | 10 |
| 50-64 | 52 | 2.2 | 5 | 1 | 3 | 4 | 3 | 5 | 8 | 12 |
| 65+ | 144 | 3.0 | 11 | 1 | 2 | 4 | 4 | 6 | 9 | 17 |
| **TOTAL SINGLE DX** | 254 | 1.1 | <1 | 1 | 1 | 1 | 1 | 2 | 2 | 3 |
| **TOTAL MULTIPLE DX** | 351 | 2.6 | 9 | 1 | 1 | 1 | 3 | 6 | 9 | 16 |
| **TOTAL** | | | | | | | | | | |
| 0-19 Years | 276 | 1.4 | 3 | 1 | 1 | 1 | 1 | 2 | 2 | 13 |
| 20-34 | 44 | 2.1 | 8 | 1 | 1 | 2 | 2 | 4 | 6 | 20 |
| 35-49 | 78 | 1.9 | 5 | 1 | 2 | 2 | 2 | 4 | 10 | 10 |
| 50-64 | 57 | 2.0 | 4 | 1 | 1 | 2 | 3 | 5 | 8 | 9 |
| 65+ | 150 | 2.9 | 10 | 1 | 2 | 4 | 4 | 6 | 8 | 17 |
| **GRAND TOTAL** | 605 | 1.9 | 6 | 1 | 1 | 1 | 2 | 4 | 6 | 13 |

## 98.1: RMVL INTRALUM FB NEC. Formerly included in operation group(s) 793.

| Type of Patients | Observed Patients | Avg. Stay | Variance | Percentiles | | | | | | |
|---|---|---|---|---|---|---|---|---|---|---|
| | | | | 10th | 25th | 50th | 75th | 90th | 95th | 99th |
| **1. SINGLE DX** | | | | | | | | | | |
| 0-19 Years | 211 | 1.2 | <1 | 1 | 1 | 1 | 1 | 2 | 2 | 3 |
| 20-34 | 6 | 2.4 | 5 | 1 | 1 | 3 | 6 | 6 | 5 | 6 |
| 35-49 | 4 | 1.2 | <1 | 1 | 1 | 1 | 1 | 2 | 2 | 2 |
| 50-64 | 3 | 1.0 | 0 | 1 | 1 | 1 | 1 | 1 | 1 | 1 |
| 65+ | 4 | 1.0 | 0 | 1 | 1 | 1 | 1 | 1 | 1 | 1 |
| **2. MULTIPLE DX** | | | | | | | | | | |
| 0-19 Years | 130 | 2.8 | 27 | 2 | 2 | 2 | 2 | 5 | 10 | 17 |
| 20-34 | 36 | 5.0 | 28 | 1 | 3 | 3 | 6 | 17 | 17 | 17 |
| 35-49 | 34 | 4.4 | 27 | 1 | 2 | 3 | 5 | 7 | 15 | 27 |
| 50-64 | 29 | 6.6 | 21 | 1 | 3 | 6 | 12 | 12 | 14 | 18 |
| 65+ | 78 | 5.4 | 16 | 1 | 2 | 5 | 8 | 10 | 12 | 16 |
| **TOTAL SINGLE DX** | 228 | 1.2 | <1 | 1 | 1 | 1 | 1 | 2 | 3 | 3 |
| **TOTAL MULTIPLE DX** | 307 | 4.3 | 26 | 1 | 1 | 2 | 6 | 11 | 13 | 18 |
| **TOTAL** | | | | | | | | | | |
| 0-19 Years | 341 | 1.8 | 11 | 1 | 1 | 1 | 2 | 3 | 4 | 13 |
| 20-34 | 42 | 4.7 | 26 | 1 | 2 | 2 | 6 | 17 | 17 | 17 |
| 35-49 | 38 | 4.1 | 25 | 1 | 1 | 2 | 5 | 9 | 15 | 27 |
| 50-64 | 32 | 6.2 | 22 | 1 | 2 | 5 | 12 | 12 | 14 | 18 |
| 65+ | 82 | 5.0 | 16 | 1 | 1 | 4 | 8 | 10 | 12 | 16 |
| **GRAND TOTAL** | 535 | 2.9 | 17 | 1 | 1 | 1 | 3 | 8 | 12 | 17 |

Length of Stay by Diagnosis and Operation, United States, 2000

# United States, October 1998–September 1999 Data, by Operation

## 98.2: RMVL OTH FB W/O INC. Formerly included in operation group(s) 793.

| Type of Patients | Observed Patients | Avg. Stay | Variance | 10th | 25th | 50th | 75th | 90th | 95th | 99th |
|---|---|---|---|---|---|---|---|---|---|---|
| **1. SINGLE DX** | | | | | | | | | | |
| 0–19 Years | 72 | 1.6 | <1 | 1 | 1 | 1 | 2 | 3 | 4 | 4 |
| 20–34 | 31 | 1.9 | 2 | 1 | 1 | 1 | 2 | 3 | 4 | 8 |
| 35–49 | 10 | 1.2 | <1 | 1 | 1 | 1 | 1 | 2 | 2 | 2 |
| 50–64 | 3 | 2.1 | <1 | 1 | 1 | 2 | 3 | 3 | 3 | 3 |
| 65+ | 1 | 1.0 | 0 | 1 | 1 | 1 | 1 | 1 | 1 | 1 |
| **2. MULTIPLE DX** | | | | | | | | | | |
| 0–19 Years | 62 | 2.6 | 4 | 1 | 1 | 2 | 3 | 7 | 7 | 11 |
| 20–34 | 58 | 3.6 | 5 | 1 | 2 | 3 | 5 | 6 | 9 | 13 |
| 35–49 | 43 | 3.7 | 10 | 1 | 1 | 3 | 5 | 8 | 10 | 13 |
| 50–64 | 39 | 3.0 | 8 | 1 | 2 | 2 | 2 | 6 | 11 | 14 |
| 65+ | 47 | 4.8 | 11 | 1 | 2 | 4 | 7 | 9 | 11 | 15 |
| **TOTAL SINGLE DX** | 117 | 1.7 | 1 | 1 | 1 | 1 | 2 | 3 | 4 | 8 |
| **TOTAL MULTIPLE DX** | 249 | 3.4 | 8 | 1 | 2 | 2 | 4 | 7 | 9 | 14 |
| **TOTAL** | | | | | | | | | | |
| 0–19 Years | 134 | 2.2 | 3 | 1 | 1 | 2 | 3 | 3 | 7 | 10 |
| 20–34 | 89 | 3.1 | 5 | 1 | 1 | 3 | 4 | 5 | 8 | 13 |
| 35–49 | 53 | 3.2 | 10 | 1 | 1 | 2 | 3 | 8 | 10 | 13 |
| 50–64 | 42 | 3.0 | 8 | 2 | 2 | 2 | 2 | 6 | 11 | 14 |
| 65+ | 48 | 4.6 | 11 | 1 | 2 | 4 | 7 | 9 | 11 | 15 |
| **GRAND TOTAL** | 366 | 3.0 | 7 | 1 | 1 | 2 | 3 | 5 | 9 | 14 |

## 98.51: RENAL/URETER/BLAD ESWL. Formerly included in operation group(s) 662.

| Type of Patients | Observed Patients | Avg. Stay | Variance | 10th | 25th | 50th | 75th | 90th | 95th | 99th |
|---|---|---|---|---|---|---|---|---|---|---|
| **1. SINGLE DX** | | | | | | | | | | |
| 0–19 Years | 23 | 2.9 | 4 | 1 | 1 | 2 | 6 | 6 | 6 | 6 |
| 20–34 | 156 | 2.0 | 1 | 1 | 1 | 2 | 2 | 6 | 6 | 6 |
| 35–49 | 224 | 1.9 | 1 | 1 | 1 | 2 | 2 | 3 | 4 | 6 |
| 50–64 | 117 | 2.0 | 3 | 1 | 1 | 2 | 2 | 3 | 4 | 14 |
| 65+ | 48 | 1.8 | 2 | 1 | 1 | 1 | 2 | 3 | 4 | 12 |
| **2. MULTIPLE DX** | | | | | | | | | | |
| 0–19 Years | 26 | 3.3 | 6 | 1 | 1 | 2 | 5 | 6 | 9 | 11 |
| 20–34 | 204 | 3.5 | 21 | 1 | 1 | 2 | 4 | 6 | 10 | 28 |
| 35–49 | 437 | 2.7 | 5 | 1 | 2 | 2 | 3 | 5 | 7 | 14 |
| 50–64 | 363 | 2.9 | 6 | 1 | 1 | 2 | 4 | 5 | 7 | 14 |
| 65+ | 413 | 3.9 | 15 | 1 | 1 | 3 | 5 | 8 | 11 | 21 |
| **TOTAL SINGLE DX** | 568 | 2.0 | 2 | 1 | 1 | 2 | 2 | 3 | 4 | 6 |
| **TOTAL MULTIPLE DX** | 1,443 | 3.2 | 11 | 1 | 2 | 2 | 4 | 6 | 9 | 17 |
| **TOTAL** | | | | | | | | | | |
| 0–19 Years | 49 | 3.1 | 5 | 1 | 1 | 2 | 5 | 6 | 6 | 11 |
| 20–34 | 360 | 2.9 | 13 | 1 | 1 | 2 | 3 | 5 | 8 | 28 |
| 35–49 | 661 | 2.4 | 4 | 1 | 1 | 2 | 3 | 4 | 5 | 9 |
| 50–64 | 480 | 2.7 | 6 | 1 | 1 | 2 | 3 | 5 | 7 | 14 |
| 65+ | 461 | 3.7 | 14 | 1 | 1 | 3 | 5 | 8 | 11 | 21 |
| **GRAND TOTAL** | 2,011 | 2.9 | 8 | 1 | 1 | 2 | 3 | 5 | 8 | 14 |

## 98.5: ESWL. Formerly included in operation group(s) 629, 662, 793.

| Type of Patients | Observed Patients | Avg. Stay | Variance | 10th | 25th | 50th | 75th | 90th | 95th | 99th |
|---|---|---|---|---|---|---|---|---|---|---|
| **1. SINGLE DX** | | | | | | | | | | |
| 0–19 Years | 23 | 2.9 | 4 | 1 | 1 | 1 | 2 | 3 | 4 | 4 |
| 20–34 | 156 | 2.0 | 1 | 1 | 1 | 1 | 2 | 3 | 4 | 8 |
| 35–49 | 225 | 1.8 | 1 | 1 | 1 | 1 | 1 | 2 | 2 | 2 |
| 50–64 | 120 | 1.9 | 3 | 1 | 1 | 2 | 3 | 3 | 3 | 3 |
| 65+ | 50 | 1.7 | 2 | 1 | 1 | 1 | 1 | 1 | 1 | 1 |
| **2. MULTIPLE DX** | | | | | | | | | | |
| 0–19 Years | 27 | 3.4 | 6 | 1 | 1 | 2 | 3 | 7 | 7 | 11 |
| 20–34 | 207 | 3.5 | 21 | 1 | 2 | 3 | 5 | 6 | 9 | 13 |
| 35–49 | 443 | 2.8 | 5 | 1 | 2 | 3 | 5 | 8 | 10 | 13 |
| 50–64 | 367 | 2.9 | 6 | 1 | 2 | 2 | 4 | 6 | 11 | 14 |
| 65+ | 414 | 3.9 | 15 | 1 | 2 | 4 | 7 | 9 | 11 | 15 |
| **TOTAL SINGLE DX** | 574 | 1.9 | 1 | 1 | 1 | 1 | 2 | 3 | 4 | 8 |
| **TOTAL MULTIPLE DX** | 1,458 | 3.2 | 11 | 1 | 2 | 2 | 4 | 7 | 9 | 14 |
| **TOTAL** | | | | | | | | | | |
| 0–19 Years | 50 | 3.2 | 5 | 1 | 1 | 2 | 5 | 6 | 6 | 11 |
| 20–34 | 363 | 2.9 | 13 | 1 | 1 | 3 | 4 | 5 | 8 | 13 |
| 35–49 | 668 | 2.4 | 4 | 1 | 1 | 2 | 3 | 6 | 8 | 13 |
| 50–64 | 487 | 2.7 | 6 | 1 | 1 | 3 | 3 | 4 | 7 | 14 |
| 65+ | 464 | 3.6 | 14 | 1 | 2 | 4 | 5 | 8 | 11 | 21 |
| **GRAND TOTAL** | 2,032 | 2.9 | 8 | 1 | 1 | 2 | 3 | 5 | 8 | 14 |

## 99.0: BLOOD TRANSFUSION. Formerly included in operation group(s) 794.

| Type of Patients | Observed Patients | Avg. Stay | Variance | 10th | 25th | 50th | 75th | 90th | 95th | 99th |
|---|---|---|---|---|---|---|---|---|---|---|
| **1. SINGLE DX** | | | | | | | | | | |
| 0–19 Years | 569 | 3.0 | 8 | 1 | 1 | 2 | 4 | 7 | 9 | 14 |
| 20–34 | 532 | 4.6 | 13 | 1 | 2 | 4 | 4 | 10 | 10 | 15 |
| 35–49 | 341 | 3.4 | 8 | 1 | 1 | 3 | 5 | 6 | 8 | 13 |
| 50–64 | 178 | 3.5 | 9 | 1 | 1 | 2 | 6 | 6 | 7 | 13 |
| 65+ | 421 | 2.3 | 7 | 1 | 1 | 2 | 2 | 5 | 7 | 13 |
| **2. MULTIPLE DX** | | | | | | | | | | |
| 0–19 Years | 5,384 | 6.2 | 74 | 1 | 2 | 4 | 7 | 12 | 18 | 51 |
| 20–34 | 5,022 | 5.5 | 25 | 1 | 2 | 4 | 7 | 11 | 14 | 26 |
| 35–49 | 9,474 | 5.3 | 30 | 1 | 2 | 4 | 7 | 11 | 14 | 28 |
| 50–64 | 13,179 | 5.5 | 25 | 1 | 2 | 4 | 7 | 11 | 15 | 25 |
| 65+ | 50,407 | 5.9 | 26 | 2 | 3 | 5 | 8 | 11 | 15 | 24 |
| **TOTAL SINGLE DX** | 2,041 | 3.4 | 10 | 1 | 1 | 2 | 5 | 7 | 10 | 14 |
| **TOTAL MULTIPLE DX** | 83,466 | 5.8 | 29 | 1 | 3 | 4 | 7 | 11 | 15 | 27 |
| **TOTAL** | | | | | | | | | | |
| 0–19 Years | 5,953 | 5.8 | 67 | 1 | 2 | 4 | 6 | 11 | 17 | 50 |
| 20–34 | 5,554 | 5.4 | 23 | 1 | 2 | 4 | 7 | 10 | 14 | 24 |
| 35–49 | 9,815 | 5.3 | 29 | 1 | 2 | 4 | 7 | 11 | 14 | 28 |
| 50–64 | 13,357 | 5.5 | 25 | 1 | 2 | 4 | 7 | 11 | 15 | 25 |
| 65+ | 50,828 | 5.9 | 26 | 2 | 3 | 5 | 7 | 11 | 15 | 24 |
| **GRAND TOTAL** | 85,507 | 5.7 | 29 | 2 | 3 | 4 | 7 | 11 | 15 | 26 |

Length of Stay by Diagnosis and Operation, United States, 2000

## 99.01: EXCHANGE TRANSFUSION. Formerly included in operation group(s) 794.

| Type of Patients | Observed Patients | Avg. Stay | Vari-ance | Percentiles | | | | | | |
|---|---|---|---|---|---|---|---|---|---|---|
| | | | | 10th | 25th | 50th | 75th | 90th | 95th | 99th |
| **1. SINGLE DX** | | | | | | | | | | |
| 0–19 Years | 32 | 1.8 | 4 | 1 | 1 | 1 | 2 | 5 | 6 | 10 |
| 20–34 | 10 | 6.6 | 26 | 1 | 4 | 4 | 7 | 15 | 15 | 19 |
| 35–49 | 1 | 4.0 | 0 | 4 | 4 | 4 | 4 | 4 | 4 | 4 |
| 50–64 | 0 | | | | | | | | | |
| 65+ | 1 | 2.0 | 0 | 2 | 2 | 2 | 2 | 2 | 2 | 2 |
| **2. MULTIPLE DX** | | | | | | | | | | |
| 0–19 Years | 247 | 7.5 | 76 | 2 | 3 | 5 | 8 | 14 | 22 | 51 |
| 20–34 | 47 | 7.4 | 32 | 2 | 4 | 5 | 9 | 15 | 23 | 24 |
| 35–49 | 18 | 9.3 | 84 | 2 | 4 | 7 | 9 | 21 | 36 | 36 |
| 50–64 | 7 | 6.7 | 25 | 1 | 2 | 7 | 8 | 18 | 18 | 18 |
| 65+ | 15 | 6.9 | 23 | 3 | 4 | 6 | 7 | 11 | 24 | 24 |
| **TOTAL SINGLE DX** | 44 | 2.2 | 4 | 1 | 1 | 2 | 2 | 3 | 5 | 15 |
| **TOTAL MULTIPLE DX** | 334 | 7.5 | 69 | 2 | 3 | 5 | 8 | 14 | 22 | 51 |
| **TOTAL** | | | | | | | | | | |
| 0–19 Years | 279 | 6.5 | 68 | 1 | 2 | 5 | 8 | 12 | 21 | 51 |
| 20–34 | 57 | 7.2 | 31 | 2 | 4 | 5 | 9 | 15 | 19 | 24 |
| 35–49 | 19 | 9.2 | 82 | 2 | 4 | 7 | 9 | 21 | 36 | 36 |
| 50–64 | 7 | 6.7 | 25 | 1 | 2 | 7 | 8 | 18 | 18 | 18 |
| 65+ | 16 | 6.6 | 5 | 2 | 2 | 6 | 7 | 3 | 6 | 11 |
| **GRAND TOTAL** | 378 | 5.9 | 54 | 1 | 2 | 4 | 7 | 11 | 19 | 43 |

## 99.03: WHOLE BLOOD TRANSFUS NEC. Formerly included in operation group(s) 794.

| Type of Patients | Observed Patients | Avg. Stay | Vari-ance | Percentiles | | | | | | |
|---|---|---|---|---|---|---|---|---|---|---|
| | | | | 10th | 25th | 50th | 75th | 90th | 95th | 99th |
| **1. SINGLE DX** | | | | | | | | | | |
| 0–19 Years | 7 | 1.3 | 1 | 1 | 1 | 1 | 1 | 1 | 2 | 7 |
| 20–34 | 3 | 4.4 | 11 | 2 | 2 | 2 | 5 | 10 | 10 | 10 |
| 35–49 | 0 | | | | | | | | | |
| 50–64 | 0 | | | | | | | | | |
| 65+ | 2 | 1.0 | 0 | 1 | 1 | 1 | 1 | 1 | 1 | 1 |
| **2. MULTIPLE DX** | | | | | | | | | | |
| 0–19 Years | 29 | 6.4 | 138 | 2 | 2 | 3 | 6 | 8 | 27 | 88 |
| 20–34 | 25 | 6.1 | 25 | 2 | 3 | 3 | 7 | 15 | 17 | 21 |
| 35–49 | 68 | 5.7 | 21 | 1 | 2 | 6 | 6 | 13 | 17 | 26 |
| 50–64 | 91 | 4.4 | 9 | 2 | 3 | 3 | 5 | 8 | 10 | 17 |
| 65+ | 361 | 5.7 | 17 | 2 | 3 | 5 | 7 | 11 | 12 | 20 |
| **TOTAL SINGLE DX** | 12 | 1.4 | 2 | 1 | 1 | 1 | 1 | 2 | 5 | 10 |
| **TOTAL MULTIPLE DX** | 574 | 5.5 | 21 | 2 | 3 | 5 | 7 | 10 | 13 | 21 |
| **TOTAL** | | | | | | | | | | |
| 0–19 Years | 36 | 3.8 | 76 | 1 | 2 | 2 | 4 | 6 | 8 | 46 |
| 20–34 | 28 | 5.9 | 24 | 2 | 3 | 3 | 7 | 15 | 17 | 21 |
| 35–49 | 68 | 5.7 | 21 | 1 | 2 | 6 | 6 | 13 | 17 | 26 |
| 50–64 | 91 | 4.4 | 9 | 2 | 3 | 3 | 5 | 8 | 10 | 17 |
| 65+ | 363 | 5.7 | 17 | 2 | 3 | 5 | 7 | 11 | 12 | 20 |
| **GRAND TOTAL** | 586 | 5.4 | 21 | 1 | 3 | 5 | 7 | 9 | 12 | 21 |

## 99.04: PACKED CELL TRANSFUSION. Formerly included in operation group(s) 794.

| Type of Patients | Observed Patients | Avg. Stay | Vari-ance | Percentiles | | | | | | |
|---|---|---|---|---|---|---|---|---|---|---|
| | | | | 10th | 25th | 50th | 75th | 90th | 95th | 99th |
| **1. SINGLE DX** | | | | | | | | | | |
| 0–19 Years | 475 | 3.3 | 8 | 1 | 1 | 2 | 4 | 7 | 9 | 14 |
| 20–34 | 496 | 4.6 | 12 | 1 | 2 | 3 | 4 | 10 | 10 | 14 |
| 35–49 | 325 | 3.5 | 8 | 1 | 1 | 3 | 5 | 6 | 8 | 15 |
| 50–64 | 156 | 3.6 | 9 | 1 | 2 | 3 | 6 | 6 | 7 | 11 |
| 65+ | 383 | 2.4 | 8 | 1 | 1 | 1 | 3 | 6 | 8 | 17 |
| **2. MULTIPLE DX** | | | | | | | | | | |
| 0–19 Years | 4,054 | 6.2 | 80 | 2 | 4 | 6 | 7 | 12 | 20 | 54 |
| 20–34 | 4,561 | 5.5 | 24 | 1 | 2 | 4 | 7 | 11 | 14 | 27 |
| 35–49 | 8,535 | 5.3 | 31 | 1 | 2 | 4 | 7 | 11 | 14 | 28 |
| 50–64 | 11,864 | 5.5 | 25 | 1 | 2 | 4 | 7 | 11 | 15 | 25 |
| 65+ | 46,785 | 5.9 | 26 | 2 | 3 | 5 | 8 | 11 | 15 | 25 |
| **TOTAL SINGLE DX** | 1,835 | 3.6 | 10 | 1 | 1 | 3 | 5 | 8 | 10 | 14 |
| **TOTAL MULTIPLE DX** | 75,799 | 5.8 | 10 | 1 | 3 | 4 | 7 | 11 | 15 | 27 |
| **TOTAL** | | | | | | | | | | |
| 0–19 Years | 4,529 | 5.9 | 73 | 1 | 2 | 4 | 6 | 11 | 18 | 50 |
| 20–34 | 5,057 | 5.4 | 23 | 1 | 2 | 4 | 7 | 10 | 14 | 24 |
| 35–49 | 8,860 | 5.2 | 30 | 1 | 2 | 4 | 6 | 11 | 14 | 28 |
| 50–64 | 12,020 | 5.5 | 25 | 1 | 2 | 4 | 7 | 11 | 15 | 25 |
| 65+ | 47,168 | 5.9 | 26 | 2 | 3 | 5 | 8 | 11 | 15 | 24 |
| **GRAND TOTAL** | 77,634 | 5.7 | 29 | 1 | 3 | 4 | 7 | 11 | 15 | 26 |

## 99.05: PLATELET TRANSFUSION. Formerly included in operation group(s) 794.

| Type of Patients | Observed Patients | Avg. Stay | Vari-ance | Percentiles | | | | | | |
|---|---|---|---|---|---|---|---|---|---|---|
| | | | | 10th | 25th | 50th | 75th | 90th | 95th | 99th |
| **1. SINGLE DX** | | | | | | | | | | |
| 0–19 Years | 22 | 2.6 | 6 | 1 | 1 | 2 | 5 | 7 | 7 | 7 |
| 20–34 | 13 | 3.1 | 3 | 1 | 3 | 3 | 4 | 5 | 7 | 7 |
| 35–49 | 10 | 2.5 | 3 | 1 | 3 | 3 | 3 | 4 | 7 | 7 |
| 50–64 | 15 | 3.8 | 17 | 1 | 3 | 3 | 3 | 13 | 13 | 13 |
| 65+ | 25 | 1.5 | 1 | 1 | 1 | 1 | 1 | 3 | 5 | 5 |
| **2. MULTIPLE DX** | | | | | | | | | | |
| 0–19 Years | 817 | 5.6 | 30 | 1 | 4 | 4 | 7 | 11 | 14 | 33 |
| 20–34 | 238 | 6.1 | 24 | 2 | 3 | 5 | 8 | 12 | 13 | 25 |
| 35–49 | 410 | 4.9 | 17 | 1 | 2 | 4 | 6 | 10 | 13 | 22 |
| 50–64 | 614 | 5.9 | 23 | 1 | 3 | 5 | 8 | 11 | 14 | 26 |
| 65+ | 1,219 | 5.9 | 24 | 1 | 2 | 5 | 8 | 12 | 15 | 22 |
| **TOTAL SINGLE DX** | 85 | 2.5 | 6 | 1 | 1 | 1 | 3 | 6 | 7 | 13 |
| **TOTAL MULTIPLE DX** | 3,298 | 5.7 | 25 | 1 | 2 | 4 | 7 | 12 | 14 | 26 |
| **TOTAL** | | | | | | | | | | |
| 0–19 Years | 839 | 5.5 | 30 | 1 | 2 | 4 | 7 | 11 | 14 | 32 |
| 20–34 | 251 | 6.0 | 24 | 2 | 2 | 5 | 8 | 12 | 13 | 21 |
| 35–49 | 420 | 4.8 | 16 | 1 | 2 | 3 | 6 | 9 | 13 | 22 |
| 50–64 | 629 | 5.8 | 23 | 1 | 3 | 5 | 8 | 11 | 14 | 26 |
| 65+ | 1,244 | 5.7 | 24 | 1 | 2 | 4 | 8 | 12 | 15 | 22 |
| **GRAND TOTAL** | 3,383 | 5.6 | 25 | 1 | 2 | 4 | 7 | 11 | 14 | 26 |

Length of Stay by Diagnosis and Operation, United States, 2000

# United States, October 1998–September 1999 Data, by Operation

## 99.06: COAG FACTOR TRANSFUSION. Formerly included in operation group(s) 794.

| Type of Patients | Observed Patients | Avg. Stay | Vari-ance | 10th | 25th | 50th | 75th | 90th | 95th | 99th |
|---|---|---|---|---|---|---|---|---|---|---|
| **1. SINGLE DX** | | | | | | | | | | |
| 0–19 Years | 17 | 1.9 | <1 | 1 | 1 | 2 | 3 | 3 | 3 | 3 |
| 20–34 | 4 | 1.9 | 2 | 1 | 1 | 1 | 1 | 4 | 4 | 4 |
| 35–49 | 0 | | | | | | | | | |
| 50–64 | 0 | | | | | | | | | |
| 65+ | 1 | 2.0 | 0 | 2 | 2 | 2 | 2 | 2 | 2 | 2 |
| **2. MULTIPLE DX** | | | | | | | | | | |
| 0–19 Years | 132 | 4.2 | 12 | 1 | 1 | 3 | 5 | 10 | 11 | 14 |
| 20–34 | 44 | 2.7 | 13 | 1 | 1 | 2 | 2 | 7 | 9 | 19 |
| 35–49 | 57 | 3.9 | 15 | 1 | 2 | 3 | 5 | 7 | 9 | 23 |
| 50–64 | 25 | 3.4 | 6 | 1 | 1 | 3 | 5 | 8 | >99 | >99 |
| 65+ | 22 | 5.5 | 8 | 2 | 2 | 6 | 8 | 9 | 10 | 11 |
| **TOTAL SINGLE DX** | 22 | 1.9 | <1 | 1 | 1 | 2 | 3 | 3 | 4 | 4 |
| **TOTAL MULTIPLE DX** | 280 | 3.9 | 12 | 1 | 1 | 3 | 5 | 8 | 11 | 21 |
| **TOTAL** | | | | | | | | | | |
| 0–19 Years | 149 | 3.9 | 11 | 2 | 2 | 3 | 5 | 10 | 11 | 14 |
| 20–34 | 48 | 2.7 | 13 | 1 | 1 | 1 | 3 | 6 | 9 | 19 |
| 35–49 | 57 | 3.9 | 15 | 1 | 2 | 3 | 5 | 7 | 9 | 23 |
| 50–64 | 25 | 3.4 | 6 | 1 | 1 | 3 | 5 | 8 | >99 | >99 |
| 65+ | 23 | 5.4 | 9 | 2 | 2 | 6 | 8 | 9 | 10 | 11 |
| **GRAND TOTAL** | 302 | 3.7 | 12 | 1 | 1 | 3 | 5 | 8 | 10 | 21 |

## 99.07: SERUM TRANSFUSION NEC. Formerly included in operation group(s) 794.

| Type of Patients | Observed Patients | Avg. Stay | Vari-ance | 10th | 25th | 50th | 75th | 90th | 95th | 99th |
|---|---|---|---|---|---|---|---|---|---|---|
| **1. SINGLE DX** | | | | | | | | | | |
| 0–19 Years | 6 | 2.7 | 31 | 1 | 1 | 1 | 1 | 2 | 22 | 22 |
| 20–34 | 3 | 6.5 | 3 | 5 | 5 | 6 | 6 | 9 | 9 | 9 |
| 35–49 | 3 | 4.9 | 18 | 1 | 1 | 3 | 10 | 10 | 10 | 10 |
| 50–64 | 5 | 1.2 | <1 | 1 | 1 | 1 | 1 | 2 | 2 | 2 |
| 65+ | 8 | 2.7 | 5 | 1 | 1 | 2 | 4 | 8 | 8 | 8 |
| **2. MULTIPLE DX** | | | | | | | | | | |
| 0–19 Years | 76 | 8.1 | 120 | 2 | 2 | 5 | 10 | 17 | 52 | >99 |
| 20–34 | 90 | 5.1 | 23 | 2 | 2 | 3 | 7 | 10 | 12 | 15 |
| 35–49 | 350 | 5.8 | 23 | 1 | 3 | 5 | 8 | 10 | 15 | 27 |
| 50–64 | 521 | 5.6 | 20 | 1 | 3 | 4 | 8 | 12 | 13 | 19 |
| 65+ | 1,838 | 5.7 | 21 | 1 | 3 | 4 | 7 | 11 | 15 | 24 |
| **TOTAL SINGLE DX** | 25 | 3.1 | 20 | 1 | 1 | 1 | 2 | 8 | 10 | 22 |
| **TOTAL MULTIPLE DX** | 2,875 | 5.7 | 24 | 1 | 2 | 4 | 8 | 11 | 14 | 25 |
| **TOTAL** | | | | | | | | | | |
| 0–19 Years | 82 | 7.2 | 110 | 1 | 1 | 5 | 8 | 17 | 52 | >99 |
| 20–34 | 93 | 5.1 | 23 | 1 | 2 | 6 | 7 | 10 | 12 | 15 |
| 35–49 | 353 | 5.8 | 23 | 1 | 2 | 5 | 8 | 10 | 15 | 27 |
| 50–64 | 526 | 5.6 | 20 | 1 | 2 | 4 | 8 | 12 | 13 | 19 |
| 65+ | 1,846 | 5.7 | 21 | 1 | 3 | 4 | 7 | 11 | 15 | 24 |
| **GRAND TOTAL** | 2,900 | 5.7 | 24 | 1 | 2 | 4 | 8 | 11 | 14 | 25 |

## 99.1: INJECT/INFUSE THER SUBST. Formerly included in operation group(s) 794.

| Type of Patients | Observed Patients | Avg. Stay | Vari-ance | 10th | 25th | 50th | 75th | 90th | 95th | 99th |
|---|---|---|---|---|---|---|---|---|---|---|
| **1. SINGLE DX** | | | | | | | | | | |
| 0–19 Years | 619 | 2.4 | 4 | 1 | 1 | 2 | 3 | 5 | 7 | 12 |
| 20–34 | 404 | 3.2 | 6 | 1 | 1 | 3 | 4 | 6 | 8 | 13 |
| 35–49 | 263 | 4.6 | 28 | 1 | 2 | 4 | 5 | 7 | 9 | 30 |
| 50–64 | 153 | 3.1 | 7 | 1 | 1 | 2 | 5 | 7 | 8 | 11 |
| 65+ | 115 | 3.8 | 19 | 1 | 1 | 3 | 5 | 8 | 8 | 10 |
| **2. MULTIPLE DX** | | | | | | | | | | |
| 0–19 Years | 3,536 | 11.0 | 184 | 1 | 2 | 5 | 15 | 28 | 42 | 63 |
| 20–34 | 1,609 | 5.2 | 26 | 1 | 2 | 4 | 7 | 11 | 14 | 27 |
| 35–49 | 2,703 | 6.9 | 58 | 1 | 2 | 5 | 9 | 15 | 17 | 37 |
| 50–64 | 3,734 | 6.3 | 38 | 2 | 3 | 5 | 7 | 13 | 18 | 31 |
| 65+ | 6,848 | 7.0 | 40 | 2 | 3 | 5 | 8 | 13 | 19 | 34 |
| **TOTAL SINGLE DX** | 1,554 | 3.2 | 11 | 1 | 1 | 2 | 4 | 6 | 8 | 13 |
| **TOTAL MULTIPLE DX** | 18,430 | 7.4 | 69 | 2 | 3 | 5 | 9 | 15 | 22 | 45 |
| **TOTAL** | | | | | | | | | | |
| 0–19 Years | 4,155 | 9.7 | 166 | 1 | 2 | 4 | 12 | 26 | 38 | 60 |
| 20–34 | 2,013 | 4.8 | 23 | 1 | 2 | 3 | 6 | 10 | 13 | 25 |
| 35–49 | 2,966 | 6.7 | 56 | 1 | 2 | 5 | 8 | 14 | 17 | 37 |
| 50–64 | 3,887 | 6.2 | 37 | 1 | 2 | 4 | 7 | 13 | 17 | 31 |
| 65+ | 6,963 | 6.9 | 39 | 2 | 3 | 5 | 8 | 13 | 18 | 33 |
| **GRAND TOTAL** | 19,984 | 7.1 | 66 | 1 | 3 | 5 | 8 | 15 | 22 | 43 |

## 99.10: INJECT THROMBOLYTIC. Formerly included in operation group(s) 794.

| Type of Patients | Observed Patients | Avg. Stay | Vari-ance | 10th | 25th | 50th | 75th | 90th | 95th | 99th |
|---|---|---|---|---|---|---|---|---|---|---|
| **1. SINGLE DX** | | | | | | | | | | |
| 0–19 Years | 2 | 1.0 | 0 | 1 | 1 | 1 | 1 | 1 | 1 | 1 |
| 20–34 | 12 | 3.6 | 7 | 1 | 1 | 3 | 6 | 8 | 8 | 8 |
| 35–49 | 30 | 4.3 | 3 | 3 | 3 | 4 | 5 | 7 | 8 | 9 |
| 50–64 | 29 | 4.2 | 3 | 1 | 1 | 4 | 6 | 6 | 6 | 9 |
| 65+ | 19 | 3.1 | 2 | 1 | 1 | 3 | 4 | 5 | 5 | 6 |
| **2. MULTIPLE DX** | | | | | | | | | | |
| 0–19 Years | 37 | 4.2 | 16 | 1 | 1 | 3 | 6 | 11 | 15 | 15 |
| 20–34 | 87 | 4.5 | 15 | 1 | 2 | 4 | 7 | 8 | 10 | 19 |
| 35–49 | 341 | 4.5 | 13 | 2 | 2 | 4 | 6 | 8 | 10 | 24 |
| 50–64 | 767 | 4.6 | 13 | 2 | 3 | 4 | 6 | 7 | 10 | 15 |
| 65+ | 1,389 | 6.2 | 16 | 2 | 4 | 6 | 7 | 11 | 15 | 23 |
| **TOTAL SINGLE DX** | 92 | 3.9 | 4 | 1 | 3 | 4 | 5 | 6 | 8 | 9 |
| **TOTAL MULTIPLE DX** | 2,621 | 5.4 | 15 | 1 | 3 | 5 | 7 | 10 | 13 | 20 |
| **TOTAL** | | | | | | | | | | |
| 0–19 Years | 39 | 4.1 | 16 | 1 | 1 | 3 | 6 | 11 | 15 | 15 |
| 20–34 | 99 | 4.4 | 14 | 1 | 2 | 4 | 7 | 8 | 10 | 17 |
| 35–49 | 371 | 4.5 | 12 | 1 | 3 | 4 | 6 | 7 | 9 | 24 |
| 50–64 | 796 | 4.6 | 13 | 1 | 3 | 4 | 6 | 7 | 9 | 15 |
| 65+ | 1,408 | 6.1 | 16 | 2 | 4 | 5 | 7 | 11 | 15 | 23 |
| **GRAND TOTAL** | 2,713 | 5.4 | 15 | 1 | 3 | 5 | 7 | 9 | 13 | 20 |

413

Length of Stay by Diagnosis and Operation, United States, 2000

# United States, October 1998–September 1999 Data, by Operation

## 99.15: PARENTERAL NUTRITION. Formerly included in operation group(s) 794.

| Type of Patients | Observed Patients | Avg. Stay | Variance | 10th | 25th | 50th | 75th | 90th | 95th | 99th |
|---|---|---|---|---|---|---|---|---|---|---|
| **1. SINGLE DX** | | | | | | | | | | |
| 0–19 Years | 49 | 4.5 | 6 | 2 | 2 | 4 | 6 | 8 | 9 | 11 |
| 20–34 | 48 | 5.7 | 14 | 2 | 3 | 5 | 7 | 9 | 16 | 16 |
| 35–49 | 26 | 10.1 | 120 | 3 | 4 | 4 | 10 | 30 | 30 | 39 |
| 50–64 | 12 | 6.4 | 9 | 4 | 4 | 4 | 8 | 11 | 13 | 13 |
| 65+ | 6 | 9.9 | 106 | 8 | 8 | 8 | 8 | 10 | 10 | 60 |
| **2. MULTIPLE DX** | | | | | | | | | | |
| 0–19 Years | 2,201 | 16.2 | 227 | 3 | 6 | 11 | 22 | 37 | 52 | 71 |
| 20–34 | 489 | 8.4 | 42 | 3 | 4 | 7 | 11 | 16 | 18 | 39 |
| 35–49 | 934 | 10.7 | 96 | 2 | 5 | 8 | 14 | 19 | 30 | 52 |
| 50–64 | 1,080 | 10.7 | 67 | 3 | 5 | 9 | 14 | 22 | 27 | 38 |
| 65+ | 1,711 | 11.7 | 87 | 4 | 6 | 9 | 14 | 22 | 32 | 47 |
| **TOTAL SINGLE DX** | 141 | 6.7 | 48 | 2 | 3 | 5 | 8 | 10 | 21 | 39 |
| **TOTAL MULTIPLE DX** | 6,415 | 12.4 | 130 | 3 | 5 | 9 | 15 | 26 | 35 | 56 |
| **TOTAL** | | | | | | | | | | |
| 0–19 Years | 2,250 | 15.9 | 224 | 3 | 5 | 11 | 21 | 37 | 51 | 71 |
| 20–34 | 537 | 8.2 | 41 | 3 | 4 | 7 | 10 | 15 | 18 | 38 |
| 35–49 | 960 | 10.7 | 97 | 4 | 4 | 8 | 14 | 19 | 30 | 51 |
| 50–64 | 1,092 | 10.7 | 67 | 3 | 5 | 9 | 14 | 22 | 27 | 38 |
| 65+ | 1,717 | 11.7 | 87 | 4 | 6 | 9 | 14 | 22 | 32 | 47 |
| **GRAND TOTAL** | 6,556 | 12.3 | 129 | 3 | 5 | 9 | 15 | 26 | 35 | 56 |

## 99.17: INJECT INSULIN. Formerly included in operation group(s) 794.

| Type of Patients | Observed Patients | Avg. Stay | Variance | 10th | 25th | 50th | 75th | 90th | 95th | 99th |
|---|---|---|---|---|---|---|---|---|---|---|
| **1. SINGLE DX** | | | | | | | | | | |
| 0–19 Years | 90 | 2.9 | 3 | 1 | 2 | 2 | 4 | 5 | 6 | 8 |
| 20–34 | 67 | 2.9 | 3 | 1 | 2 | 2 | 4 | 6 | 6 | 8 |
| 35–49 | 40 | 3.5 | 4 | 1 | 3 | 3 | 4 | 7 | 8 | 8 |
| 50–64 | 16 | 2.1 | 2 | 1 | 1 | 1 | 4 | 4 | 5 | 5 |
| 65+ | 3 | 3.4 | <1 | 3 | 3 | 3 | 4 | 4 | 4 | 4 |
| **2. MULTIPLE DX** | | | | | | | | | | |
| 0–19 Years | 212 | 3.1 | 5 | 1 | 2 | 2 | 4 | 6 | 8 | 11 |
| 20–34 | 238 | 3.5 | 5 | 1 | 2 | 3 | 4 | 6 | 8 | 10 |
| 35–49 | 347 | 3.8 | 9 | 1 | 2 | 3 | 5 | 7 | 10 | 13 |
| 50–64 | 400 | 4.2 | 12 | 1 | 2 | 3 | 5 | 8 | 10 | 17 |
| 65+ | 437 | 5.1 | 23 | 1 | 2 | 4 | 6 | 10 | 13 | 21 |
| **TOTAL SINGLE DX** | 216 | 2.9 | 3 | 1 | 2 | 2 | 4 | 6 | 6 | 8 |
| **TOTAL MULTIPLE DX** | 1,634 | 4.1 | 12 | 1 | 2 | 3 | 5 | 8 | 10 | 17 |
| **TOTAL** | | | | | | | | | | |
| 0–19 Years | 302 | 3.0 | 4 | 1 | 2 | 2 | 4 | 6 | 8 | 11 |
| 20–34 | 305 | 3.4 | 5 | 1 | 2 | 3 | 4 | 6 | 8 | 10 |
| 35–49 | 387 | 3.8 | 9 | 1 | 2 | 3 | 5 | 7 | 10 | 13 |
| 50–64 | 416 | 4.1 | 12 | 1 | 2 | 3 | 5 | 8 | 10 | 17 |
| 65+ | 440 | 5.1 | 23 | 1 | 2 | 4 | 6 | 10 | 13 | 21 |
| **GRAND TOTAL** | 1,850 | 3.9 | 11 | 1 | 2 | 3 | 5 | 7 | 9 | 16 |

## 99.11: INJECT RH IMMUNE GLOB. Formerly included in operation group(s) 794.

| Type of Patients | Observed Patients | Avg. Stay | Variance | 10th | 25th | 50th | 75th | 90th | 95th | 99th |
|---|---|---|---|---|---|---|---|---|---|---|
| **1. SINGLE DX** | | | | | | | | | | |
| 0–19 Years | 39 | 1.8 | <1 | 1 | 1 | 2 | 2 | 3 | 3 | 4 |
| 20–34 | 113 | 1.7 | <1 | 1 | 1 | 2 | 2 | 3 | 3 | 7 |
| 35–49 | 18 | 1.7 | <1 | 1 | 1 | 2 | 2 | 2 | 3 | 5 |
| 50–64 | 0 | | | | | | | | | |
| 65+ | 2 | 1.5 | <1 | 1 | 1 | 2 | 2 | 2 | 2 | 2 |
| **2. MULTIPLE DX** | | | | | | | | | | |
| 0–19 Years | 92 | 2.3 | 1 | 1 | 1 | 2 | 3 | 3 | 4 | 6 |
| 20–34 | 324 | 2.2 | 5 | 1 | 1 | 2 | 2 | 3 | 4 | 13 |
| 35–49 | 54 | 2.9 | 40 | 1 | 1 | 2 | 3 | 3 | 4 | 57 |
| 50–64 | 6 | 4.8 | 19 | 1 | 3 | 4 | 7 | 7 | 15 | 15 |
| 65+ | 5 | 5.2 | 6 | 2 | 3 | 7 | 8 | 8 | 8 | 8 |
| **TOTAL SINGLE DX** | 172 | 1.7 | <1 | 1 | 1 | 2 | 2 | 2 | 3 | 6 |
| **TOTAL MULTIPLE DX** | 481 | 2.3 | 8 | 1 | 1 | 2 | 3 | 3 | 4 | 10 |
| **TOTAL** | | | | | | | | | | |
| 0–19 Years | 131 | 2.2 | 1 | 1 | 1 | 2 | 3 | 3 | 4 | 6 |
| 20–34 | 437 | 2.0 | 4 | 1 | 1 | 2 | 2 | 3 | 4 | 9 |
| 35–49 | 72 | 2.7 | 32 | 1 | 1 | 2 | 3 | 3 | 4 | 57 |
| 50–64 | 6 | 4.8 | 19 | 1 | 1 | 4 | 7 | 7 | 15 | 15 |
| 65+ | 7 | 4.5 | 6 | 2 | 2 | 3 | 7 | 8 | 8 | 8 |
| **GRAND TOTAL** | 653 | 2.2 | 6 | 1 | 1 | 2 | 2 | 3 | 4 | 8 |

## 99.14: INJECT GAMMA GLOBULIN. Formerly included in operation group(s) 794.

| Type of Patients | Observed Patients | Avg. Stay | Variance | 10th | 25th | 50th | 75th | 90th | 95th | 99th |
|---|---|---|---|---|---|---|---|---|---|---|
| **1. SINGLE DX** | | | | | | | | | | |
| 0–19 Years | 313 | 2.1 | 4 | 1 | 1 | 2 | 2 | 3 | 5 | 12 |
| 20–34 | 21 | 2.1 | 1 | 1 | 2 | 2 | 3 | 4 | 4 | 5 |
| 35–49 | 25 | 2.9 | 3 | 2 | 2 | 2 | 4 | 5 | 8 | 8 |
| 50–64 | 23 | 1.5 | 5 | 1 | 1 | 1 | 1 | 1 | 2 | 21 |
| 65+ | 28 | 2.1 | 2 | 1 | 1 | 2 | 2 | 4 | 7 | 7 |
| **2. MULTIPLE DX** | | | | | | | | | | |
| 0–19 Years | 402 | 3.4 | 19 | 1 | 1 | 2 | 3 | 7 | 13 | 20 |
| 20–34 | 67 | 4.8 | 15 | 1 | 2 | 4 | 7 | 9 | 11 | 18 |
| 35–49 | 114 | 4.1 | 8 | 1 | 2 | 4 | 5 | 7 | 9 | 13 |
| 50–64 | 108 | 2.8 | 8 | 1 | 1 | 1 | 5 | 6 | 9 | 16 |
| 65+ | 224 | 4.6 | 17 | 2 | 3 | 4 | 5 | 7 | 12 | 23 |
| **TOTAL SINGLE DX** | 410 | 2.1 | 4 | 1 | 1 | 2 | 2 | 4 | 5 | 12 |
| **TOTAL MULTIPLE DX** | 915 | 3.8 | 16 | 1 | 2 | 3 | 5 | 7 | 11 | 20 |
| **TOTAL** | | | | | | | | | | |
| 0–19 Years | 715 | 2.8 | 13 | 1 | 1 | 2 | 3 | 5 | 9 | 20 |
| 20–34 | 88 | 4.5 | 14 | 1 | 2 | 4 | 6 | 9 | 10 | 18 |
| 35–49 | 139 | 3.9 | 7 | 1 | 2 | 4 | 5 | 7 | 9 | 12 |
| 50–64 | 131 | 2.3 | 7 | 1 | 2 | 1 | 3 | 5 | 8 | 16 |
| 65+ | 252 | 4.4 | 16 | 1 | 2 | 3 | 5 | 7 | 12 | 23 |
| **GRAND TOTAL** | 1,325 | 3.2 | 13 | 1 | 1 | 2 | 4 | 7 | 9 | 20 |

Length of Stay by Diagnosis and Operation, United States, 2000

# United States, October 1998–September 1999 Data, by Operation

## 99.18: INJECT ELECTROLYTES. Formerly included in operation group(s) 794.

| Type of Patients | Observed Patients | Avg. Stay | Variance | 10th | 25th | 50th | 75th | 90th | 95th | 99th |
|---|---|---|---|---|---|---|---|---|---|---|
| **1. SINGLE DX** | | | | | | | | | | |
| 0–19 Years | 98 | 2.1 | 3 | 1 | 1 | 2 | 3 | 3 | 5 | 11 |
| 20–34 | 66 | 2.7 | 4 | 1 | 1 | 2 | 3 | 6 | 5 | 8 |
| 35–49 | 24 | 3.1 | 7 | 1 | 1 | 2 | 4 | 8 | 8 | 9 |
| 50–64 | 7 | 2.2 | <1 | 2 | 2 | 2 | 3 | 3 | 3 | 3 |
| 65+ | 6 | 2.6 | <1 | 1 | 3 | 3 | 3 | 3 | 3 | 3 |
| **2. MULTIPLE DX** | | | | | | | | | | |
| 0–19 Years | 508 | 2.4 | 3 | 1 | 1 | 2 | 3 | 4 | 5 | 8 |
| 20–34 | 170 | 2.9 | 6 | 1 | 1 | 2 | 4 | 6 | 9 | 13 |
| 35–49 | 211 | 2.9 | 12 | 1 | 1 | 2 | 3 | 6 | 9 | 14 |
| 50–64 | 208 | 4.5 | 21 | 2 | 2 | 3 | 5 | 10 | 13 | 25 |
| 65+ | 472 | 5.0 | 28 | 2 | 2 | 3 | 6 | 9 | 15 | 31 |
| **TOTAL SINGLE DX** | 201 | 2.4 | 3 | 1 | 1 | 2 | 3 | 4 | 7 | 9 |
| **TOTAL MULTIPLE DX** | 1,569 | 3.5 | 16 | 1 | 2 | 2 | 4 | 7 | 10 | 25 |
| **TOTAL** | | | | | | | | | | |
| 0–19 Years | 606 | 2.3 | 3 | 1 | 1 | 2 | 3 | 4 | 5 | 8 |
| 20–34 | 236 | 2.9 | 6 | 1 | 2 | 2 | 4 | 6 | 8 | 13 |
| 35–49 | 235 | 2.9 | 11 | 1 | 1 | 2 | 3 | 6 | 9 | 14 |
| 50–64 | 215 | 4.4 | 20 | 2 | 2 | 3 | 5 | 10 | 12 | 25 |
| 65+ | 478 | 5.0 | 28 | 2 | 2 | 3 | 6 | 9 | 15 | 31 |
| **GRAND TOTAL** | 1,770 | 3.4 | 14 | 1 | 2 | 2 | 3 | 7 | 9 | 23 |

## 99.2: OTH INJECT THER SUBST. Formerly included in operation group(s) 794.

| Type of Patients | Observed Patients | Avg. Stay | Variance | 10th | 25th | 50th | 75th | 90th | 95th | 99th |
|---|---|---|---|---|---|---|---|---|---|---|
| **1. SINGLE DX** | | | | | | | | | | |
| 0–19 Years | 2,767 | 2.7 | 6 | 1 | 1 | 2 | 3 | 5 | 6 | 10 |
| 20–34 | 2,024 | 2.6 | 5 | 1 | 1 | 2 | 3 | 5 | 6 | 9 |
| 35–49 | 938 | 2.9 | 4 | 1 | 2 | 2 | 4 | 5 | 6 | 11 |
| 50–64 | 490 | 2.7 | 8 | 1 | 2 | 2 | 4 | 5 | 6 | 8 |
| 65+ | 298 | 3.8 | 11 | 1 | 2 | 4 | 4 | 7 | 8 | 23 |
| **2. MULTIPLE DX** | | | | | | | | | | |
| 0–19 Years | 25,087 | 3.9 | 20 | 2 | 3 | 4 | 5 | 6 | 9 | 25 |
| 20–34 | 8,383 | 4.2 | 23 | 1 | 2 | 4 | 5 | 7 | 11 | 26 |
| 35–49 | 13,520 | 4.7 | 29 | 1 | 2 | 4 | 5 | 8 | 12 | 33 |
| 50–64 | 19,352 | 5.0 | 28 | 1 | 3 | 4 | 5 | 9 | 14 | 27 |
| 65+ | 25,549 | 5.5 | 26 | 2 | 3 | 4 | 6 | 11 | 14 | 27 |
| **TOTAL SINGLE DX** | 6,517 | 2.7 | 6 | 1 | 1 | 2 | 3 | 5 | 6 | 10 |
| **TOTAL MULTIPLE DX** | 91,891 | 4.7 | 25 | 1 | 2 | 4 | 5 | 8 | 13 | 27 |
| **TOTAL** | | | | | | | | | | |
| 0–19 Years | 27,854 | 3.8 | 18 | 1 | 2 | 3 | 4 | 6 | 9 | 23 |
| 20–34 | 10,407 | 3.9 | 19 | 1 | 2 | 3 | 4 | 6 | 9 | 24 |
| 35–49 | 14,458 | 4.6 | 27 | 1 | 2 | 4 | 5 | 8 | 11 | 31 |
| 50–64 | 19,842 | 4.9 | 28 | 1 | 2 | 4 | 5 | 9 | 14 | 27 |
| 65+ | 25,847 | 5.5 | 26 | 2 | 3 | 4 | 6 | 11 | 14 | 27 |
| **GRAND TOTAL** | 98,408 | 4.6 | 24 | 1 | 2 | 4 | 5 | 8 | 12 | 26 |

## 99.19: INJECT ANTICOAGULANT. Formerly included in operation group(s) 794.

| Type of Patients | Observed Patients | Avg. Stay | Variance | 10th | 25th | 50th | 75th | 90th | 95th | 99th |
|---|---|---|---|---|---|---|---|---|---|---|
| **1. SINGLE DX** | | | | | | | | | | |
| 0–19 Years | 11 | 4.3 | 3 | 3 | 3 | 4 | 6 | 6 | 6 | 9 |
| 20–34 | 72 | 4.0 | 5 | 1 | 3 | 4 | 5 | 6 | 8 | 10 |
| 35–49 | 95 | 4.1 | 6 | 1 | 2 | 4 | 6 | 7 | 7 | 13 |
| 50–64 | 64 | 3.9 | 6 | 1 | 2 | 4 | 5 | 7 | 8 | 9 |
| 65+ | 50 | 3.4 | 5 | 1 | 1 | 3 | 5 | 7 | 8 | 9 |
| **2. MULTIPLE DX** | | | | | | | | | | |
| 0–19 Years | 54 | 5.0 | 21 | 2 | 3 | 4 | 6 | 11 | 13 | 20 |
| 20–34 | 218 | 4.1 | 7 | 2 | 2 | 4 | 6 | 7 | 9 | 11 |
| 35–49 | 689 | 4.7 | 13 | 1 | 2 | 4 | 6 | 9 | 12 | 16 |
| 50–64 | 1,163 | 4.0 | 8 | 1 | 2 | 4 | 5 | 7 | 8 | 13 |
| 65+ | 2,603 | 5.4 | 13 | 2 | 3 | 5 | 7 | 9 | 11 | 19 |
| **TOTAL SINGLE DX** | 292 | 3.9 | 6 | 1 | 2 | 3 | 5 | 7 | 8 | 10 |
| **TOTAL MULTIPLE DX** | 4,727 | 4.9 | 12 | 2 | 3 | 4 | 6 | 9 | 10 | 16 |
| **TOTAL** | | | | | | | | | | |
| 0–19 Years | 65 | 4.9 | 19 | 2 | 3 | 4 | 6 | 11 | 13 | 20 |
| 20–34 | 290 | 4.0 | 7 | 2 | 2 | 3 | 5 | 7 | 9 | 11 |
| 35–49 | 784 | 4.6 | 12 | 1 | 2 | 4 | 6 | 8 | 12 | 16 |
| 50–64 | 1,227 | 4.0 | 8 | 2 | 2 | 4 | 5 | 7 | 8 | 13 |
| 65+ | 2,653 | 5.3 | 13 | 2 | 3 | 5 | 7 | 9 | 11 | 19 |
| **GRAND TOTAL** | 5,019 | 4.8 | 12 | 2 | 3 | 4 | 6 | 9 | 10 | 16 |

## 99.21: INJECT ANTIBIOTIC. Formerly included in operation group(s) 794.

| Type of Patients | Observed Patients | Avg. Stay | Variance | 10th | 25th | 50th | 75th | 90th | 95th | 99th |
|---|---|---|---|---|---|---|---|---|---|---|
| **1. SINGLE DX** | | | | | | | | | | |
| 0–19 Years | 1,501 | 2.9 | 3 | 1 | 2 | 2 | 3 | 5 | 6 | 10 |
| 20–34 | 605 | 2.4 | 3 | 1 | 2 | 2 | 3 | 4 | 5 | 8 |
| 35–49 | 387 | 3.1 | 3 | 1 | 2 | 3 | 4 | 5 | 6 | 11 |
| 50–64 | 204 | 2.9 | 6 | 1 | 2 | 3 | 4 | 5 | 6 | 7 |
| 65+ | 115 | 3.8 | 6 | 1 | 3 | 3 | 5 | 8 | 8 | 11 |
| **2. MULTIPLE DX** | | | | | | | | | | |
| 0–19 Years | 7,001 | 4.0 | 18 | 1 | 3 | 3 | 5 | 7 | 10 | 21 |
| 20–34 | 2,468 | 4.0 | 14 | 1 | 2 | 3 | 5 | 7 | 9 | 17 |
| 35–49 | 3,127 | 4.8 | 19 | 2 | 3 | 4 | 6 | 9 | 12 | 22 |
| 50–64 | 2,818 | 5.7 | 29 | 2 | 3 | 4 | 7 | 10 | 13 | 31 |
| 65+ | 6,561 | 6.1 | 24 | 2 | 3 | 5 | 7 | 11 | 14 | 24 |
| **TOTAL SINGLE DX** | 2,812 | 2.8 | 3 | 1 | 2 | 2 | 3 | 5 | 6 | 10 |
| **TOTAL MULTIPLE DX** | 21,975 | 5.0 | 22 | 2 | 2 | 4 | 6 | 9 | 13 | 23 |
| **TOTAL** | | | | | | | | | | |
| 0–19 Years | 8,502 | 3.8 | 15 | 1 | 2 | 3 | 4 | 7 | 10 | 19 |
| 20–34 | 3,073 | 3.6 | 12 | 1 | 2 | 3 | 4 | 6 | 8 | 15 |
| 35–49 | 3,514 | 4.6 | 17 | 2 | 2 | 3 | 5 | 8 | 11 | 22 |
| 50–64 | 3,022 | 5.5 | 28 | 2 | 3 | 4 | 7 | 10 | 13 | 30 |
| 65+ | 6,676 | 6.1 | 23 | 2 | 3 | 5 | 7 | 11 | 14 | 23 |
| **GRAND TOTAL** | 24,787 | 4.8 | 20 | 2 | 2 | 4 | 6 | 9 | 12 | 21 |

Length of Stay by Diagnosis and Operation, United States, 2000

# United States, October 1998–September 1999 Data, by Operation

## 99.23: INJECT STEROID. Formerly included in operation group(s) 794.

| Type of Patients | Observed Patients | Avg. Stay | Variance | 10th | 25th | 50th | 75th | 90th | 95th | 99th |
|---|---|---|---|---|---|---|---|---|---|---|
| **1. SINGLE DX** | | | | | | | | | | |
| 0–19 Years | 359 | 2.1 | 1 | 1 | 1 | 2 | 3 | 4 | 4 | 6 |
| 20–34 | 151 | 3.0 | 2 | 1 | 2 | 3 | 4 | 4 | 5 | 6 |
| 35–49 | 175 | 3.2 | 4 | 2 | 2 | 3 | 4 | 5 | 6 | 13 |
| 50–64 | 91 | 3.1 | 2 | 2 | 2 | 3 | 4 | 6 | 6 | 6 |
| 65+ | 47 | 4.1 | 3 | 2 | 4 | 4 | 4 | 6 | 7 | 12 |
| **2. MULTIPLE DX** | | | | | | | | | | |
| 0–19 Years | 443 | 3.1 | 6 | 1 | 2 | 2 | 4 | 6 | 9 | 11 |
| 20–34 | 359 | 4.4 | 11 | 1 | 2 | 4 | 6 | 7 | 9 | 15 |
| 35–49 | 614 | 4.1 | 13 | 1 | 2 | 4 | 5 | 7 | 9 | 17 |
| 50–64 | 664 | 4.4 | 11 | 2 | 2 | 4 | 5 | 8 | 12 | 17 |
| 65+ | 1,050 | 7.1 | 25 | 3 | 4 | 5 | 9 | 14 | 16 | 20 |
| **TOTAL SINGLE DX** | 823 | 2.8 | 3 | 1 | 2 | 3 | 4 | 4 | 5 | 9 |
| **TOTAL MULTIPLE DX** | 3,130 | 5.4 | 20 | 2 | 3 | 4 | 7 | 13 | 14 | 18 |
| **TOTAL** | | | | | | | | | | |
| 0–19 Years | 802 | 2.6 | 4 | 1 | 1 | 2 | 3 | 5 | 6 | 9 |
| 20–34 | 510 | 3.9 | 8 | 1 | 2 | 3 | 5 | 7 | 7 | 15 |
| 35–49 | 789 | 3.9 | 11 | 1 | 2 | 4 | 5 | 6 | 9 | 14 |
| 50–64 | 755 | 4.3 | 10 | 2 | 2 | 3 | 5 | 7 | 12 | 16 |
| 65+ | 1,097 | 7.0 | 24 | 3 | 4 | 5 | 9 | 14 | 16 | 20 |
| **GRAND TOTAL** | 3,953 | 4.9 | 17 | 1 | 2 | 4 | 6 | 11 | 14 | 17 |

## 99.25: INJECT CA CHEMO AGENT. Formerly included in operation group(s) 794.

| Type of Patients | Observed Patients | Avg. Stay | Variance | 10th | 25th | 50th | 75th | 90th | 95th | 99th |
|---|---|---|---|---|---|---|---|---|---|---|
| **1. SINGLE DX** | | | | | | | | | | |
| 0–19 Years | 218 | 3.2 | 8 | 1 | 1 | 2 | 4 | 7 | 8 | 12 |
| 20–34 | 80 | 3.7 | 3 | 2 | 2 | 5 | 5 | 5 | 6 | 8 |
| 35–49 | 82 | 3.1 | 10 | 1 | 1 | 3 | 4 | 5 | 5 | 20 |
| 50–64 | 74 | 3.6 | 8 | 1 | 2 | 4 | 4 | 5 | 7 | 9 |
| 65+ | 54 | 4.1 | 14 | 1 | 2 | 4 | 5 | 6 | 8 | 25 |
| **2. MULTIPLE DX** | | | | | | | | | | |
| 0–19 Years | 15,709 | 4.0 | 20 | 1 | 2 | 3 | 5 | 6 | 8 | 26 |
| 20–34 | 3,444 | 4.9 | 31 | 2 | 2 | 4 | 5 | 7 | 12 | 31 |
| 35–49 | 7,911 | 4.9 | 38 | 1 | 2 | 4 | 5 | 7 | 14 | 35 |
| 50–64 | 13,721 | 5.0 | 30 | 1 | 2 | 4 | 5 | 8 | 15 | 28 |
| 65+ | 14,247 | 5.2 | 31 | 1 | 2 | 4 | 6 | 9 | 15 | 30 |
| **TOTAL SINGLE DX** | 508 | 3.4 | 8 | 1 | 2 | 3 | 5 | 7 | 8 | 12 |
| **TOTAL MULTIPLE DX** | 55,032 | 4.7 | 29 | 2 | 2 | 4 | 5 | 8 | 13 | 29 |
| **TOTAL** | | | | | | | | | | |
| 0–19 Years | 15,927 | 3.9 | 20 | 1 | 2 | 3 | 5 | 6 | 8 | 26 |
| 20–34 | 3,524 | 4.8 | 31 | 2 | 2 | 4 | 5 | 7 | 12 | 31 |
| 35–49 | 7,993 | 4.9 | 38 | 1 | 2 | 4 | 5 | 7 | 14 | 35 |
| 50–64 | 13,795 | 5.0 | 30 | 1 | 2 | 4 | 5 | 8 | 14 | 28 |
| 65+ | 14,301 | 5.2 | 31 | 1 | 2 | 4 | 6 | 9 | 15 | 30 |
| **GRAND TOTAL** | 55,540 | 4.7 | 28 | 2 | 2 | 4 | 5 | 8 | 13 | 29 |

## 99.28: INJECT BRM/ANTINEO AGENT. Formerly included in operation group(s) 794.

| Type of Patients | Observed Patients | Avg. Stay | Variance | 10th | 25th | 50th | 75th | 90th | 95th | 99th |
|---|---|---|---|---|---|---|---|---|---|---|
| **1. SINGLE DX** | | | | | | | | | | |
| 0–19 Years | 8 | 2.2 | 9 | 1 | 1 | 1 | 1 | 4 | 11 | 11 |
| 20–34 | 5 | 3.3 | 4 | 1 | 1 | 4 | 5 | 5 | 5 | 5 |
| 35–49 | 8 | 4.8 | 15 | 2 | 2 | 2 | 10 | 10 | 11 | 11 |
| 50–64 | 17 | 1.9 | 3 | 1 | 1 | 1 | 2 | 5 | 5 | 5 |
| 65+ | 10 | 2.6 | 12 | 1 | 1 | 1 | 1 | 10 | 10 | 10 |
| **2. MULTIPLE DX** | | | | | | | | | | |
| 0–19 Years | 34 | 3.4 | 4 | 1 | 1 | 4 | 5 | 5 | 6 | 12 |
| 20–34 | 76 | 4.1 | 3 | 2 | 2 | 4 | 6 | 6 | 6 | 8 |
| 35–49 | 215 | 6.5 | 47 | 2 | 3 | 5 | 7 | 11 | 13 | 40 |
| 50–64 | 364 | 5.2 | 17 | 2 | 2 | 5 | 6 | 9 | 12 | 19 |
| 65+ | 204 | 5.5 | 32 | 1 | 2 | 5 | 6 | 11 | 11 | 48 |
| **TOTAL SINGLE DX** | 48 | 2.8 | 9 | 1 | 1 | 1 | 4 | 10 | 10 | 11 |
| **TOTAL MULTIPLE DX** | 893 | 5.4 | 27 | 2 | 3 | 5 | 6 | 9 | 12 | 40 |
| **TOTAL** | | | | | | | | | | |
| 0–19 Years | 42 | 3.2 | 5 | 1 | 1 | 3 | 4 | 5 | 6 | 11 |
| 20–34 | 81 | 4.0 | 3 | 2 | 2 | 4 | 6 | 6 | 6 | 8 |
| 35–49 | 223 | 6.5 | 47 | 2 | 3 | 5 | 7 | 11 | 13 | 40 |
| 50–64 | 381 | 5.1 | 17 | 2 | 2 | 5 | 6 | 8 | 12 | 19 |
| 65+ | 214 | 5.4 | 32 | 1 | 2 | 5 | 6 | 10 | 11 | 48 |
| **GRAND TOTAL** | 941 | 5.3 | 26 | 2 | 2 | 5 | 6 | 9 | 12 | 40 |

## 99.29: INJECT/INFUSE NEC. Formerly included in operation group(s) 794.

| Type of Patients | Observed Patients | Avg. Stay | Variance | 10th | 25th | 50th | 75th | 90th | 95th | 99th |
|---|---|---|---|---|---|---|---|---|---|---|
| **1. SINGLE DX** | | | | | | | | | | |
| 0–19 Years | 657 | 2.3 | 11 | 1 | 1 | 2 | 3 | 4 | 5 | 12 |
| 20–34 | 1,168 | 2.6 | 6 | 1 | 1 | 2 | 3 | 5 | 6 | 12 |
| 35–49 | 269 | 2.4 | 4 | 1 | 1 | 2 | 3 | 4 | 5 | 9 |
| 50–64 | 97 | 2.1 | 12 | 1 | 1 | 2 | 2 | 3 | 5 | 30 |
| 65+ | 65 | 3.3 | 31 | 1 | 1 | 1 | 4 | 6 | 7 | 30 |
| **2. MULTIPLE DX** | | | | | | | | | | |
| 0–19 Years | 1,819 | 3.2 | 25 | 1 | 1 | 2 | 3 | 5 | 8 | 22 |
| 20–34 | 1,972 | 3.6 | 21 | 1 | 1 | 2 | 4 | 6 | 11 | 22 |
| 35–49 | 1,590 | 4.1 | 14 | 1 | 2 | 3 | 5 | 8 | 10 | 19 |
| 50–64 | 1,703 | 4.5 | 23 | 1 | 2 | 3 | 5 | 9 | 15 | 23 |
| 65+ | 3,337 | 4.9 | 18 | 2 | 2 | 4 | 6 | 9 | 12 | 22 |
| **TOTAL SINGLE DX** | 2,256 | 2.5 | 8 | 1 | 1 | 2 | 3 | 4 | 6 | 12 |
| **TOTAL MULTIPLE DX** | 10,421 | 4.3 | 20 | 1 | 2 | 3 | 5 | 8 | 12 | 23 |
| **TOTAL** | | | | | | | | | | |
| 0–19 Years | 2,476 | 2.9 | 21 | 1 | 1 | 2 | 3 | 5 | 7 | 21 |
| 20–34 | 3,140 | 3.2 | 15 | 1 | 2 | 3 | 3 | 5 | 8 | 19 |
| 35–49 | 1,859 | 3.7 | 13 | 1 | 2 | 3 | 5 | 8 | 10 | 17 |
| 50–64 | 1,800 | 4.3 | 22 | 1 | 2 | 3 | 5 | 9 | 14 | 23 |
| 65+ | 3,402 | 4.9 | 18 | 2 | 2 | 4 | 6 | 9 | 12 | 22 |
| **GRAND TOTAL** | 12,677 | 3.9 | 18 | 1 | 2 | 3 | 5 | 7 | 11 | 23 |

Length of Stay by Diagnosis and Operation, United States, 2000

# United States, October 1998–September 1999 Data, by Operation

## 99.3: PROPHYL VACC-BACT DIS. Formerly included in operation group(s) 794.

| Type of Patients | Observed Patients | Avg. Stay | Variance | Percentiles | | | | | | |
|---|---|---|---|---|---|---|---|---|---|---|
| | | | | 10th | 25th | 50th | 75th | 90th | 95th | 99th |
| **1. SINGLE DX** | | | | | | | | | | |
| 0–19 Years | 4 | 1.0 | 0 | 1 | 1 | 1 | 1 | 1 | 1 | 1 |
| 20–34 | 4 | 3.8 | 26 | 1 | 1 | 2 | 2 | 14 | 14 | 14 |
| 35–49 | 5 | 1.2 | <1 | 1 | 2 | 1 | 1 | 2 | 2 | 2 |
| 50–64 | 1 | 1.0 | 0 | 1 | 1 | 1 | 1 | 1 | 1 | 1 |
| 65+ | 1 | 1.0 | 0 | 1 | 1 | 1 | 1 | 1 | 1 | 1 |
| **2. MULTIPLE DX** | | | | | | | | | | |
| 0–19 Years | 30 | 4.9 | 36 | 1 | 3 | 3 | 10 | 10 | 10 | 47 |
| 20–34 | 34 | 2.7 | 2 | 1 | 2 | 2 | 3 | 4 | 6 | 8 |
| 35–49 | 29 | 2.5 | 3 | 1 | 1 | 2 | 3 | 6 | 6 | 10 |
| 50–64 | 29 | 3.3 | 5 | 2 | 2 | 3 | 4 | 6 | 6 | 12 |
| 65+ | 83 | 4.9 | 13 | 1 | 2 | 4 | 7 | 9 | 11 | 19 |
| **TOTAL SINGLE DX** | 15 | 1.7 | 7 | 1 | 1 | 1 | 1 | 2 | 2 | 14 |
| **TOTAL MULTIPLE DX** | 205 | 4.0 | 14 | 1 | 2 | 3 | 5 | 9 | 10 | 15 |
| **TOTAL** | | | | | | | | | | |
| 0–19 Years | 34 | 4.4 | 34 | 1 | 2 | 2 | 10 | 10 | 10 | 47 |
| 20–34 | 38 | 2.8 | 4 | 2 | 2 | 2 | 3 | 4 | 6 | 14 |
| 35–49 | 34 | 2.3 | 3 | 1 | 1 | 2 | 3 | 6 | 6 | 10 |
| 50–64 | 30 | 3.3 | 5 | 2 | 2 | 3 | 4 | 6 | 6 | 12 |
| 65+ | 84 | 4.9 | 13 | 1 | 2 | 4 | 7 | 9 | 11 | 19 |
| **GRAND TOTAL** | 220 | 3.9 | 14 | 1 | 2 | 3 | 5 | 9 | 10 | 14 |

## 99.4: VIRAL IMMUNIZATION. Formerly included in operation group(s) 794.

| Type of Patients | Observed Patients | Avg. Stay | Variance | Percentiles | | | | | | |
|---|---|---|---|---|---|---|---|---|---|---|
| | | | | 10th | 25th | 50th | 75th | 90th | 95th | 99th |
| **1. SINGLE DX** | | | | | | | | | | |
| 0–19 Years | 4 | 2.0 | <1 | 2 | 2 | 2 | 2 | 2 | 2 | 2 |
| 20–34 | 7 | 1.9 | <1 | 1 | 2 | 2 | 2 | 3 | 3 | 3 |
| 35–49 | 0 | | | | | | | | | |
| 50–64 | 0 | | | | | | | | | |
| **2. MULTIPLE DX** | | | | | | | | | | |
| 0–19 Years | 36 | 2.2 | 2 | 1 | 1 | 2 | 3 | 3 | 4 | 10 |
| 20–34 | 47 | 2.0 | 3 | 1 | 1 | 2 | 2 | 3 | 3 | 6 |
| 35–49 | 7 | 3.1 | 18 | 2 | 2 | 2 | 3 | 7 | 10 | 10 |
| 50–64 | 5 | 3.8 | 18 | 2 | 2 | 3 | 4 | 14 | 14 | 14 |
| 65+ | 4 | 7.4 | 25 | 3 | 3 | 4 | 13 | 13 | 13 | 13 |
| **TOTAL SINGLE DX** | 11 | 2.0 | <1 | 1 | 2 | 2 | 2 | 2 | 3 | 3 |
| **TOTAL MULTIPLE DX** | 99 | 2.4 | 5 | 1 | 2 | 2 | 2 | 3 | 5 | 13 |
| **TOTAL** | | | | | | | | | | |
| 0–19 Years | 40 | 2.1 | 1 | 1 | 1 | 2 | 2 | 3 | 3 | 10 |
| 20–34 | 54 | 2.0 | 3 | 1 | 1 | 2 | 2 | 3 | 3 | 6 |
| 35–49 | 7 | 3.1 | 7 | 2 | 2 | 2 | 3 | 7 | 10 | 10 |
| 50–64 | 5 | 3.8 | 18 | 2 | 2 | 3 | 3 | 14 | 14 | 14 |
| 65+ | 4 | 7.4 | 25 | 3 | 3 | 4 | 13 | 13 | 13 | 13 |
| **GRAND TOTAL** | 110 | 2.4 | 5 | 1 | 2 | 2 | 2 | 3 | 4 | 13 |

## 99.5: OTHER IMMUNIZATION. Formerly included in operation group(s) 794.

| Type of Patients | Observed Patients | Avg. Stay | Variance | Percentiles | | | | | | |
|---|---|---|---|---|---|---|---|---|---|---|
| | | | | 10th | 25th | 50th | 75th | 90th | 95th | 99th |
| **1. SINGLE DX** | | | | | | | | | | |
| 0–19 Years | 22,275 | 1.7 | <1 | 1 | 1 | 2 | 2 | 3 | 3 | 4 |
| 20–34 | 10 | 1.3 | <1 | 1 | 1 | 2 | 2 | 3 | 4 | 4 |
| 35–49 | 5 | 2.3 | 2 | 2 | 2 | 2 | 2 | 2 | 7 | 7 |
| 50–64 | 1 | 22.0 | 0 | 22 | 22 | 22 | 22 | 22 | 22 | 22 |
| 65+ | 0 | | | | | | | | | |
| **2. MULTIPLE DX** | | | | | | | | | | |
| 0–19 Years | 102,352 | 2.3 | 5 | 1 | 2 | 2 | 2 | 3 | 4 | 11 |
| 20–34 | 11 | 3.3 | 6 | 2 | 3 | 3 | 3 | 6 | 10 | 10 |
| 35–49 | 27 | 3.6 | 5 | 2 | 2 | 3 | 3 | 7 | 9 | 9 |
| 50–64 | 29 | 6.0 | 23 | 2 | 2 | 4 | 10 | 15 | 15 | 15 |
| 65+ | 103 | 4.5 | 15 | 1 | 2 | 4 | 6 | 7 | 8 | 28 |
| **TOTAL SINGLE DX** | 22,291 | 1.8 | <1 | 1 | 1 | 2 | 2 | 3 | 3 | 4 |
| **TOTAL MULTIPLE DX** | 102,522 | 2.3 | 5 | 1 | 1 | 2 | 2 | 3 | 4 | 11 |
| **TOTAL** | | | | | | | | | | |
| 0–19 Years | 124,627 | 2.2 | 4 | 1 | 1 | 2 | 2 | 3 | 4 | 10 |
| 20–34 | 21 | 1.7 | 2 | 1 | 2 | 2 | 2 | 3 | 4 | 10 |
| 35–49 | 32 | 3.3 | 5 | 2 | 2 | 2 | 3 | 7 | 9 | 9 |
| 50–64 | 30 | 8.0 | 48 | 2 | 2 | 5 | 15 | 22 | 22 | 22 |
| 65+ | 103 | 4.5 | 15 | 1 | 2 | 4 | 6 | 7 | 8 | 28 |
| **GRAND TOTAL** | 124,813 | 2.2 | 4 | 1 | 2 | 2 | 2 | 3 | 4 | 10 |

## 99.55: VACCINATION NEC. Formerly included in operation group(s) 794.

| Type of Patients | Observed Patients | Avg. Stay | Variance | Percentiles | | | | | | |
|---|---|---|---|---|---|---|---|---|---|---|
| | | | | 10th | 25th | 50th | 75th | 90th | 95th | 99th |
| **1. SINGLE DX** | | | | | | | | | | |
| 0–19 Years | 20,540 | 1.7 | <1 | 1 | 1 | 2 | 2 | 3 | 3 | 4 |
| 20–34 | 6 | 2.2 | 1 | 1 | 1 | 2 | 4 | 4 | 4 | 4 |
| 35–49 | 4 | 2.7 | 4 | 1 | 2 | 2 | 2 | 7 | 7 | 7 |
| 50–64 | 1 | 22.0 | 0 | 22 | 22 | 22 | 22 | 22 | 22 | 22 |
| 65+ | 0 | | | | | | | | | |
| **2. MULTIPLE DX** | | | | | | | | | | |
| 0–19 Years | 99,382 | 2.3 | 4 | 1 | 1 | 2 | 2 | 3 | 4 | 11 |
| 20–34 | 8 | 4.1 | 7 | 1 | 3 | 3 | 6 | 10 | 10 | 10 |
| 35–49 | 7 | 6.7 | 6 | 2 | 5 | 7 | 9 | 9 | 9 | 9 |
| 50–64 | 6 | 4.2 | 3 | 2 | 4 | 4 | 5 | 5 | 8 | 8 |
| 65+ | 19 | 4.5 | 4 | 2 | 4 | 5 | 5 | 7 | 8 | 8 |
| **TOTAL SINGLE DX** | 20,551 | 1.7 | <1 | 1 | 1 | 2 | 2 | 3 | 3 | 4 |
| **TOTAL MULTIPLE DX** | 99,422 | 2.3 | 4 | 1 | 1 | 2 | 2 | 3 | 4 | 11 |
| **TOTAL** | | | | | | | | | | |
| 0–19 Years | 119,922 | 2.2 | 4 | 1 | 1 | 2 | 2 | 3 | 4 | 10 |
| 20–34 | 14 | 2.9 | 4 | 1 | 1 | 2 | 4 | 6 | 6 | 10 |
| 35–49 | 11 | 5.0 | 9 | 1 | 2 | 5 | 7 | 7 | 9 | 9 |
| 50–64 | 7 | 12.1 | 82 | 2 | 4 | 5 | 22 | 22 | 22 | 22 |
| 65+ | 19 | 4.5 | 4 | 2 | 4 | 5 | 5 | 7 | 8 | 10 |
| **GRAND TOTAL** | 119,973 | 2.2 | 4 | 1 | 1 | 2 | 2 | 3 | 4 | 10 |

Length of Stay by Diagnosis and Operation

Length of Stay by Diagnosis and Operation, United States, 2000

# United States, October 1998–September 1999 Data, by Operation

## 99.59: VACC/INOCULATION NEC. Formerly included in operation group(s) 794.

| Type of Patients | Observed Patients | Avg. Stay | Variance | 10th | 25th | 50th | 75th | 90th | 95th | 99th |
|---|---|---|---|---|---|---|---|---|---|---|
| **1. SINGLE DX** | | | | | | | | | | |
| 0–19 Years | 1,724 | 2.1 | 2 | 1 | 2 | 2 | 2 | 3 | 4 | 5 |
| 20–34 | 2 | 1.8 | <1 | 1 | 2 | 2 | 2 | 2 | 2 | 2 |
| 35–49 | 1 | 2.0 | 0 | 2 | 2 | 2 | 2 | 2 | 2 | 2 |
| 50–64 | 0 | | | | | | | | | |
| 65+ | 0 | | | | | | | | | |
| **2. MULTIPLE DX** | | | | | | | | | | |
| 0–19 Years | 2,919 | 2.4 | 5 | 1 | 2 | 2 | 3 | 4 | 5 | 13 |
| 20–34 | 1 | 2.0 | 0 | 2 | 2 | 2 | 2 | 2 | 2 | 2 |
| 35–49 | 4 | 2.9 | 2 | 1 | 2 | 4 | 4 | 4 | 4 | 4 |
| 50–64 | 2 | 2.3 | 1 | 1 | 1 | 3 | 3 | 3 | 3 | 3 |
| 65+ | 11 | 4.0 | 4 | 2 | 2 | 4 | 5 | 8 | 8 | 8 |
| **TOTAL SINGLE DX** | 1,727 | 2.1 | 2 | 1 | 2 | 2 | 2 | 3 | 4 | 5 |
| **TOTAL MULTIPLE DX** | 2,937 | 2.4 | 5 | 1 | 2 | 2 | 3 | 4 | 5 | 13 |
| **TOTAL** | | | | | | | | | | |
| 0–19 Years | 4,643 | 2.3 | 4 | 1 | 2 | 2 | 2 | 3 | 4 | 10 |
| 20–34 | 3 | 1.8 | <1 | 1 | 2 | 2 | 2 | 2 | 2 | 2 |
| 35–49 | 5 | 2.3 | <1 | 2 | 2 | 2 | 2 | 4 | 4 | 4 |
| 50–64 | 2 | 2.3 | 1 | 1 | 1 | 3 | 3 | 3 | 3 | 3 |
| 65+ | 11 | 4.0 | 4 | 2 | 2 | 4 | 5 | 8 | 8 | 8 |
| **GRAND TOTAL** | 4,664 | 2.3 | 4 | 1 | 2 | 2 | 2 | 3 | 4 | 10 |

## 99.6: CARD RHYTHM CONVERSION. Formerly included in operation group(s) 794.

| Type of Patients | Observed Patients | Avg. Stay | Variance | 10th | 25th | 50th | 75th | 90th | 95th | 99th |
|---|---|---|---|---|---|---|---|---|---|---|
| **1. SINGLE DX** | | | | | | | | | | |
| 0–19 Years | 15 | 2.5 | 1 | 1 | 1 | 3 | 3 | 4 | 4 | 4 |
| 20–34 | 62 | 1.6 | 1 | 1 | 1 | 1 | 2 | 3 | 4 | 5 |
| 35–49 | 164 | 1.8 | 1 | 1 | 1 | 1 | 2 | 3 | 4 | 5 |
| 50–64 | 259 | 1.7 | <1 | 1 | 1 | 2 | 2 | 3 | 4 | 5 |
| 65+ | 364 | 1.9 | 1 | 1 | 1 | 2 | 3 | 3 | 3 | 6 |
| **2. MULTIPLE DX** | | | | | | | | | | |
| 0–19 Years | 271 | 6.5 | 150 | 1 | 1 | 3 | 6 | 14 | 23 | 70 |
| 20–34 | 299 | 2.5 | 8 | 1 | 1 | 1 | 3 | 6 | 7 | 11 |
| 35–49 | 1,071 | 3.4 | 14 | 1 | 1 | 2 | 4 | 6 | 9 | 17 |
| 50–64 | 3,636 | 3.4 | 10 | 1 | 2 | 3 | 4 | 7 | 9 | 15 |
| 65+ | 10,549 | 4.5 | 18 | 1 | 2 | 3 | 6 | 9 | 12 | 21 |
| **TOTAL SINGLE DX** | 864 | 1.8 | 1 | 1 | 1 | 2 | 2 | 3 | 4 | 5 |
| **TOTAL MULTIPLE DX** | 15,826 | 4.2 | 19 | 1 | 2 | 3 | 5 | 8 | 11 | 21 |
| **TOTAL** | | | | | | | | | | |
| 0–19 Years | 286 | 6.2 | 140 | 1 | 1 | 3 | 5 | 13 | 23 | 70 |
| 20–34 | 361 | 2.4 | 7 | 1 | 1 | 1 | 3 | 6 | 7 | 10 |
| 35–49 | 1,235 | 3.0 | 12 | 1 | 1 | 2 | 4 | 6 | 8 | 15 |
| 50–64 | 3,895 | 3.3 | 9 | 1 | 1 | 2 | 4 | 6 | 8 | 14 |
| 65+ | 10,913 | 4.4 | 18 | 1 | 2 | 3 | 6 | 9 | 12 | 21 |
| **GRAND TOTAL** | 16,690 | 4.0 | 18 | 1 | 2 | 3 | 5 | 8 | 11 | 20 |

## 99.60: CPR NOS. Formerly included in operation group(s) 794.

| Type of Patients | Observed Patients | Avg. Stay | Variance | 10th | 25th | 50th | 75th | 90th | 95th | 99th |
|---|---|---|---|---|---|---|---|---|---|---|
| **1. SINGLE DX** | | | | | | | | | | |
| 0–19 Years | 0 | | | | | | | | | |
| 20–34 | 1 | 2.0 | 0 | 2 | 2 | 2 | 2 | 2 | 2 | 2 |
| 35–49 | 0 | | | | | | | | | |
| 50–64 | 1 | 1.0 | 0 | 1 | 1 | 1 | 1 | 1 | 1 | 1 |
| 65+ | 2 | 1.4 | <1 | 1 | 1 | 1 | 2 | 2 | 2 | 2 |
| **2. MULTIPLE DX** | | | | | | | | | | |
| 0–19 Years | 76 | 14.2 | 400 | 2 | 2 | 5 | 18 | 36 | 70 | 86 |
| 20–34 | 15 | 6.3 | 28 | 2 | 2 | 6 | 7 | 8 | 10 | 34 |
| 35–49 | 54 | 8.2 | 66 | 1 | 4 | 6 | 8 | 20 | 32 | 32 |
| 50–64 | 70 | 8.4 | 62 | 2 | 4 | 7 | 9 | 19 | 37 | 37 |
| 65+ | 332 | 7.3 | 34 | 1 | 4 | 6 | 6 | 14 | 18 | 27 |
| **TOTAL SINGLE DX** | 4 | 1.3 | <1 | 1 | 1 | 1 | 2 | 2 | 2 | 2 |
| **TOTAL MULTIPLE DX** | 547 | 8.7 | 109 | 1 | 3 | 6 | 10 | 17 | 26 | 70 |
| **TOTAL** | | | | | | | | | | |
| 0–19 Years | 76 | 14.2 | 400 | 2 | 2 | 5 | 18 | 36 | 70 | 86 |
| 20–34 | 16 | 6.2 | 27 | 2 | 2 | 6 | 7 | 8 | 10 | 34 |
| 35–49 | 54 | 8.2 | 66 | 1 | 4 | 6 | 8 | 20 | 32 | 32 |
| 50–64 | 71 | 8.2 | 62 | 1 | 4 | 7 | 9 | 19 | 37 | 37 |
| 65+ | 334 | 7.2 | 34 | 1 | 4 | 6 | 6 | 14 | 18 | 27 |
| **GRAND TOTAL** | 551 | 8.6 | 109 | 1 | 3 | 6 | 10 | 17 | 26 | 70 |

## 99.61: ATRIAL CARDIOVERSION. Formerly included in operation group(s) 794.

| Type of Patients | Observed Patients | Avg. Stay | Variance | 10th | 25th | 50th | 75th | 90th | 95th | 99th |
|---|---|---|---|---|---|---|---|---|---|---|
| **1. SINGLE DX** | | | | | | | | | | |
| 0–19 Years | 6 | 2.1 | <1 | 1 | 1 | 2 | 3 | 3 | 3 | 3 |
| 20–34 | 23 | 1.4 | <1 | 1 | 1 | 1 | 2 | 2 | 2 | 5 |
| 35–49 | 76 | 1.9 | 1 | 1 | 1 | 2 | 2 | 3 | 5 | 5 |
| 50–64 | 139 | 1.8 | <1 | 1 | 1 | 2 | 2 | 3 | 3 | 5 |
| 65+ | 196 | 2.0 | 1 | 1 | 2 | 2 | 3 | 3 | 3 | 6 |
| **2. MULTIPLE DX** | | | | | | | | | | |
| 0–19 Years | 68 | 3.0 | 7 | 1 | 1 | 2 | 4 | 6 | 8 | 12 |
| 20–34 | 130 | 2.8 | 6 | 1 | 1 | 2 | 3 | 6 | 7 | 11 |
| 35–49 | 445 | 3.0 | 10 | 1 | 2 | 2 | 4 | 6 | 9 | 15 |
| 50–64 | 1,639 | 3.3 | 7 | 1 | 2 | 3 | 4 | 6 | 9 | 14 |
| 65+ | 4,642 | 4.2 | 14 | 1 | 2 | 3 | 5 | 8 | 11 | 18 |
| **TOTAL SINGLE DX** | 440 | 1.9 | 1 | 1 | 1 | 2 | 2 | 3 | 3 | 5 |
| **TOTAL MULTIPLE DX** | 6,924 | 3.8 | 12 | 1 | 2 | 3 | 5 | 8 | 10 | 17 |
| **TOTAL** | | | | | | | | | | |
| 0–19 Years | 74 | 2.8 | 7 | 1 | 1 | 2 | 4 | 5 | 8 | 12 |
| 20–34 | 153 | 2.5 | 6 | 1 | 1 | 2 | 3 | 5 | 7 | 11 |
| 35–49 | 521 | 2.7 | 8 | 1 | 1 | 2 | 3 | 5 | 8 | 15 |
| 50–64 | 1,778 | 3.2 | 7 | 1 | 2 | 3 | 4 | 6 | 8 | 14 |
| 65+ | 4,838 | 4.1 | 14 | 1 | 2 | 3 | 5 | 8 | 11 | 18 |
| **GRAND TOTAL** | 7,364 | 3.7 | 11 | 1 | 2 | 3 | 5 | 7 | 10 | 16 |

Length of Stay by Diagnosis and Operation, United States, 2000

# United States, October 1998–September 1999 Data, by Operation

## 99.62: HEART COUNTERSHOCK NEC. Formerly included in operation group(s) 794.

| Type of Patients | Observed Patients | Avg. Stay | Variance | Percentiles | | | | | | |
|---|---|---|---|---|---|---|---|---|---|---|
| | | | | 10th | 25th | 50th | 75th | 90th | 95th | 99th |
| **1. SINGLE DX** | | | | | | | | | | |
| 0–19 Years | 6 | 3.4 | 1 | 1 | 3 | 4 | 4 | 4 | 4 | 4 |
| 20–34 | 35 | 2.0 | 2 | 1 | 1 | 1 | 3 | 4 | 5 | 6 |
| 35–49 | 80 | 1.6 | 1 | 1 | 1 | 1 | 2 | 4 | 4 | 4 |
| 50–64 | 114 | 1.6 | 1 | 1 | 1 | 1 | 2 | 3 | 4 | 4 |
| 65+ | 157 | 1.9 | 1 | 1 | 1 | 2 | 2 | 3 | 3 | 7 |
| **2. MULTIPLE DX** | | | | | | | | | | |
| 0–19 Years | 82 | 3.8 | 18 | 1 | 1 | 2 | 4 | 8 | 13 | 22 |
| 20–34 | 135 | 2.2 | 6 | 1 | 1 | 1 | 2 | 6 | 7 | 9 |
| 35–49 | 520 | 3.1 | 10 | 1 | 1 | 2 | 4 | 6 | 8 | 13 |
| 50–64 | 1,802 | 3.4 | 10 | 1 | 1 | 3 | 4 | 6 | 8 | 14 |
| 65+ | 5,157 | 4.6 | 21 | 1 | 2 | 3 | 6 | 9 | 13 | 21 |
| **TOTAL SINGLE DX** | 392 | 1.8 | 1 | 1 | 1 | 1 | 2 | 3 | 4 | 6 |
| **TOTAL MULTIPLE DX** | 7,696 | 4.1 | 17 | 1 | 2 | 3 | 5 | 8 | 11 | 21 |
| **TOTAL** | | | | | | | | | | |
| 0–19 Years | 88 | 3.7 | 16 | 1 | 1 | 3 | 4 | 7 | 12 | 22 |
| 20–34 | 170 | 2.1 | 5 | 1 | 1 | 1 | 2 | 6 | 6 | 9 |
| 35–49 | 600 | 2.9 | 9 | 1 | 1 | 2 | 4 | 6 | 7 | 13 |
| 50–64 | 1,916 | 3.2 | 9 | 1 | 1 | 2 | 4 | 6 | 9 | 13 |
| 65+ | 5,314 | 4.5 | 20 | 1 | 2 | 3 | 6 | 9 | 12 | 21 |
| **GRAND TOTAL** | 8,088 | 4.0 | 17 | 1 | 2 | 3 | 5 | 8 | 11 | 21 |

## 99.7: THERAPEUTIC APHERESIS. Formerly included in operation group(s) 794.

| Type of Patients | Observed Patients | Avg. Stay | Variance | Percentiles | | | | | | |
|---|---|---|---|---|---|---|---|---|---|---|
| | | | | 10th | 25th | 50th | 75th | 90th | 95th | 99th |
| **1. SINGLE DX** | | | | | | | | | | |
| 0–19 Years | 50 | 2.3 | 2 | 1 | 1 | 2 | 3 | 4 | 5 | 6 |
| 20–34 | 41 | 3.2 | 3 | 1 | 2 | 3 | 3 | 6 | 7 | 8 |
| 35–49 | 33 | 2.5 | 7 | 1 | 1 | 1 | 4 | 7 | 8 | 15 |
| 50–64 | 18 | 9.4 | 35 | 1 | 5 | 11 | 14 | 17 | 17 | 19 |
| 65+ | 5 | 6.0 | 11 | 1 | 3 | 8 | 9 | 9 | 9 | 9 |
| **2. MULTIPLE DX** | | | | | | | | | | |
| 0–19 Years | 198 | 5.4 | 34 | 1 | 2 | 4 | 7 | 10 | 15 | 23 |
| 20–34 | 188 | 9.5 | 68 | 2 | 4 | 7 | 14 | 18 | 25 | 45 |
| 35–49 | 266 | 10.0 | 57 | 2 | 5 | 8 | 15 | 19 | 28 | 35 |
| 50–64 | 347 | 11.2 | 128 | 3 | 5 | 7 | 16 | 31 | 31 | 50 |
| 65+ | 340 | 8.6 | 48 | 3 | 4 | 7 | 11 | 17 | 22 | 33 |
| **TOTAL SINGLE DX** | 147 | 3.3 | 10 | 1 | 1 | 3 | 3 | 7 | 9 | 17 |
| **TOTAL MULTIPLE DX** | 1,339 | 9.0 | 72 | 2 | 3 | 7 | 11 | 18 | 28 | 38 |
| **TOTAL** | | | | | | | | | | |
| 0–19 Years | 248 | 4.9 | 29 | 1 | 2 | 3 | 7 | 9 | 15 | 22 |
| 20–34 | 229 | 8.0 | 60 | 2 | 3 | 5 | 11 | 16 | 24 | 45 |
| 35–49 | 299 | 9.1 | 57 | 2 | 4 | 8 | 14 | 18 | 25 | 33 |
| 50–64 | 365 | 11.1 | 124 | 2 | 3 | 7 | 15 | 31 | 31 | 45 |
| 65+ | 345 | 8.6 | 48 | 3 | 4 | 7 | 11 | 17 | 22 | 33 |
| **GRAND TOTAL** | 1,486 | 8.3 | 68 | 1 | 3 | 6 | 11 | 18 | 27 | 36 |

## 99.69: CARDIAC RHYTHM CONV NEC. Formerly included in operation group(s) 794.

| Type of Patients | Observed Patients | Avg. Stay | Variance | Percentiles | | | | | | |
|---|---|---|---|---|---|---|---|---|---|---|
| | | | | 10th | 25th | 50th | 75th | 90th | 95th | 99th |
| **1. SINGLE DX** | | | | | | | | | | |
| 0–19 Years | 3 | 1.7 | 1 | 1 | 1 | 1 | 3 | 3 | 3 | 3 |
| 20–34 | 3 | 1.0 | 0 | 1 | 1 | 1 | 1 | 1 | 1 | 1 |
| 35–49 | 8 | 1.3 | <1 | 1 | 1 | 1 | 1 | 2 | 3 | 3 |
| 50–64 | 5 | 2.7 | 8 | 1 | 1 | 2 | 3 | 9 | 9 | 9 |
| 65+ | 9 | 1.3 | <1 | 1 | 1 | 1 | 1 | 2 | 3 | 3 |
| **2. MULTIPLE DX** | | | | | | | | | | |
| 0–19 Years | 24 | 2.8 | 3 | 1 | 1 | 2 | 4 | 5 | 6 | 10 |
| 20–34 | 17 | 1.6 | 1 | 1 | 1 | 1 | 2 | 3 | 3 | 6 |
| 35–49 | 50 | 2.9 | 6 | 1 | 1 | 2 | 4 | 6 | 8 | 12 |
| 50–64 | 120 | 2.9 | 8 | 1 | 2 | 2 | 3 | 6 | 8 | 18 |
| 65+ | 390 | 4.3 | 13 | 1 | 2 | 3 | 6 | 8 | 10 | 16 |
| **TOTAL SINGLE DX** | 28 | 1.5 | 2 | 1 | 1 | 1 | 1 | 3 | 3 | 9 |
| **TOTAL MULTIPLE DX** | 601 | 3.7 | 11 | 1 | 2 | 3 | 5 | 8 | 9 | 16 |
| **TOTAL** | | | | | | | | | | |
| 0–19 Years | 27 | 2.7 | 3 | 1 | 1 | 2 | 4 | 5 | 6 | 10 |
| 20–34 | 20 | 1.5 | 1 | 1 | 1 | 1 | 2 | 3 | 3 | 6 |
| 35–49 | 58 | 2.6 | 5 | 1 | 1 | 2 | 3 | 6 | 9 | 12 |
| 50–64 | 125 | 2.9 | 8 | 1 | 2 | 2 | 3 | 6 | 8 | 18 |
| 65+ | 399 | 4.2 | 13 | 1 | 2 | 3 | 6 | 8 | 10 | 16 |
| **GRAND TOTAL** | 629 | 3.6 | 11 | 1 | 1 | 3 | 5 | 7 | 9 | 16 |

## 99.71: THER PLASMAPHERESIS. Formerly included in operation group(s) 794.

| Type of Patients | Observed Patients | Avg. Stay | Variance | Percentiles | | | | | | |
|---|---|---|---|---|---|---|---|---|---|---|
| | | | | 10th | 25th | 50th | 75th | 90th | 95th | 99th |
| **1. SINGLE DX** | | | | | | | | | | |
| 0–19 Years | 21 | 2.2 | 3 | 1 | 1 | 1 | 3 | 3 | 6 | 10 |
| 20–34 | 31 | 3.5 | 7 | 2 | 3 | 3 | 4 | 6 | 8 | 8 |
| 35–49 | 28 | 2.5 | 7 | 1 | 1 | 1 | 4 | 7 | 8 | 15 |
| 50–64 | 16 | 10.0 | 33 | 2 | 5 | 14 | 14 | 17 | 19 | 19 |
| 65+ | 5 | 6.0 | 11 | 1 | 3 | 8 | 9 | 9 | 9 | 9 |
| **2. MULTIPLE DX** | | | | | | | | | | |
| 0–19 Years | 62 | 5.3 | 33 | 1 | 1 | 4 | 8 | 10 | 15 | 33 |
| 20–34 | 127 | 10.4 | 64 | 2 | 5 | 10 | 14 | 18 | 23 | 45 |
| 35–49 | 194 | 8.8 | 49 | 3 | 5 | 8 | 11 | 17 | 21 | 38 |
| 50–64 | 231 | 13.0 | 150 | 2 | 4 | 8 | 18 | 31 | 34 | 50 |
| 65+ | 248 | 9.5 | 49 | 3 | 5 | 8 | 12 | 17 | 26 | 36 |
| **TOTAL SINGLE DX** | 101 | 3.8 | 13 | 1 | 1 | 3 | 4 | 8 | 14 | 17 |
| **TOTAL MULTIPLE DX** | 862 | 10.1 | 84 | 2 | 4 | 8 | 13 | 21 | 31 | 44 |
| **TOTAL** | | | | | | | | | | |
| 0–19 Years | 83 | 4.5 | 27 | 1 | 1 | 3 | 6 | 10 | 11 | 23 |
| 20–34 | 158 | 8.4 | 56 | 1 | 3 | 6 | 12 | 15 | 19 | 45 |
| 35–49 | 222 | 7.8 | 48 | 2 | 3 | 7 | 9 | 16 | 20 | 37 |
| 50–64 | 247 | 12.8 | 144 | 3 | 4 | 9 | 18 | 31 | 34 | 50 |
| 65+ | 253 | 9.4 | 49 | 3 | 5 | 8 | 12 | 17 | 26 | 36 |
| **GRAND TOTAL** | 963 | 9.2 | 79 | 2 | 3 | 7 | 12 | 18 | 31 | 43 |

Length of Stay by Diagnosis and Operation, United States, 2000

# United States, October 1998–September 1999 Data, by Operation

## 99.8: MISC PHYSICAL PROCEDURES. Formerly included in operation group(s) 794.

| Type of Patients | Observed Patients | Avg. Stay | Vari-ance | 10th | 25th | 50th | 75th | 90th | 95th | 99th |
|---|---|---|---|---|---|---|---|---|---|---|
| **1. SINGLE DX** | | | | | | | | | | |
| 0–19 Years | 4,499 | 1.9 | <1 | 1 | 1 | 2 | 2 | 3 | 3 | 5 |
| 20–34 | 51 | 9.4 | 244 | 1 | 2 | 5 | 10 | 17 | 37 | 86 |
| 35–49 | 38 | 5.6 | 14 | 1 | 2 | 6 | 8 | 10 | 12 | 13 |
| 50–64 | 14 | 5.3 | 41 | 1 | 2 | 2 | 8 | 19 | 19 | 19 |
| 65+ | 22 | 2.6 | 9 | 1 | 1 | 2 | 3 | 3 | 7 | 17 |
| **2. MULTIPLE DX** | | | | | | | | | | |
| 0–19 Years | 19,096 | 7.8 | 78 | 2 | 3 | 5 | 8 | 18 | 26 | 45 |
| 20–34 | 148 | 7.0 | 60 | 1 | 2 | 4 | 8 | 18 | 23 | 33 |
| 35–49 | 240 | 8.0 | 76 | 2 | 2 | 6 | 11 | 15 | 22 | 57 |
| 50–64 | 203 | 7.2 | 40 | 1 | 2 | 6 | 9 | 14 | 18 | 34 |
| 65+ | 1,245 | 7.1 | 30 | 2 | 3 | 6 | 9 | 14 | 18 | 28 |
| **TOTAL SINGLE DX** | **4,624** | **2.0** | **3** | **1** | **1** | **2** | **2** | **3** | **4** | **6** |
| **TOTAL MULTIPLE DX** | **20,932** | **7.7** | **75** | **2** | **3** | **5** | **8** | **17** | **25** | **44** |
| **TOTAL** | | | | | | | | | | |
| 0–19 Years | 23,595 | 6.3 | 65 | 1 | 2 | 4 | 7 | 14 | 23 | 41 |
| 20–34 | 199 | 7.5 | 99 | 2 | 2 | 5 | 8 | 17 | 24 | 49 |
| 35–49 | 278 | 7.7 | 69 | 2 | 2 | 6 | 10 | 15 | 20 | 57 |
| 50–64 | 217 | 7.1 | 40 | 2 | 2 | 6 | 9 | 14 | 19 | 34 |
| 65+ | 1,267 | 7.1 | 30 | 2 | 3 | 6 | 9 | 14 | 18 | 28 |
| **GRAND TOTAL** | **25,556** | **6.4** | **64** | **1** | **2** | **4** | **7** | **14** | **22** | **41** |

## 99.82: UV LIGHT THERAPY. Formerly included in operation group(s) 794.

| Type of Patients | Observed Patients | Avg. Stay | Vari-ance | 10th | 25th | 50th | 75th | 90th | 95th | 99th |
|---|---|---|---|---|---|---|---|---|---|---|
| **1. SINGLE DX** | | | | | | | | | | |
| 0–19 Years | 260 | 2.1 | 1 | 1 | 1 | 2 | 2 | 3 | 4 | 6 |
| 20–34 | 0 | | | | | | | | | |
| 35–49 | 0 | | | | | | | | | |
| 50–64 | 0 | | | | | | | | | |
| 65+ | 3 | 2.0 | 0 | 2 | 2 | 2 | 2 | 2 | 2 | 2 |
| **2. MULTIPLE DX** | | | | | | | | | | |
| 0–19 Years | 751 | 7.4 | 90 | 2 | 3 | 4 | 7 | 17 | 27 | 48 |
| 20–34 | 1 | 8.0 | 0 | 8 | 8 | 8 | 8 | 8 | 8 | 8 |
| 35–49 | 6 | 6.6 | 23 | 2 | 3 | 4 | 13 | 13 | 13 | 13 |
| 50–64 | 2 | 3.0 | 0 | 3 | 3 | 3 | 3 | 3 | 3 | 3 |
| 65+ | 9 | 3.4 | 3 | 2 | 2 | 3 | 4 | 7 | 7 | 7 |
| **TOTAL SINGLE DX** | **263** | **2.1** | **1** | **1** | **1** | **2** | **2** | **3** | **4** | **6** |
| **TOTAL MULTIPLE DX** | **769** | **7.4** | **88** | **2** | **3** | **4** | **7** | **17** | **27** | **48** |
| **TOTAL** | | | | | | | | | | |
| 0–19 Years | 1,011 | 5.8 | 69 | 1 | 2 | 3 | 5 | 12 | 21 | 41 |
| 20–34 | 1 | 8.0 | 0 | 8 | 8 | 8 | 8 | 8 | 8 | 8 |
| 35–49 | 6 | 6.6 | 23 | 2 | 3 | 4 | 13 | 13 | 13 | 13 |
| 50–64 | 2 | 3.0 | 0 | 3 | 3 | 3 | 3 | 3 | 3 | 3 |
| 65+ | 12 | 3.0 | 3 | 2 | 2 | 3 | 4 | 6 | 7 | 7 |
| **GRAND TOTAL** | **1,032** | **5.8** | **68** | **1** | **2** | **3** | **5** | **12** | **21** | **41** |

## 99.83: OTHER PHOTOTHERAPY. Formerly included in operation group(s) 794.

| Type of Patients | Observed Patients | Avg. Stay | Vari-ance | 10th | 25th | 50th | 75th | 90th | 95th | 99th |
|---|---|---|---|---|---|---|---|---|---|---|
| **1. SINGLE DX** | | | | | | | | | | |
| 0–19 Years | 4,219 | 1.9 | <1 | 1 | 1 | 2 | 2 | 3 | 3 | 5 |
| 20–34 | 0 | | | | | | | | | |
| 35–49 | 0 | | | | | | | | | |
| 50–64 | 1 | 2.0 | 0 | 2 | 2 | 2 | 2 | 2 | 2 | 2 |
| 65+ | 1 | 2.0 | 0 | 2 | 2 | 2 | 2 | 2 | 2 | 2 |
| **2. MULTIPLE DX** | | | | | | | | | | |
| 0–19 Years | 18,249 | 7.8 | 78 | 2 | 3 | 5 | 8 | 18 | 26 | 45 |
| 20–34 | 0 | | | | | | | | | |
| 35–49 | 2 | 7.2 | 12 | 2 | 2 | 9 | 9 | 9 | 9 | 9 |
| 50–64 | 0 | | | | | | | | | |
| 65+ | 2 | 8.6 | 23 | 5 | 5 | 5 | 13 | 13 | 13 | 13 |
| **TOTAL SINGLE DX** | **4,221** | **1.9** | **<1** | **1** | **1** | **2** | **2** | **3** | **3** | **5** |
| **TOTAL MULTIPLE DX** | **18,253** | **7.8** | **78** | **2** | **3** | **5** | **8** | **18** | **26** | **45** |
| **TOTAL** | | | | | | | | | | |
| 0–19 Years | 22,468 | 6.3 | 65 | 1 | 2 | 4 | 7 | 14 | 23 | 41 |
| 20–34 | 0 | | | | | | | | | |
| 35–49 | 2 | 7.2 | 12 | 2 | 2 | 9 | 9 | 9 | 9 | 9 |
| 50–64 | 1 | 2.0 | 0 | 2 | 2 | 2 | 2 | 2 | 2 | 2 |
| 65+ | 3 | 5.4 | 23 | 2 | 5 | 5 | 5 | 13 | 13 | 13 |
| **GRAND TOTAL** | **22,474** | **6.3** | **65** | **1** | **2** | **4** | **7** | **14** | **23** | **41** |

## 99.84: ISOLATION. Formerly included in operation group(s) 794.

| Type of Patients | Observed Patients | Avg. Stay | Vari-ance | 10th | 25th | 50th | 75th | 90th | 95th | 99th |
|---|---|---|---|---|---|---|---|---|---|---|
| **1. SINGLE DX** | | | | | | | | | | |
| 0–19 Years | 18 | 5.2 | 39 | 2 | 2 | 3 | 8 | 8 | 8 | 42 |
| 20–34 | 49 | 9.6 | 248 | 1 | 2 | 5 | 10 | 17 | 37 | 86 |
| 35–49 | 35 | 6.0 | 13 | 2 | 3 | 6 | 9 | 11 | 12 | 13 |
| 50–64 | 8 | 6.8 | 50 | 2 | 3 | 6 | 14 | 19 | 19 | 19 |
| 65+ | 5 | 4.9 | 23 | 3 | 3 | 3 | 3 | 17 | 17 | 17 |
| **2. MULTIPLE DX** | | | | | | | | | | |
| 0–19 Years | 89 | 6.4 | 55 | 1 | 2 | 4 | 8 | 13 | 20 | 36 |
| 20–34 | 145 | 6.4 | 54 | 1 | 3 | 4 | 7 | 17 | 25 | 33 |
| 35–49 | 225 | 8.0 | 65 | 2 | 3 | 6 | 11 | 19 | 22 | 57 |
| 50–64 | 182 | 7.5 | 42 | 2 | 3 | 6 | 15 | 15 | 19 | 34 |
| 65+ | 1,196 | 7.3 | 30 | 2 | 4 | 6 | 9 | 14 | 18 | 28 |
| **TOTAL SINGLE DX** | **115** | **7.3** | **119** | **1** | **2** | **4** | **8** | **14** | **17** | **67** |
| **TOTAL MULTIPLE DX** | **1,837** | **7.3** | **39** | **2** | **3** | **6** | **9** | **15** | **19** | **33** |
| **TOTAL** | | | | | | | | | | |
| 0–19 Years | 107 | 6.1 | 52 | 1 | 2 | 4 | 8 | 13 | 20 | 42 |
| 20–34 | 194 | 7.1 | 99 | 1 | 3 | 6 | 8 | 17 | 25 | 49 |
| 35–49 | 260 | 7.7 | 60 | 2 | 3 | 6 | 10 | 15 | 20 | 45 |
| 50–64 | 190 | 7.4 | 42 | 2 | 3 | 6 | 9 | 15 | 19 | 34 |
| 65+ | 1,201 | 7.3 | 30 | 2 | 4 | 6 | 9 | 14 | 18 | 28 |
| **GRAND TOTAL** | **1,952** | **7.3** | **44** | **2** | **3** | **6** | **9** | **14** | **19** | **33** |

Length of Stay by Diagnosis and Operation, United States, 2000

**United States, October 1998–September 1999 Data, by Operation**

## 99.9: OTHER MISC PROCEDURES. Formerly included in operation group(s) 794.

| Type of Patients | Observed Patients | Avg. Stay | Vari-ance | Percentiles | | | | | | |
|---|---|---|---|---|---|---|---|---|---|---|
| | | | | 10th | 25th | 50th | 75th | 90th | 95th | 99th |
| **1. SINGLE DX** | | | | | | | | | | |
| 0–19 Years | 5 | 1.8 | 2 | 1 | 1 | 1 | 3 | 5 | 5 | 5 |
| 20–34 | 15 | 11.2 | 31 | 4 | 5 | 14 | 14 | 17 | 19 | 19 |
| 35–49 | 12 | 6.9 | 11 | 2 | 3 | 8 | 9 | 9 | 11 | 15 |
| 50–64 | 1 | 5.0 | 0 | 5 | 5 | 5 | 5 | 5 | 5 | 5 |
| 65+ | 3 | 2.9 | 2 | 1 | 3 | 3 | 3 | 5 | 5 | 5 |
| **2. MULTIPLE DX** | | | | | | | | | | |
| 0–19 Years | 44 | 4.9 | 29 | 1 | 2 | 3 | 6 | 12 | 14 | 21 |
| 20–34 | 61 | 4.3 | 62 | 1 | 1 | 2 | 3 | 13 | 19 | 39 |
| 35–49 | 73 | 6.4 | 65 | 1 | 2 | 4 | 7 | 14 | 14 | 40 |
| 50–64 | 86 | 7.9 | 33 | 2 | 3 | 6 | 12 | 15 | 19 | 21 |
| 65+ | 646 | 6.5 | 18 | 3 | 4 | 6 | 8 | 11 | 14 | 22 |
| **TOTAL SINGLE DX** | 36 | 7.9 | 25 | 2 | 3 | 8 | 11 | 14 | 17 | 19 |
| **TOTAL MULTIPLE DX** | 910 | 6.4 | 27 | 2 | 3 | 5 | 8 | 12 | 15 | 22 |
| **TOTAL** | | | | | | | | | | |
| 0–19 Years | 49 | 4.7 | 28 | 1 | 1 | 2 | 5 | 12 | 14 | 21 |
| 20–34 | 76 | 5.1 | 63 | 1 | 1 | 2 | 5 | 17 | 19 | 39 |
| 35–49 | 85 | 6.4 | 57 | 1 | 2 | 5 | 9 | 14 | 14 | 40 |
| 50–64 | 87 | 7.9 | 32 | 2 | 3 | 6 | 12 | 15 | 19 | 21 |
| 65+ | 649 | 6.5 | 18 | 3 | 4 | 6 | 8 | 11 | 14 | 22 |
| **GRAND TOTAL** | 946 | 6.4 | 27 | 2 | 3 | 5 | 8 | 12 | 15 | 22 |

## 99.99: MISC PROCEDURES NEC. Formerly included in operation group(s) 794.

| Type of Patients | Observed Patients | Avg. Stay | Vari-ance | Percentiles | | | | | | |
|---|---|---|---|---|---|---|---|---|---|---|
| | | | | 10th | 25th | 50th | 75th | 90th | 95th | 99th |
| **1. SINGLE DX** | | | | | | | | | | |
| 0–19 Years | 5 | 1.8 | 2 | 1 | 1 | 1 | 3 | 5 | 5 | 5 |
| 20–34 | 14 | 11.4 | 31 | 4 | 6 | 14 | 14 | 17 | 19 | 19 |
| 35–49 | 12 | 6.9 | 11 | 2 | 3 | 8 | 9 | 9 | 11 | 15 |
| 50–64 | 1 | 5.0 | 0 | 5 | 5 | 5 | 5 | 5 | 5 | 5 |
| 65+ | 2 | 2.9 | 6 | 1 | 1 | 1 | 5 | 5 | 5 | 5 |
| **2. MULTIPLE DX** | | | | | | | | | | |
| 0–19 Years | 34 | 5.8 | 36 | 1 | 1 | 3 | 9 | 12 | 20 | 30 |
| 20–34 | 56 | 4.3 | 64 | 1 | 1 | 1 | 3 | 13 | 19 | 39 |
| 35–49 | 67 | 6.1 | 56 | 1 | 2 | 5 | 7 | 14 | 14 | 41 |
| 50–64 | 77 | 8.1 | 34 | 2 | 2 | 7 | 12 | 15 | 14 | 21 |
| 65+ | 628 | 6.4 | 18 | 3 | 4 | 6 | 8 | 11 | 14 | 22 |
| **TOTAL SINGLE DX** | 34 | 8.1 | 25 | 2 | 3 | 8 | 11 | 14 | 17 | 19 |
| **TOTAL MULTIPLE DX** | 862 | 6.4 | 26 | 2 | 3 | 5 | 8 | 12 | 15 | 22 |
| **TOTAL** | | | | | | | | | | |
| 0–19 Years | 39 | 5.5 | 35 | 1 | 1 | 3 | 8 | 12 | 20 | 30 |
| 20–34 | 70 | 5.1 | 65 | 1 | 1 | 2 | 4 | 17 | 19 | 39 |
| 35–49 | 79 | 6.2 | 50 | 1 | 2 | 5 | 9 | 14 | 14 | 41 |
| 50–64 | 78 | 8.1 | 34 | 2 | 2 | 7 | 12 | 15 | 14 | 21 |
| 65+ | 630 | 6.4 | 18 | 3 | 4 | 6 | 8 | 11 | 14 | 22 |
| **GRAND TOTAL** | 896 | 6.4 | 26 | 2 | 3 | 5 | 8 | 12 | 15 | 22 |

Length of Stay by Diagnosis and Operation, United States, 2000

# APPENDIX A
# Hospital Characteristics
## Short-Term, General, Nonfederal Hospitals[1]

| HOSPITAL CATEGORY | U.S. TOTAL |
|---|---|
| **Bed Size** | |
| 6–24 Beds | 511 |
| 25–49 | 1,239 |
| 50–99 | 1,391 |
| 100–199 | 1,406 |
| 200–299 | 692 |
| 300–399 | 404 |
| 400–499 | 196 |
| 500+ | 289 |
| Unknown | 15 |
| Total | **6,143** |
| **Region and Census Division** | |
| **Northeast** | **919** |
| New England | 270 |
| Middle Atlantic | 649 |
| **North Central** | **1,622** |
| East North Central | 929 |
| West North Central | 693 |
| **South** | **2,420** |
| South Atlantic | 990 |
| East South Central | 513 |
| West South Central | 917 |
| **West** | **1,182** |
| Mountain | 406 |
| Pacific | 776 |
| **Location** | |
| Urban | 3,719 |
| Rural | 2,424 |
| **Teaching Intensity** | |
| High/Medium | 455 |
| Low | 5,688 |

---

[1] For a definition of short-term, general, and nonfederal hospitals, see page vii.

# APPENDIX B
# States Included in Each Region

| Northeast | North Central | South | West |
|---|---|---|---|
| Connecticut | Illinois | Alabama | Alaska |
| Maine | Indiana | Arkansas | Arizona |
| Massachusetts | Iowa | Delaware | California |
| New Hampshire | Kansas | District of Columbia | Colorado |
| New Jersey | Michigan | Florida | Hawaii |
| New York | Minnesota | Georgia | Idaho |
| Pennsylvania | Missouri | Kentucky | Montana |
| Rhode Island | Nebraska | Louisiana | Nevada |
| Vermont | North Dakota | Maryland | New Mexico |
| | Ohio | Mississippi | Oregon |
| | South Dakota | North Carolina | Utah |
| | Wisconsin | Oklahoma | Washington |
| | | South Carolina | Wyoming |
| | | Tennessee | |
| | | Texas | |
| | | Virginia | |
| | | West Virginia | |

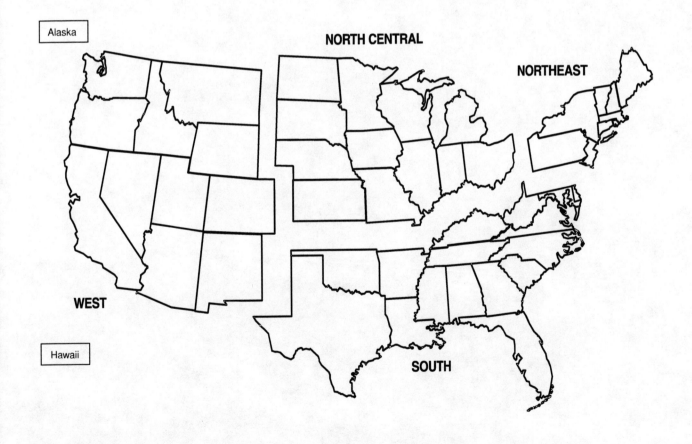

# APPENDIX C
## Operative Status of Procedure Codes

The following table lists every ICD-9-CM procedure code included in this book, its description, and its HCFA-defined operative status (*i.e.,* operative or non-operative). Operative procedures are those classified by HCFA as "operating room" procedures. HCFA physician panels classify every ICD-9-CM procedure code according to whether the procedure would, in most hospitals, be performed in the operating room. For summary (3-digit) codes that contain both operative and non-operative detail (four-digit) codes, the notation "Mixed," followed by the number of each type, will appear in the "Operative Status" column. For example, a summary code containing three operative and two non-operative detail codes will be identified as "Mixed (3, 2)."

| Code | Description | Operative Status | Code | Description | Operative Status |
|------|-------------|------------------|------|-------------|------------------|
| 01.0 | CRANIAL PUNCTURE | Non-Operative | 03.9 | SPINAL CORD OPS NEC | Mixed (5, 5) |
| 01.02 | VENTRICULOPUNCT VIA CATH | Non-Operative | 03.90 | INSERT SPINAL CANAL CATH | Non-Operative |
| 01.1 | DXTIC PX ON SKULL/BRAIN | Mixed (5, 2) | 03.91 | INJECT ANES-SPINAL CANAL | Non-Operative |
| 01.13 | CLSD (PERC) BRAIN BX | Non-Operative | 03.92 | INJECT SPINAL CANAL NEC | Non-Operative |
| 01.14 | OPEN BIOPSY OF BRAIN | Operative | 03.93 | INSERT SPINAL NEUROSTIM | Operative |
| 01.18 | DXTIC PX BRAIN/CEREB NEC | Operative | 03.95 | SPINAL BLOOD PATCH | Non-Operative |
| 01.2 | CRANIOTOMY & CRANIECTOMY | Operative | 04.0 | PERIPH NERVE INC/DIV/EXC | Operative |
| 01.24 | OTHER CRANIOTOMY | Operative | 04.01 | EXC ACOUSTIC NEUROMA | Operative |
| 01.25 | OTHER CRANIECTOMY | Operative | 04.07 | PERIPH/CRAN NERV EXC NEC | Operative |
| 01.3 | INC BRAIN/CEREB MENINGES | Operative | 04.1 | DXTIC PX PERIPH NERV | Mixed (2, 1) |
| 01.31 | INC CEREBRAL MENINGES | Operative | 04.2 | DESTR PERIPH/CRAN NERVES | Non-Operative |
| 01.39 | OTHER BRAIN INCISION | Operative | 04.3 | CRAN/PERIPH NERVE SUTURE | Operative |
| 01.4 | THALAMUS/GLOBUS PALL OPS | Operative | 04.4 | PERIPH NERV ADHESIOLYSIS | Operative |
| 01.5 | EXC/DESTR BRAIN/MENINGES | Operative | 04.41 | DECOMP TRIGEMINAL ROOT | Operative |
| 01.51 | EXC CEREB MENINGEAL LES | Operative | 04.43 | CARPAL TUNNEL RELEASE | Operative |
| 01.53 | BRAIN LOBECTOMY | Operative | 04.49 | PERIPH NERV ADHESIO NEC | Operative |
| 01.59 | EXC/DESTR BRAIN LES NEC | Operative | 04.5 | CRAN OR PERIPH NERV GRFT | Operative |
| 01.6 | EXCISION OF SKULL LESION | Operative | 04.6 | PERIPH NERVES TRANSPOS | Operative |
| 02.0 | CRANIOPLASTY | Operative | 04.7 | OTHER PERIPH NEUROPLASTY | Operative |
| 02.01 | OPENING CRANIAL SUTURE | Operative | 04.8 | PERIPHERAL NERVE INJECT | Non-Operative |
| 02.02 | ELEVATION SKULL FX FRAG | Operative | 04.81 | ANES INJECT PERIPH NERVE | Non-Operative |
| 02.06 | CRANIAL OSTEOPLASTY NEC | Operative | 04.9 | OTH PERIPH NERVE OPS | Operative |
| 02.1 | CEREBRAL MENINGES REPAIR | Operative | 04.92 | IMPL PERIPH NEUROSTIM | Operative |
| 02.12 | REP CEREBRAL MENING NEC | Operative | 05.0 | SYMPATH NERVE DIVISION | Operative |
| 02.2 | VENTRICULOSTOMY | Operative | 05.1 | SYMPATH NERVE DXTIC PX | Operative |
| 02.3 | EXTRACRANIAL VENT SHUNT | Operative | 05.2 | SYMPATHECTOMY | Operative |
| 02.34 | VENT SHUNT TO ABD CAVITY | Operative | 05.3 | SYMPATH NERVE INJECTION | Non-Operative |
| 02.4 | VENT SHUNT REV/RMVL | Mixed (2, 1) | 05.31 | ANES INJECT SYMPATH NERV | Non-Operative |
| 02.42 | REPL VENTRICLULAR SHUNT | Operative | 05.8 | OTH SYMPATH NERVE OPS | Operative |
| 02.43 | RMVL VENTRICLULAR SHUNT | Operative | 05.9 | OTHER NERVOUS SYSTEM OPS | Operative |
| 02.9 | SKULL & BRAIN OPS NEC | Mixed (5, 2) | 06.0 | THYROID FIELD INCISION | Mixed (2, 1) |
| 02.93 | IMPL IC NEUROSTIMULATOR | Operative | 06.09 | INC THYROID FIELD NEC | Operative |
| 02.94 | INSERT/REPL SKULL TONGS | Operative | 06.1 | THYROID/PARATHY DXTIC PX | Mixed (3, 1) |
| 03.0 | SPINAL CANAL EXPLORATION | Operative | 06.2 | UNILAT THYROID LOBECTOMY | Operative |
| 03.02 | REOPEN LAMINECTOMY SITE | Operative | 06.3 | OTHER PART THYROIDECTOMY | Operative |
| 03.09 | SPINAL CANAL EXPLOR NEC | Operative | 06.39 | PART THYROIDECTOMY NEC | Operative |
| 03.1 | INTRASPIN NERVE ROOT DIV | Operative | 06.4 | COMPLETE THYROIDECTOMY | Operative |
| 03.2 | CHORDOTOMY | Operative | 06.5 | SUBSTERNAL THYROIDECTOMY | Operative |
| 03.3 | DXTIC PX ON SPINAL CANAL | Mixed (2, 1) | 06.6 | LINGUAL THYROID EXCISION | Operative |
| 03.31 | SPINAL TAP | Non-Operative | 06.7 | THYROGLOSSAL DUCT EXC | Operative |
| 03.4 | EXC SPINAL CORD LESION | Operative | 06.8 | PARATHYROIDECTOMY | Operative |
| 03.5 | SPINAL CORD PLASTIC OPS | Operative | 06.81 | TOTAL PARATHYROIDECTOMY | Operative |
| 03.53 | VERTEBRAL FX REPAIR | Operative | 06.89 | OTHER PARATHYROIDECTOMY | Operative |
| 03.59 | SPINAL STRUCT REPAIR NEC | Operative | 06.9 | THYROID/PARATHY OPS NEC | Operative |
| 03.6 | SPINAL CORD ADHESIOLYSIS | Operative | 07.0 | ADRENAL FIELD EXPLOR | Operative |
| 03.7 | SPINAL THECAL SHUNT | Operative | 07.1 | OTH ENDOCRINE DXTIC PX | Mixed (7, 1) |
| 03.8 | DESTR INJECT-SPINE CANAL | Non-Operative | 07.2 | PARTIAL ADRENALECTOMY | Operative |

| Code | Description | Operative Status | Code | Description | Operative Status |
|------|-------------|------------------|------|-------------|------------------|
| 07.22 | UNILATERAL ADRENALECTOMY | Operative | 13.1 | INTRACAP LENS EXTRACTION | Operative |
| 07.3 | BILATERAL ADRENALECTOMY | Operative | 13.2 | LIN EXTRACAPS LENS EXTR | Operative |
| 07.4 | OTHER ADRENAL OPERATIONS | Operative | 13.3 | SIMP ASP LENS EXTRACTION | Operative |
| 07.5 | PINEAL GLAND OPERATIONS | Operative | 13.4 | FRAG-ASP EXTRACAPS LENS | Operative |
| 07.6 | HYPOPHYSECTOMY | Operative | 13.41 | CATARACT PHACO & ASP | Operative |
| 07.62 | EXC PIT LES-TRANSSPHEN | Operative | 13.5 | OTH EXTRACAPS LENS EXTR | Operative |
| 07.65 | TOT EXC PIT-TRANSSPHEN | Operative | 13.6 | OTH CATARACT EXTRACTION | Operative |
| 07.7 | OTHER HYPOPHYSIS OPS | Operative | 13.7 | INSERT PROSTHETIC LENS | Operative |
| 07.8 | THYMECTOMY | Operative | 13.8 | IMPLANTED LENS REMOVAL | Operative |
| 07.82 | TOTAL EXCISION OF THYMUS | Operative | 13.9 | OTHER OPERATIONS ON LENS | Operative |
| 07.9 | OTHER THYMUS OPERATIONS | Operative | 14.0 | RMVL OF POST SEGMENT FB | Operative |
| 08.0 | EYELID INCISION | Non-Operative | 14.1 | DXTIC PX POSTERIOR SEG | Operative |
| 08.1 | DXTIC PX ON EYELID | Mixed (1, 1) | 14.2 | RETINA-CHOROID LES DESTR | Mixed (5, 3) |
| 08.2 | EXC/DESTR EYELID LESION | Operative | 14.3 | REPAIR OF RETINAL TEAR | Mixed (3, 3) |
| 08.3 | PTOSIS/LID RETRACT REP | Operative | 14.4 | REP RETINA DETACH/BUCKLE | Operative |
| 08.4 | ENTROPION/ECTROPION REP | Operative | 14.49 | SCLERAL BUCKLING NEC | Operative |
| 08.5 | OTH ADJUST LID POSITION | Operative | 14.5 | OTH REPAIR RETINA DETACH | Operative |
| 08.6 | EYELID RECONST W GRAFT | Operative | 14.6 | RMVL PROSTH MAT POST SEG | Operative |
| 08.7 | OTHER EYELID RECONST | Operative | 14.7 | OPERATIONS ON VITREOUS | Operative |
| 08.8 | OTHER REPAIR OF EYELID | Non-Operative | 14.74 | MECH VITRECTOMY NEC | Operative |
| 08.81 | LINEAR REP EYELID LAC | Non-Operative | 14.9 | OTHER POST SEGMENT OPS | Operative |
| 08.9 | OTHER EYELID OPERATIONS | Operative | 15.0 | EXOC MUSC-TEND DXTIC PX | Operative |
| 09.0 | LACRIMAL GLAND INCISION | Operative | 15.1 | 1 EXOC MUSC OPS W DETACH | Operative |
| 09.1 | LACRIMAL SYSTEM DXTIC PX | Operative | 15.2 | OTH OPS ON 1 EXOC MUSCLE | Operative |
| 09.2 | LACRIMAL GLAND LES EXC | Operative | 15.3 | TEMP DETACH >1 EXOC MUSC | Operative |
| 09.3 | OTHER LACRIMAL GLAND OPS | Operative | 15.4 | OTH OPS ON >1 EXOC MUSC | Operative |
| 09.4 | LACRIMAL PASSAGE MANIP | Operative | 15.5 | EXOC MUSC TRANSPOSITION | Operative |
| 09.5 | INC LACRIMAL SAC/PASSG | Operative | 15.6 | REV EXOC MUSCLE SURGERY | Operative |
| 09.6 | LACRIMAL SAC/PASSAGE EXC | Operative | 15.7 | EXOC MUSCLE INJURY REP | Operative |
| 09.7 | CANALICULUS/PUNCTUM REP | Operative | 15.9 | OTH EXOC MUSC-TEND OPS | Operative |
| 09.8 | NL FISTULIZATION | Operative | 16.0 | ORBITOTOMY | Operative |
| 09.9 | OTH LACRIMAL SYST OPS | Operative | 16.09 | ORBITOTOMY NEC | Operative |
| 10.0 | INC/RMVL FB-CONJUNCTIVA | Operative | 16.1 | RMVL PENETR FB EYE NOS | Operative |
| 10.1 | CONJUNCTIVA INCISION NEC | Operative | 16.2 | ORBIT & EYEBALL DXTIC PX | Mixed (3, 1) |
| 10.2 | CONJUNCTIVA DXTIC PX | Operative | 16.3 | EVISCERATION OF EYEBALL | Operative |
| 10.3 | EXC/DESTR CONJUNCT LES | Operative | 16.4 | ENUCLEATION OF EYEBALL | Operative |
| 10.4 | CONJUNCTIVOPLASTY | Operative | 16.5 | EXENTERATION OF ORBIT | Operative |
| 10.5 | CONJUNCT/LID ADHESIO | Operative | 16.6 | 2ND PX POST RMVL EYEBALL | Operative |
| 10.6 | REPAIR CONJUNCT LAC | Operative | 16.7 | OCULAR/ORBITAL IMPL RMVL | Operative |
| 10.9 | OTHER CONJUNCTIVAL OPS | Operative | 16.8 | EYEBALL/ORBIT INJ REPAIR | Operative |
| 11.0 | MAGNET REMOVAL CORNEA FB | Operative | 16.82 | REPAIR EYEBALL RUPTURE | Operative |
| 11.1 | CORNEAL INCISION | Operative | 16.9 | OTHER EYE & ORBIT OPS | Mixed (4, 1) |
| 11.2 | DXTIC PX ON CORNEA | Operative | 18.0 | EXTERNAL EAR INCISION | Non-Operative |
| 11.3 | EXCISION OF PTERYGIUM | Operative | 18.1 | EXTERNAL EAR DXTIC PX | Non-Operative |
| 11.4 | EXC/DESTR CORNEAL LESION | Operative | 18.2 | EXC/DESTR EXT EAR LESION | Mixed (1, 1) |
| 11.5 | CORNEAL REPAIR | Operative | 18.29 | DESTR EXT EAR LES NEC | Non-Operative |
| 11.51 | SUTURE OF CORNEAL LAC | Operative | 18.3 | OTHER EXTERNAL EAR EXC | Operative |
| 11.6 | CORNEAL TRANSPLANT | Operative | 18.4 | SUTURE EXT EAR LAC | Non-Operative |
| 11.7 | OTHER CORNEA RECONST | Operative | 18.5 | CORRECTION PROMINENT EAR | Operative |
| 11.9 | OTHER CORNEAL OPERATIONS | Operative | 18.6 | EXT AUDIT CANAL RECONST | Operative |
| 12.0 | RMVL INOC FB ANT SEGMENT | Operative | 18.7 | OTH PLASTIC REP EXT EAR | Operative |
| 12.1 | IRIDOTOMY/SMP IRIDECTOMY | Operative | 18.9 | OTHER EXT EAR OPERATIONS | Operative |
| 12.2 | ANTERIOR SEG DXTIC PX | Operative | 19.0 | STAPES MOBILIZATION | Operative |
| 12.3 | IRIDOPLASTY/COREOPLASTY | Operative | 19.1 | STAPEDECTOMY | Operative |
| 12.4 | DESTR IRIS/CIL BODY LES | Operative | 19.2 | STAPEDECTOMY REVISION | Operative |
| 12.5 | INOC CIRCULAT FACILITAT | Operative | 19.3 | OSSICULAR CHAIN OPS NEC | Operative |
| 12.6 | SCLERAL FISTULIZATION | Operative | 19.4 | MYRINGOPLASTY | Operative |
| 12.7 | ELEVAT INOC PRESS RELIEF | Operative | 19.5 | OTHER TYMPANOPLASTY | Operative |
| 12.8 | OPERATIONS ON SCLERA | Operative | 19.6 | TYMPANOPLASTY REVISION | Operative |
| 12.9 | OTH ANTERIOR SEGMENT OPS | Operative | 19.9 | MIDDLE EAR REPAIR NEC | Operative |
| 13.0 | REMOVAL FB FROM LENS | Operative | 20.0 | MYRINGOTOMY | Mixed (1, 1) |

| Code | Description | Operative Status | Code | Description | Operative Status |
|---|---|---|---|---|---|
| 20.01 | MYRINGOTOMY W INTUBATION | Operative | 25.2 | PARTIAL GLOSSECTOMY | Operative |
| 20.1 | TYMPANOSTOMY TUBE RMVL | Non-Operative | 25.3 | COMPLETE GLOSSECTOMY | Operative |
| 20.2 | MASTOID & MID EAR INC | Operative | 25.4 | RADICAL GLOSSECTOMY | Operative |
| 20.3 | MID & INNER EAR DXTIC PX | Mixed (2, 1) | 25.5 | REPAIR OF TONGUE | Mixed (1, 1) |
| 20.4 | MASTOIDECTOMY | Operative | 25.9 | OTHER TONGUE OPERATIONS | Mixed (2, 3) |
| 20.42 | RADICAL MASTOIDECTOMY | Operative | 26.0 | INC SALIVARY GLAND/DUCT | Non-Operative |
| 20.49 | MASTOIDECTOMY NEC | Operative | 26.1 | SALIVARY GLAND DXTIC PX | Mixed (1, 2) |
| 20.5 | OTH MIDDLE EAR EXCISION | Operative | 26.2 | EXC OF SG LESION | Operative |
| 20.6 | FENESTRATION INNER EAR | Operative | 26.3 | SIALOADENECTOMY | Operative |
| 20.7 | INC/EXC/DESTR INNER EAR | Operative | 26.30 | SIALOADENECTOMY NOS | Operative |
| 20.8 | EUSTACHIAN TUBE OPS | Non-Operative | 26.31 | PARTIAL SIALOADENECTOMY | Operative |
| 20.9 | OTHER ME & IE OPS | Mixed (8, 1) | 26.32 | COMPLETE SIALOADENECTOMY | Operative |
| 21.0 | CONTROL OF EPISTAXIS | Mixed (5, 4) | 26.4 | SG & DUCT REPAIR | Operative |
| 21.01 | ANT NAS PACK FOR EPISTX | Non-Operative | 26.9 | OTH SALIVARY OPERATIONS | Mixed (1, 1) |
| 21.02 | POST NAS PACK FOR EPISTX | Non-Operative | 27.0 | DRAIN FACE & MOUTH FLOOR | Operative |
| 21.03 | CAUT TO CNTRL EPISTAXIS | Non-Operative | 27.1 | INCISION OF PALATE | Operative |
| 21.1 | INCISION OF NOSE | Non-Operative | 27.2 | ORAL CAVITY DXTIC PX | Mixed (2, 3) |
| 21.2 | NASAL DIAGNOSTIC PX | Non-Operative | 27.3 | EXC BONY PALATE LES/TISS | Operative |
| 21.3 | NASAL LESION DESTR/EXC | Non-Operative | 27.4 | OTHER EXCISION OF MOUTH | Mixed (3, 1) |
| 21.4 | RESECTION OF NOSE | Operative | 27.49 | EXCISION OF MOUTH NEC | Operative |
| 21.5 | SUBMUC NAS SEPTUM RESECT | Operative | 27.5 | PLASTIC REPAIR OF MOUTH | Mixed (6, 2) |
| 21.6 | TURBINECTOMY | Operative | 27.51 | SUTURE OF LIP LACERATION | Non-Operative |
| 21.7 | NASAL FRACTURE REDUCTION | Mixed (1, 1) | 27.54 | REPAIR OF CLEFT LIP | Operative |
| 21.71 | CLSD REDUCTION NASAL FX | Non-Operative | 27.6 | PALATOPLASTY | Operative |
| 21.8 | NASAL REP & PLASTIC OPS | Mixed (8, 1) | 27.62 | CLEFT PALATE CORRECTION | Operative |
| 21.81 | NASAL LACERATION SUTURE | Non-Operative | 27.63 | REV CLEFT PALATE REPAIR | Operative |
| 21.88 | SEPTOPLASTY NEC | Operative | 27.69 | OTHER PLASTIC REP PALATE | Operative |
| 21.9 | OTHER NASAL OPERATIONS | Mixed (1, 1) | 27.7 | OPERATIONS ON UVULA | Operative |
| 22.0 | NASAL SINUS ASP & LAVAGE | Non-Operative | 27.9 | OTH OPS ON MOUTH & FACE | Mixed (2, 1) |
| 22.1 | NASAL SINUS DXTIC PX | Mixed (1, 2) | 28.0 | TONSIL/PERITONSILLAR I&D | Operative |
| 22.2 | INTRANASAL ANTROTOMY | Non-Operative | 28.1 | TONSIL ADENOID DXTIC PX | Operative |
| 22.3 | EXT MAXILLARY ANTROTOMY | Operative | 28.2 | TONSILLECTOMY | Operative |
| 22.4 | FRONT SINUSOT & SINUSECT | Operative | 28.3 | T&A | Operative |
| 22.5 | OTHER NASAL SINUSOTOMY | Operative | 28.4 | EXCISION OF TONSIL TAG | Operative |
| 22.6 | OTHER NASAL SINUSECTOMY | Operative | 28.5 | EXCISION LINGUAL TONSIL | Operative |
| 22.62 | EXC MAX SINUS LESION NEC | Operative | 28.6 | ADENOIDECTOMY | Operative |
| 22.63 | ETHMOIDECTOMY | Operative | 28.7 | HEMOR CONTROL POST T&A | Operative |
| 22.7 | NASAL SINUS REPAIR | Operative | 28.9 | OTHER TONSIL/ADENOID OPS | Operative |
| 22.9 | OTHER NASAL SINUS OPS | Operative | 29.0 | PHARYNGOTOMY | Operative |
| 23.0 | FORCEPS TOOTH EXTRACTION | Non-Operative | 29.1 | PHARYNGEAL DXTIC PX | Non-Operative |
| 23.09 | TOOTH EXTRACTION NEC | Non-Operative | 29.11 | PHARYNGOSCOPY | Non-Operative |
| 23.1 | SURG REMOVAL OF TOOTH | Non-Operative | 29.2 | EXC BRANCHIAL CLEFT CYST | Operative |
| 23.19 | SURG TOOTH EXTRACT NEC | Non-Operative | 29.3 | EXC/DESTR PHARYNGEAL LES | Operative |
| 23.2 | TOOTH RESTOR BY FILLING | Non-Operative | 29.4 | PLASTIC OP ON PHARYNX | Operative |
| 23.3 | TOOTH RESTOR BY INLAY | Non-Operative | 29.5 | OTHER PHARYNGEAL REPAIR | Operative |
| 23.4 | OTHER DENTAL RESTORATION | Non-Operative | 29.9 | OTHER PHARYNGEAL OPS | Mixed (2, 1) |
| 23.5 | TOOTH IMPLANTATION | Non-Operative | 30.0 | EXC/DESTR LES LARYNX | Operative |
| 23.6 | PROSTHETIC DENTAL IMPL | Non-Operative | 30.09 | EXC/DESTR LARYNX LES NEC | Operative |
| 23.7 | ROOT CANAL TX & APICOECT | Non-Operative | 30.1 | HEMILARYNGECTOMY | Operative |
| 24.0 | GUM OR ALVEOLAR INCISION | Non-Operative | 30.2 | PARTIAL LARYNGECTOMY NEC | Operative |
| 24.1 | TOOTH & GUM DXTIC PX | Non-Operative | 30.3 | COMPLETE LARYNGECTOMY | Operative |
| 24.2 | GINGIVOPLASTY | Operative | 30.4 | RADICAL LARYNGECTOMY | Operative |
| 24.3 | OTHER OPERATIONS ON GUMS | Non-Operative | 31.0 | INJECTION OF LARYNX | Non-Operative |
| 24.4 | EXC OF DENTAL LES OF JAW | Operative | 31.1 | TEMPORARY TRACHEOSTOMY | Non-Operative |
| 24.5 | ALVEOLOPLASTY | Operative | 31.2 | PERMANENT TRACHEOSTOMY | Operative |
| 24.6 | EXPOSURE OF TOOTH | Non-Operative | 31.29 | OTHER PERM TRACHEOSTOMY | Operative |
| 24.7 | APPL ORTHODONT APPLIANCE | Non-Operative | 31.3 | INC LARYNX/TRACHEA NEC | Operative |
| 24.8 | OTHER ORTHODONTIC OP | Non-Operative | 31.4 | LARYNX/TRACHEA DXTIC PX | Mixed (1, 6) |
| 24.9 | OTHER DENTAL OPERATION | Non-Operative | 31.42 | LARYNGOSCOPY/TRACHEOSCPY | Non-Operative |
| 25.0 | DXTIC PX ON TONGUE | Mixed (1, 2) | 31.43 | CLSD (ENDO) BX LARYNX | Non-Operative |
| 25.1 | EXC/DESTR TONGUE LES | Operative | 31.5 | LOC EXC/DESTR LARYNX LES | Operative |

| Code | Description | Operative Status | Code | Description | Operative Status |
|------|-------------|------------------|------|-------------|------------------|
| 31.6 | REPAIR OF LARYNX | Operative | 35.22 | REPL AORTIC VALVE NEC | Operative |
| 31.69 | OTHER LARYNGEAL REPAIR | Operative | 35.23 | REPL MITRAL VALVE W TISS | Operative |
| 31.7 | REPAIR OF TRACHEA | Operative | 35.24 | REPL MITRAL VALVE NEC | Operative |
| 31.74 | REVISION OF TRACHEOSTOMY | Operative | 35.3 | TISS ADJ TO HRT VALV OPS | Operative |
| 31.9 | OTHER LARYNX/TRACHEA OPS | Mixed (4, 3) | 35.33 | ANNULOPLASTY | Operative |
| 32.0 | LOC EXC/DESTR BRONCH LES | Mixed (1, 1) | 35.4 | SEPTAL DEFECT PRODUCTION | Mixed (1, 1) |
| 32.1 | OTHER BRONCHIAL EXCISION | Operative | 35.5 | PROSTH REP HEART SEPTA | Operative |
| 32.2 | LOC EXC/DESTR LUNG LES | Mixed (3, 1) | 35.53 | PROSTH REP VSD | Operative |
| 32.21 | EMPHYSEM BLEB PLICATION | Operative | 35.6 | TISS GRFT REP HRT SEPTA | Operative |
| 32.28 | ENDO EXC/DESTR LUNG LES | Non-Operative | 35.61 | REPAIR ASD W TISS GRAFT | Operative |
| 32.29 | LOC EXC LUNG LES NEC | Operative | 35.62 | REPAIR VSD W TISS GRAFT | Operative |
| 32.3 | SEGMENTAL LUNG RESECTION | Operative | 35.7 | HEART SEPTA REP NEC/NOS | Operative |
| 32.4 | LOBECTOMY OF LUNG | Operative | 35.71 | REPAIR ASD NEC | Operative |
| 32.5 | COMPLETE PNEUMONECTOMY | Operative | 35.72 | REPAIR VSD NEC | Operative |
| 32.6 | RAD DISSECT THOR STRUCT | Operative | 35.8 | TOT REP CONG CARD ANOM | Operative |
| 32.9 | OTHER EXCISION OF LUNG | Operative | 35.81 | TOT REP TETRALOGY FALLOT | Operative |
| 33.0 | INCISION OF BRONCHUS | Operative | 35.9 | VALVES & SEPTA OPS NEC | Operative |
| 33.1 | INCISION OF LUNG | Operative | 35.94 | CREAT CONDUIT ATRIUM-PA | Operative |
| 33.2 | BRONCHIAL/LUNG DXTIC PX | Mixed (4, 5) | 35.96 | PERC VALVULOPLASTY | Operative |
| 33.22 | FIBER-OPTIC BRONCHOSCOPY | Non-Operative | 36.0 | RMVL COR ART OBSTR/STENT | Mixed (5, 2) |
| 33.23 | OTHER BRONCHOSCOPY | Non-Operative | 36.01 | 1 PTCA/ATHERECT W/O TL | Operative |
| 33.24 | CLSD (ENDO) BRONCHUS BX | Non-Operative | 36.02 | 1 PTCA/ATHERECT W TL | Operative |
| 33.26 | CLSD (NEEDLE) LUNG BX | Non-Operative | 36.05 | PTCA/ATHERECT-MULT VESS | Operative |
| 33.27 | ENDO LUNG BX (CLOSED) | Operative | 36.06 | INSERT CORONARY STENT | Non-Operative |
| 33.28 | OPEN BIOPSY OF LUNG | Operative | 36.1 | HRT REVASC BYPASS ANAST | Operative |
| 33.3 | SURG COLLAPSE OF LUNG | Mixed (2, 3) | 36.11 | AO-COR BYPASS-1 COR ART | Operative |
| 33.4 | LUNG AND BRONCHUS REPAIR | Operative | 36.12 | AO-COR BYPASS-2 COR ART | Operative |
| 33.5 | LUNG TRANSPLANTATION | Operative | 36.13 | AO-COR BYPASS-3 COR ART | Operative |
| 33.6 | HEART-LUNG TRANSPLANT | Operative | 36.14 | AO-COR BYPASS-4+ COR ART | Operative |
| 33.9 | OTHER BRONCHIAL LUNG OPS | Mixed (4, 1) | 36.15 | 1 INT MAM-COR ART BYPASS | Operative |
| 34.0 | INC CHEST WALL & PLEURA | Mixed (2, 4) | 36.16 | 2 INT MAM-COR ART BYPASS | Operative |
| 34.01 | INCISION OF CHEST WALL | Non-Operative | 36.2 | ARTERIAL IMPLANT REVASC | Operative |
| 34.02 | EXPLORATORY THORACOTOMY | Operative | 36.3 | HEART REVASC NEC | Operative |
| 34.04 | INSERT INTERCOSTAL CATH | Non-Operative | 36.9 | OTHER HEART VESSEL OPS | Operative |
| 34.09 | OTHER PLEURAL INCISION | Non-Operative | 37.0 | PERICARDIOCENTESIS | Non-Operative |
| 34.1 | INCISION OF MEDIASTINUM | Operative | 37.1 | CARDIOTOMY & PERICARDIOT | Operative |
| 34.2 | THORAX DXTIC PROCEDURES | Mixed (6, 3) | 37.12 | PERICARDIOTOMY | Operative |
| 34.21 | TRANSPLEURA THORACOSCOPY | Operative | 37.2 | DXTIC PX HRT/PERICARDIUM | Mixed (1, 7) |
| 34.22 | MEDIASTINOSCOPY | Operative | 37.21 | RT HEART CARDIAC CATH | Non-Operative |
| 34.24 | PLEURAL BIOPSY | Non-Operative | 37.22 | LEFT HEART CARDIAC CATH | Non-Operative |
| 34.25 | CLSD MEDIASTINAL BX | Non-Operative | 37.23 | RT/LEFT HEART CARD CATH | Non-Operative |
| 34.26 | OPEN MEDIASTINAL BIOPSY | Operative | 37.25 | CARDIAC BIOPSY | Non-Operative |
| 34.3 | DESTR MEDIASTINUM LES | Operative | 37.26 | CARD EPS/RECORD STUDIES | Non-Operative |
| 34.4 | EXC/DESTR CHEST WALL LES | Operative | 37.3 | PERICARDIECT/EXC HRT LES | Operative |
| 34.5 | PLEURECTOMY | Operative | 37.31 | PERICARDIECTOMY | Operative |
| 34.51 | DECORTICATION OF LUNG | Operative | 37.33 | HEART LES EXC/DESTR NEC | Operative |
| 34.59 | OTHER PLEURAL EXCISION | Operative | 37.34 | CATH ABLATION HEART LES | Operative |
| 34.6 | SCARIFICATION OF PLEURA | Operative | 37.4 | REP HEART & PERICARDIUM | Operative |
| 34.7 | REPAIR OF CHEST WALL | Mixed (3, 2) | 37.5 | HEART TRANSPLANTATION | Operative |
| 34.74 | PECTUS DEFORMITY REPAIR | Operative | 37.6 | IMPL HEART ASSIST SYST | Operative |
| 34.79 | OTHER CHEST WALL REPAIR | Operative | 37.61 | PULSATION BALLOON IMPL | Operative |
| 34.8 | OPERATIONS ON DIAPHRAGM | Operative | 37.7 | CARDIAC PACER LEAD OP | Mixed (5, 5) |
| 34.9 | OTHER OPS ON THORAX | Mixed (2, 2) | 37.71 | INSERT TV LEAD-VENTRICLE | Non-Operative |
| 34.91 | THORACENTESIS | Non-Operative | 37.72 | INSERT TV LEAD-ATR&VENT | Non-Operative |
| 34.92 | INJECT INTO THOR CAVIT | Non-Operative | 37.75 | REVISION PACEMAKER LEAD | Operative |
| 35.0 | CLOSED HEART VALVOTOMY | Operative | 37.76 | REPL TRANSVENOUS LEAD(S) | Operative |
| 35.1 | OPEN HEART VALVULOPLASTY | Operative | 37.78 | INSERT TEMP TV PACER | Non-Operative |
| 35.11 | OPN AORTIC VALVULOPLASTY | Operative | 37.8 | CARDIAC PACEMAKER DEV OP | Mixed (5, 3) |
| 35.12 | OPN MITRAL VALVULOPLASTY | Operative | 37.80 | INSERT PACEMAKER DEV NOS | Operative |
| 35.2 | HEART VALVE REPLACEMENT | Operative | 37.81 | INSERT SINGLE CHAMB DEV | Non-Operative |
| 35.21 | REPL AORTIC VALVE-TISSUE | Operative | 37.82 | INSERT RATE-RESPON DEV | Non-Operative |

| Code | Description | Operative Status | Code | Description | Operative Status |
|------|-------------|------------------|------|-------------|------------------|
| 37.83 | INSERT DUAL-CHAMBER DEV | Non-Operative | 39.53 | AV FISTULA REPAIR | Operative |
| 37.85 | REPL W 1-CHAMBER DEVICE | Operative | 39.56 | REP VESS W TISS PATCH | Operative |
| 37.86 | REPL W RATE-RESPON DEV | Operative | 39.57 | REP VESS W SYNTH PATCH | Operative |
| 37.87 | REPL W DUAL-CHAMB DEVICE | Operative | 39.59 | REPAIR OF VESSEL NEC | Operative |
| 37.89 | REV/RMVL PACEMAKER DEV | Operative | 39.6 | OPEN HEART AUXILIARY PX | Non-Operative |
| 37.9 | HRT/PERICARDIUM OPS NEC | Mixed (7, 2) | 39.8 | VASCULAR BODY OPERATIONS | Operative |
| 37.94 | IMPL/REPL AICD TOT SYST | Operative | 39.9 | OTHER VESSEL OPERATIONS | Mixed (6, 4) |
| 37.98 | REPL AICD GENERATOR ONLY | Operative | 39.93 | INSERT VESS-VESS CANNULA | Operative |
| 37.99 | OTH OPS HRT/PERICARDIUM | Operative | 39.95 | HEMODIALYSIS | Non-Operative |
| 38.0 | INCISION OF VESSEL | Operative | 39.98 | HEMORRHAGE CONTROL NOS | Operative |
| 38.03 | UPPER LIMB VESSEL INC | Operative | 40.0 | INC LYMPHATIC STRUCTURE | Operative |
| 38.08 | LOWER LIMB ARTERY INC | Operative | 40.1 | LYMPHATIC DXTIC PX | Operative |
| 38.1 | ENDARTERECTOMY | Operative | 40.11 | LYMPHATIC STRUCT BIOPSY | Operative |
| 38.12 | HEAD/NK ENDARTERECT NEC | Operative | 40.2 | SMP EXC LYMPHATIC STRUCT | Operative |
| 38.16 | ABDOMINAL ENDARTERECTOMY | Operative | 40.21 | EXC DEEP CERVICAL NODE | Operative |
| 38.18 | LOWER LIMB ENDARTERECT | Operative | 40.23 | EXC AXILLARY LYMPH NODE | Operative |
| 38.2 | DXTIC BLOOD VESSELS PX | Mixed (2, 1) | 40.24 | EXC INGUINAL LYMPH NODE | Operative |
| 38.21 | BLOOD VESSEL BIOPSY | Operative | 40.29 | SMP EXC LYMPHATIC NEC | Operative |
| 38.3 | VESSEL RESECT W ANAST | Operative | 40.3 | REGIONAL LYMPH NODE EXC | Operative |
| 38.34 | AORTA RESECTION & ANAST | Operative | 40.4 | RAD EXC CERV LYMPH NODE | Operative |
| 38.4 | VESSEL RESECT W REPL | Operative | 40.41 | UNILAT RAD NECK DISSECT | Operative |
| 38.44 | ABD AORTA RESECT W REPL | Operative | 40.5 | OTH RAD NODE DISSECTION | Operative |
| 38.45 | THOR VESS RESECT W REPL | Operative | 40.6 | THORACIC DUCT OPERATIONS | Operative |
| 38.48 | LEG ARTERY RESECT W REPL | Operative | 40.9 | LYMPHATIC STRUCT OPS NEC | Operative |
| 38.5 | LIG&STRIP VARICOSE VEINS | Operative | 41.0 | BONE MARROW TRANSPLANT | Operative |
| 38.59 | LOWER LIMB VV LIG&STRIP | Operative | 41.03 | ALLO MARROW TRANSPL NEC | Operative |
| 38.6 | OTHER VESSEL EXCISION | Operative | 41.04 | AUTLOG STEM CELL TRANSPL | Operative |
| 38.64 | EXCISION OF AORTA | Operative | 41.1 | PUNCTURE OF SPLEEN | Non-Operative |
| 38.68 | LOWER LIMB ARTERY EXC | Operative | 41.2 | SPLENOTOMY | Operative |
| 38.7 | INTERRUPTION VENA CAVA | Operative | 41.3 | MARROW & SPLEEN DXTIC PX | Mixed (1, 4) |
| 38.8 | OTHER SURG VESSEL OCCL | Operative | 41.31 | BONE MARROW BIOPSY | Non-Operative |
| 38.81 | OCCLUSION IC VESSELS NEC | Operative | 41.4 | EXC/DESTR SPLENIC TISSUE | Operative |
| 38.82 | OCCL HEAD/NECK VESS NEC | Operative | 41.5 | TOTAL SPLENECTOMY | Operative |
| 38.85 | OCCL THORACIC VESS NEC | Operative | 41.9 | OTH SPLEEN & MARROW OPS | Mixed (4, 3) |
| 38.86 | SURG OCCL ABD ARTERY NEC | Operative | 42.0 | ESOPHAGOTOMY | Operative |
| 38.9 | PUNCTURE OF VESSEL | Non-Operative | 42.1 | ESOPHAGOSTOMY | Operative |
| 38.91 | ARTERIAL CATHETERIZATION | Non-Operative | 42.2 | ESOPHAGEAL DXTIC PX | Mixed (2, 4) |
| 38.92 | UMBILICAL VEIN CATH | Non-Operative | 42.23 | ESOPHAGOSCOPY NEC | Non-Operative |
| 38.93 | VENOUS CATHETER NEC | Non-Operative | 42.24 | CLSD (ENDO) ESOPH BX | Non-Operative |
| 38.94 | VENOUS CUTDOWN | Non-Operative | 42.3 | EXC/DESTR ESOPH LES/TISS | Mixed (3, 1) |
| 38.95 | VENOUS CATH FOR RD | Non-Operative | 42.33 | ENDO EXC/DESTR ESOPH LES | Non-Operative |
| 38.98 | ARTERIAL PUNCTURE NEC | Non-Operative | 42.4 | EXCISION OF ESOPHAGUS | Operative |
| 38.99 | VENOUS PUNCTURE NEC | Non-Operative | 42.41 | PARTIAL ESOPHAGECTOMY | Operative |
| 39.0 | SYSTEMIC TO PA SHUNT | Operative | 42.5 | INTRATHOR ESOPH ANAST | Operative |
| 39.1 | INTRA-ABD VENOUS SHUNT | Operative | 42.6 | ANTESTERNAL ESOPH ANAST | Operative |
| 39.2 | OTHER SHUNT/VASC BYPASS | Operative | 42.7 | ESOPHAGOMYOTOMY | Operative |
| 39.21 | CAVAL-PA ANASTOMOSIS | Operative | 42.8 | OTHER ESOPHAGEAL REPAIR | Mixed (7, 1) |
| 39.22 | AORTA-SCL-CAROTID BYPASS | Operative | 42.9 | OTHER ESOPHAGEAL OPS | Mixed (1, 2) |
| 39.25 | AORTA-ILIAC-FEMORAL BYP | Operative | 42.92 | ESOPHAGEAL DILATION | Non-Operative |
| 39.27 | ARTERIOVENOSTOMY FOR RD | Operative | 43.0 | GASTROTOMY | Operative |
| 39.29 | VASC SHUNT & BYPASS NEC | Operative | 43.1 | GASTROSTOMY | Non-Operative |
| 39.3 | SUTURE OF VESSEL | Operative | 43.11 | PERC (ENDO) GASTROSTOMY | Non-Operative |
| 39.31 | SUTURE OF ARTERY | Operative | 43.19 | GASTROSTOMY NEC | Non-Operative |
| 39.4 | VASCULAR PX REVISION | Operative | 43.3 | PYLOROMYOTOMY | Operative |
| 39.42 | REV AV SHUNT FOR RD | Operative | 43.4 | LOC EXC GASTRIC LES | Mixed (2, 1) |
| 39.43 | RMVL AV SHUNT FOR RD | Operative | 43.41 | ENDO EXC GASTRIC LES | Non-Operative |
| 39.49 | VASCULAR PX REVISION NEC | Operative | 43.42 | LOC GASTRIC LES EXC NEC | Operative |
| 39.5 | OTHER VESSEL REPAIR | Operative | 43.5 | PROXIMAL GASTRECTOMY | Operative |
| 39.50 | PTA/ATHERECT OTH VESSEL | Operative | 43.6 | DISTAL GASTRECTOMY | Operative |
| 39.51 | CLIPPING OF ANEURYSM | Operative | 43.7 | PART GASTRECTOMY W ANAST | Operative |
| 39.52 | ANEURYSM REPAIR NEC | Operative | 43.8 | OTH PARTIAL GASTRECTOMY | Operative |

| Code | Description | Operative Status | Code | Description | Operative Status |
|------|-------------|------------------|------|-------------|------------------|
| 43.89 | PARTIAL GASTRECTOMY NEC | Operative | 46.03 | LG BOWEL EXTERIORIZATION | Operative |
| 43.9 | TOTAL GASTRECTOMY | Operative | 46.1 | COLOSTOMY | Mixed (3, 1) |
| 43.99 | TOTAL GASTRECTOMY NEC | Operative | 46.10 | COLOSTOMY NOS | Operative |
| 44.0 | VAGOTOMY | Operative | 46.11 | TEMPORARY COLOSTOMY | Operative |
| 44.01 | TRUNCAL VAGOTOMY | Operative | 46.13 | PERMANENT COLOSTOMY | Operative |
| 44.1 | GASTRIC DXTIC PX | Mixed (2, 4) | 46.2 | ILEOSTOMY | Mixed (4, 1) |
| 44.13 | GASTROSCOPY NEC | Non-Operative | 46.3 | OTHER ENTEROSTOMY | Non-Operative |
| 44.14 | CLSD (ENDO) GASTRIC BX | Non-Operative | 46.32 | PERC (ENDO) JEJUNOSTOMY | Non-Operative |
| 44.2 | PYLOROPLASTY | Mixed (2, 1) | 46.39 | ENTEROSTOMY NEC | Non-Operative |
| 44.22 | ENDO DILATION PYLORUS | Non-Operative | 46.4 | INTESTINAL STOMA REV | Operative |
| 44.29 | OTHER PYLOROPLASTY | Operative | 46.41 | SM BOWEL STOMA REVISION | Operative |
| 44.3 | GASTROENTEROSTOMY | Operative | 46.42 | PERICOLOSTOMY HERNIA REP | Operative |
| 44.31 | HIGH GASTRIC BYPASS | Operative | 46.43 | LG BOWEL STOMA REV NEC | Operative |
| 44.39 | GASTROENTEROSTOMY NEC | Operative | 46.5 | INTESTINAL STOMA CLOSURE | Operative |
| 44.4 | CNTRL PEPTIC ULCER HEMOR | Mixed (3, 3) | 46.51 | SM BOWEL STOMA CLOSURE | Operative |
| 44.41 | SUT GASTRIC ULCER SITE | Operative | 46.52 | LG BOWEL STOMA CLOSURE | Operative |
| 44.42 | SUT DUODENAL ULCER SITE | Operative | 46.6 | FIXATION OF INTESTINE | Operative |
| 44.43 | ENDO CNTRL GASTRIC BLEED | Non-Operative | 46.7 | OTHER INTESTINAL REPAIR | Operative |
| 44.5 | REVISION GASTRIC ANAST | Operative | 46.73 | SMALL BOWEL SUTURE NEC | Operative |
| 44.6 | OTHER GASTRIC REPAIR | Mixed (6, 1) | 46.74 | CLOSURE SMB FISTULA NEC | Operative |
| 44.61 | SUTURE GASTRIC LAC | Operative | 46.75 | SUTURE LG BOWEL LAC | Operative |
| 44.63 | CLOSE STOM FISTULA NEC | Operative | 46.79 | REPAIR OF INTESTINE NEC | Operative |
| 44.66 | CREAT EG SPHINCT COMPET | Operative | 46.8 | BOWEL DILATION & MANIP | Mixed (3, 1) |
| 44.69 | GASTRIC REPAIR NEC | Operative | 46.81 | INTRA-ABD SM BOWEL MANIP | Operative |
| 44.9 | OTHER STOMACH OPERATIONS | Mixed (3, 2) | 46.85 | DILATION OF INTESTINE | Non-Operative |
| 45.0 | ENTEROTOMY | Operative | 46.9 | OTHER INTESTINAL OPS | Mixed (5, 2) |
| 45.1 | SMALL BOWEL DXTIC PX | Mixed (2, 5) | 47.0 | APPENDECTOMY | Operative |
| 45.13 | SM BOWEL ENDOSCOPY NEC | Non-Operative | 47.01 | LAPSCP APPENDECTOMY | Operative |
| 45.14 | CLSD (ENDO) SM INTEST BX | Non-Operative | 47.09 | OTHER APPENDECTOMY | Operative |
| 45.16 | EGD WITH CLOSED BIOPSY | Non-Operative | 47.1 | INCIDENTAL APPENDECTOMY | Operative |
| 45.2 | LG INTESTINE DXTIC PX | Mixed (2, 7) | 47.11 | LAPSCP INCIDENTAL APPY | Operative |
| 45.22 | ENDO LG BOWEL THRU STOMA | Non-Operative | 47.2 | DRAIN APPENDICEAL ABSC | Operative |
| 45.23 | COLONOSCOPY | Non-Operative | 47.9 | OTHER APPENDICEAL OPS | Operative |
| 45.24 | FLEXIBLE SIGMOIDOSCOPY | Non-Operative | 48.0 | PROCTOTOMY | Operative |
| 45.25 | CLSD (ENDO) LG INTEST BX | Non-Operative | 48.1 | PROCTOSTOMY | Operative |
| 45.3 | LOC EXC/DESTR SMB LES | Mixed (4, 1) | 48.2 | RECTAL/PERIRECT DXTIC PX | Mixed (2, 5) |
| 45.30 | ENDO EXC/DESTR DUOD LES | Non-Operative | 48.23 | RIGID PROCTSIGMOIDOSCOPY | Non-Operative |
| 45.33 | LOC EXC SM BOWEL LES NEC | Operative | 48.24 | CLSD (ENDO) RECTAL BX | Non-Operative |
| 45.4 | LOC DESTR LG BOWEL LES | Mixed (2, 2) | 48.3 | LOC DESTR RECTAL LESION | Mixed (1, 5) |
| 45.41 | LOC EXC LG BOWEL LES | Operative | 48.35 | LOC EXC RECTAL LES/TISS | Operative |
| 45.42 | ENDO COLON POLYPECTOMY | Non-Operative | 48.36 | ENDO RECTAL POLYPECTOMY | Non-Operative |
| 45.43 | ENDO DESTR COLON LES NEC | Non-Operative | 48.4 | PULL-THRU RECT RESECTION | Operative |
| 45.5 | INTESTINAL SEG ISOLATION | Operative | 48.5 | ABD-PERINEAL RECT RESECT | Operative |
| 45.6 | OTHER SM BOWEL EXCISION | Operative | 48.6 | OTHER RECTAL RESECTION | Operative |
| 45.61 | MULT SEG SM BOWEL RESECT | Operative | 48.62 | ANT RECT RESECT W COLOST | Operative |
| 45.62 | PART SM BOWEL RESECT NEC | Operative | 48.63 | ANTERIOR RECT RESECT NEC | Operative |
| 45.7 | PART LG BOWEL EXCISION | Operative | 48.69 | RECTAL RESECTION NEC | Operative |
| 45.71 | MULT SEG LG BOWEL RESECT | Operative | 48.7 | REPAIR OF RECTUM | Operative |
| 45.72 | CECECTOMY | Operative | 48.76 | PROCTOPEXY NEC | Operative |
| 45.73 | RIGHT HEMICOLECTOMY | Operative | 48.8 | PERIRECT TISS INC/EXC | Operative |
| 45.74 | TRANSVERSE COLON RESECT | Operative | 48.81 | PERIRECTAL INCISION | Operative |
| 45.75 | LEFT HEMICOLECTOMY | Operative | 48.9 | OTH RECTAL/PERIRECT OP | Operative |
| 45.76 | SIGMOIDECTOMY | Operative | 49.0 | PERIANAL TISS INC/EXC | Mixed (3, 1) |
| 45.79 | PART LG BOWEL EXC NEC | Operative | 49.01 | INC PERIANAL ABSCESS | Operative |
| 45.8 | TOT INTRA-ABD COLECTOMY | Operative | 49.1 | INC/EXC OF ANAL FISTULA | Operative |
| 45.9 | INTESTINAL ANASTOMOSIS | Operative | 49.2 | ANAL & PERIANAL DXTIC PX | Non-Operative |
| 45.91 | SM-TO-SM BOWEL ANAST | Operative | 49.3 | LOC DESTR ANAL LES NEC | Mixed (1, 1) |
| 45.93 | SMALL-TO-LARGE BOWEL NEC | Operative | 49.39 | OTH LOC DESTR ANAL LES | Operative |
| 45.94 | LG-TO-LG BOWEL ANAST | Operative | 49.4 | HEMORRHOID PROCEDURES | Mixed (4, 4) |
| 46.0 | EXTERIORIZATION OF BOWEL | Operative | 49.46 | EXC OF HEMORRHOIDS | Operative |
| 46.01 | SM BOWEL EXTERIORIZATION | Operative | 49.5 | ANAL SPHINCTER DIVISION | Operative |

| Code | Description | Operative Status | Code | Description | Operative Status |
|------|-------------|------------------|------|-------------|------------------|
| 49.6 | EXCISION OF ANUS | Operative | 53.05 | UNILAT REP IH/GRAFT NOS | Operative |
| 49.7 | REPAIR OF ANUS | Operative | 53.1 | BILAT IH REPAIR | Operative |
| 49.79 | ANAL SPHINCTER REP NEC | Operative | 53.10 | BILAT IH REPAIR NOS | Operative |
| 49.9 | OTH OPERATIONS ON ANUS | Operative | 53.12 | BILAT INDIRECT IH REPAIR | Operative |
| 50.0 | HEPATOTOMY | Operative | 53.14 | BILAT DIRECT IH REP-GRFT | Operative |
| 50.1 | HEPATIC DXTIC PX | Mixed (2, 1) | 53.17 | BILAT IH REP-GRAFT NOS | Operative |
| 50.11 | CLSD (PERC) LIVER BIOPSY | Non-Operative | 53.2 | UNILAT FH REPAIR | Operative |
| 50.12 | OPEN BIOPSY OF LIVER | Operative | 53.21 | UNILAT FH REP W GRAFT | Operative |
| 50.2 | LOC EXC/DESTR LIVER LES | Operative | 53.29 | UNILAT FH REP NEC | Operative |
| 50.22 | PARTIAL HEPATECTOMY | Operative | 53.3 | BILAT FH REPAIR | Operative |
| 50.29 | DESTR HEPATIC LESION NEC | Operative | 53.4 | UMBILICAL HERNIA REPAIR | Operative |
| 50.3 | HEPATIC LOBECTOMY | Operative | 53.41 | UMB HERNIA REPAIR-GRAFT | Operative |
| 50.4 | TOTAL HEPATECTOMY | Operative | 53.49 | UMB HERNIA REPAIR NEC | Operative |
| 50.5 | LIVER TRANSPLANT | Operative | 53.5 | REP OTH ABD WALL HERNIA | Operative |
| 50.59 | LIVER TRANSPLANT NEC | Operative | 53.51 | INCISIONAL HERNIA REPAIR | Operative |
| 50.6 | REPAIR OF LIVER | Operative | 53.59 | ABD WALL HERNIA REP NEC | Operative |
| 50.61 | CLOSURE OF LIVER LAC | Operative | 53.6 | REP OTH ABD HERNIA-GRAFT | Operative |
| 50.9 | OTHER LIVER OPERATIONS | Non-Operative | 53.61 | INC HERNIA REPAIR-GRAFT | Operative |
| 50.91 | PERC LIVER ASPIRATION | Non-Operative | 53.69 | ABD HERNIA REP-GRFT NEC | Operative |
| 51.0 | GB INC & CHOLECYSTOSTOMY | Mixed (3, 1) | 53.7 | ABD REP-DIAPH HERNIA | Operative |
| 51.1 | BILIARY TRACT DXTIC PX | Mixed (2, 5) | 53.8 | REPAIR DH, THOR APPR | Operative |
| 51.10 | ERCP | Non-Operative | 53.80 | REP DH, THOR APPR NOS | Operative |
| 51.14 | CLSD BD/SPHINCT ODDI BX | Non-Operative | 53.9 | OTHER HERNIA REPAIR | Operative |
| 51.2 | CHOLECYSTECTOMY | Operative | 54.0 | ABDOMINAL WALL INCISION | Operative |
| 51.22 | CHOLECYSTECTOMY NOS | Operative | 54.1 | LAPAROTOMY | Operative |
| 51.23 | LAPSCP CHOLECYSTECTOMY | Operative | 54.11 | EXPLORATORY LAPAROTOMY | Operative |
| 51.3 | BILIARY TRACT ANAST | Operative | 54.12 | REOPEN RECENT LAP SITE | Operative |
| 51.32 | GB-TO-INTESTINE ANAST | Operative | 54.19 | LAPAROTOMY NEC | Operative |
| 51.36 | CHOLEDOCHOENTEROSTOMY | Operative | 54.2 | ABD REGION DXTIC PX | Mixed (4, 2) |
| 51.4 | INC BILE DUCT OBSTR | Operative | 54.21 | LAPAROSCOPY | Operative |
| 51.5 | OTHER BILE DUCT INCISION | Operative | 54.23 | PERITONEAL BIOPSY | Operative |
| 51.6 | LOC EXC BD & S OF O LES | Mixed (4, 1) | 54.24 | CLSD BX INTRA-ABD MASS | Non-Operative |
| 51.7 | REPAIR OF BILE DUCTS | Operative | 54.3 | EXC/DESTR ABD WALL LES | Operative |
| 51.8 | SPHINCTER OF ODDI OP NEC | Mixed (4, 5) | 54.4 | EXC/DESTR PERITON TISS | Operative |
| 51.84 | ENDO AMPULLA & BD DILAT | Non-Operative | 54.5 | PERITONEAL ADHESIOLYSIS | Operative |
| 51.85 | ENDO SPHINCTOT/PAPILLOT | Non-Operative | 54.51 | LAPSCP PERITON ADHESIO | Operative |
| 51.87 | ENDO INSERT BD STENT | Non-Operative | 54.59 | PERITON ADHESIOLYSIS NEC | Operative |
| 51.88 | ENDO RMVL BILIARY STONE | Non-Operative | 54.6 | ABD WALL/PERITON SUTURE | Operative |
| 51.9 | OTHER BILIARY TRACT OPS | Mixed (6, 2) | 54.61 | RECLOSE POSTOP DISRUPT | Operative |
| 51.98 | PERC OP ON BIL TRACT NEC | Non-Operative | 54.7 | OTH ABD WALL PERITON REP | Operative |
| 52.0 | PANCREATOTOMY | Operative | 54.9 | OTHER ABD REGION OPS | Mixed (4, 5) |
| 52.01 | DRAIN PANC CYST BY CATH | Operative | 54.91 | PERC ABD DRAINAGE | Non-Operative |
| 52.1 | PANCREATIC DXTIC PX | Mixed (2, 3) | 54.92 | RMVL FB PERITON CAVITY | Operative |
| 52.11 | PANC ASP (NEEDLE) BX | Non-Operative | 54.93 | CREATE CUTANEOPERIT FIST | Operative |
| 52.2 | PANC/PANC DUCT LES DESTR | Mixed (1, 1) | 54.94 | CREAT PERITONEOVAS SHUNT | Operative |
| 52.3 | PANCREATIC CYST MARSUP | Operative | 54.95 | PERITONEAL INCISION | Operative |
| 52.4 | INT DRAIN PANC CYST | Operative | 54.98 | PERITONEAL DIALYSIS | Non-Operative |
| 52.5 | PARTIAL PANCREATECTOMY | Operative | 55.0 | NEPHROTOMY & NEPHROSTOMY | Operative |
| 52.52 | DISTAL PANCREATECTOMY | Operative | 55.01 | NEPHROTOMY | Operative |
| 52.6 | TOTAL PANCREATECTOMY | Operative | 55.02 | NEPHROSTOMY | Operative |
| 52.7 | RAD PANC/DUODENECTOMY | Operative | 55.03 | PERC NEPHROSTOMY-NO FRAG | Operative |
| 52.8 | TRANSPLANT OF PANCREAS | Mixed (4, 3) | 55.04 | PERC NEPHROSTOMY W FRAG | Operative |
| 52.9 | OTHER OPS ON PANCREAS | Mixed (4, 4) | 55.1 | PYELOTOMY & PYELOSTOMY | Operative |
| 52.93 | ENDO INSERT PANC STENT | Non-Operative | 55.11 | PYELOTOMY | Operative |
| 52.96 | PANCREATIC ANASTOMOSIS | Operative | 55.2 | RENAL DIAGNOSTIC PX | Mixed (2, 3) |
| 53.0 | UNILAT IH REPAIR | Operative | 55.23 | CLSD (PERC) RENAL BIOPSY | Non-Operative |
| 53.00 | UNILAT IH REPAIR NOS | Operative | 55.3 | LOC EXC/DESTR RENAL LES | Operative |
| 53.01 | UNILAT REP DIRECT IH | Operative | 55.39 | LOC DESTR RENAL LES NEC | Operative |
| 53.02 | UNILAT REP INDIRECT IH | Operative | 55.4 | PARTIAL NEPHRECTOMY | Operative |
| 53.03 | UNILAT REP DIR IH/GRAFT | Operative | 55.5 | COMPLETE NEPHRECTOMY | Operative |
| 53.04 | UNILAT INDIRECT IH/GRAFT | Operative | 55.51 | NEPHROURETERECTOMY | Operative |

| Code | Description | Operative Status | Code | Description | Operative Status |
|------|-------------|------------------|------|-------------|------------------|
| 55.53 | REJECTED KID NEPHRECTOMY | Operative | 59.4 | SUPRAPUBIC SLING OP | Operative |
| 55.6 | KIDNEY TRANSPLANT | Operative | 59.5 | RETROPUBIC URETHRAL SUSP | Operative |
| 55.69 | KIDNEY TRANSPLANT NEC | Operative | 59.6 | PARAURETHRAL SUSPENSION | Operative |
| 55.7 | NEPHROPEXY | Operative | 59.7 | OTH URINARY INCONT REP | Mixed (2, 1) |
| 55.8 | OTHER KIDNEY REPAIR | Operative | 59.71 | LEVATOR MUSC SUSPENSION | Operative |
| 55.87 | CORRECTION OF UPJ | Operative | 59.79 | URIN INCONT REPAIR NEC | Operative |
| 55.9 | OTHER RENAL OPERATIONS | Mixed (4, 5) | 59.8 | URETERAL CATHETERIZATION | Non-Operative |
| 55.93 | REPL NEPHROSTOMY TUBE | Non-Operative | 59.9 | OTHER URINARY SYSTEM OPS | Mixed (2, 4) |
| 56.0 | TU RMVL URETERAL OBSTR | Operative | 60.0 | INCISION OF PROSTATE | Operative |
| 56.1 | URETERAL MEATOTOMY | Operative | 60.1 | PROS/SEM VESICL DXTIC PX | Mixed (5, 2) |
| 56.2 | URETEROTOMY | Operative | 60.11 | CLSD (PERC) PROSTATIC BX | Non-Operative |
| 56.3 | URETERAL DIAGNOSTIC PX | Mixed (2, 4) | 60.2 | TU PROSTATECTOMY | Operative |
| 56.31 | URETEROSCOPY | Non-Operative | 60.21 | TULIP PROCEDURE | Operative |
| 56.4 | URETERECTOMY | Operative | 60.29 | TU PROSTATECTOMY NEC | Operative |
| 56.41 | PARTIAL URETERECTOMY | Operative | 60.3 | SUPRAPUBIC PROSTATECTOMY | Operative |
| 56.5 | CUTAN URETERO-ILEOSTOMY | Operative | 60.4 | RETROPUBIC PROSTATECTOMY | Operative |
| 56.51 | FORM CUTAN ILEOURETEROST | Operative | 60.5 | RADICAL PROSTATECTOMY | Operative |
| 56.6 | EXT URIN DIVERSION NEC | Operative | 60.6 | OTHER PROSTATECTOMY | Operative |
| 56.7 | OTHER URETERAL ANAST | Operative | 60.7 | SEMINAL VESICLE OPS | Mixed (3, 1) |
| 56.74 | URETERONEOCYSTOSTOMY | Operative | 60.8 | PERIPROSTATIC INC OR EXC | Operative |
| 56.8 | REPAIR OF URETER | Operative | 60.9 | OTHER PROSTATIC OPS | Mixed (4, 2) |
| 56.9 | OTHER URETERAL OPERATION | Mixed (5, 1) | 60.94 | CNTRL POSTOP PROS HEMOR | Operative |
| 57.0 | TU BLADDER CLEARANCE | Non-Operative | 61.0 | SCROTUM & TUNICA VAG I&D | Non-Operative |
| 57.1 | CYSTOTOMY & CYSTOSTOMY | Mixed (3, 2) | 61.1 | SCROTUM/TUNICA DXTIC PX | Non-Operative |
| 57.17 | PERCUTANEOUS CYSTOSTOMY | Non-Operative | 61.2 | EXCISION OF HYDROCELE | Operative |
| 57.18 | S/P CYSTOSTOMY NEC | Operative | 61.3 | SCROTAL LES EXC/DESTR | Non-Operative |
| 57.19 | CYSTOTOMY NEC | Operative | 61.4 | SCROTUM & TUNICA VAG REP | Mixed (2, 1) |
| 57.2 | VESICOSTOMY | Operative | 61.9 | OTH SCROT/TUNICA VAG OPS | Mixed (2, 1) |
| 57.3 | BLADDER DIAGNOSTIC PX | Mixed (3, 2) | 62.0 | INCISION OF TESTIS | Operative |
| 57.32 | CYSTOSCOPY NEC | Non-Operative | 62.1 | TESTES DXTIC PX | Mixed (2, 1) |
| 57.33 | CLSD (TU) BLADDER BIOPSY | Operative | 62.2 | TESTICULAR LES DESTR/EXC | Operative |
| 57.4 | TU EXC/DESTR BLADDER LES | Operative | 62.3 | UNILATERAL ORCHIECTOMY | Operative |
| 57.49 | TU DESTR BLADDER LES NEC | Operative | 62.4 | BILATERAL ORCHIECTOMY | Operative |
| 57.5 | BLADDER LES DESTR NEC | Operative | 62.41 | RMVL BOTH TESTES | Operative |
| 57.59 | OTH BLADDER LESION DESTR | Operative | 62.5 | ORCHIOPEXY | Operative |
| 57.6 | PARTIAL CYSTECTOMY | Operative | 62.6 | REPAIR OF TESTES | Operative |
| 57.7 | TOTAL CYSTECTOMY | Operative | 62.7 | INSERT TESTICULAR PROSTH | Operative |
| 57.71 | RADICAL CYSTECTOMY | Operative | 62.9 | OTHER TESTICULAR OPS | Mixed (1, 2) |
| 57.8 | OTH URIN BLADDER REPAIR | Operative | 63.0 | SPERMATIC CORD DXTIC PX | Mixed (1, 1) |
| 57.83 | ENTEROVESICAL FIST REP | Operative | 63.1 | EXC SPERMATIC VARICOCELE | Operative |
| 57.84 | REP OTH FISTULA BLADDER | Operative | 63.2 | EXC EPIDIDYMIS CYST | Operative |
| 57.89 | BLADDER REPAIR NEC | Operative | 63.3 | EXC SPERM CORD LES NEC | Operative |
| 57.9 | OTHER BLADDER OPERATIONS | Mixed (6, 3) | 63.4 | EPIDIDYMECTOMY | Operative |
| 57.91 | BLADDER SPHINCTEROTOMY | Operative | 63.5 | SPERM CORD/EPID REPAIR | Mixed (3, 1) |
| 57.93 | CONTROL BLADDER HEMOR | Operative | 63.6 | VASOTOMY | Non-Operative |
| 57.94 | INSERT INDWELL URIN CATH | Non-Operative | 63.7 | VASECTOMY & VAS DEF LIG | Non-Operative |
| 58.0 | URETHROTOMY | Operative | 63.8 | VAS DEF & EPID REPAIR | Mixed (5, 1) |
| 58.1 | URETHRAL MEATOTOMY | Operative | 63.9 | OTH SPERM CORD/EPID OPS | Mixed (5, 1) |
| 58.2 | URETHRAL DIAGNOSTIC PX | Non-Operative | 64.0 | CIRCUMCISION | Operative |
| 58.3 | EXC/DESTR URETHRAL LES | Non-Operative | 64.1 | PENILE DIAGNOSTIC PX | Mixed (1, 1) |
| 58.4 | REPAIR OF URETHRA | Operative | 64.2 | LOC EXC/DESTR PENILE LES | Operative |
| 58.45 | HYPOSPAD/EPISPADIAS REP | Operative | 64.3 | AMPUTATION OF PENIS | Operative |
| 58.49 | URETHRAL REPAIR NEC | Operative | 64.4 | PENILE REP/PLASTIC OPS | Operative |
| 58.5 | URETHRAL STRICTURE REL | Operative | 64.5 | SEX TRANSFORMATION NEC | Operative |
| 58.6 | URETHRAL DILATION | Non-Operative | 64.9 | OTHER MALE GENITAL OPS | Mixed (7, 2) |
| 58.9 | OTHER URETHRAL OPS | Operative | 64.96 | RMVL INT PENILE PROSTH | Operative |
| 58.93 | IMPLANTATION OF AUS | Operative | 64.97 | INSERT OR REPL IPP | Operative |
| 59.0 | RETROPERITON DISSECTION | Operative | 65.0 | OOPHOROTOMY | Operative |
| 59.1 | PERIVESICAL INCISION | Operative | 65.1 | DXTIC PX ON OVARIES | Operative |
| 59.2 | PERIRENAL DXTIC PX | Operative | 65.2 | LOC EXC/DESTR OVARY LES | Operative |
| 59.3 | URETHROVES JUNCT PLICAT | Operative | 65.25 | LAPSCP OV LES EXC NEC | Operative |

| Code | Description | Operative Status | Code | Description | Operative Status |
|------|-------------|------------------|------|-------------|------------------|
| 65.29 | LOC EXC/DESTR OV LES NEC | Operative | 69.02 | D&C POST DEL OR AB | Operative |
| 65.3 | UNILATERAL OOPHORECTOMY | Operative | 69.09 | D&C NEC | Operative |
| 65.31 | LAPSCP UNILAT OOPHORECT | Operative | 69.1 | EXC/DESTR UTER/SUPP LES | Operative |
| 65.39 | UNILAT OOPHORECTOMY NEC | Operative | 69.19 | EXC UTER/SUPP STRUCT NEC | Operative |
| 65.4 | UNILATERAL S-O | Operative | 69.2 | UTERINE SUPP STRUCT REP | Operative |
| 65.41 | LAPSCP UNILATERAL S-O | Operative | 69.3 | PARACERV UTERINE DENERV | Operative |
| 65.49 | UNILATERAL S-O NEC | Operative | 69.4 | UTERINE REPAIR | Operative |
| 65.5 | BILATERAL OOPHORECTOMY | Operative | 69.5 | ASP CURETTAGE UTERUS | Mixed (2, 1) |
| 65.51 | RMVL BOTH OVARIES NEC | Operative | 69.51 | ASP CURETTAGE-PREG TERM | Operative |
| 65.6 | BILAT SALPINGO-OOPHORECT | Operative | 69.52 | ASP CURETTE POST DEL/AB | Operative |
| 65.61 | RMVL BOTH OV & FALL NEC | Operative | 69.59 | ASP CURETTAGE UTERUS NEC | Non-Operative |
| 65.62 | RMVL REM OV & FALL NEC | Operative | 69.6 | MENSTRUAL EXTRACTION | Non-Operative |
| 65.63 | LAPSCP RMVL BOTH OV/FALL | Operative | 69.7 | INSERTION OF IUD | Non-Operative |
| 65.7 | REPAIR OF OVARY | Operative | 69.9 | OTHER OPS UTERUS/ADNEXA | Mixed (4, 5) |
| 65.8 | TUBO-OVARIAN ADHESIO | Operative | 69.93 | INSERTION OF LAMINARIA | Non-Operative |
| 65.81 | LAPSCP ADHESIO OV/FALL | Operative | 69.96 | RMVL CERVICAL CERCLAGE | Non-Operative |
| 65.89 | ADHESIO OV/FALL TUBE NEC | Operative | 70.0 | CULDOCENTESIS | Non-Operative |
| 65.9 | OTHER OVARIAN OPERATIONS | Operative | 70.1 | INC VAGINA & CUL-DE-SAC | Mixed (3, 1) |
| 65.91 | ASPIRATION OF OVARY | Operative | 70.12 | CULDOTOMY | Operative |
| 66.0 | SALPINGOSTOMY/SALPINGOT | Operative | 70.14 | VAGINOTOMY NEC | Operative |
| 66.02 | SALPINGOSTOMY | Operative | 70.2 | VAG/CUL-DE-SAC DXTIC PX | Mixed (3, 2) |
| 66.1 | FALLOPIAN TUBE DXTIC PX | Operative | 70.3 | LOC EXC/DESTR VAG/CUL | Operative |
| 66.2 | BILAT ENDO OCCL FALL | Operative | 70.33 | EXC/DESTR VAG LESION | Operative |
| 66.22 | BILAT ENDO LIG/DIV FALL | Operative | 70.4 | VAGINAL OBLITERATION | Operative |
| 66.29 | BILAT ENDO OCCL FALL NEC | Operative | 70.5 | CYSTOCELE/RECTOCELE REP | Operative |
| 66.3 | OTH BILAT FALL DESTR/EXC | Operative | 70.50 | REP CYSTOCELE/RECTOCELE | Operative |
| 66.32 | BILAT FALL LIG & DIV NEC | Operative | 70.51 | CYSTOCELE REPAIR | Operative |
| 66.39 | BILAT FALL DESTR NEC | Operative | 70.52 | RECTOCELE REPAIR | Operative |
| 66.4 | TOT UNILAT SALPINGECTOMY | Operative | 70.6 | VAGINAL CONSTR/RECONST | Operative |
| 66.5 | TOT BILAT SALPINGECTOMY | Operative | 70.7 | OTHER VAGINAL REPAIR | Operative |
| 66.6 | OTHER SALPINGECTOMY | Operative | 70.71 | SUTURE VAGINA LACERATION | Operative |
| 66.61 | EXC/DESTR FALL LES | Operative | 70.73 | REP RECTOVAGINAL FISTULA | Operative |
| 66.62 | RMVL FALL & TUBAL PREG | Operative | 70.77 | VAGINAL SUSP & FIXATION | Operative |
| 66.69 | PARTIAL FALL RMVL NEC | Operative | 70.79 | VAGINAL REPAIR NEC | Operative |
| 66.7 | REPAIR OF FALLOPIAN TUBE | Operative | 70.8 | VAGINAL VAULT OBLIT | Operative |
| 66.79 | FALL TUBE REPAIR NEC | Operative | 70.9 | OTH VAG & CUL-DE-SAC OPS | Operative |
| 66.8 | FALL TUBE INSUFFLATION | Non-Operative | 70.92 | CUL-DE-SAC OPERATION NEC | Operative |
| 66.9 | OTHER FALLOPIAN TUBE OPS | Mixed (7, 1) | 71.0 | INC VULVA & PERINEUM | Operative |
| 67.0 | CERVICAL CANAL DILATION | Non-Operative | 71.09 | INC VULVA/PERINEUM NEC | Operative |
| 67.1 | CERVICAL DIAGNOSTIC PX | Operative | 71.1 | VULVAR DIAGNOSTIC PX | Operative |
| 67.12 | CERVICAL BIOPSY NEC | Operative | 71.2 | BARTHOLIN'S GLAND OPS | Mixed (4, 1) |
| 67.2 | CONIZATION OF CERVIX | Operative | 71.3 | LOC VULVAR/PERI EXC NEC | Operative |
| 67.3 | EXC/DESTR CERV LES NEC | Operative | 71.4 | OPERATIONS ON CLITORIS | Operative |
| 67.4 | AMPUTATION OF CERVIX | Operative | 71.5 | RADICAL VULVECTOMY | Operative |
| 67.5 | INT CERVICAL OS REPAIR | Operative | 71.6 | OTHER VULVECTOMY | Operative |
| 67.6 | OTHER REPAIR OF CERVIX | Operative | 71.61 | UNILATERAL VULVECTOMY | Operative |
| 68.0 | HYSTEROTOMY | Operative | 71.7 | VULVAR & PERINEAL REPAIR | Operative |
| 68.1 | UTER/ADNEXA DXTIC PX | Mixed (5, 2) | 71.71 | SUTURE VULVAR/PERI LAC | Operative |
| 68.16 | CLSD UTERINE BX | Operative | 71.79 | VULVAR/PERINEUM REP NEC | Operative |
| 68.2 | UTERINE LES EXC/DESTR | Operative | 71.8 | OTHER VULVAR OPERATIONS | Operative |
| 68.29 | UTER LES EXC/DESTR NEC | Operative | 71.9 | OTHER FEMALE GENITAL OPS | Operative |
| 68.3 | SUBTOT ABD HYSTERECTOMY | Operative | 72.0 | LOW FORCEPS OPERATION | Non-Operative |
| 68.4 | TOTAL ABD HYSTERECTOMY | Operative | 72.1 | LOW FORCEPS W EPISIOTOMY | Non-Operative |
| 68.5 | VAGINAL HYSTERECTOMY | Operative | 72.2 | MID FORCEPS OPERATION | Non-Operative |
| 68.51 | LAVH | Operative | 72.21 | MID FORCEPS W EPISIOTOMY | Non-Operative |
| 68.59 | VAGINAL HYSTERECTOMY NEC | Operative | 72.29 | MID FORCEPS OP NEC | Non-Operative |
| 68.6 | RADICAL ABD HYSTERECTOMY | Operative | 72.3 | HIGH FORCEPS OPERATION | Non-Operative |
| 68.7 | RADICAL VAG HYSTERECTOMY | Operative | 72.4 | FORCEPS ROT FETAL HEAD | Non-Operative |
| 68.8 | PELVIC EVISCERATION | Operative | 72.5 | BREECH EXTRACTION | Non-Operative |
| 68.9 | HYSTERECTOMY NEC & NOS | Operative | 72.52 | PART BREECH EXTRACT NEC | Non-Operative |
| 69.0 | UTERINE D&C | Operative | 72.54 | TOT BREECH EXTRACT NEC | Non-Operative |

| Code | Description | Operative Status | Code | Description | Operative Status |
|------|-------------|------------------|------|-------------|------------------|
| 72.6 | FORCEPS-AFTERCOMING HEAD | Non-Operative | 76.9 | OTH OPS FACIAL BONE/JT | Mixed (5, 3) |
| 72.7 | VACUUM EXTRACTION DEL | Non-Operative | 77.0 | SEQUESTRECTOMY | Operative |
| 72.71 | VED W EPISIOTOMY | Non-Operative | 77.1 | OTHER BONE INC W/O DIV | Operative |
| 72.79 | VACUUM EXTRACT DEL NEC | Non-Operative | 77.2 | WEDGE OSTEOTOMY | Operative |
| 72.8 | INSTRUMENTAL DEL NEC | Non-Operative | 77.25 | FEMORAL WEDGE OSTEOTOMY | Operative |
| 72.9 | INSTRUMENTAL DEL NOS | Non-Operative | 77.27 | TIB & FIB WEDGE OSTY | Operative |
| 73.0 | ARTIFICIAL RUPT MEMBRANE | Non-Operative | 77.3 | OTHER DIVISION OF BONE | Operative |
| 73.01 | INDUCTION LABOR BY AROM | Non-Operative | 77.35 | FEMORAL DIVISION NEC | Operative |
| 73.09 | ARTIF RUPT MEMBRANES NEC | Non-Operative | 77.37 | TIBIA/FIBULA DIV NEC | Operative |
| 73.1 | SURG INDUCTION LABOR NEC | Non-Operative | 77.39 | BONE DIVISION NEC | Operative |
| 73.2 | INT/COMB VERSION/EXTRACT | Non-Operative | 77.4 | BIOPSY OF BONE | Operative |
| 73.3 | FAILED FORCEPS | Non-Operative | 77.41 | CHEST CAGE BONE BIOPSY | Operative |
| 73.4 | MEDICAL INDUCTION LABOR | Non-Operative | 77.45 | FEMORAL BIOPSY | Operative |
| 73.5 | MANUALLY ASSISTED DEL | Non-Operative | 77.47 | TIBIA & FIBULA BIOPSY | Operative |
| 73.51 | MANUAL ROT FETAL HEAD | Non-Operative | 77.49 | BONE BIOPSY NEC | Operative |
| 73.59 | MANUAL ASSISTED DEL NEC | Non-Operative | 77.5 | TOE DEFORMITY EXC/REP | Operative |
| 73.6 | EPISIOTOMY | Non-Operative | 77.51 | BUNIONECT/STC/OSTY | Operative |
| 73.8 | FETAL OPS-FACILITATE DEL | Non-Operative | 77.6 | LOC EXC BONE LESION | Operative |
| 73.9 | OTH OPS ASSISTING DEL | Mixed (2, 3) | 77.61 | EXC CHEST CAGE BONE LES | Operative |
| 74.0 | CLASSICAL CD | Operative | 77.65 | LOC EXC BONE LES FEMUR | Operative |
| 74.1 | LOW CERVICAL CD | Operative | 77.67 | LOC EXC LES TIBIA/FIBULA | Operative |
| 74.2 | EXTRAPERITONEAL CD | Operative | 77.68 | LOC EXC LES MT/TARSAL | Operative |
| 74.3 | RMVL EXTRATUBAL PREG | Operative | 77.69 | LOC EXC BONE LESION NEC | Operative |
| 74.4 | CESAREAN SECTION NEC | Operative | 77.7 | EXC BONE FOR GRAFT | Operative |
| 74.9 | CESAREAN SECTION NOS | Operative | 77.79 | EXC BONE FOR GRAFT NEC | Operative |
| 74.99 | OTHER CD TYPE NOS | Operative | 77.8 | OTHER PARTIAL OSTECTOMY | Operative |
| 75.0 | INTRA-AMNIO INJECT-AB | Non-Operative | 77.81 | OTH CHEST CAGE OSTECTOMY | Operative |
| 75.1 | DIAGNOSTIC AMNIOCENTESIS | Non-Operative | 77.85 | PART OSTECTOMY-FEMUR | Operative |
| 75.2 | INTRAUTERINE TRANSFUSION | Non-Operative | 77.86 | PARTIAL PATELLECTOMY | Operative |
| 75.3 | IU OPS FETUS & AMNIO NEC | Mixed (1, 6) | 77.88 | PART OSTECTOMY-MT/TARSAL | Operative |
| 75.32 | FETAL EKG (SCALP) | Non-Operative | 77.89 | PARTIAL OSTECTOMY NEC | Operative |
| 75.34 | FETAL MONITORING NOS | Non-Operative | 77.9 | TOTAL OSTECTOMY | Operative |
| 75.35 | DXTIC PX FETUS/AMNIO NEC | Non-Operative | 77.91 | TOT CHEST CAGE OSTECTOMY | Operative |
| 75.4 | MAN RMVL OF RET PLACENTA | Non-Operative | 78.0 | BONE GRAFT | Operative |
| 75.5 | REP CURRENT OB LAC UTER | Operative | 78.05 | BONE GRAFT TO FEMUR | Operative |
| 75.51 | REP CURRENT OB LAC CERV | Operative | 78.07 | BONE GRAFT TIBIA/FIBULA | Operative |
| 75.6 | REP OTH CURRENT OB LAC | Mixed (1, 2) | 78.1 | APPL EXT FIXATION DEVICE | Operative |
| 75.61 | REP OB LAC BLAD/URETHRA | Operative | 78.13 | APPL EXT FIX RAD/ULNA | Operative |
| 75.62 | REP OB LAC RECTUM/ANUS | Non-Operative | 78.15 | APPL EXT FIX DEV FEMUR | Operative |
| 75.69 | REP CURRENT OB LAC NEC | Non-Operative | 78.17 | APPL EXT FIX DEV TIB/FIB | Operative |
| 75.7 | PP MANUAL EXPLOR UTERUS | Non-Operative | 78.2 | LIMB SHORTENING PX | Operative |
| 75.8 | OB TAMPONADE UTERUS/VAG | Non-Operative | 78.25 | LIMB SHORT PX FEMUR | Operative |
| 75.9 | OTHER OBSTETRICAL OPS | Mixed (2, 3) | 78.3 | LIMB LENGTHENING PX | Operative |
| 76.0 | FACIAL BONE INCISION | Operative | 78.4 | OTHER BONE REPAIR | Operative |
| 76.1 | DXTIC PX FACIAL BONE/JT | Operative | 78.5 | INT FIX W/O FX REDUCTION | Operative |
| 76.2 | DESTR FACIAL BONE LES | Operative | 78.52 | INT FIX W/O RED HUMERUS | Operative |
| 76.3 | PARTIAL FACIAL OSTECTOMY | Operative | 78.55 | INT FIX W/O RED FEMUR | Operative |
| 76.31 | PARTIAL MANDIBULECTOMY | Operative | 78.57 | INT FIX W/O RED TIB/FIB | Operative |
| 76.4 | FACIAL BONE EXC/RECONST | Operative | 78.59 | INT FIX W/O FX RED NEC | Operative |
| 76.5 | TMJ ARTHROPLASTY | Operative | 78.6 | RMVL IMPL DEV FROM BONE | Operative |
| 76.6 | OTHER FACIAL BONE REPAIR | Operative | 78.63 | RMVL IMPL DEV RAD/ULNA | Operative |
| 76.62 | OPN OSTY MAND RAMUS | Operative | 78.65 | RMVL IMPL DEV FEMUR | Operative |
| 76.64 | MAND ORTHOGNATHIC OP NEC | Operative | 78.67 | RMVL IMPL DEV TIB & FIB | Operative |
| 76.65 | SEG OSTEOPLASTY MAXILLA | Operative | 78.69 | RMVL IMPL DEV SITE NEC | Operative |
| 76.66 | TOT OSTEOPLASTY MAXILLA | Operative | 78.7 | OSTEOCLASIS | Operative |
| 76.7 | REDUCTION OF FACIAL FX | Mixed (6, 4) | 78.8 | OTHER BONE DIAGNOSTIC PX | Operative |
| 76.72 | OPEN RED MALAR/ZMC FX | Operative | 78.9 | INSERT BONE GROWTH STIM | Operative |
| 76.74 | OPEN RED MAXILLARY FX | Operative | 79.0 | CLSD FX RED W/O INT FIX | Non-Operative |
| 76.75 | CLSD RED MANDIBULAR FX | Non-Operative | 79.01 | CLSD FX RED HUMERUS | Non-Operative |
| 76.76 | OPEN RED MANDIBULAR FX | Operative | 79.02 | CLSD RED FX RADIUS/ULNA | Non-Operative |
| 76.79 | OPEN RED FACIAL FX NEC | Operative | 79.05 | CLSD FX RED FEMUR | Non-Operative |

| Code | Description | Operative Status | Code | Description | Operative Status |
|------|-------------|------------------|------|-------------|------------------|
| 79.06 | CLSD FX RED TIBIA/FIBULA | Non-Operative | 81.07 | LAT TRANS LUMBAR FUSION | Operative |
| 79.1 | CLSD FX RED W INT FIX | Operative | 81.08 | POSTERIOR LUMBAR FUSION | Operative |
| 79.11 | CRIF HUMERUS | Operative | 81.09 | REFUSION OF SPINE | Operative |
| 79.12 | CRIF RADIUS/ULNA | Operative | 81.1 | FOOT & ANKLE ARTHRODESIS | Operative |
| 79.15 | CRIF FEMUR | Operative | 81.11 | ANKLE FUSION | Operative |
| 79.16 | CRIF TIBIA & FIBULA | Operative | 81.12 | TRIPLE ARTHRODESIS | Operative |
| 79.2 | OPEN FRACTURE REDUCTION | Operative | 81.13 | SUBTALAR FUSION | Operative |
| 79.26 | OPEN RED TIBIA/FIB FX | Operative | 81.2 | ARTHRODESIS OF OTH JOINT | Operative |
| 79.3 | OPEN FX REDUCT W INT FIX | Operative | 81.4 | LOW LIMB JOINT REP NEC | Operative |
| 79.31 | ORIF HUMERUS | Operative | 81.40 | REPAIR OF HIP NEC | Operative |
| 79.32 | ORIF RADIUS/ULNA | Operative | 81.44 | PATELLAR STABILIZATION | Operative |
| 79.33 | ORIF CARPALS/METACARPALS | Operative | 81.45 | CRUCIATE LIG REPAIR NEC | Operative |
| 79.34 | ORIF FINGER | Operative | 81.47 | OTHER REPAIR OF KNEE | Operative |
| 79.35 | ORIF FEMUR | Operative | 81.5 | JOINT REPL LOWER EXT | Operative |
| 79.36 | ORIF TIBIA & FIBULA | Operative | 81.51 | TOTAL HIP REPLACEMENT | Operative |
| 79.37 | ORIF METATARSAL/TARSAL | Operative | 81.52 | PARTIAL HIP REPLACEMENT | Operative |
| 79.39 | ORIF BONE NEC X FACIAL | Operative | 81.53 | HIP REPLACEMENT REVISION | Operative |
| 79.4 | CR SEP EPIPHYSIS | Operative | 81.54 | TOTAL KNEE REPLACEMENT | Operative |
| 79.5 | OPEN RED SEP EPIPHYSIS | Operative | 81.55 | KNEE REPLACEMENT REV | Operative |
| 79.6 | OPEN FX SITE DEBRIDEMENT | Operative | 81.7 | HAND/FINGER ARTHROPLASTY | Operative |
| 79.62 | DEBRIDE OPEN FX RAD/ULNA | Operative | 81.8 | SHOULD/ELB ARTHROPLASTY | Operative |
| 79.64 | DEBRIDE OPEN FX FINGER | Operative | 81.80 | TOTAL SHOULDER REPL | Operative |
| 79.66 | DEBRIDE OPN FX TIBIA/FIB | Operative | 81.81 | PARTIAL SHOULDER REPL | Operative |
| 79.7 | CLOSED RED DISLOCATION | Non-Operative | 81.82 | REP RECUR SHOULD DISLOC | Operative |
| 79.71 | CLSD RED DISLOC SHOULDER | Non-Operative | 81.83 | SHOULD ARTHROPLASTY NEC | Operative |
| 79.75 | CLSD RED DISLOC HIP | Non-Operative | 81.84 | TOTAL ELBOW REPLACEMENT | Operative |
| 79.8 | OPEN RED DISLOCATION | Operative | 81.9 | OTHER JOINT STRUCTURE OP | Mixed (7, 2) |
| 79.85 | OPEN RED DISLOC HIP | Operative | 81.91 | ARTHROCENTESIS | Non-Operative |
| 79.9 | BONE INJURY OP NOS | Operative | 81.92 | INJECTION INTO JOINT | Non-Operative |
| 80.0 | ARTHROTOMY RMVL PROSTH | Operative | 82.0 | INC HAND SOFT TISSUE | Mixed (4, 1) |
| 80.05 | RMVL PROSTH HIP INC | Operative | 82.01 | EXPLOR TEND SHEATH HAND | Operative |
| 80.06 | RMVL PROSTH KNEE INC | Operative | 82.09 | INC SOFT TISSUE HAND NEC | Operative |
| 80.1 | OTHER ARTHROTOMY | Operative | 82.1 | DIV HAND MUSC/TEND/FASC | Operative |
| 80.11 | OTH ARTHROTOMY SHOULDER | Operative | 82.2 | EXC LES HAND SOFT TISSUE | Operative |
| 80.12 | OTH ARTHROTOMY ELBOW | Operative | 82.3 | OTH EXC HAND SOFT TISS | Operative |
| 80.14 | OTH ARTHROTOMY HAND | Operative | 82.4 | SUTURE HAND SOFT TISSUE | Operative |
| 80.15 | OTH ARTHROTOMY HIP | Operative | 82.44 | SUT FLEXOR TEND HAND NEC | Operative |
| 80.16 | OTH ARTHROTOMY KNEE | Operative | 82.45 | SUTURE HAND TENDON NEC | Operative |
| 80.2 | ARTHROSCOPY | Operative | 82.5 | HAND MUSC/TEND TRANSPL | Operative |
| 80.21 | SHOULDER ARTHROSCOPY | Operative | 82.6 | RECONSTRUCTION OF THUMB | Operative |
| 80.26 | KNEE ARTHROSCOPY | Operative | 82.7 | PLASTIC OP HND GRFT/IMPL | Operative |
| 80.3 | BIOPSY JOINT STRUCTURE | Non-Operative | 82.8 | OTHER PLASTIC OPS HAND | Operative |
| 80.4 | JT CAPSULE/LIG/CART DIV | Operative | 82.9 | OTH HAND SOFT TISSUE OPS | Mixed (2, 5) |
| 80.46 | KNEE STRUCTURE DIVISION | Operative | 83.0 | INC MUSC/TEND/FASC/BURSA | Operative |
| 80.5 | IV DISC EXC/DESTRUCTION | Mixed (3, 1) | 83.02 | MYOTOMY | Operative |
| 80.51 | IV DISC EXCISION | Operative | 83.03 | BURSOTOMY | Operative |
| 80.6 | EXC KNEE SEMILUNAR CART | Operative | 83.09 | SOFT TISSUE INCISION NEC | Operative |
| 80.7 | SYNOVECTOMY | Operative | 83.1 | MUSC/TEND/FASC DIVISION | Operative |
| 80.76 | KNEE SYNOVECTOMY | Operative | 83.12 | ADDUCTOR TENOTOMY OF HIP | Operative |
| 80.8 | OTH EXC/DESTR JOINT LES | Operative | 83.13 | OTHER TENOTOMY | Operative |
| 80.81 | DESTR SHOULDER LES NEC | Operative | 83.14 | FASCIOTOMY | Operative |
| 80.85 | DESTR HIP LESION NEC | Operative | 83.2 | SOFT TISSUE DXTIC PX | Operative |
| 80.86 | DESTR KNEE LESION NEC | Operative | 83.21 | SOFT TISSUE BIOPSY | Operative |
| 80.9 | OTHER JOINT EXCISION | Operative | 83.3 | EXC LES SOFT TISSUE | Operative |
| 81.0 | SPINAL FUSION | Operative | 83.32 | EXC LESION OF MUSCLE | Operative |
| 81.01 | ATLAS-AXIS SP FUSION | Operative | 83.39 | EXC LES SOFT TISSUE NEC | Operative |
| 81.02 | ANTERIOR CERV FUSION NEC | Operative | 83.4 | OTHER EXC MUSC/TEND/FASC | Operative |
| 81.03 | POST CERVICAL FUSION NEC | Operative | 83.45 | OTHER MYECTOMY | Operative |
| 81.04 | ANTERIOR DORSAL FUSION | Operative | 83.5 | BURSECTOMY | Operative |
| 81.05 | POSTERIOR DORSAL FUSION | Operative | 83.6 | SUTURE MUSC/TENDON/FASC | Operative |
| 81.06 | ANTERIOR LUMBAR FUSION | Operative | 83.63 | ROTATOR CUFF REPAIR | Operative |

| Code | Description | Operative Status | Code | Description | Operative Status |
|------|-------------|------------------|------|-------------|------------------|
| 83.64 | OTHER SUTURE OF TENDON | Operative | 86.28 | NONEXC DEBRIDEMENT WOUND | Non-Operative |
| 83.65 | OTHER MUSCLE/FASC SUTURE | Operative | 86.3 | OTH LOC EXC/DESTR SKIN | Non-Operative |
| 83.7 | MUSCLE/TENDON RECONST | Operative | 86.4 | RAD EXCISION SKIN LESION | Operative |
| 83.75 | TENDON TRANSF/TRANSPL | Operative | 86.5 | SKIN & SUBCU SUTURE | Non-Operative |
| 83.8 | MUSC/TEND/FASC OP NEC | Operative | 86.59 | SKIN SUTURE NEC | Non-Operative |
| 83.84 | CLUBFOOT RELEASE NEC | Operative | 86.6 | FREE SKIN GRAFT | Mixed (8, 1) |
| 83.85 | CHANGE IN M/T LENGTH NEC | Operative | 86.62 | HAND SKIN GRAFT NEC | Operative |
| 83.88 | OTHER PLASTIC OPS TENDON | Operative | 86.63 | FTHICK SKIN GRAFT NEC | Operative |
| 83.9 | OTHER CONN TISSUE OPS | Mixed (4, 5) | 86.69 | FREE SKIN GRAFT NEC | Operative |
| 83.94 | ASPIRATION OF BURSA | Non-Operative | 86.7 | PEDICLE GRAFTS OR FLAPS | Operative |
| 83.95 | SOFT TISSUE ASP NEC | Non-Operative | 86.72 | PEDICLE GRAFT ADV | Operative |
| 84.0 | AMPUTATION OF UPPER LIMB | Operative | 86.74 | ATTACH PEDICLE GRAFT NEC | Operative |
| 84.01 | FINGER AMPUTATION | Operative | 86.75 | REV PEDICLE/FLAP GRAFT | Operative |
| 84.1 | AMPUTATION OF LOWER LIMB | Operative | 86.8 | OTHER SKIN & SUBCU REP | Operative |
| 84.11 | TOE AMPUTATION | Operative | 86.82 | FACIAL RHYTIDECTOMY | Operative |
| 84.12 | AMPUTATION THROUGH FOOT | Operative | 86.83 | SIZE RED PLASTIC OP | Operative |
| 84.15 | BK AMPUTATION NEC | Operative | 86.89 | SKIN REP & RECONST NEC | Operative |
| 84.17 | ABOVE KNEE AMPUTATION | Operative | 86.9 | OTHER SKIN & SUBCU OPS | Mixed (2, 2) |
| 84.2 | EXTREMITY REATTACHMENT | Operative | 87.0 | HEAD/NECK SFT TISS X-RAY | Non-Operative |
| 84.3 | AMPUTATION STUMP REV | Operative | 87.03 | CAT SCAN HEAD | Non-Operative |
| 84.4 | IMPL OR FIT PROSTH LIMB | Mixed (3, 6) | 87.1 | OTHER HEAD/NECK X-RAY | Non-Operative |
| 84.9 | OTHER MUSCULOSKELETAL OP | Operative | 87.2 | X-RAY OF SPINE | Non-Operative |
| 85.0 | MASTOTOMY | Non-Operative | 87.21 | CONTRAST MYELOGRAM | Non-Operative |
| 85.1 | BREAST DIAGNOSTIC PX | Mixed (1, 2) | 87.3 | THORAX SOFT TISSUE X-RAY | Non-Operative |
| 85.11 | PERC BREAST BIOPSY | Non-Operative | 87.4 | OTHER X-RAY OF THORAX | Non-Operative |
| 85.12 | OPEN BIOPSY OF BREAST | Operative | 87.41 | CAT SCAN THORAX | Non-Operative |
| 85.2 | EXC/DESTR BREAST TISS | Operative | 87.44 | ROUTINE CHEST X-RAY | Non-Operative |
| 85.21 | LOCAL EXC BREAST LESION | Operative | 87.49 | CHEST X-RAY NEC | Non-Operative |
| 85.22 | QUADRANT RESECT BREAST | Operative | 87.5 | BILIARY TRACT X-RAY | Mixed (1, 4) |
| 85.23 | SUBTOTAL MASTECTOMY | Operative | 87.51 | PERC HEPAT CHOLANGIOGRAM | Non-Operative |
| 85.3 | RED MAMMOPLASTY/ECTOMY | Operative | 87.6 | OTH DIGESTIVE SYST X-RAY | Non-Operative |
| 85.32 | BILAT RED MAMMOPLASTY | Operative | 87.61 | BARIUM SWALLOW | Non-Operative |
| 85.4 | MASTECTOMY | Operative | 87.62 | UPPER GI SERIES | Non-Operative |
| 85.41 | UNILAT SIMPLE MASTECTOMY | Operative | 87.64 | LOWER GI SERIES | Non-Operative |
| 85.42 | BILAT SIMPLE MASTECTOMY | Operative | 87.7 | X-RAY OF URINARY SYSTEM | Non-Operative |
| 85.43 | UNILAT EXTEN SMP MAST | Operative | 87.73 | IV PYELOGRAM | Non-Operative |
| 85.44 | BILAT EXTEN SMP MAST | Operative | 87.74 | RETROGRADE PYELOGRAM | Non-Operative |
| 85.45 | UNILAT RAD MASTECTOMY | Operative | 87.76 | RETRO CYSTOURETHROGRAM | Non-Operative |
| 85.5 | AUGMENTATION MAMMOPLASTY | Mixed (3, 2) | 87.77 | CYSTOGRAM NEC | Non-Operative |
| 85.6 | MASTOPEXY | Operative | 87.79 | URINARY SYSTEM X-RAY NEC | Non-Operative |
| 85.7 | TOTAL BREAST RECONST | Operative | 87.8 | FEMALE GENITAL X-RAY | Non-Operative |
| 85.8 | OTHER BREAST REPAIR | Mixed (7, 1) | 87.9 | MALE GENITAL X-RAY | Non-Operative |
| 85.85 | BREAST MUSCLE FLAP GRAFT | Operative | 88.0 | SOFT TISSUE X-RAY ABD | Non-Operative |
| 85.9 | OTHER BREAST OPERATIONS | Mixed (5, 2) | 88.01 | CAT SCAN OF ABDOMEN | Non-Operative |
| 85.94 | BREAST IMPLANT REMOVAL | Operative | 88.1 | OTHER X-RAY OF ABDOMEN | Non-Operative |
| 86.0 | INCISION SKIN & SUBCU | Mixed (1, 7) | 88.19 | ABDOMINAL X-RAY NEC | Non-Operative |
| 86.01 | ASPIRATION SKIN & SUBCU | Non-Operative | 88.2 | SKEL X-RAY-EXT & PELVIS | Non-Operative |
| 86.03 | INCISION PILONIDAL SINUS | Non-Operative | 88.3 | OTHER X-RAY | Non-Operative |
| 86.04 | OTHER SKIN & SUBCU I&D | Non-Operative | 88.38 | OTHER C.A.T. SCAN | Non-Operative |
| 86.05 | INC W RMVL FB SKIN/SUBCU | Non-Operative | 88.4 | CONTRAST ARTERIOGRAPHY | Non-Operative |
| 86.06 | INSERTION INFUSION PUMP | Operative | 88.41 | CEREBRAL ARTERIOGRAM | Non-Operative |
| 86.07 | VAD INSERTION | Non-Operative | 88.42 | CONTRAST AORTOGRAM | Non-Operative |
| 86.09 | SKIN/SUBCU INCISION NEC | Non-Operative | 88.43 | PULMONARY ARTERIOGRAM | Non-Operative |
| 86.1 | SKIN & SUBCU DXTIC PX | Non-Operative | 88.45 | RENAL ARTERIOGRAM | Non-Operative |
| 86.11 | SKIN & SUBCU BIOPSY | Non-Operative | 88.47 | ABD ARTERIOGRAM NEC | Non-Operative |
| 86.2 | EXC/DESTR SKIN LESION | Mixed (3, 5) | 88.48 | CONTRAST ARTERIOGRAM-LEG | Non-Operative |
| 86.21 | EXCISION OF PILONID CYST | Operative | 88.49 | CONTRAST ARTERIOGRAM NEC | Non-Operative |
| 86.22 | EXC DEBRIDE WND/INFECT | Operative | 88.5 | CONTRAST ANGIOCARDIOGRAM | Non-Operative |
| 86.23 | NAIL REMOVAL | Non-Operative | 88.51 | VC ANGIOCARDIOGRAM | Non-Operative |
| 86.26 | LIG DERMAL APPENDAGE | Non-Operative | 88.56 | COR ARTERIOGRAM-2 CATH | Non-Operative |
| 86.27 | DEBRIDEMENT OF NAIL | Non-Operative | 88.6 | PHLEBOGRAPHY | Non-Operative |

| Code | Description | Operative Status | Code | Description | Operative Status |
|------|-------------|------------------|------|-------------|------------------|
| 88.66 | CONTRAST PHLEBOGRAM-LEG | Non-Operative | 91.4 | MICRO EXAM-FEMALE GENIT | Non-Operative |
| 88.67 | CONTRAST PHLEBOGRAM NEC | Non-Operative | 91.5 | MICRO EXAM-MS/JT FLUID | Non-Operative |
| 88.7 | DIAGNOSTIC ULTRASOUND | Non-Operative | 91.6 | MICRO EXAM-INTEGUMENT | Non-Operative |
| 88.71 | DXTIC US-HEAD/NECK | Non-Operative | 91.7 | MICRO EXAM-OP WOUND | Non-Operative |
| 88.72 | DXTIC ULTRASOUND-HEART | Non-Operative | 91.8 | MICRO EXAM NEC | Non-Operative |
| 88.74 | DXTIC ULTRASOUND-DIGEST | Non-Operative | 91.9 | MICRO EXAM NOS | Non-Operative |
| 88.75 | DXTIC ULTRASOUND-URINARY | Non-Operative | 92.0 | ISOTOPE SCAN & FUNCTION | Non-Operative |
| 88.76 | DXTIC ULTRASOUND-ABD | Non-Operative | 92.02 | LIVER SCAN/ISOTOPE FUNCT | Non-Operative |
| 88.77 | DXTIC ULTRASOUND-VASC | Non-Operative | 92.03 | RENAL SCAN/ISOTOPE STUDY | Non-Operative |
| 88.78 | DXTIC US-GRAVID UTERUS | Non-Operative | 92.04 | GI SCAN & ISOTOPE STUDY | Non-Operative |
| 88.79 | DXTIC ULTRASOUND NEC | Non-Operative | 92.05 | CV SCAN/ISOTOPE STUDY | Non-Operative |
| 88.8 | THERMOGRAPHY | Non-Operative | 92.1 | OTHER RADIOISOTOPE SCAN | Non-Operative |
| 88.9 | OTHER DIAGNOSTIC IMAGING | Non-Operative | 92.14 | BONE SCAN | Non-Operative |
| 88.91 | MRI-BRAIN & BRAIN STEM | Non-Operative | 92.15 | PULMONARY SCAN | Non-Operative |
| 88.93 | MRI-SPINAL CANAL | Non-Operative | 92.2 | THER RADIOLOGY & NU MED | Mixed (1, 8) |
| 88.94 | MRI-MUSCULOSKELETAL | Non-Operative | 92.23 | ISOTOPE TELERADIOTHERAPY | Non-Operative |
| 88.97 | MRI SITE NEC&NOS | Non-Operative | 92.24 | PHOTON TELERADIOTHERAPY | Non-Operative |
| 89.0 | DX INTERVIEW/CONSUL/EXAM | Non-Operative | 92.27 | RADIOACTIVE ELEMENT IMPL | Operative |
| 89.04 | INTERVIEW & EVAL NEC | Non-Operative | 92.28 | ISOTOPE INJECT/INSTILL | Non-Operative |
| 89.09 | CONSULTATION NOS | Non-Operative | 92.29 | RADIOTHERAPEUTIC PX NEC | Non-Operative |
| 89.1 | NERVOUS SYSTEM EXAMS | Non-Operative | 92.3 | STEREOTACTIC RADIOSURG | Non-Operative |
| 89.14 | ELECTROENCEPHALOGRAM | Non-Operative | 92.32 | MULTI-SOURCE PHOTON SURG | Non-Operative |
| 89.17 | POLYSOMNOGRAM | Non-Operative | 93.0 | DXTIC PHYSICAL TX | Non-Operative |
| 89.19 | VIDEO/TELEMETRIC EEG MON | Non-Operative | 93.01 | FUNCTIONAL PT EVALUATION | Non-Operative |
| 89.2 | GU SYSTEM-EXAMINATION | Non-Operative | 93.08 | ELECTROMYOGRAPHY | Non-Operative |
| 89.22 | CYSTOMETROGRAM | Non-Operative | 93.1 | PT EXERCISES | Non-Operative |
| 89.26 | GYNECOLOGIC EXAMINATION | Non-Operative | 93.11 | ASSISTING EXERCISE | Non-Operative |
| 89.3 | OTHER EXAMINATIONS | Non-Operative | 93.2 | OTH PT MS MANIPULATION | Non-Operative |
| 89.37 | VITAL CAPACITY | Non-Operative | 93.22 | AMB & GAIT TRAINING | Non-Operative |
| 89.38 | RESPIRATORY MEASURE NEC | Non-Operative | 93.26 | MANUAL RUPT JOINT ADHES | Non-Operative |
| 89.39 | NONOPERATIVE EXAMS NEC | Non-Operative | 93.3 | OTHER PT THERAPEUTIC PX | Non-Operative |
| 89.4 | PACER/CARD STRESS TEST | Non-Operative | 93.32 | WHIRLPOOL TREATMENT | Non-Operative |
| 89.41 | TREADMILL STRESS TEST | Non-Operative | 93.38 | COMBINED PT NOS | Non-Operative |
| 89.44 | CV STRESS TEST NEC | Non-Operative | 93.39 | PHYSICAL THERAPY NEC | Non-Operative |
| 89.5 | OTHER CARDIAC FUNCT TEST | Non-Operative | 93.4 | SKELETAL & OTH TRACTION | Non-Operative |
| 89.50 | AMBULATORY CARD MONITOR | Non-Operative | 93.44 | OTHER SKELETAL TRACTION | Non-Operative |
| 89.52 | ELECTROCARDIOGRAM | Non-Operative | 93.46 | LIMB SKIN TRACTION NEC | Non-Operative |
| 89.54 | ECG MONITORING | Non-Operative | 93.5 | OTH IMMOB/PRESS/WND ATTN | Non-Operative |
| 89.59 | NONOP CARD/VASC EXAM NEC | Non-Operative | 93.51 | PLASTER JACKET APPL | Non-Operative |
| 89.6 | CIRCULATORY MONITORING | Non-Operative | 93.53 | OTHER CAST APPLICATION | Non-Operative |
| 89.62 | CVP MONITORING | Non-Operative | 93.54 | APPLICATION OF SPLINT | Non-Operative |
| 89.64 | PA WEDGE MONITORING | Non-Operative | 93.57 | APPL OTH WND DRESSING | Non-Operative |
| 89.65 | ARTERIAL BLD GAS MEASURE | Non-Operative | 93.59 | IMMOB/PRESS/WND ATTN NEC | Non-Operative |
| 89.68 | CARDIAC OUTPUT MONIT NEC | Non-Operative | 93.6 | OSTEOPATHIC MANIPULATION | Non-Operative |
| 89.7 | GENERAL PHYSICAL EXAM | Non-Operative | 93.7 | SPEECH/READ/BLIND REHAB | Non-Operative |
| 89.8 | AUTOPSY | Non-Operative | 93.75 | OTHER SPEECH THERAPY | Non-Operative |
| 90.0 | MICRO EXAM-NERVOUS SYST | Non-Operative | 93.8 | OTHER REHAB THERAPY | Non-Operative |
| 90.1 | MICRO EXAM-ENDOCRINE | Non-Operative | 93.81 | RECREATIONAL THERAPY | Non-Operative |
| 90.2 | MICRO EXAM-EYE | Non-Operative | 93.83 | OCCUPATIONAL THERAPY | Non-Operative |
| 90.3 | MICRO EXAM-ENT/LARYNX | Non-Operative | 93.89 | REHABILITATION NEC | Non-Operative |
| 90.4 | MICRO EXAM-LOWER RESP | Non-Operative | 93.9 | RESPIRATORY THERAPY | Non-Operative |
| 90.5 | MICRO EXAM-BLOOD | Non-Operative | 93.90 | CPAP | Non-Operative |
| 90.59 | MICRO EXAM NEC-BLOOD | Non-Operative | 93.91 | IPPB | Non-Operative |
| 90.6 | MICRO EXAM-SPLEEN/MARROW | Non-Operative | 93.93 | NONMECH RESUSCITATION | Non-Operative |
| 90.7 | MICRO EXAM-LYMPH SYSTEM | Non-Operative | 93.94 | NEBULIZER THERAPY | Non-Operative |
| 90.8 | MICRO EXAM-UPPER GI | Non-Operative | 93.96 | OXYGEN ENRICHMENT NEC | Non-Operative |
| 90.9 | MICRO EXAM-LOWER GI | Non-Operative | 93.99 | OTHER RESP PROCEDURES | Non-Operative |
| 91.0 | MICRO EXAM-BIL/PANCREAS | Non-Operative | 94.0 | PSYCH EVAL & TESTING | Non-Operative |
| 91.1 | MICRO EXAM-PERITONEUM | Non-Operative | 94.08 | PSYCH EVAL & TEST NEC | Non-Operative |
| 91.2 | MICRO EXAM-UPPER URINARY | Non-Operative | 94.1 | PSYCH EVAL/CONSULT | Non-Operative |
| 91.3 | MICRO EXAM-LOWER URINARY | Non-Operative | 94.11 | PSYCH MENTAL STATUS | Non-Operative |

| Code | Description | Operative Status | Code | Description | Operative Status |
|------|-------------|------------------|------|-------------|------------------|
| 94.13 | PSYCH COMMITMENT EVAL | Non-Operative | 97.3 | RMVL THER DEV-HEAD/NK | Non-Operative |
| 94.19 | PSYCH INTERVIEW/EVAL NEC | Non-Operative | 97.4 | RMVL THOR THER DEVICE | Non-Operative |
| 94.2 | PSYCH SOMATOTHERAPY | Non-Operative | 97.49 | RMVL OTH DEV FROM THORAX | Non-Operative |
| 94.22 | LITHIUM THERAPY | Non-Operative | 97.5 | NONOP RMVL GI THER DEV | Non-Operative |
| 94.23 | NEUROLEPTIC THERAPY | Non-Operative | 97.51 | RMVL GASTROSTOMY TUBE | Non-Operative |
| 94.25 | PSYCH DRUG THERAPY NEC | Non-Operative | 97.6 | NONOP RMVL URIN THER DEV | Non-Operative |
| 94.27 | ELECTROSHOCK THERAPY NEC | Non-Operative | 97.62 | RMVL URETERAL DRAIN | Non-Operative |
| 94.3 | INDIVIDUAL PSYCHOTHERAPY | Non-Operative | 97.7 | RMVL THER DEV GENIT SYST | Non-Operative |
| 94.35 | CRISIS INTERVENTION | Non-Operative | 97.8 | OTH NONOP RMVL THER DEV | Non-Operative |
| 94.38 | SUPP VERBAL PSYCHTX | Non-Operative | 97.89 | RMVL OTH THER DEV | Non-Operative |
| 94.39 | INDIVIDUAL PSYCHTX NEC | Non-Operative | 98.0 | RMVL INTRALUM GI FB | Non-Operative |
| 94.4 | OTH PSYCHTX/COUNSELLING | Non-Operative | 98.02 | RMVL INTRALUM ESOPH FB | Non-Operative |
| 94.44 | OTHER GROUP THERAPY | Non-Operative | 98.1 | RMVL INTRALUM FB NEC | Non-Operative |
| 94.49 | OTHER COUNSELLING | Non-Operative | 98.2 | RMVL OTH FB W/O INC | Non-Operative |
| 94.5 | REFFERAL PSYCH REHAB | Non-Operative | 98.5 | ESWL | Non-Operative |
| 94.6 | ALCOHOL/DRUG REHAB/DETOX | Non-Operative | 98.51 | RENAL/URETER/BLAD ESWL | Non-Operative |
| 94.61 | ALCOHOL REHABILITATION | Non-Operative | 99.0 | BLOOD TRANSFUSION | Non-Operative |
| 94.62 | ALCOHOL DETOXIFICATION | Non-Operative | 99.01 | EXCHANGE TRANSFUSION | Non-Operative |
| 94.63 | ALCOHOL REHAB/DETOX | Non-Operative | 99.03 | WHOLE BLOOD TRANSFUS NEC | Non-Operative |
| 94.64 | DRUG REHABILITATION | Non-Operative | 99.04 | PACKED CELL TRANSFUSION | Non-Operative |
| 94.65 | DRUG DETOXIFICATION | Non-Operative | 99.05 | PLATELET TRANSFUSION | Non-Operative |
| 94.66 | DRUG REHAB/DETOX | Non-Operative | 99.06 | COAG FACTOR TRANSFUSION | Non-Operative |
| 94.67 | ALC/DRUG REHABILITATION | Non-Operative | 99.07 | SERUM TRANSFUSION NEC | Non-Operative |
| 94.68 | ALC/DRUG DETOXIFICATION | Non-Operative | 99.1 | INJECT/INFUSE THER SUBST | Non-Operative |
| 94.69 | ALC/DRUG REHAB/DETOX | Non-Operative | 99.10 | INJECT THROMBOLYTIC | Non-Operative |
| 95.0 | GEN/SUBJECTIVE EYE EXAM | Mixed (1, 7) | 99.11 | INJECT RH IMMUNE GLOB | Non-Operative |
| 95.1 | FORM & STRUCT EYE EXAM | Non-Operative | 99.14 | INJECT GAMMA GLOBULIN | Non-Operative |
| 95.2 | OBJECTIVE FUNCT EYE TEST | Non-Operative | 99.15 | PARENTERAL NUTRITION | Non-Operative |
| 95.3 | SPECIAL VISION SERVICES | Non-Operative | 99.17 | INJECT INSULIN | Non-Operative |
| 95.4 | NONOP HEARING PROCEDURE | Non-Operative | 99.18 | INJECT ELECTROLYTES | Non-Operative |
| 95.41 | AUDIOMETRY | Non-Operative | 99.19 | INJECT ANTICOAGULANT | Non-Operative |
| 95.43 | AUDIOLOGICAL EVALUATION | Non-Operative | 99.2 | OTH INJECT THER SUBST | Non-Operative |
| 95.46 | AUDITORY & VEST TEST NEC | Non-Operative | 99.21 | INJECT ANTIBIOTIC | Non-Operative |
| 95.47 | HEARING EXAMINATION NOS | Non-Operative | 99.23 | INJECT STEROID | Non-Operative |
| 96.0 | NONOP GI & RESP INTUB | Non-Operative | 99.25 | INJECT CA CHEMO AGENT | Non-Operative |
| 96.04 | INSERT ENDOTRACHEAL TUBE | Non-Operative | 99.28 | INJECT BRM/ANTINEO AGENT | Non-Operative |
| 96.05 | RESP TRACT INTUB NEC | Non-Operative | 99.29 | INJECT/INFUSE NEC | Non-Operative |
| 96.07 | INSERT GASTRIC TUBE NEC | Non-Operative | 99.3 | PROPHYL VACC-BACT DIS | Non-Operative |
| 96.1 | OTHER NONOP INSERTION | Non-Operative | 99.4 | VIRAL IMMUNIZATION | Non-Operative |
| 96.2 | NONOP DILATION & MANIP | Non-Operative | 99.5 | OTHER IMMUNIZATION | Non-Operative |
| 96.3 | NONOP GI IRRIG/INSTILL | Non-Operative | 99.55 | VACCINATION NEC | Non-Operative |
| 96.33 | GASTRIC LAVAGE | Non-Operative | 99.59 | VACC/INOCULATION NEC | Non-Operative |
| 96.35 | GASTRIC GAVAGE | Non-Operative | 99.6 | CARD RHYTHM CONVERSION | Non-Operative |
| 96.38 | IMPACTED FECES REMOVAL | Non-Operative | 99.60 | CPR NOS | Non-Operative |
| 96.4 | DIGEST/GU IRRIG/INSTILL | Non-Operative | 99.61 | ATRIAL CARDIOVERSION | Non-Operative |
| 96.49 | OTHER GU INSTILLATION | Non-Operative | 99.62 | HEART COUNTERSHOCK NEC | Non-Operative |
| 96.5 | OTHER NONOP IRRIG/CLEAN | Non-Operative | 99.69 | CARDIAC RHYTHM CONV NEC | Non-Operative |
| 96.52 | IRRIGATION OF EAR | Non-Operative | 99.7 | THERAPEUTIC APHERESIS | Non-Operative |
| 96.56 | BRONCH/TRACH LAVAGE NEC | Non-Operative | 99.71 | THER PLASMAPHERESIS | Non-Operative |
| 96.59 | WOUND IRRIGATION NEC | Non-Operative | 99.8 | MISC PHYSICAL PROCEDURES | Non-Operative |
| 96.6 | ENTERAL NUTRITION | Non-Operative | 99.82 | UV LIGHT THERAPY | Non-Operative |
| 96.7 | CONT MECH VENT NEC | Non-Operative | 99.83 | OTHER PHOTOTHERAPY | Non-Operative |
| 96.70 | CONT MECH VENT-TIME NOS | Non-Operative | 99.84 | ISOLATION | Non-Operative |
| 96.71 | CONT MECH VENT-<96 HOURS | Non-Operative | 99.9 | OTHER MISC PROCEDURES | Non-Operative |
| 96.72 | CONT MECH VENT->95 HOURS | Non-Operative | 99.99 | MISC PROCEDURES NEC | Non-Operative |
| 97.0 | GI APPLIANCE REPLACEMENT | Non-Operative | | | |
| 97.02 | REPL GASTROSTOMY TUBE | Non-Operative | | | |
| 97.05 | REPL PANC/BILIARY STENT | Non-Operative | | | |
| 97.1 | REPL MS APPLIANCE | Non-Operative | | | |
| 97.2 | OTHER NONOP REPLACEMENT | Non-Operative | | | |
| 97.23 | REPL TRACH TUBE | Non-Operative | | | |

# GLOSSARY

**Average Length of Stay:** Calculated from the admission and discharge dates by counting the day of admission as the first day; the day of discharge is not included. The average is figured by adding the lengths of stay for each patient and then dividing by the total number of patients. Patients discharged on the day of admission are counted as staying one day in the calculation of average length of stay. Patients with stays over 99 days (>99) are excluded from this calculation.

**Distribution Percentiles:** A length of stay percentile for a stratified group of patients is determined by arranging the individual patient stays from low to high. Counting up from the lowest stay to the point where one-half of the patients have been counted yields the value of the 50th percentile. Counting one-tenth of the total patients gives the 10th percentile, and so on. The 10th, 25th, 50th, 75th, 90th, 95th, and 99th percentiles of stay are displayed in days. If, for example, the 10th percentile for a group of patients is four, then 10 percent of the patients stayed four days or less. The 50th percentile is the median. Any percentile with a value of 100 days or more is listed as >99. Patients who were hospitalized more than 99 days (>99) are not included in the total patients, average stay, and variance categories. The percentiles, however, do include these patients.

**Multiple Diagnoses Patients:** Patients are classified in the multiple diagnoses category if they had at least one valid secondary diagnosis in addition to the principal one. The following codes are not considered valid secondary diagnoses for purposes of this classification:

1. Manifestation codes (conditions that evolved from underlying diseases [etiology] and are in italics in ICD-9-CM, Volume 1)

2. Codes V27.0-V27.9 (outcome of delivery)

3. E Codes (external causes of injury and poisoning)

**Observed Patients:** The number of patients in the stratified group as reported in HCIA-Sachs' projected inpatient database. Patients with stays longer than 99 days (>99) are not included. This data element does not use the projection factor.

**Operated Patients:** In the diagnosis tables, operated patients are those who had at least one procedure that is classified by HCFA as an operating room procedure. HCFA physician panels classify every ICD-9-CM procedure code according to whether the procedure would in most hospitals be performed in the operating room. This classification system differs slightly from that used in Length of Stay publications published previous to 1995, in which patients were categorized as operated if any of their procedures were labeled as Uniform Hospital Discharge Data Set (UHDDS) Class 1. Appendix C contains a list of procedure codes included in this book and their HCFA-defined operative status.

**Variance:** A measure of the spread of the data around the average, the variance shows how much individual patient lengths of stay from the average. The smallest variance is zero, indicating that all lengths of stay are equal. In tables in which there is a large variance and the patient group size is relatively small, the average stay may appear high. This sometimes occurs when one or two patients with long hospitalizations fall into the group.

# ALPHABETIC INDEX

This index provides an alphabetical listing by descriptive title for all summary (3-digit) ICD-9-CM diagnoses and procedures codes included in the book. For ease of use, titles are grouped into major classification categories (i.e., *Diseases of the Circulatory System*). These classification categories are listed for your reference below.

## ICD-9-CM Classification Categories

### Diagnosis Categories

### Procedure Categories

# Diagnosis Codes

# Diagnosis Codes

| Code | Description | Page |
|------|-------------|------|
| 220 | BENIGN NEOPLASM OVARY | 104 |
| 226 | BENIGN NEOPLASM THYROID | 107 |
| 223 | BENIGN NEOPLASM URINARY | 105 |
| 234 | CA IN SITU NEC/NOS | 111 |
| 233 | CA IN SITU BREAST/GU | 110 |
| 230 | CA IN SITU DIGESTIVE ORG | 109 |
| 231 | CA IN SITU RESPIRATORY | 109 |
| 232 | CARCINOMA IN SITU SKIN | 110 |
| 228 | HEMANGIOMA/LYMPHANGIOMA | 108 |
| 201 | HODGKIN'S DISEASE | 93 |
| 176 | KAPOSI'S SARCOMA | 75 |
| 208 | LEUKEMIA-UNSPECIF CELL | 98 |
| 214 | LIPOMA | 101 |
| 204 | LYMPHOID LEUKEMIA | 95 |
| 200 | LYMPHOSARC/RETICULOSARC | 92 |
| 189 | MAL GU NEOPL NEC/NOS | 82 |
| 156 | MAL NEOPL GB/BD | 64 |
| 170 | MAL NEOPL BONE/CART | 70 |
| 157 | MAL NEOPL PANCREAS | 64 |
| 188 | MAL NEOPL BLADDER | 80 |
| 180 | MAL NEOPL CERVIX UTERI | 76 |
| 194 | MAL NEOPL ENDOCRINE NEC | 86 |
| 150 | MAL NEOPL ESOPHAGUS | 56 |
| 184 | MAL NEOPL FE GENIT NEC | 79 |
| 174 | MAL NEOPL FEMALE BREAST | 72 |
| 148 | MAL NEOPL HYPOPHARYNX | 55 |
| 195 | MAL NEOPL ILL-DEF SITES | 86 |
| 161 | MAL NEOPL LARYNX | 66 |
| 142 | MAL NEOPL MAJOR SG | 53 |
| 175 | MAL NEOPL MALE BREAST | 75 |
| 187 | MAL NEOPL MALE GENIT NEC | 80 |
| 145 | MAL NEOPL MOUTH NEC/NOS | 54 |
| 192 | MAL NEOPL NERVE NEC/NOS | 85 |
| 160 | MAL NEOPL NOSE/ME/SINUS | 66 |
| 185 | MAL NEOPL PROSTATE | 79 |
| 154 | MAL NEOPL RECTUM/ANUS | 62 |
| 152 | MAL NEOPL SMALL BOWEL | 58 |
| 171 | MAL NEOPL SOFT TISSUE | 71 |
| 151 | MAL NEOPL STOMACH | 56 |
| 186 | MAL NEOPL TESTIS | 80 |
| 164 | MAL NEOPL THYMUS/MEDIAST | 70 |
| 162 | MAL NEOPL TRACHEA/LUNG | 67 |
| 183 | MAL NEOPL UTERINE ADNEXA | 78 |
| 179 | MAL NEOPL UTERUS NOS | 75 |
| 182 | MAL NEOPL UTERUS BODY | 77 |
| 144 | MAL NEOPLASM FLOOR MOUTH | 54 |
| 147 | MAL NEOPLASM NASOPHARYNX | 55 |
| 146 | MAL NEOPLASM OROPHARYNX | 54 |
| 158 | MAL NEOPLASM PERITONEUM | 65 |
| 172 | MALIGNANT MELANOMA SKIN | 71 |
| 181 | MALIGNANT NEOPL PLACENTA | 77 |
| 163 | MALIGNANT NEOPL PLEURA | 69 |
| 193 | MALIGNANT NEOPL THYROID | 86 |
| 141 | MALIGNANT NEOPL TONGUE | 53 |
| 199 | MALIGNANT NEOPLASM NOS | 92 |
| 191 | MALIGNANT NEOPLASM BRAIN | 83 |
| 153 | MALIGNANT NEOPLASM COLON | 58 |
| 190 | MALIGNANT NEOPLASM EYE | 83 |
| 143 | MALIGNANT NEOPLASM GUM | 53 |
| 140 | MALIGNANT NEOPLASM LIP | 52 |
| 155 | MALIGNANT NEOPLASM LIVER | 63 |
| 206 | MONOCYTIC LEUKEMIA | 97 |
| 203 | MULTIPLE MYELOMA ET AL | 95 |
| 205 | MYELOID LEUKEMIA | 96 |
| 215 | OTH BEN NEOPL SOFT TISS | 101 |
| 219 | OTH BENIGN NEOPL UTERUS | 104 |
| 211 | OTH BENIGN NEOPLASM GI | 99 |
| 159 | OTH DIGEST MAL NEOPL | 66 |
| 202 | OTH MAL NEOPL LYMPH/HIST | 93 |

| Code | Description | Page |
|------|-------------|------|
| 149 | OTH MAL NEOPL OROPHARYNX | 55 |
| 173 | OTHER MAL NEOPL SKIN | 71 |
| 207 | OTHER SPECIFIED LEUKEMIA | 98 |
| 196 | SECONDARY MAL NEOPL LN | 87 |
| 235 | UNC BEHAV NEOPL GI/RESP | 111 |
| 236 | UNC BEHAV NEOPL GU | 112 |
| 238 | UNC BEHAV NEOPL NEC/NOS | 113 |
| 237 | UNC NEOPL ENDOCR/NERV | 113 |
| 239 | UNSPECIFIED NEOPLASM | 114 |
| 218 | UTERINE LEIOMYOMA | 102 |

## ENDOCRINE, NUTRITIONAL, AND METABOLIC DISEASES, AND IMMUNITY DISORDERS (240-279)

| Code | Description | Page |
|------|-------------|------|
| 270 | AA METABOLISM DISORDER | 137 |
| 244 | ACQUIRED HYPOTHYROIDISM | 117 |
| 255 | ADRENAL GLAND DISORDERS | 131 |
| 267 | ASCORBIC ACID DEFICIENCY | 136 |
| 266 | B-COMPLEX DEFICIENCIES | 135 |
| 243 | CONGENITAL HYPOTHYROIDSM | 117 |
| 250 | DIABETES MELLITUS | 119 |
| 254 | DISEASES OF THYMUS GLAND | 131 |
| 271 | DISORD COH METABOL NEC | 137 |
| 279 | DISORD IMMUNE MECHANISM | 144 |
| 272 | DISORD LIPOID METABOL | 137 |
| 275 | DISORD MINERAL METABOL | 139 |
| 276 | FLUID/ELECTROLYTE DISORD | 139 |
| 240 | GOITER, SIMPLE/NOS | 114 |
| 274 | GOUT | 138 |
| 260 | KWASHIORKOR | 133 |
| 277 | METABOL DISORD NEC/NOS | 142 |
| 241 | NONTOXIC NODULAR GOITER | 115 |
| 261 | NUTRITIONAL MARASMUS | 133 |
| 278 | OBESITY & HYPERAL NEC | 143 |
| 246 | OTH DISORDERS OF THYROID | 118 |
| 259 | OTH ENDOCRINE DISORDERS | 133 |
| 269 | OTH NUTRITION DEFICIENCY | 136 |
| 251 | OTH PANCREATIC DISORDER | 129 |
| 262 | OTH SEVERE MALNUTRITION | 134 |
| 256 | OVARIAN DYSFUNCTION | 132 |
| 252 | PARATHYROID DISORDER | 129 |
| 253 | PITUITARY GLAND DISORD | 130 |
| 273 | PLASMA PROT METABOL PBX | 138 |
| 258 | POLYGLANDULAR DYSFUNCT | 132 |
| 263 | PROT-CAL MALNUT NEC/NOS | 134 |
| 257 | TESTICULAR DYSFUNCTION | 132 |
| 265 | THIAMINE & NIACIN DEF | 135 |
| 245 | THYROIDITIS | 118 |
| 242 | THYROTOXICOSIS | 116 |
| 264 | VITAMIN A DEFICIENCY | 135 |
| 268 | VITAMIN D DEFICIENCY | 136 |

## DISEASES OF THE BLOOD AND BLOOD-FORMING ORGANS (280-289)

| Code | Description | Page |
|------|-------------|------|
| 283 | ACQ HEMOLYTIC ANEMIA | 147 |
| 285 | ANEMIA NEC/NOS | 148 |
| 284 | APLASTIC ANEMIA | 147 |
| 286 | COAGULATION DEFECTS | 149 |
| 282 | HERED HEMOLYTIC ANEMIA | 146 |
| 280 | IRON DEFICIENCY ANEMIAS | 144 |
| 289 | OTHER BLOOD DISEASE | 153 |
| 281 | OTHER DEFICIENCY ANEMIA | 145 |
| 287 | PURPURA & OTH HEMOR COND | 150 |
| 288 | WBC DISORDERS | 152 |

## MENTAL DISORDERS (290-319)

| Code | Description | Page |
|------|-------------|------|
| 308 | ACUTE REACTION TO STRESS | 182 |
| 309 | ADJUSTMENT REACTION | 182 |
| 296 | AFFECTIVE PSYCHOSES | 165 |

# Diagnosis Codes

## DISEASES OF THE NERVOUS SYSTEM AND SENSE ORGANS (320-389)

## DISEASES OF THE CIRCULATORY SYSTEM (390-459)

# Diagnosis Codes

# Diagnosis Codes

| Code | Description | Page | Code | Description | Page |
|------|-------------|------|------|-------------|------|
| 600 | HYPERPLASIA OF PROSTATE | 398 | 666 | POSTPARTUM HEMORRHAGE | 473 |
| 588 | IMPAIRED RENAL FUNCTION | 387 | 645 | PROLONGED PREGNANCY | 436 |
| 590 | KIDNEY INFECTION | 388 | 674 | PUERPERAL COMP NEC/NOS | 479 |
| 594 | LOWER URINARY CALCULUS | 392 | 672 | PUERPERAL PYREXIA NOS | 478 |
| 606 | MALE INFERTILITY | 401 | 667 | RET PLACENTA W/O HEMOR | 475 |
| 627 | MENOPAUSAL DISORDERS | 420 | 634 | SPONTANEOUS ABORTION | 423 |
| 583 | NEPHRITIS NOS | 385 | 663 | UMBILICAL CORD COMP | 467 |
| 581 | NEPHROTIC SYNDROME | 384 | 637 | UNSPECIFIED ABORTION | 425 |
| 620 | NONINFL DISORD A.UTERINE | 413 | 671 | VENOUS COMP IN PREG & PP | 478 |
| 622 | NONINFL DISORD CERVIX | 416 | | | |
| 624 | NONINFL DISORD VULVA | 417 | | | |
| 623 | NONINFLAM DISORD VAGINA | 417 | | **DISEASES OF THE SKIN AND SUBCUTANEOUS TISSUE** | |
| 604 | ORCHITIS & EPIDIDYMITIS | 399 | | **(680-709)** | |
| 608 | OTH DISORDR MALE GENITAL | 402 | 683 | ACUTE LYMPHADENITIS | 485 |
| 616 | OTH FEMALE GENIT INFLAM | 407 | 691 | ATOPIC DERMATITIS | 487 |
| 629 | OTH FEMALE GENITAL DIS | 421 | 694 | BULLOUS DERMATOSES | 488 |
| 602 | OTH PROSTATIC DISORDERS | 399 | 680 | CARBUNCLE AND FURUNCLE | 481 |
| 599 | OTH URINARY TRACT DISORD | 396 | 681 | CELLULITIS, FINGER/TOE | 481 |
| 596 | OTHER BLADDER DISORDERS | 394 | 707 | CHRONIC ULCER OF SKIN | 493 |
| 611 | OTHER BREAST DISORDERS | 403 | 692 | CONTACT DERMATITIS | 487 |
| 601 | PROSTATIC INFLAMMATION | 398 | 700 | CORNS AND CALLOSITIES | 490 |
| 605 | REDUN PREPUCE & PHIMOSIS | 400 | 693 | DERM D/T INTERNAL AGENT | 488 |
| 586 | RENAL FAILURE NOS | 387 | 703 | DISEASES OF NAIL | 491 |
| 587 | RENAL SCLEROSIS NOS | 387 | 705 | DISORDERS OF SWEAT GLAND | 492 |
| 592 | RENAL/URETERAL CALCULUS | 389 | 690 | ERYTHEMATOSQUAMOUS DERM | 487 |
| 589 | SMALL KIDNEY | 388 | 695 | ERYTHEMATOUS CONDITIONS | 489 |
| 598 | URETHRAL STRICTURE | 396 | 704 | HAIR & FOLLICLE DISEASE | 492 |
| 597 | URETHRITIS/URETHRAL SYND | 395 | 684 | IMPETIGO | 486 |
| 615 | UTERINE INFLAMMATORY DIS | 407 | 697 | LICHEN | 490 |
| | | | 686 | OTH LOCAL SKIN INFECTION | 486 |
| | **COMPLICATIONS OF PREGNANCY, CHILDBIRTH, AND** | | 701 | OTH SKIN HYPERTR/ATROPH | 491 |
| | **THE PUERPERIUM (630-676)** | | 682 | OTHER CELLULITIS/ABSCESS | 482 |
| 641 | AP HEMOR & PLAC PREV | 427 | 702 | OTHER DERMATOSES | 491 |
| 654 | ABN PELVIC ORGAN IN PREG | 450 | 709 | OTHER SKIN DISORDERS | 495 |
| 661 | ABNORMAL FORCES OF LABOR | 464 | 685 | PILONIDAL CYST | 486 |
| 668 | COMP ANES IN DELIVERY | 475 | 698 | PRURITUS & LIKE COND | 490 |
| 639 | COMP FOLLOWING ABORTION | 426 | 696 | PSORIASIS/LIKE DISORDERS | 489 |
| 653 | DISPROPORTION | 449 | 706 | SEBACEOUS GLAND DISEASE | 493 |
| 644 | EARLY/THREATENED LABOR | 434 | 708 | URTICARIA | 494 |
| 633 | ECTOPIC PREGNANCY | 422 | | | |
| 643 | EXCESS VOMITING IN PREG | 433 | | | |
| 638 | FAILED ATTEMPTED AB | 426 | | **DISEASES OF THE MUSCULOSKELETAL SYSTEM AND** | |
| 655 | FETAL ABN AFFECT MOTHER | 452 | | **CONNECTIVE TISSUE (710-739)** | |
| 640 | HEMORRHAGE IN EARLY PREG | 426 | 735 | ACQ DEFORMITIES OF TOE | 527 |
| 630 | HYDATIDIFORM MOLE | 421 | 716 | ARTHROPATHIES NEC/NOS | 502 |
| 642 | HYPERTENSION COMPL PREG | 429 | 713 | ARTHROPATHY IN CCE | 497 |
| 636 | ILLEGAL INDUCED ABORTION | 425 | 711 | ARTHROPATHY W INFECTION | 496 |
| 675 | INFECT BREAST IN PREG | 480 | 724 | BACK DISORDER NEC & NOS | 512 |
| 647 | INFECTIVE DIS IN PREG | 439 | 712 | CRYSTAL ARTHROPATHIES | 497 |
| 635 | LEGALLY INDUCED ABORTION | 424 | 737 | CURVATURE OF SPINE | 527 |
| 662 | LONG LABOR | 466 | 710 | DIF CONNECTIVE TISS DIS | 495 |
| 670 | MAJOR PUERPERAL INFECT | 477 | 728 | DIS OF MUSCLE/LIG/FASCIA | 518 |
| 652 | MALPOSITION OF FETUS | 446 | 729 | DISORD SOFT TISS NEC | 519 |
| 632 | MISSED ABORTION | 422 | 734 | FLAT FOOT | 526 |
| 651 | MULTIPLE GESTATION | 446 | 720 | INFLAM SPONDYLOPATHIES | 506 |
| 650 | NORMAL DELIVERY | 445 | 717 | INTERNAL DERANGEMNT KNEE | 503 |
| 673 | OB PULMONARY EMBOLISM | 478 | 722 | INTERVERTEBRAL DISC DIS | 507 |
| 660 | OBSTRUCTED LABOR | 462 | 719 | JOINT DISORDER NEC & NOS | 504 |
| 658 | OTH AMNIOTIC CAVITY PROB | 456 | 731 | OSTEITIS DEFORMANS | 522 |
| 676 | OTH BREAST/LACT DIS PREG | 480 | 715 | OSTEOARTHROSIS ET AL | 498 |
| 669 | OTH COMP LABOR/DELIVERY | 476 | 732 | OSTEOCHONDROPATHIES | 523 |
| 648 | OTH CURRENT COND IN PREG | 441 | 730 | OSTEOMYELITIS | 520 |
| 656 | OTH FETAL PBX AFF MOTH | 453 | 736 | OTH ACQ LIMB DEFORMITIES | 527 |
| 659 | OTH INDICATION CARE-DEL | 458 | 733 | OTH BONE/CART DISORDER | 523 |
| 631 | OTHER ABNMAL POC | 422 | 727 | OTH DIS SYNOV/TEND/BURSA | 516 |
| 646 | OTHER COMP OF PREGNANCY | 436 | 738 | OTHER ACQUIRED DEFORMITY | 528 |
| 665 | OTHER OBSTETRICAL TRAUMA | 472 | 723 | OTHER CERV SPINE DISORD | 510 |
| 664 | PERINEAL TRAUMA W DEL | 470 | 718 | OTHER JOINT DERANGEMENT | 504 |
| 657 | POLYHYDRAMNIOS | 455 | 726 | PERIPH ENTHESOPATHIES | 514 |
| | | | 725 | POLYMYALGIA RHEUMATICA | 514 |
| | | | 714 | RA/INFLAM POLYARTHROPNEC | 498 |

# Diagnosis Codes

# Diagnosis Codes

# Diagnosis Codes

# Procedure Codes

# Procedure Codes

# Procedure Codes

# Procedure Codes

# Procedure Codes

## OPERATIONS ON THE FEMALE GENITAL ORGANS (65-71)

## OBSTETRICAL PROCEDURES (72-75)

## OPERATIONS ON THE MUSCULOSKELETAL SYSTEM (76-84)

# Procedure Codes

# Procedure Codes

| Code | Description | Page | Code | Description | Page |
|------|-------------|------|------|-------------|------|
| 90.2 | MICRO EXAM-EYE | 374 | 96.5 | OTHER NONOP IRRIG/CLEAN | 404 |
| 91.4 | MICRO EXAM-FEMALE GENIT | 377 | 97.2 | OTHER NONOP REPLACEMENT | 407 |
| 91.6 | MICRO EXAM-INTEGUMENT | 377 | 92.1 | OTHER RADIOISOTOPE SCAN | 380 |
| 90.9 | MICRO EXAM-LOWER GI | 376 | 93.8 | OTHER REHAB THERAPY | 388 |
| 90.4 | MICRO EXAM-LOWER RESP | 374 | 88.3 | OTHER X-RAY | 358 |
| 91.3 | MICRO EXAM-LOWER URINARY | 377 | 88.1 | OTHER X-RAY OF ABDOMEN | 357 |
| 90.7 | MICRO EXAM-LYMPH SYSTEM | 375 | 87.4 | OTHER X-RAY OF THORAX | 352 |
| 90.0 | MICRO EXAM-NERVOUS SYST | 373 | 93.1 | PT EXERCISES | 383 |
| 91.7 | MICRO EXAM-OP WOUND | 378 | 89.4 | PACER/CARD STRESS TEST | 369 |
| 91.1 | MICRO EXAM-PERITONEUM | 376 | 88.6 | PHLEBOGRAPHY | 361 |
| 90.6 | MICRO EXAM-SPLEEN/MARROW | 375 | 99.3 | PROPHYL VACC-BACT DIS | 417 |
| 90.8 | MICRO EXAM-UPPER GI | 375 | 94.0 | PSYCH EVAL & TESTING | 391 |
| 91.2 | MICRO EXAM-UPPER URINARY | 376 | 94.1 | PSYCH EVAL/CONSULT | 392 |
| 99.8 | MISC PHYSICAL PROCEDURES | 420 | 94.2 | PSYCH SOMATOTHERAPY | 393 |
| 89.1 | NERVOUS SYSTEM EXAMS | 367 | 94.5 | REFFERAL PSYCH REHAB | 396 |
| 96.0 | NONOP GI & RESP INTUB | 401 | 97.1 | REPL MS APPLIANCE | 407 |
| 96.3 | NONOP GI IRRIG/INSTILL | 402 | 93.9 | RESPIRATORY THERAPY | 389 |
| 96.2 | NONOP DILATION & MANIP | 402 | 98.1 | RMVL INTRALUM FB NEC | 410 |
| 95.4 | NONOP HEARING PROCEDURE | 399 | 98.0 | RMVL INTRALUM GI FB | 410 |
| 97.5 | NONOP RMVL GI THER DEV | 408 | 98.2 | RMVL OTH FB W/O INC | 411 |
| 97.6 | NONOP RMVL URIN THER DEV | 409 | 97.7 | RMVL THER DEV GENIT SYST | 409 |
| 95.2 | OBJECTIVE FUNCT EYE TEST | 399 | 97.3 | RMVL THER DEV-HEAD/NK | 407 |
| 93.6 | OSTEOPATHIC MANIPULATION | 388 | 97.4 | RMVL THOR THER DEVICE | 408 |
| 93.2 | OTH PT MS MANIPULATION | 384 | 88.2 | SKEL X-RAY-EXT & PELVIS | 358 |
| 87.6 | OTH DIGESTIVE SYST X-RAY | 354 | 93.4 | SKELETAL & OTH TRACTION | 385 |
| 93.5 | OTH IMMOB/PRESS/WND ATTN | 386 | 88.0 | SOFT TISSUE X-RAY ABD | 357 |
| 99.2 | OTH INJECT THER SUBST | 415 | 95.3 | SPECIAL VISION SERVICES | 399 |
| 97.8 | OTH NONOP RMVL THER DEV | 409 | 93.7 | SPEECH/READ/BLIND REHAB | 388 |
| 94.4 | OTH PSYCHTX/COUNSELLING | 395 | 92.3 | STEREOTACTIC RADIOSURG | 382 |
| 93.3 | OTHER PT THERAPEUTIC PX | 384 | 92.2 | THER RADIOLOGY & NU MED | 380 |
| 89.5 | OTHER CARDIAC FUNCT TEST | 370 | 99.7 | THERAPEUTIC APHERESIS | 419 |
| 88.9 | OTHER DIAGNOSTIC IMAGING | 365 | 88.8 | THERMOGRAPHY | 364 |
| 89.3 | OTHER EXAMINATIONS | 368 | 87.3 | THORAX SOFT TISSUE X-RAY | 352 |
| 87.1 | OTHER HEAD/NECK X-RAY | 351 | 99.4 | VIRAL IMMUNIZATION | 417 |
| 99.5 | OTHER IMMUNIZATION | 417 | 87.2 | X-RAY OF SPINE | 352 |
| 99.9 | OTHER MISC PROCEDURES | 421 | 87.7 | X-RAY OF URINARY SYSTEM | 355 |
| 96.1 | OTHER NONOP INSERTION | 402 | | | |